Skeletal Injury in the Child
Third Edition

Springer Science+Business Media, LLC

John A. Ogden, MD

Director of Orthopaedics, Atlanta Medical Center, Consultant,
Scottish Rite Children's Hospital, Atlanta, Georgia

Skeletal Injury in the Child

Third Edition

With Forewords by Robert N. Hensinger, MD,
and Newton C. McCollough III, MD

With 1436 Figures

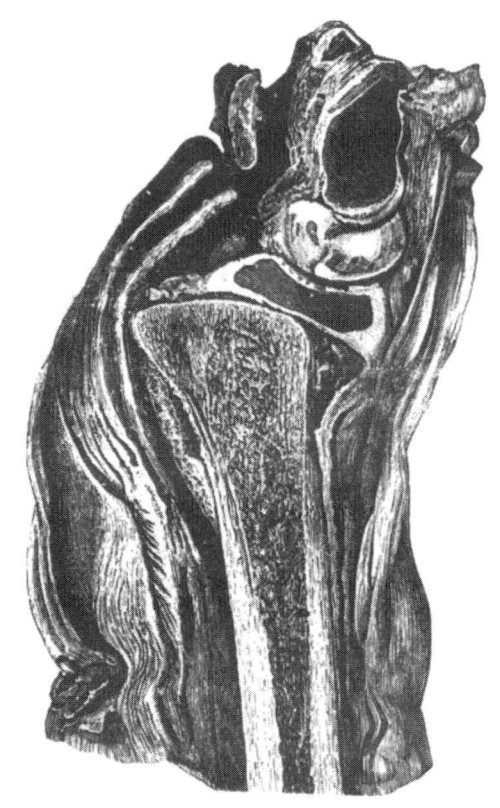

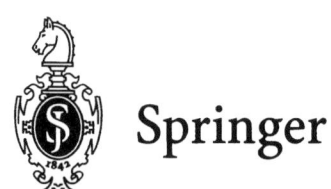
Springer

John A. Ogden, MD
Director of Orthopaedics
Atlanta Medical Center
303 Parkway Drive, NE
Atlanta, GA 30312, USA

Cover illustration: Type 2 tibial injury with a laterally based fibular metaphyseal fracture. This figure appears on p. 1048 of the text.

Library of Congress Cataloging-in-Publication Data
Ogden, John A. (John Anthony),
    Skeletal injury in the child / John A. Ogden.—3rd ed.
      p. cm.
    Includes bibliographical references and index.
    ISBN 978-1-4757-8153-3   ISBN 978-0-387-21854-0 (eBook)
    DOI 10.1007/978-0-387-21854-0

    1. Pediatric orthopedics. 2. Fractures in children. 3. Children—
Wounds and injuries. I. Title.
    [DNLM: 1. Bone and Bones—injuries. 2. Bone Development.
3. Fractures—in infancy & childhood. WE 200 034s 1999]
RD732.3.C48O36 1999
617.4'71044'083—dc21
DNLM/DLC
for Library of Congress   98-51165

Printed on acid-free paper.

The first two editions of this book were published by W. B. Saunders Company, © 1990, 1

© 2000 Springer Science+Business Media New York
Originally published by Springer-Verlag New York, Inc. in 2000
Softcover reprint of the hardcover 3rd edition 2000

All rights reserved. This work may not be translated or copied in whole or in part without the written permission of the publisher Springer Science+Business Media, LLC.
except for brief excerpts in connection with reviews or scholarly analysis. Use
in connection with any form of information storage and retrieval, electronic adaptation, computer software, or by similar or dissimilar methodology now known or hereafter developed is forbidden.
The use of general descriptive names, trade names, trademarks, etc., in this publication, even if the former are not especially identified, is not to be taken as a sign that such names, as understood by the Trade Marks and Merchandise Marks Act, may accordingly be used freely by anyone.
While the advice and information in this book are believed to be true and accurate at the date of going to press, neither the authors nor the editors nor the publisher can accept any legal responsibility for any errors or omissions that may be made. The publisher makes no warranty, express or implied, with respect to the material contained herein.

Production coordinated by Chernow Editorial Services, Inc., and managed by Terry Kornak; manufacturing supervised by Jacqui Ashri.
Typeset by Best-set Typesetter Ltd., Hong Kong.

9 8 7 6 5 4 3 2 1

ISBN 978-1-4757-8153-3   SPIN 10674738

To Dali
who has provided immense support
throughout the editions of this life work.

To Stephanie
for providing experience in the diagnosis and treatment
of the type 7 epiphyseal injury on her trampoline.

To John III
for trying hard to get a fracture
and leaving the space marbles on the stairs
so that Dad could have one instead.

To Tyler-Davis
for bringing up the rear and trying equally hard
to challenge his environment.
Perhaps you can make the next edition (hopefully not).

To Myke Tachdjian
colleague and pioneer in pediatric orthopaedics,
and most of all, a dear friend.
You are very much missed by all of us who care for children.

Foreword

It is remarkable that Dr. Ogden has created a third edition of *Skeletal Injury in the Child*. It seems just a short time since the publication of the first (1982) and second (1990) editions. The previous texts have been so comprehensive that it is difficult to imagine he could add more information to the existing chapters and create additional new chapters.

One of the new chapters concerns the multiply-injured child, who presents an increasing problem in management. More children are surviving because of modern methods of emergency transportation and resuscitation. As a consequence, a significant number with extensive head and thoracoabdominal injuries are presenting to the emergency room, posing difficult problems in the coordination of care and timing of selective aspects of management. Survival rates are improving. Most of these children have concomitant musculoskeletal injury, which must be effectively treated because of the survival potential.

There is a new chapter on abnormal healing and growth plate disruption, with particular emphasis on bony bridge resection. Our ability to recognize epiphyseal bars has greatly improved. Now, we can better anticipate and recognize growth arrest before it becomes extensive. Dr. Ogden has provided many helpful suggestions on how best to document and approach these physeal injury complications.

More and more children are intensively involved in a wide variety of high performance athletics with resultant injuries. These are not limited to acute traumatic injury but include repetitive and stress-induced problems in the immature skeleton. The new chapter on the pediatric athlete covers many of these injuries. Other injuries related not only to sports but to nonathletic injury mechanisms are covered in the regional chapters.

An overview of the operative and nonoperative approaches in fracture management is introduced early in the book. For many years surgical treatment was avoided and conservative measures were recommended. More recently, surgical reduction has become extremely popular and is ready to be placed in its proper context. Dr. Ogden has had an extensive referral practice for the management of difficult children's fractures, which brings to the text an unusual assortment of injuries and fractures and their management.

A chapter deals with the variety of new diagnostic imaging technologies such as magnetic resonance imaging, computed tomography (CT), and three-dimensional reconstruction of CT scans, all of which have been incorporated throughout this wonderfully illustrated text. Dr. Ogden has also provided new pathologic material as it applies to specific anatomic regions. His selection of illustrations helps the physician focus on these problems. A unique contribution to the text is his interesting use of material from immature animals, carefully chosen to illustrate and better understand similar injuries in the young human.

This is a huge undertaking, even when it is done by a consortium of authors. It is even more so when it is done by an individual. However, Dr. Ogden has style and consistency that provides a smooth, flowing text and lack of repetition. He is a unique individual with an excellent understanding of the effect of trauma on the immature skeleton. He has devoted his entire professional life, research, and clinical interests to the problems of skeletal injury to children, and this text continues a personal reflection of that interest and dedication.

This book is an important resource for anyone who manages musculoskeletal injuries of childhood. I think it is essential to emergency room physicians, pediatric and general orthopaedists, radiologists, pediatric residents, and students, all of whom can profit by having this text available to them. It is a wonderful correlation of anatomy, pathology, and diagnostic imaging of skeletal injury involving the child. There is no other text on fractures that has been more helpful to me or that I have found to be more comprehensive on this subject. This book is my first choice when faced with a unique or challenging problem in skeletal injury.

Dr. Ogden is to be congratulated.

Robert N. Hensinger, MD
Chairman of Orthopaedics
University of Michigan
Past President, AAOS
Ann Arbor, MI

Foreword

In the third edition of *Skeletal Injury in the Child*, Dr. Ogden enlarges the scope of the immensely comprehensive second edition of this text. New chapters covering the subjects of polytrauma, growth plate disorders and their treatment, the pediatric athlete, and an overview of nonoperative and operative approaches to children's fracture care enrich this classic text even further.

Many chapters in this new edition have been enhanced by the use of new diagnostic imaging technology, especially magnetic resonance imaging and three-dimensional reconstruction of fractures. Beyond the addition of new subjects and material, each chapter includes even more examples of rare injuries and additional pathologic material.

The third edition of this monumental work will serve as an even greater resource for those involved in the care of children's fractures. The exhaustive coverage of each topic makes this book truly unique and an invaluable source of reference.

Newton C. McCollough III, MD
Director of Medical Affairs
Shriners Hospitals for Children
Past President, AAOS
Tampa, FL

Preface to the Third Edition

Childhood and adolescence are times of individual evolution. A growing mind needs to explore the external environs and to experiment with societal challenges. Taunting wildlife as a young Maasai may seem markedly different than trying to attain a 180° flip off a skateboard ramp in Atlanta; but both youngsters are responding to specific challenges provided by the conditions under which they live. These and a multitude of other opportunities, whether a recognized environmental risk or an accident, bring about the potential for injury. Such trauma frequently involves the growing skeleton.

Writing a book such as this and subsequently revising it has been a challenging endeavor each time. Revision is necessary as diagnostic methodology, treatment techniques, and further understanding of the biology of trauma to the immature musculoskeletal system evolve. Particularly, magnetic resonance imaging (MRI) and three-dimensional imaging of both computed tomography (CT) and MRI scans have become significant diagnostic tools that allow better appreciation of the extent of intraosseous and cartilaginous injury.

A single author obviously puts forth an individual concept (hardly authoritative) concerning the many and preferred methods of diagnosis and treatment. However, my written thoughts and concepts are hardly uniquely my own. I am indebted to family, friends, students, residents, fellows, teachers and colleagues throughout the planet who have provided intellectual interchange, education, philosophy, anecdotes, and unusual cases that have coalesced to create the concept of each edition of this book.

This concept had always been dual. First, there is significant emphasis on a scientific basis, namely the inclusion of developmental and pathologic (traumatic) anatomy and histology to emphasize the nuances of musculoskeletal injury prior to skeletal maturity. Techniques of reduction, whether surgical or nonoperative, must be undertaken only after considering the biologic principles and the dynamics of childhood injury. Second, a heavy emphasis on illustrative material gives an atlas-type format to the chapters, which can visually assist the physician, no matter what his or her specialty may be, when looking for a comparable case to solve an enigmatic radiograph.

Increasing trends in operative management are evident throughout this third edition. These methods often serve to control fractures more effectively, allowing quicker rehabilitation and fewer complications than "time-honored" conservative, nonoperative approaches. Many of these "older" methods, which are often acceptable, are retained, as some readers of this book do not have ready access to the equipment that allows certain diagnostic and surgical approaches. Many parts of the world still must rely on traction and casting because of limitations within the available medical system.

John A. Ogden, MD
Atlanta, GA

Preface to the Second Edition

Since the publication of the first edition of this book, pediatric orthopaedics, including trauma, has grown immensely as a subspecialty. Appreciation of the anatomic and physiologic differences between children and adults has led to a proliferation of information in the pediatric and orthopaedic literature. The Shriners Hospitals for Crippled Children have supported my continued morphologic research into developmental skeletal biology. This particularly has allowed the study of pediatric chondroosseous injury in depth.

Updating concepts of cause, treatment, and biologic response to both continues the basic premise of this textbook—namely, the creation of a comprehensive, meaningful scientific rationale for the logical treatment of skeletal injury to the infant, child, and adolescent.

Accordingly, each chapter has been extensively revised to include pertinent new clinical and research information. Utilization of this expanding database should enable the physician to diagnose specific chondroosseous injury accurately, understand its natural history, treat the patient properly, and prevent common complications.

John A. Ogden, MD
Tampa, FL

Preface to the First Edition

Injury and the subsequent reparative response of the developing skeleton are frequently disparate from the mature skeleton. This book is an outgrowth of a desire to attain a morphologic understanding of the nuances of pediatric orthopaedic trauma. As clinicians, we have a tendency to focus on specific injuries, often ignoring trauma mechanisms and the relevance of underlying anatomy to both the initial injury and long-term consequences.

This book introduces the principles of diagnosis and treatment of fractures in children in a manner that first establishes a solid foundation of anatomy and pathomechanics on which treatment principles are based. Developmental anatomy is an overlooked facet of children's injuries, primarily because of the paucity of morphologic material available for use as source material. The unique opportunity to include the resources of the Skeletal Growth and Development Study Unit at Yale University allowed the inclusion of much material. In particular, I have attempted to translate the anatomic details into a form that has practical value. I believe that the emphasis on normal structure and function and the mechanisms of response to trauma is essential to good clinical practice.

Decision making in orthopaedics is experience-dependent in that it requires a proper mental set for what is normal for the given anatomic part at a particular age. Because of the lack of available anatomic material, the orthopaedist must rely on whatever resources he or she can muster for normal references for most of development. One can more readily accept the importance and significance of basic anatomic developmental changes if they are presented in close relation to current clinical situations in which the information is germane.

This work is primarily a clinical textbook, although discussions encompass aspects of skeletal developmental biology, particularly the response to trauma. My hope is that this book provides the medical student, the resident, and the practicing physician a logical and progressive plan of approach to children's fractures and allows ready storage retrieval and utilization of knowledge concerning each of the specific regions of injury. Because the study of orthopaedics must be a lifelong process, this book is intended to serve both as an introduction to the study of skeletal injury and a basic text for continuing study. Hopefully, it will also have import to pediatricians, general practitioners, and radiologists. The orientation is to furnish a reference book that comprehensively covers the field of musculoskeletal trauma in the child and provides adequate information for both the specialist and the resident physician.

I have tried to develop a text for the teaching of basic and applied anatomy, mechanisms, concepts, and principles that are applicable to each area of injury in the pediatric patient. The factual and patient material has been carefully selected to support an understanding of these concepts and principles. In doing so I have attempted to integrate a scientific basis with the art of medicine. The test of the value of this book will be its effectiveness in stimulating further insight into the diagnosis and care of patients who face a lifetime of challenge. If this has been achieved, the work will have been worth the effort.

John A. Ogden, MD
New Haven, CT

Acknowledgments

As is previous editions, the morphologic and histologic studies have evolved because of the progressive support of the Carl Henze Foundation, the National Easter Seals Research Foundation, the National Institutes of Health, the AO/ASIF Foundation, the Shriners Hospitals for Children, and the Skeletal Educational Association. The opportunity to assist in orthopaedic care and to assess "natural" aspects of trauma in skeletally immature animals at Busch Gardens Zoological Park in Tampa, Florida and The Disney Corporation, Orlando, Florida is also much appreciated.

The illustrations have been accomplished by Janet Barber, Patty Barber, Deby Forrester-Gyatt, and Nina Sutherland. Appreciation is extended to the National Library of Medicine for providing microfilm of Poland's classic treatise on epiphyseal injuries to produce the engravings used at the beginning of each chapter. The anatomic and histologic materials have been diligently prepared by Tim Ganey, PhD, Walter McAllister, and John Jacobs. Claire Keneally, Linda Pugh, and Fay Evatt have continued to compile comprehensive bibliographic material and patient databases. The multiple revisions have been tirelessly undertaken by Carolyn Massey. Pam Smith, RN, has been extremely helpful in getting patients back for follow-up studies. I also wish to thank my associates, G. Lee Cross, MD and Douglas F. Powell, MD for their sincere cooperation during the preparation of this text.

To cover the breadth of pediatric musculoskeletal injury, one can rely heavily on individual experience. However, no one orthopaedist has seen or will be likely to see every nuance of childhood fractures and dislocations. Accordingly, the illustrative cases in this book comprise not only my own patients but generous contributions from orthopaedic surgeons throughout the world. To each and every one of you I extend my sincere thanks and appreciation for those additional fracture examples that have made this volume as comprehensive as possible. If I have inadvertently failed to mention a contributor, please accept my apologies.

Edward Abraham, MD
R.S. Adler, MD
Jae In Ahn, MD
Michael D. Aiona, MD
Behrooz A. Akbarnia, MD
Edward Akelman, MD
Javier Albiñana, MD
Daniel Albright, MD
James Albright, MD
Benjamin L. Allen Jr., MD
Jorge Alonso, MD
Jack T. Andrish, MD
Peter F. Armstrong, MD

David Aronson, MD
James Aronson, MD
M. Azouz, MD
Thomas Bailey Jr., MD
Elhanan Bar-On, MD
Ian R. Barrett, MD
James H. Beaty, MD
Michael Bell, MD
A. Benaroya, MD
James T. Bennett, MD
Henri Bensahel, MD
Randall R. Betz, MD
R. Dale Blasier, MD

Eugene E. Bleck, MD
Walther H. Bohne, MD
G. Bollini, MD
J. Richard Bowen, MD
Christian F. Brunner, MD
Robert Bucholz, MD
Steven Buckley, MD
Stephen W. Burke, MD
Michael T. Busch, MD
Michael Cadieux, MD
Robert M. Campbell, MD
Aloysio Campos da Paz Jr., MD
S. Terry Canale, MD
Timothy P. Carey, MD
Allen Carl, MD
Henri Carlioz, MD
Norris C. Carroll, MD
William Carson, MD
Anthony Catterall, MD
Jack C.-Y. Cheng, MD
Michael Clancy, MD
Jane E. Clark, MD
William G. Cole, MD
Sherman S. Coleman, MD
Christopher L. Colton, MD
D.P. Conlan, MD
James J. Conway, MD
Daniel R. Cooperman, MD
Howard P. Cotler, MD
M.A.C. Craigen, MD
Alvin H. Crawford, MD
John C. Crick, MD
Robert J. Cummings Jr., MD
M. Dallek, MD
C. Dartoy, MD
Jon R. Davids, MD
Thomas A. DeCoster, MD
Peter A. DeLuca, MD
Julio dePablos, MD
G. Paul DeRosa, MD
Dennis P. Devito, MD
Luciano Dias, MD
Alain Dimeglio, MD
Thomas DiPasquale, DO
John P. Dormans, MD
James Drennan, MD
Denis S. Drummond, MD
D.M. Drvarich, MD
Prof. Jean Dubousset, MD
Morris O. Duhaime, MD
Michael G. Ehrlich, MD
Robert E. Eilert, MD
John C. Eldridge, MD
Marybeth Ezaki, MD
Albert B. Ferguson Jr., MD
Miguel Ferrer-Torrelles, MD
Elwyn C. Firth, BVSc
Mr. John Fixsen, F.R.C.S.
Bruce K. Foster, MD
Mark Frankel, MD

Michael Frierson, MD
James G. Gamble, MD
Timothy Ganey, PhD
Sarah J. Gaskill, MD
Seth Gasser, MD
Benjamin A. Goldberg, MD
Michael J. Goldberg, MD
J. Leonard Goldner, MD
M. Goodharzi, MD
Alfred D. Grant, MD
David Gray, MD
Neil E. Green, MD
Thomas Green, MD
Walter B. Greene, MD
J.R. Gregg, MD
Paul P. Griffin, MD
Harry J. Griffiths, MD
Kenneth J. Guidera, MD
Stephen Gunther, MD
Jeffrey F. Hassbeck, MD
John E. Hall, MD
John E. Handelsman, MD
Göran Hansson, MD
H.T. Harcke, MD
Y. Hasegawa, MD
P. Havranek, MD
Douglas M. Hedden, MD
D. Heilbronner, MD
Stephen D. Heinrich, MD
William L. Hennrikus Jr., MD
Robert N. Hensinger, MD
T. Herbert, MD
John A. Herring, MD
Frederick Hess, MD
John E. Herzenberg, MD
George Hirsch, MD
M. Mark Hoffer, MD
Louis C.S. Hsu, MD
G. Inoue, MD
R.P. Jakob, MD
Peter Jokl, MD
Eric T. Jones, MD
Lyle O. Johnson, MD
Ali Kalamchi, MD
James R. Kasser, MD
Theodore E. Keats, MD
Douglas K. Kehl, MD
Armen S. Kelikian, MD
David Keller, MD
Mr. J.A. Kenwright, F.R.C.S.
S.A. Khalil, MD
Gerhard N. Kiefer, MD
Richard E. King, MD
Thomas F. Kling Jr., MD
Steven Kopits, MD
K. Kozlowski, MD
Leon M. Kruger, MD
Ken N. Kuo, MD
Prof. Anders F. Langenskiöld, MD
Jack Lawson, MD

Acknowledgments

Louis J. Lawton, MD
David Leffers, MD
Wallace R. Lehman, MD
Edward L. Lester, MD
Mervyn R. Letts, MD
Terry R. Light, MD
Richard E. Lindseth, MD
W.E. Linhart, MD
Randall T. Loder, MD
Stephen J. Lombardo, MD
John E. Lonstein, MD
Sheila M. Love, MD
Wood Lovell, MD
John D. Lubahn, MD
John P. Lubicky, MD
G. Dean MacEwen, MD
Jay Malghem, MD
Henry J. Mankin, MD
Arthur E. Marlin, MD
Keith M. Maxwell, MD
Shirley McCarthy, MD
Newton C. McCollough, MD
J.P. McConkey, MD
Douglas W. McKay, MD
Brian McKibbin, MD
Peter L. Meehan, MD
Malcolm B. Menelaus, MD
Leslie C. Meyer, MD
Lyle J. Micheli, MD
Y. Mikawa, MD
James P. Milgram, MD
Edward A. Millar, MD
Dan Morrison, DO
Raymond T. Morrissy, MD
Colin F. Moseley, MD
Scott J. Mubarak, MD
Peter L. Munk, MD
P. Nimityongskul, MD
Roy M. Nuzzo, MD
William Obremsky, MD
William L. Oppenheim, MD
Kahlevi Österman, MD
Michael B. Ozonoff, MD
Dror Paley, MD
Arthur M. Pappas, MD
Klausdieter Parsch, MD
M.R. Patel, MD
Sir Dennis Paterson
Jaari Peltonen, MD
Hamlet A. Peterson, MD
G. Pietu, MD
A. Piña-Medina, MD
Peter Pizzutillo, MD
Ignacio V. Ponseti, MD
Shlomo Porat, MD
Jean-Gabriel Pous, MD
Andrew K. Poznanski, MD
Charles T. Price, MD
George T. Rab, MD
Ellen M. Raney, MD

Mercer Rang, MD
A.H.C. Ratliff, MD
Glen Rechtine, MD
Kent A. Reinker, MD
Thomas S. Renshaw, MD
Lee H. Riley, MD
Veijo A. Ritsila, MD
John M. Roberts, MD
Charles Rockwood, MD
Dennis R. Roy, MD
Sally Rudicel, MD
Dietrich Schlenzka, MD
Robert S. Siffert, MD
George W. Simons, MD
Nicte Shier, MD
Stephen R. Skinner, MD
James A. Slavin, MD
Clement B. Sledge, MD
John Smith, MD
Kwang S. Song, MD
Wayne O. Southwick, MD
Donald P. Speer, MD
Philip Spiegel, MD
Lynn T. Staheli, MD
Carl L. Stanitski, MD
Deborah F. Stanitski, MD
Howard Steel, MD
David B. Stevens, MD
Stephen J. Stricker, MD
Allen M. Strongwater, MD
Yoishi Sugioka, MD
J. Andy Sullivan, MD
Mark D. Suprock, MD
Michael Sussman, MD
David H. Sutherland, MD
Mihran O. Tachdjian, MD
Claudia Thomas, MD
George Thompson, MD
Vernon T. Tolo, MD
Paul D. Traughber, MD
Stephen J. Tredwell, MD
S. Troum, MD
Chester M. Tylkowski, MD
Keith D. Vanden Brink, MD
John L. VanderSchilden, MD
David Vickers, MD
Pascual Vincente, MD
Prof. Heinz Wagner
Janet Walker, MD
Arthur Walling, MD
Stephen A. Wasilewski, MD
Peter M. Waters, MD
Hugh G. Watts, MD
Dennis S. Weiner, MD
Stuart L. Weinstein, MD
Dennis R. Wenger, MD
James J. Wiley, MD
Kaye E. Wilkins, MD
Peter Williams, MD
David J. Zaleske, MD

I would also like to extend my sincere gratitude to all the residents and fellows with whom I have had the honor and pleasure to work over the past 30 years. Many of you have eagerly sought out and provided additional cases.

The staff at Springer-Verlag, ably led by Esther Gumpert, has been invaluable in putting all the pieces together.

John A. Ogden
Atlanta, GA

Contents

Foreword	vii
Robert N. Hensinger, MD	
Foreword	ix
Newton C. McCollough, III, MD	
Preface to the Third Edition	x
Preface to the Second Edition	xi
Preface to the First Edition	xii
Acknowledgments	xiii

Chapter 1
Anatomy and Physiology of Skeletal Development 1

Chapter 2
Injury to the Immature Skeleton 38

Chapter 3
The Child with Multiple Injuries 69

Chapter 4
Treatment Concepts 86

Chapter 5
Diagnostic Imaging 115

Chapter 6
Injury to the Growth Mechanisms 147

Chapter 7
Management of Growth Mechanism Injuries and Arrest 209

Chapter 8
Biology of Repair of the Immature Skeleton 243

Chapter 9
Open Injuries and Traumatic Amputations 269

Chapter 10
Complications 311

Chapter 11
Fractures in Pediatric Growth Disorders 346

Chapter 12
Pediatric Athlete 399

Chapter 13
Chest and Shoulder Girdle 419

Chapter 14
Humerus 456

Chapter 15
Elbow 542

Chapter 16
Radius and Ulna 567

Chapter 17
Wrist and Hand 650

Chapter 18
Spine 708

Chapter 19
Pelvis 790

Chapter 20
Hip 831

Chapter 21
Femur 857

Chapter 22
Knee 929

Chapter 23
Tibia and Fibula 990

Chapter 24
Foot 1091

Index 1159

13

Chest and Shoulder Girdle

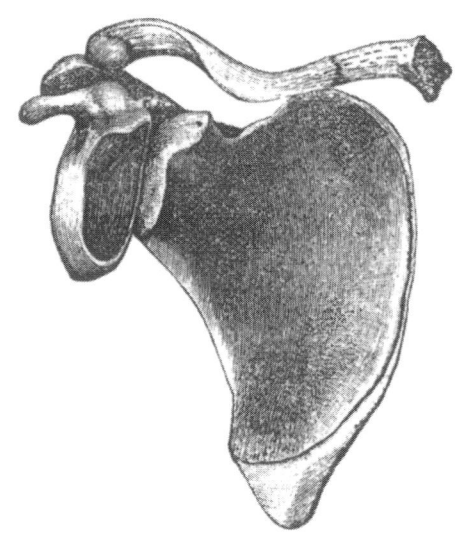

Engraving of a scapula and clavicle showing separation of the entire cartilaginous glenoid from the scapula. (From Poland J. Traumatic Separation of the Epiphysis. London: Smith, Elder, 1898)

Although the clavicle is one of the most frequently injured bones in the developing skeleton, especially before 5 years of age, the remainder of the pectoral girdle components are infrequently injured in infants and children. Prior to 10 years of age the ribs and sternum are extremely pliable and capable of much more elastic and plastic deformation than comparably skeletally aged longitudinal bones of the appendicular skeleton. The scapula is resilient, mobile, and well padded with muscles, all of which are qualities that afford it a great deal of protection from externally applied forces. In contrast, the clavicle is not as flexible as the other elements of the pectoral girdle and is extensively subcutaneous. The clavicle develops a thick cortex and multiple curves and is relatively rigid at the sternoclavicular and acromioclavicular joints, characteristics that increase its susceptibility to fracture and to sustaining proximal or distal physeal disruptions.[1,18,21]

Anatomy

Ribs

The ribs develop elongated cartilage segments anteriorly that are analogous to an epiphyseal–metaphyseal junction and a vertebral end, with two epiphyses, physes, and secondary ossification centers. The sternal ends have a growth plate that contributes to elongation of the ribs. Although no parameters of growth contribution have been derived for the rib, it is likely that more rib elongation occurs at the sternal end than from the growth plates at the spinal (posterior) end. The cartilage of the 2nd to 6th ribs forms an articulation within the sternum, with each joint being located "between" successive sternebrae. The remaining ribs have longer cartilaginous ends that generally articulate with the cartilage of the superior rib.

The sternal junction of the first rib differs from that of the other ribs. It is usually a rigid cartilaginous interposition between the manubrium and rib that subsequently ossifies to create another nonresilient "joint" compared to the lower ribs (2nd to 10th).[28] This factor probably predisposes the first rib to stress fractures.

The "chondral" (chondro-osseous) portions of the ribs are epiphyseal analogues. Eventually the proximal tissue may form multifocal calcifications or even secondary ossification centers, although this occurrence is most often present in adults. Damage to the chondro-osseous junction could hypothetically affect rib growth, although the absence of an analogous secondary ossification center makes growth arrest unlikely.

Sternum

The sternum is comprised of three anatomic regions: manubrium, sternebra, and xiphoid. The manubrium usually ossifies as a single center. In contrast, the sternal segment develops multiple, paired ossification centers that reflect both embryonic metamerism and the two longitudinal components that migrate toward the midline (Fig. 13-1). These ossific sternebra progressively arise owing to biomechanical modification within the cartilaginous anlagen.[5,15,25,27,31] The sternebra appear separate on the

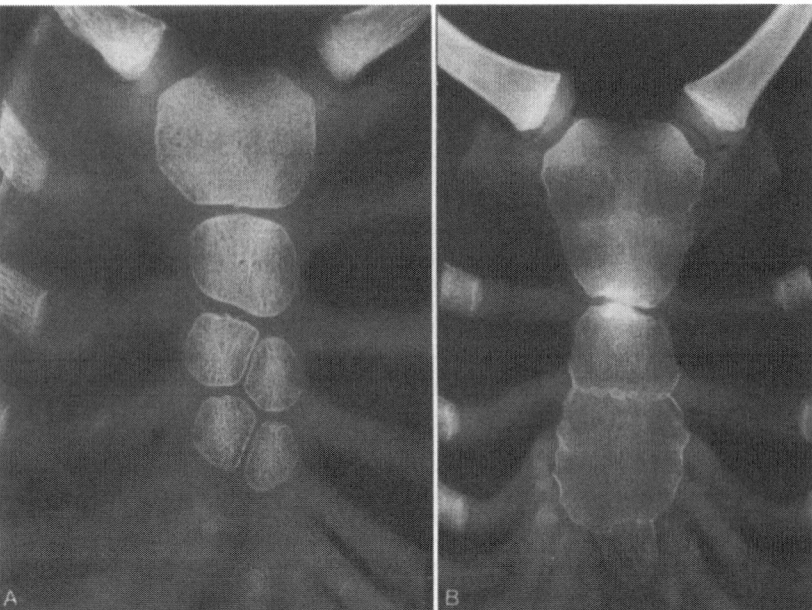

FIGURE 13-1. (A) Development showing bifid sternal ossification (3 years). (B) Fusion of the sternal units in an adolescent. The manubriosternal junction has not comparably fused.

lateral roentgenogram and may also show right/left segmentation in the anteroposterior view.[11,16] Such right/left ossification may be asymmetric or oblique, although the latter may be due to congenital variation. The intervening normal cartilaginous regions between sternebrae should not be misinterpreted as fractures. Pain or tenderness at such a chondro-osseous junction may indicate an undisplaced occult fracture through the juxtaposition of cartilage and bone. The xiphoid is the last segment of the composite sternum to ossify. Ossification is usually unifocal.

The sternum articulates with the upper ribs (2nd to 6th, sometimes the 7th) through nonsynovial joints. There is limited motion in each junction, with the resilient cartilage of the developing ribs allowing the increased chest excursion characteristic of a young child. In contrast, the 1st rib never forms a comparable "joint" with the manubrium. The cartilage of the 1st rib is anatomically continuous with the cartilage of the manubrium. This anatomic difference is a significant biomechanical factor in the development of stress fractures and nonunion of 1st rib fractures in children and adolescents.

The 8th through 10th ribs have elongated cartilage that extends cranial toward the next rib, rather than the sternum. There is no discrete articulation between rib cartilage (Fig. 13-1). Anterior cartilage is minimal on the 11th and 12th ribs.

Clavicle

The clavicle is the first fetal bone to undergo ossification, doing so initially by membranous ossification with minimal or no prior endochondral staging.[2,12,23,29] Cartilaginous growth areas subsequently develop at both ends. Normal primary ossification of clavicle begins within two mesenchymal anlagen, each with a center of ossification.[9] They appear at 6 gestational weeks and fuse approximately 1 week later. This bipartite ossification pattern may be a factor in the development of congenital pseudarthrosis (although there is still the conceptual problem of why this entity almost invariably affects the right side). The junction of the two embryonic centers of ossification are situated between the lateral and middle third of the clavicle and consequently does not correspond to the usual site of the congenital pseudarthrosis.

The clavicle extends from the manubrium to the acromial process of the scapula, serving as the only normal osseous articulation between the arm and the chest. It is constantly subjected to medially directed forces from the arm. The bone has a double curve, being convex along the medial two-thirds and concave along the lateral third (Fig. 13-2). The pattern of the curve changes during postnatal development and growth as the medial (sternal) segment elongates more rapidly than the lateral (acromial) segment (Fig. 13-3).[13,21,26] The double curve of the clavicle is a potential point of weakness in the active child. Furthermore, this double curve imitates an undisplaced clavicular fracture in some radiographic projections, especially if the nutrient artery is visualized in an unusual position.[6]

The medial end of the clavicle is concave and larger than the clavicular notch of the sternum, with which it forms an articulation. The two articulating surfaces are thus incongruent, and the joint is potentially unstable. An intraarticular meniscus partially contributes to joint stability and acts as a shock absorber. Strong ligamentous support anteriorly and posteriorly also stabilizes the joint. Virtually every motion of the upper extremity involves some motion within this joint.

The lateral third of the clavicle provides attachment for the trapezius and deltoid muscles. In the medial two-thirds, the sternocleidomastoid muscle inserts above, and the pectoralis major muscle inserts below. The subclavius muscle originates along the inferior clavicular groove. Awareness of these various muscular insertions and origins is important for understanding the directions of displacement in clavicular fractures. There are strong costoclavicular ligaments

FIGURE 13-2. Series of clavicles from subjects ranging in age from 3 months (postnatal) to 14 years. Note the medial (sternal) ends (M), lateral (acromial) ends (L), and the usual location of fractures (F).

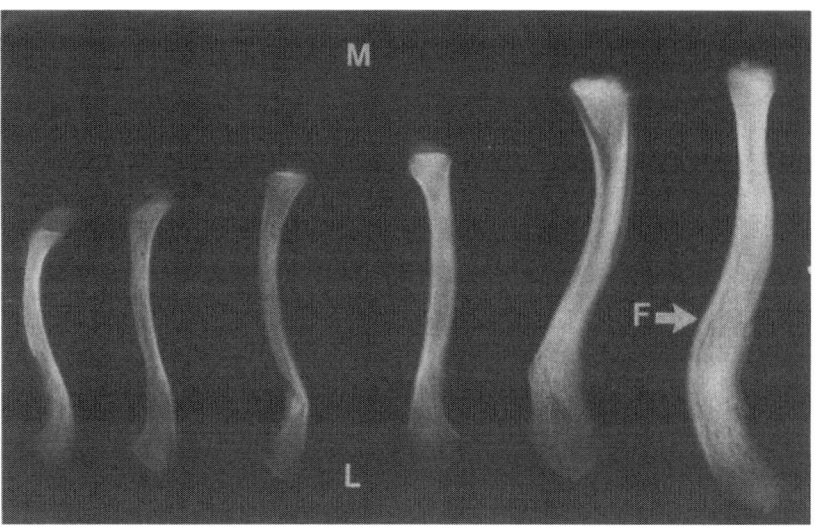

proximally, and the conoid and trapezoid ligaments connect the clavicle with the coracoid process distally. In the child these two ligaments primarily attach into the thick periosteum. As skeletal maturity is reached, Sharpey's fibers attach these ligaments more densely into the clavicular cortex.

The superior surface of the clavicle is subcutaneous throughout its entire length. This subcutaneous location potentially increases the risk of penetration of the skin in an angulated fracture, but such open fractures are rare in children and adolescents, although "tenting" of the skin often occurs. It also makes the reactive callus after a fracture quite prominent, a fact that should be emphasized to the parents at the beginning of diagnosis and treatment, not after the mass appears and the parents voice concern.

Between the ages of 15 and 18 years a secondary ossification center develops in the sternal end of the clavicle (Fig. 13-4). It is normally the last secondary center to appear. It is often difficult to visualize, even in special sternoclavicular views.[6,7] The secondary center usually fuses with the shaft by 25 years of age[14,16,26] and is the *last* epiphysis to fuse with the adjacent metaphysis. This area usually sustains a physeal fracture, rather than a sternoclavicular joint disruption, because of this unique anatomic configuration.[17]

The medial end of the clavicle is attached to the sternum and first rib by dense fibrous tissue that is difficult to disrupt in a child.[3] This joint also has a meniscus that further contributes to sternoclavicular stability (Fig. 13-5).

The distal clavicular epiphysis is relatively thin and resembles the distal epiphyses of the phalanges. Developmentally, much of the epiphyseal cartilage is replaced directly by me-

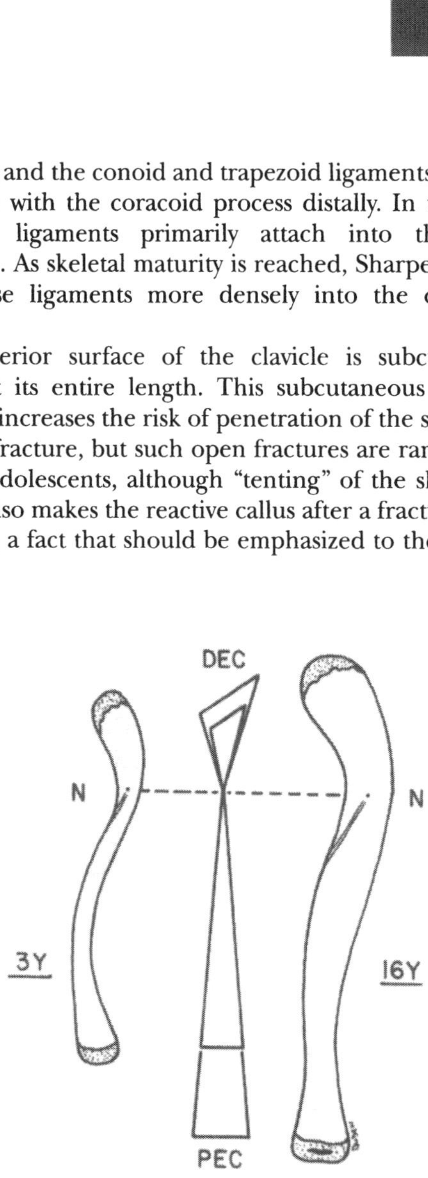

FIGURE 13-3. Clavicular growth patterns between the ages of 3 and 16 years (relative sizes derived from specimen radiographs). The endochondral cones show relative increases in length and width from the proximal (sternal) and distal (acromial) ends, with the nutrient artery used as the base reference point. Note the nutrient foramen (N) and canal, the proximal endochondral cone (PEC), and the distal endochondral cone (DEC).

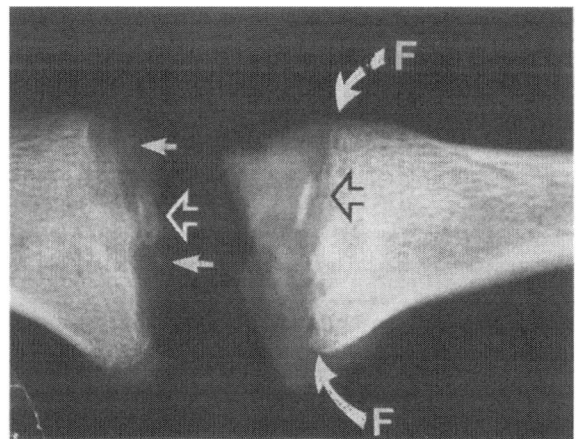

FIGURE 13-4. Sternoclavicular ends from two adolescents (15 and 17 years) show early development of proximal epiphyseal ossification centers (open arrows) and satellite ossification (small arrows). The usual location of a fracture of the medial clavicular epiphysis is shown (F, curved arrows).

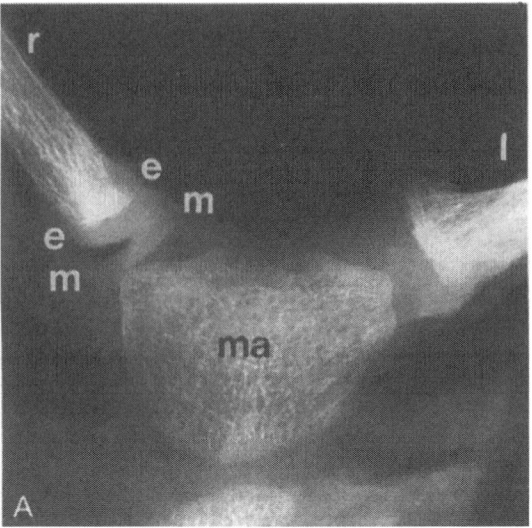
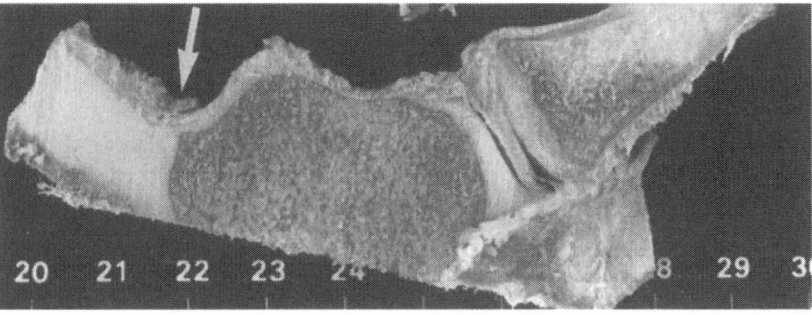

FIGURE 13-5. (A) Intact left (l) sternoclavicular joint and exploded right (r) joint show actual anatomy. Note the manubrium (ma), meniscus (m), and proximal clavicular epiphysis (e). (B) Slab section showing the meniscal articulation of the sternoclavicular joint. On the opposite side the nonarticulated synchondrosis of the first rib to the sternum (manubrium) is evident (arrow).

taphyseal bone. This small epiphysis and physis contribute only about 20–30% of the overall longitudinal growth of the clavicle.[24] Caffey did not describe secondary ossification in the distal clavicle.[4] Similarly, in an anatomic and roentgenographic study of postnatal clavicular development, no distal secondary ossification was observed.[24] In an extensive review of hundreds of specimens and radiographs, there was only one example of secondary ossification in the acromial end.[30] This may have been a pseudoepiphysis, which certainly forms in those ends of the phalanges and metatarsals that do not form a true secondary ossification center. Hence this bone resembles the longitudinal bones of the hands and feet with a secondary ossification process in one end and direct osseous expansion from the metaphysis at the other end.

The acromioclavicular joint appears to be a relatively fixed joint with minimal motion. Shoulder motion is such that the clavicle rotates in continuity with the scapula, with little motion between the clavicle and scapula.[10]

Scapula

There usually are seven scapular ossification centers.[25] One primary center occurs in the body prenatally. In contrast, six occur postnatally: two in the acromion, two (sometimes three) in the coracoid process, one along the vertebral border, and one in the inferior angle (Fig. 13-6). These postnatal ossification centers first develop in the middle of the coracoid process between 15 and 18 months of age (Fig. 13-7). A separate coracoid ossification center, sometimes called the subcoracoid bone, forms in the base between 7 and 10 years of age. This bone rapidly fuses with the scapula, but it does not fuse with the earlier-appearing midcoracoid ossification center until 14–16 years of age. A third coracoid ossification center at the tip may appear around 14 years and fuses by 18 years of age.[17,25]

Ossification of the acromial process originates from at least two (if not three) centers, one at the base and the other at the apex (at 14–16 years of age).[8] The centers form one epiphysis at about 19 years, finally fusing with the scapular spine at 22–25 years. Osseous union sometimes fails to take place between the acromion and the scapula, leaving a fibrous union that should not be misconstrued for a fracture.[19,20] The acromial metaphyseal ossification process may appear irregular.

Yazici et al. studied the morphology of the acromion in neonatal cadavers.[32] They found that the hooked-type acromion allegedly responsible for rotator cuff lesions in adults was virtually nonexistent in the neonate. Hence there does not appear to be a congenital morphologic variation that predisposes to soft tissue pathology, especially rotator cuff injuries and subacromial impingement.[22]

A secondary ossification center of the inferior scapula appears at the age of 15 years and fuses by 20 years. That of the vertebral margin appears by 17 years and fuses by 25 years.

Trauma to the Thorax and Ribs

Rib fractures in children are often associated with blunt chest trauma. Vehicular trauma and child abuse are the leading causes of chest (rib) injury (Fig. 13-8).[97,101] Rib fractures are approximately 11 times more frequent among older children and adolescents than young children, although injury to the ribs is frequent in children. Fractures are rare. The resilience of the individual ribs and the composite rib cage and sternum allow significant elastic deformation without progression to plastic deformation or fracture.[34] One needs only to observe an infant or young child with respiratory distress to appreciate the degree of elastic sternocostal deformation that is possible even without direct external pressure. Unfortunately, this elastic deformability also predisposes to severe rib cage deformation and internal injury during child abuse. Considerably more energy is required to fracture ribs in a child than in an adult.[63]

The intrinsic resilience of the ribs often results in spontaneous reduction of greenstick or complete fractures along the course of a rib after the deforming force is dissipated. Furthermore, the thick periosteum remains partially intact and contributes to the spontaneity of reduction and stability. Many of these fractures are greenstick injuries. All of these aforementioned factors make roentgenographic diagnosis extremely difficult. Often the rib injury is not diagnosed until fracture callus is evident.

Another major difference is the free movement of the mediastinum. In contrast to the relatively fixed mediastinum of the adult, that of a child is capable of wide shifts, with displacement of the heart, angulation of the great vessels, compression of the lungs, and angulation of the trachea. The cardiopulmonary consequences of such anatomic displacements following severe thoracic trauma may become life-threatening.

Most fractures involve several ribs and result from major trauma, especially as a consequence of child abuse or vehicular accidents. Fracture of a single rib from minimal trauma is less frequent. Because of the presence of a physis at the anterior (anterolateral) end of the rib, a growth plate fracture may occur. This injury may be undisplaced or spontaneously reduced once the evocative force is dissipated. Similar physeal trauma might affect the costovertebral region with major spinal or chest trauma. However, such an injury pattern has not been well described in the literature.

Kleinman et al. studied the histopathology and radiologic correlations of rib fractures in abused infants.[67–69] Fifty-one percent of osseous injuries in such circumstances involved the ribs, although only 30 of 84 rib fractures (36%) were evident on a skeletal survey. The anterior rib cartilage was highly deformable, leading to 10 injuries at the costochondral junction. Greenstick fractures within the bone were evident in 19. Most of the rib injuries were posterior, in the costotransverse region.[58]

The diagnosis of thoracic trauma is difficult, especially in the child under 2 years of age. Cardiopulmonary symptoms may not be present during the first 24 hours after injury, and there is often no correlation between evident external chest wall injury (e.g., abrasions) and underlying abnormalities. Chest radiography remains the primary evaluation of chest injuries, although it may not adequately or concisely demonstrate or may even underestimate specific abnormalities.[104]

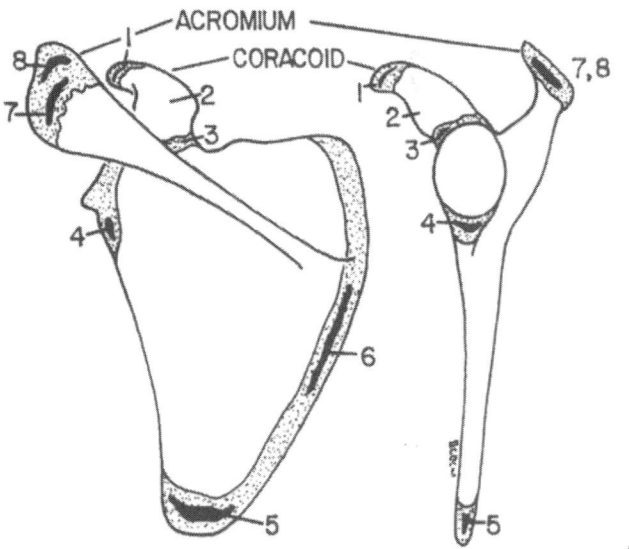

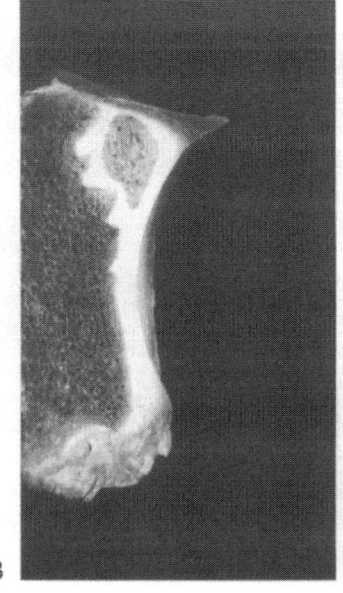

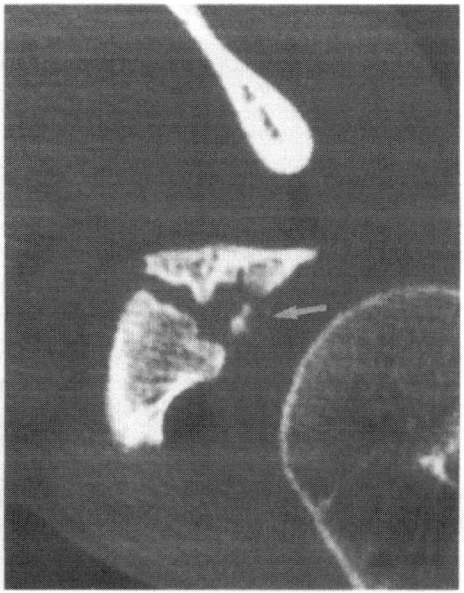

FIGURE 13-6. (A) Multiple areas of primary and secondary ossification in the scapula. 1, 3 = secondary coracoid centers; 2 = primary coracoid center; 4 = secondary infraglenoid center; 5 = secondary center at the tip of the scapula; 6 = secondary center of vertebral border; 7, 8 = secondary centers of the acromion. (B) Secondary ossification in the superior cartilage of the glenoid labrum. This is analogous to acetabular ossification (see Chapters 19, 20). (C) CT scan showing the glenoid secondary center (arrow).

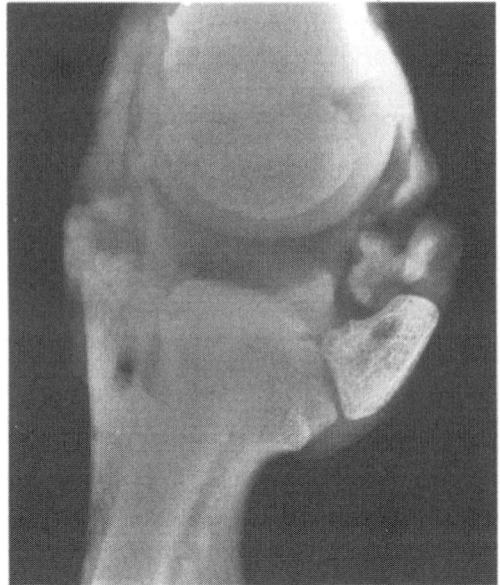
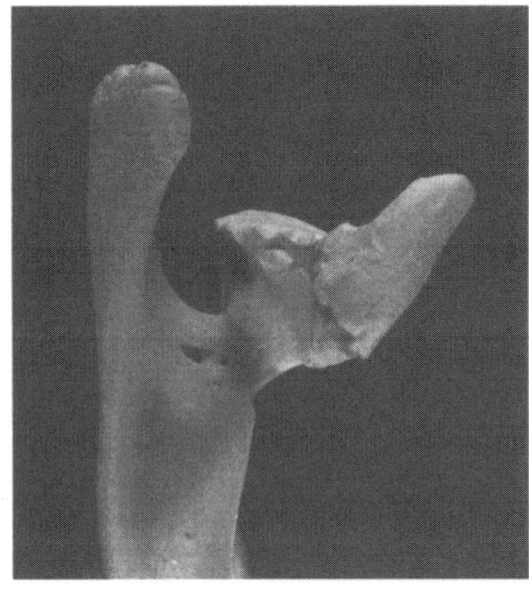

FIGURE 13-7. (A) Specimen radiograph duplicating the Y view. It shows the ossification of the coracoid process. (B) Morphologic specimen.

Healing of rib fractures is rapid and usually requires little more than symptomatic treatment. *Evaluating the possibility of internal organ injury is extremely important, as treatment of these injuries generally supersedes concern about the rib fractures.*

In the unusual circumstance in which the child sustains multiple rib fractures, the chest wall may be unstable, resulting in a flail chest with paradoxical movement of the thorax and progressive respiratory insufficiency. Lung contusion from blunt trauma contributes to the respiratory insufficiency and is a more serious component of the injury than are the rib fractures. Examination may reveal subcutaneous emphysema, palpable rib fractures, and paradoxical motion. Arterial blood gas values may indicate actual or impending respiratory failure. Treatment usually consists of stabilization using endotracheal intubation and volume-cycled respiration.

Simultaneously, assessment of thoracic and upper abdominal viscera for serious injury is mandatory.[49,70,96] Because the chest wall of a child is resilient and inwardly deformable, the intrathoracic or upper abdominal contents may be severely injured, even if the ribs are not obviously fractured. The mortality for closed-chest injuries may be higher in children without obvious rib fractures than in those with fractures. Closed-chest injuries vary significantly in severity and may be

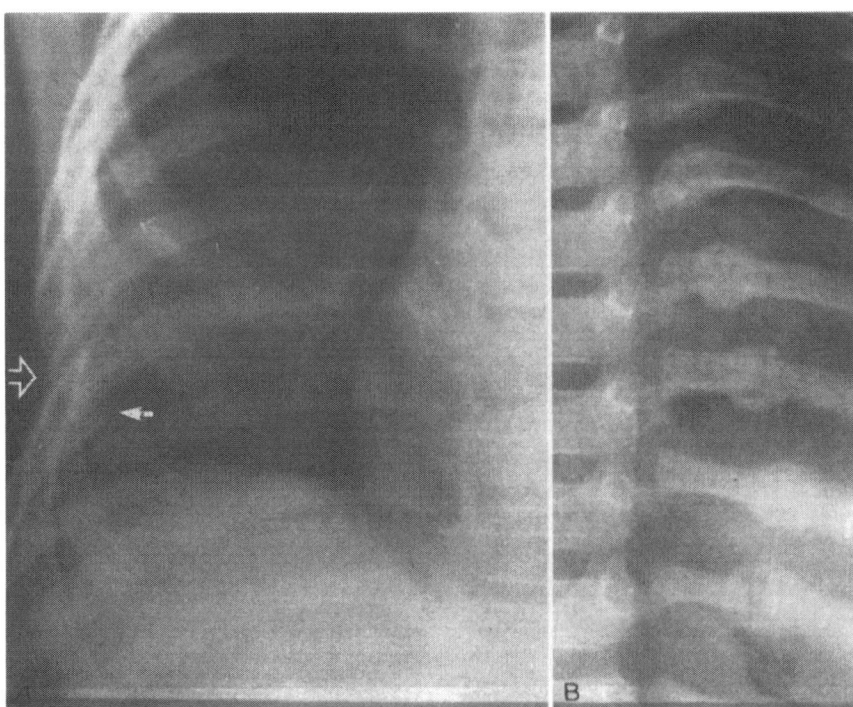

FIGURE 13-8. (A) Chest trauma in a 6-year-old boy. The open arrow indicates a concavity suggestive of a rib cage deformity; the solid arrow points to an apparently minimally displaced rib fracture. (B) Healing multiple rib fractures in a case of child abuse (the child subsequently died).

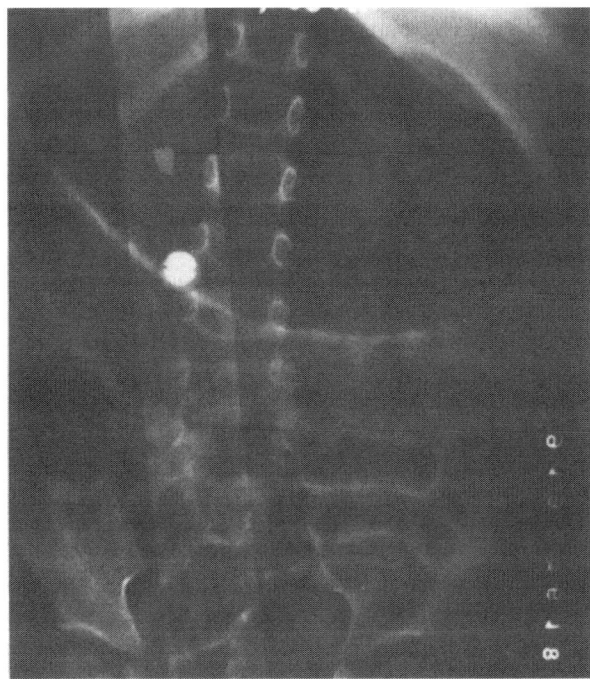

FIGURE 13-9. Aerophagia. There is massive distension of the stomach in this 2-year-old child injured in a motor vehicle accident. Decompression with a nasogastric tube relieved the acute respiratory distress.

missed in the multiply-injured child with more obvious severe trauma to the extremities or head. Closed injury to the chest wall produces few outward signs, but palpable crepitation from a rib fracture, changing level of consciousness due to hypoxia, and alteration of blood gases may be evident.

Children sustaining major trauma often experience aerophagia (Fig. 13-9). The resulting gastric dilation may compromise diaphragmatic excursion. This process is augmented by the reflex ileus often seen with pediatric trauma. Nasogastric decompression of the stomach may be necessary to protect the diaphragm and to allow the lungs to be adequately aerated.

Pediatric chest trauma is not as well documented as in adults.[51,53,66,74,103,105] Among 230 children sustaining blunt chest trauma, intrathoracic injury was observed in 29%.[52] Chest injuries are associated with the second highest mortality rate for children younger than 15 years.[52,53] The mortality associated with pediatric thoracic trauma ranges from 7% to 14%.[74,99,105]

Garcia et al. analyzed 2080 children up to 14 years of age.[62] There were 14 deaths among 33 children with multiple rib fractures (42% mortality rate). During one phase of the study, child abuse accounted for 63% of the rib injuries in children less than 3 years old. Pedestrian injuries predominated among children older than 3 years. Children with rib fractures were more severely injured and had a higher mortality rate, but no difference in morbidity, than children with blunt or penetrating trauma but without rib fractures. The mortality rate for 18 children with both rib fractures and head injury was 71%, with the risk of mortality increasing with the number of ribs fractured. They found that the presence of four or more fractured ribs identified a unique group of children who were likely to benefit from computed tomography (CT) evaluation of the head, chest, and abdomen, given the high probability of multisystem injury and the mortality associated with severe head injuries. Garcia et al.[62] undertook their study because considerable ambiguity existed owing to the fact that prevailing assumptions concerning rib fractures in children were based principally on adult experience; moreover, there was no consensus in the literature as to the frequency, significance, or severity of rib fractures sustained in pediatric trauma.[54,76,83,84,95,99,102]

First Rib Fracture

Some first rib fractures occur as a result of a large amount of energy transference to the thoracic skeleton. The force required to break the first rib often results in other serious injuries.[33] One study showed that traumatically acquired 1st rib fractures were associated with a high incidence of thoracic, vascular, abdominal, and central nervous system (CNS) injuries.[63] They described six pediatric patients with traumatic 1st rib fracture. Five patients required operative intervention. Two sustained major vascular injuries detected on physical examination (distal signs of proximal vascular injury: pulse deficit, blood pressure discordance) and confirmed by arch aortography. In view of the high percentage of patients with vascular injury, 1st rib fracture in a pediatric patient, when associated with acute, severe trauma, should prompt a search for a major vascular injury.[72] In contrast, stress fractures are not usually associated with such vascular or intrathoracic injury.[37,39,71,78–80] Begley et al. reported such fractures due to spasmodic coughing.[41,92]

Children have been included in several series of patients with traumatic 1st rib fractures,[64,85,86,91,106] and many others have been described in case reports.[60,65,89,93,95] Because a child's thorax is more compliant than that of an adult, the injury required to fracture the 1st rib acutely may also result in deep vascular or organ damage. Congenital variation of the first rib may simulate a fracture.[45]

Vascular complications may be present with 1st rib fractures.[58,60,91] Pseudoaneurysm formation is circumstantial evidence that injuries of the subclavian artery and brachial plexus may occur later, rather than concomitantly with the initial trauma.

Long-term sequelae associated with 1st rib fractures include brachioplexus injury, upper extremity arterial insufficiency, Horner syndrome, and thoracic outlet syndrome secondary to healing fractures. In Harris and Soper's study there was only one long-term complication (Horner syndrome); none of the six patients had thoracic outlet syndrome.[63] Borrelli et al. described compression of the brachioplexus consequent to a chronic pseudarthrosis.[44]

When the 1st rib is fractured in the absence of major trauma, it is usually a stress injury (Fig. 13-10).[90] In adolescents this occurs particularly during vigorous weight-training programs. Hoekstra and Binnendijk described a 1st rib fracture from a poorly fitting motocycle helmet.[64] Stress fractures of the rib have been reported in increasing numbers in adolescents who were participating in evocative sports or conditioning activities, included weight lifting, body building, repetitive throwing, and gymnastics. Proffer et al. described a 12-year-old highly competitive gymnast who had a history of shoulder pain for 2 years.[88] Conservative treatment was

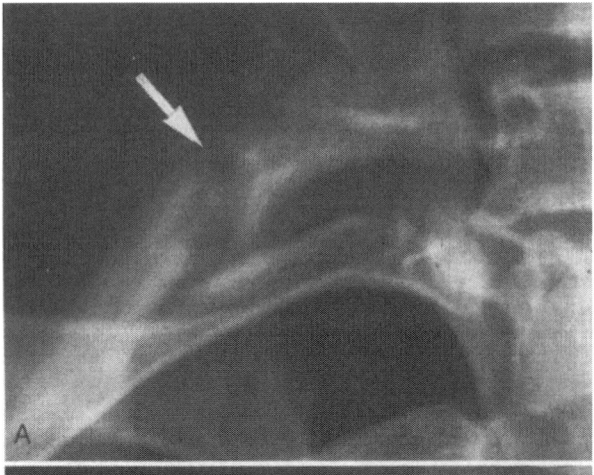
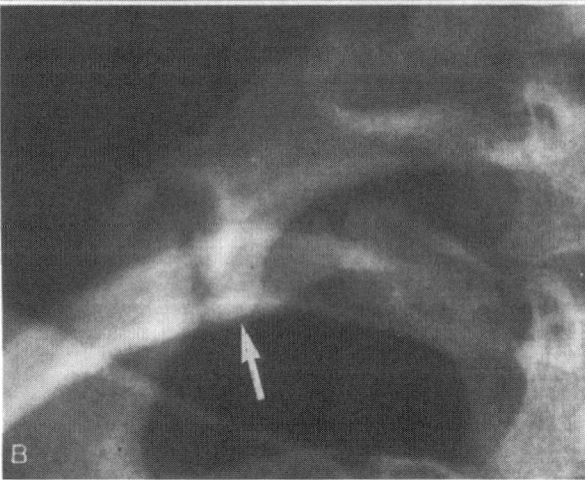

FIGURE 13-10. (A) Stress fracture (arrow) of the first rib in a 14-year-old. (B) Six months later a characteristic pseudarthrosis is present, with hypertrophy of the ends (arrow). The roentgenographic appearance changed little after this time, and the fracture was still unhealed several years later. Nineteen years later the patient, now an orthopaedist, still has a nonunion that is minimally symptomatic and a radiograph that is no different from that in 13-10B.

unsuccessful. She underwent 1st rib resection, which allowed complete return to competitive gymnastics.

Repetitive stress to the 1st rib causes stress fracture because the junction of the 1st rib and manubrium is rigid. In the young child it is a cartilaginous continuity (Fig. 13-5), and as the child grows this area increasingly ossifies. This pattern is analogous to the asymptomatic-to-symptomatic (painful) flat foot of an individual with a calcaneonavicular (tarsal) coalition. The rigidity is also a factor in failure to heal, leading to pseudarthrosis.

Gamble et al. pointed out that magnetic resonance imaging (MRI) may lead to overestimation of the seriousness and extent of the nonunion. This in turn could lead to confusion regarding the diagnosis (i.e., evaluation for tumor).[61]

Initial treatment is symptomatic immobilization of the arm and discontinuation of the evocative sports activity, especially if it is weight training. Nonunion or delayed union are common complications.[59] If pain or neurologic symptoms continue, bone grafting can be considered but may not be successful because of the intrinsic biomechanics.

Thoracic Outlet Syndrome

During the evaluation of pain over the upper anterior chest wall, stress injuries of the 1st rib assume a diagnostic priority. Yang and Letts showed that thoracic outlet syndrome may be present, especially during the rapid growth of adolescence.[107] The symptoms include aching, limb tiredness or discomfort, and occasional paresthesias.

Shoulder strengthening exercises should be tried first, although resection of a cervical rib, if demonstrable, may be necessary. The cervical rib may have a delayed appearance, similar to a calcaneonavicular coalition.

Pulmonary Contusion

Lung contusion is the most common major complication of rib fracture in the child, but it usually presents insidiously in this age group. Because of greater pulmonary reserve, a child may be completely asymptomatic, and the contusion may go unrecognized until there is blood-tinged sputum or hemoptysis or until a routine chest radiograph demonstrates parenchymal hemorrhage. Most lung contusions resolve within a week or two. Basic respiratory supportive care is usually sufficient.

Manson et al. evaluated CT for assessing blunt chest trauma.[73] They noted a propensity for pulmonary contusions to be located posteriorly or posteromedially and for them to be anatomically nonsegmental and crescentic in shape. They thought it was probably due to the relatively compliant chest in children. They also noted that for clinically significant chest trauma in children a single supine chest radiographic examination was insufficient to identify the extent of endothoracic injury.

Pulmonary contusion should be anticipated in any child with a chest injury.[43,99] Children with pulmonary contusion show a diminution in the PaO_2 and an increased intrapulmonary shunt. Swelling of the endothelial cells is followed by edema of the alveolar epithelium. Because the integrity of the capillary vessels is affected, the movement of excess fluid into the interstitial and alveolar spaces causes progressive hypoxia and increasing opacification of the lung field on the chest radiograph. Serial evaluation of the blood gases documents the increasing shunt and progressive respiratory insufficiency.

Fluid resuscitation should be performed judiciously. A Swan-Ganz catheter is useful for monitoring the pulmonary capillary wedge pressure to prevent fluid overload of the compromised lung. When pulmonary contusion is recognized clinically, fluid administration must be restricted to maintain the serum osmolarity between 290 and 300 mOsm. Diuretics may reduce excessive pulmonary interstitial fluid.

Pulmonary contusion may require endotracheal intubation and mechanical ventilation with positive end-expiratory pressure (PEEP) to improve the ventilation/perfusion ratio. Neuromuscular blockade may be effective for maximizing the benefits of the ventilator. Antibiotics lessen the chance of infection. As continuing improvement becomes evident, the patient is progressively weaned from the respirator. If continued mechanical assistance is required beyond 2 weeks, a tracheostomy may be necessary.

Pneumothorax

Pneumothorax is an uncommon pediatric thoracic injury but must be considered during evaluation of the multiply-injured child.[42] Blunt or penetrating trauma may lead to collapse of the lung and increased intrathoracic pressure. Pneumothorax may result from air leaking into the pleural space due to disruption of the lung parenchyma, a tear in the tracheobronchial tree, esophageal perforation, or penetration of the chest wall. The elasticity of the thorax in children accounts for the presence of pneumothorax in the absence of rib fractures.

Pneumothorax in a child may vary from being asymptomatic to producing severe respiratory distress. Physical examination usually shows decreased breath sounds on the involved side and a shift of the trachea to the contralateral side. Chest roentgenography confirms the diagnosis.

A pneumothorax of less than 15% in an asymptomatic child may be managed by close observation, as this amount of air usually resorbs. If a pneumothorax is suspected in a child with respiratory distress, a needle may be initially inserted to aspirate the air from the pleural space. However, proper treatment of the pneumothorax consists of subsequent insertion of a chest tube. A convenient place in the child's small chest is the anterior axillary line lateral to the pectoralis major muscle in the fourth interspace. Open wounds of the chest wall are closed to establish the integrity of the thorax so "negative" intrathoracic pressure may be maintained by thoracostomy suction. A child with chest trauma who requires general anesthesia (e.g., for fracture management) is best treated by insertion of a thoracostomy tube to prevent tension pneumothorax during the operative procedure.

Tension pneumothorax occurs because of *progressive* (continued) entry of air into the pleural space. The intrapleural pressure rises with collapse of the ipsilateral lung, shift of the mediastinum, and gradual compression of the contralateral lung. The ipsilateral diaphragm may be markedly depressed, further compromising respiratory function. Because the mediastinum in children is not fixed, wide shifts of the intrathoracic viscera may occur. Such a shift may cause angulation of the vena cava, which may incrementally decrease blood return to the right side of the heart, reduce cardiac output, and lead to cardiovascular collapse. If a thoracostomy tube is not available, an 18-gauge needle may temporarily equilibrate the intrapleural and atmospheric pressures. Thoracostomy tube drainage to water seal is usually therapeutic.

Subcutaneous Emphysema

Subcutaneous emphysema occurs when air is forced into the tissue planes of the chest and may reflect underlying injury to pleura, intercostal muscles, bronchus, trachea, or lung parenchyma. Treatment of children with subcutaneous emphysema is directed toward the primary injury, as the subcutaneous air has no physiologic effect and eventually is spontaneously absorbed.

Injuries to the Tracheobronchial Tree

Injuries to the trachea and main bronchial system are rare in the pediatric patient.[105] Disruptive injury to the airway is a consequence of blunt or penetrating trauma. The diagnosis is considered when the patient manifests a persistent air leak through a thoracostomy tube following pneumothorax, mediastinal and subcutaneous emphysema, hemoptysis, tension pneumothorax, or massive atelectasis. The side of the injury may be readily apparent from the clinical signs. The patient should undergo bronchoscopy, so laceration of the bronchial tree can be demonstrated. Once the injury is recognized, a thoracotomy with selected ventilation of the opposite lung may be lifesaving. A high tracheal injury requires repair and tracheostomy. A low tracheal or bronchial injury is usually approached directly with thoracotomy.

Hemothorax

Blood in the intrapleural space may result from vascular injury (e.g., disruption of an intercostal artery). Trauma to the major vessels is unusual in children. Parenchymal pulmonary injuries rarely bleed profusely because of the low perfusion pressure to the lung. Occult bleeding within the chest may gradually produce significant hypotension. An upright chest roentgenogram usually demonstrates an air–fluid interface.

In addition to identification and treatment of the source of bleeding, ancillary treatment requires blood and volume restoration and evacuation of blood from the intrapleural space. Thoracostomy in the posterior axillary line (seventh or eighth interspace) drains the hemothorax, reexpands the lung, and provides a means of monitoring ongoing bleeding. Autotransfusion of the aspirated blood may be possible if an appropriate collection system is available.

Cardiac Tamponade

Injury to the heart or the major intrathoracic vessels is uncommon in children. Any penetrating injury may permit blood to enter the pericardial space. The fibrous, relatively nondistensible pericardium compromises the dynamics of cardiac function by progressive pericardial tamponade. Air may dissect into the pericardium following initiation of ventilatory support with high inflation pressure and PEEP. A small volume of blood or air can severely compromise cardiac function in the child by decreasing venous return and restricting cardiac output.

Cardiac tamponade is diagnosed by recognizing specific clinical features. The child who is hypotensive despite fluid resuscitation is suspect. The association of neck vein distension with elevated central venous pressure, paradoxical pulse, and peripheral vasoconstriction in a patient in shock suggests the diagnosis.[57] Elevation of the central venous pressure is the most reliable clinical sign of tamponade.

Injuries to the Diaphragm and Abdomen

Injury to the lower rib cage may produce a ruptured diaphragm or intraabdominal damage to the liver, pancreas, kidney, or spleen.[40,48,81,94,100] Each of these potential injuries must be sought, as the consequences of a missed diagnosis may be significant.

The diaphragm may rupture from forceful blunt trauma to the lower chest or upper abdomen.[36,105] A diaphragmatic disruption, which most often involves the left side, may allow the intraabdominal contents to enter the thoracic cavity, with consequent respiratory embarrassment by lung compression. An upright chest film shows a distorted, indistinct diaphragmatic contour, with abdominal viscera in the thorax. Insertion of a nasogastric tube may facilitate the diagnosis by showing translocation of the stomach.

Brandt et al. described 13 children with diaphragmatic injury ranging in age from 1 to 15 years (average 7.5 years).[46] Eight of the patients sustained penetrating trauma, and five sustained blunt trauma; nine had associated injuries, most commonly involving the liver. All 13 patients underwent exploratory laparotomy with repair of the diaphragm. There were two deaths, both unrelated to the diaphragmatic trauma. All surviving patients recovered without sequelae. Brandt et al. believed that diaphragmatic injuries should be considered in any child suffering blunt or penetrating thoracoabdominal trauma.

Melzig et al. reported two patients: a 2-week-old infant and a 10-year-old boy.[77] They pointed out the problem of concomitant injuries masking diaphragmatic rupture. Such injuries usually involved rib fractures, splenic tears, femoral lacerations, and bowel injury.

Because of the increased compliance of the thoracic cage in children, the diaphragm may rupture without obvious signs of external injury. Morbidity and mortality may be minimized by a high index of suspicion, prompt recognition, and surgical repair of even a small diaphragmatic injury. Diaphragmatic injury occurs in 3–5% of adults with blunt trauma to the abdomen and in as many as 10–15% of patients with penetrating wounds to the lower chest. Diaphragmatic injury in children is more difficult to assess than in adults because of anatomic and physiologic differences. The child's chest wall is more compliant than that in adults. Major compression with resultant internal injury may occur without fractures or other external signs of trauma. The mediastinum of a child is more mobile than that of an adult; and venous return is more likely to be compromised by hemothorax, pneumothorax, or herniation of abdominal contents into the chest.

Virtually all children respond to trauma by swallowing air, leading to gastric distension. This may cause respiratory decompensation, particularly if the stomach is herniated into the chest through the diaphragmatic tear.

The pathophysiology of blunt diaphragmatic injury is not clearly understood. The timing of the impact within the respiratory cycle may be especially important and may explain the lack of correlation between the severity of the trauma and the occurrence of diaphragmatic rupture. In adults, pain referred to the ipsilateral shoulder is virtually always present. Unfortunately, children *seldom* describe this symptom.

Physical examination is rarely specific for diaphragmatic injury. Signs of abnormal tissue fluid in the chest, such as dullness to percussion, diminished fremitus, or decreased breath sounds, may be present. Respiratory distress is more often present in children than in adults because of the stressed child's tendency to swallow air. The presence of bowel sounds in the chest is not a reliable physical finding, as they may be transmitted from the abdomen. Furthermore, with true herniation bowel sounds may be absent because of an associated ileus.

The chest roentgenogram is the most important diagnostic study if diaphragmatic injury is suspected. However, it should be noted that in some series as many as 30–50% of the initial chest roentgenograms appeared normal. The injury became evident only subsequently with serial roentgenograms.[77]

Splenic Injury

The spleen is frequently injured when the left side of the chest is traumatized. The overlying rib cage is resilient and rarely fractures, but it allows sufficient temporary inward osseous deformation to contuse, displace, or rupture the spleen. Blood loss may be immediate or delayed if the splenic bleeding is intracapsular.

Immediate splenectomy has been advocated, but more recent clinical trials suggest that complete removal may not be necessary.[35,47,50,55,56,82] Smith et al. corroborated that splenorrhaphy in children is a significant and safe alternative to splenectomy in patients without other major injuries who appear to be hemodynamically stable.[98] Furthermore, following splenectomy many children exhibit regeneration of some splenic elements (the "born-again spleen").[73,108] Splenectomy is not without long-term complications, the most severe being inappropriate function of the immune system, often leading to sepsis.[38]

Pancreas

Pancreatic injury may lead to pancreatitis or pseudocyst formation. Osteolytic lesions have been observed in patients with traumatic pancreatitis.[81,94] These lesions are presumably due to metastatic fat necrosis.

Slipping Rib Syndrome

The eighth, ninth, and tenth costal cartilages do not attach directly to the sternum; rather, they are attached to each other by cartilage, fibrocartilage, or fibrous tissue (Fig. 13-11). This type of attachment allows greater mobility than the more rigidly attached upper ribs and makes the lower rib region susceptible to trauma. Disruption of the fibrous connections between the ribs makes the costochondral junction potentially unstable, loosening this area so there may be micromotion or macromotion.

The slipping rib syndrome is a sprain disorder in children produced by trauma to the costal cartilages of the 8th, 9th, and 10th ribs.[75,87] The symptoms are neuritic pain, autonomic symptoms, and a perception of movement of the ribs. This syndrome may be confused with intraabdominal disorders. Direct trauma from a fall or blow and indirect trauma from lifting or athletic activities are probable inciting causes. Most patients with slipping rib syndrome have pain in an upper abdominal quadrant, the epigastrium, or the inferior costal regions. Many complain of pain under the ribs. Another common presenting symptom is the perception of a "slipping" movement of the ribs.

A study of the pathology and anatomy of resected costal cartilages showed minimal changes in two patients. Examination of specimens of the 8th, 9th, and 10th ribs of cadav-

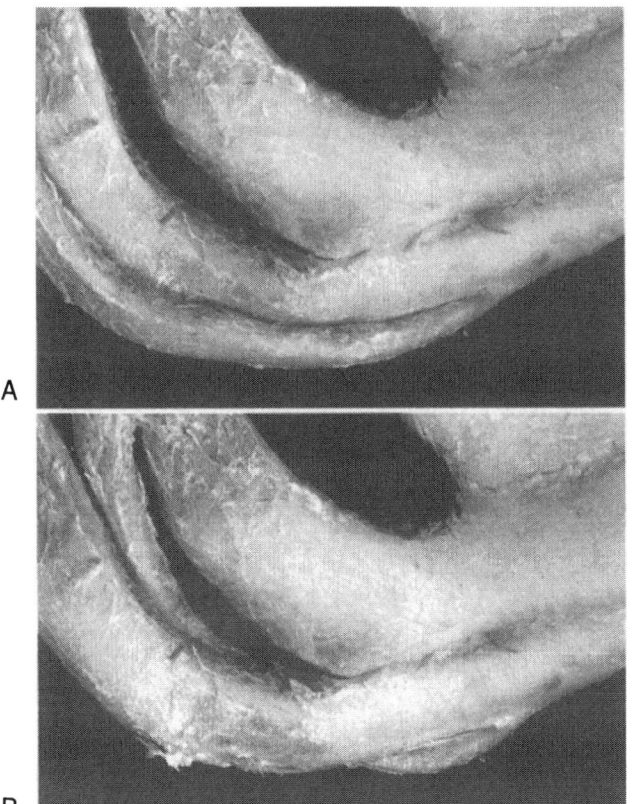

FIGURE 13-11. Rib cage to show the mechanism of slipping ribs. (A) Normal appearance in a 7-year-old child. (B) Displacement with a "slipped rib."

ers (age range 3–72 years) showed that the intercostal muscle mass was sparse at the rib tips.[75] Most often found in young, highly competitive athletes, it may follow an acute blow to the lower rib cage, although repetitive strain may also cause the symptoms.

The cartilage of these ribs was not mobile enough to allow them to come in contact with the cartilage of the ribs above or to become locked behind them. However, when the fibrous connecting tissue was incised, the cartilaginous rib tip could be subluxated, becoming trapped posterior to the rib above it.

Diagnosis is made by demonstrating tenderness of the affected cartilage. The pathognomonic finding, although not present in all cases, is a positive hooking maneuver. The examiner should place fingers under and along the inferior rib margins and pull anteriorly. Characteristically, the symptomatic child recognizes the reproduced pain or sensation of instability. Because the condition usually involves only one side of the chest, the other side may serve as the control. Diagnostic, particularly radiographic, studies are inconclusive. The use of cross-sectional tomography to evaluate patients with this disorder has not been reported.

The principal methods of treatment are reassurance, injection of the affected area with local anesthetic, and in patients with severe pain, surgical excision of the subluxating cartilaginous rib tip. Resection of the cartilage involves little morbidity if care is taken not to enter the thoracic or abdominal cavity. It may be undertaken with the adolescent patient under local anesthesia.[99]

Trauma to the Sternum

The sternum, like the ribs, is resilient in a child, and fractures are rare (Fig. 13-12). There are few reports of sternal fractures in chidlren.[109–111,114–122] The manubrium and sternum have a cartilaginous junction, allowing some motion. This manubriosternal joint may be displaced and is the most frequent region of sternal fracture in children. The cartilage between individual sternebra also represents a potential site of chondro-osseous separation, if not dislocation.

The sternum is anatomically protected from fracture by the surrounding ligaments and cartilaginous attachments from the ribs. In children these structures are even more elastic, and the ribs are more flexible. Furthermore, intercartilaginous connections between the sternebra add additional resilience to the sternum. Most injuries occur in the older child, in whom the capacity for elastic deformation, especially through the synchondroses, has lessened considerably. The primary mechanism of injury is direct violence, particularly chest compression, which may occur in sports such as wrestling in which encircling holds are a common part of the maneuvers. These injuries may occur when chest seat belt restraints are used.[110]

Bizzle reported that sternal fractures are potentially fatal injuries and stressed the need for close monitoring of cardiac

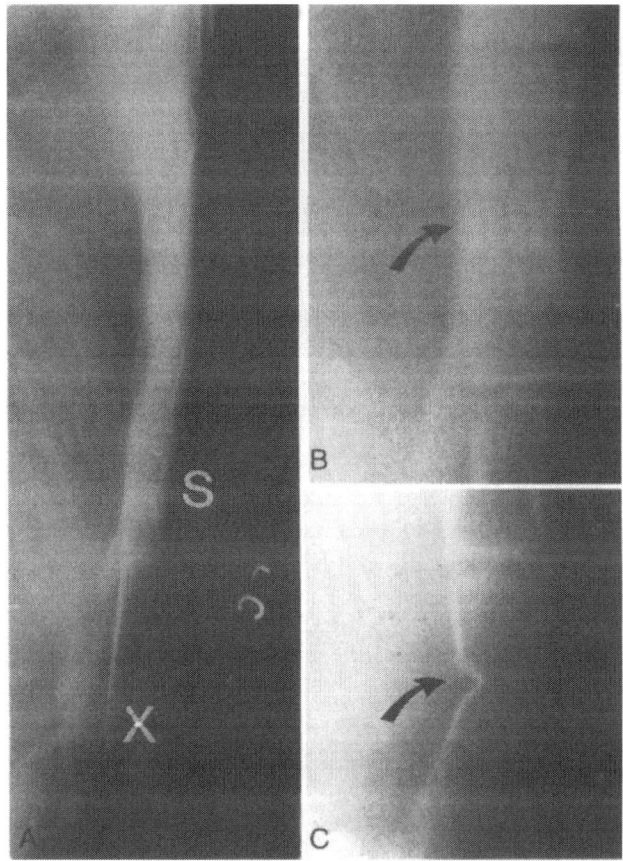

FIGURE 13-12. (A) Sternebral (S) and xiphoid (X) sternal fractures in a 15-year-old boy, sustained from a "bear hug" during a wrestling match. (B) Magnification of the sternebral fracture (arrow). (C) Magnification of the xiphoid fracture (arrow). Both injuries are incomplete (greenstick) fractures.

and respiratory status.[109] Scudamore and Ashmore noted that dislocation of a segment of the unfused sternum could occur secondary to direct or indirect trauma, osteoradionecrosis, and sickle cell anemia.[121]

Patients with isolated sternal fracture usually do not require cardiac monitoring, and patients under 4 years of age generally require short-stay observation. Only four patients out of 272 developed cardiac arrhythmias, and three of them had associated injuries.[110] There is a small association with concomitant thoracic spine fractures.

Treatment is generally symptomatic.[109,118] Most sternal fractures are symptomatically painful for a period of 2–3 weeks. Bizzle treated teenagers with a sternal brace that was similar to a clavicular brace.[109] One 16-year-old boy sustained a crushing injury to the chest and required surgical reduction and internal fixation.[120] The xiphoid may be depressed inward and may require removal or elevation if pain persists.

Haje and Bowen have shown that damage to the cartilage of the sternum may produce pectus carinatum or excavatum deformities.[112,113] Similar injuries can hypothetically or actually occur in the injured child to produce similar deformation, although most of these deformities are undoubtedly congenital failures of the embryonic midline and sternebral fusion processes.

Trauma to the Clavicle

Fractures of the clavicle occur most frequently in children during the first 10 years of life and are certainly the most prevalent skeletal injury under 5 years of age.[123–179] Fractures may occur throughout the diaphyseal region, the medial epiphyseal end, and the distal metaphyseal end (Fig. 13-13). Fractures of the midshaft, however, are most common and range from greenstick to complete. True dislocation or subluxation of proximal (sternoclavicular) or distal (acromioclavicular) joints is rare prior to skeletal maturity, which does not occur until the mid-twenties in this particular bone.

Wilkes and Hoffer found that 7% of children with a head injury had concomitant clavicular fractures; 16 of 28 children sustained mid-clavicular fractures.[178] Accordingly, the clavicle should be carefully assessed in the multiply-injured child.

The most common birth injury is a fracture of the clavicle (Fig. 13-14), occurring in approximately 5 of 1000 vertex deliveries and 160 of 1000 breech deliveries.[134,150] Oppenheim and coworkers found 58 clavicular fractures among 21,632 live births (2.7 clavicle fractures per 1000 live births).[165] Balata and associates noted an increasing incidence of perinatal fractures of the clavicle.[126] In 1977 there were 2.2 clavicular fractures per 1000 live births, and in 1980 there were 4.8 per 100 live births.[126]

Clavicular fractures in breech deliveries frequently occur when the obstetrician has difficulty delivering the extended

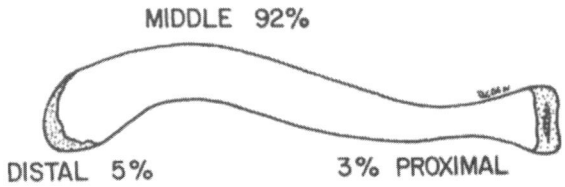

FIGURE 13-13. Usual areas and likelihood of clavicular injury.

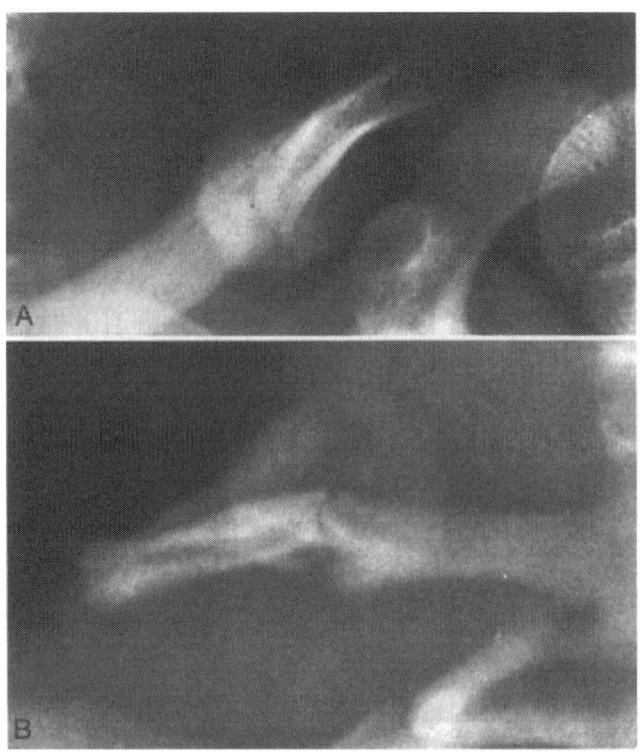

FIGURE 13-14. (A) Undisplaced fracture of the clavicle with hypertrophic callus. It was not diagnosed until 3 weeks after the injury. (B) Massive callus 3 weeks following a birth fracture.

arms and shoulders. Clavicular fractures have also been reported during cesarean section.[143,165]

Cohen and Otto analyzed the factors related to birth fractures, finding that they seemed to correlate best with birth weights over 3800 g, the level of obstetric experience of the delivering physician, and mid-forceps deliveries.[133] Oppenheim et al. found that increased birth weight and shoulder dystocia were the most predictable predisposing factors.[165]

Baskett and Allen reviewed the perinatal implications of shoulder dystocia over a 10-year period.[127] They found 254 cases of shoulder dystocia among 40,518 vaginal cephalic deliveries, with 33 cases of brachial plexus palsy and 13 clavicular fractures. They found that the incidence of dystocia was increased in the presence of a prolonged pregnancy (threefold), prolonged second stage of labor (threefold), mid-forceps delivery (tenfold), and increased birth weight. Downward traction correlated significantly with brachial plexus injury. There was only *one* case of recurrent shoulder dystocia among 80 women having 93 subsequent vaginal deliveries.

Chez et al. reviewed multiple factors in 3880 deliveries (34 fractured clavicles) and concluded that the fractured clavicle is an "unavoidable" event.[132] Roberts et al. reviewed 215 fractured clavicles among 65,091 vaginal deliveries.[168] They also concluded that *obstetric clavicular fracture was an unavoidable, unpredictable complication of an otherwise normal birth.*

Clavicular fractures in the newborn may produce little discomfort, so the fracture may not be recognized until healing callus is palpated after the neonate has been taken home. In one survey of 300 consecutive living newborns, 5 had fractured clavicles, of which *none* was suspected during the routine neonatal evaluation.[140] Conversely, neonates may present with pseudoparalysis, in which case the physician must distinguish between a fractured clavicle, birth injury to the brachial plexus, traumatic separation of the proximal humeral epiphysis (see Chapter 14), or acute osteomyelitis of the shoulder.[156,169,170] Valerio and Harmsen described osteomyelitis as a complication of perinatal clavicle fracture.[176] This infant required curettage and sequestrectomy. The infant recovered completely.

It is important to realize that brachial plexus injuries and clavicular fractures can coexist. However, temporary pseudoparalysis consequent to clavicular fracture is more likely.

Mechanism of Injury

The clavicle may be fractured neonatally during a difficult delivery.[131,135,140,154,160] Fracture of the clavicle positioned anteriorly during delivery predominates over the more posteriorly positioned clavicle. The anterior shoulder is compressed by the maternal symphysis during cephalic presentation and passage through the pelvic outlet. Another mechanism is incidental torsion, traction, and digital pressure applied to the clavicle by the obstetrician. Finally, the obstetrician may choose to fracture the clavicle deliberately to facilitate a difficult delivery, particularly if there is fetal distress.

Meghdari et al. performed an image analysis of shoulder dystocia utilizing the finite element method.[157] These studies showed that the clavicle almost always fractured under application of compressive stresses at the midshaft. It showed that a stretch of about 15–20% was necessary to damage the brachial plexus nerves. The most damaging force appeared to be shear forces. Other engineering studies have confirmed this concept.[171,172]

Once the child is ambulatory, the most common mechanism of injury is a fall. The patient may land on an outstretched arm, hand, or elbow or directly on the shoulder, directing the forces into the clavicle, which is relatively fixed and immobile at the manubrium.

Pathologic Anatomy

The most common fracture site is the junction of the middle and distal thirds of the bone. In the infant and young child the break is usually incomplete (greenstick), whereas older children and adolescents tend to have complete or comminuted fractures (Fig. 13-15), even though the fragments may not be displaced significantly. Some periosteal continuity is usually retained. Angulated, sharp fragments may pen-

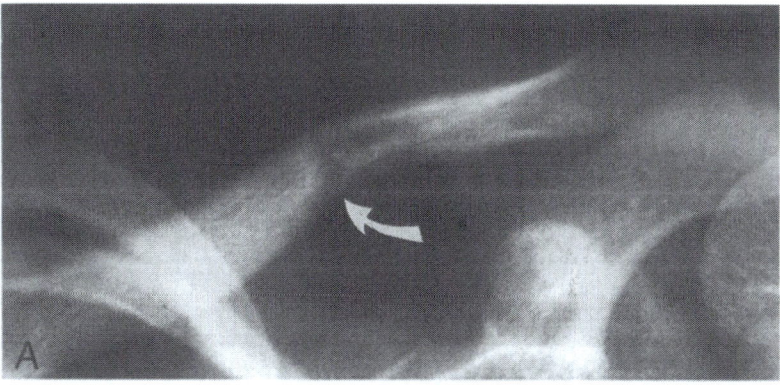
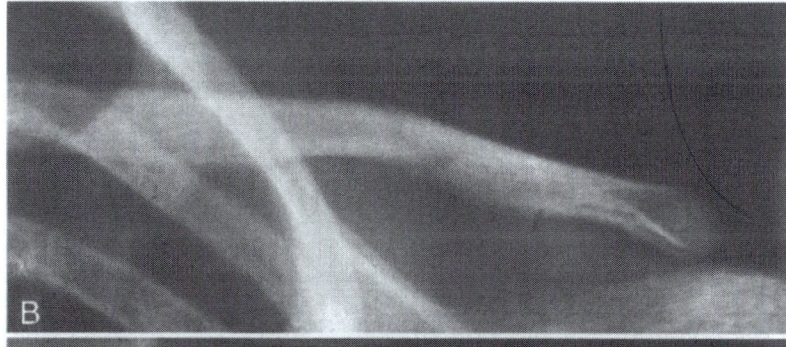
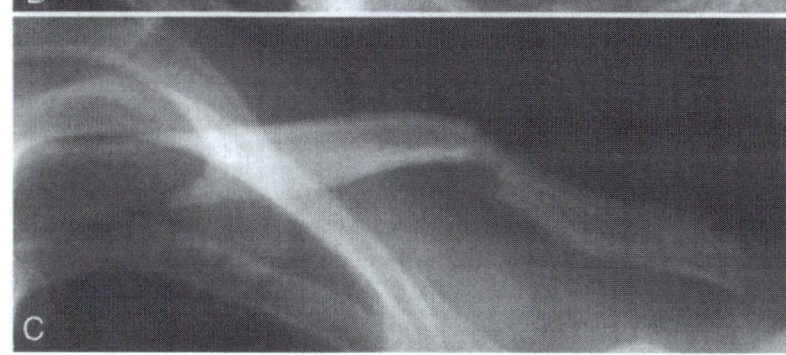

FIGURE 13-15. (A) Questionable fracture (arrow) in a child who fell on the shoulder. It is really the nutrient foramen. (B) Greenstick fracture. (C) Complete fracture with moderate displacement.

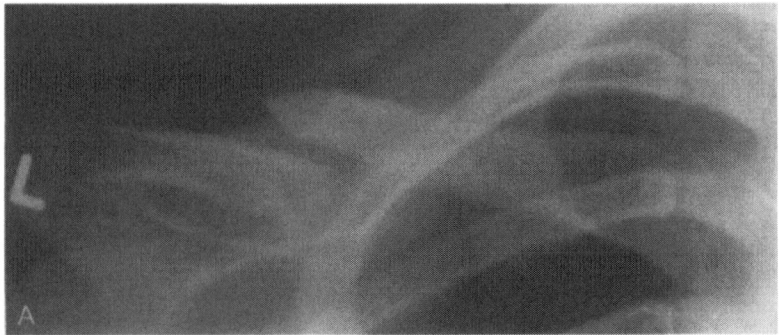
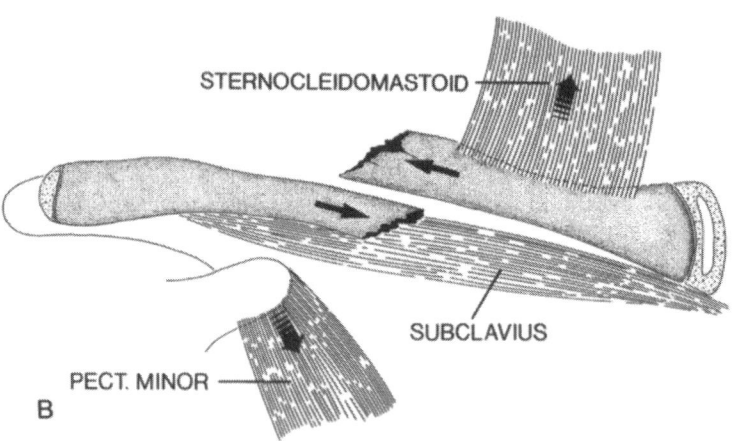

FIGURE 13-16. (A) Typical overriding of a complete clavicular fracture. (B) Muscle forces creating and maintaining this displacement pattern.

etrate the subcutaneous or cutaneous tissues and may also lacerate subclavian vessels or the brachial plexus, although these complications are infrequent in children. The clavicle does not exhibit a great capacity for plastic deformation, especially in the toddler or older child.

When the fracture is complete, muscle forces affect and maintain the subsequent deformation. The glenohumeral joint pulls the lateral fragment downward and inward. This displacement is a combination of the overall weight of the limb and the pull of the pectoralis muscles anteriorly and part of the trapezius posteriorly, with their summated forces being directed inferiorly. In contrast, the medial half is pulled upward and posteriorly by the sternocleidomastoid muscle (Fig. 13-16). The costoclavicular and sternoclavicular ligaments may act as check reins.

Diagnosis

Birth fractures are not always easy to diagnose, as they are often asymptomatic. In a roentgenographic survey of 300 consecutive live newborns, 5 had fractured clavicles (1.7%).[160] In none of these cases was the fracture suspected following the routine pediatric examination in the delivery room and the nursery. However, after each positive roentgenogram, reexamination demonstrated crepitation of the fracture site. Even in the newborn this fracture may be complete, with an overriding fragment. This should not be confused with congenital pseudarthrosis of the clavicle. Rounded ends typify the pseudarthrosis, in contrast to the sharp edges of a fracture.

Clavicular fractures may result in an *apparent* Erb's palsy (pseudoparalysis) because of the neonate's reluctance to move the arm. This pseudoparalysis clears readily and rapidly (usually within days), with no residual neurologic defect, as the fracture heals. Some patients, however, sustain both injuries, in which case the paralysis may be reduced, but slowly and not always completely.

Muscle function in the upper limb should be assessed by reflex stimulation to rule out associated brachial plexus injury. Sensation to pinprick should also be tested. This is likely to be present with pseudoparalysis but less so with true brachial plexopathy.

Infants and young children tend to be asymptomatic, and there may be no clinical evidence of the injury until the child develops callus. The callus causes marked swelling, disturbs the parents, and finally brings the antecedent injury to medical attention.

Radiography

Undisplaced fractures of the shaft and especially fractures of the medial end of the clavicle in young children may be missed on routine radiographs. The overlying second rib may obscure incomplete fractures. Normally, a soft tissue shadow parallels the superior border of the clavicle. When this shadow is absent unilaterally, more careful evaluation is recommended. Fractures in the middle third are usually depicted on routine anteroposterior roentgenograms. Demonstration of fractures of the medial and lateral ends of the clavicle often requires special oblique, lateral, or posteroanterior views. In the adolescent the diaphyseal fracture has a greater tendency to be comminuted.

The apical oblique view may be helpful for detecting a fracture of the clavicle. This particular view is obtained with the injured side of the patient angled 45° toward the x-ray tube and a 20° cephalad angulation of the x-ray beam. This view is effective for detecting nondisplaced fractures of the middle third of the clavicle in neonates and young children. Because of the normal clavicular curvature, routine radiographic views may foreshorten the central section, where most of the fractures occur. The apical oblique view has proved sensitive in cases in which the routine projection was nondiagnostic or negative.[152,177]

Occasionally, fracture of the clavicle at birth is accompanied by a physeal fracture of the proximal humeral epiphysis. Although it may not be seen on initial roentgenograms, subperiosteal new bone formation around the proximal humeral metaphysis makes it evident. Such osteoblastic reaction may be confused with osteomyelitis. Goddard et al. reported the association of clavicular fracture with atlantoaxial rotatory fixation in five patients.[145]

Treatment

Birth fractures, which are often unrecognized, do not always require treatment; they form callus rapidly and often become evident only when the mother notices the palpable callus of the healed fracture. Union usually occurs without external immobilization; and any malalignment is corrected rapidly with growth and remodeling. The infant should be handled gently, with no direct pressure over the clavicle. If

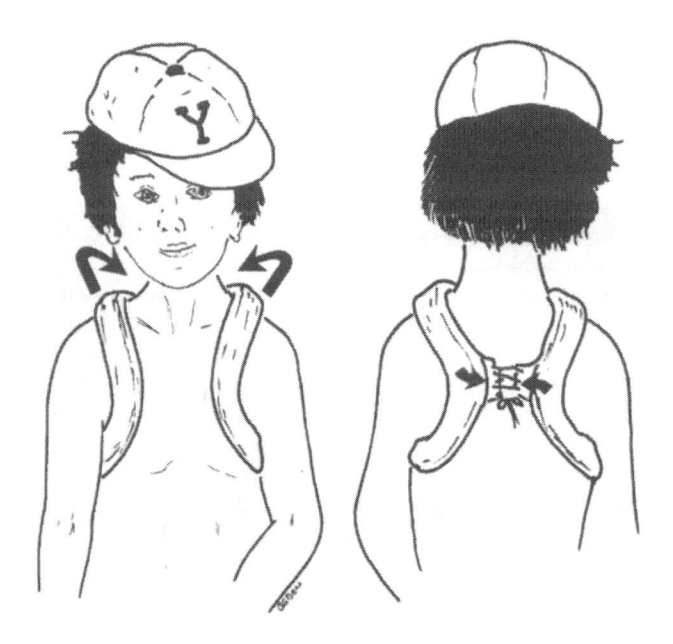

FIGURE 13-17. Figure-of-eight orthosis should pull the shoulders backward (large curved arrows) and be tightened regularly (small arrows). It should not be so tight that it impairs neurologic function of the brachial plexus.

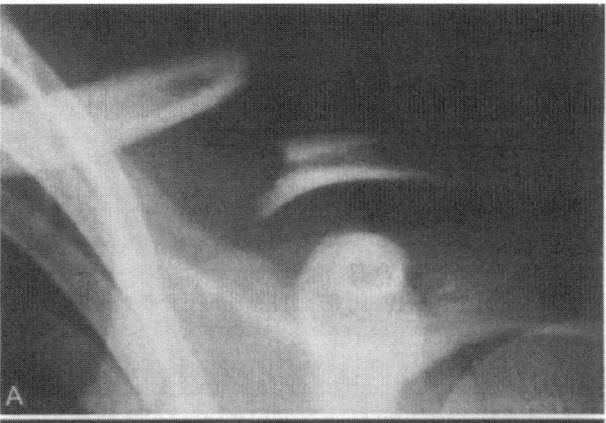

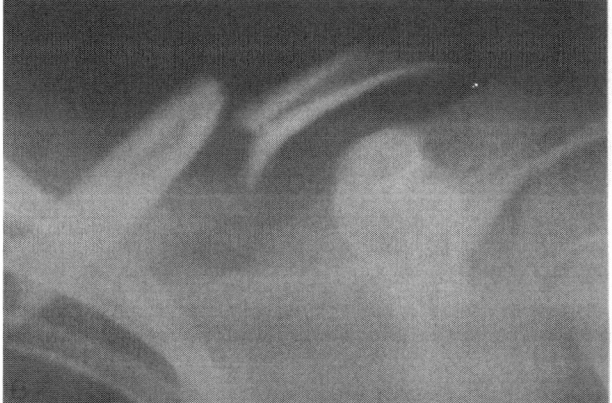

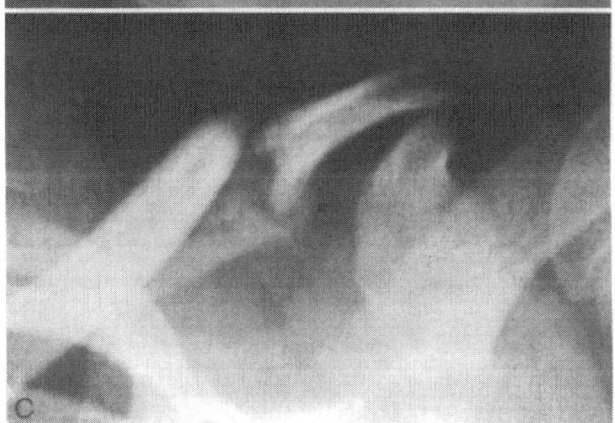

FIGURE 13-18. (A) Overriding and separated clavicular fracture. (B) Partial reduction just after application of a figure-of-eight strap. (C) Callus formation, at 3 weeks, within the intact inferior periosteal sleeve.

the fracture is painful or there is pseudoparalysis, it is best to protect the arm with a splint for 2–3 weeks. Within a week, or at most 10–14 days, the pain subsides, and the fracture begins to unite.

Children under 6 years of age with a fractured clavicle do not usually require formal, manipulative reduction. Callus formation remodels and disappears, generally within 6–9 months, a fact that should be impressed on the parents so they are not disturbed by the clinical appearance or the length of time necessary for remodeling. The child should be made comfortable by application of a figure-of-eight splint (Figs. 13-17, 13-18). The splint may be tightened slightly by the parents each evening. Immobilization should be continued for 3–4 weeks. Neuromuscular and vascular function in the arm should be checked frequently by the parents. Professional reevaluation at reasonable intervals is advisable to rule out problems.

In the older patient the figure-of-eight splint does not always adequately immobilize the fracture. Its main purpose is to remind the patient to hold the shoulders back. Accordingly, within a week it may be removed daily for hygienic purposes.

As the child gets older, the capacity for remodeling, particularly of any significant angular deformity, lessens. This factor increases the desirability of reasonable anatomic reduction. If the fracture is complete, markedly displaced, or overriding, closed reduction may be necessary. Reduction may be done after local injection of procaine or lidocaine, with great care being taken to avoid introduction of skin bacteria. The patient should sit, and the physician should be positioned behind to pull the shoulders backward while applying leverage between the scapulae. The patient may also be placed in a recumbent position, with the back over a midline sandbag and the arm over the side, which generally effects gradual reduction. In older children who require closed reduction, plaster may be added to the figure-of-eight splint to reinforce its rigidity.[141]

Even if there is significant angulation of the fracture in an adolescent, it is usually better to let the fracture heal without operative procedures and deal with the osseous prominence of the healed fracture, if clinically necessary, at a later date. Such prominences are usually remodeled, even in the adolescent patient.

Fracture of the clavicle in a child who is forced to rest in bed because of other major trauma may be managed more easily in the supine position with a small sandbag or pillow placed between the scapulae so the weight of the upper limbs gradually falls backward and reduces the fracture. For comfort, a figure-of-eight splint may be applied. If significant cosmetic deformity is present, and one does not wish to undertake an open reduction, modified lateral arm skin traction may be used, with the shoulder at 90° of abduction and 90° of external rotation.

It is unwise to complete a greenstick fracture, as is often taught with regard to other bones, inasmuch as the subclavian vessels and brachial plexus lie directly underneath the clavicle. Rupture of the subclavian vessels has been described as a cause of death.[136,138] Despite the proximity of pleura, skin, brachial plexus, and brachial vessels, complications of this fracture are rare in children. Most often the deformation in anterior and away from major neuromuscular structures. Furthermore, the injury mechanism is often a fall, rather than the more violent trauma that usually causes this bone to fracture in the adult.

Open reduction of a fractured clavicle is not generally indicated in children but may become appropriate in the adolescent.[124,149,151] If open reduction is done, a small plate is used. Alternatively, malleable plates (e.g., reconstruction plates) may be contoured to the variable anatomy of the clavicle. Small K-wires can migrate and should be avoided. If used they should be left protruding to allow removal 3–4 weeks after the injury. The fractured clavicle, like the fractured rib, heals despite almost continuous motion of the upper extremity. Nonunion is rare with closed treatment.

Remodeling

Clavicular fractures unite quickly, almost invariably with some degree of accentuated angulation. Remodeling is generally complete within a year, especially in young children. This bone remodels adequately and quickly and may be left in a reasonable degree of angular deformity. Anatomic realignment assumes more importance in adolescents, as remodeling is less active and may not correct significant loss of axial alignment.

Complications

The primary justification for exploratory surgery is to repair damaged subclavian vessels or brachial plexus. A vascular complication is suggested by a large, rapidly increasing hematoma. Surgical intervention in this case must be immediate, as the patient may die owing to extravasation of blood into the chest and shock.[124,138,148]

Subclavian vascular compression may occur owing to greenstick fracture and inferior bowing.[158,166] This complication is recognizable by venous congestion and edema of the ipsilateral arm. A chronic arteriovenous fistula has also been reported.[148]

The incidence of nonunion of clavicular fractures in patients of all ages ranges from 0.8% to 3.7%.[142,179] Nonunion of clavicular fractures in skeletally immature individuals, however, is rare. In fact, the main differential diagnoses of discontinuity of the clavicle in children and adolescents should include congenital pseudarthrosis, cleidocranial dysostosis, and neurofibromatosis, rather than nonunion following fracture.

A review of 33 patients with nonunion of a clavicular fracture included a 12-year-old and a 13-year-old, neither of whom underwent treatment of the nonunion.[179] Each had unlimited activity and hypertrophic nonunion, in contrast to the more characteristic atrophic nonunion of older patients. A third patient, 7 years of age when injured, still had a hypertrophic nonunion 6 years after the injury and underwent fixation and bone graft, which established union and restored unlimited activity. Nogi reported nonunion of the clavicle in a 12-year-old child.[162]

The treatment of discontinuity of the clavicle in children seems to be well defined. In most cases there is little functional impairment. Thus surgery may be for cosmetic purposes to eliminate the enlarged mid-clavicular mass. In patients whose presenting symptoms include pain and limited function, surgery may return the patient to full, painless activity.

Nonunion and shortening of mid-clavicle fractures, especially in young patients, does not usually occur.[139] Plate fixation for mid-clavicular fractures with gross displacement and shortening of more than 15 mm may be necessary. A one-third tubular plate is placed under the platysma to cover the plate and prevent skin discomfort. Bone grafting is rarely necessary. Mullaji and Jupiter used a low-contact dynamic compression plate that could be readily bent to contour to the specific demands of the individual clavicle.[159]

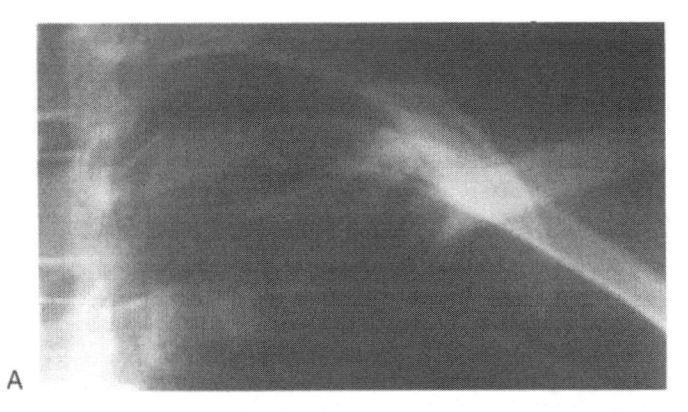

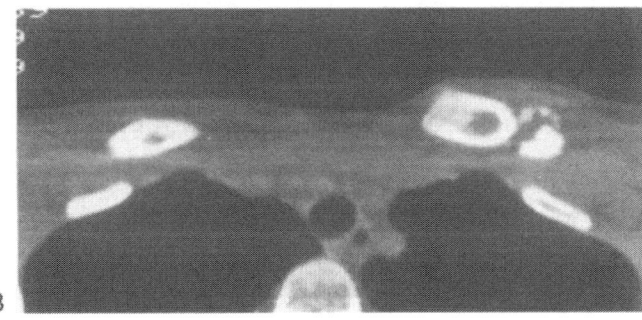

FIGURE 13-19. Complex fracture-dislocation. (A) Fracture in the junction of the proximal-middle third. The sternoclavicular region is not well visualized. (B) CT scan shows the anterior sternoclavicular disruption and the fracture.

Complex Clavicular Injury

Concomitant ipsilateral medial epiphyseal injury with fracture of the clavicular diaphysis (Fig. 13-19) during childhood is rare.[146,174] Thomas and Friedman thought that such injuries were the result of sequential trauma rather than the same traumatic incident.[174] Hardy particularly reported a 7-year-old girl who was knocked off her horse when she struck a stable door against her right shoulder as she rode past; she landed on the same shoulder. The obvious mid-clavicular fracture was treated conservatively. The sternoclavicular disruption (i.e., physeal fracture) was not noted until 12 days later, at which time the clavicular diaphyseal fracture had healed to an extent that they were able to apply external pressure to the medial end of the anteriorly displaced medial clavicle and attain full reduction.[146]

Congenital Pseudarthrosis

Congenital pseudarthrosis invariably affects the right clavicle.[180–194,197–208] It is often misinterpreted as an acute fracture. The lesion is present at birth and most likely results from failure of normal ossification patterns.[184,186,195,197] Swelling or prominence may be found at or soon after birth, although the diagnosis may be delayed for months to years. The children do not have obvious histories of birth injury, and the limb is usually painless. However, the child may be reluctant to move the arm or be unable to push it when crawling. Minor trauma often brings the deformity to medical attention. The relation of the two fragments is always the same, with the sternal fragment being larger and lying in front of and above the shorter, inferiorly directed acromial fragment (Fig. 13-20). The bone ends at the pseudarthrosis are smooth and usually overriding.

Histologic examination of the resected ends of congenital pseudarthroses of the clavicle showed cartilaginous caps and pathologic changes that were equivalent to those in epiphyses that were adding new bone.[193] This finding was confirmed by preoperative tetracyline labeling. The authors believed that the pseudarthrosis was caused by failure of the embryonic ossification centers to fuse. This is in contrast to the material discussed earlier in the anatomy section, which pointed out that the point of fusion of the two anlagen was different from the area of pseudarthrosis usually seen clinically. The difference, however, could be justified by differential growth of the two segments.[24,186] Differential growth certainly is compatible with observations that the lateral segment seems to be relatively underdeveloped when compared to the opposite clavicle.[190] This would affect the relative position of the pseudarthrosis. These studies also have shown a predominance of longitudinal growth from the proximal (sternal) end compared to the lateral (acromial) end (approximately 70–30%).[190]

Congenital pseudarthrosis should be treated as a nonunion, with careful resection and removal of the smooth cortical bone ends to expose the medullary cavity.[196,202,205] The posteroinferior periosteal continuity should be maintained. The ends may be approximated with "bone" sutures. Bone graft may not be necessary, especially in younger children. In nine cases, all done in children under 4 years of age, nonunion has not recurred.[190] All had osseous bridging within 6–8 weeks postoperatively, and all were solidly healed by 14 weeks after surgery. Interestingly, there was delayed remodeling of the callus bone that formed, and the distal

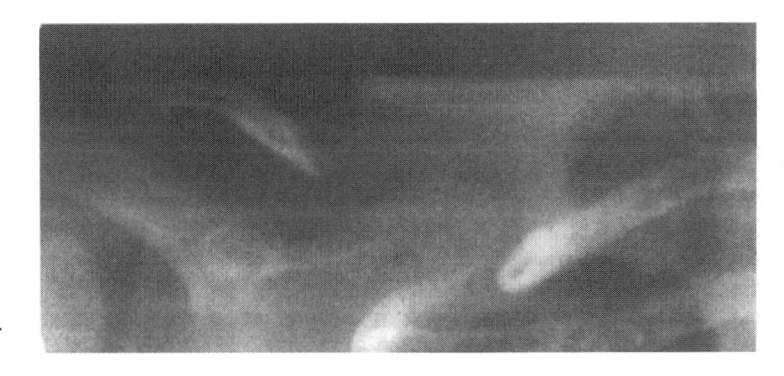

FIGURE 13-20. Congenital pseudarthrosis in a 2-month-old baby. It must be distinguished from an acute fracture.

end of the clavicle was not as well developed as that on the contralateral side.

Trauma to the Proximal (Sternal) Clavicle

Traumatic separation of the epiphysis of the sternal end of the clavicle (Fig. 13-21) occurs infrequently.[209-222,224-261] Because of the late closure of this physis, proximal physeal separation may occur even in young adults in their early twenties. The injury usually occurs with either a fall on the outstretched arm or posteriorly directed impact to the shoulder. Disruption of this region may occur during traumatic delivery (Fig. 13-22).[258]

This injury mimics sternoclavicular dislocation, which does not usually occur until the clavicle is completely mature. Any injury to this end of the clavicle in a neonate, child, adolescent, or even young adult should be considered an epiphyseal injury, not sternoclavicular joint dislocation. Infrequently, fracture of the diaphysis and sternal end may occur concomitantly, creating an unstable proximal fragment.[237]

The stability of the sternoclavicular joint is contingent on the joint capsule, the fibrocartilaginous meniscus, and the interclavicular and costoclavicular ligaments. Sternoclavicular injury is commonly caused by indirect violence, such as a fall on or blow to the shoulder, which drives the clavicle posteriorly or anteriorly. The injury is occasionally produced by direct impact to the sternoclavicular region.

Pain and swelling are usually obvious if a sternoclavicular injury is present. Posterior displacement may be associated with respiratory difficulty or dysphagia.[235] Most of the injuries are anterior, with a mass evident over the sternoclavicular region. The sternal end of the clavicle (i.e., metaphysis) may be sharply prominent and palpable immediately underneath the skin. The clavicular part of the sternocleidomastoid muscle is pulled anteriorly with the bone and is often in spasm, causing the patient's head to tilt toward the affected side. Posterior displacements, accompanied by an indentation next to the sternum, may cause intrathoracic problems, such as tracheal compression and dyspnea.[228,229,241,259]

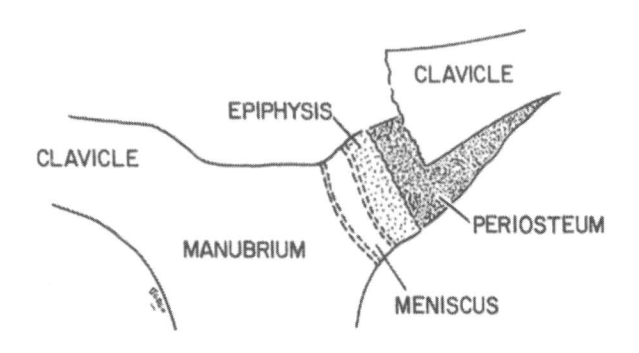

FIGURE 13-21. Epiphyseal displacement of the proximal clavicle: injury pattern.

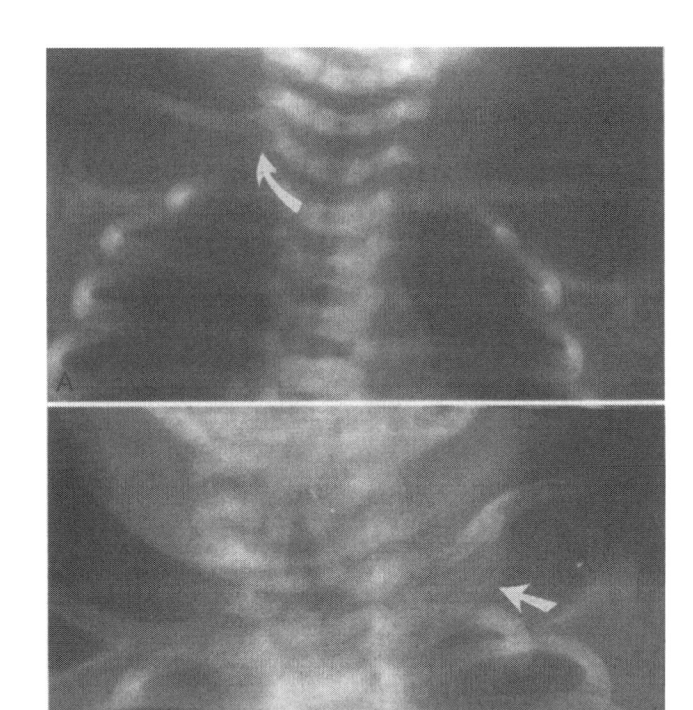

FIGURE 13-22. (A) Sternoclavicular injury (arrow) in a newborn sustained during a difficult delivery. (B) Subperiosteal new bone (arrow) filling the intact periosteal sleeve.

Radiology

Anteroposterior roentgenograms may appear normal even if sternoclavicular injury is present. Special oblique views may show the displacement of the sternal end of the clavicle. Brooks and Henning[212] recommended a 30° tangential radiograph instead of the lordotic projection, with the x-ray tube directed at a 40°–50° cephalad tilt. The Hobbs view is a superoinferior projection.[233] The Heinig view is taken with the patient recumbent and the x-ray tube parallel to the table top, approximately 30 inches away from the involved joint.[232] The grid cassette is placed perpendicular to the beam against the opposite shoulder, and the shoulder closest to the tube is abducted. If the injury occurs before ossification in the medial epiphysis, the condition is easily and often mistaken for dislocation of the sternoclavicular joint.

Cope et al. reported several radiographic projections which have been recorded as being diagnostically helpful.[217,218] These include the Rockwood or "serendipity" projection, which employs a 50° tube tilt toward the head.

Computed tomography, the optimal method for demonstrating disruption of the sternoclavicular joints, may be used not only to define the displacement (Figs. 13-23, 13-24) but also to reveal the relations of the great vessels, esophagus, and trachea to the sternoclavicular joint, the disrupted posteriorly displaced clavicular metaphysis, and any impingement on these structures.[223,224,239,240,249] CT is the best study for evaluating the extent and severity of the posterior displacement. It is also useful for follow-up studies of healing and remodeling.

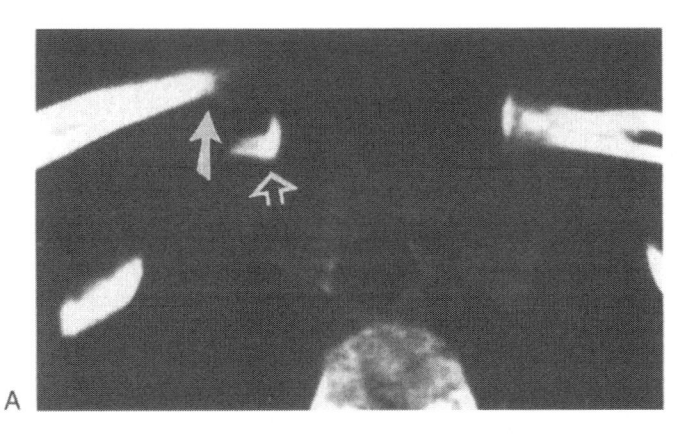

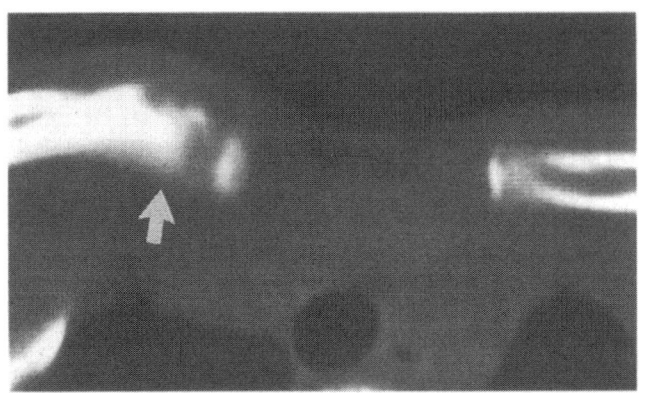

FIGURE 13-23. (A) Anterior sternoclavicular disruption (solid arrow), leaving behind an intact Thurstan Holland fragment (open arrow). (B) Healing callus (arrow) connects the displaced fragments.

Treatment

Treatment initially consists of closed, manipulative reduction and immobilization.[212,236] This approach is more effective for anterior than posterior displacement. Because a portion of the periosteal sleeve is intact, whether the displacement is anterior or posterior, complete closed reduction is not necessary in the young child. Significant amounts of subperiosteal bone fill in the "displacement defect" and progressively remodel, although the process may take several months to years.

When the proximal metaphysis is displaced anteriorly, direct pressure is placed on the osseous prominence, pushing it back into the sternoclavicular region. The periosteum should be intact posteriorly, effectively preventing overreduction into the thoracic cavity.

Posterior displacement is more difficult to reduce by closed methods. A bolster may be placed under the spine to elevate the shoulders. Direct pressure is then applied to both shoulders, forcing them backward. Application of the same force to both shoulders is more likely to move the proximal metaphysis out from behind the manubrium, where it often lies. This retrosternal location is much more difficult to reduce than one displaced directly posteriorly. If the reduction cannot be accomplished, a towel clip may be used to grasp the clavicle percutaneously to pull it forward (again with a bolster under the spine).

Open reduction may be indicated when closed, manipulative reduction fails. A *threaded* Kirschner wire may be drilled obliquely through the anterior cortex, across the epiphysis, and into the sternum to stabilize the fragments. Operative treatment with smooth pins across the fracture site or across the sternoclavicular joint is contraindicated because of the potential hazard of pin breakage or migration of the pin into the vital structures in the mediastinum (see Chapter 10). The arm must be immobilized to minimize joint motion and stress, which enhances the risk of pin breakage. The wires are removed in about 4–6 weeks. The location of the pins must be monitored closely.

Alternatively, Dacron mesh or heavy sutures using bone anchors may be used. Tricoire et al. use the tendon of the subclavian muscle to stabilize the disrupted joint.[255] All cases were posteriorly dislocated. They also found meniscal damage in three of six patients. Extensive capsular repairs may be unnecessary.

With anterior displacement, the periosteal sleeve may be pulled into the displaced region, effectively creating a membrane between the epiphysis, which is still in the joint, and the metaphysis. This situation increases the instability of the joint after closed reduction.

Eskola reviewed 12 adults and noted that primary open reduction was preferred for acute cases of proximal clavicular displacement, whether anterior or posterior.[227] Barth and Hagen also advocated surgical repair, but only for those in

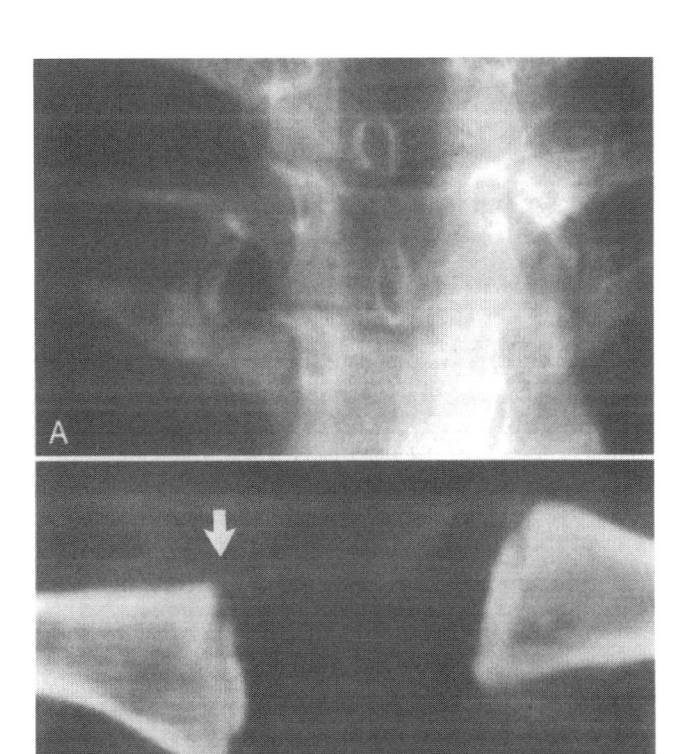

FIGURE 13-24. (A) Posterior sternoclavicular dislocation. (B) CT scan shows the dislocation (arrow).

whom an acute displacement could not be reduced by manipulation, as is the case in most children and for those in whom frequent recurrent subluxation or dislocation has occurred.[209]

Complications

Posterior displacement of the medial portion of the clavicle is potentially dangerous owing to the proximity of major anatomic structures within the chest and mediastinum. Levinsohn et al. demonstrated the proximity of the joint to vital structures in an autopsy/imaging study.[239] Death resulting from erosion of the trachea and major vessels, perforation of the esophagus, mediastinitis, thoracic outlet syndromes, syncope secondary to carotid artery compression, and arteriovenous fistula may occur.[221,229,230,252,257,259] Recurrent displacement (partial to complete) is a significant complication.

Southworth and Merritt reported complete obstruction of the innominate vein with retrograde flow up the anterior jugular vein and across the inferior thyroid vein, establishing collateral venous return.[252] A repeat venogram after closed reduction demonstrated patency of the innominate vein and normal drainage into the superior vena cava. Other complications have included tracheoesophageal fistula,[257] brachial plexus injury,[229] and intrathoracic great vessel tamponade[230] or laceration.[259] Great vessel damage is usually associated with venous distension in the neck and ipsilateral arm, hemothorax, and hemomediastinum.

Smolle-Juettner et al. described intracardiac malpositioning of a fixation wire used for sternoclavicular disruption.[251] It was in a 17-year-old boy who had a posterior subluxation. The immediate postoperative films show that the fixation wires were probably in the area of the right atrium and obviously were too deep into the chest. Unfortunately, the wires were not pulled back. Two hours later the patient went into hypovolemic shock. Emergency aortography showed bleeding into the chest and pericardium, with a tear in the anterior wall of the right atrium. The outcome was fatal.

Howard and Shafer reported that neurovascular compression fell into two groups: (1) obstruction of the carotid artery by the displaced medial end, causing syncopal symptoms; and (2) compression of the subclavian vessels or brachial plexus.[148] Another complication may be damage to the apical pleura, with subsequent pneumothorax, hemothorax, or both.[234]

Trauma to the Distal (Acromial) Clavicle

Children may sustain an injury to the distal clavicle that is analogous to a metaphyseal–epiphyseal fracture (Figs. 13-25 to 13-27) but is easily misinterpreted as an acromioclavicular separation.[262–284] The coracoclavicular ligaments usually remain intact and attached to the periosteal sleeve. Falstie-Jensen and Mikkelsen used the term "pseudodislocation" because some or all of the cartilage displaced with the periosteal sleeve.[268] Eidman et al. reported 25 children thought to have acromioclavicular joint separation; instead,

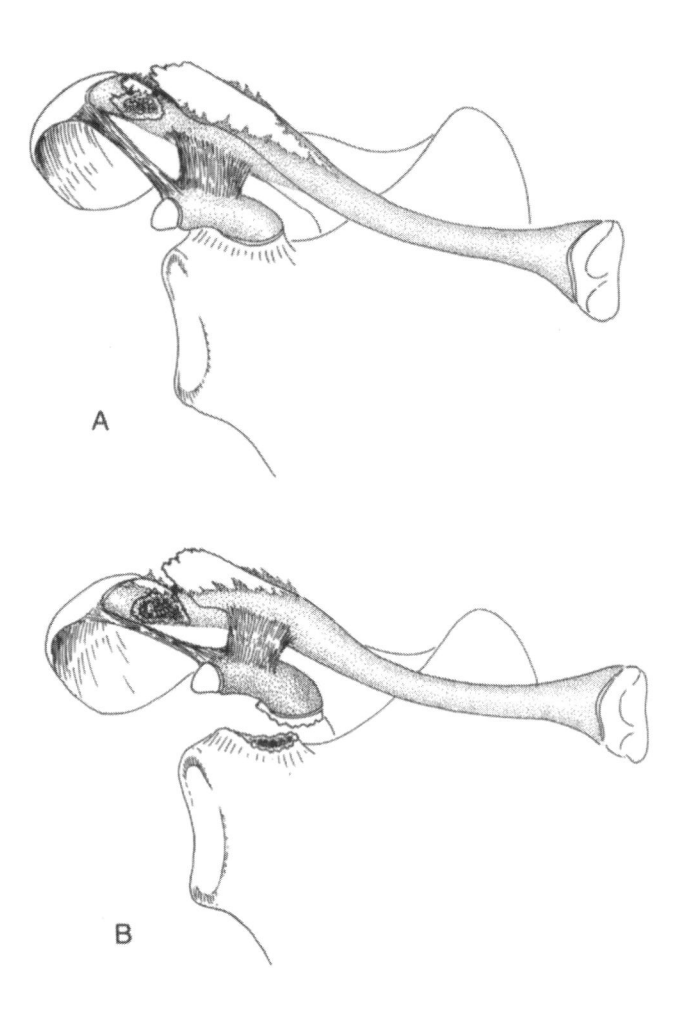

FIGURE 13-25. (A) Lateral clavicular fracture, showing the intact inferior periosteal sleeve and coracoclavicular ligaments. (B) Similar injury with concomitant fracture of the coracoid process.

each had a disruption of the distal clavicle and, in some cases, an associated fracture of the coracoid.[267] Concomitant fracture may also involve the acromion (Figs. 13-28).

These injuries, especially in the older child and adolescent, mimic acromioclavicular separation, although they are really physeal injuries in which the thin epiphysis and physis maintain their normal anatomic relation to the acromioclavicular joint, and the distal metaphysis is displaced superiorly. The periosteal sleeve is generally intact inferiorly, and the ligamentous structures connecting the clavicle with the coracoid remain attached to the periosteal sleeve. This allows rapid "reattachment" of these ligaments to the subperiosteal callus that is formed by this sleeve of tissue.

Pathology

The acromioclavicular ligaments attach densely into the perichondrium of the distal clavicular epiphysis and then subsequently blend into the periosteum. As in other regions of the developing chondro-osseous skeleton, the weakest region biomechanically is the physeal–metaphyseal interface, rendering acromioclavicular ligament disruption much less likely in the infant, child, or adolescent. Instead, the deforming forces that would cause such a separation in an adult

Trauma to the Distal (Acromial) Clavicle

invariably result in a clavicular fracture at either end or the midshaft in a child.

The pathomechanism is variable stripping of the periosteum. In severe cases, the proximal end of the clavicle is displaced superiorly, whereas the periosteal sleeve, with attached distal epiphysis, acromion, acromioclavicular joint, and coracoclavicular ligaments, remains anatomically intact (Fig. 13-29). Variations in the fracture pattern and the degree of displacement occur (Fig. 13-30). Inferior displacement also may occur. The most infrequent pattern is subcoracoid displacement.

Because the distal epiphysis retains a cartilaginous cap into the mid-twenties if not longer (similar to the delayed maturation and physiologic epiphysiodesis characterizing the proximal clavicular epiphysis), this injury pattern may occur even in the young adult. It must be distinguished from true acromioclavicular joint disruption.[279]

Diagnosis

The severity of the injury determines the clinical presentation.[282,295] There is discrete tenderness over the joint, and this pain is accentuated by motion. If fragment separation is complete, the end of the proximal segment may be prominent, tenting the skin as the weight of the arm pulls the scapula downward.

Radiology

When there is minimal disruption of the periosteal sleeve, the acromial process is in its normal position relative to the lateral end of the clavicle, whereas disruption of the sleeve leads to increasing discontinuity between the acromion and clavicle. Because the ends of the clavicle and acromion are incompletely ossified, a normal cartilage space width may be misinterpreted as widening of the acromioclavicular joint

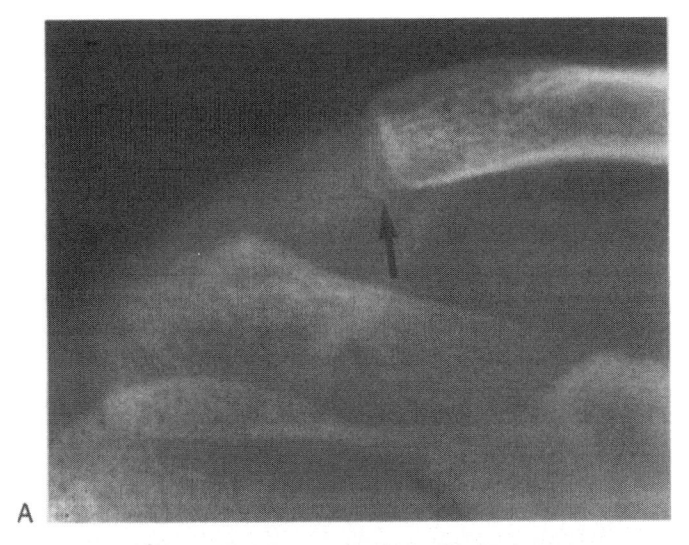

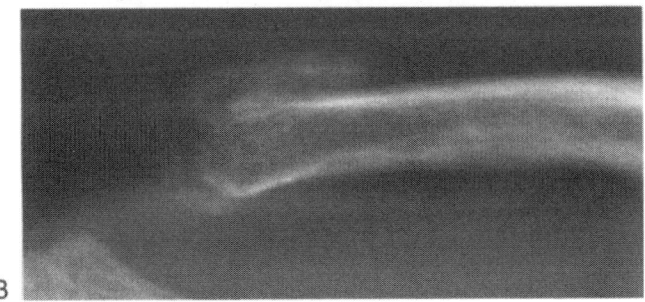

FIGURE 13-26. (A) Thin distal clavicular fracture (arrow). (B) Four weeks later.

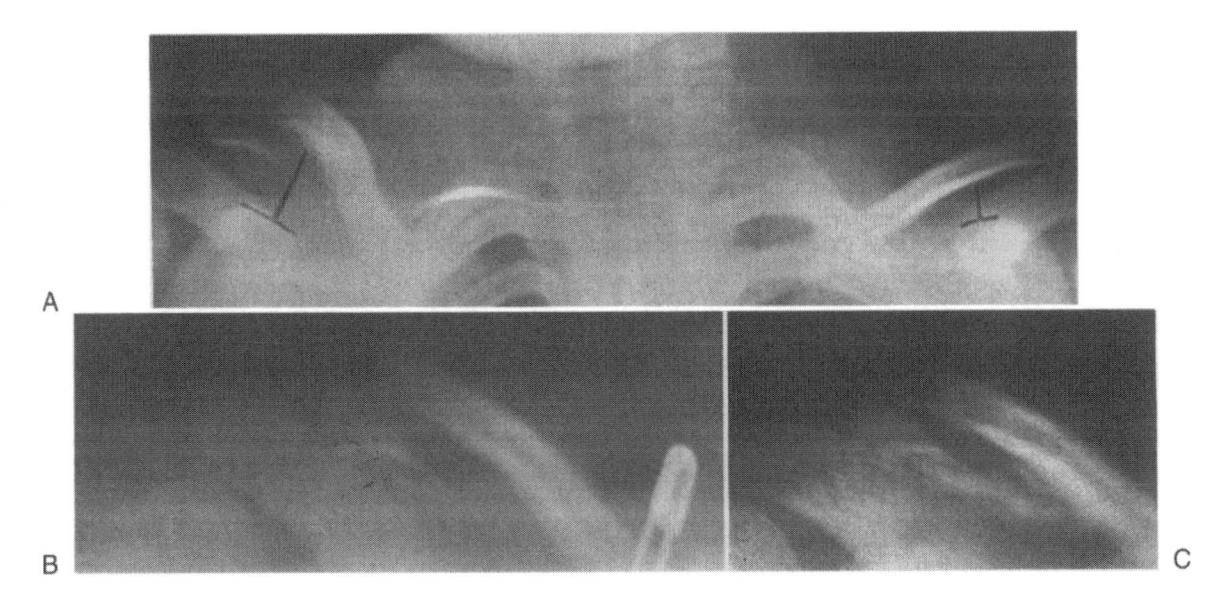

FIGURE 13-27. (A) Distal clavicular fracture. Note the separation of the coracoid from the proximal fragment compared to the opposite side. (B) Appearance after closed reduction. (C) Appearance 1 month later.

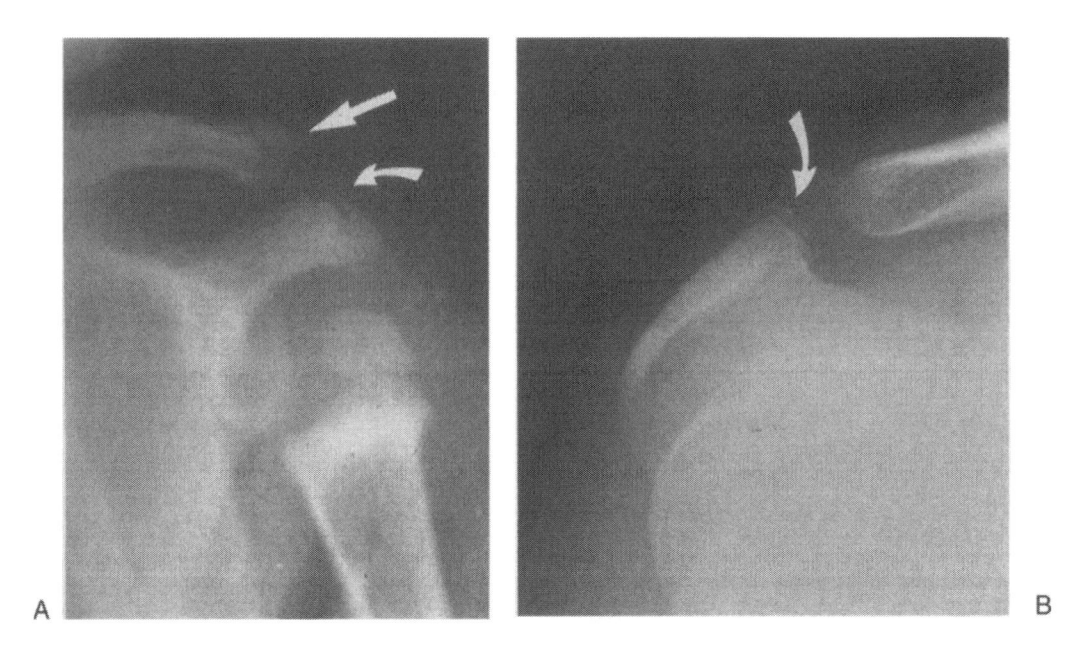

FIGURE 13-28. (A) Lateral clavicular fracture (straight arrow) with acromial fracture (curved arrow). (B) Thin avulsion of acromion (arrow) in a 10-year-old child with an acromioclavicular injury.

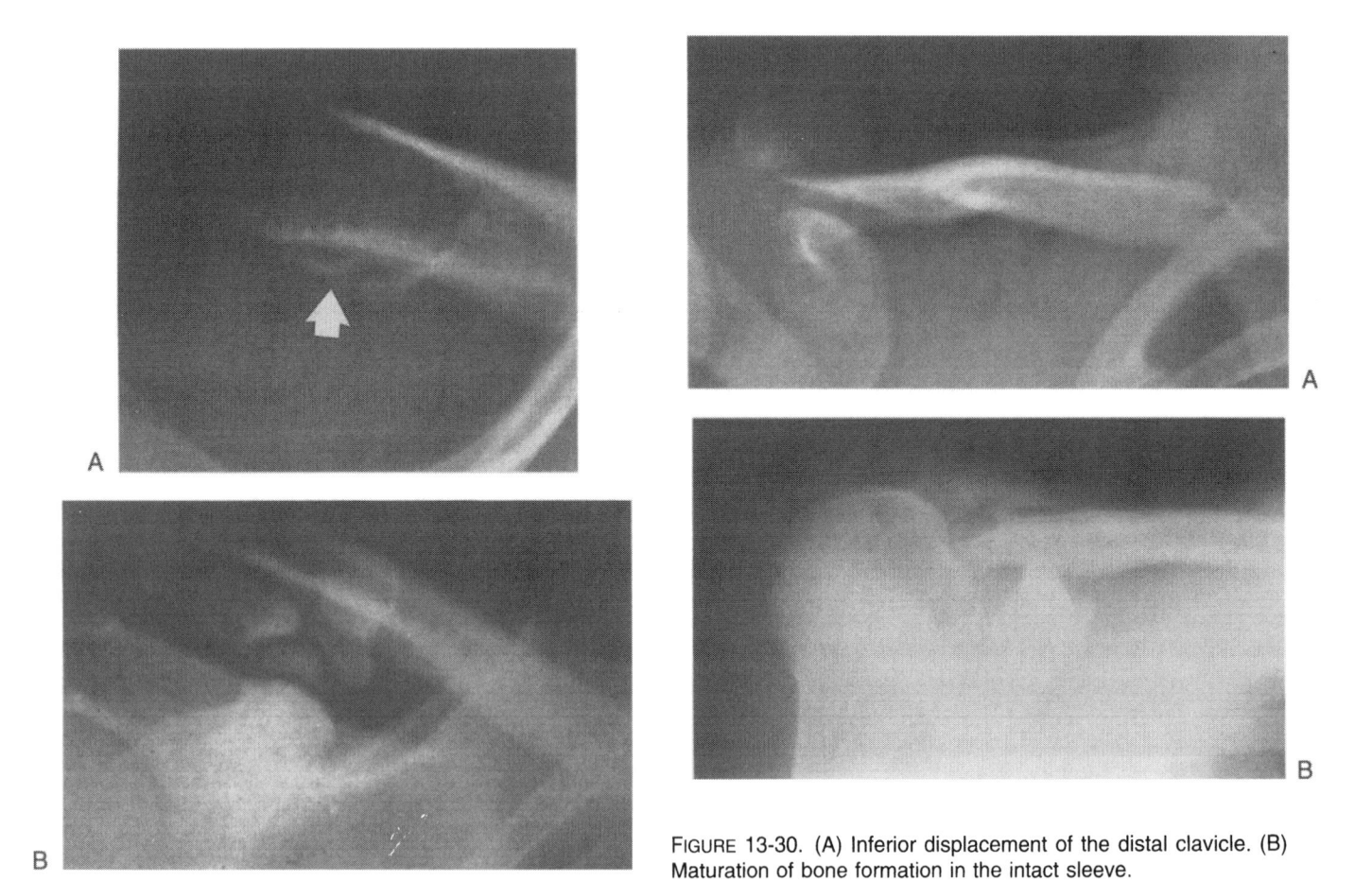

FIGURE 13-29. (A) Disruption of coracoid and trapezoid ligament bony attachments (arrow). (B) Irregular bone formation 9 years after a clavicular/coracoid injury.

FIGURE 13-30. (A) Inferior displacement of the distal clavicle. (B) Maturation of bone formation in the intact sleeve.

instead of a fracture of the lateral end of the clavicle. Displacement is variable, so stress films with the patient holding weights may accentuate the injury and help ascertain the diagnosis, as with acromioclavicular separation in the skeletally mature patient.

Associated Fractures

Avulsion fractures may be associated with distal clavicular separation.[263,267,276,280,282] These fractures undoubtedly occur because of the ligamentous attachments, with the zone of failure pulling the coracoid from its bipolar growth plate with the main body of the scapula. The bone may avulse from the clavicle or may involve some or all of the coracoid process.

Distal acromioclavicular disruption is often associated with an epiphyseal separation of the base of the coracoid process.[264] Such a fracture of the base of the coracoid is often overlooked on routine radiographs. The Stryker notch view offers the clearest profile of the entire coracoid and is the same view used to demonstrate the Hill-Sach compression fracture of the posterolateral aspect of the humeral head. This fracture is a separation of the common physis of the base of the coracoid and the upper portion of the glenoid fossa.

Scavenius and Iverson studied weight lifters and found "nontraumatic" clavicular osteolysis in these individuals.[281] The chronic repetitiveness of this injury and the changes are compatible with minimal disruption of the distal clavicular epiphysis with metaphyseal remodeling, not unlike similar instances of "widening" of the growth plate in the distal radius and proximal humerus in competitive young gymnasts and pitchers due to chronic repetitive "nontrauma" to the aforementioned regions.

Treatment

Treatment is contingent on the degree of injury, although the general principle in children and adolescents is closed reduction.[26,279] Sprains require symptomatic treatment with a sling. Undisplaced lateral clavicular fractures require symptomatic treatment with a sling, a figure-of-eight clavicle strap, or both; but they must be watched closely for subsequent displacement. Subluxation of the distal fragment may be treated with an adjustable strap going across the acromioclavicular joint. With complete displacement, the same immobilization should be employed initially; but if the reduction cannot be maintained easily, internal stabilization can be considered. The injury may be reduced by direct pressure over the distal end and then may be fixed by percutaneous pins.

Alternatively, the fracture may be opened and reduced under direct visualization. Falstie-Jensen and Mikkelsen strongly advocated open reduction.[268] When open reduction is necessary, especially for the displaced pattern, the bone should be reduced into the periosteal sleeve, which is then repaired. If the periosteal repair is not stable, threaded fixation pins may be used. The fixation wires should be removed in 4–6 weeks. The patient must be monitored closely for pin breakage. An alternative to pin fixation is the use of heavy nonabsorbable sutures with bone anchors.

If the lesion is left displaced, new bone may form within the periosteal tube, and the distal clavicle may become bifid or Y-shaped. This may lead to a deformity sufficiently uncomfortable for the patient to require subsequent reconstructive surgery (i.e., resection of the nonremodeled original distal clavicle).

Furthermore, the distal fragment may be displaced and may override, comparable to a dorsally displaced distal radial metaphyseal fracture. Such displacement may be difficult to treat by closed reduction and may be corrected more effectively by open reduction. Leaving the distal fragment overriding, especially in an older child, may result in a permanent deformity because there is a decreased tendency for metaphyseal remodeling in this region. The periosteal sleeve is usually extremely osteogenic and readily fills in any gap between the periosteum and metaphysis.

Results

Good to excellent results are seen in most cases. No children have been reported to develop growth disturbances. Acromioclavicular joint arthritis is rare, although long-term follow-up of injured children and adolescents into adult years is not available in the literature.

Clavicular "Duplication"

Partial duplication of the distal clavicle, without other abnormalities, has been termed "developmental, without clinical significance, and of purely anatomic interest."[278] Similar cases were termed "os subclaviculare" or "os acromiale."[270,274] These authors were unable to explain adequately the duplication on an embryologic basis. Oestreich suggested that at least one entity, the lateral clavicular hook, could be an acquired lesion or occur congenitally.[278] Twigg and Rosenbaum reported a case of duplication of the clavicle.[283] Montgomery and Lloyd described a similar case involving fracture of the distal epiphysis of the coracoid process and separation of the acromioclavicular joint.[276] Rather than being congenital abnormalities, it is likely that these cases represent varying degrees of unrecognized antecedent trauma in the acromioclavicular region.[265]

Following initial separation of the distal epiphysis from the metaphysis (with the acromioclavicular joint intact), the metaphysis may be displaced through a longitudinal tear of the periosteum. The patterns of healing and subsequent growth after the injury allow a partial duplication (Figs. 13-31, 13-32), limited by the extent of periosteal stripping, that may or may not remodel prior to skeletal maturation.

Subcoracoid Displacement

Gerber and Rockwood reported three cases of subcoracoid dislocation of the lateral end of the clavicle, one of which involved a 14-month-old baby.[269] There were only two previous reports of the particular injury pattern, both involving adults. The mechanism of dislocation appeared to involve forceful abduction and external rotation of the arm. The two adults reported by Derter and Rockwood had multiple injuries, including rib fractures; the infant had no other concomitant injury, although forceful abduction was a probable

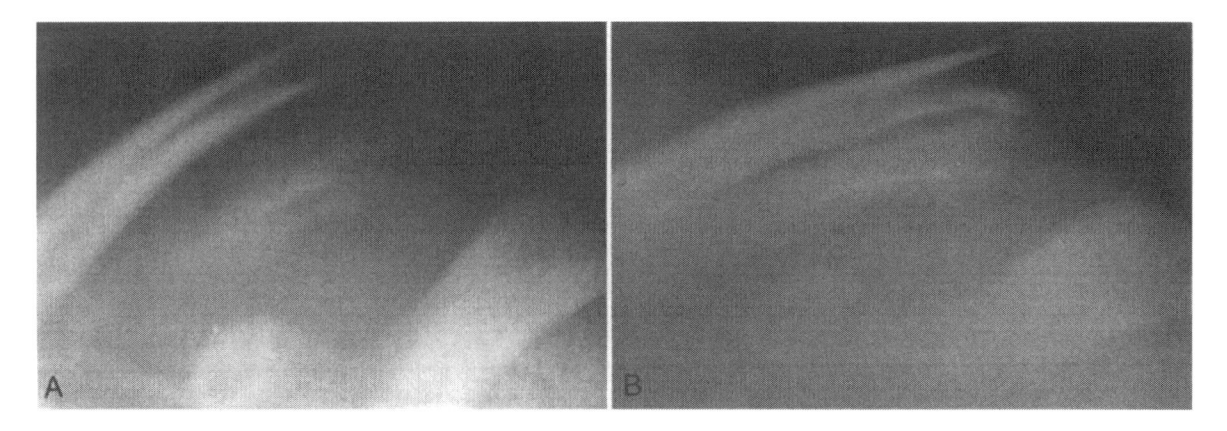

FIGURE 13-31. (A) Distal clavicular fracture in a patient with a head injury. The distal end is superiorly displaced. Bone is beginning to form in the intact, inferior periosteal sleeve. (B) Six months later, a clavicular "duplication" is evident.

mechanism. The infant underwent an open reduction and was found to have had the lateral end of the clavicle stripped from the periosteal tube in a manner somewhat similar to that of the more usual superior displacement.

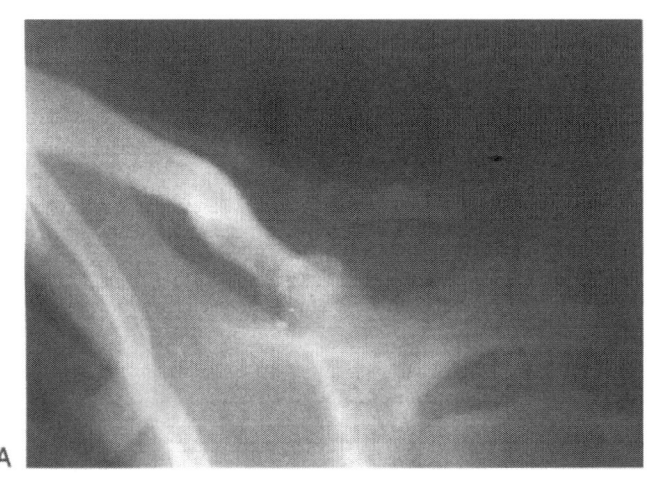

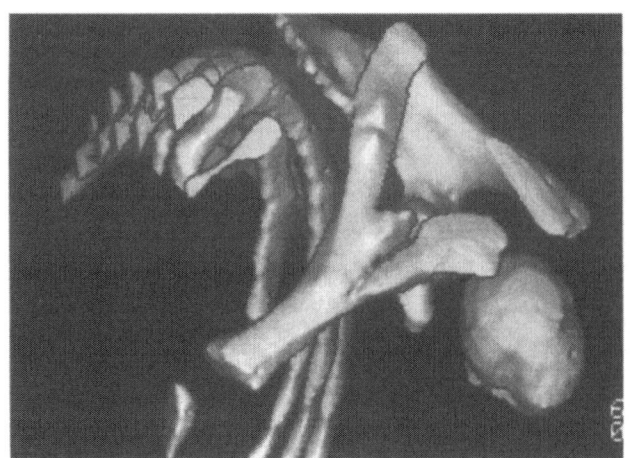

FIGURE 13-32. (A) Progressive clavicular "duplication." (B) Three-dimensional CT scan.

Acromioclavicular Dislocation

True dislocations of the acromioclavicular joint are unusual in children, primarily because the deforming forces that would cause such a separation in an adult result in a metaphyseal fracture in children. Contact sports during adolescence, however, may cause acromioclavicular dislocation. Several acromioclavicular injuries may occur: (1) ligamentous strain; (2) rupture of the acromioclavicular ligaments only; or (3) rupture of the entire ligament complex (acromioclavicular, conoid, and trapezoid).

The severity of the injury determines the clinical presentation. There is discrete tenderness over the joint that is accentuated by motion. If separation is complete, the end of the clavicle may be prominent. The patient usually complains of pain upon all movement of the shoulder, particularly forward rotation. There is specific tenderness over the acromioclavicular joint. If the joint is dislocated, the upright, prominent lateral end of the clavicle is easily palpated.

Roentgenograms are attained with the patient standing, holding weights in each hand, and a central beam passing anteroposteriorly through the joint. In subluxation the acromial process is depressed relative to the lateral end of the clavicle, whereas in dislocation there is complete discontinuity of the articular end. Because the ends of the clavicle and acromion may be incompletely ossified, a normal cartilage space width may be misinterpreted as widening of the acromioclavicular joint. An associated fracture of the lateral end of the clavicle should be ruled out.

This dislocation is primarily an "adult" injury. Therefore the reader should consult the literature on adult trauma for specific details of diagnosis and treatment.

Trauma to the Scapula

During childhood fractures of the scapula, which is highly mobile and well protected by bulky muscles, are rare.[294,299,312] Like the ribs, this thin bone is much more resilient in the child than in the adult. Until late adolescence the entire vertebral border is pliable hyaline cartilage that is equivalent to an epiphysis. Fractures usually occur along the lateral margin, including the glenoid, coracoid, and acromion.

Many of these regions have secondary ossification centers that should not be confused with fractures.[287,305,306,311]

Wilber and Evans reported 40 cases of fractured scapulae.[312] The patients ranged in age from 3 to 80 years. Most of the fractures were through nonarticular regions and did not lead to significant problems. The authors thought that open reduction was indicated only when the glenohumeral joint was involved, an unlikely event in a child. Brachial plexus and other neural injuries may accompany the fracture, and a pseudopalsy may also occur. Ada and Miller described 148 fractures involving 116 scapulae.[285]

Fractures of the body of the scapula result from direct violence, such as a crushing injury, an automobile accident, a fall, or child abuse. The blade of the scapula is often comminuted, with the fracture lines running in various directions. At times there is a small fracture along the scapular margins. The spine of the scapula may be fractured along with the body of the scapula. The infraspinous portion is more frequently fractured than the supraspinous area (Fig. 13-33). Usually the fracture fragments are minimally displaced, if at all, as they are held together by the surrounding muscles and thick periosteum of the child. Because the mechanism of injury generally involves major trauma, accompanying extensive crush injuries of the soft tissue of the thorax may be present, as well as fractures of the ribs and spinal column, pneumothorax, and subcutaneous emphysema. Rarely, the inferior tip may be dislocated between the ribs. Nettrour and associates reported a locked dislocation of the scapula when it displaced between ribs.[308]

A stress fracture may involve the scapular body in a child. Hart et al. described a 7-year-old who sustained a "minor" fall and continued to use the extremity, despite discomfort. Complete healing, after an initial 2-week period of rest, led to resolution of pain and radiologic healing 3 months later.[298]

Fractures of the scapular neck are usually caused by a direct blow to the front or back of the shoulder. The fracture line begins at the suprascapular notch and runs downward and laterally to the axillary border of the scapular neck, inferior to the glenoid, with the capsular attachments of the glenohumeral joint remaining intact. Displacement varies but is usually insignificant. Congenital deformities may mimic fracture lines.

To demonstrate these fractures adequately it is often necessary to obtain oblique or tangential views, in addition to the routine anteroposterior roentgenograms. CT scans may more effectively delineate the extent of a glenoid injury.[309]

The primary objective of treatment is to make the patient comfortable. Usually reduction of the fracture is unnecessary. Simple immobilization of the entire arm and shoulder is generally sufficient. Alternatively, the scapula may be immobilized with a sling-and-swathe dressing.

Treatment consists of support of the shoulder and arm in a sling-and-swathe dressing, with the onset of pendulum exercises about 14 days later when the patient is comfortable. Markedly displaced fractures, which are rare in children, may be treated with skeletal traction comparable to Dunlop's traction for a supracondylar fracture.

Fractures of the glenoid region are rare in children (Figs. 13-34, 13-35). They are produced by direct violence and may be associated with child abuse. They should be managed conservatively unless a large displaced fragment is present; open reduction is used as a last resort. The results of surgery are not good, although the data are derived from treatment of this injury in adults.

The acromion occasionally fractures as a result of direct violence or of indirect force transmitted vertically by the humeral head. Care must be taken when making the diagnosis, because the tip of the acromion may form a separate ossification center that is confused with a fracture line in an acutely traumatized patient. A chondro-osseous separation may occur.

Beim and Warner described a symptomatic adolescent swimmer. MRI showed an os acromiale,[287] which was treated by bone grafting and internal fixation. The pain subsided, and the patient returned to competitive swimming. Currarino and Prescott reported six similar children. A fracture was evident in four, and two were diagnosed as having an anatomic variant.[290] Morisawa et al. described acromial apophysitis in three adolescent athletes.[306] Sclerosis and osseous irregularity was evident. Conservative treatment was used. This lesion should be considered analogous to the symptomatic accessory navicular in the foot.

Edelson et al. studied the os acromiale, believing that in some cases symptomatic patients could benefit from operation.[293] Their patients were probably similar to what we have previously reported for accessory ossification of the navicular of the foot. The acrominal apophysis is a continuous cartilage, also covering the scapular spine. It may develop one or more ossification centers.

Kalideen and Satyapal described bilateral acrominal fractures in 10 of 171 neonates admitted for tetanus neonatorum.[300] The long-term results of the injury were not described. Nakae and Endo described fracture of the acromion complicating a shoulder dislocation.[307]

Fractures of the coracoid process are infrequent and may be caused by sudden muscular action of the short end of the biceps and the coracobrachialis muscles or by direct violence.[288,291,295,310] Coracoid fractures more often are associated with acromioclavicular injury or shoulder disloca-

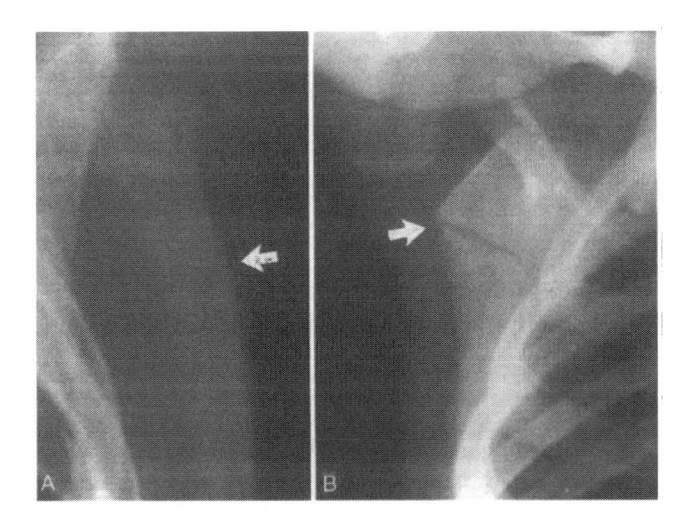

FIGURE 13-33. Scapular fractures. (A) Greenstick fracture of the margin (arrow). (B) More extensive fracture of the subglenoid region (arrow).

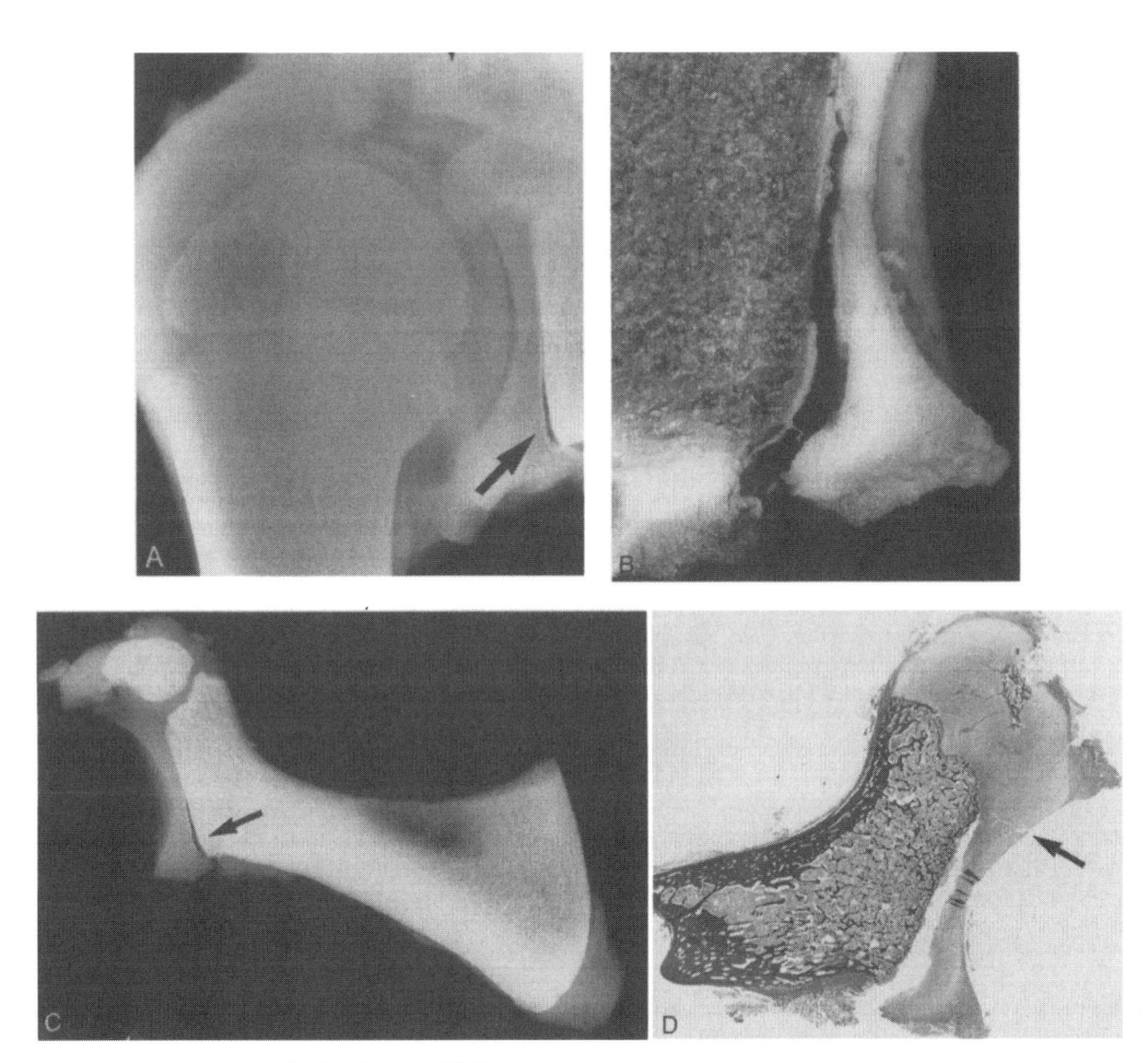

FIGURE 13-34. Glenoid growth mechanism fracture. (A) Specimen radiograph showing the fracture (arrow). (B) Morphologic view showing the injury. The glenoid cartilage is intact superiorly (analogue of greenstick fracture). (C) Radiograph of the specimen showing fracture (arrow). (D) Histology showed that a microfracture (arrow) extended into the cartilage.

tion.[313] Closed reduction and conservative treatment are indicated. Again, great care must be exercised during the roentgenographic diagnosis because of the variable ossification patterns.

Prior to epiphyseal closure, the coracoclavicular ligaments are often stronger than the epiphyseal plate, and an injury that would result in ligamentous disruption in an adult may injure only the physis of the coracoid process in a child. In addition, an accessory ossification center often develops as a shell-like, rounded ossification at the tip of the coracoid process. This area is the site of insertion of the coracoclavicular ligament. The conjoined tendon of the short head of the biceps and coracobrachialis, as well as the pectoralis minor, insert into the coracoid process anterior to the accessory physis. During adolescence, acromioclavicular separation may be accompanied by avulsion of a fragment of the coracoid epiphysis, rather than by disruption of the ligaments.

Glenoid Hypoplasia

Infrequently, children present with pain in the shoulder or apparent displacement. The possibility of glenoid dysplasia, similar to acetabular dysplasia, should be considered. Borenstein et al. reported a 12-year-old boy with symptomatic restriction of shoulder motion.[289] Lintner et al. presented a similar adolescent with sports-elicited pain.[303] Both were treated symptomatically with therapy and medication.

Scapulothoracic Dissociation

Scapulothoracic dissociation (Fig. 13-36) is a rare injury in children.[286,292] Repair of the clavicle requires internal fixation because of the extensive soft tissue disruption. The severity of brachial plexus and vascular disruptions determine the ultimate outcome. Severe scapulothoracic dissociation, in which minimal soft tissue continuity within the

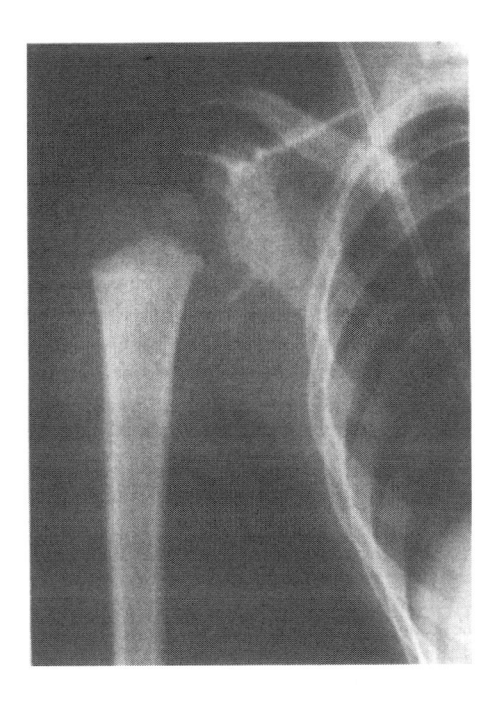

FIGURE 13-35. Glenoid fracture following child abuse.

axilla is the only bridging tissue, is not suitable for attempted replantation. Forequarter amputation is more realistic.

Lange and Noel presented several patients with traumatic lateral displacement with variable neurologic injury including neurologic compromise.[302] They proposed the term traumatic lateral scapular displacement rather than scapulothoracic dissociation, to emphasize this spectrum of possible presentations.

Scapular Winging

Mah and Otsuka reported that traumatic winging of the scapula is uncommon in children.[304] They described three cases of athletic injuries, each resolving within 6 months after conservative management. Winging probably resulted from an isolated injury of the serratus anterior muscle.[297] This muscle is innervated by the long thoracic nerve. The trauma may be acute or chronic. Trauma is probably responsible for more than 50% of scapular winging injuries. Traction played a role in the etiology in the first case, but the second case was probably due to compression of the long thoracic nerve. Usually when the traction mechanism is involved in athletic injuries, there is full return of function. No documented cases of posttraumatic scapular winging in children have required surgical intervention or muscle transfer.[296]

Kauppilä studied the anatomy and blood supply along the thoracic nerve and found that the nerve and its blood supply were vulnerable to both compression and stretching injury along the lower part of the scapula.[301] The nerve could be injured in compression rather than previously described through angulation of the nerve trunk across the second rib, subjecting it to traction during shoulder movements. Inferior movement of the scapula could result in compression of the nerve, whereas winging of the scapula might cause traction on the nerve.

Trauma to the Brachial Plexus

The incidence and long-term problems of injury to the brachial plexus have dramatically decreased since the recognition of cephalopelvic disproportion (shoulder dystocia) and improved means of managing the sequelae of neonatal Erb's palsy.[320,322,326,333,334,342,344,345,353,355,369,370] Most babies with brachial plexus injuries are products of prolonged or difficult deliveries; 10% are born in the breech position.[317]

Brachial plexus injury has also been reported in babies delivered by cesarean section.[318,319] The pattern is different from vaginal delivery, with 81% having avulsion of the upper nerve roots.[337] This type of injury cannot be treated satisfactorily by microsurgical grafting and carries a worse long-term prognosis than the more typical lower plexus injury.

Drew et al. reported a 9-year-old boy who sustained a proximal humeral fracture and experienced a slowly evolving brachial plexus injury.[332] There was no deficit noted on the initial clinical examination. Forty-eight hours later he developed progressive pain and numbness. He was explored and the nerve ends were found to be contused and under traction from the distal fragment. Variable recovery occurred

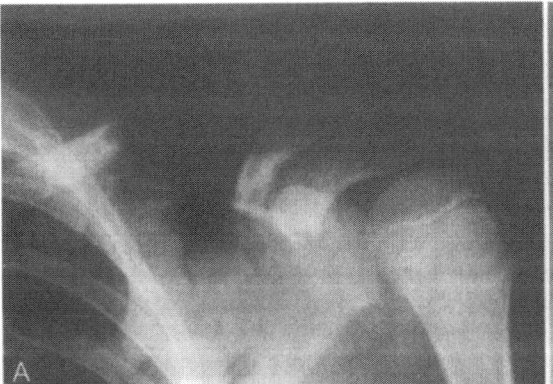

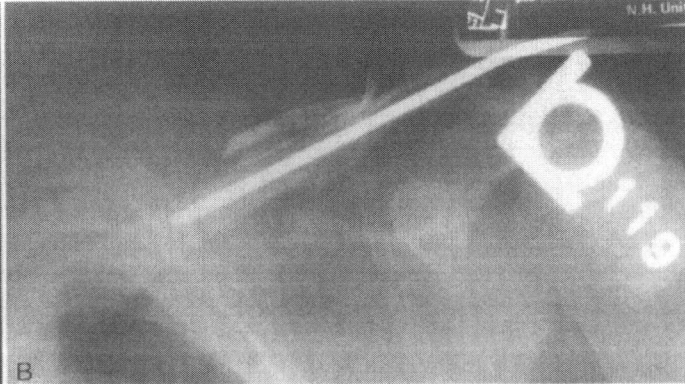

FIGURE 13-36. (A) Open clavicular fracture and scapulothoracic dissociation. This was associated with avulsion of the entire brachial plexus at the root level. Several large veins required ligation, but the artery was intact. (B) After extensive débridement, the clavicle was reduced and fixed with a medullary pin. The patient has a flail extremity 6 years later.

after the nerves were freed from the end of the humerus. Peterson and Peterson described brachial plexus injury in an infant due to a car safety seat. The child recovered completely after 8 weeks.[362]

Brachial plexus injuries may involve root avulsions combined with postganglionic nerve trunk ruptures. The site, level, and extent vary considerably. Common factors are evident. The roots most commonly injured are C5 and C6. Postganglionic nerve rupture is common in the C5 nerve root. Root avulsions are most common in the C7 and C8 nerves. Complete (global) plexus involvement is the second most common injury pattern. Kawai and coworkers, exploring experimental disruption of the brachial plexus in rabbits, found that the direction of the traction force was the determining factor.[351] Stretch injuries without nerve or root disruption (transection) may also occur.

Oppenheim et al. showed that brachial plexus injuries were associated with large neonates, shoulder dystocia, the use of forceps, and abnormal presentations, each of which results in wide separation of the head and shoulder.[165] Traction on the plexus may be lessened if the clavicle fractures. Although birth weight and general size are usually significantly greater, the complication has been reported even in normal-size neonates.

Al-Qattan et al. reviewed the prognostic value of clavicular fractures in newborns with obstetric brachial plexus palsy.[317] They found that of 13 newborn babies with palsy and concurrent clavicular fractures 2 required primary brachial plexus surgery. On the other hand, surgery was undertaken in 43 of the remaining 170 infants with palsy associated with intact clavicles. They found no prognostic value in the association of the two injuries.

Brachial plexus injury is usually diagnosed in the newborn infant when one upper extremity is not moving actively and the passive range of motion is equal on both sides.[326,369] If the active and passive motions are equally restrictive, injury to the proximal humeral epiphysis is suspected and confirmed by roentgenographic examination, although it may be difficult to interpret these roentgenograms.[356] All infants with suspected or proven Erb's palsy should be radiographed routinely to rule out concomitant osseous injury. Newborns with clavicular fractures often have a pseudoparalysis that mimics brachial plexus injury.

In newborns it is often difficult to localize the exact anatomic extent accurately. Overlap of innervation, resulting in partial loss of motor power in the muscles innervated by the various trunks of the brachial plexus, may make discrete anatomic diagnosis difficult. However, an absolutely accurate anatomic diagnosis probably has no real advantage, for either management or prognosis, in the neonate. Classification into upper (Erb), lower (Klumpke), or whole (Erb-Duchenne-Klumpke) types is useful only insofar as it conveys a general picture of the *probable* pattern and extent of involvement.[318,328]

During the neonatal period the degree of severity and the time at which spontaneous recovery may be expected are difficult to estimate. Complete, spontaneous recovery of function is hoped for in all patients, but it is impossible to predict which patients will recovery fully. Some severely involved extremities recover spontaneously after many months. The maximal time of recovery ranges from 1 to 18 months.[314,343]

Hardy reviewed more than 41,000 live births, found 36 brachial plexus injuries, and showed that 80% had a complete recovery within 13 months.[346] A wide difference in the incidence of complete recovery has been reported; Wickstrom and colleagues found an incidence of 13%, whereas Adler and Patterson reported only 7%.[314,343,374]

Because specific muscle testing is difficult in the neonate, gross movement of the shoulder, elbow, hand, and wrist should be recorded. Precise testing is not of significance, especially if a traction injury is present, as it changes over time. More precise diagnosis becomes important only if surgical intervention is being considered. Complete (global) plexus involvement is evident by a totally limp arm; scapular winging; absence of the deep tendon reflexes in the biceps, triceps, and brachioradialis; absence of the grasp reflex; torticollis; facial palsy; Horner syndrome from injury to the cervical sympathetic nerves; and diaphragmatic paralysis from phrenic nerve injury. Injury to only the C7 and C8 roots (Klumpke's paralysis) results in weakness of the wrist and finger flexors and the intrinsic muscles of the hand. The Moro reflex may be present, except for terminal fanning of the digits and flexion of the thumb and index finger. The grasp reflex is absent. Extensive sensory deficit implies a poor prognosis, but usually sensation is surprisingly intact.

Al-Qattan et al. reviewed Klumpke's palsy, finding it to occur in only 0.6% of 235 cases of obstetric plexus injury.[318] They noted that obstetric brachial plexus palsy was classified into upper (C5 or C6, ± C7 root), lower (C8–T1), and total (C5, C6, C7, or C8, ± T1) palsies. A fourth type of birth palsy, named the intermediate type, predominantly involves the C7 root.[324] The lower palsy is referred to as Klumpke's, and the paralysis is usually confined to the hand. Phrenic nerve paralysis and Horner syndrome may also be present.

Of far greater prognostic use is a clinical description, joint by joint, of the extent of involvement, particularly for patients whose care may not remain the responsibility of a single physician from year to year. Such information allows an overall plan of management to be followed.

An infant with a brachial plexus injury should be examined at 4- to 8-week intervals to further evaluate the extent of the injury and the degree of recovery. A record should be made of the range of active and passive motion of the extremities and the gross reaction to pain. Neurologic examination of the upper and lower extremities should be repeated, as brain and spinal cord injury may also occur in these children. Edema, skin changes, and trophic ulcers should be noted; and two-point discrimination and proprioception should be tested in cooperative, older children.

Hentz and Meyer reviewed brachial plexus injury in children.[347] They documented 61 cases of brachial plexus palsy in 3451 live births. Thirty-eight of these patients were followed from age 1 to 11 years; 35 patients had upper root involvement, and 3 had total palsy. The prognosis was excellent with full recovery by 1 week in 25 (66%) and by 3 months in 35 (92%); 96% of patients recovered completely. In contrast, Clarke and Curtis studied 25 patients and found that only 8 had normal upper limbs when examined 2.5–10.0 years after birth. Of the 25 patients, 10 showed abnormal abduction of the shoulder, and 7 of 25 had excessively poor upper limb function.[327] The differences probably reflect the lack of a uniform system of evaluation. They reevaluated and assessed another 44 children in whom complete recovery was possible only if the biceps and deltoid reached the M1 state (contraction without nerve) by the second month.

Marshall and DeSilva applied CT scanning to the evaluation of brachial plexus injuries in the adult.[358] It is not known whether this technology or MRI would be efficacious in a newborn for evaluating the level of the lesion—whether it is at the root from the spinal cord itself or further out peripherally. However, with current technology, and with MRI particularly, heavy sedation or an anesthetic may be necessary in the infant, which may be a contraindication to effective clinical utilization of such an evaluation.

Urabe et al. studied a 2-month-old baby with brachial plexus palsy by MRI.[373] They demonstrated traumatic pseudoparalysis involving an avulsion injury. They noted that MRI provided accurate information for evaluating the type and level of the brachial plexus injury, thereby improving the choice of subsequent treatment. They also noted that it was superior to myelography or CT. In view of the newer approaches to brachial plexus surgery, Francel et al. evaluated the efficacy of fast spin-echo MRI.[335] The method is highly effective for delineating pathologic anatomy.

Boome and Kaye showed that if beginning recovery is not evident by 3 months, a significant residual (permanent) functional deficit is likely.[323] They also thought that infants without evidence of recovery at 3 months were candidates for root grafting. Jackson et al. studied two brachial plexus injuries.[349] There was full recovery at an average of 3 months (range 2 weeks to 12 months). A small number had residual paralysis at more than 26 months. They concluded that the newborn usually has a favorable prognosis for recovery. Others have supported this conclusion.[331,360]

Regardless of the incidence of spontaneous recovery and the transient quality of the paralysis in some patients, contractures and deformities may occur rapidly. Therefore every child in whom birth palsy is diagnosed or suspected should receive early therapy. One should not await spontaneous recovery, as limitation of motion and deformity may persist, despite complete return of muscle power, if therapy is delayed.

Frequent, diligent, gentle exercises that put all the joints of the involved extremity through a full range of passive motion are the cornerstone of early management of the patient with obstetric palsy. It is hoped that such therapy can prevent or decrease contractures. If some degree of paralysis persists, prevention of contracture allows more latitude in the choice of subsequent reconstructive procedures. As for deformities complicating poliomyelitis, it is a basic axiom of treatment that fixed deformity must be overcome before tendon or muscle transfers are performed in order to produce more normal function.

Braces, strapping, splints, and pinning the arm to the head of the crib have been recommended. These procedures are attractive because they supposedly prevent the most obvious deformity of an internally rotated and adducted shoulder.

It is more important, however, that the parents be taught how to apply gentle motion to the shoulder, elbow, and wrist joints with each diaper change. The parents should hold the top of the shoulder and lift the patient's arm gently for effective, passive exercises at the glenohumeral joint. If there are supination contractures of the forearm or adduction contractures of the thumb, the parents should stretch them carefully. Occasionally, posterior plaster splints at the elbow and wrist can prevent palmar flexion contractures. The physician should review the performance at each follow-up visit.

Kennedy reported early suture of brachial plexus injuries in 1903, but virtually nothing further was done in the way of surgical intervention until a recent resurgence of interest.[316,352,354,364] Advances such as refined electroneuromyographic methods for early assessment of brachial plexus lesions and encouraging results from microsurgical reconstruction of peripheral nerves and brachial plexus in adults have led to application of this technology to the newborn.[339,357,368,371] Solonen and associates operated on three patients with brachial plexus palsy from birth injury within 3 months of birth.[368] Reconstruction of part of the torn brachial plexus was accomplished with free nerve grafts. They noted that the improvement found an average of 2 years or more after surgery was much better than that which could have been achieved without surgery. Many patients end up with permanent incapacity; and if surgical intervention can diminish the disability without undue risk, it is justified. The primary improvement in the cases reported by Solonen and associates was in the function of the deltoid and biceps, which are important to overall shoulder and elbow function, especially to position the hand for adequate function. Repair may involve direct neurorrhaphy or, if it is not possible, reconstruction with free nerve grafts.

The patient with global palsy and no return of neurologic function after 3–4 months of age is probably the best candidate for nerve transfer (neurotization).[336] This procedure attempts to restore partial function through nerve transpositions, such as using branches of the intercostal nerves.

Gilbert et al. reviewed 21 cases of brachial (Erb's) palsy explored between 7 weeks and 9 years of age.[340,341] They found that ruptures of the upper root junction of C5–6 were frequent and could be repaired by nerve graft. Avulsion from the spinal cord was more frequent in the lower roots. They concluded that exploration and attempted repair should be done early, preferably at the age of 2–3 months, in the absence of spontaneous recovery.

Sloof reviewed repairs followed for at least 2 years and noted that good results were achieved with an upper plexus lesion. On the other hand, in those with root avulsion and subtotal lesions the final result was less positive, particularly when those children had been breech deliveries.[367]

Kawabata et al. described neurotization of the accessory nerve with transfer to multiple brachial plexus injuries (mean age at surgery 5.9 months).[350] Altogether 67% of the patients regained deltoid function, 88% in the infraspinatus and 100% in the biceps. Wrist dorsiflexion and triceps was the least (25%) successful. There was no functional compromise in the trapezius. Chuang et al. have reported similar good results in 99 patients.[325]

The problems of later management and consequences of operative procedures to restore function are well described in articles by Adler and Patterson,[314] Wickstrom and colleagues,[374] Marshall et al.,[359] and others.[329,375] Phipps and Hofer used latissimus dorsi and teres major transfer to the rotator cuff.[363] They found that the procedure provided active external rotation and, less frequently, shoulder abduction.

It is important to follow these children through to skeletal maturity, as their abnormally innervated muscle may lead to differences in the growth of the bones, particularly the shoulder and elbow.[315,321,330,359,361,365] Undoubtedly, these differences are due to abnormal growth stimulation from muscle imbalance. Attitudinal posturing of the shoulder may lead to a posterior dislocation.[372] The overall shape of the humeral head may be different from that of the opposite side. Posteromedial dislocation or subluxation at the elbow is common.

These children are subject to fractures. In children with severe muscular insufficiency there usually is concomitant osteopenia and osteoporosis, increasing the susceptibility to pathologic fractures. Because of the lack of appropriate sensory perception, they may not be aware of either bone or joint injury. Delayed union and nonunion may occur because of the sensory neuropathy. Charcot arthropathy may develop. In instances of flail shoulder or breakdown from a Charcot arthropathy, a glenohumeral fusion may be appropriate.

Hernandez and Dias emphasized the use of CT to evaluate the shoulder in children with brachial plexopathy.[348] They found a significant number of patients with subluxation and glenoid or humeral head deformity.

Trophic ulceration may lead to loss of portions of the digits. Rossitch et al. presented a 1-year-old who began to self-mutilate digits following brachial plexus injury.[366] They thought that this process was probably motivated by subjective pain in an effort to relieve the pain, a concept that has relevance to deafferentation animal models.

References

Anatomy

1. Abbott LC, Lucas DB. The function of the clavicle. Ann Surg 1954;140:583–589.
2. Anderson H. Histochemistry and development of the human shoulder and acromioclavicular joints with particular reference to the early development of the clavicle. Acta Anat (Basel) 1963;55:124–151.
3. Bearn JG. Direct observations of the function of the capsule of the sternoclavicular joint in clavicular support. J Anat 1967;101:159–170.
4. Caffey J. Pediatric X-ray Diagnosis, 8th ed. Chicago: Year Book, 1985.
5. Chen JM. Studies on the morphogensis of the mouse sternum: experiments on the closure and segmentation of the sternal bands. J Anat 1953;87:1413–1427.
6. Corrigan GE. The neonatal clavicle. Biol Neonate 1959;2:713–792.
7. Destouet JM, Gillula LA, Murphy WA, Sagel SS. Computed tomography of sternoclavicular joint and sternum. Radiology 1981;138:123–128.
8. Edelson JG, Zuckerman J, Hershkovitz I. Os acromiale: anatomy and surgical implications. J Bone Joint Surg Br 1993;75:551–555.
9. Fawcett J. The development and ossification in the human clavicle. J Anat Physiol 1913;47:225–252.
10. Flatow EL. The biomechanics of the acromioclavicular, sternoclavicular and scapulothoracic joints. AAOS Instr Course Lect 1993;42:237–245.
11. Forland M. Cleidocranial dysostosis. Am J Med 1962;33:792–796.
12. Gardner E. The embryology of the clavicle. Clin Orthop 1968;58:9–16.
13. Guidera KJ, Grogan DP, Pugh L, Ogden JA. Hypoplastic clavicles and lateral scapular redirection. J Pediatr Orthop 1991;11:523–526.
14. Jit I, Kulkarni M. Times of appearance and fusion of epiphysis at the medial end of the clavicle. Indian J Med Res 1976;64:773–782.
15. Klima M. Early development of the human sternum and the problem of homologization of the so-called suprasternal structures. Acta Anat (Basel) 1968;69:473–484.
16. Koch AR. Die Fruhentwicklung der Clavicula beim Menschen. Acta Anat (Basel) 1960;42:177–185.
17. Kuhns LR, Sherman MP, Poznanski AK, Holt JF. Humeral head and coracoid ossification in the newborn. Radiology 1973;107:145–149.
18. Ljunggren AE. Clavicular function. Acta Orthop Scand 1979;50:261–268.
19. McClure JG, Raney RB. Anomalies of the scapula. Clin Orthop 1975;110:22–31.
20. Morrison DS, Bigliani LU. The clinical significance of variations in acromial morphology. Orthop Trans 1986;11:234.
21. Moseley HF. The clavicle: its anatomy and function. Clin Orthop 1968;58:17–27.
22. Mudge MK, Bernardino L, Wood VE, Frykman GK, Linda L. Rotator cuff tears associated with os acromiale. J Bone Joint Surg Am 1990;66:427–429.
23. Ogata S, Uhthoff HK. The early development and ossification of the human clavicle; an embryologic study. Acta Orthop Scand 1990;61:330–334.
24. Ogden JA, Conlogue GJ, Bronson ML: Radiology of postnatal skeletal development. III. The clavicle. Skeletal Radiol 1979;4:196–203.
25. Ogden JA, Conlogue GJ, Bronson ML, Jensen PS. Radiology of postnatal skeletal development. II. The manubrium and sternum. Skeletal Radiol 1979;4:189–195.
26. Ogden JA, Phillips SB. Radiology of postnatal skeletal development. IV. The scapula. Skeletal Radiol 1983;9:157–169.
27. O'Neal M, Dwornik JJ, Ganey T, Ogden JA. Postnatal development of the human sternum. J Pediatr Orthop 1998;18:398–405.
28. O'Neal M, Ganey T, Ogden JA. Anatomical development of the first rib and the manubrium. J Pediatr Orthop, accepted.
29. Rönning O, Kantomää T. The growth pattern of the clavicle in the rat. J Anat 1988;159:173–179.
30. Todd TW, DiErrico J. The clavicular epiphyses. Am J Anat 1928;41:25–37.
31. Wong M, Carter DR. Mechanical stress and morphologic endochondral ossification of the sternum. J Bone Joint Surg Am 1988;70:992–1000.
32. Yazici M, Kopuz C, Gülman B. Morphologic variants of acromion in neonatal cadavers. J Pediatr Orthop 1995;15:644–647.

Thoracic and Rib Trauma

33. Albers JE, Rath RK, Glaser RS. Severity of intrathoracic injuries associated with first rib fractures. Ann Thorac Surg 1982;6:614–618.
34. Alp M, Yurdakl Y, Gurese A, Saylam A, Aytac A. Symptomatic cervical rib in childhood. Turk J Pediatr 1982;24:121–115.
35. Aronson DZ, Scherz AW, Einhorn AH, Becker JM, Schneider KM. Nonoperative management of splenic trauma in children: a report of six consecutive cases. Pediatrics 1977;60:482–485.

References

36. Ashbing GF. Rupture of the diaphragm from blunt trauma. Arch Surg 1968;97:801–804.
37. Bailey P. Surfer's rib: isolated first rib fracture secondary to indirect trauma. Ann Emerg Med 1985;14:346–349.
38. Balfanz JR. Overwhelming sepsis following splenectomy for trauma. J Pediatr 1976;88:458–460.
39. Barrett GR, Shelton WR, Miles JW. First rib fractures in football players: a case report and literature review. Am J Sports Med 1988;16:674–676.
40. Bass BL, Eichelberger MR, Schisgall RM. Nonoperative therapy for stable liver injury in children. In: Brooks BF (ed) The Injured Child. Austin, TX: University of Texas Press, 1985, pp 44–52.
41. Begley A, Wilson DS, Shaw J. Cough fracture of the first rib. Injury 1995;26:565–566.
42. Bergmann L. Ermüdungsfrakturen der ersten Rippe und ihre Kombination mit einem Spontanpneumothorax. Z Erkr Atmungsorgane 1984;163:75–79.
43. Bonadio WA, Hellmich T. Post-traumatic pulmonary contusion in children. Ann Emerg Med 1989;18:1050–1052.
44. Borrelli J, Merle M, Hubert J, Grosdidier G, Wack B. Compression du plexus brachial par pseudarthrose de la premiere côte. Ann Clin Main 1984;3:266–268.
45. Bowie ER, Jacobson HG. Anomalous development of the first rib simulating isolated fracture. AJR 1945;58:161–165.
46. Brandt ML, Luks FI, Spigland NA, DiLorenzo M, Laberge JM, Ouimet A. Diaphragmatic injury in children. J Trauma 1992;32:298–301.
47. Burrington JD. Surgical repair of a ruptured spleen in children: report of eight cases. Arch Surg 1977;112:417–419.
48. Canty TG, Aaron WS. Hepatic artery ligation for exsanguinating liver injuries in children. J Pediatr Surg 1975;10:693–700.
49. Cobb LM, Vinocur MD, Waagner CW, et al. Intestinal perforation due to blunt trauma in children in an era of increased nonoperative treatment. J Trauma 1986;26:461–463.
50. Cooney DR. Splenic and hepatic trauma in children. Surg Clin North Am 1981;61:1165–1180.
51. Drew R, Perry JF, Fischer R. The expediency of peritoneal lavage for blunt trauma in children. Surg Gynecol Obstet 1977;145:885–888.
52. Eichelberger MR, Mangubat EA, Sacco WJ. Outcome analysis of blunt injury in children. J Trauma 1988;28:1108–1117.
53. Eichelberger MR, Randolph JG. Thoracic trauma in children. Surg Clin North Am 1981;61:1181–1197.
54. Feldman KW, Brewer DK. Child abuse, cardiopulmonary resuscitation and rib fractures. Pediatrics 1984;73:3313–342.
55. Feliciano PD, Mulling RJ, Trunkey DD, et al. A decision analysis of traumatic splenic injuries. J Trauma 1992;33:340–348.
56. Fischer KC, Eraklis A, Rossello P, Treves S. Scintigraphy in the follow-up of pediatric splenic trauma treated without surgery. J Nucl Med 1978;19:3–9.
57. Fisher GW, Scherz RG. Neck vein catheters and pericardial tamponade. Pediatrics 1973;52:868–871.
58. Fisher RD, Rienhoff WF. Subclavian artery laceration resulting from fracture of the first rib. J Trauma 1966;6:571–581.
59. Frieberger RH, Mayer V. Ununited bilateral fatigue fractures of the first ribs. J Bone Joint Surg Am 1964;46:615–618.
60. Galbraith NF, Urschel HC, Wood RE, Razzuk MA, Paulson DL. Fracture of the first rib associated with laceration of subclavian artery. J Thorac Cardiovasc Surg 1973;65:641–643.
61. Gamble JG, Comstock C, Rinsky LA. Erroneous interpretation of magnetic resonance images of a fracture of the first rib with non-union. J Bone Joint Surg Am 1995;77:1883–1887.
62. Garcia VF, Gotschall CS, Eichelberger MR, Bowman LM. Rib fractures in children: a marker of severe trauma. J Trauma 1990;30:695–700.
63. Harris GJ, Soper RT. Pediatric first rib fractures. J Trauma 1990;30:343–345.
64. Hoekstra HJ, Binnendijk B. Geisoleerde beiderzijdse fractuur van de eerste rib, verband houdend met een niet goed passende integraalhelm. Ned Tijdschr Geneeskd 1982;126:891–893.
65. Jones D. Bilateral fracture of the first rib with bilateral pneumothorax. Injury 1974;5:255–256.
66. Kilman JW, Charnock E. Thoracic trauma in infancy and childhood. J Trauma 1969;9:863–873.
67. Kleinman PK, Marks SC, Adams VI, Blackbourne BD. Factors affecting visualization of posterior rib fractures in abused infants. AJR 1988;150:635–638.
68. Kleinman PK, Marks SC, Nimkin K, Rayder SM, Kessler SC. Rib fractures in 31 abused infants: post-mortem radiologic-histologic study. Radiology 1996;200:807–810.
69. Kleinman PK, Marks SC, Spevak MR, Richmond JM. Fractures of the rib head in abused infants. Radiology 1993;185:1113–1123.
70. Langer JC, Winthrom JC, Wesson DE, et al. Diagnosis and incidence of cardiac injury in children with blunt thoracic trauma. J Pediatr Surg 1989;24:1091–1094.
71. Lankenner PA, Micheli LJ. Stress fracture of the first rib. J Bone Joint Surg Am 1985;67:159–169.
72. Lazrove S, Harley DP, Grinnell VS, White RA, Nelson RJ. Should all patients with first rib fracture undergo arteriography? J Thorac Cardiovasc Surg 1982;83:532–537.
73. Manson D, Babyn PS, Palder S, Bergman K. CT of blunt chest trauma in children. Pediatr Radiol 1993;23:1–5.
74. Mayer T, Matlak M, Johnson D. The modified injury severity scale in pediatric multiple trauma patients. J Pediatr Surg 1980;15:713–726.
75. McBeath AA, Keene JS. The rib-tip syndrome. J Bone Joint Surg Am 1975;57:795–797.
76. Meller JL, Little AG, Shermeta DW. Thoracic trauma in children. Pediatrics 1984;74:813–819.
77. Melzig EP, Swank M, Salzberg AM. Acute blunt traumatic rupture of the diaphragm in children. Arch Surg 1976;111:1003–1011.
78. Mikawa Y, Kobori M. Stress fractures of the first rib in a weight lifter. Arch Orthop Trauma Surg 1991;110:121–122.
79. Mintz AC, Albano A, Reisdorff EJ, Choe KA, Lillegard W. Stress fracture of the first rib from serratus anterior tension: an unusual mechanism of injury. Ann Emerg Med 1990;19:411–414.
80. Moore RS. Fracture of the first rib: an uncommon throwing injury. Injury 1991;22:1413–150.
81. Never FS, Roberts FF, McCarthy V. Osteolytic lesions following traumatic pancreatitis. Am J Dis Child 1977;131:738–741.
82. Pearl RH, Wesson DE, Spence LJ, et al. Splenic injury: a 5-year update with improved results and changing criteria for conservative management. J Pediatn Surg 1988;24:121–125.
83. Peclet MH, Newman KD, Eichelberger MR, et al. Patterns of injury in children. J Pediatr Surg 1990;25:85–91.
84. Peclet MH, Newman KD, Eichelberger MR, Gottschall CS, Garcia VF, Bowman LF. Thoracic trauma in children: an indicator of increased mortality. J Pediatr Surg 1990;25:961–966.
85. Phillips EH, Rogers WF, Gaspar MR. First rib fractures: incidence of vascular injury and indications for angiography. Surgery 1981;89:42–47.
86. Poole GV, Myers RT. Morbidity and mortality rates in major blunt trauma to the upper chest. Ann Surg 1981;193:70–75.
87. Porter GE. Slipping rib syndrome: an infrequently recognized entity in children; a report of three cases and review of the literature. Pediatrics 1985;76:810–813.
88. Proffer DS, Patton JJ, Jackson DW. Non-union of a first rib fracture in a gymnast. Am J Sports Med 1991;19:198–201.

89. Rademaker M, Redmond AD, Barber PV. Stress fracture of the first rib. Thorax 1983;38:312–313.
90. Regoort M, Raaymakers EL. Fractur van de eerste rib als gevolg van een triviaal ongeval. Ned Tijdscher Geneeskd 1990;134:813–821.
91. Richardson JD, McElvein RB, Trinkle JK. First rib fractures: hallmark of severe trauma. Ann Surg 1975;181:251–254.
92. Roberge RJ, Morgenstern MJ, Osborn H. Cough fractures of the rib. Am J Emerg Med 1984;2:513–517.
93. Sacchetti AD, Beswick DR, Morse SD. Rebound rib: stress-induced first rib fracture. Ann Emerg Med 1983;12:177–179.
94. Schackelford PG. Osseous lesions in pancreatitis. Am J Dis Child 1977;131:731–732.
95. Schweich P, Fleisher G. Rib fractures in children. Pediatr Emerg Care 1985;1:187–189.
96. Sivit CJ, Taylor GA, Eichelberger MR. Chest injury in children with blunt abdominal trauma: evaluation with CT. Radiology 1989;171:815–818.
97. Smeets AJ, Robber SGF, Meradji M. Sonographically detected costo-chondral dislocation in an abused child: a new sonographic sign to the radiological spectrum of child abuse. Pediatr Radiol 1990;20:566–567.
98. Smith JS, Wengrovitz MA, DeLong BS. Prospective validation of criteria, including age, for safe, nonsurgical management of the ruptured spleen. J Trauma 1992;33:363–369.
99. Smyth BT. Chest trauma in children. J Pediatr Surg 1979;14:41–47.
100. Stone HH, Ansley JD. Management of liver trauma in children. J Pediatr Surg 1977;12:3–10.
101. Strouse PJ, Owings CL. Fractures of the first rib in child abuse. Radiology 1995;197:763–765.
102. Thomas PS. Rib fractures in infancy. Ann Radiol (Paris) 1977;20:115–122.
103. Velcek FT, Weiss A, DiMaio D, et al. Traumatic death in urban children. J Pediatr Surg 1977;12:375–384.
104. Vyas PK, Sivit CJ. Imaging of blunt pediatric thoracic trauma. Emerg Radiol 1997;4:16–25.
105. Welch KJ. Thoracic injuries. In: Randolph JG (ed) The Injured Child. Chicago: Year Book, 1980.
106. Wilson JM, Thomas AN, Goodman PC, Lewis FR. Severe chest trauma: morbidity implications of first and second rib fractures in 120 patients. Arch Surg 1978;113:846–849.
107. Yang J, Letts SM. Thoracic outlet syndrome in children. J Pediatr Orthop 1996;16:514–517.
108. Zachary RB, Emergy JL. Abdominal splenosis following rupture of a spleen in a boy aged 10 years. Br J Surg 1959;46:415–416.

Sternum

109. Bizzle PG. Sternal bracing: an approach to the treatment of sternal fractures. Orthopaedics 1983;6:129–132.
110. Brookes JG, Dunn RJ, Rogers IR. Sternal fractures: a retrospective analysis of 272 cases. J Trauma 1993;35:46–54.
111. Gibson LD, Carter R, Hinshaw DB. Surgical significance of sternal fracture. Surg Gynecol Obstet 1962;114:443–446.
112. Haje SA. Iatrogenic pectus carinatum: a case report. Int Orthop 1995;19:370–373.
113. Haje SA, Bowen JR. Preliminary results of orthotic treatment of pectus deformities in child and adolescents. J Pediatr Orthop 1992;12:795–800.
114. Helal B. Fracture of the manubrium sterni. J Bone Joint Surg Br 1964;46:602–604.
115. Holderman HH. Fracture and dislocation of the sternum. Ann Surg 1928;88:252–254.
116. Mitchell EA, Elliott RB. Spontaneous fracture of the sternum in a youth with cystic fibrosis. J Pediatr 1980;97:789–790.
117. Ostremski I, Wilde BR, Morsa JL, et al. Fracture of the sternum in motor vehicle accidents and its association with mediastinal injury. Injury 1990;21:81–83.
118. Perez FL Jr, Coddington TC. A fracture of the sternum in a child. J Pediatr Orthop 1983;3:513–515.
119. Robertson DH. Kyphosis and fracture of the manubrium in tetanus. J Bone Joint Surg Br 1955;37:466–467.
120. Scott ML, Arens JF, Ochsner JL. Fractured sternum with flail chest and post-traumatic pulmonary insufficiency syndrome. Ann Thorac Surg 1973;15:386–393.
121. Scudamore CH, Ashmore PG. Spontaneous sternal segment dislocation: a case report. J Pediatr Surg 1982;17:61–66.
122. Wojcite JB, Morgan AS. Sternal fracture: the natural history. Ann Emerg Med 1988;17:912–914.

Clavicle

123. Acker DB, Sachs BP, Friedman EA. Risk factors for the shoulder dystocia in the average weight infant. Obstet Gynecol 1986;67:614–618.
124. Alkalaj I. Internal fixation of a severe clavicular fracture in a child. Isr J Med Sci 1960;9:306–309.
125. Al-Qattan MM, Clarke HM, Curtis CG. The prognostic value of concurrent clavicular fractures in newborns with obstetrical brachial plexus injuries. J Hand Surg [Br] 1994;19:7213–7730.
126. Balata A, Olzai MG, Porcu A, et al. Fracture of the clavicle in the newborn. Pediatr Med Chir 1984;6:125–129.
127. Baskett TF, Allen AC. Perinatal implications of shoulder dystocia. Obstet Gynecol 1995;86:14–17.
128. Bonnet J. Fracture of the clavicle. Arch Chir Neerl 1975;27:143–148.
129. Brown BL, Lapinski R, Berkowitz GS, Holzman I. Fractured clavicle in the neonate: a retrospective three-year review. Am J Perinatol 1994;11:331–333.
130. Burke SW, Jameson VP, Roberts JM, Johnstone CE, Willis J. Birth fractures in spinal muscular atrophy. J Pediatr Orthop 1986;6:34–36.
131. Calandi C, Bartolozzi G. On 110 cases of fracture of the clavicle in the newborn. Clin Pediatr 1975;64:264–267.
132. Chez RA, Carlan S, Greenberg SL, Spellacy WN. Fractured clavicle is an unavoidable event. Am J Obstet Gynecol 1994;171:797–798.
133. Cohen AW, Otto SR. Obstetric clavicular fractures. J Reprod Med 1980;25:119–122.
134. Corrigan GE. The neonatal clavicle. Biol Neonate 1959;2:79–86.
135. DeBlasio A, Iafusco F. Fracture of the clavicle in newborn infants. Pediatria (Napoli) 1960;68:815–826.
136. Dickson JW. Death following fractured clavicle. Lancet 1952;2:666–667.
137. Enzler A. Die Claviculafraktur ab geburtsverletzung des Neugeborenen. Schweiz Med Wochenschr 1960;80:1280–1283.
138. Editorial. The death of Sir Robert Peal. Lancet 1850;2:113–114.
139. Faithful DK. Lam P. Dispelling the fears of plating midclavicular fractures. J Shoulder Elbow Surg 1993;2:314–316.
140. Farkas R, Levine S. X-ray incidence of fractured clavicle in vertex presentation. Am J Obstet Gynecol 1950;59:204–209.
141. Fitisenko I. On the treatment of clavicular fracture in children. Khirurgiia (Mosk) 1963;39:36–43.
142. Ghormley RK, Black JR, Cherry JH. Ununited fractures of the clavicle. Am J Surg 1941;51:343–348.
143. Gilbert WM, Tchabo J. Fractured clavicle in the newborn. Int Surg 1988;73:123–129.
144. Gitsch G, Schatten C. Frequency and potential causal factors of clavicular fractures in obstetrics. Zentralbl Gynakol 1987;109:9013–9912.

145. Goddard NJ, Stabler J, Albert JS. Atlanto-axial rotatory fixation and fracture of the clavicle. J Bone Joint Surg Br 1990;72:72–75.
146. Hardy JRW. Complex clavicular injury in childhood. J Bone Joint Surg Br 1991;74:154.
147. Hernandez C, Wendel GD. Shoulder dystocia. Clin Obstet Gynecol 1990;33:526–534.
148. Howard F, Shafer S. Injuries to the clavicle with neurovascular complications. J Bone Joint Surg Am 1965;47:1335–1346.
149. Jablon M, Sutker A, Post M. Irreducible fractures of the middle-third of the clavicle. J Bone Joint Surg Am 1979;61:295–296.
150. Joseph PR, Rosenbeld W. Clavicular fractures in neonates. Am J Dis Child 1990;144:165:5–9.
151. Klein P, Sommerer G, Link W. Schultergurtelverletzung im Kindesalter: Operation oder konservatives Vorgehen? Unfallchirurgie 1991;17:14–18.
152. Kornguth PJ, Salazer AM. The apical oblique view of the shoulder: its usefulness in acute trauma. AJR 1987;149:113–116.
153. Kreisinger V. Sur le traitement des fractures de la clavicule. Rev Chir Paris 1927;46:376–384.
154. Lehmacher K, Lehmann C. Clavicular fractures in newborn infants after spontaneous delivery in the occipital position. Z Geburtshilfe Gynakol 1962;158:134–137.
155. Levine MG, Holroyde J, Woods JR, Siddiqi RA, Scott M, Miodornik M. Birth trauma: incidence and predisposing factors. Obstetrics 1984;63:792–795.
156. Madsen ET. Fractures of the extremities in the newborn. Acta Obstet Gynecol Scand 1955;34:41–74.
157. Meghdari A, Davoodi R, Masbah F. Engineering analysis of shoulder dystocia in the human birth process by the finite element method. Proc Inst Mech Eng 1992;206:243–250.
158. Mital M, Aufranc O. Venous occlusion following greenstick fracture of the clavicle. JAMA 1968;206:1301–1302.
159. Mullaji AB, Jupiter JB. Low-contact dynamic compression plating of the clavicle. Injury 1994;25:41–45.
160. Nasso S, Verga A. La frattura della clavicola del neonato. Minerva Pediatr 1954;6:593–599.
161. Nocon JJ, McKenzie DK, Thomas LJ, Hansell RS. Shoulder dystocia: an analysis of risks and obstetric maneuvers. Am J Obstet Gynecol 1992;168:1732–1739.
162. Nogi J. Non-union of the clavicle in a child: a case report. Clin Orthop 1975;110:19–21.
163. Ohel G, Haddad S, Fischer O, Levit A. Clavicular fractures of the neonate: can it be predicted before birth? Am J Perinatol 1993;10:441–443.
164. O'Leary JA, Leonotti UB. Shoulder dystocia: prevention and treatment. Am J Obstet Gynecol 1990;162:5–9.
165. Oppenheim WL, Davis A, Growdon WA, Dorey FJ, Davlin LB. Clavicle fracture in the newborn. Clin Orthop 1990;250:176–180.
166. Penn I. The vascular complications of fractures of the clavicle. J Trauma 1964;4:811–815.
167. Ralis ZA. Birth trauma to babies born by breech delivery and its possible fatal consequences. Arch Dis Child 1975;50:4–13.
168. Roberts S, Hernandez C, Adams M, et al. Neonatal clavicular fracture: an unpredictable event. Am J Obstet Gynecol 193;168:433–437.
169. Rubin A. Birth injuries: incidence, mechanism and end result. Obstet Gynecol 1964;23:218–221.
170. Sanford HN. The Moro reflex as a diagnostic aid in fracture of the clavicle in the newborn infant. Am J Dis Child 1931;41:1304–1307.
171. Sharma V. Applications of finite element and expert systems methods: a study of shoulder dystocia. MSc thesis, University of Houston, 1988.
172. Soral J. Design amd development of engineering aids to evaluate the birthing process. MSc thesis, University of Houston, 1988.
173. Swartz DP. Shoulder girdle dystocia in vertex delivery. Obstet Gynecol 1960;15:194–206.
174. Thomas CB, Friedman RJ. Ipsilateral sternoclavicular dislocation and clavicle fracture. J Orthop Trauma 1989;3:355–357.
175. Turnpenny PD. Fractured clavicle of the newborn in a population with high prevalence of grand-multiparity: analysis of 78 consecutive cases. Br J Obstet Gynaecol 1993;100:338–341.
176. Valerio PG, Harmsen P. Osteomyelitis as a complication of perinatal fracture of the clavicle. Eur J Pediatr 1995;154:497–502.
177. Weinberg B, Seife B, Alonso P. The apical oblique view of the clavicle: its usefulness in neonatal and childhood trauma. Skeletal Radiol 1991;20:201–203.
178. Wilkes JA, Hoffer MM. Clavicle fractures in head injured children. J Orthop Trauma 1987;1:55–58.
179. Wilkins RM, Johnston RM. Ununited fractures of the clavicle. J Bone Joint Surg Am 1983;65:773–778.

Congenital Pseudarthrosis

180. Adelaar RS, Urbaniak JR. Congenital pseudarthrosis of the clavicle: a case presentation and review of the literature. Interclin Information Bull 1974;11:1–6.
181. Ahmadi B, Steel HH. Congenital pseudarthrosis of the clavicle. Clin Orthop 1977;126:130–134.
182. Alldred AJ. Congenital pseudarthrosis of the clavicle. J Bone Joint Surg Br 1963;45:312–319.
183. Barger WL, Marcus RE, Lttleman FP. Late thoracic outlet syndrome secondary to pseudarthrosis of the clavicle. J Trauma 1984;24:857–859.
184. Behringer BR, Wilson FC. Congenital pseudarthrosis of the clavicle. Am J Dis Child 1972;123:51–71.
185. Brooks S. Bilateral congenital pseudarthrosis of the clavicle. Br J Clin Pract 1984;38:432–433.
186. Burkus JK, Ogden JA. Bipartite primary ossification in the developing human femur. J Pediatr Orthop 1982;2:63–65.
187. Fechter JD, Kuschner SH. The thoracic outlet syndrome. Orthopedics 1993;16:1243–1251.
188. Fitzwilliam DCL. Hereditary cranio-cleido-dystosis. Lancet 1910;2:1466–1475.
189. Gibson DA, Carroll N. Congenital pseudarthrosis of the clavicle. J Bone Joint Surg Br 1970;52:621–643.
190. Grogan DP, Love SM, Guidera KJ, Ogden JA. Operative treatment of congenital pseudarthrosis of the clavicle. J Pediatr Orthop 1991;11:176–180.
191. Hagen LJ. Congenital pseudarthrosis of the clavicle. Acta Orthop Scand 1980;51:858–859.
192. Herman S. Congenital bilateral pseudarthrosis of the clavicle. Clin Orthop 1973;91:162–163.
193. Hirata S, Miya H, Mizuno K. Congenital pseudarthrosis of the clavicle. Clin Orthop 1995;315:242–245.
194. Höcht B, Gay B, Arbogast R. Die Behandlung der kongenitalen Klavikulapseudarthrosis of the clavicle. J Bone Joint Surg Br 1975;57:24–27.
195. Jinkins WJ. Congenital pseudarthrosis of the clavicle. Clin Orthop 1969;62:183–186.
196. Legaye J, Noel H, Lokietek W. La pseudarthrose congenitale de la clavicule: à propos d'une observation et revue de la literature. Acta Orthop Belg 1991;57:203–212.
197. Lloyd-Roberts GC, Apley AG, Owen R. Reflections upon the aetiology of congenital pseudarthrosis of the clavicle. J Bone Joint Surg Br 1975;57:24–29.
198. Manashil G, Laufer S. Congenital pseudarthrosis of the clavicle: report of 3 cases. AJR 1979;132:678–679.

199. March HC. Congenital pseudarthrosis of the clavicle. J Can Assoc Radiol 1982;33:35–36.
200. Owen R. Congenital pseudarthrosis of the clavicle. J Bone Joint Surg Br 1970;52:644–652.
201. Quinlan WR, Brady PG, Regan BF. Congenital pseudarthrosis of the clavicle. Acta Orthop Scand 1980;51:483–492.
202. Richter H. Die angeborene Klavikulapseudarthrose. Zentralbl Chir 1991;116:151–154.
203. Rossignol SC. Bilateral congenital pseudarthrosis of the clavicle treated with costo-scapular fusion. J Bone Joint Surg Br 1948;30:220.
204. Sakellarides H. Pseudarthrosis of the clavicle. J Bone Joint Surg Am 1971;43:130–138.
205. Schnall SB, King JD, Marrero G. Congenital pseudarthrosis of the clavicle: a review of the literature and surgical results of 6 cases. J Pediatr Orthop 1988;8:316–321.
206. Toledo L, MacEwen GD. Severe complications of surgical treatment of congenital pseudarthrosis of the clavicle. Clin Orthop 1979;139:64–67.
207. Wall JJ. Congenital pseudarthrosis of the clavicle. J Bone Joint Surg Am 1970;52:1003–1009.
208. Wechselberg K. Untersuchungen zur Diagnose und Prognose der geburtstraumatischen Claviculafraktur. Med Monatsschr 1972;26:498–500.

Proximal (Sternoclavicular) Injury

209. Barth E, Hagen R. Surgical treatment of dislocations of the sternoclavicular joint. Acta Orthop Scand 1983;54:740–747.
210. Benson LS, Donaldson JS, Carrol NC. Use of ultrasound in management of posterior sternoclavicular dislocation. J Ultrasound Med 1991;10:115–118.
211. Borowiecki B, Charow A, Cook W, Rozycki D, Thaler S. An unusual football injury. Arch Otolaryngol 1972;95:185–187.
212. Brooks A, Henning G. Injury to the proximal clavicular epiphysis. J Bone Joint Surg Am 1972;54A:1347–1348.
213. Burnstein MI, Pozniak MA. Computed tomography with stress maneuver to demonstrate sternoclavicular joint dislocation. J Comput Assist Tomogr 1990;14:1513–160.
214. Burrows HJ. Tenodesis of subclavius in the treatment of recurrent dislocation of the sternoclavicular joint. J Bone Joint Surg Br 1915;33:240–243.
215. Butterworth RD, Kirk AA. Fracture dislocation sternoclavicular joint: case report. Va Med Monthly 1952;79:98–100.
216. Clark RL, Milgram JW, Yawn DH. Fatal aortic perforation and cardiac tamponade due to a Kirschner wire migrating from the right sternoclavicular joint. South Med J 1974;67:316–318.
217. Cope R. Dislocations of the sternoclavicular joint. Skeletal Radiol 1993;22:233–238.
218. Cope R, Riddervold HO, Shore JL, Sistrom CL. Dislocations of the sternoclavicular joint: anatomic basis, etiologies, and radiologic diagnosis. J Orthop Trauma 1991;5:373–384.
219. Dans GP, Dnez D, Newton BB Jr, Kober R. Migration of a Kirschner wire from the sternum to the right ventricle. Am J Sports Med 1995;21:321–322.
220. Dartoy C, Fenoll B, Paule R, LeNen D, Colin D, Thoma M. Particularités des fractures des extrémités de la clavicule chez l'enfant. Acta Orthop Belgica 1994;60:296–299.
221. Deepak M, Gangahar MD, Flogartes T. Retro-sternal dislocation of the clavicle producing thoracic outlet syndrome. J Trauma 1978;8:363–372.
222. Denham RH Jr, Dingley AE. Epiphyseal separation of the medial end of the clavicle. J Bone Joint Surg Am 1967;49:1173–1178.
223. Destouet JM, Gilula LA, Murphy WA, Sagel SS. Computed tomography of the sternoclavicular joint and sternum. Radiology 1981;138:123–128.
224. Deutsch AL, Resnick D, Mink JH. Computed tomography of the glenohumeral and sternoclavicular joints. Orthop Clin North Am 1985;16:497–511.
225. Docquier J, Soete P, Twahirwa J. La luxation retrosternale de la clavicule. Acta Orthop Belg 1982;48:947–950.
226. Elliott AC. Tripartite injury of the clavicle: a case report. So Afr Med J 1986;70:115–116.
227. Eskola A. Sternoclavicular dislocation: a plea for open treatment. Acta Orthop Scand 1986;57:227–228.
228. Ferry AM, Rook FW, Masterson JH. Retrosternal dislocation of the clavicle. J Bone Joint Surg Am 1957;39:905–910.
229. Gangahar DM, Flogaite T. Retrosternal dislocation of the clavicle producing thoracic outlet syndrome. J Trauma 1978;18:363–372.
230. Gardner MAH, Bidstrup BP. Intrathoracic great vessel injury resulting from blunt chest trauma with posterior dislocation of the sternoclavicular joint. Aust NZ J Surg 1983;53:427–430.
231. Hardy JRW. Complex clavicular injury in childhood. J Bone Joint Surg Br 1992;74:154.
232. Heinig CF. Retrosternal dislocation of the clavicle: early recognition, x-ray diagnosis and management. J Bone Joint Surg Am 1968;50:830.
233. Hobbs DW. Sternoclavicular joint: a new axial radiographic view. Radiology 1968;90:801.
234. Howard FM, Shafer SJ. Injuries to the clavicle with neurovascular complications. J Bone Joint Surg Am 1965;47:1335–1346.
235. Jougon JB, Lepront DJ, Cromer CEH. Posterior dislocation of the sternoclavicular joint leading to mediastinal compression. Ann Thorac Surg 1996;61:711–713.
236. Karlen MA. Tratamiento quirurgivo de la epifiseolosis clavicular. Bol Soc Cir Uruguay 1943;14:94–103.
237. Lemire L, Rosman M. Sternoclavicular epiphyseal separation with adjacent clavicular fracture. J Pediatr Orthop 1984;4:118–120.
238. Leonard JW, Gifford RW. Migration of a Kirschner wire from the clavicle into the pulmonary artery. Am J Cardiol 1965;16:598–600.
239. Levinsohn EM, Bunnell WP, Yuan HA. Computed tomography in the diagnosis of dislocations of the sternoclavicular joint. Clin Orthop 1979;140:12–16.
240. Lewonowski K, Bassett GS. Complete posterior sternoclavicular epiphyseal separation: a case report and review of the literature. Clin Orthop 1992;281:84–88.
241. Lucas GL. Retrosternal dislocation of the clavicle. JAMA 1965;193:850–852.
242. Lucet L, Le Loët X, Ménard JF, et al. Computed tomography of the normal sternoclavicular joint. Skeletal Radiol 1996;25:237–241.
243. Nettles JS, Linscheid RL. Sternoclavicular dislocations. J Trauma 1968;8:158–164.
245. Penn I. The vascular complications of fractures of the clavicle. J Trauma 1964;4:819–831.
246. Poland J. Traumatic Separation of the Epiphyses. London: Smith, Elder, 1889.
247. Rockwood CA. Dislocations of the sternoclavicular joint. AAOS Instruct Course Lect 1975;24:144–152.
248. Rodrigues HM. Case of dislocation inwards of the internal extremity of the clavicle. Lancet 1843;1:3013–3015.
249. Selesnik FH, Jablon M, Frank C, Post M. Retrosternal dislocation of the clavicle. J Bone Joint Surg Am 1984;66:287–291.
250. Simurda M. Retrosternal dislocation of the clavicle: a report of four cases with a method of repair. Can J Surg 1968;11:487–490.
251. Smolle-Juettner FM, Hofer PH, Pinter H, Friehs G, Szyskowitz R. Intracardiac malpositioning of a sternoclavicular fixation wire. J Orthop Trauma 1992;6:102–105.

252. Southworth SR, Merritt TR. Asymptomatic innominate vein tamponade with retromanubrial clavicular dislocation: a case report. Orthop Rev 1988;17:789–791.
253. Steenberg RE, Raviteh MM. Cervicothoracic approach for subclavian vessel injury from compound fracture of the clavicle: considerations of subclavian-axillary exposures. Ann Surg 1963;157:833–846.
254. Swischuk LE. Pain and decreased movement of left arm. Pediatr Emerg Care 1991;7:163–170.
255. Tricoire JL, Colombier JA, Chiron P, Puget J, Utheza G. Les luxations sterno-claviculaires posterieures. Rev Chir Orthop 1990;76:313–344.
256. Tyler H, Sturrock W, Callow F. Retrosternal dislocation of the clavicle. J Bone Joint Surg Br 1963;45:132–137.
257. Wasylenko MJ, Busse EF. Posterior dislocation of the clavicle causing fatal tracheoesophageal fistula. Can J Surg 1981;24:626–627.
258. Wheeler ME, Laaveg SJ, Sprague BL. S–C joint disruption in an infant. Clin Orthop 1979;139:68–69.
259. Worman LW, Leagus C. Intrathoracic injury following retrosternal dislocation of the clavicle. J Trauma 1967;7:416–423.
260. Worrell J, Fernandez GN. Retrosternal dislocation of the clavicle: an important injury easily missed. Arch Emerg Med 1986;3:133–135.
261. Yang J, Al-Etani H, Letts M. Diagnosis and treatment of posterior sternoclavicular joint dislocations in children. Am J Orthop 1996;2:565–569.

Distal (Acromioclavicular) Injury

262. Allman FL Jr. Fractures and ligamentous injuries of the clavicle and its articulation. J Bone Joint Surg Am 1967;49:774–784.
263. Bernard TN, Brunet ME, Haddad RJ. Fractured coracoid process in acromioclavicular dislocations. Clin Orthop 1983;175:227–232.
264. Combalia A, Arandes JM, Alemany X, Ramón R. Acromioclavicular dislocation with epiphyseal separation of the coracoid process: report of a case and review of the literature. J Trauma 1995;38:812–815.
265. Dartoy C, Fenoll B, Hra B, LeNan D, et al. Le fracturer décollement épiphysaire de l'extrémité distale de la clavicule. Ann Radiol (Paris) 1993;36:125–128.
266. Dewar FP, Barrington TW. The treatment of chronic acromioclavicular dislocation. J Bone Joint Surg Br 1965;47:32–35.
267. Eidman DK, Siff SJ, Tullos HS. Acromioclavicular lesions in children. Am J Sports Med 1981;9:150–154.
268. Falstie-Jensen S, Mikkelsen P. Pseudodislocation of the acromioclavicular joint. J Bone Joint Surg Br 1982;64:368–369.
269. Gerber C, Rockwood CA Jr. Subcoracoid dislocation of the lateral end of the clavicle: a report of three cases. J Bone Joint Surg Am 1987;69:924–927.
270. Golthamer C. Duplication of the clavicle. Radiology 1957;68:576–578.
271. Gurd FB. The treatment of complete dislocation of the outer end of the clavicle: a hitherto undescribed operation. Ann Surg 1941;113:1094–1096.
272. Havranek P. Injuries of distal clavicular physis in children. J Pediatr Orthop 1989;9:213–215.
273. Katznelson A, Nerubay J, Oliver S. Dynamic fixation of the avulsed clavicle. J Trauma 1976;16:841–844.
274. Liberson R. Os acromiale: a contested anomaly. J Bone Joint Surg 1937;19:683–689.
275. Luzcano MA, Anzell SH, Kelly P. Complete dislocation and subluxation of the acromioclavicular joint: end results in 73 cases. J Bone Joint Surg Am 1961;43:379–891.
276. Montgomery SP, Lloyd RD. Avulsion fracture of the coracoid epiphysis with acromioclavicular separation. J Bone Joint Surg Am 1977;59:963–965.
277. Nordqvist A, Petersson C, Redlund-Johnell I. The natural course of lateral clavicular fracture: 15 (11–21) year follow-up of 110 cases. Acta Orthop Scand 1993;64:87–91.
278. Oestreich AE. The lateral clavicle hook: an acquired as well as a congenital anomaly. Pediatr Radiol 1981;11:147–150.
279. Ogden JA. Distal clavicular physeal injury. Clin Orthop 1984;188:68–73.
280. Protass JJ, Stampfli FV, Osmer JC. Coracoid process fracture diagnosis in acromioclavicular separation. Radiology 1975;116:61–64.
281. Scavenius M, Iverson BF. Nontraumatic clavicular osteolysis in weight lifters. Am J Sports Med 1992;20:463–467.
282. Taga I, Uoneda M, Ono K. Epiphyseal separation of the coracoid process associated with acromioclavicular sprain. Clin Orthop 1986;207:138–141.
283. Twigg HL, Rosenbaum RC. Duplication of the clavicle. Skeletal Radiol 1981;6:281.
284. Weber BG, Brunner C, Freuler F. Die Frakturenbehandlung bei Kindern und Jugendlichen. Berlin: Springer, 1978.

Scapula

285. Ada JR, Miller ME. Scapular fractures: analysis of 113 cases. Clin Orthop 1991;269:174–179.
286. An HS, Vonderbrink JP, Ebraheim NA, Shiple F, Jackson WT. Open scapulothoracic dissociation with intact neurovascular status in a child. J Orthop Trauma 1988;2:36–38.
287. Beim GM, Warner JJP. Symptomatic os acromiale: recognition and treatment. Pittsburgh Orthop J 1996;7:46–51.
288. Benton J, Nelson C. Avulsion of the coracoid process in an athlete. J Bone Joint Surg Am 1971;53:356–358.
289. Borenstein ZC, Mink J, Oppenheim W, Rimoin DL, Lachman RS. Case report 655. Skeletal Radiol 1991;20:134–136.
290. Currarino G, Prescott P. Fractures of the acromion in young children and a description of a variant in acromial ossification which may mimic a fracture. Pediatr Radiol 1994;24:231–233.
291. DeRosa G, Kettelkamp D. Fracture of the coracoid process of the scapula. J Bone Joint Surg Am 1977;59:696–697.
292. Ebraheim NA, An HS, Jackson WT, et al. Scapulothoracic dissociation. J Bone Joint Surg Am 1988;70:428–432.
293. Edelson JG, Zuckerman J, Hershkovitz I. Os acromiale: anatomy and surgical implications. J Bone Joint Surg Br 1993;74:551–555.
294. Euler E, Habermeyer P, Kohler W, Scheweilberer L. Skapulafrakturen: Klassifikation und Differentialtherapie. Orthopade 1992;21:158–162.
295. Goldberg RP, Betsy V. Oblique angled view for coracoid fractures. Skeletal Radiol 1983;9:195–197.
296. Gonza GR, Harris WR. Traumatic winging of the scapula. J Bone Joint Surg Am 1979;61:1230–1233.
297. Gregg JR, Labosky D, Harty M, et al. Serratus anterior paralysis in the young athlete. J Bone Joint Surg Am 1979;61:825–832.
298. Hart RA, Diamandakis V, El-Khoury G, Buckwalter JA. A stress fracture of the scapular body in a child. Iowa Orthop J 1994;15:228–232.
299. Imatani R. Fractures of the scapula: a review of 53 fractures. J Trauma 1975;15:473–478.
300. Kalideen JM, Satyapal KS. Fractures of the acromium in tetanus neonatorum. Clin Radiol 1994;49:563–565.
301. Kauppila LI. The long thoracic nerve: possible mechanisms of injury based on autopsy study. J Shoulder Elbow Surg 1993;2:244–248.

302. Lange RH, Noel SH. Traumatic lateral scapular displacement: an expanded spectrum of associated neurovascular injury. J Orthop Trauma 1993;7:361–366.
303. Lintner DM, Sebastianelli WJ, Hanks GA, Kalenak A. Glenoid dysplasia. Clin Orthop 1992;283:145–148.
304. Mah JY, Otsuka NY. Scapular winging in young atheletes. J Pediatr Orthop 1992;12:245–247.
305. McClure JG, Raney RB. Anomalies of the scapula. Clin Orthop 1975;110:22–31.
306. Morisawa K, Umemura A, Kitamura T, et al. Apophysitis of the acromion. J Shoulder Elbow Surg 1996;5:153–156.
307. Nakae H, Endo S. Traumatic posterior dislocation of the shoulder with fracture of the acromion in a child. Arch Orthop Trauma Surg 1996;115:238–139.
308. Nettrour LF, Krufky EL, Mueller RE, Raycroft JF. Locked scapula: intrathoracic dislocation of the inferior angle. J Bone Joint Surg Am 1972;54:413–416.
309. Ng GPK, Cole WG. Three-dimensional CT reconstruction of the scapula in the management of a child with a displaced intraarticular fracture of the glenoid. Injury 1994;25:671–680.
310. Ogawa K, Yoshida A, Takahashi M, Michimasa U. Fractures of the coracoid process. J Bone Joint Surg Br 1996;78:17–19.
311. Pettersson H. Bilateral dysplasia of the neck of the scapula and associated anomalies. Acta Radiol Diagn (Stockh) 1981;22:81–84.
312. Wilber MC, Evans EB. Fractures of the scapula: an analysis of forty cases and a review of the literature. J Bone Joint Surg Am 1977;59:358–362.
313. Wong-Pack W, Bobechko P, Becker E. Fractured coracoid with anterior shoulder dislocation. J Can Assoc Radiol 1980;31: 278–279.

Brachial Plexus Injury

314. Adler JB, Patterson RL. Erb's palsy: long-term results of treatment in eighty-eight cases. J Bone Joint Surg Am 1967;49: 1052–1064.
315. Aitken J. Deformity of the elbow joint as a sequel to Erb's obstetrical paralysis. J Bone Joint Surg Br 1952;34:352–365.
316. Alanen M, Halonen JP, Katevuo K, Vilkki P. Early surgical exploration and epineural repair in birth brachial palsy. Z Kinderchir 1986;14:335–337.
317. Al-Qattan MM, Clarke HM, Curtis CG. The prognostic value of concurrent clavicular fractures in newborn with obstetric brachial plexus palsy. J Hand Surg [Br] 1994;19:721–730.
318. Al-Qattan MM, Clarke HM, Curtis CG. Klumpke's birth palsy: does it really exist? J Hand Surg [Br] 1995;20:113–123.
319. Al-Qattan MM, El-Sayed AAF, Al-Kharfy TM, Al-Jurayan NAM. Obstetrical brachial plexus injury in newborn babies delivered by caesarean section. J Hand Surg [Br] 1996;21:263–265.
320. Aston JW. Brachial plexus birth palsy. Orthopaedics 1979;2: 594–601.
321. Babbitt DP, Cassidy RH. Obstetrical paralysis and dislocation of the shoulder in infancy. J Bone Joint Surg Am 1968; 50:1447–1452.
322. Baskett TF, Allen AC. Perinatal implications of shoulder dystocia. Obstet Gynecol 1995;86:14–17.
323. Boome RS, Kaye JC. Obstetric traction injuries of the brachial plexus: natural history, indications for surgical repair and results. J Bone Joint Surg Br 1988;70:571–576.
324. Brunelli GA, Brunelli GR. A fourth type of brachial plexus lesion: the intermediate (C7) palsy. J Hand Surg [Br] 1991; 16:492–494.
325. Chuang DC, Lee GW, Hasham F, Wei FC. Restoration of shoulder abduction by nerve transfer in avulsed brachial plexus injury: evaluation of 99 patients with various nerve transfers. Plast Reconstr Surg 1995;96:122–128.
326. Chung SMK, Nessenbaum MM. Obstetrical paralysis. Orthop Clin North Am 1975;6:393–400.
327. Clarke HM, Curtis CG. An approach to obstetrical brachial plexus injuries. Hand Clin 1995;11:563–580.
328. Comtet JJ, Sedel L, Fredenucci JF, Herzberg G. Duchenne-Erb palsy. Clin Orthop 1988;237:17–23.
329. Covey DC, Riordan DC, Milstead ME, Albright JA. Modification of the L'Episcopo procedure for brachial plexus birth palsies. J Bone Joint Surg Br 1992;74:897–901.
330. Cummings RJ, Jones ET, Reed FE, Mazur JM. Infantile dislocation of the elbow complicating obstetric palsy. J Pediatr Orthop 1996;16:589–593.
331. Donn SM, Faix RG. Long-term prognosis for the infant with severe birth trauma. Clin Perinatol 1983;10:507–520.
332. Drew SJ, Giddins GEB, Birch R. A slowly evolving brachial plexus injury following a proximal humeral fracture in a child. J Hand Surg [Br] 1995;20:24–25.
333. Eng GD. Brachial plexus injuries in newborn infants. Pediatrics 1971;78:18–28.
334. Erb WH. Über eine eigenthumliche Localisation von Lahmungen im Plexus brachialis. Verh Naturhist Med Ver Heidelberg NF 1874;2:130–154.
335. Francel PC, Koby M, Park TS, et al. Fast spin-echo magnetic resonance imaging for radiological assessment of neonatal brachial plexus injury. J Neurosurg 1995;83:461–466.
336. Friedman AH. Neurotization of elements of the brachial plexus. Neurosurg Clin North Am 1991;2:165–174.
337. Gentjens G, Gilbert A, Helsen K. Obstetric brachial plexus palsy associated with breech delivery: a different pattern of injury. J Bone Joint Surg Br 1996;78:303–306.
338. Gilbert A. Long-term evaluation of brachial plexus surgery in obstetrical palsy. Hand Clin 1995;11:583–594.
339. Gilbert A, Khouri N, Carlioz H. Exploration chirurgicale du plexus brachial dans la paralysie obstetricale: constellations anatomiques chez 21 malades operes. Rev Chir Orthop 1980; 66:33–42.
340. Gilbert A, Khouri N, Carlioz H. Exploration chirurgicale du plexus brachial dans la paralysie obstétricale. Rev Chir Orthop 1980;66:33–41.
341. Gilbert A, Whitaker I. Obstetrical brachial plexus lesions. J Surg 1991;16B:481–491.
342. Gonik B, Hollyer VL, Allen R. Shoulder dystocia recognition: differences in neonatal risks for injury. Am J Perinatol 1991; 8:31–34.
343. Gordon M. The immediate and long-term outcome of obstetric birth trauma. I. Brachial plexus paralysis. Am J Obstet Gynecol 1973;117:51–56.
344. Greenwald AG, Schute PC, Shiveley JL. Brachial plexus palsy: a 10-year report on the incidence and prognosis. J Pediatr Orthop 1984;4:681–692.
345. Hankins GDV, Clark SL. Brachial plexus palsy involving the posterior shoulder at spontaneous vaginal delivery. Am J Perinatol 1995;12:44–45.
346. Hardy AE. Birth injuries of the brachial plexus: incidence and prognosis. J Bone Joint Surg Br 1981;63:98–101.
347. Hentz VR, Meyer RD. Brachial plexus microsurgery in children. Microsurgery 1991;12:175–185.
348. Hernandez RJ, Dias L. CT evaluation of the shoulder in children with Erb's palsy. Pediatr Radiol 1988;18:333–336.
349. Jackson ST, Hoffer MM, Parrish N. Brachial-plexus palsy in the newborn. J Bone Joint Surg Am 1988;70:1217–1220.
350. Kawabata H, Kawai H, Masatomi T, Yasui N. Accessory nerve neurotization in infants with brachial plexus birth palsy. Microsurgery 1994;15:768–772.
351. Kawai H, Ohta I, Masatomi T, Kawabata H, Masada K, Ono K. Stretching of the brachial plexus in rabbits. Acta Orthop Scand 1989;60:635–638.

References

352. Kennedy R. Suture of the brachial plexus in birth paralysis of the upper extremity. BMJ 1903;1:298–301.
353. Klumpke A. Contribution a l'etude des paralysies radiculaires du plexus brachial: paralysies radiculaires totales; paralysies radiculaires inferieures; de la participation des filets sympathiques oculo-pupillaires dans ces paralysies. Rev Med 1885; 5:591, 739.
354. Laurent JP, Lee R, Shenaq S, et al. Neurosurgical correction of upper brachial plexus birth injuries. J Neurosurg 1993;79:197–203.
355. Leffert RD. Brachial Plexus Injuries. New York: Churchill Livingstone, 1985.
356. Liebolt FL, Furey JG. Obstetrical paralysis with dislocation of the shoulder. J Bone Joint Surg Am 1953;35:227–230.
357. Magalon G, Bordeaux J, Legre R, Aubert JP. Emergency versus delayed repair of severe brachial plexus injuries. Clin Orthop 1988;237:32–35.
358. Marshall RW, DeSilva RD. Computerized axial tomography in traction injuries of the brachial plexus. J Bone Joint Surg Br 1986;68:734–738.
359. Marshall RW, William DH, Birch R, Bonney G. Operations to restore elbow flexion after brachial plexus injuries. J Bone Joint Surg Br 1988;70:577–582.
360. Michelon BJ, Clarke HM, Curtis CG, Zucker RM, Seifu Y, Andrews DF. The natural history of obstetrical brachial plexus palsy. Plast Reconstr Surg 1993;93:675–680.
361. Narakas AO. Injuries to the brachial plexus. In: Bora FW (ed) The Pediatric Upper Extremity: Diagnosis and Management. Philadelphia: Saunders, 1986.
362. Peterson CR, Peterson CM. Brachial plexus injury in an infant from a car safety seat. N Engl J Med 1991;325:1587–1588.
363. Phipps GJ, Hoffer HM. Latissimus dorsi and teres major transfer to rotator cuff for Erb's palsy. J Shoulder Elbow Surg 1995;4:124–129.
364. Platt JH Jr. Neurosurgical management of birth injuries of the brachial plexus. Neurosurg Clin North Am 1991;2:175–185.
365. Pollock AN, Reed MH. Shoulder deformities from obstetrical brachial plexus paralysis. Skeletal Radiol 1989;18:295–197.
366. Rossitch E Jr, Oakes WJ, Ovelmen-Levitt J, Nashold BS Jr. Self-mutilation following brachial plexus injury sustained at birth. Pain 1992;50:201–211.
367. Sloof ACJ. Obstetric brachial plexus lesions and their neurosurgical treatment. Clin Neurol Neurosurg 1993;95(suppl):873–877.
368. Solonen KA, Telaranta T, Ryöppy S. Early reconstruction of birth injuries of the brachial plexus. J Pediatr Orthop 1981;1:367–374.
369. Specht EE. Brachial plexus injury in the newborn: incidence and prognosis. Clin Orthop 1975;110:32–34.
370. Stevens JH. Brachial plexus paralysis. Clin Orthop 1988;237:4–8.
371. Taylor AS. Results from the surgical treatment of brachial birth palsy. JAMA 1907;48:96–99.
372. Troum S, Floyd WE, Waters PM. Posterior dislocation of the humeral head in infancy associated with obstetrical paralysis. J Bone Joint Surg Am 1993;75:1370–1375.
373. Urabe F, Matsuishit, Kouinis K, et al. MR imaging of birth brachial palsy in a two-month-old infant. Brain Dev 1991; 13:130–131.
374. Wickstrom J, Haslam ET, Hutchinson RH. The surgical management of the residual deformities of the shoulder following birth injuries of the brachial plexus. J Bone Joint Surg Am 1955;37:27–36.
375. Zancolli EA, Zancolli ER Jr. Palliative surgical procedures in sequelae of obstetrical palsy. Hand Clin 1988;4:643–669.

14

Humerus

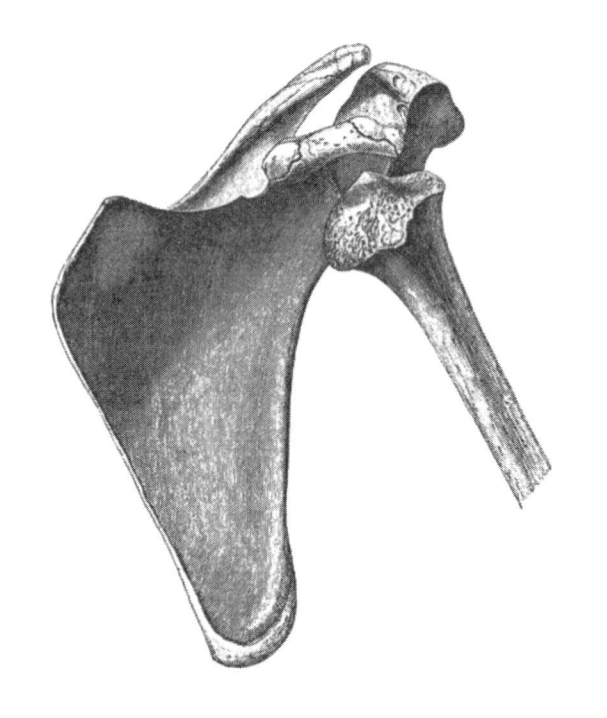

Engraving of a type 1 physeal injury of the proximal humerus. (From Poland J. Transmatic Separation of the Epiphyses. London: Smith, Elder, 1898)

At birth the initial contour of the **proximal humeral physis** has a transverse orientation, similar to the proximal femur. However, during subsequent postnatal development, this physeal contour is progressively modified into the conical (pyramidal) shape that characterizes the adolescent.[19] A medial growth zone under the humeral head usually is subjected to compression stresses, and the lateral region is subjected to both compression and tension forces, depending on the position and functional activity of the various shoulder muscles (Figs. 14-1 to 14-3). Variations in glenoid development may also affect the morphology of the proximal humerus.[6,15]

As the proximal humerus matures, the anatomic structures of the physis and contiguous metaphysis play a major role in the overall resistive strength and patterns of fracture. The progressively conical apex has a posteromedial position that resists forces directed posteriorly and axially. The apex of the cone is medial to a plane drawn from the anterior to the posterior insertions of the rotator cuff musculature. This plane includes a small portion of the medial metaphysis anteriorly but more of it posteriorly, and it is probably a significant anatomic factor predisposing the proximal humerus to the common type 2 growth mechanism fracture in the older child.

The epiphyseal (secondary) ossification center of the proximal humerus may not be present at birth, except in its formative (preosseous) stage. Approximately 20% of neonates have a radiologically evident epiphyseal ossification center at birth. By 4 months this ossification center becomes radiologically evident. The ossification center in the greater tuberosity appears between 6 and 18 months, and an ossification center for the lesser tuberosity occurs later, although this structure is highly variable and frequently does not appear as an independent ossification center. The ossification centers of the greater tuberosity and humeral head form osseous connections at the microscopic level as early as 10–14 months, although it depends on individual rates of development. Coalescence of these two osseous centers usually becomes radiologically evident at 4–7 years. The physis undergoes histologic closure at approximately 12–14 years in girls and 15–17 years in boys (Fig. 14-4).

The periosteum plays a significant role in the strength of the proximal humeral growth plate and its susceptibility to injury. The periosteum is thicker posteriorly than anteriorly. This anatomic variation plays a significant role in preventing posterior displacment of the metaphysis. In contrast, displacement of the metaphysis is relatively easily produced through the thinner anterior portion of the periosteum. This anatomic variation in thickness remains throughout skeletal maturation. When the periosteum gives way, it tends to disrupt lateral to the intertubercular groove under the long head of the biceps. The bicipital tendon and osseous groove appear to be predisposing factors to the development of the medial metaphyseal fragment in type 2 growth mechanism injuries.

The proximal humeral physis is significant to both humeral and overall arm length, contributing approximately

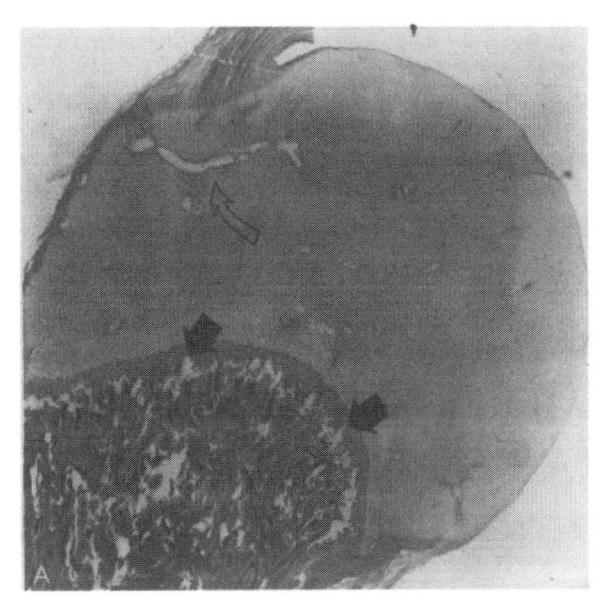

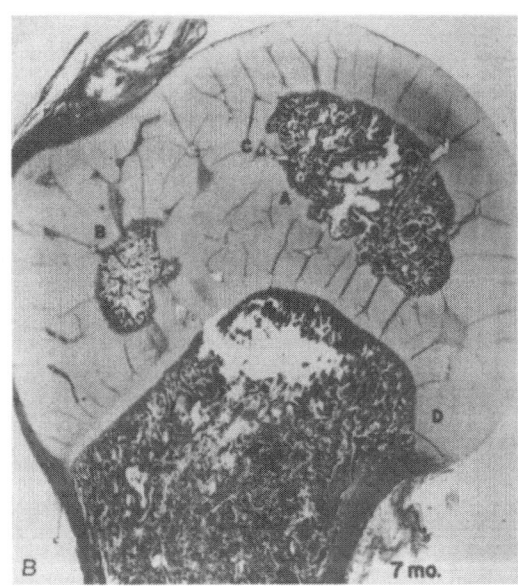

FIGURE 14-1. Development of the proximal humerus. (A) Neonatal humerus showing a vascular cartilage canal penetrating from the greater tuberosity (open arrow). The solid arrows indicate the plane of separation in a birth injury or child abuse. Such an injury invariably involves a fracture, rather than a shoulder dislocation. (B) At 7 months, secondary ossification centers are present in the capital humerus, A, and greater tuberosity, B. A vascular channel, C, enters the capital humeral center. The medial physis curves distally at D, creating a contour similar to that of the early proximal femur.

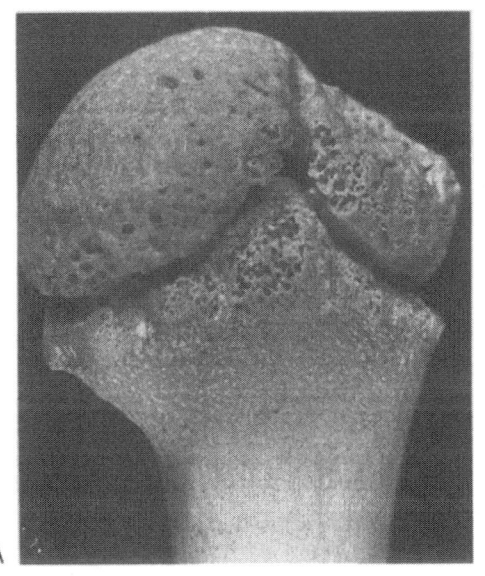

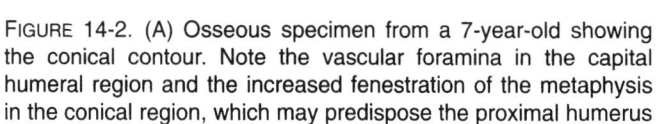

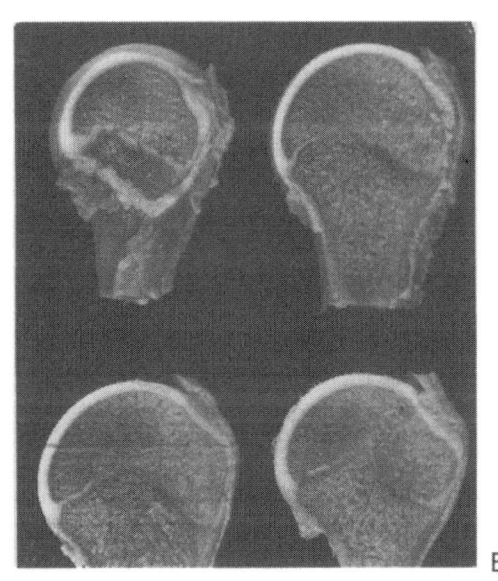

FIGURE 14-2. (A) Osseous specimen from a 7-year-old showing the conical contour. Note the vascular foramina in the capital humeral region and the increased fenestration of the metaphysis in the conical region, which may predispose the proximal humerus to certain failure patterns. (B) Serial sections of proximal humerus from a 12-year-old show the variable contour of the physis depending on the anteroposterior depth. This varied contour affects fracture patterns.

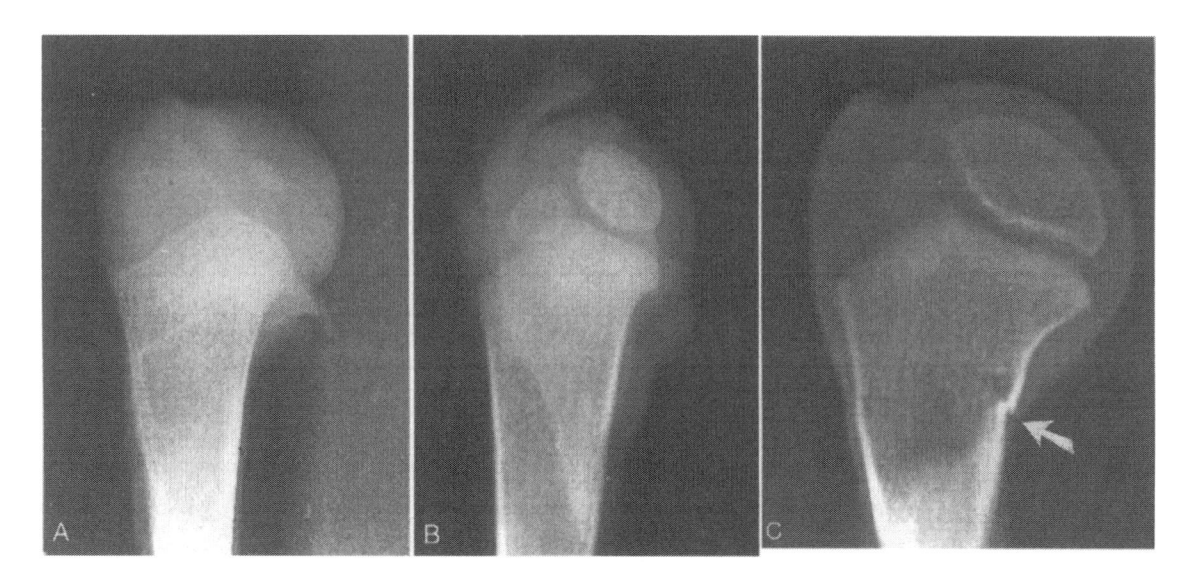

FIGURE 14-3. Air/cartilage roentgenograms demonstrating cartilage and bone. (A) Two months. (B) Seven months. (C) Three years. Note also the acute metaphyseal fracture (arrow).

80% of the longitudinal growth of the humerus. Impairment of this normal growth process may have a major effect on the overall length of the involved limb.

The **metaphysis** is initially flat at its interface with the physis. With growth, the central area extends upward, creating a pyramidal shape. Several large muscles attach to this area; such attachment may affect metaphyseal cortical development, creating irregularities (Fig. 14-5). This situation is similar to the cortical variants described for the medial distal femoral metaphysis (see Chapter 21).

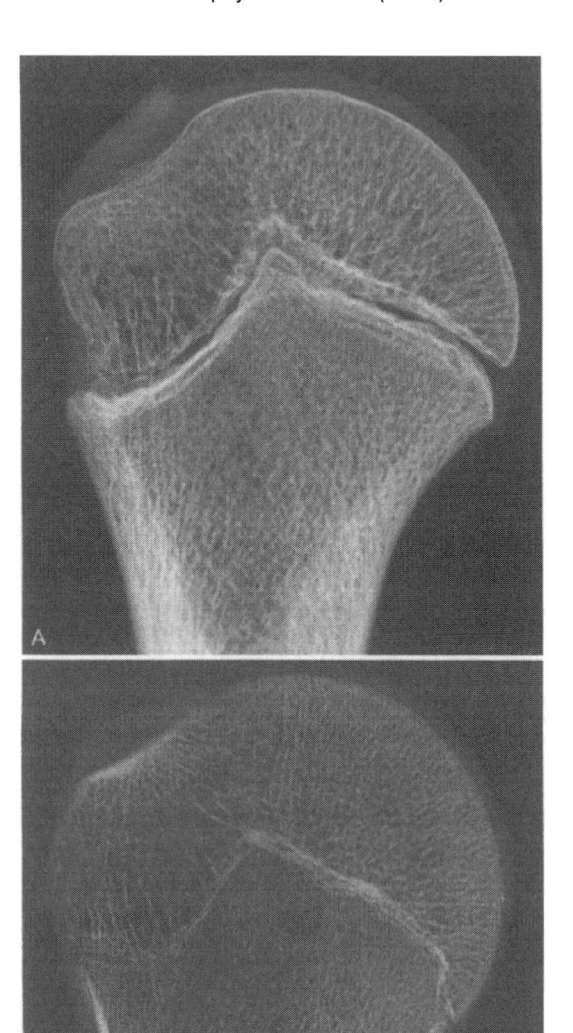

FIGURE 14-4. (A) Roentgenogram from a 13-year-old boy, showing subchondral sclerosis preceding final physeal closure. (B) Slab section from a 15-year-old showing almost complete physeal closure with coalescence of subchondral plates.

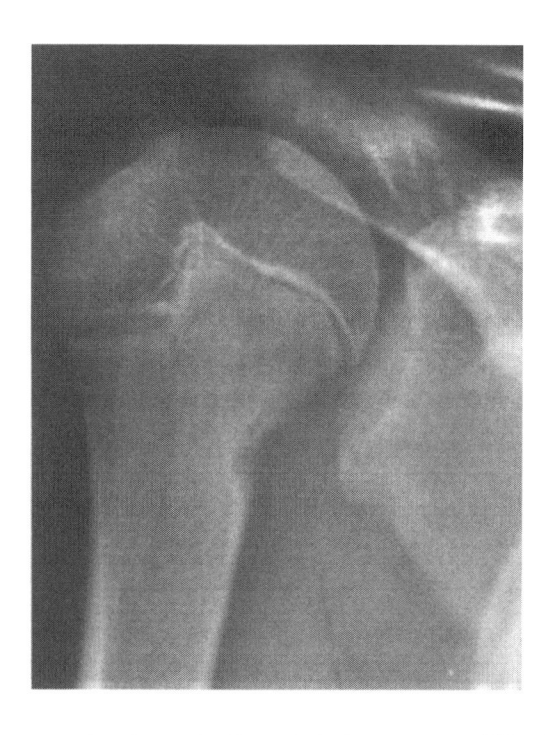

FIGURE 14-5. Medial cortical irregularity in a 14-year-old boy being evaluated for shoulder pain. This is a normal radiologic variant, similar to the medial irregularity often seen in the distal femur.

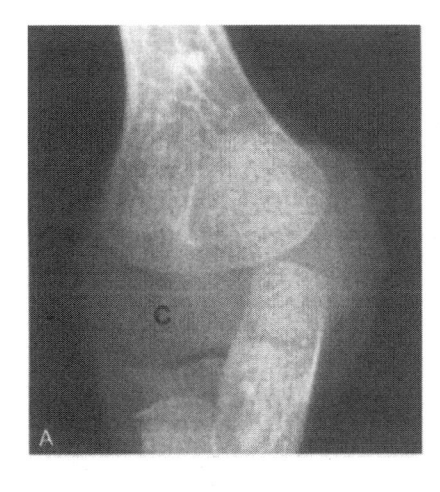

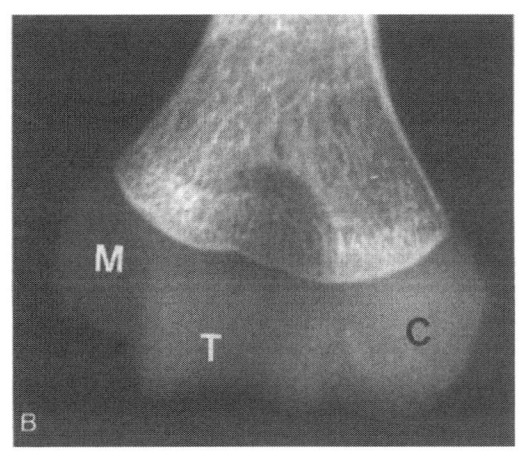

FIGURE 14-6. Distal humeral development in a 6-month-old baby. (A) Intact elbow joint with air outlining the radiohumeral portions of the joint. Note the capitellum (C). (B) Air/cartilage contrast showing cartilaginous epiphyseal contours. Note the medial epicondyle (M), trochlea (T), and capitellum (C).

As a rough definition, the **diaphysis** extends from the upper border of the insertion of the pectoralis major to the supracondylar ridge. This area has multiple muscular attachments, which, depending on the level of the fracture, significantly affect the displacement of the fragments. The humeral shaft is roughly cylindrical in its upper half but becomes gradually broadened and flattened distally.

The major nerves variably traverse along the humeral shaft. The most serious likelihood of potential injury is to the radial nerve, which lies adjacent to the posterolateral surface of the shaft. It traverses obliquely and laterally as it passes from the axilla to the anterolateral epicondylar region. It may be injured acutely or be subsequently entrapped in fracture callus. Nerve entrapment may occur even with greenstick diaphyseal fractures.

The supracondylar process is a normal variation in approximately 1% of patients.[3] It is usually located 5–7 cm above the medial epicondyle at skeletal maturity. Obviously, this distance may be less in the younger child, as growth increases the position (distance) of the process from the physis. It may be connected distally with a tendinous band extending to the medial epicondyle and may provide an anomalous insertion for the pronator teres. When this tendinous band is calcified or ossified, it may outline a foramen. When the median nerve and artery pass through this structure, increased traction from growth or compression or swelling following trauma may cause arterial or nerve dysfunction. On rare occasions, this supracondylar process is fractured.[7,13,16]

In the supracondylar region of the **distal humerus**, the osseous septum separating the olecranon fossa from the coronoid fossa varies in thickness (see Fig. 14-8, below). Roentgenographically, it has variable radiodensity. Occasionally, there is complete osseous perforation, although fibrous tissue still separate the anterior and posterior portions of the fossa. The variability of the radiographic appearance must be considered when evaluating a patient.[7,25] The foramen (fossa) essentially divides the supracondylar metaphysis into two columns.[1,14] This is an important feature in the instability of a fracture in this region. The two-column structure also affects surgical fixation.

Diagnosis of distal humeral injuries is rendered particularly difficult because of the variable extent of secondary ossification (Figs. 14-6 to 14-12).[8,9,11,12,17,20,21,23] Significant injury may occur with deceptively little roentgenographic evidence.[5] The overall joint contours and separation of capitellar and trochlear surfaces are present at birth and do not change significantly with subsequent development. Disruption of these relations with medial or lateral condylar fractures may alter joint contours, mechanics, and circulatory dynamics.[10] The ossification centers appear in the following sequence: capitellum (at 3–4 months), medial epicondyle (at 4–6 years), medial condyle (at 8–9 years), and lateral epicondyle (at 9–11 years). The trochlear center consistently develops from multiple foci (Fig. 14-9). A small, medial accessory ossification center of the trochlea may appear after the major foci have fused. These variations may simulate a fracture fragment.[23–25] There may be considerable variation

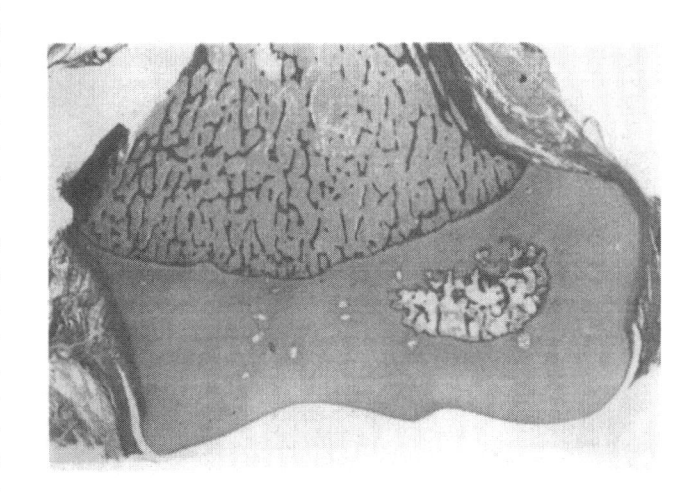

FIGURE 14-7. Distal humeral development in a 2-year-old.

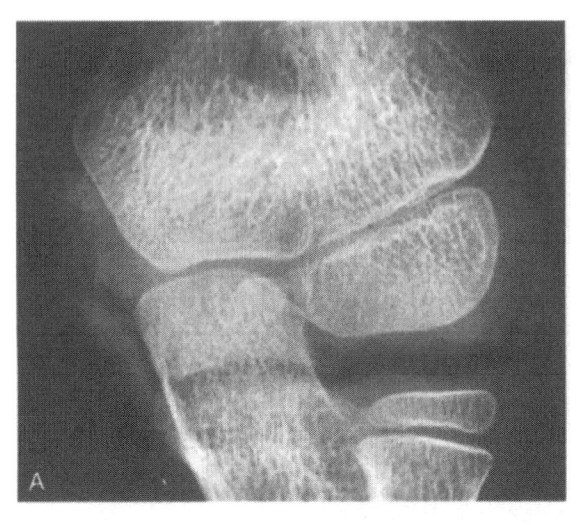

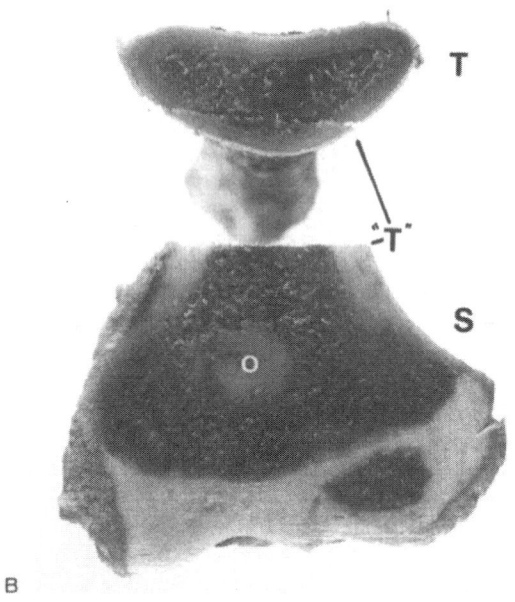

FIGURE 14-8. Distal humeral development in a 6-year-old. (A) Air outlines the joint and epiphyseal contours. (B) Sagittal (S) section of chondro-osseous epiphysis and transverse (T) section of shaft at the level of "T". Above the olecranon fossa (O), the anatomic configuration of the shaft is more stable than the transverse contour at the fossa.

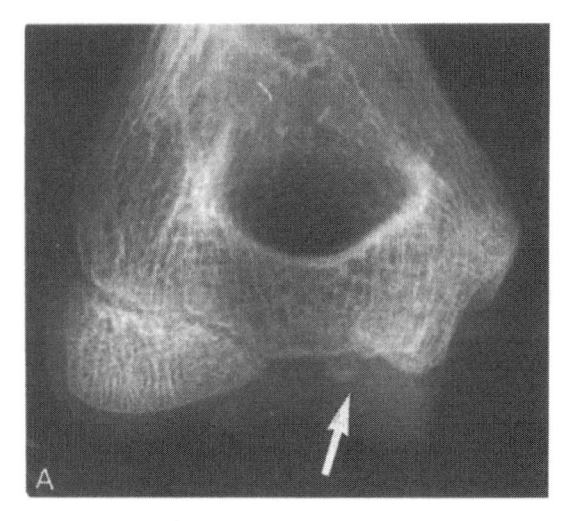

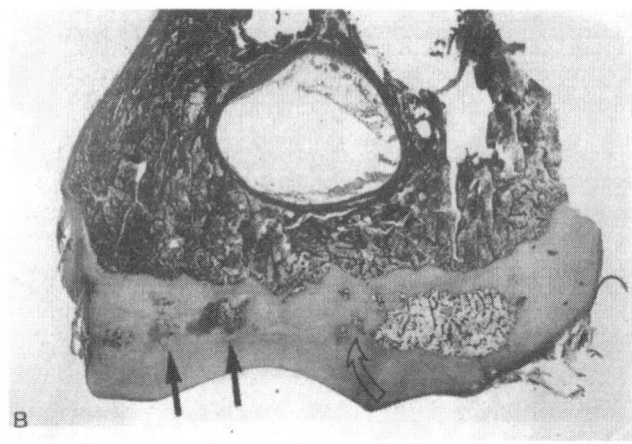

FIGURE 14-9. Distal humeral development in an 8-year-old. (A) Roentgenogram shows that trochlear ossification is beginning (arrow). (B) Histologic section. Note the multifocal ossification of the trochlea (solid arrows) and the satellite ossification of the capitellum (open arrow).

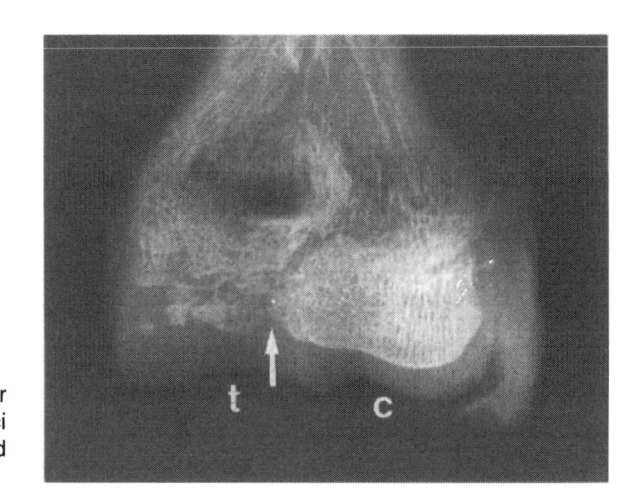

FIGURE 14-10. Distal humeral development in a 10-year-old. The trochlear ossification center is beginning to coalesce with the multiple ossific foci and the capitellar ossification center (arrow). Note the trochlea (t) and capitellum (c).

Humerus

The ulnar nerve runs in a groove along the posterior aspect of this epicondyle, an anatomic relation responsible for the frequency of ulnar nerve injury, especially contusion, with a medial epicondylar fracture, The medial epicondyle is often considered an epiphysis that does not contribute to the longitudinal growth of the humerus. This is a misconception. This particular region initially develops as an integral part of the medial condyle. With growth it becomes a functionally, though not anatomically, separate entity; and it appears to be unassociated with the major histologic changes characteristic of a traction-responsive physis, such as the tibial tuberosity. Injury to the medial epicondyle, if it occurs in a young child, may lead to growth alteration because it causes disruption of the physis as it curves around the main portion of the condyle. The older the child at the time of a distal humeral injury, the less likely it is that any significant growth disturbance will follow.

A supratrochlear dorsale accessory ossicle may develop behind the supracondylar fossa.[18,27] It may be excised if the patient is symptomatic.

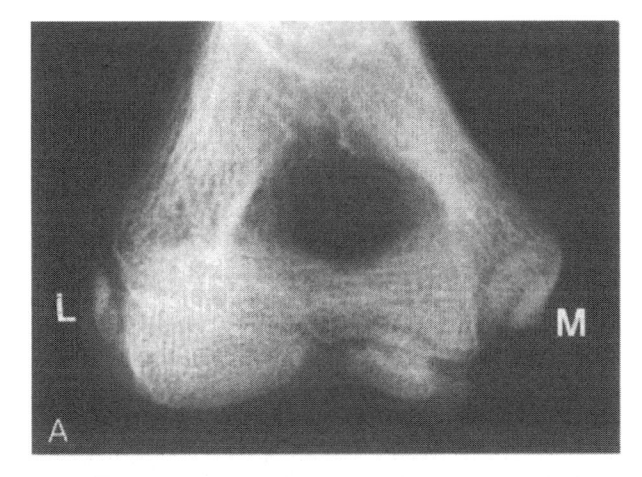

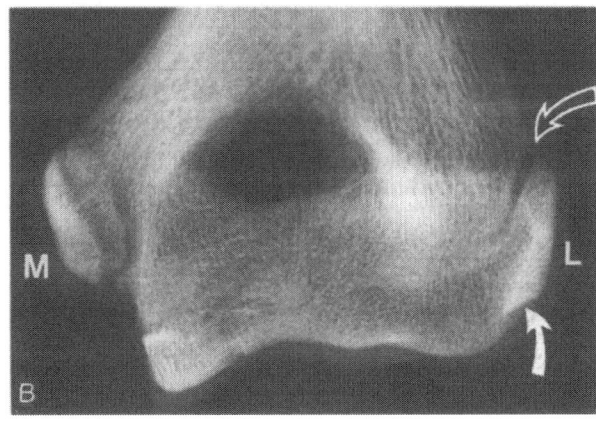

FIGURE 14-11. (A) Distal humeral development in a 12-year-old. Both epicondyles have developed secondary centers (L = lateral epicondyle; M = medial epicondyle). (B) Distal humerus of a 14-year-old. The lateral epicondyle has fused with the capitellum (solid arrow) but not with the metaphysis (open arrow).

of secondary ossification from right to left. Comparison views are not totally reliable for symmetry to rule out injury.

The lateral epicondyle serves as the origin of the radial collateral ligament, the supinator muscle, and the common extensor muscle tendon. Irregular or multifocal ossification is typical in the immature lateral epicondyle of the humerus and may be misdiagnosed as an avulsion.[11]

Comparison to the opposite side is not always helpful, as asymmetric epiphyseal ossification is relatively common, most likely due to differing muscular activity and strength in dominant versus nondominant arms. The ossification center of the lateral epicondyle appears at about 12 years of age and fuses with the lateral condyle at age 14 years. The lateral epicondyle does not fuse directly with the humeral metaphysis as does the medial epicondyle. Instead, it fuses first with the contiguous epiphyseal ossification center of the capitellum at 14–16 years (Fig. 14-12); then the combined ossific mass fuses with the distal humeral metaphysis.

The ossification center of the medial epicondyle appears about 5 years of age and unites with the metaphysis between 14 and 16 years.[19] The common tendon of the flexor muscles of the forearm originates from the medial epicondyle, which also attaches to the ulnar collateral ligament of the elbow.

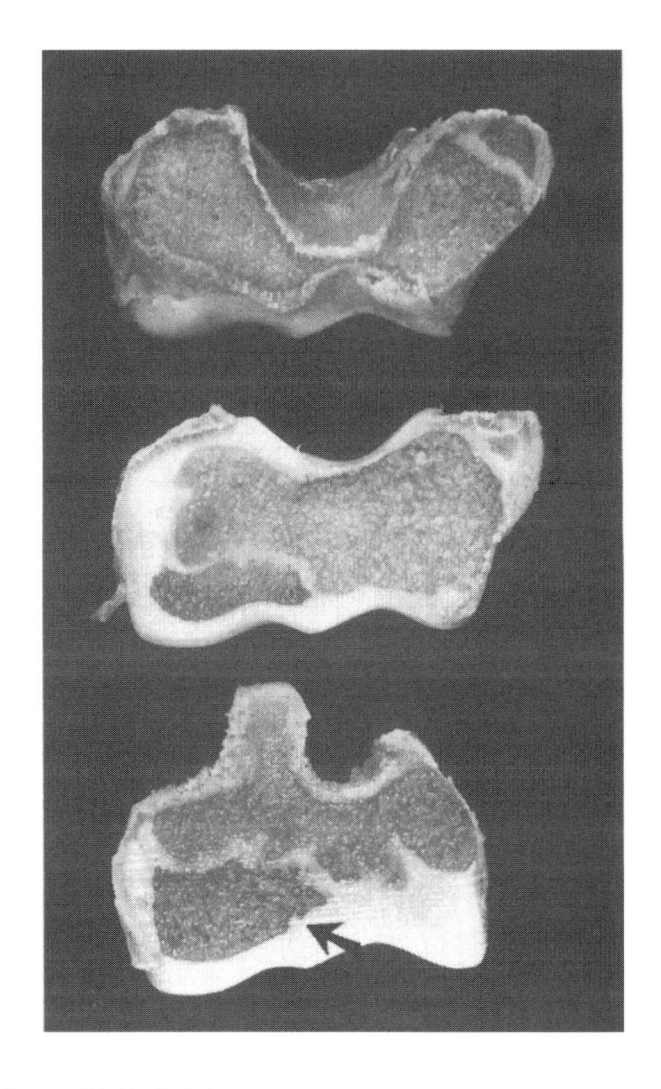

FIGURE 14-12. Serial transverse sections of the distal humerus. Because of the anterior tilt of the distal epiphysis (see Figure 14-13) portions of the epiphysis and metaphysis are evident in the same transection. The capitellar ossification center is readily evident (arrow). The bicolumnar morphology is also evident.

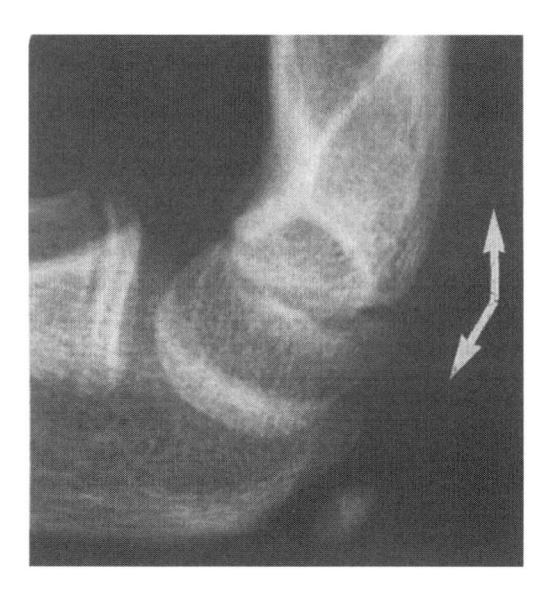

FIGURE 14-13. Normal lateral view showing anterior angulation of the capitellum (arrow). This angulation must be restored in fracture reductions.

The carrying angle of the elbow does not have a significant gender difference, but it does have an age difference in that there is a gradual increase in the carrying angle with progressive skeletal maturation.[4] The mean carrying angle is 15° in the 0- to 4-year age group and increases to 17.8° by the time of skeletal maturity.[4] This contrasts with a reported slight gender difference of the mean carrying angle of 13° in women and 11° in men.[2,26]

The distal humerus has a normal forward angulation that is most evident when supracondylar or capitellar (lateral condylar) fractures are being evaluated (Fig. 14-13). Realignment of this anatomic configuration should be attempted during any fracture reduction, as misalignment (usually a relative hyperextension) may affect elbow mechanics, especially the ability to flex or extend completely.[22] Capitellar misalignment may also significantly affect the ability to supinate or pronate.

Glenohumeral Joint Dislocation

Subluxation and dislocation of the shoulder are rare in an infant or young child but become more common during adolescence.[30,33,34,35,44] Instability may occur as a complication of various types of neurologic abnormalities, particularly brachial plexus injuries (see Chapter 13). Developmental anterior capsular redundancy predisposes certain individuals to progressively unstable shoulders.[42] Subluxation and dislocation may develop slowly.[46–50]

Congenital morphologic differences may predispose to shoulder instability. Glenoid dysplasia, although much less common than acetabular dysplasia, certainly may be associated with a chronically painful shoulder.[15] The patient shown in Figure 14-14 was referred for bilateral "chronically dislocated" shoulders, but evaluation revealed intact glenohumeral joints and redirection of the scapulae almost 90°, such that they were rotated onto the sides of the rib cage. The underlying deficit appeared to be hypoplasia of the clavicles.[32]

The anatomic structure and extent of functional motion predispose the proximal humerus to epiphyseal separation in the child and adolescent in response to forces that, in contrast, may lead to glenohumeral dislocation in an adolescent or young adult.[36,39,43] Rowe and Sakellarides reviewed 500 cases of shoulder dislocation and found that only 8 involved patients between the ages of 6 months and 10 years.[40] Almost 20% of the cases occurred during the second decade of life, usually in those ages 17–20 years (generally after skeletal maturity had been attained). The highest recurrence rates were in patients under 20 years of age, rather than adults. They also showed that many young adults with habitual voluntary dislocation of the shoulder probably commenced the process during early adolescence, at a time when the growth plate was undergoing physiologic closure and the laxity of the ligamentous structures around the shoulder was normally decreasing.

Huber and Gerber reviewed 25 children with voluntary (habitual) subluxation (36 shoulders).[35] Eighteen children were managed by "skillful neglect." Only two required shoulder surgery as adults; the others were satisfied with the function of the shoulder. Seven children (10 shoulders) underwent stabilizing procedures, but only three patients were satisfied with the results. None of the patients had emotional or psychiatric problems. Huber and Gerber thought there was no indication for prophylactic surgical intervention. None of the patients developed osteoarthritis during the follow-up ranging from 6 to 26 years.

The capsule of the shoulder joint has an intrinsic laxity that allows some displacement during stress. This may be documented arthrographically in a child with chronic shoulder discomfort or pain (Fig. 14-15). It may also be seen in pseudosubluxation of the proximal humerus when there is a fracture with hemarthrosis or reactive joint effusion (Fig. 14-16). The intrinsic capsular elasticity and joint volume contribute little to anterior shoulder instability.[41] Rather, instability probably relates to damage to the surrounding muscular stabilizing structures.

In an assessment of 75 children (150 joints), signs of instability were found in 57% of the boys and 48% of the girls.[30] The most frequent sign was a positive posterior drawer test (63 shoulders). Seventeen patients had multidirectional instability. Generalized joint laxity was not a feature of these subjects.

Dislocation in the skeletally immature patient is usually anteroinferior (Fig. 14-17), probably due to an intrinsic area of laxity and the common mechanism of hyperabduction and extension. The affected child's appearance is comparable to that of the adult. The arm is usually in slight abduction and external rotation. An anterior bulge may be seen from the side. In the case of subluxation or persistent pain after reduction, translation should be tested in the anterior and posterior directions. The "apprehension test" should also be used, wherein external rotation and abduction elicits concern that the shoulder is about to displace.

The radiologic diagnosis of displacement of the developing shoulder is usually readily evident. Any patient should be radiographed prior to reduction to be certain that the more

Glenohumeral Joint Dislocation

FIGURE 14-14. (A) This boy was referred for evaluation of "bilateral congenital shoulder dislocations." His mother had the same "problem." (B) CT scan shows redirection of the scapula into lateral positions, rather than glenohumeral dislocations.

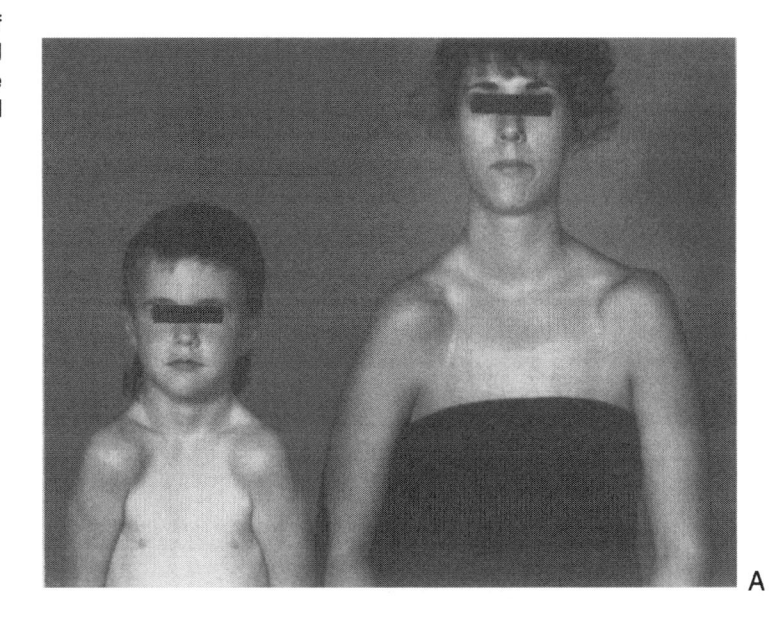

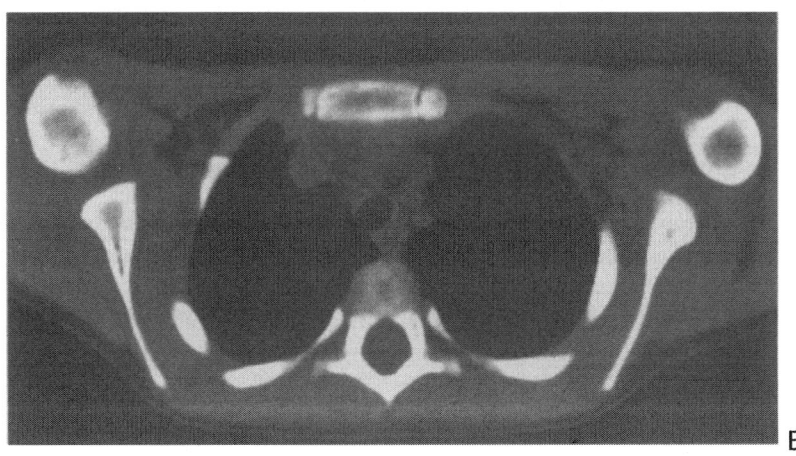

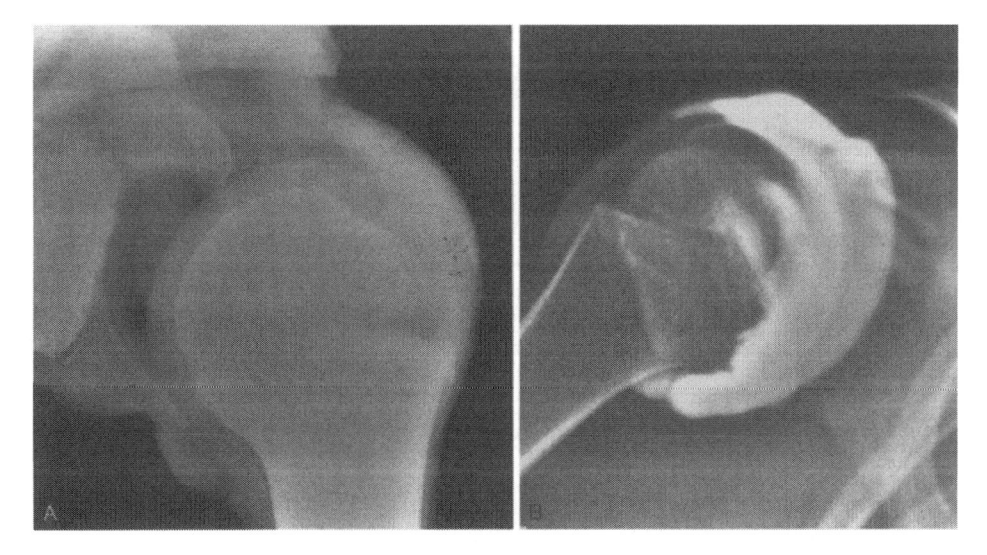

FIGURE 14-15. (A) Laxity was present in a 7-year-old, demonstrated in a specimen from a forequarter amputation. (B) Motion evident in an arthrogram. This patient had chronic shoulder pain due to pitching in the Little League.

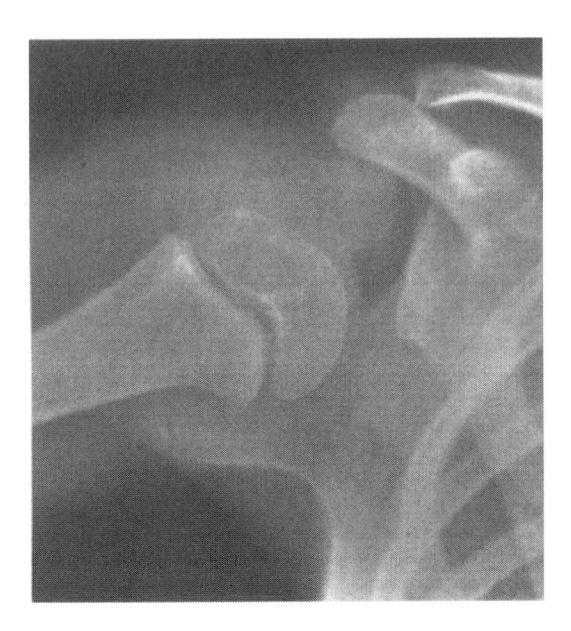

FIGURE 14-16. Traction creates a vacuum arthrogram that outlines the extent of subluxation and thickness of the humeral head cartilage.

common injury, proximal humeral physeal fracture, has not occurred. Other diagnostic imaging modalities may be helpful. A computed tomography (CT) scan can corroborate chronic residual subluxation after a documented dislocation that has been acutely reduced. Magnetic resonance imaging (MRI) may delineate areas of internal trabecular damage that are part of the progressive biologic changes leading to a Hill-Sachs lesion (Fig. 14-18).[31] A classic Hill-Sachs lesion is evident in Figure 14-19.

Treatment of this injury is similar in adults and children. Longitudinal traction is applied to the arm, concomitant with countertraction. The arm initially is held in an internally rotated position. External rotation is applied gradually. Adequate muscle relaxation facilitates the maneuvers. Many children have generalized joint laxity, which makes reduction relatively easy. Great care must be taken not to use excessive force (particularly rotatory), as it could theoretically cause a complicating traumatic epiphysiolysis, similar to a slipped capital femoral epiphysis associated with reduction of a hip dislocation. However, I am unaware of any reported patient with this potential complication.

The arm should be immobilized in a sling-and-swathe dressing. Pendulum exercises may be started at 10–14 days. If the patient develops pain during the postinjury period, MRI may be useful to delineate soft tissue (i.e., labrum, capsule) damage that may contribute to chronic instability or subluxation. Rotator cuff injury does not commonly occur in this age group.[85,86]

Redislocation may occur. Wagner and Lyne reported that traumatic shoulder dislocations were rare in adolescents when the epiphyses were open. In 8 of 10 of their affected patients, however, the dislocation recurred and ultimately required operative intervention and capsular repair.[43]

The Bankart lesion is an avulsion of the glenohumeral ligament–labral complex.[45] These ligaments may be disrupted from the cartilaginous humeral head as well. Children may sustain a chondro-osseous glenoid rim fracture as a comparable injury (see section on scapular injury in Chapter 13).

Operative approaches are comparable to those used in the adult. Because capsular redundancy is common, soft tissue procedures should be emphasized. No child or adolescent should have surgery, though, without an intense period of rehabilitation.[37,38]

Coracoid transfer may be used for recurrent anterior instability of the shoulder in adolescents. Placement of the screw through the coracoid process does not appear to affect subsequent development of that region adversely.[28] The youngest patient was 14 years,[28] and the procedure is *not* recommended for boys younger than that; it should *not* be considered in boys or girls under 12 years of age.

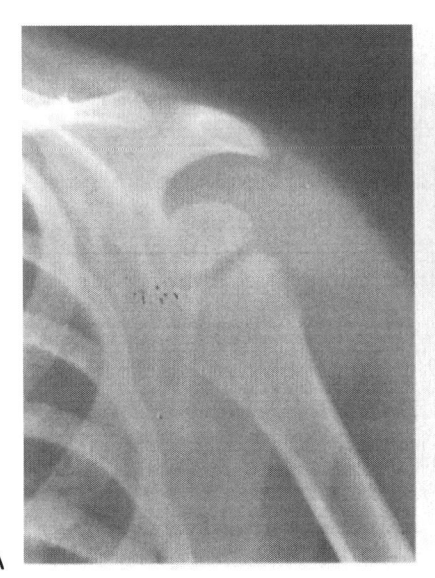

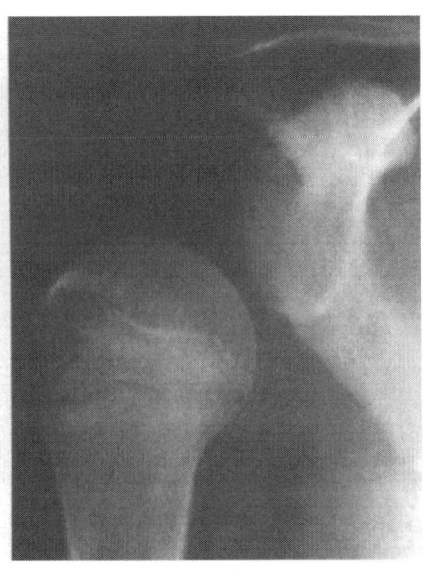

FIGURE 14-17. (A) Dislocation (anterior) in a 5-year-old. (B) Dislocation in a 12-year-old girl.

Glenohumeral Joint Dislocation

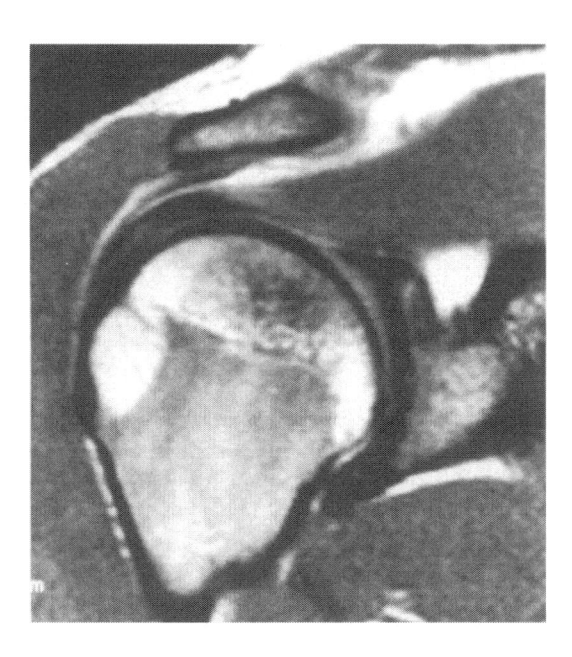

FIGURE 14-18. Bone bruising in the humeral head after a dislocation that required reduction in the emergency room. Would this create the preconditions necessary to lead to an area of collapse (Hill-Sachs lesion)?

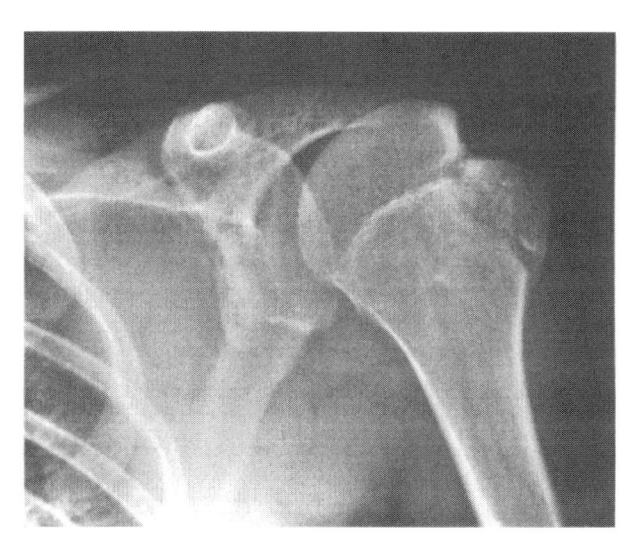

FIGURE 14-19. Severe chondro-osseous deformity in a 15-year-old boy with multiple dislocations.

Brachial Plexus Injury

A chronic subluxation or dislocation of the shoulder may be associated with a childhood brachial plexus injury.[46,47,49,50] Several years may elapse before such instability becomes a clinical problem. Acquired disorders such as a septic shoulder during infancy may cause a similar problem.[48]

Luxatio Erecta

Luxatio erecta is an infrequent condition that may occur during a difficult delivery (Fig. 14-20A).[23,29] The arm is held in an overhead position and is externally rotated and abducted. The humeral head becomes locked below the inferior glenoid margin. Capsular laxity due to the effect of maternal hormones may be a predisposing factor, similar to developmental hip dysplasia.

The same infrequent pattern of inferior dislocation with the arm overhead may occur in older children (Fig. 20B). The tendency for children to hang from heights (e.g., monkey bars, tree limbs) may play a role in the causation.

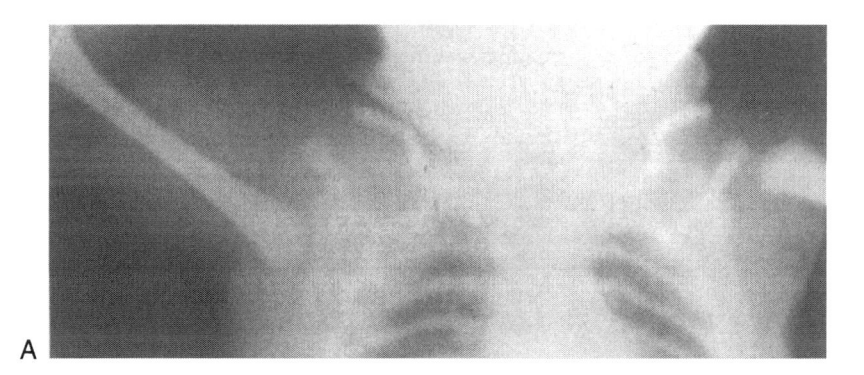

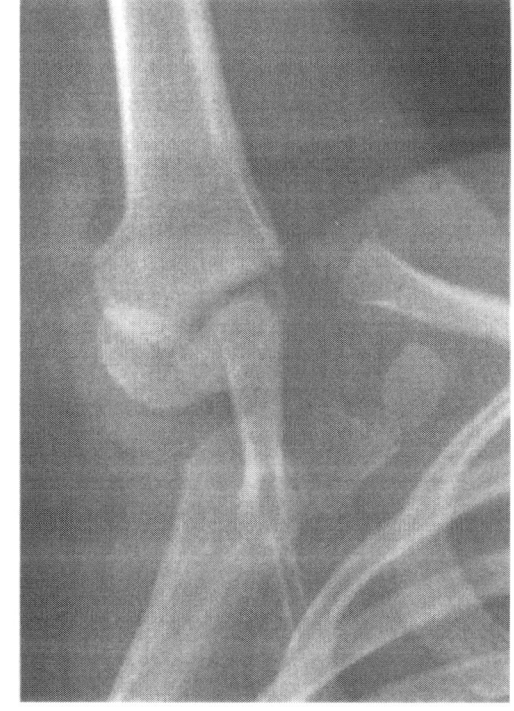

FIGURE 14-20. (A) Luxatio erecta in a neonate following traumatic delivery. It must be distinguished from a physeal fracture. (B) Luxatio erecta in a 5-year-old boy.

Closed reduction should be attempted for luxatio erecta. Adequate anesthesia and muscle relaxation should be undertaken to avoid complications such as a proximal humeral physeal disruption. The need for open reduction is rare.

Obstetric Injury

Congenital "dislocation" of the shoulder has been described as a birth injury.[51-64] It is usually associated with difficult delivery and must be differentiated from a proximal humeral physeal fracture. Many cases are not diagnosed until several months after birth. When diagnosed acutely, closed reduction should be undertaken. If the infant presents several weeks to months after delivery, soft tissue contractures may necessitate open reduction.

Great caution should be taken before rendering such a diagnosis of dislocation. The proximal humerus is more likely to be fractured as a transphyseal injury (Fig. 14-21), an injury that usually leads to anteromedial displacement of the shaft and an *apparent* dislocation roentgenographically.[65-85]

During the perinatal period the usual mechanism of injury is a difficult delivery consequent to shoulder-pelvic disproportion (dystocia).[66,74,77,80] The injury has been reported following cesarean section.[72] In actuality, the proximal humerus is still contained within the joint, and the proximal metaphysis is laterally displaced.

Clinical diagnosis may be difficult. A neonate with a fracture consequent to the birth injury may have a relative "paralysis" (pseudoparalysis) of the arm, so the injury may be misinterpreted as a brachial plexus palsy.[49,65] It is usually possible to stimulate the child to move the major part of the arm and forearm musculature. Crepitation and discomfort (crying, irritability) contrast a fracture from a brachial plexus palsy. The type of trauma that causes a brachial plexus injury also may cause chondro-osseous injury.

About 20% of newborns have an ossification center that is radiologically evident. This assists in making a definite diagnosis. A shoulder arthrogram may be used to make the diagnosis (Fig. 14-21), or ultrasonography can be useful.[41,67,71,83]

The arm should be splinted to the body with some type of wrap. Confirmation of a fracture is possible by repeat films 7-10 days after birth, when metaphyseal callus usually becomes evident.

Although often alluded to as an injury that heals quickly without problems, these fractures are not inconsequential. Children sustaining these fractures should be followed closely throughout skeletal maturation so growth abnormalities, particularly humerus varus (Fig. 14-22), may be detected.[73,75,79] These growth discrepancies may lead to altered anatomy and significant arm length inequality.

Unusual deformities of the shoulder may predispose to neonatal fracture. In the patient illustrated in Figure 14-23 a "snap" was felt during birth. The child subsequently became asymptomatic. Follow-up showed a glenohumeral fusion with an established nonunion at the site of a probable transphyseal fracture. This went on to create a pseudarthrosis as a substitute for the absence of glenohumeral motion.

Proximal Humeral Physeal Fracture

Epiphyseal fractures constitute the major injury pattern to the shoulder and proximal humerus prior to skeletal maturity.[87-168] Neer and Horwitz reported a 3% incidence of proximal humeral epiphyseal injuries in their series of all epiphyseal fractures.[141] If metaphyseal fractures are also considered (including the commonly encountered unicameral or aneurysmal bone cyst with pathologic fracture), the incidence of proximal humeral injuries in children and adolescents is probably reasonably comparable to the incidence in adults.

Injuries to the proximal humerus occur infrequently during the neonatal period, more frequently during the first decade, and relatively frequently between 11 and 16 years of age. Any such injury in a child under 18 months of age should raise the possibility of child abuse in the differential diagnosis. The oldest reported patient with a proximal humeral epiphyseal injury was a 23-year-old with pituitary dysfunction, although Poland mentioned the injury in a 26-year-old.[149,163] In most involved age groups boys outnumber girls 3:1 or 4:1. Participation in structured athletics is a significant predisposing factor.[93,103,156] As with neonatal fractures, these injuries may be associated with a slowly evolving brachial plexus palsy.

Mechanism of Injury

During infancy a child may be injured by a fall. However, the battered child syndrome always must be considered, as injury to the proximal humerus is unusual in an infant. The injury during later childhood and adolescence is associated with two major causal mechanisms. First, a falling child throws the arm into an abducted, extended, and externally rotated position to break a fall. This transmits the force toward the shoulder joint, at which point the most structurally weak anatomic area fails: the metaphysis in the young child and the physis in the older child. Second, the child or adolescent may fall directly on the lateral side of the shoulder, in which case the major deforming force is imparted directly into the epiphysis, growth plate, and metaphysis. After the initial deforming forces cease, maintenance or worsening of the deformity is contingent on the interplay of the muscular forces and the extent of osseous and periosteal disruption.

Pathologic Anatomy

Several types of fracture may be encountered. A type 1 physeal injury is characteristic of neonates, infants, and young children up to the age of 4-5 years (Fig. 14-24). In older children and adolescents the characteristic growth mechanism injury shifts to type 2, with a posteromedial metaphyseal fragment remaining attached to the physis (Figs. 14-25, 14-26). Other types of physeal injury are encountered infrequently because of the mobility of the glenohumeral joint and the anatomy of the proximal humerus. In particular, because the humeral head is much larger than the associated glenoid and less anatomically restricted, the mechanical forces that may be applied usually are not

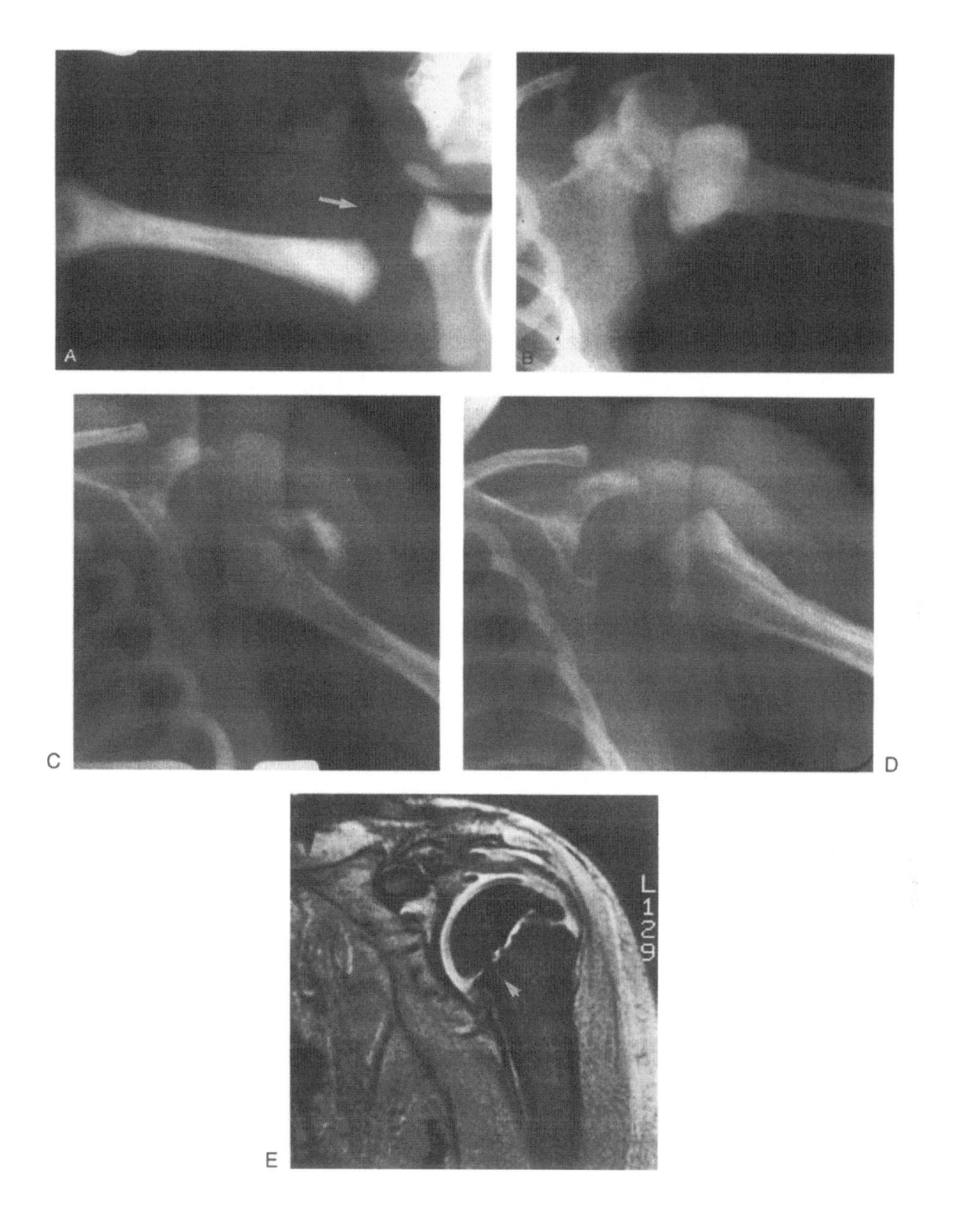

FIGURE 14-21. (A) Apparent dislocation of the shoulder following traumatic delivery. Instead, it was a physeal fracture. A small metaphyseal fragment (arrow) remained with the humeral head. (B) Arthrography confirms the located humeral head and the displaced shaft. (C) Reactive metaphyseal bone 8 days after the birth injury. (D) Six months later. (E) Nine years later there is medial growth arrest. MRI shows the bone bridge (arrow).

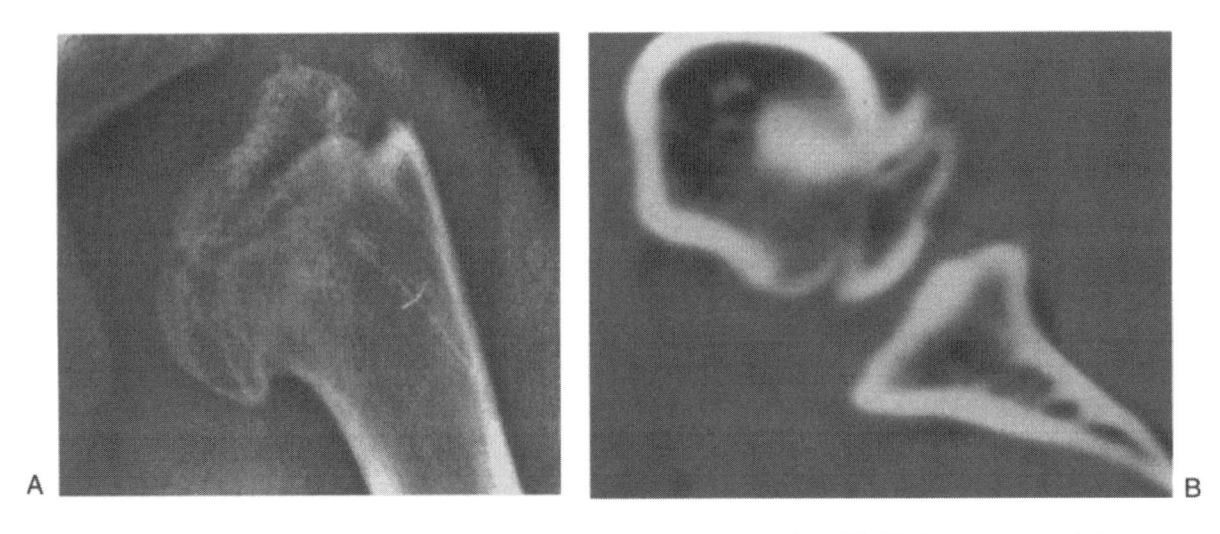

FIGURE 14-22. (A) Humerus varus at age 8 years. A "snap" was felt at birth. (B) CT shows the bone bridge.

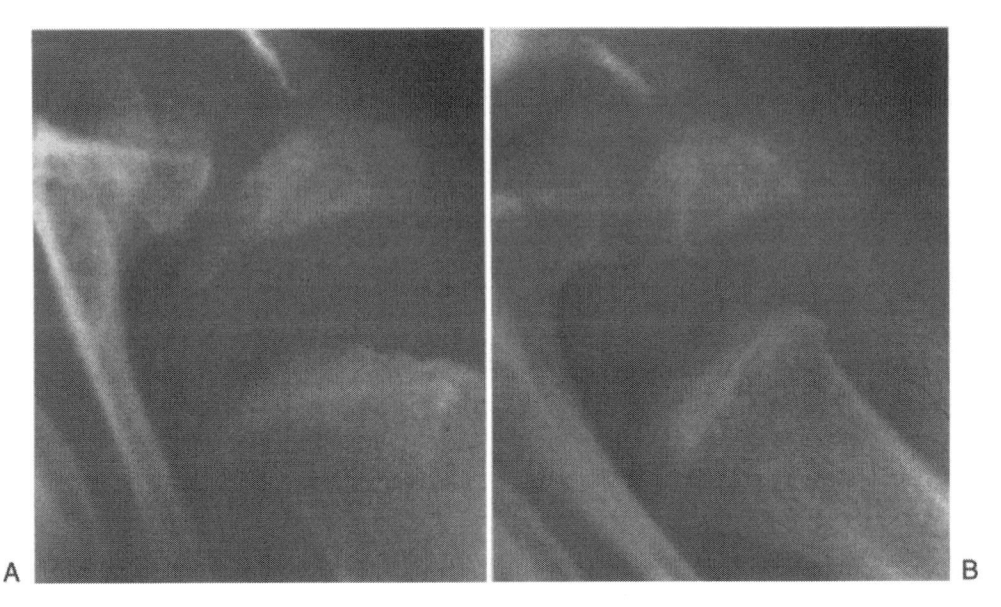

FIGURE 14-23. This child was being evaluated for abnormal shoulder motion. (A) Anteroposterior view shows an abnormally wide space between the humeral ossification center and the metaphysis. The glenoid is hypoplastic. (B) Abduction showed motion through this space, which was a pseudarthrosis that developed because of congenital fusion of the glenoid to the proximal humeral epiphysis.

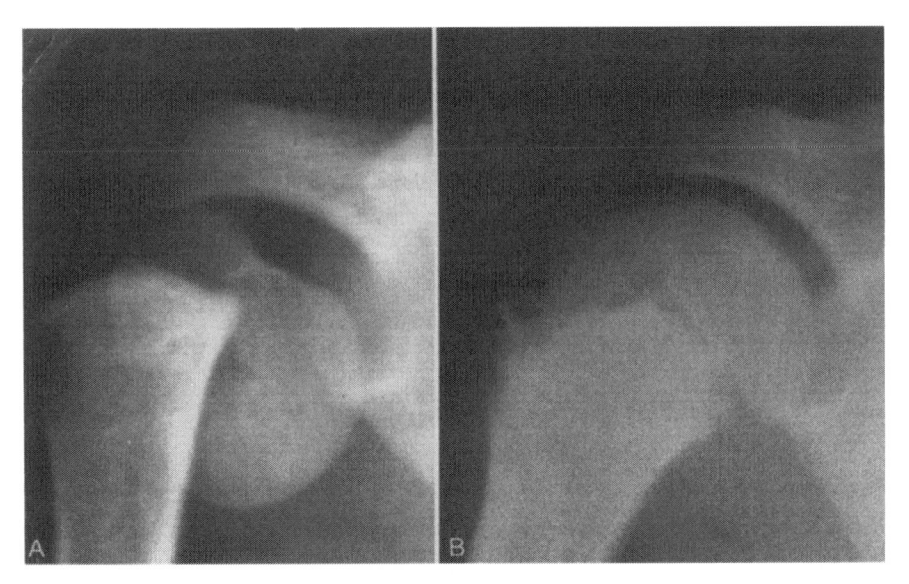

FIGURE 14-24. Type 1 injury in a 6-year-old. (A) Displaced epiphysis. (B) Reduced.

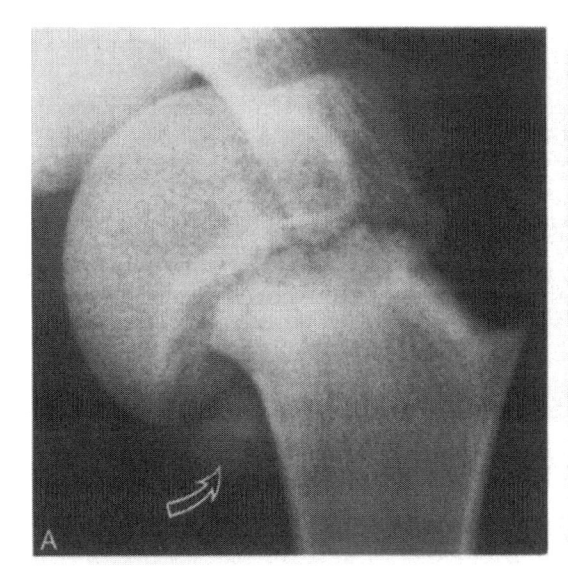

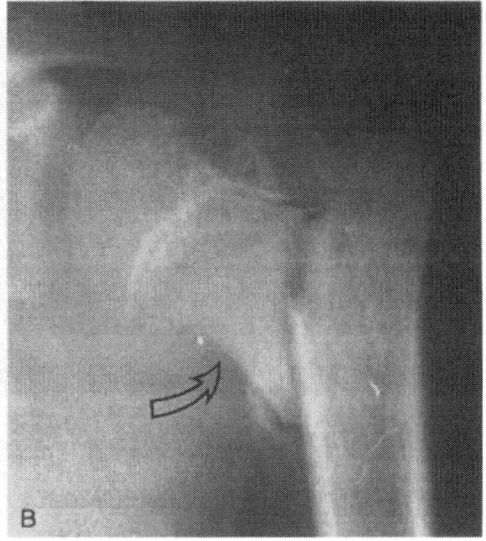

FIGURE 14-25. Type 2 injuries. (A) Small medial metaphyseal fragment (arrow). (B) Large metaphyseal fragment (arrow), more characteristic of the injury during adolescence.

capable of introducing shear forces comparable to those that cause type 3 and 4 injuries in other epiphyseal regions. However, type 5 microinjuries or bone bruises may accompany type 1 or 2 injuries as a result of the adduction nature of the injury mechanism. This explains some of the growth abnormalities (e.g., humerus varus) and limb length inequalities. Type 3 injuries may occur in the older adolescent undergoing closure of the physis.[37,101,158]

With these aforementioned fracture types, partial displacement is much more common than complete displacement. The fracture-producing mechanism and the deforming muscle forces usually cause an adduction deformity of the proximal fragment relative to the distal fragment, although abduction (valgus) angulation may occur.[136]

During the neonatal and early childhood periods, when children are more susceptible to type 1 than type 2 injury, the contour of the growth plate tends to be more transverse than conical. As the child grows, the underlying metaphyseal region assumes an increasingly asymmetric configuration, with the apex tending to be posteromedial. As this pyramidal pattern becomes more prominent, the child becomes more susceptible to a type 2 rather than a type 1 growth mechanism injury.

With type 2 growth mechanism injuries the fracture begins in the lateral portion of the physis (tension failure), propagates medially, and turns distally to continue into the metaphysis, leaving a variable-sized metaphyseal fragment. The periosteum tends to be stripped from the more lateral portions of the humeral metaphysis while remaining intact medially in the area of the metaphyseal fragment.[112] The distal (metaphyseal) portion of the fracture may displace through a rent (buttonhole) in the periosteum (Fig. 14-27). The portion of intact periosteum extending from the metaphyseal fragment to the more distal portions of the diaph-

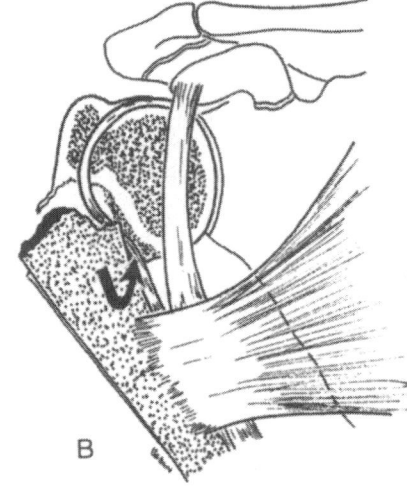

FIGURE 14-26. Mechanism of a medial fragment caused by the path of the biceps tendon (long head). (A) Normal anatomic relations of the long head (arrow). (B) The tendon may be displaced behind the distal fragment (arrow), which may prevent anatomic reduction.

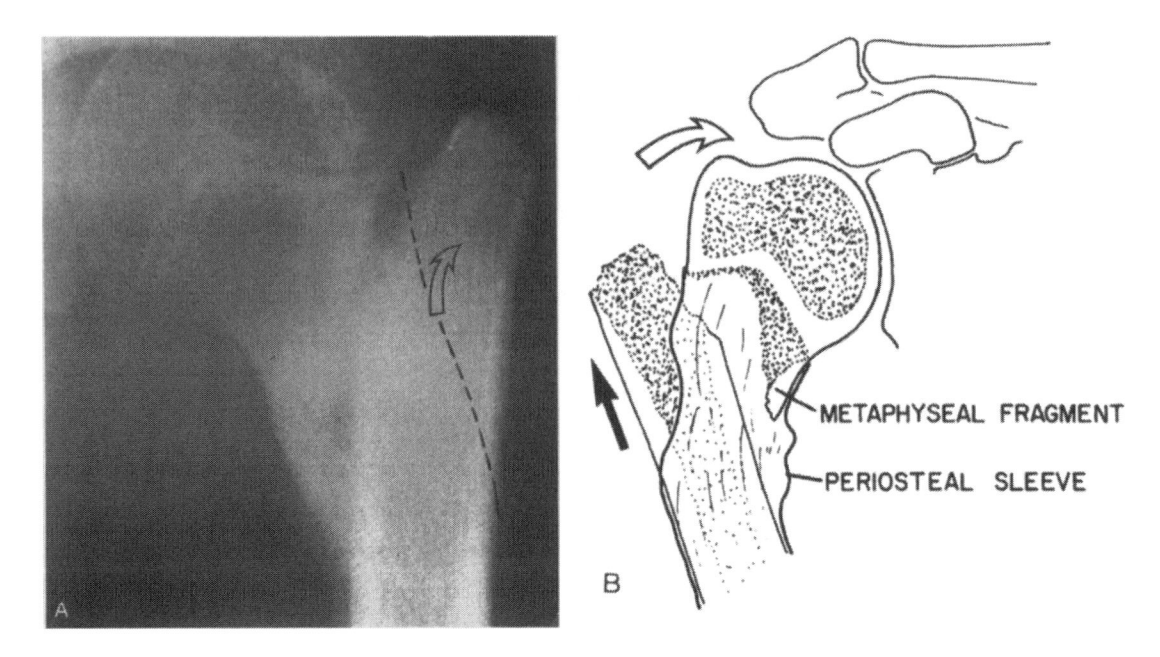

FIGURE 14-27. (A) Distal fragment has probably displaced through a periosteal rent. (B) The injury.

ysis tends to contract, making reduction difficult after a few days.[106] Periosteal continuity also allows some control over the formation of membranous new bone (callus).

As previously discussed, the degree of displacement of the fragments is contingent on three factors: the deforming forces that cause the initial displacement, the morphologic extent of the fracture, and the muscle pulls that maintain angulation and displacement or worsen them. Displacement may be graded into three types: (1) displacement less than one-half the diameter of the metaphyseal shaft; (2) displacement more than one-half the metaphyseal diameter; and (3) complete displacement. With grades 2 and 3 there usually is an accompanying varus angular deformity. When there is angular displacement, the epiphysis tends to be adducted and posteriorly displaced, while the remaining metaphysis and shaft are comparably adducted but anteriorly displaced. Although some displacement relates to the primary mechanism of the injury, the epiphysis tends to be rotated into mild adduction and external rotation by the pull of attached muscles, and the shaft is drawn forward by the combined pulls of the pectoralis major, latissimus dorsi, and teres major muscles. Lateralization and cephalad displacement of the distal fragment tend to be accentuated by the pull of the deltoid muscle (Fig. 14-28). When the fracture initially is minimally displaced, an inherent stability is imparted by the contour of the epiphyseal plate and the surrounding periosteum. This tends to negate any effect from muscular attachments and the directions of pull. However, when the separation is grade 2 or 3, the fracture becomes less stable, and muscular deforming forces tend to play a more dominant role, often converting partial displacement to complete displacement.

Displacement is a highly variable factor in injuries to the proximal humerus and, along with a patient's age and anticipated growth (Fig. 14-29), is taken into account when deciding on therapy. The younger the child, the less important is aggressive, accurate correction of the displacement. However, as the child approaches adolescence, significant displacements become much less acceptable and must be reduced to being as anatomically correct as possible.

The main neurovascular bundle is anteromedial to the joint. The axillary nerve courses inferior to the glenohumeral joint, wrapping around it to supply the deltoid muscle. It is adjacent to the fragment of the metaphysis with a type 2 injury and near the apex of the injury with a type 1 injury. Complete paralysis of the deltoid may accompany injury. Because the mechanism of injury is often a direct fall on the shoulder, a contusion to the nerve may occur as it tranverses between the deltoid and the proximal humerus.

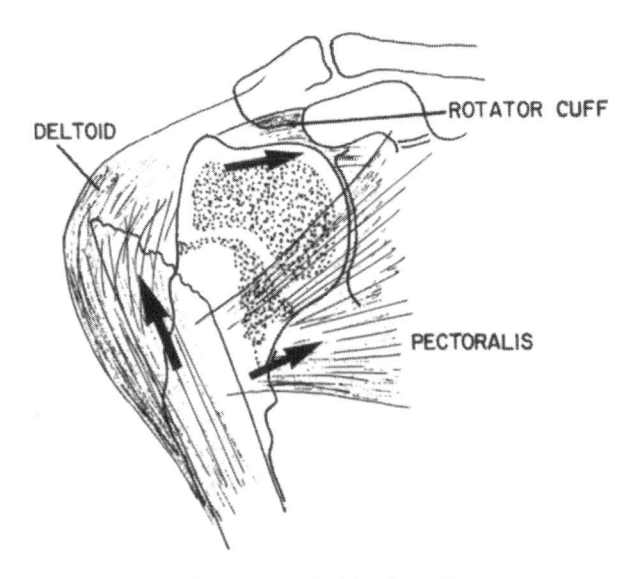

FIGURE 14-28. Muscle pull.

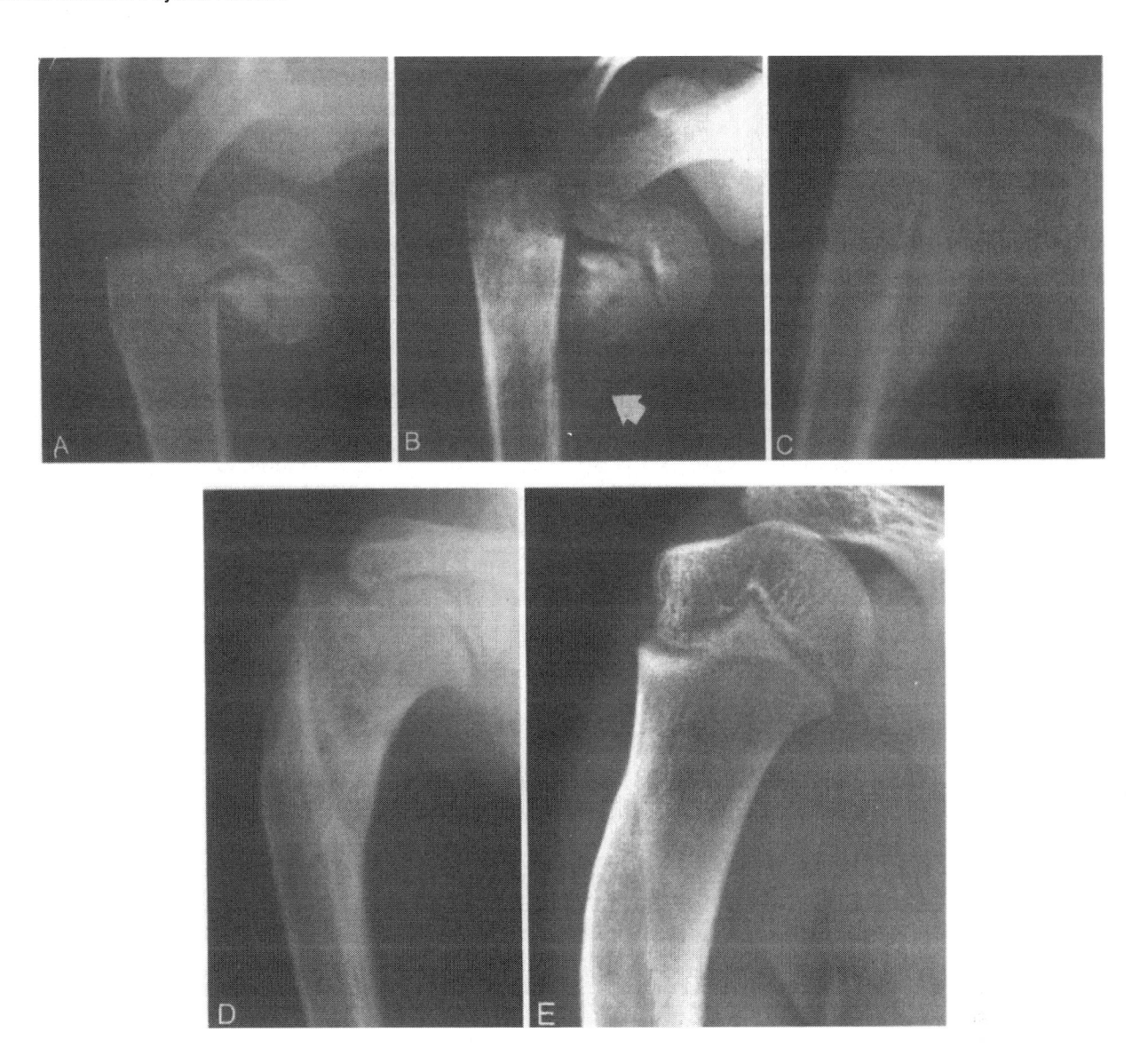

FIGURE 14-29. (A) Initial injury in a 3-year-old, with medial displacement of the proximal fragment and overriding. Multiple attempts at closed reduction under general anesthesia were unsuccessful. (B) Four weeks later new bone formation is evident in the periosteal sleeve (arrow). (C) Eight weeks later the medially displaced sleeve is filling. (D) Four months after injury longitudinal growth and remodeling have taken place. (E) Four years after the injury.

Most of these neural injuries are transient and recover spontaneously.

Proximal humeral epiphyseal fractures may be associated with glenohumeral dislocation.[109,144] The dislocation may be missed.

Diagnosis

Swelling and localized tenderness around the shoulder joint enhance the likelihood of a shoulder fracture. Ecchymosis may appear 2–3 days after the injury. Because displacement is often not a major part of these injuries, relative shortening of the arm is infrequent, although the presence of such a physical sign certainly helps in the diagnosis. False motion and crepitus between the fracture fragments may be detected, but searching for such findings should be kept to a minimum to avoid risking injury to the axillary or any other nerve. Diagnosis is best made on the basis of roentgenographic, rather than physical, findings.

Roentgenographic Findings

The evidence for a proximal humeral fracture depends on the age of the child, the extent of the ossification of the humeral head and greater tuberosity, and the presence of any pathologic conditions. Pathologic changes are reasonably obvious in the adolescent, the age at which they are most likely to be encountered. Similarly, fractures of either the metaphysis or growth plate tend to be reasonably obvious because of their characteristic anatomic changes, particularly the displacement and the contiguous metaphyseal fragment. In the infant or young child, diagnosis may be difficult because of the small amount of epiphyseal cartilage that has undergone ossification.

Areas such as the acromion may be injured concomitantly. Adequate radiologic evaluation should include the entire pectoral girdle.

Treatment

In general, treatment of injuries to the proximal humerus utilize closed methods, with open reduction saved for difficult cases and for older patients in whom the initial nonoperative methods are unsatisfactory.[99,105,106,115,122,134,167] The fracture usually heals satisfactorily and has a high propensity to remodel, despite displacement (Fig. 14-29). The extent of remaining growth potential must always be kept in mind.

The arm is brought out to length by gentle longitudinal traction and then placed in a comfortable position. The use of a general anesthetic may not be necessary, as perfect anatomic reduction usually is not required. Most series have shown that young children treated in a conservative fashion, with minimal efforts at reduction and with significant displacement of the proximal humerus relative to the shaft, have virtually no significant long-term functional disabilities or abnormal morphology. Even in adolescents sufficient longitudinal growth and remodeling capacity remain to justify leaving the fragments overriding or in mild varus.

In older children and adolescents the fracture is usually a type 2 injury, generally accompanied by a grade 1 (mild) displacement. This fracture is stable, and manipulation is not usually necessary. With grade 2 and 3 injuries, in which angulation and displacement are greater, it is recommended that the humeral fragments be manipulated into a more acceptable position, although absolute anatomic reduction is still unnecessary.

The use of various anesthetic agents should be based on the experience of the surgeon and the cooperativeness of the patient. It may be better to perform such a reduction under a general anesthetic, as the use of an analgesic/amnesic agent (e.g., diazepam) may not allow enough muscle relaxation to gain adequate reduction. As the time interval from onset of injury to attempted reduction increases, so do the amount of soft tissue swelling, the degree of contracture (especially in the damaged periosteum), and the involuntary muscle activity, which makes reduction increasingly difficult. It is difficult to control the proximal epiphyseal fragment, as it is a relatively mobile structure and almost impossible to stabilize completely during manipulation.

The arm is brought into approximately 90° of abduction, flexion, and mild external rotation to accomplish the reduction. The arm is then brought back into a position adjacent to the body. This maneuver gives an idea of the degree of stability of the reduction and if it is possible to treat the patient with shoulder immobilization. Whenever possible, the physician should avoid treatment in a forced abduction position, as it would increase the deforming forces applied through the pectoralis major and may affect the stability of the fracture. If there is any angular deformity, even with a grade 1 fracture, a gentle closed reduction may be attempted. Absolute anatomic reduction is usually unnecessary, as gradual growth and remodeling correct most mild to moderate displacements.

The shoulder and arm should be immobilized by whatever method the physician prefers to use.[123] My preference is a shoulder immobilizer.

Should the fracture prove unstable, Nilsson and Svartholm have reported successful use of a hanging cast, with gradual spontaneous reduction of the displaced, angulated proximal fragment.[143] The shoulder also may be placed in a spica cast with the arm in abduction, forward flexion, and neutral rotation. The exact position may be determined using image intensification. The arm should be abducted only as far as necessary to ensure stability of reduction. Placement in the extreme positions (e.g., "Statue of Liberty") may cause problems, such as incomplete brachial plexus palsy, and are to be avoided. If that is the only stable position, percutaneous pin fixation should be used. When casting, splinting, or a sling is used, reduction should be confirmed.

The patient may be placed in traction using skin traction or, if necessary, skeletal traction with an olecranon pin. This method of treatment, however, may stretch the capsule and subluxate the humeral head, rather than disengaging the fragments. Increasing emphasis on reduced hospitalization (costs) makes this treatment one to reserve for children needing a few days of observation. This applies particularly to the polytraumatized patient.

Whether a sling, cast, or traction is chosen as the primary method of nonoperative treatment, it is imperative that periodic roentgenograms be obtained because the reduction may be lost anytime within the first 2–3 weeks. By the end of 3 weeks, however, there usually is sufficient cartilaginous and ossifying callus to impart intrinsic stability. Solid union should be present by 3–4 weeks, and the child may then be progressively allowed out of immobilization. Early motion, the mainstay of therapy in adults, is relatively unnecessary in children because of their intrinsic ability to restore function rapidly after an injury.

Open reduction or closed reduction with percutaneous fixation (Fig. 14-30) should be reserved for the older or difficult to treat patient in whom there is concern over persistent deformity and shortening. The inability to control fracture fragments because of severe multisystem injury, particularly head injury, is also an indication for open reduction or closed reduction with percutaneous pinning. The long head of the biceps may be caught between the fragments and impede adequate reduction.[106] This condition is difficult to diagnose and should not be used as the primary indication for open reduction. A child whose presenting problem, many days after injury, is a prominent segment of bone (the lateral metaphysis) is not necessarily a candidate for an operation either, as remodeling usually leads to gradual disappearance of such a protuberance and improved shoulder abduction.

Other than children with a head injury and uncontrolled rigidity, I have encountered few patients who seemed to fit the criteria for open reduction. One such patient had multiple injuries, including a Monteggia fracture-dislocation of the ipsilateral elbow. Following reduction of the elbow, he was placed in traction. What appeared to be a type 2 epiphyseal injury of the proximal humerus did not respond effectively. Because of inability to control the additional metaphyseal fragment, the injury was explored. The segment was a large portion of the anterolateral metaphysis that had fractured completely free from the remainder of the shaft and from the adjacent metaphyseal fragment, which was still attached to the epiphysis. In contrast, the free fragment had been denuded of all soft tissue attachments during the acute

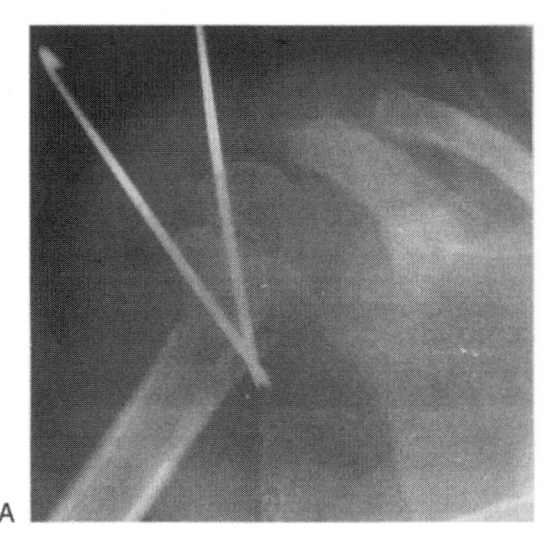

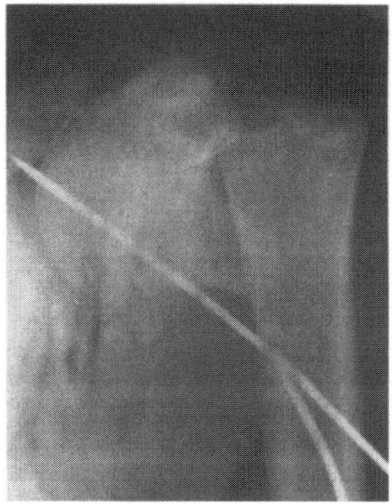

FIGURE 14-30. (A) Percutaneous pins through a large metaphyseal fragment. (B) Percutaneous fixation, which is inappropriate because the pin penetrates too far and the fracture has not been reduced. This solution should not have been accepted.

injury. The fragment was placed back in an anatomic position underneath the biceps tendon, which was preventing its reduction. It was stabilized with tension-band wire fixation.

Results

Most believe that proximal humeral injuries heal well, even in instances of serious displacement, and that a normal shoulder may be expected at the completion of skeletal growth.[88,89] However, Neer and Horwitz showed that the long-term results are not as benign as most authors have described, with a high incidence of subtle to overt longitudinal growth impairment being the main complication.[141]

Complications

The usual problems encountered with adult shoulder injuries, such as joint stiffness, malunion, avascular (ischemic) necrosis, nonunion, myositis ossificans, and extraarticular calcification, are rare in children. The major complications in children are (1) limb length inequalities and (2) varus deformity. Mild angular growth deformities are more readily tolerated in this joint than any other because of the degrees of freedom of motion and scapular mobility.

Neer and Horwitz found a large number of patients who had shortening whether associated with displacement of less than one-third the shaft diameter or total displacement.[141] This shortening appeared to affect mainly patients who sustained their injury after the age of 11 years. Patients younger than 11 years did not have major growth abnormalities and, in fact, appeared to make up for the initial shortening through a process comparable to femoral overgrowth following fracture. The same criteria appeared to apply to angular deformity: Children over age 11 had less correction and maintained some varus deformity. The major factor to consider in any decision for treatment thus appears to be the anticipated remaining longitudinal growth in the physis.

Baxter and Wiley reviewed 57 patients with proximal humeral epiphyseal fractures. They found that, regardless of treatment, the maximum shortening of the humerus averaged 2 cm and residual varus angulation was insignificant.[94]

Varus deformity complicating proximal humeral fractures in adults is a well acknowledged clinical occurrence, but it is virtually ignored as a significant complication during childhood.[69] Most authors state that such an angular deformity corrects spontaneously with subsequent growth. Similarly, varus deformity sustained during the neonatal period, when diagnosis of a fracture is difficult, is also considered to have minimal long-term consequences.

Posttraumatic humerus varus may develop gradually and not as a result of immediate angulation of the humeral head. It most likely occurs as a result of undetectable microtrauma to the medial side of the proximal humeral growth plate, eventually resulting in the formation of a small osseous bridge followed by a significant radiologic deformity. If a patient presents early with such a beginning deformity, he or she should be followed at least annually, as physeal fusion may eventually occur, and the apparent radiolucent defect (in reality filled with articular and epiphyseal cartilage) does not appear to represent a major risk to fracture. If the abnormality is encountered at a relatively early age (before 6–7 years of age), it may be possible to resect the osseous bridge. If any significant functional limitations occur during the late adolescent period, acromionectomy may be more beneficial than a valgus osteotomy of the surgical neck.

An infrequent complication is injury to the circumflex or axillary nerve adjacent to the region of the fracture. This usually results in transient paralysis of the deltoid and resolves within a few weeks or months.

Stress Injury

Barnett described "Little League shoulder syndrome" as a chronic proximal humeral epiphysiolysis in adolescent baseball pitchers.[93] Characteristic of this chronic lesion is widening of the growth plate with metaphyseal cystic changes.[93]

These abnormalities may be encountered in a number of increasingly popular childhood and adolescent highly competitive sports, including swimming, tennis, and gymnastics. As described in Chapters 4 and 12, repetitive force to a

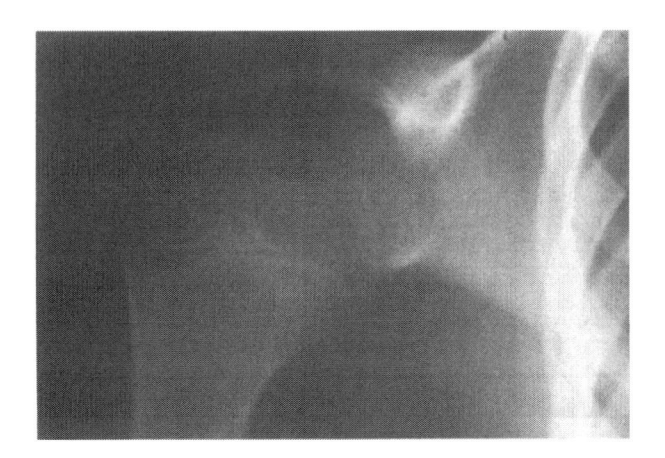

FIGURE 14-31. Apophysitis in an adolescent tennis player. Note the widening of the lateral physeal region.

growth plate may cause microfailure and a degree of osteolysis in the juxtaphyseal metaphysis, which causes widening of the physeal region (Fig. 14-31).

Lesser Tuberosity Avulsion

Lesser tuberosity avulsions are rare.[129] Unrecognized acute avulsion of the attachment of the pectoralis may result in the subsequent formation of an exostosis (Fig. 14-32).

Shoulder Fusion

Pruitt et al. described shoulder arthrodesis in 17 patients. All were undertaken for neuromuscular deficiencies (polio, posttraumatic).[146] The position of fusion was not important, although excessive abduction or forward flexion should be avoided.

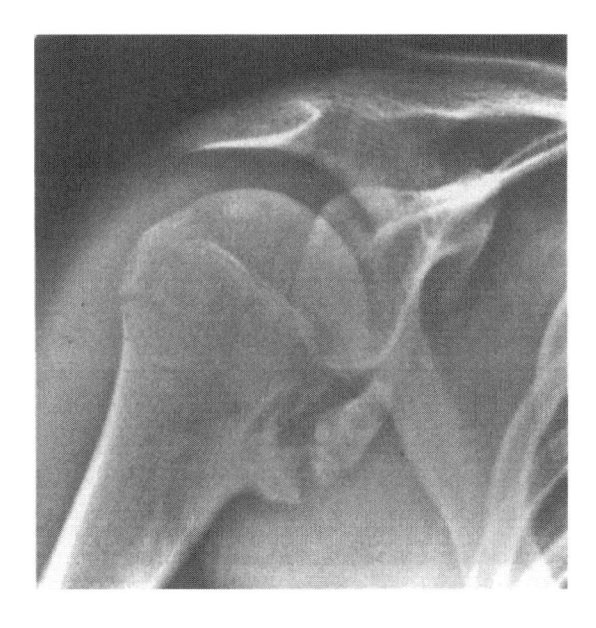

FIGURE 14-32. Old fracture of the lesser tuberosity.

Proximal Metaphysis

The proximal metaphysis is highly susceptible to fracture in the 5- through 11-year range, during which period such injuries may be more frequent than proximal epiphyseal fractures. The susceptibility of the metaphysis to these fractures probably relates to the rapid elongation and the structural changes and remodeling that take place in the cortex and spongiosa. Pathologic fractures through cystic lesions are also quite common in this age group.[170] Two basic fracture patterns occur: (1) a transverse fracture with or without loss of cortical continuity; and (2) a torus fracture with maintenance of much of the cortical integrity despite the buckling (Figs. 14-33, 14-34).

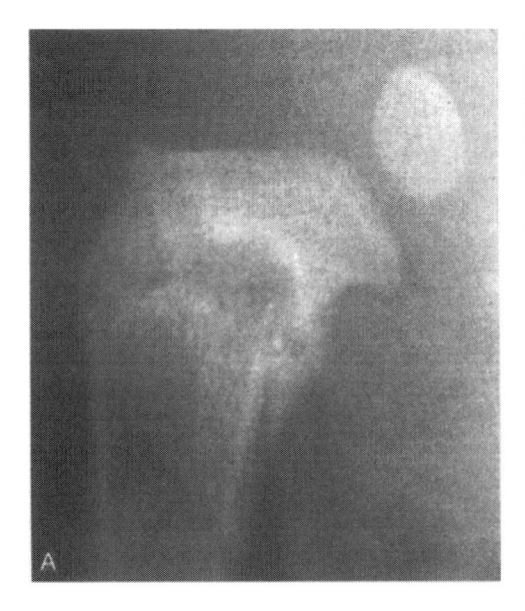

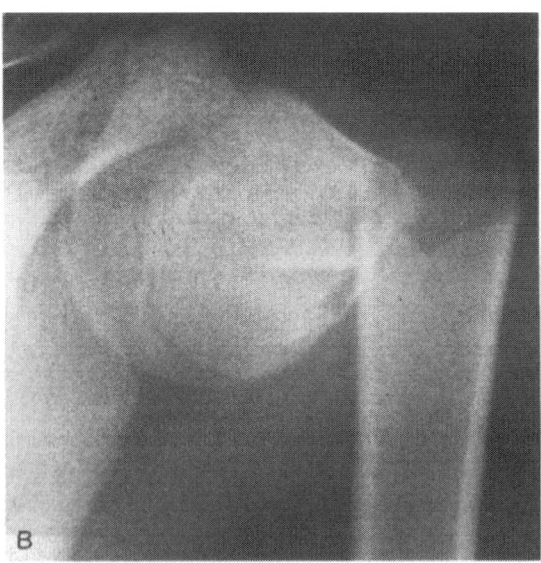

FIGURE 14-33. (A) Metaphyseal fracture in a 5-month-old. Strong periosteal attachments maintain the alignment. (B) Proximal metaphyseal fracture in a 12-year-old. It is anatomically comparable to a physeal fracture. The shaft is displaced laterally and the proximal fragment rotated 90°. It must be corrected.

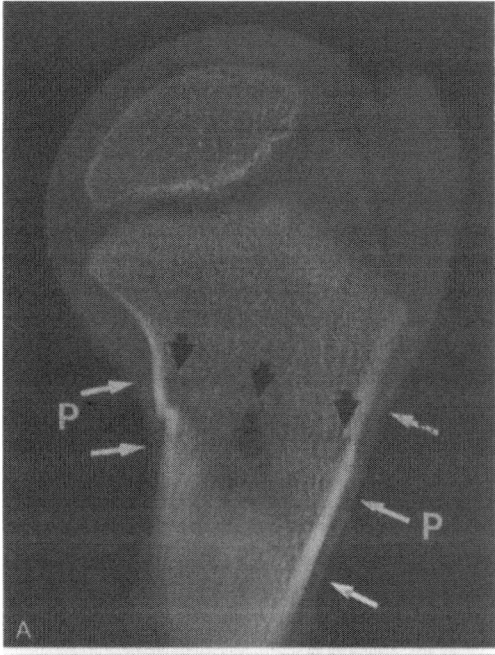

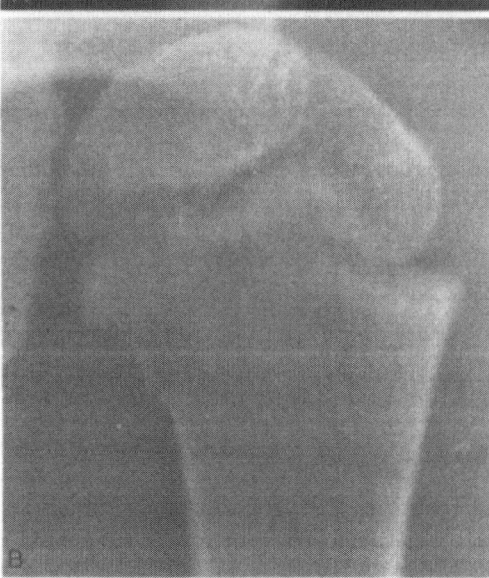

FIGURE 14-34. (A) Metaphyseal fracture in a 3-year-old who had been fatally injured in an auto accident. The fracture crosses the metaphysis transversely; the periosteum (P, white arrow) remained intact and prevented significant displacement. This fracture is primarily a compression failure, a mechanism that is more likely in a young child. (B) Undisplaced transverse metaphyseal fracture with minimal medial torus injury.

Greenstick fractures are common but seldom occur with significant angular deformity. They are usually torus fractures. Completely displaced metaphyseal fractures may be much more difficult to manage than type 2 physeal injuries. The shaft may penetrate the deltoid muscle and lie subcutaneously, making reduction difficult because of the interposed muscle.

The use of a hanging cast may align the fragments effectively over a few days. Roentgenograms must be attained to assess any displacement, as it may result in delayed union or malunion (Fig. 14-35).

Fracture of the proximal metaphysis may lead to temporary ischemia of the juxtaphyseal bone (Fig. 14-35), the mechanism of which is described in Chapters 1 and 6. The area is well vascularized, and quickly reestablishes the normal peripheral and central metaphyseal circulatory patterns. Because of the rapid rate of growth of the proximal humeral physis, the cartilage may become relatively thick until the invasive metaphyseal circulation is re-established.

Pathologic fractures may be treated as metaphyseal fractures are, with immobilization in a sling for several weeks until the acute fracture healing is completed, after which time primary treatment of the cyst can be undertaken, if indicated.[170] However, treatment of the cyst with bone graft at the time of fracture is not absolutely contraindicated. The fracture region often has collapsed into a varus position, and while an attempt should be made to correct this, it is often difficult (see Chapter 11). Steroids should *not* be injected at the time of an acute pathologic fracture, as they may adversely affect the normal inflammatory component of the healing response. Allow any pathologic fracture to heal spontaneously before attempting steroid eradication of a bone cyst.

Diaphyseal Fractures

Diaphyseal injuries are relatively uncommon in children.[171-205] The proximal and distal humeral chondroosseous structures are more likely to fail. Significant segments of the periosteum remain intact, lessening degrees of displacement and facilitating treatment (Fig. 14-36). Transverse humeral shaft fractures generally result from a direct blow (tapping fracture), whereas spiral fractures are produced by twisting injuries, although muscular violence without an associated fall may also do this. In children under 18 months child abuse must be considered in the differential diagnosis. The incidence of child abuse is approximately 20% in children under 3 years, and even higher in infants under eighteen months.

Mechanism of Injury

Most fractures of the shaft of the humerus are caused by indirect violence, such as a twisting or fall, rather than direct impact. This mechanism tends to cause oblique or comminuted fractures (Fig. 14-37). When the child lands on the elbow or hand with a twisting motion to the remainder of the body, the incidence of spiral or oblique fractures is greater. Less commonly, athletic activities such as throwing may cause a spiral injury. However, if a child sustains an injury in such situations, the possibility of a pathologic fracture must be closely assessed. Transverse fractures tend to be associated more frequently with obstetric injury or direct blows, often by landing on the upper arm or shoulder. In contrast to adults, segmental (comminuted) diaphyseal fractures are infrequent in children.

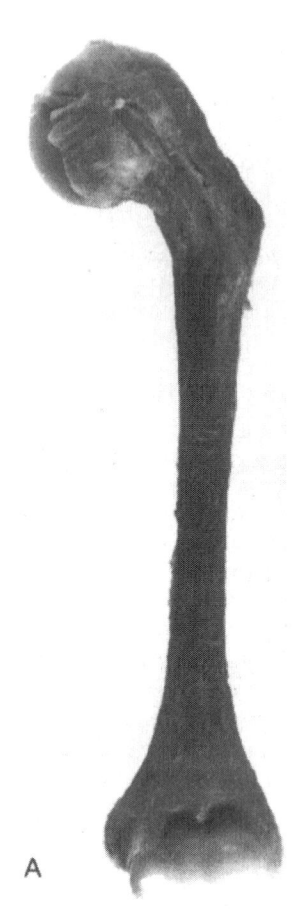

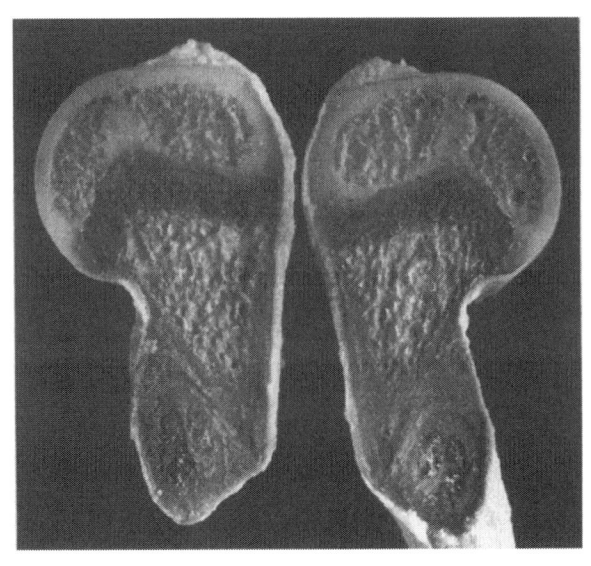

FIGURE 14-35. Malunion of a proximal humeral fracture in a 14-year-old. (A) Anterior view. (B) Specimen was sectioned to produce the slabs. Little remodeling has taken place between the proximal and distal cortices. The darker metaphysis reflects temporary ischemia and physiologic slowdown of growth and remodeling.

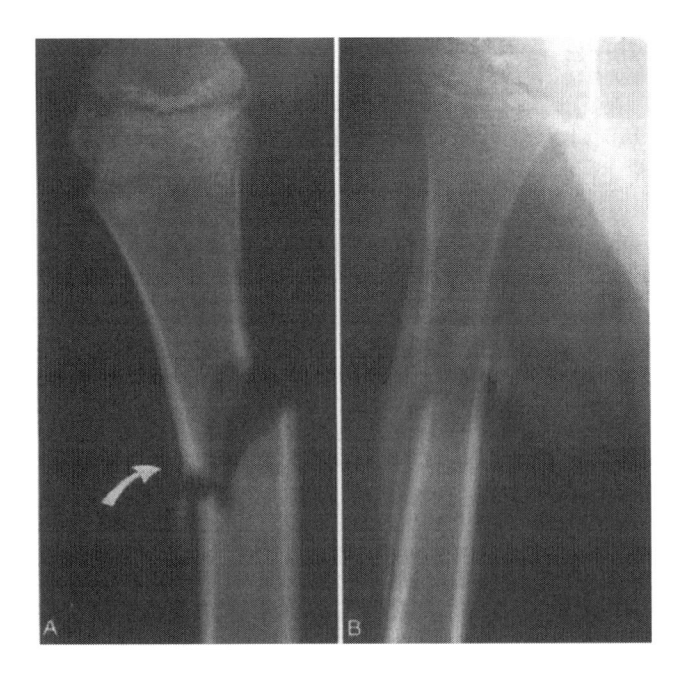

FIGURE 14-36. Diaphyseal fracture. (A) Three weeks after reduction early bone formation is evident along the periosteal tube, which remained intact along one side of the fracture (arrow). (B) By six weeks, extensive callus formation is evident along the side with intact periosteum; the side with periosteal rupture shows much less formation of new bone.

Pathologic Anatomy

The direction of displacement of fracture fragments is contingent on the level of the fracture relative to the levels of muscular insertion, especially the deltoid muscle. Fractures involving the lower third of the shaft below the level of deltoid insertion generally exhibit anterolateral displacement of the proximal fragment due to the combined pull of the supraspinatus, deltoid, and coracobrachialis muscles. The distal fragment usually is displaced proximally and medially by the spasm and contraction of the biceps and brachialis muscles (Fig. 14-38). If the fracture involves the diaphysis or metaphysis proximal to the insertion of the deltoid, but distal to the insertion of the pectoralis major, the deltoid muscle displaces the distal fragment laterally and upward. At the same time, the pectoralis major, latissimus dorsi, and teres major muscles and the rotator cuff musculature of the shoulder joint adduct and internally rotate the proximal fragment (Fig. 14-38).

The proximal humerus is usually retroverted relative to the supracondylar region. Therefore when treating these injuries in children, particularly those with significant displacement, an attempt should be made to restore this normal anatomic configuration. Rotation of the fragments does not usually correct itself following fracture. Therefore it must be assumed that treatment of the arm with significant internal rotation of the lower fragment may, if the upper fragment is at all displaced or externally rotated,

FIGURE 14-37. Diaphyseal fracture patterns. (A) Transverse, with some of periosteum intact. (B) Transverse, with complete periosteal rupture. (C) Oblique. (D) Spiral.

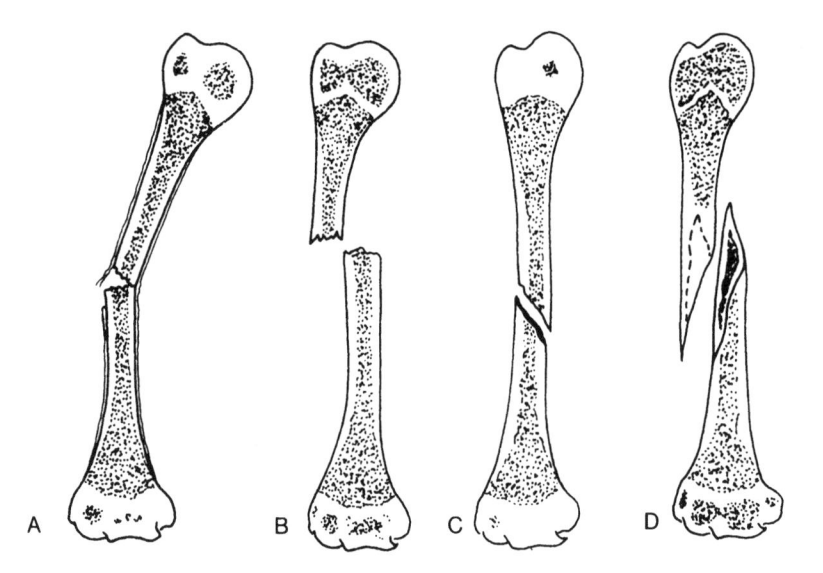

cause decreased retroversion and predisposes the shoulder to subsequent subluxation anteriorly. Because, the more powerful forces deforming the proximal fragment tend to be those that represent the rotator cuff and internal rotators of the shoulder, it usually cannot be sufficiently internally rotated to have a major effect on the normal degree of retroversion.

Diagnosis

The clinical diagnosis is usually obvious because of deformity, local swelling, and pain. Roentgenographic studies can establish the fracture pattern.

The close relation of the radial nerve to the humeral shaft along the musculospiral groove makes it particularly vulnerable to injury (contusion, neurotmesis, axonotmesis). Furthermore, injury to the nerves may occur consequent to their deformation by the fracture fragments, either during the original injury or with subsequent manipulation. Careful assessment of nerve function, both sensory and motor, is absolutely essential before *and* after any manipulation. If the radial nerve is paralyzed, the dorsum of the hand between the first and second metacarpals is commonly anesthetic, and a variable amount of motor power is lost in the extensors of the wrist, fingers and thumb, and the forearm supinators.

Treatment

Treatment of children requires an appreciation that their normal state of activity is greater than that of adults and that once pain subsides they are less willing to be quiet and properly utilize such methods of treatment as hanging casts. If there is marked displacement of the fragments, the initial step must be reduction of the fracture, which should be accomplished by closed means unless there is an open injury. Priority should be given to nonoperative treatment.[169,190]

The initial reduction maneuver is application of downward traction to correct overriding, disengage the fracture fragments, and displace them from muscular interpositions. The proximal fragment must be put in continuity with the distal fragment. Roentgenograms following reduction must be obtained in both anteroposterior and lateral views. Overriding of 1 cm may be accepted because the humerus exhibits overgrowth, similar to the femur. Angulation of 15°–20° is the most that should be accepted. This is particularly true if the angulation is at the middle or lower third because the bulk of the corrective growth occurs proximally; hence there is not the same amount of remodeling in this area as with an angularly displaced fracture involving the more proximal regions (Fig. 14-39). In the more proximal regions, a 20°–25° angular deformation is likely to be corrected by growth and remodeling. The only exception might be in the neonate, in whom fractures that seem innocuous initially may rapidly deform to significant malunion during treatment but remodel with equal rapidity.

In infants and young children, the fracture requires immobilization for 4–6 weeks, usually by the use of a modified Velpeau bandage or sling-and-swathe.[172] If the fracture is unstable, traction may be indicated. In small children this probably can be accomplished with skin traction. In the older child it may be necessary to use skeletal traction with

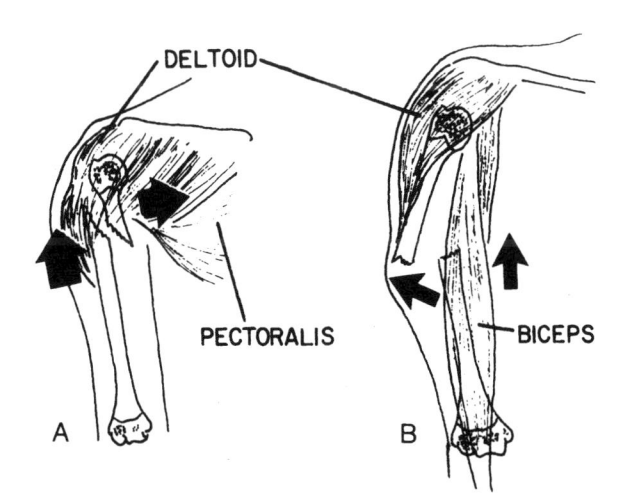

FIGURE 14-38. (A) Effects of muscle pulls on displacing fracture fragments when the fracture is above the deltoid insertion. (B) Effects of muscle pulls on displacing fracture fragments when the fracture is below the deltoid insertion.

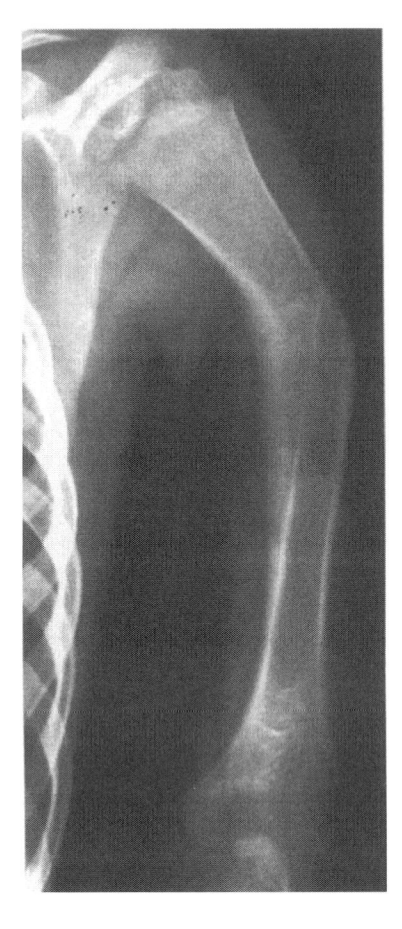

FIGURE 14-39. Retention of angulation.

an olecranon pin, especially if the fracture is extremely unstable or if there is any suggestion of neurovascular compromise. A shoulder spica also may be used in the older child with a relatively unstable fracture that can be reduced only in abduction.

It is possible that older children will cooperate enough to allow utilization of a device such as the hanging cast (Fig. 14-40) or cast-brace.[198] The supinating force of the biceps is lost by a fracture at this level, and the elbow joint is held in pronation by the unopposed action of the pronators. Because the joint is relatively fixed in pronation, attempts to place the forearm in supination may result in varus deformity at the fracture site. A collar and cuff are attached to a plaster loop at the wrist and passed around the patient's neck. The cast should be light, so distraction of the fracture fragments does not occur, although continuity of at least some of the thick periosteum tends to prevent this problem. The forearm should be transverse to the longitudinal axis of the body when the patient is standing. The length of the suspension collar is adjusted to allow the arm to be in this position. The patient should sleep in a semirecumbent position, rather than totally supine. As soon as pain subsides, the patient may be treated with range of motion exercises (circumduction and pendulum).

The use of internal or external fixation should be considered for unstable fractures or children with multiple management problems (e.g., head injury, polytrauma). Internal fixation with flexible intramedullary nails has been recommended.[200] Plating may also be considered. The use of external fixation must be approached cautiously, as the distal pins may be near the radial nerve.

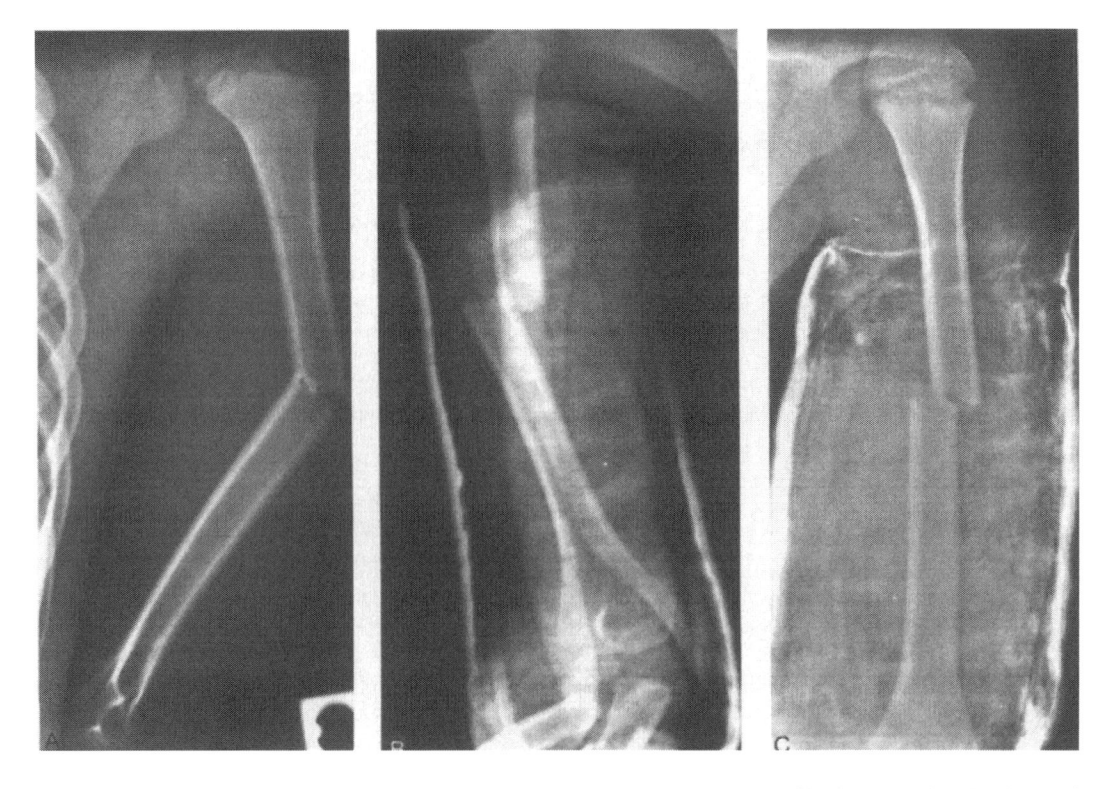

FIGURE 14-40. (A) Angulated diaphyseal fracture. (B) Initial cast treatment without reduction. (C) After closed reduction and molded cast.

Diaphyseal Fractures

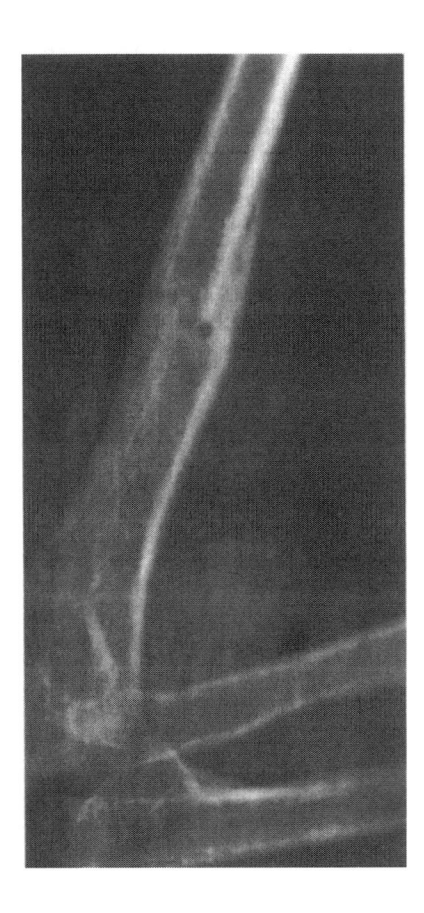

FIGURE 14-41. This patient had a radial nerve injury accompanying the fracture. It was elected to see if spontaneous recovery would occur, rather than explore the region. Three months after the injury a "Matev" sign is evident. Exploration revealed an entrapped radial nerve, which was carefully extricated by unroofing the tunnel. Radial nerve function returned completely within 4 months.

MacFarlane and Mushayt reported a 5-year-old girl who had a proximal physeal fracture and a mid-shaft fracture.[191] Closed manipulation was not successful. The proximal fracture was opened, reduced from herniated muscle, and pinned. The diaphyseal fracture was plated. This injury might be termed a floating shoulder.

Complications

Malunion may result if too much angulation is accepted or if pathologic circumstances (e.g., cerebral palsy) are present. Cerebral palsy may also lead to exuberant callus because of muscle. Because the humerus exhibits preferential proximal growth (80% of overall humeral length), angulation in the middle and distal thirds of the diaphyseal/metaphyseal shaft has little likelihood of correction. Furthermore, if the malunion is at the level of the deltoid tuberosity, normal muscular forces may help maintain the deformity.

Torode described a humeral fracture in a newborn (cesarean section)[202] that had not healed at 3 years. The patient underwent internal fixation and bone grafting. The bone and arm appeared normal at 15 months.

Nerve injury is particularly likely to occur with fractures of the junction of the middle and lower thirds of the shaft. Furthermore, the nerve may become entrapped at the time of fracture between reduced fracture fragments or subsequently in the developing callus (Fig. 14-41).[191,205]

Permanent radial nerve paralysis is infrequent in children.[185] Complete transection of the nerve is unlikely with a closed fracture. Nerve function is usually recovered completely. If the damage appears to be a major contusion of the nerve that will take a long time to recover, the hand and wrist are splinted in positions of function as part of the treatment. Follow-up includes electromyographic evaluation to determine the level and extent of injury and the chances for recovery. So long as continued improvement occurs, there is no indication for exploration. However, if, after the fracture has satisfactorily healed without evidence of neurologic improvement, exploration of the nerve and appropriate surgery are indicated. In some instances the nerve is trapped in scar tissue or even in callus; if so, it must be carefully removed and transposed to prevent recurrence of the injury.

Supracondylar Process

The supracondylar process (Fig. 14-42) usually is connected to the medial epicondyle by a fibrous band referred to as the ligament of Struthers.[206,209] The pronator teres muscle may partially originate from the ligament. The median nerve and brachial artery may pass between this ligament and the underlying humerus. A compressive neuropathy may occur either chronically or acutely following distal humeral fractures.[207,208,211] The process may be fractured.[210,212,213] If neuropathy occurs in a patient with a combined distal humeral

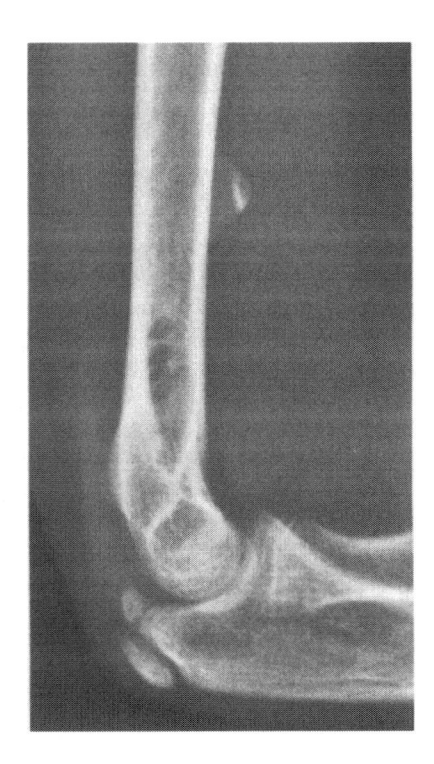

FIGURE 14-42. Supracondylar process. It was found incidental to a healing olecranon fracture.

injury and an evident supracondylar process, prophylactic resection of the process and ligament is recommended.[208]

Al-Nail described a 10-year-old boy who fell and presented with compression of the median nerve and brachial artery.[206] Radiography revealed a fracture of the supracondylar process. He was treated by excision of the process and ligament. Full recovery followed.

Distal Metaphysis (Supracondylar) Injuries

Supracondylar humeral fracture is the most common elbow injury in the developing skeleton, accounting for approximately 50–60% of injuries to this area.[214–576] It is also a relatively common fracture in immature animals (Fig. 14-43). It occurs most frequently in children between the ages of 3 and 10 years. It is associated with a high incidence of complications consequent to both (1) malunion resulting from inadequate reduction and maintenance and (2) growth mechanism injuries. Angular malunion has minimal chance of correcting spontaneously in the varus/valgus plane and should be corrected during the initial reduction. In contrast, anterior or posterior angulation usually improves, if it does not correct completely. The potential for neurovascular

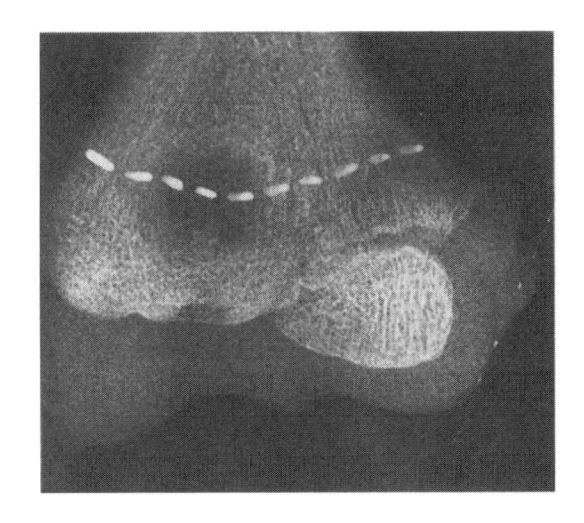

FIGURE 14-44. Specimen of distal humerus showing the characteristic region of fracture (dotted line) relative to the epiphyseal region and articular surface. Note how the fracture traverses the supracondylar foraminal region.

compromise, both acute and chronic, may also lead to serious dysfunction in the forearm and hand.

Classification

Supracondylar fractures may be classified into four types, all basically involving the foraminal region (Fig. 14-44): (1) flexion type (which probably accounts for 1–2% of these fractures) and the extension types (each representing about one-third of the fractures); (2) pure extension type; (3) extension-abduction, which is usually easy to treat, especially in traction, because the osseous instability lies on the lateral side where soft tissue stability is available and where traction tends to reduce the fracture; and (4) extension-adduction, which constitutes the source of most posttreatment varus deformities, especially when the fracture line lies in the oblique plane and is comminuted on the medial side.

Pathologic Anatomy

Extension Type

Viewed from the sagittal plane, the fracture line traverses obliquely upward and backward. Viewed from the coronal (frontal) plane it usually appears relatively transverse. The more transverse the fracture is in both planes, the more stable is the injury. Although the fracture is usually complete, greenstick injuries do occur (Fig. 14-45). The latter may be deceptive. Impaction or widening may lead to acute, often unrecognized, cubitus varus (Fig. 14-46) or valgus deformation at the time of acute injury. The distal fragment may be displaced proximally and posteriorly by transmission of the fracture force upward through the bones of the forearm. Rotation of the fragments is usually evident on the radiograph (Fig. 14-47).

The distal end of the proximal fragment projects anteriorly and may pierce the periosteum as it is stripped from

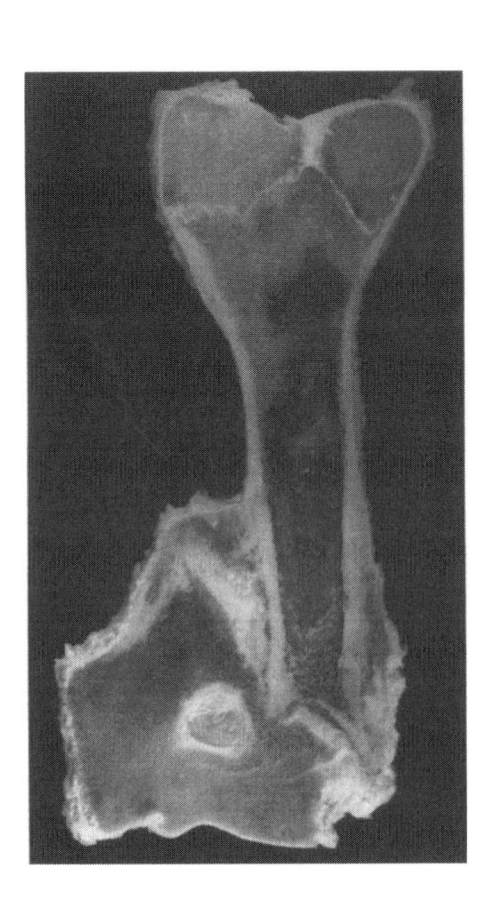

FIGURE 14-43. Supracondylar fracture in a skeletally immature giraffe.

Distal Metaphysis (Supracondylar) Injuries

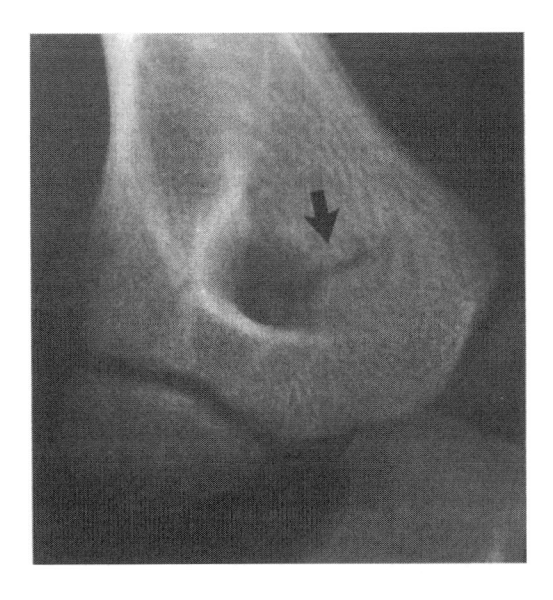

FIGURE 14-45. Greenstick supracondylar fracture.

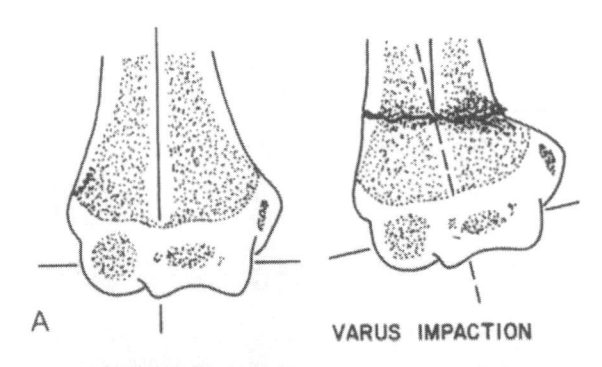

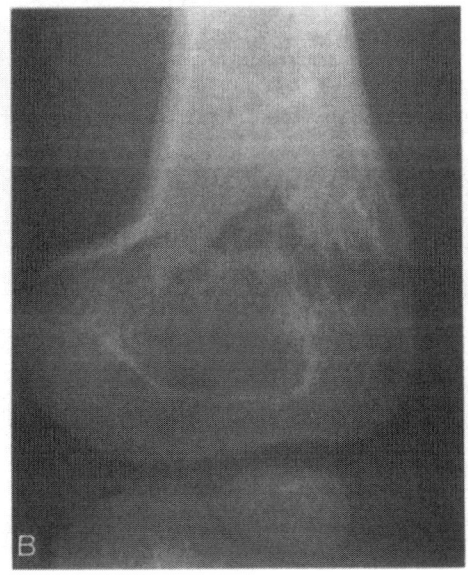

FIGURE 14-46. (A) Greenstick fracture causing medial trabecular/cortical compression leading to cubitus varus. It must be corrected with manipulation. (B) Acute cubitus varus in a 5-year-old. This was not corrected.

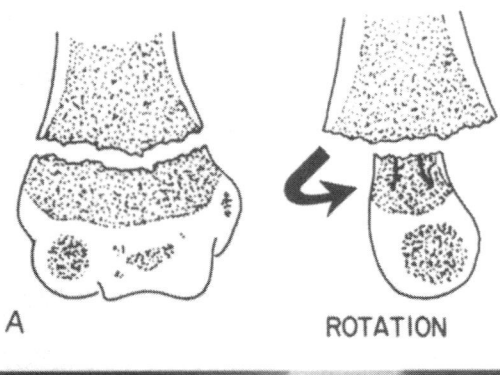

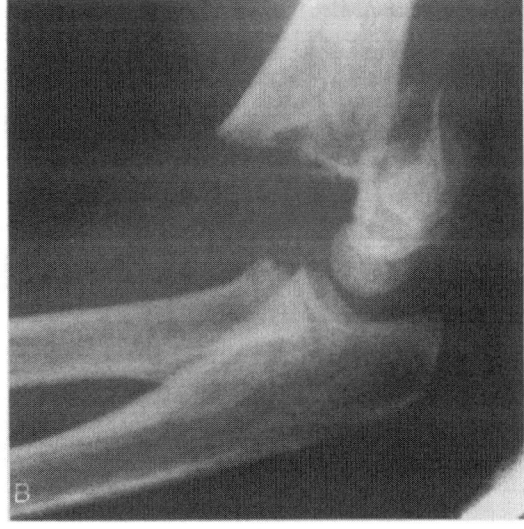

FIGURE 14-47. (A) Rotation. (B) Roentgenogram of acute injury showing an anteroposterior view of the proximal fragment and a lateral view of the distal fragment forearm.

both the anterior surface of the lower fragment and the posterior surface of the upper fragment (Fig. 14-48). With severe displacement, the proximal fragment may penetrate the skin, creating an open injury. The displacement of fracture fragments is somewhat limited by the extent of periosteal stripping, as this structure is rarely disrupted completely.[236]

There may be considerable extravasation of blood from the open marrow cavity and disrupted periosteum, causing associated swelling and accumulation of fluid in the elbow region. Because this compartment is fairly tight, it is essential to observe closely the extent of swelling and decide if surgical release is indicated. The nerves and blood vessels may be contused or lacerated by the osseous fragments or by the dissecting hematoma that infiltrates the antecubital region.

Flexion Type

The fracture line in the sagittal plane generally courses upward and forward, with the proximal fragment being displaced posteriorly and the distal fragment anteriorly and upward. Again, the degrees of varus, valgus, tilting, and rotation vary. The periosteum is disrupted on the posterior

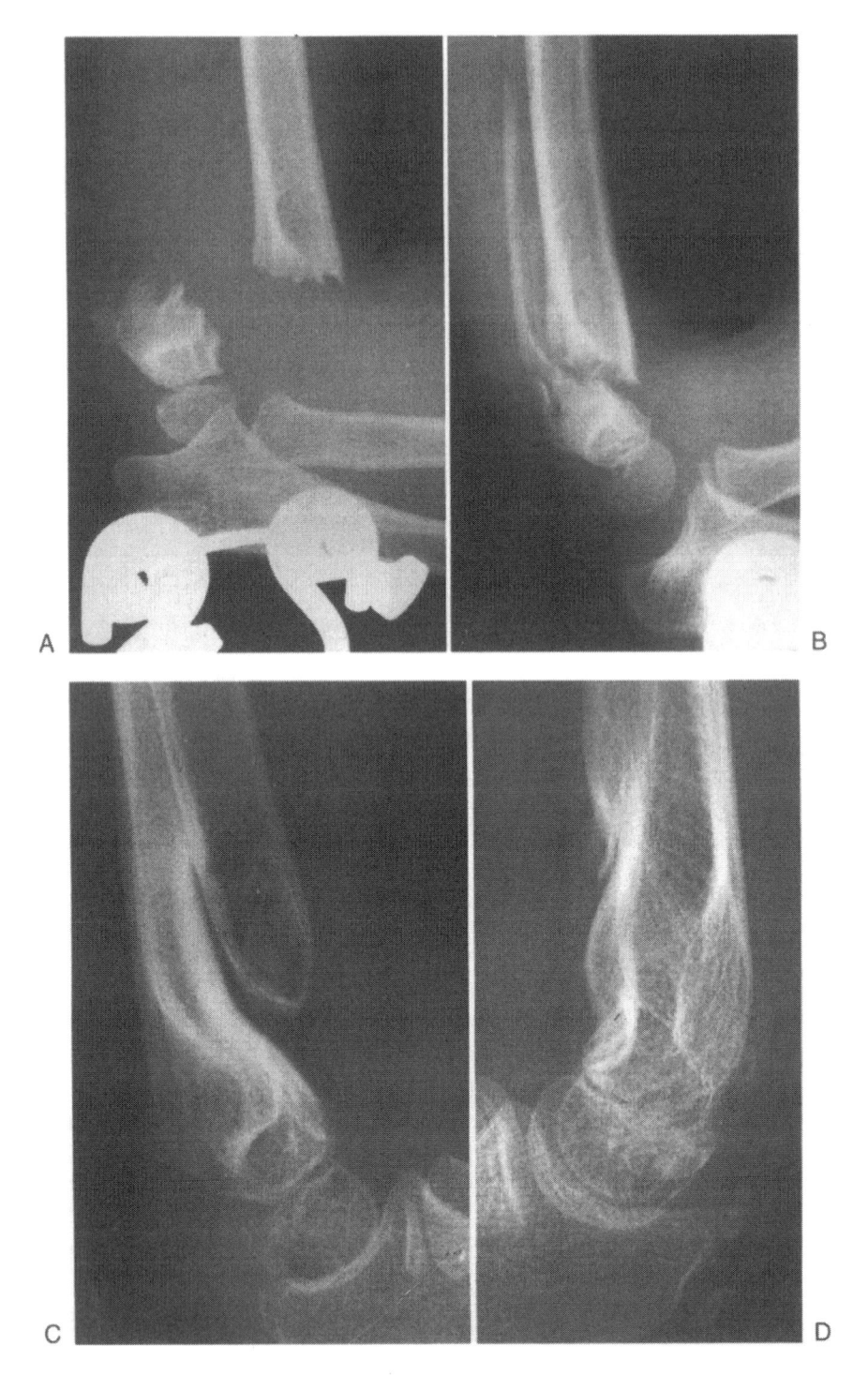

FIGURE 14-48. (A) Posterior displacement and overriding when first placed in traction. The proximal fragment is subcutaneous due to posterior displacement of muscle. (B) Distal fragment settled into a better anatomic position. (C) Similar case showing how further growth gradually corrects the deformity. Note the extensive posterior callus, complete lack of anterior callus, and porotic change in the anterior fragment. (D) There is minimal evidence of the injury 4 years later.

surface of the distal fragment and stripped from the anterior surface of the proximal fragment. Soft tissue swelling and damage are usually less than with the extension type, and neurovascular complications are rare.

Displacement

In general, three main types of displacement occur with a supracondylar fracture. The first type is loss of the normal anterior tilt of the distal end of the humerus. This is usually a greenstick fracture and probably requires no reduction. With the second type, the distal fragment is displaced and tilted posteriorly. In addition, there may be a medial or lateral shift. With the third type, the distal fragment is completely displaced in a posterior direction, with medial or lateral shift and usually some medial or lateral angulation.

The displacement may be such that the distal end of the shaft projects through the skin or deep fascia. If it projects through the deep fascia, ecchymosis may be evident in the antecubital fossa in addition to the gross deformity and marked swelling. Antecubital ecchymosis means that the deep fascia has been punctured and signifies that reduction of the fracture may be difficult owing to the interposition and redirection of soft tissues.

Because the muscles around the elbow are ensheathed in dense fascia and reinforced by the lacertus fibrosis, these vessels are held down tightly as they traverse the antecubital fossa. If there is marked posterior displacement of the distal fragment, the neurovascular bundle may be stretched over the distal end of the shaft fragment. This may occlude the venous or arterial blood supply (or both) by causing attenuation, direct compression, or irritation of the adventitia and sympathetic nerve fibers, causing spasm at the level of or distal to the injury and even in the collateral circulatory branches.

Graham studied adult cadavers to better comprehend the problems encountered with a supracondylar fracture and found that soft tissue stability was provided on the lateral side of the fracture by expansion of the triceps, the brachioradialis, and the extensor carpi radialis longus.[346] Similar tissue stability was *not* evident on the medial side. The expansion of the triceps provided some posterior soft tissue stability, but the muscle mass spanning the fracture site anteriorly was insufficient to provide such stability. Except for a few clinically insignificant fibers arising from the medial supracondylar ridge, the pronator teres arises only from the medial epicondyle and therefore is part of the forearm. This muscle did not reliably influence rotation of the distal fragment.[347] Experimental work in primates suggests muscular soft tissue and periosteal hinging have little effect on fracture stability.[217]

When the fracture is forcibly rotated, the sharp corner of the proximal fragment may tear the periosteum, permitting gross displacement. The rent in the periosteum leaves some of the periosteum around the fracture intact to form a useful hinge that may aid the attempted reduction. The periosteum may be stripped from the shaft for several inches proximally, depending on the degree of displacement at the time of injury. The extent of stripping becomes evident 2–3 weeks later by observing the length of the posterior callus.

The anatomic cause of fracture instability relates not only to the obliquity of the fracture surfaces but to the bicolumnar nature of this region (Fig. 14-49). The supracondylar foramen effectively creates two divergent columns, each of which must be anatomically reduced. However, the pattern of fracture obliquity in each column often differs.

Diagnosis

Supracondylar fractures may be diagnosed by history, clinical findings, and roentgenographic studies. Swelling may be minimal if the injury is seen shortly after occurrence or when displacement has been minimal. The more the displacement, the more swelling and deformity are likely to be evident. The forearm is usually held in pronation during examination. Note the degree of pronation or supination, as it may help to determine the varus/valgus instability.

Whereas examination of the fracture site is important, careful assessment of the distal neurovascular function in the injured limb is mandatory (Fig. 14-50). Radial and ulnar nerve injuries are recognized relatively easily. Median nerve involvement is generally incomplete and often overlooked. It may result in loss of flexion of the distal interphalangeal joint of the index finger, loss of flexion of the interphalangeal joint of the thumb, or numbness of the tip of the index finger. Any neurovascular deficit must be assessed completely and followed carefully.

Failure to detect vascular injuries may be disastrous and lead to permanent deformity and disability of the forearm musculature.[101] Signs of vascular compartment syndrome may include pain, pallor, cyanosis, absence of pulse, coldness, paresthesia or paralysis, any of which may indicate the possibility of impending Volkmann's ischemia. The arm should be checked also for possible concomitant fractures of the proximal or distal radius (Fig. 14-51) or proximal humerus.

Roentgenographic Evaluation

Roentgenographic examination confirms the diagnosis. The limb must be splinted adequately (well above the elbow) and comfortably before the patient is sent for radiographic evaluation. The elbow should be in some flexion, although excessive flexion of the elbow must be avoided to minimize possible neurovascular compromise by edematous tissue and displaced fragments.

Instructions to the technician must indicate that true anteroposterior and lateral projections of the distal humerus and elbow joint be obtained *without* simply rotating the forearm. If instructions are not given to move the entire upper extremity as a unit, the technician may simply rotate the forearm through the fracture site and give two views of the distal fragment rotated 90°, with the proximal fragment remaining the same. An anteroposterior view of the elbow can reveal whether the fracture line is transverse or oblique and whether the distal fragment is medially or laterally angulated. A lateral view of the elbow shows whether the distal fragment is displaced posteriorly or anteriorly and the extent to which normal anteroposterior angulation is lost.

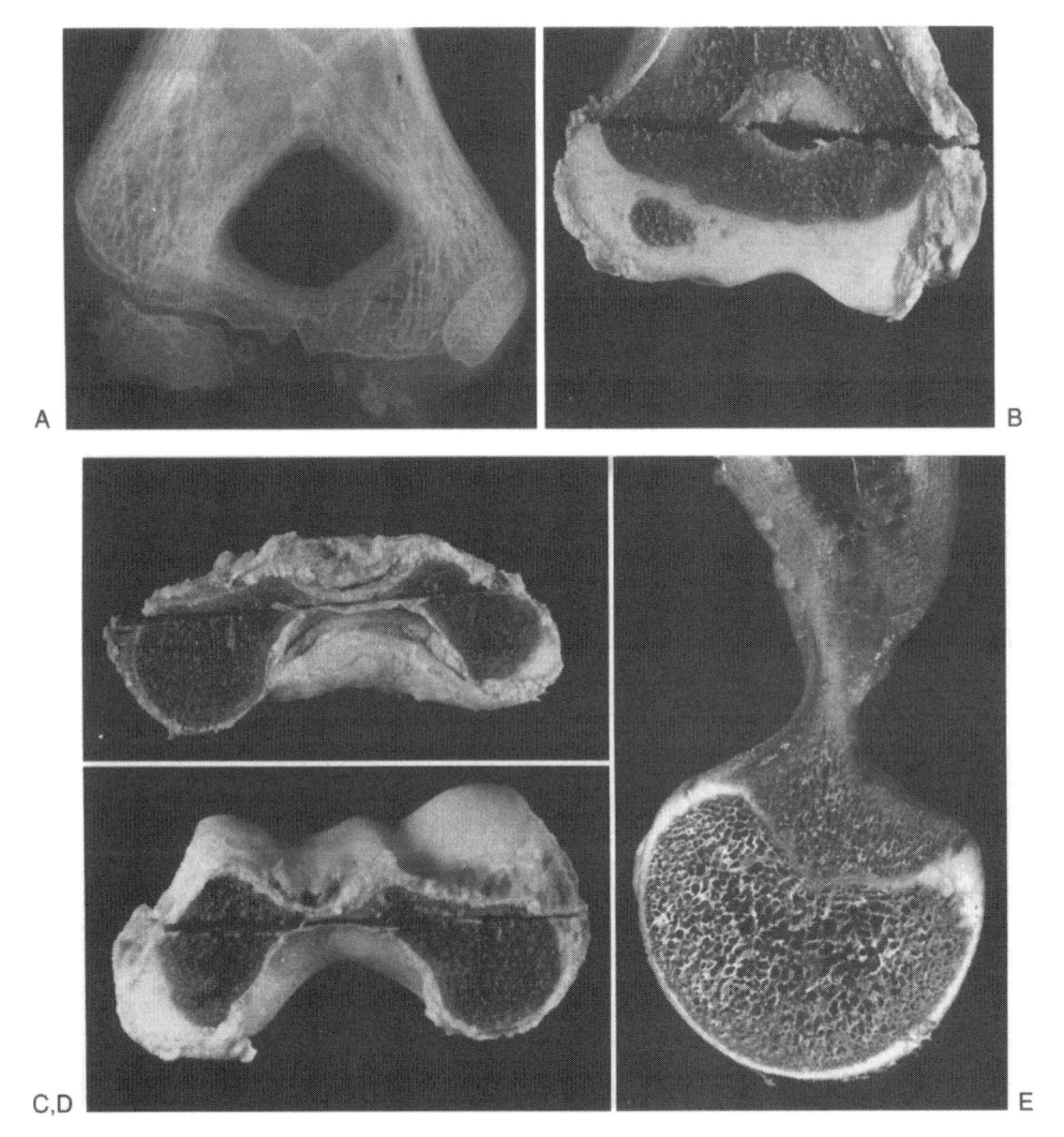

FIGURE 14-49. (A) Radiograph of foramen dividing the distal humerus into columns. (B) If a cut is made through the supracondylar foramen, the "bicolumnar" nature of this region becomes evident, as seen in (C) looking proximally, and (D) looking distally. (E) Lateral slab emphasizes the "precarious" nature of the central region, which cannot be counted on for any stability. (E) is from our genetically closest relative, the chimpanzee.

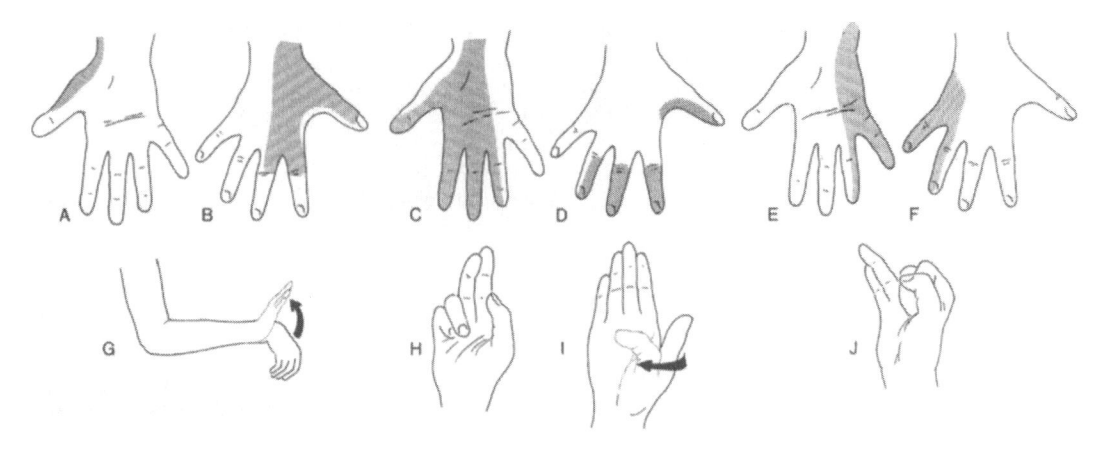

FIGURE 14-50. Sensory and motor functions of the radial nerve (A, B, G), median nerve (C, D, H, I), and ulnar nerve (E, F, J).

Distal Metaphysis (Supracondylar) Injuries

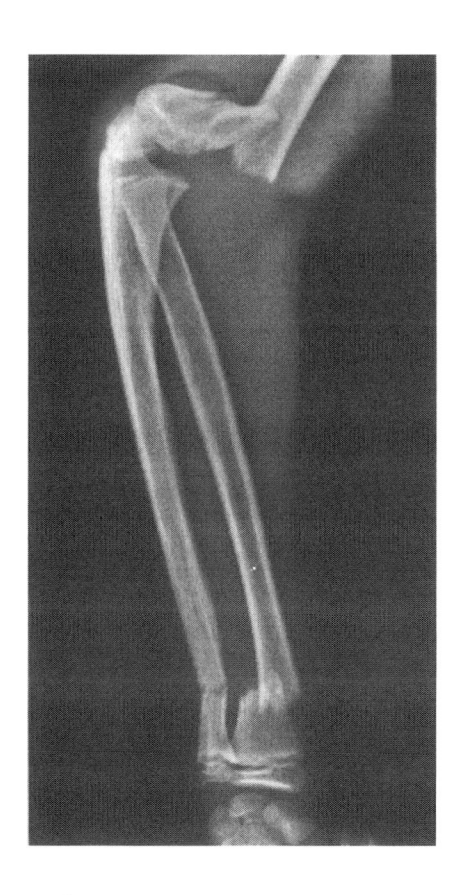

FIGURE 14-51. Concomitant fractures of supracondylar and wrist regions.

Treatment

Millis et al. presented an algorithm for management of supracondylar fracture; it is an excellent review for anyone treating these particular injuries.[450] Of 108 consecutive children with supracondylar fracture in this study, an initial attempt at closed reduction was undertaken in 101 cases. The attempt was successful in only 61. Any fracture with persistent vascular defects should be explored, reduced, and pinned without delay. Traction is never considered a substitute for reduction, though it may be useful to allow swelling to subside over a short period of time (e.g., 24–48 hours), after which reduction is attempted. Finally, open reduction should be considered whenever closed reduction cannot be achieved gently.

The direction of the fracture line is a major factor in the success or failure of closed reduction treatment. Generally, fracture fragments separated by a long, oblique line are more difficult to reduce and more likely to slip after closed reduction than those separated by a relatively transverse fracture line.

Treatment of undisplaced or minimally displaced extension-type fractures consists of fixing the arm with the elbow flexed to 90° (less if possible) and the forearm in a neutral or pronated position. This positioning is continued for 3–4 weeks. Follow-up roentgenograms are obtained after a few days to be certain the fracture has not displaced or angulated (especially into varus).

Cubitus varus may occur even following minimally displaced fractures. *One always must be cautious that a minimally displaced fracture is not of more magnitude than seems evident.* A belief that no reduction is necessary may be inappropriate (Fig. 14-46). If there has been compression on the medial side or widening laterally with an incompletely broken medial cortex, the fracture may be carefully manipulated and the medial or lateral tilting of the distal fragment corrected. The carrying angle of the elbow is matched to the normal side whenever feasible. However, a stable impacted fracture should not be converted to a grossly unstable one merely to correct varus.

Compression forces from normal muscle tone and elasticity of soft tissues surrounding the fracture fragments also may tilt the distal fragment, even during immobilization. In the presence of mild medial or lateral displacement, these factors may further a deformity that is already present or has been unrecognized.

The moderately displaced extension-type supracondylar fracture with some residual bone continuity should be treated by closed reduction under general anesthesia, provided there is no neurovascular compromise. The techniques are as follows (Figs. 14-52, 14-53). Length is restored by traction and countertraction with the elbow in extension, not hyperextension, to prevent excessive traction on the brachial vessels and nerves. Next, while maintaining traction with the forearm pronated and the elbow in slight flexion, the posterior displacement of the distal fragment is reduced. This is done by lifting it anteriorly while pushing the proximal fragment posteriorly. Then the lateral displacement is reduced by pushing the distal fragment medially. Any rotational deformity is corrected at this time. The elbow is then flexed to 90° to tighten the posterior periosteum and to maintain the reduction. With supracondylar fractures the biceps temporarily loses its supinating action.

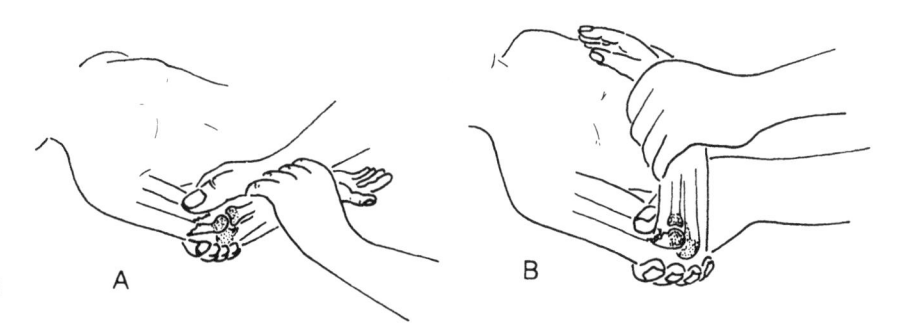

FIGURE 14-52. Reduction utilizing flexion methods.

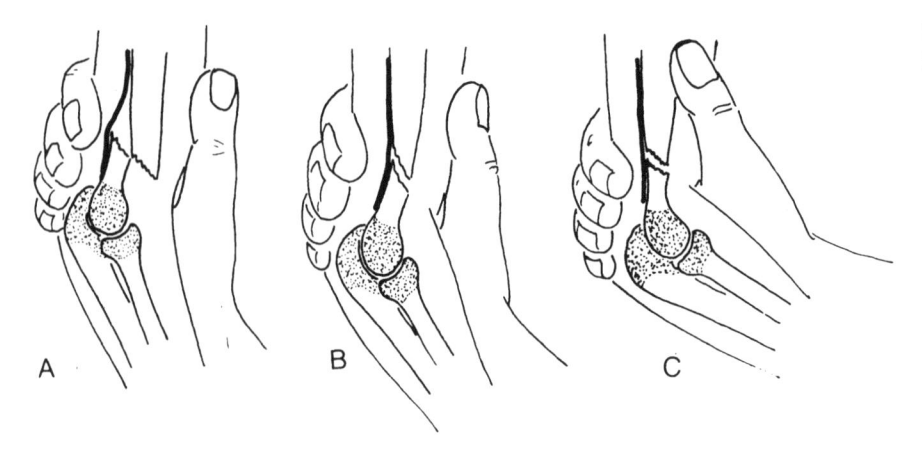

FIGURE 14-53. Reduction utilizing extension methods.

Because of the discontinuity of the humerus, the unopposed action of the strong pronator teres muscle may swing the proximal radioulnar joint into pronation. Because the joint is fixed by the pronators, varus deformity of the fracture site may gradually result from unopposed muscular force, even with a properly applied cast.[315]

The direction of the original displacement of the distal fragment is also considered when deciding on the position in which the forearm is to be immobilized in a cast (Fig. 14-54). If the distal fragment is displaced medially, the forearm is pronated to tighten the medial hinge, close the fracture line on the lateral side, and decrease the tendency to cubitus varus deformity. If the distal fragment is displaced laterally, supination of the forearm tightens the lateral periostal hinge, closes the fracture line on the medial side, and prevents cubitus valgus. With a posteriorly displaced fracture a posterior hinge of the periosteum is present. The use of intact periosteal hinges to aid in and maintain reduction is part of successful closed reductions.

The effect of various types of displacement of the distal fragment on the carrying angle was studied by simulating transverse supracondylar fractures by osteotomy.[517] Medial and lateral displacement of the distal fragment *without* concomitant angular deformity did not change the carrying angle. Internal rotation of the distal fragment also had no effect on the degree of the carrying angle.[517]

The osseous relations of the medial and lateral epicondyles and the olecranon process may be assessed through the Lyman Smith triangle or Bauman's angle. With the elbow flexed to a right angle, three osseous points make a fairly symmetric equilateral triangle and tend to lie in a plane parallel with the plane of the posterior surface of the upper arm. In some children the capitellum becomes quite prominent in 90° of flexion and disturbs the symmetry of the lateral segment of the triangle. When the elbow is in complete extension, the three osseous points are almost in a straight line.

Circulation must be assessed frequently within the first 48 hours after injury. The family should be made aware of the signs of circulatory compromise so they can watch the child carefully at home. If there is a mildly displaced fracture but a moderate amount of swelling with a suggestion of vascular compromise, overnight hospitalization should be considered for close observation and elevation of the extremity.

The displaced fracture is reduced under general anesthesia because of the difficulty of reduction and the importance of trying to obtain reduction on the first attempt. Repetitive manipulations should be minimized because of the possibility of injury to vessels and nerves during each manipulative attempt. Once the fracture has been reduced satisfactorily, the peripheral circulation must be assessed again. If it is normal, a long arm cast or splint may be applied. The cast

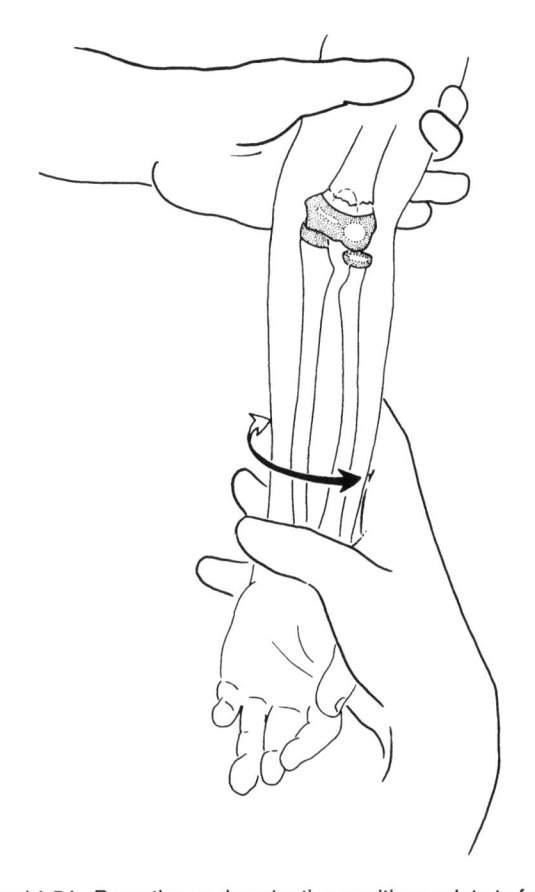

FIGURE 14-54. Pronation and supination positions relate to fracture obliquity and which soft tissues are intact. This may be assessed by stress testing under fluoroscopy while attempting closed reduction.

Distal Metaphysis (Supracondylar) Injuries

should not constrict the soft tissues of the antecubital area. A window cut in the wrist region of the radial artery allows the distal circulation to be checked.

About 120° of flexion may be necessary to ensure stability. The radial pulse may disappear for a few minutes after initial reduction. If the fingers are pink, this may be satisfactory; but if the fingers become white, the degree of flexion is reduced. If flexion to a right angle is not possible without circulatory impairment, check to see if the posterior displacement is corrected. If the moderately displaced fracture is anatomically reduced but the vascular status remains questionable, several options are available: (1) fixation with percutaneous K-wires; (2) casting in this position, then increasing the flexion when the swelling is less, usually in 3–7 days; (3) placement in traction; (4) open reduction and internal fixation, with or without direct exploration of the vessels. When in doubt, obtain a vascular surgical consultation.

Roentgenograms in the anteroposterior and lateral projections determine the adequacy of reduction (Fig. 14-55). Any lateral or medial tilting must be corrected *completely*. Appositional alignments are less significant, as they usually correct spontaneously through remodeling and have little or no effect on the carrying angle or the final range of motion of the elbow. Posterior angulation and flexion deformities are in the plane of motion of the elbow and usually correct themselves. Rotation of the distal fragment is not corrected by remodeling and may appear unusual on the roentgenograms. Although this rotation is well compensated clinically by the degree of rotation at the shoulder, this should not be an excuse to fail to observe and attempt to correct rotational malalignment as much as possible.

In the presence of marked swelling, closed reduction is carried out just as outlined, but the patient is placed in Dunlop's skin or skeletal traction for several days until the swelling subsides. If it is difficult or impossible to maintain adequate skin traction, it may be necessary to apply skeletal traction with a pin inserted through the proximal ulna. In general, however, skeletal traction is reserved for a severely displaced fracture, one that cannot be reduced satisfactorily, or one that proves unstable. Prolonged traction is used decreasingly because of hospital costs, although its use in other parts of the world may be necessary and effective.

After swelling subsides, the arm may be removed from traction and immobilized. The overall degree of stability is checked before and after application of a cast. Roentgenograms are obtained at short intervals following the injury to verify maintenance of the reduction. These films are best obtained 5–10 days following the injury and 2–4 weeks later. These roentgenograms are important because muscular forces may reintroduce deformity during the first 10–14 days after injury, particularly if a crushing injury has occurred to the medial or lateral side with loss of cortical integrity.

Flexion Injury

The flexion injury usually is relatively simple to treat. Closed reduction is carried out by traction and flexion, followed by correction of the lateral tilting and displacement by manual pressure. The elbow then is immobilized in "extension," although 20°–30° of flexion may be more comfortable for the patient.

Unstable Fractures

A completely displaced supracondylar fracture is treated best by closed manipulative reduction, followed by skeletal traction or some type of internal fixation (e.g., percutaneous pins). Because of increasing emphasis on the cost of hospitalization, traction is often bypassed in favor of skeletal fixation. However, for the severely swollen elbow with a variable pulse or a question of compartment syndrome, 24–48 hours may make a big difference in the ease and safety of a closed or open reduction. Extended placement in traction (2–3 weeks) is probably best avoided for most children.

The basic traction technique is as follows. Under general anesthesia a Kirschner wire is inserted through the proximal ulna about 2–3 cm distal to the tip of the olecranon process and *beyond the physis*. Osseous landmarks about the elbow are carefully identified, and the wire is drilled from the medial to the lateral side to avoid tethering of the ulnar nerve. Because considerable swelling is often present, great care must be taken to ensure insertion of the pin into the metaphyseal bone. A threaded Kirschner wire has less chance of becoming loose and causing skin tract infection but is more uncomfortable during removal.[276,373] As an alternative, screws are available for placement directly into the olecranon.

Once the pin is in place the surgeon must decide on the most efficacious method of traction. Traction may be directed to the side (Fig. 14-56) or overhead (Fig. 14-57).[308,313] If used properly and diligently, neither method is superior to the other. When setting up the traction, medial

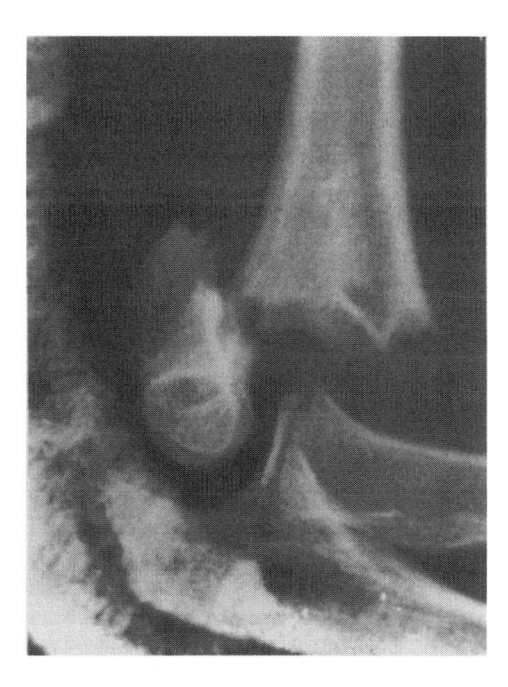

FIGURE 14-55. Attempted reduction. It has been *incompletely* corrected for rotation and so the "reduction" is unacceptable.

FIGURE 14-56. (A) Side-directed (Dunlop's) traction. Control of pronation and supination is not easy. (B) Additional traction may be applied to the proximal fragment.

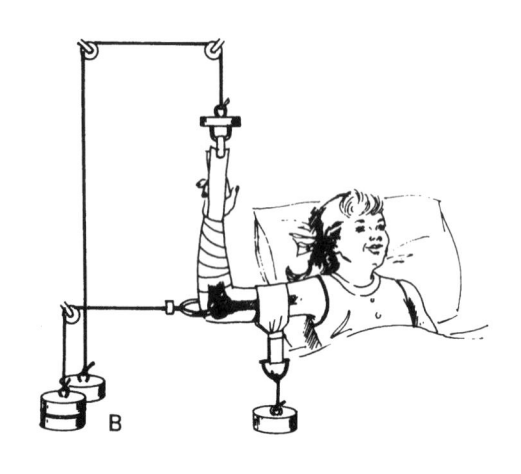

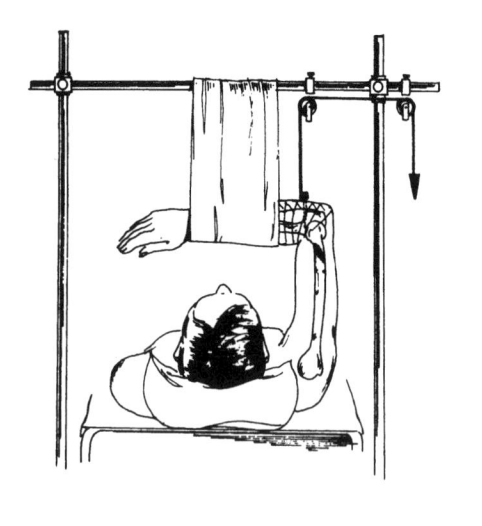

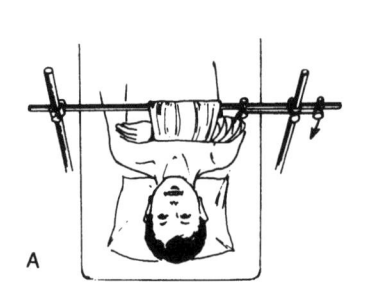

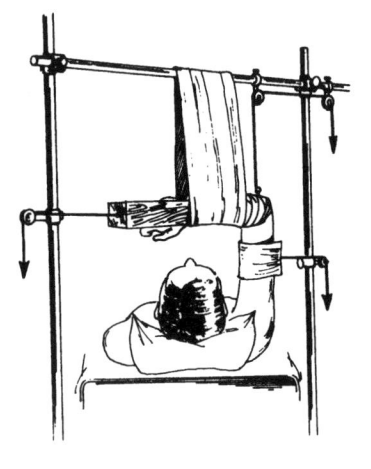

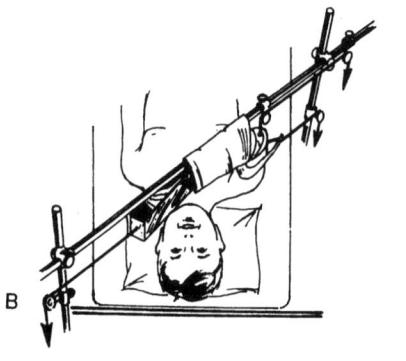

FIGURE 14-57. (A) Placement of a patient in bed relative to overhead traction. (B) Angulation of the traction may control rotation.

Distal Metaphysis (Supracondylar) Injuries

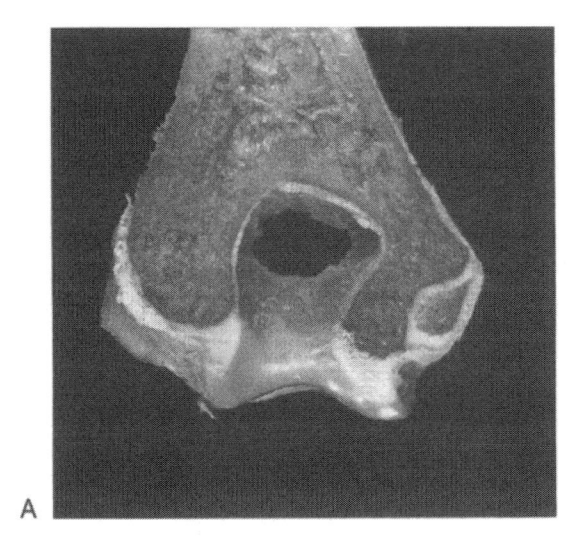

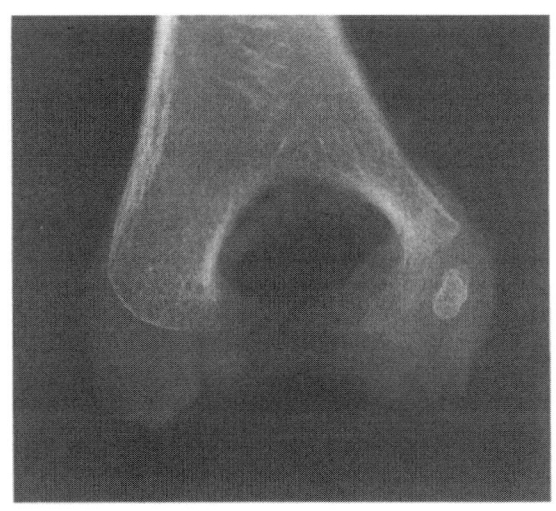

FIGURE 14-58. Bicolumnar nature of the distal humerus in a 7-year-old boy. The supracondylar fossa may be large. (A) Slab section. (B) Radiograph.

and lateral tilting of the distal fragment must be assessed and carefully corrected. Roentgenograms are made to determine the accuracy of reduction.

Lateral traction may be applied with the shoulder abducted 60° and the arm elevated 20° from the horizontal, a position that improves venous drainage of the upper limb and limits patient movement. Overhead traction does not always provide optimum control of the proximal fragment as the patient moves about in bed. However, if the child is placed in overhead traction with his head against the headboard, he can only move downward and rotate externally, thereby minimizing rotational abnormality. It is possible for the child to force the elbow into acute flexion and cause circulatory embarrassment.[527] A 3- to 5-pound weight is applied to the lateral traction bow, and the forearm is suspended. For fractures in which the proximal fragment is anteriorly displaced, a sling with a 1-pound weight is applied to the upper arm, pulling it posteriorly to try to reduce this angular displacement.[356]

The maintenance of reduction is determined by serial roentgenograms. The fracture is removed from traction when it proves stable enough to be casted (usually 10–14 days).

Rotation and varus or valgus deformities do not always correct spontaneously in traction and may require remanipulation. If deformity exists after 3–4 weeks, corrective osteotomy may have to be considered; but it should be postponed until maximum improvement of function has been obtained. The functional result may be such that late osteotomy may be unnecessary.

When considering any fixation, whether inserted percutaneously or under direct vision, the unique bicolumnar nature of the distal humerus must be considered (Fig. 14-58). The pins should be either driven obliquely along the anatomic curve of each column (Fig. 14-59) or directed

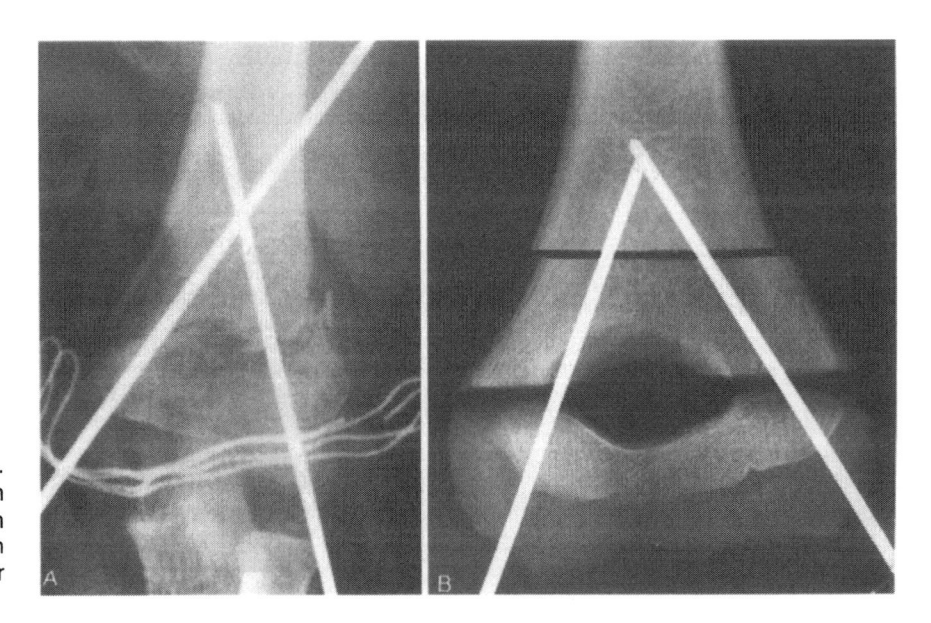

FIGURE 14-59. Techniques of pin fixation. (A) Reduction allows anatomic restoration and accurate pin placement. (B) Proper pin placement: one in each osseous column medial and lateral to the supracondylar foramen.

more transversely across the cortical bone of the supracondylar forearm. The latter method may give three or four cortex fixations per pin.

Closed reduction may be performed and percutaneous K-wires introduced (Fig. 14-60) to prevent redisplacement, particularly when the elbow cannot be flexed beyond a right angle.[354,531] After the fracture has been reduced by closed methods, one K-wire is inserted through the medial epicondyle and another through the lateral epicondyle. This is best done using the image intensifier. Alternatively, two pins may be introduced from the lateral side (Fig. 14-61). Transfixing the ulna and condylar fragment by traversing the elbow joint is unnecessary and may lead to stiffness. Any pin must adequately cross the fracture and stabilize it.

Open reduction is indicated if the fracture is markedly unstable or if there is significant neurovascular compromise. In the latter case, it may be necessary to explore the artery or increase the amount of space through which the vessels traverse at the level of the lacertus fibrosus.[328,352,374,485,511,558,559,567] Open reduction and internal fixation have been condemned because of elbow stiffness. However, a careful open reduction with minimal soft tissue dissection should not

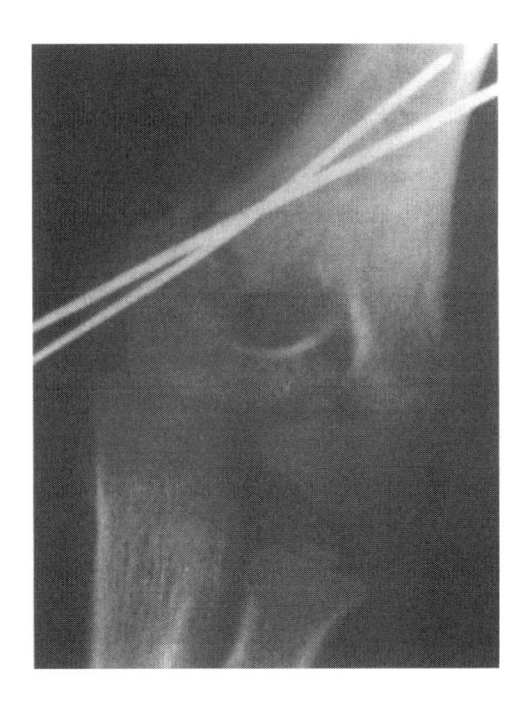

FIGURE 14-61. Closed reduction with percutaneous pin fixation. Two pins have been placed in the lateral epicondyle to maintain reduction and control rotation.

create any more problems than multiple attempts at closed reduction. Certainly for older adolescents, especially those with T-shaped intercondylar fractures, open reduction is indicated.

A posterior approach may be used for open reduction.[339] The triceps aponeurosis is incised as an inverted V and turned distally. The ulnar nerve is isolated and protected. Kirschner wires then may be introduced retrogradely through the fracture site into the medial and lateral epicondyles, emerging through the skin, but avoiding the ulnar nerve. Under direct vision the fracture is reduced, and the Kirschner wires are passed into the proximal fragment. Rotational correction is checked before passing a second Kirschner wire.

Results

Most minimally to moderately displaced fractures heal without significant problems (Fig. 14-62), and function is fully returned within 3 months after the injury. If displacement is severe, the recovery time is longer, but return of function is usually complete. However, complete return of flexion may take from several months to several years because of prominence of the anteriorly directed metaphysis. Remodeling generally corrects this problem.

The child is allowed to set his or her own pace of rehabilitation and to determine any physical limitations. In most instances, there are minimal or no residual contractures, especially if the child is followed for more than a year after the fracture. Weights and aggressive physical therapy are never used to stretch the elbow into full extension. In fact, it may be impossible depending on the direction of the distal

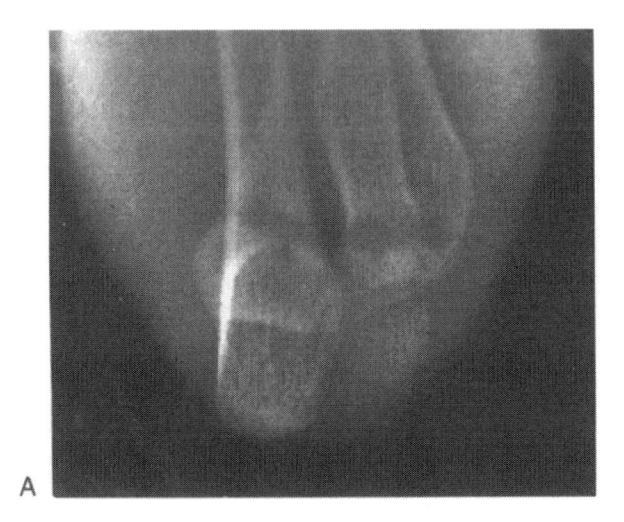

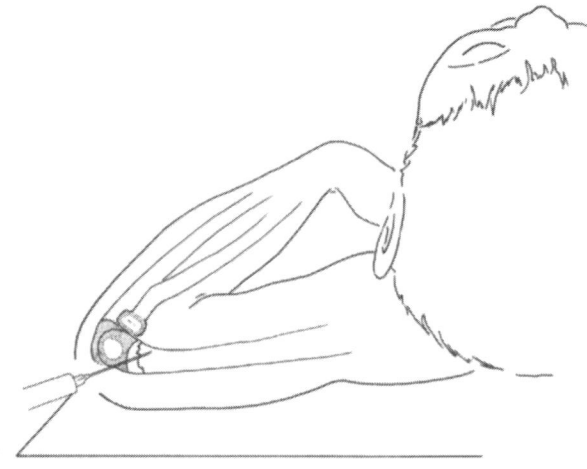

FIGURE 14-60. Reduction may be verified by flexing the forearm. (A) With the arm still on the fluoroscope. (B) Pins may be inserted percutaneously under direct fluoroscopic vision.

FIGURE 14-62. Displaced distal fragment usually has posteromedial attachment of the periosteum, but the periosteum strips away from the proximal fragment. Anteroposterior (A) and lateral (B) views show the extensive subperiosteal new bone that forms if the fragment is not reduced.

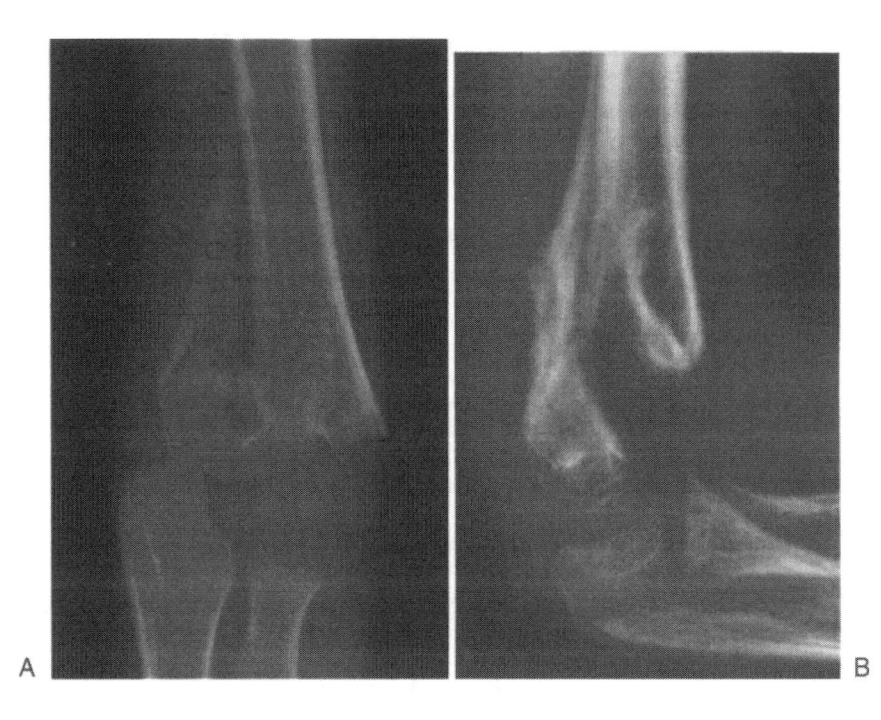

fragment. Growth and redirection of the distal humerus may be necessary to restore some range of motion.

Complications

Varus-Valgus

The "carrying angle" is the lateral angle made by the longitudinal axis of the fully supinated forearm and the longitudinal axis of the upper arm when the elbow is completely extended but not hyperextended. If the forearm is pronated or the elbow is flexed, this carrying angle cannot be evaluated adequately. However, if the flexed elbow is examined posteriorly and compared with the opposite uninjured elbow, changes in the carrying angle become more apparent.

It is important to remember that the carrying angle is subject to considerable normal individual variation. In 150 normal children it averaged 6.1° in girls (range 0°–12°) and 5.4° in boys (range 0°–11°).[518] Some children (9%) have no carrying angle (cubitus rectus), and 48% have a carrying angle of 5° or less.[518]

The complication of reversed carrying angle (gunstock deformity; cubitus varus) has several causes: (1) incomplete correction of displacement of the distal fragment at the time of original reduction (Figs. 14-63, 14-64); (2) growth disturbance of the trochlear portion of the physis; and (3) vascular-mediated stimulation of the capitellar physis, creating eccentric overgrowth (similar to tibia valgum following a proximal metaphyseal fracture). This reversed carrying angle rarely causes significant loss of elbow joint function but may create an unappealing cosmetic deformity.[245,323,331,396,412]

Ippolito et al. presented a long-term follow-up into young adult years, finding that the carrying angle remained the same in 18 patients, decreased in 22 patients, and increased in 13 compared to the value present at the time of initial fracture healing several weeks after the injury.[377] They thought that this indicated there was a potential for growth imbalance of the physis of the distal humerus and that it might be comparable to the phenomenon occurring in the proximal tibia due to vascular variation.

The mediolateral variability of blood supply to the proximal tibia is described in Chapter 23. Particularly, it seems to stimulate medial physeal growth in the proximal tibial physis preferentially, causing postinjury angulation (tibia valga). The advanced maturation of the capitellum versus the trochlea is associated with a greater circulation laterally than medially. Temporary asymmetric hyperemia as part of the generalized fracture healing response could certainly occur and contribute to varus angulation.

The varus angulation may be mild, moderate, or severe. Depending on the age at the time of injury, it may lead to deformation of the forearm as a secondary response. Although uncommon, physeal damage may occur, leading to progressive deformity.

If treated properly, there should be minimal varus as an immediate complication.[129] However, this type of injury is deceptive, particularly if there is minimal displacement. Malunion or angular deformity noted after acute treatment (i.e., 4–6 weeks) is most likely due to malunion, *not* to a growth disturbance.

If the varus or valgus deformity of the elbow is severe and stable (i.e., not related to growth injury but to static deformity from the original injury), correction may be indicated by supracondylar osteotomy of the humerus.[226,316,387,449] If there has been injury to the nerve or perhaps involvement with the fracture callus, it can be corrected at the same time.

Corrective supracondylar osteotomy is not always an easy operation. It is best to use a closing wedge osteotomy. Care must be taken during the placement of internal fixation, as false aneurysm formation, nerve injury, and bone infection may occur.

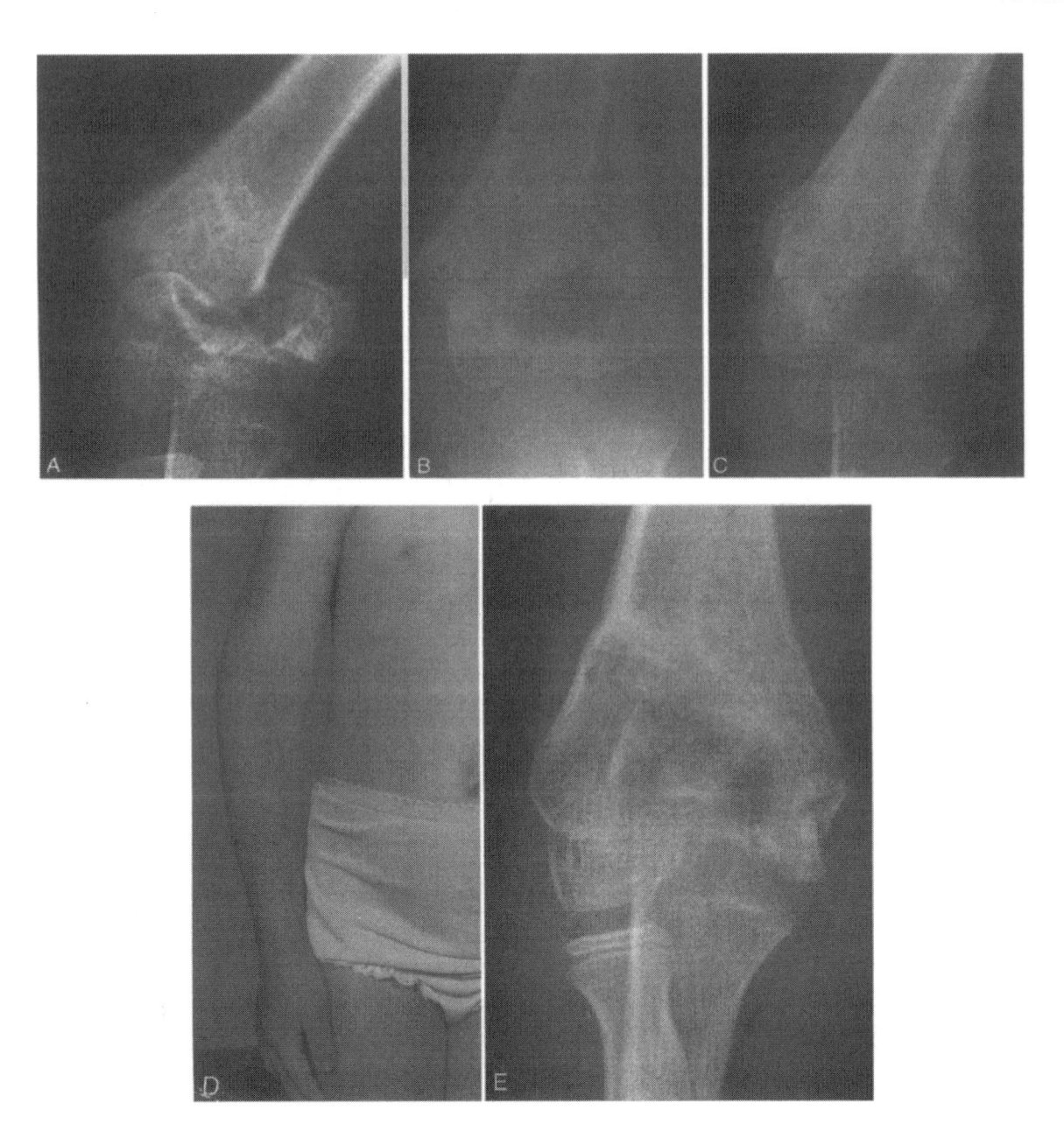

FIGURE 14-63. (A) Acute fracture with primary varus impaction. (B) Reduction failed to correct the varus angle, although the position appeared good from the lateral view. (C) One year later the varus has not corrected at all. (D) Clinical appearance of the cubitus varus. (E) Appearance after corrective osteotomy.

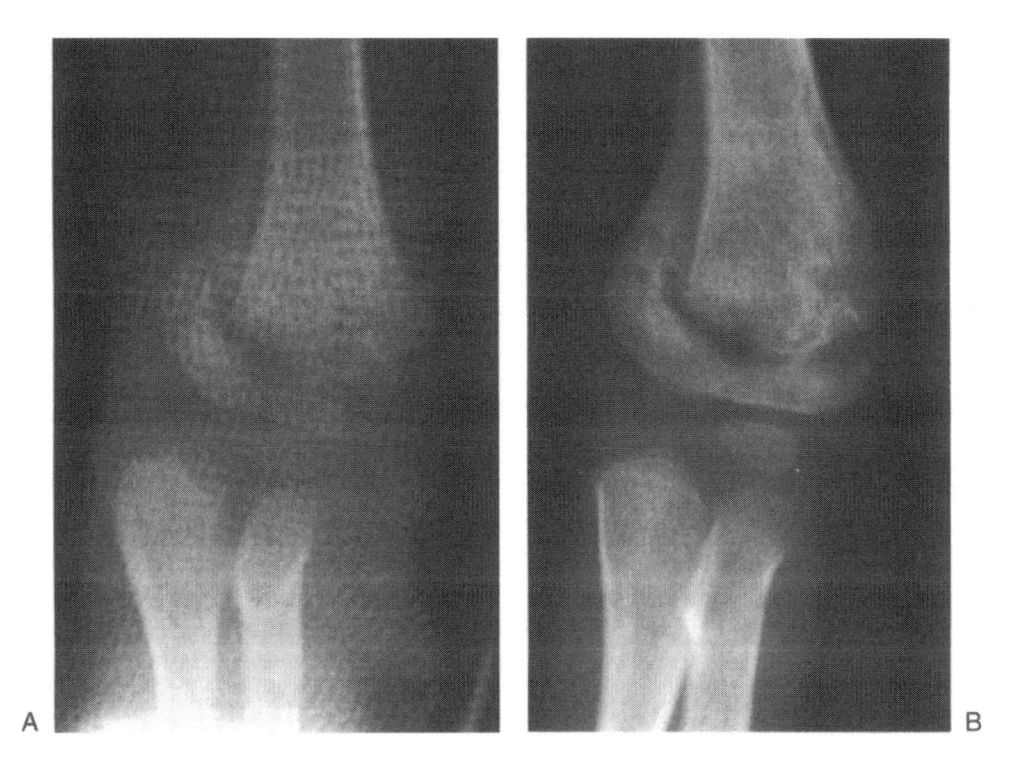

FIGURE 14-64. (A) Varus deformity was not corrected when the patient was placed in a cast. (B) After-casting the deformity.

Oppenheim et al. reviewed 45 corrective supracondylar osteotomies performed for posttraumatic cubitus varus in 43 children.[468] Excellent results were obtained in only 33 patients, with unsatisfactory results in 12. The operation, though seemingly simple, had a significant complication rate of almost 25%; the complications included neuropraxia, sepsis, and cosmetically unacceptable scarring. The authors believed that a comprehensive preoperative plan and a lateral closing wedge osteotomy, leaving the medial cortex intact and ignoring the rotational deformity in the correction, were the best ways to avoid complications.

Lateral condylar or transcondylar fractures may occur in patients who have a cubitus varus following supracondylar fracture. I have seen this in five patients (Fig. 14-65). The varus configuration should not be arbitrarily termed a "cosmetic" deformity. The mechanics of the elbow are variably disrupted. When patients attempt to protect themselves during a fall by using the arm, the varus position excessively loads the lateral side, enhancing the varus forces and causing lateral condylar fracture.

Volkmann's Ischemia (Compartment Syndrome)

As awareness of compartment syndrome has increased, the incidence of the complication has decreased.[322,423,500,506,571] The five classic warning signs of Volkmann's ischemia are pain, pallor (cyanosis), pulselessness, paresthesia, and paralysis. *The most important is pain.* Ischemia should always be suspected when increasing pain develops in the forearm following injury to the elbow and forearm or following treatment for such injury. A characteristic physical finding is exaggeration of the pain upon passive extension of the fingers, followed by taut, progressive swelling and firmness of the lower compartment of the forearm. The radial pulse may be absent or present. The presence of a normal radial pulse does *not* absolutely rule out Volkmann's ischemia. There may be a varying degree of sensory loss, with the median nerve almost always involved and the ulnar nerve involved in many cases.

The pathophysiology is as follows. The ischemia initially produces anoxia in the muscles. The increasing intramuscular edema causes a progressive increase in the intrinsic pressure within the muscles. Circular, relatively unyielding dressings of the limb and limited expansion of the taut fascia around the muscles of the forearm increase the venous compression and intramuscular compression, further increasing the intrinsic compartmental pressure. Pressor receptors within the forearm compartment and within the muscle itself stimulate reflex vasospasm, which subsequently affects the vessels. This vasospasm further aggravates and worsens the initial vascular compromise, setting up a destructive ischemia–edema cycle.

If the process persists, the next stage is necrosis of muscle, with eventual secondary fibrosis and possible development of heterotopic calcification. The time frame necessary to go from pressure increase to necrosis is not firmly established. The infarct is ellipsoid shaped and is along the axis of the distribution of the anterior interosseous artery. The flexor digitorum profundus and pollicus brevis muscles and the median nerve are most commonly and severely affected. If during the acute stage the palmar compartment of the forearm is surgically exposed, the deep fascia is taut and

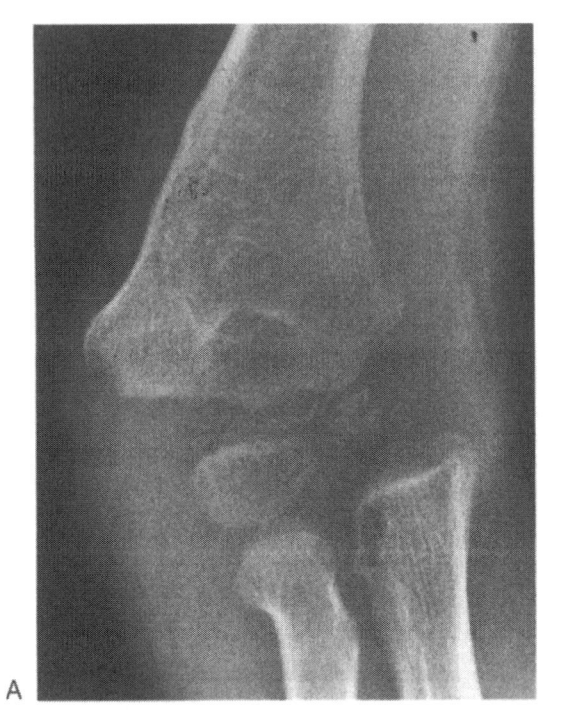

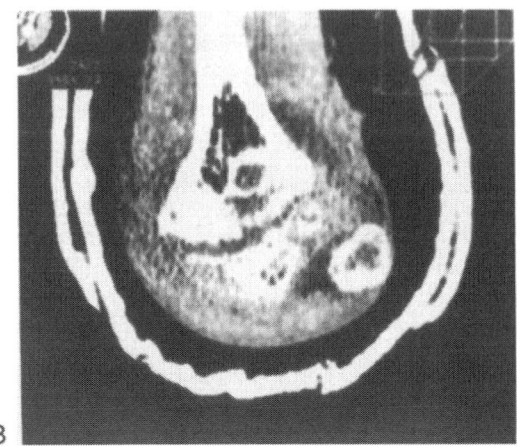

FIGURE 14-65. This boy had a cubitus varus following a supracondylar fracture. He fell, reinjuring the elbow. (A) Radiograph was interpreted as a lateral condylar fracture. (B) However, the MRI showed it to be a transphyseal injury. During the open reduction a corrective wedge was taken from the metaphysis.

spread widely when split. The muscles may be pale or blueblack due to extravasation of blood resulting from the altered hemodynamics.

This circulatory embarrassment may occur if the brachial artery is (1) caught and kinked at the fracture site (Fig. 14-61), (2) the artery is contused and in spasm at the moment of fracture, (3) a tight encircling cast is compressing the brachial vessels, (4) there is rapidly progressive swelling in the taut fascial compartment, or (5) a subintimal hematoma is present.[291,455,522,528] Distal to the lacertus fibrosus, the brachial artery branches into the radial and ulnar arteries. The radial artery is superficially located, whereas the ulnar artery is situated more deeply, traversing deep to the pronator teres. The ulnar artery gives origin to the common interosseous artery, which divides into anterior and posterior interosseous branches. The flexor digitorum profundus and flexor pollicis longus receive their blood supply from the anterior interosseous artery. The median nerve is particularly vulnerable to damage because of its course deep to the lacertus fibrosus and through the substance of the pronator teres muscle.

The acute destructive processes of Volkmann's ischemia are progressive and generally reach a peak (i.e., irreversibility) within 8–12 hours after the injury. If untreated, the swelling and sensitivity gradually subside, even if ischemia has been present, and the muscles of the flexor compartment undergo progressive fibrosis leading to contractural deformity. The elbow becomes fixed, the forearm pronated, the wrist flexed, the metacarpophalangeal joint hyperextended, and the interphalangeal joint flexed.

A decision must be made whether to continue observation or consider surgical decompression. The situation can be assessed by measuring compartment pressures at appropriate intervals to see if the pressure in the palmar (volar) compartment is increased. During the acute ischemic stage, treatment should be urgent. If the various signs and symptoms cannot be relieved within a few hours after pressure measurement by extending the elbow, removing tight encircling bandages, or reducing the fracture, arteriography should be considered. If the brachial artery is only in spasm, a stellate ganglion block may lead to relief. If this does not improve the situation, fasciotomy of the forearm and exploration of the brachial artery are indicated. The major vessels are often intact with compartment syndrome.

Surgical Release

A longitudinal incision is made at the flexor crease of the elbow, medial to the biceps tendon. It is extended along the middle of the palmar surface of the forearm to the flexor crease of the wrist. Proximally, the incision may be extended to expose the brachial artery without crossing the flexor crease. The subcutaneous tissues are divided and the antebrachial fascia sectioned longitudinally throughout the entire length. The fascial sheath of each muscle (the epimysium or perimysium) is carefully divided from its lower to upper margin. Muscle fibers should not be sectioned. Usually circulation returns immediately. If these measures do not lead to improvement, the brachial artery should be explored or arteriography performed. The fascia must be left open. Muscle edema may prevent approximation of the skin edges, in which case the wound is left open and closed several days later after the edema has subsided. A skin graft may be necessary. Postoperatively, the wrist and hand must be splinted to prevent deformation.

Treatment of established Volkmann's ischemia is contingent on the severity of the deformity and the length of time since the original injury. The contracted flexor muscles in the forearm may be lengthened at their muscle junction, along with neurolysis of the median and ulnar nerves. In severe cases it is possible to shorten both bones of the forearm to gain relative length of the contracted muscles. Myocutaneous transplants may be considered.

Intercondylar Injuries

Osseous Vascular Changes

Graham et al. reported avascular necrosis of the trochlea in one child with supracondylar injury.[345]

Neurologic Complications

At any given time the radial, ulnar, or median nerve may be injured at the time of fracture, during attempted reduction, by compression from Volkmann's ischemia, or by entrapment in the fracture callus.[244,370,371,428,479,523,532,544] Entrapment may be evident as the Matev sign (Fig. 14-66). The radial nerve is most commonly injured because of its position relative to the fracture line. Siris reported 11 nerve injuries in 330 supracondylar fractures (7 radial, 4 ulnar).[514] Brown et al. found a nerve injury incidence of 7% (16 of 207) with 7 ulnar, 4 radial, 4 median, and 1 combined ulnar-median.[271] In another review of 162 supracondylar fractures, there were 23 neural injuries: 12 radial, 6 ulnar, 5 median, 4 ulnar, 1 radial, and 1 iatrogenic from percutaneous pins. All deficits resolved within 2–6 months.

Lipscomb and Burleson described selective anterior interosseous nerve compression.[423] It is of major importance to assess the arm carefully for the possibility of damage to this particular nerve, although the findings are often subtle. A significant number of nerve injuries are isolated to the anterior interosseous branch. The physical finding is an inability to flex the distal phalanges of the thumb and index finger without associated sensory deficits. This problem usually resolves within a few weeks of the injury. A review of 101 supracondylar fractures found 6 cases of isolated anterior interosseous nerve palsy.[290]

With a few exceptions most nerve injuries accompanying supracondylar fractures recover full activity within 6–10 weeks, although a time lapse of as much as 5–6 months has been reported. Observation and supportive therapy comprise the preferred initial approach to neural injury.[293] If there is no evidence of recovery by 5–6 months, evaluation by electromyography, exploration, and neurolysis may be necessary.

Elbow Dislocation

Failure to correct the normal anterior angulation of the entire distal epiphysis after hyperextension injuries based on the assumption that this type of malunion will correct with time may alter elbow mechanics. Recurrent posterior dislocation following supracondylar fracture has been reported.[419]

Myositis

Spinner et al. described an 18-year-old man who sustained blunt elbow trauma.[524] He had developed decreased elbow motion over the next year, followed by acute onset of pain after another fall. Radiography revealed a fracture of the base of a myositis ossificans lesion.

Intercondylar Injuries

Intercondylar (T) fractures of the distal humeral condyles are unusual during childhood, tending to occur more frequently in older children and adolescents.[577–584] They represent type 4 growth mechanism injuries involving each of the distal columns (Figs. 14-67 to 14-69). It is possible even to have an undisplaced intercondylar fracture (Fig. 14-70).[628] Most of these injuries are unstable.

Diagnosis is often difficult with standard views. Lateral condylar fractures commonly remain undiagnosed until

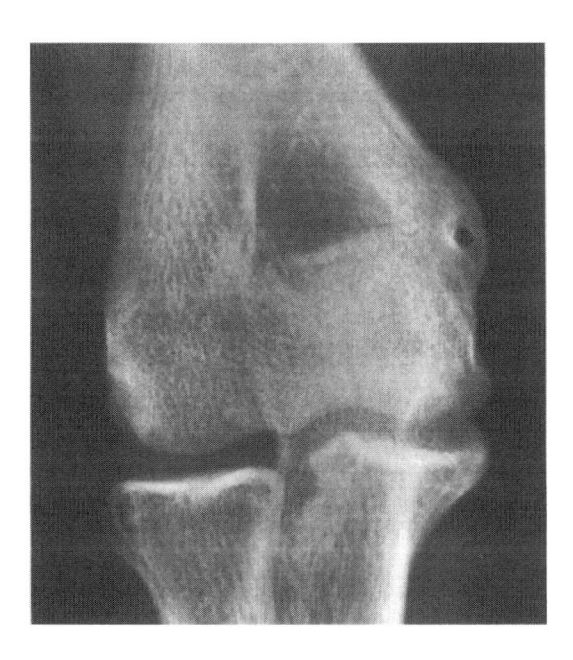

FIGURE 14-66. Matev sign due to entrapment of the ulnar nerve.

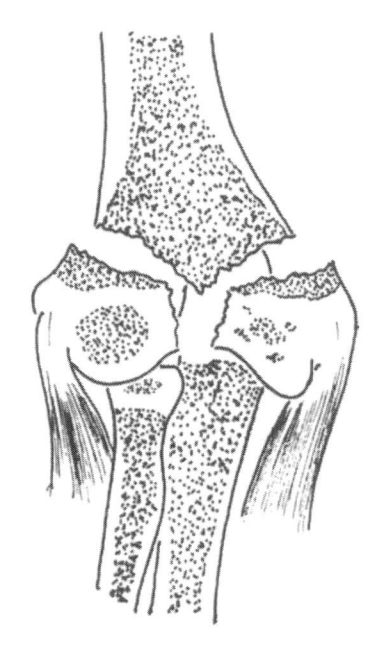

FIGURE 14-67. Intercondylar T fracture, creating a type 4 growth mechanism injury of each column.

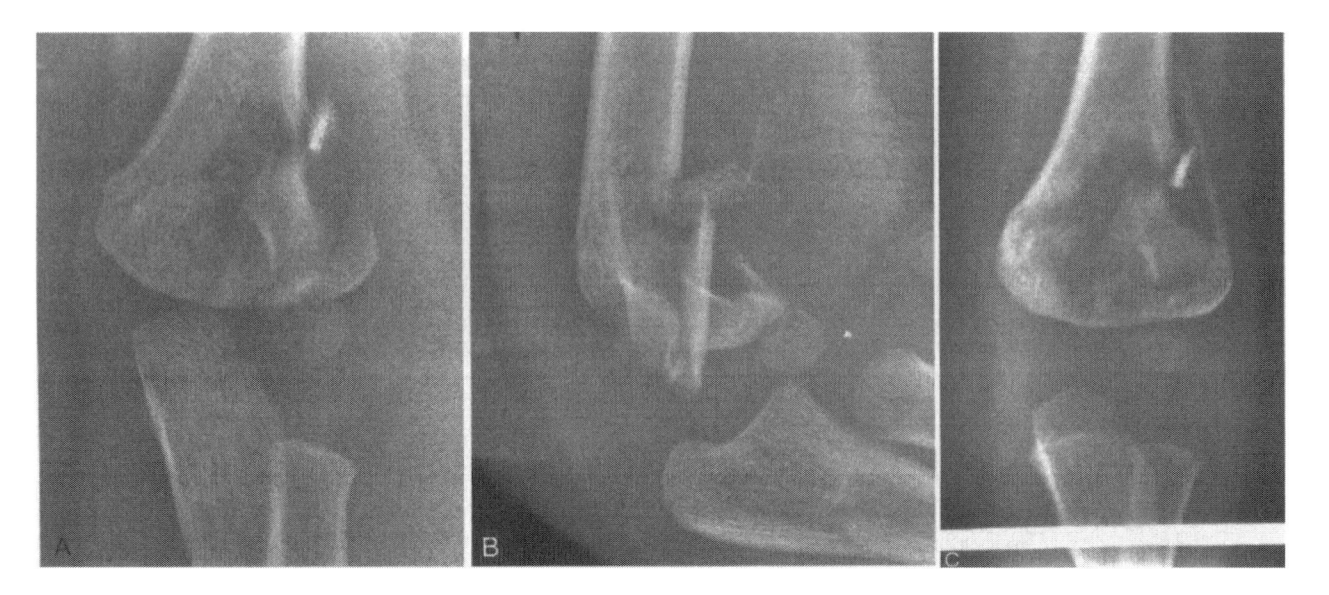

FIGURE 14-68. Anteroposterior (A) and lateral (B) views of a severely comminuted intercondylar fracture. (C) Appearance after 6 weeks in traction. The fracture is anatomically reduced. Note the subperiosteal new bone laterally.

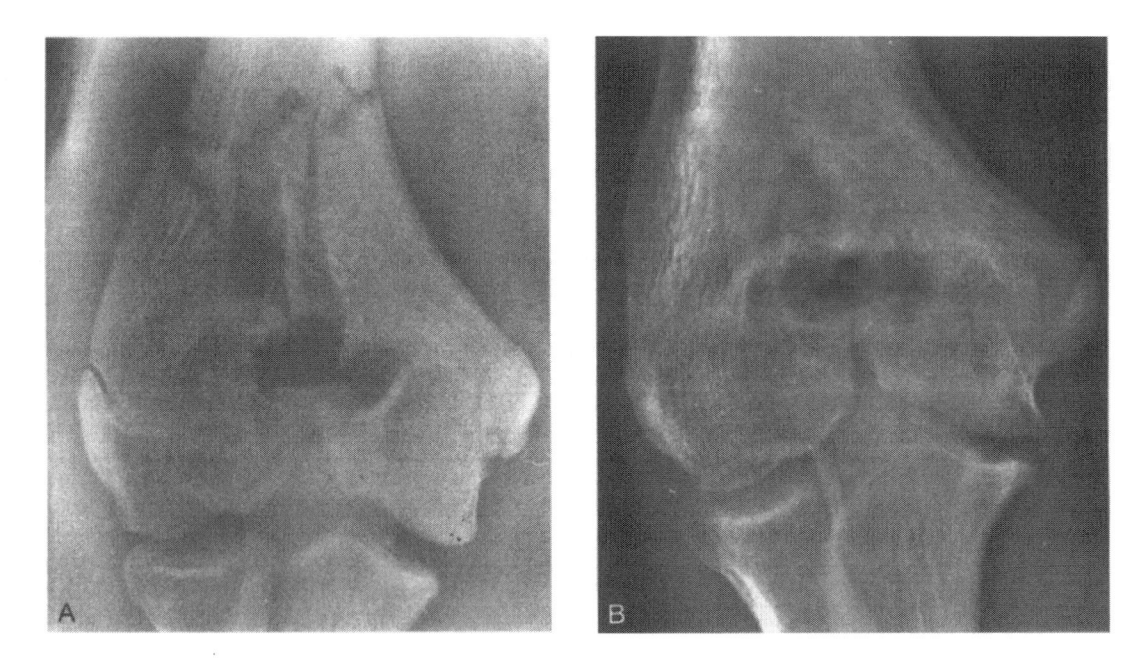

FIGURE 14-69. (A) Comminuted intercondylar fracture in an adolescent. It was treated by open reduction and multiple pin fixation. (B) Appearance 3 months later, with all pins removed.

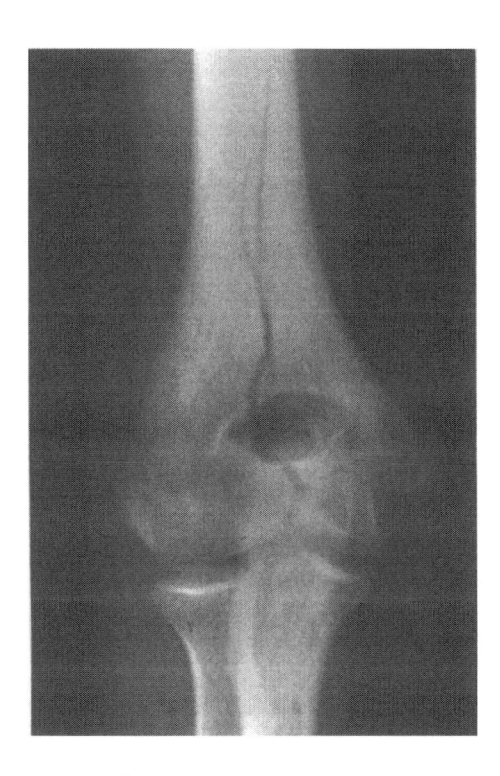

FIGURE 14-70. Undisplaced intercondylar fracture in a 15-year-old boy.

oblique films reveal the medial condylar fragment. An MRI scan may better delineate the fracture components (Fig. 14-71).

Treatment depends on the extent of soft tissue and osseous injury. If swelling or comminution is severe, olecranon traction is appropriate. If unstable fragments are present, some type of internal fixation may be necessary (Fig. 14-72). The recommended surgical approach is a posterior (triceps splitting) method.[632] Factors affecting the outcome include accuracy of reduction, development of ischemic necrosis of the trochlea or capitellum, and the degree of initial displacement.

A growth plate fracture pattern of a metaphyseal fracture (e.g., supracondylar) may have additional linear longitudinal propagation toward the physis. This pattern may propagate along the physeal–metaphyseal interface or into the epiphysis, creating a variation of intercondylar injury.

Transcondylar Injuries

Transcondylar injury of the entire distal humeral physis and epiphysis (Fig. 14-73) may be a much more common injury than is fully appreciated.[583-634] Smith is credited with the first description, in 1850.[628] It is often misdiagnosed as a dislocated elbow because of the difficulty interpreting the roentgenogram, particularly in neonates, infants, and young children.[588,601,605,610] The entire distal epiphysis of the humerus is displaced posteriorly, laterally, or forward, depending on the mechanism of the injury (Figs. 14-74, 14-75). The violence may be direct or indirect. Separation of the entire distal humeral epiphysis is a relatively common injury during difficult deliveries and the battered child syndrome (Fig. 14-76).

DeLee et al. described three categories of transcondylar distal humeral fracture.[596] Group A (0–9 months of age) had no capitellar ossification center visible and generally no or a minimal metaphyseal fragment. Group B (ages 7 months to 3 years) had a capitellar ossification center and usually a small metaphyseal fragment. Group C (ages 3–7 years) had a well developed capitellar ossification center and generally

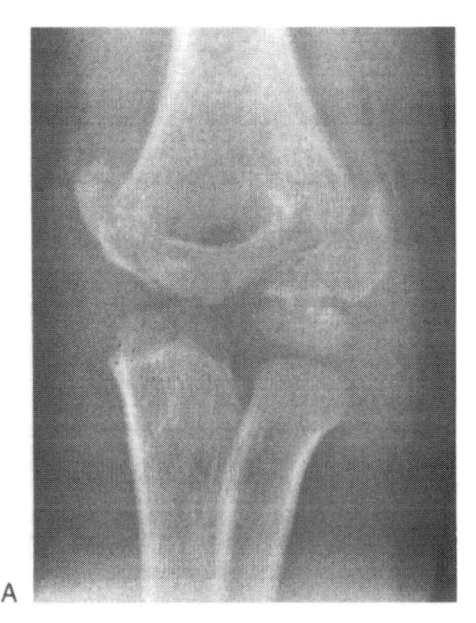

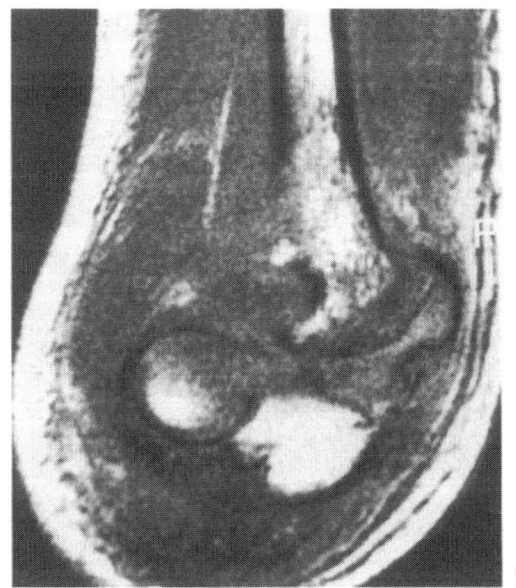

FIGURE 14-71. (A) Intercondylar fracture with two type 4 condylar fractures. (B) MRI shows the displacement.

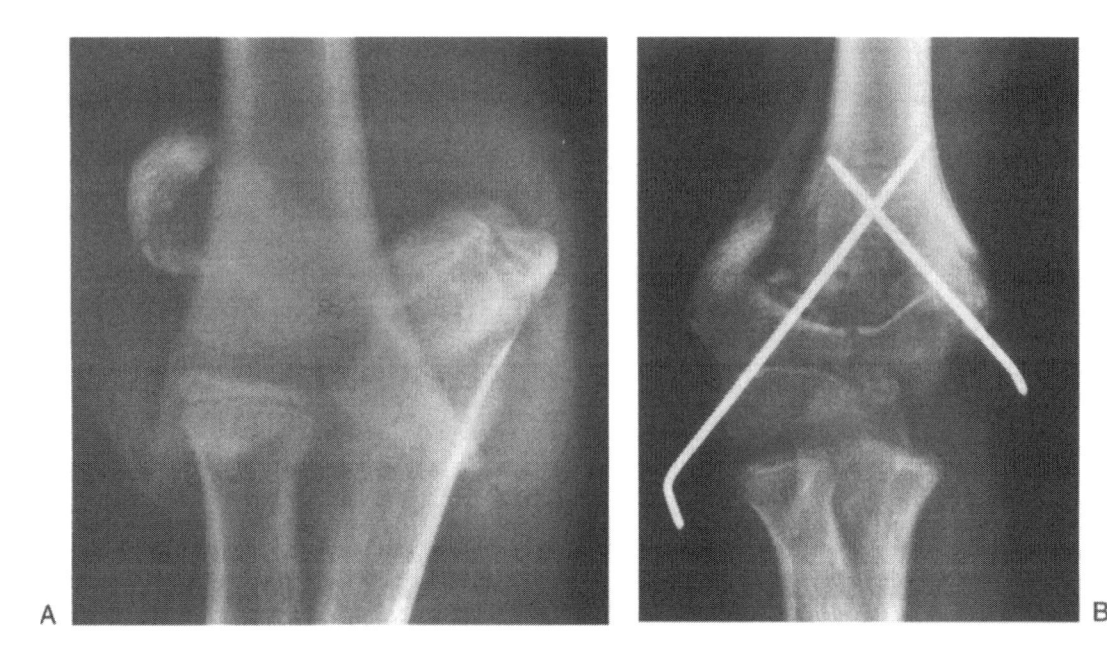

FIGURE 14-72. (A) Intercondylar fracture in a 9-year-old-boy. (B) It was reduced and pinned.

a large metaphyseal fragment.[319] Thus there was an age-related shift from a type 1 to a type 2 growth mechanism injury.

These fractures may be difficult to diagnose. The most important distinguishing feature is the normal relation of the ossification center of the capitellum to the proximal radius, although in the small infant child it may not be readily evident. A longitudinal line drawn through the shaft of the radius normally passes through the capitellum, but with dislocation of the elbow or radial head, it does not. The latter indicates some type of disruption of the radiohumeral joint.

A type 2 physeal injury of the entire epiphysis must be differentiated from a fracture of the lateral condyle of the

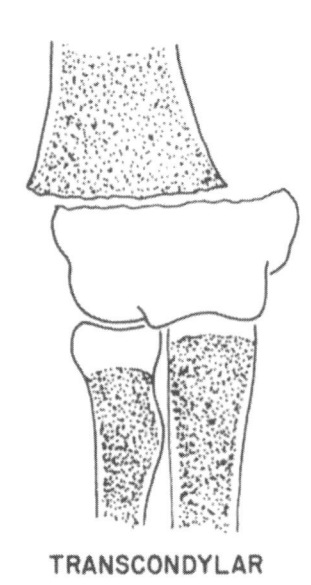

FIGURE 14-73. Transcondylar fracture, an injury of the entire distal humeral physis.

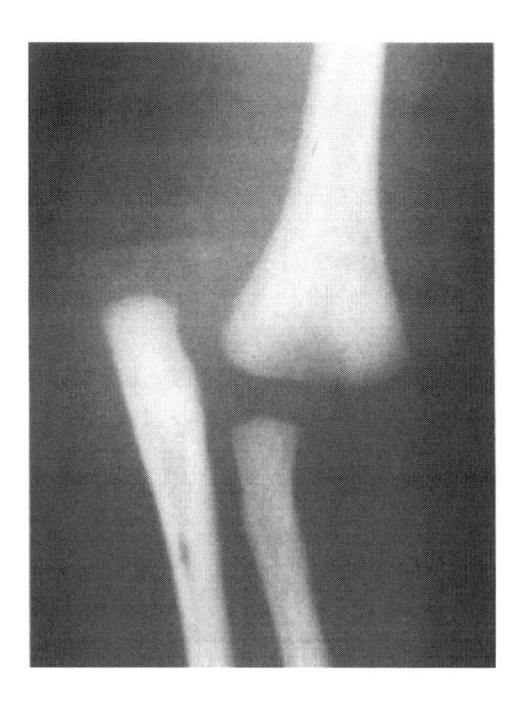

FIGURE 14-74. Apparent elbow dislocation. The medial displacement should make one consider a complete distal humeral fracture.

Transcondylar Injuries

FIGURE 14-75. Transcondylar fractures. Note the thin plate of metaphyseal bone (arrow). Another clue was the lateral view of the radius and ulna versus the anteroposterior view of the humerus.

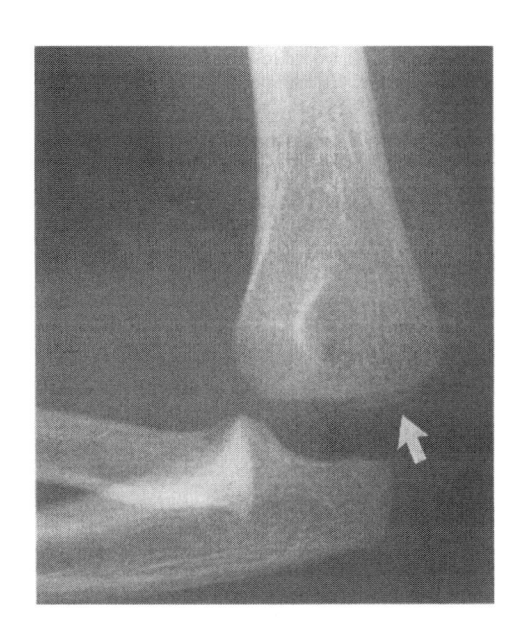

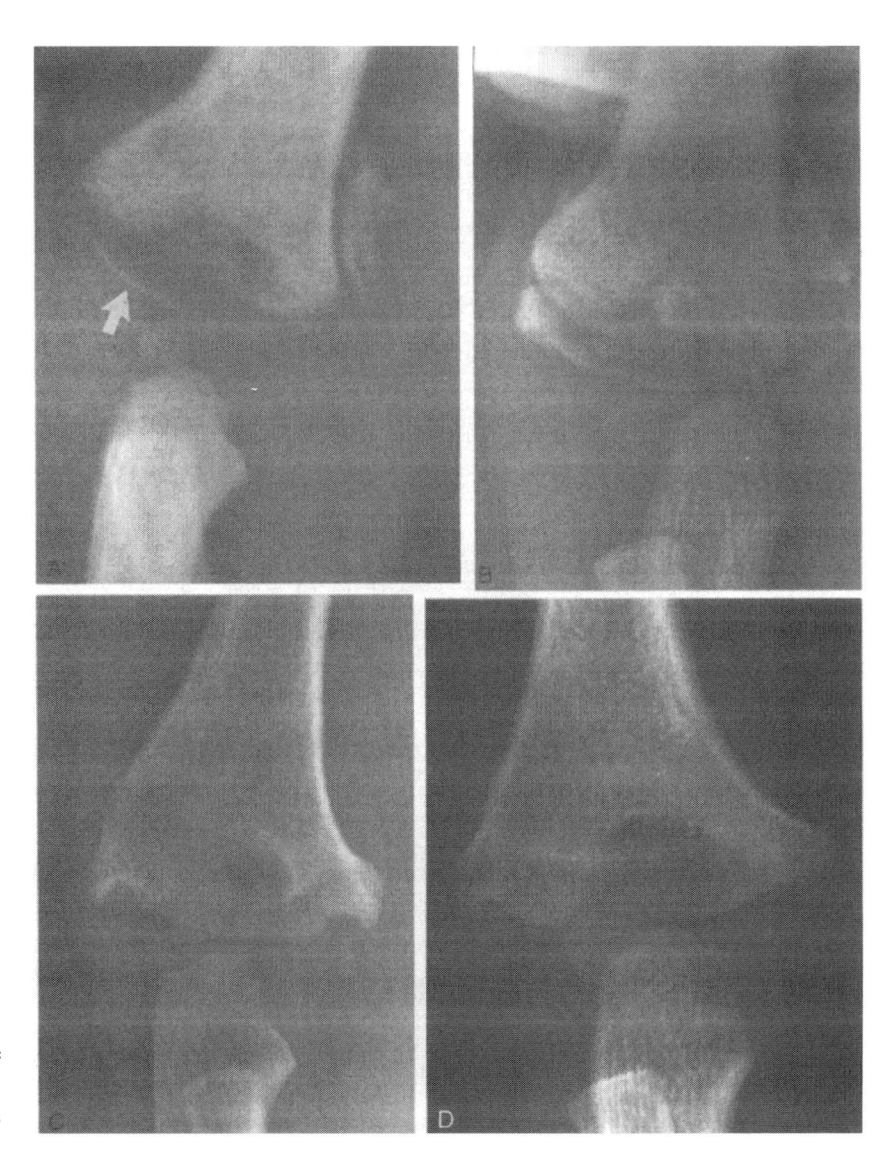

FIGURE 14-76. Child abuse. (A) Appearance of transcondylar fracture 3 weeks after injury. Note the thin metaphyseal bone (arrow). It was treated by closed reduction. (B) Six weeks. (C) Five months. (D) Two years.

humerus, which is a type 3 or 4 physeal injury. With type 3 or 4 physeal injuries the fracture fragment is often displaced by the pull of the common extensor muscles of the forearm, with subsequent loss of the normal relation of the radial head. Transcondylar epiphyseal separations usually displace medially, whereas elbow dislocations are usually lateral. Other fractures (e.g., olecranon) may also occur (Fig. 14-77).

Stricker et al. described a 3-year-old child with an unusual variation of a transcondylar fracture.[629] The fracture was a coronal fracture, as described for the lateral condyle (see Lateral Condyle Injuries, below) but also including the trochlea. An anterior portion of the metaphysis had led to a diagnosis of lateral condyle fracture. The olecranon was also fractured.

If the diagnosis cannot be made accurately, the child should be treated empirically. However, if there is any question, particularly regarding the possibility of deformity, it is feasible to use arthrography to help diagnose the injury (Fig. 14-78). Sonography also may be used.[589,623]

Closed reduction is the initial treatment of choice. Reduction is performed by traction on the forearm and, most importantly, gentle correction of the medial displacement and varus tilt of the epiphyseal fragment. Because the cross-sectional area at the physis (level of the fracture) is greater than that in the supracondylar area, the tendency to tilt and displace is less. Malrotation should be corrected. The elbow is flexed to 90° and the forearm pronated.

The distal epiphysis is usually displaced medially, and the medial portion of the periosteal hinge remains intact. Therefore by pronating the forearm, the intact periosteal sleeve may be used as a hinge to maintain the reduction.

Corroborative roentgenograms should be obtained to ensure the adequacy of reduction (Fig. 14-79). A posterior splint is applied for 3–4 weeks. Admission to the hospital following reduction allows monitoring of the circulation.

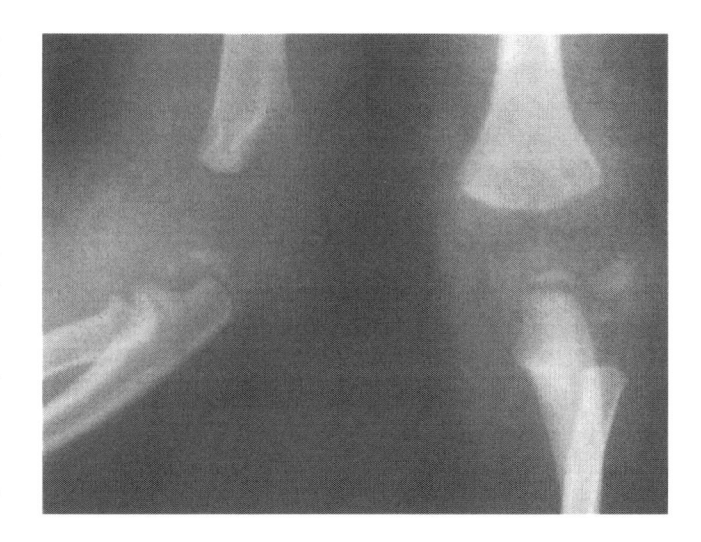

FIGURE 14-77. Combined transcondylar and olecranon fractures.

When there is a delay between the time of injury and the institution of medical care, there may be massive swelling about the elbow. It may necessitate traction following reduction to reduce the swelling.

Open reduction may be indicated, although closed reduction with percutaneous pinning is also an acceptable approach (Fig. 14-80). If the patient is not seen until several weeks have elapsed since the initial injury, reduction is not attempted. Any residual deformity may be corrected by osteotomy. In the case shown in Figure 14-81, no acute reduction was done. Several months later the altered anatomy was still impossible to define accurately. The entire condylar unit apparently has shifted medially, forming a large area of new

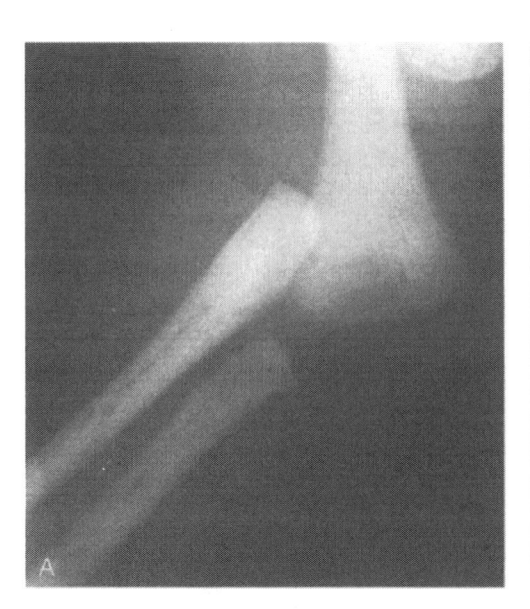

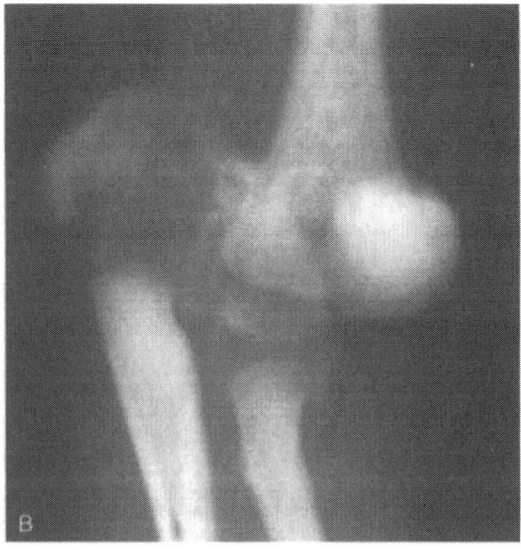

FIGURE 14-78. (A) Medial shift of radius and ulna. This is *not* a dislocation. (B) Arthrography outlines the displaced distal epiphysis.

Transcondylar Injuries

FIGURE 14-79. Closed reduction. Rotation, however, has *not* been corrected.

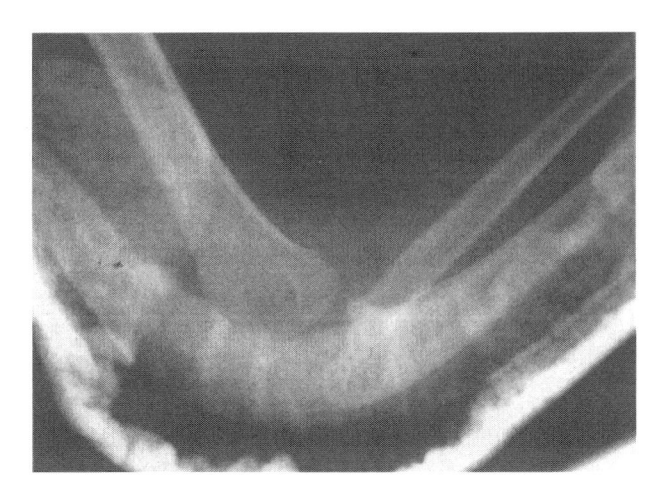

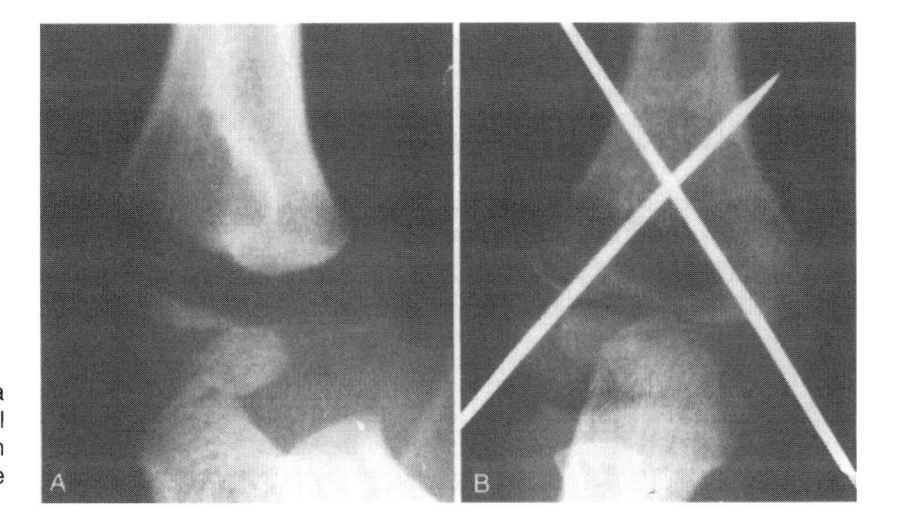

FIGURE 14-80. (A) Transcondylar fracture in a 2-year-old showing the complete metaphyseal plate. (B) This fracture was treated with open reduction and pin fixation (note air outlining the capitellum).

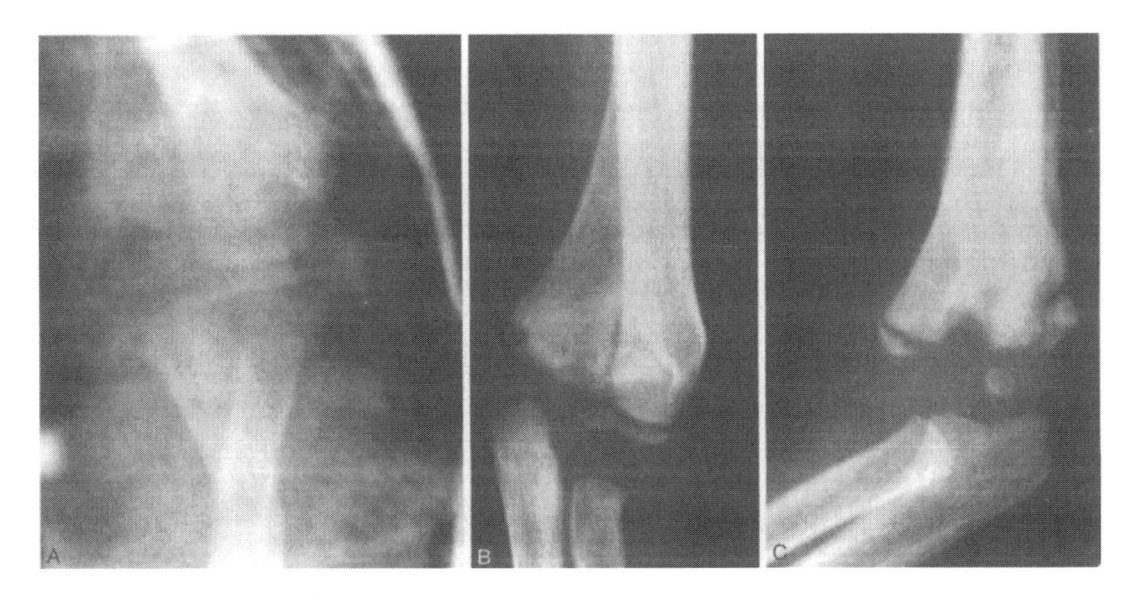

FIGURE 14-81. Unusual transcondylar fracture in an infant. Note the massive subperiosteal new bone formation. Apparently, the fracture left the lateral epicondyle attached to the proximal fragment. (A) Appearance early during initial treatment. (B, C) Large subperiosteal new bone segment medially, with irregular bone in the region of the presumptive lateral epicondyle.

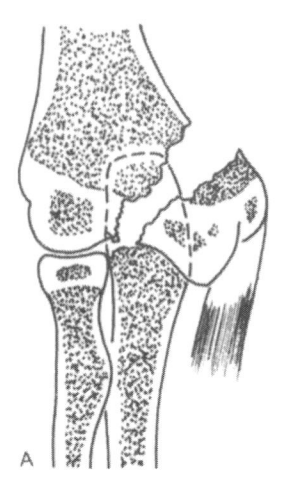

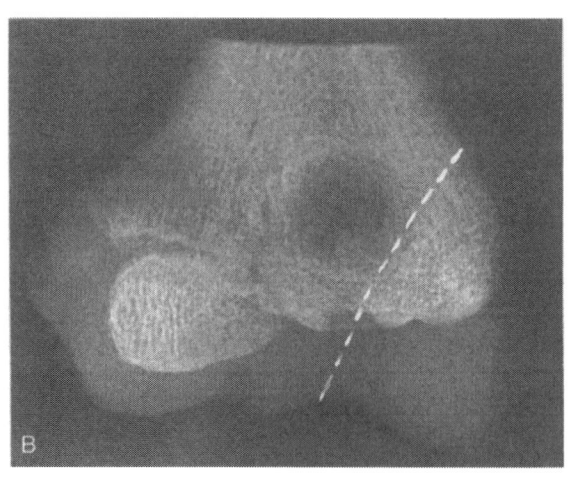

FIGURE 14-82. Type 4 injury of medial condyle. (A) The injury. (B) Typical fracture pattern (dotted line) on the specimen roentgenogram.

bone subperiosteally. Some of the lateral epicondyle was probably left behind and has subsequently ossified.

Cubitus varus occurs less frequently with transcondylar fractures than with supracondylar fractures, but growth deformity due to focal premature epiphysiodesis is a significant complication. Abe et al. found that 15 of 21 children with transcondylar fracture developed varus deformity following treatment.[585] One was progressive owing to a definite physeal injury. Neurovascular complications also appear infrequently.

Medial Condyle Injuries

Medial condyle injuries have been reported infrequently.[635–665] The fracture is comparable to the lateral condyle fracture, with a type 4 growth mechanism injury being the most common pattern (Fig. 14-82). Type 3 growth mechanism injuries also may occur. Epiphyseal propagation of the fracture probably remains within the trochlea. This injury may be confused with displacement of the medial epicondyle (Fig. 14-83), particularly if it occurs at a time when there is minimal ossification within the trochlear portion of the epiphysis.[638,642,651] Differentiation between condylar versus epicondylar is essential because treatment is quite different.

As part of the differential diagnosis, one must consider congenital abnormalities. Tanabu et al. described two cases of the hypoplasia of the trochlea that resulted in a progressive cubitus varus and ulnar nerve palsy.[663] Sato and Miura described several cases of hypoplasia of the trochlea.[661] Several other abnormalities were also present (hypoplastic capitellum, hypoplastic radial head). None of the patients had well-documented childhood injury.

In a review of fractures of the medial condyle, children less than 5 years of age tended to have undisplaced fractures that could be treated with closed methods and generally gave good results, whereas older children tended to have more

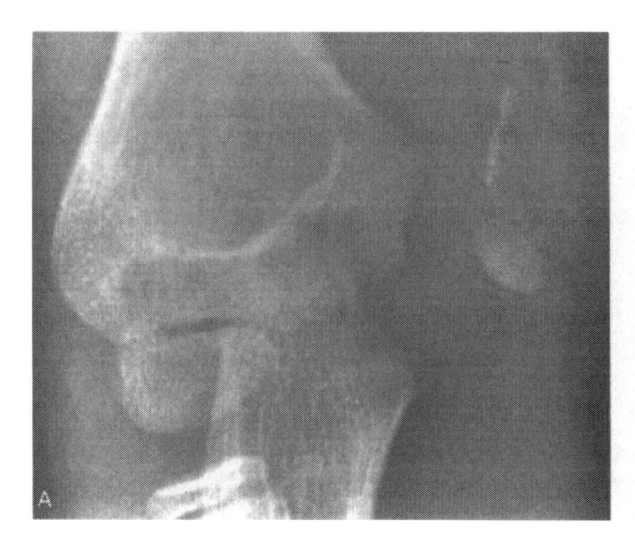

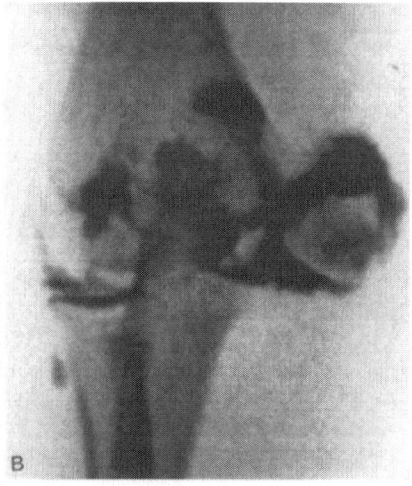

FIGURE 14-83. (A) Apparent displaced medial epicondylar injury. (B) Arthrogram shows the medial condylar component.

Medial Epicondyle Injuries

severely displaced fractures that required open reduction.[635] Good results were obtained when the patients were seen early after injury and when there was adequate reduction of their fractures.

Medial condylar fractures are usually unstable, with both physeal and articular surface disruption. In general, they should be treated with open reduction and accurate restoration of the joint congruency (Fig. 14-84). A posterior approach through or around the triceps is effective. Release of the ulnar nerve may be necessary to mobilize the fragment.

Significant complications have not been reported. Extensive dissection of the fragment should be avoided because it might predispose the patient to ischemic necrosis of the trochlea. A neglected medial condyle fracture may develop a nonunion (Fig. 14-85). Growth injury also may occur, leading to cubitus varus deformation.

Eighteen years after an original injury, Hanspal reviewed the case originally reported by Cothay.[638,649] This patient had a loss of 15° of full flexion, 15° of full extension, and a 10° decrease in the carrying angle compared to the opposite side. She was not complaining of any significant problems.

Repetitive stress injuries may involve the trochlea. They may lead to ischemic changes (Fig. 14-86) or fragmentation with a loose body (Fig. 14-87). Ferretti and Papandres described a trochlear stress fracture in a 14-year-old male gymnast.[644]

Medial Epicondyle Injuries

Fractures of the medial epicondyle usually occur between 7 and 15 years of age and constitute about 10% of all fractures of the elbow region in children.[666–714] This injury is unusual in young children. The mechanism is generally a valgus strain of the elbow joint that produces traction on the medial epicondyle through the flexor muscles (Fig. 14-88). The epicondyle may be variably displaced or even dislocated into the elbow joint owing to the opening up of the joint by a marked valgus stress.[666,697] There may be displacement in association with posterolateral dislocation of the elbow. Many of the cases are associated with partial or complete dislocation of the elbow (see Chapter 15).

Several patterns of epicondylar fracture are possible (Figs. 14-89 to 14-92). Epicondylar fractures represent type 3 or 4 growth mechanism injuries: Part of the fracture propagates through the epiphyseal cartilage between the epicondyle and condyle, disrupting the normally continuous distal humeral growth plate. Articular cartilage is not normally disrupted in this injury.

Physical findings often depend on the degree of displacement. The elbow usually is partially flexed for comfort.

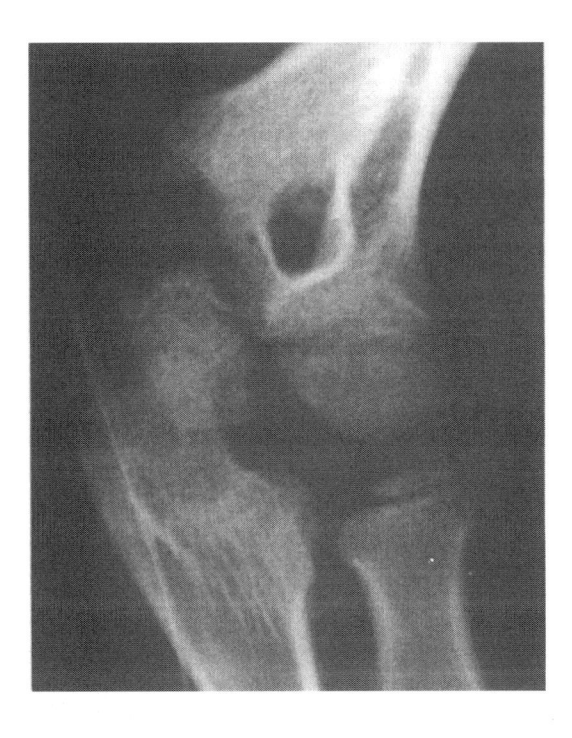

FIGURE 14-85. Untreated medial condyle fracture with established nonunion.

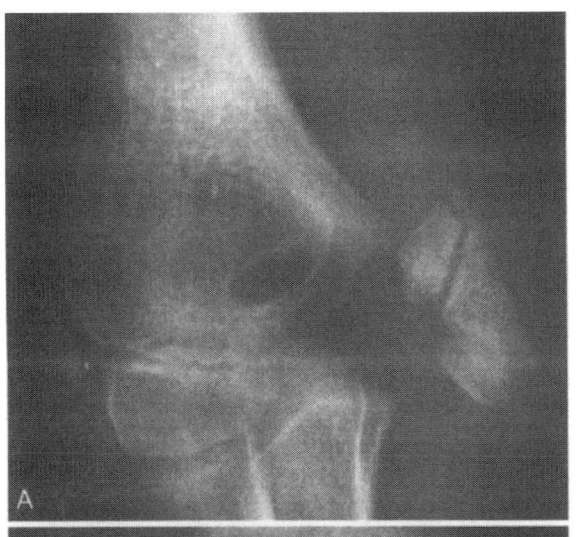

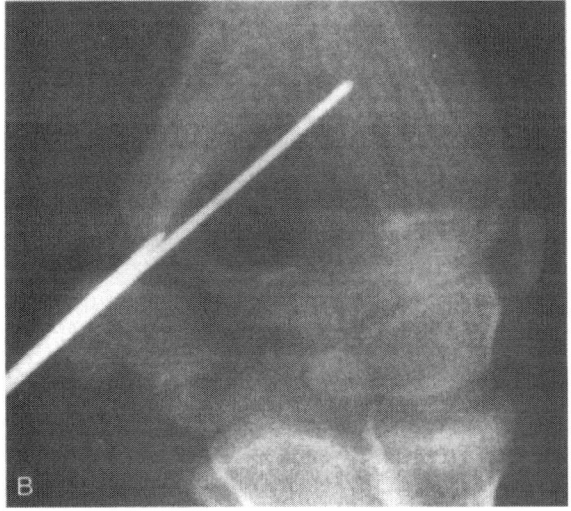

FIGURE 14-84. (A) Anteroposterior view of a type 4 injury with 90° of rotation of the fragment. (B) Appearance following open reduction.

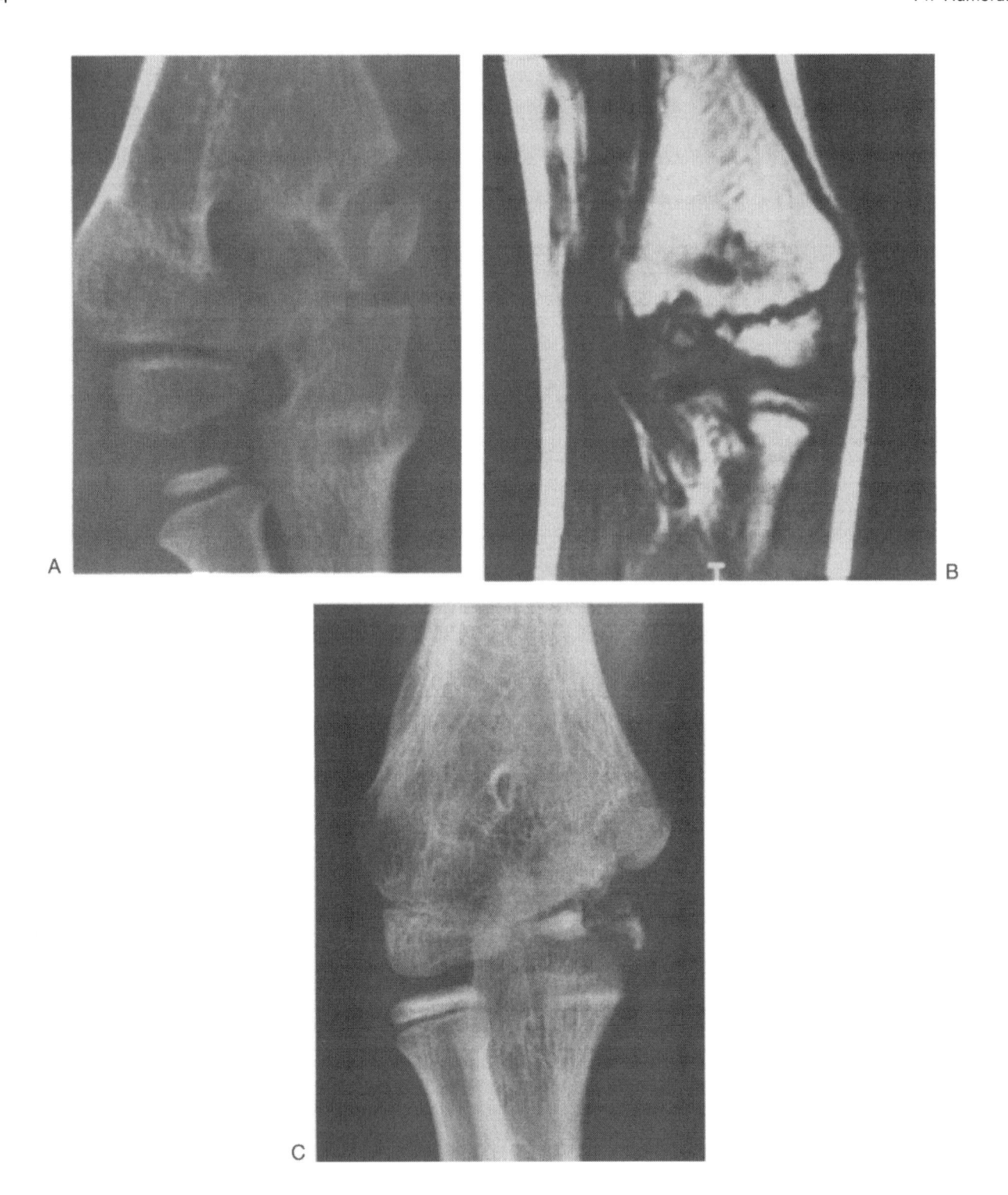

FIGURE 14-86. (A) Trochlear osteochondritis in a competitive gymnast. The patient had intermittent elbow pain. (B) MRI shows irregularity of the metaphysis and epiphysis. (C) Result 2 years later.

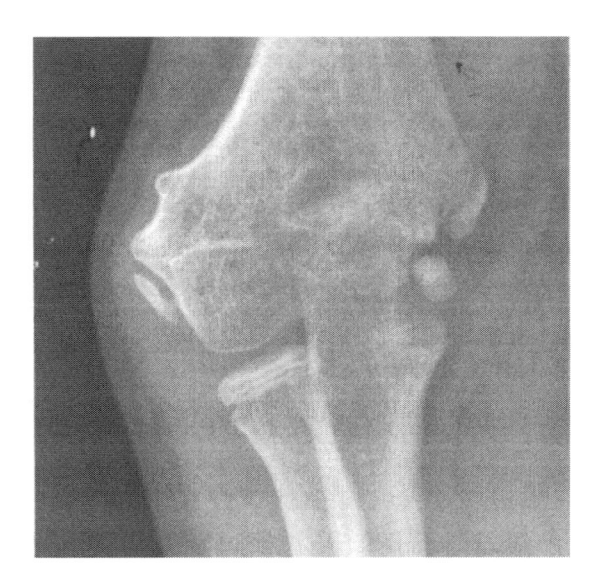

FIGURE 14-87. Chronic medial condylar injury due to pitching. There is sclerosis in some of the trochlear ossification and an osteochondritic fragment.

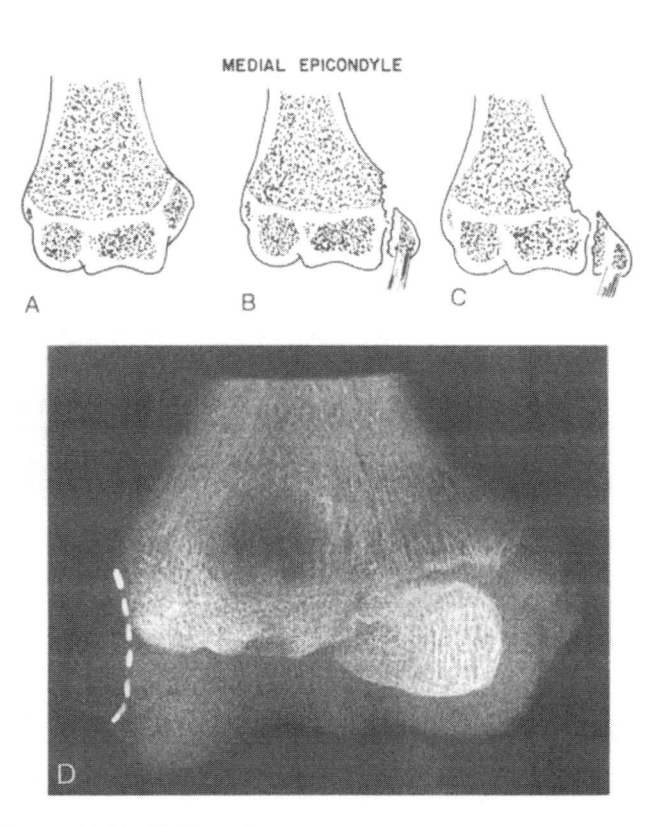

FIGURE 14-88. Medial epicondylar injury. (A) Normal. (B) Type 3. (C) Type 4. (D) Typical pattern of fracture (dotted line) depicted on a specimen.

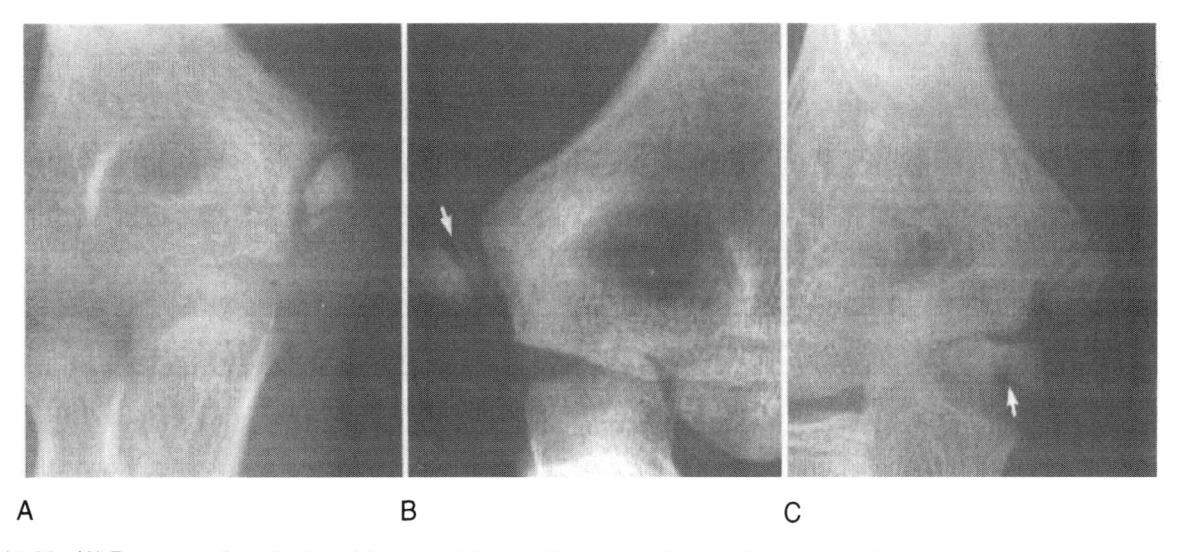

FIGURE 14-89. (A) Fragmented, undisplaced fracture of the medial epicondyle. (B) Displaced fracture showing a small metaphyseal fragment (arrow). (C) Propagation of a fracture into the medial condylar physis (arrow). This was an undisplaced "greenstick" injury. (D) Transversely directed fracture (arrow). (E) Sleeve fracture of the medial epicondyle.

D   E

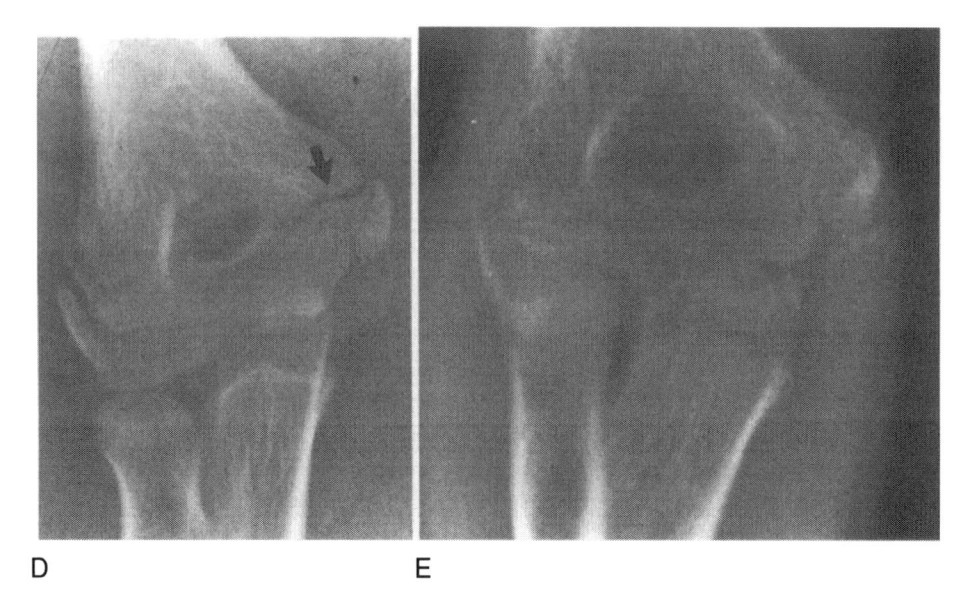

FIGURE 14-89. (*Continued*)

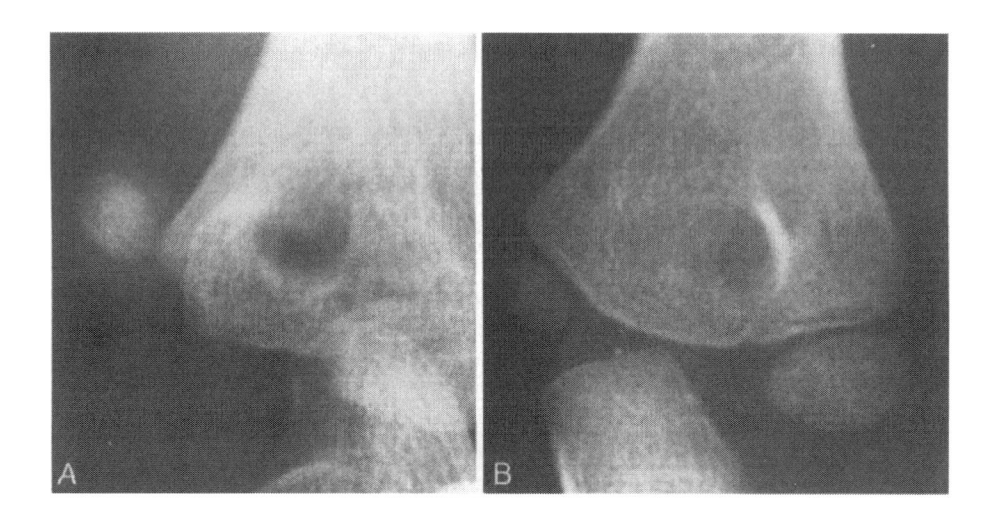

FIGURE 14-90. (A) Superior displacement. (B) Inferior displacement.

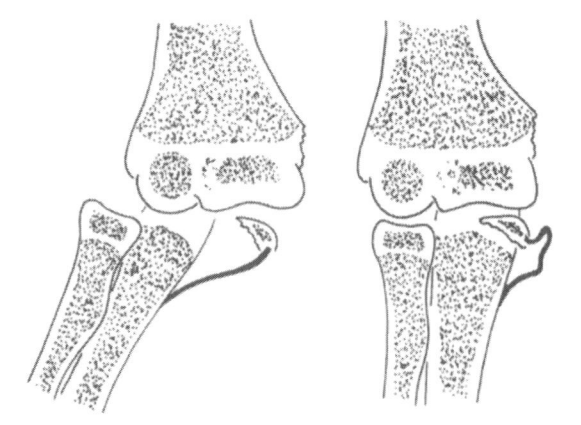

FIGURE 14-91. Intraarticular displacement.

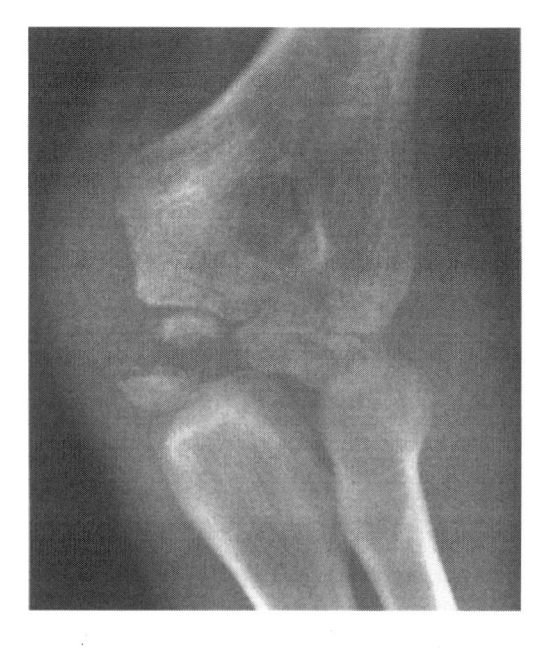

FIGURE 14-92. Intraarticular entrapment of the medial epicondyle. It was removed by arthrotomy.

Motion is painful, particularly to a valgus stress or pronation of the forearm. The medial joint line is tender. There are some diagnostic problems. The unossified region in a child less than 5 years of age is not easily diagnosed radiographically. Separation of the medial condyle may seem to be an epicondylar separation (Fig. 14-83).

The clinical signs of medial hematoma and pain may be more obvious than any radiographically evident separation of the epicondyle. The degree of displacement must be assessed as accurately as possible and the presence of concomitant injury noted. Concomitant fracture of the radial neck may occur as a result of the injury mechanism (see Chapter 16). The ulnar nerve frequently is traumatized by the force and direction of displacement.

Roentgenograms may disclose the absence of the medial epicondyle from its normal position or widening of its physis compared to the physis of the opposite side. The displaced fragment may be seen in the lateral and posterior-oblique projections. If the diagnosis is in doubt, roentgenograms of the opposite elbow are obtained in the same degree of rotation (remember, asymmetry may be normal). When the medial epicondyle is displaced into the joint space the articular cartilage space may be widened, although in a young child with a large mass of unossified cartilage in the trochlear region this is often not readily evident. When the elbow is dislocated posterolaterally, the medial epicondyle is usually located posterior to the trochlea. Stress views may be necessary to establish the true stability or instability of the lesion (Fig. 14-93).

If the medial epicondyle is displaced, the joint should be immobilized for 3 weeks in a long arm cast with the elbow in moderate flexion and the forearm in pronation. If the epicondyle is moderately displaced but the elbow is stable on valgus strain, treatment again consists of immobilization in a long arm cast for 3 weeks. According to some authors, the functional result may be excellent, even if the fracture heals by fibrous union.[667] Occasionally, the fragment fails to heal, and symptoms of ulnar nerve damage and irritation occur. If such symptoms supervene, the fragment should be excised. If closed treatment is chosen for treatment, the elbow is radiographed again in 4–5 days to see if the pull of the attached flexor musculature has caused subsequent or further displacement.

In a review of a large number of patients treated operatively, it was noted that if the fracture was displaced more than 2 mm consistently good results were obtained with closed reduction and percutaneous pinning.[687] If the medial epicondyle is markedly displaced (i.e., more than 5 mm) and rotated 90° or if the elbow joint is unstable on application of valgus strain, open reduction and internal fixation are indicated (Fig. 14-94).

A longitudinal incision placed slightly posteriorly allows visualization of the ulnar nerve. There often is significant hematoma throughout the subcutaneous tissue, and dissection must be carried out carefully down to the level of fracture. Any joint hematoma is evacuated. Some physicians recommend ignoring the ulnar nerve by not dissecting it. My impression has been that significant swelling and contusion are present, and neurolysis and decompression of the tunnel in which the ulnar nerve traverses usually results in alleviating symptoms in patients who had mild to moderate preop-

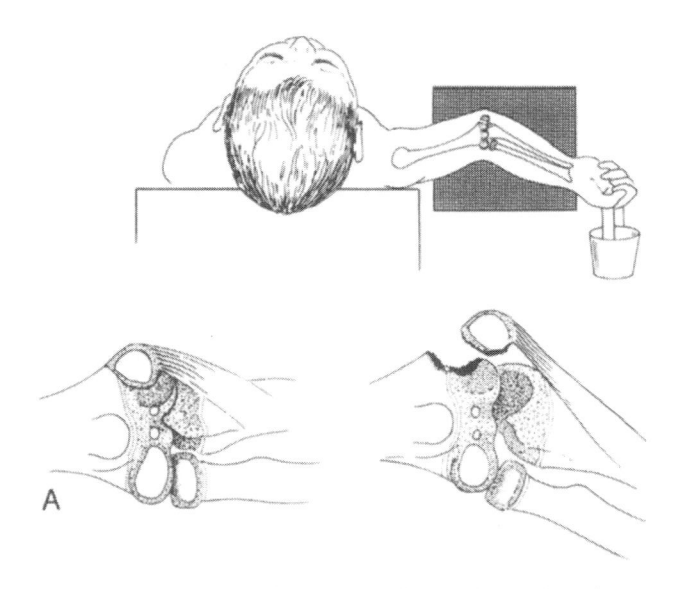

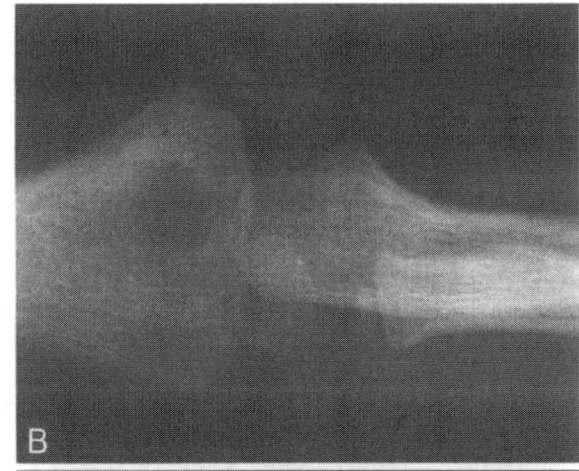

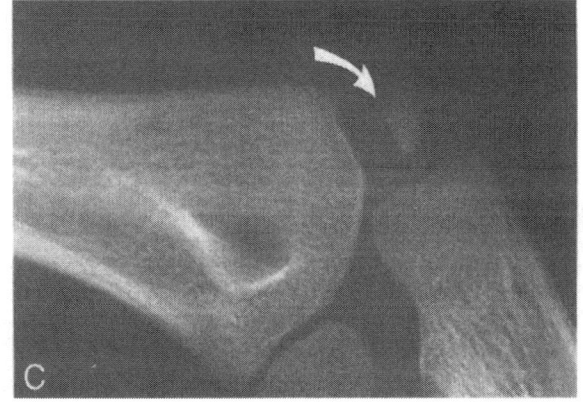

FIGURE 14-93. (A) Positioning for stress radiography. (B) Three-year-old child with pain over the medial epicondyle and apparent separation. (C) Application of valgus stress (arrow) pulled the epicondyle inferiorly.

erative ulnar compression symptomatology. This procedure also allows evaluation of the nerve, and in virtually every case some degree of contusion of the nerve has been evident. This explains some of the problems that develop as part of the normal healing phenomenon following closed reduction. To attribute all postoperative nerve injuries to surgical

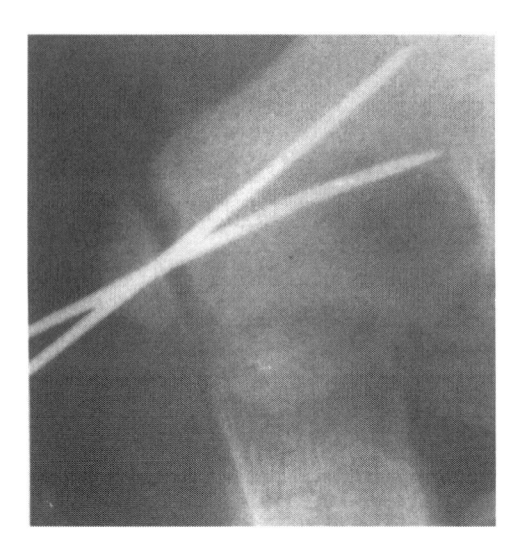

FIGURE 14-94. Open reduction with pin fixation of an unstable elbow.

trauma is probably inaccurate, inasmuch as these children are frequently operated on immediately after arrival at the hospital, sometimes without an adequate neurologic examination to ascertain the damage preoperatively. Furthermore, it might take a few days, or at least a few more hours, for the signs of neurologic damage from a contusion to develop. If the ulnar nerve has been displaced into the joint with the fragment, it must be extricated during open reduction.

The elbow is flexed and held in neutral rotation to minimize traction in the flexor muscles. Rotation may be checked by lining up the flexor muscle fibers. The fragment is secured by Kirschner wires: Two wires lessen the chance for rotation. The arm should be in a cast for 4–6 weeks, at which time the pins are removed and early motion is started. A small compression screw may also be used. Premature epiphysiodesis is unlikely to cause any long-term problems.

Skak et al. reviewed 24 displaced medial epicondylar fractures,[703] all but one of which had been treated by an open procedure. They were reviewed 2–13 years later. Five types of deformity were found: pseudarthrosis, ulnar sulcus, double-contoured epicondyle, hypoplasia, or hyperplasia. None of the deformities interfered seriously with daily activities, but there were symptoms and signs that made a difference between a good and an excellent result. The patients thought that their athletic ability was compromised. Skak et al. noted that some deformities occurred through the use of rigid internal fixation in the young child.

There are few reports of long-term follow-up of medial epicondylar fractures.[667] Treatment of medial epicondyle fractures purportedly produces good results. Flexion contractures of 40°–45° may occur if the patient is immobilized more than 3–4 weeks. Early immobilization of the elbow following medial epicondyle fractures within 3 weeks or less should be encouraged, although it may lead to delayed union or fibrous nonunion if the fracture has been treated nonoperatively.

Ulnar nerve paresis is a common complication of this injury but may not occur until several months or years after the initial injury.[714] It is probably more common with moderately displaced fractures that are allowed to heal by fibrous union and then develop an irritative pseudarthrosis. Excision of the fragment and neurolysis are usually sufficient treatment in such cases. Translocation of the nerve anterior to the epicondyle may also be necessary.

This injury is not usually associated with any major growth problems, primarily because it tends to occur at a time when physiologic physeal closure is commencing. Therefore premature epiphysiodesis generally does not result in any major growth deformity. Full extension may be slow to return and incomplete when it does, although this occurs in only a few cases.

Nonunion of medial epicondylar fractures may lead to pain (see Fig. 14-116, below). Josefsson and Danielsson followed 56 nonoperatively treated medial epicondylar fractures in children ranging in age from 7 to 17 years.[689] These patients and displacement ranging from 1 to 15 mm. They were examined an average of 35 years (range 21–48 years) after their injuries. Pseudarthrosis had developed in 31 patients, but only 3 had mild ulnar nerve symptoms. The function and range of motion of the elbow was good in all cases. The authors did not describe any significant radiologic changes of degenerative arthritis. If the epicondyle is painful, however, excision of the fragment may be undertaken.

Degenerative arthritis is an underemphasized, but real, long-term consequence of nonunion of the epicondyle with chronic elbow instability (Figs. 14-95, 14-96).

Woods and Tullos showed that the tendency of forward rotation of the medial epicondyle could interfere with collateral ligament function in certain positions, particularly if this is the dominant arm in a young athlete.[713] Chronic microdisruption of the medial epicondyle from repetitive stress may lead to radiographic changes (Fig. 14-97).

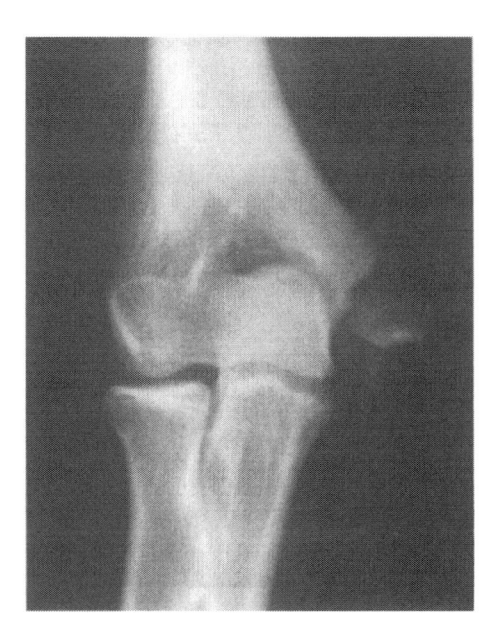

FIGURE 14-95. Displacement of fragments 2 years after a "normal" radiograph. This elbow was painful.

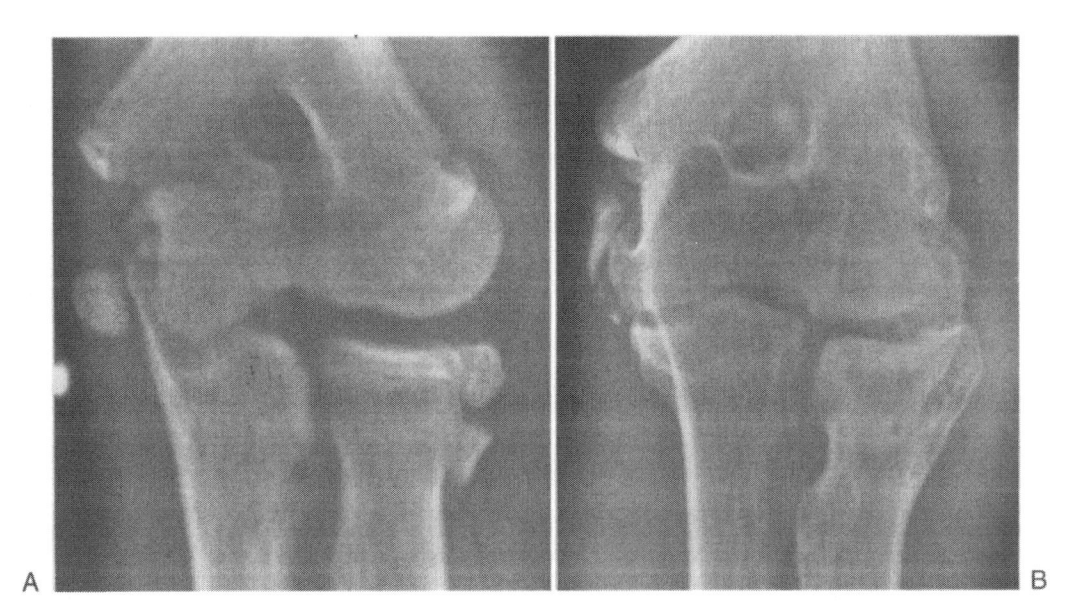

FIGURE 14-96. (A) Displaced medial epicondylar fracture and radial head fracture. Both were treated conservatively. (B) Similar combination of injuries. This patient is 27 years old and has incapacitating elbow pain.

Zaltz et al. found a high incidence of subluxation or dislocation of the ulnar nerve in patients.[714] Inoue described a 13-year-old boy who underwent closed reduction for an elbow dislocation. Six months later he presented because of restricted elbow motion. At arthrotomy the entrapped medial epicondylar fragment was removed.[688]

Lateral Condyle Injuries

Fractures of the lateral condyle are relatively common, constituting approximately 10–15% of all fractures in the region of the elbow.[715-807] These injuries occur in children between the ages of 3 and 14 years but seem to be most common between 6 and 10 years of age.

Classification

The injury is usually a type 4 physeal injury, although it also may be a type 3 injury if there is minimal or no extension of the fracture into the metaphysis (Fig. 14-98). In most instances however, there is a thin plate metaphysis where the fracture has propagated; therefore, by definition, a type 4 injury exists. The thin metaphyseal bone plate may be cen-

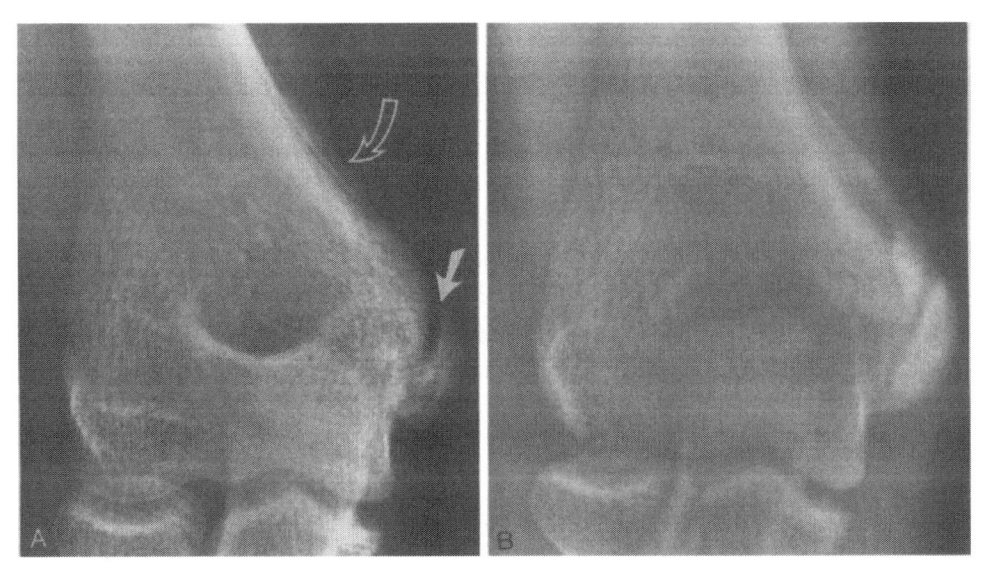

FIGURE 14-97. This Little League pitcher complained of a painful elbow. (A) Presenting film shows reactive bone (open arrow) and mild separation (solid arrow). (B) Healing 7 weeks later.

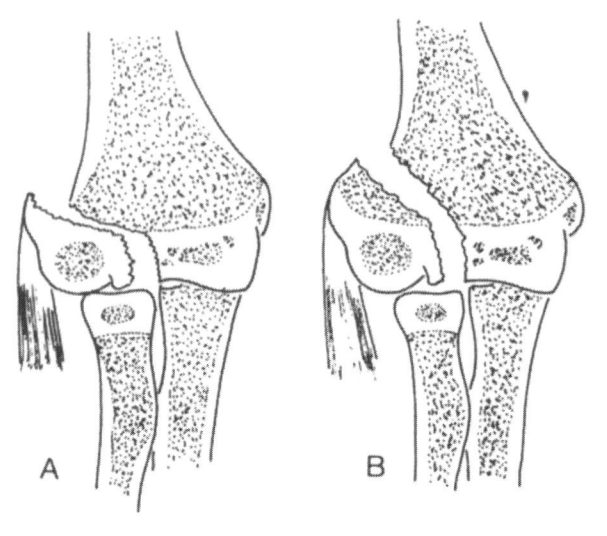

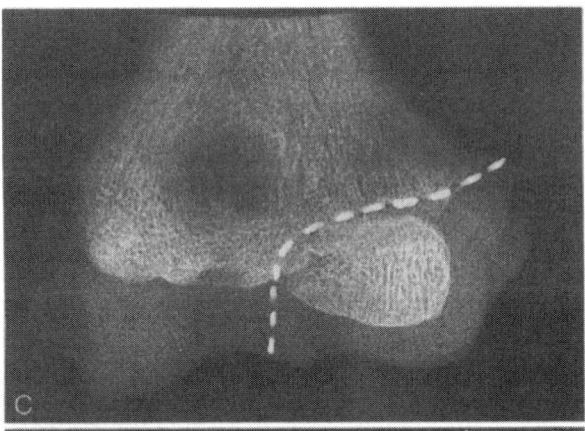

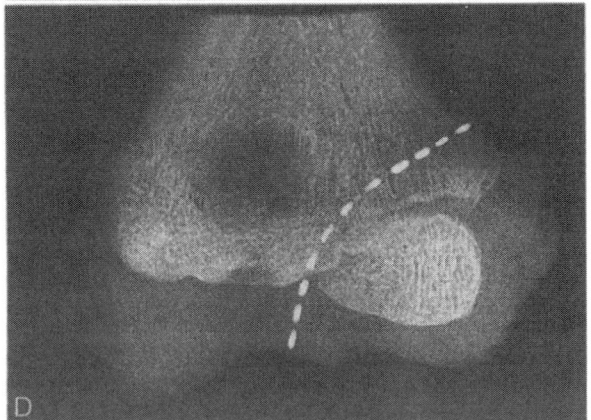

FIGURE 14-98. Type 3 (A) and type 4 (B) lateral condyle fractures. Note how the fracture does not involve just the capitellum but extends through part of the trochlear cartilage. (C, D) Specimen roentgenograms depicting these two patterns.

trally located because of the lappet contour of the physis. This fracture is both an intraarticular injury, and a disruption of a major portion of the physeal growth mechanism of the distal humerus (Figs. 14-99, 14-100). Propagation of the fracture through the epiphysis rarely occurs exactly at the junction between the trochlea and the capitellum. Most often the fracture extends into the trochlea to disrupt the trochlear articular surface. The capitellar articular surface is usually intact.

The condylar fragment usually includes the physis and secondary ossification center of the capitellum, cartilaginous portions of the trochlea (including physis), the lateral epicondyle, and part of the lateral metaphysis with the radial collateral ligament and the common tendon of the extensor muscles attached to it. The fracture fragment may be undisplaced or variably displaced and rotated by the pull of the extensors of the wrist and fingers (Figs. 14-101, 14-102).

The degree of the rotation of the fragment varies. It may be turned 90° so the articular surface faces inward (toward the remaining trochlea) and the fracture surface laterally (Fig. 14-103). In its extreme form, it is rotated 180° around both horizontal and vertical axes, with the distal articular surface facing outward and the lateral surface inward. If left in these malrotated positions, the apposition of joint surface cartilage to the remaining fracture surfaces of the metaphysis and trochlea invariably results in a nonunion and subsequent deformity, as the articular tissue is not associated with a normal process of ossification (see Chapter 1).

Less frequently there is a fracture through part of the capitellar ossification center (Fig. 14-104) (sleeve or shell fracture concept).[382] With such fractures only the capitellum and extreme lateral portions of the physis (especially the epicondyle) are involved.

Fractures of the lateral condyle of the humerus may also be associated with partial or complete medial dislocation of the elbow or with olecranon fractures (Fig. 14-105).

Lateral humeral condyle fractures have been classified into three types: (1) Incomplete fracture in which a hinge of articular cartilage is present, allowing some lateral angulation at the elbow, with no other displacement evident. (2) Complete fracture of the condyle in which the initial lateral displacement may be slight. The fracture fragment is free to move, and the displacement may be proximal, lateral, rotatory, or a combination.[779] (3) Complete fracture in which the fragment is displaced and rotated. Type 1 fractures are stable. Type 2 fractures are prone to progressive displacement, delayed union, or nonunion. Type 3 fractures do not unite unless they are reduced and fixed, which usually requires open reduction.[779]

Pathomechanics

The fracture usually results from indirect violence, such as a fall on the outstretched hand with the forearm abducted and the elbow extended. The force is transmitted through the radius. The lesion also may be produced by a traction force that thrusts the elbow into a varus position (Fig. 14-106). In such instances the fracture may begin at different points. When there is indirect force, as from a fall on the hand, the fracture may start as an intraarticular fracture propagating toward the physis. In contrast, a varus stress to the region

Lateral Condyle Injuries

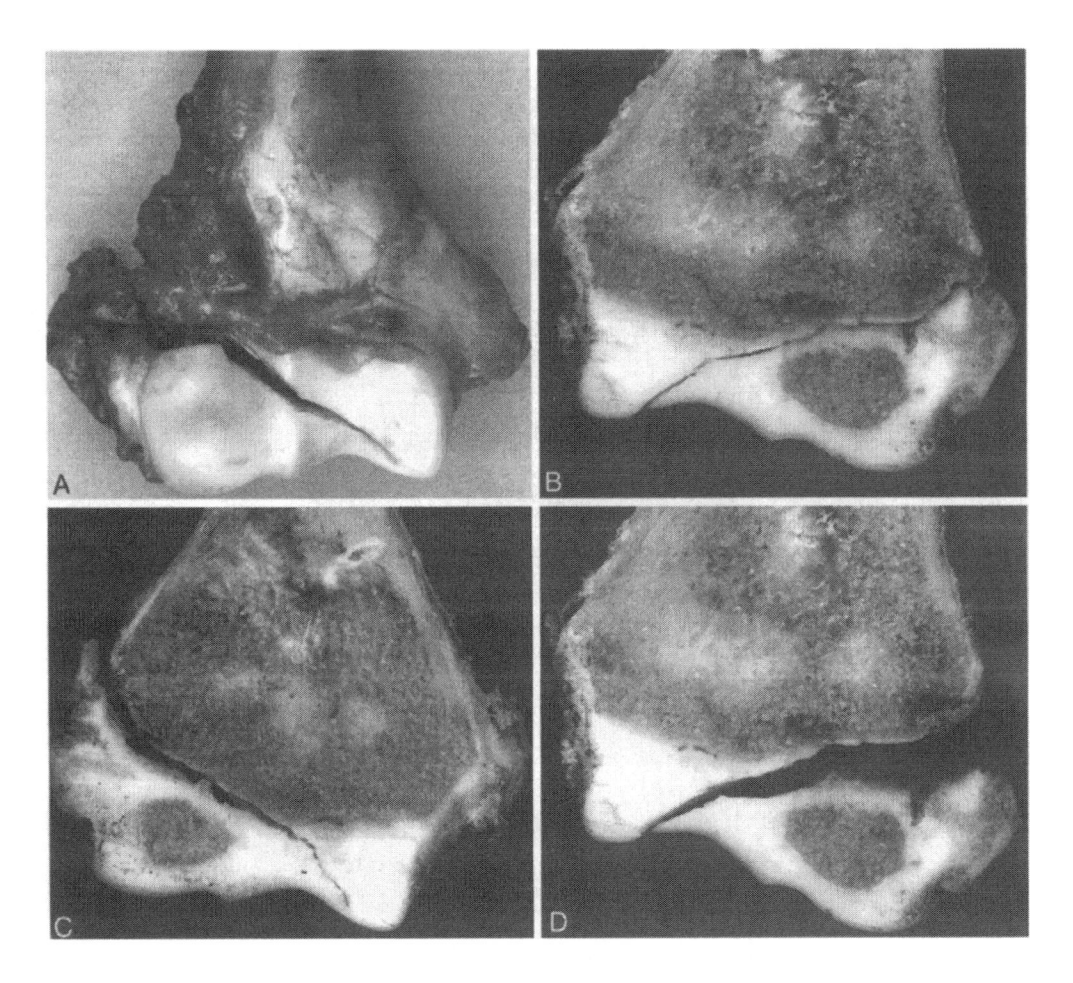

FIGURE 14-99. Lateral condyle fracture in a child sustaining a traumatic forequarter amputation. (A) Disruption of the articular surface of the trochlea. Note that the fracture is incomplete. (B, C, D) Variable displacements of the lateral condylar fracture.

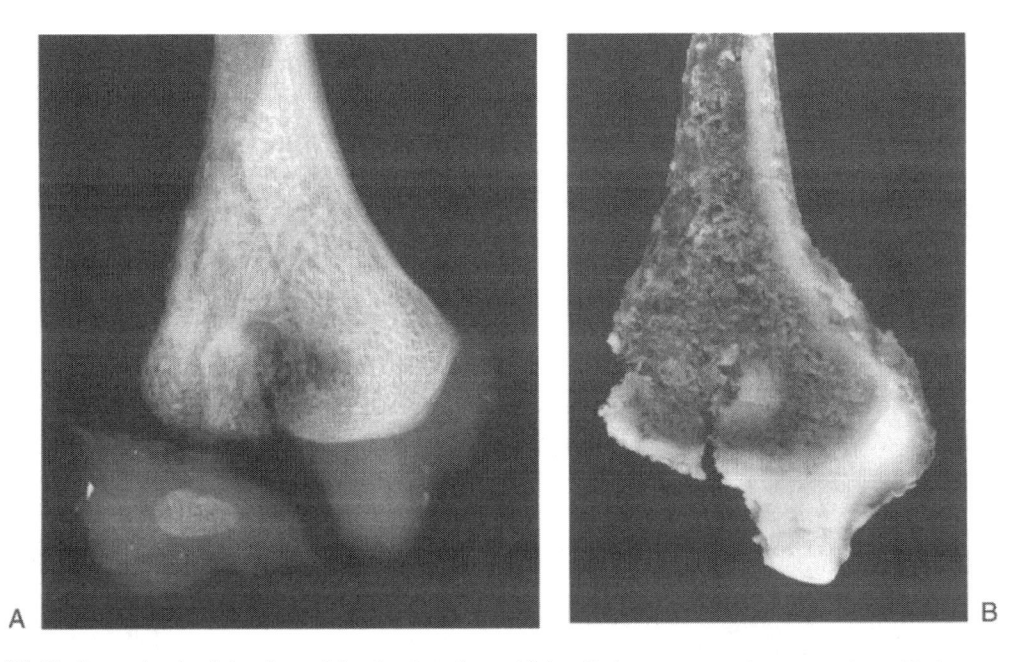

FIGURE 14-100. (A) Radiograph of a lateral condylar fracture in a child suffering a traumatic amputation. (B) Slab section showing a section of the capitellar physis on the "wrong" side of the fracture and additional longitudinal propagation into the supracondylar foramen.

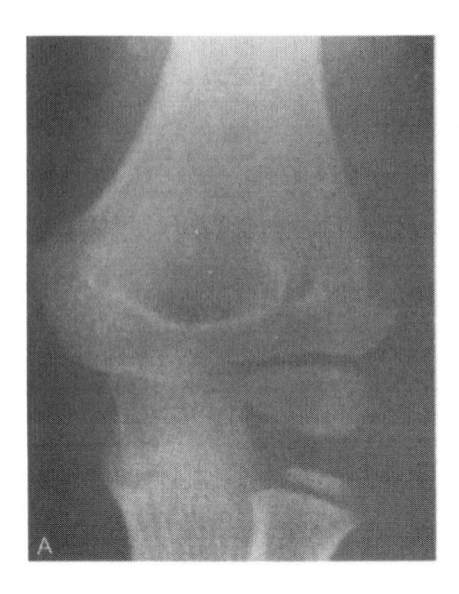

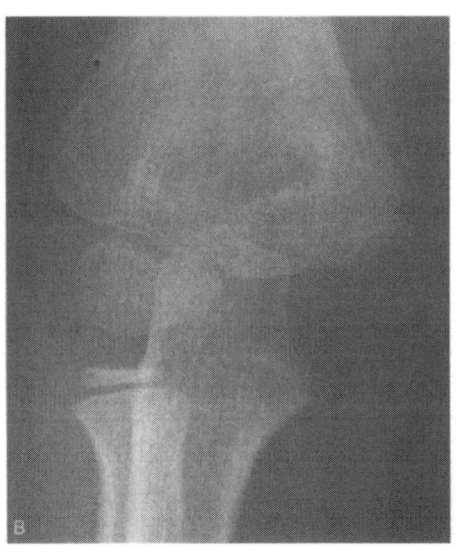

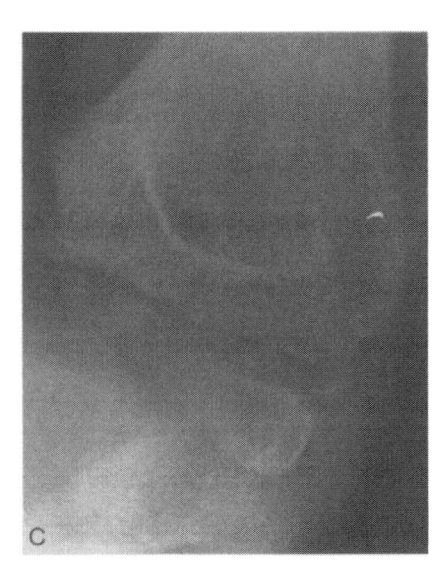

FIGURE 14-101. Undisplaced fractures through the lateral. (A) Metaphyseal disruption should alert one to condylar injury. (B) Thin metaphyseal (juxtaphyseal) remnant indicates the presence of a condylar injury. (C) Thin metaphyseal plate with propagation into the trochlear ossification center.

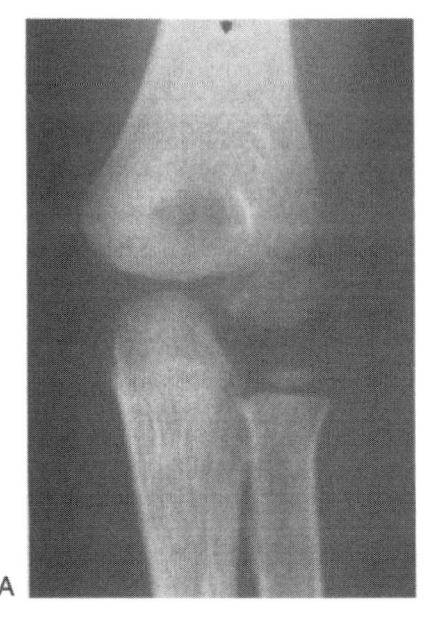

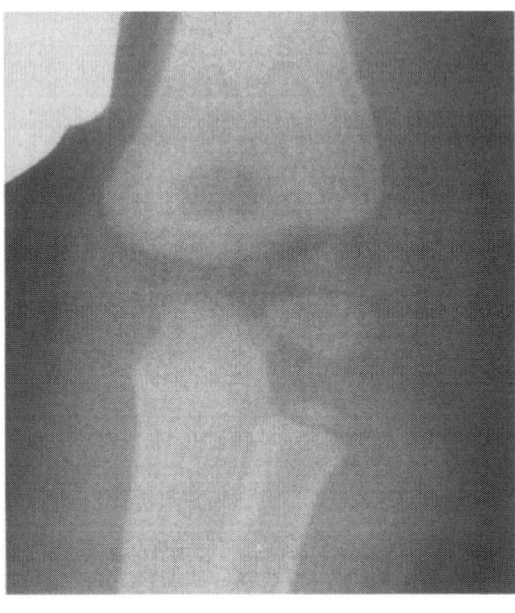

FIGURE 14-102. (A) Seemingly minimally displaced lateral condylar fracture. (B) Two weeks later separation is evident.

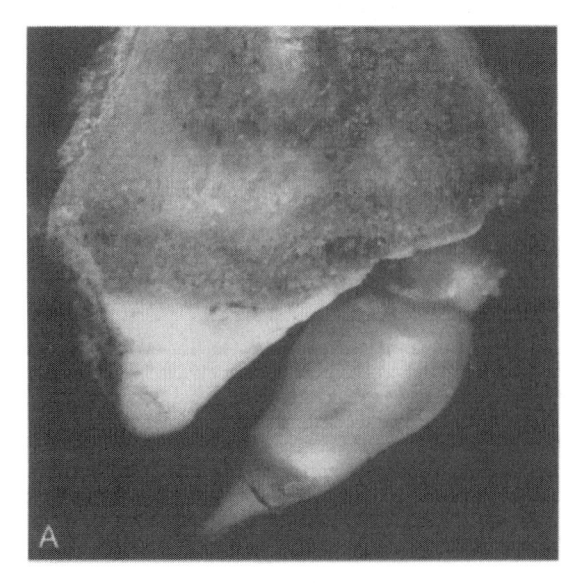

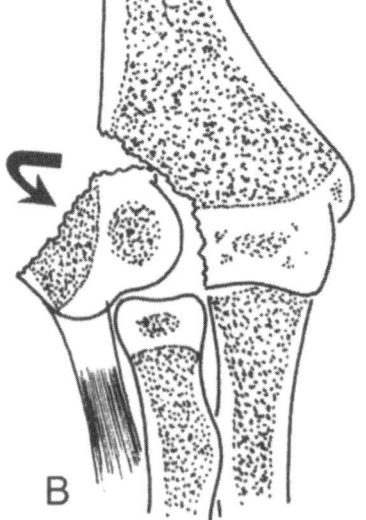

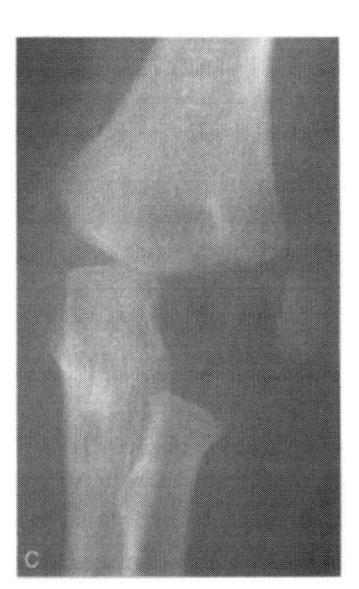

FIGURE 14-103. (A) Rotated lateral condylar fracture in a specimen. (B) Fragment rotation. (C) Clinical example.

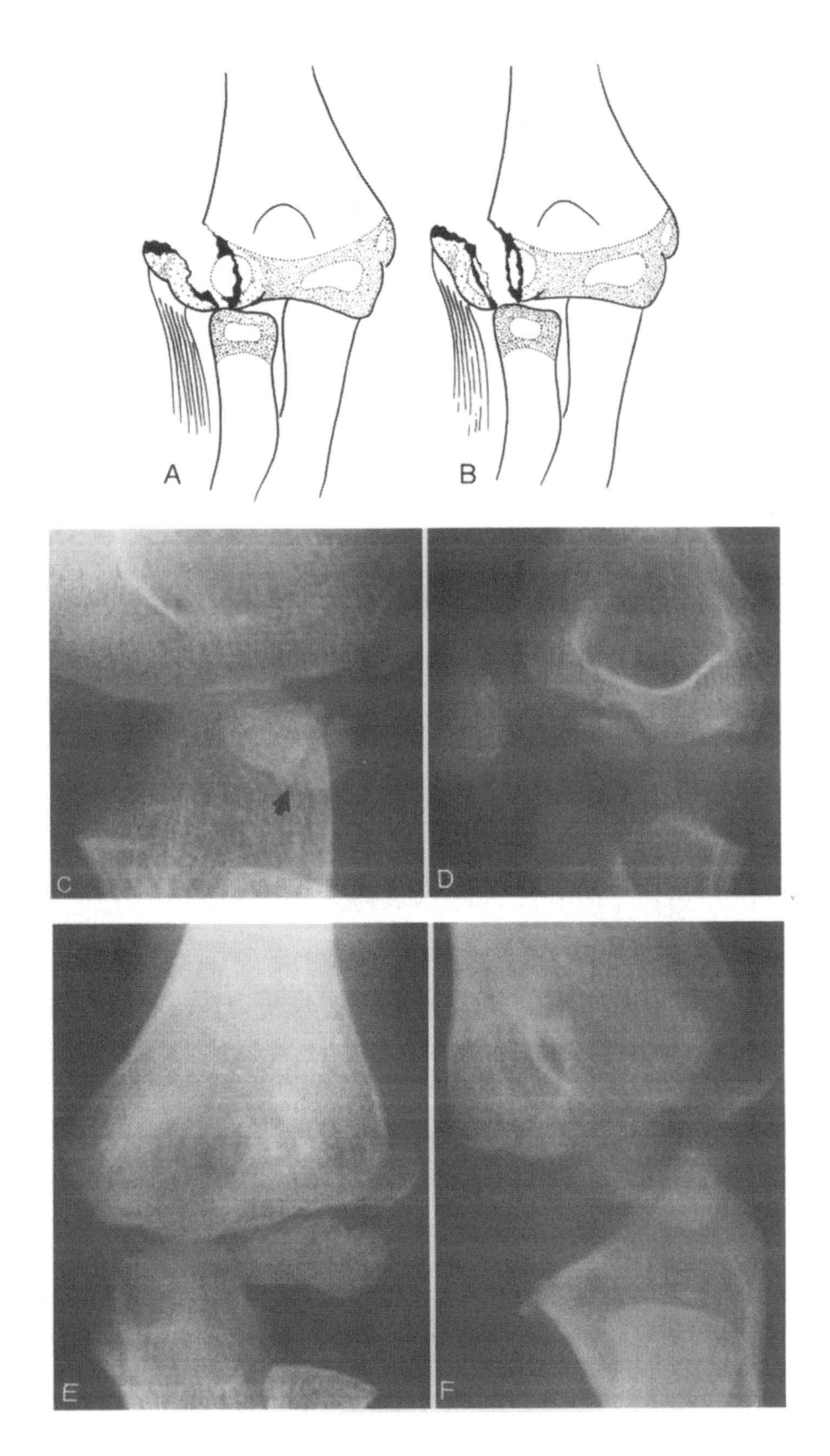

FIGURE 14-104. (A, B) Patterns of fractures *through* the capitellar ossification center. (C) Undisplaced (arrow). (D) Displaced. (E) Oblique view shows a metaphyseal fragment. (F) Stress view shows extension into the capitellum.

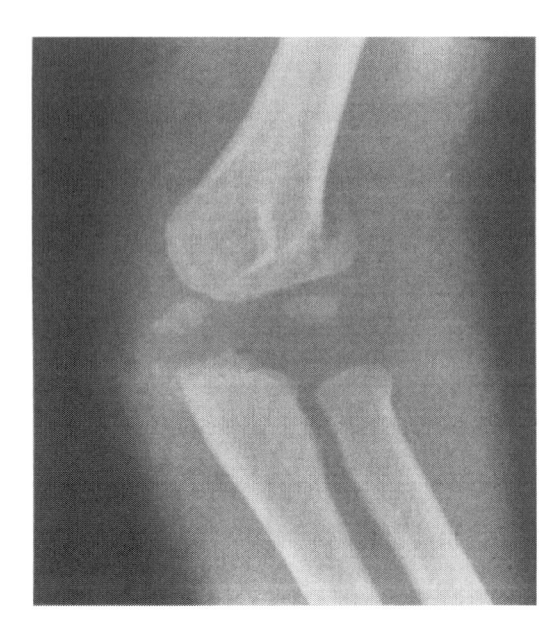

FIGURE 14-105. Combined lateral condyle and olecranon fractures. Is this medial epicondyle or olecranon?

may be associated with disruption of the peripheral zone of Ranvier and propagation across the physis to the junction of the capitellum and trochlea. The biomechanics of the cartilage probably change because of the variable appearance and size of the capitellar and trochlear ossification centers.

Jakob et al. produced this fracture experimentally by applying a varus strain to the extended elbow.[765] In this anatomic study, the only deforming force that produced a fracture of the lateral condyle was forced varus angulation with the elbow extended and the forearm supinated. This caused a fracture in four of seven elbows. The children, all of whom had died from injury, were between 2.5 and 10 years of age at the time of death. In one case there was an associated transverse adduction fracture of the olecranon, as seen in the clinical situation. In three of the four elbows the lateral condylar fragment was attached to the trochlea by a substantial bridge of cartilage. When the arm was repositioned, this bridge acted as a hinge, guiding the fragment back into position, preventing significant displacement, and maintaining an intact articular surface enclosing the fracture line. Whether this occurs in the clinical situation is difficult to say. However, the case shown in Figure 14-99 shows that an incomplete (hinged) fracture may occur clinically. Arthrography may help delineate this situation, particularly if there is any question about whether to go ahead with an open reduction. The trochlear ridge on the ulna behaves as a fulcrum for avulsion of the lateral condyle by the lateral fragment. The bone separates, but some epiphyseal and articular cartilage may remain intact as a hinge. As soon as this hinge is divided, the fracture becomes highly unstable, and the condyle can be easily displaced and rotated. The hinged fracture reduces when the varus angulation is corrected. If deforming angulation is increased, the cartilage hinge may tear, which may lead to fracture displacement and dislocation of the elbow (type 4 injury). The incomplete and complete injury patterns have been encountered in traumatically amputated arms.

Some of the blood supply to the lateral condyle enters by its soft tissue attachments, particularly posteriorly at the origin of the long extensor muscles.[754] However, the important intracartilaginous vessels traverse between trochlea and capitellum and are disrupted by the transepiphyseal nature of the fracture. Extensive dissection during open reduction may affect the remaining vascularity beyond the initial traumatic disruption.

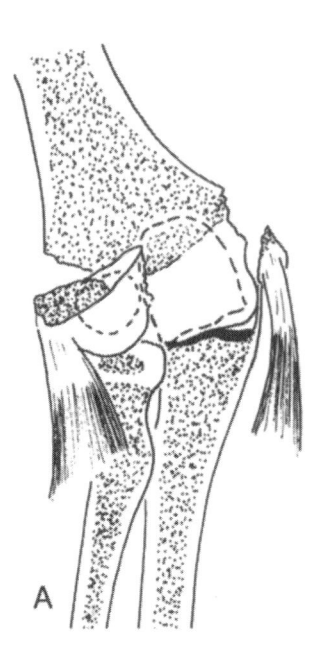

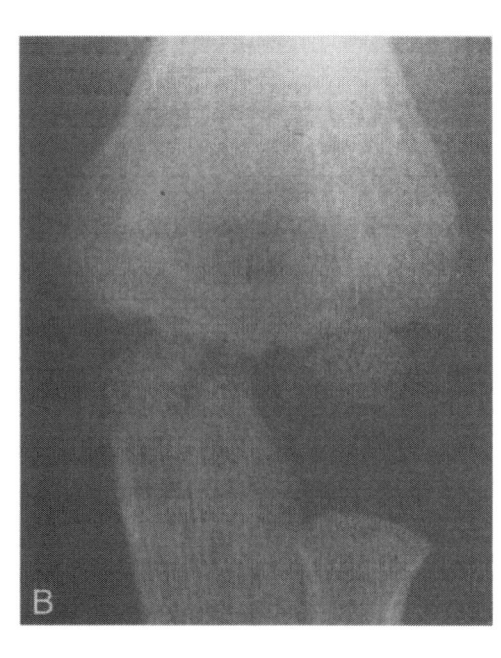

FIGURE 14-106. (A) Formation of a fracture by "locking" of the olecranon and concomitant fracture of the olecranon. (B) Example of the injury pattern with concomitant olecranon and lateral condylar fractures.

Diagnosis

These patients generally have severe pain following injury, with marked swelling, ecchymosis, and local tenderness over the lateral portion of the elbow. Rotation of the forearm is often unrestricted, especially with undisplaced fractures, but it may be quite painful. In most cases the diagnosis can be made easily by the roentgenographic findings. Sometimes only the oblique view discloses either displacement or evidence of the undisplaced fracture line. A true lateral view, particularly when compared to the opposite side, may show loss of the normal anterior tilt of the capitellum, suggesting the diagnosis.

Lateral condylar fractures are serious injuries. The fracture is often diagnosed merely as a chip fracture on the outer margin of the elbow (i.e., the metaphysis) and is not recognized as being half of the distal humerus. This leads to undertreatment, allowing fracture motion and increasing the likelihood of delayed union or nonunion.

Grossly displaced fractures are usually obvious on radiographs, but undisplaced ("hairline") fractures are easy to miss. When there is clinical evidence of a fracture but no radiographic signs, further views should be obtained, particularly oblique views, until the fracture is evident or ruled out as unlikely. Stress films may be used to show this fracture (Fig. 14-107). In the particularly young child, the ossification center may not be present, and the true nature of the injury may not be completely comprehended. An arthrogram may help (Fig. 14-108). The younger the child and the less well developed the ossification centers, the greater is the likelihood that this injury will be overlooked. MRI may better define the fracture morphology (Fig. 14-109).

Treatment

With lateral condyle fractures, it is recognized that displacement is almost always underestimated on routine radiographic studies. At surgery one is often surprised by the instability of these fractures. Surgical techniques must be minimally aggressive to preserve the soft tissues essential to condylar vascularization. One should not hesitate to incise

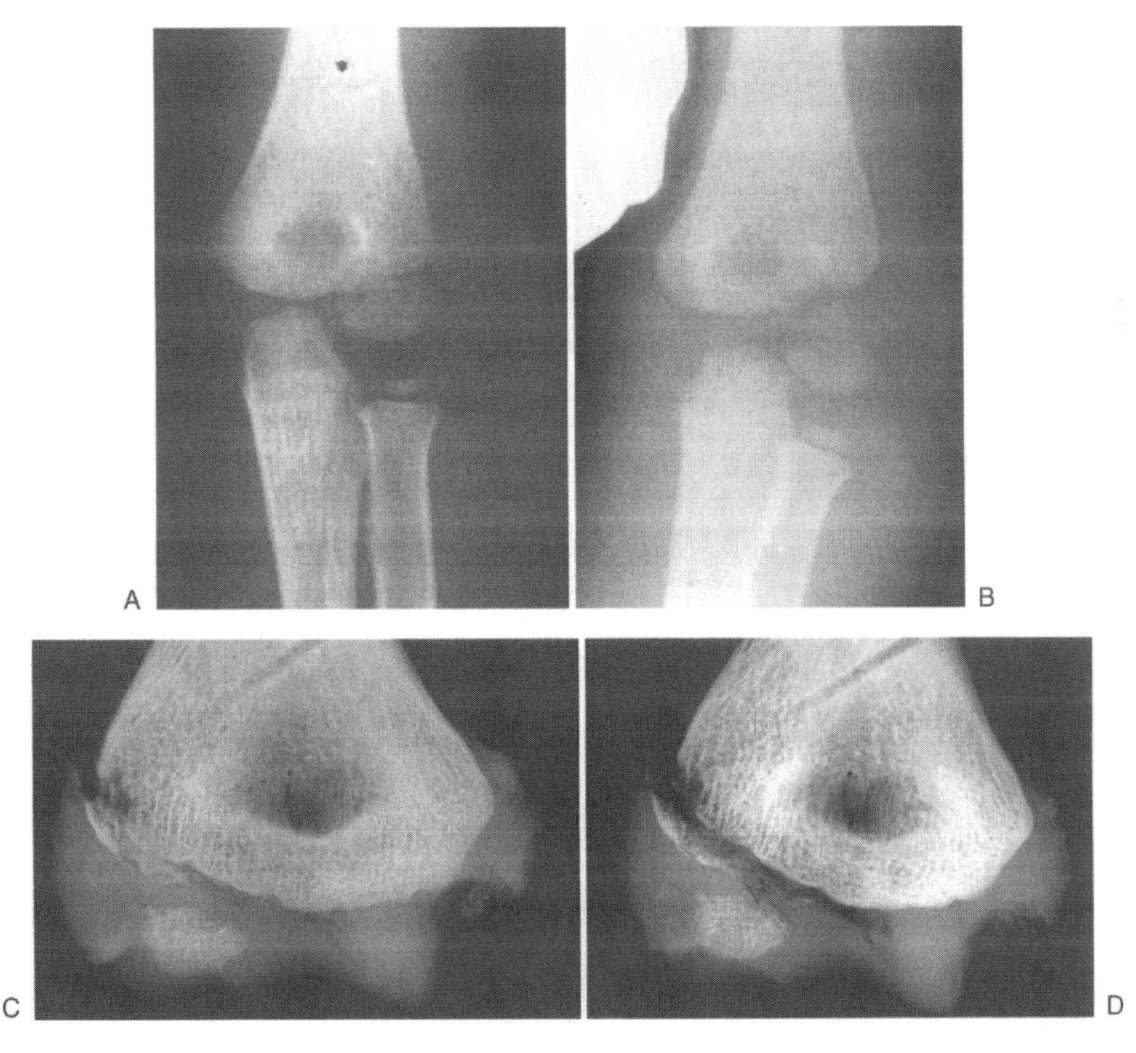

FIGURE 14-107. (A) Seemingly undisplaced lateral condylar fracture. (B) Stress film opens the fracture, emphasizing its latent instability. (C, D) Reduced and stress opening of fracture.

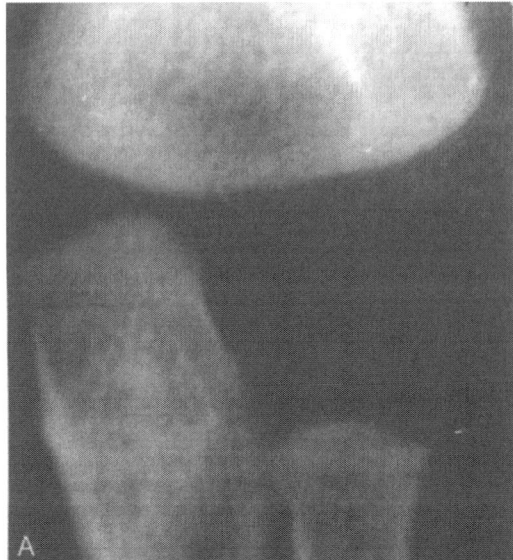

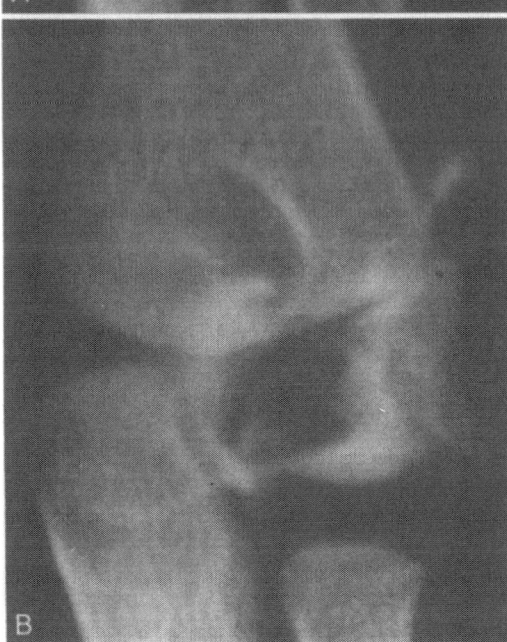

FIGURE 14-108. (A) Diagnosis is impossible on standard films in the young infant without capitellar ossification. (B) Arthrography helps with the diagnosis. The dye has surrounded the capitellar fragment.

ensured. Repeat roentgenograms should be obtained within the first 5–10 days to detect any subsequent displacement that may require open reduction (Fig. 14-110).

Even these undisplaced fractures must be considered unstable, as they tend to become displaced, *even with immobilization*, because of the pull of the common extensors. Because the fracture line crosses the physis, accurate anatomic repositioning is imperative to decrease the likelihood of growth damage. Furthermore, the congruity of the joint must be restored.

Badelon et al. noted that during surgery slight pronation or supination movements of the forearm mobilized the condylar fragment, despite the use of pins or sutures. They thought that slight movement of the hand could affect the fracture despite open reduction and internal fixation.[720] They also thought that this explained the delayed union of the lateral condyle when closed treatment and casting were used and moted that a minimum of 6 weeks of immobilization in a cast was necessary. Wiggling the fingers, which is usually encouraged in children, causes some fracture site motion in the child treated by closed methods and a long arm cast.

Flynn et al. emphasized that all minimally displaced fractures of the lateral condylar epiphysis should be watched closely for increasing displacement and delayed healing.[741] When there is a small area of osseous fracture compared to a large surface area of cartilaginous fracture (physis), the amount of bone/bone healing ratio is small, and the healing of the cartilaginous areas may take significantly longer. If an undisplaced fracture is unstable, as seen by stress film or arthrography, percutaneous fixation or open reduction is appropriate. The undisplaced or minimally displaced lateral condyle is more likely to have displacement, delayed union, or nonunion because of closed reduction and an assumption that it will readily heal.

Any evidence of acute or delayed displacement is an indication for open reduction and internal fixation (Figs. 14-111, 14-112). It should be done by fixation across the entire

small remnants of capsule and synovium to control the intraarticular reduction. The vasculature is usually not entering through this region; and if the fracture is not being operated on until several days after the original injury, this tissue may contract significantly.

The undisplaced fracture may be treated by immobilization in a long arm cast with the elbow in 90° of flexion and the forearm in full supination to minimize the pull of the extensor muscles. *Even undisplaced fractures of the lateral condyle are potentially unstable and may become displaced while immobilized.* With an undisplaced lateral condylar fracture, if the adjacent soft parts are intact, a satisfactory outcome is usually

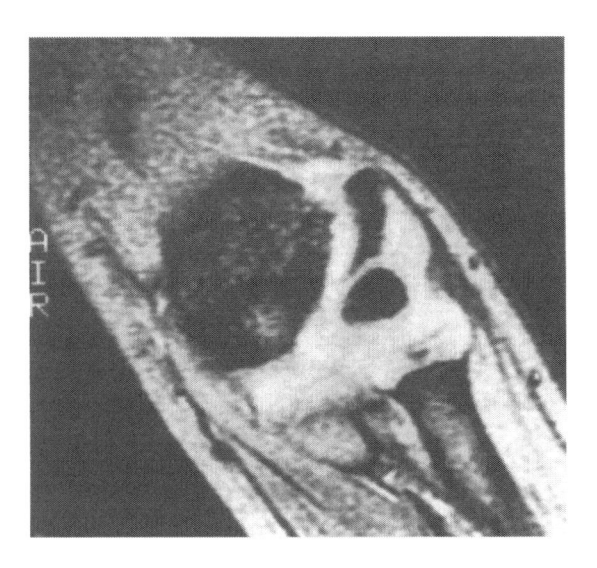

FIGURE 14-109. MRI of a lateral condylar fracture.

FIGURE 14-110. (A) Presenting radiograph. The patient was treated with a long arm cast. (B) Three weeks later a widened fracture gap is evident. It was treated by removing the fibrous tissue down to the physis, bone grafting, and percutaneous pins.

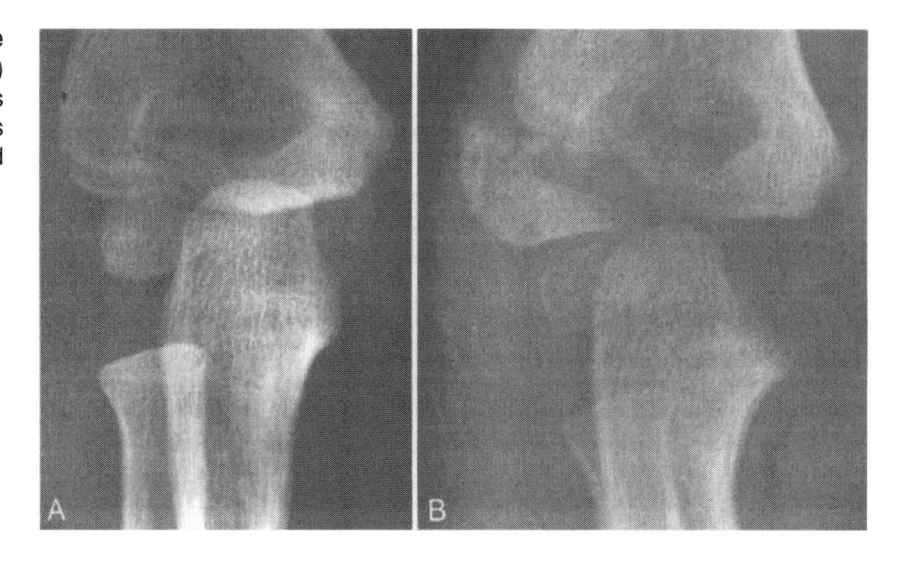

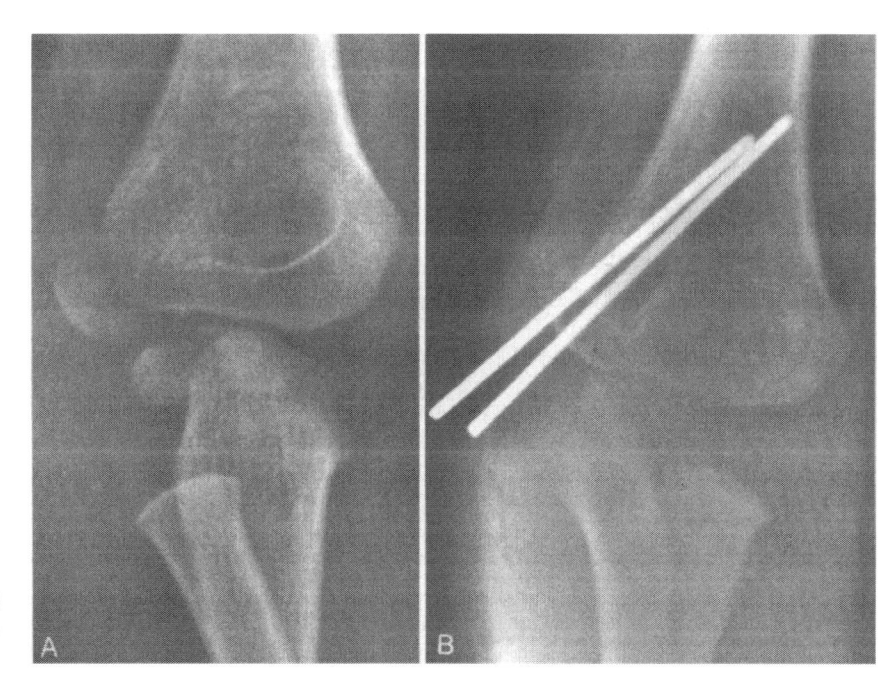

FIGURE 14-111. (A) Moderately displaced lateral condylar fracture. (B) Open reduction with internal fixation.

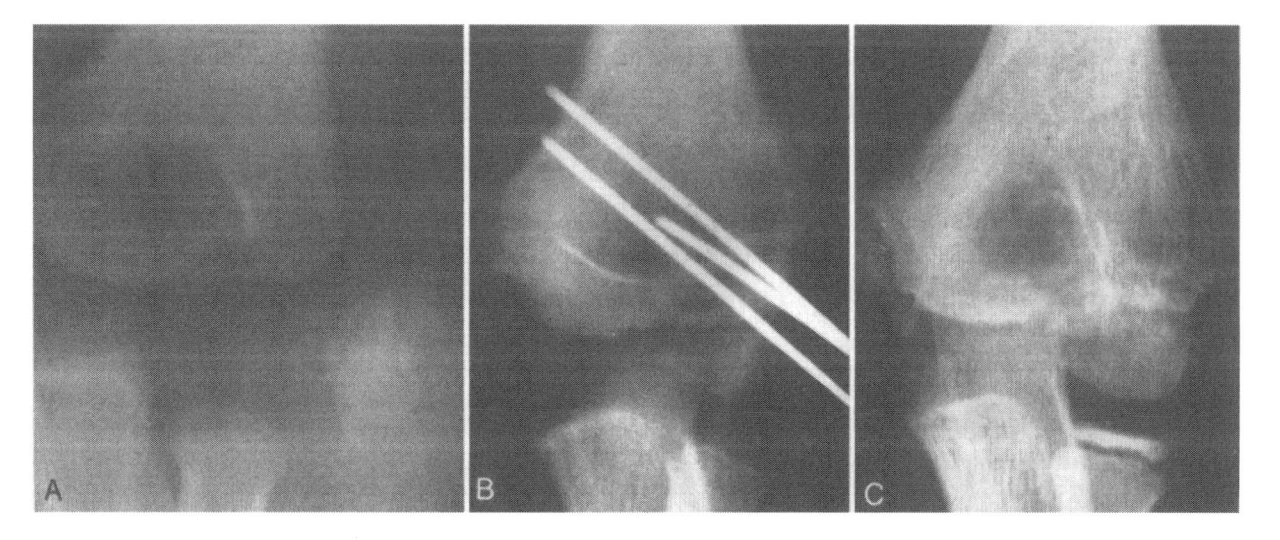

FIGURE 14-112. (A) Completely displaced and rotated capitellar fragment. (B) Open reduction and pin fixation. (C) Three years later.

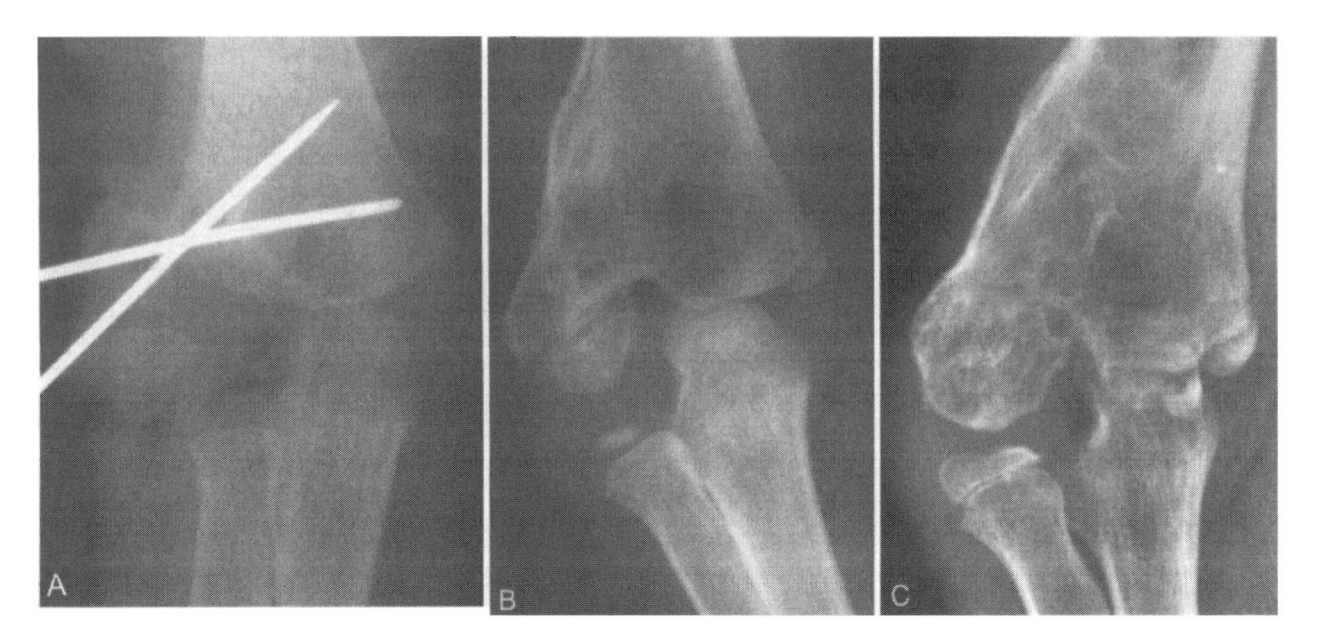

FIGURE 14-113. (A) Inappropriate reduction. Air outlines the disrupted radiohumeral joint. No attempt was made to reduce this further. (B) Healing 5 months later. (C) Three years later. The elbow is painful.

epiphysis and fixation of the fragments of the metaphysis if they are sufficiently large. If possible, pins crossing the physis are avoided. Image intensification may be used, but it is probably wise to treat these injuries with an open reduction, as part of the concept of reduction is adequate restoration of the various articular surfaces. Any intraarticular fragments of cartilage or bone are removed and the joint thoroughly irrigated.

Open reduction and internal fixation is done under tourniquet, with an incision made directly over the lateral condyle. The joint is irrigated to obtain a clear view of the articular surfaces. the fragment is minimally dissected free of soft tissue attachments but should be visualized sufficiently to see if it is rotated in different planes. The periosteum may be herniated into the region between the fragments and should be removed. The fracture must be reduced anatomically, at the fracture line in the metaphysis and at the joint surface. Failure to do so may create an abnormal elbow joint (Fig. 14-113). Kirschner wires, which should be smooth, are placed across the region. Fluoroscopy, image intensification, or biplane radiographs are obtained to ensure reduction.

When opening and reducing the fracture one must not detach all the muscles from the lateral epicondyle, because these carry some of the blood supply to the condylar fragment. If detachment is undertaken, the condyle may undergo partial to complete aseptic necrosis and premature epiphysiodesis.

The Late Case

A patient with a relatively undisplaced fracture and no clinical or roentgenographic union may not seek treatment until several weeks or months after injury (Figs. 14-114, 14-115).

Flynn et al. reported a series of nonunited minimally displaced fractures.[740,741] They noted that with unrecognized fractures the results of the nonunion were the symptoms that brought the child to the attention of the surgeon. Jeffrey pointed out that: (1) nonunion may originate in a fracture with relatively minor displacement and little or no rotation; (2) the orthopaedist may be unaware that union has failed; and (3) the nonunion may not be discovered until some later date.[766]

Flynn et al. believed that early roentgenographic evidence of nonunion was seen best in the anteroposterior view as a "high collar-like projection" of the posterolateral metaphyseal fragment attached to the epiphysis.[741] There was lateral shifting and blunting of the fracture edges of the metaphyseal fragment, little or no callus formation, and a still distinct fracture gap. If this phenomenon is observed after the fifth week, it should be recognized as a delayed union. If it persists after the third month, nonunion is definite, and appropriate surgical treatment should be carried out.

This delayed union pattern may respond effectively to pin stabilization, even several months after the injury. Minimal resection of fibrous callus is needed. Bone grafting may be unnecessary if the metaphyseal subchondral plate adjacent to the nonunion is fenestrated with two or three drill holes; the fragment is immobilized by pin or screw fixation. The epiphyseal segment of the fracture should not be débrided of fibrous tissue.

Jakob et al. found that the results of open reduction performed more than 3 weeks after the fracture are no better than the results of no treatment at all.[765] Reduction may infarct the lateral condylar fragment by damaging the blood supply. The degree of displacement seems to be significant. The greater the displacement, the more likely it is that surgery will lead to complications.

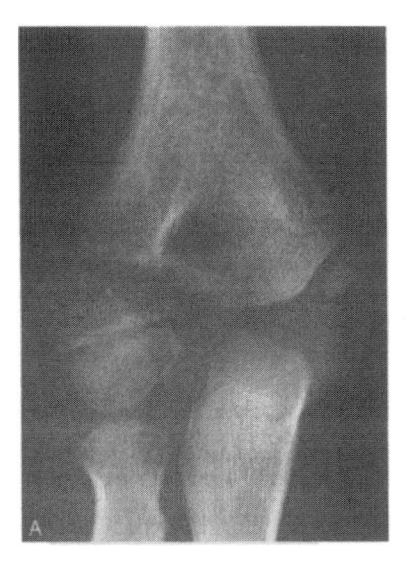

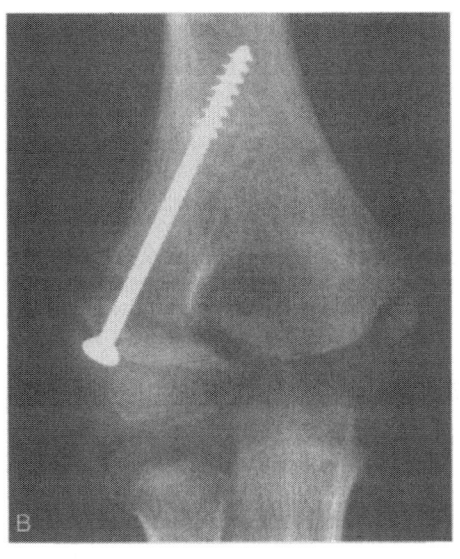

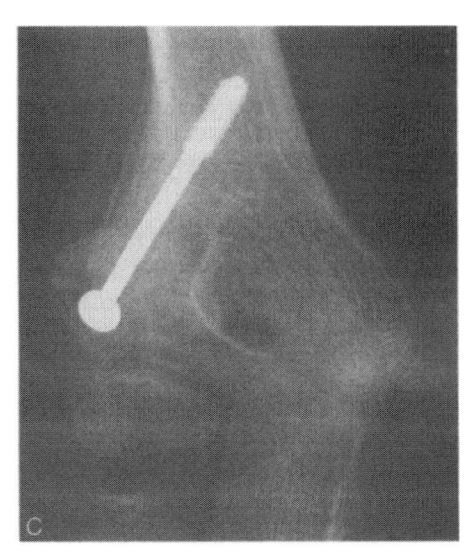

FIGURE 14-114. Delayed union. (A) Appearance 5 months after an "undisplaced" fracture. (B, C) The child was subsequently treated by excision of the fibrous nonunion and internal fixation. Healing was rapid.

Occasionally, a parent seeks treatment several weeks after the original injury for a significantly displaced fracture of the lateral condyle. Should it be accepted or corrected? Late surgery often causes stiffness and osteonecrosis. Some authors recommend a "hands-off" policy for any displaced fracture that has gone untreated for more than 4 weeks.[769] However, if it is still reasonably early (within a few weeks of the injury), open reduction, careful dissection, and anatomic reduction may still be recommended. It may be necessary to carefully currette some healing callus to obtain accurate anatomic reduction. Ununited fractures beyond a few weeks of age, in which nonunion is established, probably are difficult to treat by any method. However, an effort should be made to create bone-to-bone apposition of metaphyseal fragments in the displaced position. Once solid union is established and there is no evidence of growth arrest, a corrective osteotomy may be done.

The child who presents with a several-month delay and established nonunion still should be treated. An anatomic reduction is not the goal. Instead, the osseous metaphyseal portion of the fracture is exposed, carefully curretted, and if necessary packed with bone graft. Pin or screw stabilization is also used. The epiphyseal and articular portions are not exposed.

Results

Flynn and Richards studied the healing responses of fractures with less than 4 mm displacement, most of which were treated with closed reduction. They recognized three patterns of healing.[740] The first, which comprised almost half of the lesions, healed rapidly in 6 weeks with reasonably abundant callus and subperiosteal new bone. The second group (38%) healed slowly over 8–12 weeks, mostly by endosteal

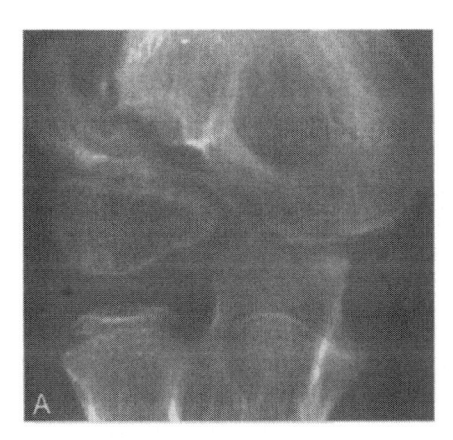

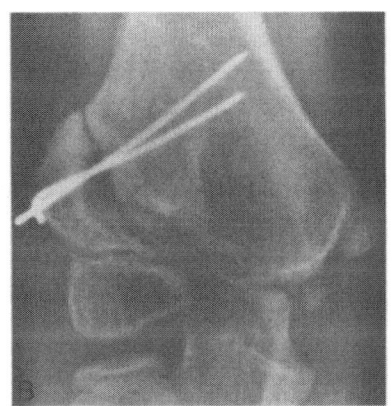

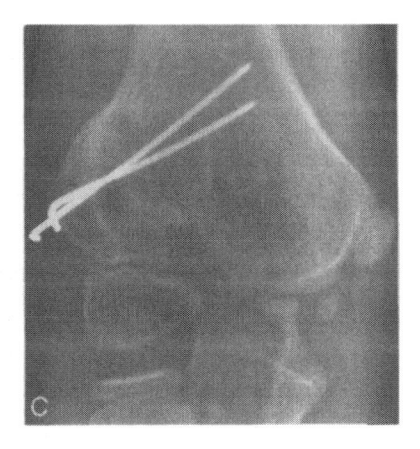

FIGURE 14-115. (A) Nonunion 6 months after injury. (B) Three weeks after pin fixation and bone graft. There was no attempt to take down the fibrous union completely. (C) Four months after surgery. Union is complete.

union with little peripheral callus. The remaining 13% displayed progressive displacement of the fragment in the cast and required subsequent surgery to prevent nonunion. These elbows were salvaged with fixation or bone grafting, sparing the physis of the condylar fragment. Flynn and Richards[740] also noted that if the fracture was displaced less than 2 mm the union was usually adequate. If the displacement was 3 mm or more, however, the incidence of delayed union, malunion, and nonunion was much higher.

Jakob et al. reviewed 48 children: 20 with minimally displaced fractures and 28 with displaced fractures requiring open reduction and internal fixation.[765] Four patients had a fracture line crossing the capitellar epiphysis and entering the joint lateral to the trochlea. The rest had injuries in which the fracture fragment included the capitellum and lateral part of the trochlea. Three of the patients developed avascular necrosis, and in two the lateral part of the distal humeral growth plate closed prematurely.

Complications

Nonunion

Severe, unrecognized injuries may progress to nonunion and marked elbow deformity (Fig. 14-116).[766] Smith recently reported an 84-year follow-up of a patient with nonunion.[792] The functional disability was minimal, but complete ulnar nerve palsy was present.

Nonunion and growth arrests result from minimally displaced fractures more commonly than from markedly displaced and rotated fractures, probably because the severe fractures are treated more adequately with surgery.[740,741] Minimally displaced fractures may displace more (in millimeters) by continued motion but rarely rotate to the degree significantly displaced injuries do. The continual motion creates a bridge of fibrocartilage between the osseous and cartilaginous fragments.

Nonunion subsequently results in progressive cubitus valgus due to retardation and growth arrest of the lateral condylar physis and continued normal growth of the medial condylar region of the physis. Eventually, degenerative changes supervene.

Suggested causes for delayed union and nonunion have included lack of immobilization, synovial fluid bathing the fracture, and soft tissue interposition. Continued micromotion is probably the most significant factor. In many cases the fracture has rotated 90° in at least one, if not two, planes, causing articular cartilage to appose epiphyseal cartilage or metaphyseal bone. It is unlikely that this articular cartilage surface will heal to the remaining osseous portions of the distal humerus.

Flynn and Richards argued that nonunion in a good position was acceptable but that it may become symptomatic, especially in athletic children.[740] Furthermore, careful distinction must be made between what is considered nonunion in good position and nonunion in poor position. Early surgery is recommended for established nonunion when the condylar fragment is in good position. If the united fragment is in poor position, unless the surgeon is skilled and familiar with the area, particularly the contours of the growth plate, it is advisable to refer the patient to another surgeon or leave the fracture fragment as is. An attempt to replace it anatomically may traumatize the physis of the fragment; and although the remainder of the elbow continues to grow, the physeal plate of the fragment may close and growth potential is lost. This in turn leads to valgus deformity, and little benefit is derived from the semiacute surgery.

Extensive bone grafting to obtain union before completion of growth is not recommended because functional disability is not usually significant in the presence of nonunion. If the fracture has been treated by closed reduction, the presence of nonunion is a strong indication that the fragments have not been adequately stabilized or that they may have rotated 90° or 180° and only seem to be reduced. In such a

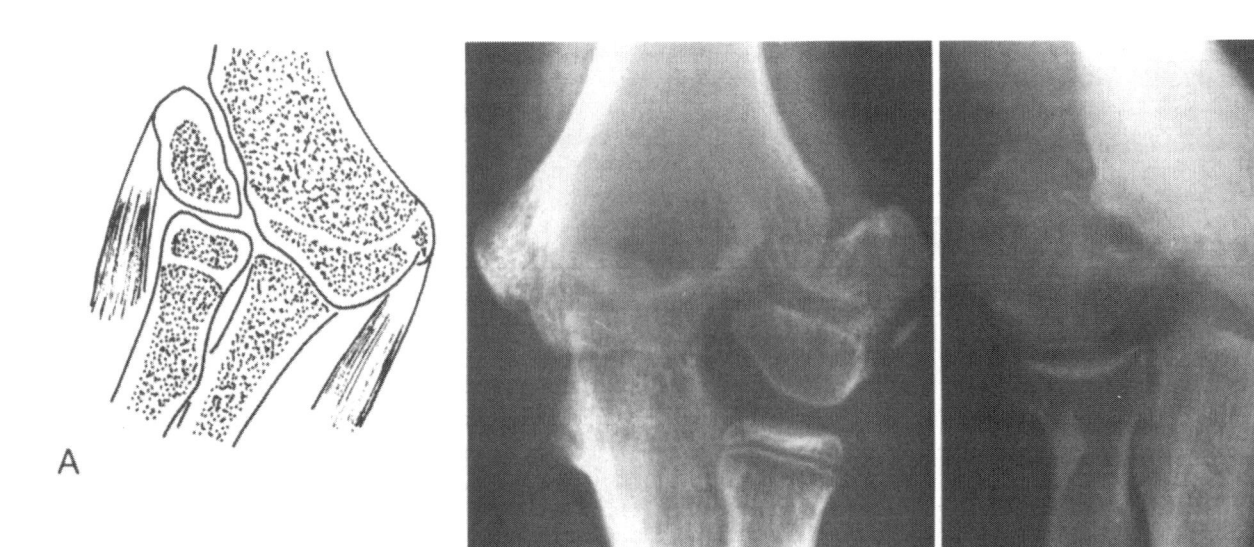

FIGURE 14-116. (A) Condylar nonunion. (B, C) Development of a nonunion from 4 to 17 years of age in an untreated patient.

situation, open reduction and exploration are indicated, despite the fact that the fracture may be several weeks old. Surgery may reveal that there is a rotation or that there is unopposed tissue that can be removed with firm reduction and Kirschner wire fixation. Bone graft from the metaphyseal fragment to the remainder of metaphysis may be helpful.

A patient with established nonunion in which the epiphyseal cartilage plate of the lateral condylar fragment is already closed is not a good candidate for surgery. Surgery may achieve union, but the condyle is unable to grow with the remainder of the elbow. Thus surgery may not prevent recurrent valgus deformity and may not yield a satisfactory elbow. Such a patient may be better left untreated until growth is complete, with later transfer of the ulnar nerve if tardy ulnar palsy occurs. In the adult, when the site of nonunion is painful, the fragment can be fixed (with or without bone graft) or excised, but only after careful consideration of the effect it may have on elbow function. The fragment should never be excised in the immature elbow because the same sequelae that follow excision of the radial head would ensue. Osteotomy of the distal part of the humerus at maturity may be necessary to correct the deformity.

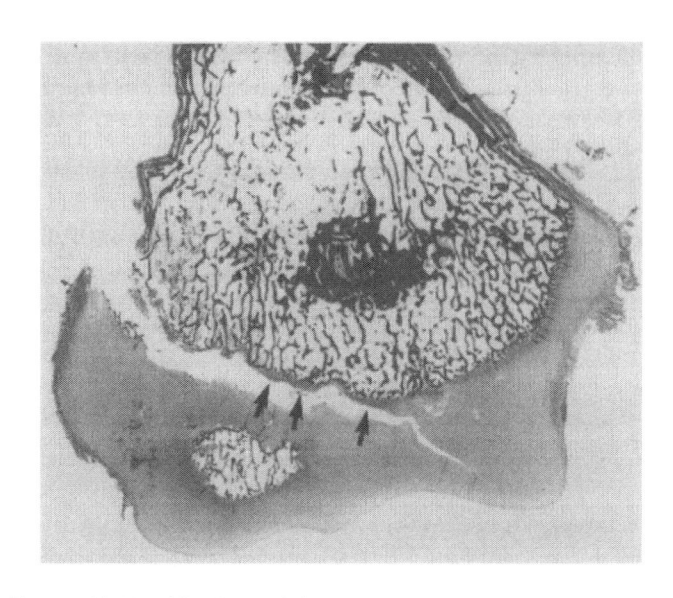

FIGURE 14-117. Histology of physeal damage in a lateral condylar fracture. Arrows indicate segments of physis that are completely separated from the epiphysis. They included germinal cells devoid of physeal blood supply.

Growth Damage

Lateral condylar fractures generally are type 4 injuries, with most passing through the cartilaginous trochlear epiphysis. They are thus likely to affect subsequent growth, although to a *highly variable* and *unpredictable* degree. Because they do go through an area that subsequently ossifies, there may be premature fusion between the trochlea and capitellar ossification centers, limiting latitudinal development and osseous bridging across the physis. If the fracture involves the margins of the secondary ossification of the capitellum, the likelihood of subsequent growth arrest increases. Should there be growth arrest, it increases the cubitus valgus deformity. As shown in Figure 14-117, microscopic physeal disruption may occur and predispose to physeal arrest, even with excellent closed or open reduction techniques.

Figures 14-99, 14-100, 14-101, and 14-117 show anatomic specimens of lateral condylar fractures that had significant damage to the physis. Particularly, segments of physis were on the wrong side of the fracture, attached to the metaphysis instead of remaining with the epiphysis, rendering the segment ischemic. Presumably, this fragmentation occurs in a number of children and may be the real reason for premature bridging. Accordingly, the treating physician must warn the parents of the risk regardless of whether closed or open treatment is used.

Malunion and premature growth arrest (Fig. 14-118) to the lateral condyle also may cause progressive cubitus valgus. This deformity of the elbow may be corrected by osteotomy of the distal humerus; but if it is corrected in the face of premature growth arrest, the deformity may recur because of the localized growth injury. If a specific localized defect can be observed, it may be possible to treat it with resection and fat interposition.

Wadsworth studied 28 children with fractures of the capitellum.[799,800] He distinguished two types of premature epiphyseal fusion. With the first type the capitellar secondary ossification center fused to the metaphysis; with the second type the capitellum and trochlea ossifications fused together and then fused subsequently to the metaphysis at the apex of the original fracture. Delayed union results in prolonged hyperemia and possible stimulation of growth on the lateral side of the elbow producing a cubitus varus. If there is damage to the growth plate, an osseous bridge inevitably forms across the plate. In addition to the obvious premature growth arrest and fusion, an additional 11 of the remaining 22 patients had narrowing of the distal humeral epiphyseal plate, implying some loss of appositional growth.[424]

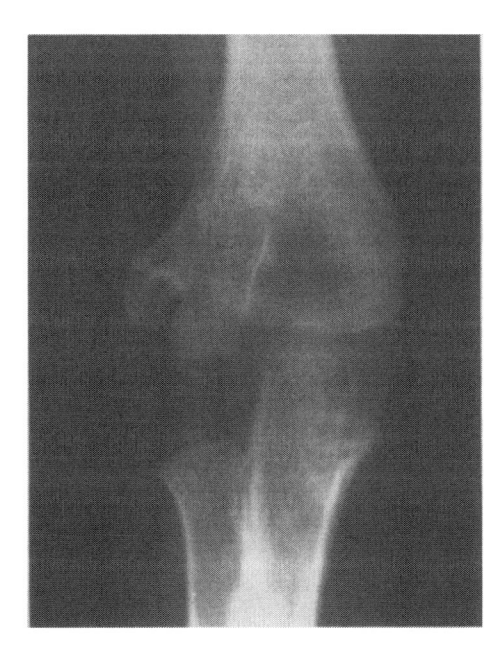

FIGURE 14-118. Abnormal growth after lateral condylar fracture (treated closed).

Another complication is poor articulation of the ulna with the trochlea, which impairs elbow movement.[778] Because the fracture usually extends through a significant portion of the trochlea, it is easy to understand how inadequate apposition of the joint surfaces creates this complication.

An infrequent radiologic finding is the "fishtail" deformity of the distal end of the humerus. This deformity is probably due to damage of the growth plate immediately adjacent to the fracture line (Fig. 14-119). The abnormality may produce cubitus valgus with limitation of movement, or it may even progress to degenerative arthritis.[799,803] None of the three patients with this abnormality reported by Jakob et al. had a deviation of the carrying angle, nor did they lose any mobility of the elbow.[765]

This phenomenon may occur in well reduced as well as poorly reduced fractures, and it may be due to deficient development of part of the trochlea or to fibrous union not unlike that shown in Chapter 6, in which there is fibrocartilage rather than true hyaline cartilage. This deformity is always most marked when the capitellum united in a rotational deformity and in cases with overgrowth of the lateral condyle.

Another infrequent complication of lateral condyle fractures is radioulnar synostosis, although great care must be taken when ascribing this particular deformity to the fracture. The possibility of preexistent synostosis must be considered.

One of the more important complications of injury to the capitellar epiphysis is ulnar neuritis, which is usually due to progressive cubitus valgus.[749,756,761,781] Neuritis may be due to simple compression by the band bridging the two heads of the flexor carpi ulnaris when the capacity of the cubital tunnel is less than normal.

The ulnar nerve is repeatedly stretched by motion of the elbow at the apex of the deformity and by the increasing valgus deformation; and it may become progressively irritated in its course behind the medial epicondyle.[715] At the earliest signs of neuritis, either the ulnar nerve should be transferred anterior to the medial epicondyle or the epicondyle should be removed and the nerve allowed to move over the remaining area. Use of the latter approach is contingent on the degree of deformity and the age of the child; it should not be used prior to skeletal maturity.

Split Capitellar Fracture

As previously alluded to, a variant of the lateral condylar fracture goes through the capitellar ossification center[735,736,783] rather than extending to the trochlear region. These fractures may be undisplaced (Fig. 14-120) or variably disrupted (Figs. 14-121, 14-122). In some instances the separation is at

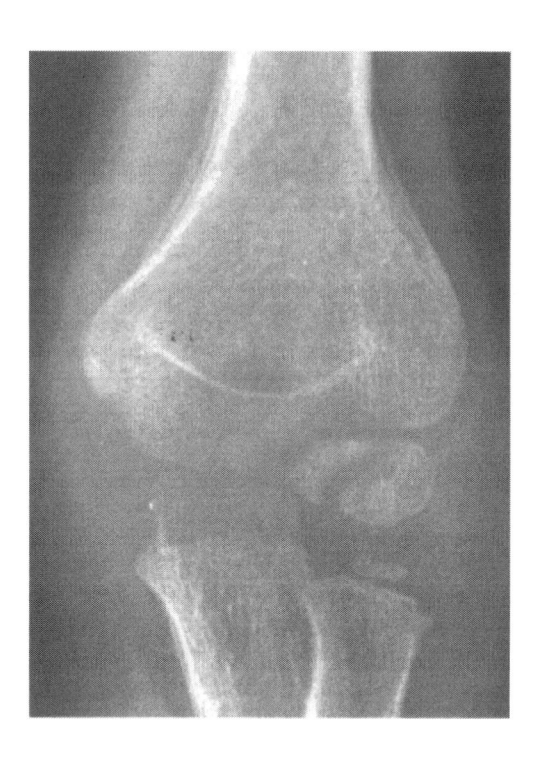

FIGURE 14-120. Split capitellar fracture.

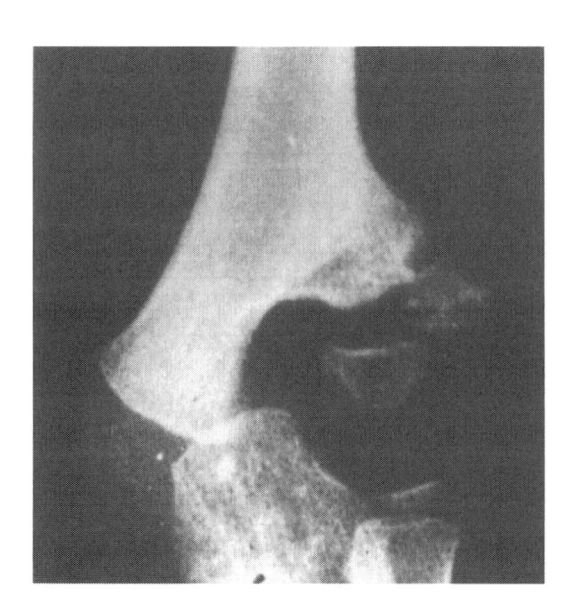

FIGURE 14-119. Fishtail deformity.

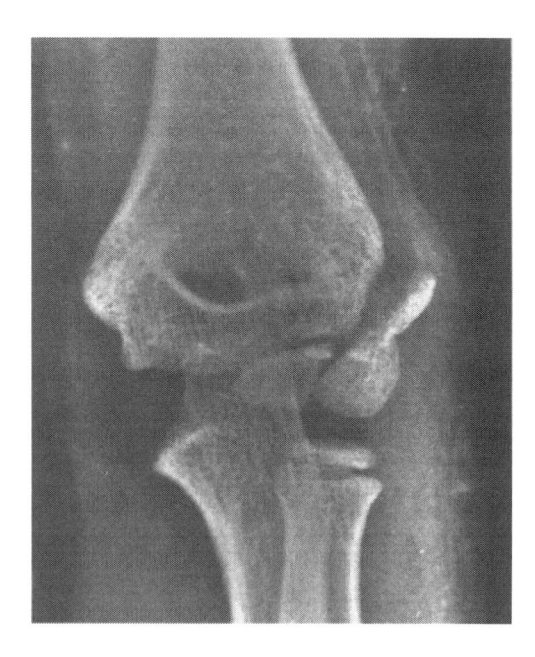

FIGURE 14-121. Type 4 displaced split capitellar fracture treated with open reduction with internal fixation.

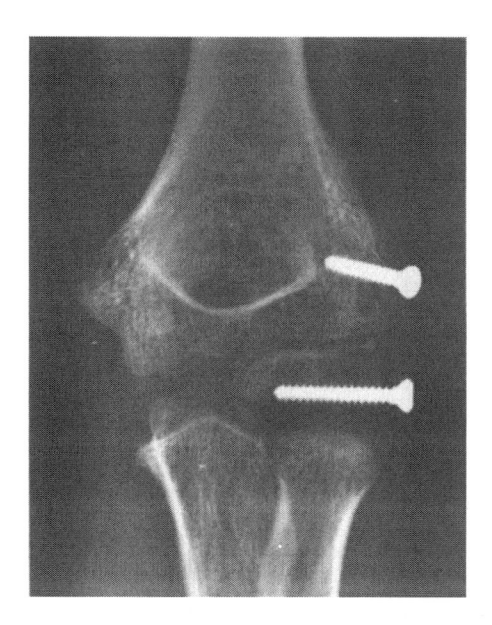

FIGURE 14-122. Split fracture.

or near the maturing chondro-osseous interface. This pattern may leave only a thin shell of subchondral bone attached to the displaced fragment (Fig. 14-123).

As with more typical lateral condylar fracture patterns, the injury may appear to be stable. Such a fracture must be observed closely for displacement as hydrostatic pressures dissipate. Most of these fractures require careful open reduction and internal fixation.

Lateral Epicondyle Injuries

The lateral epicondylar ossification center often is irregular and easily confused with a fracture. Injury to this particular epicondyle, compared to the medial epicondyle, is infrequent (Figs. 14-124 to 14-127).[808,809] Most often the injury

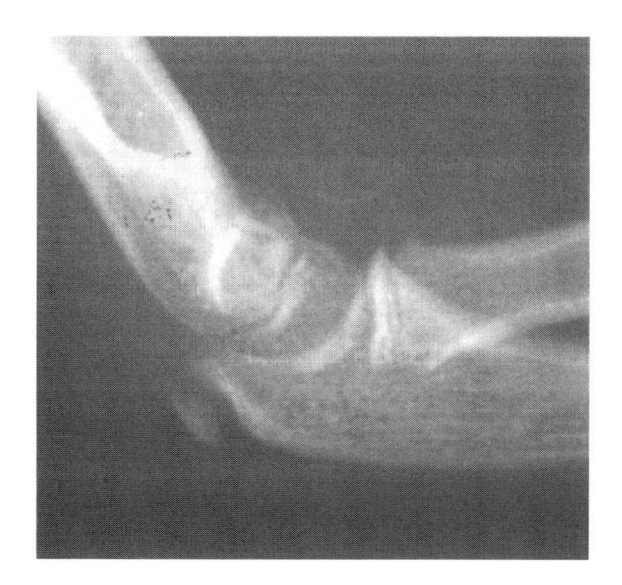

FIGURE 14-123. Sleeve fracture of the capitellum. It was repositioned and held with polyglycolic pins.

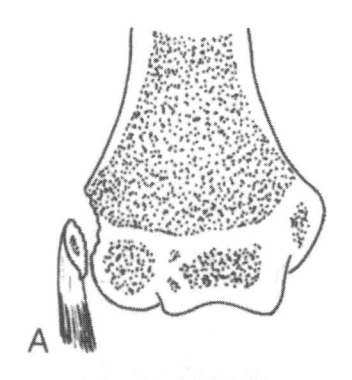

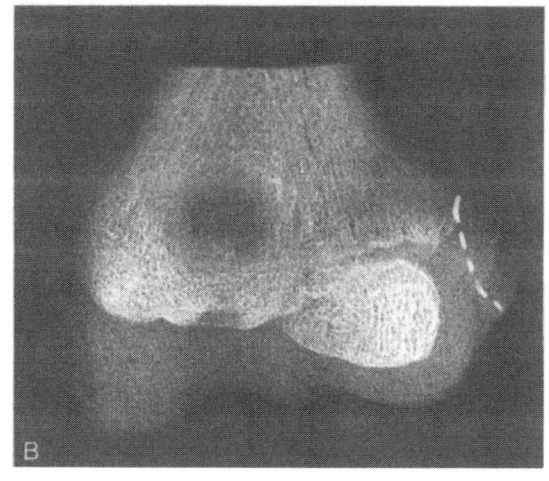

FIGURE 14-124. (A) Fracture of the lateral epicondyle. (B) Roentgenographic depiction of a specimen.

accompanies elbow dislocation. Chronic avulsion may occur as a repetitive athletic injury.

In most cases there is relatively little displacement of the fragment. Immobilization of the elbow for 3–4 weeks may be sufficient. If the fragment is displaced more than 2–3 mm, open reduction should be considered. Because these injuries tend to occur in children approaching skeletal maturity, the risk of associated growth arrest is minimal.

Floating Elbow

A distal humeral fracture and an ipsilateral forearm fracture or fractures (Fig. 14-128) create a difficult combination of injuries.[810-814] Closed treatment of both usually leads to unacceptable reduction of at least one of the injuries.

The distal humeral injury should be stabilized by closed reduction and percutaneous pinning or open reduction and internal fixation. The forearm fractures are then treated by closed reduction and casting.

The distal humeral injury may be a supracondylar, transcondylar, lateral condylar, or medial condylar fracture. Similarly, a variety of forearm injuries may be present, such as an olecranon fracture, a radial neck fracture, a Monteggia equivalent, or diaphyseal radioulnar fractures.

As many as 10–15% of all supracondylar fracture patients also have a second injury involving the ipsilateral radius and

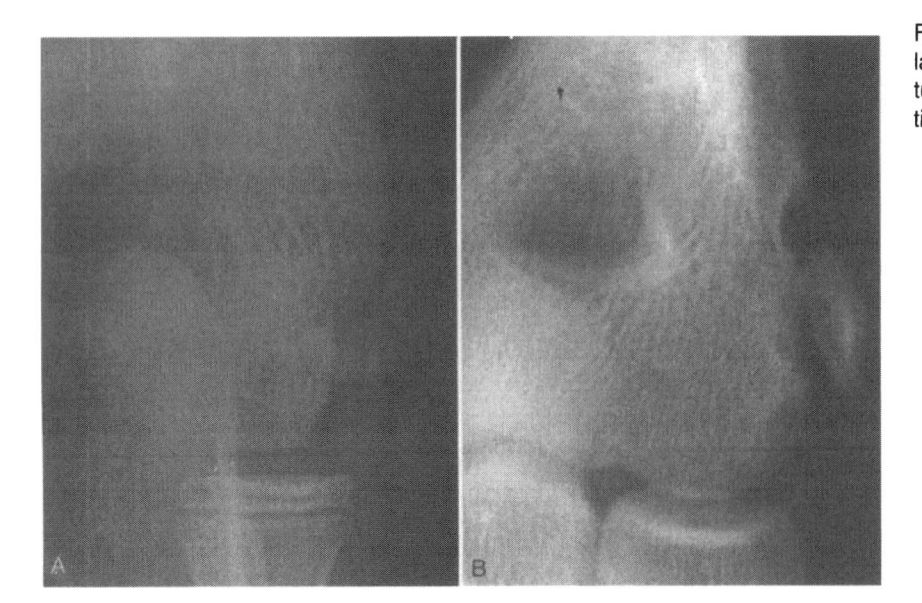

FIGURE 14-125. (A) Acute fracture of the lateral epicondyle. (B) Appearance of the fracture 5 years later, following skeletal maturation. Fibrous nonunion had occurred.

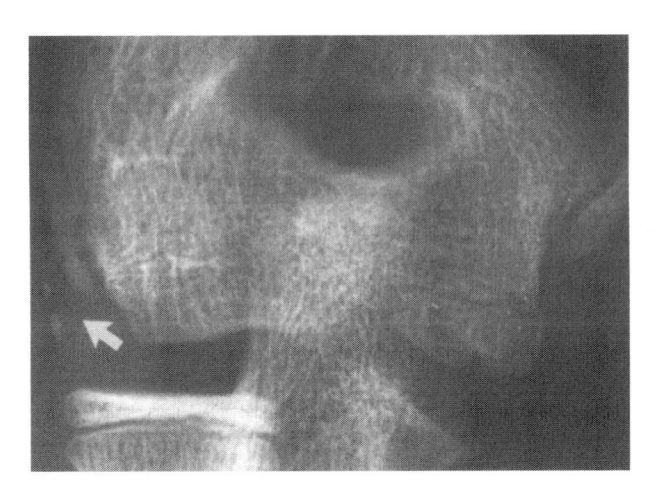

FIGURE 14-126. Lateral epicondylar avulsion injury (arrow) in a 14-year-old boy who fell directly on his elbow. There was mild varus instability. The fracture was treated by closed reduction and immobilization at 90° of elbow flexion.

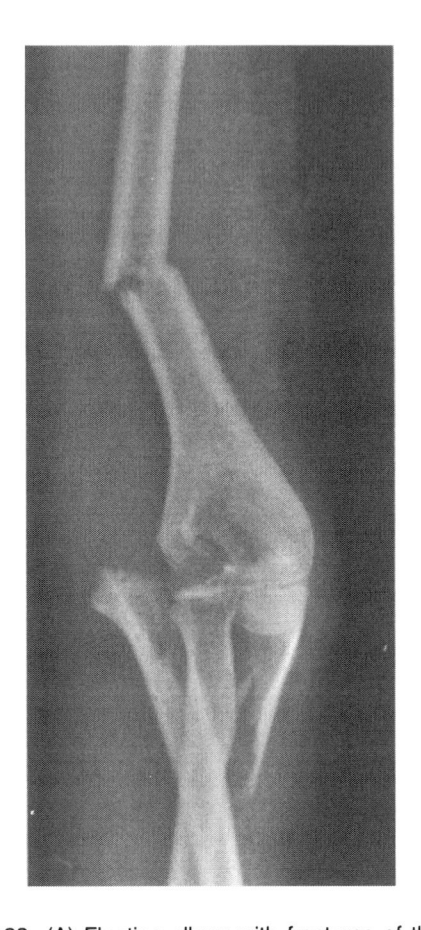

FIGURE 14-128. (A) Floating elbow with fractures of the humeral diaphysis and ulnar metaphysis. (B) The cast has not effectively treated the fractures.

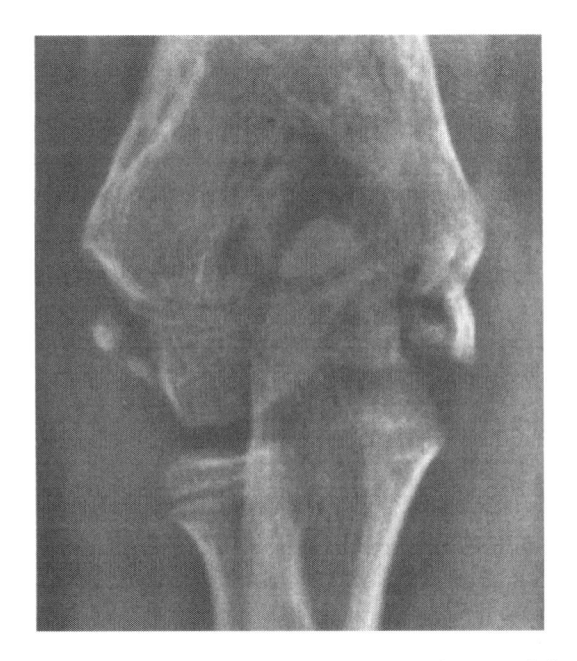

FIGURE 14-127. Medial and lateral epicondylar fractures following elbow dislocation.

ulna. The distal radius/ulna is the most likely site of radioulnar injury.

Elbow swelling is a significant problem. The potential for the development of compartment syndrome or ischemia may be higher with combined injuries than with either injury alone.

References

Anatomy

1. Aebi H. Der Ellbogenwinkel, seine Beziehungen zu Geschlect, Korperbay und Huftbrate. Acta Anat (Basel) 1947;3:228–237.
2. Atkinson WB, Elftman H. The carrying angle of the human arm as a secondary sex character. Anat Rec 1945;91:49–58.
3. Barnard LB, McCoy SM. The supracondyloid process of the humerus. J Bone Joint Surg 1946;28:845–846.
4. Beals RK. The normal carrying angle of the elbow. Clin Orthop 1976;119:194–199.
5. Brodeur AE, Silberstein MJ, Graviss ER, Luisiri A. The basic tenets for appropriate evaluation of the elbow in pediatrics. Curr Probl Diagn Radiol 1983;12:1–7.
6. Gardner E, Gray DJ. Prenatal development of the human shoulder and acromioclavicular joints. Am J Anat 1953;106:219–246.
7. Genner B. Fracture of the supracondyloid process. J Bone Joint Surg Am 1959;41:1333–1334.
8. Greenspan A, Norman A, Rosen N. Radial head-capitellum view in elbow trauma: clinical application and radiographic-anatomic correlation. AJR 1984;143:355–359.
9. Gudmundsen E, Ostensen H. Accessory ossicles in the elbow. Acta Orthop Scand 1987;58:130–132.
10. Haroldson S. The intraosseous vasculature of the distal end of the humerus with special reference to capitulum. Acta Orthop Scand 1957;27:81–93.
11. Hoffman AD. Radiography of the pediatric elbow. In: Morrey BF (ed) The Elbow and Its Disorders. Philadelphia: Saunders, 1985.
12. Hudson TM. Elbow arthrography. Radiol Clin North Am 1981;19:227–242.
13. Kolb LW, Moore RD. Fractures of the supracondylar process of the humerus. J Bone Joint Surg Am 1967;49:532–538.
14. Le Floch P. The distal humerus: a structure with two pillars. Anat Clin 1982;4:235–241.
15. Linter DM, Sebastianelli WJ, Hanks GA, Kalenak A. Glenoid dysplasia: a case report and review of the literature. Clin Orthop 1992;283:145–148.
16. Lund HJ. Fracture of the supracondyloid process of the humerus: report of a case. J Bone Joint Surg 1930;12:925–926.
17. McCarthy SM, Ogden JA. Roentgenography of postnatal skeletal development. V. The distal humerus. Skeletal Radiol 1982;7:239–249.
18. Oberman WR, Loose HWC. The os supratrochleare dorsale: a normal variant that may cause symptoms. AJR 1983;141:123–127.
19. Ogden JA, Conlogue GJ, Jensen P. Radiology of postnatal skeletal development: the proximal humerus. Skeletal Radiol 1978;2:153–161.
20. Page AC. Critical evaluation of the radial head-capitellum view in elbow trauma. AJR 1986;146:81–86.
21. Resnick CS, Hartenberg MA. Ossification centers of the pediatric elbow: a rare normal variant. Pediatr Radiol 1986;16:254–257.
22. Sempe M. Skeletal growth and maturation of the elbow: kinetic study. Ann Radiol (Paris) 1976;19:733–742.
23. Silberstein MJ, Brodeur AE, Graviss ER. Some vagaries of the capitellum. J Bone Joint Surg Am 1979;61:244–247.
24. Silberstein MJ, Brodeur AE, Graviss ER. Some vagaries of the lateral epicondyle. J Bone Joint Surg Am 1982;64:444–448.
25. Silberstein MJ, Brodeur AE, Graviss ER, Luisiri A. Some vagaries of the medial epicondyle. J Bone Joint Surg Am 1981;63:524–528.
26. Steel FLD, Tomlinson JDW. The "carrying angle" in man. J Anat 1958;92:315–321.
27. Wood VE, Campbell GS. The supratrochleare dorsale accessory ossicle in the elbow. J Shoulder Elbow Surg 1994;3:395–397.

Glenohumeral Dislocation

28. Barry TP, Lombardo SJ, Kerlan RK, et al. The coracoid transfer for recurrent anterior instability of the shoulder in adolescents. J Bone Joint Surg Am 1985;67:383–387.
29. Davids JR, Talbott RD. Luxatio erecta humeri. Clin Orthop 1990;252:144–149.
30. Emery RJH, Mullaji AB. Glenohumeral joint instability in normal adolescents. J Bone Joint Surg Br 1991;73:406–408.
31. Gudinchet F, Naggar L, Ginalski JM, Dutoit M, Schnyder P. Magnetic resonance imaging of nontraumatic shoulder instability in children. Skeletal Radiol 1992;21:19–21.
32. Guidera KJ, Grogan DP, Pugh LI, Ogden JA. Hypoplastic clavicle and lateral scapular redirection. J Pediatr Orthop 1991;11:523–526.
33. Heck CC. Anterior dislocation of the glenohumeral joint in a child. J Trauma 1981;21:174–175.
34. Hovelins L. Anterior dislocation of the shoulder in teenagers and young adults: five year prognosis. J Bone Joint Surg Am 1987;69:393–399.
35. Huber H, Gerber C. Voluntary subluxation of the shoulder in children. J Bone Joint Surg Br 1993;76:118–122.
36. Laskin RS, Sedlin EO. Luxatio erecta in infancy. Clin Orthop 1971;80:126–129.
37. Marans HJ, Angel KR, Shemitsch EH, Wedge JH. The fate of traumatic anterior dislocation of the shoulder in children. J Bone Joint Surg Am 1992;74:1242–1244.
38. Mizuma K, Itakura Y, Muratsu H. Inferior capsular shift for inferior and multi directional instability of the shoulder in young children: report of two cases. J Shoulder Elbow Surg 1992;1:200–206.
39. Rockwood CA. Subluxation and dislocations of the glenohumeral joint. In: Rockwood CA, Wilins K, King R (eds) Fractures in Children, 2nd ed, vol 3. Philadelphia: Lippincott, 1984.
40. Rowe CR, Sakellarides HT. Factors related to recurrences of anterior dislocations of the shoulder. Clin Orthop 1961;20:40–51.
41. Sperber A, Wredmark T. Capsular elasticity and joint volume in recurrent anterior shoulder instability. Arthroscopy 1994;10:598–601.
42. Uhthoff HK, Piscopo M. Anterior capsular redundancy of the shoulder: congenital or traumatic? An embryological study. J Bone Joint Surg Br 1985;67:363–366.
43. Wagner KT, Lyne ED. Adolescent traumatic dislocations of the shoulder with open epiphyses. J Pediatr Orthop 1983;3:61–66.
44. Whitman R. The treatment of congenital and acquired luxations at the shoulder in childhood. Ann Surg 1905;42:114–115.
45. Wolf EM, Chen JC, Dickeson K. Humeral avulsion of glenohumeral ligaments as a cause of anterior shoulder instability. Arthroscopy 1995;11:600–607.

Brachial Plexus

46. Dunkerton MC. Posterior dislocation of the shoulder associated with obstetric brachial plexus injury. J Bone Joint Surg Br 1989;71:764–766.
47. Fairbank HAT. A lecture on birth palsy: subluxation of the shoulder joint in infants and young children. Lancet 1913; 1:1217–1223.
48. Green NE, Wheelhouse WW. Anterior subglenoid dislocation of the shoulder in an infant following pneumococcal meningitis. Clin Orthop 1978;135:125–127.
49. Liebolt FL, Furey JG. Obstetrical paralysis with dislocation of the shoulder. J Bone Joint Surg Am 1953;35:227–230.
50. Troum S, Floyd WE III, Waters PM. Posterior dislocation of the humeral head in infancy associated with obstetrical paralysis. J Bone Joint Surg Am 1993;75:1370–1375.

Congenital Dislocation

51. Cozen L. Congenital dislocation of the shoulder and other anomalies: report of a case and review of the literature. Arch Surg 1937;35:956–966.
52. Edwards H. Congenital displacement of shoulder joint. J Anat 1928;62:177–182.
53. Frosch L. Congenital subluxation of shoulders. Klin Wochenschr 1923;4:701–702.
54. Greig DM. True congenital dislocation of the shoulder. Edinb Med J 1923;30:157–175.
55. Heilbronner DM. True congenital dislocation of the shoulder. J Pediatr Orthop 1990;10:408–410.
56. Kuhn D, Rosman M. Traumatic, nonparalytic dislocation of the shoulder in a newborn infant. J Pediatr Orthop 1984;4:121–123.
57. Lichtblau PD. Shoulder dislocation in the infant: case report and discussion. J Fla Med Assoc 1977;64:313–320.
58. Peterson H. Bilateral dysplasia of the neck of the scapula and associated anomalies. Acta Radiol Diagn 1981;22:81–84.
59. Phelps AM. Report of a case of congenital dislocation of the shoulder backward. Trans Am Orthop Assoc 1896;8:239–245.
60. Roberts JB. A case of excision of the head of the humerus for congenital subacromial dislocation of the humerus. Am J Med Sci 1905;130:1001–1007.
61. Robinson D, Aghasi M, Helperin N, Kopilowicz L. Congenital dislocation of the shoulder: case report and review of the literature. Contemp Orthop 1989;18:595–598.
62. Scudder CL. Congenital dislocation of the shoulder joint: a report of two cases. Arch Pediatr 1890;7:260–269.
63. Valentin B. Die kongenitale schulterluxation, bericht über drei falle in einer familie. Z Orthop Chir 1931;55:239–240.
64. Wolff G. Über einen fall von kongenitaler Schulterluxation. Z Orthop Chir 1929;51:199–209.

Obstetric Injury

65. Babbit DP, Cassidy RH. Obstetrical paralysis and dislocation of the shoulder in infancy. J Bone Joint Surg Am 1968;50:1447–1452.
66. Bonelli A, Schiavetti E. Considerazioni su alcuni aspetti delle fratture di gomito nel bambino. Chir Organi Mov 1963;52:286–294.
67. Broker FHL, Burbach T. Ultrasonic diagnosis of separation of the proximal humeral epiphysis in the newborn. J Bone Joint Surg Am 1990;72:187–191.
68. DeSimone DP, Morwessel RM. Diagnostic arthrogram of a Salter I fracture of the proximal humerus in a newborn. Orthop Rev 1988;17:782–785.
69. Ellefsen BK, Frierson MA, Raney EM, Ogden JA. Humerus varus: a complication of neonatal and childhood injury and infection. J Pediatr Orthop 1994;14:479–486.
70. Haliburton RA, Barber JR, Fraser RL. Pseudodislocation: an unusual birth injury. Can J Surg 1967;10:455–457.
71. Howard CB, Shinwell E, Nyska M, Meller I. Ultrasound diagnosis of neonatal fracture separation of the upper humeral epiphysis. J Bone Joint Surg Br 1992;74:471–472.
72. Kellner KR. Neonatal fracture and cesarean section. Am J Dis Child 1982;136:865–868.
73. Langenskiöld A. Adolescent humerus varus. Acta Chir Scand 1953;105:353–362.
74. Lemberg R, Liliequist B. Dislocation of the proximal epiphysis of the humerus in newborns. Acta Paediatr Scand 1970;59:377–380.
75. Lucas L, Gill JH. Humerus varus following birth injury to the proximal humerus. J Bone Joint Surg 1947;29:367–369.
76. Marino-Zuco C. Sul trattamento incruento delle fratture sovracondiloidee dell'omero nei bambini. Ortop Traumatol App Mot 1930;3:29–34.
77. Michel L. Le decollement obstetrical de l'epiphyse superieure de l'humerus. Orthop Rev 193;24:201–203.
78. Ogden JA, Weil UH, Hampton RF. Developmental humerus varus. Clin Orthop 1976;116:158–166.
79. Paneva-Holevitch E, Yankov E. Humerus varus congenitus. Rev Chir Orthop 1979;65:45–48.
80. Scaglietti O. The obstetrical shoulder trauma. Surg Gynecol Obstet 1938;66:868–873.
81. Slesarev SP. Dysplasia and birth injury of the shoulder joint. Ortop Travmatol Protez 1983;1:32–37.
82. Spissak L, Kirnak J, Vojtko M. Therapeutic results in proximally dislocated epiphyseolyses of the humerus. Acta Chir Orthop Traumatol Cech 1980;47:438–443.
83. Van den Broek JAC, Vegter J. Diagnose van Epifysiolyse van her proximale deel van de humerus by een pasgeborne met echografie. Ned Tijdshcr Geneeskd 1988;132:1015–1017.
84. White SJ, Blane CE, DiPietro MA, Kling TF Jr, Hensinger RN. Arthrography in evaluation of birth injuries of the shoulder. J Can Assoc Radiol 1987;38:113–116.

Rotator Cuff

85. Nutton RW. Acute calcific supraspinatus tendinitis in a three-year-old child. J Bone Joint Surg Br 1987;69:148.
86. Thunjhunwala HR. Abduction contracture of the deltoid muscle in children. Int Orthop 1995;19:289–290.

Proximal Epiphysis and Physis

87. Adams JE. Little league shoulder: osteochondritis of the proximal humeral epiphysis in boy baseball pitchers. Calif Med 1966;105:22–25.
88. Aitken AP. End results of fractures of proximal humeral epiphysis. J Bone Joint Surg 1936;18:1036–1047.
89. Aitken AP. Fractures of the proximal humeral epiphysis. Surg Clin North Am 1963;43:1575–1583.
90. Ansorg P, Graner G. Behandlung und Ergebnisse nach Sultergelenknahen Oberarmbrüchen in Wachstumsalter. Beitr Orthop Traumatol 1978;25:653–659.
91. Aufranc OE, Jones WN, Butler JE. Epiphyseal fracture of the proximal humerus. JAMA 1970;213:1476–1477.
92. Austin LJ. Fractures of the morphological neck of the humerus in children. Can Med Assoc J 1939;40:546–549.

References

93. Barnett LS. Little league shoulder syndrome: proximal humeral epiphyseolysis in adolescent baseball pitchers. J Bone Joint Surg Am 1985;67:495–496.
94. Baxter MP, Wiley JJ. Fractures of the proximal humeral epiphysis. J Bone Joint Surg Br 1986;68:570–575.
95. Beck E. Epiphysealösungen am proximalen Oberarmende. Arch Orthop Unfallchir 1965;57:26–36.
96. Beebe AC, Bell DF. The management of severely displaced fractures of the proximal humerus in children. Tech Orthop 1989;4:1–4.
97. Böhler J. Behandlung der subkapitalen Oberarmbrüche Jugendlichen. Klin Med 1965;20:136–147.
98. Bourdillon JF. Fracture-separation of the proximal epiphysis of the humerus. J Bone Joint Surg Br 1950;32:35–37.
99. Bouyala JM, Chrestian P, Jacquemier M. La voie axillaire dans l'abord chirurgical de l'epaule et de l'extremite superieure de l'humerus. Chir Pediatr 1980;21:287–294.
100. Budig H. Endergebnisse bei Epiphysenlösungen und Oberarmbrücher am proximalen Ende von Kinder und Jugenlichen. Arch Orthop Unfallchir 1958;49:521–531.
101. Burgos-Flores J, Gonzalez-Herranz P, Lopez-Monde JG, et al. Fractures of the proximal humeral epiphysis. Int Orthop 1993;17:16–19.
102. Butterworth RD, Carpenter EB. Bilateral slipping of the proximal epiphysis of the humerus. J Bone Joint Surg Am 1948;30:1003–1005.
103. Chaill BR, Tullos HS, Fain RH. Little league shoulder. J Sports Med 1974;2:150–155.
104. Campbell J, Almond GA. Fracture-separation of the proximal humeral epiphysis. J Bone Joint Surg Am 1977;59:262–263.
105. Cauchoix J, Duparc J, Boulez P. Traitement des fractures ouvretes de jambe. Mem Acad Chir 1957;83:811–815.
106. Charry V. Un cas de fracture irreductible du col chirurgical de l'humerus chez un adolescent. Orthop Rev 1937;24:244–246.
107. Ciaramella G, Rulfoni R. Le complicazioni neurologiche nelle fratture dell'artro superiore. Chir Ital 1962;14:569–572.
108. Clément JL, Cahuzac JP, Ganbert J, Bollini G, Bonyala JM. Fractures et décollements épiphysaires de l'extrémité supérieure de l'humerus. Rev Chir Orthop 1988;74(suppl 2):139–144.
109. Cohn BT, Froimson AI. Salter III fracture dislocation of glenohumeral joint in a 10 year old. Orthop Rev 1986;15:403–405.
110. Conwell HE. Fractures of the surgical neck and epiphyseal separations of upper end of humerus. J Bone Joint Surg 1926;8:508–510.
111. Curtis RJ Jr. Operative management of children's fractures of the shoulder region. Orthop Clin North Am 1990;21:315–324.
112. Dameron TB Jr, Reibel DB. Fractures involving the proximal humeral epiphyseal plate. J Bone Joint Surg Am 1969;51:289–297.
113. DeMourgues G, Fischer L. Résultat lointain des décollements épiphysaires de l'extrémité supérieure de l'huméus de l'adolescent. Rev Chir Orthop 1971;57:241–246.
114. Divis G. Epiphysiolysis humeri unter beträchtlicher Dislokation des Gelenkskopfes: unblütige Reposition. Arch Orthop Unfallchir 1927;25:342–346.
115. Doliveux P. Traitement chirurgical des fractures hautes de l'humerus a gros deplacement chez le grand enfant. Ann Orthop Ouest 1970;2:49–54.
116. Dotter WE. Little Leaguers' shoulder: a fracture of the proximal epiphyseal cartilage of the humerus due to baseball pitching. Guthrie Clin Bull 1953;23:68–72.
117. Drew SJ, Giddens GEB, Birch R. A slowly evolving brachial pleuxus injury following a proximal humeral fracture in a child. J Hand Surg [Br] 1995;20:24–25.
118. Evrard H, Deltour D, Hubert M. Capital and diaphyseal fractures of the humerus in children. Acta Orthop Belg 1982;48:739–744.
119. Fraser R, Haliburton R, Barber J. Displaced epiphyseal fractures of the proximal humerus. Can J Surg 1967;10:427–432.
120. Frey C, Klöti J. Spätresultate der subkapitalen Humerus fraktur im Kindesalter. Z Kinderchir 1989;44:280–282.
121. Friedlaender HL. Separation of the proximal humeral epiphysis. Clin Orthop 1964;35:163–169.
122. Gerard Y, Segal P. Traitement chirurgical des decollements epiphysaires de l'extremité supérieure de l'humerus chez l'adolescent. Rev Chir Orthop 1973;59:205–209.
123. Gilchrist D. A stockinette-velpeau for immobilization of the shoulder girdle. J Bone Joint Surg Am 1963;45:1382–1388.
124. Gouin JL. A propos des fractures de l'extremite superieure de l'humerus chez l'enfant. Paris: Thesé, 1955.
125. Guibert L. Allouis M, Bourdelat D, Cater P, Gabut JM. Fractures et décollements éiphysaires de l'extrémité supérieure de l'humérus chez l'enfant: place et modalités du traitment chirurgical. Chir Pediatr 1983;24:197–200.
126. Hartigan JW. Separation of the lesser tuberosity of the head of the humerus [letter]. New York Med J 1895;61:276–277.
127. Hohn JC. Fractures of the humerus in children. Orthop Clin North Am 1976;7:557–571.
128. Jeffrey CC. Fracture separation of the upper humeral epiphysis. Surg Gynecol Obstet 1953;96:205–208.
129. Klasson SC, Vander Schilden JL, Park JP. Late effect of isolated avulsion fractures of the lesser tubercle of the humerus in children. J Bone Joint Surg Am 1993;75:1691–1694.
130. Kohler R, Trillaud JM. Fracture and fracture separation of the proximal humerus in children: report of 136 cases. J Pediatr Orthop 1983;3:326–330.
131. Koszlam. [Fractures of the surgical neck of the humerus in children.] Chir Narz Ruchu 1975;40:327–333.
132. Languepin A. Evaluation pendant la croissance des cas de fractures de l'extrémité de l'humérus. Ann Orthop Ouest 1974;3:61–62.
133. Larsen CF, Kiaer T, Lindquist S. Fractures of the proximal humerus in children: a nine year follow-up on 64 unoperated cases. Acta Orthop Scand 1990;61:255–257.
134. Lee HG. Operative reduction of an unusual fracture of the upper epiphyseal plate of the humerus. J Bone Joint Surg 1944;26:401–404.
135. LePelley M, Jolly A, Cuny C, Wack B, Bean A. Fractures de l'extrémité supérieure de l'humérus chez l'enfant: a propos de 50 cas. Ann Med Nancy 1981;20:411–414.
136. Levin GD. A valgus angulation fracture of the proximal humeral epiphysis. Clin Orthop 1976;116:155–158.
137. Lohite GM, Riley LH Jr. Isolated avulsion of the subscapularis insertion in a child: a case report. J Bone Joint Surg Am 1985;67:635–636.
138. Mah JY, Hall JE. Arthrodesis of the shoulder in children. J Bone Joint Surg Am 1990;72:582–586.
139. Makin M. Early arthrodesis for a flail shoulder in young children. J Bone Joint Surg Am 1977;59:317–321.
140. McBride ED, Sisler J. Fractures of the proximal humeral epiphysis and the juxta-epiphyseal humeral shaft. Clin Orthop 1965;38:143–149.
141. Neer CS II, Horwitz BS. Fractures of the epiphyseal plate. Clin Orthop 1965;41:24–30.
142. Neviaser RJ. Injuries to and developmental deformities of the shoulder. In: Bora FW Jr (ed) The Pediatric Upper Extremity Philadelphia: Saunders, 1986.
143. Nilsson S, Svartholm F. Fractures of the upper end of the humerus in children. Acta Chir Scand 1965;130:433–449.
144. Obremsky W, Routt MLC. Fracture-dislocation of the shoulder in a child: case report. J Trauma 1994;36:137–140.

145. Olszewski W, Sokolowski J, Swiecicki M. [Fractures and epiphysedyses of the proximal end of the humerus in children.] Chirurg Narz Ruchu 1974;39:569–573.
146. Pruitt DL, Hulsey RE, Fink B, Menske PR. Shoulder arthrodesis in pediatric patients. J Pediatr Orthop 1992;12:640–645.
147. Razemon JP, Baux S. Des fractures et les fractures-luxations de l'extrémité supériure de l'humérus. Rev Chir Orthop 1969; 55:387–496.
148. Reisig J, Vinz H, Grobler B. Differenzierte Behandlung der proximalen Humerusfraktur im Kindesalter. Z Chir 1980;105: 25–31.
149. Robin GC, Kedar SS. Separation of the upper humeral epiphysis in pituitary gigantism. J Bone Joint Surg Am 1962;44: 189–192.
150. Roche AE. The ultimate result of a case of separated upper epiphysis of the humerus. Clin J 1926;55:478–480.
151. Seijfarth G, Hemicke W. Proximale Oberarmbrüche bei Kindern und Jugendlichen. Beitr Orthop Traumatol 1975;22: 469–476.
152. Sherk H, Probst C. Fractures of the proximal humeral epiphysis. Orthop Clin North Am 1975;6:401–412.
153. Shibuya S, Ogawa K. Isolated avulsion fracture of the lesser tuberosity of the humerus: a case report. Clin Orthop 1984;2 11:215–218.
154. Siebler G. Zur operativen behandlung proximaler humerusfrakturen bei kindern und jugendlichen. Unfallchirurgie 1984;10:237–246.
155. Smith FM. Fracture-separation of the proximal humeral epiphysis. Am J Surg 1956;91:627–631.
156. Strauss RH, Lanese RR. Injuries among wrestlers in school and college tournaments. JAMA 1982;248:2016–2018.
157. Sullivan CA, Berman J. Blunt axillary artery injury in children: case reports. Vasc Surg 1988;22:60–65.
158. Te Slaa RL, Nollen AJG. A Salter type 3 fracture of the proximal epiphysis of the humerus. Injury 1987;18:429–431.
159. Thornheer W. Epiphysenlösung und Epiphysenfraktur am proximalen Humerusende. Ther Umsch 1969;26:129–133.
160. Tondeur G. Les fractures recentes de l'epanie. Acta Orthop Belg 1964;30:5–11.
161. Torg JS, Pollack H, Sweterlisch P. The effect of competitive pitching on the shoulders and elbows of preadolescent baseball players. Pediatrics 1972;49:267–272.
162. Tullos HS, King JW. Lesions of the pitching arms in adolescents. JAMA 1972;220:264–271.
163. Van Hove. Decollement epiphysaire du coude: recul de trentesix ans. Acta Orthop Belg 1951;17:289–292.
164. Visser JD, Rietberg M. Interposition of the long head of the biceps in fracture separation of the proximal humeral epiphysis. Neth J Surg 1980;32:1–3.
165. Vivian DN, Janes JM. Fractures involving the proximal humeral epiphysis. Am J Surg 1954;87:211–215.
166. Wahl D. Frakturen am proximalen Humerusende bei Kindern. Beitr Orthop Traumatol 1982;29:379–388.
167. Whitman R. A treatment of epiphyseal displacements and fractures of the upper extremity of the humerus designed to assure definite adjustment and fixation of the fragments. Ann Surg 1908;47:706–708.
168. Zanolli R. Fracture dell epifisi superiore del omero. Chir Organi Mov 1928;12:445–447.

Proximal Metaphysis

169. Ballard T, Marsh JL. Non-operative treatment of a completely displaced and shortened proximal humeral metaphysis fracture in a child. Iowa Orthop J 1991;12:80–84.
170. Stropeni L. L'omero varo da rottura spontanea di cisti ossea metafisari. Chirurgie 1938;12:531–534.

Diaphysis

171. Allen ME. Stress fracture of the humerus: a case study. Am J Sports Med 1974;12:244–245.
172. Astedt B. A method for the treatment of humerus fractures in the newborn using the S. von Rosen splint. Acta Orthop Scand 1969;40:234–236.
173. Balfour GW, Mooney V, Ashby ME. Diaphyseal fractures of the humerus treated with a ready-made fracture brace. J Bone Joint Surg Am 1982;64:11–13.
174. Bostman O, Bakalim G, Vainionpaa S, Wilppula E, Patiala H, Rokkanen P. Radial palsy in shaft fracture of the humerus. Acta Orthop Scand 1986;57:316–319.
175. Bouyala JM, Christian P, Jacquemier M, Ramaherisson P. La voie axillaire dans l'abord chirurgical de l'épaule et de l'éxtremité supérieure de l'humérus chez l'enfant. Chir Pediatr 1980;21:287–288.
176. Desbrosses J, Rebouillat J, Bosser C, Guilleminet M. Quelques reflexions sur le traitement des fractures des os longs chez l'enfant. Presse Med 1958;86:1929–1932.
177. Duthie HL. Radial nerve in osseous tunnel at humeral fracture site diagnosed radiographically. J Bone Joint Surg Br 1957; 39:746–747.
178. Eitenmüller J, David A, Scott A, Muhr G. Die operative Behandlung von Schaftfrackturen der oberen Extremität im Kindesalter, Indikation, zeitpunkt und verfahren swahl. Hefte Unfallheilkd 1990;212:377–380.
179. Filipe G, DuPont GY, Carlioz H. Les fractures itératives des deux os de l'avant bras de l'enfant. Chir Pediatr 1979;20:421–426.
180. Gainor BJ, Metzler M. Humeral shaft fracture with brachial artery injury. Clin Orthop 1986;204:154–161.
181. Gilchrist KK. A stockinette-velpeau for immobilization of the shoulder girdle. J Bone Joint Surg Am 1949;49:750–751.
182. Guibert L, Allouis M, Bourdelat D, Catier P, Babut JM. Fractures et décollements épiphysaires de l'extrémité supérieure de l'humérus chez l'enfant: place et modalités du traitment chirurgical. Chir Pediatr 1983;24:197–200.
183. Gupta A, Sharma S. Volar compartment syndrome of the arm complicating a fracture of the humeral shaft: a case report. Acta Orthop Scand 1991;62:77–78.
184. Hendrich V. Technik und Ergebnisse der Osteosynthese kindlicher Schaftfrakturen an der oberen Extremität. Hefte Unfallheilkd 1990;212:382–384.
185. Holstein A, Lewis GB. Fractures of the humerus with radial-nerve paralysis. J Bone Joint Surg Am 1963;45:1382–1396.
186. Judet J, Rigault P, Plumerault J. Fracture des deux os de l'avant bras chez l'enfant: etude critique à propos de 213 cas. Presse Med 1965;73:833–838.
187. Judet J, Rigault P, Plumerault J. Fracture diaphysaire des deux os l'avant bras chez les enfants: technique et résultat du traitment par fixateur externe de R et J Judet. Presse Med 1966; 74:2583–2588.
188. Lange RH, Foster RJ. Skeletal management of humeral shaft fractures associated with forearm fractures. Clin Orthop 1985;195:173–177.
189. MacFarlane I, Mushayt K. Double closed fractures of the humerus in a child. J Bone Joint Surg Am 1990;72:443.
190. Machan F-G, Vinz H. Die Oberarmschaftfraktur in Kindesalter. Unfallchirurgie 1993;19:166–174.
191. MacNichol MF. Roentgenographic evidence of median-nerve entrapment in a greenstick humeral fracture. J Bone Joint Surg Am 1978;60:998–1000.
192. Paitevin R, Pouliquen JC, Langlais J. Fractures des deux os de l'avant-bras chez l'enfant. Rev Chir Orthop 1986;72:41–43.

193. Pollock FH, Drake D, Bovill EG, Day L, Trafton PG. Treatment of radial neuropathy associated with fractures of the humerus. J Bone Joint Surg Am 1981;63:239–243.
194. Postacchini F, Morace GB. Fractures of the humerus associated with paralysis of the radial nerve. Ital J Orthop Traumatol 1989;14:455–464.
195. Rettig AC, Beltz, HF. Stress fracture in the humerus in an adolescent tennis tournament player. Am J Sports Med 1985;13:55–58.
196. Rigault P. Fracture de l'avant bras chez l'enfant. Ann Chir 1980;34:814–816.
197. Samardzic M, Grujicic D, Milinkovic ZB. Radial nerve lesions associated with fractures of the humeral shaft. Injury 1990;21:220–222.
198. Sarmiento A, Kinman PB, Galvin EG, Schmitt RH, Phillips JG. Functional bracing of fractures of the shaft of the humerus. J Bone Joint Surg Am 1977;59:596–601.
199. Schärli AF, Winiker H. Schaftfrakturen des Kleinkindesalters. Z Unfallchir 1989;82:216–226.
200. Sessa S, Lascombes P, Prevot J, Gayneux E, Blanquart D. Embrochage centro-médullaire dans les fractures de l'extrémité supérieure de l'humérus chez l'enfant et l'adolescent. Chir Pediatr 1990;31:43–46.
201. Strait RT, Siegel RM, Shapiro RA. Humeral fractures without obvious etiologies in children less than 3 years of age: when is it abuse? Pediatrics 1995;96:667–671.
202. Torode IP. Pseudarthrosis of the humerus in an infant: a case report. J Orthop Surg 1994;2:89–94.
203. Welz K. Individual isierendes Vorgehen bei Osteosynthese im Wachstumsalter. Beitr Orthop Trauma 1984;31:437–446.
204. Whitson RO. Relation of the radial nerve to the shaft of the humerus. J Bone Joint Surg Am 1954;36:85–88.
205. Wolfe JS, Eyring EJ. Median-nerve entrapment within a greenstick fracture. J Bone Joint Surg Am 1974;56:1270–1272.

Supracondylar Process

206. Al-Nail I. Humeral supracondylar spur and Struthers' ligament: a rare case of neurovascular entrapment in the upper limb. Int Orthop 1994;18:393–394.
207. Al-Qattan MM, Husband JB. Median nerve compression by the supracondylar process: a case report. J Hand Surg [Br] 1991;16:101–103.
208. Burczak JR. Median nerve palsy after operative treatment of intra-articular distal humerus fracture with intact supracondylar process. J Orthop Trauma 1994;8:252–254.
209. Cunningham DJ. Supra-condyloid process in the child. J Anat Physiol 1899;33:357–358.
210. Doane CP. Fractures of the supracondylar process of the humerus. J Bone Joint Surg Am 1936;18:757–759.
211. Laha RK, Dijouvny M, DeCastro SC. Entrapment of median nerve by supra-condylar process of the humerus. J Neurosurg 1977;46:252–259.
212. Newman A. The supracondylar process and its fracture. AJR 1969;105:844–849.
213. Spinner RJ, Lins RE, Jacobson SR, et al. Fractures of the supracondylar process of the humerus. J Hand Surg [Am] 1994;19:1038–1041.

Supracondylar Injury

214. Aamodt A, Grønmark T. Suprakondylaere humerus frakturer hos born. Tidsskr Nor Laegeforen 1991;111:1240–1241.
215. Abe M, Ishizu T, Nagaoka T, Oromuro T. Recurrent posterior dislocation of the head of the radius in post-traumatic cubitus varus. J Bone Joint Surg Br 1995;77:582–585.
216. Abe M, Ishizu T, Shirai H, et al. Tardy ulnar nerve palsy caused by cubitus varus deformity. J Hand Surg [Am] 1995;20:5–9.
217. Abraham E, Powers T, Witt P, Ray RD. Experimental hyperextension supracondylar fractures in monkeys. Clin Orthop 1982;171:309–314.
218. Abulfotooh M. Reduction of displaced supracondylar fracture of the humerus in children by manipulation in flexion. Acta Orthop Scand 1978;49:39–45.
219. Adams J, Rizzoli H. Tardy radial and ulnar nerve palsy. J Neurosurg 1959;16:342–346.
220. Aebi H. Der elbogenwinkel, seine beziehungen zu geschlect, köerperbau und hüftbreite. Acta Anat (Basel) 1947;3:229–237.
221. Alburger PD, Weidner PL, Betz RR. Supracondylar fractures of the humerus in children. J Pediatr Orthop 1992;12:16–19.
222. Alcott WH, Bowden BW, Miller PR. Displaced supracondylar fractures of the humerus in children: long-term follow-up of 69 patients. J Am Osteopath Assoc 1977;76:914–915.
223. Ali E. Supracondylar fracture of the numerus in children in Guyana. West Indian Med J 1981;30:34–37.
224. Allenborough CG. Remodeling of the humerus after supracondylar fractures in childhood. J Bone Joint Surg Br 1953;35:386–395.
225. Alonso-Llames M. Bilaterotricipital approach to the elbow: its application in the osteosynthesis of supracondylar fractures of the humerus in children. Acta Orthop Scand 1972;43:479–483.
226. Alonso-Llames M, Diaz-Peletier R, Moro Martin A. The correction of post-traumatic cubitus varus by hemi-wedge osteotomy. Int Orthop 1978;2:215–218.
227. Altchek M. Cubitus varus deformity following supracondylar fractures of the humerus. J Pediatr Orthop 1983;3:622–626.
228. Amspacher J, Merssenbaugh J. Supracondylar osteotomy of the humerus for correction of rotational and angular deformities of the elbow. South Med J 1964;57:846–850.
229. An KN, Morrey BF, Chao EYS. Carrying angle of the human elbow joint. J Orthop Res 1984;1:369–373.
230. Andressi A. Sulla contenzione con doppio filo transcutaneo delle fratture sovracondiloidee dell'omero del bambini. Arch Orthop 1962;74:406–412.
231. Andressi A. Studio comparativo sui metodi di osteomitesi percutanea con fili di kirschner nelle fratture sovracondiloidee scomposte dell'omero del bambina. Minerva Orthop 1985;36:295–300.
232. Arbogast RB, Gay G, Hochst B. Behandlungsergebnisse nach supracondylaren Humerusfrakturen im Kindesalter. Unfallheilkunde 1980;148:456–463.
233. Archibald DA, Roberts JA, Smith MG. Transarticular fixation for severely displaced supracondylar fractures in children. J Bone Joint Surg Br 1991;73:147–149.
234. Arino VL, Lluch EE, Ramirez AM, Ferrer J, Rodriguez L, Baixauli F. Percutaneous fixation of supracondylar fractures of the humerus in children. J Bone Joint Surg Am 1977;59:914–916.
235. Arnala I, Paananen H, Lindel-Iwan L. Supracondylar fractures of the humerus in children. Eur J Pediatr Surg 1991;1:27–29.
236. Arnold JA, Nasca RJ, Nelson CL. Supracondylar fractures of the humerus: the role of dynamic factors in prevention of deformity. J Bone Joint Surg Am 1977;59:386–390.
237. Aronson DC, van Vollenhoven E, Meeuwis JD. K-wire fixation of supracondylar humeral fractures in children: results of open reduction via a ventral approach in comparison with closed treatment. Injury 1993;24:179–181.
238. Aronson DD, Prager BI. Supracondylar fractures of the humerus in children: a modified technique for closed pinning. Clin Orthop 1987;219:174–177.
239. Ashbell TS, Kleinert HE, Kutz JE. Vascular injuries about the elbow. Clin Orthop 1967;50:107–121.

240. Ashhurst APC. An Anatomical and Surgical Study of Fractures of the Lower End of the Humerus. Philadelphia: Lea & Febiger, 1910.
241. Ating'a JEO. Conservative management of supracondylar fractures of the humerus in Eastern Provincial General Hospital, Machokos. East Afr Med J 1984;61:557–561.
242. Avellan WH. Uber Frakturen des unteren Humerusendes bei Kindern. Acta Chir Scand 1933;(suppl 27):1–49.
243. Babut JM, Guillaumat M, Vertrand JP, Mourot M. Complications vasculo-nerveuses des fractures supracondyliennes chez l'enfant sur une serie de 293 cas. Ann Med Nancy 1972;9: 605–611.
244. Bailey GG Jr. Nerve injuries in supracondylar fractures of the humerus in children. N Engl J Med 1939;221:260–263.
245. Bakalim G, Wilppula E. Supracondylar humerus fractures in children: causes of changes in the carrying angle of the elbow. Acta Orthop Scand 1972;43:366–371.
246. Bamford DJ, Stanley D. Anterior interosseous nerve paralysis: an underdiagnosed complication of supracondylar fracture of the humerus in children. Injury 1989;20:294–295.
247. Banskota A, Volz RG. Traumatic laceration of the radial nerve following supracondylar fracture of the elbow. Clin Orthop 1984;184:150–154.
248. Barac M, Gujic M, Hranilovic B. Behandlungen der Bruche am distalen Teil des Oberarms. Hefte Unfallheilkd 1974;114: 26–32.
249. Basom W. Supracondylar and transcondylar fractures in children. Clin Orthop 1953;1:43–54.
250. Baumann E. Beitrage zur Kenntnis der Frakturen am Ellbogengelenk. Unter besonderer Berucksichtigung der Spatfolgen. I. Allgemeines und Fractura supracondylica. Beitr Klin Chir 1929;146:1–23.
251. Baumann E. Die Behandlung von Oberarm bruchen mittels Vertikalextension. Beitr Klin Chir 1931;152:260–268.
252. Baumann E. Zur Behandlung der Brüche des distalen Humerusendes beim Kind. Chir Praxis 1960;4:317–319.
253. Beck A. Therapy of supracondylar fractures in children. Zentralbl Chir 1933;60:2242–2247.
254. Bellemore MG, Barrett IR, Middleton RW, Scougall JS, Whiteway DW. Supracondylar osteotomy of the humerus for correction of cubitus varus. J Bone Joint Surg Br 1984;66:566–572.
255. Bender J. Cubitus varus after supracondylar fracture of the humerus in children: can this deformity be prevented? Reconstr Surg Traumatol 1979;17:100–105.
256. Bender J, Busch CA. Results of treatment of supracondylar fractures of the humerus in children with special reference to the cause and prevention of cubitus varus. Arch Chir Neerl 1978;30:29–36.
257. Berghausen T, Leslie BM, Ruby LK, Zimbler S. The severely displaced pediatric supracondylar fracture of humerus. Orthop Rev 1986;15:510–513.
258. Berndt V, Klemke KH, Furtenhofer K. Indikationen und Ergebnisse der operativen Versorgung ellenbogennaher Oberarmbrüche im Kindesalter. Unfallheilkunde 1980;148: 459–467.
259. Bertola L. On supracondylar fractures of the humerus in childhood. Minerva Ortop 1959;10:543–550.
260. Bhuller GS, Connolly JF. Ipsilateral supracondylar fractured humerus and fractured radius: case presentation. Nebr Med J 1982;67:85–87.
261. Bieh L, Gradinger R. Ellenbogengelenkshafte frakturen beim kind. Fortschr Med 1983;101:226–237.
262. Biyanni A, Gupta SP, Sharma JC. Determination of medial epicondylar epiphyseal angle for supracondylar humeral fractures in children. J Pediatr Orthop 1993;13:94–97.
263. Blount WP, Schulz I, Cassidy RH. Fractures of the elbow in children. JAMA 1951;146:699–705.
264. Bongers KF, Ponsen RJG. Use of Kirschner wires for percutaneous stabilization of supracondylar fractures of the humerus in children. Arch Chir Neerl 1979;31:203–206.
265. Bosanquet JS, Middleton RW. The reduction of supracondylar fractures of the humerus in children treated by traction-in-extension: a review of 18 cases. Injury 1983;14:373–377.
266. Bour P. L'embrochage descendant dans le traitment des fractures supracondyliennes de conde chez l'enfant. Nancy: Thèse Médecine, 1983, pp 108–120.
267. Boyd HB, Altenberg AR. Fractures about the elbow in children. Arch Surg 1944;49:213–220.
268. Brewster AH, Karp M. Fractures in the region of the elbow in children: an end-result study. Surg Gynecol Obstet 1940;71: 643–648.
269. Bristow WR. Myositis ossificans and Volkmann's paralysis: notes on two cases illustrating the rarer complications of supracondylar fracture of the humerus. Br J Surg 1923;10:475–479.
270. Broudy AS, Jupiter J, May JW Jr. Management of supracondylar fractures with brachial artery thrombosis in a child: case report and literature review. J Trauma 1979;19;540–542.
271. Brown IC, Zinar DM. Traumatic and iatrogenic neurologic complications after supracondylar humerus fractures in children. J Pediatr Orthop 1995;15:440–443.
272. Buhl O, Hellberg S. Displaced supracondylar fractures of the humerus in children. Acta Orthop Scand 1982;53:67–74.
273. Bulle G, Bay V. Beitrag zu konservativen behandlung der supracondylaren humerusfrakturen im kindesalter. Der Unfall im Kindesalter. Kinderchirurgie 1972;11:749–753.
274. Camp J, Ishizue K, Gomez M, Gelberman R, Akeson W. Alteration of Baumann's angle by humeral position: implications for treatment of supracondylar humerus fractures. J Pediatr Orthop 1993;13:521–525.
275. Carcassone M, Bergoin M, Hornung H. Results of operative treatment of severe supracondylar fractures of the elbow in children. J Pediatr Surg 1972;7:676–681.
276. Carli C. Wire traction for supracondylar fracture of the elbow in children. Chir Organ Mov 1933;18:311–316.
277. Carlson CS, Rosman MA. Cubitus varus: a new and simple technique for correction. J Pediatr Orthop 1982;2:199–202.
278. Casiano E. Reduction and fixation by pinning, "banderillero" style, fractures of the humerus in children. Milit Med 1960;125:363–365.
279. Celiker O, Pestilci FI, Tuzuner M. Supracondylar fractures of the humerus in children: analysis of the results in 142 patients. J Orthop Trauma 1990;4:265–269.
280. Chatterji ML. Observations on supracondylar fractures of humerus: its pathomechanism and management. Indian J Orthop 1979;13:152–158.
281. Chattopadhyay A. A suggested method of fixation in supracondylar fracture. J Indian Med Assoc 1984;82:204–206.
282. Cheng JCY, Lam TP, Shen WY. Closed reduction and percutaneous pinning for type III displaced supracondylar fractures of the humerus in children. J Orthop Trauma 1995;9:511–515.
283. Chess DG, Leshy JL, Hyndman JC. Cubitus varus: significant factors. J Pediatr Orthop 1994;14:190–192.
284. Clavert JM, Lecerf C, Mathieu JC, Buck P. La contention en flexion de la fracture supra-condylienne de l'humerus chez l'enfant. Rev Chir Orthop 1984;70:109–115.
285. Clement DA. Assessment of a treatment plan for managing acute vascular complications associated with supracondylar fractures of the humerus in children. J Pediatr Orthop 1990; 10:97–100.
286. Copley LA, Dormans JP, Davidson RS. Vascular injuries and their sequelae in pediatric supracondylar humeral fractures: toward a goal of prevention. J Pediatr Orthop 1996;16:99–103.
287. Corkery PH. The management of supracondylar fractures in the humerus in children. Br J Clin Pract 1964;18:583–589.

References

288. Cotta H, Puhl W, Martini AK. Über die Behandlung knöchen Verletzungen des Ellenbogengelenkes im Kindesalter. Unfallheilkunde 1979;82:41–46.
289. Coventry MB, Henderson CC. Supracondylar fractures of the humerus: 49 cases in children. Rocky Mt Med J 1956;53:458–461.
290. Cramer KE, Green NE, Devito DP. Incidence of anterior interosseous nerve palsy in supracondylar humerus fractures in children. J Pediatr Orthop 1993;13:502–505.
291. Cregan JCF. Prolonged traumatic arterial spasm after supracondylar fracture of the humerus. J Bone Joint Surg Br 1951; 33:363–364.
292. Cuendet MC. Supracondylar fractures of the humerus in children. Am Fam Physician 1973;12:176–183.
293. Culp RW, Osterman AL, Davidson RS, Skirven T, Bora FW. Neural injuries associated with supracondylar fractures of the humerus in children. J Bone Joint Surg Am 1990;72:1211–1215.
294. Dacol M. L'ostéotomie de valgisation supracondylienne de l'humerus dans les cals vicieux de l'enfant. Nice: Thèse Méd, 1979.
295. Dallek M, Mommsen U, Jungbluth KH, Kahl HJ. Die supracondylare humerusfraktur im kindesalter, ihre behandlung und ergebnisse nach der methode von Blount. Unfallchirurgie 1985;11:912–920.
296. D'Ambrosia RD. Supracondylar fractures of humerus: prevention of cubitus varus. J Bone Joint Surg Am 1972;54:60–66.
297. D'Ambrosia R, Zink W. Fractures of the elbow in children. Pediatr Ann 1982;11:541–543.
298. Damsin JP, Langlais J. Fractures supracondyliennes: symposium sur les fractures du coude chez l'enfant, sous la direction de J C Pouliquen. Rev Chir Orthop 1987;73:421–436.
299. Danielson L, Pettersson H. Open reduction and pin fixation of severely displaced supracondylar fractures of the humerus in children. Acta Orthop Scand 1980;51:249–255.
300. D'Arienzo M, Innocenti M, Pennisi M. The treatment of supracondylar fractures of the humerus in childhood (cases and results). Arch Putti Chir Organi Mov 1983;33:261–264.
301. Davids JR, Maguire MF, Mubarek SJ, Wenger DR. Lateral condylar fracture of the humerus following post traumatic cubitus varus. J Pediatr Orthop 1994;14:466–470.
302. DeBoeck H, DeSmet P, Penders W, DeRydt D. Supracondylar elbow fractures with impaction of the medial condyle in children. J Pediatr Orthop 1995;15:444–448.
303. Decoulx J. Les atteintes traumatiques et orthopédiques des membres et des ceintures comportant un risque vasculaire. Rev Chir Orthop 1974;60:27–32.
304. Della-Torre P, Roscini P, Mancini GB, Fiacca C. Supracondylar fractures of the humerus in children: bloodless treatment; review after more than 5 years. Arch Putti Chir Organi Mov 1984;34:217–223.
305. DeRosa GP, Graziano GP. A new osteotomy for cubitus varus. Clin Orthop 1988;236:160–165.
306. Deutschlander K. Zur Behandlung der suprakondylaren Uberstreckungsbruchen des Oberarmes. Chirurg 1934;6:733–738.
307. Divis G. Epiphyseolysis Humeri unter Betrachtlicher Dislokation des Gelenkskopfes: Unblutige Reposition. Arch Orthop Unfallchir 1927;25:342–349.
308. Dodge HS. Displaced supracondylar fractures of the humerus in children: treatment by Dunlop's traction. J Bone Joint Surg Am 1972;54:1408–1418.
309. Dormans JP, Squillante R, Sharf H. Acute neurovascular complications with supracondylar humerus fractures in children. J Hand Surg [Am] 1995;20:1–4.
310. Dowd GS, Hopcroft PW. Varus deformity in supracondylar fractures of the humerus in children. Injury 1979;10:297–303.
311. Duben W. Frakturen des Ellenbogengelenkes. Kinderchirург 1972;(suppl BII):736–752.
312. Ducret H. Traitment chirurgical du cubitus varus post traumatique de l'enfant (a propos de 20 cas). Lyon: These, 1987.
313. Edman P, Lohr G. Supracondylar fractures of the humerus treated with olecranon traction. Acta Chir Scand 1963;126:505–509.
314. Eid AM. Reduction of displaced supracondylar fracture of the humerus in children by manipulation in flexion. Acta Orthop Scand 1978;49:39–44.
315. Ekesparre WV. Treatment of supracondylar fractures of the humerus in the child. Ann Chir Infant 1970;11:213–219.
316. El-Ahwany MD. Supracondylar fractures of the humerus in children with a note on the surgical correction of late cubitus varus. Injury 1973;6:45–52.
317. El-Sharkawi A, Fattah H. Treatment of displaced supracondylar fractures of the humerus in children in full extension and supination. J Bone Joint Surg Br 1965;47:273–279.
318. Elstrom JA, Pankovich AM, Kassab MT. Irreducible supracondylar fracture of the humerus in children: a report of two cases. J Bone Joint Surg Am 1975;57:680–681.
319. Fearn CB, Goodfellow JW. Anterior interosseous nerve palsy. J Bone Joint Surg Br 1965;47:91–93.
320. Felsenreich F. Kindliche suprakondylare frakturen und post traumatische deformitaten des ellenbogengelenkes. Arch Orthop 1931;29:555–561.
321. Felsenreich F. Behandlungsergebnisse nach schweren supracondylären Oberarmbrüchen der kinder im "gefensterten thorax-Armgrips." Chirurg 1936;8:128–132.
322. Fevre M, Judet J. Traitment de sequelles de la maladie de Volkmann. Rev Chir Orthop 1957;43:437–445.
323. Finochietto R, Ferre RL. Fractures del codo: cubito aro posttraumatico. Prensa Med Argent 1937;12:598–605.
324. Florio L, Maurizo E. Meccanismo di produzione delle fratture sovracondiloidee del'omero: contributo su 24 fratture rare. Arch Putti Chir Organi Mov 1965;20:171–178.
325. Flynn JC. Deformity following supracondylar fracture of the humerus. J Fla Orthop Soc 1986;4:17–19.
326. Flynn JC, Matthews JG, Benoit RL. Blind pinning of displaced supracondylar fractures of the humerus in children: sixteen years experience with long-term follow-up. J Bone Joint Surg Am 1974;56:263–272.
327. Foster BK, Sandow M, Southwood RT. Supracondylar fractures of the humerus in childhood. J Bone Joint Surg Br 1983;65:674.
328. Fowles JV, Kassab MT. Displaced supracondylar fractures of the humerus in children: a report on the fixation of extension and flexion fractures by two lateral percutaneous pins. J Bone Joint Surg Br 1974;56:490–500.
329. France J, Strong M. Deformity and function in supracondylar fractures of the humerus in children variously treated by closed reduction and splinting, traction and percutaneous pinning. J Pediatr Orthop 1992;12:489–494.
330. Franke C, Reilmann H, Weinreich S. Langzeitergebnisse der Behandlung von suprakondylären Humerusfrakturen bei Kindern. Unfallchirurgie 1992;95:401–404.
331. French PR. Varus deformity of the elbow following supracondylar fractures of the humerus in children. Lancet 1959;1:439–441.
332. Fujioka H, Nakabayashi Y, Hirata S, et al. Analysis of tardy ulnar palsy associated with cubitus varus deformity after a supracondylar fracture of the humerus: a report of four cases. J Orthop Trauma 1995;9:435–440.
333. Furrer M, Mark G, Rüedi T. Management of displaced supracondylar fractures of the humerus in children. Injury 1991;22:259–262.

334. Gaddy BC, Manske PR, Pruitt DL, Schoenecker PL, Rouse AM. Distal humeral osteotomy for correction of post-traumatic cubitus varus. J Pediatr Orthop 1994;14:214–219.
335. Galindo E, Merchán ECR, Martin T, et al. Pseudoartrosis de una fractura supracondiles del húmero en an niño: a propósito de un case. Rev Ortop Trauma 1984;28:237–241.
336. Gao GX. A simple technique for correction of cubitus varus. Clin Med J 1986;99:853–854.
337. Garbuz DS, Leitch K, Wright JG. The treatment of supracondylar fractures in children with an absent radial pulse. J Pediatr Orthop 1991;16:594–596.
338. Gartland JJ. Management of supracondylar fractures of the humerus in children. Surg Gynecol Obstet 1959;109:145–152.
339. Gates DJ. Supracondylar fracture of humerus: problem in children managed with open reduction. Orthop Rev 1982;11: 91–96.
340. Gehling H, Gotzen L, Granna Dakis K, Hessman M. Behandlung and Ergebnisse bei suprakondylären Humerus Frakturen im Kindesalter. Unfallchirugie 1995;98:88–97.
341. Gerardi JA, Houkom JA, Mack GR. Treatment of displaced supracondylar fractures of the humerus in children by closed reduction and percutaneous pinning. Orthop Rev 1989;18: 1089–1095.
342. Gerstner CH, Hartmann C, Jaschke W, et al. Perkutane Bohrdrahtosteosynthese bei der suprakondylären Humerusfraktur beim kind. Zentralbl Chir 1981;106:603–608.
343. Gøjerloff C, Søjbjerg JO. Percutaneous pinning of supracondylar fractures of the humerus. Acta Orthop Scand 1978; 49:597–603.
344. Gouber MA, Healy WA III. The posterior approach to the elbow revisted. J Pediatr Orthop 1996;16:215–219.
345. Graham B, Tredwell SJ, Beauchamp RD, Bell HM. Supracondylar osteotomy of the humerus for correction of cubitus varus. J Pediatr Orthop 1990;10:228–231.
346. Graham HA. Supracondylar fractures of the elbow in children. Part I. Clin Orthop 1967;54:85–92.
347. Graham HA. Supracondylar fractures of the elbow in children. Part II. Clin Orthop 1967;54:93–99.
348. Grant HW, Wilson LE, Bisset WH. A long-term follow-up study of children with supracondylar fractures of the humerus. Eur J Pediatr Surg 1993;3:284–286.
349. Griffin PP. Supracondylar fractures of the humerus: treatment and complications. Pediatr Clin North Am 1975;22:477–489.
350. Griffin PP. Supracondylar fracture of the humerus in children. Orthop Surg 1982;1:2–7.
351. Groppo G, Angelini C, Bertone A. Percutaneous pinning of displaced supracondylar fractures of the humerus in children. Ital J Orthop Traumatol 1982;18:479–484.
352. Gruber MA, Hudson OC. Supracondylar fractures of the humerus in childhood: end-result study of open reduction. J Bone Joint Surg Am 1964;46:1245–1252.
353. Guetjens GG. Ischaemic anterior interosseous nerve injuries following supracondylar fractures of the humerus in children. Injury 1994;26:343–344.
354. Haddad RJ Jr, Saer KJ, Riordan DC. Percutaneous pinning of displaced supracondylar fractures of the elbow in children. Clin Orthop 1970;71:112–119.
355. Hadlow AT, Devane P, Nicol RO. A selective treatment approach to supracondylar fracture of the humerus in children. J Pediatr Orthop 1996;16:104–106.
356. Hagen R. Skin-traction-treatment of supracondylar fractures of the humerus in children. Acta Orthop Scand 1964;35:138–146.
357. Harris IE. Supracondylar fractures of the humerus in children. Orthopedics 1992;15:811–817.
358. Hart GM, Wilson DW, Arden GP. The operative management of the difficult supracondylar fracture of the humerus in the child. Injury 1977;9:30–35.
359. Hart VL. Reduction of supracondylar fracture in children. Surgery 1942;11:33–39.
360. Havranek P, Hajkova H. Treatment of supracondylar fractures of the humerus in children. Acta Chir Orthop Traumatol Cech 1984;51:65–72.
361. Henrikson B. Supracondylar fracture of the humerus in children: a late review of end-results with special reference to the cause of deformity, disability and complications. Acta Chir Scand 1966;(suppl 369):1–146.
362. Hernandez MA III, Roach JW. Corrective osteotomy for cubitus varus deformity. J Pediatr Orthop 1994;14:487–491.
363. Hesoun P. Die suprakondyläre Oberarmfraktur im Kindesalter: Auswertung von 99 suprakondylären Oberarmfrakturen aus den Jahren 1965 bis 1975. Unfallheilkunde 1976;79: 213–218.
364. Higaki T, Ikuta Y. The new operation method of the domed osteotomy for 4 children with varus deformity of the elbow joint. J Jpn Orthop Assoc 1982;31:30–35.
365. Hindman BW, Schreiber RR, Wiss FA, Ghilarducci MJ, Avolio RE. Supracondylar fractures of the humerus: prediction of the cubitus varus deformity with CT. Radiology 1988;168:513–515.
366. Hirt HJ, Vogel W, Reichmann W. Die suprakondylare Humerusfraktur im Kindesalter. Munch Med Wochenschr 1976;118:705–711.
367. Hofmann V. Behandlung der suprakondylaren Humerusfraktur im Kindesalter. Zentralbl Chir 1968;93:1678–1683.
368. Höllwarth M, Hausbrandt D. Supracondyläre Frakturen im Kindesalter. Unfallheilkunde 1980;148:452–457.
369. Holmberg L. Fractures of the distal end of the humerus in children. Acta Chir Scand 1945;(suppl 103):1–117.
370. Holmes JC, Skolnick MD, Hall JE. Untreated median-nerve entrapment in bone after fracture of the distal end of the humerus: postmortem findings after forty-seven years. J Bone Joint Surg Am 1979;61:309–310.
371. Hordegen KM. Neurologische Komplikationen bei kindlichen suprakondylaren Humerusfrakturen. Arch Orthop Unfallchir 1970;68:294–299.
372. Hovelius L, Tuvesson T. Anterior interosseous nerve paralysis as a complication of supracondylar fractures of the humerus in children. Arch Orthop Trauma Surg 1980;96:59–63.
373. Høyer A. Treatment of supracondylar fracture of the humerus by skeletal traction in an abduction splint. J Bone Joint Surg Am 1952;34:623–637.
374. Huegel A, Bijan A. Zur dringlichen primar-operativen Versorgung kindlicher suprakondylarer Oberarmfrakturen. Bruns Beitr Klin Chir 1974;221:633–638.
375. Infranzi A, Trillat A. Une nouvelle technique pour le traitement des fractures sus-condyliennes de l'humerus. Lyon Chir 1960; 55:90–94.
376. Ingelrans P, Lacheretz M, Barberis D. Les fractures de l'extremite supérieure de l'humerus chez l'enfant. Lille Chir 1970;25:297–304.
377. Ippolito E, Caterini R, Scola E. Supracondylar fractures of the humerus in children. J Bone Joint Surg Am 1986;68:333–344.
378. Ippolito E, Moneta MR, D'Arrigo C. Post-traumatic cubitus varus: long-term follow-up of corrective supracondylar humeral osteotomy in children. J Bone Joint Surg Am 1990;72: 757–765.
379. Izadpanah M. Die modifizierte Blountsche Methode bei suprakondylaren Humerusfrakturen im Kindesalter. Arch Orthop Unfallchir 1973;77:348–353.
380. Jacobus DA. Supracondylar fractures of the humerus in children: operative treatment. J Am Osteopath Acad Orthop 1982;1:5–11.
381. Jaffe L. Supracondylar fractures of the humerus in children: an emphasis on the extension type and its complications. Contemp Orthop 1981;3:828–832.

References

382. Jazayeri M, Rodda T. Ipsilateral fractures of distal radius and supracondylar of elbow. Orthop Rev 1980;9:85–89.
383. Jefferyss CD. "Straight lateral traction" in selected supracondylar fractures of the humerus in children. Injury 1977;8:213–216.
384. Jones ET, Louis DS. Median nerve injuries associated with supracondylar fractures of the humerus in children. Clin Orthop 1980;150:181–186.
385. Judet J. Traitement des fractures épiphysaires de l'enfant par broche trans-articulaire. Mem Acad Chir 1947;73:562–566.
386. Judet J. Traitement des fractures sus-condyliennes transversales de l'humérus chez l'enfant. Rev Chir Orthop 1953;39:199–212.
387. Kagan N, Herold HZ. Correction of axial deviations after supracondylar fractures of the humerus in children. Int Surg 1953;58:735–739.
388. Kamal AS, Austin RT. Dislocation of the median nerve and brachial artery in supracondylar fractures of the humerus. Injury 1980;12:161–163.
389. Kanaujia RR, Ikuta Y, Muneshige H, et al. Dome osteotomy for cubitus varus in children. Acta Orthop Scand 1988;59:314–318.
390. Kasser JR, Richards K, Millis M. The triceps dividing approach to open reduction of complex distal humeral fractures in adolescents: a Cybex evaluation of triceps function and motion. J Pediatr Orthop 1990;10:93–96.
391. Katthagen BD, Mittelmeier H, Schmitt E. Korrekturosteotomie des distalen humerus nach kindlichen ellenbogenverletzungen. Unfallheilkunde 1983;86:349–353.
392. Keenan WNW, Clegg J. Variations of Bauman's angle with age, sex and side: implications for its use in radiological monitoring of supracondylar fracture of the humerus in children. J Pediatr Orthop 1996;16:97–98.
393. Kekomaki M, Luoma R, Rikalainen H, Vikki P. Operative reduction and fixation of a difficult supracondylar extension fracture of the humerus. J Pediatr Orthop 1984;4:13–17.
394. Khadzhiev K. Treatment of supra- and transcondylar fractures of the humerus in children. Ortop Travmatol Protez 1985;4:32–37.
395. Khare GN, Gautam VK, Kochhar VL, Anand C. Prevention of cubitus varus deformity in supracondylar fractures of the humerus. Injury 1991;22:202–206.
396. King D, Secor C. Bow elbow (cubitus varus). J Bone Joint Surg Am 1951;33:572–576.
397. Kirz PH, Marsh HO. Supracondylar fractures of the humerus in children. Orthop Rev 1981;10:85–91.
398. Klassen RA. Supracondylar fractures of the elbow in children. In: Morrey BF (ed) The Elbow and Its Disorders. Philadelphia: Saunders, 1985.
399. Klems H, Weigert M. Die supracondylare Humerusfraktur des kindes: zur wahl des behandlungsverfahrens. Akt Traumatol 1975;5:117–122.
400. Klissoon N, Galpin R, Gayle M, et al. Evaluation of the role of comparison radiographs in the diagnosis of traumatic elbow injuries. J Pediatr Orthop 1995;15:449–453.
401. Kotwal PP, Mani GV, Dave PK. Open reduction and internal fixation of displaced supracondylar fractures of the humerus. Int Surg 1989;74:119–122.
402. Kramhoft M, Keller IL, Solgaard S. Displaced supracondylar fractures of the humerus in children. Clin Orthop 1987;221:215–220.
403. Kurer MHJ, Regan MW. Completely displaced supracondylar fracture of the humerus in children: a review of 1708 comparable cases. Clin Orthop 1990;256:205–212.
404. Kutscha-Lissberg K, Rauhs R. Frische Ellenbogen-verletzungen im Wachstumsalter. Hefte Unfallheilkd 1974;118:26–32.
405. Labelle H, Bunnell WP, Duhaime M, Poitras B. Cubitus varus deformity following supracondylar fractures of the humerus in children. J Pediatr Orthop 1982;2:539–546.
406. Laer L von. Die supracondylare Humerusfraktur im Kindesalter. Arch Orthop Traumatol Surg 1979;95:123–129.
407. LaGrange J, Rigault P. Les fractures de l'extremite inferieure de l'humerus chez l'enfant. Rev Chir Orthop 1962;48:4–9.
408. LaGrange J, Rigault P. Fractures supracondyliennes. Rev Chir Orthop 1962;48:337–342.
409. Lal GM, Bhan S. Delayed open reduction for supracondylar fractures of the humerus. Int Orthop 1991;15:189–191.
410. Lalanandham T, Laurence WN. Entrapment of the ulnar nerve in the callus of a supracondylar fracture of the humerus. Injury 1984;16:129–130.
411. Landin LA, Danielsson LG. Elbow fractures in children: an epidemiological analysis of 589 cases. Acta Orthop Scand 1986;57:309–314.
412. Langenskiöld A, Kivilaakso R. Varus and valgus deformity of the elbow following supracondylar fracture of the humerus. Acta Orthop Scand 1967;38:313–324.
413. Languepin A. Evolution pendant la croissance des cals des fractures de l'extremite superieure de l'humerus. Ann Orthop Ouest 1974;6:69–73.
414. Laupattarakasen W, Mahaisavariya B, Kowsuwon W, Saengnipathkul S. Pentalateral osteotomy for cubitus varus: clinical experience of a new technique. J Bone Joint Surg Br 1989;71:667–670.
415. Laurent D, Accary D. Complication vasculaire d'une fracture supra-condylienne de l'humerus: arteriographie trompeuse. Rev Chir Orthop 1981;67:495–497.
416. Lawrence W. Supracondylar fractures of the humerus in children: a review of 100 cases. Br J Surg 1956;44:143–148.
417. Lefort G, Miscault GD, Gillier P, Coppeaux J, Daoud S. Lesions artérielles au cours des fractures supracondyliennes de l'humérus chez l'enfant. Chir Pediatr 1986;27:100–102.
418. Lefort L. Fractures supra-condyliennes de l'humerus chez l'enfant. Ann Chir 1982;36:293–298.
419. Levai JP, Tanguy A, Collin JP, Teinturier P. Un cas de luxation posterieure recidivante du conde liee a un cal vicieux de la palette humerale. Rev Chir Orthop 1979;65:457–459.
420. Levine MJ, Horn B, Pizzutillo PD. Treatment of cubitus varus in the pediatric population with humeral osteotomy and external fixation. J Pediatr Orthop 1996;16:597–601.
421. Liddell WA. Neurovascular complications in widely displaced supracondylar fractures of the humerus. J Bone Joint Surg Br 1967;49:806.
422. Link W, Henning F, Schmid J, Baranowski D. Die suprakondyläre Oberarmfraktur im Kindesalter. Akt Traumatol 1986;16:17–20.
423. Lipscomb PR, Burleson RJ. Vascular and neural complications in supracondylar fractures of the humerus in children. J Bone Joint Surg Am 1955;37:487–492.
424. Lonroth H. Measurement of rotational displacement in supracondylar fractures of the humerus. Acta Radiol 1962;57:65–70.
425. Lorge F. Les fractures supracondyliennes de l'humérus chez l'enfant: a propos de 376 cas. Lyon: Thèse Méd, 1978.
426. Louvelle H, Bunnel WP, Duhaime M, et al. Cubitus varus deformity following supracondylar fractures of the humerus in children. J Pediatr Orthop 1982;2:539–545.
427. Lubinus HH. Über den Entstehungsmechanismus und die Therapie der supracondylären Humerusfraktur. Dtsch Z Chir 1924;186:289–306.
428. Lugnegard H, Walheim G, Wennberg A. Operative treatment of ulnar nerve neuropathy in the elbow region. Acta Orthop Scand 1977;18:176–199.
429. Lund-Kristenson J, Vibald D. Supracondylar fractures of the humerus in children. Acta Orthop Scand 1976;47:375–380.

430. Macafee AL. Infantile supracondylar fracture. J Bone Joint Surg Br 1967;49:768–770.
431. Macioce D, Leardi G, Colombo A, Oldani M. La nostra esperienza nel traitamento delle fratture sovracondiloidee di omero nell' infanzia. Minerva Ortop 1987;38:37–41.
432. Madsen E. Supracondylar fractures of the humerus in children. J Bone Joint Surg Br 1955;37:241–245.
433. Maffei SG, Girolami M, Ceccarelli F. The treatment of supracondylar fractures of the humerus in children by closed reduction and fixation with percutaneous Kirschner wires. Ital J Orthop Traumatol 1983;19:181–187.
434. Mahaisavariya B, Laupattarakasem W. Supracondylar fracture of the humerus; malrotation versus cubitus varus deformity. Injury 1993;24:416–418.
435. Mann TS. Prognosis in supracondylar fractures. J Bone Joint Surg Br 1963;45:516–522.
436. Marburger R, Burgess RC. Delayed high median neuropathy after supracondylar humeral fracture. Clin Orthop 1995;315:246–250.
437. Marck KW, Koolman AM, Buninen Dijk B. Brachial artery rupture following supracondylar fracture of the humerus. Neth J Surg 1986;38:81–84.
438. Marion J, LaGrange J, Faysse R, et al. Les fractures de l'extremité inférieure de l'humérus chez l'enfant. Rev Chir Orthop 1962;48:333–490.
439. Marquis GP, Binns FG. A rare cause of brachial artery injury. J Bone Joint Surg Br 1990;72:319–320.
440. Martin DF, Tolo VT, Sellers DS, Weiland AJ. Radial nerve laceration and retraction associated with a supracondylar fracture of the humerus. J Hand Surg [Am] 1989;14:542–545.
441. Mastragostino S, Stella G, Valle GM, Boero S. Le fratture sovracondiloidee di omero nell' età evolutiva. Giarn Ital Ortop Traum 1991;17:161–168.
442. Maylahn DJ, Fahey JJ. Fractures of the elbow in children. JAMA 1958;116:220–225.
443. McCoy GF, Piggot J. Supracondylar osteotomy for cubitus varus: the value of the straight arm position. J Bone Joint Surg Br 1988;70:283–286.
444. McDonnell DP, Wilson JC. Fractures of the lower end of the humerus in children. J Bone Joint Surg Am 1948;30:347–358.
445. McGraw JJ, Akbarnia BA, Hanel DP, Keppler L, Burdge RE. Neurological complications resulting from supracondylar fractures of the humerus in children. J Pediatr Orthop 1986;16:647–651.
446. Mehserle WL, Meehan PL. Treatment of the displaced supracondylar fracture of the humerus (type III) with closed reduction and percutaneous cross-pin fixation. J Pediatr Orthop 1991;11:705–711.
447. Merchant ECR. Supracondylar fractures of the humerus in children: treatment by overhead skeletal traction. Orthop Rev 1992;21:475–482.
448. Meya R, Hacke W. Anterior interosseous nerve syndrome following supracondylar lesions of the median nerve: clinical findings and electrophysiological investigations. J Neurol 1983;129:91–94.
449. Milch H. Treatment of humeral cubitus valgus. Clin Orthop 1965;38:120–125.
450. Millis MB, Singer IJ, Hall JE. Supracondylar fracture of the humerus in children: further experience with a study in orthopaedic decision-making. Clin Orthop 1984;188:90–97.
451. Mitchell WJ, Adams JP. Effective management for supracondylar fractures of the humerus in children. Clin Orthop 1962;23:197–204.
452. Mitchell WJ, Adams JP. Effective management for supracondylar fractures of the humerus in children: a ten year review. JAMA 1961;175:573–577.
453. Moehring HD. Irreducible supracondylar fracture of the humerus complicated by anterior interosseous nerve palsy. Clin Orthop 1986;206:228–230.
454. Mohammed S, Rymaszewski LA. Supracondylar fractures of the distal humerus in children. Injury 1995;267:487–489.
455. Montgomery AH, Ireland J. Traumatic segmentary arterial spasm. JAMA 1935;105:1741–1743.
456. Monticelli G. Indicazioni e risultati nella cura delle fratture sovracondiloidee recenti dell'omero nei bambini. Ortop Traumat App Mot 1949;17:235–238.
457. Monticelli G. Le fratture metaepifisarie del gomito nei bambini consolidate in deformita. Loro evoluzioni in rapporto all'accrescimento. Ortop Traumat App Mot 1958;26:13–17.
458. Monticelli G. Il gomito varo post-traumatico. Ortop Traumatol App Mot 1958;26:475–480.
459. Morger R. Frakturen und luxationen am kindlichen Ellenbogen. Basel-New York: Karger, 1965.
460. Morger R. Verletzungen am kindlichen Ellbogen. Z Kinderchir 1972;11:717–726.
461. Mourgues G, Fischer LP. Resultats lointains des decollements epiphysaires de l'extremite superieure de l'humerus chez l'adolescent. Rev Chir Orthop 1971;53:241–247.
462. Nacht J, Ecker M, Chung S, Lotke P, Das M. Supracondylar fractures of the humerus in children treated by closed reduction and percutaneous pinning. Clin Orthop 1983;177:203–208.
463. Nand S. Management of supracondylar fractures of the humerus in children. Int Surg 1977;57:893–899.
464. Nassar A. Correction of varus deformity following supracondylar fracture of the humerus. J Bone Joint Surg Br 1974;56:573–578.
465. Niemann KMW, Gould JS, Simmons B, Bora FW Jr. Injuries to and developmental deformities of the elbow in children. In: Bora FW Jr (ed) The Pediatric Upper Extremity. Philadelphia: Saunders, 1986.
466. Norman O. Roentgenological studies on dislocation in supracondylar fractures of the humerus. Ann Radiol (Paris) 1975;18:395–399.
467. Omer GE Jr, Simmons JW. Fracture of the distal humeral metaphyseal growth plate. South Med J 1968;61:651–653.
468. Oppenheim WL, Clader TJ, Smith C, Bayer M. Supracondylar humeral osteotomy for traumatic childhood cubitus varus deformity. Clin Orthop 1984;188:34–39.
469. Ormandy L. Olecranon screw fixation for skeletal traction of the humerus. Am J Surg 1974;127:656–661.
470. Ottolenghi CE. Prophylaxie du syndrome de Volkmann dans des fractures supracondyliennes du coude chez l'enfant. Rev Chir Orthop 1971;57:517–523.
471. Palmer EE, Niemann KM, Vesely D, Armstrong JH. Supracondylar fracture of the humerus in children. J Bone Joint Surg Am 1978;60:653–656.
472. Parmeggiani G, Lommi G. Le fratture sovracondiloidee dell'omero nell' infanzia. Minerva Ortop 1965;16:490–494.
473. Peh WCG, Sayampanathan SRE, Balachandran N. Presentation of supracondylar fractures of the humerus in Singapore children. Singapore Med J 1984;25:424–428.
474. Peters CL, Scott SM, Stevens PM. Closed reduction and percutaneous pinning of displaced supracondylar humerus fractures in children: description of a new closed reduction technique for fractures with brachialis muscle entrapment. J Orthop Trauma 1995;9:430–434.
475. Piggot J, Graham HK, McCoy GF. Supracondylar fractures of the humerus in children: treatment by straight lateral traction. J Bone Joint Surg Br 1986;68:577.
476. Pirone AM, Graham HK, Krajbich JI. Management of displaced extension-type supracondylar fractures of the humerus in children. J Bone Joint Surg Am 1988;70:641–650.

References

477. Pirot P, Gharib M, Langer I. Supracondylar humeral fractures in infants and small children. Z Kinderchir 1981;32:347–362.
478. Poitras B, Labelle H, Tchelebi H, et al. Supracondylar fractures of the humerus in children: review of 217 cases. Un Med Can 1983;112:325–329.
479. Poli G, Dal-Monte A. Supracondylar fractures of the humerus in children. Chir Organi Mov 1984;69:31–35.
480. Post M, Haskell SS. Reconstruction of the median nerve following entrapment in supracondylar fracture of the humerus. J Trauma 1974;14:252–257.
481. Pouliquen JC. Fractures supra-condyliennes de l'enfant. J Chir 1976;112:165–172.
482. Powell PJW. Arterial occlusion in juvenile humeral supracondylar fracture. Injury 1974;6:254–257.
483. Prévot J, Lascombes P, Métzizeau JP, Blanquart D. Fractures supra-condyliennes de l'humérus de l'enfant: traitement par embrochage descendant. Rev Chir Orthop 1990;76:191–197.
484. Prietto CA. Supracondylar fractures of the humerus. J Bone Joint Surg Am 1979;61:425–428.
485. Ramsey RH, Griz J. Immediate open reduction and internal fixation of severely displaced supracondylar fractures of the humerus in children. Clin Orthop 1973;90:130–135.
486. Raux P, Rigault P, Cirotteau Y, Guyonvarch G. Traitement du cubitus varus post-traumatique de l'enfant: a propos de 32 cas. Rev Chir Orthop 1975;61:141–146.
487. Ravaglia P, Saveriano G, Zara C. 251 Fratture sovracondiloidee di gomito in età pediatrica. Minerva Ortop 1984;35:741–752.
488. Razemon JP, Baux S. Les fractures de l'extremite superieure de l'humerus: rapport de la XLIIIe reunion annuelle de la SOFCOT. Rev Chir Orthop 1969;55:388–392.
489. Reinaerts HHM, Cheriex EC. Assessment of dislocation in the supracondylar fracture of the humerus, treated by overhead traction. Reconstr Surg Traumatol 1979;17:92–96.
490. Resch H, Helweg G. Die Bedeutung des Rotationsfehlers bei der suprakondylären Oberarmfraktur des Kindes. Akt Traumatol 1987;17:65–72.
491. Rettig H. Frakturen im Kindesalter. Munich: Verlag-Bergmann, 1957.
492. Ribault L. Le cubitus varus post-traumatique chez l'enfant (à propos de 8 cas chez l'enfant Africain). Acta Orthop Belg 1992;58:183–187.
493. Rigault P, Padovani JP, Chapuis B. Fractures et decollements epiphysaires de l'extrémité supérieure de l'humerus chez l'enfant. Forum Chir 1977;7:27–34.
494. Rogers LF, Malave S Jr, White H, Tachdjian MO. Plastic bowing, torus and greenstick supracondylar fractures of the humerus: radiographic clues to obscure fractures of the elbow in children. Pediatr Radiol 1978;128:145–148.
495. Rona G, Eltz A, Kuderna H, Turek S. Ergebnisse der nachuntersuchung kindlicher suprakondylarer oberarmbruche nach konservativer und operativer Behandlung. Unfallheilkunde 1980;148:447–452.
496. Rosman M. A fracture board to facilitate the management of supracondylar humeral fractures in children. J Trauma 1975;15:153–154.
497. Rowell PJW. Arterial occlusion in juvenile humeral supracondylar fracture. Injury 1975;6:254–265.
498. Royce RO, Duthowsky JP, Kasser JP, Rand FR. Neurologic complications after K-wire fixation of supracondylar humerus fractures in children. J Pediatr Orthop 1991;11:191–194.
499. Royle SG, Burke D. Ulna neuropathy after elbow injury in children. J Pediatr Orthop 1990;10:495–496.
500. Sabate AF, Rubio I, Olivares M. Desprendimentos epifisarios graves del cuello humeral. Barcelona Quirurg 1974;18:329–332.
501. Salter RB. Supracondylar fractures in childhood. J Bone Joint Surg Br 1959;41:881.
502. Sandegard E. Fracture of the lower end of the humerus in children: treatment and end results. Acta Chir Scand 1943;(suppl 89):1–184.
503. Satter P, Schulte HD, Dorr B. Die ergebnisse der behandlung supracondylärer Oberarmfrakturen bei Kindern unter besonderer berucksichtigung der Methode nach Blount. Zentralbl Chir 1971;96:125–137.
504. Schantz ZK, Riegels-Nielsen P. The anterior interosseous nerve syndrome. J Hand Surg [Br] 1992;17:514–512.
505. Schickendanz H, Schramm H, Herrmann K, Jager S. Fractures and dislocations in the elbow in childhood. Am Fam Physician 1973;13:176–183.
506. Schink W. Die Fractura supracondylica humeri und die ischämische Kontraktur im Kindesalter. Chirurg 1968;39:417–423.
507. Schlag G, Hable W. Die gedeckte Bordhrah osteosynthese des stark verschoberen Kindlichen suprakondylären Oberarmbruches. Monatsscher Unfallheilkd 1971;74:97–120.
508. Schoenecker PL, Delgado E, Rotman M, Sicard GA, Capelli AM. Pulseless arm in association with totally displaced supracondylar fracture. J Orthop Trauma 1996;10:414–415.
509. Schück R, Bartsch M, Link W. Die chirurgische Behandlung distaler Humerusfrakturen im Kindesalter. Z Kinderchir 1989;44:283–285.
510. Setton D, Khouri N. Paralysie de nerf radial et fractures supracondyliennes de l'humérus chez l'enfant. Rev Chir Orthop 1992;78:28–33.
511. Shifren PG, Gehring HW, Iglesias LJ. Open reduction and internal fixation of displaced supracondylar fractures of the humerus in children. Orthop Clin North Am 1976;7:573–582.
512. Sibley TF, Briggs PJ, Gibson MJ. Supracondylar fractures of the humerus in childhood: range of movement following the posterior approach to open reduction. Injury 1991;22:456–458.
513. Sigge W, Behrens K, Roggenkamp K, Wurtenberger H. Comparison of Blount's sling and Kirschner wire fixation in the treatment of a dislocated supracondylar humeral fracture in childhood. Unfallchirurgie 1987;13:82–88.
514. Siris IE. Supracondylar fracture of the humerus: an analysis of 330 cases. Surg Gynecol Obstet 1939;68:201–216.
515. Skolnick MD, Hall JE, Micheli LJ. Supracondylar fractures of the humerus in children. Orthopedics 1980;3:395–399.
516. Smeets RJC. Supracondylaire humerus fracturen bij kinderen. Thesis, University of Amsterdam, 1976.
517. Smith FM. Children's elbow injuries: fractures and dislocations. Clin Orthop 1967;50:7–17.
518. Smith L. Supracondylar fractures of the humerus treated by direct observation. Clin Orthop 1967;50:37–42.
519. Smyth EHJ. Primary rupture of brachial artery and median nerve in supracondylar fracture of the humerus. J Bone Joint Surg Br 1956;38:736–741.
520. Sorrel E. A propos des fractures supracondyliennes de l'humerus chez l'enfant. Rev Chir Orthop 1946;32:383–386.
521. Sorrel E, Longuet Y. La voie trans-brachial anterieure dans la chirurgie des fractures supra-condyliennes de l'humerus chez l'enfant (indication et technique). Rev Chir Orthop 1946;32:3–8.
522. Spear HC, Janes JM. Rupture of the brachial artery accompanying dislocation of the elbow or supracondylar fracture. J Bone Joint Surg Am 1951;33:889–894.
523. Spinner M, Schreiber S. Anterior interosseous nerve paralysis: a complication of supracondylar fracture of the humerus in children. J Bone Joint Surg Am 1969;51:1584–1590.

524. Spinner RJ, Jacobson SR, Nunley JA. Fracture of a supracondylar humeral myositis ossificans. J Orthop Trauma 1995; 9:263–265.
525. Spitzer AG, Patterson DC. Acute nerve involvement in supracondylar fractures of the humerus in children. J Bone Joint Surg Br 1973;55:227.
526. Staples OS. Supracondylar fracture of the humerus in children. JAMA 1958;168:730–733.
527. Staples OS. Complications of traction treatment of supracondylar fracture of the humerus in children. J Bone Joint Surg Am 1959;41:369.
528. Staples OS. Dislocation of the brachial artery: a complication of supracondylar fracture of the humerus in childhood. J Bone Joint Surg Am 1965;47:1525–1532.
529. Sutton WR, Greene WB, Georgopoulos G, Dameron TRB Jr. Displaced supracondylar humeral fractures in children: a comparison of results and costs in patients treated by skeletal traction versus percutaneous pinning. Clin Orthop 1992;278: 81–87.
530. Sweeney J. Osteotomy of the humerus for malunion of supracondylar fractures. J Bone Joint Surg Br 1975;57: 117.
531. Swenson AL. The treatment of supracondylar fractures of the humerus by Kirschner-wire fixation. J Bone Joint Surg Am 1948;30:993–997.
532. Symeonides PP, Paschaloglou C, Pagalides T. Radial nerve enclosed in the callus of a supracondylar fracture. J Bone Joint Surg Br 1975;57:523–524.
533. Te Slaa RL, Faber WM, Nollen AJG, Ven Straaten T. Supracondylar fractures of the humerus in children: a long term follow-up study. Neth J Surg 1988;40:100–103.
534. Thomas AP. Entrapment of the proximal fragment of supracondylar fractures. J Bone Joint Surg Br 1990;72:321–322.
535. Thompson VP. Supracondylar fractures of the humerus in children. JAMA 1951;146:609–612.
536. Thorleifsson R, Karlsson J, Thorsteinsson T. Median nerve entrapment in bone after supracondylar fracture of the humerus: case report. Arch Orthop Trauma Surg 1984;107: 183–185.
537. Toledano B, Price AE. Constructing a bracket for fixation of supracondylar fractures in children. Orthop Rev 1990;19: 1026–1029.
538. Tongio J. Damages vasculaires au cours des lesions orthopediques et traumatiques des membres: etude radiologique. Rev Chir Orthop 1974;60:45–53.
539. Topping RE, Blanco JS, Davis TJ. Clinical evaluation of crossed-in versus lateral pin fixation in displaced supracondylar humerus fractures. J Pediatr Orthop 1995;15:435–439.
540. Uchida Y, Ogata K, Sugioka Y. A new three-dimensional osteotomy for cubitus varus deformity after supracondylar fracture of the humerus in children. J Pediatr Orthop 1991;11: 327–331.
541. Uchida Y, Sugioka Y. Ulnar nerve palsy after supracondylar humerus fracture. Acta Orthop Scand 1990;61:118–119.
542. Urlus M, Kestelijn P, VanLommel E, et al. Conservative treatment of displaced supracondylar humerus fractures of the extension type in children. Acta Orthop Belg 1991;57:382–389.
543. Vahvanen V, Aalto K. Supracondylar fracture of the humerus in children. Acta Orthop Scand 1978;49:225–230.
544. Vanderpool DW, Chalmers J, Lamb DW, Whiston TB. Peripheral compression lesions of the ulnar nerve. J Bone Joint Surg Br 1968;50:792–803.
545. Van Egmond DB, Tavenier D, Meeuwis JD. Anatomical and functional results after treatment of dislocated supracondylar fractures of the humerus in children. Neth J Surg 1985; 37:45–51.
546. Vasili LR. Diagnosis of vascular injury in children with supracondylar fractures of the humerus. Injury 1988;19:11–13.
547. Virenque J, LaFage J. Les fractures supra-condyliennes du conde chez l'enfant: resultats compares des traitments orthopedique et chirurgical, a propos de 163 observations. Ann Chir 1967;21:544–549.
548. Voss FR, Kasser JR, Trepman E, Simmons E Jr, Hall JE. Uniplanar supracondylar humeral osteotomy with preset Kirschner wires for post traumatic cubitus varus. J Pediatr Orthop 1994;14:471–478.
549. Vugt AB, Severijnen RM, Festen C. Neurovascular complications in supracondylar humeral fractures in children. Arch Orthop Trauma Surg 1988;107:203–205.
550. Wade FV, Batdorf J. Supracondylar fracture of the humerus in a child: a twelve year review with follow-up. J Trauma 1961;1: 269–271.
551. Wagner M. Operationsindikation bei Frakturen am distalen Humerusende im Wachstumsalter. Unfallheilkunde 1980;148: 433–438.
552. Wahl D. Post-traumatic cubitus varus. Zentralbl Chir 1983; 108:1086–1089.
553. Wahl D, Lent G, Kurth C. Über die Einteilung der kindlichen supracondylaren Humerusfrakturen und ihr praktischer Wert. Zentralbl Chir 1979;104:1393–1397.
554. Waldron VD. Supracondylar elbow fixture in the growing child. Orthop Rev 1990;11:437–439.
555. Walle W, Egungd N, Eikelug L. Supracondylar fracture of the humerus in children: review of closed and open reduction leading to a proposal for treatment. Injury 1985;16:296–302.
556. Webb AJ, Sherman FC. Supracondylar fractures of the humerus in children. J Pediatr Orthop 1988;8:87–92.
557. Webb AJ, Sherman FC. Supracondylar fractures of the humerus in children. J Pediatr Orthop 1989;9:315–325.
558. Weiland AJ, Meyers S, Tolo VT, Berg HL, Mueller J. Surgical treatment of displaced supracondylar fractures of the humerus in children. J Bone Joint Surg Am 1978;60:657–661.
559. Weller S. Konservierte oder operative Behandlung von suprakondylaren Oberarmfrakturen. Akt Traumatol 1974;2: 79–84.
560. Wilkins KE. The management of severely displaced supracondylar fractures of the humerus. Techn Orthop 1989;4:5–24.
561. Wilkins KE. The operative management of supracondylar fractures. Orthop Clin North Am 1990;21:269–289.
562. Wilkins KE. Residuals of elbow trauma in children. Orthop Clin North Am 1990;21:291–314.
563. Williamson DM, Coates CJ, Miller RK, et al. The normal characteristics of the Bauman (humero-capitellar) angle: an aid in the assessment of supracondylar fractures. J Pediatr Orthop 1992;12:696–698.
564. Williamson DM, Cole WG. Treatment of ipsilateral supracondylar and forearm fractures in children. Injury 1992;23: 159–161.
565. Williamson DM, Cole WG. Treatment of selected extension supracondylar fractures of the humerus by manipulation and strapping in flexion. Injury 1993;24:249–252.
566. Wilppula E, Bakalim G. Late results in supracondylar humeral fractures in children. Arch Orthop Trauma Surg 1985;104: 23–28.
567. Windfeld P, Pilgaard S. Osteosyntese af suprakondylaere humerus frakturer hos born. Nord Med 1961;66:1266–1271.
568. Wong HK, Balasubramanian P. Humeral torsional deformity after supracondylar osteotomy for cubitus varus: its influence on the post osteotomy carrying angle. J Pediatr Orthop 1992; 12:490–493.
569. Worlock P. Supracondylar fractures of the humerus: assessment of cubitus varus by the Baumann angle. J Bone Joint Surg Br 1986;68:755–757.

570. Worlock PH, Colton CL. Displaced supracondylar fractures of the humerus in children treated by overhead olecranon traction. Injury 1984;15:316–320.
571. Worlock PH, Colton C. Severely displaced supracondylar fractures of the humerus in children: a simple method of treatment. J Pediatr Orthop 1987;7:49–51.
572. Wray J. Management of supracondylar fracture with vascular insufficiency. Arch Surg 1965;90:279–283.
573. Yamamoto I, Ishii S, Usui M, Ogino T, Kaneda K. Cubitus varus deformity following supracondylar fracture of the humerus. Clin Orthop 1985;201:179–184.
574. Zanella FE. Injuries of the elbow and forearm in children. Rontgenblatter 1984;37:111–115.
575. Zilioli E, Ottaviani C, Maridati C, Morandi A. Le fratture sovracondiloidee scomposte di omero nel bambina. Minerva Ortop 1989;40:403–406.
576. Zionts LE, McKellop HA, Hathaway R. Torsional strength of pin configurations used to fix supracondylar fractures of the humerus in children. J Bone Joint Surg Am 1994;76:253–256.

Intercondylar

577. Beghin JL, Bucholz RW, Wenger DR. Intercondylar fractures of the humerus in young children. J Bone Joint Surg Am 1982;64:1083–1087.
578. Gabel GT, Barnes DA, Tullos HS. Greenstick intercondylar fracture of the distal humerus. Clin Orthop 1988;235:272–274.
579. Godette GA, Gruel CR. Percutaneous screw fixation of intercondylar fracture of the distal humerus. Orthop Rev 1993;12:466–468.
580. Jarvis JG, D'Astous JL. The pediatric T-supracondylar fracture. J Pediatr Orthop 1984;4:697–701.
581. Jupiter JB, Barnes KA, Goodman LJ, Saldaña AE. Multiplane fracture of the distal humerus. J Orthop Trauma 1993;7:216–220.
582. Kasser J, Richards K, Millis M. The triceps-dividing approach to open reduction of complex distal humeral fractures in adolescents. J Pediatr Orthop 1990;10:93–96.
583. Miller OL. Blind nailing of the "T" fracture of the lower end of the humerus which involves the joint. J Bone Joint Surg Am 1939;21:933–938.
584. Papavasiliou VA, Beslikas TA. T-Condylar fractures of the distal humeral condyles during childhood: an analysis of six cases. J Pediatr Orthop 1986;6:302–305.

Distal Physis (Transcondylar)

585. Abe M, Ishizu T, Nagaoka T, Onamura T. Epiphyseal separation of the distal end of the humeral epiphysis: a follow-up note. J Pediatr Orthop 1995;15:426–434.
586. Akbarnia BA, Silberstein MJ, Rende RJ, et al. Arthrography in the diagnosis of fractures of the distal end of the humerus in infants. J Bone Joint Surg Am 1986;68A:599–602.
587. Allen PD, Gramse AE. Transcondylar fractures of the humerus treated by Dunlop traction. Am J Surg 1945;67:217–221.
588. Barrett WP, Almquist EA, Staheli LT. Fracture separation of the distal humeral physis in the newborn. J Pediatr Orthop 1984;4:617–619.
589. Bergenfeldt E. Über schaden an der epiphysenfuge bei operativer behandlung von frakturen am unteren humerusende. Acta Chir Scand 1932;71:103–106.
590. Berman JM, Weiner DS. Neonatal fracture-separation of the distal humeral chondroepiphysis: a case report. Orthopedics 1980;3:875–876.
591. Camera U. Sul distacco traumatico totale puro dell'epifisi omerale inferiore. Chir Organi Mov 1926;10:294–297.
592. Chand K. Epiphyseal separation of distal humeral epiphysis in an infant. J Trauma 1974;14:521–523.
593. Cothay DM. Injury to the lower medial epiphysis of the humerus before development of the ossific center. J Bone Joint Surg Br 1967;49:766–767.
594. Dameron TB Jr. Transverse fractures of distal humerus in children. AAOS Instr Course Lect 1981;30:224–227.
595. DeJager LT, Hoffman EB. Fracture-separation of the distal humeral epiphysis. J Bone Joint Surg Br 1991;73:143–146.
596. DeLee JC, Wilkinson KE, Roger LF, Rockwood CA. Fracture-separation of the distal humeral epiphysis. J Bone Joint Surg Am 1980;62:46–51.
597. Dias JJ, Lamont AC, Jones JM. Ultrasonic diagnosis of neonatal separation of the distal humeral epiphysis. J Bone Joint Surg Br 1988;70:825–828.
598. Downs DM, Wirth CR. Fracture of the distal humeral chondroepiphysis in the neonate: a case report. Clin Orthop 1982;169:155–157.
599. Dunlop J. Transcondylar fractures of the humerus in childhood. J Bone Joint Surg 1939;21:59–73.
600. Ekengren K, Bergdahl S, Ekstrom G. Birth injuries to the epiphyseal cartilage. Acta Radiol Diagn 1978;19:197–206.
601. Ellis P, Grogan DP, Ogden JA. Fractures of the distal humerus in children. Orthop Update 1986;4:2–8.
602. Grantham SA, Tietjen R. Transcondylar fracture: dislocation of the elbow. J Bone Joint Surg Am 1976;58:1030–1031.
603. Hanson PE, Barne DA, Tullos HS. Arthrographic diagnosis of an injury pattern in the distal humerus of an infant. J Pediatr Orthop 1982;2:569–572.
604. Heuter C. Anatomische Studien an der Extremitatengelenken Neugeborner und Erwachsener. Virchows Arch 1862;25:572–587.
605. Holda ME, Manoli A, LaMont RL. Epiphyseal separation of the distal end of the humerus with medial displacement. J Bone Joint Surg Am 1980;62:525–527.
606. Jensenius H. Efterundersogelse af fratura humeri supracondylica hos born. Nord Med 1948;37:19–22.
607. Johansson J, Rosman M. Fracture of the capitulum humeri in children: a rare injury, often misdiagnosed. Clin Orthop 1980;146:157–160.
608. Judet J. Traitment des fractures epiphysaires de l'enfant par broche transarticulaire. Mem Acad Chir 1947;73:562–565.
609. Judet J. Traitment des fractures sus-condyliennes transversales de l'humerus chez l'enfant. Rev Chir Orthop 1953;39:199–203.
610. Kaplan SS, Reckling FW. Fracture separation of the lower humeral epiphysis with medial displacement. J Bone Joint Surg Am 1971;53:1102–1104.
611. Macafee AL. Infantile supracondylar fracture. J Bone Joint Surg Br 1967;49:768–770.
612. Marmor L, Bechtol CO. Fracture separation of the lower humeral epiphysis: report of a case. J Bone Joint Surg Am 1960;42:333–336.
613. Mauer I, Kolovos D, Loscos R. Epiphyseolysis of the distal humerus in a newborn. Bull Hosp Joint Dis 1967;28:109–111.
614. McIntyre WM, Wiley JJ, Charette RJ. Fracture-separation of the distal humeral epiphysis. Clin Orthop 1984;188:98–100.
615. Menniti D, Rossi A. I Distacchi epifisari Obstetrici. Arch Putti Chir Organi Mov 1966;21:192–194.
616. Menon TJ. Fracture separation of the lower humeral epiphysis due to birth injury: a case report. Injury 1982;14:168–169.
617. Merten DF, Kirks DR, Ruderman RJ. Occult humeral epiphysis fracture in battered infants. Pediatr Radiol 1981;10:151–154.
618. Mizuno K, Hirohata K, Kashiwagi D. Fracture-separation of the distal humeral epiphysis in young children. J Bone Joint Surg Am 1979;61:570–573.

619. Moroz PF. Results of surgical treatment of ununited transcondylar fractures of the humerus in children. Ortop Travmatol Protez 1983;1:30–33.
620. Omer JE, Simmons JW. Fracture of the distal humeral metaphyseal growth plate. South Med J 1968;61:651–652.
621. Paige ML, Port RB. Separation of the distal humeral epiphysis in the neonate. Am J Dis Child 1985;139:1203–1205.
622. Peiro A, Mut T, Aracil J, Martos F. Fracture-separation of the lower humeral epiphysis in young children. Acta Orthop Scand 1981;52:295–298.
623. Peterson HA. Triplane fracture of the distal humeral eipiphysis. J Pediatr Orthop 1983;3:81–84.
624. Peterson HA. Physeal injuries of the distal humerus. Orthopedics 1992;15:799–808.
625. Rogers LF, Rockwood CA Jr. Separation of the entire distal humeral epiphysis. Radiology 1973;106:393.
626. Ruo GY. Radiographic diagnosis of fracture-separation of the entire distal humeral epiphysis. Clin Radiol 1987;38:635–637.
627. Siffert RS. Displacement of the distal humeral epiphysis in the newborn infant. J Bone Joint Surg Am 1963;45:165–169.
628. Smith RW. Observations on disjunction of the lower epiphysis of the humerus. Dublin Q J Med Sci 1850;9:63–64.
629. Stricker SJ, Thomson JD, Kelly RA. Coronal-plane transcondylar fracture of the humerus in a child. Clin Orthop 1993;294:308–311.
630. Valdiserri L, Kelescian G. Su un caso di distacco epifisario osterico dell'estremita distale dell'omero. Osp Ital Chir 1965;13:407–410.
631. Welk LA, Adler RS. Case report 725. Skeletal Radiol 1992;21:198–200.
632. Willem SB, Stuyck J, Hoogmartens M, et al. Fracture-separation of the distal humeral epiphysis. Acta Orthop Belg 1987;53:109–111.
633. Yngve DA. Distal humeral epiphyseal separation. Orthopedics 1985;8:102–104.
634. Yoo CH, Kim YJ, Suh JT, et al. Avascular necrosis after fracture-separation of the distal end of the humerus in children. Orthopedics 1992;15:959–963.

Medial Condyle

635. Bensahel H, Csukonyi Z, Badelon O, Badaoui S. Fractures of the medial condyle of the humerus in children. J Pediatr Orthop 1986;6:430–433.
636. Brock HD, Casteleya PP, Opdecam P. Fracture of the medial humeral condyle: report of a case in an infant. J Bone Joint Surg Am 1987;69:1442–1444.
637. Chacha PB. Fracture of the medial condyle of the humerus with rotational displacement. J Bone Joint Surg Am 1970;52:1453–1458.
638. Cothay DM. Injury to the lower medial epiphysis of the humerus before development of the ossific centre: report of a case. J Bone Joint Surg Br 1967;49:766–767.
639. Dahl-Iverson E. Fracture condylienne humerale interne: reduction simple, sanglante. Lyon Chir 1936;33:234–237.
640. Dangles C, Tylowski C, Pankovich AM. Epicondylotrochlear fracture of the humerus before appearance of the ossification center: a case report. Clin Orthop 1982;171:161–163.
641. De Boeck H, Casteleyn PP, Opdecam P. Fracture of the medial humeral condyle. J Bone Joint Surg Am 1987;69:1442–1444.
642. Fahey J, O'Brien E. Fracture separation of the medial humeral condyle in a child confused with fracture of the medial epicondyle. J Bone Joint Surg Am 1971;53:1102–1104.
643. Faysse R, Marion J. Fractures du condyle interne de l'humerus. Rev Chir Orthop 1962;48:337–340.
644. Ferretti A, Papandres P. Stress fracture of the trochlea in an adolescent gymnast. J Shoulder Elbow Surg 1994;3:399–401.
645. Fowles JV, Kassab MT. Displaced fractures of the medial humeral condyle in children. J Bone Joint Surg Am 1980;62:1159–1163.
646. Ghawabi M. Fracture of the medial condyle of the humerus. J Bone Joint Surg Am 1975;57:677–680.
647. Granger B. On a particular fracture of the inner condyle of the humerus. Edinb Med J 1818;14:196–197.
648. Grant IR, Miller JH. Osteochondral fracture of the trochlea associated with fracture dislocation of the elbow. Injury 1974;6:257–260.
649. Hanspal RS. Injury to the medial humeral condyle in a child reviewed after 18 years. J Bone Joint Surg Br 1985;67:638–644.
650. Harrison RB, Keats TE, Frankel CJ, et al. Radiographic clues to fractures of the unossified medial humeral condyle in young children. Skeletal Radiol 1984;11:209–212.
651. Hasner E, Husby J. Fracture of epicondyle and condyle of humerus. Acta Chir Scand 1951;101:195–199.
652. Higgs S. Fractures of the internal epicondyle of the humerus. BMJ 1936;2:666–668.
653. Ingersoll RE. Fractures of the humeral condyles in children. Clin Orthop 1965;41:32–39.
654. Kilfoyle RM. Fractures of the medial condyle and epicondyle of the elbow in children. Clin Orthop 1965;41:43–50.
655. Martel W, Abell MR. Post-traumatic necrosis ("osteochondritis dissecans") supratrochlear fossa distal end of humerus. Skeletal Radiol 1978;2:173–176.
656. Murakami Y, Komiyama Y. Hypoplasia of the trochlea and the medial epicondyle of the humerus associated with ulnar neuropathy: report of two cases. J Bone Joint Surg Br 1978;60:225–227.
657. Papavasiliou V, Nenopoulos S, Venturis T. Fractures of the medial condyle of the humerus in childhood. J Pediatr Orthop 1987;7:421–425.
658. Pollosson E, Arnulf G. Fracture du condyle interne—reposition sanglante. Lyon Chir 1937;34:337–339.
659. Potter CMC. Fracture-dislocation of the trochlea. J Bone Joint Surg Br 1954;36:250–253.
660. Saraf SK, Tuli SM. Concomitant medial condyle fracture of the humerus in a childhood posterolateral dislocation of the elbow. J Orthop Trauma 1989;3:352–354.
661. Sato K, Miura T, Hypoplasia of the humeral trochlea. J Hand Surg [Am] 1990;15:1004–1007.
662. Speed JS, Macey HB. Fractures of the humeral condyles in children. J Bone Joint Surg 1933;15:903–919.
663. Tanabu S, Yamauchi Y, Fukushima M. Hypoplasia of the trochlea of the humerus as a cause of ulnar-nerve palsy. J Bone Joint Surg Am 1985;67:151–154.
664. Vanthournout I, Rudelli A, Valenti P, Montagne JP. Osteochondritis dissecans of the trochlea of the humerus. Pediatr Radiol 1991;21:600–601.
665. Yoo CH, Suh JT, Suh KT, et al. Avascular necrosis after fracture-separation of the distal end of the humerus in children. Orthopedics 1992;15:959–963.

Medial Epicondyle

666. Aitken AP, Childress HM. Intraarticular displacement of internal epicondyle following dislocation. J Bone Joint Surg 1938;20:161–166.
667. Bede WB, Lefebvre AR, Rosman MA. Fractures of the medial humeral epicondyle in children. Can J Surg 1975;18:137–141.
668. Bensahel H, Csukonyi, Badelon O, Badaoui S. Fractures of the medial condyle of the humerus in children. J Pediatr Orthop 1986;6:430–433.
669. Bernstein SM, King JD, Sanderson RA. Fractures of the medial epicondyle of the humerus. Contemp Orthop 1981;3:637–640.

670. Chessare JW, Rogers LF, White H, Tachdjian MO. Injuries of the medial epicondylar ossification center of the humerus. AJR 1977;129:49–54.
671. Childress HM. Recurrent ulnar-nerve dislocation at the elbow. J Bone Joint Surg Am 1956;38:978–984.
672. Cole RJ, Jenison M, Hayes CW. Anterior elbow dislocation following medial epicondylectomy: a case report. J Hand Surg [Am] 1994;19:614–616.
673. Cothay DM. Injury to the lower medial epiphysis of the humerus before development of the ossific centre: report of a case. J Bone Joint Surg Br 1967;49:766–767.
674. Dangles C, Tylkowski C, Pankovich AM. Epicondylotrochlear fracture of the humerus before appearance of the ossification center: a case report. Clin Orthop 1982;171:161–163.
675. Dias JJ, Johnson GV, Hoskinson J, Sulaiman K. Management of severely displaced medial epicondyle fractures. J Orthop Trauma 1987;1:59–63.
676. Driessen AP, Binnendijk B. Frakturen des medialen Epicondylus humeri und des lateralen condylus humeri bei Kindern. Z Kinderchir Suppl 1972;11:756–762.
677. Eid AM. Displacement of the medial epicondyle into the elbow joint. Egypt Orthop J 1975;10:160–172.
678. Eklöf O, Nordstrand A, Skog P-A. Avulsion fracture of the medial humerus epicondyle: results of treatment. Z Kinderchir 1970;9:114–117.
679. Fahey JJ, O'Brien ET. Fracture-separation of the medial humeral condyle in a child confused with fracture of the medial epicondyle. J Bone Joint Surg Am 1971;53:1102–1104.
680. Fairbank HAT, Buxton SJD. Displacement of the internal epicondyle into the elbow joint. Lancet 1934;2:218–219.
681. Févre M, Roudatis A. La réduction non sanglante des fractures de l'épitrochlée avec interposition de ce fragment dans l'interligne articulaire du conde. Rev Orthop 1993;20:300–314.
682. Fowles JV, Kassab MT, Moula T. Untreated intra-articular entrapment of the medial humeral epicondyle. J Bone Joint Surg Br 1980;66:562–565.
683. Fowles JV, Slimane N, Kassab MT. Elbow dislocation with avulsion of the medial humeral epicondyle. J Bone Joint Surg Br 1990;72:102–104.
684. Granger B. On a particular fracture of the inner condyle of the humerus. Edinb Med Surg J 1818;14:196–201.
685. Haw DW. Avulsion fracture of the medial epicondyle of the elbow in a young javelin thrower. Br J Sports Med 1081;15:47–48.
686. Higgs SL. Fractures of the internal epicondyle of the humerus. BMJ 1936;2:666–667.
687. Hines RF, Herndon WA, Evans JP. Operative treatment of medial epicondyle fractures in children. Clin Orthop 1987;223:170–174.
688. Inoue G. Neglected intra-articular entrapment of the medial epicondyle after dislocation of the elbow. J Shoulder Elbow Surg 1994;3:320–322.
689. Josefsson PO, Danielsson LG. Epicondylar elbow fracture in children: 35-year follow-up of 56 unreduced cases. Acta Orthop Scand 1986;57:313–319.
690. Mandat K, Marcickiewicz A, Wieczorkiewicz B, et al. Leczenie zlamán nadklykciowych kosci ramiennej u dzieci. Chir Narzad Ruchu I Orthoped Polska 1987;54:139–144.
691. Marion J, Faysse R. Fractures de l'épitrochlée. Rev Chir Orthop 1962;48:447–470.
692. Martini M, Hallaj N, Daoud A, Descamps L. Les luxations traumatiques récentes du conde: a propros de 94 observations. Acta Orthop Belg 1978;44:542–54.
693. Masse P. Technique de réduction des luxations due conde avec fracture ou interposition de l'épitrochlée. Rev Prat 1955;5:1038–1041.
694. Moon MS, Kim I, Han IH, et al. Arm wrestler's injury: report of seven cases. Clin Orthop 1980;147:219–221.
695. Papavasiliou VA. Fracture-separation of the medial epicondylar epiphysis of the elbow joint. Clin Orthop 1982;171:172–174.
696. Nyska M, Peiser J, Lukiec F, Katz T, Liberman N. Avulsion fracture of the medial epicondyle caused by arm wrestling. Am J Sports Med 1992;20:347–350.
697. Patrick J. Fracture of the medial epicondyle with displacement into the elbow joint. J Bone Joint Surg 1946;28:143–146.
698. Robert M, Moulies D, Alain JL. Les fractures de l'épitrochlée chez l'enfant. Chir Pediatr 1985;26:175–179.
699. Roberts NW. Displacement of the internal epicondyle into the elbow-joint. Lancet 1934;2:78.
700. Rosendahl B. Displacement of the medial epicondyle into the elbow joint: the final result in a case where the fragment has not been removed. Acta Orthop Scand 1959;28:212–219.
701. Schmier AA. Internal epicondylar epiphysis and elbow injuries. Surg Gynecol Obstet 1945;9:416–421.
702. Silberstein MJ, Brodeur AE, Graviss ER, Lusiri A. Some vagaries of the medial epicondyle. J Bone Joint Surg Am 1991;62:524–528.
703. Skak SV, Grossman F, Wagn P. Deformity after internal fixation of fracture separation of the medial epicondyle of the humerus. J Bone Joint Surg Br 1994;76:297–302.
704. Smith FM. Medial epicondyle injuries. JAMA 1972;142:396–400.
705. Tayeb AA, Shiveley RA. Bilateral elbow dislocations with intraarticular displacement of the medial epicondyles. J Trauma 1980;20:332–334.
706. Van Niekerk JLM, Severijnen RS. Medial epicondyle fractures of the humerus. Neth J Surg 1975;37:141–144.
707. Vecsei V, Perneczky A, Poltezauer P. Therapy of fractures of epicondylus medialis humeri. Arch Orthop Unfallchir 1975;82:233.
708. Walker HB. A case of dislocation of the elbow with separation of the internal epicondyle and displacement of the latter into the joint cavity. Br J Surg 1828;15:677–680.
709. Weber BG. Epiphysenfugen verletzungen. Helv Chir Acta 1964;31:103–108.
710. Wilkins KE. Fracture of the medial epicondyle in children. AAOS Instr Course Lect 1991;40:3–10.
711. Wilson JN. The treatment of fractures of the medial epicondyle of the humerus. J Bone Joint Surg Br 1960;42:778–781.
712. Wilson NI, Ingam R, Rhyaszewski L, Miller JH. Treatment of fractures of the medial epicondyle of the humerus. Injury 1988;19:342–344.
713. Woods G, Tullos H. Elbow instability and medial epicondyle fractures. Am J Sports Med 1977;5:23–29.
714. Zaltz I, Waters PM, Kasser JR. Ulnar nerve instability in children. J Pediatr Orthop 1996;16:567–569.

Lateral Condyle

715. Adams J, Rizzoli H. Tardy radial and ulnar nerve palsy. J Neurosurg 1959;16:342–347.
716. Agins HJ, Marcus NW. Articular cartilage sleeve fracture of the lateral humeral condyle capitellum: a previously undescribed entity. J Pediatr Orthop 1984;4:620–622.
717. Akbarnia BA, Silberstein MJ, Rende RJ, Graviss ER, Lusiri A. Arthrography in the diagnosis of fractures of the distal end of the humerus in infants. J Bone Joint Surg Am 1986;68:599–602.

718. Alvarez E, Patel MR, Nimberg G, Pearlman HS. Fracture of the capitulum humeri. J Bone Joint Surg Am 1975;57:1093–1096.
719. Amgwerd P, Sacher P. Behandlung der condylus radialis humeri Fraktur beim Kind. Unfallchirurgie 1990;830:49–53.
720. Badelon O, Bensahel H, Mazda K, Vie P. Lateral humeral condylar fractures in children: a report of 47 cases. J Pediatr Orthop 1988;8:31–36.
721. Badelon O, Vie P, Mazda K, Bensahel H. Fracture du condyle externe de l'humerus chez l'enfant: a propos d'une serie de 46 cas. Rev Chir Orthop 1986;72:66–71.
722. Badger FG. Fractures of the lateral condyle of the humerus. J Bone Joint Surg Br 1954;36:147.
723. Baumann E. Permanent damage after fracture of the condylis humeri radialis in children and its prevention. Helv Chir Acta 1958;25:4–5.
724. Beck E. Brüche des radialen oberarmcondyls bei Kindern. Arch Orthop Unfallchir 1966;60:340–356.
725. Beltran J, Rosenberg S, Kawelblum M, et al. Pediatric elbow fractures; MRI evaluation. Skeletal Radiol 1994;23:277–281.
726. Broca A. Décollments épiphysaires et fractures de la région condylienne externe. J Prax (Paris) 1944;97:117–119.
727. Conner AN, Smith MGH. Displaced fractures of the lateral humeral condyle in children. J Bone Joint Surg Br 1970;52:460–464.
728. Contargyris A. Paralysie tardive post-traumatique du nerf cubital: ostéotomie supra-condylienne. Rev Chir Orthop 1953;39:97–101.
729. Crabbe W. The treatment of fracture-separation of the capitular epiphysis. J Bone Joint Surg Br 1963;45:722–726.
730. Dallek M, Jungbluth KH. Histomorphologische Untersuchungen zur Entstehung der condylus-radialis-humeri-Fraktur im Wachstumsalter. Unfallchirurgie 1990;16:57–62.
731. Davis JR, Maguire MF, Mubarek SJ, Wenger DR. Lateral condylar fracture of the humerus following post-traumatic cubitus varus. J Pediatr Orthop 1994;14:466–470.
732. DeBoeck H. Surgery for non-union of the lateral humeral condyle in children. 6 cases followed for 1–9 years. Acta Orthop Scand 1995;66:401–402.
733. Dhillon KS, Sengupta S, Singh BJ. Delayed management of fracture of the lateral humeral condyle in children. Acta Orthop Scand 1988;59:419–424.
734. Dormans JP, Armstrong PF. Lateral condylar fracture in children: treatment of the acute fracture or the established nonunion. Techn Orthop 1989;4:25–29.
735. Dorvaric DM, Rooks MD. Anterior sleeve fracture of the capitellum. J Orthop Trauma 1990;4:188–192.
736. Duguet B, LeSauot J. Fractures du capitellum chez l'enfant. Chir Pediatr 1980;21:331–333.
737. Dunoyer JC. Déformations squelettiques consécutives aux fractures du condyle externe. Ann Orthop Quest 1974;6:82–87.
738. Fineschi G. Thérapeutique des fractures du condyle externe. Arch Putti Chir Org Moviment 1951;27:36–45.
739. Finnbogason T, Karlsson G, Lindberg L, Mortensson W. Nondisplaced and minimally displaced fractures of the lateral humeral condyle in children: a prospective radiographic investigation of fracture stability. J Pediatr Orthop 1995;15:422–425.
740. Flynn JC, Richards JF Jr. Non-union of minimally displaced fractures of the lateral condyle of the humerus in children. J Bone Joint Surg Am 1971;53:1096–1101.
741. Flynn JC, Richards JF Jr, Saltzman RT. Prevention and treatment of non-union of slightly displaced fractures of the lateral humeral condyle in children. J Bone Joint Surg Am 1975;57:1087–1092.
742. Fontanetta P, MacKenzie DA, Rosman M. Missed, maluniting, and malunited fractures of the lateral humeral condyle in children. J Trauma 1978;18:329–335.
743. Foster DE, Sullivan JA, Gross RH. Lateral humeral condylar fractures in children. J Pediatr Orthop 1985;5:16–22.
744. Fournet-Fayard J. Fractures du condyle externe. Rev Chir Orthop 1987;73:451–456.
745. Fowles JV, Kassab MT. Fracture of the capitulum humeri: treatment by excision. J Bone Joint Surg Am 1974;56:794–798.
746. Fowles JV, Rizkallah R. Intra-articular injuries of the elbow: pitfalls of diagnosis and treatment. Can Med Assoc J 1976;114:125–129.
747. Freeman RH. Fractures of the lateral humeral condyle. J Bone Joint Surg Br 1959;41:631.
748. Gaur SC, Varma AN, Swarup A. A new surgical technique for old united lateral condyle fractures of the humerus in children. J Trauma 1993;334:68–69.
749. Gay JR, Love JG. Diagnosis and treatment of tardy paralysis of the ulnar nerve: based on a study of 100 cases. J Bone Joint Surg 1947;29:1087–1097.
750. Grantham SA, Norris TR, Bush DC. Isolated fractures of the humeral capitellum. Clin Orthop 1981;161:262–269.
751. Grogan DP, Ogden JA. Pediatric elbow fracture need not be your nemesis. J Musculoskel Med 1986;3:64–68.
752. Hahn NF. Fall von eine besondere Variet der Frakturen des Ellenbogens. Z Kinder Geburtshilfe 1853;6:185–189.
753. Hansen PE, Barnes DA, Tullos HS. Case report: arthrographic diagnosis of an injury pattern in the distal humerus of an infant. J Pediatr Orthop 1982;2:569–571.
754. Haraldsson S. An osteochondrosis deformans juvenilis capituli humeri including investigation of intraosseous vasculature in distal humerus. Acta Orthop Scand 1959;(suppl 38):1–214.
755. Hardacre J, Nahigian S, Froimson A, Brown J. Fractures of the lateral condyle of the humerus in children. J Bone Joint Surg Am 1971;53:1083–1095.
756. Harrison MJG, Nurick S. Results of anterior transposition of the ulnar nerve for ulnar neuritis. BMJ 1970;1:27–32.
757. Hefti E, Jakob RP, von Laer L. Frakturen des condylus radialis humeri bei Kindern und Jugendlichen. Orthopade 1981;10:274–279.
758. Hennrikus WL, Millis MB. The dinner fork technique for treating displaced lateral condylar fractures of the humerus in children. Orthop Rev 1995;24:1278–1280.
759. Herring JA. Lateral condylar fracture of the elbow. J Pediatr Orthop 1986;6:724–728.
760. Heyl JH. Fractures of the external condyle of the humerus in children. Ann Surg 1935;101:1069–1074.
761. Holmes JC, Hall JE. Tardy ulnar nerve palsy in children. Clin Orthop 1978;135:128–132.
762. Holst-Nielsen F, Ottsen P. Fractures of the lateral condyle of the humerus in children. Acta Orthop Scand 1974;45:518–523.
763. Inoue G, Horii E. Combined shear fractures of the trochlea and capitellum associated with anterior fracture-dislocation of the elbow. J Orthop Trauma 1992;6:373–375.
764. Ippolito E, Tudisco C, Farsetti P, Caterini R. Fracture of the humeral condyles in children: 49 cases evaluated after 18–45 years. Acta Orthop Scand 1996;67:173–178.
765. Jakob R, Fowles J, Rang M, Kassab M. Observations concerning fractures of the lateral humeral condyle in children. J Bone Joint Surg Br 1975;57:430–436.
766. Jeffrey CC. Non-union of the epiphysis of the lateral condyle of the humerus. J Bone Joint Surg Br 1958;40:396–405.
767. Johansson J, Rosman M. Fracture of the capitulum humeri in children: a rare injury, often misdiagnosed. Clin Orthop 1980;146:157–163.
768. Kalenak A. Ununited fracture of the lateral condyle of the humerus: a fifty year follow-up. Clin Orthop 1977;124:181–185.
769. Kini MG. Fractures of the lateral condyle of the lower end of the humerus with complications: a simple technique for

closed reduction of the capitellar fracture. J Bone Joint Surg 1942;24:270–280.
770. Krö A, Genelin F, Obrist J, Zirknitzer J. Fehlheilungen und Wachstunsstörungen nach: Frakturen des condylus radialis humeri im Kindersalter. Unfallchirurgie 1989;15:113–121.
771. Lagrange J, Rigault P. Fractures du condyle externe. Rev Chir Orthop 1962;48:415–420.
772. Liberman N, Katz T, Howard CB, Nyska M. Fixation of capitellar fractures with the Herbert screw. Arch Orthop Trauma Surg 1991;110:155–157.
773. Lorenz H. Zur kenntnis der fractura capitulum humeri (eminential capitätae). Dtsch Z Chir 1905;1:531–534.
774. Magilligan DJ. Unusual regeneration of bone in a child. J Bone Joint Surg 1946;28:873–876.
775. Mäkelä EA, Böstman O, Kekomäki, et al. Biodegradable fixation of distal humeral physeal fractures. Clin Orthop 1992;283:237–243.
776. Marzo JM, d'Amato C, Strong M, Gillespie R. Usefulness and accuracy of arthrography in management of lateral humeral condyle fractures in children. J Pediatr Orthop 1990;10:317–321.
777. Masada K, Kawai H, Kawabata H, et al. Osteosynthesis for old, established non-union of the lateral condyle of the humerus. J Bone Joint Surg Am 1990;72:32–40.
778. McLearie M, Merson RD. Injuries to the lateral condyle epiphysis of the humerus in children. J Bone Joint Surg Br 1954;36:84–89.
779. Milch H. Fractures of the external humeral condyle. JAMA 1956;160:641–644.
780. Mouchet A. Fracture du condyle externe. Paris: Thèse, 1898.
781. Mouchet A. Paralysies tardines du nerf cubital a la suite des fractures du condyle externe de l'humerus. J Chir (Paris) 1914;12:437–449.
782. Ogino T, Minami A, Fukuda K. Tardy ulnar nerve palsy caused by cubitus varus deformity. J Hand Surg [Br] 1986;11:352–355.
783. Peterson HA. Triplane fracture of the distal humerus. J Pediatr Orthop 1983;3:81–84.
784. Reinders JF, Lens J. A missed opportunity: two fractures of the lateral humeral condyle in a girl aged 5 years. Neth J Surg 1983;35:78–80.
785. Robert M, Longis B, Moulies D, Alain JL. Les fractures du condyle externe chez l'enfant. Ann Chir 1984;38:621–626.
786. Röhl L. On fractures through the radial condyle of the humerus in children. Acta Chir Scand 1953;104:74–79.
787. Roye DP Jr, Bini SA, Ionfosino A. Late surgical treatment of lateral condylar fractures in children. J Pediatr Orthop 1991;11:195–199.
788. Rutherford A. Fractures of the lateral humeral condyle in children. J Bone Joint Surg Am 1985;67:851–856.
789. Schneider G, Pouliquen JC. Old ununited and malunited fractures of the lateral humeral condyle in children. J Orthop Surg 1993;1:34–41.
790. Silberstein MJ, Brodeur AE, Graviss ER. Some vagaries of the capitellum. J Bone Joint Surg 1979;61:244–247.
791. Simpson LA, Richards RR. Internal fixation of a capitellar fracture using Herbert screws. Clin Orthop 1986;209:166–170.
792. Smith FM. An eighty-four year follow-up on a patient with ununited fracture of the lateral condyle of the humerus. J Bone Joint Surg Am 1973;55:378–380.
793. Smith MGH. Osteochondritis of the humeral capitulum. J Bone Joint Surg Br 1964;46:50–54.
794. So YC, Fang D, Leong JCY, Bong SC. Varus deformity following lateral humeral fractures in children. J Pediatr Orthop 1985;5:569–972.
795. Thönell S, Mortensson W, Thomasson B. Prediction of the stability of minimally displaced fractures of the lateral humeral condyle. Acta Radiol 1988;29:367–370.
796. Van Vugt AB, Severijnen RV, Festern C. Fractures of the lateral humeral condyle in children: late results. Arch Orthop Trauma Surg 1988;107:206–209.
797. Von Laer L, Pagels P, Schroeder L. The treatment of fractures of the radial condyle of the humerus during the growth phase. Unfallheilkunde 1983;86:503–508.
798. Voshell AF, Taylor KPA. Regeneration of the lateral condyle of the humerus after excision. J Bone Joint Surg 1939;21:421–424.
799. Wadsworth TG. Premature epiphyseal fusion after injury to the capitulum. J Bone Joint Surg Br 1964;46:46–49.
800. Wadsworth TG. Injuries of the capitular (lateral humeral condylar) epiphysis. Clin Orthop 1972;85:127–133.
801. Ward WG, Nunley JA. Concomitant fractures of the capitellum and radial head. J Orthop Trauma 1988;2:114–116.
802. Wilson JN. Fractures of the external condyle of the humerus in children. Br J Surg 1955;43:88–92.
803. Wilson PD. Fracture of the lateral condyle of the humerus in childhood. J Bone Joint Surg 1936;18:301–318.
804. Yates C, Sullivan JA. Arthrographic diagnosis of elbow injuries in children. J Pediatr Orthop 1987;7:54–58.
805. Zanella FE, Piroth P. Prognosis of condylus-radialis-humeri fractures in children following conservative and osteosynthesis treatment. Akt Traumatol 1984;14:115–119.
806. Zeier FG. Lateral condylar fracture and its many complications: shall it be truth or consequences? Orthop Rev 1981;10:49–52.
807. Zeier FG. Complications of fractures of growing lateral humeral condyles. Contemp Orthop 1982;5:87–92.

Lateral Epicondyle

808. Capla D, Kundrat J. Surgical therapy for fractures of the lateral épicondyle of the humerus (Czech). Acta Chirurg Orthop Traumatol Cech 1977;44:539–544.
809. Koudela K, Kavan Z. Fracture of the lateral epicondyle of the humerus with elbow dislocation inward and detachment of the medial epicondyle (Czech). Acta Chirurg Orthop Traumatol Cech 1977;44:553–556.

Floating Elbow

810. Biyani A, Gupta SP, Sharma JC. Ipsilateral supracondylar fractures of humerus and forearm bones in children. Injury 1987;20:203–207.
811. Papavsilou V, Nenopoulos S. Ipsilateral injuries of elbow and forearm in children. J Pediatr Orthop 1986;6:58–61.
812. Stanitski CL, Micheli LJ. Simultaneous ipsilateral fracture of the arm and forearm in children. Clin Orthop 1980;153:218–220.
813. Templeton PA, Graham HK. The floating elbow in children. J Bone Joint Surg Br 1995;77:791–796.
814. Williamson DM, Cole WG. Treatment of ipsilateral supracondylar and forearm fractures in children. Injury 1992;23:159–161.

15

Elbow

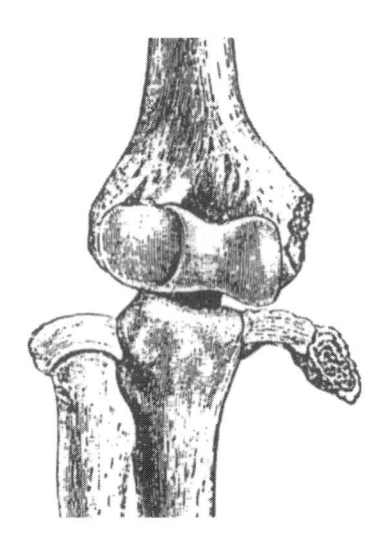

Engraving of dislocation of the elbow and concomitant medial epicondylar fracture. (From Poland J. Traumatic Separation of the Epiphyses. *London: Smith, Elder, 1898)*

Much of the chondro-osseous anatomy of the elbow, particularly the variable development of the epiphyseal ossification centers, is dealt with in Chapter 14 (humerus) and Chapter 16 (radius and ulna). The development and chondro-osseous transformation of each of these ossification centers may be irregular and often asymmetric (which must be remembered when assessing comparison films). The changes should not be confused with acute fracture, osteochondritis, or any other elbow lesions frequently encountered in childhood and adolescent athletes.[1,5,7,10,11]

The elbow has a complex geometry with three integrated joints (radiocapitellar, trochleoulnar, proximal radioulnar). It is a hinge joint tightly constrained by the contiguous ligamentous and capsular tissues.[3,4] These soft tissues attach proximally to various points around the distal humeral metaphysis and epiphysis, including the epicondyles. The distal attachments are primarily to the ulnar metaphysis, both medially and laterally (Fig. 15-1). The ligamentous attachments of the proximal radius do not add appreciably to stability laterally. In the child these ligaments often exhibit sufficient laxity prior to skeletal maturity that subluxation, dislocation, spontaneous reduction, and manipulative reduction are relatively easy compared to that in the adult. Such laxity also predisposes to nursemaid's elbow. The high incidence of concomitant medial epicondylar fracture when the child's elbow dislocates suggests that the medial collateral ligament is a significant constraining factor compared to other ligaments. Both the ulnar and radial ligaments principally attach to the ulna. No major collateral arm-to-forearm stabilizing structures attach directly to the proximal radius. The soft tissues stabilizing the medial side of the elbow consist of the anterior and posterior fibrous groupings of the medial collateral ligament and the medial capsule located between these bands. The anterior portion of the medial collateral ligament is a primary stabilizer of the elbow, both in extension and when subjected to valgus stress.[2] The relative contribution of the posterior ligament to elbow stability is minimal. The lateral ligament complex consists of the lateral collateral ligament, the annular ligament, and the accessory posterior annular ligament.[9]

Compromise of the anterior portion of the medial collateral ligament renders the elbow grossly unstable except in full extension. The anterior capsule provides primary stability, augmented by the lateral and medial ligaments.[6] In the skeletally mature patient posterior dislocation of the elbow invariably disrupts the anterior portion of the medial collateral ligament.[8] *However,* the rarity of redislocation or chronic instability following posterior elbow dislocation in children attests to the ultimate functional integrity of the medial collateral ligament and suggests that the ligament may not be significantly disrupted in elbow dislocations. In children the frequent concomitant fracture of the medial epicondyle allows chondro-osseous failure and extensive subperiosteal stripping, rather than discrete medial ligament failure. So long as the fracture heals, elbow stability is usually maintained. However, if the epicondyle undergoes nonunion or displaced fibrous malunion, variable elbow instability may occur, similar to the residual functional weakness in the anterior cruciate ligament seen with tibial spine injuries in children (see Chapter 23). This may predispose to degenerative osteoarthritis at an early age. There are no studies in children or adolescents with epicondylar injury to ascertain

Dislocation

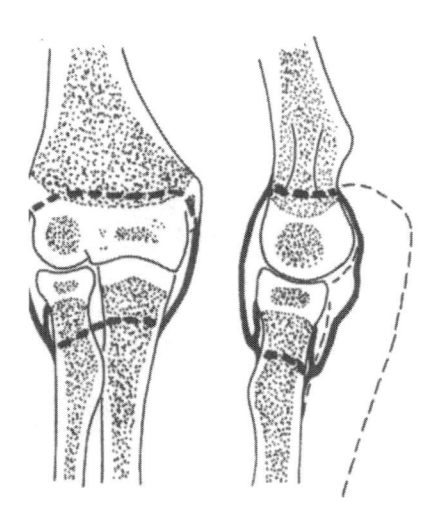

FIGURE 15-1. Elbow capsular and ligamentous attachments in an 8-year-old. These attachments may change with progressive chondro-osseous development. The medial and lateral capsules and ligaments are relatively taut in extension but become relaxed in flexion. The anterior and posterior ligaments have more redundancy to allow flexion and extension. The ulna is outlined by the narrow dashed line in the lateral view.

whether concomitant ligament damage also occurs (similar to the concomitance of cruciate injury associated with tibial spine avulsion).

In an experimental study of ligamentous injuries using cadaver elbows from adults, posterior dislocation of the elbow could be produced only when combined valgus and external rotatory torque was applied.[9] These investigators were unable to dislocate elbows with varus and internal rotatory torque forces or in extreme positions. In the elbow specimens that had an experimentally produced posterior dislocation, there usually was simultaneous rupture of the anterior part of the medial collateral ligament along with the annular ligament. In contrast, a lateral collateral ligament tear was evident in only 2 of 10 specimens.

Dislocation

Elbow dislocation, which constitutes about 5% of elbow injuries in children, appears to be the most common joint dislocation in children.[12-111] It is increasingly frequent after 8 years of age, reaching a peak during adolescence. This injury usually follows a fall on the outstretched hand with the elbow incompletely flexed, but dislocation also may occur as a hyperextension injury. Deforming forces, however, tend to be transmitted away from the joint to the proximal third of the radial and ulnar shafts or to the distal humerus; and they usually cause radioulnar shaft, supracondylar metaphyseal, or transcondylar physeal fractures, rather than elbow joint dislocations, much like the injury pattern at the knee.

The direction of displacement varies with the direction of the applied deforming force. Posterior displacement, which is usually accompanied by lateral displacement, is most common. Medial displacement should arouse suspicion of a transcondylar (physeal) fracture, rather than an elbow dislocation. Rotatory luxation with total displacement of one forearm bone and part of the other may occur with the posterior type when only one collateral ligament is torn. Divergent dislocation of the radius and ulna is rare in the child, as is anterior dislocation.

The complex association of axial and rotatory forces may cause not only capsular and ligamentous disruptions but a wide variety of concomitant chondro-osseous injuries.[13,42,61,82,86,94,95,99,100] Pure dislocation, unaccompanied by fracture, is relatively uncommon in children. *Always look for an associated fracture*, many of which are subtle (e.g., occult type 1 physeal injury or a chondro-osseous sleeve fracture), and be cognizant of cartilaginous epicondylar injuries that may not be evident radiographically. Multiple injuries may occur in the same arm, with distal radioulnar fractures being relatively common (Fig. 15-2). Complete examination of the injured extremity and sufficiently detailed pre- and postreduction films are essential to the diagnosis of these associated injuries. In the young child (under 5 years) evidence of condylar displacement may not be obvious until an extended period of time has elapsed following the acute injury.

Dislocation of the elbow is unusual in children under 2 years of age. Instead, they usually sustain a fracture of the entire distal humeral physis (transcondylar). This usually leads to a posteromedial shift of the radiolucent distal humeral epiphysis that is often misinterpreted as an elbow dislocation. The diagnosis must be accurate, as the treatment for elbow region fractures and an elbow dislocation differ significantly (see Chapters 14, 16).

Because of the hazard of concomitant neurovascular injuries, reduction frequently may have to be urgent.[32,71,74,87,97,108] The complete neurovascular status at and distal to the injured elbow must be ascertained *before* reduction, particularly in view of the potential for entrapping the median nerve or stretching the ulnar nerve. The same, careful neurovascular evaluation must also be carried out *after* reduc-

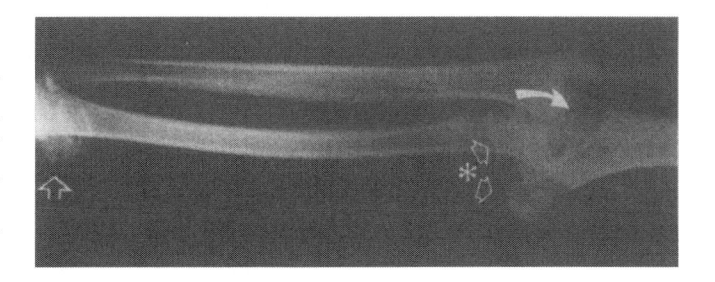

FIGURE 15-2. Dislocated elbow in a 10-year-old boy. This roentgenogram focused on the open injury. The solid curved arrow indicates the intraarticular air present because of the open wound. Note how the air–cartilage interface has outlined the cartilaginous components of the capitellum and trochlea (*arrows). A concomitant fracture of the distal radius was also present (open arrow) but was barely visible on the roentgenogram, which had been centered specifically on the supracondylar region.

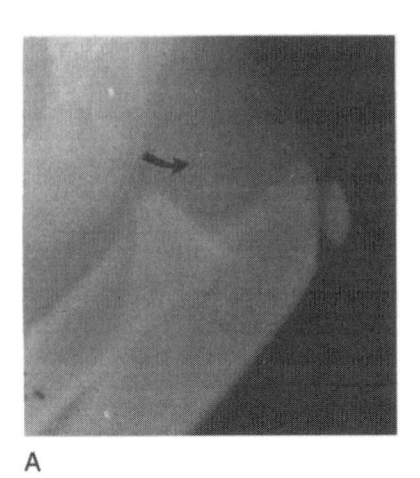

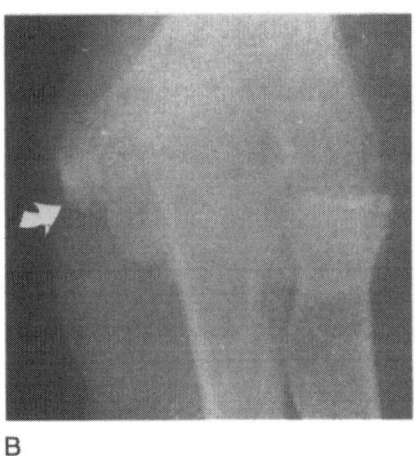

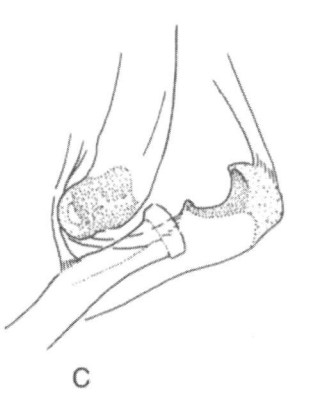

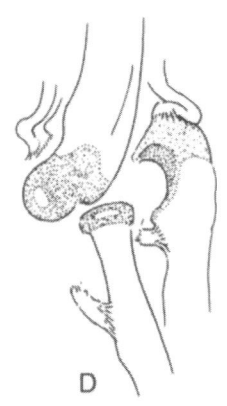

FIGURE 15-3. Lateral (A) and anterior (B) views of a posterolateral dislocation (black arrow) in a 7-year-old. The medial epicondyle is fractured but undisplaced (white arrow). (C, D) Posterior dislocation in flexion (C) and hyperextension (D), which has a higher risk of capsular disruption.

tion, as a potential complication of closed reduction is nerve entrapment within the joint.

Classification

Several patterns of elbow dislocation occur in children.

1. Posterior dislocation of the radius and ulna without other *obvious* osseous injury (Fig. 15-3).
2. Posterior dislocation with a fracture of the coronoid process (Fig. 15-4). There may be a shell separation of the unossified portion.
3. Posterior dislocation with a separation of part or all of the medial epicondyle (Fig. 15-5). This epicondylar fragment may be completely displaced into the elbow joint.
4. Posterior displacement with a fracture of the radial head or neck (Figs. 15-6, 15-7).
5. Posterior dislocation with a fracture of the olecranon (Fig. 15-8).
6. Lateral dislocation with a fracture of the lateral epicondyle of the humerus (Fig. 15-9).
7. Dislocation with a medial or lateral condylar fracture (Fig. 15-10).
8. Anterior dislocation, which is rare in children.
9. Divergent dislocation of the proximal radius and ulna (Fig. 15-11).
10. Convergent dislocation with translocation of the radius and ulna (Fig. 15-12).
11. Anterior or anterolateral displacement of the radius with a fracture of the ulna, the Monteggia fracture-dislocation, or a variant of it (see Chapter 16 for a complete discussion of this pattern).

Pathomechanics

Posterior dislocation usually results from a fall on the outstretched hand with the forearm supinated and the elbow extended or partially flexed. The force of the fall is transmitted along the forearm to the coronoid process. The coronoid process, which resists posterior displacement of the ulna, is more readily temporarily deformed in children because it is incompletely ossified. The laterally sloping surface of the inner two-thirds of the trochlea converts the

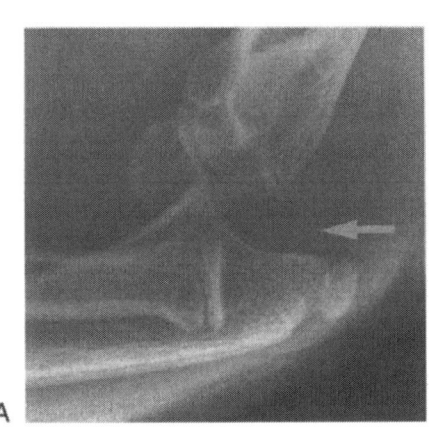

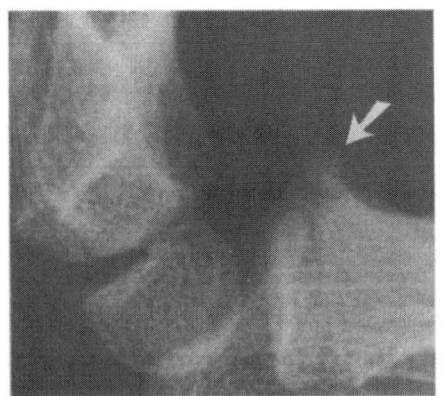

FIGURE 15-4. (A) Posterior elbow dislocation with an osseous fragment (arrow). The point of origin of the fragment cannot be readily determined. (B) Reduced dislocation shows that this fragment was a concomitant fracture of the coronoid process (arrow) of the ulna.

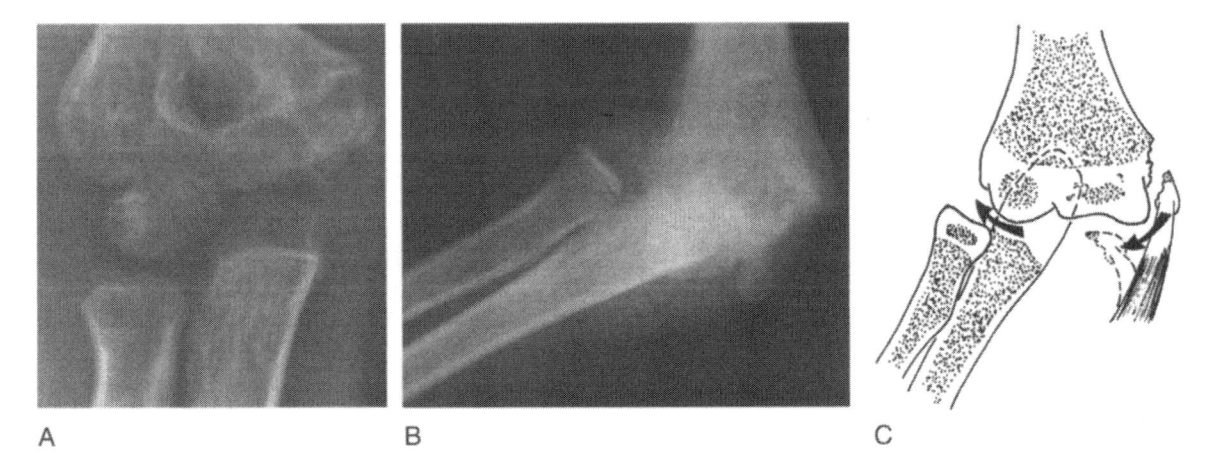

FIGURE 15-5. (A) Posterolateral dislocation with a displacement of the medial epicondyle. Such mild displacement may be missed on the initial evaluation. The additional fragments are multifocal trochlear ossification. (B) Posterior displacement of the medial epicondyle. Posteromedial soft tissue attachments are intact and may allow a satisfactory closed reduction without the need for fixation of the epicondyle. (C) Posterior dislocation with concomitant avulsion of the medial epicondyle, which may be pulled into the joint.

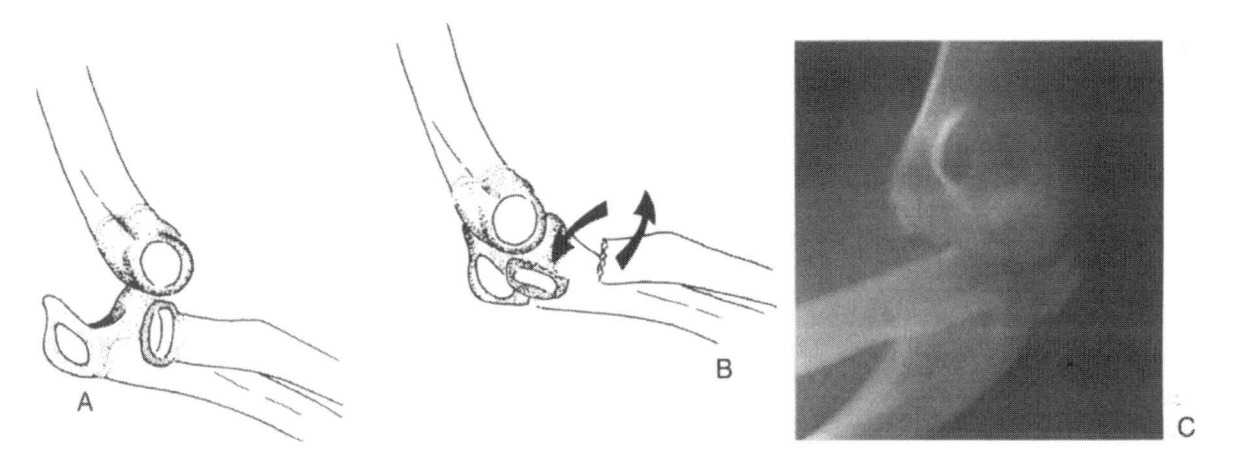

FIGURE 15-6. (A, B) Mechanism of displacing the radial epiphysis during injury or reduction. The radial head may impact posteriorly against the capitellum during attempted reduction. (C) Elbow dislocation with a displaced and rotated radial head fracture.

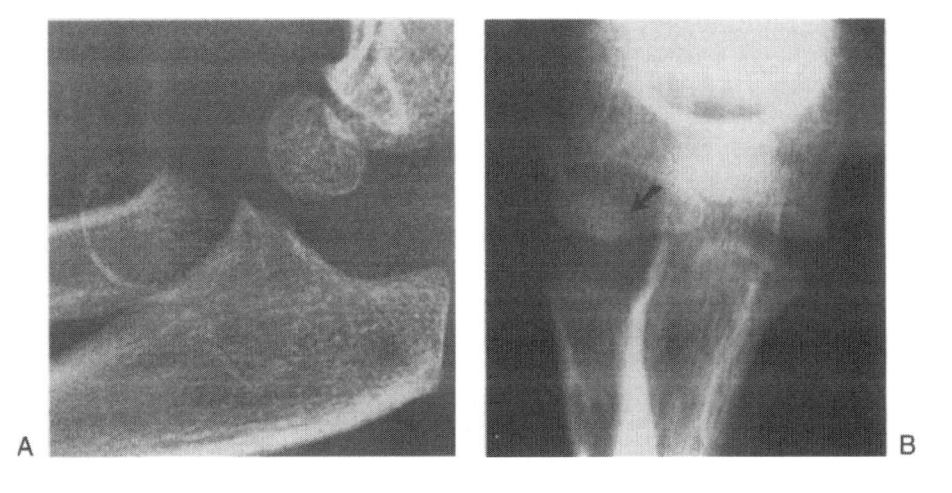

FIGURE 15-7. (A) Radial head displacement with a dislocation of the elbow. (B) Following reduction the radial head is displaced (arrow).

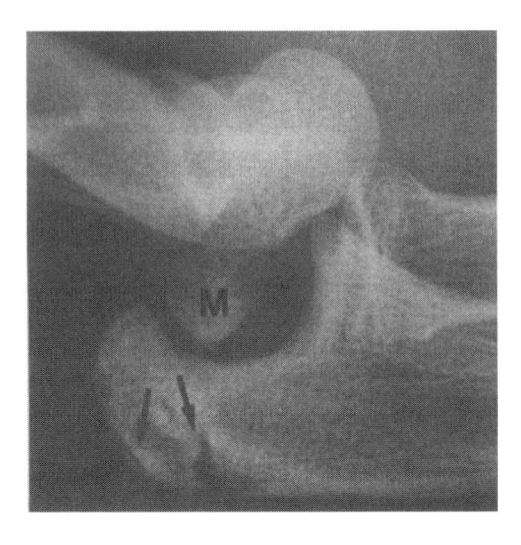

FIGURE 15-8. Posterior dislocation in a 14-year-old with concomitant olecranon fractures (arrows). One fracture line initially involved the closing physis but then extended into the joint. The medial epicondyle (M) has been displaced posteriorly.

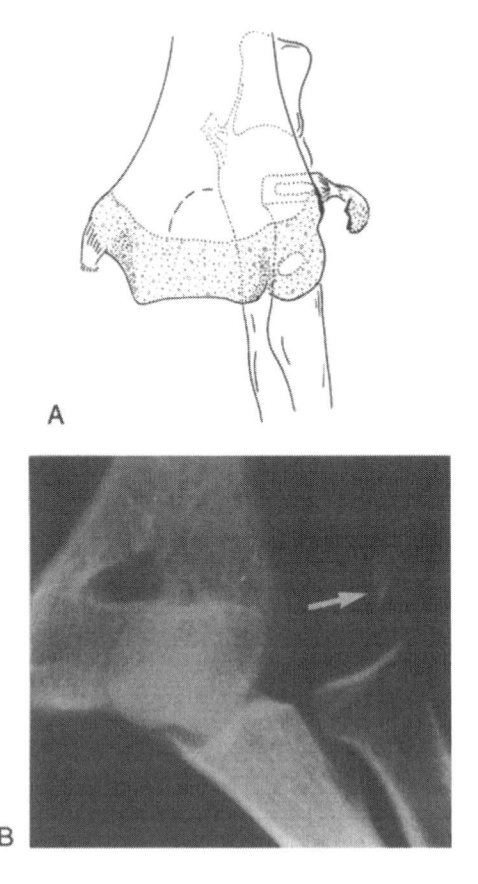

FIGURE 15-9. (A) Lateral displacement (arrow) with concomitant fracture of the lateral epicondyle. (B) Dislocation and lateral epicondylar fracture (arrow) in a 15-year-old girl.

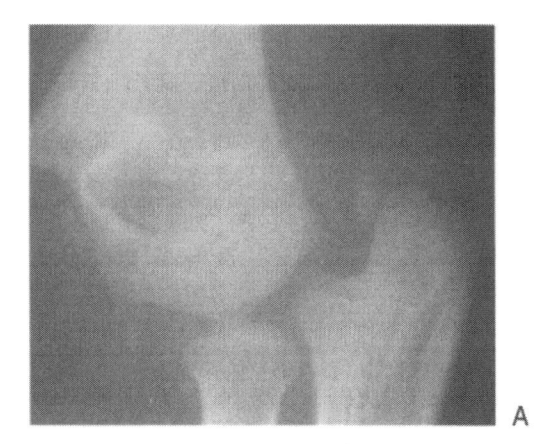

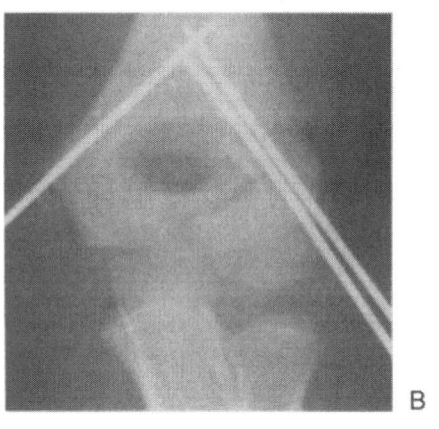

FIGURE 15-10. (A, B) Elbow dislocation complicated by displaced medial epicondylar and lateral condylar fractures that required open reduction and internal fixation.

applied vertical thrust to a lateral rotation and partial valgus strain. The anterior capsule of the elbow joint is stretched by the force of the impact. The upper end of the ulna is displaced backward and then laterally. Collateral ligaments are stretched or ruptured (Fig. 15-13). On the outer side of the joint, the lateral ligament and capsule are attenuated or stripped superiorly. The posterolateral capsule is torn, and the posterior periosteum is often stripped in a distal to proximal direction. The biceps tendon is the rotational valgus fulcrum. This muscle, along with the triceps, then contracts, effectively "locking" the posterior dislocation.

With posterolateral dislocations, damage also occurs to the medial side of the joint, with considerable bruising and swelling often evident. Most often the medial epicondyle is detached in children; it is unlikely that the medial ligament is stretched or ruptured. After reduction, especially pin fixation of the medial epicondyle, it is not usually possible to stress the joint into valgus. The ligaments retain relative continuity with the periosteum, even though the attachment may have been stripped from the underlying bone.

The forearm bones may be laterally or medially displaced to varying degrees, depending on the extent of injury to the radial and ulnar collateral ligaments and contiguous musculotendinous tissues. Without damage to the ulnar collateral ligament, continued valgus stress may avulse the medial epicondyle, displacing this fragment along with the forearm bones. The lateral ligament may be torn at its upper attachment; frequently there is accompanying detachment of a fragment of the lateral epicondyle. The posterior part of the capsule, particularly the part behind the lateral ligament, may be torn from its superior attachment.

Classification

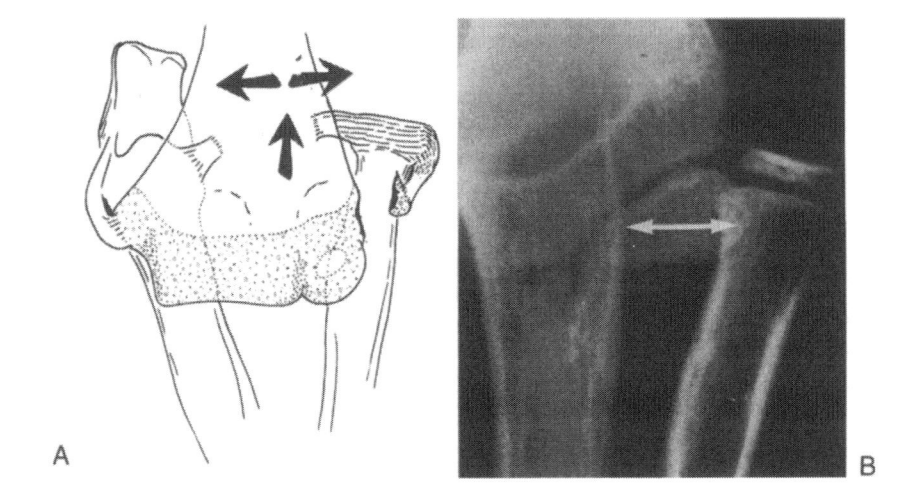

FIGURE 15-11. (A) Divergent dislocation. There is dislocation not only of the elbow joint but also of the proximal radioulnar joint (up arrow), leading to separation of the radius and ulna. This may disrupt or displace the annular ligament significantly and may require open reduction and repair or reduction of the ligament. This injury is analogous to a Monteggia injury. (B) Demonstrative case of divergent dislocation (arrows).

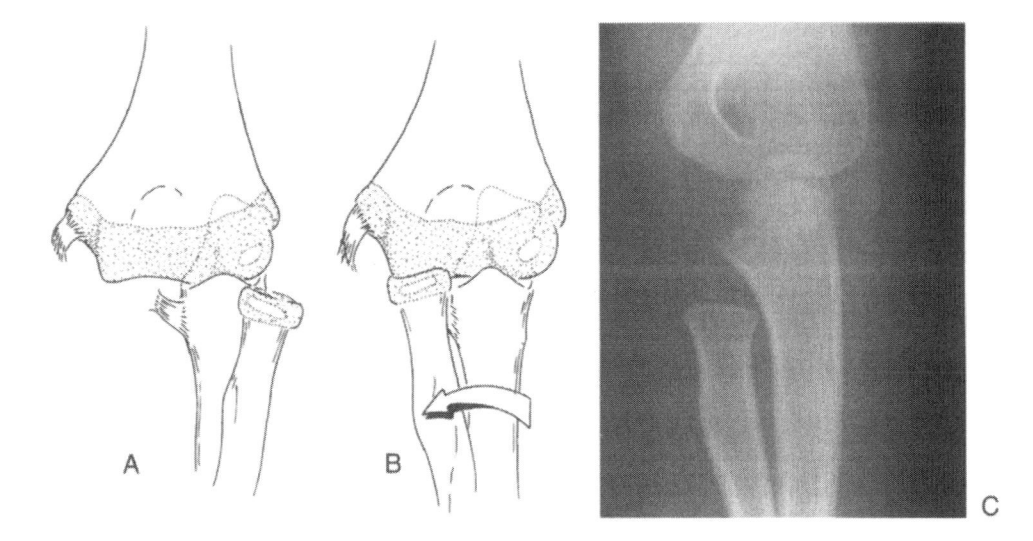

FIGURE 15-12. Translocation (convergent dislocation) of radius and ulna following dislocation. (A) Initial posterolateral displacement. (B) Translocation of the radius to "articulate" with the trochlea. (C) Convergent dislocation in a five-year-old girl.

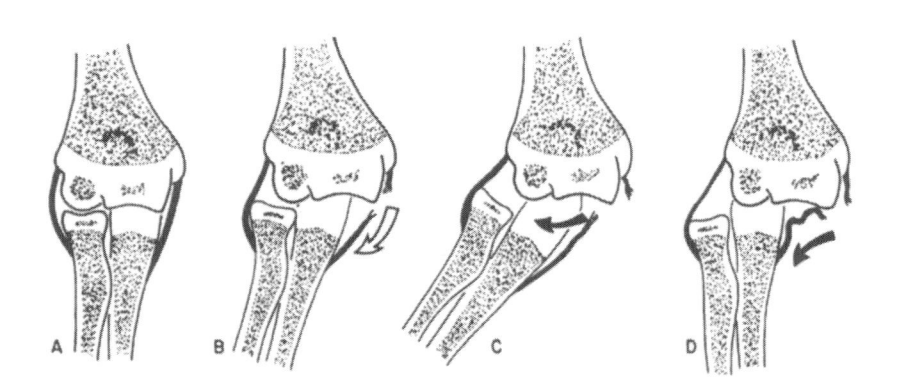

FIGURE 15-13. Mechanics of an elbow dislocation. See text for details.

The radius and ulna, being firmly bound together by the annular ligament and interosseous membrane, are usually displaced posteriorly in unison. Infrequently, however, the two bones may be separated when the annular ligament is displaced over the radial head or disrupted (divergent dislocation). The coronoid process of the ulna may become locked in the olecranon fossa of the posterior distal humerus.

Diagnosis

The differential diagnosis of an elbow dislocation basically consists of distinguishing a dislocation from the various fractures that may involve the variably radiolucent elbow region, especially supracondylar fracture, lateral condylar fracture, or transcondylar fracture, all of which may superficially or clinically appear to be a dislocation. It is important to realize that a dislocated elbow may spontaneously reduce when the evocative forces dissipate, further complicating the diagnosis. A careful history helps diagnose this injury.

The child usually presents with a painful, swollen, deformed elbow that is held in partial flexion and often supported by the opposite hand because of extreme discomfort. Attempted motion of the elbow may be painful, restricted, and associated with marked muscle spasm. The forearm appears shortened. Many physical findings are obscured by the marked soft tissue swelling. It is imperative that the neurovascular function of the forelimb be closely assessed to determine variable damage to the brachial artery and the major nerves.

Because the child is often apprehensive, noncontact observation or simply encouraging the child to move the fingers are ways to initiate the examination until cooperation can be gained. Sensation must be gently tested in the three major nerve distributions, including the anterior and posterior interosseous divisions. The child should be encouraged to make the O sign with the index finger and thumb. If it cannot be done, injury to the anterior interosseous nerve has probably occurred, causing paralysis of the flexor pollicis longus. This is usually a traction-type injury, with recovery likely.

Dislocation is diagnosed most easily roentgenographically. Except when there is a serious vascular injury requiring "immediate" reduction, roentgenograms are obtained prior to treatment to rule out the presence of associated fractures of the epicondyles, coronoid process, proximal radius and ulna, or lateral condyle. Furthermore, an apparent dislocation may be a transcondylar fracture of the distal humerus (especially in children under 2 years of age). A child should never be sent for diagnostic imaging without adequate splintage, both for comfort and to prevent further soft tissue injury and osseous displacement. Insist that the entire arm be rotated as a unit for the radiographic views; otherwise the technologist may inadvertently rotate only the forearm through the dislocation.

A significant problem in the young child is determination of avulsion of a *non*ossified medial or lateral epicondyle. If palpation evinces significant tenderness or there is a palpable mass, avulsion has probably occurred. Stress radiography that opens the medial joint is also most likely to be accompanied by epicondylar damage. Arthrography may be helpful in the small child with an unossified medial epicondyle. Diagnosis is important because this fracture, and others, may require reduction and skeletal fixation. Furthermore, an apparent medial epicondylar fracture, may instead be a larger, medial condylar injury of the nonossified trochlear epiphysis (remember, this is radiolucent for most of the first decade of life). Medial epicondylar injury is more likely than lateral epicondylar injury.

Spontaneous reduction of a dislocated elbow is common. Often the child presents with a history of a fall and the physical finding of a swollen, edematous elbow but without obvious radiographic evidence of injury. However, if one looks carefully at the radiograph, signs of antecedent dislocation may be present: avulsion of the coronoid process, avulsion of the medial epicondyle, or fracture of the radial epiphysis. The avulsion indicates that the elbow most likely has been transiently out of the joint, with the brachialis muscle often avulsing the coronoid process. On spontaneous reduction or with reduction in the emergency room, the capitellum may cause a fracture of the radial epiphysis, resulting in posterior or anterior displacement of the epiphysis upon reduction (Figs. 15-9, 15-10). With posterior dislocations the radial head is usually displaced posteriorly and dorsally, whereas with an anterior dislocation the radial head is displaced onto the palmar surface of the radius.

Treatment

An acute posterior dislocation can often be reduced without general anesthesia. Reduction in children under age 12, however, is probably best done with relaxation and an analgesic to prevent complications such as an iatrogenic fracture of the radial head. Prior knowledge of lateral rotation and displacement is useful for the reduction, as initial hypersupination may be necessary to free the head of the radius and the coronoid process.

A gentle, effective reduction method is as follows. Place the patient in the prone position with the injured limb hanging over the edge of the table. The weight of the arm usually provides sufficient distal traction. Encircle the arm to give countertraction and push the olecranon downward and forward (Fig. 15-14). Following reduction, the elbow should be acutely flexed as much as swelling permits without causing neurocirculatory impairment. An alternative method of reduction comprises extension to slight hyperextension, subsequent downward traction, and finally flexion (Fig. 15-15). The hyperextension should be as little as possible because it increases reduction forces and may lead to anterior muscular injury. Open reduction is indicated if closed reduction is unsuccessful to anatomically reduce or stabilize a chondro-osseous fragment or in a chronic dislocation that is several days to weeks old. *Always assess neurovascular function after the manipulative reduction.*

In most cases the presence of the epicondyle in the joint is an indication for open reduction to reduce the epicondyle satisfactorily and fix it with pins. The fragment is removed from the joint, as it may impede reduction and subsequent function. More importantly, the ulnar nerve may and should be explored, as it also may have been displaced, stretched, or otherwise compromised. Valgus stress and closed manipulation occasionally succeed in displacing the epicondyle

Classification

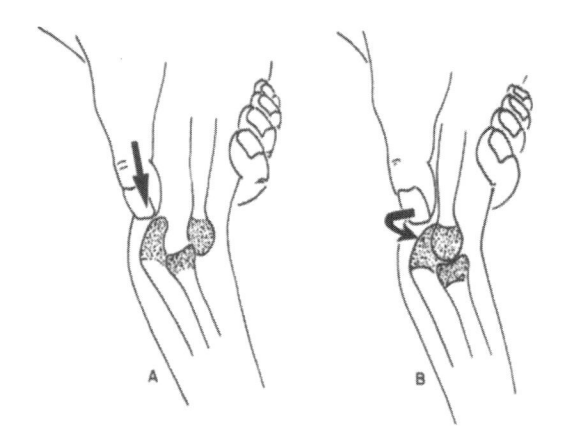

FIGURE 15-14. Reduction utilizing mild elbow flexion. Posterior pressure has been applied directly to the olecranon.

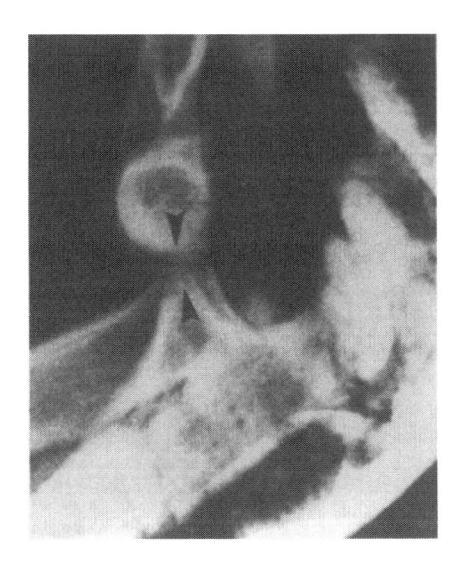

FIGURE 15-16. Postreduction film showing failure to obtain adequate reduction. The distal humerus is locked on the coronoid process of the ulna (arrowheads). Subsequent closed reduction was successful.

from the joint. If the medial epicondyle remains displaced more than 2–3 mm, it should be fixed in place to add to the stability of the elbow.

Once the elbow is reduced, the integrity of the medial and lateral collateral ligaments is tested and the elbow moved through a full range of motion to ensure that no fragment, particularly the medial epicondyle, is caught within the joint where it may impinge on joint surfaces. Roentgenographic confirmation of reduction is essential, as swelling may lead to a false impression that complete reduction has been attained (Fig. 15-16). This also allows further assessment of the associated fractures. An adequate preoperative assessment should have revealed any accompanying fractures that must be reevaluated after closed reduction or that necessitate open reduction as the primary treatment (e.g., a completely displaced radial head).

Fowles et al. reported on 28 children with combined elbow dislocation and avulsion of the medial epicondyle.[43] Nineteen underwent a successful closed reduction. Eleven had a normal elbow at follow-up, but eight had lost an average of 15° of flexion. Nine children required open reduction and internal fixation of the epicondylar fragment (one for an open injury, three for displacement of the epicondyle, and six for intraarticular entrapment of the fragment). Five of these children had ulnar nerve contusion, and four required anterior transposition of the nerve. Of these nine patients, only three had normal elbows; six had lost an average of 37° of flexion. Fowles et al. thought that surgery was indicated only for those children in whom the epicondyle was trapped within the joint or significantly displaced after closed reduction.

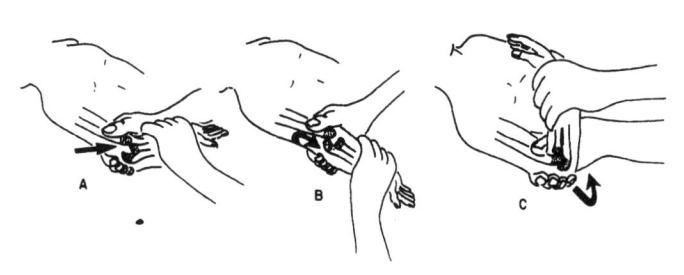

FIGURE 15-15. Reduction utilizing mild elbow hyperextension.

Greiss and Massias reported a patient in whom a posterolateral elbow dislocation proved irreducible because the radial head was caught in a buttonhole tear of the lateral collateral ligament and capsule. It necessitated open reduction.[46]

Divergent Dislocation

During elbow dislocation the annular ligament may be damaged or displaced over the radial head. This causes additional dislocation of the proximal radioulnar joint, creating complex joint disruption referred to as divergent elbow dislocation (Fig. 15-11). Clinical descriptions of divergent dislocation were reported as early as 1854 by Warmont[107] and 1893 by Wright.[110] There have been several radiographically verified cases.[16,26,34,57,96] With one exception all cases of transverse divergent dislocation of the elbow have occurred in children, undoubtedly because of the ligamentous laxity normally present. This pattern could be considered a variant of the Monteggia injury (see Chapter 16).

Closed reduction has been possible in most reported cases, either by traction alone or in combination with direct pressure to the upper ends of the radius and ulna.[96] Reduction requires reducing the ulna in routine fashion and at the same time applying medial pressure over the radial head. If left untreated (Fig. 15-17), the radial head remains displaced, creating a situation analogous to a chronic Monteggia injury.

Reduction is accomplished under sedation with longitudinal traction to reduce the ulna, followed by lateral elbow compression and flexion to partially reduce the radial head, and finally continued supination to completely reduce the radial head. The elbow should allow immediate full range of motion. If not, suspect interposed tissue. Surgery may be necessary to reduce and stabilize the proximal radioulnar joint, as the annular ligament must be torn or completely displaced (similar to the Monteggia injury).

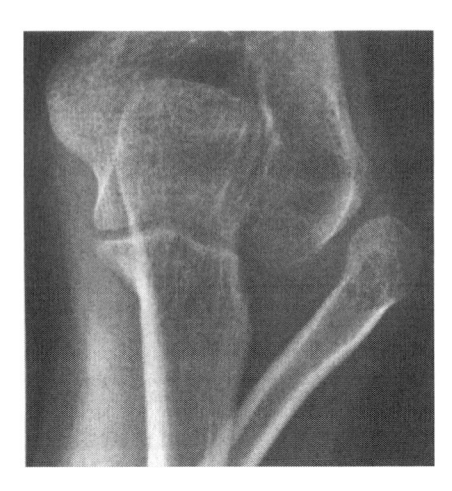

FIGURE 15-17. Chronic divergent elbow dislocation 11 years after the original injury.

Translocation (Convergent Dislocation)

An unusual elbow dislocation is proximal radioulnar translocation (Fig. 15-18; also see Fig. 15-12). During dislocation, the proximal radioulnar soft tissue interrelations (especially the annular ligament) are dislocated, disrupted, or both to the extent that the two bones become "unlinked" and then cross (hyperpronation mechanism).[68] In a case of convergent dislocation, the upper radius and ulna were dislocated posteriorly in a reversed relation due to extreme pronation.[26] This dislocation is usually irreducible by closed means because of the interposition of the annular ligament.

The reversed anatomic relation may remain after reduction. The radial head then articulates with the trochlea and the ulna with the capitellum. In one reported case of this complication, open reduction and restoration of the anatomic relations were undertaken. It required ulnar osteotomy. Ischemic necrosis of the proximal radial epiphyseal ossification complicated the reduction.[49]

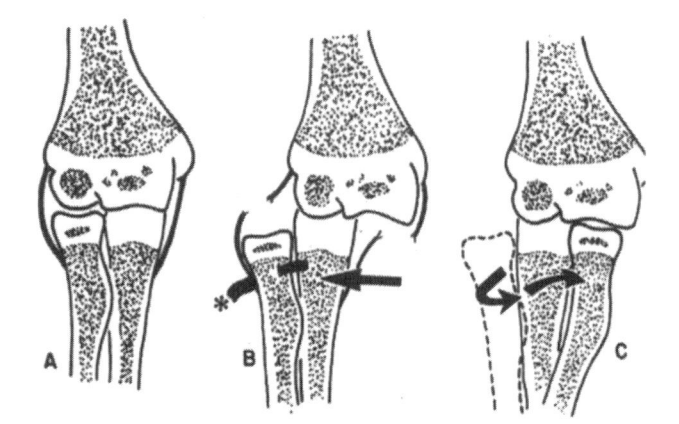

FIGURE 15-18. Translocation mechanism. *Annular ligament disruption. The arrow in (B) indicates the lateral shift. The arrows in (C) show the subsequent anteromedial displacement and "reduction" of the radial head in the trochlear joint.

Complications

Vascular Complications

Vascular injury is rare if a simple dislocation occurs, but becomes more likely if a fracture is also present.[52,53,56,62,63,67] Hemorrhage into the closed antecubital space may produce sufficient tension to cause forearm ischemia. Volkmann's ischemic contracture also may complicate posterior dislocation of the elbow when the brachial artery has been injured. Following closed reduction, depending on the severity of the trauma, the extent of soft tissue swelling, and the diminished pulse (e.g., found by examination, Doppler study), it may be wise to admit the child to the hospital overnight to allow close observation.

When assessing vascular integrity in a child's arm, caution must be advised against placing too much reliance on "capillary filling." Collateral circulation may be sufficient to provide excellent superficial and digital capillary filling but insufficient to ensure adequate muscle physiology, especially as the young child grows into a mature adolescent. Doppler flow evaluation studies along the course of the vessel are more reliable noninvasive indicators of vascular integrity. Arteriography may also be considered.

Wheeler and Linscheid reported vascular complications in 8 of 110 elbow dislocations.[109] They are generally associated with the more violent injuries, particularly open ones. The severity of injury to the brachial artery may vary from simple contusion or spasm to laceration, rupture, or subintimal hemorrhage. Any discrete vascular injuries should be repaired, as indicated, following diagnosis by direct observation (if the wound is open) or arteriography (see Chapter 7 for generalities of the vascular injury).

Neurologic Complications

Neural injury appears to be more frequent than vascular injury.[32,40,45,48,70,71,75,87,88,90,97,98,108] Wheeler and Linscheid reported neurologic complications in 24 of 110 elbow dislocations (three times more neurologic complications than vascular complications).[109] The ulnar nerve was involved in 16 of 24 patients, the median nerve in 3, and both ulnar and median nerves in 4; the remaining patient sustained a brachial plexus injury. Most injuries are contusions or stretching injuries, without gross disruption of nerve continuity.

The ulnar nerve appears to be the most frequently injured nerve. The common posterolateral dislocation of the elbow results in a stretch injury to the medially based ulnar nerve. The tight constraints on the nerve at the medial epicondylar level affect the risk of injury (e.g., contusion, interstitial hemorrhage).

Hallet described three types of ulnar nerve injury. In type I the nerve is caught between the humerus and ulna. In type II the nerve runs through a healed fracture in the medial epicondyle. In type III the nerve is looped into the humeralulnar joint anteriorly.[48] Types I and III are the most common. Early removal of the entrapped nerve is the treatment of choice. A type II injury often escapes notice. If a palsy or any type of neuropathy exists, entrapment should be considered, with a diagnosis by type undertaken. A fracture of the medial epicondyle with an otherwise normal radiograph and a full range of joint motion should alert the examiner to the possibility of type II entrapment.

Because most capsular damage, even when medial and lateral ligaments are involved, is anterior to the epicondyles, and the medial epicondyle stays attached to the posterosuperior periosteal/perichondrial tissue (which may be stripped extensively from the distal humeral metaphysis), the ulnar nerve rarely is mobile enough to be displaced into the joint. Even when the epicondyle is displaced into the joint, the ulnar nerve usually stays attached to the less-displaced soft tissues.

Close observation of radiographs may document the fracture callus-forming Matev's sign, which is the sclerosis-rimmed osseous tunnel caused by passage of the median nerve through the maturing callus.[74]

The median nerve may be injured, displaced into the joint, and associated with delayed diagnosis. Interestingly, intraarticular entrapment of the median nerve has been reported only in children. Persistent pain or increasing median nerve dysfunction should alert one to the possibility of such entrapment. Median nerve exploration must be undertaken once such entrapment has been diagnosed. If the nerve is functionally intact, which may be demonstrated by nerve stimulation, its removal from the joint is sufficient treatment. If, however, the nerve is severely damaged, crushed, or scarred and is seemingly nonfunctional, resection of the damaged section with end-to-end reanastomosis or interposition graft may be necessary or appropriate.

Intraarticular entrapment of the median nerve may occur during dislocation or reduction.[88,90,97] Because the medial epicondylar attachments are usually intact, it is assumed that the median nerve loops into the trochleoulnar joint through the torn medial capsule as the forearm is forced into valgus and extension during acute dislocation.[65] It is then trapped in this location, during reduction, by the flare of the medial condyle of the trochlea. To avoid such a rare neurologic complication, Watson-Jones suggested gentle traction on the forearm while it is in the flexed position, with no hyperextension of the joint preliminary to reduction.[108] Hyperextension is a potentially dangerous reduction procedure, predisposing the median nerve to intraarticular displacement. However, all nerves displaced into the elbow joint had good return of function after open reduction and removal of the nerve from the joint.[71]

The treatment of neurologic complications should be conservative because most are stretch injuries that recover spontaneously. Persistent ulnar nerve paralysis should be treated by neurolysis and, if necessary, anterior transposition. Any intraarticular entrapment should be treated by open release of the nerve from the joint whenever the diagnosis is made. Surprising recovery of nerve function may occur even many months after entrapment.

Contractures

As in adults, joint stiffness is often encountered following dislocation and reduction of the elbow in children. Both the child and the parents should be informed that the major difficulty is regaining full motion in the joint. Complete extension may never be recovered in older children, although the loss of the last 5°–10° of extension usually is not associated with a significant functional deficit. To prevent contractures, elbow immobilization usually is no longer than 4 weeks in the child over 10 years of age. Younger children can probably tolerate longer immobilization.

Capsular tearing is responsible for the prolonged stiffness that often follows dislocation of the elbow. The capsular attachment to the ulna is frequently torn. The posterior capsule may also be torn at its attachment to the humerus, although it is more likely that it is stripped away because of the contiguity of the capsule with the posterior periosteum.

Manipulation or passive physiotherapy is seldom required for joint stiffness.[35] In fact, this approach may be detrimental because it may be accompanied by further joint irritation, capsular tearing, and hematoma formation. A year may be required to regain full motion in the child's elbow. The child is usually his or her own best physiotherapist.

Correction of posttraumatic flexion contracture of the elbow by limited anterior capsulotomy may effectively decrease the posttraumatic flexion contracture in properly selected patients.[103] However, whether such procedures are necessary or appropriate in young children is still open to discussion. Similarly, lack of flexion may be treated by V-Y advancement of the triceps aponeurosis.

Heterotopic Bone

Myositis ossificans is uncommon with a simple dislocation, but when it occurs it usually restricts motion (Figs. 15-19, 15-20). Reactive bone around chondro-osseous disruptions and capsular tears may also restrict motion.

Although heterotopic bone formation occurs less frequently in children than in adults, it is frequent enough to be of concern in children who dislocate an elbow. If such ossification occurs, it may restrict elbow motion. In one series, this complication occurred in 32 of 110 dislocations.[101] Formation of heterotopic bone usually occurs below the medial or lateral epicondyle along the course of the collateral ligaments (Fig. 15-21) or the posterior capsule (Fig. 15-22). It is often evident within 3–4 weeks after the initial injury. Bone also may form in damaged muscle as myositis

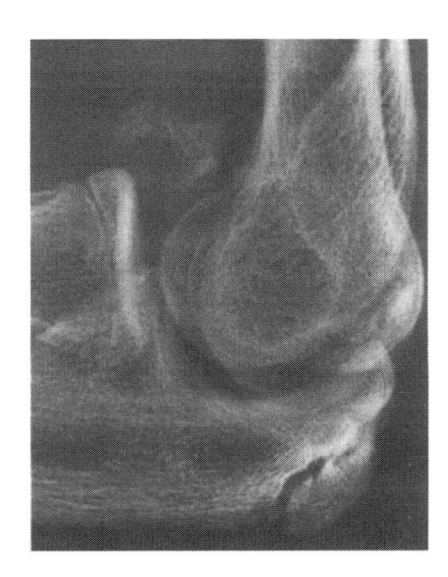

FIGURE 15-19. Ossification around the radial head allowed a range of motion of only 40°–90°. Over a 6-month period, however, this increased to 15°–160°, with diminution of the ossification.

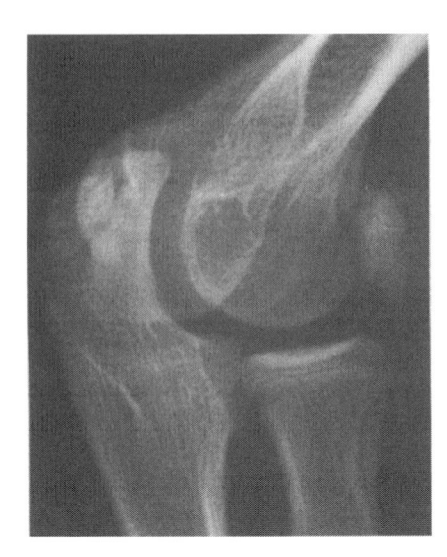

FIGURE 15-20. Excessive anterior heterotopic bone following dislocation. It moved with the radius and ulna and blocked flexion beyond 105°. The proximal radius also shows evidence of reactive bone where the capsule and periosteum were stripped.

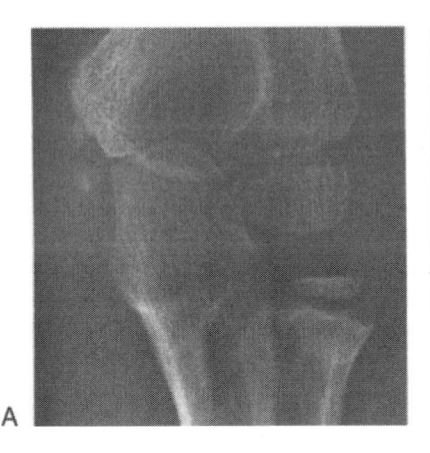

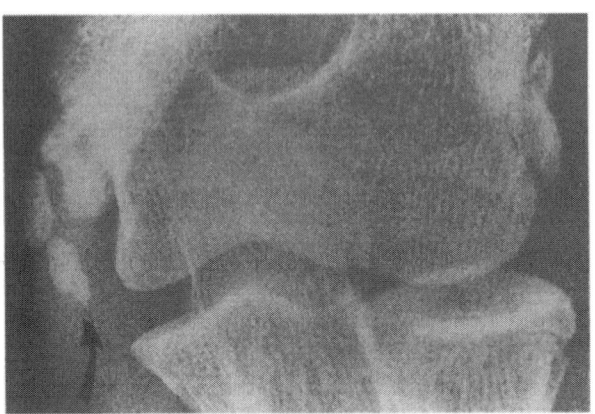

FIGURE 15-21. (A) Heterotopic bone (arrow) in the "medial collateral ligament." It was probably due to chondro-osseous failure of a portion of the medial epicondyle as a sleeve fracture, rather than a true ligamentous injury. The radial head is still subluxated and exhibits some altered physeal growth. (B) Five years later the avulsed bone (arrow) is still evident.

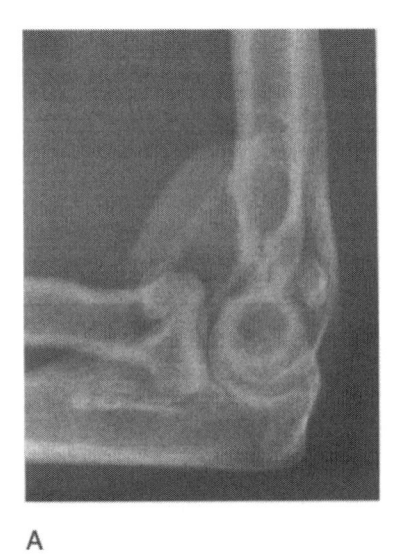

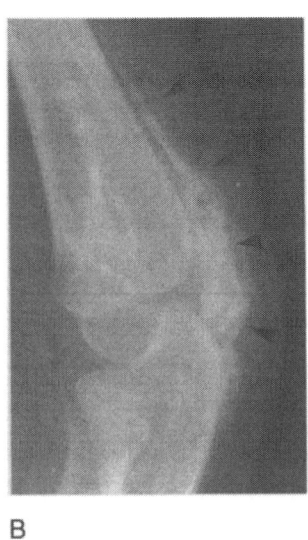

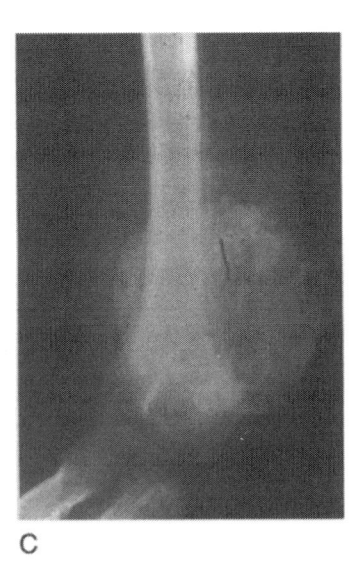

FIGURE 15-22. (A) Anterior heterotopic bone formation. (B) Extensive heterotopic ossification in the posterior capsular, subperiosteal, and muscular regions following dislocation. (C) Massive heterotopic bone following elbow dislocation.

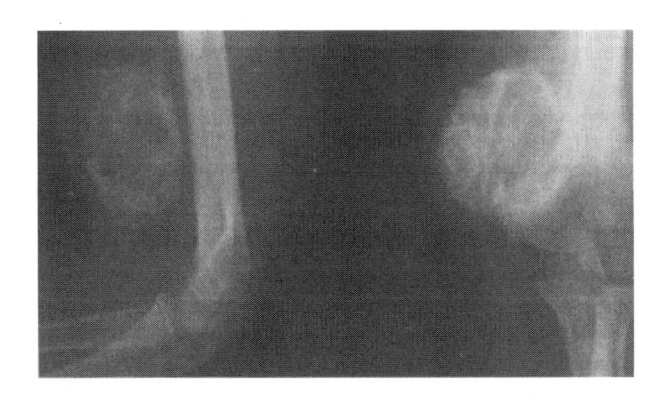

FIGURE 15-23. Complete lateral dislocation of the elbow in an 8-year-old. Note the extensive myositis ossificans in the biceps of this child 5 months later.

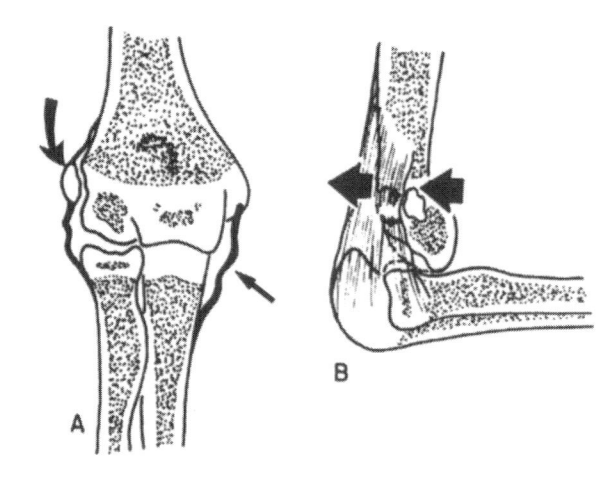

FIGURE 15-24. Recurrent dislocation. (A) The ligaments are attenuated (small arrow), and the lateral epicondyle did not heal (large arrow). (B) This allows chronic posterior displacement (arrows) and may lead to progressive deformation of the capitellum and radial head.

ossificans (Fig. 15-23). Large deposits of bone may impair normal joint function. Children show a tendency to resorb ectopic calcification and ossification before it becomes mature bone, although it may not occur until 6–8 months after the injury (see Chapter 10). If surgical excision is necessary, the best results occur in skeletally immature patients. Excision should be done only after 6–9 months have elapsed since the injury and only when the ectopic ossification appears mature, with well defined peripheral sclerosis. A "cold" bone scan, reasonably indicative of cessation of bone-forming activity, is a favorable prognostic study for the timing of resection but cannot be absolutely correlated with a lessened risk of recurrence.

Recurrent Dislocation

Recurrent elbow dislocation is rare in children.* Linscheid and Wheeler found only two recurrent cases in 110 children with elbow dislocations.[66] The pathologic defect is usually a laxity of the posterolateral ligamentous capsular structures consequent to the failure of any spontaneous repair or reattachment.[84] The medial or lateral epicondyle may also develop nonunion, contributing to micro- or macroinstability. Lateral nonunion allows displacement of the radius from its normal articulation with the capitellum (Fig. 15-24). The intact lateral ligament normally prevents this displacement; but if its superior attachments have been stripped or if it is more lax than normal, the head of the radius no longer closely apposes the contour of the capitellum, and at some point in extension backward slipping of the radial head may occur.

Ejsted et al. described two cases of habitual recurrent dislocation of the elbow.[37] Both patients had a mental disorder, which presumably was a contributory factor, just as for recurrent shoulder dislocation. The elbows in both patients were stabilized surgically.

Not all patients with recurrent dislocation have complete dislocation. Instead, the radial head may subluxate into a capitellar defect or capsular pocket and be reduced easily by the child, who may complain only of a sensation of locking. Progressive damage to the osteochondral surfaces is often significant. As the head of the radius displaces backward, it may abrade the posterolateral margin of the capitellum. An osteochondral fracture may occur. A permanent defect in the posterolateral margin of the capitellum may result, and the edge of the radial head may be damaged. The ulna, especially the coronoid process, may be deformed; and the olecranon process may be deficient. Anterior capsular instability may also contribute to chronic dislocation. Arthrography may be useful for diagnosing these lesions and delineating the pathoanatomy.[38,59] In the older child or adolescent three dimensional computed tomography (CT) reconstruction may help define morphology and assist in preoperative planning.

Trias and Comean strongly advocated the concept that chondro-osseous changes, such as congenital hypoplasia of the olecranon, were secondary to ligamentous instability, which was the primary cause of chronic dislocation.[102] The normal hyperlaxity of the ligaments of children may also be a significant causal factor. Certainly, subtle, if not overt, subluxation due to ligament instability may affect acetabular development, so there is no reason comparable cartilaginous changes could not occur in the unossified elbow components.

Because recurrent dislocation is infrequent, one should try to refrain from any operative ligament reconstruction during childhood. The normal process of growth is associated with a gradual tightening of ligaments and may lead to improved overall stability. Operative treatment is indicated if the dislocation recurs following minimal injury in the older child or adolescent. Reattachment of the capsule and ligaments to the lateral epicondyle (Fig. 15-25) is the most important step in repairing this complication.[18] Other available methods include transfer of the bicipital tendon to the coronoid process by an intraarticular bone graft (which cannot be used effectively in the skeletally immature child in whom this area is still cartilaginous), and repair or reinforcement of soft tissues around the elbow joint using fascial or tendon strips to reinforce the collateral ligaments. Zeier repaired both the medial and lateral ligaments using fascia lata slings.[111]

---
*Refs. 36,37,47, 50,55,58,73,75,84,102,111.

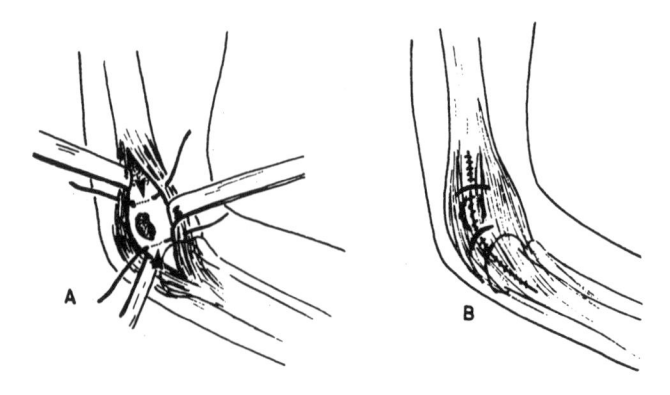

FIGURE 15-25. Described repair for recurrent elbow dislocation.

Unreduced Dislocations

Allende and Freytes reported a series of chronic, untreated dislocations of the elbow.[14] They thought that any acute elbow dislocation that had not been reduced by 3 weeks could not be reduced satisfactorily by closed, manipulative reduction. They described 31 cases of chronic dislocations of the elbow in children and reported various operative methods for reduction. The major impediment to reduction is soft tissue contracture, particularly in the triceps, as the elbow has usually been held in extension.[93] Often it is impossible to reduce these dislocations adequately and maintain the full length in the triceps. The tendinous portion usually must be lengthened. There often is fibrous pannus within the joint, which must be removed from the olecranon region to permit adequate reduction.

If the dislocation remains for several months to years, the distal humerus may progressively deform, as may the proximal radius and the ulna (Figs. 15-26 to 15-29). Undoubtedly, such deformations result from the lack of normal joint reaction forces, as with hip dysplasia. The younger the child, the more likely it is that an alteration of morphology will occur. The longer the elbow remains dislocated, the greater is the likelihood that reduction will be unstable or impossible owing to both altered morphology and soft tissue contractures.[21] Even if reduction can be attained, normal mobility (function) may not be possible, and instability subluxation and dislocation become more likely.

Volkov and Oganesian used the Ilizarov device to mobilize chronic elbow joint contractures progressively and to reduce old dislocations.[106] The basic concept for correcting the contracture is first to distract the joint surfaces and maintain a space between them to prevent excessive pressure and then to produce gradual, controlled passive flexion and extension of the joint until adequate (not necessarily normal) function is restored.

Fowles et al. studied 15 children with untreated posterior dislocations of the elbow.[41] Three had a useful range of painless flexion and were not treated by surgery. Twelve had a stiff elbow and underwent open reductions between 3 weeks and 3 years after the original injury. The triceps was lengthened whenever it prevented reduction. Kirschner wires were sometimes necessary to stabilize the elbow temporarily. Complications included transient paralysis of the hand in one patient and myositis ossificans with a rigid elbow in another. These authors followed the patients for 1–6 years after surgery. In 11 of the patients the average range of flexion was increased fourfold; and in all children who underwent surgery the elbow had a useful range through 90° of flexion. Eleven of the children thought that the function of the arm was improved. Four had been operated on within 6 weeks of the original accident and probably were in a better position to do well. Fowles et al. noted that open reduction was always worth trying, at least in children.

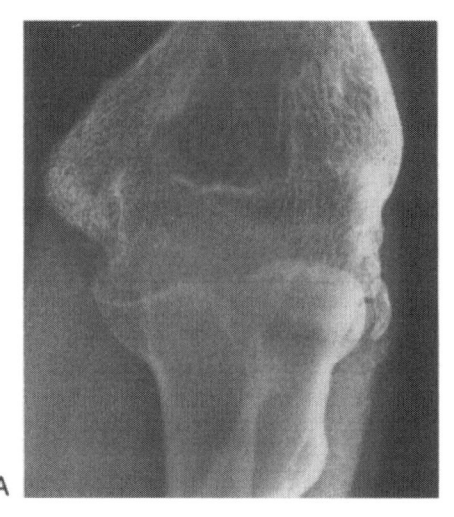

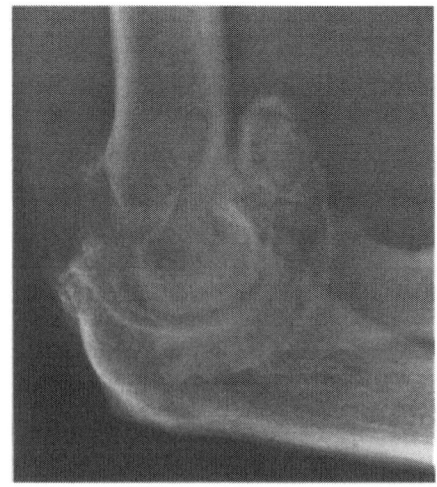

FIGURE 15-26. (A) Appearance of the elbow in a 23-year-old man who had had an elbow dislocation at 9 years of age. The radius was never reduced. Morphologic change is evident. (B) Severe heterotopic bone in a 20-year-old woman who dislocated her elbow at 10 years of age.

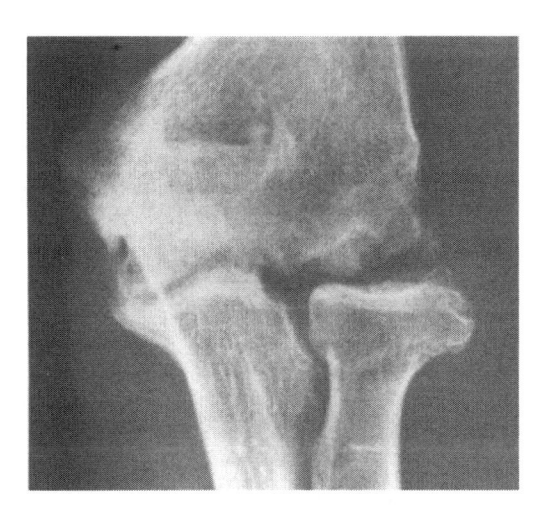

FIGURE 15-27. Incompletely reduced old elbow dislocation (16 years previously at 8 years of age). The radial head remains subluxated. Osteoarthritic changes are evident.

Pulled Elbow

One of the most common elbow injuries encountered in infants and young children is the "pulled" elbow.[112-154,156-172] This term is used to identify an entity in which the radial head is traumatically "locked" because of sudden traction on the hand or forearm when the elbow is extended and the forearm hyperpronated. This entity has various eponyms, such as nursemaid's elbow and temper tantrum elbow. It may occur when pulling a child as he or she stumbles, when swinging the child, or when forcefully pulling the child away from something enticing. It is one of the most common injuries to the elbow in children under 4 years of age; it rarely occurs after age 5, with a peak incidence between 1 and 3 years.

High incidences of this injury have been reported.[132,160,172] Quan and Marcuse showed that 0.5% (4.6/1000) of the total visits to one hospital's emergency department were attributable to pulled elbow.[157] These patients constituted 22% of all young children presenting for evaluation of an elbow injury.

Most studies show that radial head subluxation occurs predominantly in the left elbow. This observation is logical, as most parents or caretakers are right-handed and when walking naturally hold the child by their left hand. The condition is rarely bilateral.

Pathomechanics

The suspected pathophysiology and clinical presentation have not changed from the early description by Lindeman[142] in 1885. Radial head subluxation occurs when there is sudden traction on the wrist or hand while the elbow is extended and the forearm is hyperpronated. It cannot occur when the elbow is flexed or when the forearm is supinated.

One of the early theories reported that the head of the radius was not fully developed and that the periphery of the cartilaginous end was smaller than or equal to the neck, such that the head was not firmly held in place by the annular lig-

ament. This is a *misinterpretation* of a statement attributed to Piersol.[155] Ryan examined the upper end of the radius in 15 fetal specimens and found that the radial head, even at birth, was definitely larger than the neck and that the ratio of the two (head/neck) does not differ greatly from that of an adult.[158] Salter and Zaltz found that the diameter of the radial head was larger than the neck by 30–60%.[160] Similar studies (unpublished) in our skeletal developmental laboratory of 29 prenatal and 54 postnatal specimens support this observation that the radial head, from before birth through adolescence, is *always* larger than the metaphysis.[115] Thus the concept that the radial head is easily pulled through the annular ligament because it is smaller than or equal in width to the radial neck is erroneous.

Stone studied the mechanism of injury in 12 anatomic specimens and was able to produce the lesion in 6 of the elbows.[167] He observed that the annular ligament slipped partially over the radial head *only* when the forearm was pronated. He also observed that the radial head was slightly oval, rather than circular, and that when the forearm was supinated the anterior aspect of the radial head was relatively elevated from the neck. Conversely, in pronation the anterior aspect of the radial head is tilted slightly downward. Salter and Zaltz also observed that the superior surface of the radial head, viewed from above, was slightly more oval than circular and, with forearm supination, the sagittal diameter of the radial head is consistently greater than the coronal diameter.[160]

My studies have shown that the plane of the articular surface is not completely perpendicular to the longitudinal axis of the radius (similar to the proximal tibia). Laterally and posteriorly the radial head "rises" gradually, so when traction is applied with the forearm in pronation the annular

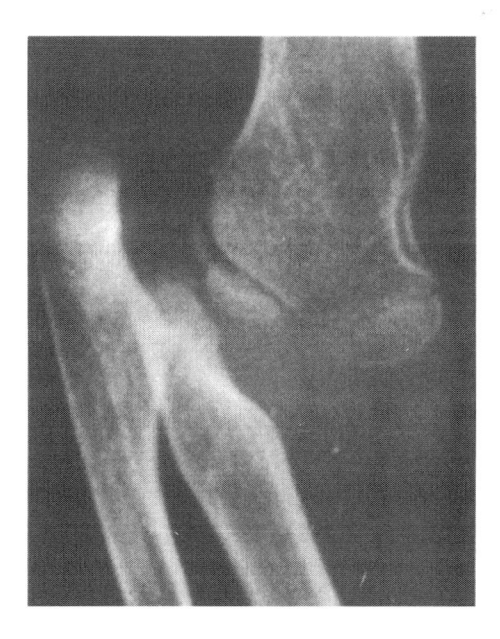

FIGURE 15-28. Chronic elbow dislocation in a 9-year-old boy who had sustained an "injury" to the elbow 4 years earlier. It had never been treated. The lateral view shows posterior displacement of radius and ulna. Ossification is evident in the capitellum, trochlea, and medial epicondyle.

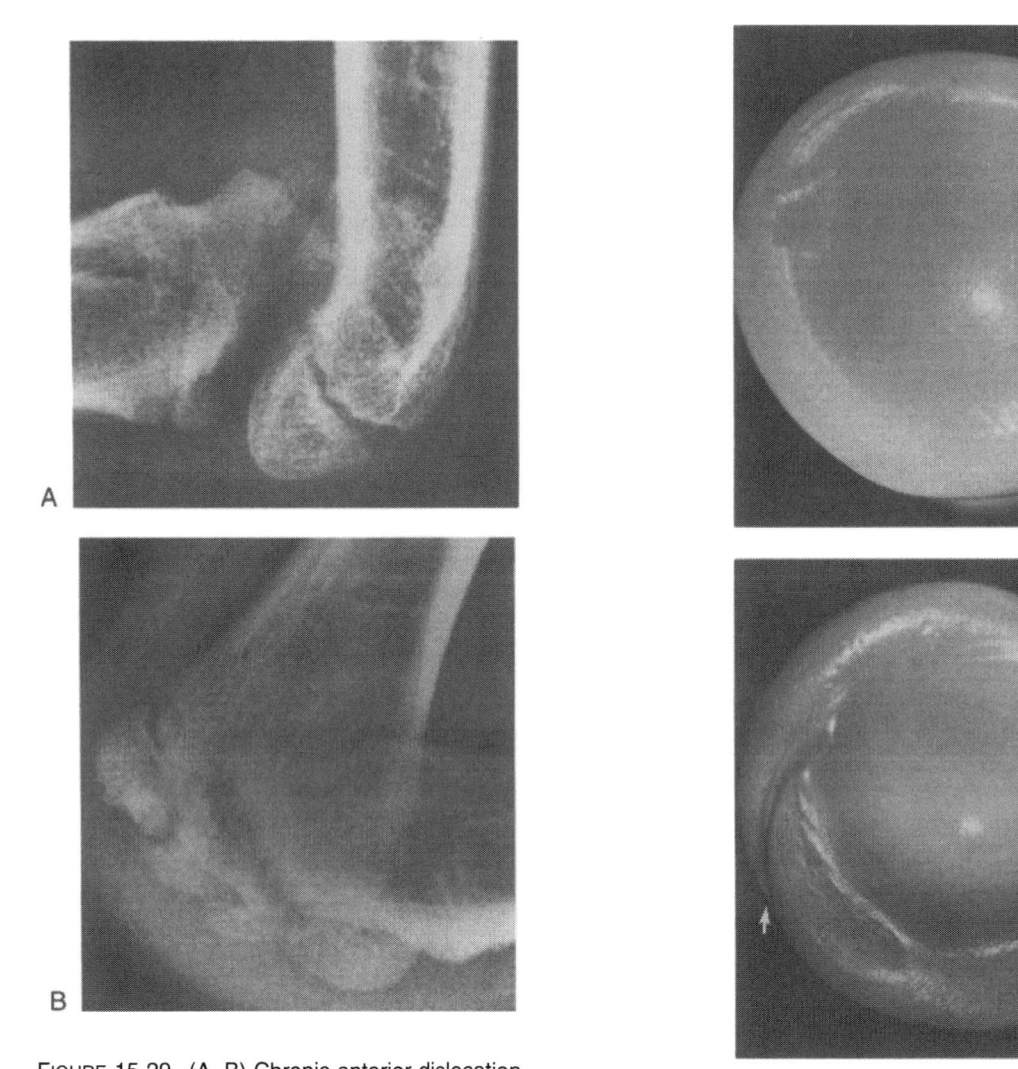

FIGURE 15-29. (A, B) Chronic anterior dislocation.

FIGURE 15-30. (A) Normal radial head showing slightly eccentric central depression. (B) Effect of hyperpronation prior to tissue fixation. The annular ligament partially displaced over the anterior margin and indented the biologically plastic cartilage (arrows).

ligament must lie over the less prominent (i.e., "lower") portion, which also has a straighter side angle relative to the longitudinal axis. The annular ligament may stretch and slip over a portion of the radial head (Figs. 15-30 to 15-33). In full supination the radius, at the site of the annular ligament, is outflared, so it is difficult for the annular ligament to displace onto the edge of the epiphysis or further onto a portion of the articular surface. However, when the arm is fully pronated, this portion of the metaphysis and epiphysis assumes a much straighter position that more easily allows the annular ligament to be displaced in a proximal (upward) direction, allowing the ligament to cover a portion of the radial head. This effectively "locks" the radial head, preventing rotation.

McRae and Freeman studied 25 elbows from stillborns and concluded that a pulled elbow was caused by the annular ligament slipping partially over the radial head.[145] Salter and Zaltz anatomically duplicated the mechanism of displacement with sudden, firm, steady traction on the extended elbow, first in supination and then in pronation.[160] They were not able to subluxate the radial head in any of the specimens when the traction was applied with the forearm in supination, but when traction was applied in pronation, a transverse tear was produced in the thin distal attachment of the annular ligament, allowing it to displace over the radial head.

Our studies show that displacement may occur without tearing the annular attachments of the annular ligament (Figs. 15-32, 15-33). When the proximal edge of the annular ligament did not extend beyond the diametric (midportion) of the radial head, the interposed ligament could be repositioned to its normal anatomic position by simple supination of the forearm. In specimens from older children, a comparable tear or displacement could not be produced because of the thicker, stronger attachments. In operative cases and one traumatic amputation with a Monteggia injury, we found that the annular ligament may remain intact and yet slip

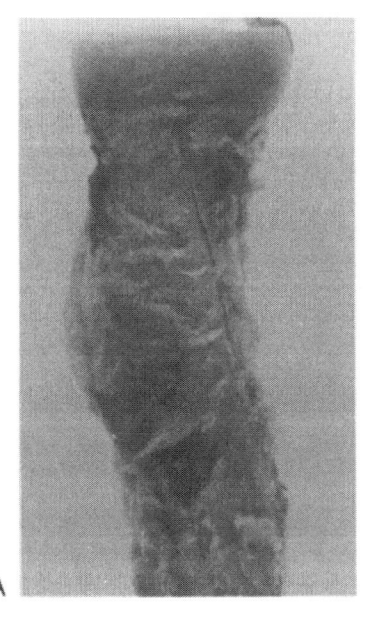

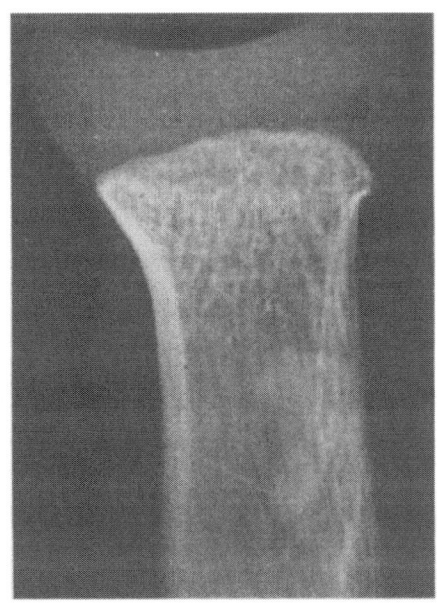

FIGURE 15-31. Proximal radius from a 17-month-old toddler. (A) Morphological specimen. (B) Radiograph of specimen. There are subtle contour differences in the metaphyseal-epiphyseal flaring. In pronation the more gradual flare is presented to the annular ligament. In contrast, supination presents the more angulated contour to the annular ligament.

completely over and off the radial head. This ligament is highly mobile in the infant and young child.

Diagnosis

The diagnosis of a pulled elbow is usually based on both the history and clinical findings. The parent, caretaker, or child describes an activity in which the forearm was subjected to significant traction while extended and pronated (Fig. 15-34). Occasionally a click is felt or heard. The child is usually in discomfort or pain and refuses to use the affected arm. The pain is generally at the elbow, mainly over the radial head, although a few children complain of pain in the wrist or the shoulder. The arm remains in pronation and either hangs limp in slight flexion or is cradled on the chest by the other hand and guarded from manipulation by appropriately concerned adults. Bobrow stated that fewer than 50% of physicians in one family practice residency program were able clinically to recognize a typical case of nursemaid's elbow.[115]

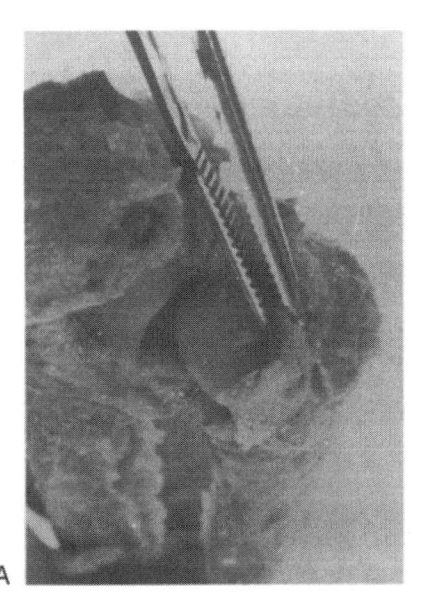

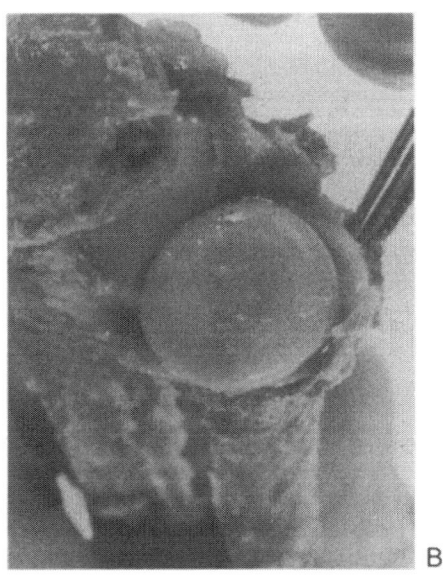

FIGURE 15-32. Mechanism of a pulled elbow. (A) In pronation the radial head subluxates slightly away from the ulna, and the annular ligament displaces onto the radial head. (B) With supination, however, the radial head relocates into the radioulnar joint, and the annular ligament relocates below the radial head.

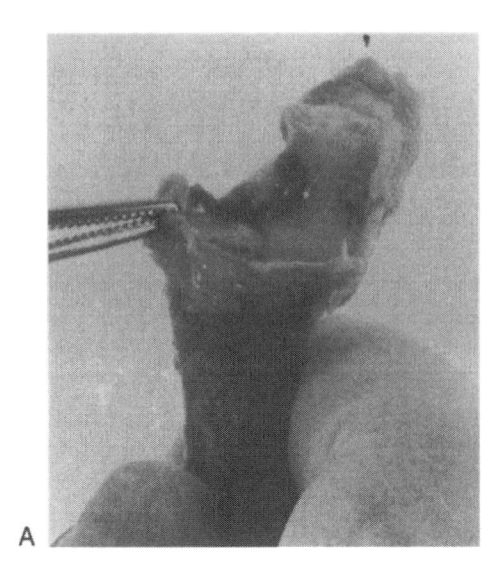

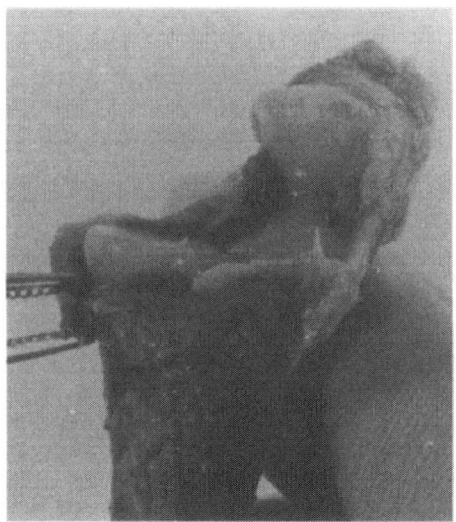

FIGURE 15-33. Anatomy of the pulled elbow. (A) In pronation the annular ligament slips over the anterolateral radial margin. (B) With supination the higher, more flared side of the radial head forces the annular ligament back into anatomic position.

Radiographs are usually reported as normal.[123,128,136,165] One textbook noted that "although we have examined the elbows radiographically in scores of such cases, we have not been able to demonstrate the dislocation. The radiography technicians probably reduce the dislocation consistently before the film is exposed to their manipulations of the elbow by positioning the patient. In an attempt to obtain an adequate anteroposterior film of the joint, the technician routinely supinates the forearm, much to the child's momentary opposition. The arm then no longer hurts and is usually mobile after the radiograph.

Salter and Zaltz identified Stone's 1916 report as the only existing radiographic demonstration of displacement of the proximal end of the radius in relation to the capitellum in this entity, but they believed the evidence to be unconvincing as a *reliable* radiographic demonstration of nursemaid's elbow.[160,167] Frumkin believed that nursemaid's elbow could be demonstrated radiographically by a line drawn through the longitudinal axis of the radius that fails to bisect the capitellar ossification center (Fig. 15-35).[128] Many authors do not advocate obtaining radiographs if the clinical presentation and response to reduction are typical.[160] A roentgenogram may be useful for ruling out actual or associated fractures, which are rare. Ultrasonography has been used for the diagnosis but has not been found overly useful.[140]

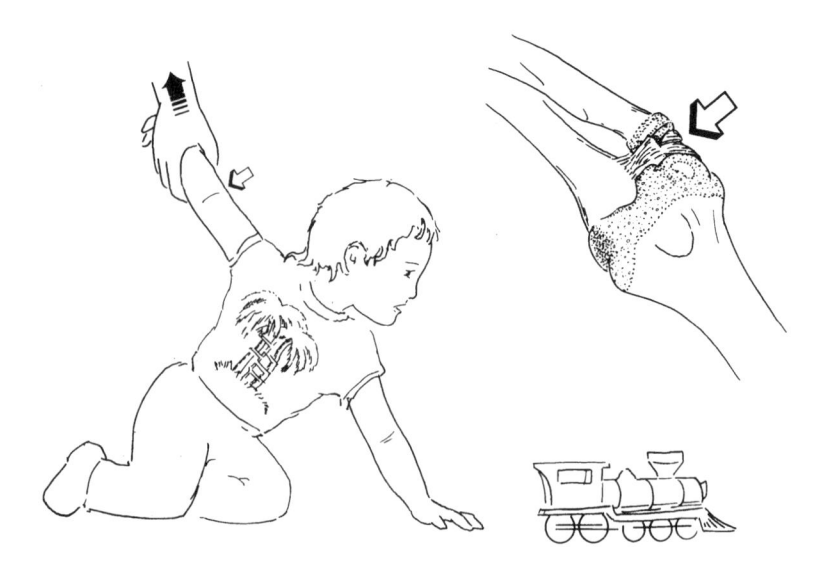

FIGURE 15-34. Hyperpronation mechanism of a pulled elbow sustained as the child forces the elbow into a direction opposite to the person holding him, causing the annular ligament to subluxate (arrow).

FIGURE 15-35. Nineteen-month-old girl with a pulled elbow. The metaphysis appears laterally (A) and posteriorly (B) subluxated relative to the capitellar ossification center. The radial longitudinal axis does not bisect the capitellum.

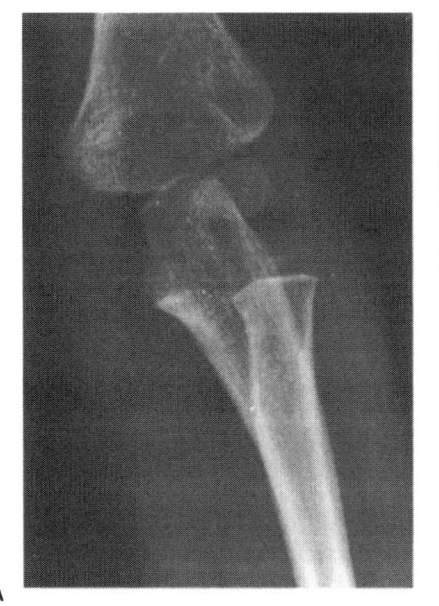

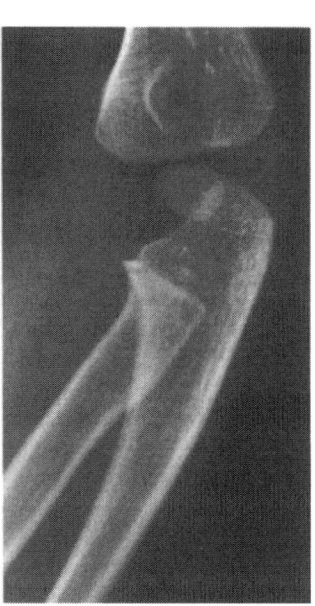

Treatment

Reduction, in virtually all patients, is easily accomplished by rapid supination. The preferred method of reduction is to flex the elbow to 90° and place the thumb over the radial head while exerting mild pressure to the radial head (Fig. 15-36). Using the other hand, the child's forearm is then rapidly and firmly rotated into full supination. As reduction is achieved, a palpable, sometimes audible, click may be felt in the region of the radial head. The child generally evinces instantaneous relief of pain, stops crying, and begins, almost immediately, to use the arm in a normal fashion. Some children take a longer time, sometimes 2–3 days, to recover.

Immobilization, other than the use of a sling for comfort, is not usually necessary unless the displacement is a repeat occurrence. Immobilization with a sling for several days to a week or more has been suggested to protect the ligament from further stress and to allow it to heal. The efficacy of this treatment has never been evaluated statistically.

Treatment failures are rare and are usually associated with not feeling or hearing a click. Occasionally, several attempts at reduction are necessary before a full range of motion is restored.

If the subluxation is irreducible (a rare situation), open reduction is indicated.[170] Although it may require dividing the annular ligament, usually small nerve hooks are used to grasp and pull the ligament over the radial head and allow appropriate reduction to the neck (metaphysis) without transection of the annular ligament. I have never encountered a case that required open reduction.

Results

Restoration of motion and function is usually instantaneous following pronation to supination manipulation. Recurrence of the injury, however, is relatively common (my daughter experienced four episodes within a 10-month period). Salter and Zaltz,[160] Snellman,[165] and Quan and Marcuse[157] each noted an almost 40% incidence of recurrent injury. However, there are no long-term studies of the consequences. A long-term effect may be chronic mild subluxation. No documented cases of subsequent complete radial head dislocation have been reported.

Little League Elbow

The overhead throwing of a baseball or other object is a relatively abnormal activity for the developing arm and puts an unusual, repetitious strain on the wrist, shoulder, and elbow.[173] The overhead serve in tennis creates a similar motion. The elbow joint is whipped forcefully from acute flexion into complete extension with either pronation or supination of the forearm and ulnar flexion of the wrist.[174] Throwing a curve ball puts additional traction strain on the medial epicondyle, which is the point of attachment of the pronator and flexor muscles of the forearm. The epiphyses are still open in boys of the age groups involved in most

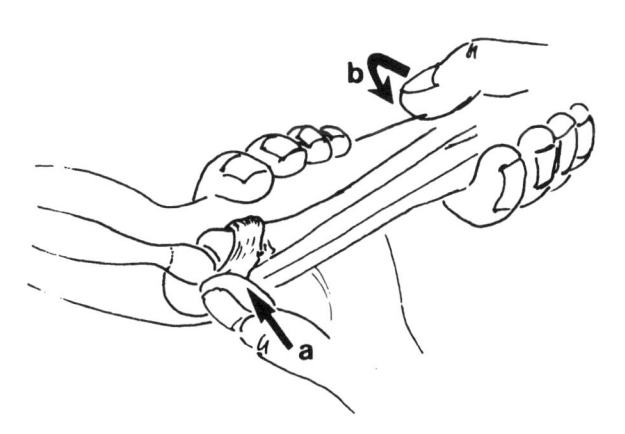

FIGURE 15-36. Mechanism for reducing a pulled elbow. The thumb is placed directly over the radial head (a) while the forearm is supinated (b).

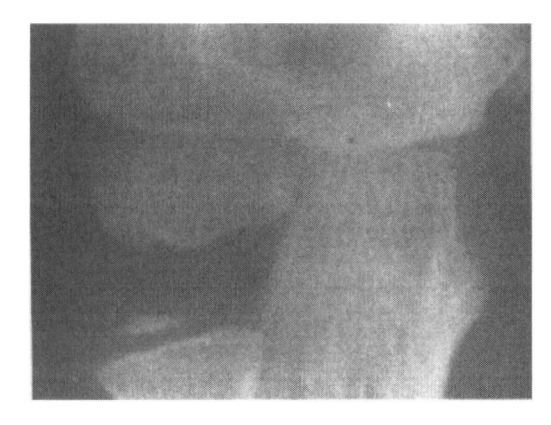

FIGURE 15-37. Small Panner's lesion (arrow) of the capitellum.

organized baseball, so the epicondyle is often subjected to the repetitive forceful pull of these muscles.[182] Little league elbow reaches its peak in boys at the age of 13–14 years.[175,178,185,188,189,198,199] Other sports, such as tennis, are also capable of causing these lesions in skeletally immature athletes.[191]

This condition classically has been restricted to boys playing organized baseball and involves the dominant elbow almost exclusively. Girls are being diagnosed with increasing frequency, however, with tennis and gymnastics being the more likely evocative sports. Most of the patients are first evaluated between 9 and 15 years of age, when they usually complain of a dull ache, effusion, and restricted elbow extension.

Singer and Roy reported seven cases of osteochondrosis of the capitellum in five high-performance female gymnasts between the ages of 11 and 13 years.[196] They thought that this injury was potentially an increasing problem in girls put through exercise regimens that placed major stress on the elbow. In gymnasts the arm often functions as a weight-bearing extremity under considerable stress. In contrast to the comparable lesion in young baseball players who are just potentially beginning their careers, young female gymnasts are basically reaching the peak of their sport when they acquire this injury. They are also likely to be approaching skeletal maturity. Others have reported this problem.[191]

Adams studied both elbows of 162 boys 9–14 years of age, dividing them into three categories: pitchers, nonpitchers, and a control group who had never played organized baseball.[173] Changes involving the medial epicondylar epiphysis and opposing articular surfaces of the capitellum and the head of the radius in the throwing arm appeared to be directly proportional to the amount and type of throwing. The most striking changes were in the arms of pitchers. Some degree of accelerated growth, separation, and fragmentation of the medial epicondylar epiphysis was noted in the throwing arm of all eight pitchers in the study. Five cases of traumatic osteochondritis of the capitellum and the head of the radius were also found among the pitchers. Because these conditions invariably develop only in the pitching (throwing) arms, the major cause undoubtedly is the excessive, repetitious microtrauma.

Studies of the mechanics of the pitching motion using accelerometers showed there was no difference in the patterns of muscle activity during acceleration with different delivery styles, even when trying to throw breaking pitches. The main factors causing an elbow injury were not the method of delivery but, rather, the *amount* of throwing and the *force* with which the ball was thrown.[174,184] The same applies to repetitive use in the overhand tennis serve and various impact and swinging routines in gymnastics.

Many coaches and managers argue that most sore arms are due to incorrect throwing motions or failure to warm up properly, which is often true in adults. In youngsters, however, regardless of the throwing motion, the physes are continually subjected to the pull of the attached muscles. Structurally and histologically the epicondylar physes do not seem to be as specifically adapted to excessive, forceful, traction stress as is the tibial tuberosity. The opposing articular surfaces of the joint are also subjected to repetitive trauma from excessive throwing. Trauma of this kind may eventually cause osteochondritic changes and chronic widening of the physes (similar to that reported in the wrist and shoulder in response to repetitive athletic activity).

In a survey of 120 pitchers aged 11 and 12 years, 20% were found to have elbow symptoms, 10% had flexion contractures, and 23% had radiographic changes related to traction stresses on the medial side of the elbow.[188] Five percent had more serious lateral compression findings related to either the radial head or the capitellum. However, none of the boys with lateral joint compartment problems had significant symptoms. Radiographic changes in the medial epicondyle include fragmentation, irregularity, mild separation, enlargement or beaking, and sclerosis (Figs. 15-37, 15-38). These are all various stages of the same reactive process.

Capitellum

The pathogenesis of osteochondral lesions of the elbow still is not completely understood. The sex and age of the patient and the location and laterality of the lesion suggest repetitive trauma as the most probable cause. Underlying this rationale are the possibilities of epiphyseal cartilage failing

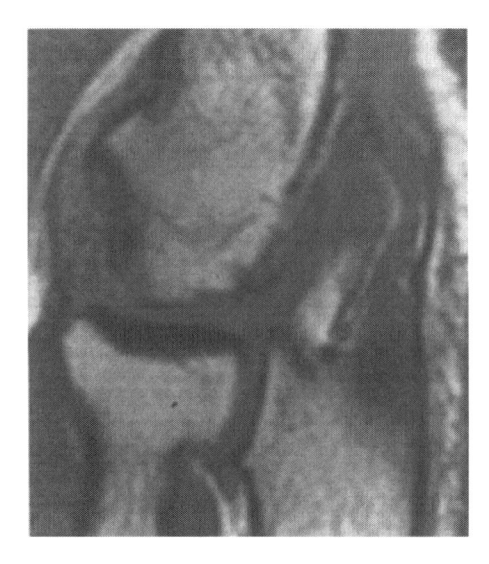

FIGURE 15-38. Panner's lesion. MRI shows a large defect in the capitellum.

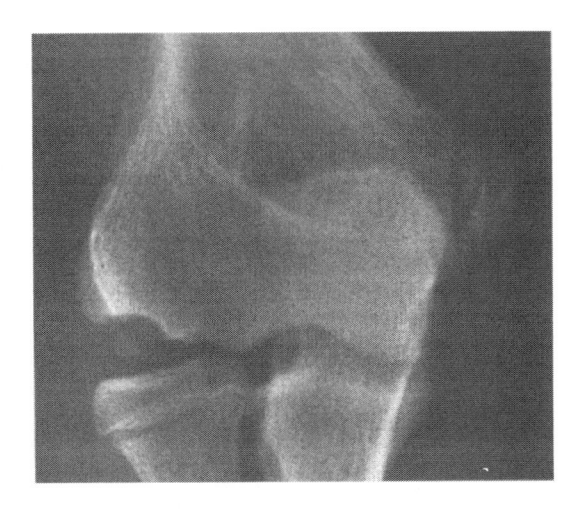

FIGURE 15-39. Capitellar defect in a 12-year-old baseball pitcher.

to ossify, chronic vascular deficiencies, or defective repair mechanisms.[175–177,179–181,185–187,190,192–197,200] This involvement of the capitellum is usually referred to as Panner's disease. In some cases congenital deformities predispose to the development of these lesions.

The capitellum of the humerus is most frequently involved (Fig. 15-39), and the radial head less frequently. The earliest radiologically evident lesion is usually a minimal radiolucency of the convexity of the capitellar epiphyseal ossification center adjacent to the radial articulation. Tomography may show the defect, which eventually becomes apparent on plain radiographs. Magnetic resonance imaging (MRI) is also useful for demonstrating the lesion, often before it becomes radiologically evident. Arthrography may show the articular cartilage to be normal or irregular, and it is helpful for determining the mobility of a fragment and the indications for surgery. The edges of the fossa may be ragged and are sometimes sclerotic. If the chondro-osseous fragment is significantly displaced, it may become free within the joint, leading to chronic damage (Fig. 15-40).

Mitsunaga et al. divided the lesions into type I (in which the fragments were still attached) and type II (in which the loosened fragments were lying free and floating within the joint).[190] Residual limitations were highest in the type II lesions that had been treated nonsurgically or surgically after a long delay. The best surgical results occurred with excision of the osteochondral defect or loose body or bodies along with drilling or curettage of the subchondral bone.

The prognosis for healing and recovery is good once any loose fragments have been removed. If all loose bodies are not removed, overgrowth, secondary reactive sclerosis, and cystic changes may be evident in the condyle, and normal motion may be compromised (Fig. 15-41). Long-term followup (averaging 23 years) showed impaired motion and pain on effort. More than half of the patients had degenerative osteoarthritis in the elbow.

Epicondyle

Epicondylar trauma often occurs without roentgenographically apparent separation. Chronic traction may lead to increased underlying bone formation, effectively enlarging the medial epicondyle. It is essentially the self-induced focal equivalent of chondrodiatasis limb lengthening. Accordingly, the diagnosis must be made on clinical grounds. Radiographic evidence may occur later (Fig. 15-42).

Demonstrable epicondylar separation may be associated with capitellar fragmentation of the ossification center or, in cases of violent motion, dislocation of the elbow joint. Soft tissue injury may be evident. Roentgenograms of the contralateral elbow may be helpful for diagnosing minimal separation, but beware of asymmetry due to the excessive use of the involved arm. Such minimal epicondylar separation may heal by fibrous union. Consequently, roentgenographically demonstrable callus is not always encountered. Sclerosis of the epicondylar center may also occur (Fig. 15-43). Clinical pain (on examination) may indicate a need to intervene. Initial treatment should be cessation of the evocative activity. Closed (percutaneous) or open fixation is indicated in rare cases.

Treatment

Treatment for these various conditions is *primarily preventive*. The following steps are recommended: (1) Alert parents, coaches, administrators, and family physicians that these conditions exist and that the presenting symptoms of soreness or pain in this age group indicate "epiphysitis." Moreover, it should *not* be treated as muscle soreness or "pointer." (2) Encourage youngsters to report elbow pain or soreness *immediately* and reassure them that doing so does not always mean they can no longer participate in the sport. (3) Discourage youngsters from excessive practice, as such excessive activity invites trouble rather than perfection. (4) Abolish evocative activities, such as curve ball throwing for the younger age groups, as it not only places additional strain on the elbow but encourages excessive practice to perfect it.

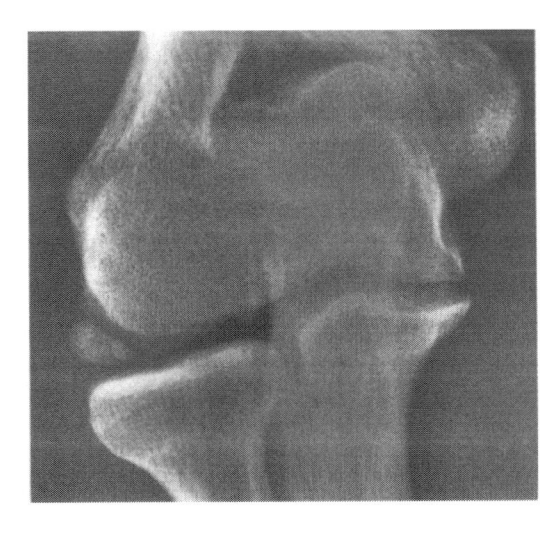

FIGURE 15-40. Loose body in the elbow joint of a teenage high-performance throwing athlete.

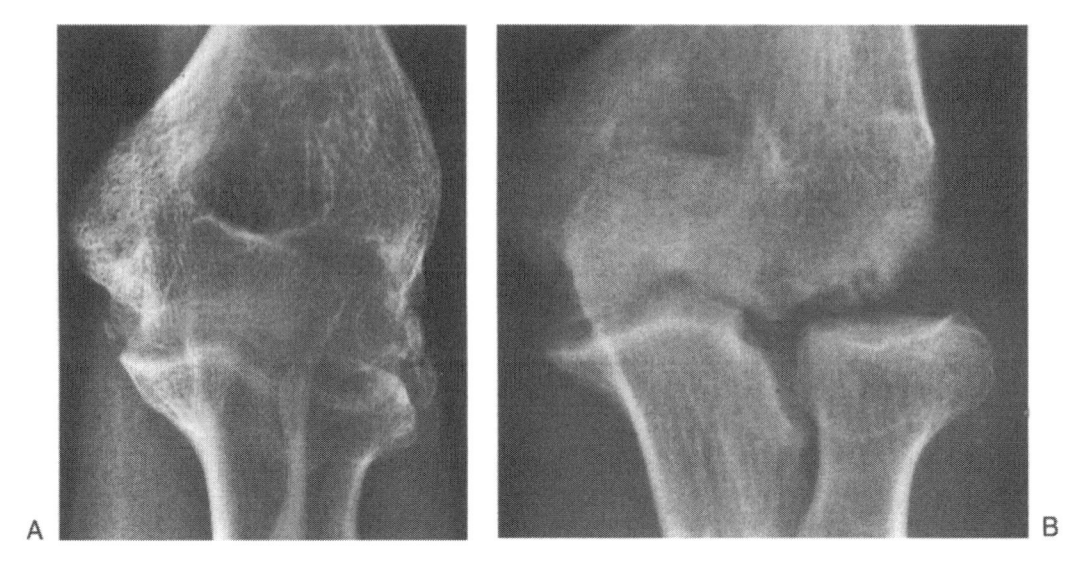

FIGURE 15-41. (A) Some fragmentation may remain "separate" but reasonably in place, yet cause pain by micromotion. (B) Postoperative appearance following fragment removal.

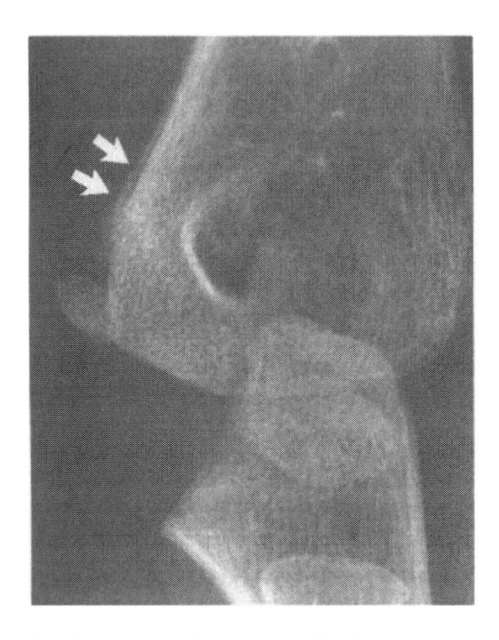

FIGURE 15-42. Chronic medial epicondylitis in a young gymnast. Subperiosteal new bone formation (arrow) has occurred owing to the repetitive application of stress, loosening the chondro-osseous interface.

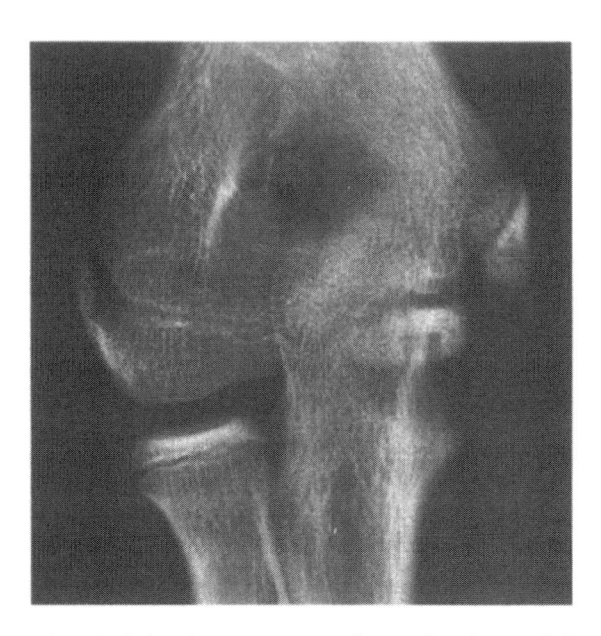

FIGURE 15-43. Sclerotic appearance of a portion the medial epicondyle in an adolescent baseball pitcher. An irregularity is also present in the trochlear ossification center.

References

Anatomy

1. Gunn G. Patella cubiti. Br J Surg 1927;15:612–615.
2. Habernak H, Ortner F. The influence of anatomic factors in elbow joint dislocation. Clin Orthop 1992;274:226–230.
3. Hotchkiss RN, Weiland AJ. Valgus stability of the elbow. J Orthop Res 1987;5:372–377.
4. London JT. Kinematics of the elbow. J Bone Joint Surg Am 1981;63:529–535.
5. McCarthy SM, Ogden JA. Radiology of postnatal skeletal development. VI. Elbow joint, proximal radius and ulna. Skeletal Radiol 1982;9:17–26.
6. Morrey BF, An KN. Articular and ligamentous contributions to the stability of the elbow joint. Am J Sports Med 1983;11:315–319.
7. Resnick CS, Hartenberg MA. Ossification centers of the pediatric elbow: a rare normal variant. Pediatr Radiol 1986;16:254–256.
8. Schwab GH, Bennett JB, Woods GW, Tullos HS. Biomechanics of elbow instability: role of the medial collateral ligament. Clin Orthop 1980;146:42–52.
9. Sojerg JO, Lelmig P, Kjaersgaard-Anderson P. Dislocation of the elbow: an experimental study of the ligamentous injuries. Orthopaedics 1989;12:461–463.
10. Souvegrain J, Nahum H, Bronstein H. Etude de la maturation osseuse du coude. Ann Radiol (Paris) 1962;5:542–550.
11. Zeitlin A. The traumatic origin of accessory bones at the elbow. J Bone Joint Surg 1935;17:933–938.

Dislocation

12. Ainsworth SR, Aulicino PL. Chronic posterolateral dislocation of the elbow in a child. Orthopedics 1993;16:212–215.
13. Aitken AP, Childress HM. Inter-articular displacement of the internal epicondyle following dislocation. J Bone Joint Surg 1938;20:161–166.
14. Allende G, Freytes M. Old dislocation of the elbow. J Bone Joint Surg 1944;26:691–706.
15. Al-Qattan MM, Zuker RM, Weinberg MJ. Type 4 median nerve entrapment after elbow dislocation. J Hand Surg [Br] 1994;19:613–615.
16. Andersen K, Mortensen AC, Gron P. Transverse divergent dislocation of the elbow: a report of two cases. Acta Orthop Scand 1985;56:442–443.
17. Aufranc OE, Jones WN, Turner RH, Thomas WH. Dislocation of the elbow with fracture of the radial head and distal radius. JAMA 1967;202:897–900.
18. Barr LL, Babcock DS. Sonography of the normal elbow. AJR 1991;157:793–798.
19. Beaty JH, Donati NL. Recurrent dislocation of the elbow in a child: case report and review of the literature. J Pediatr Orthop 1990;11:392–396.
20. Berquist TH. The elbow and wrist. Top Magn Reson Imag 1989;1:15–27.
21. Billett DM. Unreduced posterior dislocation of the elbow. J Trauma 1979;19:186–188.
22. Blance CE, Kling TF, Andrews JC, DiPietro MA, Hensinger RN. Arthrography in the post-traumatic elbow in children. AJR 1984;143:17–21.
23. Blatz DJ. Anterior dislocation of the elbow: findings in a case of Ehlers-Danlos syndrome. Orthop Rev 1981;10:129–131.
24. Bock GW, Cohen MS, Resnik D. Fracture-dislocation of the elbow with inferior radioulnar dislocation: a variant of the Essex-Lopresti injury. Skeletal Radiol 1992;21:315–317.
25. Bruce C, Laing P, Dorgan J, Klenerman L. Unreduced dislocation of the elbow. J Trauma 1993;35:962–965.
26. Caravias DE. Forward dislocation of the elbow without fracture of the olecranon. J Bone Joint Surg Br 1957;39:334.
27. Carey RP. Simultaneous dislocation of the elbow and the proximal radioulnar joint. J Bone Joint Surg Br 1984;66:254–256.
28. Carl A, Prado S, Teixiera K. Proximal radioulnar transposition in an elbow dislocation. J Orthop Trauma 1992;6:106–109.
29. Ciaudo O, Guerin-Surville H. Importance de la lesion du faisceau moyen du ligament lateral externe dans le mecanisme des luxations du coude. J Chir 1980;117:237–239.
30. Ciaudo O, Huguenin P, Bensahel H. Un cas de luxation recidivante du coude chez l'enfant: incidence pathogenique. Rev Chir Orthop 1982;68:207–210.
31. Cohn I. Forward dislocation of both bones of the forearm at the elbow. Surg Gynecol Obstet 1922;35:77–79.
32. Cotten FJ. Elbow dislocation and ulnar nerve injury. J Bone Joint Surg 1929;11:348–352.
33. Cummings RJ, Jones ET, Reed FE, Mozur JM. Infantile dislocation of the elbow complicating obstetric palsy. J Pediatr Orthop 1996;16:589–593.
34. DeLee JC. Transverse divergent dislocation of the elbow in a child: case report. J Bone Joint Surg Am 1981;63:322–323.
35. Dickson RA. Reversed dynamic slings: a new concept in the treatment of post-traumatic elbow flexion contractures. Injury 1976;8:35–38.
36. Dryer R, Buckwalter J, Sprague B. Treatment of chronic elbow instability. Clin Orthop 1980;148:254–255.
37. Ejsted R, Christensen FA, Nielson WB. Habitual dislocation of the elbow. Arch Orthop Trauma Surg 1986;105:187–190.
38. Eto RT, Anderson PW, Harley JD. Elbow arthrography with the application of tomography. Radiology 1975;115:283–288.
39. Fazzi UG, Ryaszewski LA. Recurrent dislocation of the elbow in identical twins. J Shoulder Elbow Surg 1996;5:401–403.
40. Fourrier P, Levai JP, Collin JP. Incarceration du nerf median au cours d'une luxation du coude. Rev Chir Orthop 1977;63:13–16.
41. Fowles JV, Kassab MT, Douik M. Untreated posterior dislocation of the elbow in children. J Bone Joint Surg Am 1984;66:91–92.
42. Fowles JV, Rizkallah R. Intra-articular injuries of the elbow: pitfalls of diagnosis and treatment. Can Med Assoc J 1976;114:125–131.
43. Fowles JV, Slimane N, Kassab M. Elbow dislocation with avulsion of the medial humeral epicondyle. J Bone Joint Surg Br 1990;72:102–104.
44. Grant IR, Miller JH. Osteochondral fracture of the trochlea associated with fracture-dislocation of the elbow. Injury 1975;6:257–260.
45. Green NE. Entrapment of the median nerve following elbow dislocation. J Pediatr Orthop 1982;3:384–386.
46. Greiss M, Messias R. Irreducible posterolateral elbow dislocation: a case report. Acta Orthop Scand 1987;58:421–422.
47. Hall RM. Recurrent posterior dislocation of the elbow joint in a boy. J Bone Joint Surg Br 1953;35:56.
48. Hallet J. Entrapment of the median nerve after dislocation of the elbow. J Bone Joint Surg Br 1981;63:408–412.
49. Harvey S, Tchelebi H. Proximal radio-ulnar translocation. J Bone Joint Surg Am 1979;61:447–449.
50. Hassman GC, Brunn F, Neer CS II. Recurrent dislocation of the elbow. J Bone Joint Surg Am 1975;57:1080–1084.
51. Heilbronner DM, Manoli A II, Little RE. Elbow dislocation during overhead skeletal traction therapy. Clin Orthop 1981;154:185–187.

52. Henderson RS, Robertson IM. Open dislocation of the elbow with rupture of the brachial artery. J Bone Joint Surg Br 1952; 34:636–637.
53. Hennig K, Franke D. Posterior displacement of the brachial artery following closed elbow dislocation. J Trauma 1980;20: 96–98.
54. Henriksen BM, Gehrchen PM, Jørgensen MB, Gerner-Schmidt H. Treatment of traumatic effusion in the elbow joint: a prospective, randomized study of 62 consecutive patients. Injury 1995;26:475–478.
55. Herring JA, Sullivan J. Instructional case: recurrent dislocation of the elbow. J Pediatr Orthop 1989;9:483–484.
56. Hofmann KE III, Moneim MS, Omer GE, Ball WS. Brachial artery disruption following closed posterior elbow dislocation in a child: assessment with intravenous digital angiography. Clin Orthop 1984;184:145–149.
57. Holbrook JL, Greene NE. Divergent pediatric elbow dislocation. Clin Orthop 1988;234:72–74.
58. Jacobs RL. Recurrent dislocation of the elbow: a case report and review of the literature. Clin Orthop 1971;74:151–154.
59. Johannson O. Capsular and ligament injuries of the elbow joint: a clinical and arthrographic study. Acta Chir Scand 1962; suppl 287:1–159.
60. Kapel O. Operation for habitual dislocation of the elbow. J Bone Joint Surg Am 1951;33:707–710.
61. Kaplan SS, Reckling RW. Fracture separation of the lower humeral epiphysis with medial displacement. J Bone Joint Surg Am 1971;53:1105–1108.
62. Kerin R. Elbow dislocation and its association with vascular disruption. J Bone Joint Surg Am 1969;51:756–758.
63. Kilburn P, Sweeny JG, Silk FF. Three cases of compound posterior dislocation of the elbow with rupture of the brachial artery. J Bone Joint Surg Br 1962;44:119–121.
64. Krisnamoorthy S, Bose K, Wong KP. Treatment of old unreduced dislocation of the elbow. Injury 1976;8:39–42.
65. Letts M. Dislocations of the child's elbow. In: Morrey BF (ed) The Elbow and Its Disorders. Philadelphia: Saunders, 1985.
66. Linscheid RL, Wheeler DK. Elbow dislocations. JAMA 1965; 194:1171–1176.
67. Louis DS, Ricciardi J, Sprengler DM. Arterial injuries: a complication of posterior elbow dislocation. J Bone Joint Surg Am 1974;56:1631–1636.
68. MacSween WA. Transposition of radius and ulna associated with dislocation of the elbow in a child. Injury 1976;10: 314–316.
69. Mahaisavariya B, Laupattlaokasen W, Supachutikul A, et al. Late reduction of dislocated elbow: need triceps be lengthened? J Bone Joint Surg Br 1993;75:426–428.
70. Malkawi H. Recurrent dislocation of the elbow accompanied by ulnar neuropathy: a case report and review of the literature. Clin Orthop 1981;161:270–274.
71. Mannerfelt L. Median nerve entrapment after dislocation of the elbow. J Bone Joint Surg Br 1968;50:152–155.
72. Manquel M, Minkowitz B, Shimotsu G, et al. Brachial artery laceration with closed posterior elbow dislocation in an eight year old. Clin Orthop 1993;296:109–112.
73. Mantle J. Recurrent posterior dislocation of the elbow. J Bone Joint Surg Br 1966;48:590.
74. Matev I. A radiological sign of entrapment of the median nerve in the elbow joint after posterior dislocation: a report of two cases. J Bone Joint Surg Br 1976;58:353–355.
75. McKellar-Hall R. Recurrent posterior dislocation of the elbow joint in a boy. J Bone Joint Surg Br 1953;35:56.
76. Meyn MA, Quibley TB. Reduction of posterior dislocation of the elbow by traction on the dangling arm. Clin Orthop 1974; 103:106–108.
77. Mih AD, Wolf FG. Surgical release of elbow-capsular contracture in pediatric patients. J Pediatr Orthop 1994;14:458–461.
78. Milch H. Bilateral recurrent dislocation of the ulna at the elbow. J Bone Joint Surg 1936;18:777–780.
79. Mintzer CM, Walters PM. Late presentation of a ligamentous ulnar collateral ligament injury in a child. J Hand Surg [Am] 1994;19:1048–1049.
80. Naidoo KS. Unreduced posterior dislocations of the elbow. J Bone Joint Surg Br 1982;64:603–606.
81. Nakano A, Tanaka S, Hirofujie, et al. Transverse divergent dislocation of the elbow in a six-year-old boy: case report. J Trauma 1992;32:118–119.
82. Niemann KMW, Gould JS, Simmons B, Bora FW Jr. Injuries to and developmental deformities of the elbow in children. In: Bora FW Jr (ed) The Pediatric Upper Extremity: Diagnosis and Management. Philadelphia: Saunders, 1986.
83. Noonan KJ, Blair WF. Chronic median-nerve entrapment after posterior fracture-dislocation of the elbow. J Bone Joint Surg Am 1995;77:1572–1575.
84. Osborne GB, Cotterill P. Recurrent dislocation of the elbow. J Bone Joint Surg Br 1966;48:340–346.
85. Oury JH, Roe RD, Laning R. A case of bilateral anterior dislocations of the elbow. J Trauma 1972;12:170–173.
86. Patrick J. Fracture of the medial epicondyle with displacement into the elbow joint. J Bone Joint Surg 1946;28:143–147.
87. Pritchard DJ, Linscheid RL, Svien HJ. Intra-articular median nerve entrapment with dislocation of the elbow. Clin Orthop 1973;90:100–103.
88. Pritchett JW. Entrapment of the median nerve after dislocation of the elbow. J Pediatr Orthop 1984;4:752–753.
89. Protzman RR. Dislocation of the elbow joint. J Bone Joint Surg Am 1978;60:539–541.
90. Rana NA, Kenwright J, Taylor RG, Rushworth G. Complete lesion of the median nerve associated with dislocation of the elbow joint. Acta Orthop Scand 1974;45:365–369.
91. Robert M, Aubard Y, Dixneuf B, Moulies D, Alain JL. Posterior luxations of the elbow in children. Acta Orthop Belg 1984;50: 750–757.
92. Saraf SK, Tuli SM. Concomitant medial condyle fracture of the humerus in a childhood posterolateral dislocation of the elbow. J Orthop Trauma 1989;3:352–354.
93. Silva JF. The problems relating to old dislocation and the restriction of the elbow movement. Acta Orthop Belg 1975;41: 399–411.
94. Smith FM. Displacement of the medial epicondyle of the humerus into the elbow joint. Ann Surg 1946;124:410–425.
95. Smith FM. Children's elbow injuries: fractures and dislocations. Clin Orthop 1967;50:7–30.
96. Sovio OM, Tredwell SJ. Divergent dislocation of the elbow in a child. J Pediatr Orthop 1986;6:96–97.
97. St. Clair-Strange FG. Entrapment of the median nerve after dislocation of the elbow. J Bone Joint Surg Br 1982;64: 224–225.
98. Steiger RN, Larrick RB, Meyer TL. Median nerve entrapment following elbow dislocation in children. J Bone Joint Surg Am 1969;51:381–385.
99. Sysa NF. Perelomy skeiki luchevoi kosti, sochetaiushchiesia s vyvikhom v plecheloktevom sustave u detei [Fractures of the radius neck associated with dislocation of the elbow joint in children]. Vestn Khir 1989;143:82–84.
100. Tayob AA, Shively RA. Bilateral elbow dislocations with intraarticular displacement of the medial epicondyle. J Trauma 1980;20:332–335.
101. Thompson HC, Garcia A. Myositis ossificans: aftermath of elbow injuries. Clin Orthop 1967;50:129–134.
102. Trias A, Comeau Y. Recurrent dislocation of the elbow in children. Clin Orthop 1974;100:74–77.

References

103. Urbaniak JR, Hansen PE, Beissinger SF, Aitken MS. Correction of post-traumatic flexion contracture of the elbow by anterior capsulotomy. J Bone Joint Surg Am 1985;67:1160–1164.
104. Van Haaren ERM, van Vaught AB, Bode PJ. Posterolateral dislocation of the elbow with concomitant fracture of the lateral humeral condyle: case report. J Trauma 1994;35:288–295.
105. Vicente P, Orduña M. Transverse divergent dislocation of the elbow in a child. Clin Orthop 1993;294:312–313.
106. Volkov MV, Oganesian OV. Restoration of functions in the knee and elbow with a hinge-distractor apparatus. J Bone Joint Surg Am 1975;57:591–600.
107. Warmont A. Luxation simultanee du cubitus en dedans et du radius en dehors, compliquee de fracture de l'avant-bras. Mon Hop J Prog Med Chir Prat 1854;1:961–963.
108. Watson-Jones R. Primary nerve lesions in injuries of the elbow and wrist. J Bone Joint Surg 1930;12:121–140.
109. Wheeler DK, Linscheid RL. Fracture-dislocations of the elbow. Clin Orthop 1967;50:95–106.
110. Wright JS. Dislocation of the bones of the right forearm backwards, the radius being outward and ulna being inward and the head of the radius being dislocated from the base of the ulna. Phys Surg 1893;15:67–70.
111. Zeier FG. Recurrent traumatic elbow dislocation. Clin Orthop 1982;169:211–214.

Pulled Elbow

112. Amir D, Frankl U, Pogrund H. Pulled elbow and hypermobility of joints. Clin Orthop 1988;257:94–99.
113. Anderson SA. Subluxation of the head of the radius, a pediatric condition. South Med J 1942;35:286–287.
114. Beagel PM. "Slipped elbow" in children. Maine Med Assoc 1906;45:293–296.
115. Bobrow RS. Childhood radial head subluxation: physician unfamiliarity with "nursemaid's" or "pulled" elbow. NY State J Med 1977;77:908–909.
116. Bourquet J. Memoire sur les luxations dites incompletes de l'extremite. Rev Med Chir Soc Med Nat Iasi 1854;15:287–289.
117. Boyette BP, Ahoskie NC, London AH Jr. Subluxation of the radius, "nursemaid's elbow." J Pediatr 1948;32:278–281.
118. Bretland PM. Pulled elbow in childhood. Br J Radiol 1994;67:1176–1185.
119. Broadhurst RW, Buhr AJ. The pulled elbow. BMJ 1959;1:1018.
120. Caldwell CE. Subluxation of the radial head by elongation. Cincinnati Lancet Clin 1891;66:496–497.
121. Choung W, Heinrich SD. Acute annular ligament interposition into the radiocapitellar joint in children (nursemaid's elbow). J Pediatr Orthrop 1995;15:454–456.
122. Corrigan A. The pulled elbow. Med J Aust 1965;2:187–189.
123. Costigan PG. Subluxation of the annular ligament at the proximal radioulnar joint. Alberta Med Bull 1952;17:7–10.
124. Cushing HW. Subluxation of the radial head in children. Boston Med Surg J 1886;114:77–78.
125. David ML. Radial head subluxation. Am Fam Physician 1987;35:143–146.
126. Davis JH. Subluxation of the radial head in children (nursemaid's elbow). Med Times 1865;13:1379–1380.
127. Dubuc JE, Rombouts JJ, Vincent A. Luxations of the proximal end of the radius in children. Acta Orthop Belg 1984;50:815–836.
128. Frumkin K. Nursemaid's elbow: a radiographic demonstration. Ann Emerg Med 1985;14:690–693.
129. Gardner J. On an undescribed displacement of the bones of the forearm in children. London Med Gaz 1837;20:878–879.
130. Gatrell CB. Radiologic findings in radial head subluxation. Am J Dis Child 1986;140:856.
131. Green JT, Gay FH. Traumatic subluxation of the radial head in young children. J Bone Joint Surg Am 1954;36:655–662.
132. Griffin ME. Subluxation of the head of the radius in young children. Pediatrics 1955;15:103–106.
133. Hamer AJ, Monaghan D, Steiner GM. Investigation of "pulled elbow" in children by ultrasound scan. J Pediatr Orthop 1993;2:159–160.
134. Hart GM. Subluxation of the head of the radius in young children. JAMA 1959;169:1734–1736.
135. Hutchinson J. On certain obscure sprains of the elbow occurring in young children. Ann Surg 1885;2:90–97.
136. Illingworth CM. Pulled elbow: a study of 100 patients. BMJ 1975;2:672–674.
137. James JB. Partial dislocation of the head of the radius peculiar to children. BMJ 1886;2:1058–1059.
138. Jongshaap HCN, Youngson GG, Beattie TF. The epidemiology of radial head subluxation ("pulled elbow") in the Aberdeen City area. Health Bull 1990;48:58–61.
139. Kanter AJ, Bruton OC. Subluxation of the head of the radius. Am Practitioner 1952;31:39–42.
140. Kosuwon W, Mahaisavariya B, Saengnipanthkul S, et al. Ultrasonography of pulled elbow. J Bone Joint Surg Br 1993;75:421–422.
141. Lamont AC, Dias JJ. Ultrasonic diagnosis of dislocation of the radius in an infant with Down's syndrome. Br J Radiol 1991;64:849–851.
142. Lindeman SH. Partial dislocation of the radial head peculiar to children. BMJ 1885;2:1058–1059.
143. Magill HK, Aitken P. Pulled elbow. Surg Gynecol Obstet 1954;98:753–756.
144. Matles AL, Eliopoulous K. Internal derangement of the elbow in children. Int Surg 1967;48:259–263.
145. McRae R, Freeman P. The lesion in pulled elbow. J Bone Joint Surg Br 1965;47:808.
146. McVeagh TC. The slipped elbow in young children. Calif Med 1951;74:260–262.
147. Mehara AK, Bhan S. A radiologic sign in pulled elbows. Int Orthop 1995;19:174–175.
148. Mehta L. Subluxation of radial head in children with reference to radial head and neck diameters. J Indian Med Assoc 1972;59:238–239.
149. Meyer RJ, Roelofs HA, Bluestone J. Accidental injury to the preschool child. J Pediatr 1963;63:95–105.
150. Michelman B. Recurrent radial head subluxation in a 3 year old child: case report. West Eng Med J 1991;106:44–45.
151. Miles KA, Finlay DBL. Disruption of the radiocapitellar line in the normal elbow. Injury 1989;20:365–367.
152. Miller TO, Insall J. Radial head subluxation in adolescence. NY State J Med 1975;75:80–82.
153. Moore EM. Subluxation of the radius from extension in young children. Trans NY Med Assoc 1886;3:18–19.
154. Newman J. "Nursemaid's elbow" in infants six months and under. J Emerg Med 1985;2:403–404.
155. Piersol GA. Human Anatomy, 9th ed. Philadelphia: Lippincott, 1930.
156. Piroth P, Gharib M. Die traumatische subluxation des radiuskopfchens (Chassaignac). Dtsch Med Wochenschr 1976;101:1520–1523.
157. Quan L, Marcuse EK. The epidemiology and treatment of radial head subluxation. Am J Dis Child 1985;139:1194–1197.
158. Ryan JR. The relationship of the radial head to radial neck diameters in fetuses and adults with reference to radial-head subluxation in children. J Bone Joint Surg Am 1969;51:781–783.

159. Sachetti A, Ramoska EE, Glascow C. Non-classic history in children with radial head subluxation. J Emerg Med 1990;8:151–153.
160. Salter R, Zaltz C. Anatomic investigations of the mechanism of injury and pathologic anatomy of "pulled elbow" in children. Clin Orthop 1971;77:134–143.
161. Schunk JE. Radial head subluxation: epidemiology and treatment of 87 episodes. Ann Emerg Med 1990;19:1019–1023.
162. Silquini PL. La pronazione dolorosa. Minerva Ortop 1963;14:481–483.
163. Silver CM, Simon SD. Subluxation of head of the radius ("pulled elbow") in children. RI Med J 1960;43:772–773.
164. Smith EE. Subluxation of the head of the radius in children. Ohio State Med J 1949;45:1080–1081.
165. Snellman O. Subluxation of the radial head in children. Acta Orthop Scand 1959;28:311–315.
166. Snyder HS. Radiographic changes with radial head subluxation in children. J Emerg Med 1990;8:265–269.
167. Stone CA. Subluxation of the head of the radius: report of a case and anatomical experiments. JAMA 1916;1:28–29.
168. Sweetman R. Pulled elbow. Practitioner 1959;182:487–489.
169. Tesch SJ, Schutzman SA. Prospective study of recurrent radial head subluxation. Arch Pediatr Adolesc Med 1996;150:164–166.
170. Triantafyllou SJ, Wilson SC, Rychale JS. Irreducible "pulled elbow: in a child. Clin Orthop 1992;284:153–155.
171. Van Arsdale WW. On subluxation of the head of the radius in children: with a resume of one-hundred consecutive cases. Ann Surg 1889;9:401–423.
172. Van Santvoord R. Dislocation of the head of the radius downward (by elongation). NY State Med J 1987;45:63–64.

Little League Elbow

173. Adams JE. Injury to the throwing arm: a study of traumatic changes in the elbow joints of boy baseball players. Calif Med 1965;102:127–132.
174. Albright JA, Jokl P, Shaw R, Albright JP. Clinical study of baseball pitchers: correlation of injury to the throwing arm with method of delivery. Am J Sports Med 1978;6:15–21.
175. Antoni R, Robert DR. Juvenile osteochondritis of the radial head. J Bone Joint Surg Am 1963;45:576–582.
176. Bauer M, Jonsson K, Josefsson PO, Lindén B. Osteochondritis dissecans of the elbow: a long-term follow-up study. Clin Orthop 1992;284:156–160.
177. Bianco AJ. Osteochondritis dissecans. In: Morrey B (ed) The Elbow and Its Disorders. Philadelphia: Saunders, 1985.
178. Brogdon BG. Little league elbow. AJR 1960;83:671–675.
179. Brown R, Blaxina ME, Kerlan RK, et al. Osteochondritis of the capitellum. J Sports Med 1974;2:27–46.
180. Chiroff RT, Cook CP III. Osteochondritis dissecans: a histological and microradiographic analysis of surgically excised lesions. J Trauma 1975;15:689–696.
181. Elzenga P. Juvenile osteochondrosis deformans of the capitulum humeri (Panner's disease). Arch Chir Neerl 1969;21:67–75.
182. Godshall RW, Hansen CA. Traumatic ulnar neuropathy in adolescent baseball pitchers. J Bone Joint Surg Am 1971;53:359–361.
183. Gugenheim JJ, Stanley RF, Woods GW, Tullos HS. Little league survey: the Houston study. Am J Sports Med 1976;4:189–200.
184. Hang YS, Lippert FG III, Spolek GA, Harrington RM. Biomechanical study of the pitching elbow. Int Orthop 1979;3:217–223.
185. Haraldsson S. On osteochondrosis deformans juvenilis capituli humeri including investigation of intra-osseous vasculature in distal humerus. Acta Orthop Scand 1959;suppl 38:1–147.
186. Heller CJ, Wiltse LL. Avascular necrosis of the capitellum humeri (Panner's disease): a report of a case. J Bone Joint Surg Am 1960;42:513–516.
187. Klein EW. Osteochondrosis of the capitellum (Panner's disease). AJR 1962;88:466–469.
188. Larson RL, Singer KM, Bergstrom R, Thomas S. Little league survey: the Eugene study. Am J Sports Med 1976;4:201–209.
189. Lipscomb AB. Baseball pitching injuries in growing athletes. J Sports Med 1975;3:25–34.
190. Mitsunaga MM, Adishian DA, Bianco AJ Jr. Osteochondritis dissecans of the capitellum. J Trauma 1982;22:53–55.
191. Nocini S, Silvij S. Clinical and radiological aspects of gymnast's elbow. J Sports Med 1982;22:54–59.
192. Osebold WR, El-Khoury G, Ponseti IV. Aseptic necrosis of the humeral trochlea: a case report. Clin Orthop 1977;127:161–163.
193. Panner HJ. An affection of the capitulum humeri resembling Calve-Perthes disease of the hip. Acta Radiol 1927;8:617–625.
194. Pritsch M, Engel J, Ganel A, Farin I. Osteochondrosis of the elbow. Orthop Rev 1981;10:89–92.
195. Roberts N, Hughes R. Osteochondritis dissecans of the elbow joint: a clinical study. J Bone Joint Surg Br 1950;32:348–360.
196. Singer KM, Roy SP. Osteochondritis of the humeral capitellum. Am J Sports Med 1984;12:351–360.
197. Smith MGH. Osteochondritis of the humeral capitellum. J Bone Joint Surg Br 1964;46:50–54.
198. Torg JS, Pollack H, Sweterlitsch P. The effect of competitive pitching on the shoulders and elbows of pre-adolescent baseball players. Pediatrics 1972;49:267–272.
199. Tullos HS, King JW. Lesions of the pitching arm in adolescents. JAMA 1972;220:264–271.
200. Woodward AH, Bianco AJ Jr. Osteochondritis dissecans of the elbow. Clin Orthop 1975;110:35–41.

16

Radius and Ulna

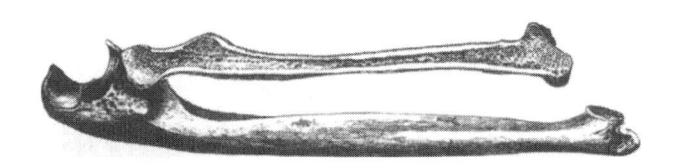

Engraving of a complication of a distal radial physeal fracture leading to premature growth arrest and radial shortening. (From Poland J. Traumatic Separation of the Epiphysis. *London: Smith, Elder, 1898)*

The development of secondary ossification of the proximal ulna may make interpretation of injury difficult, as variations of normal radiographic findings are frequently misinterpreted as a fracture (especially an avulsion fracture).[2] Consequently, the characteristics and variations of secondary ossification of the olecranon process must be learned so false-positive diagnoses are avoided.[17]

There are two functional ulnar prominences, the olecranon and the coronoid, with epiphyseal and articular cartilage connecting them (Fig. 16-1). It is important to realize that an epiphysis and physis are present under the articular cartilage, even if some of the epiphyseal region extending toward the coronoid process does not develop a distinct secondary ossification center. The secondary ossification process is essentially confined to the olecranon segment, although a small anatomically separate ossification center, may develop infrequently in the coronoid. The distal portion of the proximal ulna and the coronoid process are formed by the ulnar metaphysis, and the proximal portion is formed by the olecranon epiphysis (Fig. 16-1). The secondary ossification center does not usually appear in the olecranon until the ninth to tenth year (Figs. 16-1 to 16-3). This secondary ossification center is usually unifocal, although it is bipartite or multipartite in some children (Fig. 16-4). When bipartite, the accessory center is usually located near the tip of the olecranon.[10,17] A variation, the patella cubitus, is defined radiographically as a sesamoid bone in the triceps tendon. The accessory bones, however, are not anatomically separate from the rest of the olecranon. It is likely that a patella cubitus represents partial avulsion of the epiphysis as it is ossifying, not unlike the Osgood-Schlatter lesion in the proximal tibia. Pain may indicate an occult chondro-osseous injury, similar to the painful accessory navicular (see Chapters 6, 24). These osseous variations often must be distinguished from fractures. A bone scan may be useful for such differentiation, with a positive scan strongly indicative of acute injury.

Closure of the ulnar physis occurs from the juxtaarticular side outward, so when a boy is about 13 years old the inner portion of the olecranon physis is closed, and the outer (most external) portion may still be evident as a radiolucent line. The normal open or fusing physis of the olecranon has a well-defined sclerotic margin, which is *not* present with an acute fracture. Girls experience similar closure patterns, but earlier than boys, usually between 11 and 12 years.

An olecranon bursa is not usually present in children younger than 6–7 years of age. With increasing use of the arm and progressive ossification, this gliding structure progressively develops.[4] Formation of the bursa during late childhood explains the relatively low incidence of olecranon bursitis consequent to trauma in children. An older child may injure the bursa by a direct blow, leading to acute swelling or, less likely, to chronic inflammation.

The anatomy of the proximal radius also affects injury patterns.[10,22] The discoid-shaped head of the radius is *always* of greater diameter than the neck (even during fetal development). The head and neck of the radius are well defined, the head is larger than the neck, and a radial notch appears in the ulna. Although not as distinct during the fetal stage, the radial head, even during the first year, shows the same eccentric concavity and defined anterolateral rim as in the adult.[10]

The plane of the articular surface is tilted relative to the longitudinal axis of the radius. This tilt varies depending on the rotation. The exact degree of tilting and shifting may be measured only on films obtained at proper angles to the plane of angulation (Fig. 16-5). The changing tilt affects the up-and-down sliding motion of the annular ligament. Because one of the problems of proximal radial fractures is increased angulation, during reduction one should remember that there is normally a mild tilt. The concavity within the proximal radius that articulates with the capitellum may

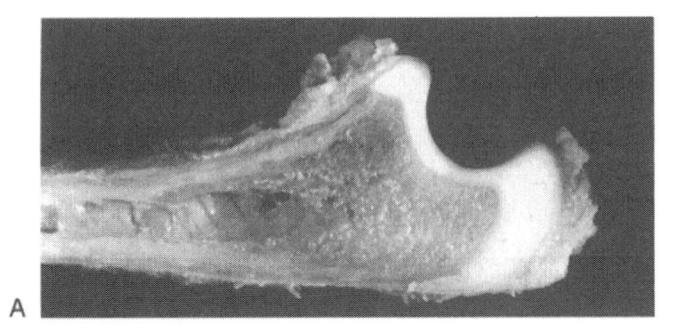

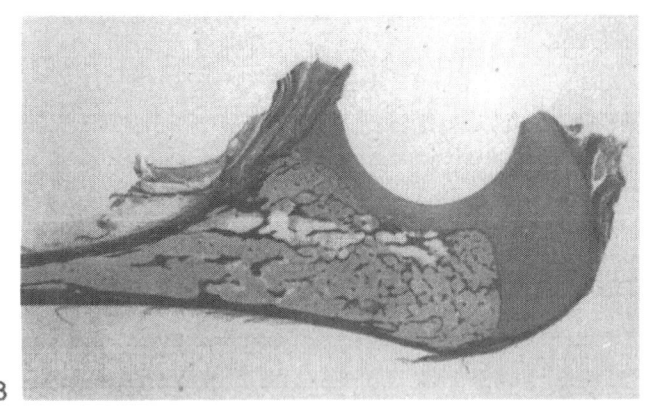

FIGURE 16-1. (A) Section of the proximal ulna from a 2-year-old girl. Epiphyseal cartilage is present from the olecranon to the coronoid process. (B) Histologic section. There is a continuous growth plate all along this cartilage.

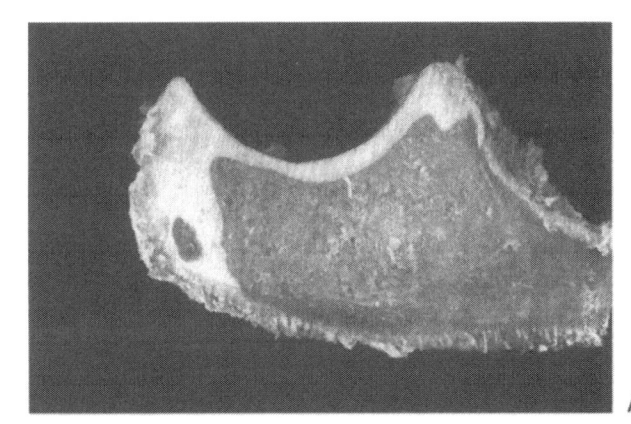

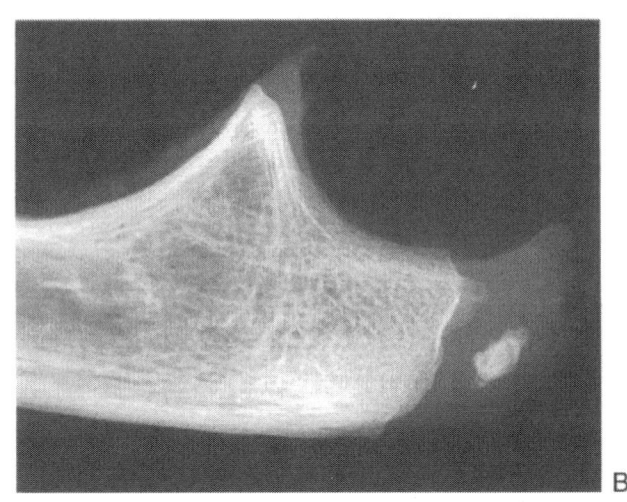

FIGURE 16-2. (A) Sagittal section of the proximal ulna from a 5-year-old child. The olecranon ossification center is well established. (B) Radiograph of the specimen.

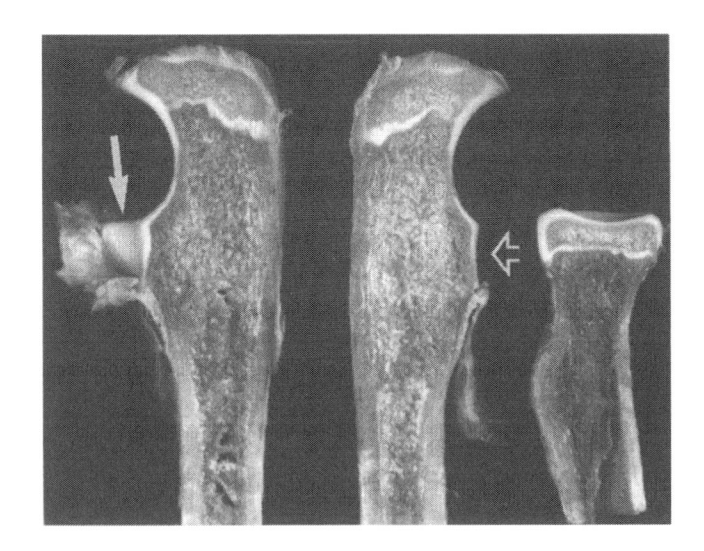

FIGURE 16-3. Slab sections of the ulna and radius of a 13-year-old boy. The olecranon ossification center is well developed. Note the coronoid process (solid arrow) is part of the proximal radioulnar joint (open arrow).

be eccentric (Fig. 16-5), which affects rotational dynamics and the tautness within the annular ligament.

The epiphysis of the radial head is covered extensively by articular cartilage. It is present not only over the end of the radius but circumferentially around the sides to allow radioulnar movement. There is no perichondrium on this particular epiphysis. The epiphyseal blood supply has a short intraarticular course along the metaphysis, which is surrounded by the annular ligament. This situation creates a susceptible intracapsular epiphyseal blood supply similar to that of the capital femoral epiphysis (Fig. 16-6). The blood supply may be damaged by epiphyseal or metaphyseal separation. Because the usual level of injury through the metaphysis is near the entry of the vessels, ischemic necrosis must be considered a potential complication. However, there is often hyperemia of the fracture site, causing overgrowth of the radial head, rather than significant growth limitation.

The proximal radial epiphysis may not ossify until a child is 5–7 years old and usually unites between 12 and 15 years of age. It generally ossifies symmetrically. Because of the epiphyseal tilt, however, ossification may be asymmetric and may resemble a triangle rather than an ellipse in certain positions.[10,11,16] An angular shape may also indicate a problem of abnormal radiohumeral joint stress, such as a radioulnar synostosis or Panner's disease. Because these conditions are not diagnosed in many children until an episode of trauma, the

FIGURE 16-4. Normal variations of the formation of the olecranon secondary ossification center. They could easily be interpreted as a fracture during the evaluation of acute trauma.

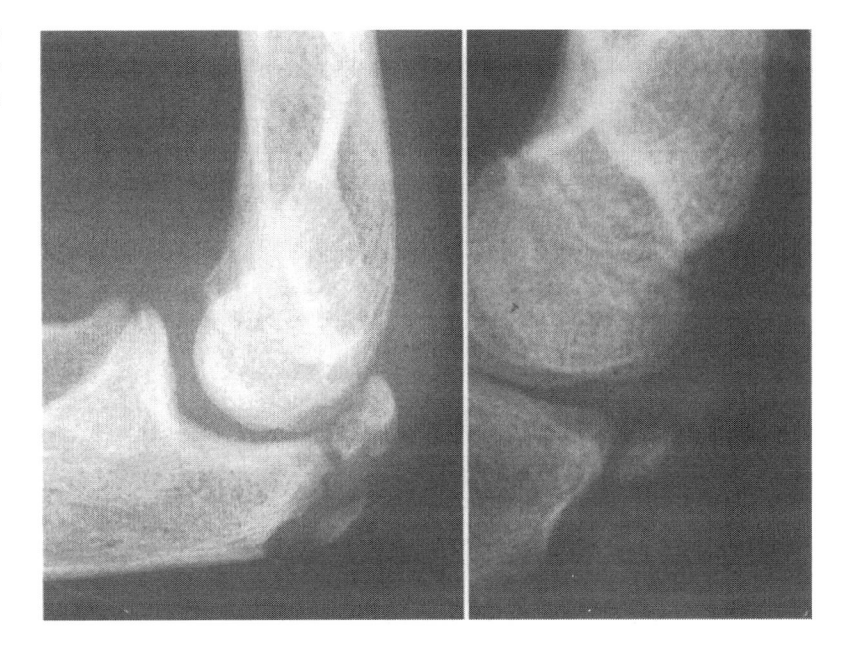

physician should be aware of these potential problems of differential diagnosis as related to normal anatomic development and maturation.

The upper end of the ulna articulates with the trochlea of the distal humerus and provides primary flexion-extension of the elbow. It also articulates with the head of the radius through an extension of the joint proximally on both the radius and the ulna (Fig. 16-7). The proximal and distal radioulnar joints tend to be clinically ignored articulations, although they are especially important in the Monteggia injury, pulled elbow, and the Galeazzi injury.

The radial head is tightly constrained by the capitellar and ulnar articular surfaces. This anatomic construction permits rotation and flexion-extension while creating intrinsic stability. Both articular relations are disrupted during a Monteggia injury. The annular ligament holds the radial metaphysis against the shaft of the ulna and the ulnar articular extension. The annular ligament further restrains the radioulnar joint. This ligament has some laxity, which allows displacement in radial head subluxation and may permit displacement of the radial head without significant tearing, especially in younger children. The ligament may be torn or displaced in Monteggia injuries. A synovial recess usually extends under the ligament.

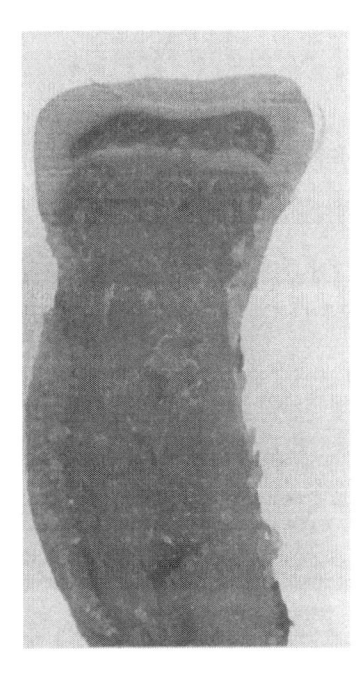

FIGURE 16-5. Sagittal section through the radial head and bicipital tuberosity. The radial head concavity is eccentric and slightly tilted relative to the longitudinal axis of the radial shaft.

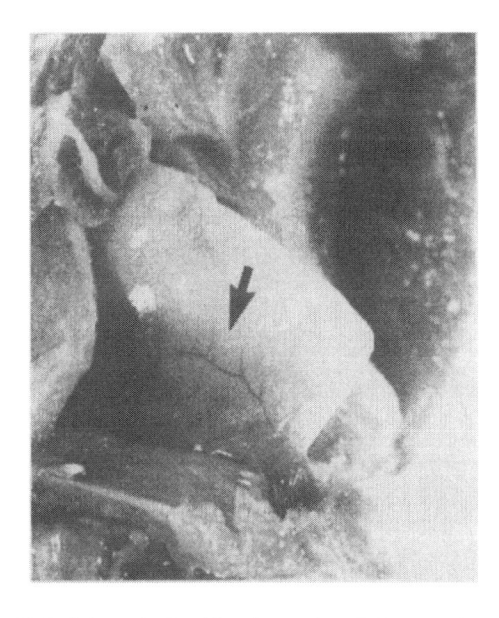

FIGURE 16-6. Intraarticular blood supply of the proximal radius. Several small vessels (arrow) extend transversely and longitudinally under the annular ligament, which has been pulled down.

ficiently to allow adequate roentgenographic evaluation.[3] By the time a child is 5 years of age, the tuberosity begins to have enough prominence to be visible roentgenographically (Fig. 16-8). Prior to this age, forearm fractures are infrequent and are generally greenstick, with the intact cortex and the thick periosteal sleeve maintaining longitudinal continuity and minimizing any rotational misalignment.

The sagittal and coronal cross-sectional diameters of the radius and ulna change with age and anatomic level. Proximally, both have a circular appearance, although for much of the diaphysis the two bones have a cam (pear) shape. As such, rotational deformities often are detected by the differences in the widths of the apposed fragments.

The radius and ulna are bound together firmly by the interosseous membrane, which provides a hinge mechanism for integrated rotatory movements.[5,8,9] This interosseous ligament attaches along the tip of the "cam" of both the radius and the ulna. Correction of the rotational deformity is directed at restoring the interosseous ligament mechanics, which are important in pronation and supination. Specialized ligaments are present at each end. The annular ligament holds the proximal radioulnar joint together. The distal radioulnar and radiocarpal joints are connected by the

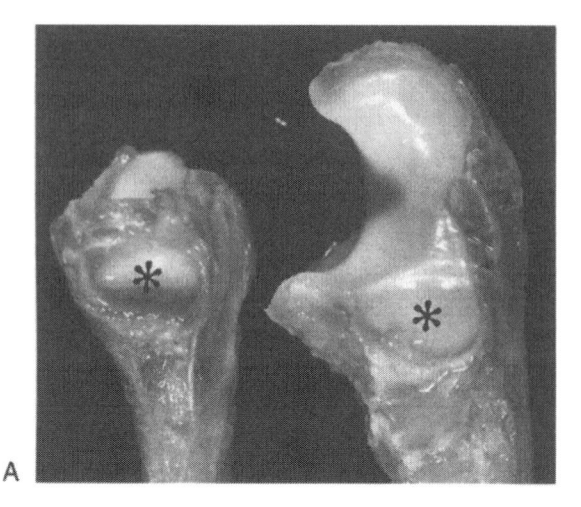

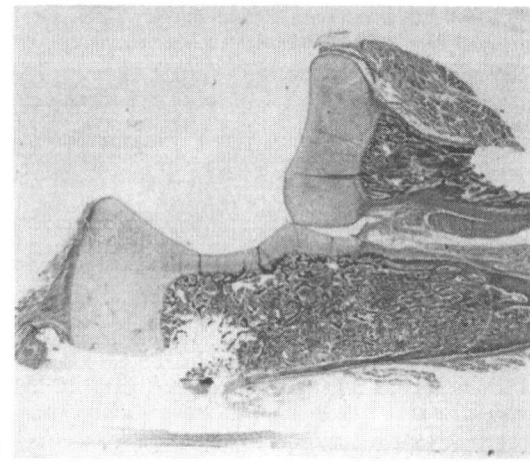

FIGURE 16-7. (A) Proximal and distal ulna showing the articular surfaces (*) for the radius. These joints are important and must be considered during the evaluation and treatment of wrist and elbow trauma. These joints remain throughout skeletal maturation, and the correct structural relationships are necessary for forearm rotation. (B) Histology of the proximal radioulnar relations.

The proximal radioulnar joint is stable in supination because (1) the radial head is not circular but slightly oval, and with the forearm in supination the greatest diameter of the head comes in contact with the proximal radioulnar joint; (2) the margin of the radial head is not the same width around the head, so in full supination the broadest portion of the margin of the radial head comes in contact with the proximal notch of the ulna and gives the broadest articular contact; (3) in full supination the interosseous membrane is most taut; (4) the annular ligament is reinforced by the anterior and posterior components of the radial collateral ligaments; and (5) in full supination the anterior, thicker fibers of the quadrate ligament of Denuce stabilize the radial head more strongly into the proximal radioulnar joint.[18,19]

The biceps tendon inserts onto the radial tuberosity. This osseous prominence becomes progressively larger as the child grows. Evans stressed its potential use for assessing the relative rotation of the proximal fragments in forearm fractures.[7] Its usefulness is contingent on its being developed suf-

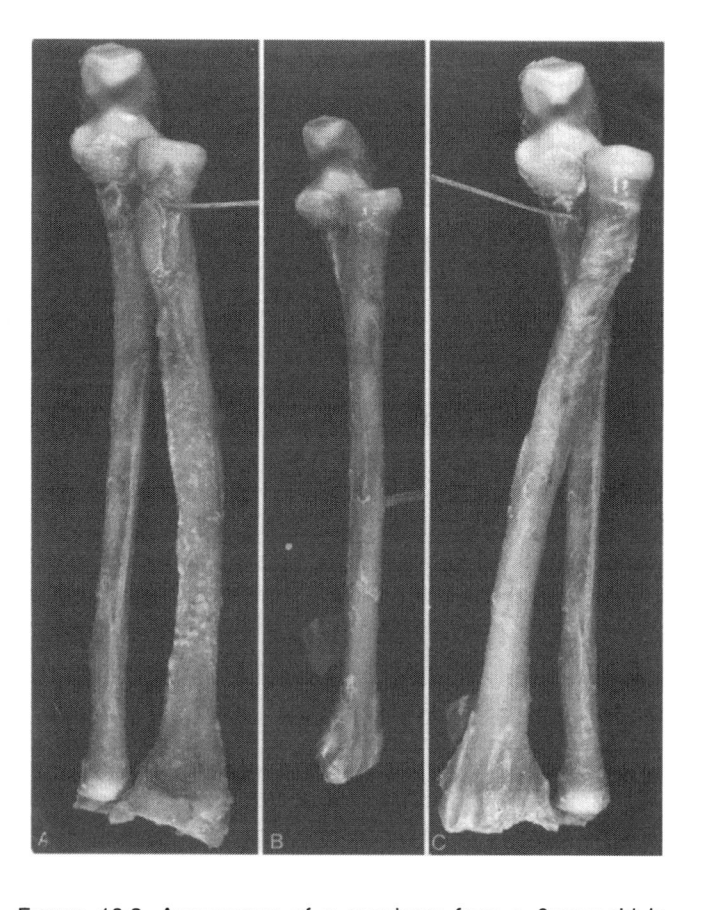

FIGURE 16-8. Appearance of a specimen from a 6-year-old in supination (A), neutral position (B), and pronation (C). In supination the bicipital tuberosity (probe) faces anteriorly, whereas in pronation it rotates posteriorly. Again, note that in supination the radial "flare" is prominent but that it decreases in pronation. This lessens the mechanical block to proximal migration of the annular ligament.

dorsal and palmar radiocarpal ligaments and by a meniscus (triangular fibrocartilaginous complex, or TFCC) bridging the distal radius to the ulnar styloid. The TFCC effectively separates portions of the interarticulations. The TFCC should be intact in the normal child, although anatomic variations may occur.

Throughout the diaphyses, the radius and ulna exhibit gentle curves (Fig. 16-8). The radiologist and orthopaedist should be familiar with these patterns, as they allow detection of mild to excessive bowing (plastic deformation) without evident fracture. Such a pattern of deformation, rather than a complete fracture, is characteristic of these bones in infants and young children and should alert the physician to be aware of other problems, such as the Monteggia injury.

When these gentle curve patterns are present along the shafts of both the radius and the ulna, basic forearm rotation (supination-pronation) follows a relatively simple conical pattern when analyzed mathematically.[3] The essential feature is paired joint motion at both the proximal and distal radioulnar joints. The mechanical axis of the forearm is a line connecting the rotational center of the proximal radius and the similar rotational center of the distal ulna. This line is the stable side of a right triangle, of which the hypotenuse is the radial longitudinal axis and the rotating leg is the transverse axis of the distal radius and triangular ligament. Rotation of the radius about the ulna thus normally generates a half-cone (Fig. 16-9).

If the effective mechanical rotational axis is disrupted, as with angulation of the radius, ulna, or both following injury, paired joint motion is variably disrupted, and a simple rotational cone becomes mechanically or geometrically impossible. Radial angular deformity is more significant, as this bone essentially generates the rotational half-cone. Angular deformity introduces nonaxial torsion of the segment distal to the fracture.

When there is a fracture of one or both of the forearm bones, the direction and extension of displacement of the fragments are contingent on the initial deforming force, the level of fracture, and the degree of muscle action. During reduction and immobilization of these fractures, the origin, insertion, and action of the various forearm muscles must be considered. The biceps and supinator muscles insert into the proximal third of the radius and are powerful supinators of the forearm. The pronator teres inserts into the middle third of the radius, and the pronator quadratus is located on the anterior aspect of the lower forearm and inserts into the distal third of the radius. The brachioradialis originates from the lower end of the humerus and inserts on the lateral surface of the distal radius immediately above the styloid process. Depending on the position of the arm, this muscle assists in pronation or supination, bringing it from either position to neutral. The extensors of the wrist and digits have a less deforming influence on forearm fractures than does the brachioradialis. The extensors may also act as a dynamic posterior splint when under tension. The extensor and abductors of the thumb are synergistic with the brachioradialis and tend to pull the distal fragment of the radius proximally. The flexor muscles of the forearm usually pull the distal fragments anteriorly and produce dorsal bowing of the radius and ulna.

With fractures involving the upper third of the forearm above the insertion of the pronator teres, the proximal fragment is often supinated and flexed because of the relatively unopposed action of the biceps and supinator. The distal fragment is pronated by the action of the pronator teres and quadratus muscles. Therefore to align the fracture properly, during reduction and treatment the distal fragment usually should be supinated.

For fractures of the middle third (i.e., below the insertion of the pronator teres), the proximal fragment of the radius is held in neutral rotation by the action of the biceps. The distal fragment is pronated and drawn toward the ulna by the pronator quadratus. When achieving anatomic reduction, the distal fragment is brought into neutral rotation. Failure to correct excessive angular deformities of childhood fractures may limit normal rotational mechanics during adulthood.

The distal radioulnar joint is a double-pivot joint that unites the distal ulnar epiphysis, ulnar notch of the radius, and distal radial epiphysis by the TFCC.[6,15,21] The distal radius develops a biconcave contour to accommodate the scaphoid and lunate (Fig. 16-10). However, as the secondary ossification center enlarges, it rarely duplicates the undulating articular contour. The distal ulnar articular cartilage surface is completely covered by this disc, so normally the ulna never articulates directly with the proximal carpal row.[20] The distal ulnar surface glides against the articular disc of triangular cartilage.[1] This triangular cartilage is attached by a thick apex to the base of the ulnar styloid (Fig. 16-11). The thinner base of the triangular ligament is attached to the leading edge of the radius just proximal to the carpal articular surface.

The dorsal portion of the triangular fibrocartilage and the dorsal radiocarpal ligament tend to be taut in pronation. The slight dorsal displacement in pronation, with the ulnar

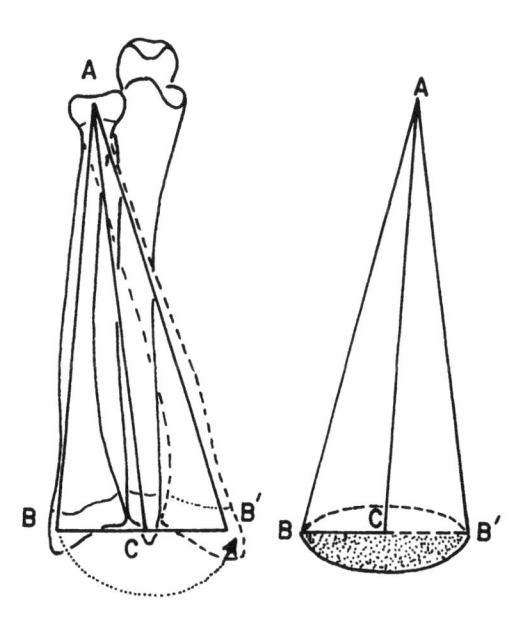

FIGURE 16-9. Rotation of the radius on the ulna. The mechanical triangle of rotation (ABC) has an axis from the center of the radial head (A) to the ulnar styloid (C). The radial styloid (B) rotates around to a pronated position (B'), subtending a semicircular conical base (stippling).

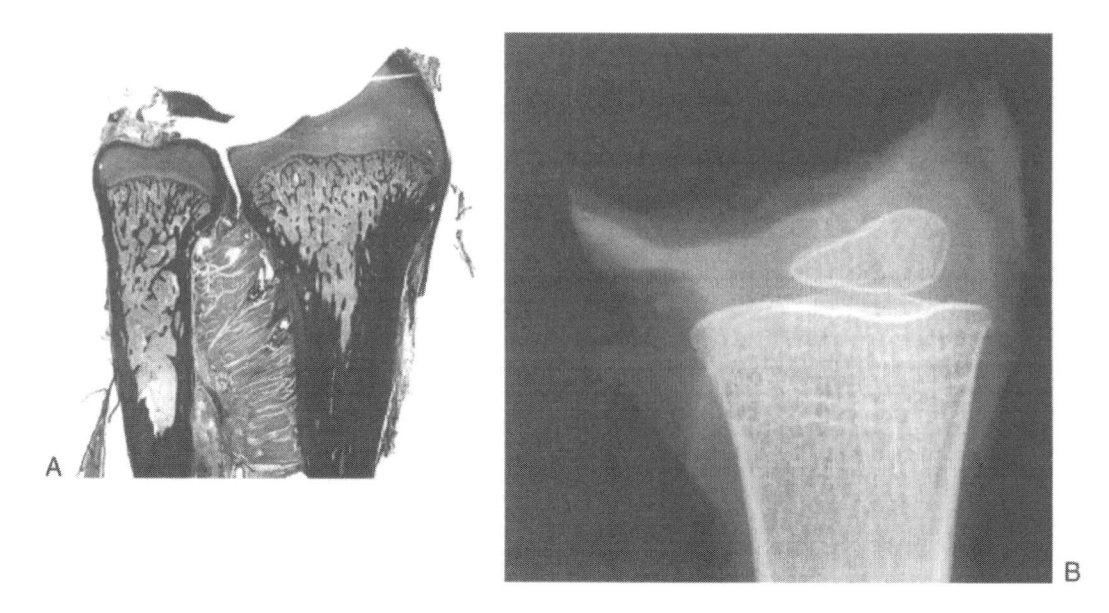

FIGURE 16-10. Histologic specimen (A) and radiograph (B) showing the biconcave shape of the distal radius to accommodate the scaphoid and lunate.

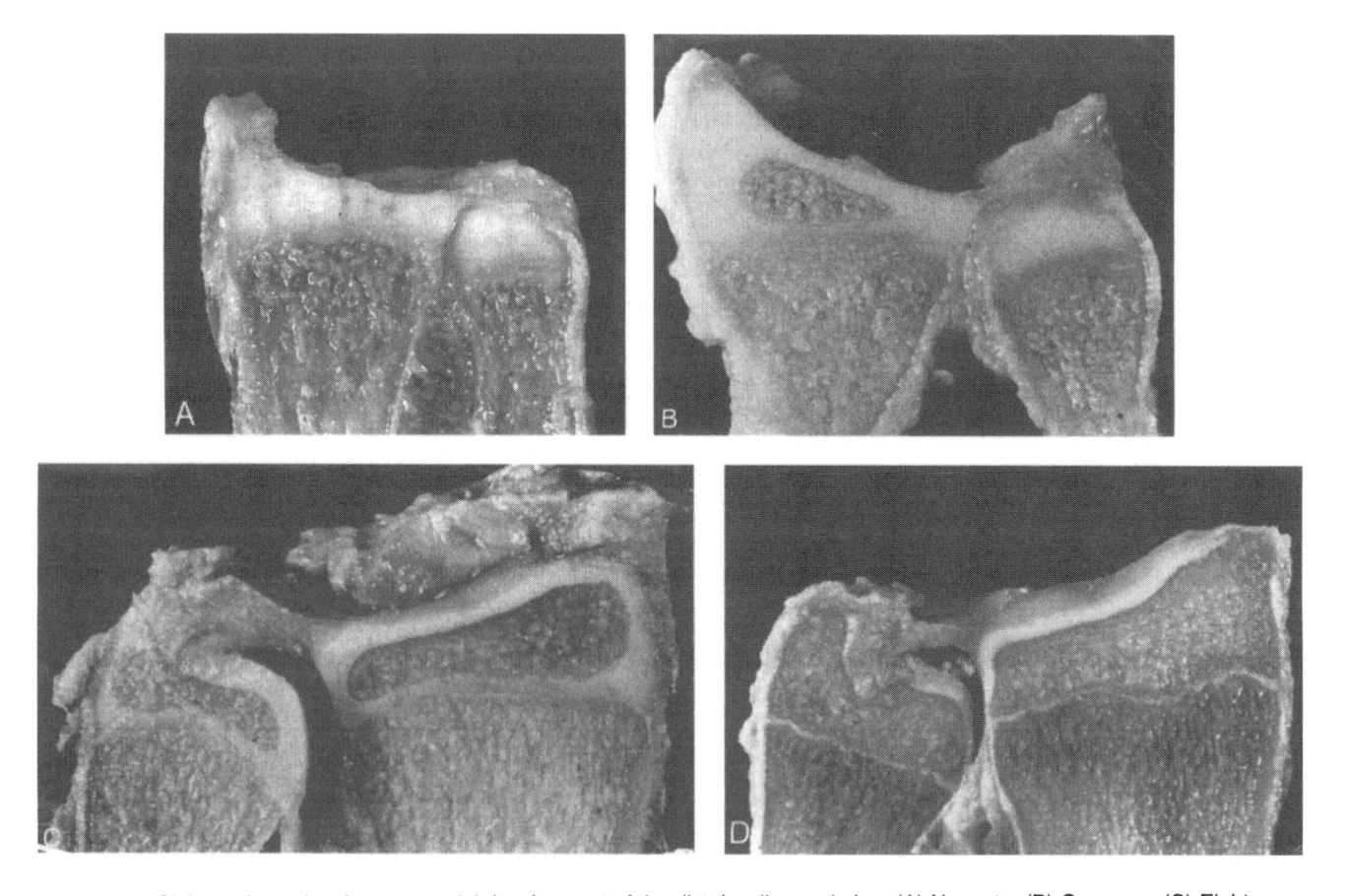

FIGURE 16-11. Slab sections showing sequential development of the distal radius and ulna. (A) Neonate. (B) One year. (C) Eight years. (D) Twelve years.

styloid relatively fixed, explains the tendency of the fracture to propogate through the ulnar styloid, even in children in whom the entity may not be recognized because the area is completely cartilaginous. As this area ossifies, radiologic nonunion often becomes evident. Permanent radiologic "nonunion" is much less frequent.

The distal radial ossification center appears at 6–12 months. In contrast, the distal ulna does not initially ossify until 5 years (Figs. 16-11, 16-12). The radial and ulnar centers then progressively expand. The radial center is initially spherical but becomes triangular.[13] The distal radial and ulnar physes are the major contributors to elongation of these two bones.[13,14] Physiologic epiphysiodesis occurs at 14 years in girls and 16 years in boys. The metaphyseal cortex changes significantly during development, as does the thickness of the hypertrophic zone of the physis. Both factors undoubtedly play a role in the age-related changing patterns of distal radial injury.

The radial styloid is one of the last areas to ossify and does so by the extension of the secondary center. Accessory bones

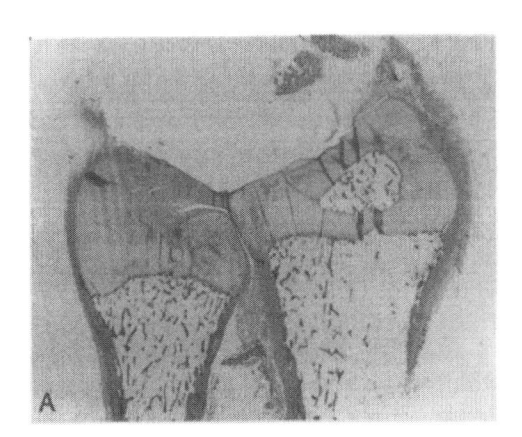

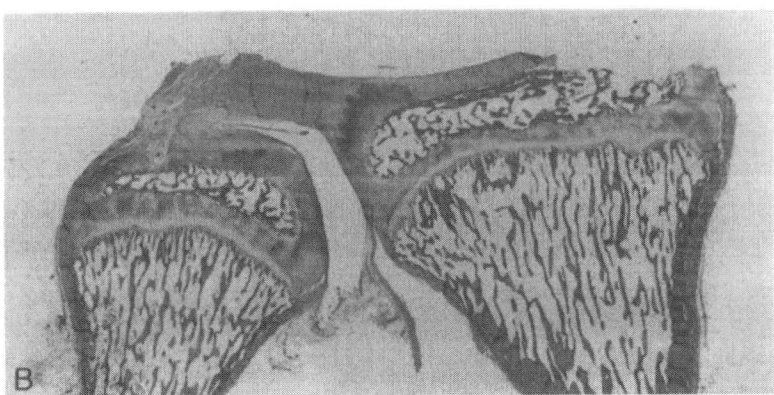

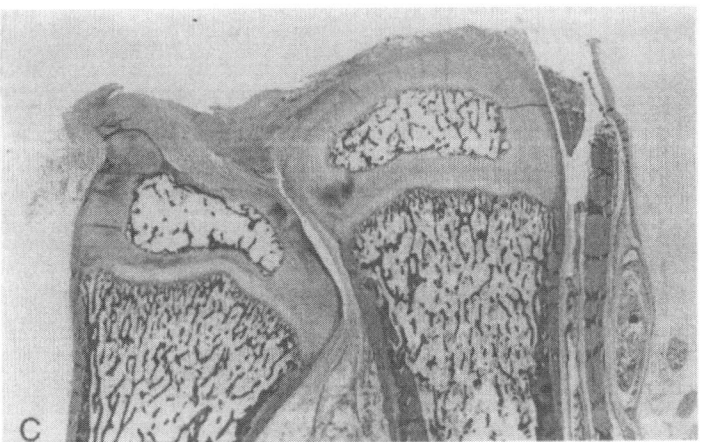

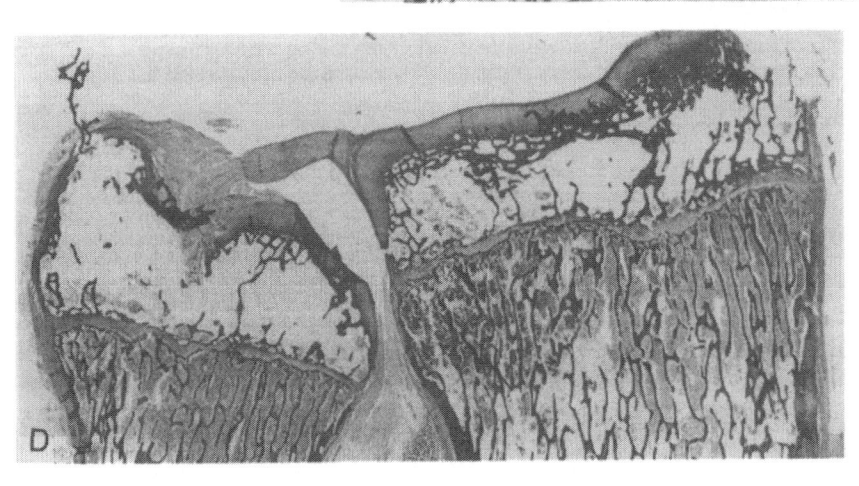

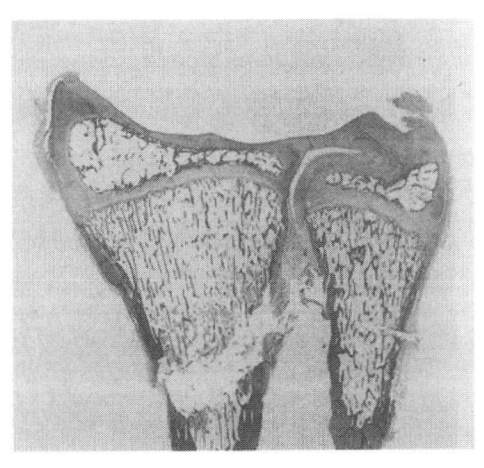

FIGURE 16-12. Sequential histologic development of the distal radius and ulna. (A) One year. (B) Seven years. (C) Ulna minus variant. (D) Thirteen years. (E) Fourteen years. The biconcave radial articular contour is readily evident.

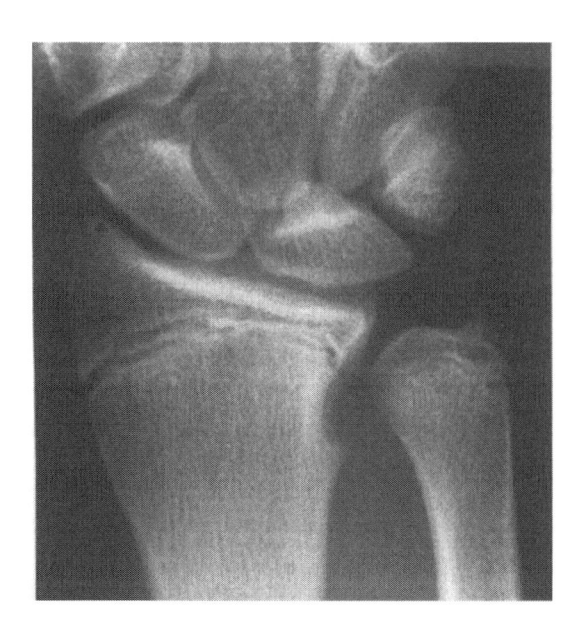

FIGURE 16-13. Radiologic variant of the distal radioulnar joint.

have not been reported in this styloid. A fracture is more likely if a lucency is seen in this area. The ulnar styloid is the last region to ossify. A cartilaginous fracture of the ulnar styloid may accompany a distal radial fracture and may not become evident until a radiographically separate secondary center eventually appears in the styloid. This is not a variation of ossification. A truly separate (accessory) ossification center for the ulnar styloid is rare.

Variations of the ulnar side of the distal radial metaphysis may occur and have the appearance of a peripheral cystic "defect" (Fig. 16-13). They should be considered a normal radiologic variant. Irregular development of the physis in this area may lead to a Madelung's deformity, which should be considered comparable to Blount's disease in young children.

Before and during adolescence many children show longitudinal osseous striations in the physis between the metaphysis and the distal epiphyseal ossification centers, both radial and ulnar (Fig. 16-14).[12] These striations are normal calcifications or ossifications in the portions of cartilage contiguous to the channels of the transepiphyseal arteries. They probably represent areas of microtrauma that lead to minimal or incomplete physeal bridge formation but do not lead to restriction of growth. The hydraulic pressures generated by continued growth probably constantly microfracture these bridges. In some instances a sclerotic line is evident in the marrow following the orientation of the longitudinal axis. This may be considered, conceptually, as microcallatosis.

Fracture Incidence

Forearm fractures are common in children. Problems of treatment vary considerably with the age of the patient and the level and displacement of the fracture. Generally, there is less comminution, union is more rapid, and residual deformities tend to be corrected by subsequent growth, compared with similar injuries in an adult.[23-39]

From the standpoint of the age relation to injury, the average ages of children with radioulnar fractures are 6.1 years for upper third fractures, 6.7 years for middle third, 6.9 years for lower third, 8.5 years for lower sixth, and 9.8 years for distal epiphyseal fractures.[32] Gandhi and colleagues reported that only 20% of distal fractures were in children under 5 years of age.[32] The susceptibility of the lower radial epiphysis to injury in children older than 10 years may be related to the increased growth rate that occurs about that time and the consequent microscopic changes at the level of the physis.[23] Data from our skeletal development laboratory suggest there are changes in physeal thickness, the zone of Ranvier, and metaphyseal cortical density during these various age-susceptibility periods.[13]

One series of 375 forearm fractures included 23 fractures of the radial head and neck, 8 fractures of the upper third, 28 fractures of the middle third, 54 fractures of the lowest third, 195 fractures of the distal metaphysis, and 67 juxtaepiphyseal injuries.[37] Gandhi and colleagues studied more than 1700 fractures of the forearm in children under 12 years of age.[32] The incidence of the fractures (excluding

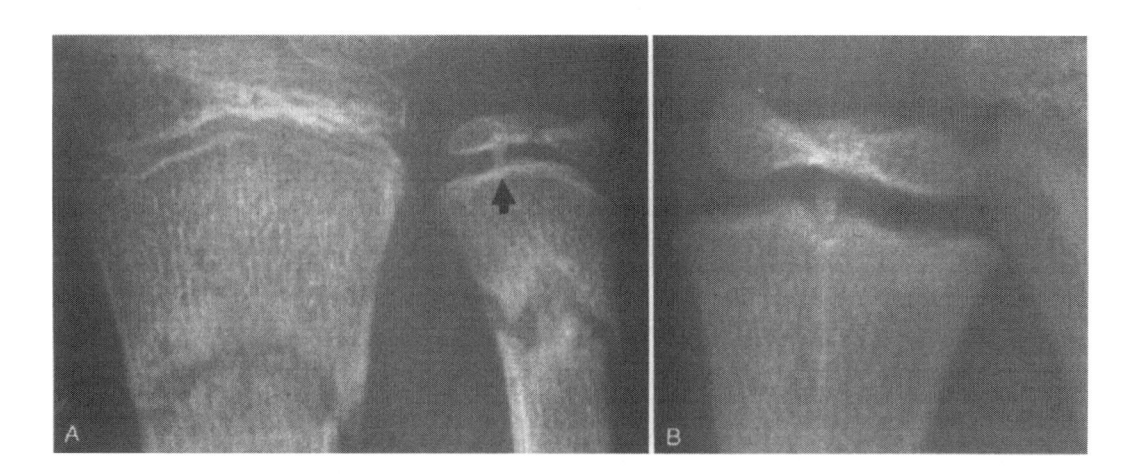

FIGURE 16-14. (A) Transphyseal longitudinal ossification pattern (arrow) in a 10-year-old child detected during evaluation of a metaphyseal fracture. (B) Longitudinal striation accompanied by linear striation within the endosteal metaphyseal bone.

those of the olecranon and the head and neck of the radius) was as follows: 0.4% Monteggia's fracture dislocation; 1.0% fracture of the upper third; 2.6% complete fracture in the middle third involving both bones; 0.9% complete fracture of the middle third of both bones; 42.0% greenstick fracture in the lower third of one bone; 24.6% greenstick fracture of the lower third of both bones, 5.2% complete fracture of the lower third of the radius with or without complete or greenstick fracture of the lower third of the ulna, and 14% involving a fracture separation of the lower radial epiphysis.

Most fractures of the radius and ulna in children are either distal compression fractures or undisplaced, angulated greenstick fractures. They present few treatment problems. However, there tends to be complacency about reducing some deformities. Significant problems may occur if any bowing (plastic deformation) remains, even in the undisplaced greenstick fracture. The goal of treatment of any radial or ulnar fracture should be restoration of full function as soon as possible, with prevention of loss of supination and pronation.

Rotational deformities should not exist at any forearm fracture site after manipulative reduction. Loss of pronation of up to 30° may be hidden by abduction of the shoulder. In contrast, loss of supination is not as easy to conceal.

Some authors have stated that angular deformity of up to 35° remodels in fractures of the distal third, but that more than 15° of residual angulation for more proximal fractures probably leads to diminished function. Because the extent of correction of malunion depends on further longitudinal bone growth, it is influenced also by the distance of the fracture from the metaphysis. The closer the fracture is to the metaphysis (especially the distal one), the greater the potential for spontaneous correction. *The nearer the fracture is to the midshaft, the more likely there will be a residual problem. Therefore angulation in the midshaft of the bone should be accepted with caution.*

The usual outcome of forearm fractures in children appears to be complete functional recovery in most patients when manipulative closed anatomic reduction and immobilization are used. However, in one series, fractures of the upper third showed unsatisfactory results in 50% of the patients, with the major problem being loss of supination and pronation, although the children did not complain of any significant functional disability.[37] By the end of 4 years, only nine children had any problems when judged by the same standards. Thomas and associates stressed that the patients with a poorer outcome were usually treated by open reduction and fixation.[37] Among 67 patients with juxtaphyseal fractures, 5 developed a Madelung-type deformity that was probably due to an unsuspected or undetected physeal injury.

Some authors believe that open reduction of radioulnar fractures is unnecessary.[24–26] Although open reduction and internal fixation are not usually indicated, they should not be discounted totally as treatment modalities *when deemed necessary*. With the improved methods of internal fixation and anesthesia, there is an increasing tendency to use closed and open reduction for young children and adolescents—treatments that are extremely successful for forearm fractures in adults.

Refracture at the same site after an apparently solid union may occur with forearm fractures in children.[25] Bosworth encountered six cases in a study of 54 fractures.[27] In another series, refractures occurred in only nine patients, representing 0.5%, at intervals varying from 2 to 6 months from the time of presumed radiologic union.[32]

Olecranon Fractures

Fractures involving the olecranon physis are infrequent in children.[41–47,51,53,55–62,64,65] Mahlahn and Fahey reported only 19 such patients in a series of 300 elbow fractures in children.[58] Newell reviewed 40 cases in children ranging in age from 15 months to 11 years and found that olecranon physeal fractures usually occurred around the age of 5 years.[59] Mahlahn and Fahey found the average age was 8.5 years.[58]

Papavasiliou et al. reviewed 58 fractures of the olecranon in children; 43 were associated with other injuries to the elbow, and 15 were isolated fractures of the olecranon.[60] They particularly studied the latter 15 and described a classification that basically subdivided them into group A (isolated intraarticular fractures of the olecranon) and group B (isolated extraarticular fractures of the olecranon, or a greenstick fracture). The latter injuries were generally metaphyseal and distal to the coronoid process. The authors did note a case of pseudarthrosis developing approximately 1 year after injury. Recommended open reduction had been refused by the parents in this case.

Suprock and Lubahn reported a case of olecranon fracture through the physis accompanying a radial shaft fracture, essentially a reverse of a Monteggia lesion.[62] It required open reduction of the olecranon fracture for stability.

Classification

The olecranon physeal fracture is often undisplaced or incomplete. Usually the fracture is approximately perpendicular to the longitudinal axis of the ulna, probably because of a locking into the olecranon fossa. The longitudinal split fracture, which appears in approximately 10% of adult cases, is atypical in children.

These fractures usually occur through the metaphyseal bone adjacent to the olecranon physis (Fig. 16-15). Occasionally, there is a fracture through the chondro-osseous

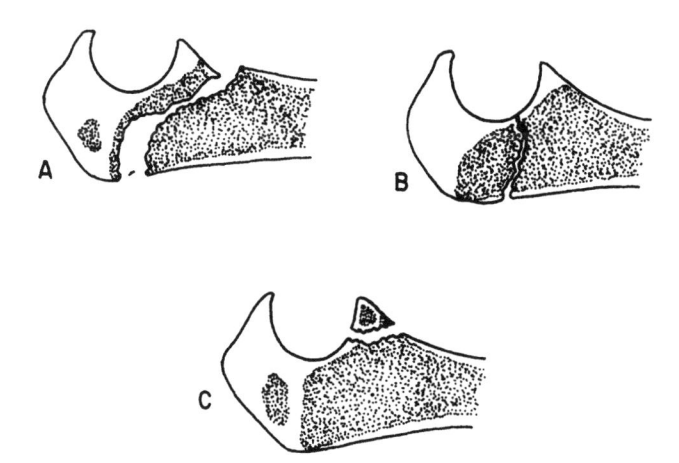

FIGURE 16-15. Fracture patterns in the proximal ulna. (A) Fracture through the entire metaphysis. (B) Fracture into the joint. (C) Coronoid fracture.

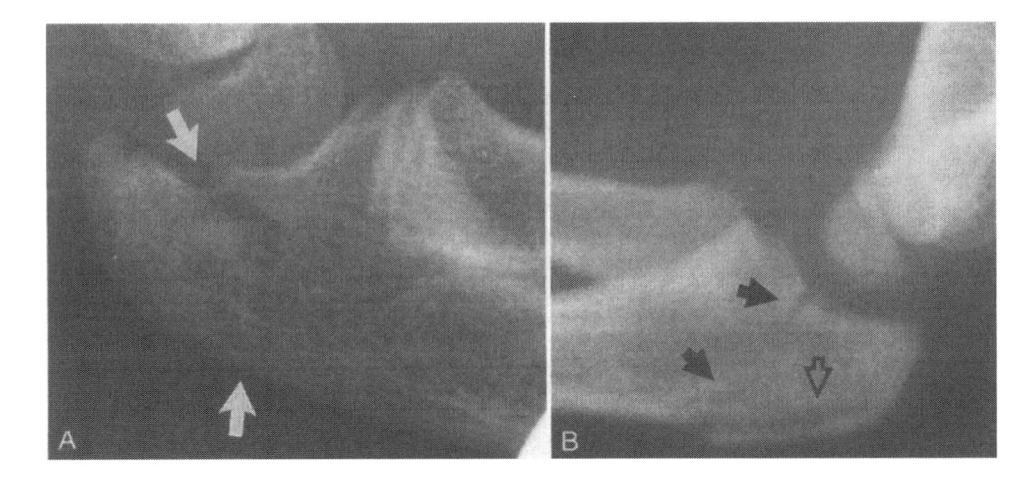

FIGURE 16-16. Patterns of fracture within the metaphysis, most likely due to valgus force rather than avulsion. (A) Mild displacement with comminution (arrows). (B) Greenstick injury (solid arrows) with comminution of cortex (open arrow).

junction in a child (under the age of 10 years) before the olecranon secondary ossification center appears. Often the fracture is incomplete and does not encroach on the joint surface, as the fracture has not propagated through the cartilage (Fig. 16-16). There may be minimal widening of the space between the olecranon ossification center and the metaphysis. Follow-up radiographs may reveal the true nature of the injury as an undisplaced physeal fracture (Fig. 16-17).

A sleeve fracture may occur, separating the unossified (cartilaginous) proximal ulnar epiphysis from the ossification center. A fracture may also occur through the ossification center. These patterns are rare.

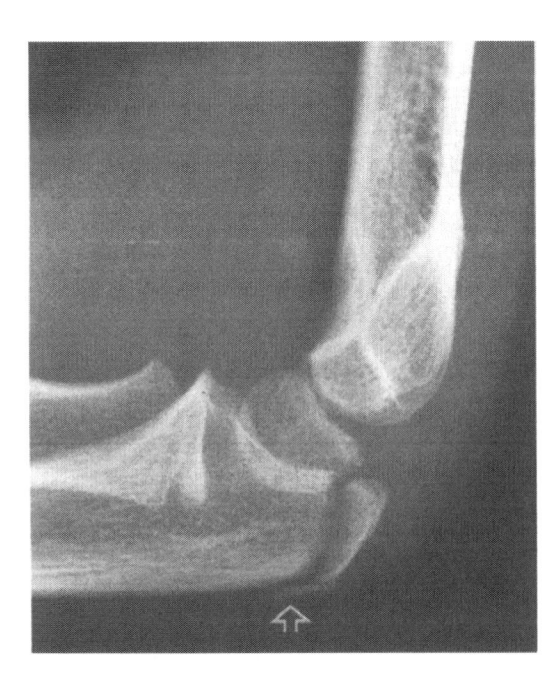

FIGURE 16-17. Minimally displaced olecranon fracture. Periosteal continuity probably prevented further displacement and is making new bone (arrow).

Pathomechanics

The structure of the olecranon in a child differs significantly from that in an adult. The bone is more trabecular, and fractures may be difficult to identify. Articular cartilage and epiphyseal cartilage layers are thick and permit osteochondral fractures. The transversely oriented subchondral bone of the metaphysis tends to direct fractures into the metaphysis rather than the physis. In one series, 20 of 33 children in whom the olecranon fracture was the only injury had a direct blow to the elbow from a fall, rather than a fall on the hand while the elbow was hyperextended.[59]

If the elbow is extended, the olecranon is locked in the olecranon fossa of the distal humerus. When a varus or valgus force is then applied (Fig. 16-18), the olecranon levers against the fossa margins, and the deforming strain is absorbed by the metaphyseal region located at the level of the joint. With a valgus force, the radial head or medial epicondyle may also fracture. Always look for these potential associated injuries.

Once the fracture occurs through the metaphysis, the contractile force of the triceps may further displace the fragment, pulling it proximally (Fig. 16-19). A simple evocative test of stability is to obtain lateral films in extension and flexion (Fig. 16-20). Widening of any gap mandates open reduction and fixation.

The metaphyseal fragment may be small and the equivalent of a patellar sleeve fracture. The displaced fragment may become locked within the elbow joint (Fig. 16-21).

Diagnosis

In most cases the diagnosis is readily evident on the lateral film. However, if the fragments are undisplaced or the fracture is through the physeal-metaphyseal interface of an epiphysis with no secondary ossification center, the diagnosis is sometimes empirical or based on careful examination. Palpation of the fracture gap may not be easy because of soft tissue swelling.

Ossification variations may also affect the interpretation of fractures.[40,42,48,49,52,54,66] Burge and Benson reported a case of

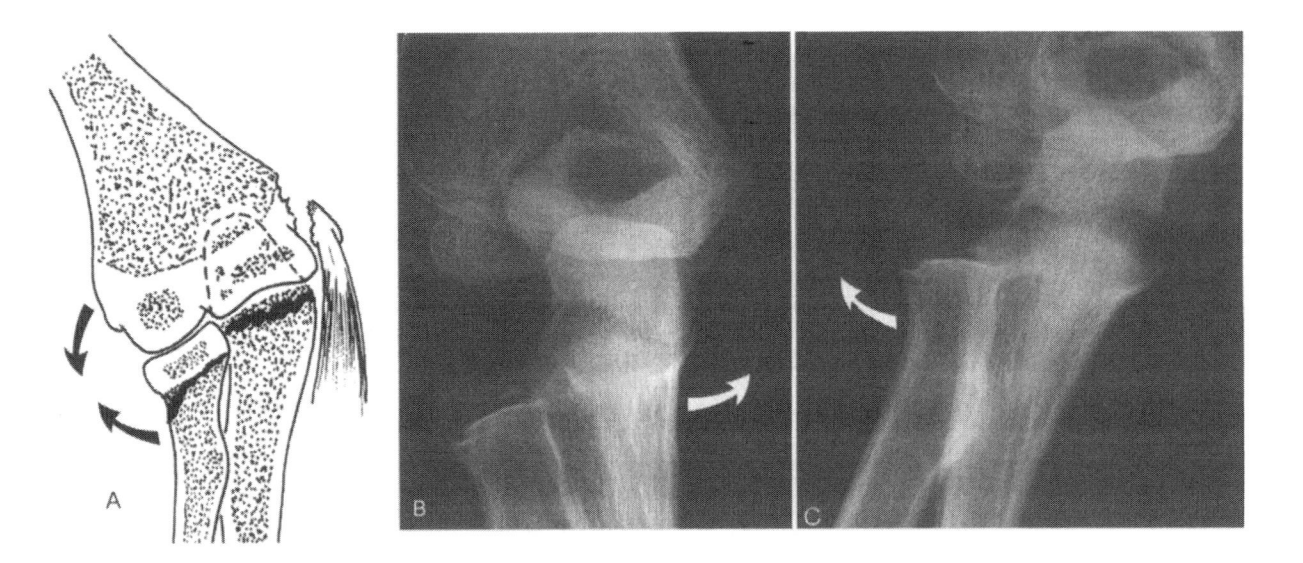

FIGURE 16-18. (A) Common fracture mechanism. (B, C) Roentgenograms showing how the olecranon pivots (arrows) in the humeral fossa in varus (B) and valgus (C) deformations.

bilateral congenital pseudarthrosis of the olecranon, which must be distinguished from fracture of the olecranon and patella cubiti.[42] Habbe reported a fracture through a patella cubiti.[49] Whether such lesions are a congenital anomaly, an ununited epiphysis of the olecranon, or a posttraumatic process is still subject to debate.[66] Most of the patients described in the literature are male. Because boys are more apt to be involved in injuries and are more likely to have radiologic studies of the elbow, the apparent difference in sex predisposition may not be significant.

The absence of soft tissue swelling and joint effusion is usually incompatible with the presence of a fracture of the olecranon, especially one extending directly into the joint space. Occasionally, however, difficulty arises when a patient has a positive fat pad sign and the physeal line extends into the joint space. A comparison radiograph may be indicated in these patients. Occasionally fractures of the proximal tip of the olecranon are not associated with a joint effusion, as the joint capsule and synovial tissue do not always extend to the tip. The proximal part of the olecranon and the radial neck are the two areas of the elbow in which a fracture may occur without displacement of the fat pads.

There may be a normally wide space between the early ossification of the epiphysis and the adjacent metaphysis. This separation is larger than 5 mm in some patients and should not be mistaken for an epiphyseal separation. Figures 16-19 and 16-20 show metaphyseal avulsion fractures of the olecranon. One can assume that the olecranon epiphysis, although not yet ossified, is displaced proximally along with the avulsed metaphysis. This type of injury, although often referred to as a chip fracture, is far more serious and a great deal more complicated. This fracture really represents separation of a nonossified (radiolucent) epiphysis of the olecranon with an associated metaphyseal avulsion. With such fractures, the separation occurs because of the pull of the

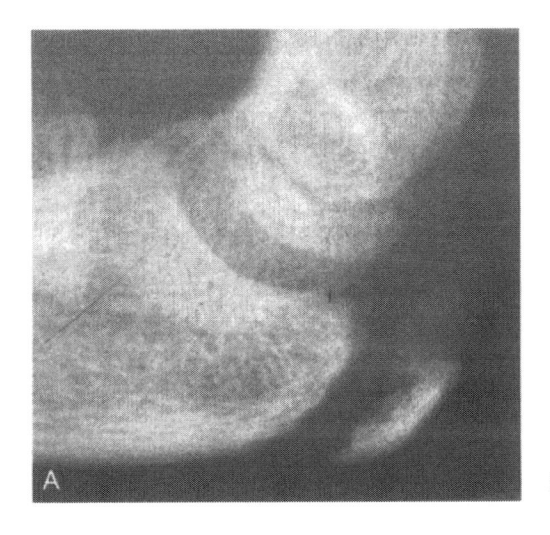

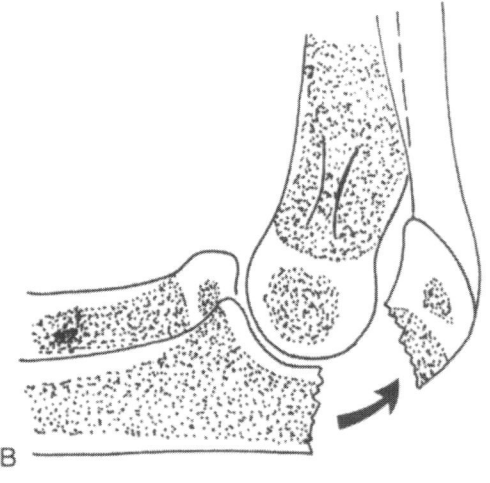

FIGURE 16-19. (A) Fracture of proximal ulna. The fragment is a portion of the metaphysis, not the secondary ossification center. (B) Displaced fracture pattern.

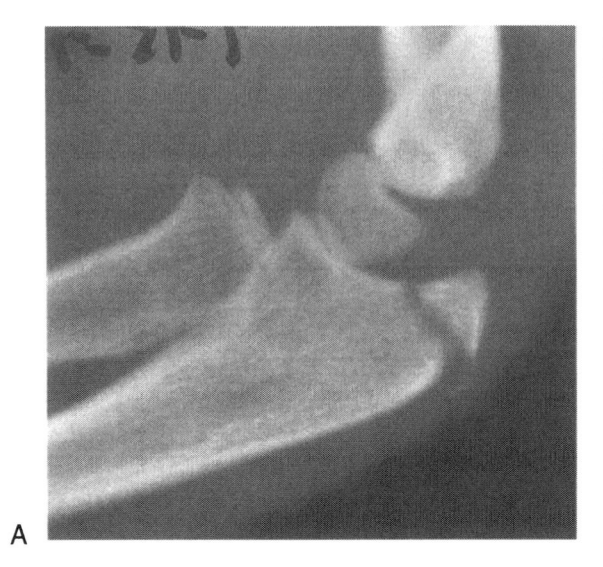

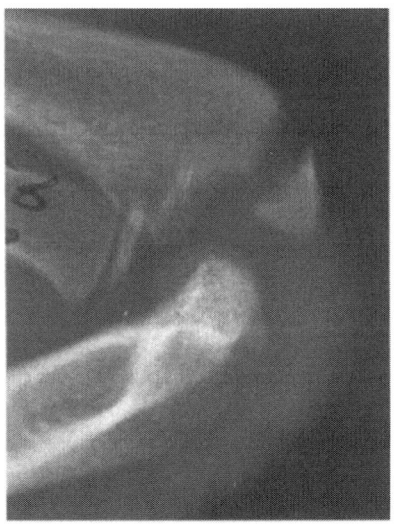

FIGURE 16-20. (A) Seemingly minimally displaced olecranon fracture. (B) Flexion (a simple stress test) shows the fracture to be at risk for further displacement. This fracture needs to be treated with tension band wiring.

attached triceps muscle (as when the elbow is suddenly flexed against the opposing triceps muscle).

Treatment

Closed reduction should be the initial method of treatment, as many olecranon fractures are greenstick fractures with some cortical and epiphyseal integrity (especially if the fracture is acquired by locking the olecranon during a varus or valgus stress). The fracture usually occurs in extension with this pathomechanism. The greenstick deformity may be hyperextended relative to the rest of the ulna and should be pushed back with the elbow flexed. The elbow should be splinted and a repeat roentgenogram obtained to be sure the fracture fragments are still in continuity.

Although immobilization in a cast with the elbow at approximately 90° for 3–4 weeks is recommended, the results indicate that in the usual undisplaced, incomplete fracture a period of 3 weeks in a sling may be the only treatment necessary.

The displaced olecranon fracture during childhood is best treated by open reduction with internal fixation of the fracture, repair of any triceps aponeurotic tear, and external immobilization (Figs. 16-22 to 16-24). Methods of fixation include transfixing the epiphysis to the metaphysis with smooth pins and annular wire or suture fixation. Pins should be small and are removed when healing is evident (at least 4–6 weeks, as this is a slowly growing physeal unit, and new formation of metaphyseal bone on the proximal side of the fracture is limited). Annular fixation has the advantage of avoiding the physis. The wire should loop through the triceps aponeurosis as it attaches to the olecranon and a transverse tunnel in the metaphysis just distal to the joint to avoid physeal damage. Minimum soft tisse stripping (i.e., periosteum) should lessen the risk of peripheral physeal damage. A transfixation screw should not be used, as it may permanently damage the physis. Pins should not be removed prematurely, or the injury may recur. Small diameter pins are unlikely to cause any physeal arrest, especially in a slow-growing physis.

An and Loder reported intraarticular entrapment of a displaced olecranon fracture in a 4-year-old.[41] It required open reduction and internal fixation.

Results

Olecranon fractures usually heal without any limitation of function or growth deformity, especially when a greenstick injury is involved. With displaced injuries, healing may be delayed, especially if a thin layer of metaphyseal bone must fuse to the rest of the metaphysis.

Complications

Growth arrest is unusual after an olecranon fracture, primarily because this region does not contribute significantly to the overall longitudinal growth of the ulna. In the young child, growth arrest could lead to disparate development of

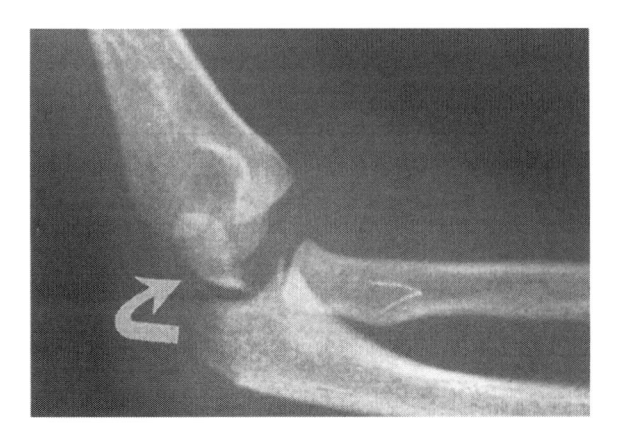

FIGURE 16-21. Intraarticular displacement (arrow) of the olecranon epiphysis.

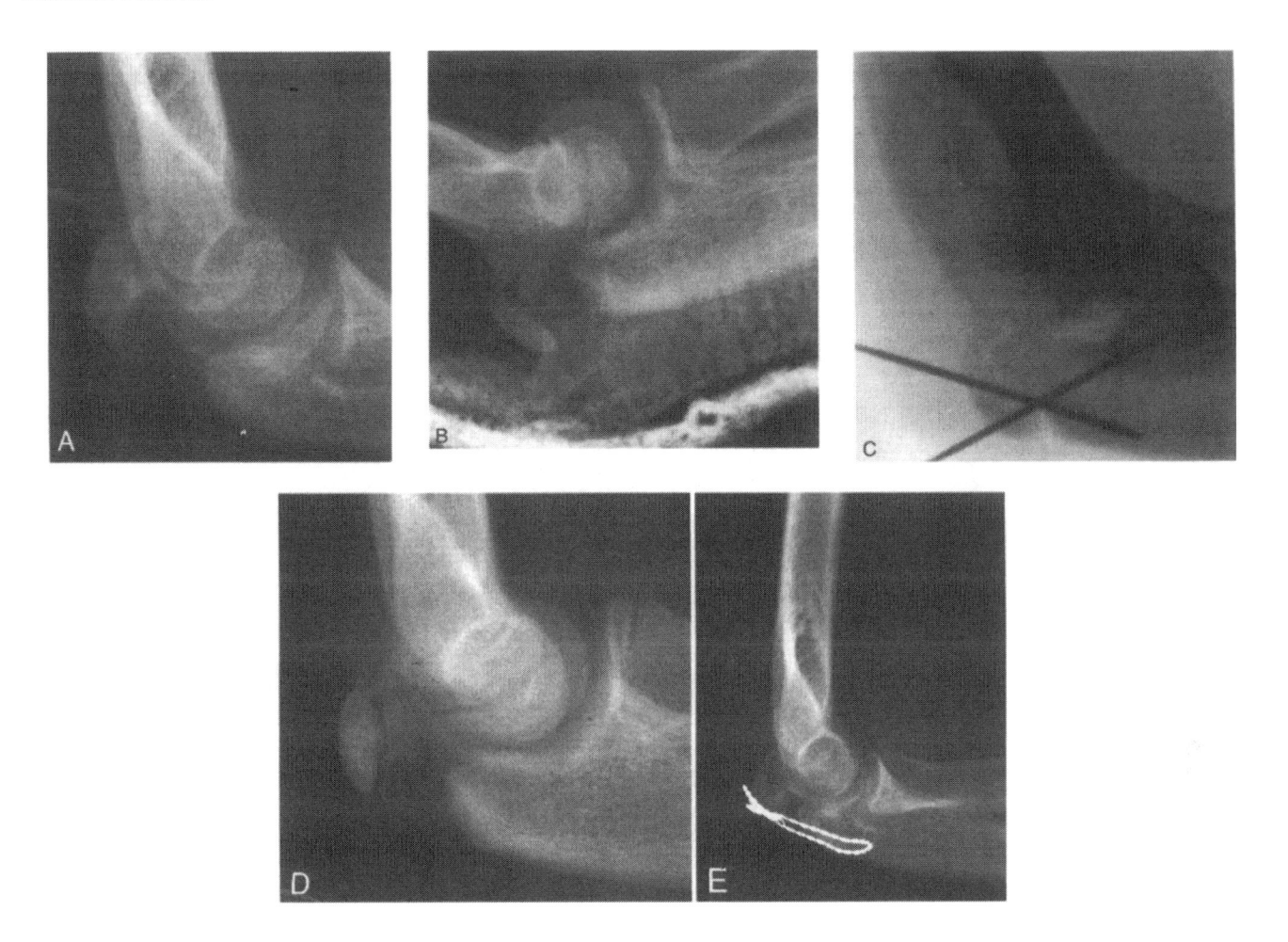

FIGURE 16-22. (A) Fracture of the proximal ulna of a 9-year-old child. The triceps has displaced the fragment. (B) Closed reduction in extension failed to reduce the fragment. (C) This fragment was fixed with crossed Kirschner (K) wires, which were removed 6 weeks later. (D) Three days after removal of the wires the fragment redisplaced during normal activity. (E) This was fixed by cerclage wiring.

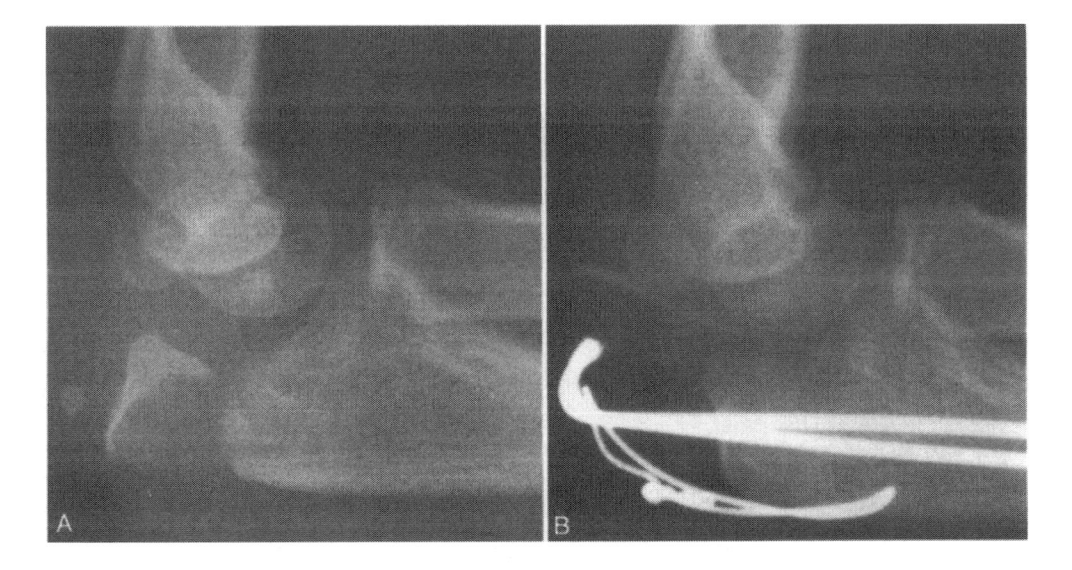

FIGURE 16-23. (A) Displaced sleeve fracture of the olecranon. (B) Result of longitudinal pin and cerclage wire fixation. No secondary ossification is present in the olecranon.

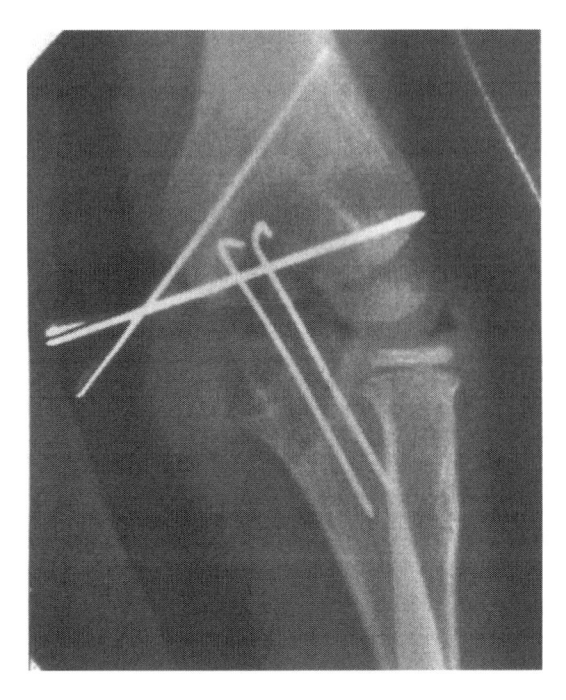

FIGURE 16-24. Combined injury of the olecranon and medial epicondyle. Both were treated with open reduction and pin fixation. A tension band suture also was used on the olecranon.

the proximal ulna relative to the proximal radius and thereby affect varus or valgus position and limit elbow function.

Matthews observed a patient who sustained nonunion following an olecranon fracture that was fixed with a suture.[57] Pavlov et al. reported two cases of nonunion of the olecranon epiphysis in adolescent baseball pitchers.[61] Figure 16-25 shows a patient treated conservatively (with a cast in 90° of flexion) who developed a fibrous union.

Figure 16-26 shows the elbow of a 10-year-old girl who had sustained an "elbow injury" 6 years earlier but was told there was no fracture evident on the radiograph. She had progressive loss of elbow motion. In retrospect, she had avulsed the unossified region of the olecranon away from the ossification center (shell fracture). Repetitive motion continued to pull the area proximally, and it subsequently ossified. It was removed, and the triceps aponeurosis was repaired. Function improved but did not equal that on the other side.

Heterotopic bone may complicate this injury pattern. Because of the hinge mechanism of the injury (see previous section), delayed healing of the olecranon and radial head abnormalities may occur.

Gymnastic Injury

Avulsions of the olecranon through the physis may occur in competitive gymnasts. The spectrum of abnormalities ranged from widening of the olecranon physis to fragmentation of the epiphyseal ossification center. The appearances are similar to that of the Osgood-Schlatter lesion.

Typical of gymnastics is a sudden extension of the elbow through the action of the triceps that results in traction and shearing forces on the olecranon. It can act at two sites: (1) the insertion of the triceps tendon into the olecranon, creating a situation on the developing ossification center similar to the patellar tendon on the tibial tuberosity, and (2) the olecranon physis itself.

Coronoid Process

Coronoid process fractures may be classified as follows: type I, avulsion of the tip of the coronoid process; type II, a single or comminuted fragment involving 50% of the process or less; and type III, a single or comminuted fragment involving more than 50% of the process. They may be subclassified with regard to the absence (a) or presence (b) of an associated dislocation of the elbow. There is an increased incidence of complications associated with elbow dislocation and fewer optimal results than with type III.

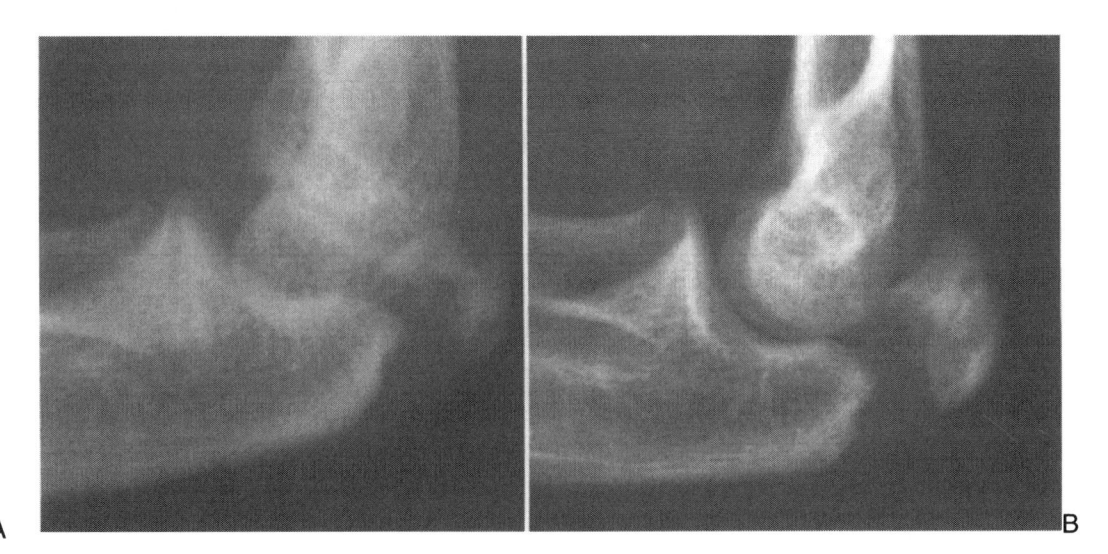

FIGURE 16-25. (A) Displaced olecranon fracture. This was splinted. (B) Ten weeks later nonunion was evident.

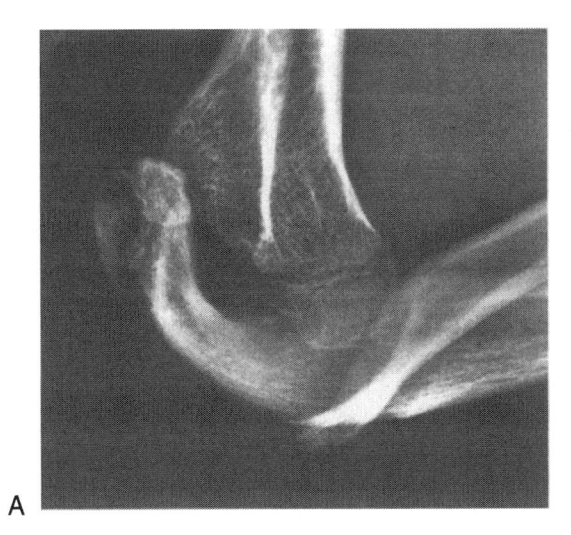

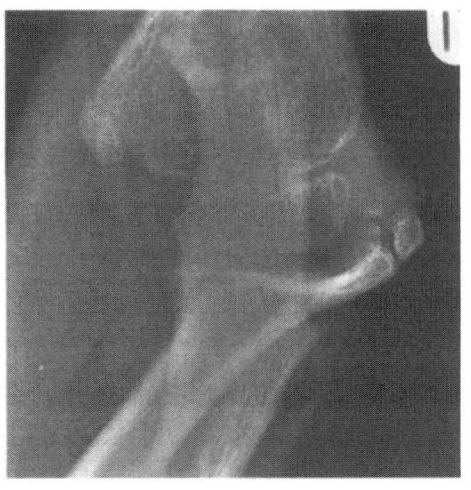

FIGURE 16-26. (A, B) This 10-year-old girl had an "elbow injury" at age 4 years that went untreated. It probably was an olecranon fracture coupled with dislocation of the radial head. An attenuated olecranon is evident, along with a deformed proximal radius.

Coronoid process fractures certainly occur in children (Figs. 16-27, 16-28). Fractures of the coronoid region may be missed in children during routine lateral radiographs of the elbow, as the radial head may overlie the coronoid process. Accordingly, an oblique radiograph may be necessary to visualize the fracture if suspected.

The anterior portion of the epiphysis, including the coronoid process and its subchondral bone, may flip 180° and displace into the joint. This injury is treated by arthrotomy and replacement of the fragment.

Hanks and Kottmeier reported a fracture involving the entire coronoid process of the ulna[50] that was treated with open reduction and internal fixation. The patient also had a fracture of the distal radius. The authors noted that most fractures of the coronoid process are small, they are often associated with dislocation of the elbow, and the suggested treatment is to "ignore them," as they usually have no effect on the final outcome. Open reduction and internal fixation is recommended for fractures that interfere with joint motion. The stability of the elbow is dependent on the stability of the collateral ligaments and on the coronoid process. The natural history of a large, displaced coronoid process fracture is not well known, but data suggest that these patients are at risk for developing chronic instability of the elbow.

Tanzman and Kaufman described a similar coronoid injury in a 12-year-old girl who also sustained a right wrist fracture.[63] When the arm was immobilized in a cast at 90°, the fracture was further displaced. The arm was taken out of the cast and the limb immobilized in full extension, with the concept that the tension induced in the brachialis tendon would reduce the fracture. It led to accurate and complete reduction of the fracture. Immobilization was maintained for 4 weeks, after which active mobilization was begun. The authors thought that this injury occurred because of hyperextension or as a result of abutment of the coronoid against

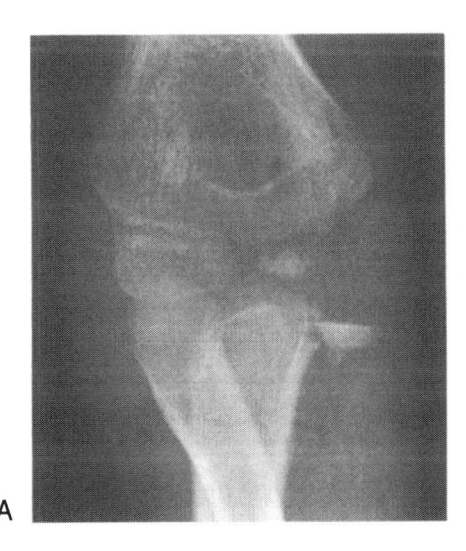

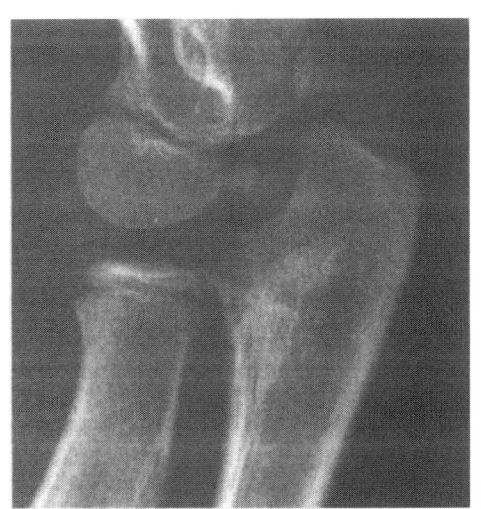

FIGURE 16-27. (A) Anteroposterior view of a coronoid fracture. (B) Oblique view. The "intraarticular fragment" is rarely the early trochlear ossification center (according to the radiology report).

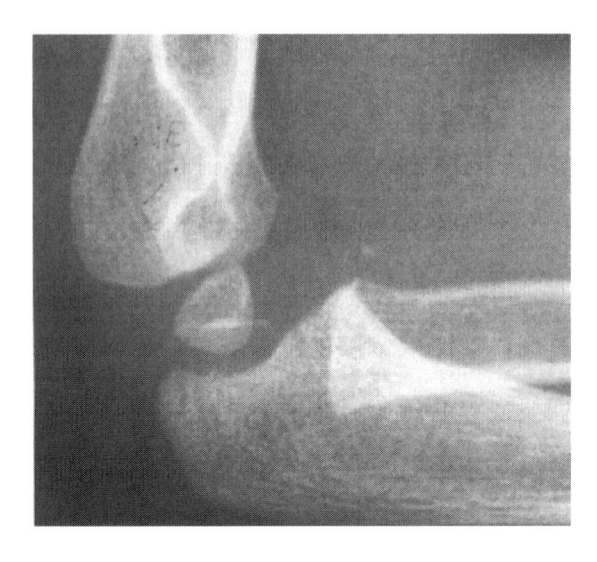

FIGURE 16-28. Intraarticular displacement of a sleeve fracture of the coronoid process.

the trochlea during forceful posterior displacement of the ulna. In this particular patient they believed that a dislocation had not occurred. This method of reduction was in contrast to the usual suggestion of maximum flexion.

The surgical approach to the ulnar coronoid process is usually medial, involving sharp dissection of the flexor carpi ulnaris and flexor digitorum profundus muscles from the medial side of the ulna. These muscles are reflected superiorly to protect the ulnar nerve and its motor branches. By continued dissection, the coronoid process and distal tendon of the brachialis muscle are exposed.

Proximal Radial Fractures

Proximal radial fractures are common in the developing elbow.[67-154] Radial head and neck fractures account for 5–10% of injuries to the elbow region.[101] Newman described 48 displaced radial neck fractures in children 4–13 years old.[121] In two children, the fracture occurred before ossification appeared and was recognized only by a thin, displaced piece of metaphysis (Thurstan Holland sign). In 38 cases the pattern of injury was lateral or valgus angulation. In all cases, the angulation of the radial head was at least 30° from the normal axis. Henrikson found 55 fractures of the proximal radius, which included 50 fractures of the neck (metaphyseal injury) and 5 fractures through the epiphysis and apophysis.[94]

O'Brien reviewed 125 cases.[122] He found only four that classified as a type 1 or 2 growth mechanism injury, believing that most proximal radial injuries were fractures through the juxtaphyseal metaphysis. There were 40 patients (almost one-third of his patients) who had early closure of the epiphysis and increased carrying angles up to 25°, although none was severe enough to require osteotomy. A complicating proximal radiohumeral synostosis developed in six patients.

Fractures commonly occur when children are 10–13 years of age, with the range beginning at about 5 years, when the ossification center first appears. Whether these injuries occur before that time is difficult to ascertain because of the absence of the ossification center. Approximately 75% of the cases occur in children 9 years of age or older.

Multiple injuries may occur.[79,112,121] In one series, 11 of 38 patients had associated avulsion injuries of the medial side of the elbow, 5 had olecranon fractures, 4 had avulsed medial epicondyles, and 2 had ruptured medial collateral ligaments. Other injury patterns include the following: (1) radial head dislocation and fracture; (2) rupture of the annular ligament; (3) elbow dislocation; (4) capitellar fracture; (5) dislocated radial head; (6) navicular fracture; and (7) radial nerve palsy. The wrist also must be assessed carefully. Children may get Essex Lopresti injuries or their equivalents. As in adults they may be difficult to diagnose and may be present as variants because of the presence of physeal fractures instead of cortical fractures.

Classification

Fractures vary from growth mechanism involvement to injuries through the metaphysis with angular deformity. The fracture line may appear to be through the epiphysis, but it usually is a compression of the epiphyseal head into the metaphyseal expansion of the narrow neck. Thus these fractures tend to be impaction or greenstick injury patterns. With either injury pattern the fragment may be completely displaced.

A fracture of the metaphyseal neck of the radius should be differentiated from a true physeal or epiphyseal fracture of the head of the radius, which occurs less frequently during childhood. McBride and Monnet believe that a true slipped epiphysis is unusual.[113] However, in one report of 34 cases, 50% were in the radial neck proper and 50% were type 2 fractures involving the proximal radial physis and metaphysis.[139]

Growth mechanism injuries range from type 1 to 4 (Figs. 16-29 to 16-31). The type 1 and 2 pattern injuries are often difficult to differentiate from adjacent metaphyseal injuries, although treatment and prognosis are virtually the same. Type 3 and 4 injuries require accurate diagnosis and open reduction. Because of the limited vascularity to the radial head, these small fragments carry a high risk of ischemic necrosis and physeal bridging (premature closure). Type 7 injuries (intraepiphyseal) are infrequent.

The most common injury pattern involves a fracture through the metaphyseal neck (Figs. 16-32 to 16-34). These fractures are often greenstick angulations (compactions) with some intrinsic stability. Fractures may be defined as (1) mild: less than 30° of angular deformity; (2) moderate: 30°–60° of angulation; or (3) severe: greater than 60° of

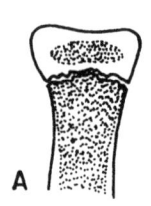

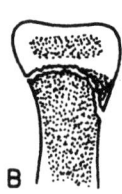

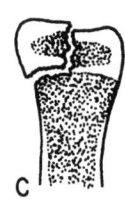

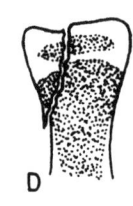

FIGURE 16-29. Growth mechanism injuries of the proximal radius. (A) Type I. (B) Type 2. (C) Type 3. (D) Type 4 transphyseal injuries.

Proximal Radial Fractures

FIGURE 16-30. (A) Type 3 fracture of the proximal radius in a 13-year-old girl during the final stages of epiphysiodesis (similar to a Tillaux fracture). (B) Type 4 fracture (arrow). Both of these fractures should be anatomically reduced.

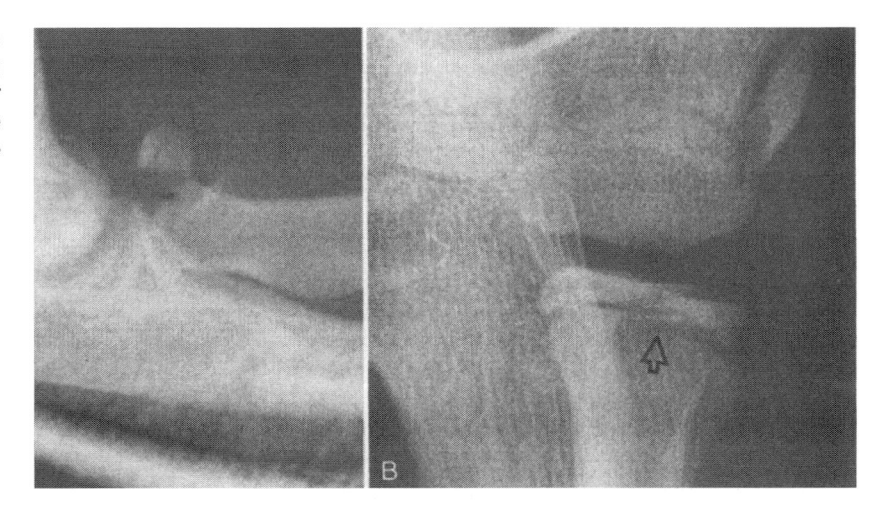

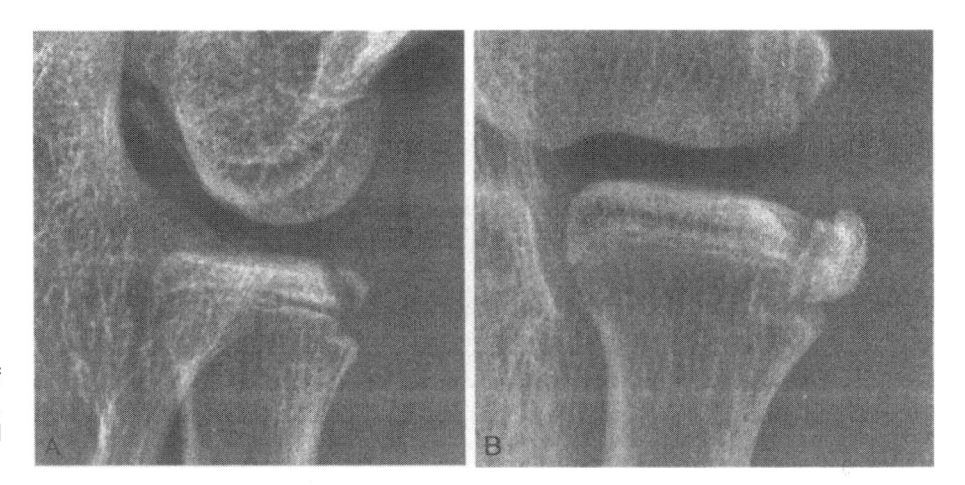

FIGURE 16-31. (A) Type 4 fracture of the radial head. (B) Seven months later. Further ossification led to physeal bridging.

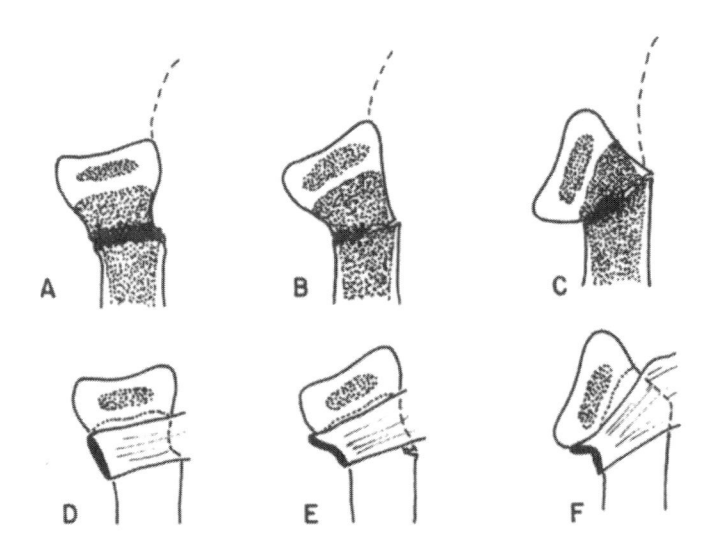

FIGURE 16-32. (A–C) Metaphyseal injuries, showing patterns of angular deformation. (D–F) Presentation of injury relative to the annular ligament.

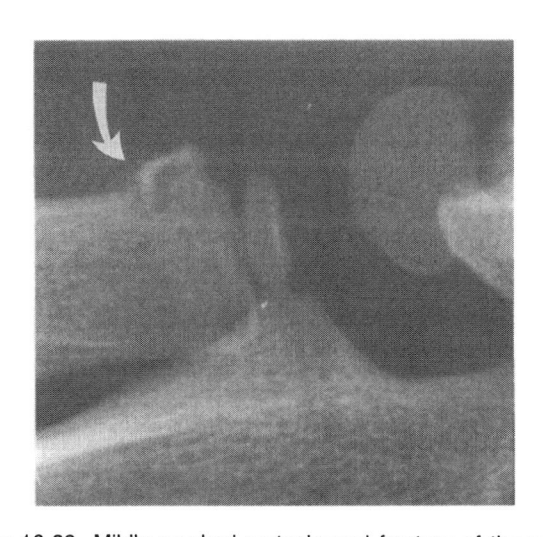

FIGURE 16-33. Mildly crushed metaphyseal fracture of the proximal radius (arrow).

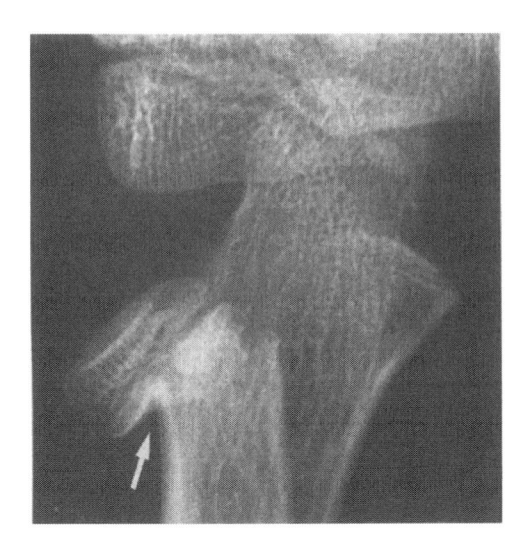

FIGURE 16-34. Severely angulated proximal radial fracture. Note the deformed metaphyseal cortex (arrow).

angulation. The fracture may also be completely displaced (Figs. 16-35 to 16-37).

Pathomechanics

The normal carrying angle of the elbow makes valgus injury more likely in a fall on the outstretched arm. The position of the elbow at impact determines whether the ulna is also fractured. In full extension, the tight ligaments around the elbow direct the olecranon into the fossa of the distal humerus, so varus and valgus movements are minimized. In this position, continued valgus strain fractures the radial neck. The olecranon frequently sustains a concomitant oblique fracture. If there is some flexion, the olecranon is not held as firmly within the olecranon fossa and may rotate, so a solitary fracture of the radial neck results from the force. If a child sustains a dislocation of the elbow, a displaced fracture of the radial neck may also occur.

The mechanism of injury, a fall on the outstretched hand, drives the capitellum against the outer side of the head of the radius, tilting and displacing it outward. Such a mechanism applies a valgus strain to the elbow at the moment of

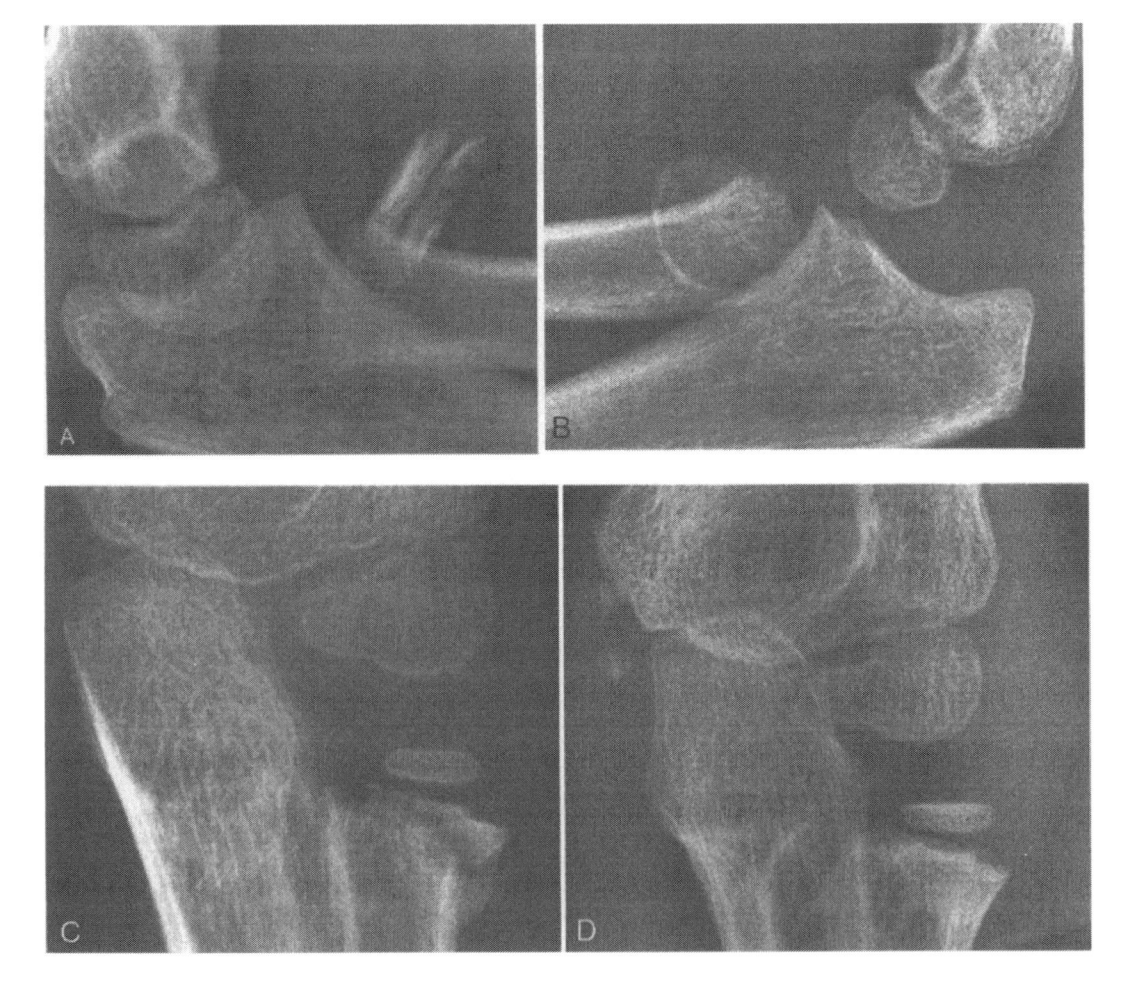

FIGURE 16-35. (A) Completely displaced metaphyseal fracture in a 9-year-old child. (B) Similar injury in a 6-year-old child. (C) Two months after open reduction. (D) Four months later. Note the bipartite medial epicondylar ossification, indicating injury to that area also.

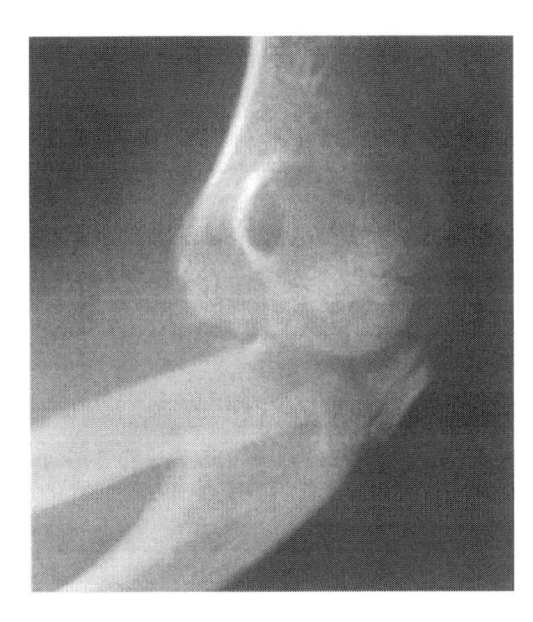

FIGURE 16-36. Mechanistically many of these fractures occur with an elbow dislocation or Monteggia injury in which the posteriorly/inferiorly displaced radial head is subsequently knocked off by spontaneous or attempted reduction. Probably some failure of the physis has occurred in the original injury that makes completion of the fracture likely during reduction.

injury. Accordingly, one may find an associated traction lesion of the inner side of the joint, which may take the form of a medial epicondyle avulsion or, much less likely in a child, rupture of the medial collateral ligament.

The direction of tilting of the displaced head of the radius relative to the shaft of the radius varies with the rotational position of the radius at the time of injury. Thus, if the forearm is supinated at the moment of impact, the displacement of the capital epiphysis is outward (lateral). This displacement is shown in the usual anteroposterior radiograph taken in supination. If the forearm is in midposition, the adjacent posterior quadrant of the radial head is subjected to the greatest violence; and when the forearm is returned to a position of full supination, the head may be tilted backward relative to the radial shaft.

According to Jeffrey, another mechanism of injury is when the patient first falls on the hand and sustains a temporary posterior dislocation or subluxation of the elbow joint.[96,97] The resulting upward force of the flexed elbow displaces the radial head posteriorly almost 90° by the impact against the inferior aspect of the capitellum. Spontaneous reduction of the elbow dislocation leaves the separated radial head underneath the capitellum.[96,122,153] This particular form of injury is discussed further in Chapter 11.

Diagnosis

The injured elbow is usually held in moderate flexion, with the forearm in neutral rotation. There may be local swelling and ecchymosis over the lateral aspect of the elbow. Palpation of the radial head and neck may elicit tenderness. There may be occasional crepitation of the fragments when motion is attempted. Pain may be referred distally to the wrist. Flexion and extension are restricted; pronation and supination are painful and restricted.

Roentgenograms initially are obtained in anterior and lateral views (Figs. 16-34, 16-35). When clinical findings are suggestive, but the standard roentgenograms are inconclusive, it is advisable to examine several views of the proximal radius in various degrees of rotation or evaluate the proximal radius under fluoroscopy. Sometimes small metaphyseal fragments are visible. A dislocated proximal fragment may be projected into the shadow of the ulna. As a result, the structural changes may be missed on routine films. In such cases, oblique or tangential projections may be useful. The maximal degree of the tilting of the radial head should be determined, which, again, may require nonstandard views or fluoroscopy. Fat pad signs may be the only indication of an undisplaced injury.

A child with a fracture of the radial head may present with more distally referred pain, even in the wrist.[67] As with any injury in which there is rather diffuse or even selective pain in a child, it is important to radiograph the *entire* involved bone. As many as 50% of patients with a fracture of the radial head or neck have an associated injury, such as fracture of the olecranon, avulsion of the medial epicondyle, or dislocation of the elbow.

The degree of angulation may be accurately determined only by an anteroposterior radiograph obtained with the forearm in the position of rotation at the moment of impact.[152] Jeffrey has advocated obtaining radiographs in various degrees of forearm rotation.[97] A more practical method is to assess the child with fluoroscopy by pronating and supinating the forearm to find the maximal extent of angulation. Alternatively, if a well-formed secondary ossification center is present, it appears as a rectangle when the bone is in the maximal degree of angulation. Comparison views are less appropriate, as there are normal variations in the radiographic appearance of the proximal radius.

Treatment

For the undisplaced or minimally displaced fracture of the radial head or neck, treatment consists of immobilizing the

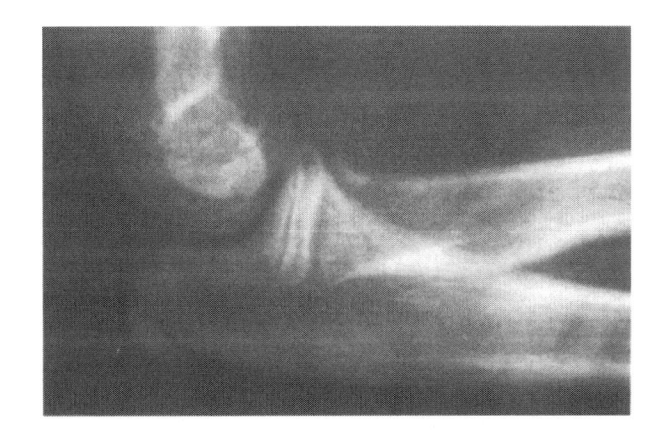

FIGURE 16-37. This radial head flipped 180° during spontaneous reduction. The articular surface faces the metaphysis.

elbow with a posterior splint in 90° of flexion and neutral rotation of the forearm for approximately 10–14 days. Movement should be started when the injury is no longer painful.[90] Early mobilization is recommended but is not used if there is residual pain at the fracture site on either motion or direct palpation. Initial movements include flexion-extension and pronation-supination exercises; the arm should be protected in a sling because of the normal state of activity of a child.

The basic aim of treatment is to restore the normal range of forearm supination and pronation. Tilting of the radial head 20°–30° may be compatible with this aim in a young child with remodeling potential. However, this observation is not an excuse to leave this degree of angular deformity because it may *not* improve with time. Every attempt should be made to achieve an optimal degree of angular correction. Lateral tilting of up to 30° is probably acceptable, as there is usually spontaneous correction through remodeling. This correction is less likely with the older child (over 10 years) because the proximal radius has much less growth potential than does the distal physis. Furthermore, with a crushing metaphyseal injury one cannot be certain there is no concomitant physeal injury that may lead to growth slowdown or arrest and that may cause further angular deformity and tilting of the radial head. Permanent malunion may result.

Closed reduction is usually accomplished by partial to complete extension of the elbow to provide some fixation of the ulna relative to the humerus, followed by adduction of the forearm to correct or overcorrect the carrying angle and widen the radiohumeral articulation, a maneuver designed to create a space into which the displaced radial head may be reduced.[90] This position is held, and the forearm is rotated to bring the radial head into a position from which it may be pushed by direct pressure into correct alignment (Fig. 16-38). As a prelude to manipulation it is important to determine the direction of displacement of the radial head. Manipulative reduction is carried out with the forearm in the degree of rotation that brings the most prominent part of the displaced head farthest laterally. If it is done under image intensification, it is often possible to determine the position of supination or pronation that best emphasizes the fracture in such a way that the thumb may be applied to produce a correction force. Firm digital pressure is applied in an upward and inward direction to complete the reduction. If roentgenography proves that the reduction is satisfactory, the arm is immobilized in a posterior splint.

When there is angulation of 30°–60°, closed reduction under anesthesia is appropriate and usually successful. Some accept an initial angulation of less than 30°, but even this should be treated with an attempted reduction. If the angulation is more than 60°, closed reduction is usually unsuccessful and open reduction or the toggle maneuver is indicated. The proximal humerus of the affected limb is stabilized by an assistant. The elbow is flexed to 90°. The forearm is held by the surgeon's ipsilateral hand (i.e., the left hand for the left forearm and vice versa) in maximum possible supination. No varus strain is applied. Pressure is then applied by the thumb of the surgeon's other hand over the anterolateral aspect of the head of the radius, just distal and lateral to the cubital fossa. At the same time the affected forearm is gradually but steadily rotated to a neutral position and then into a position of full pronation. This maneuver rotates the displaced and tilted radial head under the external pressure; and with the elbow flexion providing a lax capsule, the radial head is usually reduced. Reduction and stability may be confirmed fluoroscopically.

For moderately displaced fractures (i.e., 30°–60° of angular deformity), closed reduction with the patient under general anesthesia is attempted first.[124] If satisfactory reduction is achieved, a long arm cast is applied with the elbow held at 70°–90° of flexion, neutral rotation, and three-point fixation with the medial elbow as the fulcrum; a slight varus stress is then applied to the cast to lessen pressure at the radiohumeral joint. Usually, a period of 3–4 weeks is sufficient to achieve healing. It should be remembered that this area does not normally have a dense cortex and is not accustomed to assuming significant joint reaction forces, so it might collapse if the arm is used and pronation-supination movement is started. Repeat roentgenograms during the first 2 weeks ensure that reduction is maintained.

Open reduction may be undertaken when the radial epiphysis is displaced completely from the shaft or when manipulative reduction has been unsuccessful. It should be done as soon as possible after the injury, as extended periods are sometimes associated with a higher incidence of myositis ossificans and ischemic necrosis.[124,146]

Even if it is completely separated, the radial head should be replaced anatomically, as revascularization may occur (but is unlikely after 24 hours). The head and neck of the radius normally are relatively poorly vascularized (i.e., dependent on only a few vessels), so ischemic change is a likely complication. In cases with major dislocation of the fragments, the periosteum may be completely severed. Extensive stripping of the periosteum should not be undertaken. Removal may result in significant relative differences of growth rates between the radius and ulna.[108] Silastic

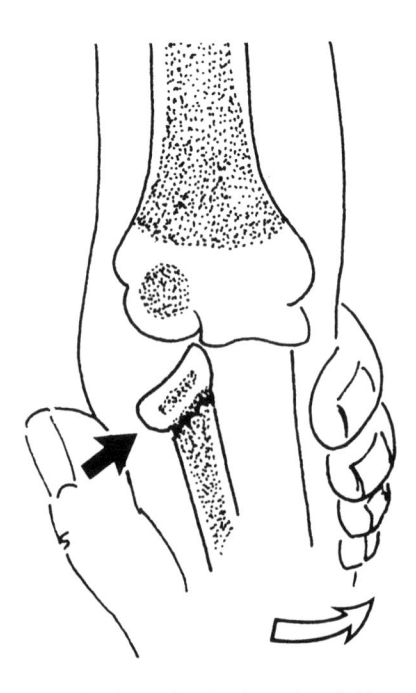

FIGURE 16-38. Mechanism of reduction of radial head angulation. The thumb is pressed against the radial head (black arrow) while the forearm is directed into a varus position (open arrow).

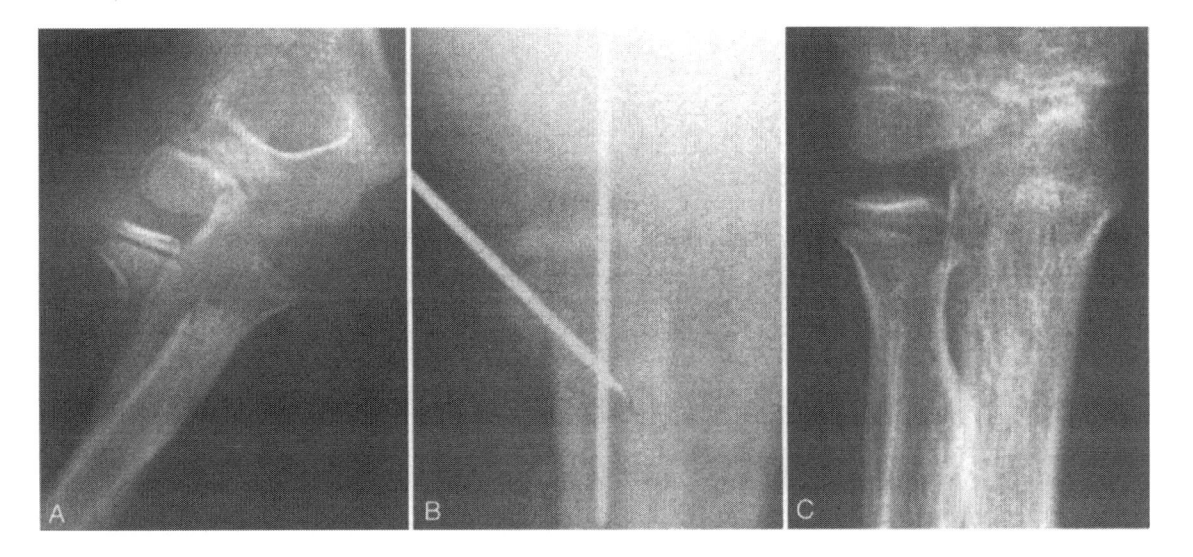

FIGURE 16-39. (A) Completely displaced proximal radial head fracture. (B) Open reduction with pin fixation. (C) Seven months later.

spacers should be avoided in children. The annular ligament is not sectioned unless it is absolutely necessary to achieve reduction. Every effort should be made to protect the annular ligament; if it is damaged, it should be repaired. The forearm should be fully pronated and supinated to test the stability of the reduction.

When necessary, fixation may be accomplished by angular placement of wires through the margin of the radial head into the metaphysis (Fig. 16-39). Placing the wire through the capitellum into the center of the radial head and along the radial shaft with the elbow flexed at 90° and the forearm in midrotation is less desirable and rarely necessary if it is possible to achieve fixation without involving the articular surfaces.

Fowles and Kassab described the breaking of two transarticular K-wires from the humerus to the radius.[86] This method should be avoided. Oblique placement of K-wires through the radial head is the best approach.

I recommend peripheral placement of the fixation wires. The ends of the wires are left subcutaneously or penetrating the skin so they can be easily removed. The ends are bent 90° to prevent migration. A well-padded dressing is applied, followed by a posterior shell that can be converted after 3–4 days to a formal long arm cast when swelling subsides.

Other authors have recommended various methods of fixation. Key used sutures in the periosteum of the neck and sutured the annular ligament about it.[102,103] Reidy and Van Gorder did not use any internal fixation, except for an occasional suture.[131] O'Brien occasionally used a Kirschner wire.[122] Jones and Esah used K-wires introduced behind and lateral to the lateral condyle of the humerus, crossing the radial head obliquely into the shaft.[98]

Merchan thought that displacement of more than 2 mm, rather than 5 mm, was an indication for open reduction.[114] He also recommended K-wires for transfixing the joint, but the risk of breakage is significant. He reported 36 children: 18 with a good result, 8 a fair result, and 10 a poor result. He believed that the risk of poor results was associated with severe displacement and that use of open reduction per se was not the causal factor. In six cases the K-wire bent, and in two cases it broke. In one instance it could not be removed, remaining permanently in the medullary cavity.

Carl and Ain described a complex fracture of the radial neck in a child that involved fractures of the radial neck, the olecranon, and the medial epicondyle.[75] Medial and lateral fixation were necessary to control the three planes of instability. They thought that the combination of the two injuries (olecranon or medial epicondyle), which often singularly accompany the radial head fracture, created the unstable situation.

Care must be taken to protect the posterior interosseous nerve. This nerve may be exposed by separating the fibers of the supinator muscle. Wide exposure may prevent neuropraxia of the posterior interosseous nerve and facilitates positioning of the radial head on its neck.

Metaizeau and colleagues described an interesting technique in which a K-wire was passed from the distal end of the radius through the medullary canal.[115,116] By toggling it under fluoroscopy, they manipulated the radial head into place without having to undertake open reduction of the radial head. The K-wire was then left in place until healing occurred. They thought that inadequate reduction of radial head fractures led to long-term limitation of elbow and forearm movements. They also believed that these complications could be alleviated by distal-to-proximal placement of a Kirschner wire with a toggle maneuver to flip the radial head into place if closed reduction with the thumb did not work.[115,116]

Metaizeau et al. used their technique of intramedullary reduction and pinning in 31 fractures with a tilt between 30° and 80° and 16 fractures with a tilt of more than 80°.[115,116] Altogether 30 of 31 in the first group and 11 of 16 in the second group had excellent or good functional results. Their technique is to bend a Kirschner wire 1.2–2.0 mm in diameter, depending on the patient's age; the last 3 mm are bent more sharply. Four of the lesions that were more than 80° could not be reduced satisfactorily with this technique and were subsequently treated with open reduction. The authors thought that a residual angulation of more than 10°–15° in the 10- to 12-year range or an angulation of more than 20°–30° in a younger child would not be remodeled by subsequent growth and would therefore lead to variable subluxation of the joint, depending on the position of the forearm.

Bernstein et al. used a technique of percutaneous reduction under image intensification,[71] generally for significantly displaced radial neck fractures. Eighteen patients were so treated. Steele and Graham described use of the same technique.[143]

With type 3 or 4 growth mechanism injuries, closed reduction should be attempted first, although open reduction is frequently necessary. Most of these injuries result in premature closure of the epiphysis and may accentuate valgus angulation, depending on the amount of remaining growth.

The type 4 physeal injury produces a dilemma. The displaced fragment is often too small to be fixed effectively. In some cases it can be excised. The result may not be good, but the loss of motion after this fracture may be due to other factors because the injury is usually produced by considerable violence.

When treating markedly displaced and fragmented fractures, many authors believe that only two methods are likely to give satisfactory results: excision of the capital fragment or open reduction. However, the radial head usually should not be excised in a child because marked growth disturbance can occur. A Madelung-type deformity may also develop at the wrist, with radial deviation of the hand, depending on the amount of growth remaining. In a patient close to skeletal maturity, with a severely comminuted injury of the proximal radius, it is probably best to treat the adolescent as an adult and excise the radial head.

If the fracture is diagnosed late, radial head tilting may be corrected by an osteotomy and, if necessary, bone graft. If the patient is skeletally mature, the radial head may be excised.

Immobilization following open reduction is as described for closed treatment and should be continued for 2–4 weeks. If K-wires have been used, they should be removed before active rehabilitation.

Results

Full return of supination and pronation may take several months, although there is little permanent disability. Restriction of motion of the elbow may also occur. Rotation of the forearm is most often affected. Pronation was limited in 21 elbows, supination in 14, and both motions in 13.[37] Flexion and extension, in contrast, were infrequently limited. When the upper radial epiphysis has been completely displaced from the shaft, some permanent loss of movement is anticipated, even when accurate reduction has been secured by open operation.[96]

McBride and Monnet reported nine patients with a follow-up that ranged from 3 to 15 years.[113] In general, the results were good. They were negative about the results of open reduction in these injuries but did recommend that after disruption or transection of the annular ligament, reduction could be maintained by a small K-wire through the center of the head and into the neck and by a good repair of the annular ligament. Nonunion developed in two patients treated by open reduction, and eventually resection of the radial head was undertaken because of persistent pain.[113]

In another study the carrying angle was increased 5°–10° in six cases and 15°–20° in three; 17 patients had no change in the carrying angle.[126] Only two patients showed an increased valgus angle of more than 10° in the injured arm, compared with the unaffected arm. The carrying angle increased in about 30% of the children owing to premature closure of the growth plate of the radius.

Steinberg and associates, in a long-term review (more than 4 years) of fractures of the neck of the radius in children, showed that 31% had a poor result.[144] Primary angulation appeared to be the most important factor affecting the results. Periarticular ossification, ischemic necrosis, and enlargement of the radial head were the most important causes of poor results. They thought that more accurate reduction was mandatory to improve the final outcome. The prognosis is good, with the fractures often giving a usable, but seldom normal, elbow.[86,144] In the Steinberg et al. series, a good reduction at surgery did not always guarantee a good result at follow-up examination.[144]

D'Souza et al. studied 100 patients with radial neck fractures.[80] Excellent and good results were obtained consistently after closed manipulation. Open reduction was often followed by a fair or poor result. They thought that operative correction should not be attempted unless the radial head is displaced 45°.

Complications

The complications of radial neck fracture include synostosis, avascular or ischemic necrosis (Fig. 16-40), premature fusion of the physis (Fig. 16-41), enlargement of the radial head or neck, deformed epiphysis (Fig. 16-42), ectopic calcification, nonunion (Fig. 16-43), vascular or peripheral nerve injury, and impaction injury to the articular surface, with loss of motion and abnormal wear of the cartilage.

There is a slightly higher incidence of complications following open reduction than after closed reduction. Synostosis, though rare, is a hazard even of closed reduction and may result in cubitus varus. Heterotopic ossification may also occur and reduce rotation; it is more likely after open reduction.

Key described an elbow dislocation with posterior displacement of the radius.[102] Roentgenograms showed an irregularity of the epiphyseal plate a year later. There was also an indentation of the capitellum, suggestive of irregular joint reaction forces across the radiohumeral joint. Wood reported two similar cases of posterior displacement of the epiphysis.[153] One patient was treated with open reduction and 6 years later had good function and a normal radiograph. The second patient was also treated with open reduction; and when the patient was seen 2 years after injury, radiographs showed distortion of the growth of the proximal end of the radius and limitation of pronation and supination.

Synostosis between the proximal radius and ulna has been reported.[79,84,122] In three patients in Henrikson's study,

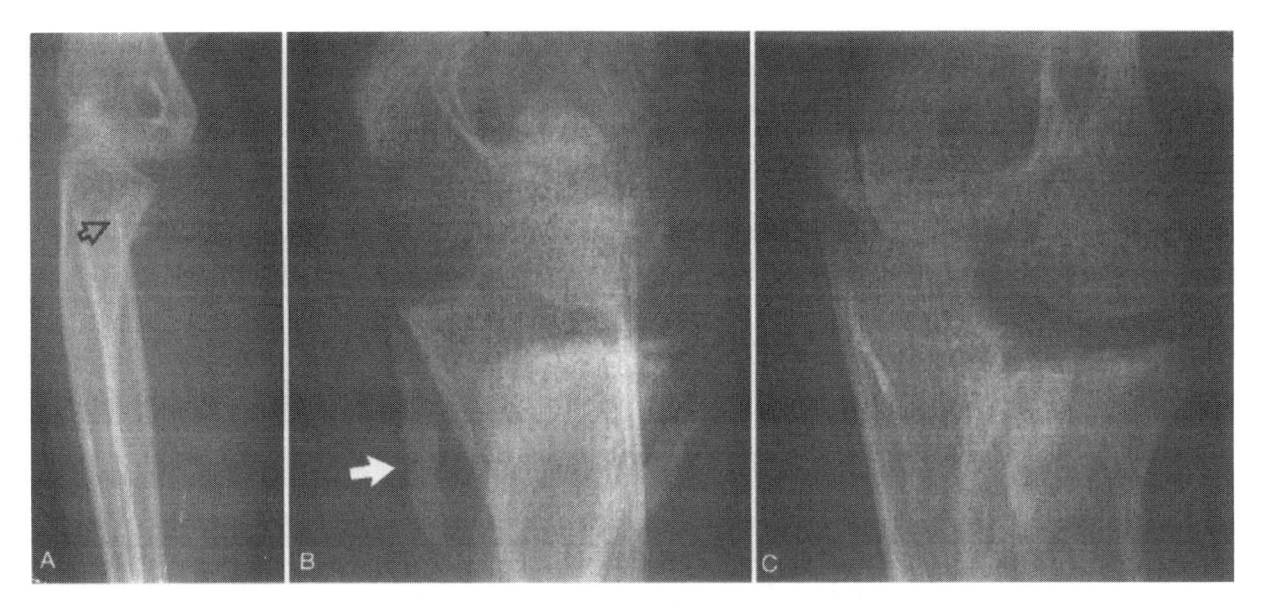

FIGURE 16-40. (A) Complete displacement of the radial head (arrow). It was placed back on the shaft by open reduction. Anteroposterior (B) and oblique (C) views showing ischemic necrosis and premature epiphysiodesis 18 months later. (B) Ectopic bone is also evident (solid arrow).

a synostosis developed between the radius and the ulna.[94] In one, a radioulnar synostosis developed consequent to osteotomy.[113] Fielding reported radioulnar cross-union following displacement of the proximal radial epiphysis in an 11-year-old boy who was treated with closed reduction.[84] Fibrous adhesions between the radius and ulna were also noted.[98] Such adhesions block rotation of the forearm comparable to synostosis.

Nonunion is infrequent. It results from failure to achieve adequate reduction and maintain it (Fig. 16-43).

Premature fusion of the upper radial epiphysis occurs often with moderately and markedly displaced fractures and may cause shortening of the radius and increased cubitus valgus, contingent on the age of the child at the time of the injury and the severity of the cartilaginous damage. Premature fusion occurred in about one-third of O'Brien's patients, but in none of them was the ensuing cubitus valgus severe enough to require osteotomy.[122]

Ischemic necrosis of the radial head may occur. It does not appear to be related to the degree of initial displacement or to the age at the time of injury. The results are poor.[98] Ischemic necrosis of the whole head is rare, even when the head is completely reduced. Partial ischemic necrosis is seen more frequently. Irregularity of the radial head and premature closure of the proximal radial physis are common. In one series premature fusion occurred in 11 of 30 cases.[131]

Other complications have been noted. New bone formation (heterotopic bone) and deformity of the radial head with enlargement occur in some cases and may restrict elbow motion. O'Brien reported a notch in the radial neck in 6 of 125 cases, and believed it due to scarring and damage to the annular ligament.[122] Colton showed a patient with a 180° flip of the radial head during closed reduction (Fig. 16-37). Follow-up showed significant growth arrest and irregular overgrowth with decreased function. Failure to correct displacement or angulation may affect the rotation of the radial head in the ulnar notch, producing a cam effect, rather than a rotation.

Dislocation of the Head of the Radius

Isolated dislocation of the head of the radius (Figs. 16-44, 16-45) with no other congenital abnormality in the elbow is infrequent.[155–203] White suggested that some of the cases reported as congenital dislocations of the radial head may have been caused by trauma during delivery or early

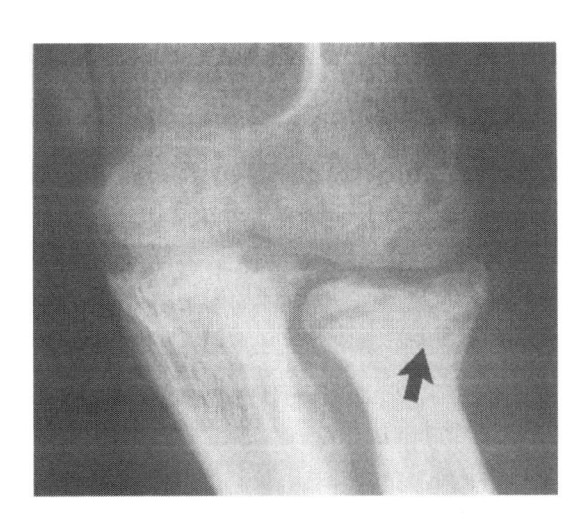

FIGURE 16-41. Premature fusion of the physis (arrow).

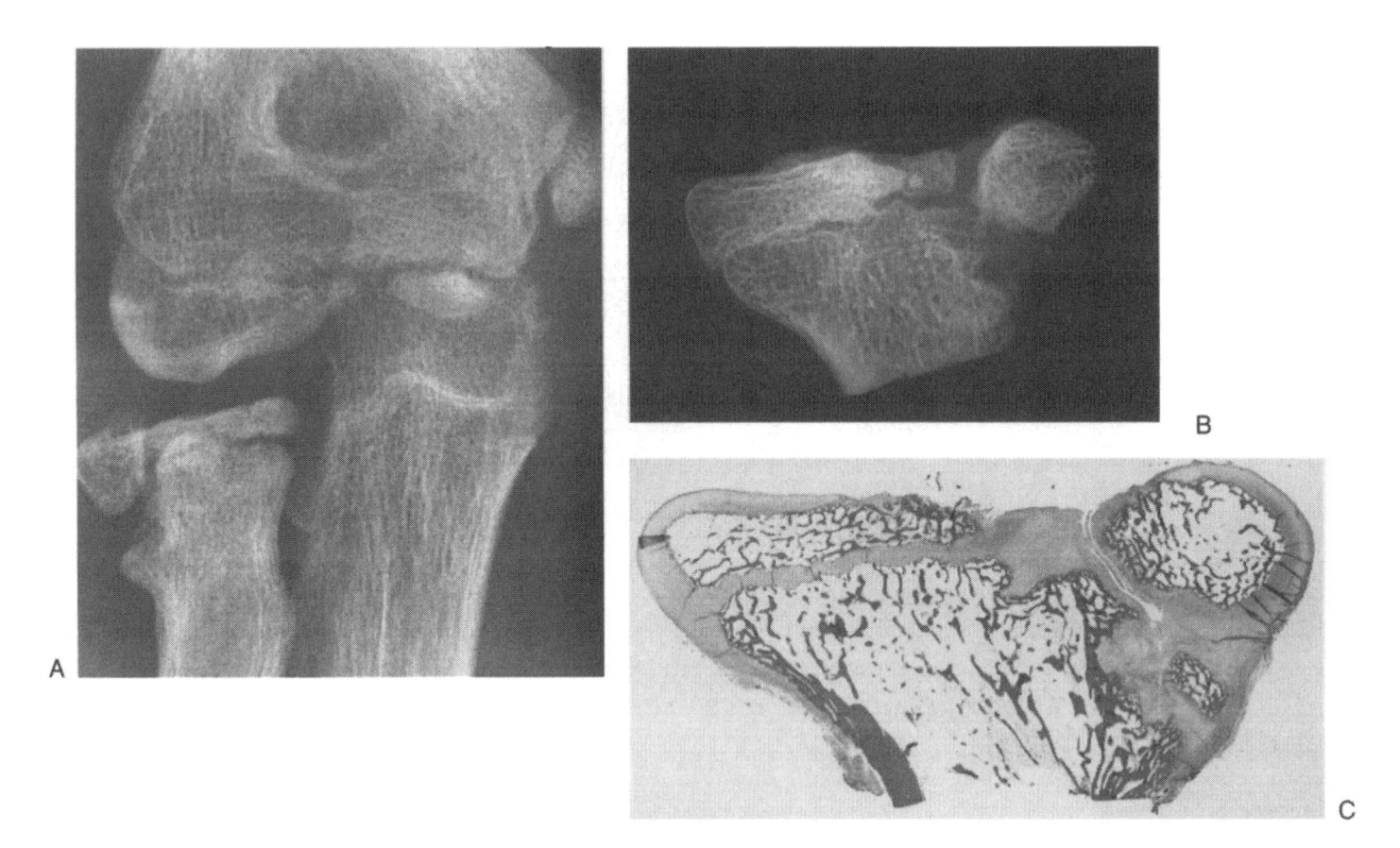

FIGURE 16-42. (A) Nonunion of type 4 injury of the radial head. The parents opted for radial head excision because of severe pain. (B) Radiograph of the specimen. (C) Histology shows loss of central articular cartilage and nonunion of the fragment.

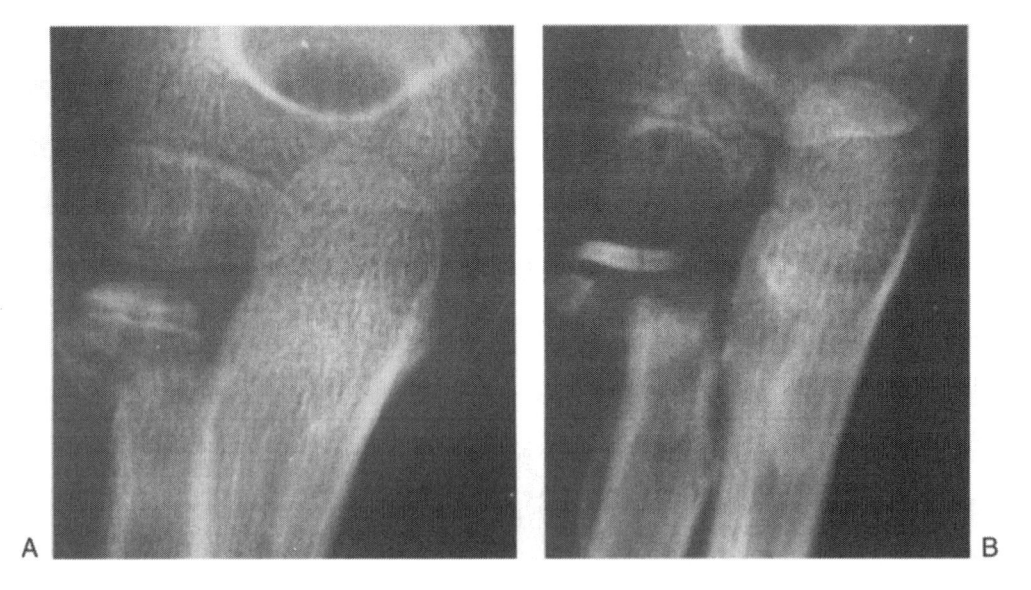

FIGURE 16-43. (A) Fracture treated by closed reduction. Delayed union is evident at 6 weeks. (B) Nonunion and ischemic necrosis at 14 weeks.

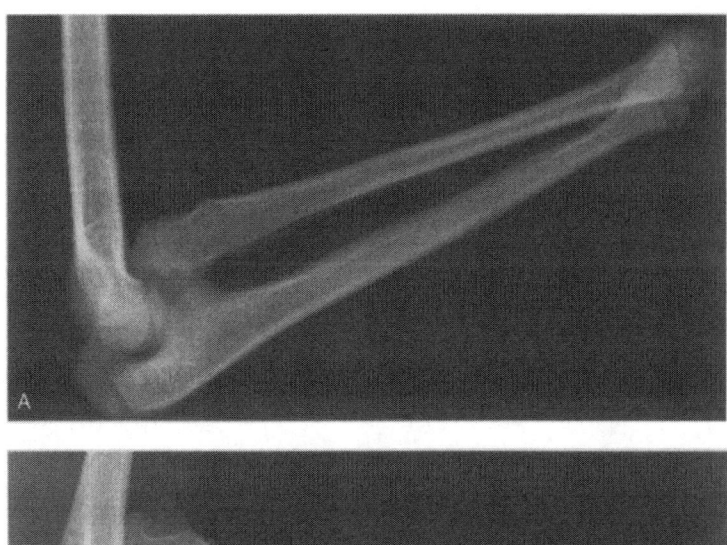

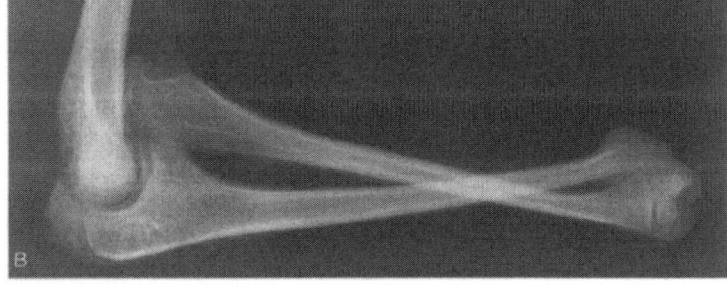

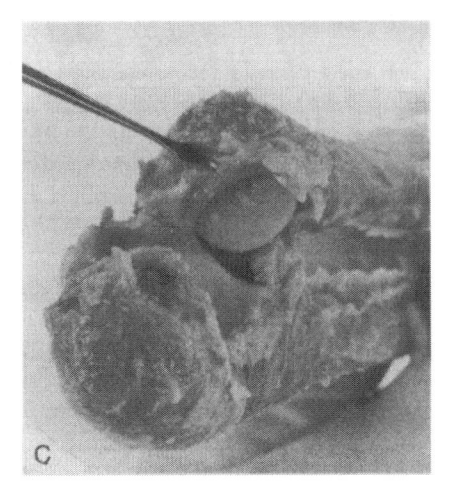

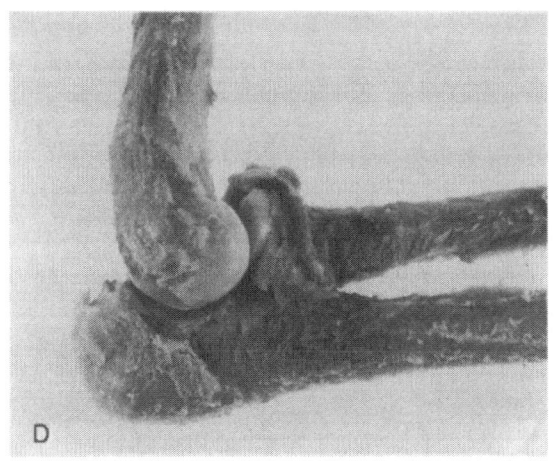

FIGURE 16-44. Progressive, nontraumatic subluxation of the radial head in cadaver specimens. The child had severe cerebral palsy with elbow contractures that undoubtedly led to progressive displacement of the proximal radius, similar to the progressive appearance of subluxation and dislocation of the hip in these severely spastic children. (A) Roentgenogram of the right side. This side could be reduced in some positions. (B) More severe involvement of the left side. This could not be reduced because of severe capsular distortion. (C) Annular ligament over the radial head of the specimen shown in (A). After dissection freed this from the capsule, it could be reduced. (D) Intact, back around the metaphysis.

infancy.[199] For distinguishing between congenital and traumatic dislocations, one of the most reliable signs is the condition of the capitellum. If it is significantly underdeveloped, a congenital dislocation is likely, although early postnatal subluxation or dislocation (i.e., infantile "nursemaid's" elbow) might lead to secondary joint deformation on both sides of the joint, as with developmental hip disease. Confusion may arise when a child with a congenital or pathologic dislocation falls on his or her elbow. The ensuing radiographs may mimic an acute injury.

With congenital dislocation of the radial head, there is no capsular inclusion and a poorly developed radial head with a convex shape (Fig. 16-46). Vesely explored radial heads in cases of congenital dislocation and described capsular distortion and displacement of the annular ligament.[198] These findings were similar to those of the case shown in Figure 16-44.

The annular ligament is quite mobile in infants. Accordingly, it may completely displace over and off the radial head and not be recognized because of the limited ossification in

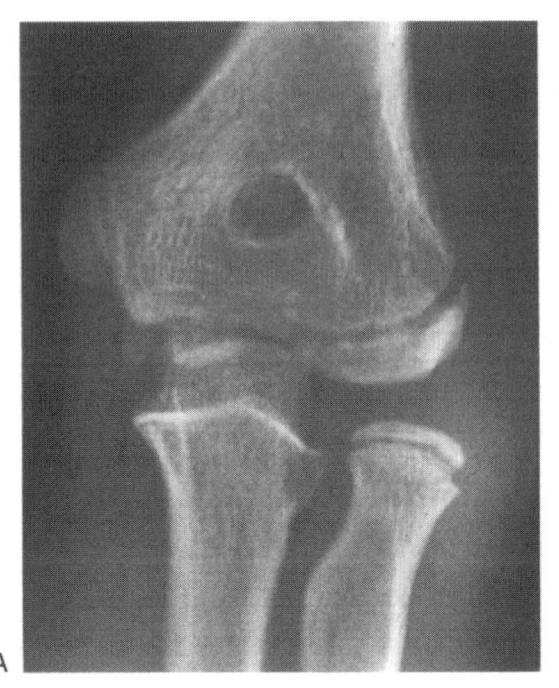

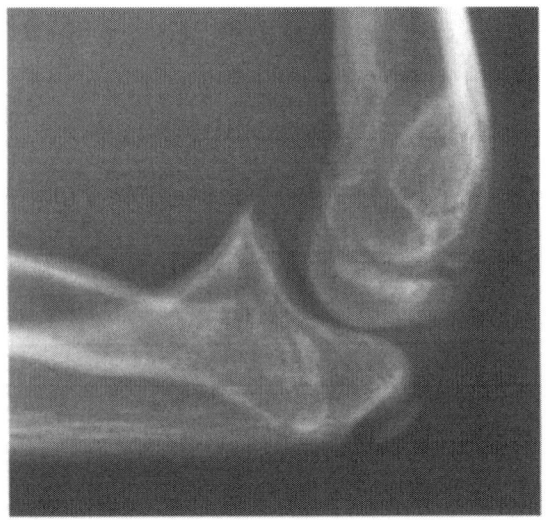

FIGURE 16-45. (A) This child had an elbow injury 3 years earlier. No fracture was seen on the radiograph according to the dictated radiology report. The child, now 9 years old, had painful, restricted motion made worse by pitching a baseball. (B) Although the anteroposterior view seemed unremarkable (according to the radiologist), the lateral view readily shows the posterior displacement.

the infant's elbow epiphyses. It is the equivalent of nursemaid's elbow in toddlers.

Isolated traumatic dislocation of the radial head has been regarded as a "pseudo-Monteggia" lesion (Fig. 16-45). The absence of the concomitant ulnar fracture is due in part to the plasticity of the ulna in infants and young children, which permits transient bowing of the bone without progression to fracture. However, the "weakness of the annular ligament" that predisposes certain children to nursemaid's elbow may allow a rare individual to develop complete dislocation of the radial head.

Caravias reported acute radial head dislocation that resembled classic "congenital" dislocation of the head of the radius. The first case was treated with closed reduction, but anatomic restoration was not attained. During follow-up, after skeletal maturation had been obtained the head of the radius was completely displaced from its radiohumeral articulation. Caravias' second case was a 36-year-old woman who had injured her elbow at the age of 5 years. The head of the radius was lateral to the capitellum but not as high-riding as some cases of congenital dislocation. His third case was a girl of 18 years who apparently had a lesion that was first recognized when she was approximately 2 weeks old, although it had not been associated with any known birth trauma.[159]

For distinguishing isolated radial head dislocation due to trauma from a congenital deformity, Mardam-Bey and Ger

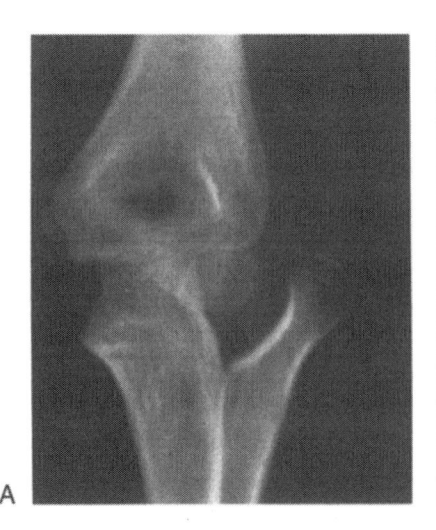

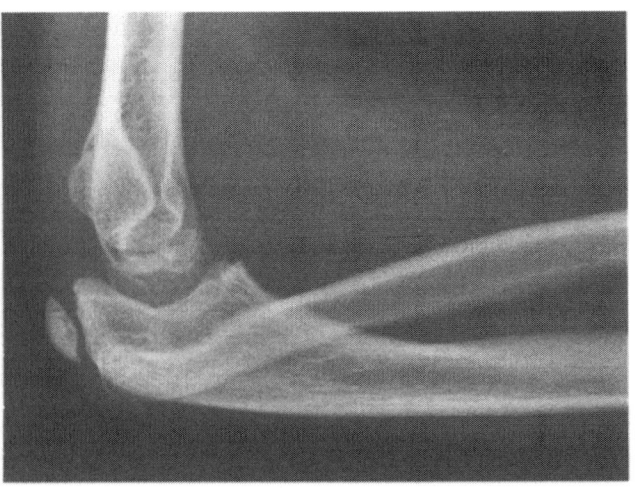

FIGURE 16-46. Anteroposterior (A) and lateral (B) views of a congenitally dislocated proximal radius.

found that congenital radial head dislocation *never* occurred as an isolated anomaly.[182] It was ordinarily associated with a misshapen metaphysis and epiphyseal ossification center (when the latter finally appeared). With true acute isolated dislocation of the radial head, the radial head is usually shaped normally. Unfortunately, because these cases are often in infants the radiolucent anatomic shape may be ascertained only by arthrography or arthroscopy.

Schubert described a case of a dislocated radial head in a newborn who was treated with the arm in supination; the infant had an uneventful recovery.[190] Cockshott and Omololu described a 6-day-old baby with bilateral dislocations that seemed to reduce easily in full supination and dislocate in pronation.[161] Some radial head dislocations in the presence of Erb's palsy may be due to unrecognized accidental subluxation or dislocation in the newborn (i.e., neonatal "nursemaid's" elbow) or progressive postnatal displacement resulting from muscle imbalance.

Vesely described isolated traumatic dislocations of the radial head in children.[198] He reviewed 17 cases and found 2 with concomitant fractures of the radial head; 13 of the dislocations were anterior, 3 were lateral, and 1 was posterior; 4 were treated with open reduction. Chronic dislocation developed in two cases, including one case that was not reduced until 8 months after the injury. A synostosis developed in one case.

Neviaser and LeFevre reported an isolated dislocation of the radius in a 7-year-old child.[185] They treated the child with open reduction because of irreducibility and found a transverse tear in the anterior capsule, exactly where one might expect it if this were a mechanism somewhat similar to that of nursemaid's elbow. The proximal portion of the capsule was lying in the normal anatomic bed of the radial head, precluding reduction. The constricting buttonhole effect of the tear was relieved by a capsular incision; and when the capsule was withdrawn from the joint, the radial head was easily reduced.

Lloyd-Roberts and Bucknill believed that many of these cases represented perinatal or infantile radial head subluxation that progressively deformed.[266] They believed that open reduction and reconstruction of the annular ligament were indicated to reestablish radiohumeral and radioulnar rotational mechanics. I have treated a similar case in a boy with generalized joint laxity. He was found to have sternoclavicular and radial head "dislocations" at birth, but no treatment was given. Figure 16-47 shows the roentgenographic appear-

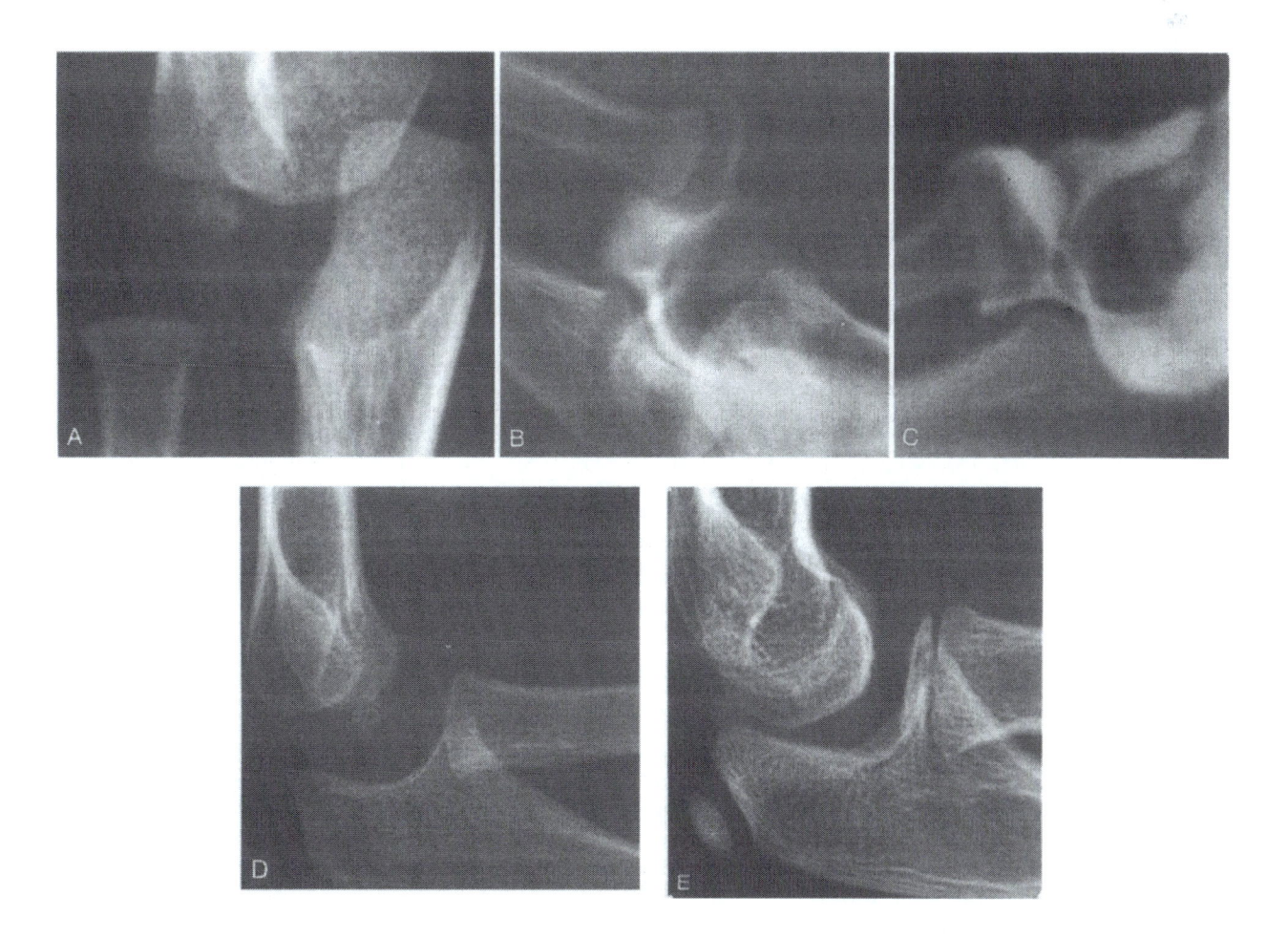

FIGURE 16-47. (A) Appearance of the elbow in a 4-year-old boy with "congenital" dislocation of the proximal radius. (B) Arthrogram showing maximal displacement. (C) Arthrogram of "reduction," which was incomplete because of soft tissue interposition. The patient subsequently underwent exploratory surgery. The annular ligament was displaced completely over the radius, sitting in the space between the radius and the ulna. It was dissected free of the capsule, divided, and reattached in anatomic position. (D) Appearance 6 months later. (E) Eight years later.

ance when he was examined at 4 years of age. He lacked full rotation and was having elbow pain localized to the radial head. The annular ligament was displaced over the radial head (between the radius and ulna), similar to the case shown in Figure 16-44. The ligament segments were dissected free anterior and posterior to the ulnar attachments. The ligament was then divided, the ends were replaced in their encircling anatomic position around the neck, and the ligament was repaired. The capitellum was mildly deformed and permitted some continued subluxation. The reduction was maintained with a pin for 6 weeks. He has complete flexion and extension 10 years postoperatively, but a mild subluxation is present in full pronation.

Whether the management should be conservative or surgical depends on the ease of reduction, maintenance of the reduction, and the delay in diagnosis. An acute reduction may be possible through traction and full supination, with application of direct pressure over the radial head. The elbow should be flexed to 90° and the forearm held in full supination. This position diminishes the pull of the biceps and tenses both the interosseous membrane and the quadrate ligament. In the series of Hudson and Beer, five of the six cases were easily reduced by closed means.[175] The duration of immobilization following a closed reduction is 3–6 weeks.

Armstrong and McLaren reported a case in which the biceps tendon wrapped around the displaced radial head and prevented closed reduction.[157]

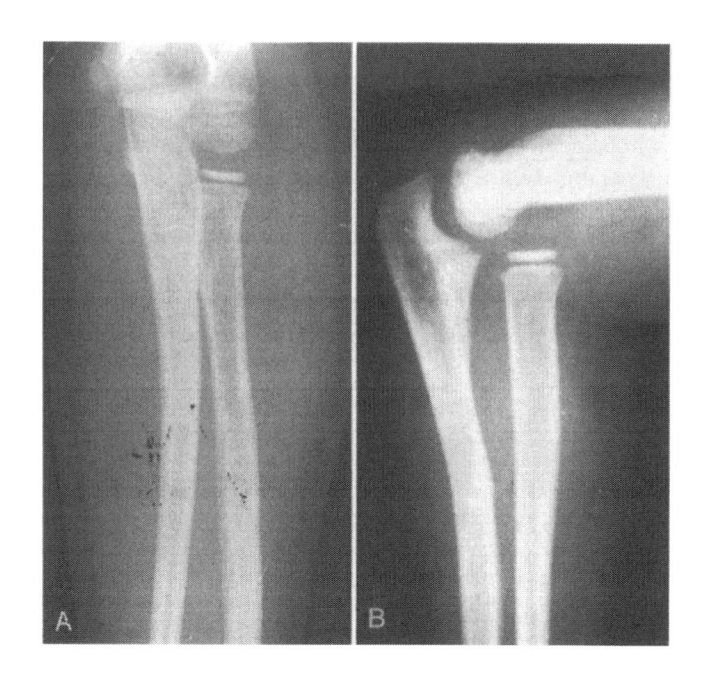

FIGURE 16-48. (A) Be wary of the seemingly normal-appearing anteroposterior view. (B) In the lateral view of this 8-year-old girl, the Monteggia injury is evident. The ulna had only a plastic deformation (bowing).

Monteggia Lesions

Classically, the Monteggia injury involves a fracture of the proximal third of the ulna in association with dislocation of the radial head. However, the injury must be suspected whenever there is any pattern of injury (bowing, greenstick injury, fracture) anywhere along the ulna *without* an obvious associated fracture of the radius[204–321]; and, in fact, the radial head may not be completely dislocated. It may be subluxated such that normal function is subsequently compromised if left untreated.

The level of the fracture of the ulna varies. In approximately two-thirds of patients it is located at the junction of the proximal and middle thirds of the shaft, in 15% it is located in the middle third, and in the remainder it is equally distributed between the distal third of the shaft and the olecranon region. The ulnar fracture may be greenstick (Figs. 16-48, 16-49) or subtle bowing, and the apparent mildness of the ulnar injury may deter accurate appreciation of the entire injury. It is important to remember that the appearance of the latter two ulnar injury patterns does not reveal the extent of angular deformation at the movement of maximal injury; spontaneous, incomplete reduction is common. Fractures of both bones combined with dislocation of the radial head may also occur, although this pattern is infrequent. Such variations of injury have led to classic patterns of injury and variants, which are more likely in children.

Theodorou described three patients in whom the radial head dislocation was associated with fracture of the distal radius and ulna, a combination not usually found in adults.[308] Because of the mechanism of a falling injury, wrist injuries often accompany Monteggia fracture-dislocations in children. It is imperative that the wrist be accurately assessed at the same time the elbow and midforearm are being roentgenographically examined.

The age of incidence has been reported as 2 months to adulthood, but the injury occurs most frequently in children between 7 and 10 years.

Classification

There are three basic types of Monteggia fracture-dislocations: type 1 (extension type), in which the head of the radius is dislocated anteriorly, with palmar (volar) angulation of the fractured shaft of the ulna (Figs. 16-50, 16-51); type 2 (flexion type), in which the radial head is dislocated posteriorly, with dorsal angulation of the fractured shaft of the ulna (Fig. 16-52); and type 3, in which the radial head is dislocated laterally along with the fractured shaft of the ulna (Fig. 16-53). A type 4 injury essentially has a type 1 pattern with an additional fracture through the radius in its proximal third (Fig. 16-54). It is a physeal injury in some children, a Monteggia variant.

In one series, type 1 was the most common (85%), followed by type 2 (10%) and type three (5%).[236] Bado described an incidence of 1.7% in 3200 forearm fractures, with 57% being type 1, 15% type 2, 19% type 3, and the others scattered through the various equivalents of type 4 and subtle variations of the previous types.[208]

There are equivalents to these basic types, such as dislocation of the head of the radius without evident fracture of the ulna, which may occur because of the capacity of the ulna to deform elastically or plastically and to return, variably,

Monteggia Lesions

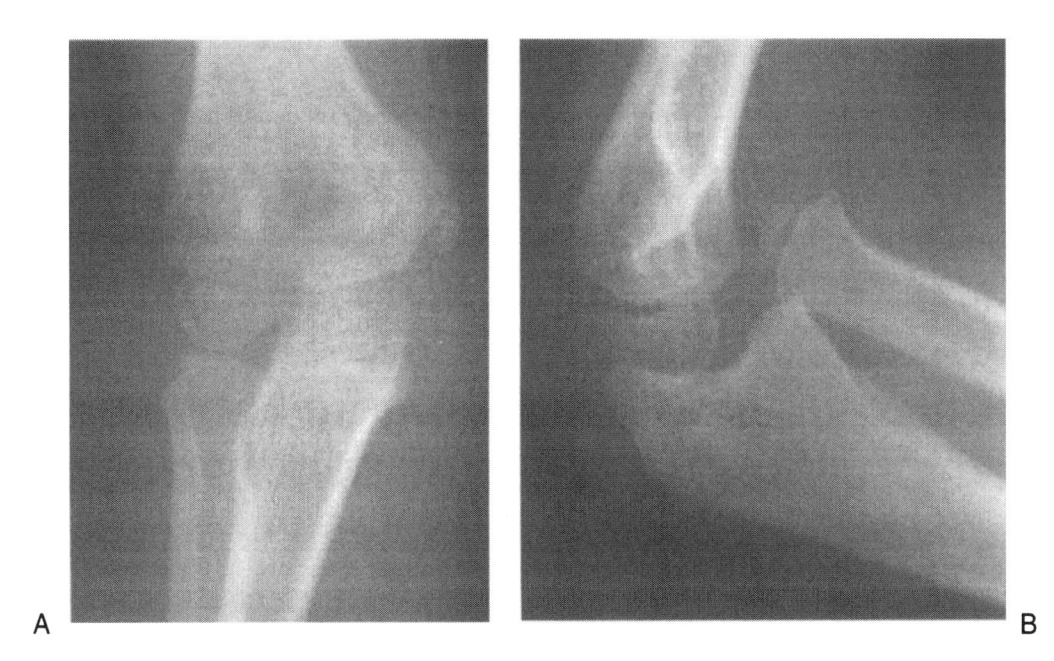

FIGURE 16-49. In this 6-year-old boy with an ulnar diaphyseal angulated greenstick fracture, the anteroposterior view (A) looked "normal," whereas the lateral view (B) showed the medial head dislocation.

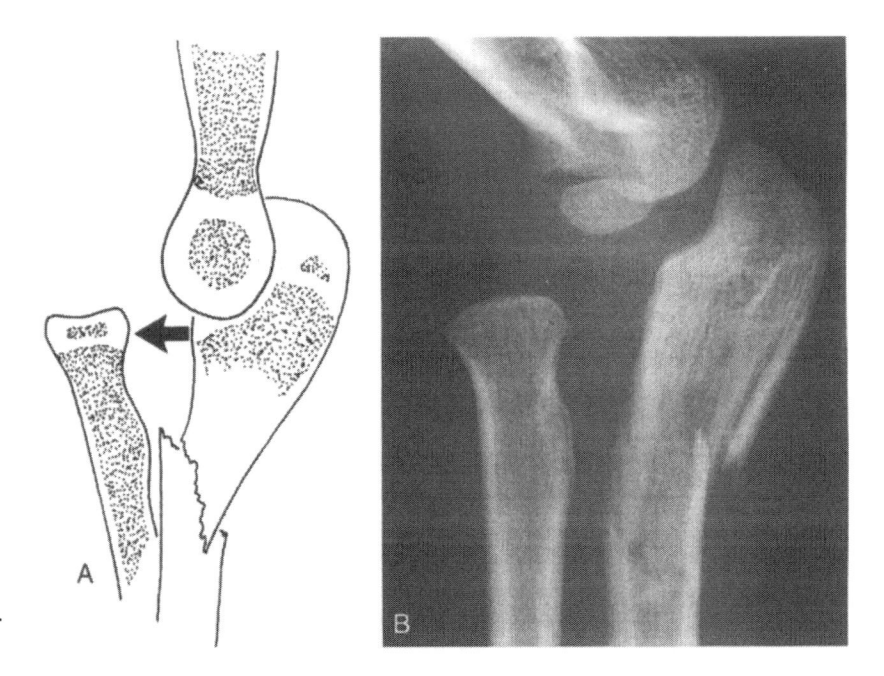

FIGURE 16-50. (A) Anterolateral Monteggia injury. (B) Roentgenographic appearance.

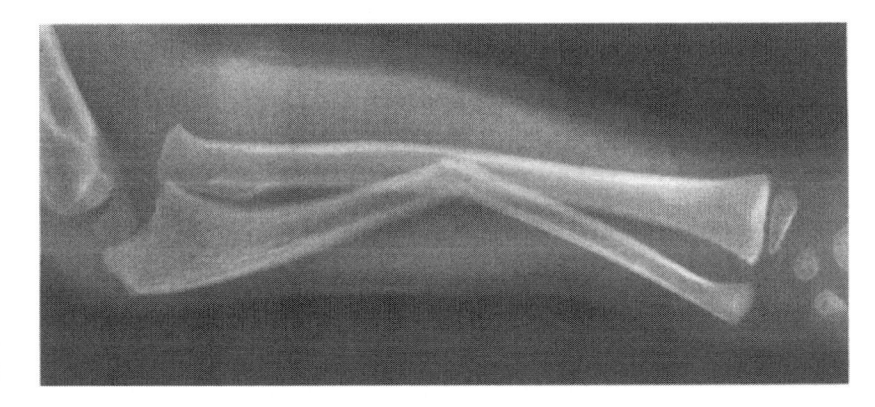

FIGURE 16-51. Angulated ulnar diaphyseal fracture associated with anterior dislocation of the radial head.

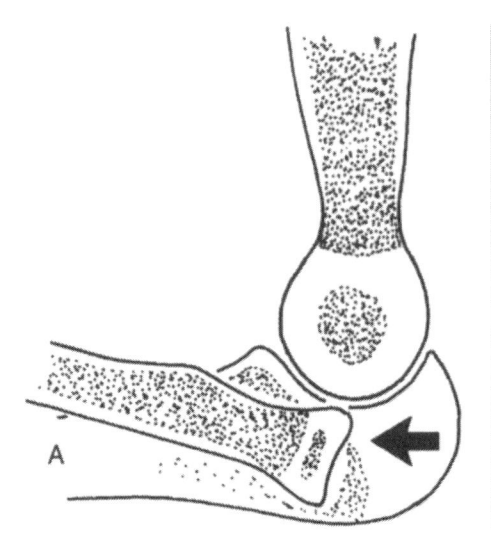

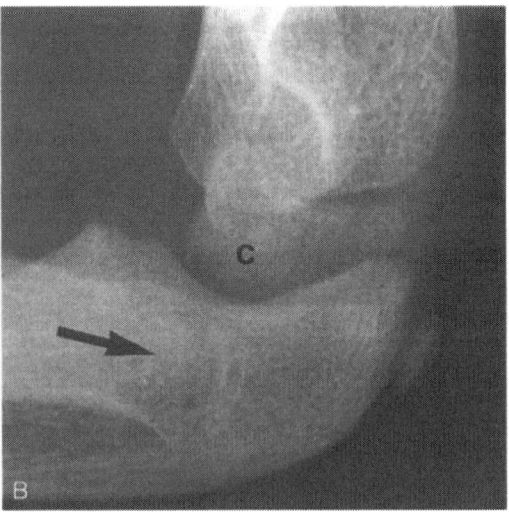

FIGURE 16-52. (A) Posterior Monteggia injury. (B) Roentgenographic appearance. The arrow shows the radius pointing away from the capitellum (c).

almost to the original shape (Fig. 16-55). Other variants include fracture of the ulna associated with (1) a located radial epiphysis but a displaced radial shaft or (2) a dislocated radial epiphysis associated with a radial shaft in its normal anatomic alignment with the capitellum.

The type 3 Monteggia lesion with lateral dislocation, which occurs in both children and adults, has a higher incidence of associated radial nerve injury. Lateral dislocation of the head of the radius associated with incomplete fracture of the olecranon producing varus deformity is considered an unusual Monteggia fracture.[210,317,319]

Pathomechanics

When a child falls forward on an outstretched hand, the forearm is usually pronated; and at the moment of impact the hand becomes relatively fixed to the ground. Because of the downward momentum of the falling body, a rotational

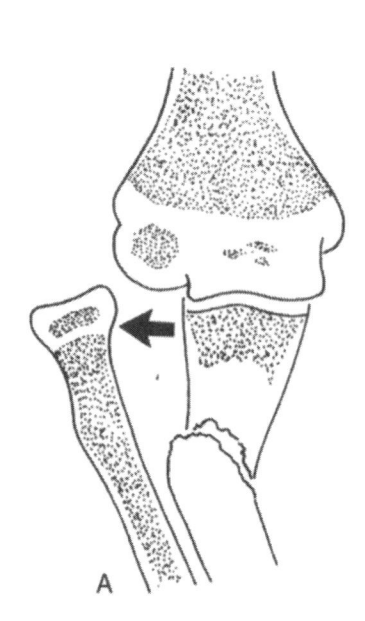

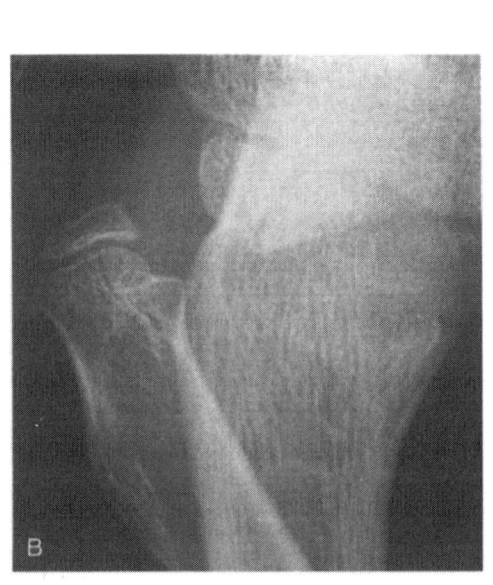

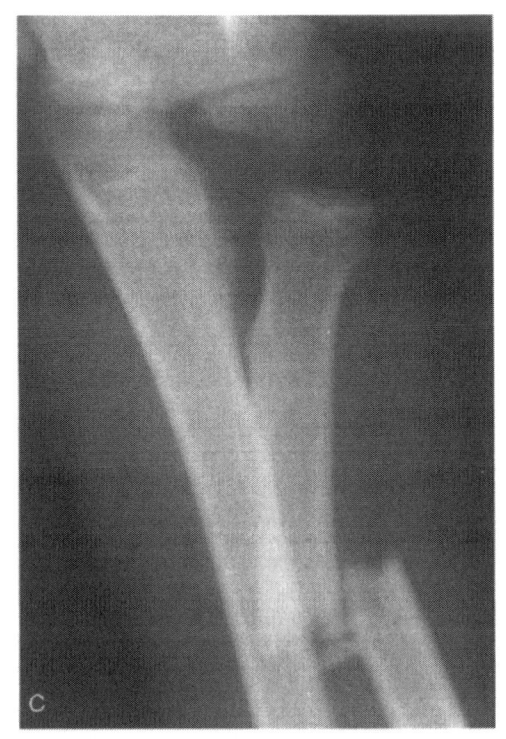

FIGURE 16-53. (A) Lateral Monteggia injury. (B) Roentgenographic appearance. (C) Lateral subluxation associated with fracture of both bones. Note the widening of the proximal radioulnar joint, which should be a warning sign of disruption of this joint.

FIGURE 16-54. Anterolateral dislocation of the radial head associated with diaphyseal fractures of *both* radius and ulna. It is considered a Monteggia variant or equivalent.

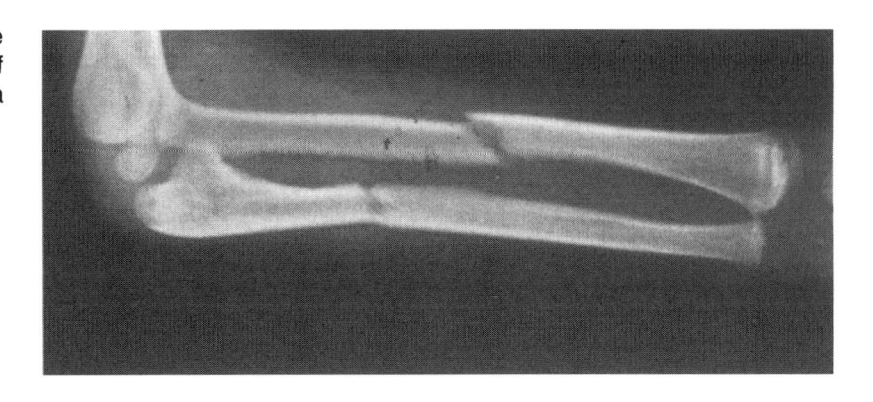

force is added when twisting of the trunk causes external rotation of the humerus and ulna. If this force continues until the normal limit of pronation at the proximal radioulnar joint is reached, something must give. The ulna is liable to deform or fracture. At the same time, the radius is forced into extreme pronation and lies across the ulna at the junction of the upper and middle thirds. Evans believes that as the ulna fractures the two bones come in contact, and at that point a fulcrum is formed over which the upper end of the radius is forced forward.[236] As the pronation force continues, the radius is either levered forward out of the superior radioulnar joint (probably after disruption of the annular ligament) or is fractured in its upper third. Contact is not necessary, as hyperpronation places the radial head and radiocapitellar morphologic relationships in a position whereby the relatively lax annular ligament may be displaced but stays intact, allowing dislocation (Figs. 16-56, 16-57).

Speed and Boyd reported that a direct blow over the posterior aspect of the proximal ulna could produce this injury.[302] This hypothesis was accepted until evidence gained from 18 cadavers and clinical observations suggested hyperpronation as a mechanism of injury. Speed and Boyd stated that the bicipital tuberosity was most posterior in hyperpronation and that this position made the radius subject to the greatest force from the biceps tendon during violent contraction of the muscle. Evans[236] and Penrose[282] produced Monteggia's lesions by pronation in cadavers.

Both hypotheses were challenged by Tompkins, who presented evidence that hyperextension with the forearm in a neutral position was also an acceptable pathomechanism for type 1 injuries.[310] He based this assertion on clinical and radiologic examinations of acutely injured patients that showed type 1 Monteggia's lesions with the forearm in a neutral or slightly supinated position. With open type 1 fractures, the proximal ulnar fragment usually penetrates the palmar skin on the ulnar side of the forearm. Biomechanical investigations of the moments and components of force suggest, theoretically at least, that with the hand fixed in pronation and the elbow in full extension or hyperextension, contraction of the biceps pulls the head of the radius into the lesser sigmoid notch. A neutral position of the forearm tends to lift the radius slightly out of the confines of the annulus.

Hume described three cases of anterior dislocation of the head of the radius associated with an undisplaced fracture of the olecranon in children.[251] Hume appears to have been the first to describe this particular mechanism, although Speed and Boyd suggested that a hyperextension injury to the elbow may cause displacement of the olecranon epiphysis associated with anterior dislocation of the radial head.[302]

Evans showed that with the anterior Monteggia injury, forced hyperpronation first ruptures the capsular and annular ligaments, then fractures the shaft of the ulna, and finally rotates the head of the radius so it lies in front of the capsule.[7] Having prevented reduction of the radial head, the interposed capsule then acts as a mechanical block to full flexion.

Because of the ease with which the radial head is often reduced in children, especially if treated early, and the excellent long-term results, it is possible that the annular ligament is not disrupted longitudinally. Rather, it may tear transversely along its more distal insertion and incompletely herniate into the radiocapitellar joint, similar to the mechanism for a nursemaid's elbow in a young child (see Chapter 11).

With a greenstick ulnar injury, the most probable mechanism is a fall on the outstretched hand during which the forearm is supinated, as it might be if the child were falling backward. The direction of the angulation of the ulna is determined by the exact direction of the fall, which may produce a varus, valgus, or hyperextension strain in the forearm.

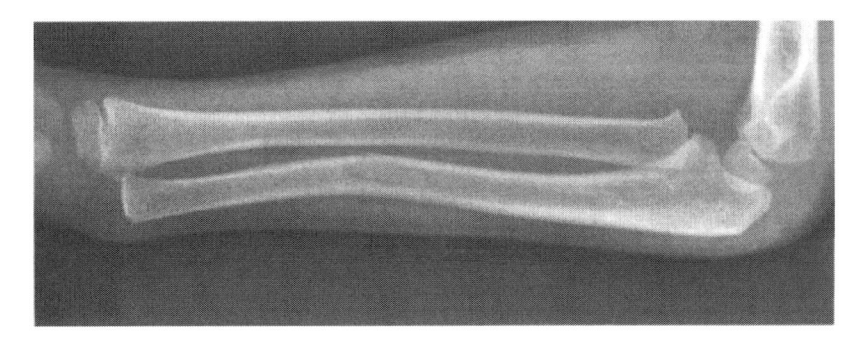

FIGURE 16-55. Greenstick fracture of the ulna with anterior dislocation of the radial head.

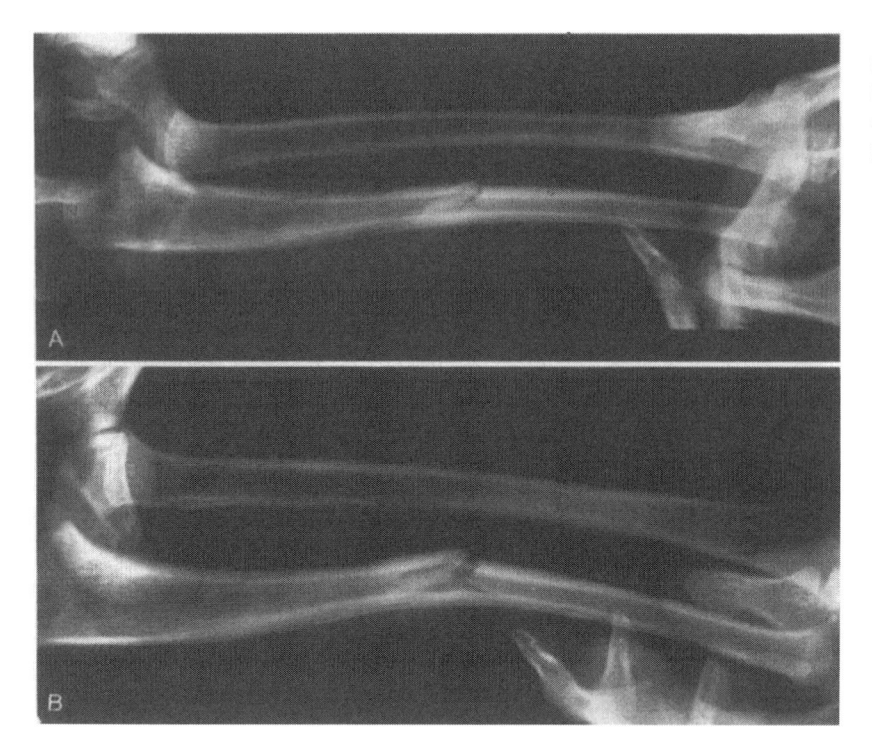

FIGURE 16-56. Monteggia injury in a child suffering a traumatic forequarter amputation. (A) Radiograph showing a greenstick ulnar fracture. (B) Duplication of the probable fracture force displaces the radial head.

Figures 16-56 and 16-57 show the mechanism in a boy who sustained a traumatic forequarter amputation. There was a greenstick ulnar injury. By accentuating the deformity, it was possible to duplicate the radial head dislocation (Fig. 16-56). An important observation was that the annular ligament had *not* been torn but, instead, had been displaced over the radial head and lodged between the proximal radius and ulna. Such displacement of the ligament may certainly occur in the clinical situation and may be more common than a ligament tear (Fig. 16-58), which is less likely in any joint injury in a skeletally immature individual.

Diagnosis

For practical purposes, there is never an isolated fracture of the ulna (Fig. 16-59). The radius must be closely examined clinically and roentgenographically for injury to the proximal radiohumeral joint. Some fractures in Evans' series were greenstick, and the mildness of this injury may have prevented accurate interpretation and appreciation of the actual severity.[236] Wright also reported the combination of greenstick ulnar fracture with Monteggia injury.[319] A fracture of the ulna with angulation or overriding and without an accompanying fracture of the radius makes dislocation of the radial head suspect until proved otherwise. Proof may be obtained by including the elbow in all radiographs of suspected fractures of the ulna. In children it is significant that with a Monteggia lesion a high percentage of ulnar fractures are greenstick or even excessive bowing, lulling one into a false sense of security regarding the possible subluxation or dislocation of the proximal radius. Furthermore, it is often difficult to distinguish the exact location of the radial head, as it may not be ossified. Great care must be taken not to miss this particular diagnosis.

A patient with a Monteggia injury usually holds the elbow partially flexed, with the forearm in pronation (not unlike a young child with "nursemaid's elbow"). Any rotation of the forearm or flexion-extension of the elbow is painful and restricted. The dislocated radial head may be palpable. In the presence of soft tissue swelling or deformity of the forearm or elbow, a dislocated radial head may be difficult to demonstrate clinically.

The arm should be splinted in a position of comfort. The dislocated radial head may severely limit flexion or extension. Accordingly, anteroposterior views of the humerus, radius, and ulna and a lateral view of the elbow should be obtained.

Roentgenograms of the forearm must include the elbow and the wrist to rule out injuries at both the proximal and the distal ends of the radial head. Normally, the longitudinal axis of the radius passes through the ossification center of the capitellum of the humerus (in the lateral view). If it does not, the radial head may be subluxated or dislocated. A line drawn through the long axis of the radius should pass through the capitellum in *all* lateral views, from full extension to full flexion. Because of extension of ossification from capitellum into the trochlea, the location of the longitudinal axis in the anteroposterior view is not as reliable as it is in the lateral view. The radial head may be displaced anteriorly, laterally, or occasionally posteriorly.

If the roentgenographic beam is centered over the midforearm, as it often is, the elbow is included toward the edge of the radiograph, especially if the ulna is fractured at the mid- or distal shaft. Distortion may make the radiohumeral relation seem normal. The fractured ulna may be the predominant clinical and radiographic finding that focuses attention on the ulnar lesion. Accurate anteroposterior and lateral views must center on the elbow to give the best chance to delineate subtle injuries.

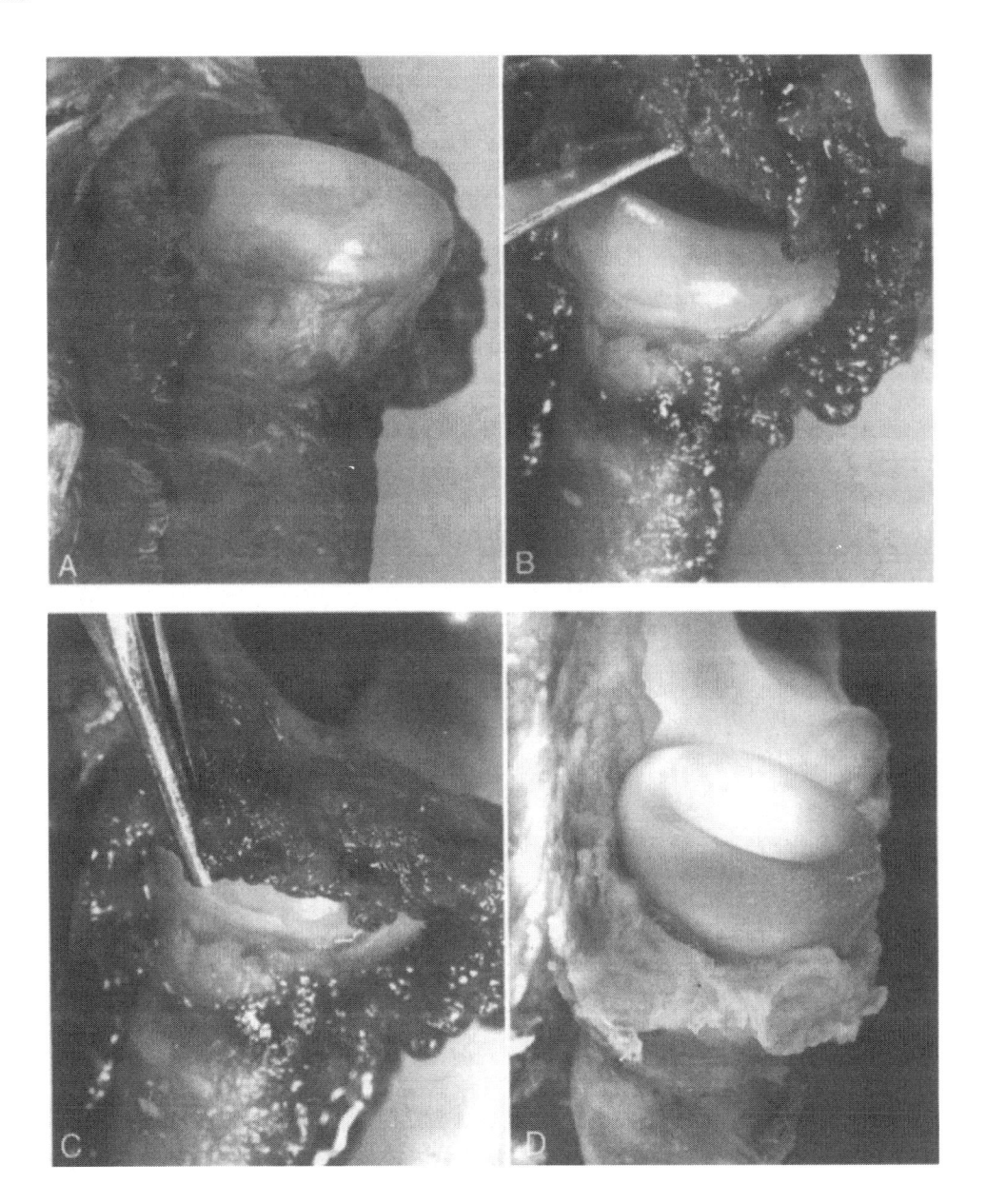

FIGURE 16-57. Specimen of the ulna and radial head shown radiographically in Figure 16-56. (A) Dislocated radial head. The annular ligament is between the radius and ulna. (B, C) The ligament is pulled onto the radial head. (D) Annular ligament back in its anatomic position. (Also see Figure 16-73.)

Treatment

To reduce the anterior Monteggia dislocation the forearm is placed in full supination, and longitudinal traction is applied. The elbow is gently flexed 90°–120° to relax the biceps. The radial head is repositioned by direct manual pressure. The angulated ulnar shaft is then reduced, which may not be difficult once the radial head has been repositioned. Following reduction, the radial head is usually stable, so long as the elbow is kept in acute flexion and the annular ligament is in its normal position (Fig. 16-60). Radiographic proof of reduction is essential (Fig. 16-61).

Tompkins pointed out that the ulnar fracture tends to develop an increased radial bow during immobilization.[310] This bowing is caused by the normal slight bowing of the ulna and the isometric contraction of the flexor muscles in the forearm. The forearm should be immobilized in neutral rotation or only slight supination, with the cast carefully molded over the lateral side of the ulna at the level of the fracture. So long as the elbow is in acute flexion of 110° or more, the biceps is relaxed and it is unnecessary to keep the forearm in full supination to maintain the reduction.

A posterior Monteggia fracture is usually reduced by applying traction to the forearm with the elbow in full extension. The radial head is reduced manually, and the posterior angulation of the ulnar fracture is anatomically aligned. The arm should be positioned in almost full extension, with a cast or splint then applied.

Once the radial head is reduced completely, the elbow should be flexed, extended, and then flexed again. If there

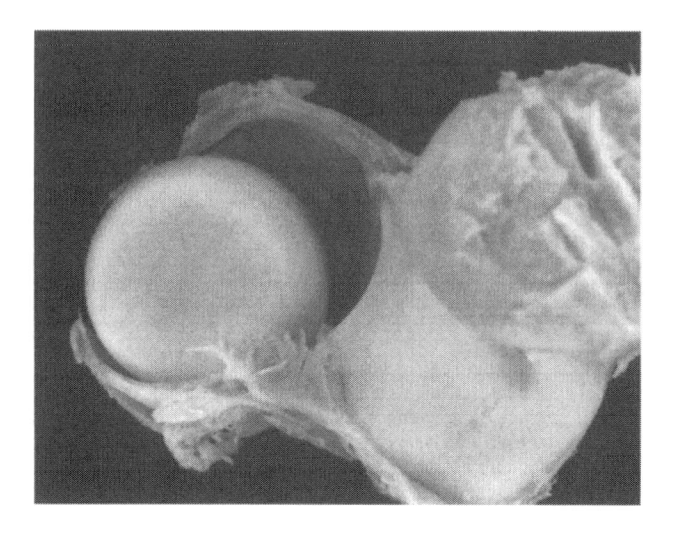

FIGURE 16-58. Specimen from an 11-year-old boy showing displacement of the radius after transection of the annular ligament.

Late Case

In instances in which the diagnosis is delayed or missed, open surgery may be necessary to reduce the radial head. Bell Tawse reported six children with undiagnosed Monteggia fractures.[211] Malunited fractures of the ulna with persistent dislocation of the radial head, restricted flexion, and increased cubitus valgus developed in all of these patients. These children originally had greenstick fractures of the ulna. Five were treated successfully by open reduction and reconstruction of the annular ligament. One patient experienced recurrence of the dislocated radial head.

Bell-Tawse constructed a new ulnar ligament by dissecting a slip of the triceps tendon, leaving it attached to the ulna,

is no interposition of the annulus, the radial head should remain reduced, especially if the reduced ulnar fragments are also reasonably stable. In children it is more important to reduce the radiocapitellar dislocation accurately than to gain absolute anatomic reduction of the ulnar fracture, as remodeling corrects minor ulnar angulations of 5°–10°. Residual angulation beyond 10° may enhance the risk of recurrent subluxation or dislocation. Confirming roentgenograms should be obtained at intervals to be certain that the radial head has not redislocated during the postreduction period.

Open reduction may be necessary, particularly when the radial head cannot be returned to its normal position by closed manipulation. Interposition of the annular ligament may prevent reduction of the radial head. Interposition is of three types: partial, in which portions of the ligament are interposed between the radial head and the ulna; complete, in which the radial head pulls out of the ligament, leaving it intact, an injury that accounts for most failures of reduction; or fragmentary, in which small cartilaginous or osteocartilaginous fragments may be present, most frequently associated with type 2 lesions. If open reduction is undertaken, great care must be taken during the postoperative assessment to avoid *inadequate* reduction (Fig. 16-62).

Open reduction of the radial head and repair of the annular ligament always carry the risk of subsequent ectopic ossification. Although closed reduction of the radial head displacement may be successful, open reduction may still be necessary for the accompanying ulnar injury.

Immobilization is maintained until there is union of the ulna, which ordinarily requires 3–8 weeks, depending on the patient's age. The patient's elbow is then progressively mobilized. Emphasis should be on flexion-extension exercises, followed by supination-pronation exercises.

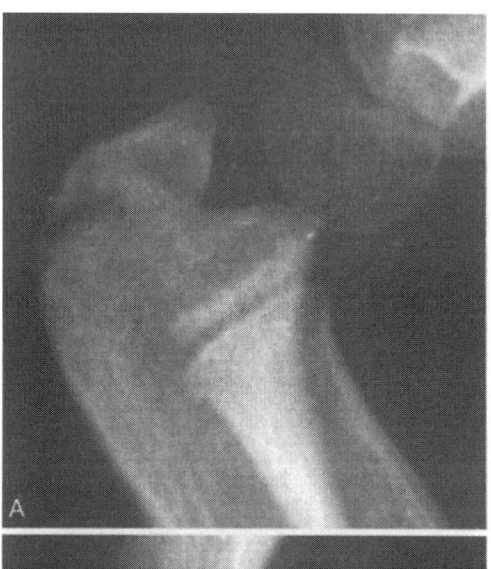

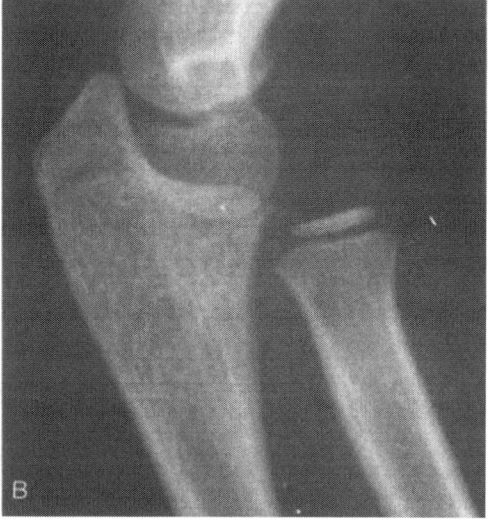

FIGURE 16-59. (A) Lateral view of an olecranon fracture associated with radial head dislocation. It was "reduced," casted, and allowed to heal. (B) Seven weeks later the olecranon fracture has healed, but the radial head is still dislocated. Such a divergent fracture-dislocation is a variation of the Monteggia injury.

FIGURE 16-60. (A) Mid-shaft ulnar fracture associated with proximal radial dislocation. As the distal radius and ulna are displaced dorsally (open arrow), the radial head levers out anteriorly (solid arrow). (B) Closed reduction of the dislocated radial head allowed closed reduction of the ulnar fracture.

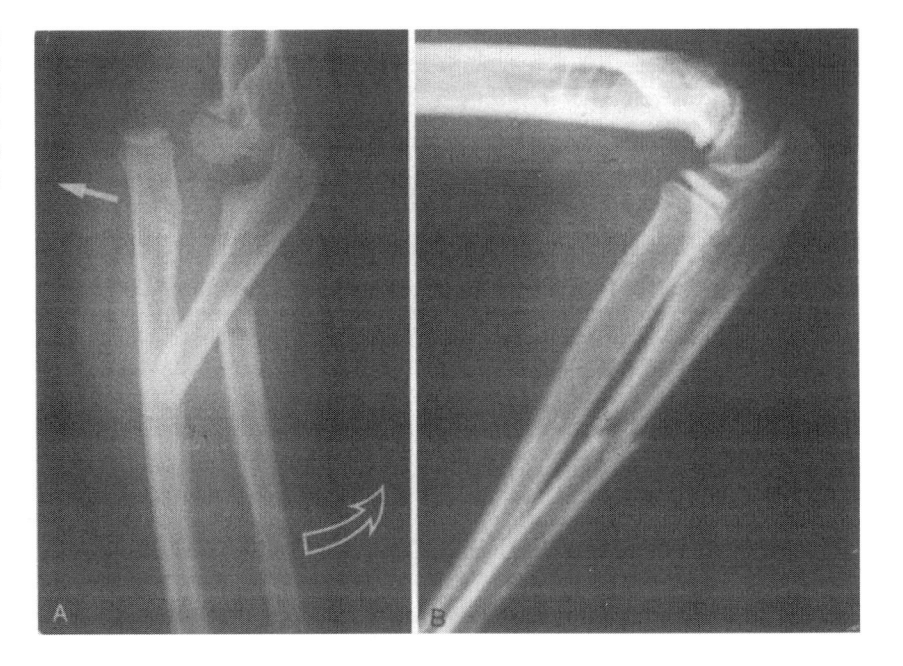

passing it around the neck of the radius, and securing it through a hole in the ulna.[211] Accurate dissection of the damaged or displaced annular ligament allows direct repair instead (Fig. 16-63). The radioulnar joint and the radiohumeral joint must be accurately reduced. The arm should be held in extension and supination probably for at least 6 weeks after open repair.

The triceps fascia may not grow or elongate as the child grows. Accordingly, the still enlarging (widening) radial neck may have to grow around the tissue, which can lead to a constrictive deformity of the radial neck (Fig. 16-64).

If reduction of the radial head is difficult because of ulnar shortening or angulation, it is better to lengthen the proximal ulna with an oblique (overlapping) osteotomy, rather than shortening the radial neck. It is not always necessary to fix the ulnar osteotomy internally.

There is no absolute time interval between injury and open reduction. If more than a year has elapsed since the injury, however, the chances of a good result decrease. I have performed the procedure on several children 19–26 months after injury (Fig. 16-63) and 4 years later for a "congenital" injury (Fig. 16-47), all with acceptable functional results, although none had anatomically normal radiographs.

A major factor influencing the possibility of reduction and the risk of recurrence of subluxation or dislocation postoperatively is the extent of biologic deformation of the radial head and the capitellum. I recommend an arthrogram with videotaped range of motion. A computed tomography (CT)

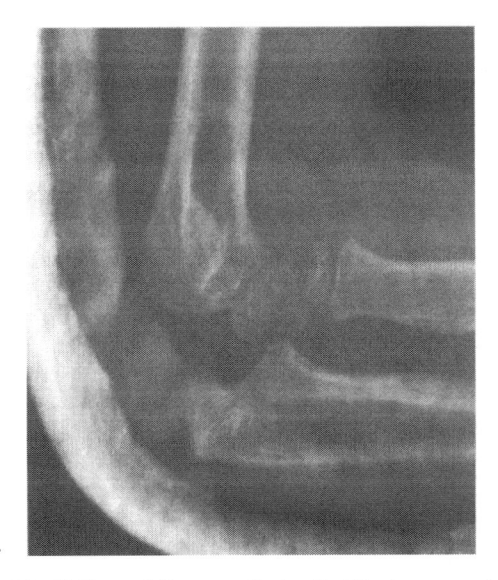

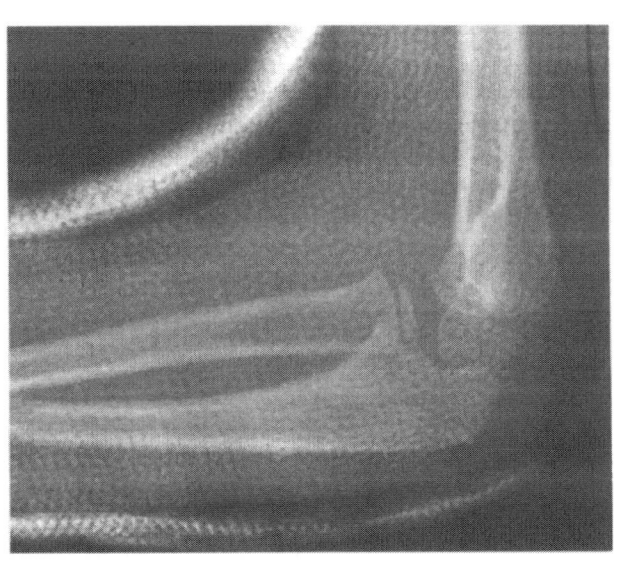

FIGURE 16-61. Neither of these patients (A, B) shows postreduction evidence of successful reduction of the radial head dislocation. Unfortunately, both were accepted as being adequately "reduced."

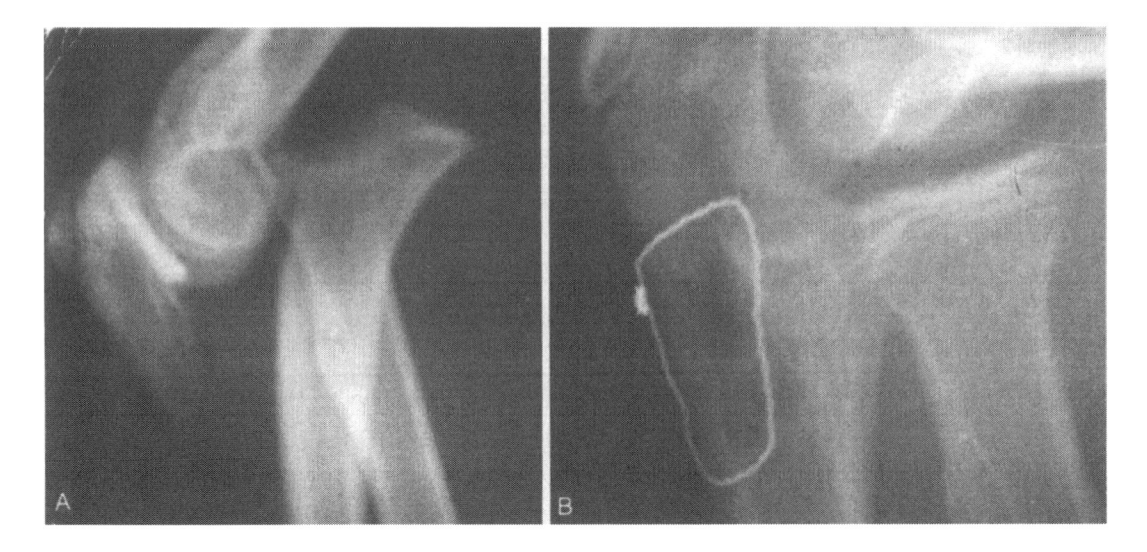

FIGURE 16-62. (A) Anterior Monteggia injury accompanying a proximal ulnar fracture. (B) The ulna was reduced and stabilized with a tension band wire; the radius was reduced without opening the radiohumeral joint.

or magnetic resonance imaging (MRI) scan with three-dimensional reconstruction also may provide essential information. A bullet-shaped radial head or a major indentation of the capitellum may presage a poor result. If a period of more than 3 months has elapsed, the possibility of postoperative heterotopic ossification causing ankylosis or fibrosis of the elbow following surgery must be considered.

In a child, a dislocated radial head is resected only if no other treatment is possible, as it may lead to cubitus valgus, prominence of the distal end of the ulna, and radial deviation of the head. Removing the radial head should be deferred until the completion of skeletal growth and then done only if decreased function or symptoms, especially pain, make it necessary. Individual circumstances, however, may necessitate removal of the radial head prior to skeletal maturation.

Results

In most reported series, children have fewer sequelae from a reduced Monteggia lesion than do adults. The major complications generally occur in adult patients, with usually no significant healing problems of the ulnar fracture in children and full return of elbow function. Redislocation of the radial head is rare. The incidence of residual subluxation has not been well documented.

Complications

Complications, although infrequent in children, may include the following: (1) Chronic dislocation and malposition as a result of misdiagnosis (Fig. 16-65), which is probably the most frequent complication. (2) Recurrent subluxation or dislocation of the radial head after initial closed reduction. (3) Posterior interosseous nerve neuropathy, which is most common in the type 3 injury pattern, although it has also been reported in type 1 and 2 patterns. Because spontaneous recovery usually occurs, exploration should not be attempted prior to 6 weeks after the injury. (4) Fracture of the radial head may occur with type 2 lesions and may lead to premature epiphysiodesis of the proximal radial physis. If the fractured radial head is displaced in the child, it should be reduced and kept in place, as removing the radial head in a child usually is not indicated. (5) Distal radioulnar joint disturbance may occur but is not believed to be significant. (6) Open wounds may cause infection. (7) Myositis ossificans (Fig. 16-66). (8) Radiohumeral ankylosis. (9) Radioulnar synostosis (Fig. 16-67). (10) Radioulnar dysfunction.

According to Thompson and Hamilton, the development of myositis ossificans is usually associated with dislocation of the entire elbow, rather than just the radial head.[309] The time lapse between injury and operation has been implicated as a predisposing factor in the formation of myositis.

Spinner and coworkers described posterior interosseous nerve palsy as a complication of Monteggia injuries in children.[303] The posterior interosseous nerve is the motor branch of the radial nerve. In 25% of all individuals the nerve lies in direct contact with the radius during its passage to the supinator, and in 30% a fibrous band (arch) is formed by the muscle insertion, by which the nerve is held close to the bone. This area may easily be injured during dislocation of the radial head. The area where the nerve passes around the proximal radius is most susceptible to a traction- or compression-type injury. With radial head dislocation, a lesion in continuity (stretching) is created at this level. Two of Spinner et al.'s cases were transitory, with neuropraxia-type lesions.[303] Stein and colleagues also described posterior interosseous nerve compression at the proximal edge of the supinator muscle through the fibrous arch of Frohse.[304]

Morris reported a case in which the radial head dislocation was irreducible because of entrapment of the radial nerve between the radial head and the ulna.[271] Jessing described nerve injuries in 6 of 14 patients.[255] Of the three children in his series, one had a type 1 lesion with complete

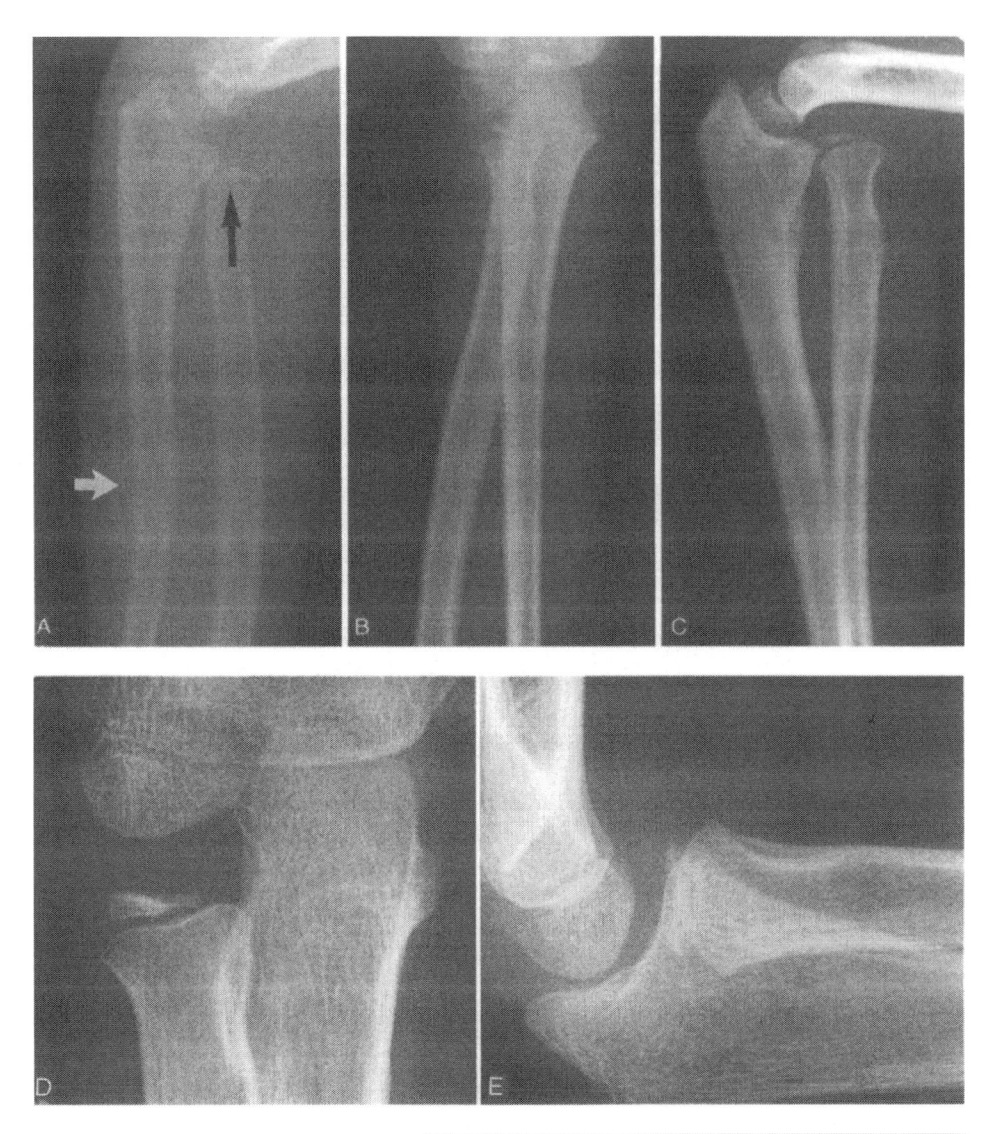

FIGURE 16-63. (A) Original injury. Treatment was directed to the greenstick ulnar fracture (white arrow). The dislocated radial head was missed at the time of injury and in several postreduction films (black arrow). (B, C) Two years later a secondary ossification center has developed in the proximal radius but not in the normal side. It may be due to injury-induced hyperemia. Open reduction and internal fixation were performed. The annular ligament, which was torn, displaced, and scarred, was dissected sharply from the anterior and posterior capsules. It was anatomically intact on the ulna. The damaged ends were repaired, restoring it to an annular configuration. (D, E) Appearance 6 months after operation. The radius is stable, and there is full return of motion. (F) Seven years after open reduction.

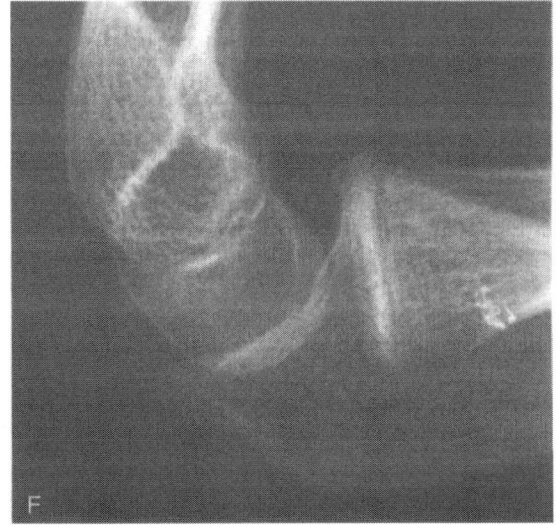

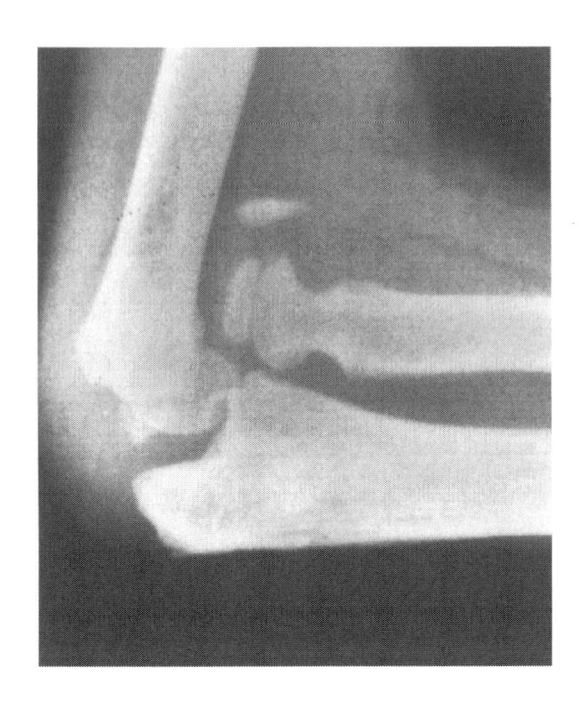

FIGURE 16-64. Bell-Tawse repair 3 years previously. The graft did not grow or elongate, causing indentation of the neck. There is also heterotopic bone formation.

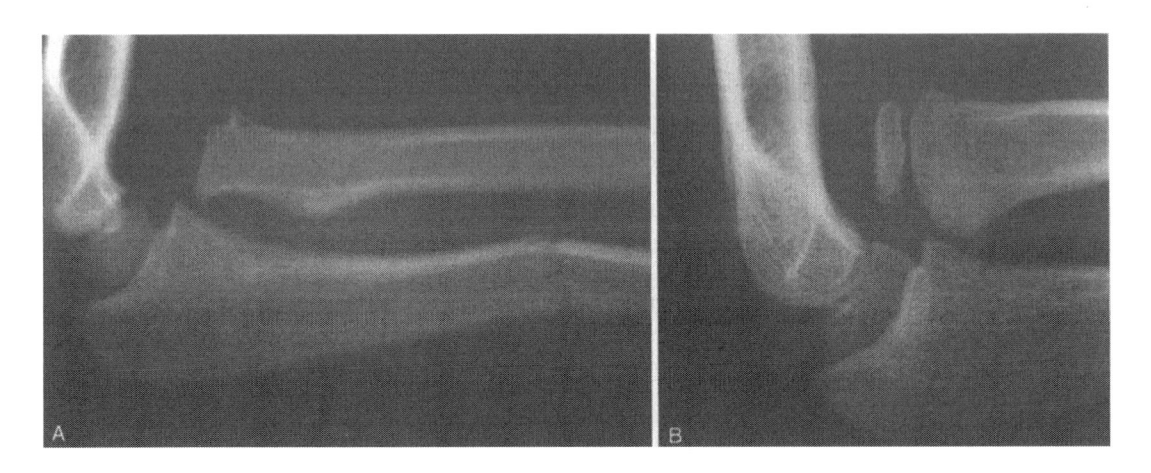

FIGURE 16-65. (A) Acute Monteggia injury. Unfortunately, the "reading" of this radiograph was "ulnar greenstick fracture." (B) Appearance 3 years later. The parents chose not to attempt reduction.

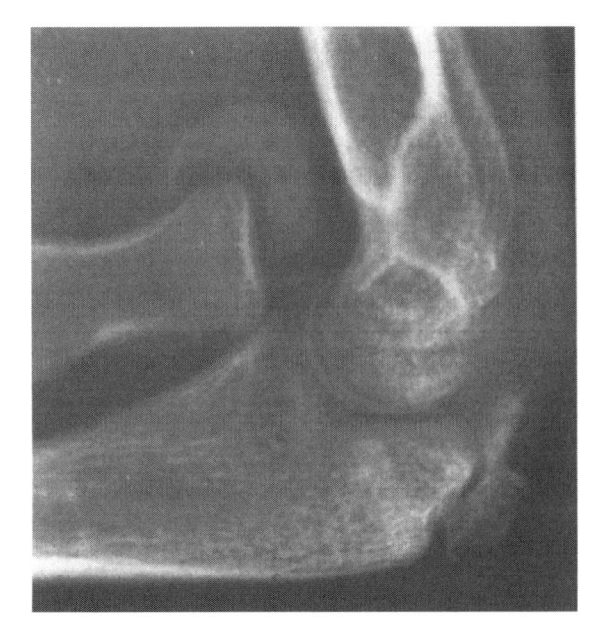

FIGURE 16-66. Ectopic bone around a redislocated radial head that had been treated by open reduction.

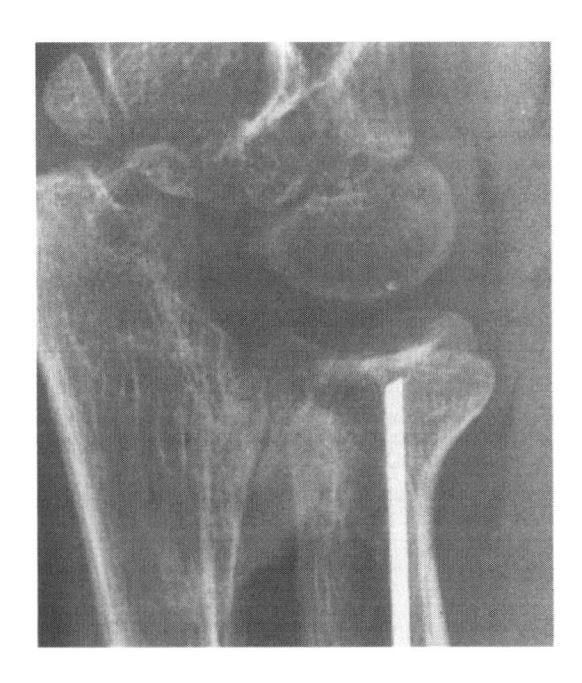

FIGURE 16-67. Synostosis after a Monteggia injury. This patient had a transarticular temporary fixation. The K-wire broke.

Diaphyseal Injuries

FIGURE 16-68. (A) Delayed healing of a Monteggia injury in a girl with an Erb's palsy. The radial head readily dislocated when the nonunion was angulated. (B) As healing slowly occurred, the radial head subluxated.

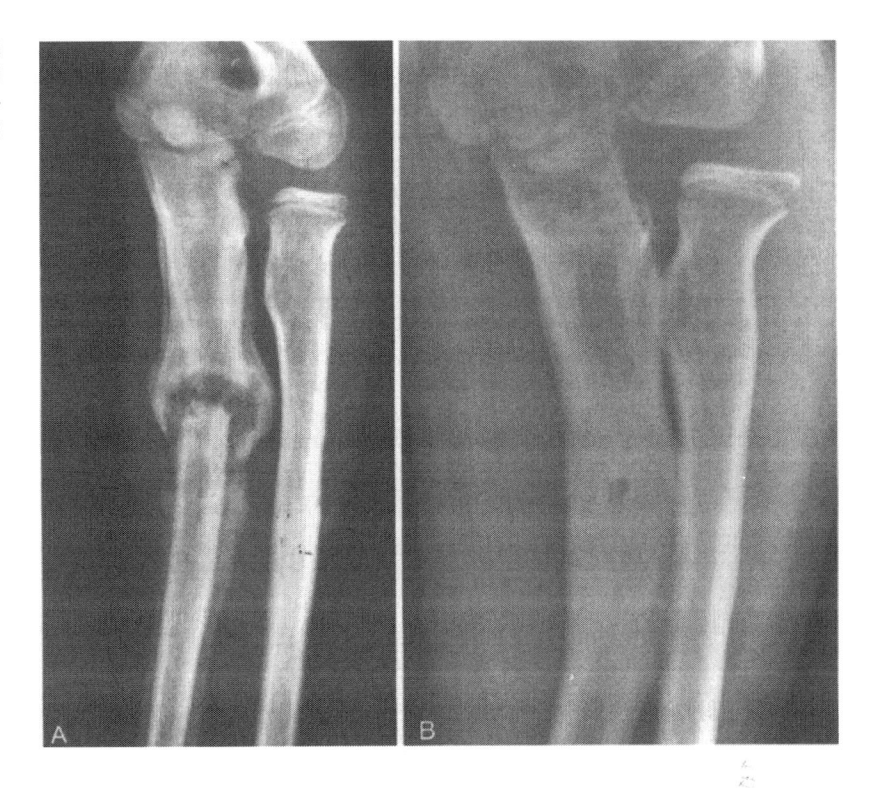

paralysis of the deep branch of the radial nerve. Beginning functional improvement was evident 8 weeks after the injury. Bado's 55 cases included 4 with radial nerve injuries, 2 with ulnar nerve injuries, and 1 with both ulnar and median nerve injuries.[207]

Preexistent neurologic deficits may create problems. The presence of neuromuscular imbalance from an Erb's palsy may allow chronic motion at the fracture site. In the case shown in Figure 16-68, the ulnar fracture was readily diagnosed, but disruption of the lateral and annular ligaments was not originally appreciated. The delayed union of the fracture eventually healed after surgical intervention, but the radiocapitellar joint remained unstable.

Chronic dislocation is sometimes compatible with normal use of the elbow. Many patients have no symptoms and are able to use the arm in sports and daily activities.

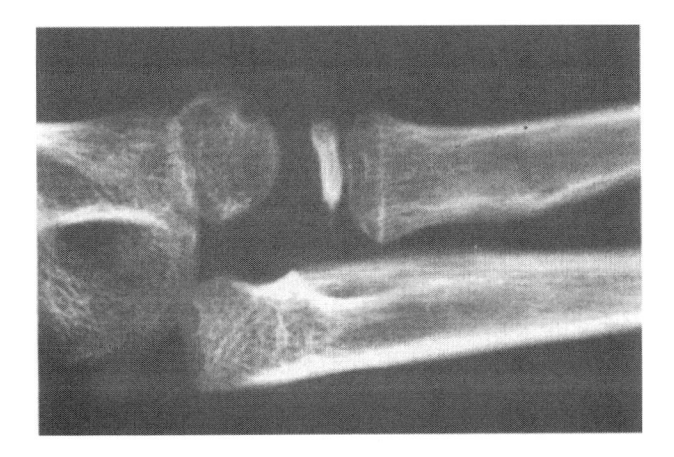

FIGURE 16-69. Ischemic necrosis of the radial head. Capitellar change is evident.

A rare complication of the Monteggia injury is ischemic necrosis (Fig. 16-69). The infrequent occurrence of this complication is probably related to the variability of the circulation to the radial head.

Another infrequent complication arises with transarticular temporary stabilization. If the patient decides to "mobilize" the joint, a K-wire may be bent. If repetitive motion is attempted, it may lead to pin failure (Fig. 16-67).

Diaphyseal Injuries

Diaphyseal injuries of the radius, ulna, or both are common in children.[24–38,322–437] The severity may vary from pure bowing to greenstick to complete fracture with displacement. The diaphyseal level of the fracture varies. In children there is a greater tendency for the radius and ulna to deform or fracture (whether greenstick or complete) at the same level, rather than at significantly different levels. There is also a likelihood of complete fracture of one bone, with plastic deformation or greenstick injury or the other. The thick periosteum allows maintenance of some skeletal tissue continuity, even when both bones are displaced. This highly osteogenic tissue also allows excellent healing of both fractures by closed means. When the adolescent is approaching skeletal maturity, the periosteum loses some of this capacity, increasing the risk of delayed union or nonunion.

Classification

Radioulnar fractures follow many patterns. There may be simple plastic deformation (bowing), greenstick injury, or complete fracture. The bones may be angulated or displaced, with or without significant overriding. The bones may be fractured at different levels, or only one bone may be fractured. However, one must look carefully for bowing or greenstick failure of the seemingly noninjured bone or a Monteggia or Galeazzi injury. Greenstick fractures are often evident only in one projection, whereas a view at 90° may slow a seemingly intact, uninjured bone. Oblique views may even be necessary to delineate the injury pattern specifically.

Plastic deformation is a failure pattern affecting tubular bones such as the fibula, radius, and ulna (see Chapters 2, 5, 6). The deformation is often difficult to diagnose. Because of microstructural failure, permanent deformation may be introduced (Figs. 16-70). Stress fracture may also occur (Fig. 16-71). More often there is definite evidence of a greenstick injury (Figs. 16-72, 16-73). Cortical failure may be minimal. The radius often sustains a greenstick failure, whereas the ulna, instead, undergoes plastic deformation (Fig. 16-74). The ulna may also sustain a greenstick fracture without apparent radial injury. Both bones may sustain greenstick injuries (Fig. 16-75).

Angular deformation varies. The radius may deform 30°–40° without concomitant ulnar injury. The periosteum is disrupted on the tensile failure side in such angulation but is usually intact along the compression side, a factor that should be considered during any reduction manipulation. Even when both bones are fractured, only *one* may be angulated. Angulation varies from mild to severe. The true degree of angulation may require oblique views. Mid-shaft angulation should be defined as accurately as possible and subsequently corrected, as osseous remodeling is least likely in the mid-shaft. Similarly, overriding varies significantly.

Diagnosis

Roentgenograms should include both the wrist and elbow joints to be certain there is no dislocation of either the proximal (Monteggia injury) or the distal (Galeazzi injury) radioulnar joint. It is possible to have a Monteggia injury with a fracture of the radius or plastic deformation of the ulna, as well as the typical pattern of a fracture of the ulna. Initial roentgenograms should be true anteroposterior and lateral views. Nonstandard angles and degrees of rotation may complicate interpretation but may eventually be necessary to better define fracture patterns and the extent of traumatic deformation.

The radius is a curved bone that is cam-shaped in cross section at several levels. Malrotation of the radius may be recognized by a break in the smooth curve of the bone or a difference in the width of the cortices of the apposed fracture fragments. In fractures of the forearm, palmar or flexor bowing (i.e., of the apex) is usually a sign of pronation deformity, whereas dorsal or extensor bowing (at the apex) usually signifies a supination deformity.

Evans drew attention to the bicipital tuberosity roentgenographic sign.[7] The problem in the younger child is that this region of the tuberosity may be minimally developed and may not suffice as an accurate indicator, as it does in older children, adolescents, and adults. The tuberosity normally lies medially when the forearm is fully supinated (i.e., it faces the ulna). It lies posteriorly in midposition and laterally in full pronation. If there is any question about this positioning, a similarly rotated view of the normal, uninvolved arm may be obtained. The estimated degree of proximal rotation may be used as a guideline to determine the best treatment position in which to place the distal fragments relative to the proximal fragments.

In infants and young children under 3 years of age (especially under 18 months), child abuse must be considered as part of the differential diagnosis, especially when the fracture already has callus or when metachronous, multiple fractures are present (see Chapter 11).

Neurovascular Injury

Because nerves and blood vessels are infrequently injured in children's forearm fractures, there is a tendency to overlook the possibility of such damage. Detailed, well documented examination is essential. The median nerve is protected from the radius by intervening layers of muscle. The ulnar nerve is close to bone and is occasionally damaged, especially with open fractures near the lower end. Warren described two cases of anterior interosseous nerve palsy.[432] In both cases there was complete, but temporary, paralysis of the flexor pollicis longus and index finger segment of the flexor digitorum profundus. Both patients made a full, spontaneous recovery without exploration of the nerve. The anterior interosseous nerve branches from the median nerve distal to the neck of the radius and passes along with the anterior interosseous vessels extending along the interosseous membrane. Because of the proximity of the nerve to the radius, it is subject to injury in a displaced forearm fracture.

Davis and Green reported six nerve injuries: four median, one ulnar, and one posterior interosseous.[31] All cleared spontaneously within 3 weeks, suggesting that each was a neuropraxia. The possibility of nerve injury is particularly important in distal third fractures; adequate assessment of the median nerve must be done. Although it happens infrequently, the medial nerve may be traumatized when the distal fragment is dorsally displaced and the forearm is shortened.

Compartment Syndrome

Despite the presence of closed fascial spaces in the forearm, the frequency of compartment syndrome followed by ischemic (Volkmann's) contracture is low in children, especially when compared to the risk in supracondylar fractures. The fractures, particularly when complete, tend to allow dissipation of intracompartmental pressure into the more superficial area and throughout other compartments. Care must be taken to watch for increased pressure in the anterior compartment. Clinical monitoring of pressure is appropriate. If signs warrant such a diagnosis, the child should be admitted, the cast bivalved, and the arm elevated. If symptoms of excessive pain and pain with finger motion do not rapidly dissipate, increased pressure is likely and should be addressed with fasciotomies or, better yet, direct measurement of compartment pressures. This complication is discussed in detail in Chapter 10.

Rotation

Before discussing treatment, it is essential to consider rotation (supination-pronation), as restoration of this function

Diaphyseal Injuries

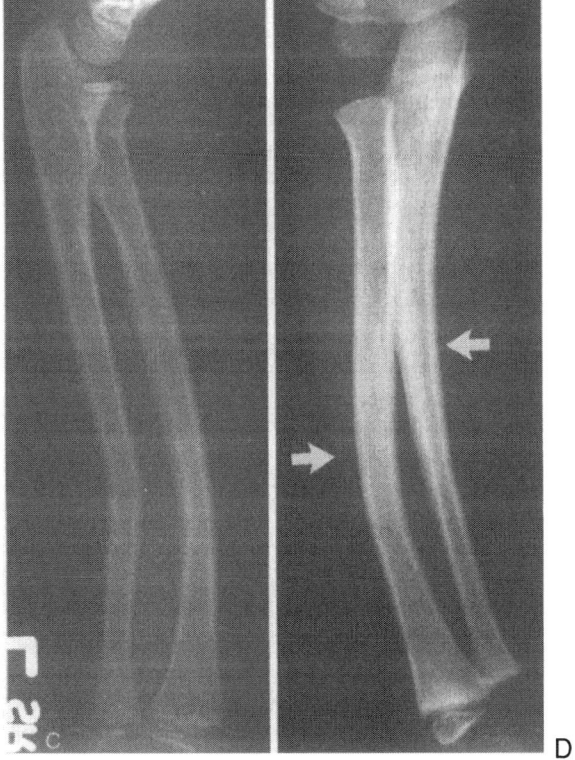

FIGURE 16-70. (A) Plastic deformation of the ulna (arrow). (B) Contralateral side. This girl lacks full supination and pronation. (C) Plastic deformation of the radius with ulnar fracture. (D) Greenstick bowing of both bones (arrows) in a 4-year-old.

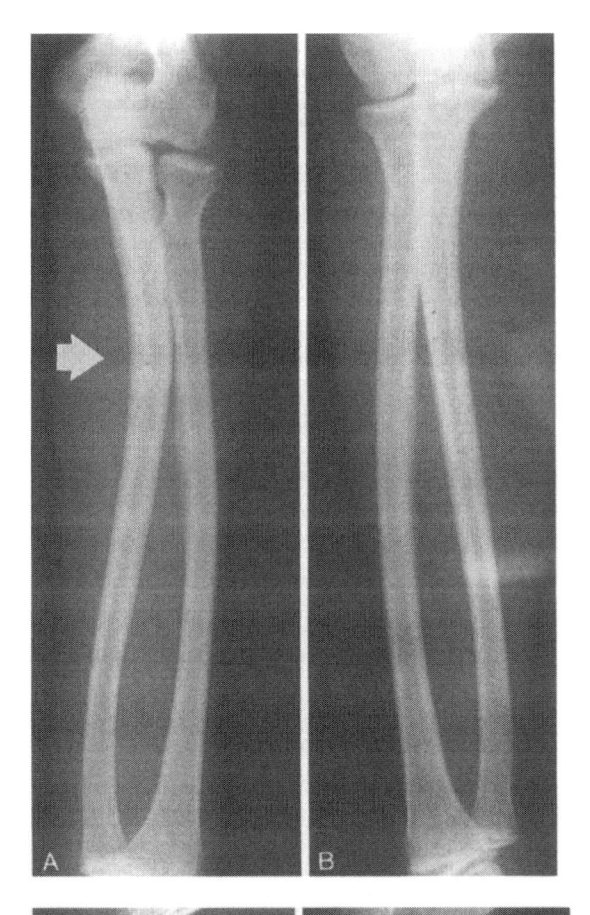

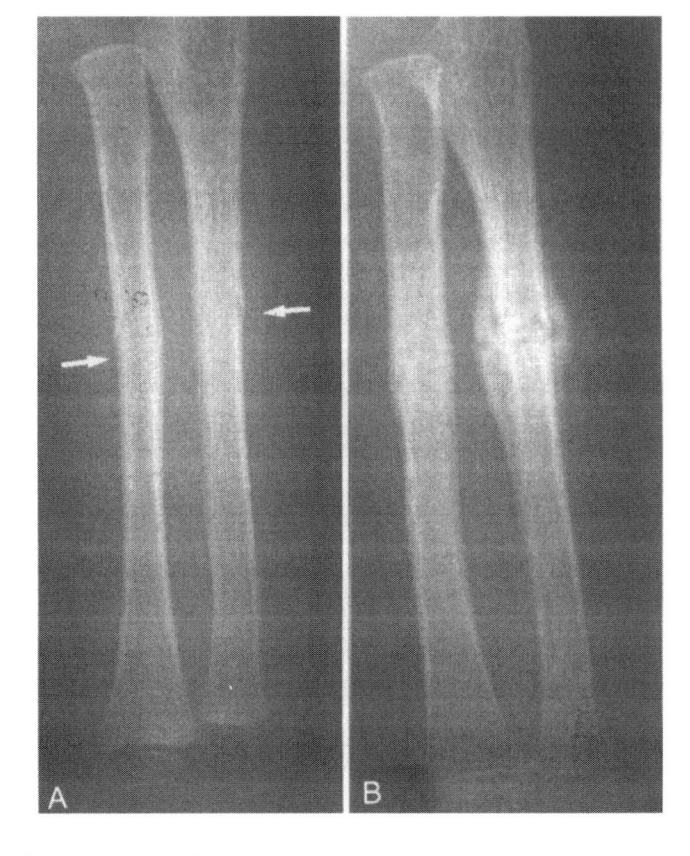

FIGURE 16-71. (A) Nondisplaced stress injury (arrows) of the radius and ulna. (B) Eight weeks later.

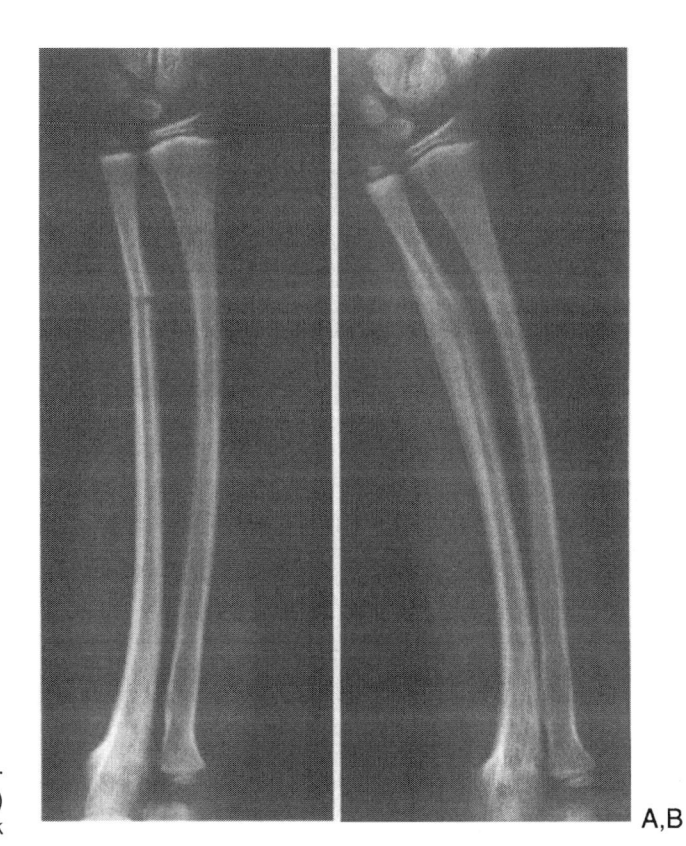

FIGURE 16-72. (A) Greenstick fracture of the ulna. (B) Four months later.

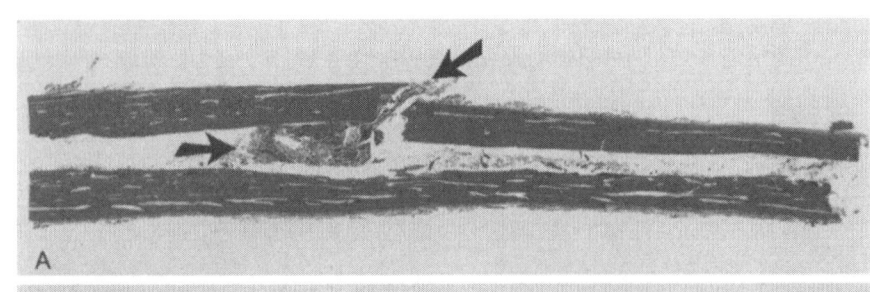

FIGURE 16-73. Greenstick injury shown radiographically in Figures 16-56 and 16-57. (A) Histologic view showing entrapped muscle (arrows). (B) Duplication of bending to fracture one cortex.

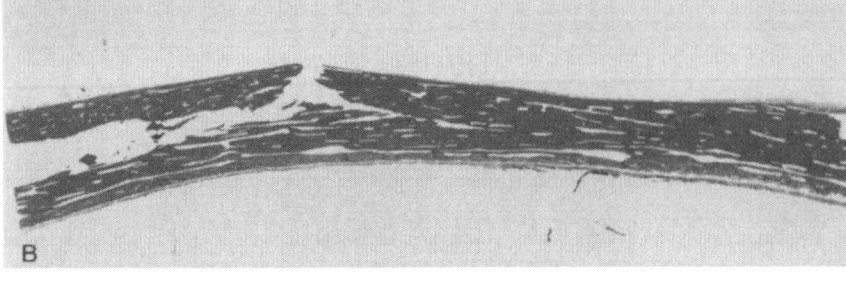

is an important aspect of treatment. Forearm rotation normally has a range of 180°.[15,398,405] The vertically paired proximal and distal radioulnar joints move synchronously. Normal radial bowing is essential to the rotational axis of the radius about the ulna and should be maintained in any reduction. Failure to do so potentially disrupts the rotational cone (Fig. 16-76).

Although a child may adapt functionally to a decrease in rotational motion up to 50%, forearm fractures should be treated in a manner that avoids, as much as possible, any significant loss of normal supination and pronation.[424] Rotation is lost with loss of longitudinal alignment of one or both bones. This causes variable widening and narrowing of the interosseous membrane during attempted rotatory movements.

Loss of rotation is a common problem after forearm fractures, no matter what the level of fracture.[348] Knight and Purvis found a residual rotational deformity between 20° and 60° in 60% of their patients.[373] Evans found a malrotation deformity of more than 30° in 56% of the cases.[7,349] The

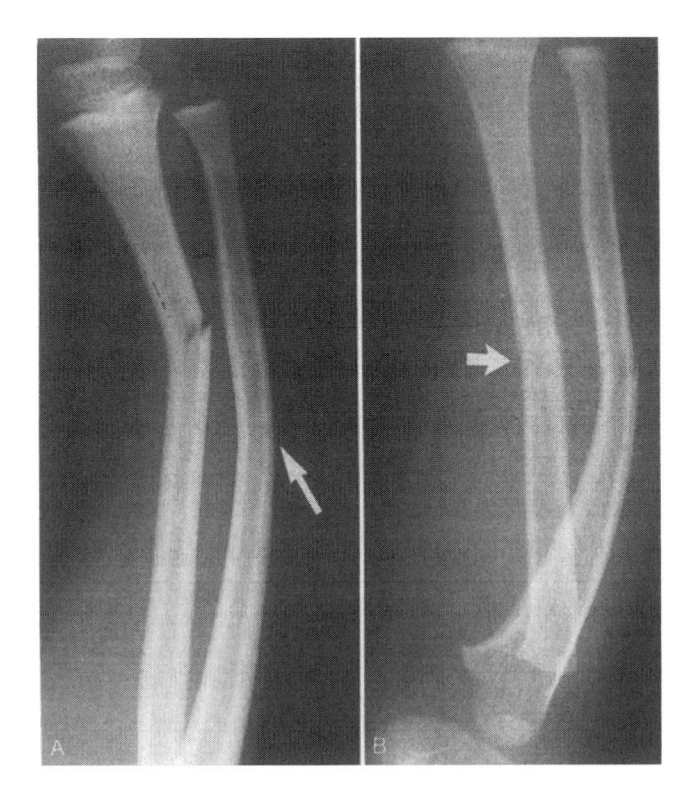

FIGURE 16-74. (A) Radial greenstick and ulnar plastic failure pattern. Ulnar failure is proximal (arrow) to the radial fracture. (B) Ulnar greenstick fracture with barely discernible radial injury (arrow). It was a hyperpronation injury.

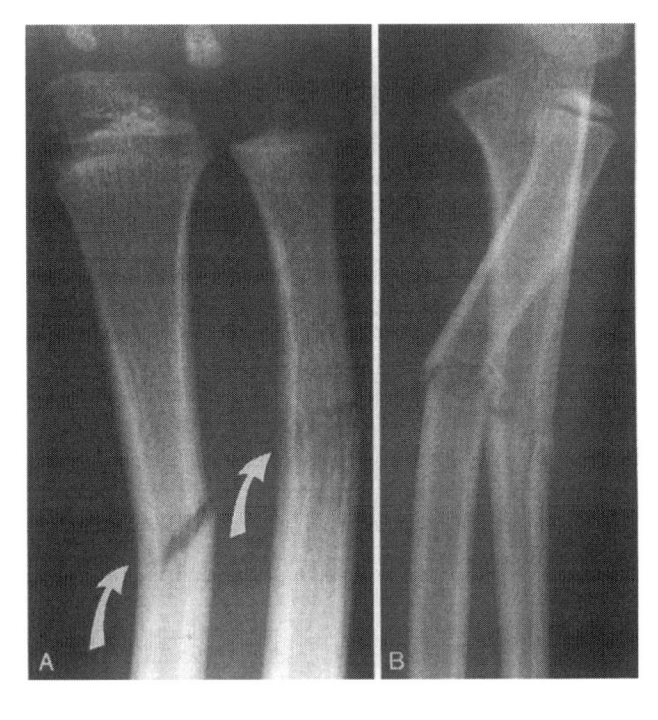

FIGURE 16-75. (A) Greenstick injury of both radius and ulna. The lateral cortex is intact on both (arrows). (B) Greenstick fractures of both bones. The radius is angulated, and the ulna is spontaneously reduced.

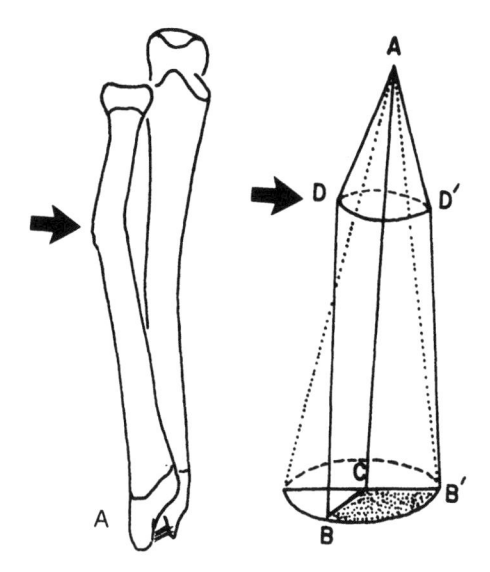

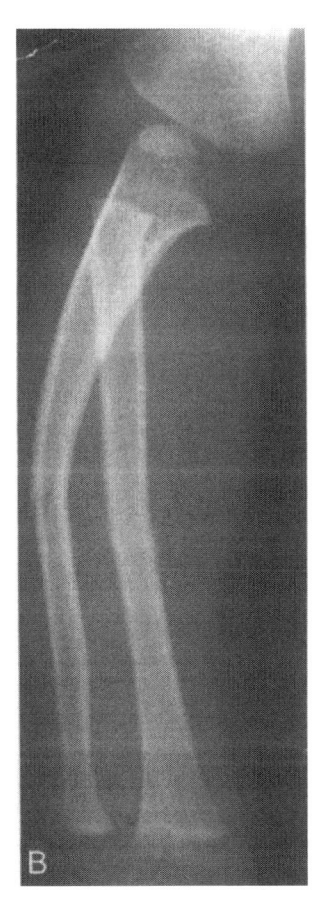

FIGURE 16-76. (A) Angular malunion introduces a frustrum (D) into the normal cone of rotation, thereby limiting the area (stippling) of the cone base. In this example, residual pronation of the distal radius restricts full supination. (B) Type of angulation that may seriously impair forearm rotation. See Figure 16-9 for normal rotational axis cone.

distal fragment is usually pronated, so supination is primarily affected.

Fractures have been produced in skeletally mature cadavers to determine the effects of various degrees of angular malunion.[349] Malrotation of 10° limited rotation by 10°, but 10° of angular malunion limited rotation by 20°. Bayonet apposition did not limit rotation. Pure narrowing of the interosseous space was important in proximal fractures. Narrowing impeded rotation by causing the bicipital tuberosity to impinge on the ulna. Malalignment of the fractures of the ulnar metaphysis increased articular tension so the head of the radius was not free to rotate. These observations probably are readily applicable to children.

Matthews and colleagues tested specimens for the effect of residual angulation from simulated fractures of both bones of the forearm.[386] Ten- and twenty-degree angulations were selected for testing. With 10° of malunion there was little significant functional loss of forearm rotation, but with 20° of angulation, in any direction, there was statistically significant and functionally important loss of forearm rotation.[386]

Christensen and colleagues tried to ascertain why there is a difference of opinion in the literature concerning the proper positions of immobilizing the forearm that would ensure separation of the radius and ulna and prevent cross-union.[5] They studied 36 adult cadaver forearms. The smallest interosseous distance was in pronation. The greatest distance was in midposition. The widest base was on the middle-third of the forearm. They further showed that the interosseous membrane was tense in 30° of supination but became increasingly relaxed with further supination or pronation.

It is usually possible to recognize these rotational deformities and correct them when treating the fracture. The variability of supination and pronation of the proximal and distal fragments may be demonstrated radiographically. If the upper part of the arm lies in supination and the distal part looks as if it is pronated, supination should be the major reduction direction to move the fracture back to anatomic position. Infrequently, the fracture reduction is sufficiently stable to allow testing of the range of movement. Of course, a full range of movement indicates an accurate reduction. Determination of the correct rotational position in which to immobilize fractures of both bones of the forearm is important to prevent a corresponding limitation of rotational movement.

Significant rotational deformity may be created at the time of reduction of complete fractures if they are manipulated improperly. The concept of pronating all distal third fractures, supinating all proximal third fractures, and leaving middle third fractures in neutral has been repeatedly recommended as the proper method of reduction since Evans' original article on the rotatory nature of forearm fractures.[349] *The "rule of the thirds," however, should not be applied rigidly to these fractures.* Reduction of the complete distal third fracture by forcible pronation may in fact result in malrotation of the fracture site, a deformity that usually does not completely correct with growth, regardless of the age of the child.

Accurate reduction of the bone ends is best accomplished when the rotational deformity is corrected and fluoroscopically assessed. Even a small inaccuracy can prevent the interlocking of the bone ends, on which stability depends. The orthodox position in which to immobilize these fractures is that of full supination for the upper third and of midposition (neutral rotation) for fractures of the middle and lower thirds. These positions are based on the anatomic arrangement and function of the pronator and supinator muscles in the forearm. It is unreasonable to suppose that all fractures at a given level present the same degree of rotational deformity. Other factors may also be involved, such as variations in the direction and leverage of muscle pull with varying degrees of angulation of the fragments, differences in the tension of the biceps with flexion and extension of the elbow, and the effect of the interosseous membrane. The position, with respect to rotation, in which such fractures should be immobilized is governed by the degree of rotation of the upper radial fragment, the upper fragment of the ulna being stable because of the type of elbow articulation.

It has been standard teaching that fractures of the upper third of the radius and ulna be immobilized in full supination because the proximal fragment may be pulled into supination by the biceps and supinator muscles.[339,346,348] Some suggest that this arbitrary concept is a mistake because cases in which the fully supinated position is used may have a significant incidence of malunion. In full pronation the brachioradialis muscle may act as a bowstring to increase the dorsal tilt of the distal fragment and cause angulation or redisplacement. However, flexing the wrist may counteract this deformity. An accurate study of the radiograph is required to decide whether these lesions are pronation or supination injuries, and the degree of rotation should be assessed to determine the position of greatest stability. Gainor and Hardy recommended immobilizing these fractures in full extension to control rotation.[358] Manipulation under fluoroscopy is often helpful to determine the optimum position of stability.

Although remodeling often corrects 30°–40° of angular displacement of a distal metaphysis in a child with sufficient remaining growth, remodeling usually does *not* do anything more than round off the ends of malunited fractures of the diaphysis, and it never corrects rotational deformity accompanying the malunion. It must always be remembered that angular fractures of the forearm are associated with some degree of rotational deformity. Any loss of motion due to mid-shaft or proximal fractures tends to be permanent.

Treatment

When treating fractures of the radius and ulna in children, longitudinal (axial) and rotational alignments are the most important goals of reduction. Reduction may be more difficult when the radial fracture is proximal to the ulnar fracture. Reduction of these fractures may be more difficult to maintain with the elbow in flexion. Sometimes they are more stable in extension. Overriding is acceptable so long as longitudinal alignment and the interosseous spacing are maintained.

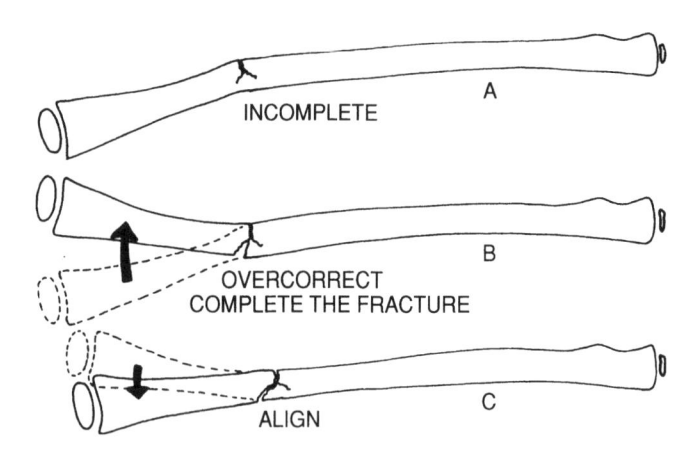

FIGURE 16-77. Completion of the fracture in greenstick injuries of the radius and ulna.

The completion of greenstick fractures may be necessary. Failure to do so may predispose to recurrent displacement or angular deformation. Reangulation may be prevented by placing the arm in the correct degree of pronation or supination and holding this position in the cast. In general, greenstick fractures should be slightly overcorrected by slow manipulation to take the plastic deformation out of the fracture (Fig. 16-77). Overcorrection may complete the fracture and may be accompanied by an audible or palpable crack. If this is not done, the plastic deformation may reappear, even in a cast (Fig. 16-78). This observation applies primarily to mid-shaft fractures.

Sanders and Heckman reported 14 cases of plastic deformation of the radius and ulna and suggested a method of pressure application over a period of several minutes to lessen the plastic deformation.[414] They thought this reduced the clinical deformity, allowed treatment of any accompanying fractures, and led to earlier return of full supination and pronation in the forearm. Certainly, their method of prolonged pressure should be attempted prior to considering open reduction or osteoclasis.

Complete fractures of the radius and ulna may be troublesome. The following guidelines should be used: (1) Good reductions must be attained and held with a well-molded cast. (2) Cortical apposition, even if bayonet, is adequate so long as rotation is correct, the interosseous space is preserved, and there is no longitudinal axial angulation. (3) Immobilize the fracture in the position—*any position*—in which the alignment is correct and the reduction feels (and

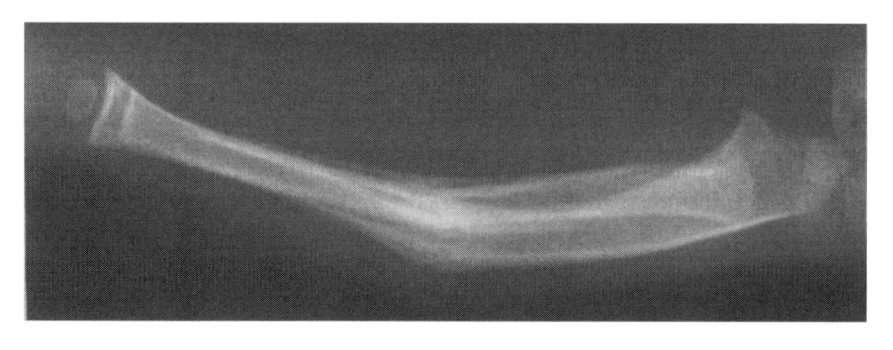

FIGURE 16-78. Residual angular malunion complicating greenstick fractures in which the injury was not "completed."

fluoroscopically appears) stable. (4) Minor improvements can and should be made through remanipulation up to 3–4 weeks after injury, at which time the fracture becomes mechanically firm. *Do not be afraid to remanipulate.* (5) Be prepared to carry out either closed reduction with percutaneous intramedullary rodding or open reduction and internal fixation, even in children under the age of 10 years, rather than accept a poor position. Skin traction is a method that may be used to try to attain a reduction during the first few days after significant injury, subsequently attempting another closed reduction. (6) Always warn the parents about the possibilities of remanipulation of short-term recurrent deformity to prevent long-term deformity and loss of function.

The method of reduction advocated for complete fractures of the radius alone or the radius and ulna together precludes the possibility of a rotational deformity. After enough analgesia, anesthesia, or both have been administered to provide adequate muscle relaxation, the arm may be suspended by finger traps and a counterweight of 10–15 pounds applied across the upper arm. Enough time should elapse to allow the fracture to be brought out to length and to correct the overriding of the distal fragment, although a toggle maneuver is often necessary to connect the cortices. After length has been restored in this fashion, the fracture is allowed to seek its own level of rotation, rather than manipulating the distal fragment into any preconceived position of theoretically correct rotation. With the forearm suspended in fingertip traction, the two fragments usually spontaneously assume correct rotational alignment. Such fractures usually attain a neutral or slightly pronated position.

No rotatory manipulation of the fracture should be done once the overriding has been corrected and the cortices engaged. The examiner should check to see if there is adequate rotational correction by assessing the width of the cortices of the two fragments, which is usually easily recognized by the disparity of width between the two fracture fragments. Remodeling may correct the cortical width difference, but it does *not* correct the rotational (or angular) deformity.

The width of the interosseous space often can be restored by manual pressure to the soft tissue between the bones, provided swelling is not excessive. If swelling is present, attempts to reduce the fracture may be deferred several days and overhead traction or splinting used until the soft tissue swelling subsides. When traction is maintained, a long arm cast is applied with the elbow in 90° of flexion and the forearm fully supinated. The cast must be molded well over the palmar aspect of the radius. Again, pressure is applied to maintain the interosseous space while the cast material is consolidating.

Failure to restore normal alignment, with regard to both longitudinal and rotational deformation, may cause restriction of pronation and supination of the forearm after fracture healing. Bayonet or side-to-side apposition with some overriding is acceptable, provided the ulna and radius do not deviate toward one another and that the interosseous space is maintained (Figs. 16-79, 16-80). Reduction of

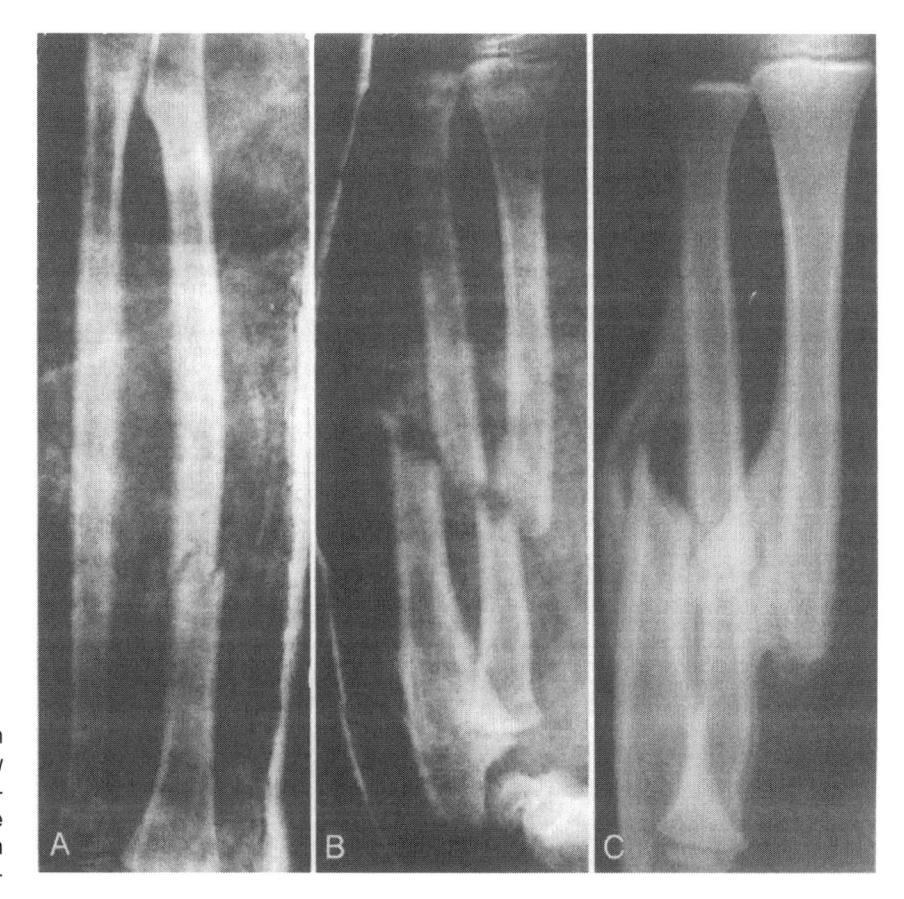

FIGURE 16-79. Satisfactory closed reduction of both bones. (A) The anteroposterior view shows longitudinal alignment and good maintenance of the interosseous space. (B) The lateral view shows mild overriding but with adequate longitudinal alignment. (C) Subperiosteal new bone.

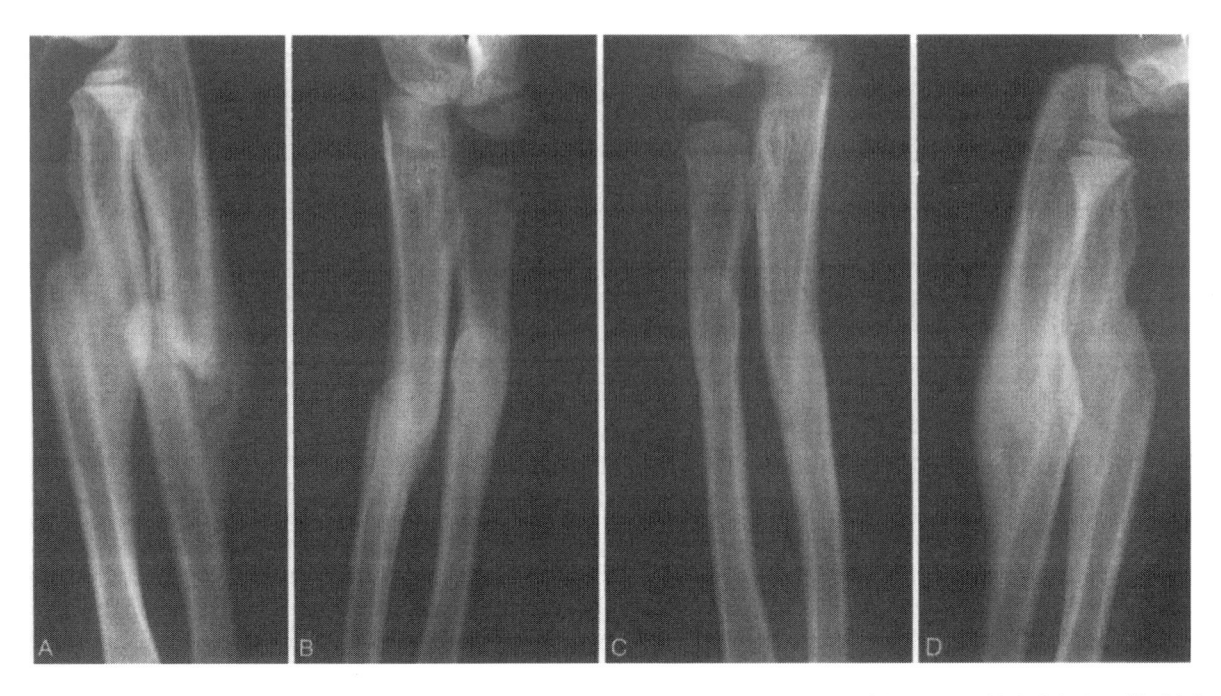

FIGURE 16-80. (A, B) Appearance 4 months after injury of displaced, overriding fractures in a child with multiple injuries. (C, D) Appearance 16 months later. Extensive remodeling has occurred.

one bone with continued overriding of the other is not usually an acceptable reduction. To determine if this condition exists, it is best to obtain true anteroposterior and lateral films. Any obliquity in the film may be deceptive in terms of the degree of angular deformation (longitudinal malalignment).

These fractures must be maintained in an immobilized position in a well-molded cast with three-point fixation (Fig. 16-81) for longer than most children's fractures (about 6–8 weeks), to allow satisfactory callus formation. The cast should be changed as necessary to compensate for decreased swelling.

Because deformation and angular malalignment may occur at a much later time after the initial injury, it is imperative that serial roentgenograms be examined to detect any loss of position. If closed manipulation is unsuccessful, open surgical reduction may be indicated, especially in the older child (over 10 years) or the patient who is close to skeletal maturity. A well-padded cast that acts as a compression dressing may be applied and combined with elevation. The fracture should be remanipulated 5–7 days later. Skeletal traction may also be applied.

Open reduction of both bone fractures in young children may be necessary. There is a belief that open reduction is forbidden in children, but not all fractures of both bones can be successfully managed by closed reduction (Figs. 16-82 to 16-84). Internal fixation is preferable to malunion. High oblique fractures in teenagers are likely to require open reduction.

There is an increasing acceptance of percutaneous pinning of one or both bones. With this technique flexible rods (of which several varieties are available: Rush rods) and the Nancy nail are inserted through small metaphyseal fenestrations. The radius is best approached in a distal to proximal method. The ulna is easier to approach in a proximal to distal direction. Because of relatively early maturation and growth of the proximal end of the ulna, a rod or nail may be inserted through an epiphyseal drill hole. However,

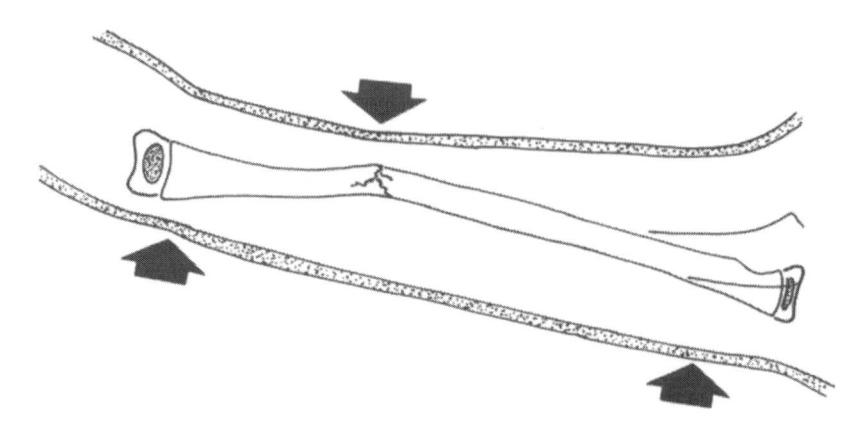

FIGURE 16-81. Principle of three-point fixation (arrows) of the greenstick fracture to prevent reangulation while the arm is in the cast.

Diaphyseal Injuries

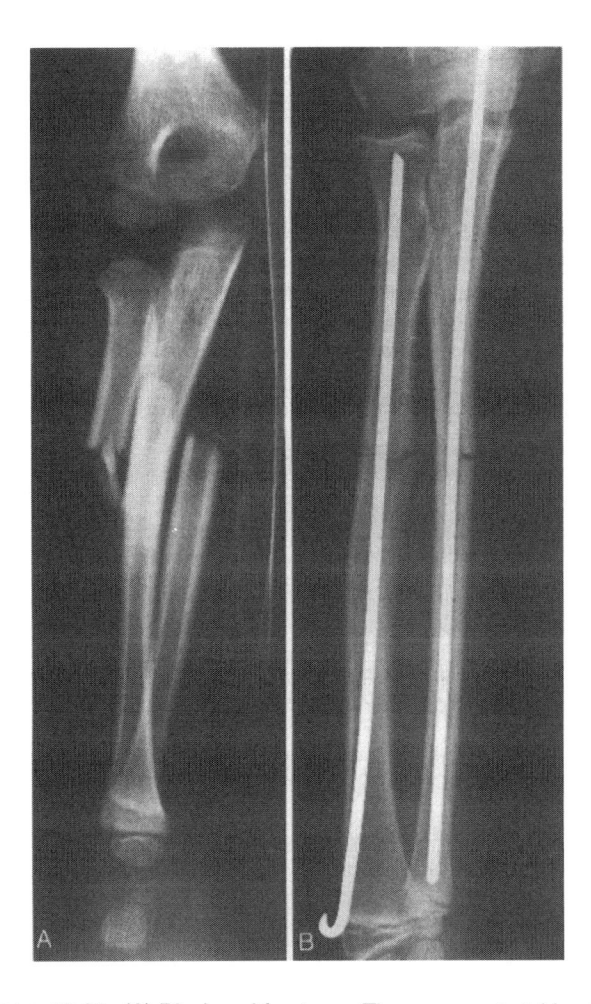

FIGURE 16-82. (A) Displaced fractures. They were not stable after closed reduction. (B) Similar fractures of the radius and ulna in an adolescent. These fractures were treated with intramedullary rods. If this technique is used, it is recommended that the ulnar rod be placed through the proximal metaphysis if the adjacent physis is still functional. In this patient the proximal radius and ulna had undergone physiologic epiphysiodesis. The distal ends were still functional, and rod placement in the radial metaphysis did not interfere with growth.

my preference is a fenestration just distal to the proximal epiphysis.

Results

In a series of 88 greenstick fractures, the only complication was recurrent palmar angulation of the fracture. When encountered during the first 3 weeks after injury, they were remanipulated.[31] Beyond this time, remanipulation is decreasingly successful. Of greenstick fractures of the distal third of the radius and ulna, there were 8 complications in 62 patients; all developed recurrent palmar angulation of 15°–30°. This loss of position, which resulted in up to 30° of palmar angulatipn, occurred witin the first week in five patients, all of whom experienced improvement by remanipulation. A gradual increase in angulation over 4–6 weeks may occur in these patients but usually does not increase beyond 15°.

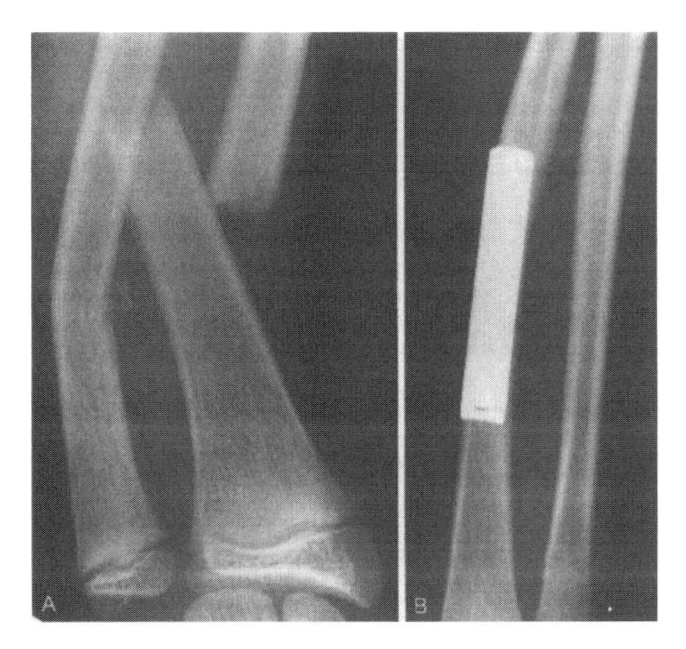

FIGURE 16-83. (A) Radial fracture combined with torus injury to the ulna in an 11-year-old child. Closed reduction was impossible. (B) Tubular plate was applied.

During the first decade of life there is usually complete correction of angular (longitudinal axis) deformity up to 20°–25°, but beyond this age or this degree of malposition the likelihood of spontaneous correction decreases.[367] The correction occurs principally at the distal physis and less so at the proximal physis and by cortical drift and remodeling at the fracture site. The longitudinal angulation may remain.

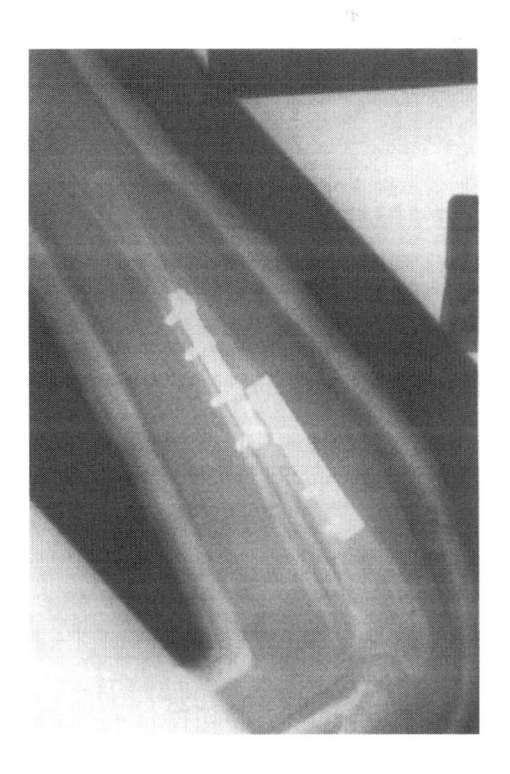

FIGURE 16-84. Bilateral plating. Use the smallest plates possible that can stabilize the fracture.

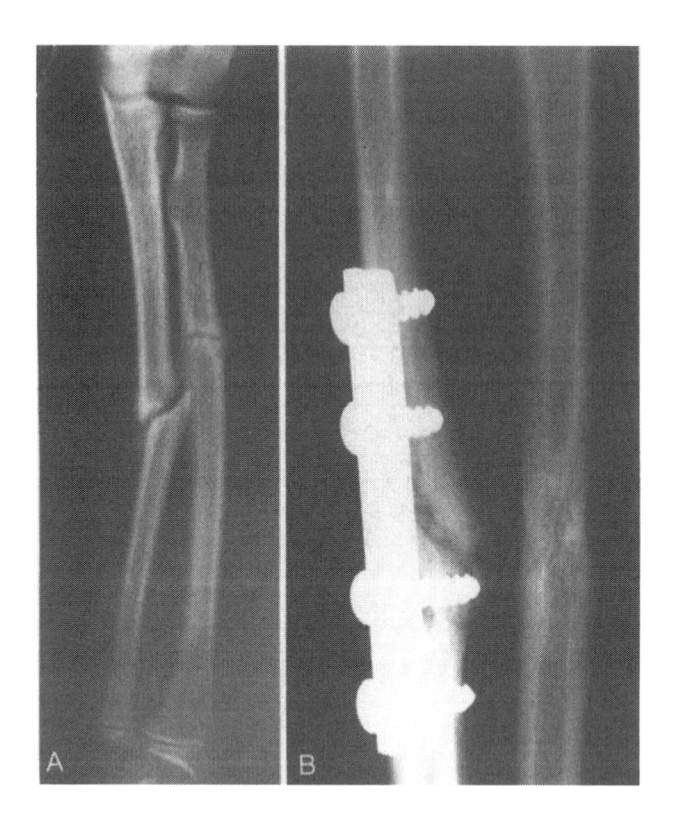

FIGURE 16-85. (A) Delayed union and malunion of the ulna with delayed union of radius. The radius had healed by 4 months after the injury. (B) One year later the patient still had a tender ulnar malunion. She was treated with a compression plate. Four weeks postoperatively, the fracture is healing. Note that the radius has healed well.

Complications

Complications are infrequent but often difficult to manage. Although delayed union or nonunion is rare in young children because of the highly osteogenic periosteum, older children and adolescents are increasingly susceptible to this complication. One bone may unite, albeit delayed, and delayed union or nonunion may develop in the other bone (Figs. 16-85 to 16-87). This delayed union or nonunion occurs because of rotational micromotion of the slower healing fracture once the other fracture heals. These complications should be treated with compression plating and localized bone grafting. Extensive bone grafting is usually unnecessary once the fracture is internally immobilized.

Angular union (malunion) is also infrequent (Fig. 16-88). When present, it should be allowed to mature and then be treated by appropriate corrective osteotomy. Fuller and McCullough believed that in children with malunited fractures of the forearm little useful correction of deformity could be anticipated with diaphyseal fractures when the child was older than 8 years.[356]

Synostosis may occur, especially when the fractures are at the same level (Fig. 16-89). Removal of the synostosis is not easy and should not be attempted until the process is mature (at least 6 months). An important technical point is to remove the synostosis segment by an extraperiosteal dissection. Otherwise, a possible periosteal continuity may remain and enhance the likelihood of recurrence. Interposition of soft tissue, fat, muscle, or Silastic membrane may prevent recurrence, although recurrence is probable in the highly osteogenic immature skeleton.

Allowing children out of immobilization too early may result in a stress or complete fracture through the original fracture and new callus (Fig. 16-90). One way to prevent this is gradual remobilization. At 4–6 weeks the long arm cast is converted to a short arm cast. This conversion allows elbow movement and limited supination-pronation and begins to stimulate some corrective remodeling of the trabecular and cortical bone. A protective splint or orthosis for 2–3 months in an active child is often appropriate, especially for fractures that have healed slowly or in the child insistent on returning rapidly to a structured sport.

In one series, 3 of the 547 fractures were open, and 1 was subsequently complicated by gas gangrene, even though adequate débridement had been carried out at the time of presentation.[31] Osteomyelitis of closed forearm fractures has also been reported (see Chapter 9).

Rayan and Hayes described a case of fracture of both bones of the forearm in which the flexor digitorum profundus was trapped within the ulnar fracture.[406] The complication was not recognized until 2 years after the fracture, when it healed with a lytic defect in the ulna. Release of the muscle belly from its entrapment and release of the adhesions allowed full restoration of function. As shown in Figure 16-73 the greenstick fracture undoubtedly opened up enough

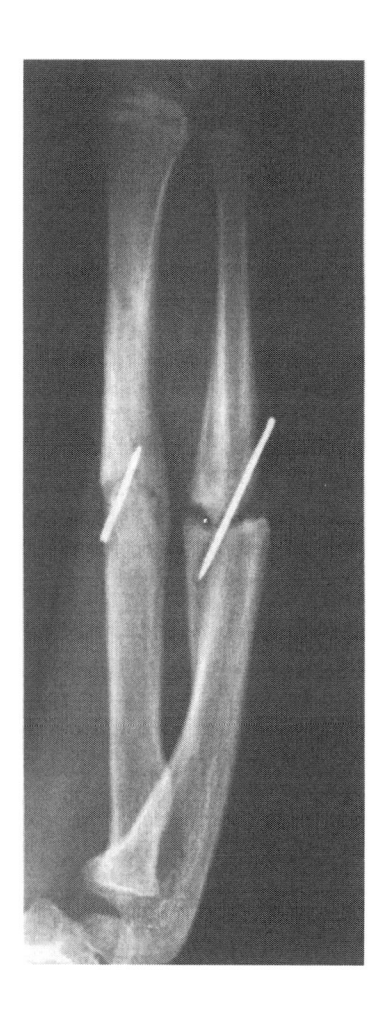

FIGURE 16-86. Less acceptable method of treating delayed union or nonunion using small percutaneous pins.

FIGURE 16-87. Delayed union following closed reduction. (A) Delayed union of both bones. (B) Delayed union of the ulna.

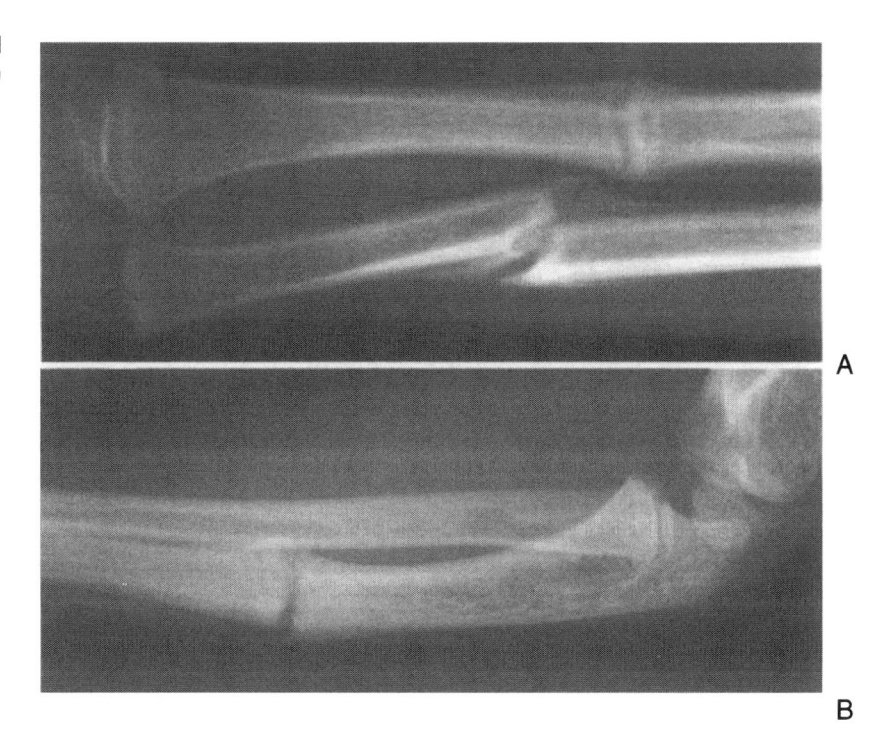

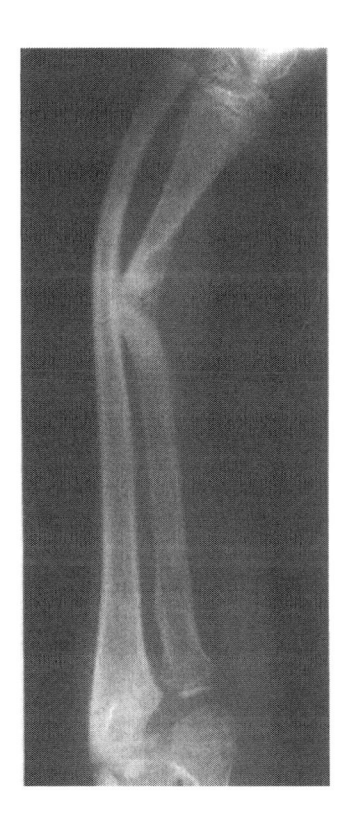

FIGURE 16-88. Angular malunion and delayed union with accompanying severe plastic deformation of the ulna. Correction required osteotomy of both bones.

at maximum deformation to allow some muscle tissue to become lodged in the open fracture gap of the damaged cortex. As the fracture "closed" with the dissipation of the deforming force, this muscle tissue became entrapped within the fracture. This phenomenon may happen more frequently than realized in these fractures. However, functional problems do not seem to be common.

Distal Radial and Ulnar Metaphyseal Injuries

The distal radius and ulna are among the most commonly injured regions of the developing skeleton.[438–527] One of the most frequent types of fracture is the greenstick injury, which may take several forms. A torus fracture (Fig. 16-91) is variable buckling of the cortical bone of the radius, with minimal evidence of trabecular disruption.[479] This pattern is common in young children. The diagnosis is often made in a film taken weeks after the original injury because the original roentgenogram did not disclose the injury. Careful attention must be paid to both anteroposterior and lateral views to look for subtle metaphyseal deformation. If the wrist is tender and swollen, consider oblique views if a torus injury is not evident on the standard views. It is a type 8 growth mechanism injury that results in temporary ischemia of the metaphysis distal to the fracture and subsequent sclerosis during immobilizatior and normalization of bone density with subsequent revascularization (see Chapter 6). The ulna may be (seemingly) uninvolved or may sustain variably severe injury (beware the ulnar styloid injury and late-appearing "nonunion"). The other pattern is a classic greenstick injury with buckling of the palmar cortex, angulation, and loss of dorsal cortical integrity (Fig. 16-92), which may also be associated with a crushing injury with some cortical displacement.

FIGURE 16-89. (A, B) Progressive development of radioulnar synostosis complicating proximal third fractures of both bones.

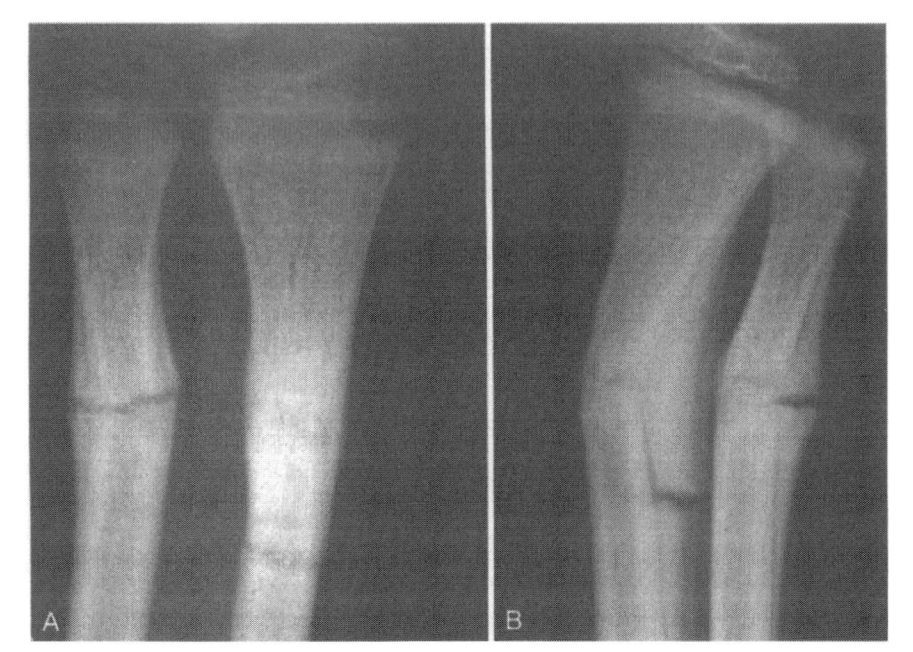

FIGURE 16-90. Refracture following injury to the distal third. The ulna has fractured through the callus at the level of the original injury, and the radial callus has fractured proximal to the original injury. (A) Anteroposterior view. (B) Lateral view.

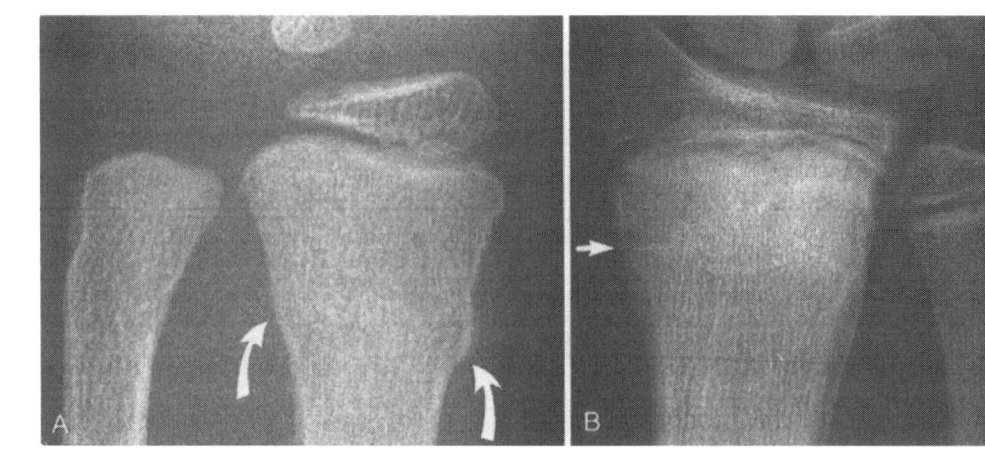

FIGURE 16-91. (A) Typical distal radial torus fracture (arrows). (B) Similar injury in an older child. There is mild sclerosis in the distal metaphysis and subperiosteal new bone proximal to the fracture. The ulnar styloid is fractured, with the fracture still minimally evident (arrow).

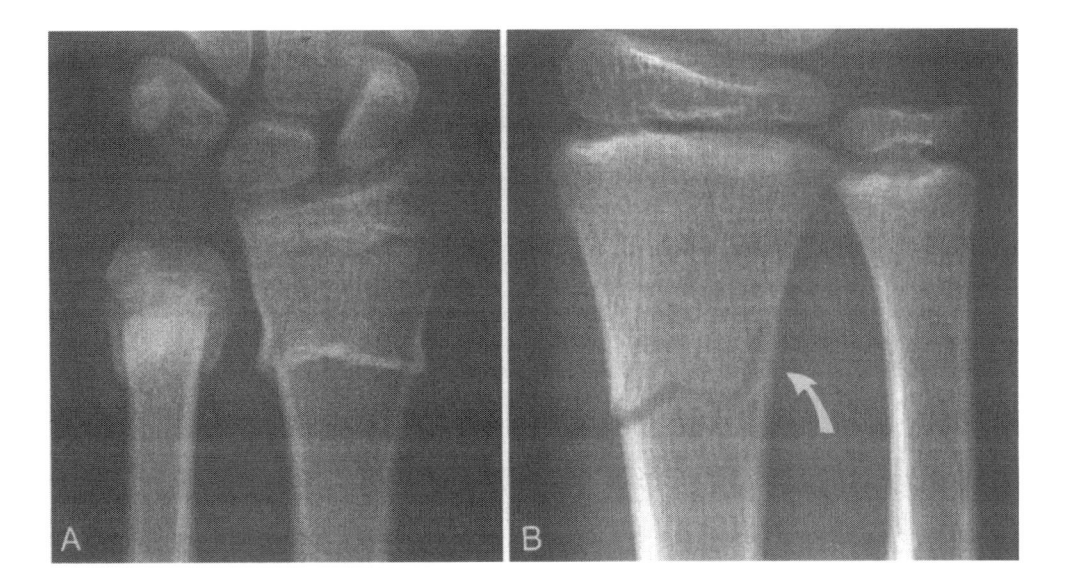

FIGURE 16-92. (A) Buckling of the entire radial cortex with a concomitant ulnar fracture. Cortical integrity and overlap are present on the dorsal (compression) side. The ulna was intact in this patient. (B) Greenstick distal radial fracture with intact cortex on the "ulnar side" (arrow).

In a more severe greenstick injury, the fracture may be dorsally angulated, with disruption of the palmar cortex and an intact, but deformed, dorsal cortex (Fig. 16-93). The fracture may also exhibit complete loss of cortical integrity. If the fracture is undisplaced, the periosteal sleeve is usually intact and imparts a significant degree of stability.

In the most severe injury pattern, the distal fragments are displaced dorsally and radially with various degrees of overriding (Fig. 16-94). The fracture of the radius is usually complete, although fractures of the ulna may be complete and similarly displaced, greenstick, or minimally involved, with injury to the styloid process, similar to a Colles' fracture in an adult.

There is an injury pattern with longitudinal propagation toward the physis. This increases the risk that the physis has absorbed some of the fracture energy and so is at risk for growth alteration. This pattern, a variant of a type 8 growth mechanism injury, is discussed in detail in Chapter 6.

Pathomechanics

With a greenstick injury, the impact of indirect violence of a fall on the outstretched hand coupled with a rotational strain crumples the dorsal cortex, but the palmar cortex remains intact. The distal fragment in a torus fracture may be angulated dorsally or may be displaced minimally. Because the greenstick injury absorbs a large amount of energy that is not dissipated by a complete cortical fracture or displacement of fragments, the compression force may be transmitted into the physis as a type 5 injury, which is difficult to diagnose at the time of original injury but must be sought at the follow-up examinations.

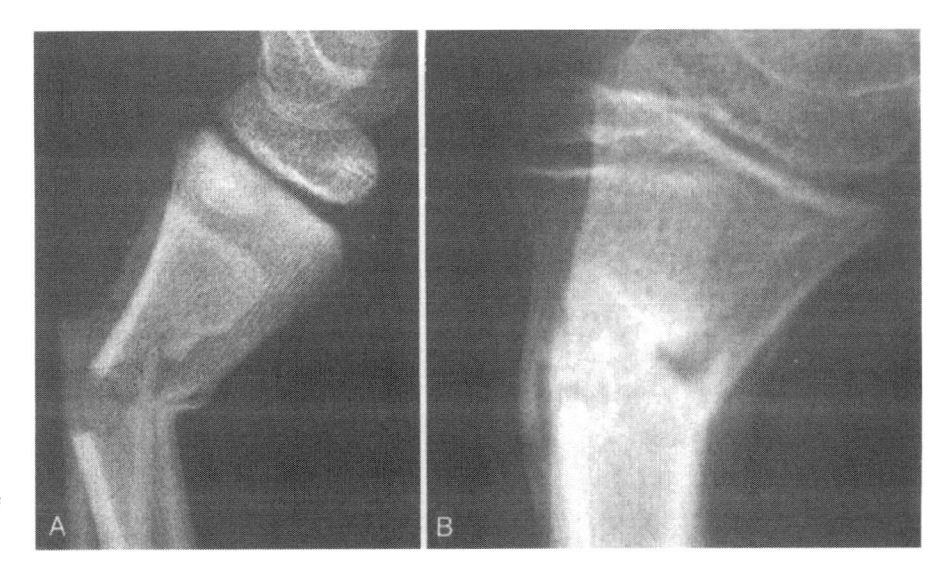

FIGURE 16-93. (A) Angular deformity of a distal radial metaphyseal fracture. (B) Nine weeks later.

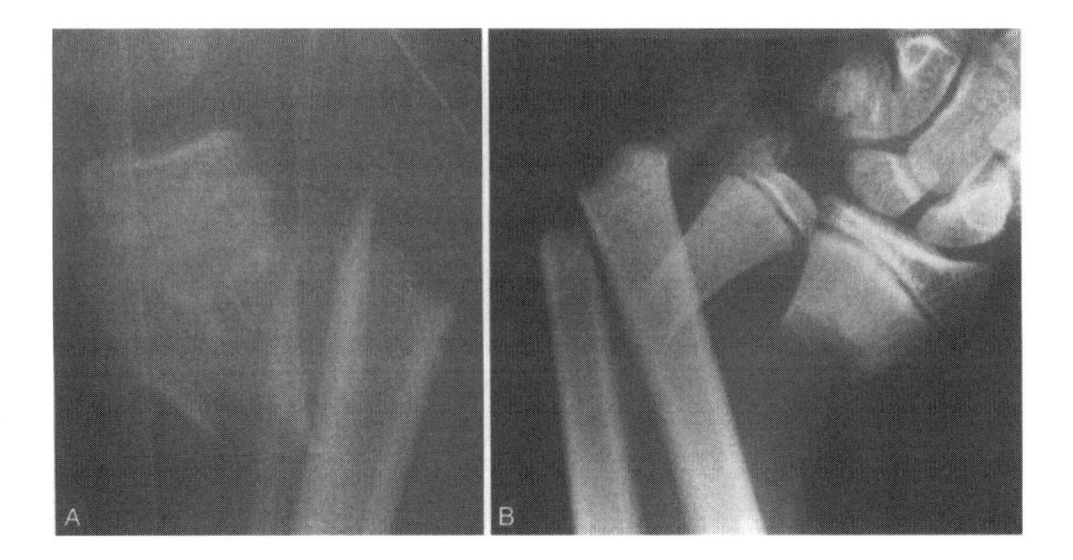

FIGURE 16-94. Displaced distal metaphyseal fractures. (A) Lateral view of characteristic dorsal displacement. (B) Severe displacement and angular deformity.

Even when there is no displacement of the radial fracture, the ulnar styloid is often fractured, which occurs because of the integrated relation of the distal radius and ulna through the triangular fibrocartilage (Figs. 16-11, 16-12). However, because the ulnar styloid is often unossified in those who are in the usual age range for this fracture, the diagnosis is not ordinarily evident until several weeks to months after the injury, when the area finally ossifies and appears radiographically as nonunion.

Diagnosis

The diagnosis is usually evident clinically. The child presents with a painful, swollen wrist. If there is dorsal displacement, the classic "silver fork" deformity may be evident. Roentgenography confirms the injury in most instances, although in some cases the initial roentgenograms may not show any evidence of injury. In these cases the diagnosis must be made empirically on the basis of clinical findings. It is still wise to treat the patient, even in the absence of obvious radiologic findings, because subsequent use of the unprotected extremity may lead to an obvious, sometimes completely displaced fracture.

The neurovascular status should be assessed carefully. With the dorsally displaced fracture, the median nerve is particularly susceptible to acute injury (especially stretching) from the fracture fragment and more chronic injury from the swelling and compromise of the tunnel by the displacement of soft tissue and skeletal elements. Posttraumatic carpal tunnel syndrome is rare in children.

Treatment

A torus fracture is an undisplaced injury that usually involves only the distal metaphysis and does not necessitate reduction, merely immobilization in a well-fitting splint or cast for 3–4 weeks. Hughston advocated using a cast that includes the wrist and elbow, believing that if this type of cast is not used there may be angulation during the healing process.[367]

Onne and Sandblom defined the angular deformity of the distal third fracture but did not define an absolute number of degrees to use as a guideline.[395] If the angle exceeds 25°–30° in infants or 15°–20° in children beyond the second year, closed reduction with completion of the fracture by reversal of the deformity is usually indicated. Like greenstick fractures of the mid-shaft, torus fractures may deform because of powerful muscles acting across the wrist, coupled with intrinsic deforming plasticity in the remaining intact bone.

A greenstick fracture of the radius at the junction of the metaphysis and diaphysis with some supination is common and problematic because angulation tends to recur, even after reduction. The forearm should be held in full pronation in an above-elbow cast with three-point fixation. If the deformity is severe, it may be necessary to complete the fracture, as previously described for fractures. However, casting in full pronation with an above-elbow cast allows the intact periosteum to lock the fracture in place and usually stops a supination deformity from developing.

Complete fractures should be reduced with the patient under an anesthetic, as relaxation is an essential part of the reduction and is rarely obtained without complete muscular relaxation.[282,454,459] The technique of reduction is to re-create and overexaggerate the deformity (Fig. 16-95). First, the extremity is subjected to longitudinal traction in the line of the deformity, with countertraction at the elbow. The surgeon pushes the fragments into normal position, and the distal radius and ulna are pressed to restore the width of the interosseous space. It is desirable to achieve anatomic alignment (Fig. 16-96) in the longitudinal and rotational directions, but the cortices may overlap in the lateral view. Bayonet apposition usually should not be accepted

Distal Radial and Ulnar Metaphyseal Injuries

FIGURE 16-95. Method for reducing a dorsally displaced distal radial or radioulnar fracture. R = radius; U = ulna. (A) Initial deformity. (B) Hyperextend the distal unit. (C) Push or "walk" the fractured ends until they lock. (D) Bring the wrist back to its neutral position. Although complete anatomic reduction is not essential, longitudinal and rotational alignments must be attained and maintained.

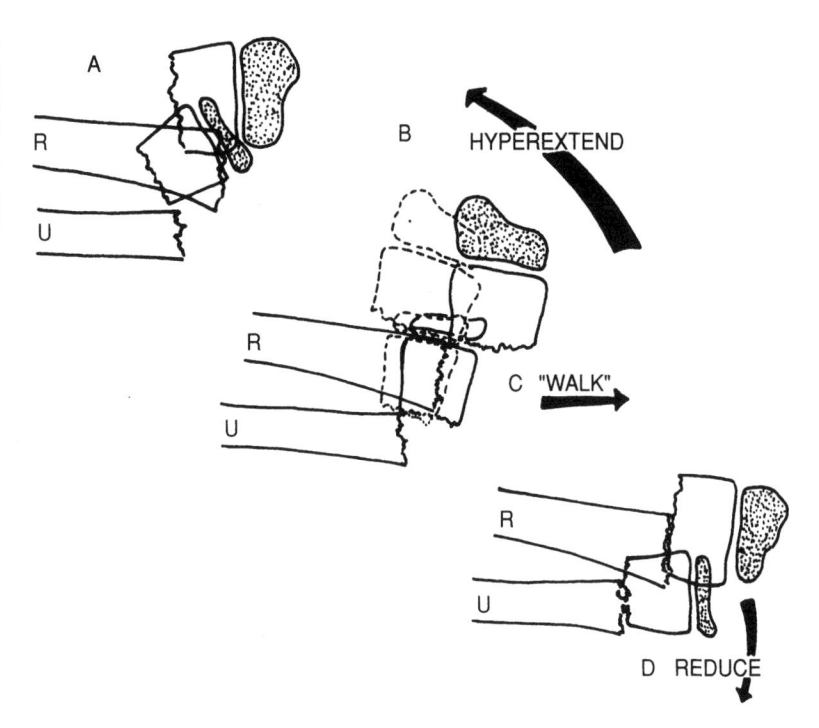

(Fig. 16-97). Encroachment of the interosseous space by the fragments should be corrected, as it may restrict the rotation of the forearm, although with growth there may be sufficient remodeling to overcome this problem. Minimal overriding may be remodeled. Marked overriding occasionally requires skeletal traction through the metacarpals to stretch soft tissues enough to allow manipulative correction.

An above-elbow cast may be applied for immobilization and should be maintained for 6 weeks. Again, it is imperative to check the injury at adequate intervals to assess any subsequent redisplacement. A splint should be used for several additional weeks, especially in children with complete fractures.

Open reduction is infrequently indicated in children (Fig. 16-98). In my experience, it has been necessary in only a few cases among several hundred examples of this injury. In these cases the pronator quadratus muscle had been disrupted, with the proximal fragment of the radius buttonholed into or through the muscle; it was impossible, except under direct vision, to free the fragments and replace them on the palmar side of the forearm because some of the muscle had been displaced onto the dorsal aspect of the proximal fragment.

A totally unstable distal radial fracture in a child who is approaching skeletal maturity can probably be treated more like a fracture in an adult: Open reduction and internal fixation with pins or plates is undertaken.

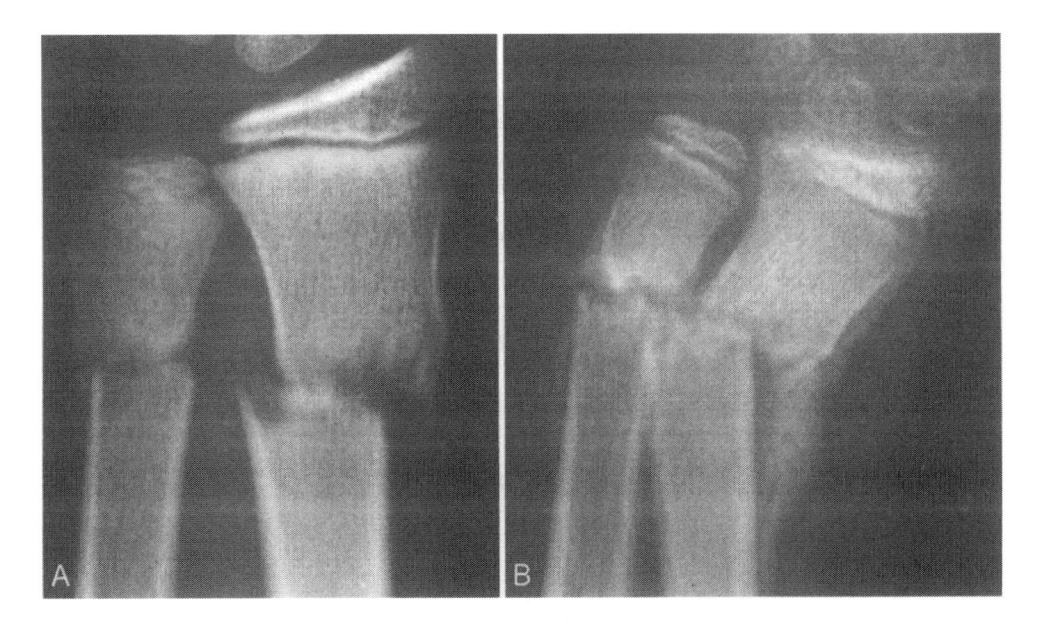

FIGURE 16-96. (A) Successful closed reduction. (B) It was not held well in the cast, however, and progressively angulated.

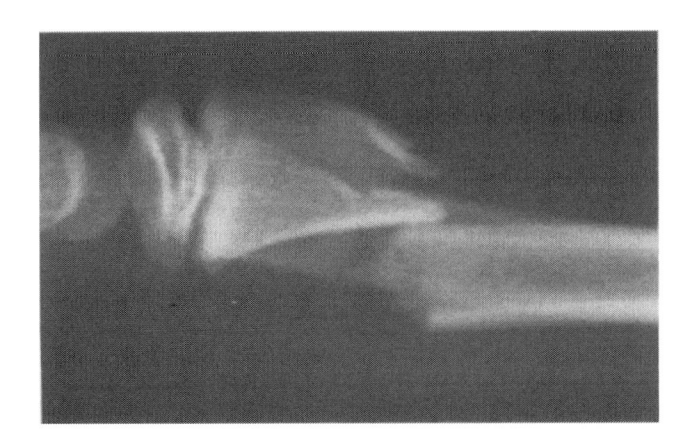

FIGURE 16-97. Dorsally displaced distal radial fracture (the ulna is not displaced). This fracture does not always or adequately remodel.

Treatment Problems

These fractures may appear simple to treat, but they are often more difficult to take care of adequately than can be appreciated initially and may be less than ideally managed because of certain concepts. The following are areas that lead to poor results.

Failure to Attain Adequate Initial Reduction

The more accurate the initial reduction, the less is the potential for loss of alignment. Reduction of displaced, overriding fractures of the distal forearm is particularly difficult in the presence of marked local swelling. Unless neurovascular compromise is present, there is no emergency in treating these fractures. Compression is applied with a splint and the child treated by elevating the extremity (hospital or home); adequate reduction is then undertaken once the swelling has receded. Reduction with the patient under anesthesia is less traumatic, as the fracture may be manipulated under optimal conditions and with the use of an image intensifier.

Failure to Immobilize the Forearm in a Position of Stability

The degree of rotation of the forearm in which fractures of the radius and ulna should be immobilized has been the subject of some controversy. The forearm should be immobilized in that position of rotation (i.e., supination, pronation, neutral) in which the reduction appears to be most stable. This position may be determined best using an image intensifier. A standard routine practice has been full pronation in lower third fractures, but it should be approached only as a relative guideline and not an absolute indication for positioning the wrist and forearm. If the reduction is stable, full supination is recommended to allow the radius and ulna to parallel each other. If an adequately applied cast is maintained during this period, the pull of the muscles should not cause malalignment of the satisfactorily reduced stable fracture. Stability of reduction may be determined clinically and by a roentgenographic examination.

Failure to Break the Cortex Completely in Angulated Greenstick Fractures

Failure to break the cortex completely in angulated greenstick fractures is one of the most common pitfalls. Merely to straighten the bone is not sufficient. The intact cortex must be completely broken. In some instances when there is no

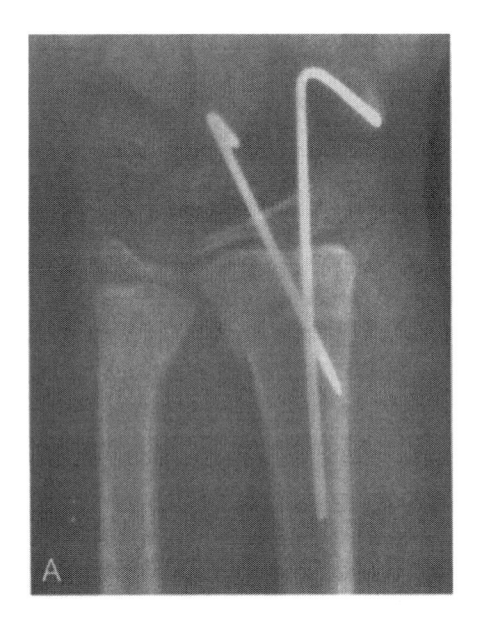

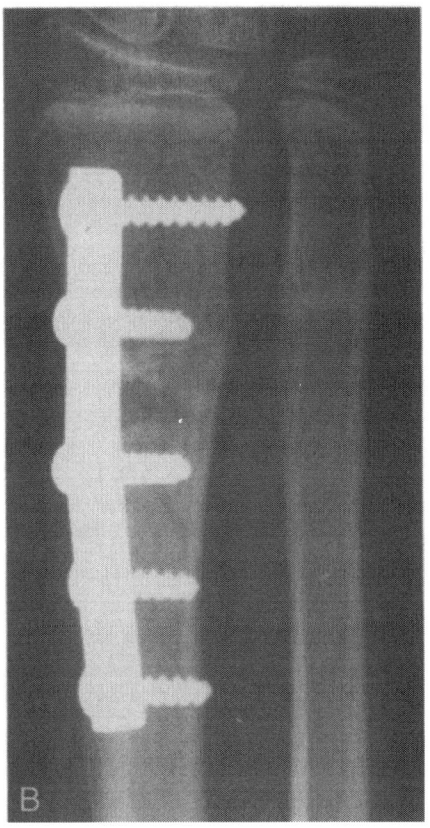

FIGURE 16-98. (A) Open reduction of a distal metaphyseal fracture. (B) Open reduction and plate fixation.

apparent fracture of the ulna, there may be significant greenstick bowing in association with the complete fracture or a true greenstick fracture of the radius. These fractures are deceptive. The fracture of the radius should be completed in such an instance, as the intrinsic plastic deformation of the ulna makes it bow the potentially unstable radius.

Loose Cast

To maintain reduction, external compression by the cast must be secure. As swelling around the fracture site subsides and muscles atrophy, the cast may become loose and the fracture fragments are subsequently displaced or are in loose alignment. A loss of position may occur as late as 3–4 weeks following reduction. A loose cast may be detected by roentgenography, as can the possibility of angular deformation. It is important that the fracture be radiographed within a week after initial reduction. If there is any evidence of loosening of the cast or beginning angular deformity, particularly toward the original deformity, the cast should be removed and replaced with a snug, well-fitting, three-point fixation cast. The type of cast is, of course, the preference of the individual surgeon. One cannot overemphasize the importance of a snug, but not constricting, cast or splint for preventing loss of alignment and frequent cast changes, as necessitated by the subsidence of swelling. Sugar tong (incomplete) casts accommodate swelling during the early stages but should usually be followed by a well-molded circumferential cast after the swelling dissipates.

Displaced fractures of the radius and ulna are immobilized in a sturdy long arm cast that extends from the upper arm to the metacarpal heads, with the elbow in 90° of flexion. Stiffness of joints from prolonged immobilization is generally not a problem in children. For unstable fractures of the distal third of the radius, the plaster should include the proximal phalanges to immobilize the metacarpophalangeal joints. Secure fixation of the proximal phalanx is particularly important; otherwise children tend to use the thumb and fingers and may cause redeformation in an anatomically unstable fracture.

Failure to Detect and Correct Loss of Position

The fracture must be roentgenographed at appropriate intervals. By 10–14 days some radiolucent callus may begin to appear. This biologically plastic callus may enhance the stability of a re-reduction, but it may also impede attempts to improve angulation. Adequate roentgenograms are essential. In particular, anteroposterior and true lateral views must be obtained, as oblique views may be misleading and may make the fracture appear more or less deformed than it is.

Results

In general, the results of treating distal metaphyseal fractures are good to excellent. Because many are undisplaced greenstick injuries, there is minimal rotational or angular deformity requiring extensive remodeling. Even with displaced fractures, the results are good when a satisfactory reduction has been attained. Problems arise when the fracture reangulates or is left dorsally displaced.

Complications

A relatively high incidence of complications occur with complete fracture of the distal third of the radius and ulna. Of 47 patients in one series, 22 had complications, including angular deformity, rotational deformity, gas gangrene, medial nerve injury, and refracture. In another series, recurrent dorsal angulation at the fracture site was the most common complication, occurring in 43 of 547 patients.[31] The incidence of the complication after greenstick fractures of the distal third of the radius alone or after fractures of the radius and ulna together was 10%, and after complete fractures of the distal radius and ulna it was 25%.[31] An intact ulna apparently helps stabilize a complete fracture of the distal radius alone, as the incidence of reangulation of this fracture pattern was only 10%. This significant difference in the incidence of reangulation between greenstick and complete fractures of the distal third suggests that breaking the intact cortex, thereby converting the greenstick distal fracture into a complete fracture, may not be the best method of reduction. As seen radiographically, greenstick fractures appear to be angulated. I agree with the concept and believe that greenstick fractures may be satisfactorily managed by the technique of converting the greenstick fracture into a complete fracture when appropriate and indicated. However, Evans pointed out that the apparent angulation deformity seen with greenstick fractures in children is often a rotational deformity.[7] By rotating the forearm under an image intensifier, one can observe that the apparent angulation disappears or lessens as the forearm reaches the proper plane of rotation. Rotational correction may be easier and more efficacious than trying to convert the angulated greenstick fracture into a complete fracture.[493] Evans showed that distal-third greenstick fractures reduce relatively easily by maximal pronation of the forearm.[7]

Circulatory compromise and its major consequence, Volkmann's ischemia, may occur with fractures of both bones of the forearm when the forearm is swollen or when a displaced fracture that requires repeated manipulation is present. The more extensive the soft tissue trauma, particularly from a direct blow or wringer injury, the more likely is the possibility of enough swelling to create forearm compartment problems. Compartment pressure monitoring should be considered.

One of the "complications" of least concern is radiographically delayed union, nonunion, or overgrowth of the ulnar styloid, which represents a type 7 growth mechanism injury (Fig. 16-99). This injury occurs because of the anatomic relations, especially the triangular cartilage. The injury often occurs through a completely cartilaginous styloid, making diagnosis roentgenographically difficult. Subsequently, as the styloid ossifies the nonunion becomes evident. Nonunion probably occurs because of the difficulty of epiphyseal cartilage healing and chronic tensile stresses. Onne and Sandblom found two cases with follow-up problems relative to the ulnar styloid, with pain on maximal supination caused by a pseudarthrosis of the styloid process or by a fibrous union between the styloid and the remainder of the ulnar secondary ossification center.[395] My experience has been similar. A radiographic nonunion is not necessarily an anatomic nonunion, nor is it usually symptomatic.

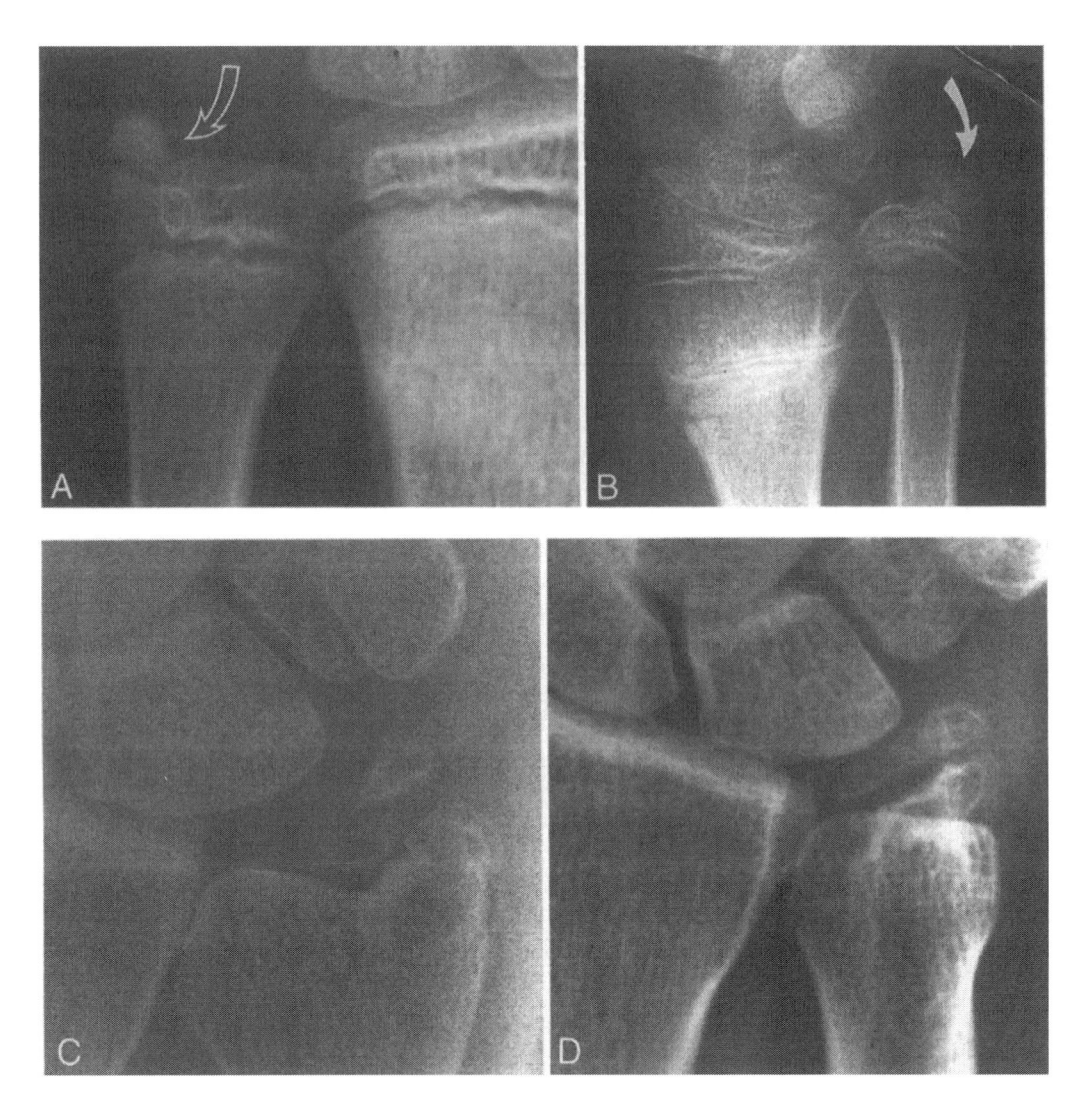

FIGURE 16-99. (A) Ulnar styloid nonunion (arrow). It accompanied a torus radial injury. (B) Hypertrophic overgrowth (arrow) of the ulnar styloid fracture. (C, D) Progressive ossification in the styloid nonunion.

These fractures usually heal rapidly with extensive callus formation. However, severe periosteal injury or possible vascular disruption may be associated with delayed healing. The child must be protected until the fracture is completely healed.

Disrupted periosteum may not heal completely. A fragment that is displaced beyond the confines of the periosteum may not remodel completely and may lead to formation of an exostosis.

In the series described by Davis and Green, most of the 16 distal-third greenstick fractures that reangulated were treated initially in neutral rotation; only two were reduced in pronation.[31] It appears that, although reduction of a greenstick fracture of the distal third by pronation of the forearm does not entirely eliminate the possibility of reangulation, recurrent palmar angulation is less likely to occur if this method of reduction is used. Palmar angulation is probably not of significant consequence in a child under 10 years of age, as the growing bone adequately remodels the deformity. In the child over 12 years, angulation cannot be accepted because of the limited amount of remodeling. The most difficult clinical problem then arises: How much angulation is acceptable in the child between the ages of 10 and 12 years?

There were 36 fractures with significant deformities in the series of Gandhi and colleagues.[32] They believed that angulation as great as 35° in the distal third of the radius would correct itself within 5 years; but they emphasized that knowing that this bone has "correcting power" is not an excuse for leaving the fracture unreduced or for not attempting to secure an adequate reduction (Fig. 16-100). At the same time, these results suggest that there is no justification for carrying out repeated manipulations or open reduction of such fractures. Despite reassurance, parents naturally are anxious if there is a clinical or radiographic deformity when the cast is removed, and they require an answer to the question of how long it will persist. In my experience, it appears that most deformities of the distal third of the radius are corrected fully in 2–3 years (Fig. 16-101). There should be a reluctance to accept an angular deformity of more than 20° in a child over 10 years old who has less capacity for full correction, particularly if the child is a girl who undergoes early fusion at 12–14 years of age.

Open fractures that involve the distal radius are relatively common, especially if the mechanism of injury is a fall on

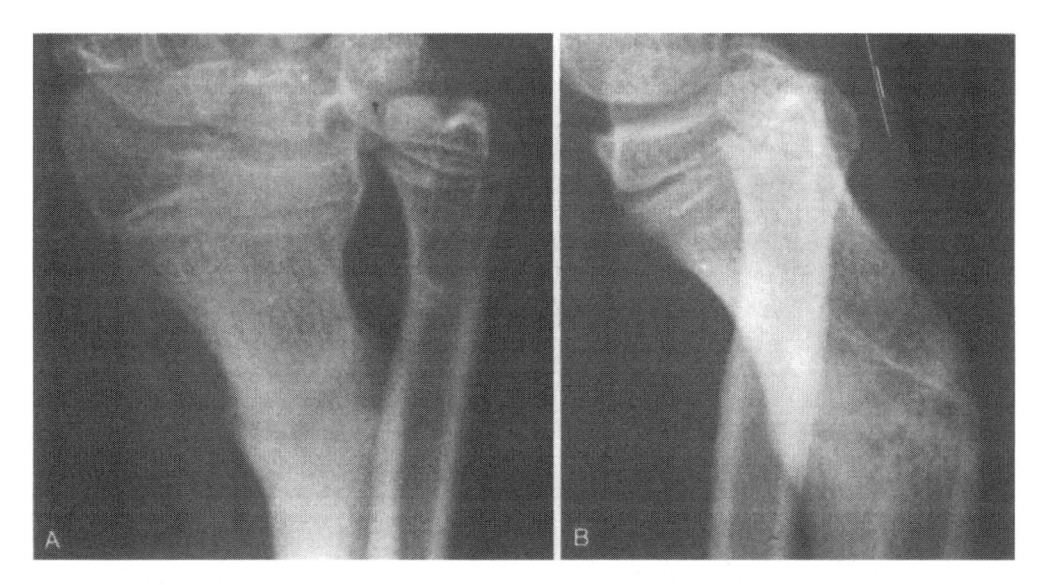

FIGURE 16-100. Anteroposterior (A) and lateral (B) views of residual malunion in a 12-year-old girl. Insufficient growth was left in the distal radius after a fracture 8 months previously. The radius was left angulated, resulting in decreased rotational capacity and relative ulnar lengthening. A corrective osteotomy is necessary.

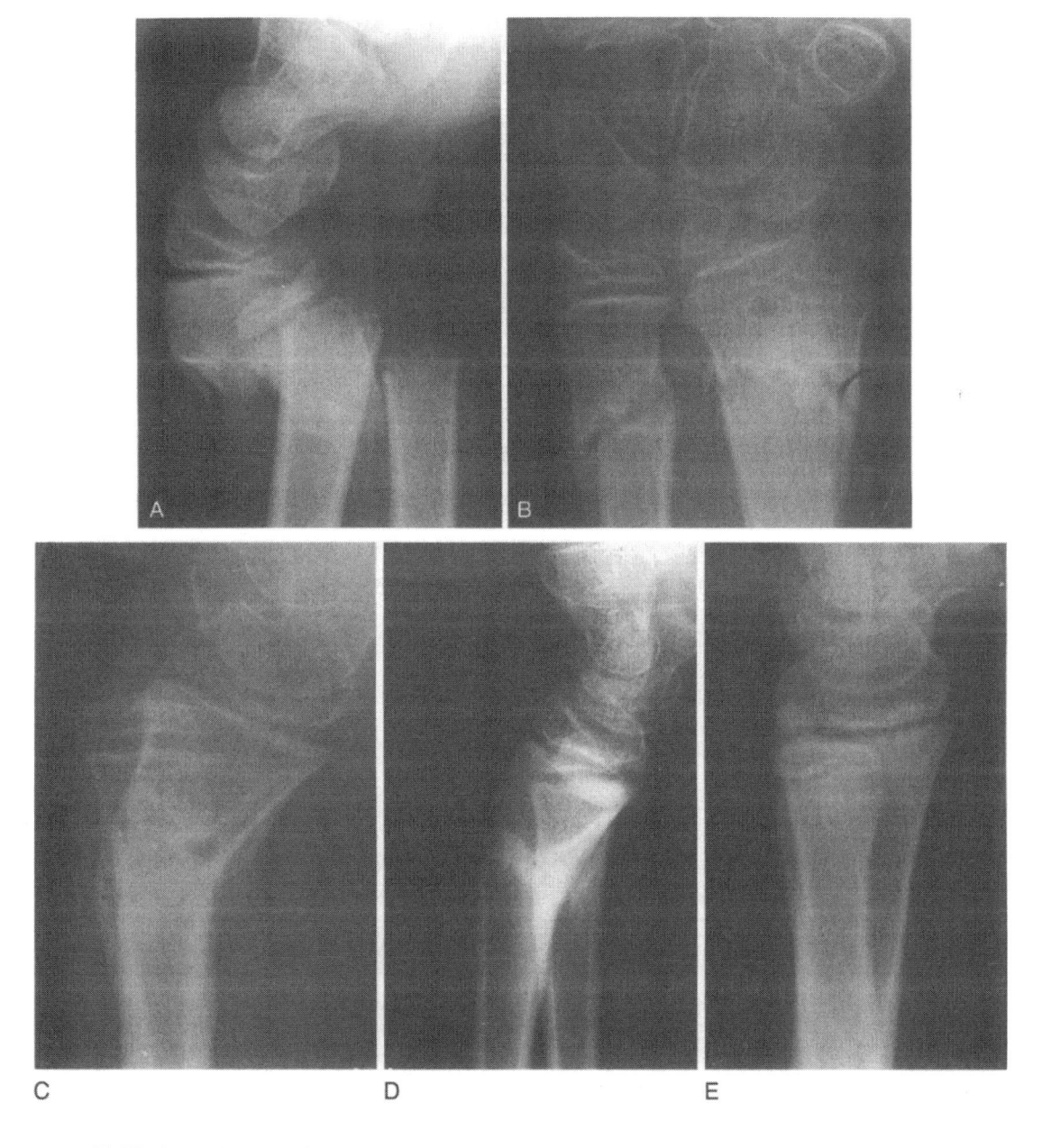

FIGURE 16-101. (A) Displaced fracture of the distal third of the radius. (B) Appearance of the fracture 3 weeks after reduction. (C) At 6 weeks there was further reangulation. (D) One year later remodeling is evident. (E) Three years later the malunion is fully corrected.

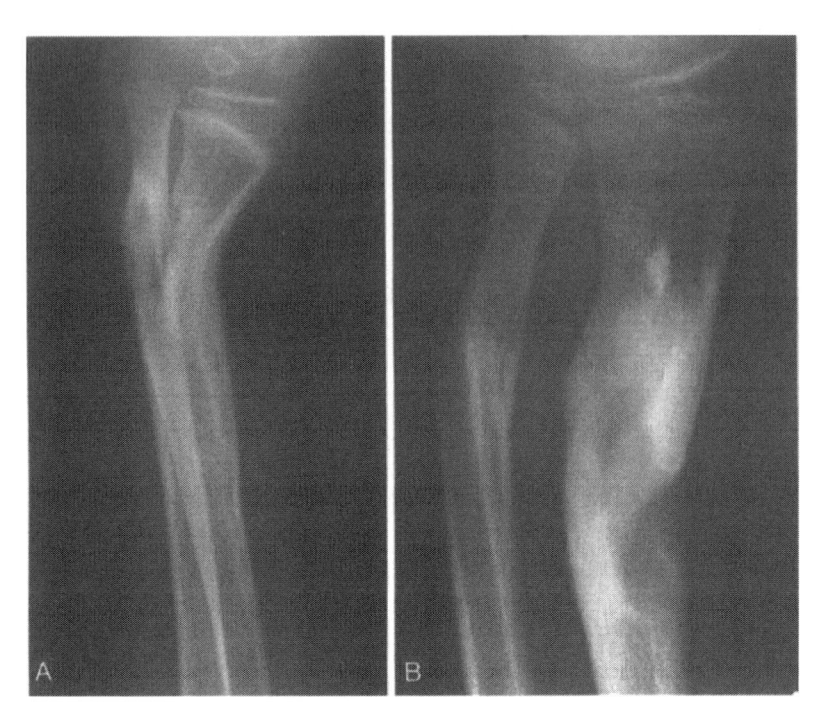

FIGURE 16-102. (A) Malunion after an open fracture complicated by infection. (B) Two years later the angular malunion is markedly improved, and the sclerotic bone at the sites of the fracture and the osteomyelitis is remodeling.

the wrist. If this fall occurs in dirt, the risk of contamination with soil microorganisms is significant (and may include *Clostridium*). These injuries must be treated aggressively with débridement and left open to heal by secondary granulation or subjected to delayed closure. Even with appropriate treatment, osteomyelitis may supervene (Fig. 16-102). Failure to appreciate fully the severity of such open injuries may lead to significant damage and loss of cartilage and bone.

The possibility of growth arrest with distal radial metaphyseal or physeal fractures has been minimized in the past. However, a study by Lee et al. showed that some type of an important growth disturbance developed in 7% of the children.[476] Four of the seven patients had a significant compression mechanism according to the history. Premature closure of the growth plate of the distal ulna, leading to disparity, did not occur in any of the children in the study of Lee et al. The correction of the deformity is contingent on the specific anatomic changes. Growth arrest may complicate even a torus fracture.[440]

Although the Madelung deformity is considered a congenital abnormality, Vender and Watson described a case of bilateral closure of the ulnar side of the distal radius in a patient with a history of high-level gymnastic training.[500] They thought that cumulative microtrauma to the ulnar side of the growth plate was responsible.

Distal Radial Epiphyseal and Physeal Injuries

Classification

Every type of growth mechanism injury may affect the distal radius (Fig.16-103).[440–444,446,447,451,452,460,467,470,476,477,481,484,485,487,488,]

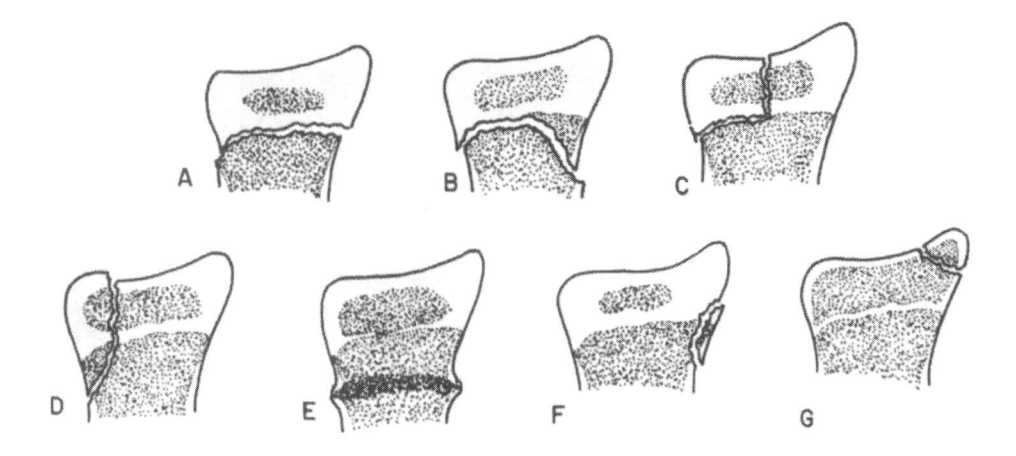

FIGURE 16-103. Growth mechanism injuries. A. Type 1. B. Type 2. C. Type 3. D. Type 4. E. Type 8. F. Type 6. G. Type 7.

Distal Radial Epiphyseal and Physeal Injuries

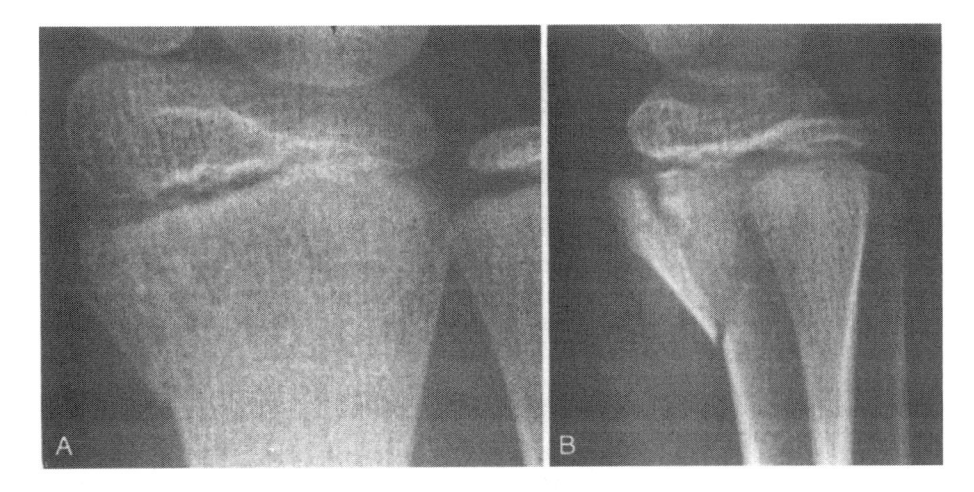

FIGURE 16-104. Type 2 injury. (A) Anteroposterior view shows minimal metaphyseal injury. (B) Lateral view shows more extensive cortical disruption. The possibility that a type 4 injury is present, rather than the type 2 injury, must be considered.

[495,498–500,505,506] The distal ulnar physis, however, is less frequently involved. Because of the crushing, twisting nature of many of these injuries, localized physeal damage (type 5) may occur and is probably more frequent than realized.

Type 2 injuries are the most common, especially in older children (more than 10 years of age) and are usually associated with posterior (dorsal) displacement of the metaphyseal fragment. They are often accompanied by a fracture through the ulnar styloid (Figs. 16-104 to 16-106).

Type 1 injury patterns are the next most common (Figs. 16-107, 16-108). The epiphysis may be significantly displaced (Fig. 16-109). Type 3 and type 4 injuries also occur but are infrequent (Fig. 16-110). Type 7 injuries usually involve the radial styloid (Fig. 16-111).

The radial fracture may be associated with a greenstick fracture of the ulnar metaphysis, separation of the distal ulnar epiphysis, or fracture of the ulnar styloid process.[465] The ulnar injury usually does not involve the ulnar physis.

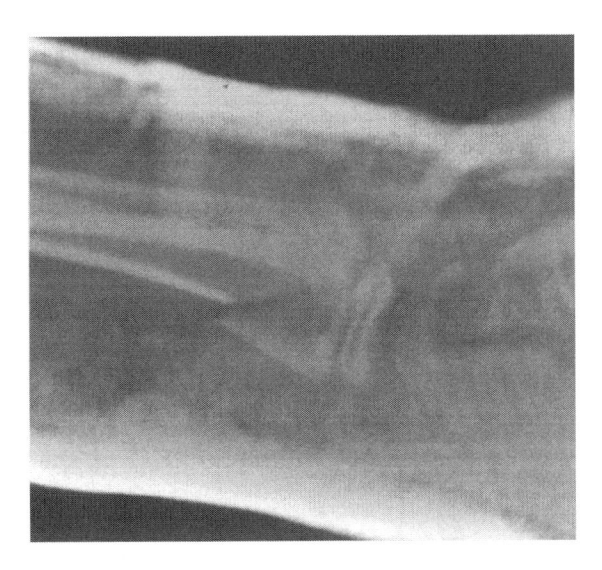

FIGURE 16-105. Barton's fracture. This volar displacement is rare in children, who usually have a dorsal displacement because of the frequent mechanism of falling on the extended or hyperextended hand.

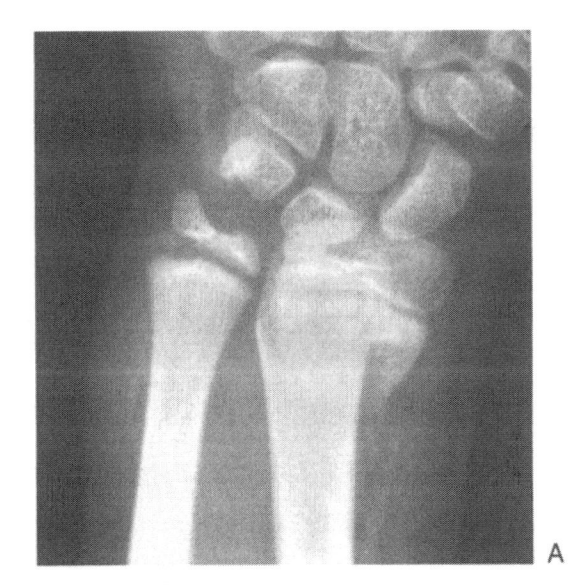

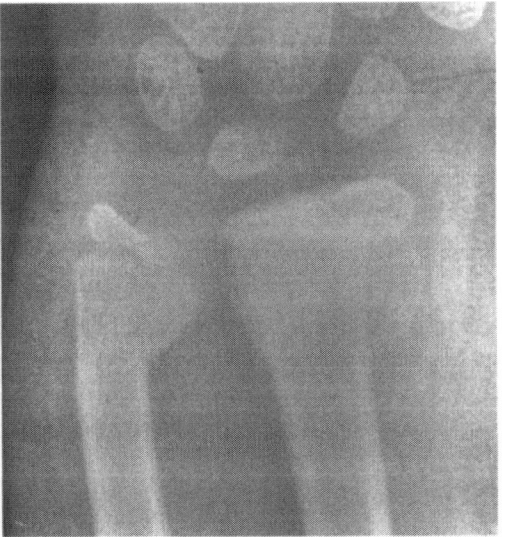

FIGURE 16-106. (A) Type 2 radial fracture with a type 2 ulnar fracture. (B) Type 2 radial fracture with a type 1 ulnar fracture.

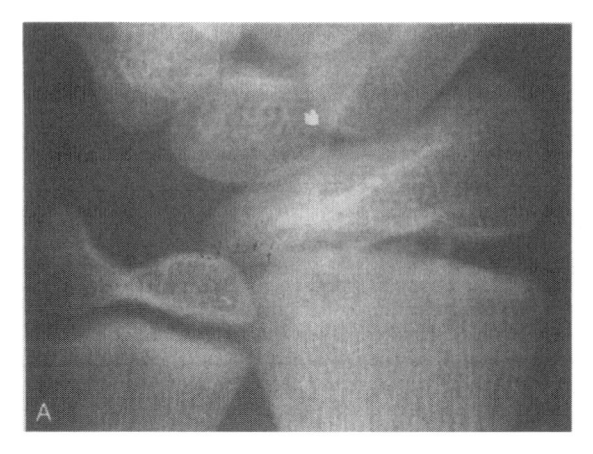

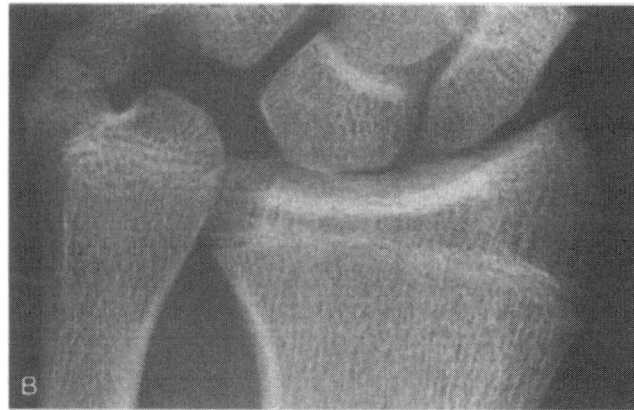

FIGURE 16-107. (A) Distal radial fracture (type 1). This fracture is open on the "radial" side and compressed on the "ulnar" side. Such a fracture must be watched closely for growth arrest. (B) Two years later the patient, who did not have proper follow-up examinations, returned complaining of pain over the ulnar styloid. The distal ulna had overgrown, and the distal radius closed prematurely. An ulnar styloid nonunion is evident. There was no indication of the ulnar injury on the initial film.

Pathomechanics

Injuries to the distal radial epiphysis and physis usually result from a fall on the outstretched hand. The forces are dorsally and longitudinally displaced and produce a combination of impaction and shearing at the level of the physis. Because of the triangular fibrocartilaginous complex (TFCC), the ulnar styloid frequently is fractured concomitantly (Fig. 16-112). The shearing forces of hyperextension and supination displace the distal radial epiphysis dorsally. The periosteum is stripped from the dorsal metaphysis but remains attached to the physis and epiphysis. If the transverse vector is greater and more shearing is present, the likelihood of physeal damage decreases. However, when the longitudinal vector increases, the tendency for damage to the physis and the potential rate of growth disturbance increase.

Diagnosis

The fracture is usually dorsally displaced, and the child may present with pain and swelling. There are rarely signs of neurologic or vascular deficiency, but they must be adequately

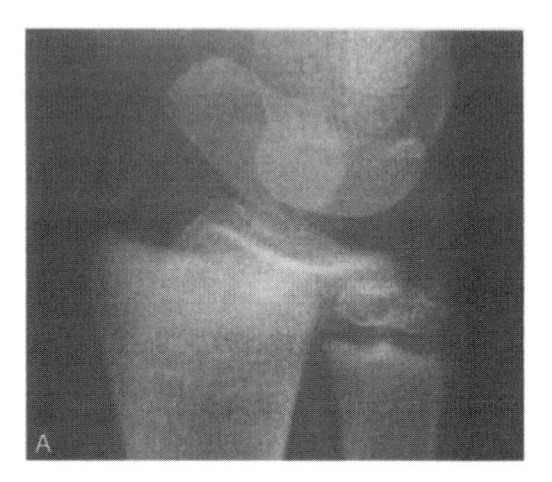

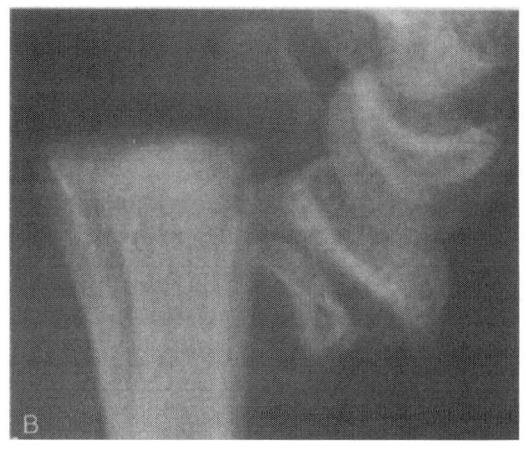

FIGURE 16-109. Dorsally displaced physeal injury. (A) Anteroposterior view. (B) Lateral view.

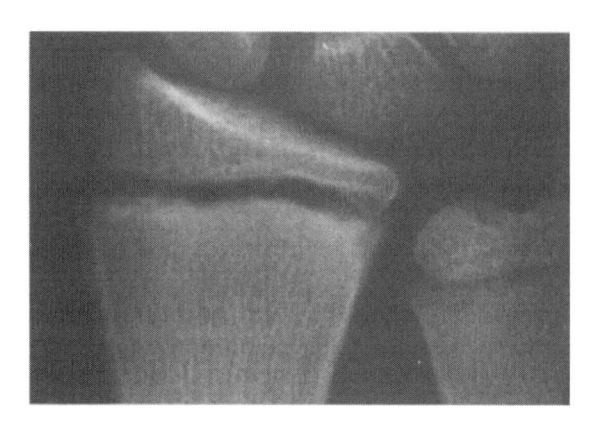

FIGURE 16-108. Type 1 injury. Mild displacement with widening of the physis.

Distal Radial Epiphyseal and Physeal Injuries

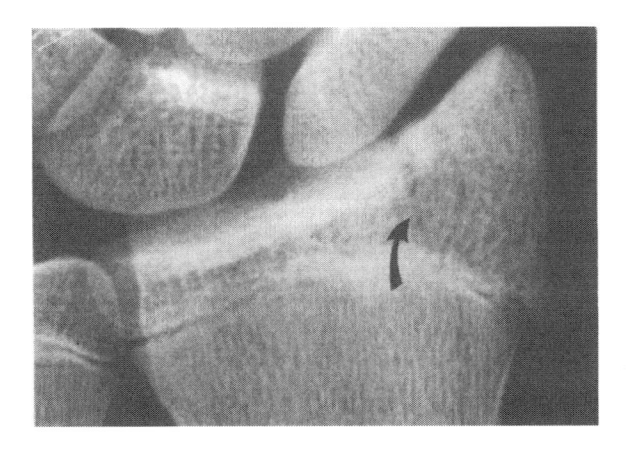

FIGURE 16-110. Undisplaced type 3 injury (arrow).

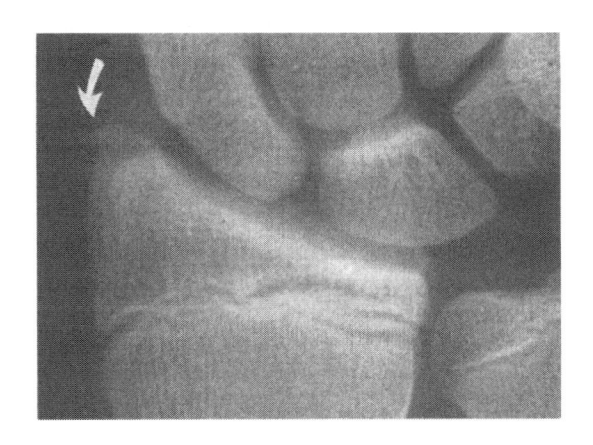

FIGURE 16-111. Type 7 injury of the radial styloid (arrow).

sought, as they do sometimes occur. Finger motion, though painful, is ordinarily present and may appear normal. Sometimes only pain and swelling are present, with apparently normal roentgenographic findings.

Roentgenograms establish the diagnosis, which is best visualized in the lateral projection. Often the dorsal metaphyseal fragment is small, but it is pathognomonic of the type 2 injury pattern, even if there is no epiphyseal displacement.

The lack of ossification in the ulnar styloid makes diagnosis of the usual accompanying fracture difficult. Pain over the styloid is usually indicative of concomitant injury. Because of fibrous union, direct expansion of ossification cannot occur across this tissue to unite with ossification within the fragment.

Treatment

The injury usually is easily reduced by direct pressure (with the patient under appropriate anesthesia and muscle relaxation). Wrist flexion does not help to hold the reduction, because the wrist joint easily flexes to 80° before the capsule tightens enough to exert any influence on the distal frag-

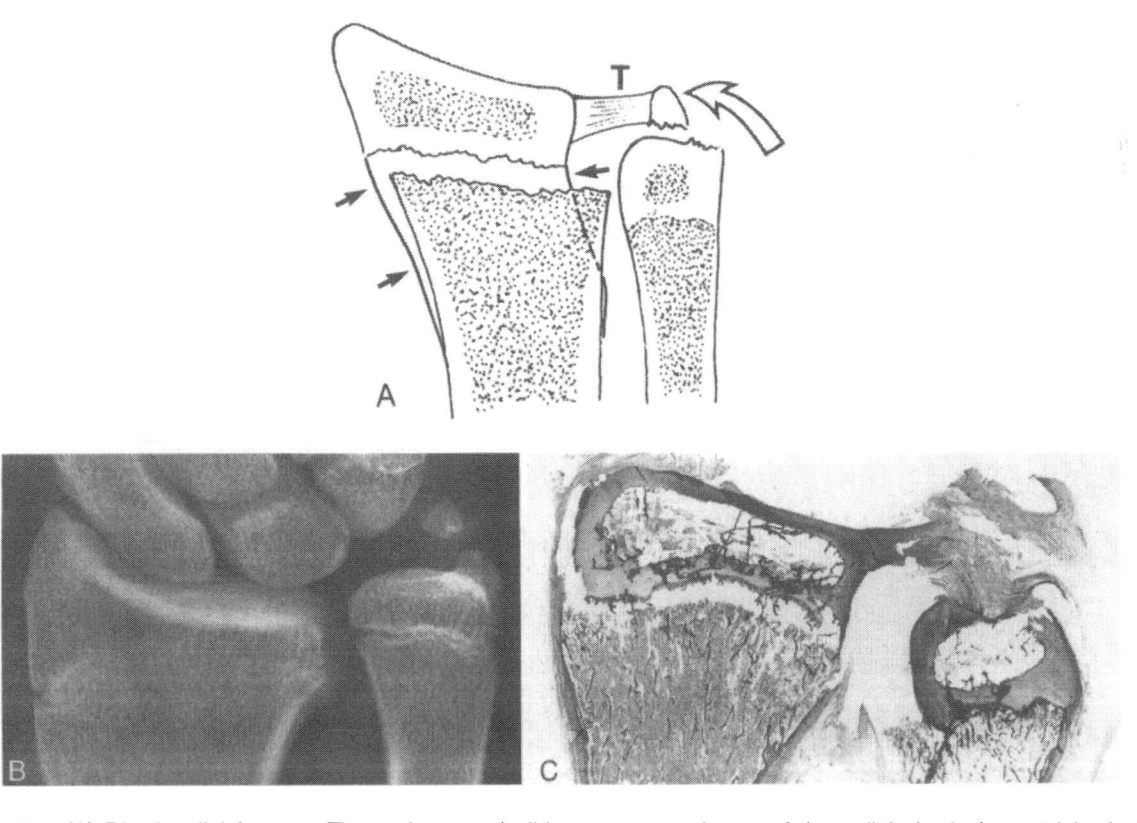

FIGURE 16-112. (A) Distal radial fracture. The periosteum (solid arrows) strips away and may be used to stabilize the reduction. The triangular cartilage (T) causes avulsion of the ulnar styloid (open arrow). (B) Nonunion following combined fracture. Note the premature closure of the radial physis (type 1 injury) and open ulnar physis. (C) Histologic specimen showing a type 1 fracture of the distal radius. Note that the triangular fibrocartilage complex is pulling on the ulnar styloid.

ment. This position is unacceptable. Therefore the wrist should be left in a neutral position once an epiphyseal separation has been reduced, and one must rely on three-point molding of the cast. After closed reduction, immobilization is maintained for 3–4 weeks.

Repeated, forceful manipulations must be avoided because of the potential for further damage to the physis.[444,474] Bragdon reported a case of premature closure of the distal radius consequent to forceful, repetitive manipulation.[452]

Malposition does not persist, as was well demonstrated by Aitken.[441,442] Within a maximal period of 2–3 years, but more usually within 6–12 months, the distal radial epiphysis assumes its normal relation to the radial metaphysis through remodeling and longitudinal growth. New subperiosteal bone forms on the dorsum and side of the distal radius (Fig. 16-113), and the palmar portion of the metaphysis is gradually absorbed. If repeated attempts at closed reduction fail, it is wise to leave the epiphysis partially displaced and count on extensive metaphyseal remodeling, rather than risk further physeal injury (Fig. 16-114).

Closed reduction is accomplished readily in most instances owing to the type 1 and type 2 lesions with an intact dorsal periosteum. Rarely are they totally displaced, as with comparable fractures of the distal metaphysis. Despite the usual ease of reduction, it is not always possible to reduce the

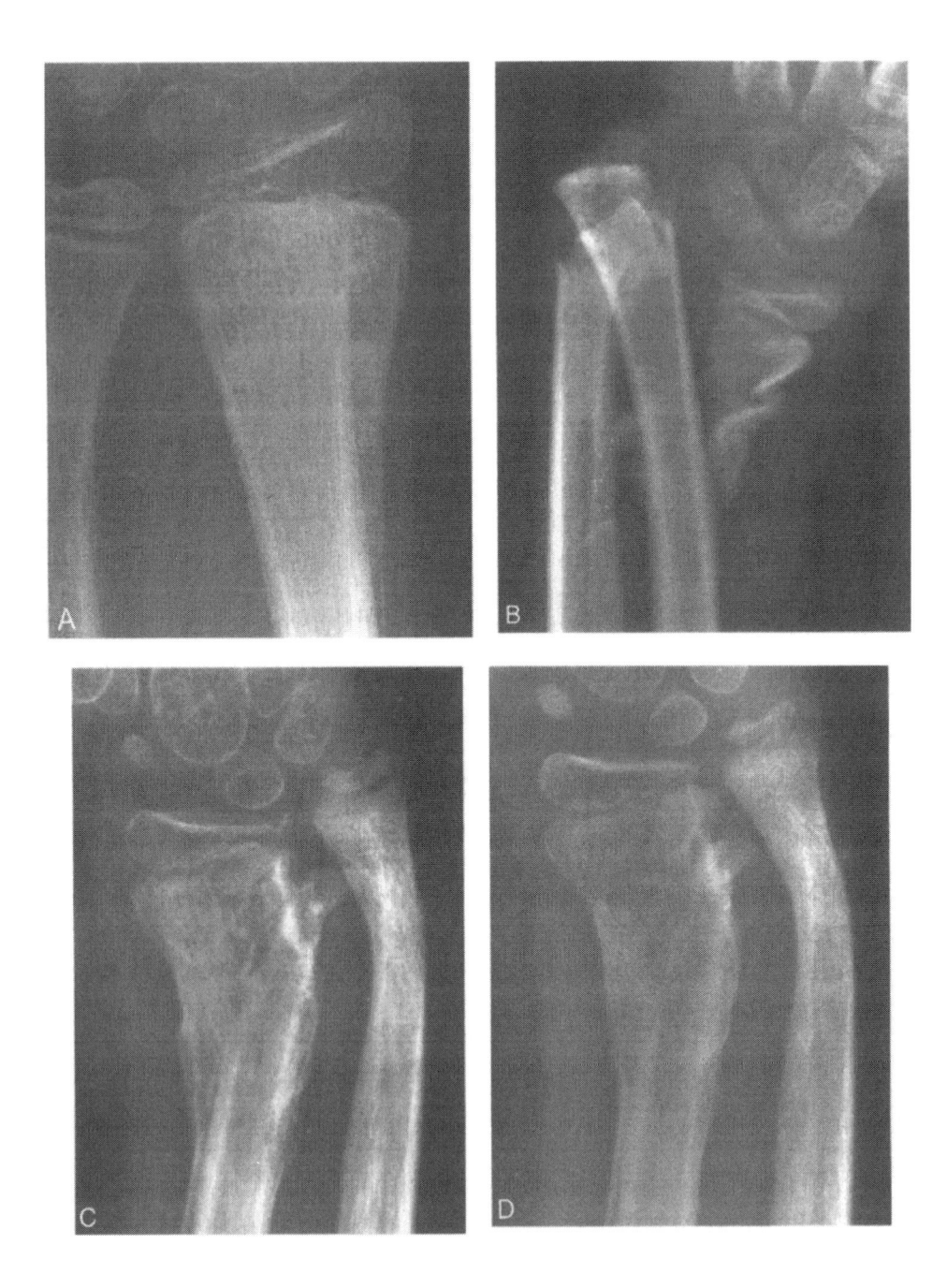

FIGURE 16-113. (A) Extensive new subperiosteal bone formation after a type 2 injury. (B–D) Progressive formation and remodeling of a type 2 physeal injury.

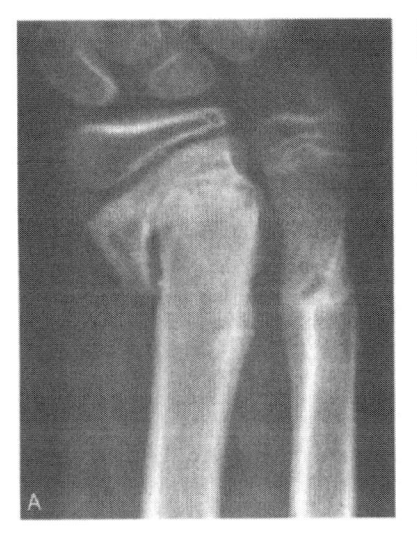

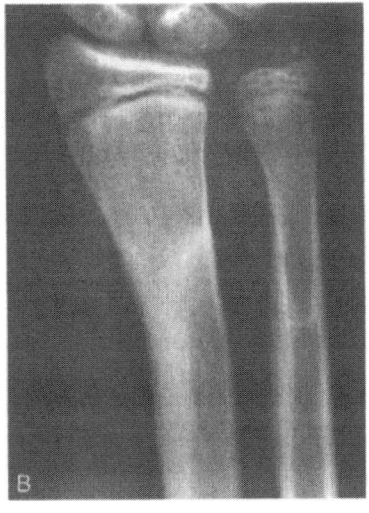

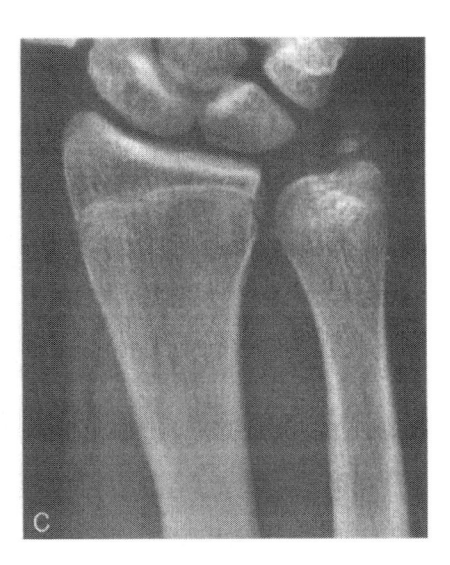

FIGURE 16-114. (A) Type 2 fracture. (B) Two years later. (C) Four years later. Note the nonunion of the ulnar styloid.

dorsal displacement fully. However, repeated, forceful manipulations are not necessary, provided that approximately 50% apposition of the fragments has been attained.

Open reduction of the markedly displaced epiphysis is usually not indicated, although type 3 or type 4 injuries require open reduction (Fig. 16-115). Soft tissue interposition may also prevent closed reduction.[472,477,481,505]

Results

In general, results are good to excellent. These injuries tend to occur in older children; and if growth arrest supervenes, the amount of remaining growth may not be enough to cause significant angular deformity or ulnar overgrowth. Functional limitation is minimal within a few weeks.

Complications

Neurologic Problems

Sterling and Habermann reported a case of posttraumatic median nerve compression in a 10-year-old boy who experienced immediate alleviation of many of his symptoms following initial reduction.[497] The initial sensory decrease took several more days to return to normal. The boy did not require an open reduction or carpal tunnel release. The association of median nerve compression with Colles' fractures in adults is well known, but there have been few reports of this associated phenomenon in children.[438,483] Sterling and Habermann, were able to reduce the symptoms with the fracture reduction. In one of my cases, traction and elevation after reduction did not relieve the symptoms, and exploration and carpal tunnel release were finally necessary. The median nerve was contused. It appears that carpal tunnel anatomic relations do not change significantly with age. Consequently, compression of the median nerve in the carpal tunnel may occur at any age. It is important to examine the child carefully and recognize the condition of the medial nerve prior to as well as after reduction.

Growth Disturbance

Of 53 patients with fractures of the distal radial epiphysis, only one patient in the Davis and Green series had a growth disturbance.[31] However, I have encountered a significant number of patients with distal radial growth deformities.

The distal end of the radius is an infrequent site for growth disturbance due to injury (Figs. 16-116 to 16-120). Several articles have emphasized the possibility of growth damage.[467] The distal ulna may also be involved, which may be due to a localized type 5 injury initially diagnosed as a sprain because there is no significant fracture evident radiographically.

Occasionally, longitudinal forces of the impact damage some of the germinal cells of the physis, producing a localized type 5 physeal injury (Fig. 16-119). This microinjury pattern cannot be detected immediately but is often evident 6–12 months following injury. If the injury is detected early, the possibility of resecting the osseous bridge may be considered.

A Madelung-type deformity may appear, although radiographically it does not resemble the congenital deformity

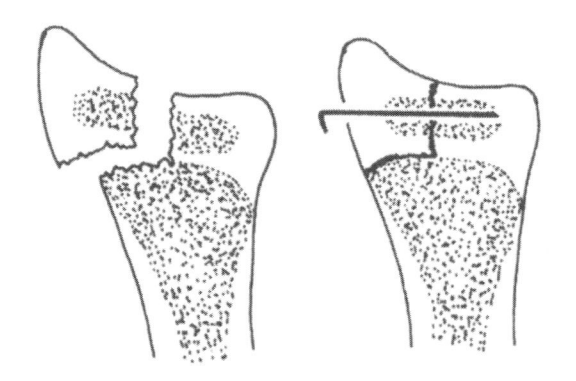

FIGURE 16-115. Type 3 injury of the distal radius with recommended transverse pin or small screw placement.

630

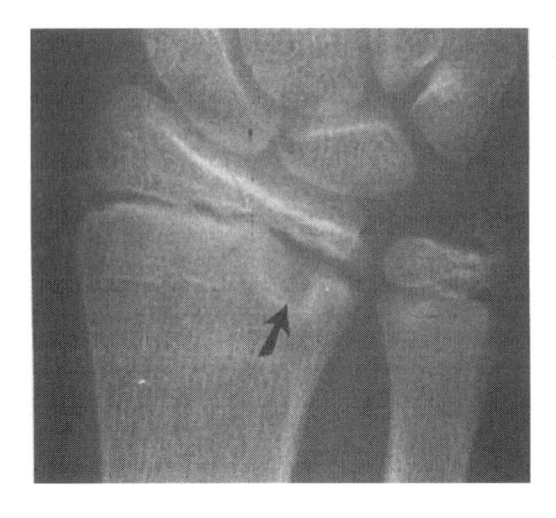

FIGURE 16-116. Partial physeal damage (arrow).

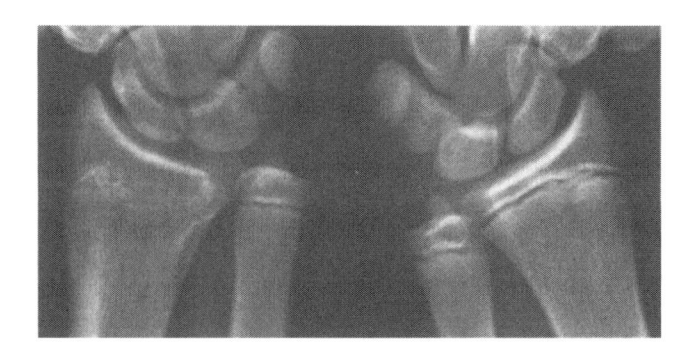

FIGURE 16-117. Premature growth arrest of the radius after type I injury.

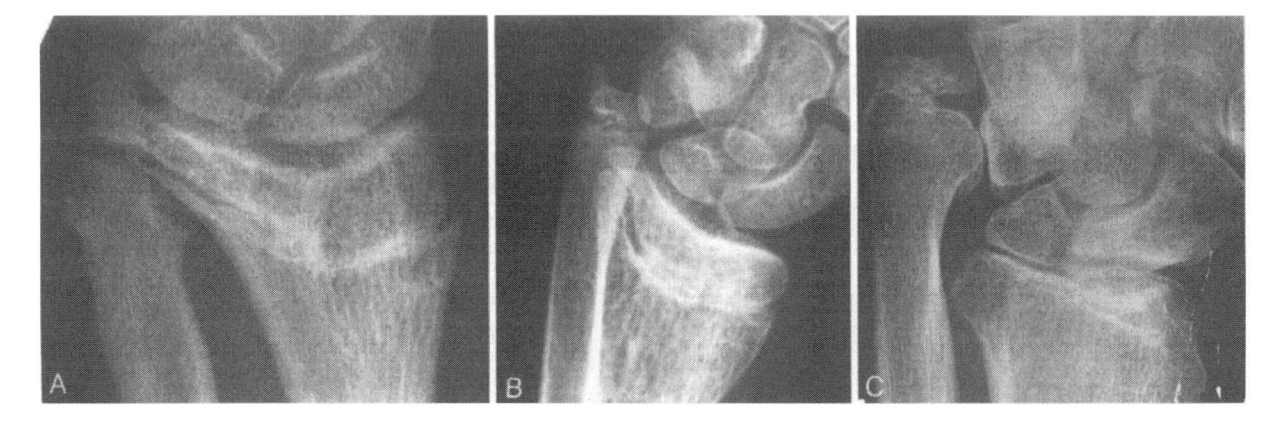

FIGURE 16-118. (A) Premature arrest of the entire distal radius following type 2 injury. Note the styloid nonunion. (B) Growth arrest of the "radial" side of the distal radius, with continued growth on the "ulnar" side. (C) Complete growth arrest of the distal radius with overgrowth of the distal ulna.

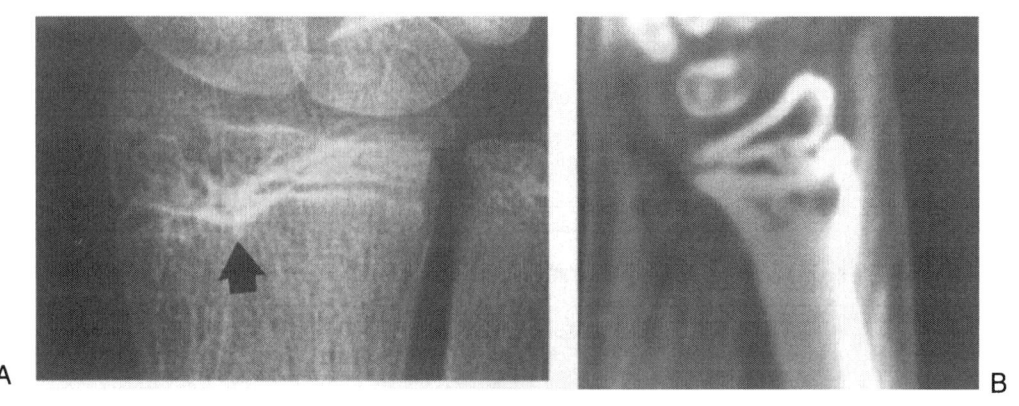

FIGURE 16-119. (A) Localized osseous bridge (arrow) following type 1 injury. (B) Computed tomography shows such bridging.

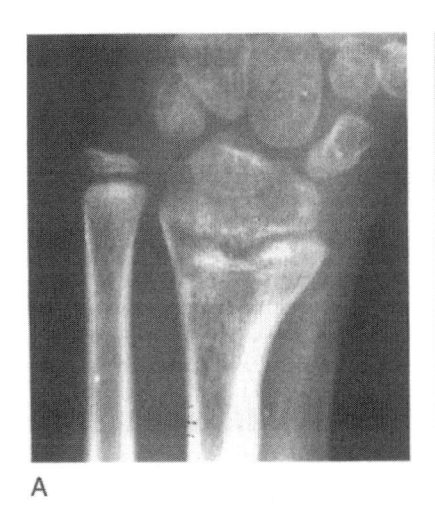

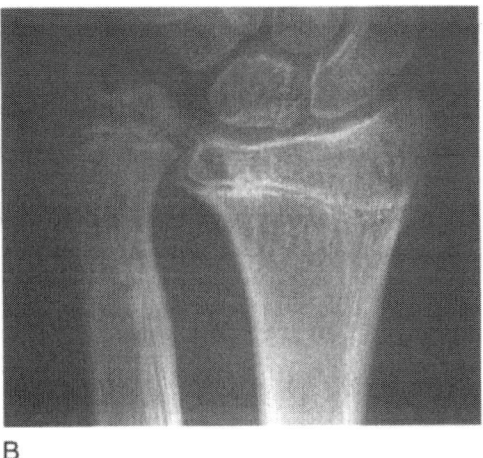

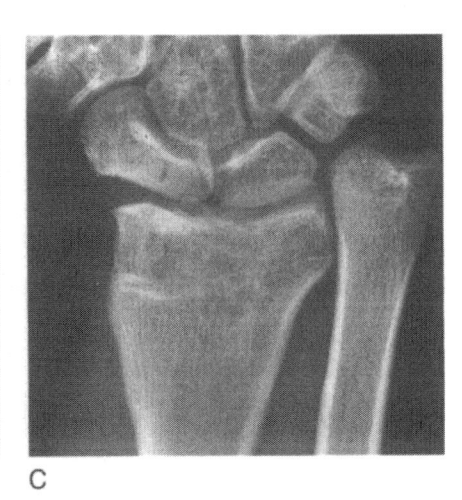

FIGURE 16-120. Radial growth arrest. (A) Slowdown of growth at 7 years. (B) Premature bridging at 10 years. (C) Premature growth arrest at 14 years.

(Fig. 16-121). The Madelung-like deformity occurs because of premature partial fusion of the distal radial epiphysis.[37,491]

Synostosis

Disruption of periosteum and soft tissues around the distal radioulnar joint may lead to excessive bone formation in the interosseous membrane region. The reactive process may proceed to a discrete synostosis (Fig. 16-122). Resection of this complication must await maturation of the reactive process.

Exostosis

An exostosis may form (Fig. 16-123). It is probably due to localized type 6 damage to the periphery of the physis.

Ulnar Styloid

Onne and Sandblom found that two patients had follow-up problems relative to the ulnar styloid, having pain on maximal supination because of a pseudarthrosis of the styloid process or at least a fibrous union between the styloid and the remainder of the ulnar secondary ossification center.[395] This fracture was not evident roentgenographically at the time of the original injury because of the extent of cartilage in that area. The physician must always be careful to consider the possibility of an ulnar styloid cartilaginous fracture, even when ossification does not extend out to that region. The patient and parents should be warned about it and follow-up roentgenograms obtained to determine if it is present as ossification progresses into the region. The likelihood of long-term problems such as pain are rare.

The anatomic interrelation of the ulna and the carpus is important for understanding the high incidence of associated styloid fractures and the uncommon nature of ulnar physeal injury. The distal ulnar epiphysis articulates with the ulnar notch of the radius and, through the TFCC, with the

FIGURE 16-121. Localized growth arrest with Madelung-like deformity.

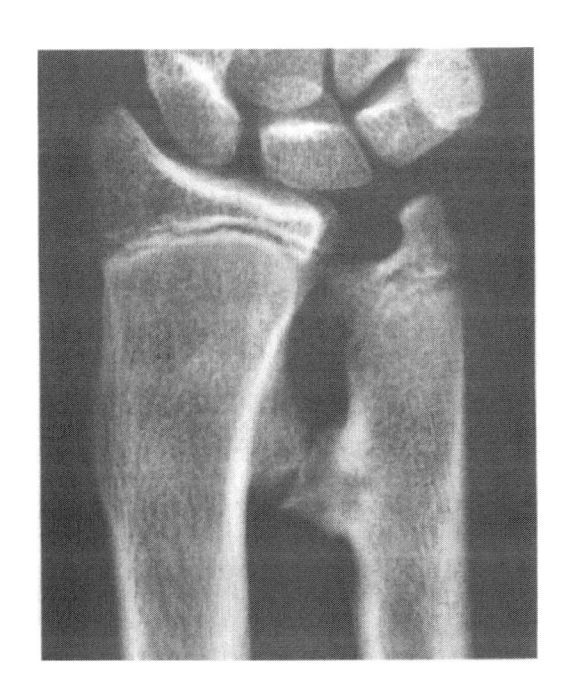

FIGURE 16-122. Synostosis with ulnar growth damage.

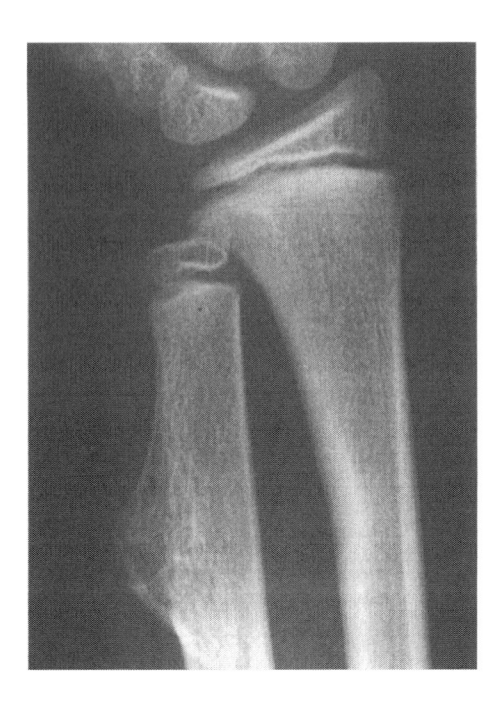

FIGURE 16-123. Ulnar exostosis following an injury that occurred 3 years previous to this film.

distal radial epiphysis. The thick base of this fibrocartilage complex attaches to the ulnar styloid.

Distal Ulnar Physeal Injuries

Injuries to the distal ulnar physis are infrequent but may lead to significant deformity (Figs. 16-124 to 16-128). Most of these injuries accompany distal radial fractures. Most often the distal ulnar injury is a type 7 (styloid) injury. However, discrete ulnar physeal fractures may also occur, as solitary lesions or accompanying a distal radial fracture.[528-540]

Fractures of the distal ulnar physis are an associated injury in fewer than 4% of distal radial injuries. Specific ulnar physeal injuries are clinically distinct and merit differentiation from styloid injuries. Ulnar epiphyseal injuries may also occur in the presence of an ulnar metaphyseal fracture or fractures of both bones of the forearm. They are sometimes listed as the childhood equivalent of the Galeazzi injury.

The low incidence of distal ulnar physeal fracture may be explained in part by the cushioning effect imparted by the interposition of the meniscus between the ulna and the proximal carpal row and propagation of deforming forces through the triangular cartilage directly into the styloid process. These styloid fractures, classified as a type 7 growth mechanism injury, do not usually extend to the primary ulnar physis.

Roentgenographic diagnosis of ulnar physeal and epiphyseal injuries may be difficult. The distal ulnar epiphysis appears later than the radius, not usually ossifying until the sixth year. A separate ossification center for the styloid process has been described but generally occurs at the same level as the main ossification center at its ulnarmost border, rather than at the distal tip of the styloid. A true accessory ossification center for the distal ulnar styloid is infrequent. When present, antecedent trauma with a fibrous union should be suspected. A fracture of the ulnar styloid prior to ossification may not be evident until a radiographic, but not necessarily anatomic, nonunion appears.

In our study, type 1 growth mechanism fractures were the most common physeal pattern.[533] There were six of type 3 growth mechanism injury and one each of types 2 and 4. The specific ulnar physeal injury pattern was not recognized initially in two patients, both of whom developed premature physeal closure. No obvious fracture was present radiographically in either of the anatomic dissections of traumatically avulsed arms, although, microscopic type 1 injuries

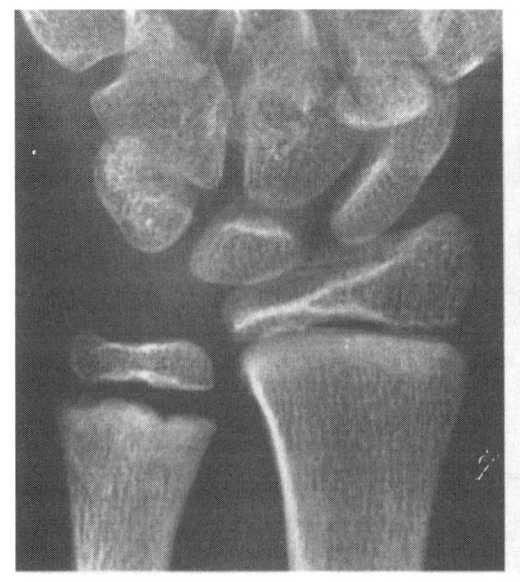

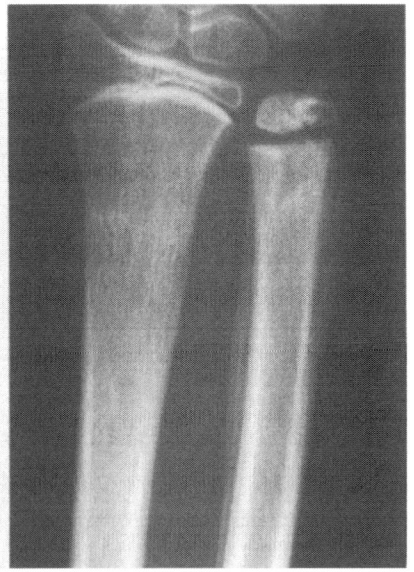

FIGURE 16-124. (A) Widening of the distal ulnar physis indicates a type 1 injury. (B) Subperiosteal reactive bone 5 weeks later confirms the injury.

Distal Ulnar Injuries

FIGURE 16-125. Completely displaced type 2 physeal injury of the distal ulnar physis.

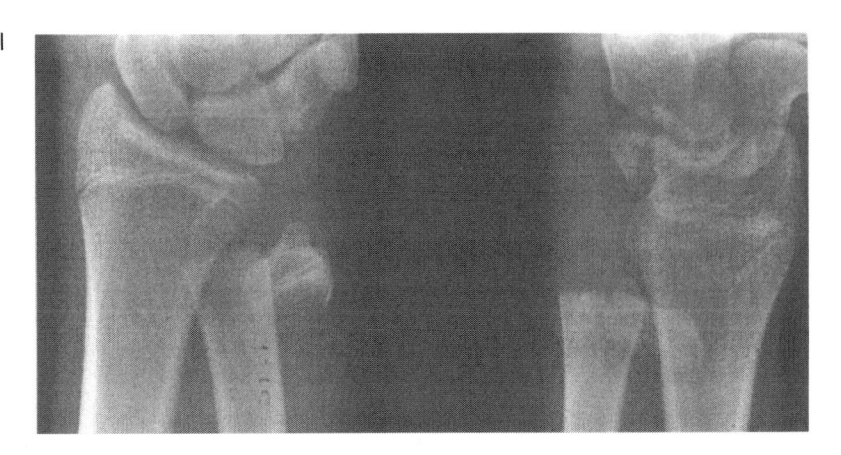

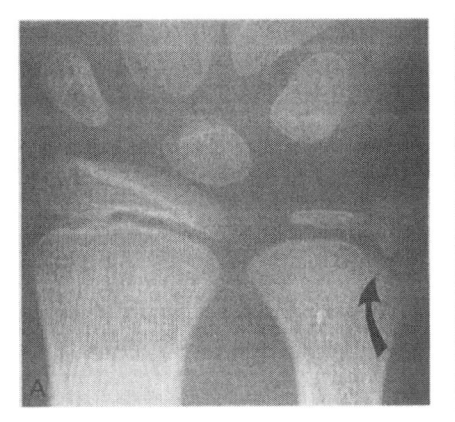

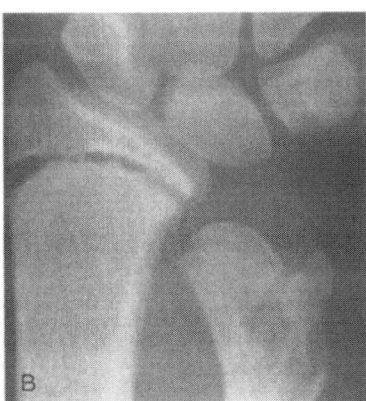

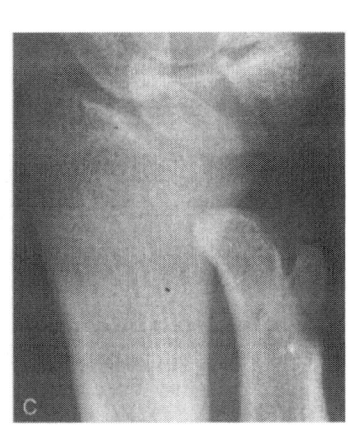

FIGURE 16-126. Growth deformity (arrow), probably due to type 4 ulnar injury (original films unavailable). (A) Six months. (B) Two years. (C) Four years after the injury.

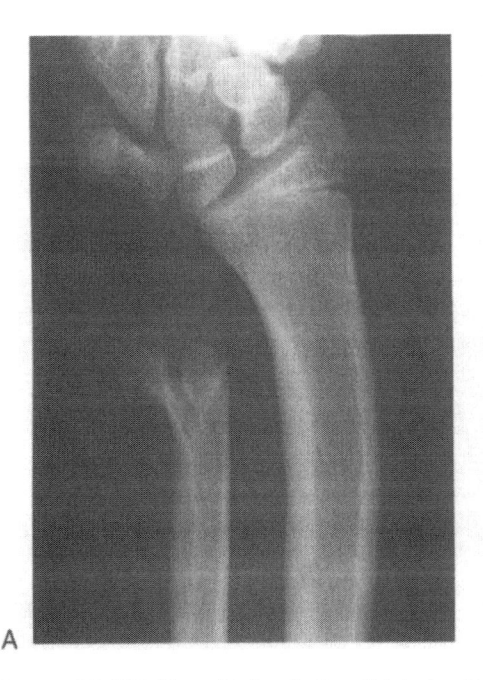

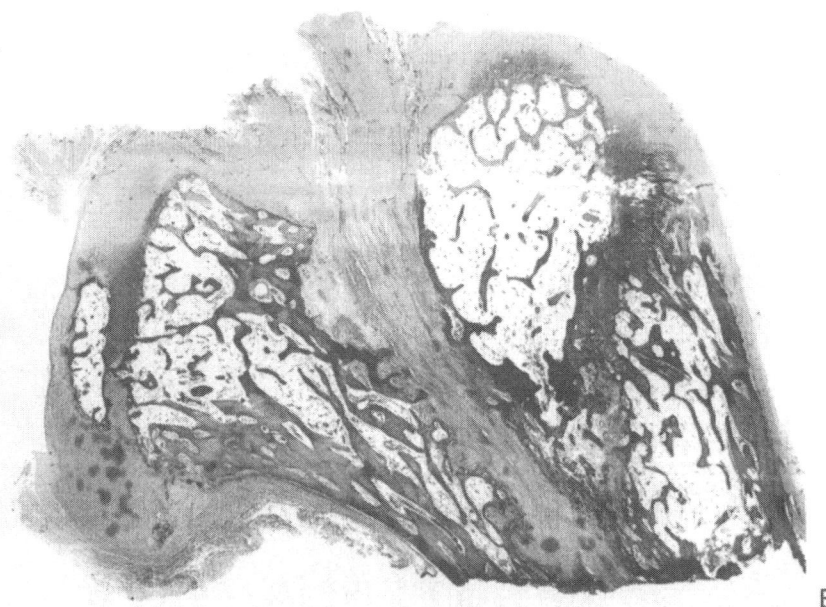

FIGURE 16-127. Type 4 injury to the distal ulna 5 years earlier. (A) Radiograph. (B) Pathologic specimen after resection and release of soft tissue tethering.

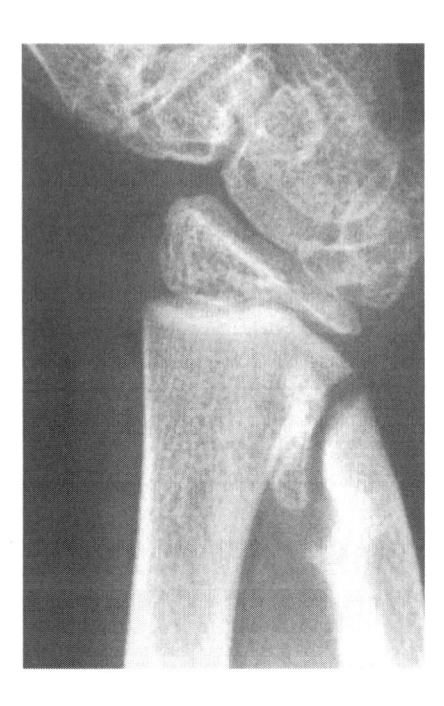

FIGURE 16-128. Angular deformity due to physeal damage.

were present in both ulnas. These two patients, who had sustained traumatic amputations, had a greenstick ulnar diaphyseal fracture associated with a Monteggia dislocation of the radial head and displaced radial and ulnar mid-diaphyseal fractures in addition to a torus fracture of the distal radial metaphysis. Eleven patients sustained distal radial metaphyseal fractures, four of which were incomplete torus injuries. The remaining seven patients sustained distal radial physeal injuries.

Fractures of the distal ulnar physis have been most commonly reported as a type 2 growth mechanism injury pattern. The high incidence of type 1 growth mechanism injuries in our series has not been described previously.[533]

The distal ulna that was resected in one case was examined histologically (Fig. 16-127). The region underneath the ulnar styloid had growth arrest of the physis. In contrast, the region adjacent to the radius had continued to grow, albeit in a deformed manner. A fibrovascular bridge separated the two portions and was probably the remnant of the original type 3 or type 4 injury.

Displacement may be minimal and difficult to diagnose, with the injury being evident only as widening of the physis. In five of our cases the ulnar injury was not apparent initially and was diagnosed only retrospectively with the development of distal ulnar growth impairment.[533]

Initial treatment for displaced ulnar physeal injuries should be directed at anatomic reduction. Fourteen patients were treated with closed reduction, although open reduction was offered (and refused) in three of the fourteen.[533] Operative reduction was necessary after failed attempts at closed reduction in four of our patients (Fig. 16-129). As seen in our cases even with anatomic (open) reduction, there was a high incidence of physeal closure, which most likely reflects the significant disruptive force, ischemia, and soft tissue damage that accompanies these injuries.

Evans et al. described an irreducible type 2 injury of the distal ulna *without* an accompanying radial fracture.[532] At surgery the extensor carpi ulnaris was trapped between the epiphysis and metaphysis. Sumner and Khuri also described tendon and nerve interposition that prevented closed reduction.[539]

There has not been long-term follow-up of a sufficient number of patients with distal ulnar physeal injuries to outline accurately the prevalent natural history of the injury pattern. Of 183 reported cases, adequate long-term follow-up was documented in only 17 cases. Eleven of these patients had premature growth arrest of the distal ulna.

Growth arrest with creation of an ulnar minus variant may occur relatively frequently. Peinado showed that experimental impairment of distal ulna growth in the rabbit had a major effect on deforming the distal radial growth patterns and causing displacement to the ulnar side.[485]

Bell et al. reported on the phenomenon of ulnar impingement syndrome, in which a shortened ulna was impacted against the distal radius and caused a painful, disabling pseudarthrosis.[448] Ten of the eleven cases resulted from excision of the distal ulna after injury to the wrist. However, one was due to growth arrest after fracture of the distal ulna in a child. The symptoms are a painful, clicking wrist and a weak grip. Clinical examination reveals a narrow wrist with pain on compression of the radius and ulna and on forced supination. Radiographs may show scalloping of the distal radius at the site of impingement. The best treatment for symptoms of distal radial ulnar problems after injury in young, active patients is reconstruction, not excision.

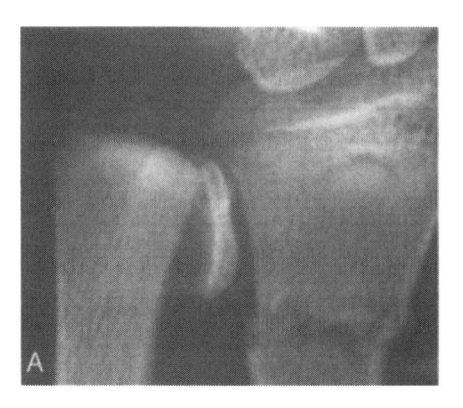

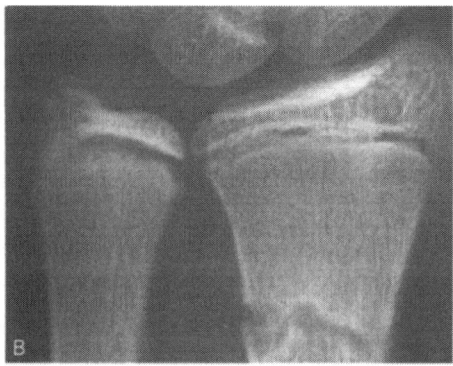

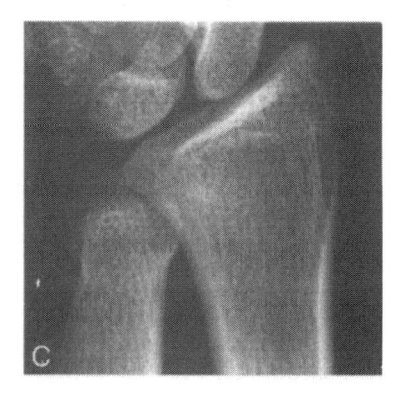

FIGURE 16-129. (A) Type 1 injury of the distal ulna associated with a radial metaphyseal fracture. (B) Fracture was treated with open reduction and a transplanted fixation pin. (C) Patient came back 3 years later because of wrist pain. The ulnar physis had closed prematurely, and the radial articular surface was deformed angularly.

Long-term clinical and radiographic follow-up data were obtained for 18 patients.[533] Follow-up ranged from 1 to 14 years, with an average follow-up of 3.5 years. Premature physeal closure occurred in 10 of these patients (55%). The degree of ulnar minus variance ranged from 2 to 30 mm. For comparing the ulnas we preferred this measurement to additional x-ray exposure of routine contralateral films. Secondary changes of the distal radius and carpus were evident on the radiographs of seven patients. No patient has developed Kienbock's disease.

Despite the radiographic findings, patients with posttraumatic growth arrest have surprisingly few symptoms. In fact, most are asymptomatic. Cosmetic appearance was the most common complaint. Radial deviation was limited, but it was generally not the patients' concern.

Nelson et al. reported four cases of posttraumatic distal ulnar growth arrest with ulnar shortening of 22–39 mm and secondary changes in the radius and carpus.[535] They noted that the progression of deformity was greatest during adolescence. No patient in their study had significant pain or functional impairment, but the cosmetic appearance was displeasing.

The ulna derives 70–80% of its longitudinal growth from the distal epiphysis. Accordingly, longitudinal growth slowdown or arrest could be expected to result in significant deformity. Premature physeal closure is an uncommon complication of forearm fractures, reported to occur in fewer than 7% of distal radial epiphyseal injuries. The exact incidence of premature closure of the ulnar physis is unknown, but it occurred in 55% of our cases with long-term follow-up and in a significant number of cases in the literature. This high incidence of premature physeal closure undoubtedly reflects the force required to overcome the protective anatomy of the wrist before sustaining a distal ulnar physeal injury. All distal ulnar physeal injuries should be followed closely for possible premature physeal closure.

Follow-up radiographs of the skeletally immature wrist may show multiple longitudinal osseous striations crossing the physis of both the radius and ulna. These striations were originally thought to be anatomic variants (i.e., calcification surrounding transepiphyseal vessels). However, recent radiographic and histologic analysis of these striations indicate that they most likely represent a microscopic response to antecedent minor wrist trauma.[12]

Premature closure of the distal ulnar physis may result in several changes at the distal radioulnar joint. Shortening results in the development of an ulnar minus wrist. Ulnar shortening from posttraumatic or other causes, such as hereditary multiple exostoses, may cause a tethering effect on the radius, producing characteristic secondary changes related to the degree of shortening. These changes include lateral bowing of the radial diaphysis, ulnar angulation of the distal radial epiphysis, and ulnar translation of the carpus. There may be tethering and contracture of the soft tissues on the ulnar side of the wrist. Radioulnar convergence also causes loss of the radioulnar joint buttress. Laboratory studies producing impairment of distal ulnar growth in rabbits have demonstrated similar deforming forces on distal radial growth patterns.

Treatment for the posttraumatic ulnar minus wrist is similar to that for other causes of postaxial longitudinal deficiencies and ulnar clubhands. Surgical intervention may be indicated for cosmetic deformity, progressive ulnar subluxation of the carpus, pain, and restricted range of motion at the wrist. Options include resection of the soft tissue tethering, distal radial epiphysiodesis, lateral stapling of the physis for selective partial epiphysiodesis, opening or closing wedge osteotomies of the radius, and ulnar callotasis or chondrodiatasis. Reconstructive procedures, rather than excision of the distal ulna, are preferred whenever feasible.

Galeazzi Fracture-Dislocation

The Galeazzi injury was originally described by Sir Astley Cooper in 1822 but did not receive its eponym until reported by Galeazzi in 1934. The significance of recognizing the Galeazzi-equivalent fracture is (1) appreciation of the presence of a physeal injury and the possible risk of growth plate arrest, and (2) maintenance of stability of the distal radioulnar joint by accurate reduction of the distal ulna. The TFCC usually remains intact. In adults the Galeazzi injury is more common than the Monteggia combination. It is the reverse in the pediatric group. The pediatric injury also has less soft tissue injury or tearing of the interosseous membrane than in the adult.

The Galeazzi injury is a fracture of the shaft of the radius combined with dislocation of the distal radioulnar joint (Figs. 16-130 to 16-133).[541–563] This definition does not include those rare injuries in which there is a fracture of the radial neck and head associated with dislocation of the distal radioulnar joint (Essex-Lopresti injuries).

Schneiderman et al. anatomically studied the interosseous membrane of the forearm with a particular concern for evaluating its structure in the Roland-Galeazzi fracture-dislocation.[561] They thought that the term "interosseous membrane" was a misnomer, and because the structure was a complex of multiple elements with a significant role in force transmission across the forearm, they believed that the term "interosseous ligamentous complex" would be more descriptive. With the Galeazzi fracture-dislocation, this complex may act as a constraint to radial shortening, but it may also act as a stress riser for radial fracture. Anatomic reduction and internal fixation of the radius with early mobilization of the extremity are probably indicated for treatment of most Galeazzi fracture-dislocations in adults and adolescents, and they should be considered in children.

Mikic described 125 patients, including 14 children with the classic lesion and 25 patients with a special type comprising fractures of both bones as well as dislocation of the distal radioulnar joints.[554] Of the children in Mikic's series, there was only 1 patient under 10 years of age and 13 patients between 10 and 16 years.

Landfried et al. studied variants of Galeazzi fracture-dislocation.[549] They thought that a fracture of the radial shaft or metaphysis associated with a fracture through the ulnar growth plate with the epiphysis still attached to the TFCC and accompanied by displacement of the shaft and metaphysis created the equivalent. They described three cases, all of which were treated by open reduction and internal fixation. The distal ulnar epiphysis is more likely to avulse before rupture of the triangular fibrocartilage complex.

Letts and Rowahani reviewed Galeazzi equivalent injuries of the wrist in children and found that the variant—separation of the distal ulnar growth plate with displacement of the ulnar metaphysis—was much more common than the

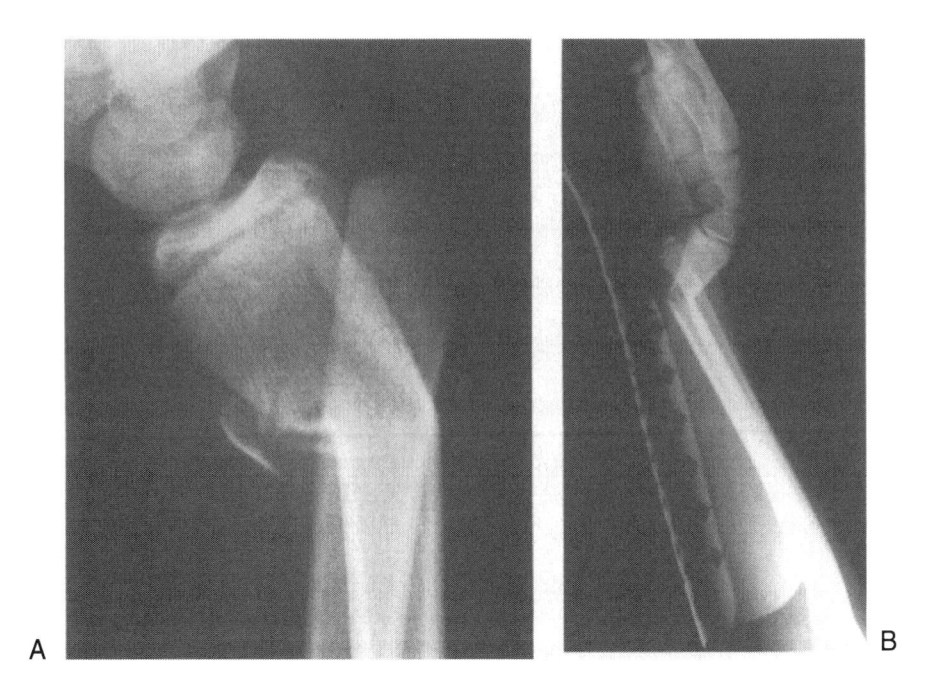

FIGURE 16-130. (A, B) Galeazzi injuries accompany distal radial metaphyseal fractures.

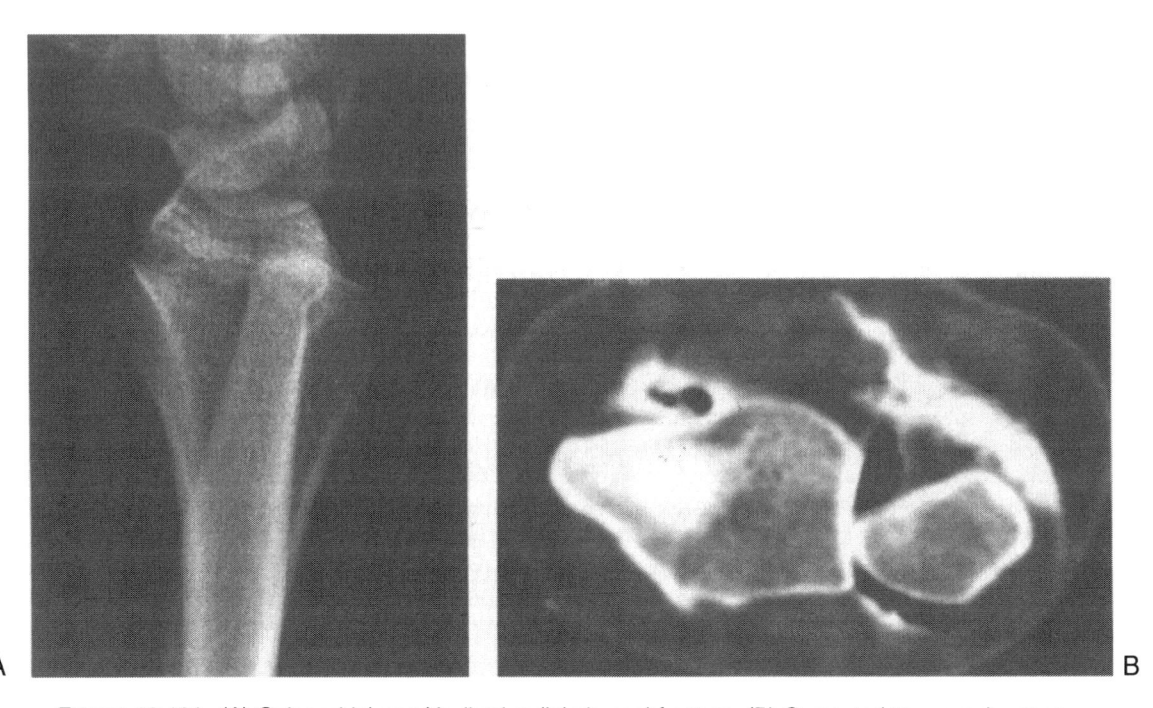

FIGURE 16-131. (A) Galeazzi injury with distal radial physeal fracture. (B) Computed tomography scan.

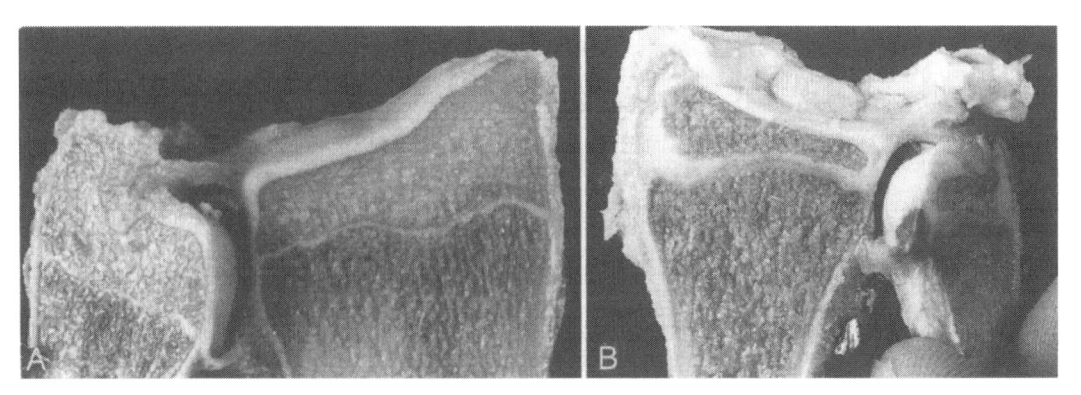

FIGURE 16-132. Re-creation of a Galeazzi injury in specimens, showing how the ulna rotates out from under the triangular cartilage. (A) Beginning rotation. (B) More pronounced rotation.

FIGURE 16-133. Isolated Galeazzi injury.

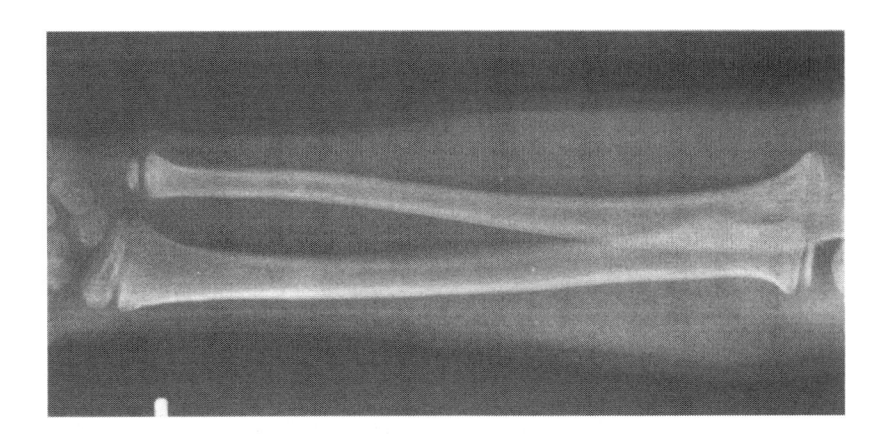

classic Galeazzi fracture-dislocation.[551] They found that the outcome of the equivalent fractures compared to classic Galeazzi injuries was less favorable. One child sustained complete growth plate arrest of the distal ulna.

Involved children frequently have greenstick-type fractures with angular displacement. Most of the time the dislocation of the distal radioulnar joint is evident clinically and roentgenographically (Fig. 16-130). However, sometimes the ulnar head is only subluxated, which is more evident clinically than roentgenographically (Fig. 16-131).

The distal radioulnar joint is stabilized by various structures, such as the ulnar collateral ligament, the anterior and posterior radioulnar ligaments, and the pronator quadratus. The most important stabilizing force is the TFCC. There can be no dislocation of the distal radioulnar joint without some damage to this strong intraarticular fibrocartilaginous ligament. The specific function of the TFCC is to limit the rotational movements of the radius and ulna relative to one another. However, in the skeletally immature patient, avulsion of the ulnar styloid process is the equivalent of rupture of the TFCC and was noted in 30% of the patients in Mikic's series.[554]

There is disagreement over the exact mechanism producing the Galeazzi injury. Most likely, the mechanism is a fall on the outstretched hand combined with extreme pronation of the forearm. The forces cross the radiocarpal articulation, initially producing the dislocation and forced shortening of the radial shaft as the displacement discontinues. Dislocation of the distal ulna causes tearing of the TFCC, which then loses its stabilizing influences on the wrist. Rotational stresses on the forearm also seem essential for dislocation of the distal radioulnar joint. It has been demonstrated clinically and experimentally that a tear or detachment of the triangular articular disc is the first step to dislocation and occurs at the extreme of pronation and extension of the wrist.

Although diagnosis of the Galeazzi fracture-dislocation should not be difficult, it is often missed. The radial fracture is always noted, but the disruption of the distal joint may be easily overlooked, and the ulnar head may seem to protrude and be slightly more mobile than usual. Every roentgenographic examination of an isolated fracture of the radius must include the inferior radioulnar joint. Mikic advocated the use of arthrography to ascertain the presence of the Galeazzi lesion.[554] An abnormal arthrogram showing passage of contrast medium from the wrist into the inferior radioulnar joint cannot be specifically diagnostic of a triangular disc rupture because there may be perforation of the normal disc. However, this perforation is usually present in older patients, not in children, so arthrography can probably be used diagnostically when indicated in younger patients (Fig. 16-134). MRI offers a noninvasive technique for assessing the distal radioulnar joint.

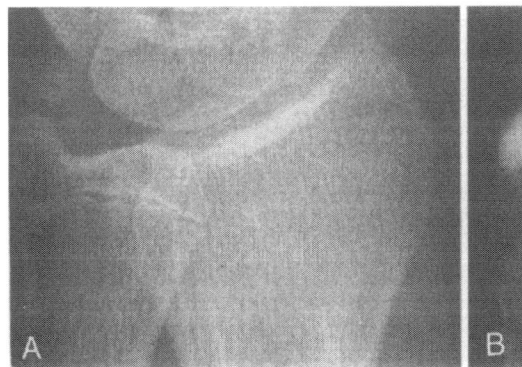

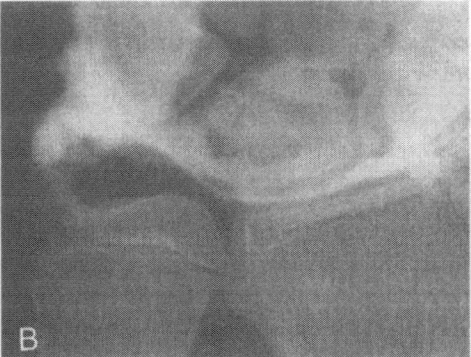

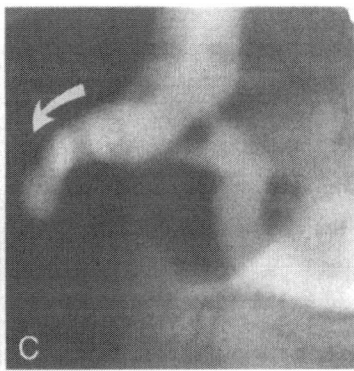

FIGURE 16-134. (A) Premature growth arrest of the distal radius 1 year after bilateral type 1 injuries. The ulnar styloid exhibits nonunion. This patient subsequently had her wrist "twisted" and had chronic, unremitting pain for 3 months prior to this film. (B) Arthrography was performed. Dye surrounds the styloid ossicle, but the triangular cartilage is intact. (C) Extrusion of dye through the capsular defect (arrow). Exploration showed that the triangular cartilage was subluxated from the ulnar articular surface. There was extensive synovitis. It was thought to be an incomplete Galeazzi injury. Treatment consisted of excising the triangular cartilage and styloid fragment, with capsular repair. Eight months after treatment the patient was asymptomatic.

Disruption of the distal radioulnar joint, particularly low grade versions of a Galeazzi injury, can probably be analyzed by CT through this joint (Fig. 16-131).

In Mikic's group, 12 patients were treated nonoperatively.[554] Adequate, stable reduction was easily achieved by manipulation in all cases, probably because most of the fractures were subperiosteal (greenstick). In nine patients the results were excellent, and in only one 15-year-old boy was there redisplacement of the radial fragments with palmar angulation. Closed reduction failed in one patient, and he was subsequently treated with internal fixation and had a fair result. In one 16-year-old boy, percutaneous pinning yielded an excellent result. The patient shown in Fig. 16-134 was treated by resection of the triangular cartilage.

Once the radial fracture is anatomically reduced and the forearm supinated, the subluxation or dislocation of the distal radioulnar joint generally reduces spontaneously and becomes stable. Open reduction is required in some children.

Walsh et al. reviewed 41 children under 15 years of age with a fracture of the radius and probable "disruption" of the distal radioulnar joint.[562] In 41% of the cases the second injury to the radioulnar joint had not been recognized initially. The results of conservative management were generally good; the authors found that the more distal the radial fracture, the greater were the problems encountered. They were able to obtain an initial reduction in all except two patients, both of whom required open reduction. None of these patients had associated fractures of the ulna. They were true disruptions along the joint. Thirty-six of the patients had excellent or fair results after simple manipulation and immobilization. Walsh et al. stressed the importance of obtaining a true lateral radiograph during the evaluation of these injuries, both before and after treatment.

References

Anatomy

1. Acosta R, Huat W, Scheker LR. Distal radio-ulnar ligament motion during supination and pronation. J Hand Surg [Br] 1993;18:502–505.
2. Brodeur AE, Silberstein MJ, Graviss ER. Radiology of the Pediatric Elbow. Boston: GK Hall, 1981.
3. Burman M. Primary torsional fracture of the radius or ulna. J Bone Joint Surg Am 1953;35:665–674.
4. Chen J, Alk D, Eventov I, Wientroub S. Development of the olecranon bursa: an anatomic cadaver study. Acta Orthop Scand 1987;58:408–409.
5. Christensen JB, Cho KO, Adams JP. A study of the interosseous distance between the radius and ulna during rotation of the forearm. J Bone Joint Surg Br 1965;46:778–779.
6. Ekenstam FA. Anatomy of the distal radioulnar joint. Clin Orthop 1992;275:14–18.
7. Evans EM. Rotational deformity in the treatment of fractures of both bones of the forearm. J Bone Joint Surg Br 1951;31:548–553.
8. Hollister AM, Gellman H, Waters RL. The relationship of the interosseous membrane to the axis of rotation of the forearm. Clin Orthop 1994;298:272–276.
9. Hotchkiss RN, An KN, Sowa DT, et al. An anatomic and mechanical study of the interosseous membrane of the forearm: pathomechanics of proximal migration of the radius. J Hand Surg [Am] 1989;14:256–261.
10. McCarthy SM, Ogden JA. Radiology of postnatal skeletal development. VI. Elbow joint, proximal radius and ulna. Skeletal Radiol 1982;9:17–26.
11. Nussbaum AJ. The off-profile proximal radial epiphysis: another potential pitfall in the x-ray diagnosis of elbow trauma. J Trauma 1983;23:40–46.
12. Ogden JA. Transphyseal linear ossific striations of the distal radius and ulna. Skeletal Radiol 1990;19:173–180.
13. Ogden JA, Beall JK, Conlogue GJ, Light TR. Radiology of postnatal skeletal development. IV. Distal radius and ulna. Skeletal Radiol 1981;6:255–266.
14. Pritchett JW. Growth and development of the distal radius and ulna. J Pediatr Orthop 1996;16:575–577.
15. Salter N, Dareus HD. The amplitude of forearm and of humeral rotation. J Anat 1953;87:407–416.
16. Silberstein MJ, Brodeur AE, Graviss ER. Some vagaries of the radial head and neck. J Bone Joint Surg Am 1982;64:1153–1156.
17. Silberstein MJ, Brodeur AE, Graviss ER, Luisiri A. Some vagaries of the olecranon. J Bone Joint Surg Am 1981;63:722–725.
18. Spinner M. The arcade of Frohse and its relationship to posterior interosseous nerve paralysis. J Bone Joint Surg Br 1968;50:809–812.
19. Spinner M, Kaplan EB. The quadrate ligament of the elbow: its relationship to the stability of the proximal radioulnar joint. Acta Orthop Scand 1970;41:632–647.
20. Thiru-Pathi RG, Ferlic DC, Clayton ML, McClure DC. Arterial anatomy of the triangular fibrocartilage of the wrist and its surgical significance. J Hand Surg [Am] 1986;11:258–263.
21. Vesely DG. The distal radio-ulnar joint. Clin Orthop 1967;51:75–91.
22. Weiss APC, Hastings H II. The anatomy of the proximal radioulnar joint. J Shoulder Elbow Surg 1992;1:193–199.

General

23. Alexander CJ. Effect of growth rate on the strength of the growth plate shaft junction. Skeletal Radiol 1976;1:67–76.
24. Blount WP. Fractures of the forearm in children. Ind Med Surg 1963;32:9–16.
25. Blount WP. Forearm fractures in children. Clin Orthop 1967;51:93–107.
26. Blount WP, Schaeffer AA, Johnson JH. Fractures of the forearm in children. JAMA 1942;120:111–116.
27. Bosworth BM. Fractures of both bones of the forearm in children. Surg Gynecol Obstet 1941;72:667–674.
28. Buck P, Folscheiller J, Jenny G. Über die Behandlung von 376 Vorderarmschaft-bruchen bei Kindern. Hefte Unfallheilkd 1976;89:51–60.
29. Carlioz H, Coulon JP. Fracture metaphysaire et diaphysaire de l'enfant. Ann Chir 1980;34:491–498.
30. Dau W. Behandlung von Unterarmbruchen im Kindesalter. Chir Prax 1976;4:485–492.
31. Davis DR, Green DP. Forearm fractures in children: pitfalls and complications. Clin Orthop 1976;120:172–183.
32. Gandhi RK, Wilson P, Mason-Brown JJ, MacLeod W. Spontaneous correction of deformity following fractures of the forearm in children. Br J Surg 1963;50:5–12.
33. Koncz M. Spätergebnisse bei Unterarmfrakturen im Kindesalter. Arch Orthop Unfallchir 1973;76:300–315.

34. Lindholm R, Puronvarsi U, Lindholm S, Leiviska T. Vorderarmschaft-bruche bei Kindern und Erwachsenen. Beitr Orthop Traumatol 1972;7:369–374.
35. Papavasiliou V, Nenopoulos S. Ipsilateral injuries of the elbow and forearm in children. J Pediatr Orthop 1986;6:58–60.
36. Steinert VF. Unterarm-frakturen im Kindersalter. Beitr Klin Chir 1966;212:170–176.
37. Thomas EM, Tuson KWR, Browne PSH. Fractures of the radius and ulna in children. Injury 1975;7:120–124.
38. Tischer W. Forearm fractures in childhood. Zentralbl Chir 1982;107:138–148.
39. Wilson P. Fractures and dislocation in the region of the elbow. Surg Gynecol Obstet 1933;53:335–354.

Proximal Ulna (Olecranon)

40. Ahlgren SA, Rydholm A. Patella cubiti: report of a case. Acta Orthop Scand 1975;46:931–933.
41. An HS, Loder RT. Intraarticular entrapment of a displaced olecranon fracture: a case report. Orthopedics 1989;12:289–290.
42. Burge P, Benson M. Bilateral congenital pseudarthrosis of the olecranon. J Bone Joint Surg Br 1987;69:460–462.
43. Cotton FJ. Separation of the physis of the olecranon. Boston Med Surg J 1900;2:692–694.
44. Donati D, Martini A, Chitoni G. Il distacco epifisans di olecrano; descrizione di un caso. Chir Organi Mov 1992;77:303–306.
45. Fan GF, Wn CC, Shin CH. Olecranon fractures treated with tension band wiring techniques—comparisons among three different configurations. Chang Gung Med J 1993;16:231–238.
46. Florio L, Barile L. La frattura isolata dell' olecrano nell' età infantile. Studio clinics e problemi diagnostici. Osp Ital Chir 1983;36:265–274.
47. Grantham S, Kiernan HA. Displaced olecranon fracture in children. J Trauma 1975;15:197–204.
48. Gunn DR. Patella cubiti. Med J Malaysia 1965;19:314–317.
49. Habbe JE. Patella cubiti: a report of four cases. AJR 1942;48:513–516.
50. Hanks GA, Kottmeier SA. Isolated fracture of the coronoid process of the ulna: a case report and review of the literature. J Orthop Trauma 1990;4:193–196.
51. Hunter LY, O'Connor GA. Traction apophysitis of the olecranon. Am J Sports Med 1980;8:51–54.
52. Ishikawa H, Hirohota K, Kashiwagi D. A case report of patella cubiti. Z Rheumatol 1976;35:407–411.
53. Kovach J, Baker BE, Mosher JF. Fracture separation of the olecranon ossification center in adults. Am J Sports Med 1985;13:105–111.
54. Levine MA. Patella cubiti. J Bone Joint Surg Am 1950;32:686–687.
55. Lowery WD, Kurzweil PR, Forman SK, Morrison DS. Persistence of the olecranon physis: a cause of "Little League elbow." J Shoulder Elbow Surg 1995;4:143–147.
56. Macko D, Szabo RM. Complications of tension-band wiring of olecranon fractures. J Bone Joint Surg Am 1985;67:1396–1401.
57. Matthews JG. Fractures of the olecranon in children. Injury 1981;12:207–212.
58. Maylahn DJ, Fahey JJ. Fractures of the elbow in children. JAMA 1958;166:220–228.
59. Newell RLM. Olecranon fractures in children. Injury 1975;7:33.
60. Papavasiliou VA, Beslikas TA, Nenopoulos S. Isolated fractures of the olecranon in children. Injury 1987;18:100–102.
61. Pavlov H, Torg JS, Jacobs B, Vigorita V. Nonunion of olecranon epiphysis: two cases in adolescent baseball pitchers. AJR 1981;136:819–820.
62. Suprock MD, Lubahn JD. Olecranon fracture with ipsilateral closed radial shaft fracture in a child with open epiphysis. Orthopedics 1990;13:463–465.
63. Tanzman M, Kaufman B. Fracture of the coronoid process of the ulna requiring reduction in extension. J Hand Surg [Am] 1988;13:741–742.
64. Torg JS, Moyer RA. Nonunion of a stress fracture through the olecranon epiphyseal plate observed in an adolescent baseball pitcher: a case report. J Bone Joint Surg [Am] 1977;59:264–265.
65. Turtel AH, Andrews JR, Schob CJ, et al. Fractures of unfused olecranon physis: a re-evaluation of this injury in three athletes. Orthopedics 1995;18:390–394.
66. Van Demark RE, Anderson TR. Fractured patella cubiti: report of case with pathologic findings. Clin Orthop 1967;53:131–134.

Proximal Radius

67. Anderson TE, Breed AL. A proximal radial metaphyseal fracture presenting as wrist pain. Orthopedics 1982;5:425–427.
68. Aufranc OE, Jones WN, Turner RH, Thomas WH. Radial neck fractures in a child. JAMA 1967;202:1140–1142.
69. Baehr FH, Hathaway LE Jr. Removal of separated upper epiphysis of the radius. N Engl J Med 1932;24:1263–1266.
70. Benz G, Roth H. Frakturen im Bereich des Ellenbogens im Kindes und Jugendalter. Unfallchirurg 1985;11:128–135.
71. Bernstein S, McKeever P, Bernstein L. Percutaneous reduction of displaced radial neck fractures in children. J Pediatr Orthop 1993;13:85–88.
72. Bohler J. Die konservative Behandlung von bouchen des radiushalse. Chirurg 1950;21:687–688.
73. Bohrer JV. Fractures of the head and neck of the radius. Ann Surg 1933;97:204–208.
74. Borde J, Dayot P. Fracture de l'extrémité supérieure du radius. Ann Orthop Ouest 1975;7:31–36.
75. Carl AL, Ain MC. Complex fracture of the radial neck in a child: an unusual case. J Orthop Trauma 1994;8:255–257.
76. Chauveaux D, Khouri N. Fracture de l'extrémité supérieure du radius chez l'enfant. J Orthop Pediatr Hop Trousseau Paris 1981;2:27–39.
77. Cotta H, Puhl W, Maritini K. Über die Behandlung knocherner Verletzungen des Ellenbogen gelenkes im Kindesalter. Unfallheilkunde 1979;82:41–46.
78. Dormans JP, Rang M. Fractures of the olecranon and radial neck in children. Orthop Clin North Am 1990;21:257–268.
79. Dougall A. Severe fractures of the neck of the radius in children. J R Coll Surg Edinb 1969;14:220–225.
80. D'Souza S, Vaishya R, Klenerman L. Management of radial neck fractures in children: a retrospective analysis of one hundred patients. J Pediatr Orthop 1993;13:232–238.
81. Ellman H. Anterior angulation deformity of the radial head. J Bone Joint Surg Am 1975;57:776–778.
82. Fasol P, Schedl R. Percutaneous repositioning of fractures of the radial head in children with a Steinman pin. Wien Klin Wochenschr 1976;88:135.
83. Feray C. Methode originale de reduction "peu sanglante" des fractures graves de la tete radiale chez l'enfant. Presse Med 1969;77:2155–2157.
84. Fielding JW. Radio-ulnar crossed union following displacement of the proximal radial epiphysis. J Bone Joint Surg Am 1964;46:1277–2378.
85. Fogarty EE, Blake NS, Regan BF. Fracture of the radial neck with medial displacement of the shaft of the radius. Br J Radiol 1983;56:486–487.

86. Fowles JV, Kassab MT. Observations concerning radial neck fractures in children. J Pediatr Orthop 1986;6:51–57.
87. Fraser KE. Displaced fracture of the proximal end of the radius in a child. J Bone Joint Surg Am 1995;77:782–783.
88. Gaston SR, Smith FM, Baab O. Epiphyseal injuries of the radial head and neck. Am J Surg 1953;85:266–276.
89. Gille P, Mourot M, Aubert D, Lecuyer F, Djebar A. Fracture par torsion du col du radius chez l'enfant: note concernant le mecanisme de cette fracture. Rev Chir Orthop 1978;64:247–248.
90. Goldenbert RR. Closed manipulation for the reduction of fractures of the neck of the radius in children. J Bone Joint Surg 1945;27:267–273.
91. Grindes JP. Les fractures du col du radius chez l'enfant. Thesis No. 4. Univ Toulouse, 1981.
92. Harward E. Anterior angulation deformity of the radial head. J Bone Joint Surg Am 1975;57:776–778.
93. Hassle M, Mellerowicz FH. Frakturen des proximalen Radius im Wachstumsalter. Unfallchirurg 1991;17:24–33.
94. Henrikson B. Isolated fractures of the proximal end of the radius in children: epidemiology, treatment and prognosis. Acta Orthop Scand 1969;40:246–260.
95. Herndon JH, Williams JJ, Weidman CD. Radial growth and function of the forearm after excision of the radial head. J Bone Joint Surg Am 1990;72:736–741.
96. Jeffrey CC. Fractures of the head of the radius in children. J Bone Joint Surg Br 1950;32:314–324.
97. Jeffrey CC. Fractures of the neck of the radius in children: mechanism of causation. J Bone Joint Surg Br 1972;54:717–719.
98. Jones ERL, Esah M. Displaced fractures of the neck of the radius in children. J Bone Joint Surg Br 1971;53:429–439.
99. Judet J, Judet R, Lefranc J. Fracture du col radial chez l'enfant. Ann Chir 1962;16:1377–1385.
100. Kaplan EB. Surgical approach to the proximal end of the radius and its use in fractures of the head and neck of the radius. J Bone Joint Surg 1941;23:86–92.
101. Kaufman B, Rinott MG, Tanzman M. Closed reduction of fractures of the proximal radius in children. J Bone Joint Surg Br 1989;71:66–67.
102. Key J. Survival of the head of the radius in a child after removal and replacement. J Bone Joint Surg 1946;28:148–152.
103. Key JA. Treatment of fractures of the head and neck of the radius. JAMA 1939;96:101–106.
104. Kohler R, James J, Brigand T, Michel CR. Traitement des fractures du radius chez l'enfant par poinconnage percutané (19 cas). Rev Chir Orthop 1991;27(suppl 1):140.
105. Kraus J. Läsionen der Epiphysenfuge am Radiusköpfchen. Akt Traumatol 1975;5:127–131.
106. Krösl W. Operative Behandlung der kompletten Epiphysenlösung am proximalen Speichenende. Chir Praxis 1960;4:49–54.
107. Leung KS, Tse PYT. A new method of fixing radial neck fractures: brief report. J Bone Joint Surg Br 1989;71:326–327.
108. Lewis RW, Thibodeau AA. Deformity of the wrist following resection of the radial head. Surg Gynecol Obstet 1937;64:1079–1082.
109. Lindham S, Hugosson C. The significance of associated lesions including dislocation in fractures of the neck of the radius in children. Acta Orthop Scand 1979;50:79–83.
110. MacEwan DW. Changes due to trauma in the fat plane overlying the pronator quadratus muscle: a radiologic sign. Radiology 1964;82:879–886.
111. Maheshwer CB, Pryor GA. Herbert screw fixation of a Salter Harris type III epiphyseal injury of the radial head. Injury 1994;25:475–476.
112. Manoli A. Medial displacement of the shaft of the radius with a fracture of the radial neck. J Bone Joint Surg Am 1979;61:788–789.
113. McBride ED, Monnet JC. Epiphyseal fractures of the head of the radius in children. Clin Orthop 1960;16:264–271.
114. Merchan ECR. Percutaneous reduction of displaced radial neck fractures in children. J Trauma 1994;37:812–814.
115. Metaizeau JP, Lascombes P, Lemelle JL, Fintayson D, Prevot J. Reduction and fixation of displaced radial neck fractures by closed intramedullary pinning. J Pediatr Orthop 1993;13:355–360.
116. Metaizeau JP, Prevot J, Schmitt M. Reduction et fixation des fractures et decollements epiphysaires de la tete radiale par broche centro-medullaire. Rev Chir Orthop 1980;66:47–49.
117. Mommsen U, Sauer JD, Bethke K, Schontag H. Der Bruch des proximalen Radius im Kindersalter. Langenbecks Arch Chir 1980;351:111–118.
118. Morrey BF, Chao EY, Hui FC. Biomechanical study of elbow following excision of the radial head. J Bone Joint Surg Am 1979;61:63–68.
119. Mouchet A. Fractures of the neck of the radius. Rev Chir 1900;22:596–603.
120. Murray RC. Fractures of the head and neck of the radius. Br J Surg 1940;28:109–118.
121. Newman JH. Displaced radial neck fractures in children. Injury 1977;9:114–121.
122. O'Brien PE. Injuries involving the proximal radial epiphysis. Clin Orthop 1965;41:51–58.
123. Oppolzer RV. Zur reposition des angebrachenen Radius Kopfchens. Zentralbl Chir 1939;66:94.
124. Patterson RF. Treatment of displaced fracture of the neck of the radius in children. J Bone Joint Surg 1934;16:695–698.
125. Pennegot GF. Fracture du col et de la tête du radius. Rev Chir Orthop 1987;73:473–480.
126. Perrin J. Les Fractures du Cubitus Accompagnees de Luxation de l'Extremité Supérieur du Radius. Paris: These de Paris, G Steinheil, 1909.
127. Pesudo JV, Aracil J, Barcelo M. Leverage method in displaced fractures of the radial neck in children. Clin Orthop 1982;169:215–218.
128. Peters CL, Fuchs G. Zur Behandlung der dislozierten Radiushalsfraktur im Kindersalter. Z Kinderchir 1974;15:332–337.
129. Raisch D. Zur Behandlung der Frakturen des Radiushöpfchens im Kindesalter. Z Kinderchir 1967;4:71–76.
130. Rebattu I. Fractures du col du radius chez l'enfant: Place de la technique de reduction par poincon percutané. Thesis No. 121. Lyon, 1985.
131. Reidy JA, Van Gorder GW. Treatment of displacement of the proximal radial epiphysis. J Bone Joint Surg Am 1963;45:1355–1372.
132. Renné J. Zur Therapie frischer, kindlicher Radiusköpfchenfrakturen und in luxationen. Akt Traumatol 1974;4:1–15.
133. Robert M, Moulies D, Longis B, Alain JL. Fractures of the upper part of the radius in children. Chir Pediatr 1986;27:318–321.
134. Rokito SE, Anticevic D, Strongwater AM, Lehman WB, Grant AD. Chronic fracture-separation of the radial head in a child. J Orthop Trauma 1995;9:259–262.
135. Roy DR. Radioulnar synostosis following proximal radial fracture in child. Orthop Rev 1986;15:67–72.
136. Rūcleert K, Fūchs G. Zur Behandlung der dislozierten Radiusholssfraktur im Kindesalter. Z Kinderchir 1974;15:332–237.
137. Schwartz RP, Young F. Treatment of fractures of the head and neck of the radius and slipped radial epiphysis in children. Surg Gynecol Obstet 1933;57:528–534.

138. Scullion JE, Miller JH. Fracture of the neck of the radius in children: prognostic factors and recommendations for management. J Bone Joint Surg Br 1985;67:491.
139. Sessa S, Lascombes P, Prevot J, Gagneux E. Fractures of the radial head and associated elbow injuries in children. J Pediatr Orthop Part B 1996;5:200–209.
140. Speed K. Fractures of the head of the radius. Am J Surg 1924;38:157–162.
141. Speed K. Traumatic lesions of the head of the radius. Surg Clin North Am 1924;4:651–655.
142. Stankovic P, Emmerman H, Burkhardt K, Kurtsch U. Die Frakturen des proximalen Radius im Kindesalter. Z Kinderchir 1975;72(suppl 6):77–85.
143. Steele JA, Graham HK. Angulated radial neck fractures in children. J Bone Joint Surg Br 1992;74:760–764.
144. Steinberg EL, Golomb D, Salama R, Wientroub S. Radial head and neck fractures in children. J Pediatr Orthop 1988;8:35–40.
145. Strong ML, Kropp M, Gillespie R. Fracture of the radial neck and proximal ulna with medial displacement of the radial shaft: report of two cases. Orthopedics 1989;12:1577–1579.
146. Svinukhov NP. The outcomes of operative treatment of fractures of the neck of the radius in children. Ortop Travmatol Protez 1965;26:13–29.
147. Tibone JE, Stoltz M. Fractures of the radial head and neck in children. J Bone Joint Surg Am 1981;63:100–106.
148. Träger KH. Zur Behandlung der dislozierten Radiushalsfraktur im Kindersalter. Arch Orthop Unfallchir 1974;80:25–30.
149. Vahvanen V, Gripenberg L. Fracture of the radial neck in children. Acta Orthop Scand 1978;49:32–38.
150. Van Rhijn LW, Schuppers HA, van der Eijken JW. Reposition of a radial neck fracture by a percutaneous Kirschner wire. Acta Orthop Scand 1995;66:177–179.
151. Vostal O. Fractures of the neck of the radius in children. Acta Chir Orthop Traumatol Cech 1970;37:294–301.
152. Wedge JH. Fractures of the neck of the radius in children. In: Morrey (ed) The Elbow and Its Disorders. Philadelphia: Saunders, 1985, p 237.
153. Wood SK. Reversal of the radial head during reduction of fracture of the neck of the radius in children. J Bone Joint Surg Br 1969;51:707–710.
154. Wray CC, Harper WM. The upside-down radial head: brief report. Injury 1989;20:241–242.

Radial Head Dislocation

155. Almquist EE, Gordon LH, Blue AI. Congenital dislocation of the head of the radius. J Bone Joint Surg Am 1969;51:1118–1127.
156. Amako M, Masada K, Ohhno H, et al. Developmental dislocation of the radial head. J Shoulder Elbow Surg 1994;3:169–172.
157. Armstrong RD, McLaren AC. Biceps tendon blocks reduction of isolated radial head dislocation. Orthop Rev 1987;16:104–108.
158. Bucknill TM. Anterior dislocation of the radial head in children. Proc R Soc Med 1977;70:620–624.
159. Caravias DE. Some observations on congenital dislocation of the head of the radius. J Bone Joint Surg Br 1957;39:86–90.
160. Cavlak Y, Kindel H. Irreponible isolierte dislokation des radiukopfchens. Unfallchirurgie 1984;10:89.
161. Cockshott WP, Omololu A. Familial posterior dislocation of both radial heads. J Bone Joint Surg Br 1958;40:483–486.
162. Danielsson LG, Theander G. Traumatic dislocation of the radial head at birth. Acta Radiol [Diagn] (Stockh) 1981;22:379–382.
163. Ellman H. Anterior angulation deformity of the radial head. J Bone Joint Surg Am 1975;57:776–778.
164. Exahou EL, Antoniou NK. Congenital dislocation of the head of the radius. Acta Orthop Scand 1970;41:551–556.
165. Fox KW, Griffin LG. Congenital dislocation of the radial head. Clin Orthop 1960;18:234–243.
166. Futami T, Tsukamoto Y, Fujita T. Rotation osteotomy for dislocation of the radial head. Acta Orthop Scand 1992;63:455–456.
167. Gallo J, Moreau C. Luxation isolée de la tête radiale. Ann Orthop Oeust 1971;3:31–34.
168. Gattey PH, Wedge JH. Unilateral posterior dislocation of the radial head in identical twins. J Pediatr Orthop 1986;6:220–221.
169. Good CJ, Wicks MA. Developmental posterior dislocation of the radial head. J Bone Joint Surg Br 1983;65:64–65.
170. Green JT, Gay FH. Traumatic subluxation of the radial head in young children. J Bone Joint Surg Am 1954;36:655–662.
171. Gunn DR, Pilley VK. Congenital dislocation of the head of the radius. Clin Orthop 1964;84:108–113.
172. Hamilton W, Parkes JC II. Isolated dislocation of the radial head without fracture of the ulna. Clin Orthop 1973;97:94–96.
173. Heidt RS, Stern PJ. Isolated posterior dislocation of the radial head. Clin Orthop 1982;168:136–138.
174. Hirayama T, Takemitsu Y, Yagihara K, Mikita A. Operation for chronic dislocation of the radial head in children. J Bone Joint Surg Br 1987;69:639–642.
175. Hudson DA, Beer JD. Isolated traumatic dislocation of the radial head in children. J Bone Joint Surg Br 1986;68:378–381.
176. Jaspers PJT. Late treatment of radial head dislocations. Reconstr Surg Traumatol 1979;17:107–112.
177. Kelikian H. Dislocations of the radial head. In: Congenital Deformities of the Hand and Forearm. Philadelphia: Saunders, 1974.
178. Kelly Agnew D, Davis RJ. Congenital unilateral dislocation of the radial head. J Pediatr Orthop 1993;13:526–528.
179. Kuebler JU, Suter A, Exner GU. Luxation "congenitale" de la tête radiale. Ann Chir Main 1992;11:153–156.
180. Lancaster S, Horowitz M. Lateral idiopathic subluxation of the radial head: case report. Clin Orthop 1987;214:171–173.
181. Linhart WE. Die Therapie der persistierenden Radius köpfchen luxation bei Kindern. Beitr Orthop Traumatol 1989;367:176–179.
182. Mardam-Bey T, Ger E. Congenital radial head dislocation. J Hand Surg 1979;4:316–320.
183. McFarland B. Congenital dislocation of the head of the radius. Br J Surg 1936;24:41–49.
184. Mizuno K, Usui Y, Kohnana K, Hirohata K. Familial congenital unilateral anterior dislocation of the radial head: differentiation from traumatic dislocation by means of arthrography. J Bone Joint Surg Am 1991;73:1086–1090.
185. Neviaser RJ, LeFevre GW. Irreducible isolated dislocation of the radial head. Clin Orthop 1971;80:72–74.
186. Novotny F, Florian M. Pourazove isolovane vyklougeni hlavicky radia. Acta Chir Orthop Cech 1970;37:284–287.
187. Peeters FL. Radiological manifestations of the Cornelia de Lange syndrome. Pediatr Radiol 1975;3:41–46.
188. Pletcher D, Hoffer MM, Koffman DM. Nontraumatic dislocation of the radial head in cerebral palsy. J Bone Joint Surg Am 1976;58:104–105.
189. Salama R, Weintroub S, Weissman SL. Recurrent dislocation of the radial head. Clin Orthop 1977;125:156–158.
190. Schubert JJ. Dislocation of the radial head in the newborn infant. J Bone Joint Surg Am 1965;47:1019–1022.
191. Southmayd W, Parks JC. Isolated dislocation of the radial head without fracture of the ulna. Clin Orthop 1973;97:94–96.

192. Stelling FH, Cote RH. Traumatic dislocation of the head of the radius in children. JAMA 1956;160:732–735.
193. Stìren G. Traumatic dislocation of the radial head as an isolated lesion in children. Acta Chir Scand 1959;116:144–147.
194. Svend-Hansen H, Jensen B. Luksation of capitulum radii hos born. Ugeskr Laeger 1977;139:1226–1228.
195. Tait GR. Sulaiman SK. Isolated dislocation of the radial head: a report of two cases. Br J Accid Surg 1988;19:125–127.
196. Thompson JD, Lipscomb AB. Recurrent radial head subluxation treated with annular ligament reconstruction. Clin Orthop 1989;246:131–135.
197. Travaglini F. La Lussazione traumatica isolata del capitello radiale. Arch Chir Moviment 1972;16:422–441.
198. Vesely DG. Isolated traumatic dislocations of the radial head in children. Clin Orthop 1967;50:31–36.
199. White JRA. Congenital dislocation of the head of the radius. Br J Surg 1943;30:377–379.
200. Wiley JJ, Pegington J, Horwich JP. Traumatic dislocation of the radius at the elbow. J Bone Joint Surg Br 1974;56:501–507.
201. Yamamoto M, Futami T, Yamashita Y, Taba H, Yo S. Supination osteotomy of radial shaft for congenital and traumatic dislocation of the radial head. Rinsho Shinkeigaku 1976;11:27–29.
202. Yasuwaki Y, Itagane H, Nagata Y, et al. Isolated lateral traumatic dislocation of the radial head in a boy: case report. J Trauma 1993;35:312–313.
203. Zivkovic T. Traumatic dislocation of the radial head in a 5-year-old boy. J Trauma 1978;18:289–290.

Monteggia Lesion

204. Attarian DE. Annular ligament reconstruction in chronic posttraumatic radial head dislocation in children. Contemp Orthop 1993;27:259–264.
205. Aufranc OE, Jones WN, Bierbaum BE. Late traumatic dislocation of the radial head. JAMA 1969;208:2465–2467.
206. Austin R. Tardy palsy of the radial nerve from a Monteggia fracture. Injury 1976;7:202–204.
207. Bado JL. The Monteggia Lesion. Springfield, IL: Charles C Thomas, 1962.
208. Bado J. The Monteggia lesion. Clin Orthop 1967;50:71–86.
209. Bär W, Vick J. Behandlung ergebnisse bei Monteggia-Frakturen. Beitr Orthop Trauma 1968;15:347–353.
210. Beddow FH, Corkery PH. Lateral dislocation of the radiohumeral joint with greenstick fracture of the upper end of the ulna. J Bone Joint Surg Br 1960;42:782–784.
211. Bell Tawse A. The treatment of malunited anterior Monteggia fractures in children. J Bone Joint Surg Br 1965;47:718–723.
212. Bensahel H. Fractures de Monteggia. Rev Prat 1972;22:1679-1684.
213. Bensahel H, Desgrippes Y. Luxations residuelles de la tete radiale dans la fracture de Monteggia. Ann Chir Infant 1973;14:229–237.
214. Best TN. Management of old unreduced Monteggia fracture dislocations of the elbow in children. J Pediatr Orthop 1994;14:193–199.
215. Bhandari N, Jindal P. Monteggia lesion in a child: variant of a Bado type-IV lesion. J Bone Joint Surg Am 1996;78:1252–1253.
216. Biyani A. Ipsilateral Monteggia equivalent injury and distal radial and ulnar fracture in a child. J Orthop Trauma 1994; 8:431–433.
217. Blasier RD, Trussell A. Ipsilateral radial-head dislocation and distal fractures of both forearm bones in a child. Am J Orthop 1995;24:498–500.
218. Bouyala JM, Bollini G, Jacquemier M, et al. Le traitement des luxations anciennes de la tête radial chez l'enfant. Chir Pediatr 1976;17:96–103.
219. Bouyala JM, Chrestian P, Ramaherison P. L'osteotomie haute du cubitus dans le traitement de la luxation anterieure residuelle aprés fracture de Monteggia. Chir Pediatr 1978;19:201–203.
220. Boyd HB. Treatment of fractures of the ulna with dislocation of the radius. JAMA 1940;115:1699–1703.
221. Boyd HB, Boals JC. The Monteggia lesion: a review of 159 cases. Clin Orthop 1969;66:94–100.
222. Braq H. Fractures de Monteggia. Rev Chir Orthop 1987;73: 481–483.
223. Bruce H, Harvey JP Jr, Wilson J. Monteggia fractures. J Bone Joint Surg Am 1974;56:1563–1576.
224. Bryan RS. Monteggia fracture of the forearm. J Trauma 1971;11:992–998.
225. Bucknill TM. Anterior dislocation of the radial head in children. Proc Soc Med 1977;70:620–624.
226. Chen WS. Late neuropathy in chronic dislocation of the radial head: report of two cases. Acta Orthop Scand 1992;63:343–344.
227. Creer WS. Some points about the Monteggia fracture. Proc R Soc Lond 1947;40:241–242.
228. Cunningham SR. Fracture of ulna with dislocation of head of radius. J Bone Joint Surg 1934;16:351–354.
229. Curry GJ. Monteggia fracture. Am J Surg 1947;73:613–621.
230. Delcourt P. Réfection du ligament de Denucé dans la fracture de Monteggia négligée de l'enfant. Acta Orthop Belg 1972; 38:359–363.
231. Dormans JP, Rang M. The problem of Monteggia fracture-dislocations in children. Orthop Clin North Am 1990;21:251–256.
232. Dubuc JE, Romborets JJ, Vincent A. Les luxations de l'extrémité proximale du radius chez l'enfant. Acta Orthop Belg 1984;50:815–836.
233. Duverney JG. Traite des Maladies des Os. Paris: De Bure l'Aine, 1751.
234. Eady JL. Acute Monteggia lesions in children. J SC Med Assoc 1975;71:107–111.
235. Eady JL. Acute Monteggia lesions in children. Orthop Dig 1976;4:15–20.
236. Evans EM. Pronation injuries of the forearm with special reference to the anterior Monteggia fracture. J Bone Joint Surg Br 1949;31:578–588.
237. Fahmy NRM. Unusual Monteggia lesions in children. Injury 1981;12:399–404.
238. Fournier D. L'Oeconomic Chirurgical. Paris: Francoise Clouzier & Cie, 1671.
239. Fowles JR, Sliman N, Kassab MT. The Monteggia lesion in children: fracture of the ulna and dislocation of the radial head. J Bone Joint Surg Am 1983;65:1276–1283.
240. Frazier JL, Buschmann WR, Insler HP. Monteggia type 1 equivalent lesion: diaphyseal ulna and proximal radius fracture with a posterior elbow dislocation in a child. J Orthop Trauma 1991;5:373–379.
241. Freedman L, Luk K, Leong JCY. Radial head reduction after a missed Monteggia fracture: brief report. J Bone Joint Surg Br 1988;70:846–847.
242. Germain JP. Fracture de Monteggia avec luxation laterale de la tête radiale. Un Med Can 1976;105:56–60.
243. Gibson W, Timperlake R. Operative treatment of a type IV Monteggia fracture-dislocation in a child. J Bone Joint Surg Br 1992;74:780–781.
244. Giustra P, Killoran P, Furman R. The missed Monteggia fracture. Radiology 1974;110:45–47.

245. Givon U, Pritsch M, Levy O, et al. Monteggia and equivalent lesions. Clin Orthop 1997;337:208–215.
246. Gottschalk E. Zur osteosynthese Kindlicher Vorderarmfrakturen unter Einschluss von Radiusköpfchen, olecranon und Monteggia-Schaden. Beitr Orthop Traumatol 1980;27:78–95.
247. Guilleminet M, Faysse R. Traitement chirurgicale de la fracture de Monteggia chez l'enfant. Lyon Chir 1957;53:412–415.
248. Hertl P, Verdenhalven T. Monteggia-Verletzungen. Orthopade 1988;17:328–335.
249. Hirayama T, Takemitsu Y, Yagihara K, Mikita A. Operation for chronic dislocation of the radial head in children. J Bone Joint Surg Br 1987;69:639–642.
250. Höllworth M, Hansbrandt D. Die Monteggia-Fraktur im Kindersalter. Unfallheilkunde 1978;81:77–80.
251. Hume AC. Anterior dislocation of the head of the radius associated with undisplaced fracture of the olecranon in children. J Bone Joint Surg Br 1957;39:508–512.
252. Hunt GH. Fracture of the shaft of the ulna with dislocation of the head of the radius. JAMA 1939;112:1241–1244.
253. Hurst LC, Dubrow EN. Surgical treatment of symptomatic chronic radial head dislocation: a neglected Monteggia fracture. J Pediatr Orthop 1983;3:227–230.
254. Iselin F, Rigault P, Judet J. Fractures de Monteggia chez l'enfant. Presse Med 1966;74:2898–2901.
255. Jessing P. Monteggia lesions and their complicating nerve damage. Acta Orthop Scand 1975;46:601–609.
256. Judet R, Lord G, Roy-Camille R. Osteotomy of the cubital diaphysis in old dislocations of the radial head in the child. Presse Med 1962;70:1307–1308.
257. Kalamchi A. Monteggia fracture-dislocation in children. J Bone Joint Surg Am 1986;68:615–619.
258. Kamali M. Monteggia fracture: presentation of an unusual case. J Bone Joint Surg Am 1974;56:841–843.
259. Kini MG. Dislocation of the head of the radius associated with fracture of the upper third of the ulna. Antiseptic 1940;37:1059–1062.
260. Kristiansen B, Erikson AF. Simultaneous type II Monteggia lesion and fracture separation of the lower radial epiphysis. Injury 1986;17:51–52.
261. Leconte D, Abdulwahed O, Mouterde P. Traitement chirurgical de la fracture récente de Monteggia chez le nourrisson. Chir Pediatr 1989;30:213–214.
262. Lehfuss H. A propos de la fracture de Monteggia chez l'enfant. Monatsschr Unfallheilkd 1974;77:59–65.
263. Leitner B. Behandlungsergebnisse der Brüche der Elle mit begleitender Speichenköpfchen verrenkung (Monteggia-Verletzung). Hefte Unfallheilkd 1953;46:102–139.
264. Letts M, Locht R, Wiens J. Monteggia fracture-dislocations in children. J Bone Joint Surg Br 1985;67:724–727.
265. Lichter RL, Jacobsen T. Tardy palsy of the posterior interosseous nerve with a Monteggia fracture. J Bone Joint Surg Am 1975;57:124–125.
266. Lloyd-Roberts GC, Bucknill RM. Anterior dislocation of the radial head in children. J Bone Joint Surg Br 1977;59:402–407.
267. Mandaba JL, Desgrippes Y, Bensahel H. Reflexion a propos d'une serié de 38 fractures de Monteggia chez l'enfant. J Chir (Paris) 1979;116:573–576.
268. Mehta SD. Flexion osteotomy for untreated Monteggia fracture in children. Indian J Surg 1985;47:15–19.
269. Molnar J, Kovalkovits I. Operative Behandlung der Monteggia-Frakturen. Beitr Orthop Traumatol 1969;16:501–507.
270. Monteggia GB. Istituzione Chirurgiche, 2nd ed. Milan: G Maspero, 1813–1815.
271. Morris AH. Irreducible Monteggia lesion with radial-nerve entrapment. J Bone Joint Surg Am 1974;56:1744–1746.
272. Mullick S. The lateral Monteggia fracture. J Bone Joint Surg Am 1977;59:543–545.
273. Nand S. Clinical study of Monteggia fracture-dislocation. J Bone Joint Surg Br 1966;48:198.
274. Naylor A. Monteggia fractures. Br J Surg 1942;29:323–326.
275. Nishio A, Toguchida K, Kuwahara K, Otsuki K. Treatment of the old Monteggia fracture-dislocation by osteotomy of the ulna. Sangyo Igaku 1965;8:67–72.
276. Olney BW, Menelaus MB. Monteggia and equivalent lesions in children. J Pediatr Orthop 1989;9:219–223.
277. Oner FC, Diepstraten AFM. Treatment of chronic posttraumatic dislocation of the radial head in children. J Bone Joint Surg Br 1993;75:577–581.
278. Oveson O, Brok KE, Arreskøv J, Bellstrom T. Monteggia lesions in children and adults: an analysis of etiology and long-term results of treatment. Orthopedics 1990;13:529–534.
279. Papavasiliou V, Nemopoulos SP, Monteggia-type elbow fractures in childhood. Clin Orthop 1988;233:230–233.
280. Peiro A, Andres F, Fernandez-Esteve F. Acute Monteggia lesions in children. J Bone Joint Surg Am 1977;59:92–97.
281. Peltier LF. Eponymic fractures: Giovanni Battista Monteggia and Monteggia's fracture. Surgery 1957;42:585–591.
282. Penrose JH. The Monteggia fracture with posterior dislocation of the radial head. J Bone Joint Surg Br 1951;33:65–73.
283. Picard JJ, Caire SC. Les luxations résiduelles de la tête radial après fracture de Monteggia chez l'enfant. Lyon Chir 1962;58:773–780.
284. Poinsot G. Dislocations of the head of the radius downward (by elongation). NY State J Med 1885;41:8–12.
285. Polonsky AD. Monteggia fracture. J Bone Joint Surg Br 1956;38:593.
286. Ramsey RH, Pedersen HE. The Monteggia fracture-dislocation in children. JAMA 1962;182:1091–1098.
287. Rao SBN, Patrick J. Isolated fracture-dislocation of the proximal radius: a previously undescribed injury. Injury 1991;22:484–485.
288. Raux P. Fracture de Monteggia chez l'enfant: étude de 57 cas. Ann Chir Infant 1975;16:423–435.
289. Ravessoud FA. Lateral condylar fracture and ipsilateral ulnar shaft fracture: Monteggia equivalent lesions? J Pediatr Orthop 1985;5:364–366.
290. Reckling FW, Cordell LD. Unstable fracture-dislocations of the forearm (Monteggia and Galeazzi). J Bone Joint Surg Am 1982;64:857–863.
291. Renné J, Bäuerle E. Therapeutische Mäglichkeiten nach ungenügend behandelten Monteggia-Verletzungen. Z Orthop 1976;114:659–663.
292. Ring D, Waters PM. Operative fixation of Monteggia fractures in children. J Bone Joint Surg Br 1996;78:734–739.
293. Rodgers WB, Smith B. A type IV Monteggia injury with a distal diaphyseal fracture in a child. J Orthop Trauma 1993;7:84–86.
294. Rodgers WB, Waters PM, Hall JE. Chronic Monteggia injuries in children: complications and results of reconstruction. J Bone Joint Surg Am 1996;78:1322–1329.
295. Salem GI, Göber W, Kreuzer W, Wense G. Über den Verrenkungsbouch im Ellenbogengelenk. Unfallheilkunde 1974;77:49–54.
296. Schultiz KP. Die operative Behandlung der veralteten Radiusköpfchen-luxation im Kindesalter. Arch Orthop Unfallchir 1975;225–229.
297. Shonnard PY, Decoster TA. Combined Monteggia and Galeazzi fractures in a child's forearm. Orthop Rev 1994;23:755–759.
298. Simpson JM, Andreshak TG, Patel A, Jackson WT. Ipsilateral radial head dislocation and radial shaft fracture. Clin Orthop 1991;266:205–208.
299. Smith FM. Monteggia fractures: analysis of 25 consecutive fresh injuries. Surg Gynecol Obstet 1947;85:630–640.

300. Soin B, Hunt N, Hollingdale J. An unusual forearm fracture in a child suggesting a mechanism for the Monteggia injury. Injury 1995;26:407–408.
301. Solcard R. Fracture de Monteggia vicieusement consolidee avec synostose radiocubitale. Rev Chir Orthop 1932;19:36–39.
302. Speed JS, Boyd HB. Treatment of fractures of the ulna with dislocations of the radius. JAMA 1940;115:1699–1705.
303. Spinner M, Freundlich BD, Teicher J. Posterior inter-osseous nerve palsy as a complication of Monteggia fractures in children. Clin Orthop 1968;58:141–145.
304. Stein F, Grabias SL, Deffer PA. Nerve injuries complicating Monteggia lesions. J Bone Joint Surg Am 1971;53:1432–1436.
305. Stelling FH, Cote RH. Traumatic dislocation of head of radius in children. JAMA 1956;169:732–736.
306. Stoll TM, Willis RB, Paterson DC. Treatment of the missed Monteggia fracture in the child. J Bone Joint Surg Br 1992; 74:436–440.
307. Tajima T, Yoshizu T. Treatment of long-standing dislocation of the radial head in neglected Monteggia fractures. J Hand Surg [Am] 1995;20:591–594.
308. Theodorou SD. Dislocation of the head of the radius associated with fractures of the upper end of the ulna in children. J Bone Joint Surg Br 1969;51:700–706.
309. Thompson HA, Hamilton AT. Monteggia fracture: internal fixation of fractured ulna with intramedullary pin. Am J Surg 1950;73:579–584.
310. Tompkins DG. The anterior Monteggia fracture. J Bone Joint Surg Am 1971;53:1109–1114.
311. Trillat A, Marsan C, Lapeyre B. Classification et traitement des fractures de Monteggia a propos de 36 observations. Rev Chir Orthop 1969;55:639–657.
312. Van Sanvoordt R. Dislocation of the radial head downward. NY State J Med 1887;45:63–64.
313. Verneret C, Langlais J, Pouliquen JC, Rigault P. Luxations anciennes post-traumatiques de la tête radiale chez l'enfant. Rev Chir Orthop 1989;75:77–89.
314. Wiener R, Scheier HJG, Grummont P, et al. Veraltete Radiusköpfchen-luxation bei Kindern nach Monteggia Verletzungen. Orthopade 1981;10:307–310.
315. Wiley JJ, Galey JP. Monteggia injuries in children. J Bone Joint Surg Br 1985;67:728–731.
316. Winklemann W, Schulitz KP, Küster HH. Der meta-epiphysäre Typ der Monteggia-Fraktur. Chirurg 1978;49:452–456.
317. Wise A. Lateral dislocation of the head of the radius with fracture of the ulna. J Bone Joint Surg 1941;23:379–381.
318. Wisniewski T, Hac B. Ocena loyników leczenia zlamán typn Monteggia. Chir Narzad Ruchu Ortop Polska 1970;35:579–584.
319. Wright PR. Greenstick fracture of the upper end of the ulna with dislocation of the radiohumeral joint or displacement of the superior radial epiphysis. J Bone Joint Surg Br 1963; 45:727–731.
320. Yamamoto M, Futani T, Yamashita Y, Taba H, Amari S. Supination osteotomy for congenital and traumatic dislocation of radius head. Rinsho Seikeigeka 1976;11:27–35.
321. Yoshizu T. Treatment of neglected Monteggia fracture-dislocations. Rinsho Seikeigeka 1987;22:165–174.

Diaphysis

322. Alpar EK, Thompson K, Owen R, Taylor JF. Midshaft fractures of forearm bones in children. Injury 1981;13:153–158.
323. Amit Y, Salai M, Chechick A, et al. Closed intramedullary nailing for the treatment of diaphyseal forearm fractures in adolescence: a preliminary report. J Pediatr Orthop 1985; 5:143–146.
324. Anderson LD. Complications of forearm fractures. I. Malunion. Complications Orthop 1988;3:39–41.
325. Anderson LD. Complication of forearm frctures. II. Delayed union and non-union. Complications Orthop 1988;3:78–82.
326. Ashhurst AC, John RL. The treatment of fractures of the forearm with notes of the end results. Episcopal Hosp Rep 1913;1:224–230.
327. Bagley CH. Fractures of both bones of the forearm. Surg Gynecol Obstet 1926;42:95–103.
328. Bjelland JC. Radiology case of the month: acute plastic bowing fracture of the ulna. Ariz Med 1976;33:653–655.
329. Blackburn N, Ziv I, Rang M. Correction of the malunited forearm fracture. Clin Orthop 1984;188:54–57.
330. Blankstein A, Liberty E, Itay S, et al. Biomechanical aspect of traumatic bowing of the forearm in children. Orthop Rev 1985;14:217–221.
331. Blasier RD, Salamon PB. Pediatric adolescent forearm fractures. Oper Tech Orthop 1993;3:128–133.
332. Blount WP, Schaefer AA, Johnson JH. Fractures of the forearm in children. JAMA 1942;120:111–116.
333. Borden S. Traumatic bowing of the forearm in children. J Bone Joint Surg Am 1974;56:611–616.
334. Borden S. Roentgen recognition of acute plastic bowing of the forearm in children. AJR 1975;125:524–530.
335. Buch J, Leixnering M, Hintringer W, Poigenfürst J. Markdrähtung instabiler unterarm Schaft brüche bei Kindern. Unfallchirurg 1991;17:253–258.
336. Calati A, Poli A. Il fenomeno dell' iperallungamento osseo consequente a fratture diafisarie di ossa lunghe riportate nell'infanzia e nel d'adolescenza. Minerva Ortop 1959;10:827–846.
337. Carey PJ, Alburger PD, Betz RR, et al. Both-bone forearm fractures in children. Orthopedics 1992;15:1015–1019.
338. Chigot PL, Esteve P. Traitement des fractures diaphysaires de l'avant-bras chez l'enfant. Rev Prat 1972;221:1615–1635.
339. Creasman C, Zaleske DJ, Ehrlich G. Analyzing forearm fractures in children: the more subtle signs of impending problems. Clin Orthop 1984;188:40–53.
340. Crowe JE, Swischuk LE. Acute bowing fractures of the forearm in children: a frequently missed injury. AJR 1977;128:981–984.
341. Davis DR, Green DP. Forearm fractures in children: pitfalls and complications. Clin Orthop 1976;120:172–184.
342. Davis MW, Litman T, Barnett RM. Plastic deformation of the forearm in children following trauma. Minn Med 1977;60: 635–636.
343. Demos TC. Radiologic case study: traumatic (plastic) bowing of the ulna. Orthopedics 1980;3:1108–1109.
344. DePablos J, Franzeb M, Barrios C. Longitudinal growth patterns of the radius after forearm fractures conservatively treated in children. J Pediatr Orthop 1994;14:492–495.
345. Destot E. De las perte des mouvements de pronation et de supination dans les fractures de l'avant bras. Lyon Med 1909;112:61–72.
346. Destot E. Pronation and supination of the forearm in traumatic lesions. Presse Med 1913;21:41–48.
347. Dietz JM. Contribution à l'étude de la prono-supination chez l'enfant après fracture de'avant-bras traitée orthopédiquement. Strasbourg: Theses Médecine, 1980, no. 153.
348. Duruwalla J. Study of radioulnar movements following fractures of the forearm in children. Clin Orthop 1979;139:114–120.
349. Evans EM. Fractures of the radius and ulna. J Bone Joint Surg Br 1951;33:548–561.

References

350. Fatti JF, Mosher JF. An unusual complication of fracture of both bones of the forearm in a child. J Bone Joint Surg Am 1986;68:451–453.
351. Feldkamp G, Daum R. Langzeitergebnisse kindlicher Unterarmschaftbruche. Unfallheilkdunde 1978;132:389–392.
352. Filipe G, Dupont JY, Carlioz H. Les fractures iteratives des deux os de l'avant bras de l'enfant. Chir Pediatr 1979;20:421–426.
353. Finsterbush A, Stein H, Robin GC, et al. Recent experiences with intravenous regional anesthesia in limbs. J Trauma 1972;12:81–84.
354. Firica A, Popescu R, Scarlat M, et al. De ostéosynthèse stable élastique, nouveau concept biomécanique: étude expérimentale. Rev Chir Orthop 1981;67(suppl II):82–91.
355. Flynn JM, Waters PM. Single-bone fixation of both-bone forearm fractures. J Pediatr Orthop 1996;16:655–659.
356. Fuller DJ, McCullough CJ. Malunited fractures of the forearm in children. J Bone Joint Surg Br 1982;64:364–367.
357. Gainor BJ, Olson S. Combined entrapment of the median and anterior interosseous nerves in a pediatric both-bone forearm fracture. J Orthop Trauma 1990;4:197–199.
358. Gainor JW, Hardy JH III. Forearm fractures treated in extension: immobilization of fractures of the proximal bones of the forearm in children. J Trauma 1968;9:167–171.
359. Gandhi RK, Wilson P, Mason Brown JJ, MacLeod W. Spontaneous correction of deformity following fractures of the forearm in children. Br J Surg 1962;50:5–10.
360. Glorion B, Delplace J, Boucher M. Déformation squelettique de l'avant-bras après traumatisme des deux os chez l'enfant. Ann Orthop Ouest 1974;6:91–95.
361. Guzzanti V, Di Lazzaro A, Lembo A, Gigante A. Il trattamento chirurgico delle fratture diafisarie dell' avambraccio in et à evolutivà. Arch Putt Chir Organi Mov 1991;39:93–100.
362. Haasbeek JF, Cole WG. Open fractures of the arm in children. J Bone Joint Surg 1995;77:575–581.
363. Hackethal KH. Vollapparative gaschlouene Fraktur reposition und percutane Markraum-Schienung bei Kindern. Arch Klin Chir 1963;304:621–626.
364. Harbison JS, Stevenson TM, Lipert JR. Forearm fractures in children. Aust NZ J Surg 1978;48:84–88.
365. Hogstrom H, Nilsson BE, Willner S. Correction growth following diaphyseal forearm fracture. Acta Orthop Scand 1976;47:299–303.
366. Holdsworth BJ, Sloan JP. Proximal forearm fractures in children: residual disability. Injury 1982;14:174–179.
367. Hughston JC. Fractures of the forearm in children. J Bone Joint Surg Am 1962;44:1678–1693.
368. Jenny G. Traitement des fractures des deux os de l'avant bras chez l'enfant daprès une série continue de 463 cas. Strasbourg Med J 1966;26:236–242.
369. Judet J, Rigault P, Plumerault J. Fracture diaphysaire des deux os de l'avant bras chez les enfants: technique et resultat du traitement par fixateur externe. Presse Med 1966;74:2583–2588.
370. Karger C, Dietz JM, Heckel T, et al. Devenir des cals vicieux diaphysaires de l'avant-bras chez l'enfant. Rev Chir Orthop 1986;72(suppl II):44–47.
371. Kay S, Smith C, Oppenheim WL. Both bone midshaft forearm fractures in children. J Pediatr Orthop 1986;6:306–310.
372. Kersley JB, Scott BW. Restoration of forearm rotation following malunited fractures: Baldwin's operation. J Hand Surg [Br] 1990;15:421–424.
373. Knight RA, Purvis GD. Fractures of both bones of the forearm in adults. J Bone Joint Surg Am 1949;31:755–764.
374. Kramhøft M, Solgaard S. Displaced diaphyseal forearm fractures in children: classification and evaluation of the early radiographic prognosis. J Pediatr Orthop 1989;9:586–589.
375. Kumar VP, Satku K, Helm R, Pho RWU. Radial reconstruction in segmental defects of both forearm bones. J Bone Joint Surg Br 1988;70:815–817.
376. Kurz W, Lange D. Operative Behandlung von Verderarmschaft bone chen bei Kindern. Chir Praxis 1971;15:287–293.
377. Kurz W, Vinz H, Wahl D. Spätergebnisse nach osteosynthese von Unterarmschaftfrakturen im Kindesalter. Zentralbl Chir 1982;107:149–155.
378. Lascombes P, Poncelet T, Prevot J. Fractures itératives de l'avant-bras chez l'enfant. Rev Chir Orthop 1988;74(suppl II):137–139.
379. Lascombes P, Prevot J, Ligier JN, et al. Elastic stable intramedullary nailing in forearm shaft fractures in children: 85 cases. J Pediatr Orthop 1990;10:167–171.
380. Levinthal DH. Fractures of the lower one third of both bones of the forearm in children. Surg Gynecol Obstet 1933;57:790.
381. Ligier JN, Métaizeau JP, Lascombes P, Oncelet T, Prévot J. Traitement des fractures diaphysaires des deux os de l'avant-bras de l'enfant par embrochage élastique stable. Rev Chir Orthop 1987;73(suppl II):149–151.
382. Lin HH, Strecleer WB, Manske PR, et al. A surgical technique of radioulnar osteoclasis to correct severe forearm rotation deformities. J Pediatr Orthop 1995;15:53–58.
383. London PS. Observations on the treatment of some fractures of the forearm by splintage that does not include the elbow. Injury 1971;2:252–270.
384. Lorthior J. Traitement des fractures chez l'enfant. Acta Orthop Belg 1965;31:611–618.
385. Mantout JP, Metaizeau JP, Ligier JN, Prevot J. Embrochage centro-medullaire des fractures des deux os de l'avant-bras chez l'enfant: techniques, indications. Ann Med Nancy Est 1984;23:149–151.
386. Matthews LS, Kaufer H, Garver DF, Sonstegard DA. The effect on supination-pronation of angular malalignment of fractures of both ones of the forearm. J Bone Joint Surg Am 1982;64:14–17.
387. Metaizeau JP. L'osteosynthese chez l'enfant: techniques et indications. Rev Chir Orthop 1983;69:495–503.
388. Metaizeau JP, Ligier JN. Le traitement chirurgical des fractures des os longs chez l'enfant: interferences entre l'osteosynthese et les processus physiologiques de consolidation. Indications therapeutiques. J Chir (Paris) 1984;121:527–537.
389. Miller JH, Osterkamp JA. Scintigraphy in acute plastic bowing of the forearm. Radiology 1972;142:742.
390. Moesner J, Östergaard AH. Diaphysefrakturer høs born. Nord Med 1966;75:355–357.
391. Naga AH, Broadrick GL. Traumatic bowing of the radius and ulna in children. NC Med J 1977;38:452–456.
392. Nielsen AB, Simonsen O. Displaced forearm fractures in children treated with AO plates. Injury 1984;15:393–396.
393. Nilsson BOE, Obrant K. The range of motion following fracture of the shaft of the forearm in children. Acta Orthop Scand 1977;48:600–602.
394. Nunley JA, Urbaniak JR. Partial bony entrapment of the median nerve in a greenstick fracture of the ulna. J Hand Surg [Am] 1980;5:557–559.
395. Onne L, Sandblom P. Late results in fractures of forearm in children. Acta Orthop Scand 1949;98:549–567.
396. Ortega R, Loder RT, Louis DS. Open reduction and internal fixation of forearm fractures in children. J Pediatr Orthop 1996;16:651–654.
397. Parsch K. Die Morote-Drahtung bei proximalen und mittlerun Underarmschaftfaldüren des Kindes. Operat Orthop Traumatol 1990;2:245–255.
398. Patrick J. A study of supination and pronation with special reference to the treatment of forearm fractures. J Bone Joint Surg 1946;28:737–748.

399. Poitevin R, Pouliquen JC, Langlais J. Fractures of both bones of the forearm in children: apropos of 162 cases. Rev Chir Orthop 1986;72(suppl II):41–43.
400. Poli G, Zucchi M, Assiso J, Dal Monte A. Le fratture d'avanbraccio nel bambini. Chir Organi Mov 1984;49:349–354.
401. Ponet M, Jawish R. Embrochage élastique stable des fractures des deux os de l'avant-bras de l'enfant. Chir Pediatr 1989;30:117–120.
402. Posman CL, Little RE. Radioulnar synostosis following an isolated fracture of the ulnar shaft. Clin Orthop 1986;213:207–210.
403. Price CT, Scott DS, Kurzner ME, Flynn JC. Malunited forearm fractures in children. J Pediatr Orthop 1990;10:705–712.
404. Prosser AJ, Hooper G. Entrapment of the ulnar nerve in a greenstick fracture of the ulna. J Hand Surg [Br] 1986;11:211–212.
405. Ray RD, Johnson RJ, Jameson RM. Rotation of the forearm. an experimental study of pronation and supination. J Bone Joint Surg Am 1951;33:993–996.
406. Rayan GM, Hayes M. Entrapment of the flexor digitorum profundus in the ulna with fracture of both bones of the forearm. J Bone Joint Surg Am 1986;68:1102–1103.
407. Reisch RB. Traumatic plastic bowing deformity of the radius and ulna in a skeletally mature adult. J Orthop Trauma 1994;8:258–262.
408. Rigault P. Fracture de l'avant bras chez l'enfant. Ann Chir 1980;34:810–816.
409. Roberts JA. Angulation of the radius in children's fractures. J Bone Joint Surg Am 1986;68:751–754.
410. Roy DR, Crawford AH. Operative management of fractures of the shaft of the radius and ulna. Orthop Clin North Am 1990;21:245–250.
411. Roy-Camille R, Honnart F. Les fractures des deux os de l'avant-bras, leurs complications, leur traitement. Nouv Presse Med 1972;1:1029–1032.
412. Royle SG. Compartment syndrome following forearm fracture in children. Injury 1990;21:73–76.
413. Rydholm U, Nilsson JE. Traumatic bowing of the forearm. Clin Orthop 1979;139:121–124.
414. Sanders WE, Heckman JD. Traumatic plastic deformation of the radius and ulna. Clin Orthop 1984;188:58–67.
415. Schwarz N, Pienaar S, Schwarz AF, et al. Refracture of the forearm in children. J Bone Joint Surg Br 1996;78:740–744.
416. Simon L. Mark drahtossteosynthese bei Kindlichen Unterarmschaftfrakturen. Akt Traumatol 1975;5:133–139.
417. Stanitski CL, Micheli LJ. Simultaneous ipsilateral fractures of the arm and forearm in children. Clin Orthop 1980;153:218–222.
418. Tarr R, Garfinkel A, Sarmiento A. The effects of angular and rotational deformities of both bones of the forearm. J Bone Joint Surg Am 1984;66:65–70.
419. Theil A. Diskussion der Indikation der operativen Behandlung kindlicher Unterarmschaftbrüche. Sportverl Sportschad 1992;6:133–134.
420. Thorndike A Jr, Simmler CL Jr. Fractures of the forearm and elbow in children. N Engl J Med 1941;225:475–480.
421. Thomas EM, Tuson KWR, Browne RSH. Fractures of the radius and ulna in children. Injury 1975;7:120–124.
422. Torpey BM, Pess GM, Kircher MT, et al. Ulnar nerve laceration in a closed both bone forearm fracture. J Orthop Trauma 1996;10:131–134.
423. Tredwell SJ, Van Peteghem K, Clough M. Pattern of forearm fractures in children. J Pediatr Orthop 1984;4:604608.
424. Undeland K. Rotational movements and bony union in shaft fractures of the forearm. J Bone Joint Surg Br 1962;44:340–348.
425. Vainionpää S, Bostman O, Patiala H, Rokkanen P. Internal fixation of forearm fractures in children. Acta Orthop Scand 1987;58:121–123.
426. Verstreken L, Delronge G, Lamoureux J. Shaft forearm fractures in children: intramedullary nailing with immediate motion: a preliminary report. J Pediatr Orthop 1988;8:450–453.
427. Victor J, Mulier T, Faboy G. Refracture of radius and ulna in a female gymnast. Am J Sports Med 1993;21:753–754.
428. Vince KG, Miller JE. Cross-union complicating fracture of the forearm. J Bone Joint Surg Am 1987;69:651–660.
429. Voto SJ, Weiner DS, Leighley B. Redisplacement after closed reduction of forearm fractures in children. Orthopedics 1990;10:79–84.
430. Voto SJ, Weiner DS, Leighley B. Use of pins "and plaster" in the treatment of unstable pediatric forearm fractures. J Pediatr Orthop 1990;10:85–89.
431. Walker JL, Rang M. Forearm fractures in children: cast treatment with the elbow extended. J Bone Joint Surg Br 1991;73:299–301.
432. Warren JD. Anterior interosseous nerve palsy as a complication of forearm fractures. J Bone Joint Surg Br 1963;45:511–512.
433. Wilson J. Fractures of the forearm. Pediatr Clin North Am 1967;14:664–683.
434. Wolfe JS, Eyring EJ. Median nerve entrapment within a greenstick fracture. J Bone Joint Surg Am 1974;56:1270–1272.
435. Wright J, Rang M. Internal fixation for forearm fractures in children. Tech Orthop 1989;4:44–47.
436. Wyrsch B, Mencio GA, Green NE. Open reduction and internal fixation of pediatric forearm fractures. J Pediatr Orthop 1196;16:644–650.
437. Younger AS, Tredwell SJ, Mackenzie WG, et al. Accurate prediction of outcome after pediatric forearm fracture. J Pediatr Orthop 1994;14:200–206.

Distal Radius and Ulna

438. Abbott LE, Saunders JB. Injuries of median nerve in fractures of the lower end of the radius. Surg Gynecol Obstet 1933;57:507–510.
439. Abe M, Shirai H, Okamoto M, Onomura T. Lengthening of the forearm by callus distraction. J Hand Surg [Br] 1996;21:151–163.
440. Abram LJ, Thompson GH. Deformity after premature closure of the distal radial physis following a torus fracture with a physeal compression injury. J Bone Joint Surg Am 1987;69:1450–1453.
441. Aitken AP. The end results of the fractured distal radial epiphysis. J Bone Joint Surg 1935;17:302–308.
442. Aitken AP. Further observations on the fractured distal radial epiphysis. J Bone Joint Surg 1935;17:922–927.
443. Aminian A, Schoenecker PL. Premature closure of the distal radial physis after fracture of the distal radial metaphysis. J Pediatr Orthop 1995;15:495–498.
444. Ansorg P, Graner G. Effectiveness of conservative treatment following distal radius epiphyses injuries. Zentralbl Chir 1985;110:360–365.
445. Aufaure P, Bendjeddou M, Gilbert A. Les fractures du poignet et de la main chez l'enfant. Ann Chir 1982;36:499–506.
446. Bailey DA, Wedge JH, McCulloch RG, et al. Epidemiology of fractures of the distal end of the radius in children as associated with growth. J Bone Joint Surg Am 1989;71:1225–1231.
447. Beals RK. Premature closure of the physis following diaphyseal fractures. J Pediatr Orthop 1990;10:717–720.

References

448. Bell MJ, Hill RJ, McMurtry RY. Ulnar impingement syndrome. J Bone Joint Surg Br 1985;67:126–129.
449. Bellemere P, Badelon O, Bensahel H. Trois cas rares de fracture basse du radius associée a un decollement epiphysaire du cubitus. Ann Chir Main Memb Super 1992;11:147–152.
450. Borton D, Masterson E, O'Brien T. Distal forearm fractures in children: the role of hand dominance. J Pediatr Orthop 1994;14:496–497.
451. Boyden EM, Peterson HA. Partial premature closure of the distal radial physis associated with Kirschner wire fixation. Orthopedics 1991;14:585–588.
452. Bragdon R. Fractures of the distal radial epiphysis. Clin Orthop 1965;41:59–63.
453. Caine D, Roy S, Singer KM, Broekhoff J. Stress changes of the distal radial growth plate. Am J Sports Med 1992;20:290–298.
454. Carr CR, Tracy HW. Management of fractures of the distal forearm in children. South Med J 1964;57:540–550.
455. Chess DG, Hyndman JC, Leahey JL, et al. Short arm plaster cast for distal pediatric forearm fractures. J Pediatr Orthop 1994;14:211–213.
456. Crawford AH. Pitfalls and complications of fractures of the distal radius and ulna in childhood. Hand Clin 1988;4:403–413.
457. Dicke TE, Nunley JA. Distal forearm fractures in children: complications and surgical indications. Orthop Clin North Am 1993;24:333–340.
458. Doczi J, Springer G, Renner A, Martsa B. Occult distal radial fractures. J Hand Surg [Br] 1995;20:614–617.
459. Eichler J. Spätschaden an den Radioulnargelenken nach Unterarmverletzungen am Wachsenden Skeletal. Chir Praxis 1966;4:437–440.
460. Evans DL, Stauber M, Frykman GK. Irreducible epiphyseal plate fracture of the distal ulna due to interposition of the extensor carpi ulnaris tendon. Clin Orthop 1990;251:162–165.
461. Friberg KSI. Remodeling after distal forearm fractures in children. I. The effects of residual angulation on the spatial orientation of the epiphyseal plates. Acta Orthop Scand 1979;50:537–546.
462. Friberg KSI. Remodeling after distal forearm fractures in children. II. The final orientation of the distal and proximal epiphyseal plates of the radius. Acta Orthop Scand 1979;50:731–739.
463. Friberg KSI. Remodeling after distal forearm fractures in children. III. Correction of residual angulation of fractures of the radius. Acta Orthop Scand 1979;50:740–749.
464. Gibbons CL, Woods DA, Pailithorpe C, et al. The management of isolated distal radius fractures in children. J Pediatr Orthop 1994;14:207–210.
465. Grimault L, Leonhart E. De collément epiphysáire de l'extrémites inférieure du radius. Rev Chir (Orthop) 1925;12:261–266.
466. Gupta RP, Danielsson LG. Dorsally angulated solitary metaphyseal greenstick fractures in the distal radius: results after immobilization in pronated, neutral and supinated position. J Pediatr Orthop 1990;10:90–92.
467. Hernandez J Jr, Peterson HA. Fracture of the distal radial physis complicated by compartment syndrome and premature physeal closure. J Pediatr Orthop 1986;6:627–630.
468. Hodgkinson PD, Evans DM. Median nerve compression following trauma in children. J Hand Surg [Br] 1993;18:475–477.
469. Holmes JR, Louis DS. Entrapment of pronator quadratus in pediatric distal radius fractures: recognition and treatment. J Pediatr Orthop 194;14:498–500.
470. Horil E, Tamura Y, Nakamura R, Miura T. Premature closure of the distal radial physis. J Hand Surg Br 1993;18:11–16.
471. Kapandji AI, Delaunay C. Une dislocation inférieure rare de la radio-cubitale inférieure par épiphyseodèse post-fracturaire spontané du radius. Ann Chir Main Memb Super 1993;12:140–147.
472. Karlsson J, Appelqvist R. Irreducible fracture of the wrist in a child. Acta Orthop Scand 1987;58:280–281.
473. Kohler R, Walch G, Noyer D, Chappuis JP. Main bote post-traumatique: problems thérapeutiques (à propos de 5 cas). Rev Chir Orthop 1982;68:333–342.
474. Kramer W, Neugebauer W, Schönemann B, Maier G. Results of conservative treatment of distal radius fractures. Langenbecks Arch Chir 1986;367:247–251.
475. Larsen E, Vittas D, Torp-Pederson S. Remodeling of angulated distal forearm fractures in children. Clin Orthop 1988;237:190–195.
476. Lee BS, Esterhai JL, Das M. Fracture of the distal radial epiphysis. Clin Orthop 1984;185:90–96.
477. Lesko PD, Georgis T, Slabaugh P. Irreducible Salter-Harris type II fracture of the distal radial epiphysis. J Pediatr Orthop 1987;7:719–721.
478. Lettin AWF. Carpal tunnel syndrome in childhood. J Bone Joint Surg Br 1965;47:556–559.
479. Light TR, Ogden DA, Ogden JA. The anatomy of metaphyseal torus fractures. Clin Orthop 1984;188:103–108.
480. Mani GV, Hui PW, Cheng JCY. Translation of the radius as a predictor of outcome in distal radial fractures of children. J Bone Joint Surg Br 1993;75:808–811.
481. Manoli A. Irreducible fracture-separation of the distal radial epiphysis. J Bone Joint Surg Am 1982;64:1095–1096.
482. Martin C, Massé P. Le syndrome du canal carpien chez l'enfant. Arch Fr Pediatr 1958;15:930–940.
483. Meadoff N. Median nerve injuries in fractures in the region of the wrist. Calif Med 1949;70:252–256.
484. Mischkowksy T, Daum R, Rof W. Injuries of the distal radial epiphysis. Arch Orthop Trauma Surg 1980;96:16–17.
485. Peinado A. Distal radial epiphyseal displacement after impaired distal ulnar growth. J Bone Joint Surg Am 1979;61:88–92.
486. Perona PG, Light TR. Remodeling of the skeletally immature distal radius. J Orthop Trauma 1990;4:356–361.
487. Peterson HA. Triplane fracture of the distal radius: case report. J Pediatr Orthop 1996;16:192–194.
488. Pritchett JW. Does pinning cause distal radial growth plate arrest? Orthopedics 1994;17:550–551.
489. Proctor MT, Moore DJ, Peterson JMH. Redisplacement after manipulation of distal radial fractures in children. J Bone Joint Surg Br 1993;65:453–454.
490. Pruitt DL, Gilula LA, Manske PR, Vannier MW. Computed tomography scanning with image reconstruction in evaluation of distal radius fractures. J Hand Surg [Am] 1994;19:720–727.
491. Ranawat CS, DeFirore J, Straub LR. Madelung's deformity: an end-result study of surgical treatment. J Bone Joint Surg Am 1975;57:772–775.
492. Ray TD, Tessler RH, Dell PC. Traumatic ulnar physeal arrest after distal forearm fractures in children. J Pediatr Orthop 1996;16:195–200.
493. Roberts JA. Angulation of the radius in children's fractures. J Bone Joint Surg Br 1986;68:751–754.
494. Roy Dr. Completely displaced distal radius fractures with intact ulnas in children. Orthopedics 1989;12:1089–1092.
495. Santoro V, Mara J. Compartment syndrome complicating Salter-Harris type II distal radius fracture. Clin Orthop 1988;233:226–228.
496. Seriat-Gauthier B, Jouve JL. Le décollements: fractures de l'extrémité inférieure du radius à déplacement antérieure chez l'enfant. Chir Pediatr 1988;29:265–268.

497. Sterling AP, Habermann ET. Acute post-traumatic median nerve compression associated with a Salter II fracture dislocation of the wrist. Bull Hosp Joint Dis Orthop Inst 1963; 34:161–171.
498. Sumner JM, Khuri SM. Entrapment of the median nerve and flexor pollicis longus tendon in an epiphyseal fracture-dislocation of the distal radial-ulnar joint. J Hand Surg [Am] 1984;9:711–714.
499. Valverde JA, Albinana J, Certucha JA. Early post-traumatic physeal arrest in distal radius after a compression injury. J Pediatr Orthop Part B 1996;5:57–60.
500. Vender MI, Watson HK. Acquired Madelung-like deformity in a gymnast. J Hand Surg [Am] 1988;13:19–21.
501. Vickers D, Nielsen G. The Madelung deformity: surgical prophylaxis (physiolysis) during the late growth period by resection of the dyschondrosteosis lesion. J Hand Surg [Br] 1992;17:401–407.
502. Vuhov V, Ristic K, Stevanovic, Bumbasirevic M. Simultaneous fractures of the distal end of the radius and scaphoid bone. J Orthop Trauma 1988;2:120–123.
503. Waters PM, Kolettis GJ, Schwend R. Acute median neuropathy following physeal fractures of the distal radius. J Pediatr Orthop 1994;14:173–177.
504. Woodbury DF, Fischer B. An overriding radius fracture in a child with an intact ulna: management considerations. Orthopedics 1985;8:763–765.
505. Young TB. Irreducible displacement of the distal radial epiphysis complicating a fracture of the lower radius and ulna. Injury 1984;16:166–168.
506. Zehntner MK, Jakob RP, McGanity PL. Growth disturbance of the distal radial epiphysis after trauma: operative treatment by corrective radial osteotomy. J Pediatr Orthop 1990;10:411–415.

Stress Injury

507. Albanese SA, Palmer AK, Kerr DR, et al. Wrist pain and distal growth plate closure of the radius in gymnasts. J Pediatr Orthop 1989;9:23–28.
508. Aldbridge MJ. Overuse injuries of the distal growth epiphysis. In: Hoshizeki TB, Salmala JH, Petiot B (eds) Diagnostics, Treatment and Analysis of Gymnastic Talent. Montreal: Sports Psyche Editions, 1987.
509. Caine D, Roy S, Singer KM, Broekhoff J. Stress changes of the distal radial growth plate: a radiographic survey and review of the literature. Am J Sports Med 1992;20:295–298.
510. Carter SR, Aldridge MJ, Fitzgerald R, et al. Stress changes of the wrist in adolescent gymnasts. Br J Radiol 1988;61:109–112.
511. Chang CY, Shih C, Pedd JW. Wrist injuries in adolescent gymnasts of a Chinese opera school: radiographic survey. Radiology 1995;195:861–864.
512. DeSmet L, Classens A, Fàbry G. Gymnast wrist. Acta Orthop Belg 1993;59:377–380.
513. DeSmet L, Fabry G. Growth arrest of the distal radial epiphysis in a javelin thrower: reversed Madelung? J Pediatr Orthop Part B 1995;4:116–117.
514. Dobyns JH, Gabel GT. Gymnasts wrist. Hand Clin 1990;6:493–505.
515. Fagg P. Reversed Madelung's deformity with nerve compression. J Hand Surg [Br] 1987;13:23–27.
516. Fliegel CP. Stress related widening of the radial growth plate in adolescents. Ann Radiol (Paris) 1986;29:374–376.
517. Mandelbaum BR, Bartolozzi AR, Davis CA, et al. Wrist pain syndrome in the gymnast, pathogenic, diagnositic and therapeutic considerations. Am J Sports Med 1989;17:305–317.
518. Read MTF. Stress fractures of the distal radius in adolescent gymnasts. Br J Sports Med 1981;15:272–276.
519. Resnick DL. Case 6: a 12-year-old gymnast with intermittent pain in the wrist. Radiographics 1988;8:246–248.
520. Roy S, Caine D, Singer KM. Stress changes in the distal radial epiphysis in young gymnasts: a report of twenty-one cases and a review of the literature. Am J Sports Med 1985;13:301–308.
521. Ruggles DL, Peterson HA, Scott SG. Radial growth plate injury in a female gymnast. Med Sci Sports Exerc 1991;23:393–396.
522. Ryan JR, Salciccioli GG. Fractures of the distal radial epiphysis in adolescent weight lifters. Am J Sports Med 1976;4:26–27.
523. Shih C, Chang CY, Penn JW, et al. Chronically stressed wrists in adolescent gymnasts: MR imaging appearance. Radiology 1995;195:855–859.
524. Tolat A, Sanderson P, DeSmet L, Stanley J. Acquired positive ulnar variance following chronic epiphyseal injury deformity in the gymnast. J Hand Surg [Am] 1988;13:19–21.
525. Vender MI, Watson HK. Acquired Madelung-type deformity in a gymnast. J Hand Surg [Am] 1988;13:19–21.
526. Weiss APC, Sponseller PD. Salter-Harris type I fracture of the distal radius due to weight lifting. Orthop Rev 1989;18:233–235.
527. Yong-Huig K, Wedge JH, Bowen CV. Chronic injury to the distal ulnar and radial growth plates in an adolescent gymnast. J Bone Joint Surg Am 1988;70:1087–1088.

Distal Ulna

528. Bell MJ, Hill RJ, McMurty RY. Ulnar impingement syndrome. J Bone Joint Surg Br 1985;67:126–129.
529. Biyani A, Mehara A, Bhan S. Morphologic variations of the ulnar styloid process. J Hand Surg [Br] 1990;15:352–354.
530. Burgess RC, Watson HK. Hypertrophic ulnar styloid nonunions. Clin Orthop 1988;228:215–217.
531. Engber WD, Keene MD. Irreducible fracture-separation of the distal ulnar epiphysis. J Bone Joint Surg Am 1985;67:1130–1132.
532. Evans DL, Stanber M, Frykman GK. Irreducible epiphyseal plate fracture of the distal ulna due to interposition of the extensor carpi ulnaris tendon: a case report. Clin Orthop 1990;251:162–165.
533. Golz RJ, Grogan DP, Greene TL, Belsole RJ, Ogden JA. Distal ulnar physeal injury. J Pediatr Orthop 1991;11:318–326.
534. Minani A, Ishikawa J, Kondo E. Painful unfused separate ossification center of the ulnar styloid: a case report. J Hand Surg [Am] 1994;19:1045–1047.
535. Nelson OA, Buchanan JR, Harrison CS. Distal ulnar growth arrest. J Hand Surg [Am] 1984;9:164–171.
536. Paul AS, Kay PR, Haines JF. Distal ulnar growth plate arrest following a diaphyseal fracture. J R Coll Surg Edinb 1992;37:347–348.
537. Peinado A. Distal radial epiphyseal displacement after impaired distal ulnar growth. J Bone Joint Surg Am 1979;61:88–92.
538. Ray T, Tessler RH, Dell PC. Traumatic ulnar physeal arrest after distal forearm fractures in children. J Pediatr Orthop 1996;16:195–200.
539. Sumner JM, Khuri SM. Entrapment of the median nerve and flexor pollicis longus tendon in an epiphyseal fracture-dislocation of the distal radioulnar joint: a case report. J Hand Surg [Am] 1984;9:711–713.
540. Watson HK, Brown RE. Ulnar impingement syndrome after Darrach procedure: treatment by advancement lengthening osteotomy of the ulna. J Hand Surg [Am] 1989;14:302–306.

References

Galeazzi Injury

541. Albert MJ, Engber WD. Dorsal dislocation of the distal radioulnar joint secondary to plastic deformation of the ulna. J Orthop Trauma 1990;4:466–469.
542. Albert SM, Wohl MA, Rechtman AM. Treatment of the disrupted radio-ulnar joint. J Bone Joint Surg Am 1963:45:1373–1381.
543. Bednar JM, Osterman AL. The role of arthroscopy in the treatment of traumatic triangular fibrocartilage injuries. Hand Clin 1994;10:605–614.
544. Chidgey LK. The distal radioulnar joint: problems and solutions. J Am Acad Orthop Surg 1995;3:95–109.
545. Coleman HM. Injuries of the articular disc at the wrist. J Bone Joint Surg Br 1960;42:522–529.
546. DeSmet L. The distal radio-ulnar joint: pathology evaluation interactions-treatment. Thesis, Katholieke University, Leuven, 1994.
547. Galeazzi R. Di una particolare sindrome traumatica dello scheletro dell' avambracchio. Atti Mem Soc Lombardi Chir 1934;2:12–27.
548. Itoh Y, Woriuchi Y, Takahashi M, et al. Extensor tendon involvement in Smith's and Galeazzi's fractures. J Hand Surg [Am] 1987;12:535–540.
549. Landfried MJ, Stenchik M, Susi JG. Variant of Galeazzi fracture-dislocation in children. J Pediatr Orthop 1991;11:332–335.
550. Lechner J, Steiger R, Ochsner P. Die Operative Behandlung der Galeazzi-Fraktur. Unfallchirurg 1993;96:18–23.
551. Letts M, Rowahani N. Galeazzi-equivalent injuries of the wrist in children. J Pediatr Orthop 1993;13:561–566.
552. Leung PC, Hung LK. An effective method of reconstructing post-traumatic dorsal dislocated distal radioulnar joints. J Hand Surg [Am] 1990;15:925–928.
553. Maculé Beneyto F, Arandes Renú JM, Ferreres Claramunt A, Ramón Soler R. Treatment of Galeazzi fracture-dislocations. J Trauma 1994;36:352–355.
554. Mikic Z. Galeazzi fracture-dislocations. J Bone Joint Surg 1975;8:1071–1080.
555. Moore TM, Lester DK, Sarmiento A. The stabilizing effect of soft-tissue constraints in artificial Galeazzi fractures. Clin Orthop 1985;194:189–194.
556. Palmer AK. Triangular fibrocartilage complex lesions: a classification. J Hand Surg [Am] 1989;14:594–606.
557. Reckling FW. Unstable fracture-dislocations of the forearm (Monteggia and Galeazzi lesions). J Bone Joint Surg Am 1982;64:857–863.
558. Reckling FW, Cordell LD. Unstable fracture-dislocations of the forearm: the Monteggia and Galeazzi lesions. Arch Surg 1968;96:999–1007.
559. Reckling FW, Peltier LF. Riccardo Galeazzi and Galeazzi's fracture. Surgery 1965;58:453–459.
560. Rose-Innes AP. Anterior dislocation of the ulna at the inferior radio-ulnar joint. J Bone Joint Surg Br 1960;42:515–521.
561. Schneiderman G, Meldrum RD, Bloebaum RD, Tarr R, Sarmiento A. The interosseous membrane of the forearm: structure and its role in Galeazzi fractures. J Trauma 1993;35:879–885.
562. Walsh HPJ, McLaren CAN, Owen R. Galeazzi fractures in children. J Bone Joint Surg Br 1987;69:730–733.
563. Wechsler RJ, Wehbe MA, Rifkin MD, Edeiken, Branch HM. Computed tomography diagnosis of distal radioulnar subluxation. Skeletal Radiol 1987;16:1–5.

17

Wrist and Hand

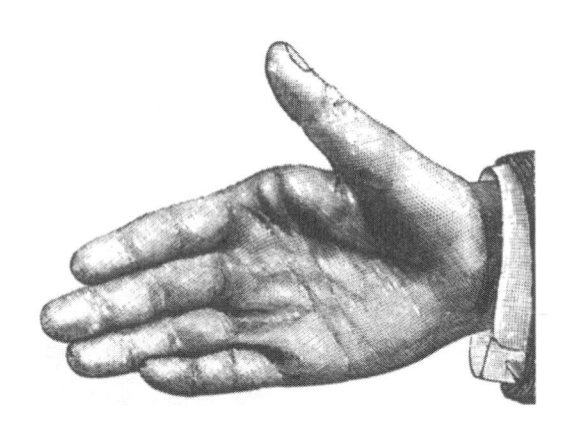

Engraving of a complex metacarpophalangeal dislocation. (From Poland J. Traumatic Separation of the Epiphyses. *London: Smith, Elder, 1898)*

The changing osseous anatomy of the hand and wrist is probably better known than the rest of the child's skeleton, as this region is evaluated so frequently for skeletal injuries. However, virtually all studies are based on roentgenographic data and have minimal if any substantiation with specific chondro-osseous anatomic studies.[4,18]

Anatomy

Development

Prenatally, each carpal bone assumes a basic morphologic shape as a cartilaginous anlage that is reasonably comparable to the final ossified adult shape. During postnatal development there are minimal changes in the general contours of these cartilaginous components. Garn et al. studied 138 embryos and fetuses and showed that carpal metacarpal and phalangeal fusions arose from incomplete separation of these cartilaginous precursors.[7]

Carpal primary ossification is minimally present at birth. Each primary ossification center gradually proceeds from a relatively small focus out to the peripheral contours, which are comprised of articular cartilage, perichondrium, or periosteum (Fig. 17-1). The immature, enlarging osseous contours are variable and changing, and they do not always reflect the actual contour of the unossified cartilage prior to adolescence. Longitudinal growth deformity in the distal radius or ulna or abnormal muscle forces exerted across the wrist may cause mild to moderate structural changes in the cartilaginous portions of the carpal bones. Ossification basically follows any preexistent cartilaginous shape, whether normal or a deformation.

The scaphoid is the largest bone in the proximal carpal row. Ossification begins when the child is between the ages of 4 and 6 years and is complete by 13–15 years of age.[4,5] Ossification begins in the more distal portion and progressively extends into the more proximal segment (Fig. 17-2). This developmental pattern may be a factor predisposing to delayed union and nonunion in the adolescent and young adult. How this pattern is affected by intraosseous blood flow is unknown. The retrograde blood supply of the scaphoid is such that waist fractures endanger the vascularity of the proximal pole, and ischemic necrosis may accompany nonunion, although to a lesser extent in children than in adults. Disruption of the venous system may be a significant factor in the altered vascular physiology of the injured scaphoid.[10]

Until ossification is complete, the scaphoid is almost entirely cartilaginous circumferentially, which increases the cushioning effect during trauma and thus lessens the susceptibility to fracture throughout skeletal maturation. The susceptibility of the scaphoid to being fractured changes commensurate with this increasing chondro-osseous transformation and with the changing stiffness of the individual bone and the entire carpal region.

Gelberman and Menonn studied the extraosseous and intraosseous vascularity of the carpal scaphoid in adults.[8] Most of the intraosseous vascularity and the entire proximal pole come from branches of the radial artery entering through the dorsal ridge, whereas the bone of the distal tuberosity receives its blood supply from palmar radial artery branches. There is collateral circulation to the scaphoid by way of the dorsal and palmar branches of the anterior interosseous artery. The palmar operative approach appears

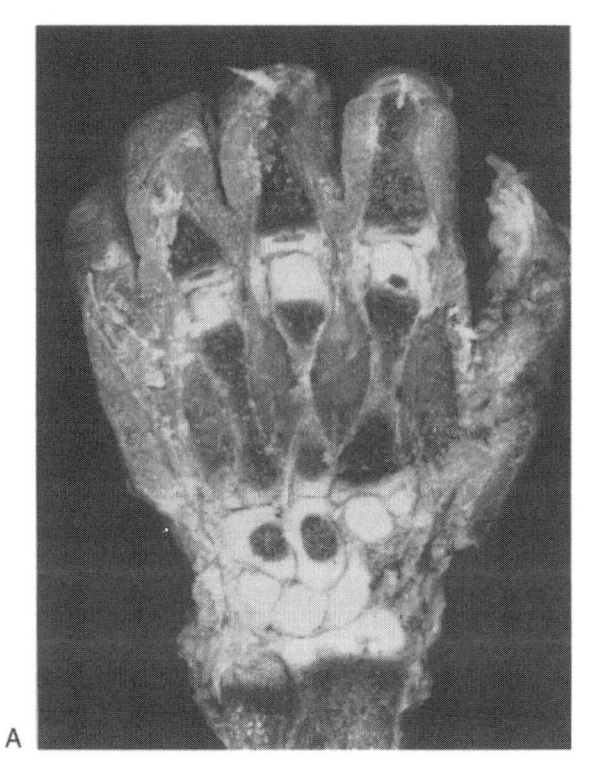

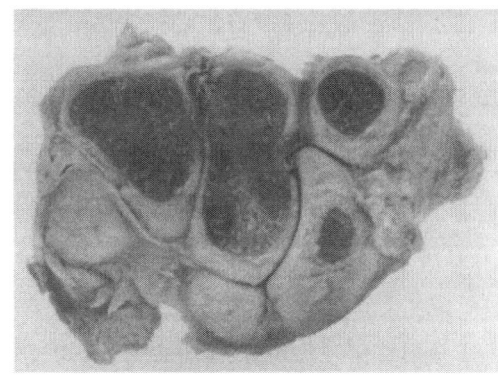

FIGURE 17-1. Anatomic sections. (A) Three-year-old. (B) Ossification within the carpus at 6 years.

to be the least traumatic to the blood supply of the proximal pole. In the child, because the ossification center develops more distally and then proceeds into the proximal portion, it appears that there may be selective dominance of the distal supply initially and a progressive "takeover" from the proximal supply to reach the adult pattern. This would certainly explain the pattern of ischemic damage. However, both vessels may participate in the formation of the ossification center.

The lunate may develop two ossification centers that subsequently fuse, although rarely separation persists. Sometimes the lunate fuses incompletely with an adjacent carpal bone, giving rise to a spurious "fracture line." Kobayashi et al. described complete congenital absence of the lunate bilaterally in a young adult who presented for evaluation of pain in the left forearm.[12] Interestingly, there was shell-like ossification of the left lunate but none of the right lunate. Computed tomographic (CT) scans showed that there was cartilaginous tissue present in the radiolucent areas. Bipartite ossification has also been described for the trapezium and trapezoid. The pisiform, the smallest carpal bone and the last to ossify, often does so from multiple foci.

Irregular or multifocal ossification should not be misinterpreted as chondro-osseous trauma, although unrecognized damage to carpal bones during progressive maturation may be the cause of many radiologic variants about the wrist. Furthermore, as shown with variations of the patella, foot, and ankle, what appears to be a separation on radiologic examination may actually have complete cartilaginous continuity.

In the proximal phalanx of the thumb and the proximal and middle phalanges of the fingers, small, sharply defined linear "defects" are often visible on routine radiographs.[1,4] They are the diaphyseal nutrient foramina, which are less frequent in the distal phalanges (except the thumb). These defects should not be confused with incomplete cortical fractures.

Chondroepiphyses are initially located at the proximal and distal ends of each phalanx (see Chapter 1), although only one epiphysis in each phalanx and metacarpal eventually forms a secondary ossification center.[9,15,16] In such areas the associated physis is transversely oriented. The secondary center forms in the proximal epiphysis of each phalanx. In contrast, the secondary centers of the metacarpal epiphyses are distal, except for the thumb in which it is proximal. At the opposite end of each of these developing bones the epiphyseal cartilage is rapidly replaced by endochondral ossification until only a thin layer of cartilage exists. This layer is composed of articular cartilage, germinal epiphyseal cartilage, and a slow-growing physis that contributes little to longitudinal growth but does allow continued hemispheric growth of the end of the bone as the joint enlarges.

There may be an apparent epiphysis and physis at the nonepiphyseal end of a metacarpal or phalanx. Such pseudoepiphyseal ossification centers are common in the distal first metacarpal (Fig. 17-3). Caffey believed that the term pseudoepiphysis was a misnomer and that there is no such anatomic entity. Histologically, there definitely is such a structure that results when metaphyseal ossification mushrooms into the epiphyseal region (see Chapter 1).[4,8,15]

The developmental morphology of secondary ossification in the "nonepiphyseal" ends of small longitudinal bones is characterized by formation of the pseudoepiphysis.[14–16] Both direct ossification extension from the metaphysis into the epiphysis and pseudoepiphysis formation proceed and continue to be more mature than formation and expansion of the classic epiphyseal (secondary) ossification center at the opposite end of each specific bone. Direct metaphyseal to epiphyseal ossification usually starts centrally and expands hemispherically, replacing physeal and epiphyseal cartilage simultaneously. Three basic patterns of pseudoepiphysis formation may occur. First, the aforementioned central osseous bridge extends from the metaphysis across the physis into the epiphysis and subsequently expands to create a mushroom-like osseous structure. In the second pattern, a peripheral osseous bridge forms, creating an osseous ring or an eccentric bridge between the metaphysis and the epiphysis. In the third pattern, multiple bridging occurs. In each situ-

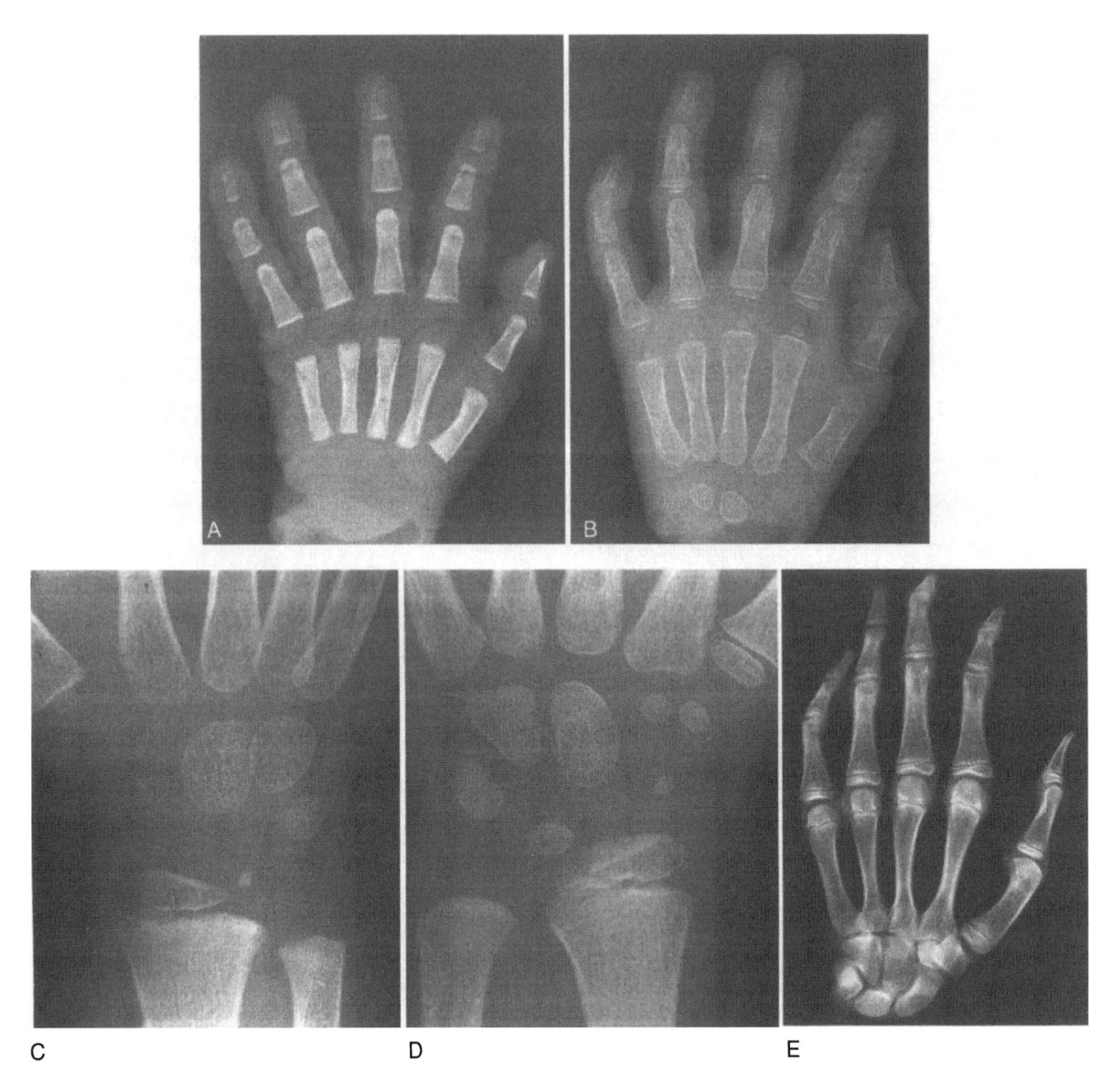

FIGURE 17-2. Sequential development of the wrist and hand. Early development in the neonate (A) and at 14 months (B). Note the variable development of the secondary ossification centers of the metacarpals in (B). The second metacarpal epiphysis ossifies first, followed in order, by the third, fourth, and fifth metacarpals. The last metacarpal epiphysis to ossify is the first (thumb). (C–E) Subsequent developmental sequence into adolescence. The scaphoid does not completely ossify until relatively late in skeletal maturation, a factor that may minimize readily recognizable fractures during childhood and adolescence.

ation the associated remnant physis lacks typical cell columns and is incapable of contributing to the postnatal longitudinal growth of the involved bone. Pseudoepiphyses are well formed by 4–5 years of age and coalesce with the rest of the bone months to years before skeletal maturation occurs at the opposite epiphyseal end, which ossifies in the typical pattern with formation of a secondary center completely within the cartilaginous epiphysis.

Solitary pseudoepiphyseal involvement should not be misinterpreted as a fracture line or as indicative of systemic disease. Multiple pseudoepiphyses may indicate an underlying illness or dysplasia. In particular, hypothyroidism may be associated with such developmental chondro-osseous variations.

The precise origin and insertion of collateral ligaments into the metacarpals and phalanges prior to physeal closure are not clearly described.[3,11] Middle and distal phalangeal attachments are into the epiphyses and metaphyses, not unlike what is seen in the long bones. In contrast, attachments at the metacarpophalangeal joint are only into the epiphyses of the metacarpals and proximal phalanges. These attachments affect fracture and displacement patterns.

Anatomy

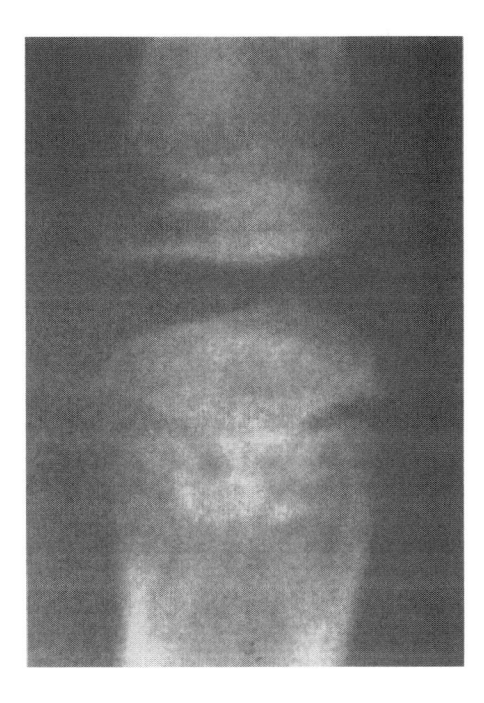

FIGURE 17-3. Pseudoepiphysis of the distal end of the thumb metacarpal in a 3-year-old. The lucency extends across most of the transverse diameter of the shaft. Metaphyseal ossification "mushrooms" into the cartilage and leaves peripheral cartilage remnants that appear roentgenographically like peripheral physeal cartilage during physiologic epiphysiodesis. (See Chapter 1 for a more detailed discussion of this process.)

Berger and Landsmeer studied the palmar radiocarpal ligaments in 54 adult cadaver wrists and 23 fetuses.[2] They identified three palmar radiocarpal ligaments. The radioscaphocapitate ligament originates from the radial styloid process and inserts into the radial aspect of the waist of the scaphoid. It spreads over the distal pole of the scaphoid and interdigitates with fibers of the triangular fibrocartilage. The long radiolunate ligament originates just ulnar to the radioscaphocapitate ligament and is separated from it by an interligamentous sulcus. A short radiolunate ligament inserts as a flat sheet of fibers into the proximal margin of the palmar surface of the lunate. Each ligament is intracapsular and is enveloped within a continuous superficial fibrous stratum and deep synovial stratum. Palmar radiocarpal ligaments as a group are a major structural component of the palmar wrist from fetal development through skeletal maturation. These ligaments are intracapsular.

Pulley positions are relatively constant throughout postnatal development, with the gross anatomic characteristics correlating closely to those of the adult hand.[6] Flake et al. particularly showed the relation of certain pulleys, such as the "a" pulley of the thumb, to the growth plates and physes. Interestingly, the physes appear to be relatively free of attachments of pulleys, which is compatible with allowing continued growth of the pulley attached to areas that are "static" compared to the region of growth.

Functional Anatomy

Proper hand splinting after an injury is extremely important, even though complications from inappropriate positioning are less likely to develop in a child than in an adult. Because of the overall amount of ligamentous laxity usually present, permanent joint contractures are not as common a residual problem in children as they are in adults. Furthermore, injuries to the hand produce bleeding and swelling in the surrounding soft tissues. The inflammatory process, an essential part of healing during the early stages, may create adhesions between complex gliding tissue planes. Such adhesions are often inevitable and necessary for complete healing, and their formation cannot be prevented. Their effect, however, may be minimized by appropriate positioning during treatment and controlled, progressive mobilization. Even in the child, stiffness and swelling after injury may last several months; but unlike that in the adult, it usually dissipates.

The classic "position of function" for the hand is better termed the "ready-to-grasp position" or the "position of rest" (Fig. 17-4). Children's fingers, particularly the fleshy hand of an infant or toddler, may become temporarily stiff in this position. In view of better concepts of hand anatomy and rehabilitation, this is not the optimal position.

The metacarpophalangeal joint is a biaxial, ball-and-socket joint. In acute flexion the collateral ligaments are at their greatest length and tension because of the eccentric origin of the ligament on the metacarpal and the flare of the metacarpal epiphysis. If the metacarpophalangeal joint is in extension, the collateral ligaments may become stiff in the shortened position. Therefore the preferred functional position of splinting for the metacarpophalangeal joint in the injured hand appears to be full 90° flexion (Fig. 17-4).

FIGURE 17-4. (A) Classic position of function for immobilization of the adult hand. (B) More appropriate intrinsic-plus position of function for immobilizing hand injuries in children.

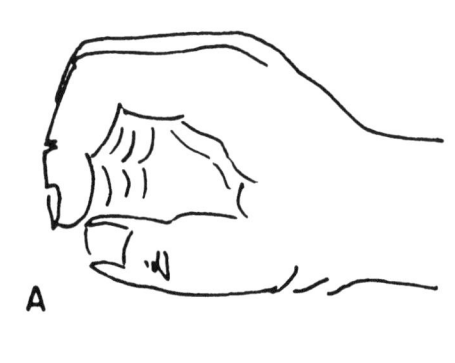

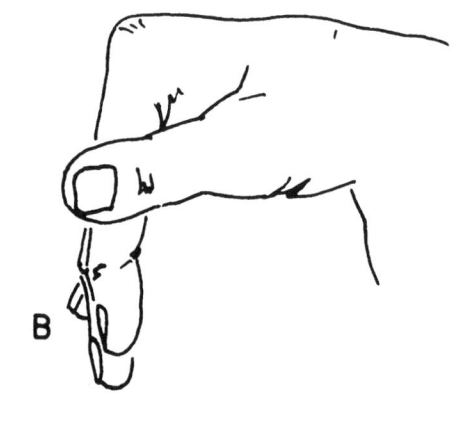

The ligamentous morphology becomes different at the proximal interphalangeal joint,[13] a hinge joint without significant lateral motion capacity. The palmar plate is less mobile than that of the metacarpophalangeal joint. It is attached firmly to the epiphysis of the middle phalanx. In flexion the palmar plate folds like an accordion. If the palmar plate is left in the flexed position, portions of it may become adherent to each other, leading to a stiff joint. The checkreins appear to be the primary pathologic structure causing proximal interphalangeal joint contracture.[19] The collateral ligaments of the proximal interphalangeal joint are under the greatest tension (length) in the lateral aspect of the condyle of the proximal phalanx.[13] Consequently, proximal interphalangeal joints should be splinted in 15°–20° of flexion to prevent shortening of the collateral ligaments and palmar plate.

Edema after surgery or trauma is a significant concomitant and plays a role in stiffness of the hand.[17] Local venous return is a causal factor in edema formation and plays a role in its management. There are three functional independent venous systems: superficial palmar, deep palmar, and dorsal veins. These systems act synergistically, producing the greatest velocity increase when concurrently activated during fist-clenching. There is a large perforator in the first interosseous space and a relatively constant one in the fourth interosseous space. They transmit significant volumes of blood from deep palmar veins to the dorsal superficial venous system, where variable cutaneous tension continues the pumping mechanism. This pumping mechanism is just as important in the child as it is in the adult.

Injury Incidence

Because of the activity level of children, the hand is one of the most frequent areas of trauma, although not necessarily specific chondro-osseous injury.[20–75] Bhende et al. reviewed 364 patients (187 boys and 177 girls; median age 10 years) with hand injuries.[24] The most common types of injury were lacerations (38%), soft tissue injuries (28%), fractures (20%), and sprains (8%). About 60% of the injuries were sustained in the home. The little finger was the most commonly fractured digit (37%) and the fifth metacarpal the most commonly fractured bone.

Beaton et al. studied 1003 patients with hand injuries; only 58 of these patients were less than 16 years of age.[22] They found that among both left- and right-handers injuries to the right hand were more common than to the left hand. The exception was accidents to right-handers at work, in which group there were more injuries to the left hand.

Unfortunately, many trauma studies involving children specifically preclude the incidence of hand or wrist injury. Carpal injuries and multiple unstable fractures of the metacarpals are certainly infrequent in children, whereas other hand fractures, especially phalangeal fractures and interphalangeal dislocations, are common. Probably the most frequent fracture is a crush injury to the distal phalanx and the fingertip. The spontaneous exploration of the surrounding enviroment by any child predisposes to such injuries. Various hand fractures in children, which often seem like minor injuries, may have serious consequences because of aberrant growth and occult infection. Unfortunately, many of these fractures are treated according to guidelines established for comparable adult injuries.

Hastings and Simmons reviewed 354 pediatric hand fractures and found that the incidence of epiphyseal injury was much higher than that reported elsewhere in the skeleton,[41] but growth disturbances were rare. Fractures were most common in the border digits, with displacement within a given digit being most common in the metacarpal, next most common in the proximal and distal phalanges, and least common in the middle phalanx. Malunion most often was associated with failure to obtain adequate lateral and anteroposterior roentgenograms of the individual digits, failure to evaluate postreduction alignment, and the erroneous assumption that growth would correct deficient reduction.

Children's finger ligaments are strong and resilient. Because they are stronger than the associated physes, the sudden extension of a ligament generally results in chondroosseous, rather than ligamentous, damage (Figs. 17-5, 17-6). To a lesser extent, this is also true of the fibrous joint capsules.

Leonard and Dubravicik collected 276 fractures involving a child's hand; 41% were physeal fractures. However, these children's hand fractures constituted only 0.45% of their overall practice. Of these fractures, 10% required open reduction for adequate restoration of normal anatomy.[49]

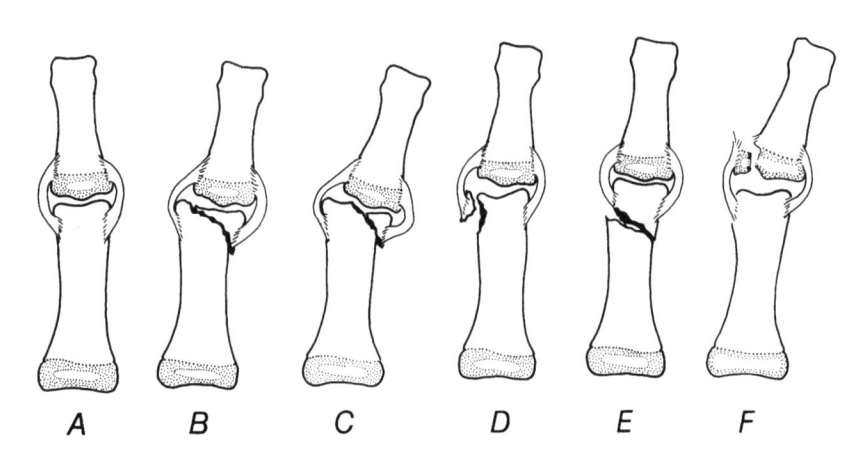

FIGURE 17-5. Interphalangeal injuries caused by osseous failure prior to ligament failure. (A) Normal anatomy. (B) Unicondylar. (C) Partial condylar. (D) Lateral avulsion. (E) Bicondylar. (F) Type 3 epiphyseal.

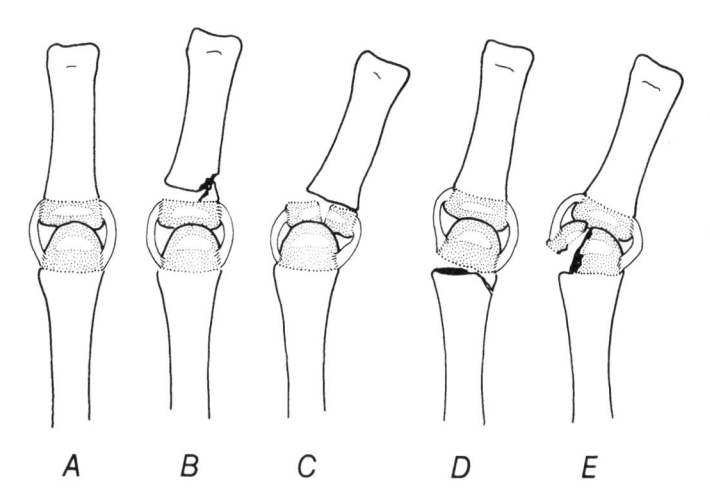

FIGURE 17-6. Metacarpophalangeal injuries caused by osseous failure prior to ligament failure. (A) Normal anatomy. (B) Type 2 physeal. (C) Type 3 physeal. (D) Type 2 physeal. (E) Type 3 physeal.

Bora and colleagues reviewed 100 patients with epiphyseal fractures of the hand; 90 fractures were closed and 10 were open.[25] Of the 90 closed fractures, 80 were treated successfully with closed manipulation. Seven of the other ten were treated with closed reduction and percutaneous pin fixation; three were old fractures that had healed in an unacceptable (malaligned) position.

Almost all metacarpal and phalangeal fractures heal sufficiently by 3–4 weeks to allow active range of motion. In children, radiologic union is not necessarily a prerequisite to starting protected motion. Fractures should probably not be immobilized in children longer than 6 weeks, unless there is an obvious delay in healing. If such is evident, a change in treatment (e.g., open reduction and internal fixation) may have to be considered.

There is definite conservatism in the treatment of children's hand fractures. Greater degrees of displacement and deformity seem to be tolerated on the assumption that the patient's young age and potential for further growth will correct the deformity. Although remodeling usually occurs, a deformity may not correct spontaneously unless the angulation or displacement is within a plane of anatomically permitted motion.

Diagnostic Imaging

Roentgenograms in at least two planes (anteroposterior and lateral) are essential to assess any hand fracture adequately. It is imperative that a true lateral view of the involved digit be obtained. Superimposition of other fingers in the lateral view may obscure significant details. The fourth and fifth metacarpals may be brought into lateral view with 10° of supination; and the second and third metacarpals may be brought into lateral view with 10° of pronation. Alternatively, lateral tomography of a specific digit may delineate the anatomy of the injury. Perhaps the most common cause of missed or improper diagnosis of fractures in children's fingers is failure to obtain a true lateral view of the involved finger. Additional oblique views may also be necessary to evaluate joint injuries properly, particularly to assess small, juxtaarticular fractures.

Magnetic resonance imaging (MRI) of the hand and wrist has lagged behind its use for larger joints. It is the procedure of choice in children with chronic wrist pain. Intercarpal ligament tears, although uncommon, may occur, along with triangular fibrocartilage complex (TFCC) lesions. Ischemic necrosis may also occur. Chondro-osseous separation is probably an underdiagnosed entity in the immature carpus. MRI can help delineate tendon abnormalities.

General Treatment Guidelines

Initial evaluation and primary care of the injured hand are critical. One of the greatest pitfalls in treating these injuries is that the primary focus is the fracture, and the damage to soft tissues is overlooked. Both open and closed injuries must be examined meticulously for damage to tendons, nerves, and blood vessels. Maximal functional recovery must be the goal of treatment for every hand injury.

Immobilization of a child's hand always presents a challenge. Well-fitting plaster casts and splints are notoriously difficult to apply in the small child. Bulky, soft dressings may be used for immobilizing the infant's hand. In older children, gutter splints incorporating at least one adjacent uninjured digit may be used to help control rotational deformity.

The true "position of safety" is the *intrinsic-plus position*, with 90° of flexion at the metacarpophalangeal joints and almost complete extension in the proximal interphalangeal joints (Fig. 17-4). The thumb is best held in an abducted, opposed position.

Placing the fingers in a banjo splint, in which the fingers are extended and divergent, is rarely acceptable. Wrapping the hand around a gauze bandage over which all the fingers may stiffen is also poor practice. Universal splints rarely fit children. Because of the ease with which the small child's hand can slip backward, the universal splint may cause fingers to assume a suboptimal position.

A solitary finger should rarely be immobilized in a child. When a single finger is immobilized, there is an increased possibility that angulation or malrotation will develop by the time the cast or splint is removed.

For fractures of the metacarpals and phalanges, it is important to recognize and correct rotational malalignment. Remodeling never corrects rotational deformity of a digit. Accordingly, it is imperative to reduce all fractures of the phalanges and metacarpals in proper rotational alignment. This practice is not always easy, as subtle degrees of malrotation that are not recognized during the period of immobilization may result in significant functional impairment after full range of motion has been regained. The best way to monitor rotational alignment is to study the planes of the fingernails in the splint carefully, comparing the injured digit with the adjacent normal fingers and the counterpart in the opposite hand (Fig. 17-7). Assessing malrotation of the thumb is more difficult. True lateral radiographs are helpful. Normally, a true lateral radiograph provides simultaneous lateral views of the interphalangeal joints of a finger and the metacarpophalangeal and interphalangeal joints of the thumb.

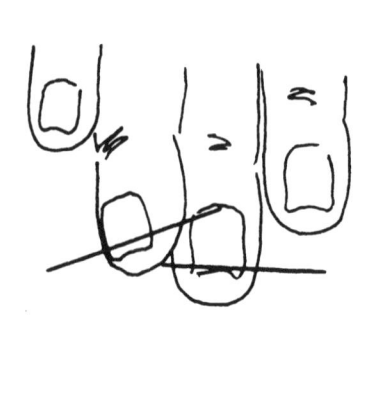

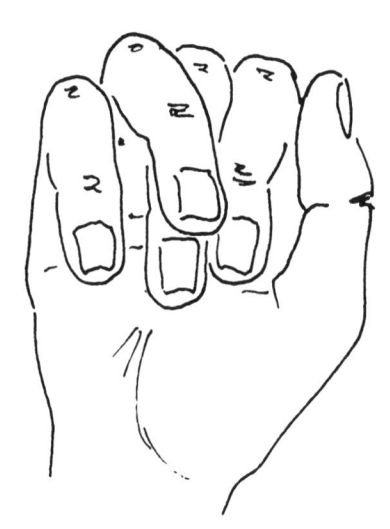

FIGURE 17-7. Fingernails should be coplanar, and all of the flexed fingers should be reasonably parallel. In malrotation, whether involving a metacarpal or phalanx, the uniform plane of the fingernails is disrupted, and the involved digit overlaps the normal digits.

Davis and Stothard reviewed 678 finger fractures seen in an emergency department.[31] They noted that of 624 initially treated by nonhand surgeons, 169 (27%) had inappropriate treatment. Many of the management errors were simple: failure to prescribe antibiotics for open injuries, failure to reduce displaced fractures accurately, and unsatisfactory splintage. They strongly recommended that all finger fractures be assessed and treated by surgeons with sufficient training in the management of hand injuries. Although the title of their article implied that all fractures should be referred to a hand surgery service, their comment that such fractures should be treated by surgeons with training in the management of hand injuries suggests review and treatment by an orthopaedic surgeon. Their recommendation that treatment not be undertaken by emergency room physicians with no or minimal training in the nuances of hand injuries deserves support.

Johnson et al. surveyed two time periods during the early and the late 1980s and found that 8.2% of child abuse injuries involved the hands during the earlier time period and that it increased to 13.4% during the late 1980s.[44] Of 94 patients, 19 sustained injury only to the hand: 8 burns, 2 bruises, 2 human bites, 3 lacerations, and 4 fractures. Children with burns to the hand alone were significantly younger than those with other types of injuries. They thought that the hand was frequently the primary or incidental target of child abuse and must be considered for any child with such injuries, particularly in the age range of high child abuse incidence.

Rankin et al. described acquired rotational digital deformity as a result of digital sucking.[56] It was usually radial rotation of the index finger. In most cases rotational deformities spontaneously resolved once finger sucking ceased. However, in a few cases, particularly when the habit is unduly prolonged, deformities may persist and cause functional impairment. Surgical intervention may be indicated in such a patient, possibly rotational osteotomy of the metacarpal or the proximal phalanx depending on where the deformity seems to be most obvious.

Ryan and Turner also described hand complications in children due to digital sucking.[57] They noted that digital sucking is common among children and often regarded as a harmless habit. However, the effects of prolonged or vigorous digital sucking on the development of orthodontic abnormalities certainly have been described. Reports of hand complications are much less frequent. Stone and Mullins found that thumb sucking was the most frequent predisposing factor for chronic paronychia in children.[68] They described five patients with significant rotational abnormalities and were able to rectify all of the problems with corrective splintage. None required surgery. Four of the five patients had a history of digital infection.

Carroll and associates reported a case of acute calcific deposition adjacent to a metacarpal in an 11-year-old child.[29] This patient participated actively in gymnastics but denied any specific injury. The mass was injected with methylprednisolone acetate and lidocaine, resulting in complete relief. The deposition may have been caused by chronic trauma.

Closed phalangeal fractures in children are usually treated by simple methods, with a return to normal or almost normal function expected. The exceptional case requires open reduction. The most common exception is a fracture through the distal end of the phalanx, with rotatory displacement of the head of the phalanx in relation to the more distal phalangeal base.

Fractures of the phalanges and metacarpals heal rapidly, and remodeling of angulation often occurs in fractures in the metaphyseal region. Little remodeling may be expected for fractures distant from the epiphyseal end containing the secondary ossification center. For example, in the distal end of a phalanx, growth is primarily from a spherical rather than a transverse physis, which is nonlongitudinal growth. Accordingly, malunion usually requires operative correction.

Greene et al. have described a simple technique of composite wiring for various oblique and transverse fractures in the phalanges and metacarpals.[38] These methods are readily applicable to children. Parsons et al. recommended the use of micro external fixators for unstable fracture patterns in the phalanges.[55] These devices should be used carefully in children, avoiding the growth plate and secondary ossification centers whenever possible.

Wrist

Carpal Subluxation and Dislocation

Injury to the wrist joint is unusual prior to skeletal maturity.[79,95,112] Except in children with significant ligamentous laxity, such as those with Larsen or Ehler-Danlos syndrome (see Chapter 11), subluxation or dislocation of the wrist is almost nonexistent. Because of the density of ligamentous and capsular attachments from the carpus into the distal radial and ulnar epiphyses, injurious forces invariably cause distal radiolunar epiphyseal and metaphyseal fractures.

The wrist joint capsule may be partially damaged during a fall; and because of the proximity of extensor tendon compartments, a communication may develop, leading to progressive symptoms of chronic, painful tenosynovitis (Fig. 17-8). These injuries may be accurately diagnosed by wrist joint arthrography or MRI and subsequently treated by operative closure of the capsular defect.

Gilula presented an excellent review of various geometric principles of parallelism and overlapping articular surfaces for the analysis of carpal injuries.[98,99] These lines are principally described for skeletally mature individuals, and their complete applicability to the skeletally immature child is limited.

Cooney et al. described TFCC tears in 33 patients,[85] including 3 patients under 15 years of age. They found that open repair of the peripheral tear produced excellent results, particularly in the younger patients. This certainly should be considered in children, rather than resection of portions of the TFCC.[85] Arthroscopy also should be used as the initial approach for analysis and repair.[88]

Dautel et al. studied 26 patients with arthroscopy who had otherwise normal static or dynamic radiographs.[88] They found five patients with true scapholunate instability; none was a child.

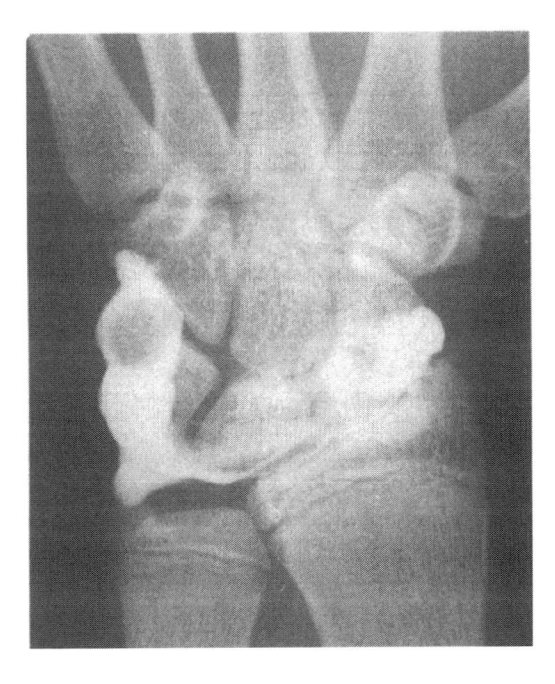

FIGURE 17-8. Ulnar pain in a gymnast. A capsular and intercarpal defect is evident distal to the ulnar styloid.

Carpal Fractures

Nafie reviewed carpal fractures in children.[127] The scaphoid was involved in 71, the triquetrum in 5, the trapezium in 3, the hamate in 2, and the trapezoid in 1.

Scaphoid Fractures

Fracture of the scaphoid (Figs. 17-9 to 17-11) is the most common carpal injury in the child.* It has been reported in children less than 7 years of age.[110] Bloem reported a 4-year-old patient with fractures of the capitate and the third, fourth, and fifth metacarpals; a scaphoid fracture, however, was not evident at the age of 4 years. Instead, nonunion of the scaphoid fracture was diagnosed only when the patient was 11 years old. This nonunited scaphoid fracture was presumed to have occurred when the patient was 4 years of age.[81] Greene et al. reported a patient, injured at 6 years of age, whose subsequent radiographs usually showed a nonunited fracture through the ossific nucleus of the scaphoid.[102]

Horii et al. described scaphoid fractures following repetitive punching.[105] They found that the location of the fracture was comparable to a scaphoid fracture caused by wrist extension injuries.

Mussbichler reviewed more than 3000 hand and wrist injuries in children and noted that injuries of the scaphoid were relatively common, finding 107 with roentgenologically evident damage to the carpal bones, 100 of which had a fracture through the scaphoid.[126] They included 15 injuries through the waist, 33 in the distal aspect, and 52 avulsions of the radiodorsal aspect. There were no fractures through the proximal part of the bone. In another series of 108 scaphoid fractures, 49% of the patients had distal third fractures and 38% had avulsion fractures, with all fractures except one being on the dorsoradial surface of the distal pole.[150] Avulsion fractures really represent sleeve fractures, similar to type 7 growth mechanism injuries in long bones (see Chapter 6).

In one report of 64 patients with a mean age of 11 years, only one patient had a concomitant injury (fracture of the neck of the fifth metacarpal in the same hand), and the most frequently fractured area was in the distal third (60%), primarily involving the scaphoid tuberosity.[83] The waist of the scaphoid was fractured in 24 cases (33%). Displacement was present in only five cases. In four patients the displacement was visible on the initial radiograph, and in the fifth it became apparent 6 weeks after injury during the course of treatment with a cast (this was the only patient in whom the bone eventually failed to unite).[83]

When evaluating the child with distal radial fracture, it is important to rule out the potential complication of associated fracture of the carpal scaphoid.[83,94,102,126,139,150] Lahoti et al. described an associated fracture of the scaphoid accompanying the distal radial physeal fracture.[109] Trumble et al. described six patients with ipsilateral fractures of the scaphoid and radius,[148] including one skeletally immature

---

* Refs. 77–83,87,89,93,94,100–102,104–106,109,110,113–115,117,118, 120,121,123,125–129,133,137–139,141,142,144,145,147,148,150,154.

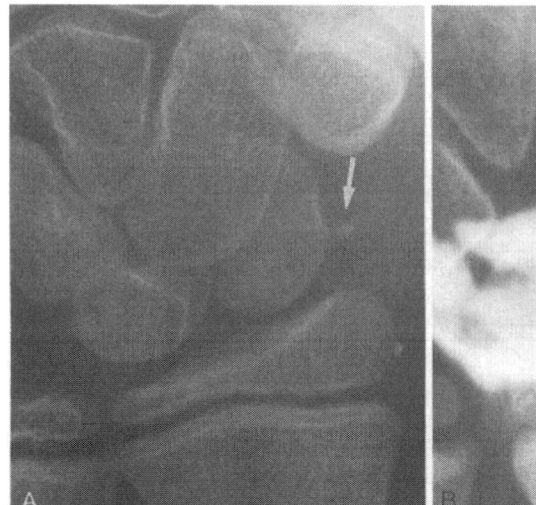

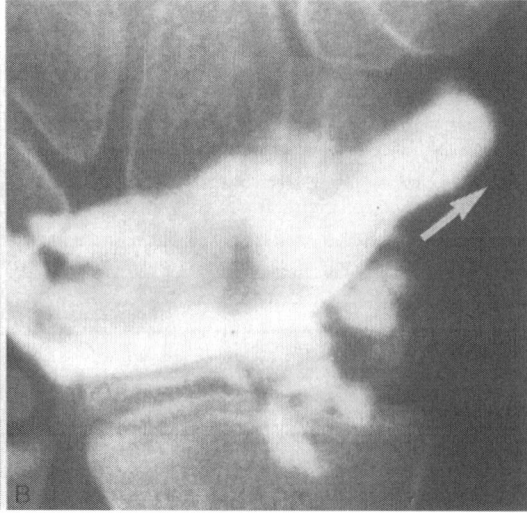

FIGURE 17-9. (A) Chondro-osseous avulsion fracture (arrow) of the scaphoid in an 11-year-old child. (B) Arthrography showed a diverticulum near this fracture (arrow). At surgery, the capsule was damaged, and nonunion was evident. The small fragment was removed and the capsule reattached to the scaphoid perichondrium.

individual. Coexistence of the two injuries is infrequent (Fig. 17-12) but must be assessed in any case involving a distal radial fracture. Other carpal bones may be fractured concomitantly.

Early, appropriate treatment obviously depends on an accurate diagnosis. The diagnosis is difficult when the fracture involves the primarily cartilaginous scaphoid. Arthrography, CT, or MRI might delineate this fracture at an earlier time.

Tiel-Van Buul et al. evaluated the role of radiography and scintigraphy for diagnosing a suspected scaphoid fracture.[147] They believed that the best diagnostic strategy and the management of clinically suspected scaphoid fractures consisted of initial radiography followed by bone scintigraphy in patients who had seemingly negative radiographs. The positive predictive value for initial radiographs was 0.76 and decreased to 0.15 for follow-up. The sensitivity of radiographs decreased from 64% to 30%. In contrast, the specificity of the bone scan was 98%.

Finkenberg et al. studied the diagnosis of occult scaphoid lesion in fractures by ultrasound vibration.[93] Whether this methodology is applicable to children is unknown because cartilage may have different vibratory rates from the fully ossified bone of an adult.

As discussed in Chapters 1 and 6, the carpal and tarsal epiphyses may have a unique failure pattern in which there

FIGURE 17-10. Distal pole scaphoid fracture in a 14-year-old. This pattern of injury is common prior to skeletal maturation.

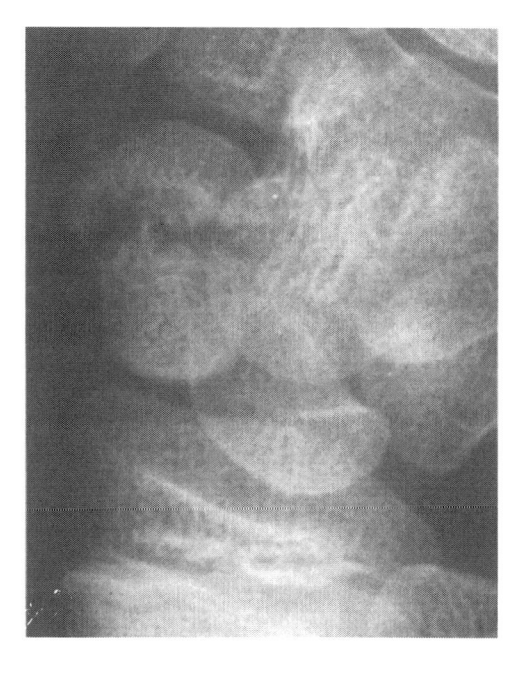

FIGURE 17-11. Waist fracture. Delayed union with widening of the fracture line due to repetitive motion in a child being initially evaluated 9 weeks after a wrist injury. The radiodensity of the two sides is similar, suggesting that the vascularity to the proximal half is intact.

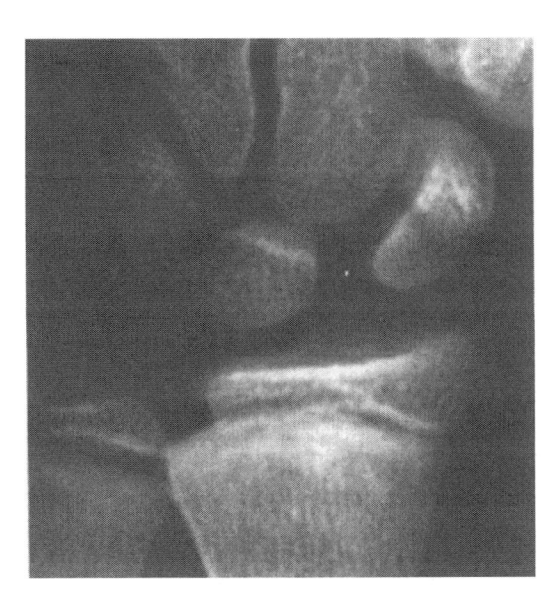

FIGURE 17-12. Concomitant scaphoid and distal radial epiphyseal fractures. The "widening" of the scapholunate gap must be assessed carefully. It was normal in this child because of incomplete chondro-osseous transformation.

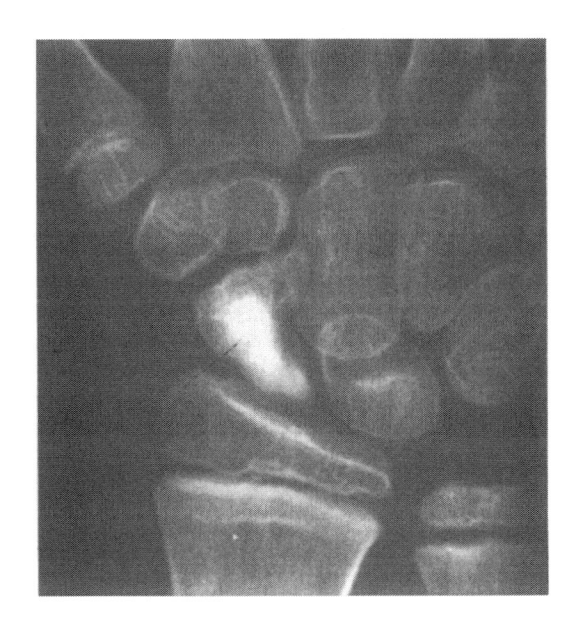

FIGURE 17-13. Sclerotic appearance of the carpal scaphoid, suggesting an ischemic complication.

is separation of some of the unossified cartilage from the expanding primary or secondary ossification center (sleeve or shell fracture pattern). Actual separation (displacement) may be minimal and not associated with fracture propagation into the cartilage to create a loose fragment. The true extent of such an injury pattern in the scaphoid or any other carpal bone is unknown. The increased application of MRI in children with wrist pain may help ascertain the specific morphologic diagnosis. Eventual ossification of the cartilaginous region, coupled with fibrous or fibrocartilaginous nonunion, is a likely cause of the eventual development of a bipartite carpal bone.

As with the young adult, the child who presents with a painful wrist following even low-energy trauma and with pain in the anatomic snuffbox, but shows normal radiographs, should be treated until a fracture is either confirmed or refuted by follow-up clinical and radiographic examinations.

Scaphoid fractures in children usually heal with closed treatment. A short arm-thumb spica cast is recommended for avulsion and incomplete fractures in children. For transverse fractures, 4–8 weeks of immobilization is recommended. In cases in which the injury was neglected, the diagnosis was delayed, or in which there is apparent bone resorption, a longer period of immobilization, often 8–16 weeks, may be necessary.

One of the major concerns with adult scaphoid fractures is ischemic necrosis.[146] It does not appear to be a frequent complicating factor in children's fractures (Fig. 17-13), but children must still be followed closely for such a complication. Grundy reported irregularity of the margin of the scaphoid at the site of the healed fracture in four cases.[104] However, this irregularity might have been a change consequent to micromotion of the injury and not necessarily indicative of a vascular complication. Letts and Esser showed that there is a separate small artery supplying the distal portion of the scaphoid that is usually intact in the avulsed fragment, thus supporting healing of the area.[111]

Cristiani et al. evaluated ischemic necrosis of carpal bones by MRI and found that the MRI was more sensitive than scintigraphy.[87] It certainly should be considered in patients with unusual pain following injury to the wrist, particularly to look for potential separations at a chondro-osseous interface.

Because of the high incidence of avulsion and distal third fractures in children, rather than waist fractures, the incidence of nonunion in scaphoid fractures (Figs. 17-14 to 17-16) is considerably lower in pediatric patients than

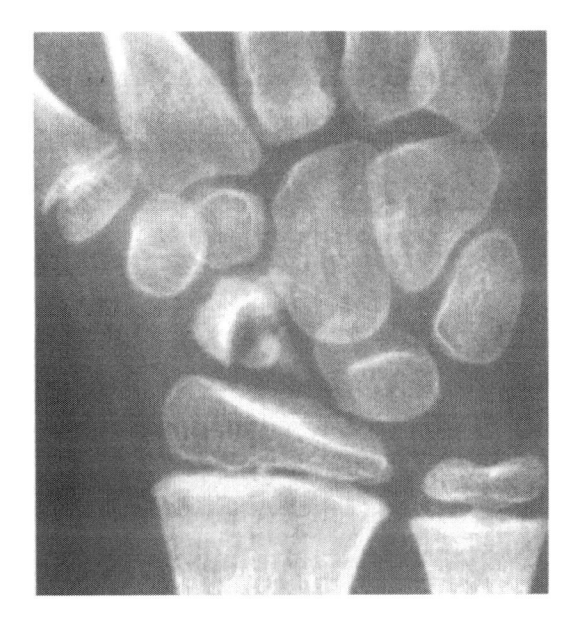

FIGURE 17-14. Well-established nonunion of a carpal scaphoid fracture in an 11-year-old child.

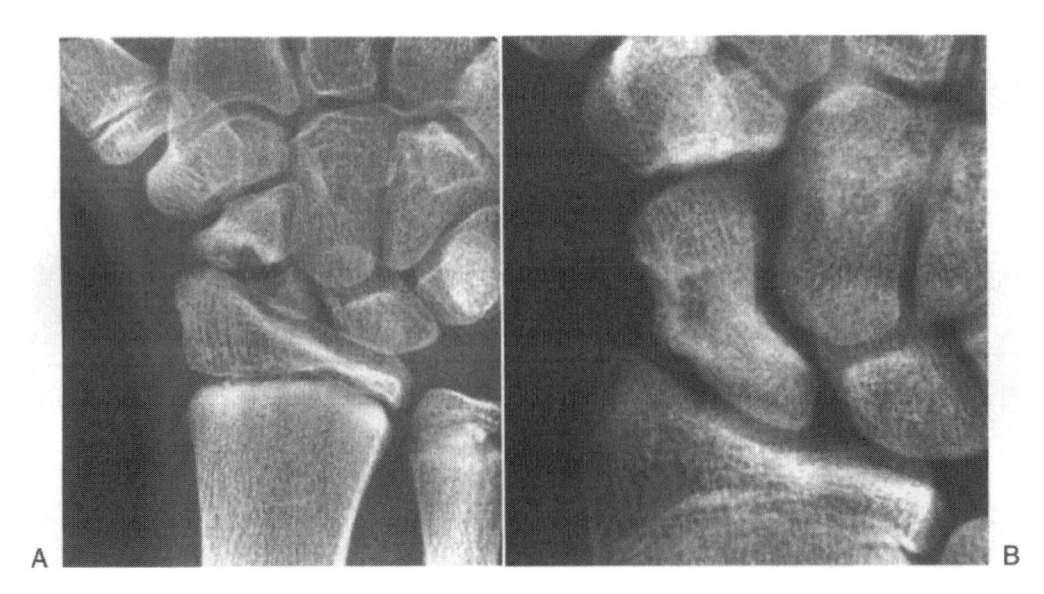

FIGURE 17-15. (A) Appearance of a scaphoid fracture 5 weeks after a wrist injury. The radiograph obtained at the time of the acute injury was read as negative, and the youngster was not casted. Open reduction and internal fixation were done. An allograft was also used. (B) Appearance 8 months after surgery. The fracture is healed, but there is altered carpal morphology.

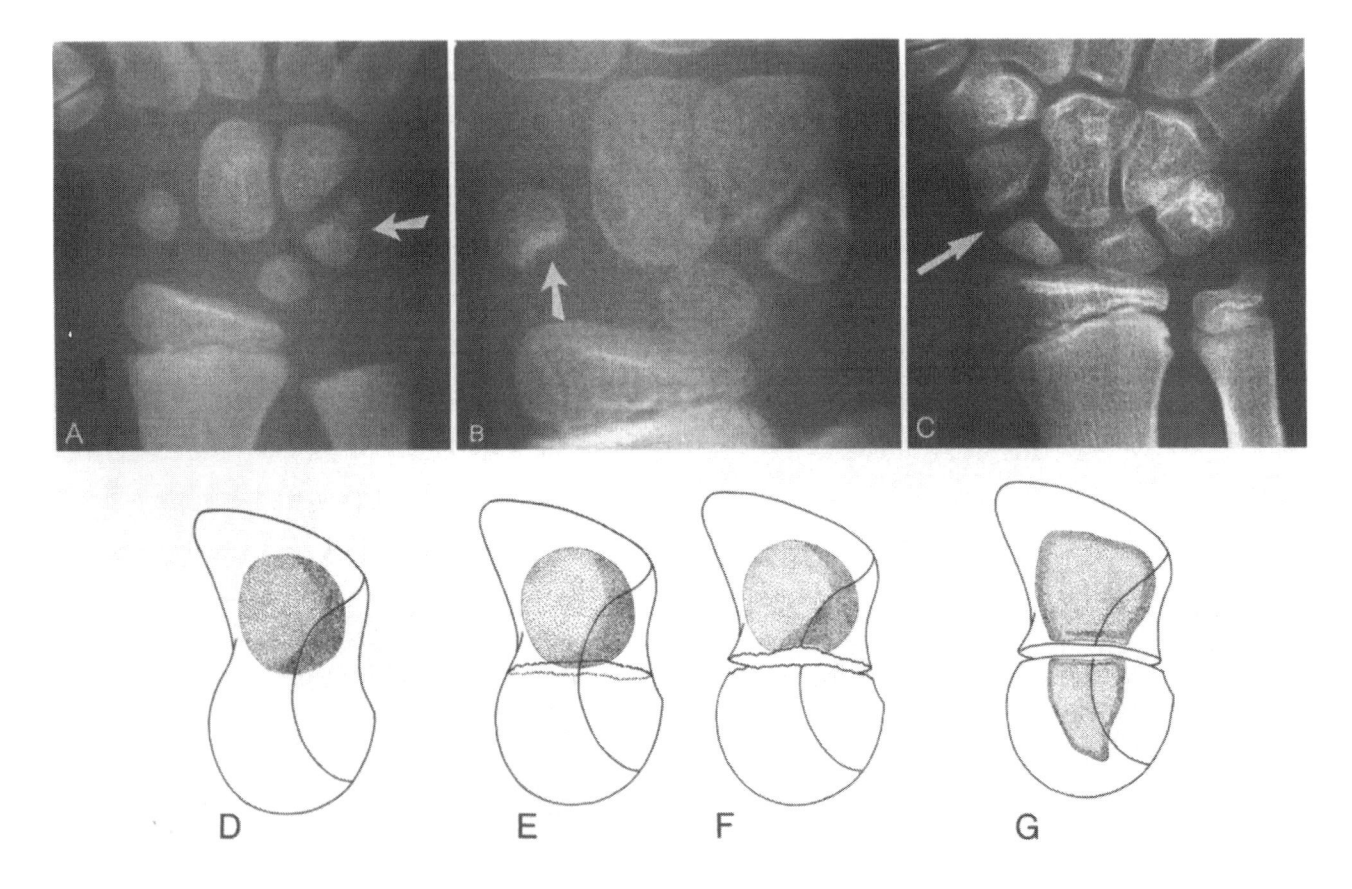

FIGURE 17-16. (A) Initial radiograph shows an obvious triquetral fracture (arrow) but no evidence of a scaphoid fracture. (B) Several weeks later the triquetral fracture is healing. Sclerosis and irregularity are evident along the proximal edge of the navicular ossification center (arrow). (C) Radiologic nonunion (arrow) several months later. This was interpreted by the radiologist as a bipartite scaphoid. Because the patient had no pain the family refused surgery. A fibrous union was most likely present. (D–G) Drawings depicting this case. (D) Preinjury. (E) Fracture at the chondro-osseous junction. (F) Micromotion widens the fracture gap. (G) Nonunion is evident as the proximal fragment ossifies.

in adults.[123,129,138] Mussbichler[126] reported two cases of scaphoid nonunion in children, Southcott and Rosman[142] reported eight cases, Maxted and Owen[120] reported two cases, and Pick and Segal[133] reported one case.[120,127,133,142] All nonunions were grafted with autogenous bone, which led to good clinical and radiologic results. Nonunion in children is best managed by bone grafting through the palmar approach.[142,154]

In the case shown in Figure 17-16 radiologic nonunion was most likely due to motion, rather than intrinsic damage to the blood supply. It should be noted that Mazet and Hohl referred to neglected scaphoid fractures; they stated that vacuolation and pseudocyst formation appear earlier in the proximal fragment, and sclerotic changes do not usually appear for a year.[121] In contrast, Kohler and Zimmer suggested that posttraumatic cystic changes developed mainly in the distal fragment because of the better blood supply.[108]

DeBoeck et al. described nonunion of a carpal scaphoid fracture in an 8.5-year-old.[89] The original injury occurred 7 months prior to roentgenograms that showed nonunion of the scaphoid with sclerosis of the distal portion and cyst formation at the fracture site. The child healed with conservative treatment.

Kerlinke and McCabe analyzed the literature on scaphoid fractures and union and concluded that the natural history of nonunion of the scaphoid was not as severe as had been reported.[106] They noted, however, that there is much variability in the studies, and absolute recommendations could not be derived from this study. In contrast, Lingström and Nyström reviewed 32 patients 2–37 years of age following scaphoid trauma.[113] They found a 100% incidence of progressive radiocarpal osteoarthritis. They thought that an effort to attain reduction should be attempted. The only exception was the patient in whom the radiocarpal joint was already severely deteriorated by advanced degenerative arthritis.

The rationale for operative treatment of scaphoid nonunion in the adult is well established. It has been shown that the altered kinematics of the nonunited scaphoid predictably lead to late intercarpal and radiocarpal degenerative arthritis. The validity of these conclusions has not been proved in children. Although it is technically possible to fuse scaphoid nonunions in skeletally immature patients,[92,114,141] previous reports have generally dealt with adolescents who have waist fractures. Furthermore, a radiographic "nonunion" in a child (Fig. 17-16) may not be an anatomic nonunion. The tarsal navicular/accessory navicular is an excellent example of such disparity (see Chapter 24).

Mintzer and Waters described open reduction and internal fixation in a 9-year-old.[125] It was undertaken because of significant deformity and displacement of the child's initial presentation. Suzuki and Herbert also described a 10-year-old boy treated with open reduction and internal fixation with bone grafting.[145] Nakamura et al. reviewed 10 patients with symptomatic scaphoid malunion.[128] All suffered from pain, restricted range of motion, and decreased grip strength. In another study seven patients underwent corrective osteotomy, grafting, and internal fixation. Refracture of a proximal pole scaphoid fracture may occur, as it did in two skeletally immature patients.[80]

The existence of a "congenital" bipartite scaphoid continues to be questioned.[92,103,108,110,116,140] It is possible that some children fracture the ossifying scaphoid, present minimal or no symptoms, and eventually develop a scaphoid that appears to be bipartite.[101,133] If this is true, the assumption supports the concept that bipartition is secondary to trauma.[116] This bipartite entity may result from an undiagnosed fracture of the scaphoid early in its distal to proximal ossification sequence (see Fig. 17-16 above). Similar phenomena are now recognized as potential etiologic factors in cases of bipartite patella and accessory tarsal navicular bone (see Chapters 22, 24). Morphologic and histologic studies have definitely shown that epiphyseal cartilage bridges the radiolucent gap between the ossification centers in these two conditions and that this gap may continue into adult years or gradually disappear when the ossification centers coalesce.

Doman and Marcus studied a patient with congenital bilateral bipartite scaphoid with MRI.[92] They showed the presence of contiguous cartilage between the seemingly "separated" bones and no evidence of significant signal changes in the adjacent bone that would indicate a previous injury or reparative process. They thought this case supported the congenital nature of some of these bipartite bones, although they did not preclude trauma as a factor in other cases, particularly the unilateral one.

Injuries to Other Carpal Bones

Injuries of the other carpal bones are infrequent in children.[84,91,96,97,111,119,122,124,135,136,143,152,155] It has been suggested that the cartilaginous covering of the juvenile bones imparts a certain resilience that renders the enclosed osseous centrum less susceptible to fracture than the comparable mature bone.

The diagnosis may be missed because of a lack of suspicion and the difficulty of assessing minimal radiographic change in the acutely injured child. The diagnosis of a lunate or capitate fracture in a young child may be supported by findings of pain, swelling, and limited motion at the wrist (Figs. 17-17, 17-18). Other bones are involved infrequently (Figs. 17-19). These fractures may not be easily demonstrable on initial radiographs; and like adult fractures they may not appear until weeks following the injury.[122,143] Treatment with immobilization should begin when a suspected diagnosis is rendered. They usually heal without consequence.

The carpal tunnel view is helpful for unrecognized fractures of the carpus, especially those involving the pisiform and hamate.[76,143] The hook of the hamate shows quite well in this view (if it is ossified). The carpal tunnel view is obtained by placing the pronated forearm against the film cassette and having the patient manually dorsiflex the hand by pulling the fingertips dorsally with the opposite hand. The central x-ray beam is angled approximately 25°–35° and directed at the palmar surface of the carpus. If the patient is unable to dorsiflex the hand secondary to pain, the angulation of the x-ray tube may be varied to achieve a good view of the carpal tunnel.

Letts and Esser thought that fractures of the triquetrum in children (Fig. 17-19) were more common than fully appre-

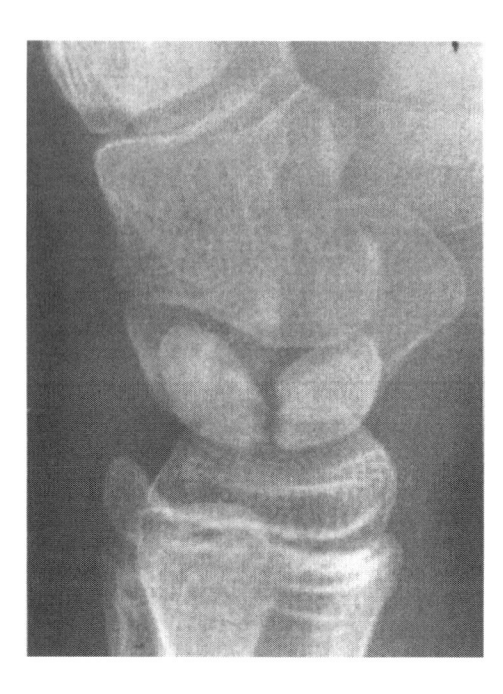

FIGURE 17-17. Lunate fracture. While the anteroposterior view showed no evidence of injury, the lateral view readily revealed the fracture.

ciated.[111] The fractures were often subtle, often appearing as a flake avulsion that required a good oblique radiograph to diagnose. Fifteen patients were reviewed; all but three were missed initially. Follow-up, averaging 4 years, showed only two patients with complaints of wrist stiffness and discomfort. Three fractures involved the body.

Light noted that Keinbock's disease has been reported in skeletally immature individuals in children as young as 7-8 years of age[112,136] A patient with a lunate fracture (11-year-old boy) treated by open reduction and K-wire fixation, developed fragmentation and collapse ("genuine" Kienbock's disease) 1 year after the injury.[91] Trumble and Irving showed that MRI could be used for early evaluation of Keinbock's disease, especially in young patients.[149] Viegas and Ampar also emphasized the usefulness of MRI for early assessment of revascularization of Keinbock's disease.[151]

Peyton and Moore described a fracture through a trapezoid-capitate congenital coalition.[132] Such fusions are infrequent, and fractures through them are rare.

Compson described associated transcarpal injuries with distal radial physeal fractures in three children.[84] Two cases involved simultaneous fractures of both the scaphoid and the capitate. The third case involved the scaphoid and the triquetrum. Compson emphasized that the full extent of these injuries is not always recognized on the initial radiographs. He cited the study of Nafie of radiographs of proven carpal fractures in 82 children[127]: 71 fractures were isolated to the scaphoid, whereas all the other carpal bones accounted for only 11 fractures. He noted that others had described isolated fractures of the capitate.[135,155] In each study he pointed out the delay in diagnosis, noting that no radiograph obtained before 3 weeks showed the fracture on the same view. In fact, fractures of the capitate were seen only on oblique views and did not show on the standard anteroposterior projections.

DeCoster et al. described an unusual pediatric carpal fracture dislocation in a 10-year-old child who sustained a type 3 fracture of the distal radius associated with fractures across the scaphoid, lunate, and triquetrum[90] (Fig. 17-20). The fractures were treated with open reduction and internal fixation with ligamentous repair to combine dorsal and palmar approaches. At follow-up there was good wrist function but abnormal carpal development.

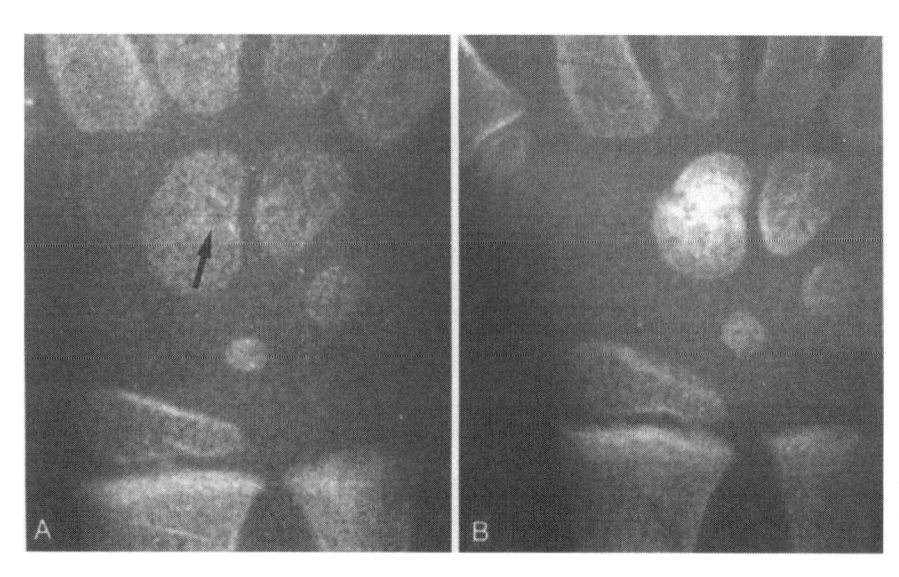

FIGURE 17-18. (A) Minimal evidence of capitate injury (arrow). (B) Healing made the capitate fracture more evident because of reactive sclerosis.

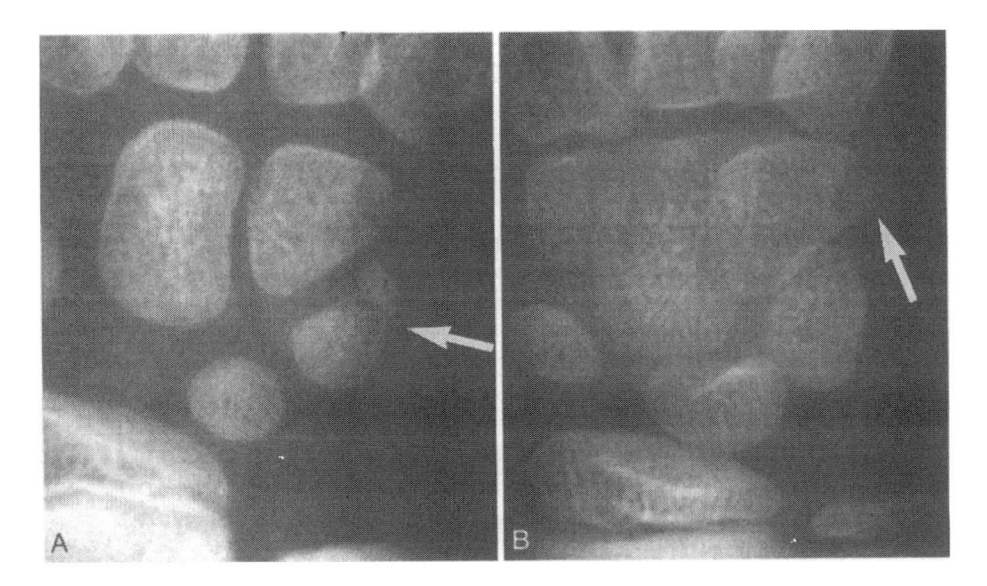

FIGURE 17-19. (A) Triquetral fracture (arrow). (B) Hamate fracture (arrow).

Intercarpal Disruptions

Traumatic intercarpal instability (Figs. 17-21, 17-22) in the young child presents problems of diagnosis and management because of variable degrees of carpal ossification.[86,107,131,153] The scaphoid and lunate do not ossify until a child is 4 years of age. Peiro and associates documented transscaphoid, perilunate dislocation in a 10-year-old boy.[130] The mechanism of injury undoubtedly is similar to that in the adult. Fluoroscopy and arthrography may be useful.[134]

Children with ligamentous laxity may be predisposed to perilunate instability. Prospective evaluation using stress views and motion fluoroscopy can disclose the problem much more easily than static radiographs.

Craigan described a 10-year-old-girl with a complaint of thumb dislocation.[86] Radiographs, however, revealed dorsal subluxation at the midcarpal joint. Gerard reported a 7-year-old girl who had fallen from a table at 3 months of age.[95] She did not use her hand when crawling. Radiography revealed osteopenia in the carpus. The capitate was displaced into the proximal row, and the entire carpus was displaced with collapse into a palmar flexion deformity.

Gidden and Shaw reported a combined physeal fracture of the distal radius with lunate subluxation.[97] The patient was initially treated with closed methods for the radial fracture. The lunate subluxation was not diagnosed until 4 weeks later; because of continued clinical and radiologic evidence of instability, he underwent surgery. The lunate subluxation was corrected by longitudinal traction, following which the dorsal ligaments were repaired.

Letts and Esser[111] noted only two reports of scapholunate dissociation in the skeletally immature patient secondary

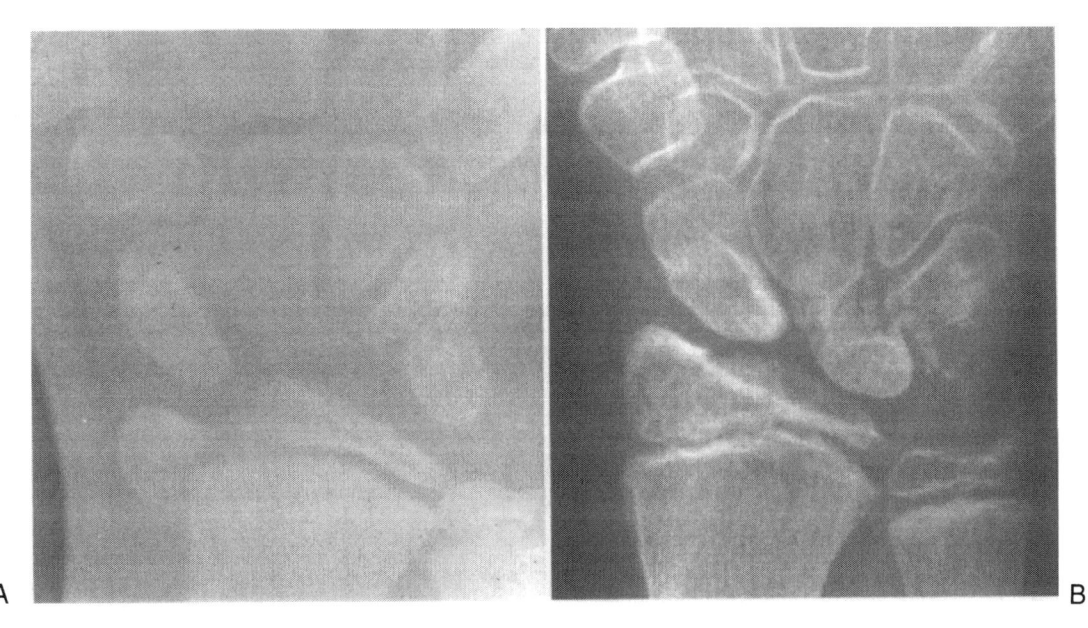

FIGURE 17-20. (A) Original injury. (B) Three months later. It is a complex fracture-dislocation of the wrist.

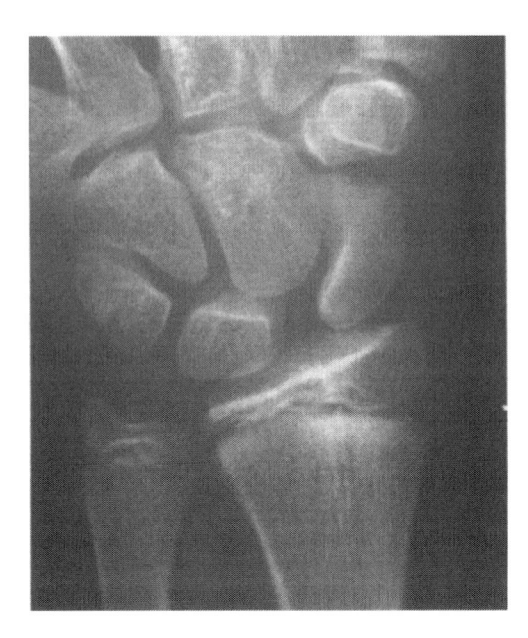

FIGURE 17-21. "Terry Thomas" sign. This patient had a painful wrist 7 weeks after acute injury without treatment. This is a scapholunate dissociation. Such widening, in the absence of pain, may be due to patterns of chondro-osseous maturation.

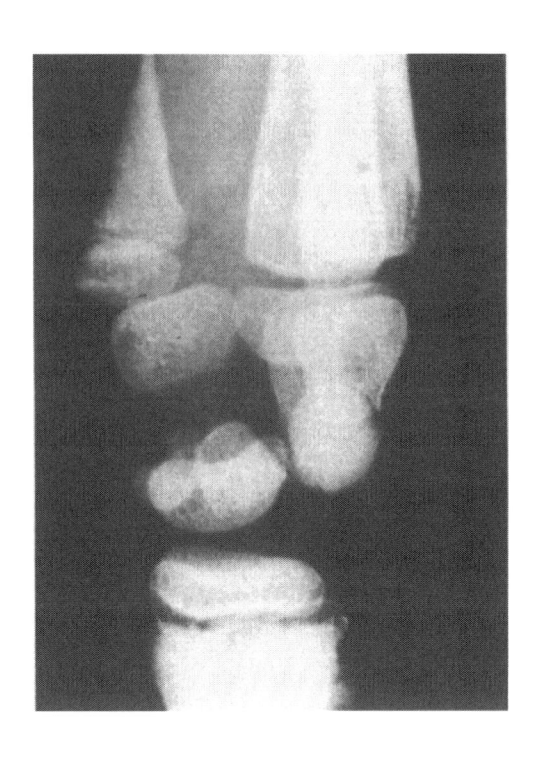

FIGURE 17-22. Transscaphoid perilunate dislocation. The distal radius was also fractured (type 1 physeal injury).

to ligamentous disruption. They were by Zimmerman and Weiland[156] and Gerard.[95]

Closed reduction should be attempted first. Even when scapholunate dissociation is suspected and is treated by immobilization, the outcome is based on the patient's symptoms and skeletal maturity. Any operative treatment is directed toward achieving a stable, painless wrist. In a young child another important treatment goal must be to prevent the development of structural deformities. For long-term treatment a protective orthosis should be used. So long as these bones have a significant amount of cartilage, remodeling may occur.

Carpometacarpal Joint Dislocation

Dislocation or subluxation of the carpometacarpal joints are rare in children. Such an injury is usually associated with crushing and fracture of one or more metacarpals. The thumb carpometacarpal joint is the most likely to be involved.

Kleinman and Grantham described multiple carpometacarpal joint dislocations.[107] This injury was associated with physeal fractures of the middle and ring fingers. This patient is similar to the case shown in Figure 17-23. The

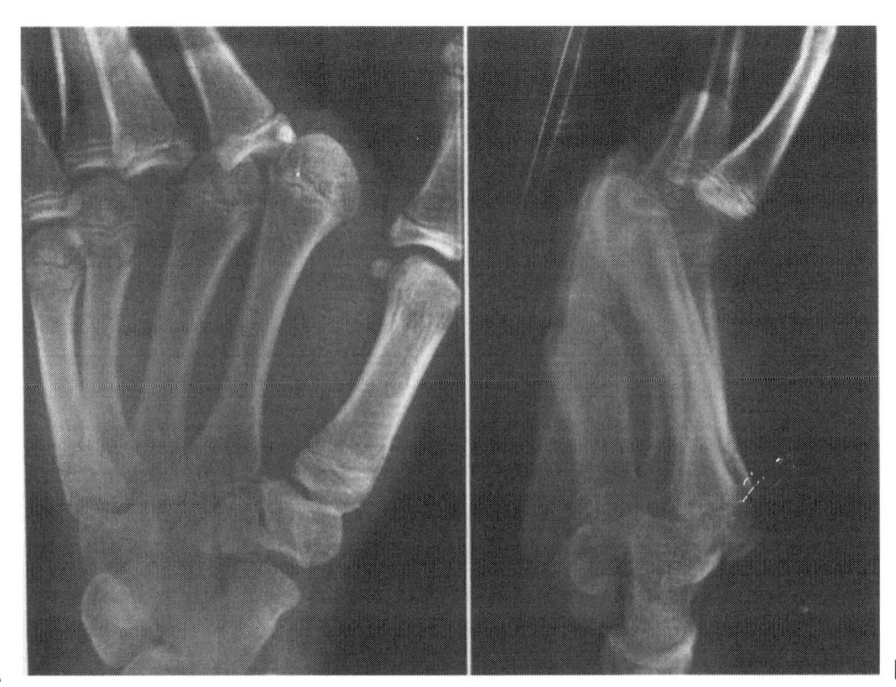

FIGURE 17-23. Carpometacarpal (CMC) fracture-dislocation and concomitant metacarpophalangeal (MCP) dislocations. (A) Anteroposterior view shows CMC disruption and MCP dislocations of the index and long fingers. (B) Lateral view shows dorsal CMC displacement and MCP displacement.

FIGURE 17-24. Dislocation of the thumb MCP joint in a 5-year-old child that was reduced and stabilized. There is a slight shift of the epiphysis of the proximal phalanx, suggesting an occult type 1 growth mechanism injury.

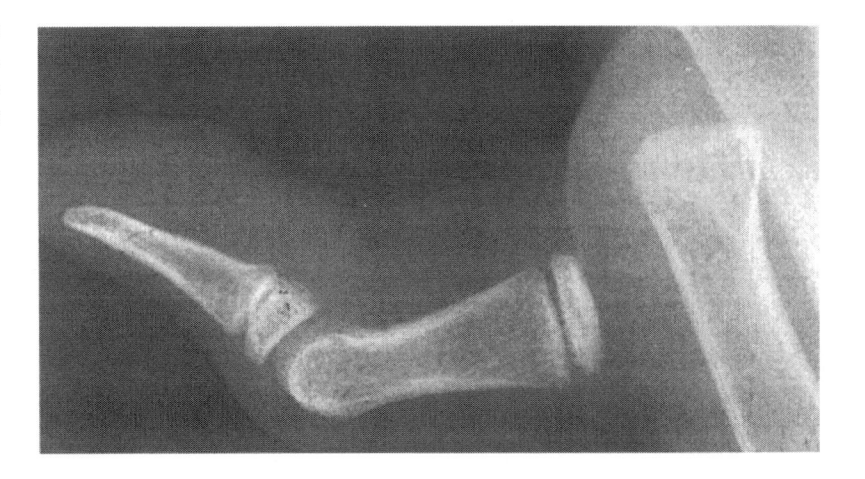

patient was treated with open reductions. A 10-week follow-up described good appearance and function. Unfortunately, further follow-up was not available.

Whitson described a 10-year-old boy who fell and sustained fracture-dislocations of the medial four metacarpal-carpal joints.[153] A 4-week follow-up showed partial recurrence of the luxation and some sclerosis in the proximal end of the third metacarpal. Further follow-up was not described.

Thumb

Dislocation

Dislocation of the thumb usually involves the metacarpophalangeal joint (Fig. 17-24). The metacarpal head is pushed through the thumb musculature, especially the flexor pollicis brevis, and may also buttonhole through the joint capsule (Fig. 17-25). Such structures may partially entrap the metacarpal head. In contrast to digital metacarpophalangeal dislocations, however, complete, constricting encirclement of the metacarpal neck does not occur, thereby increasing the likelihood of closed reduction. The intrinsic muscles retain their insertion with the sesamoids and serve to guide the plate palmarward, keeping it from being irreducibly displaced into the joint. The sesamoids, which may not be roentgenographically evident in younger children, indicate the position of the palmar plate.

The initial treatment is closed reduction, which is usually successful. Reduction may be simplified by first flexing the metacarpal to reduce intrinsic muscle tightness while concomitantly applying longitudinal traction. Flexion with continued traction completes the reduction. If capsular or muscular interposition is present, an open reduction may be necessary (Fig. 17-26). Because the digital nerves of the thumb may be displaced by the traumatic anatomy, care must

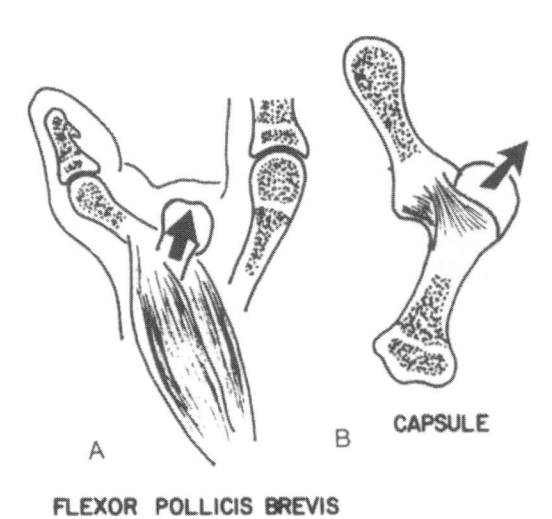

FIGURE 17-25. Displacement of the metacarpal head through the flexor pollicis brevis (A) or capsule (B).

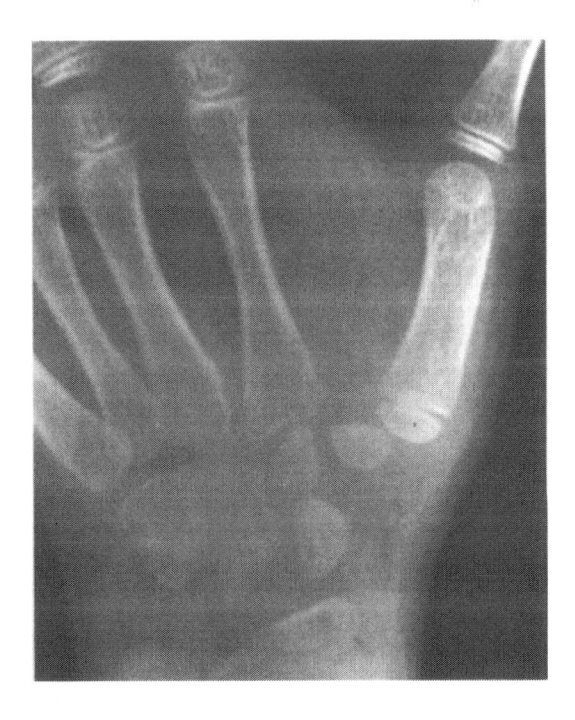

FIGURE 17-26. Dislocation of the thumb MCP joint that required open reduction and stabilization.

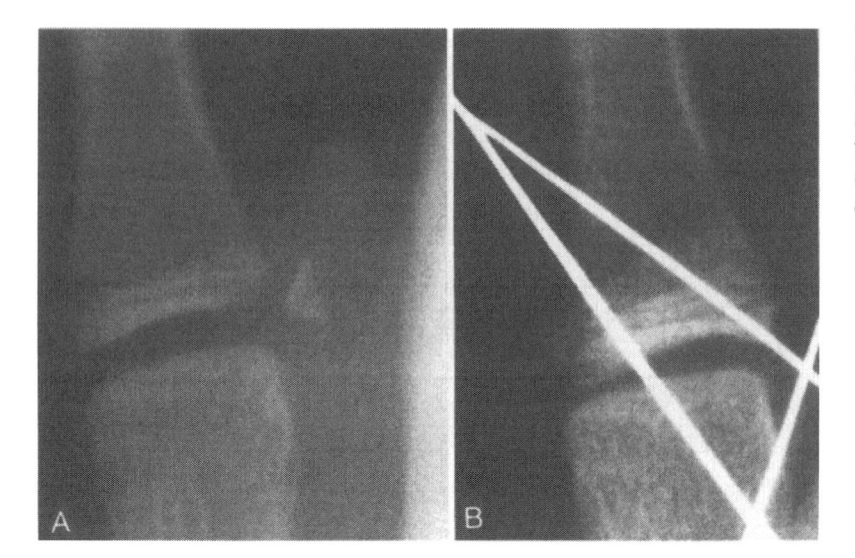

FIGURE 17-27. Gamekeeper's thumb in a 12-year-old child. (A) Type 3 avulsion fracture with 90° of rotation of the epiphyseal fragment. The articular surface faces the epiphyseal fracture line. (B) It was treated by multiple K-wires that fixed the fragment and buttressed and immobilized both the fragment and the phalanx.

be taken to visualize them adequately prior to, as well as following, any open reduction.

Interphalangeal Dislocation

Interphalangeal dislocation of the thumb is less frequent than dislocation of the thumb metacarpophalangeal joint. Closed reduction is usually successful. Small avulsion fractures (type 7 injuries) may accompany the dislocation and may require internal fixation if joint stability is compromised.

Rath and Kotwal described an unusual injury with a closed dislocation of the interphalangeal joint of the thumb accompanied by dislocation of the secondary ossification center of the proximal phalanx in an 8-year-old-boy.[161] It became infected and following débridement was thought to be totally necrotic and ischemic. They maintained the length of the thumb with an external fixator and incorporated a bone graft from the ipsilateral ulna to maintain the length of the thumb without significant loss of function.

Collateral Ligament Injury

Gamekeeper's thumb of the metacarpophalangeal joint results from partial or total disruption of the ulnar collateral ligament in the adult. In a child, ulnar and radial collateral ligament "tears" of the thumb are usually type 3 or 4 chondro-osseous injuries (Figs. 17-27, 17-28), although type 2 injuries may also occur (Fig. 17-29).[157] These corner fractures of the epiphysis are equivalent to collateral ligament injuries in adults.[164] If the articular surface is involved, these fractures should be accurately corrected by open reduction and pinning. Failure to treat them adequately may cause permanent deformity and instability.

Winslet et al. reported three adolescents with open physes who sustained fractures of the ulnar side of the proximal

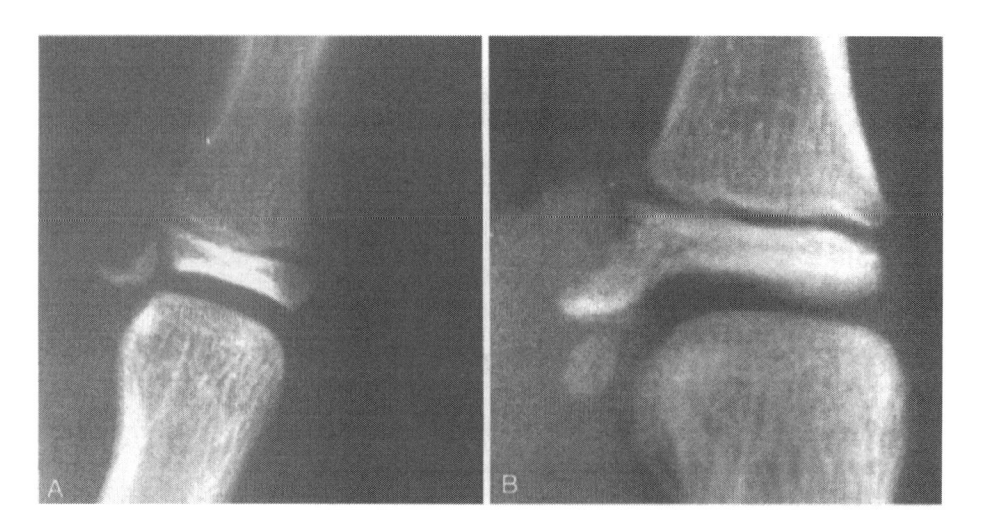

FIGURE 17-28. (A) Displaced type 3 injury. (B) Seven weeks later there is malunion and joint deformity.

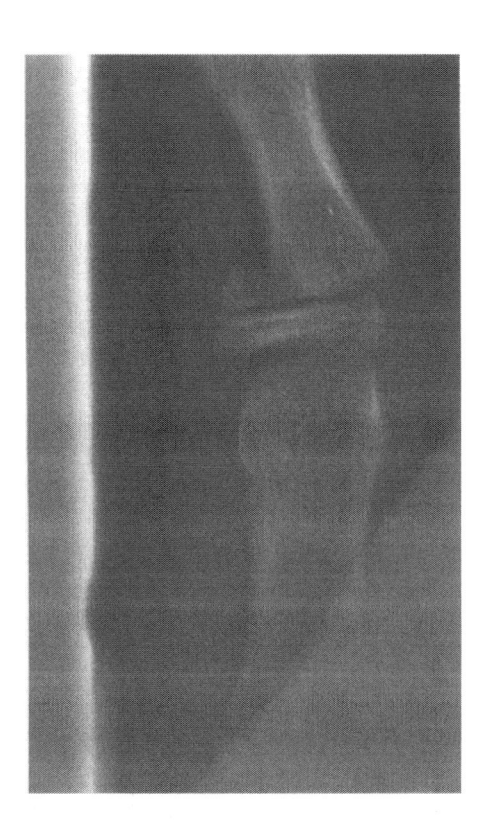

FIGURE 17-29. Displaced, angulated type 2 injury.

phalanx while break-dancing.[167] All had ligamentous laxity and at least 90° rotation of the fragment, requiring open reduction.

A pure ligamentous avulsion of the ulnar collateral ligament of the thumb of a 12-year-old child with open epiphyses has been described.[159,165,166] There was no reported evidence of cartilaginous injury in any of these patients.

Bennett's Fracture Analogue

Impacted fractures of the base of the thumb metatarsal (Bennett's fracture) usually occur in children as a physeal injury, with the most frequent pattern being type 2 (Fig. 17-30).[158,162] An analogous fracture may involve the metaphyseal–diaphyseal junction. The anterior oblique ligament that anchors the first metacarpal to the trapezium is strong.

The two primary variables of childhood Bennett's fracture are the size of the metaphyseal fragment and the amount of displacement of the shaft from the epiphysis. The base of the metacarpal is pulled proximally and radially by the abductor pollicis longus, which inserts at the base; and the insertion of the adductor further distally levers the base radially (abduction). The periosteal sleeve is usually partially intact and may be used effectively for stabilization during closed reduction.

Minimally displaced fractures require protection with a cast. In a young child, up to 30° of angulation may be acceptable at the base of the thumb, although reduction to a lesser degree of malalignment should be attempted. Angulation of more than 30° should be corrected by manipulation. Pressure is applied to the base of the thumb, and counterpressure is placed over the head of the metacarpal. A common error is to hyperextend the metacarpal joint by applying pressure too far distally, which does nothing to correct the deformity.

Occasionally, complete displacement may buttonhole through the periosteal sleeve. Although a closed reduction may look easy and is worth attempting, many of these injuries require open reduction to maneuver the metaphysis back into position through the periosteal tear.

Radial displacement of the thumb may be corrected by manipulation and cast immobilization. Ulnar displacement, however, usually defies attempts at closed reduction and frequently requires open reduction with internal (wire) fixation. Even if an ulnar displacement is treated by closed reduction, this type must be followed closely because redisplacement may occur in the cast.

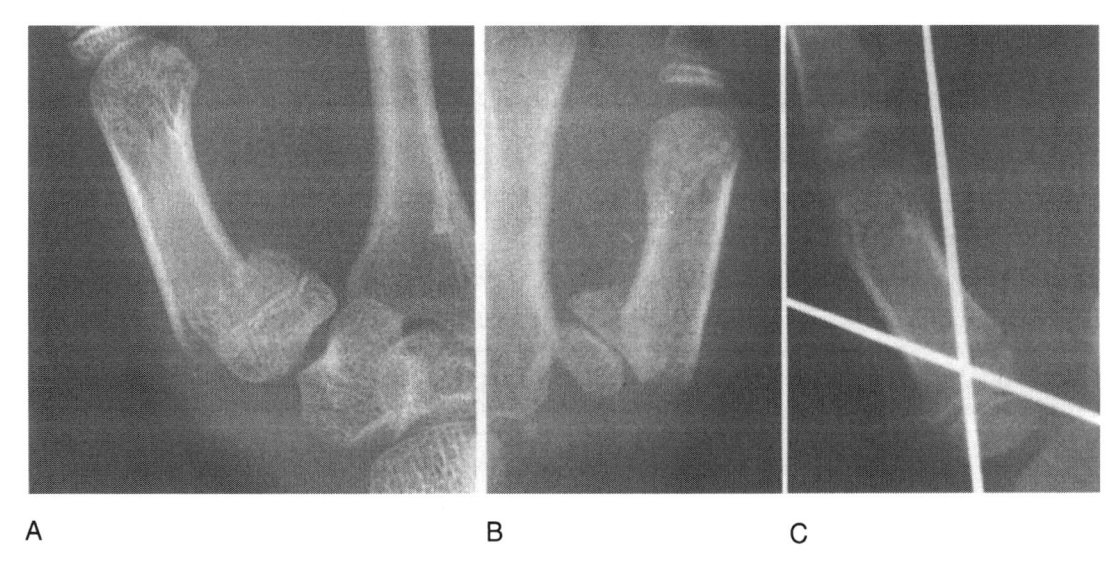

A   B   C

FIGURE 17-30. (A) Mildly displaced Bennett's fracture leaving an ulnar metaphyseal fragment and adduction angulation of the rest of the thumb. (B) Displaced Bennett's fracture analogue. (C) It should be reduced and internally stabilized.

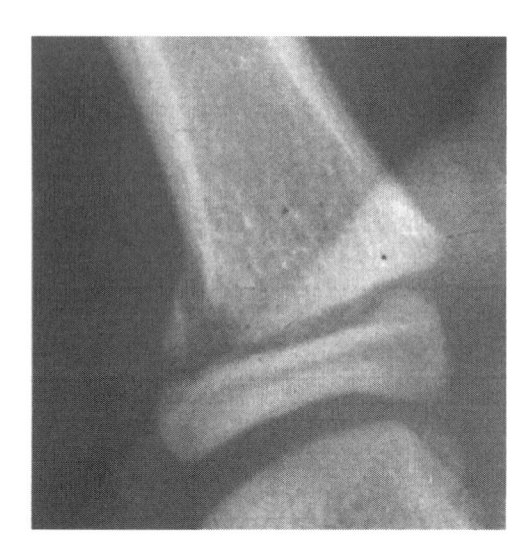

FIGURE 17-31. Type 2 fracture of the proximal phalanx. The Thurstan Holland fragment is usually on the radial side. Radial angulation of the rest of the thumb is common.

Fracture of the Phalanges

The proximal bases of the proximal phalanx and the thumb metacarpal of the thumb are common sites of epiphyseal injury. A closed injury at the thumb metacarpophalangeal joint that results in ulnar or radial instability is probably an epiphyseal fracture of the proximal phalanx, rather than the ligamentous injury commonly seen in the adult. Stress views may be necessary to delineate the undisplaced fracture or the small fragment.

The proximal phalanx most often sustains a physeal fracture compared to a diaphyseal or phalangeal neck (distal) fracture (Fig. 17-31). This fracture may be a type 1, 2, 3, or 4 injury, depending on the mechanism and the degree of skeletal maturity. There is usually an associated radial angulation. Treatment for type 1 and 2 injuries is closed reduction with adduction to correct the radial angulation. Types 3 and 4 usually require open reduction and accurate restoration of joint surface anatomy.

Posttraumatic angular deformity of the base of the proximal phalanx of the thumb may be corrected by epiphyseal distraction using a minidistractor.[160]

The proximal phalanx may sustain a distal (condylar) fracture (Fig. 17-32). This fracture may be acutely or progressively unstable, despite an initial innocuous appearance. There may be complete rotation of 180°, directing the articular surface at the fracture. Delayed union may occur, especially if the original injury is not splinted, necessitating closed or open reduction and pin fixation. Remodeling is not extensive in this end of the bone, and malunion may result in permanent deformity.

Fracture of the distal phalangeal epiphysis of the thumb is relatively common (Figs. 17-33, 17-34). It is often a crushing injury associated with an open fracture and must be handled carefully so as not to lose soft tissue or cause complicating osteomyelitis, which could result in premature epiphysiodesis in a young child. The flexor tendon attaches to the palmar shaft surface, and the extensor slip primarily attaches into the epiphysis. Accordingly, the epiphysis may retain a normal relation to the proximal phalanx, whereas the remainder of the distal phalanx is flexed. This angular deformity must be corrected during closed reduction. Open reduction may be necessary for a type 3 injury.

Shibu and Gault reported a 12-year-old girl with sequential crush injury to the tip of the thumb at 18 and 36 months.[163] She had overgrowth of the tip of the phalanx.

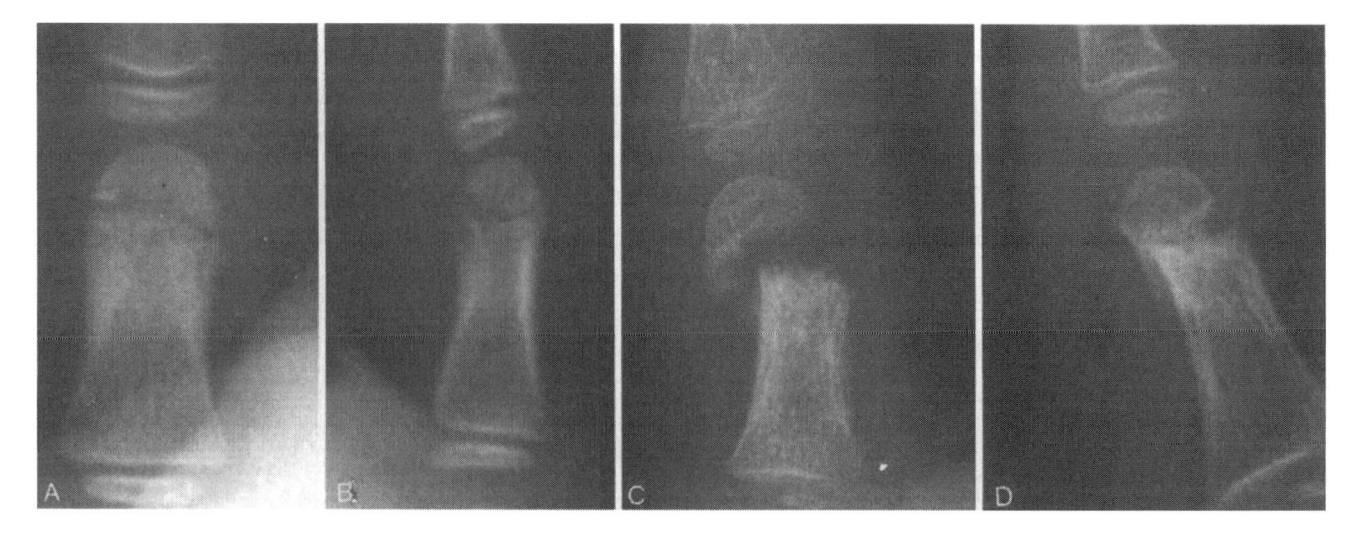

FIGURE 17-32. (A, B) Anteroposterior and lateral views of a fracture of the distal end of the proximal phalanx of the thumb in a 7-year-old child. This fracture was undisplaced, and healing was uneventful. (C) A similar injury in a 4-year-old child had this appearance 7 weeks after injury (splinted for 2 weeks, with no roentgenogram at the time of splint removal). The child was subsequently treated by open reduction. (D) Three weeks after open reduction, the fracture shows osseous healing.

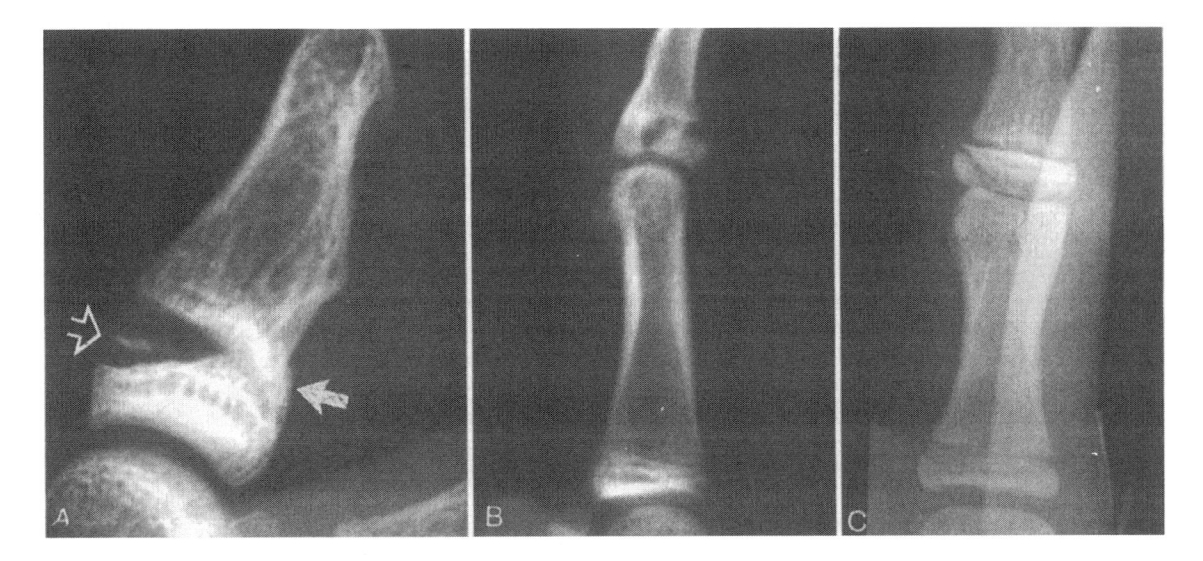

FIGURE 17-33. (A) Type 2 fracture of the distal phalanx of the thumb. Note the transverse remnant of the subchondral metaphyseal plate (Werenskiöld fragment) on the tension failure side (open arrow) and the Thurstan Holland fragment on the compression failure side (closed arrow). (B) Type 3 injury pattern. (C) Type 7 (intraepiphyseal) injury pattern.

Metacarpals

Proximal Injury

The proximal area is likely to be injured when the hand is crushed (Fig. 17-35). Closed reduction and attention to soft tissue swelling and damage are essential.

Isolated fractures of the base of the metacarpals are infrequent.[171] The fourth and fifth metacarpals are most often involved (Fig. 17-36). Fractures involving the second metacarpal usually involve the radial side. That in the boy shown in Figure 17-37 involved the ulnar side and displaced the fragment into the palmar space in contrast to the usual dorsal displacement. Open reduction may be necessary.

Diaphyseal Fracture

Fractures of the metacarpal shaft (diaphysis) are less common in children than in adults (Fig. 17-38).[177] Transverse fractures of the metacarpals are usually the result of direct blows. They angulate dorsally because of the original deformation and the palmar force subsequently exerted by the interosseous muscles. Oblique fractures of the metacarpal shafts result from a torque force, with the finger acting as the long lever; and they tend to shorten and rotate (Fig. 17-39), rather than angulate. Fractures of the third and fourth metacarpals tend to shorten less because of the tethering effect of the deep transverse metacarpal ligament, whereas fractures of the second and fifth metacarpals tend to have more pronounced shortening and rotation.

A stress fracture of the index metacarpal has been described in a highly competitive tennis player.[179] Other metacarpals may also sustain comparable stress fractures.

Royle reviewed 98 metacarpal fractures for rotational deformity.[175] Approximately 25% had minor malrotation of less than 10°. Only five had more than 10° of malrotation. In only 2 of 98 patients did such rotary malunion require operative intervention.[174]

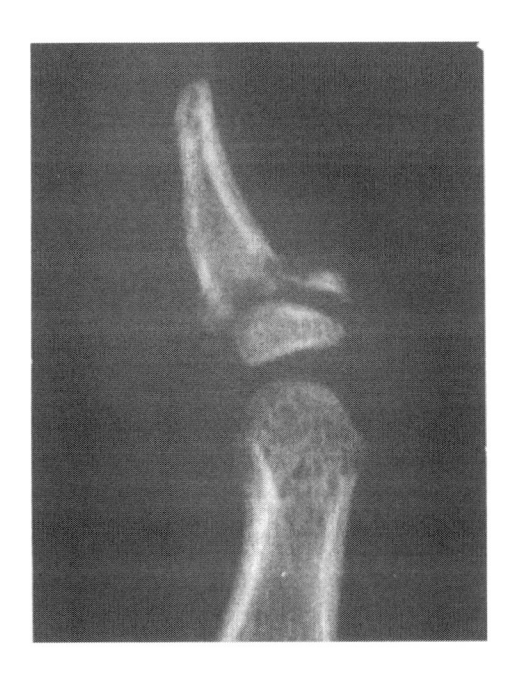

The same principles apply to these fractures in both children and adults. Most fractures are correctly treated by simple immobilization. Dorsal "bowing" may be corrected by relaxing the wrist extensors, the long finger flexors, and the interosseous muscles. If the hand is properly posi-

FIGURE 17-34. Displaced type 2 injury of the thumb.

tioned with a splint, these fractures usually heal with little difficulty.

Nonunion may occur.[169] It usually heals satisfactorily after adequate fixation and does not require extensive grafting (Figs. 17-40, 17-41). A synostosis may complicate a crushing or blast injury (Fig. 17-42).

Distal Fractures (Epiphyseal)

With the exception of the fifth metacarpal, fractures involving the distal metacarpal heads (Figs. 17-43, 17-44) appear to be relatively infrequent in children and adolescents.[170,172,177] They must be analyzed carefully to determine the actual or potential extent of damage to the interrelated mechanisms of longitudinal or latitudinal growth as well as disruption of the articular surface. Shortening of the metacarpal is the most significant complication and may occur after a seemingly innocuous injury. Brown described a boy who sustained a fracture through the neck and epiphysis of the third metacarpal (a type 2 injury).[168] Three years later roentgenograms showed a slowdown in growth of the third metacarpal. Figure 17-45 shows a similar fracture of the distal metacarpal of the index finger, with accompanying diaphyseal injury. Three years later roentgenograms showed a slowdown in growth of the third metacarpal.

Type 3 growth mechanism injuries may occur (Fig. 17-46).[173] Growth arrest is a potential complication of

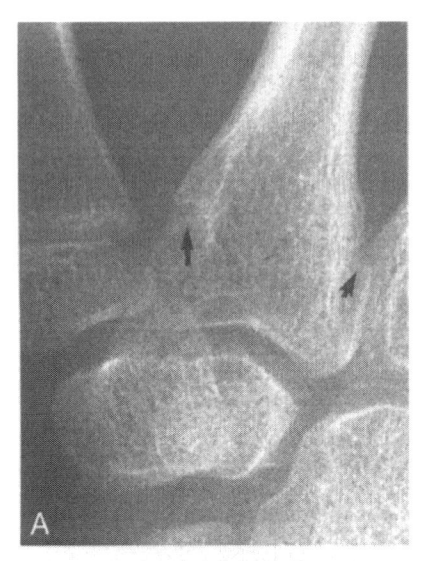

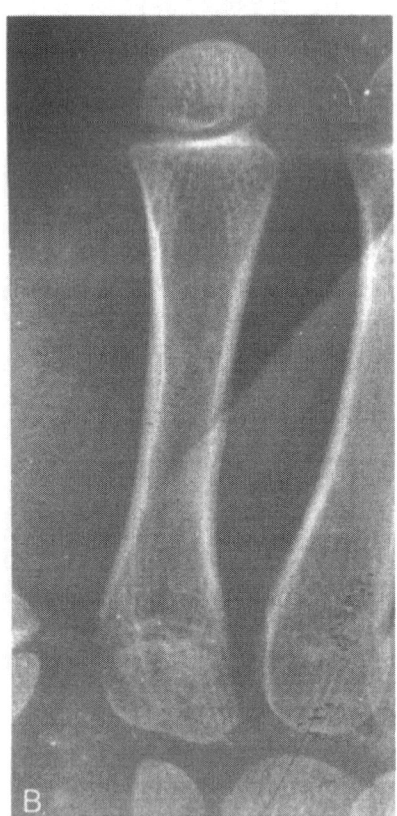

FIGURE 17-35. (A) Minimally evident proximal metacarpal fracture (arrow). This injury may be confused with a pseudoepiphysis (which is painless). (B) It was not treated, and the patient subsequently presented for evaluation of carpal pain, undoubtedly due to the pseudarthrosis that has developed.

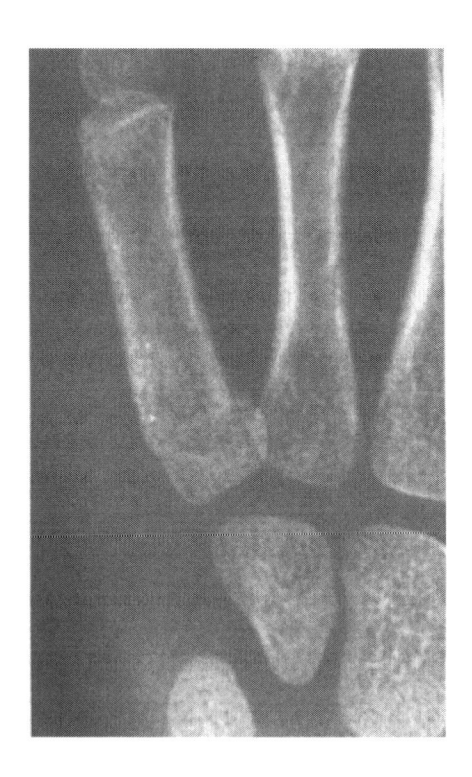

FIGURE 17-36. Fracture of the proximal end of the fifth metacarpal.

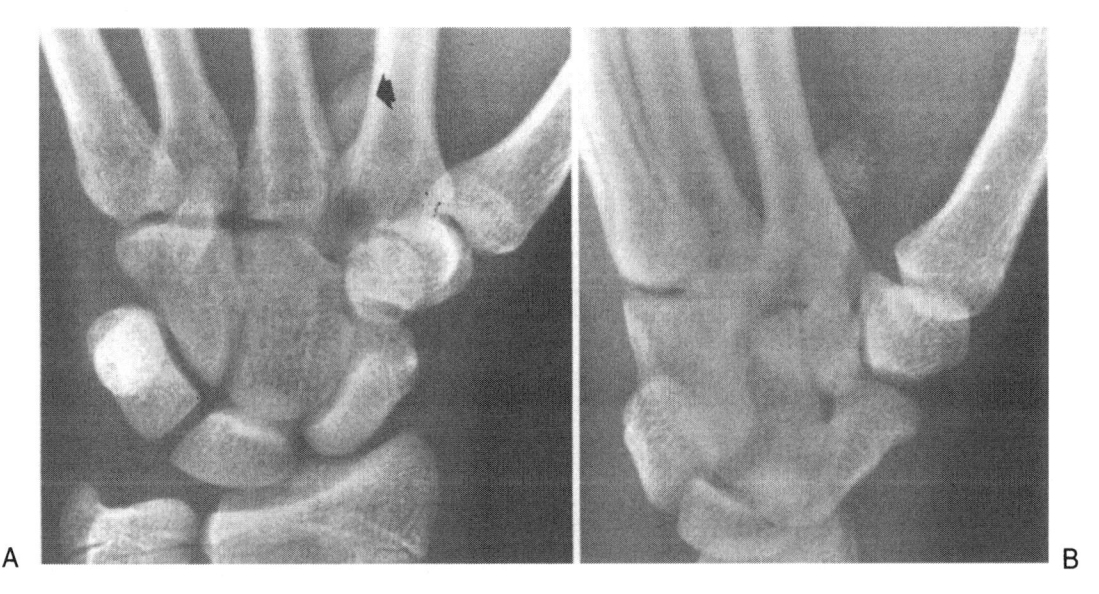

FIGURE 17-37. (A) Fracture of the ulnar side of the second metacarpal (arrow). (B) Oblique view showing palmar displacement of the fragment.

type 3 and 4 growth mechanism injuries. Schiund reported a case of locked metacarpophalangeal joint due to an intraarticular fracture of the metacarpal head that was not readily evident on standard radiographs.[176] It proved to be an osteochondral fracture, splitting the head as a type 3 injury.

Open reduction and internal fixation of the fracture may be necessary. As Hastings and Simmons have indicated, however, open reduction does *not* guarantee a good result in displaced, intraarticular hand fractures in children.[41]

The probability that vascular injury plays a role in growth deformity must be considered. Because of the extensive

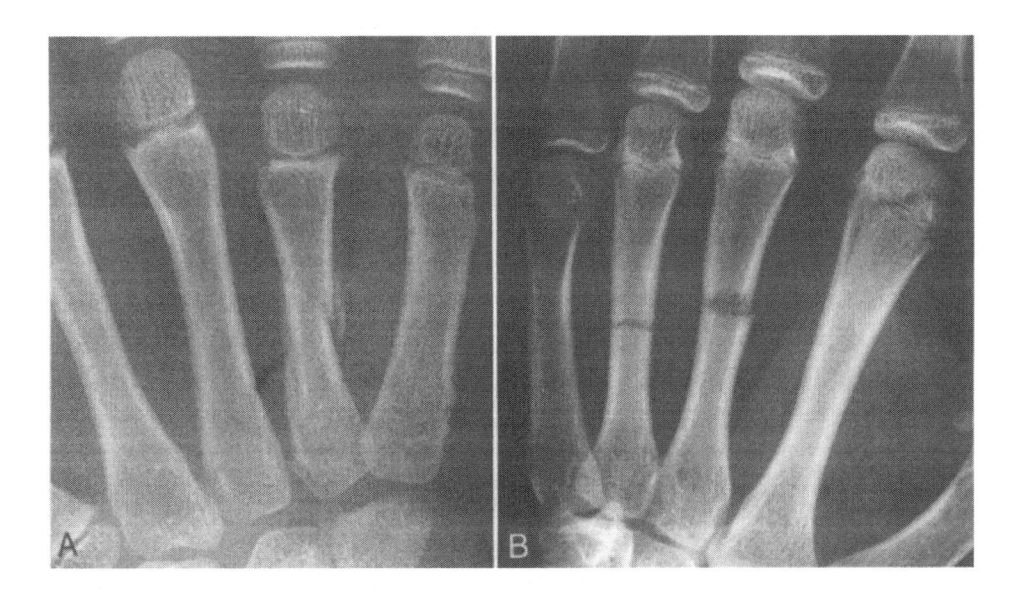

FIGURE 17-38. (A) Diaphyseal fracture of the fourth metacarpal. (B) Undisplaced transverse diaphyseal fractures of the third and fourth metacarpals.

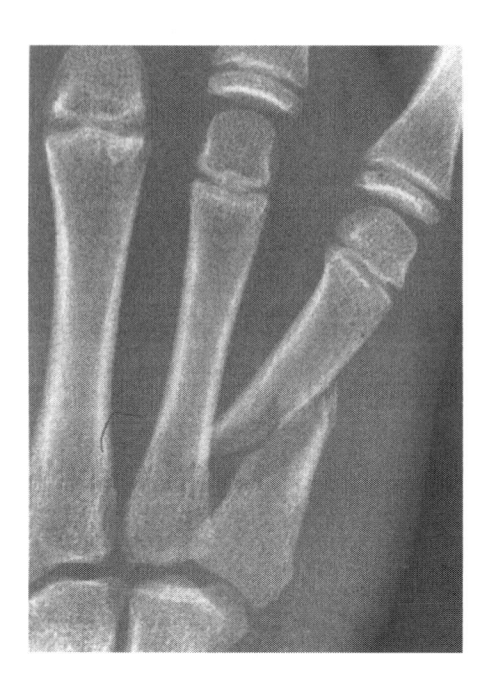

FIGURE 17-39. Fracture of the diaphysis of the fifth metacarpal.

articular surface and joint capsular attachments, there is a limited intracapsular course of the epiphyseal and physeal vessels, making these regions potentially as susceptible to temporary ischemia as the radial and femoral heads. The temporary vascular interruption could lead to decreased longitudinal growth and premature closure. However, the posttraumatic revascularization would allow enlargement of the metacarpal head and peripheral growth through the zone of Ranvier, a well-recognized phenomenon in Legg-Calvé-Perthes disease. Wright and Dell described ischemic necrosis and the vascular anatomy of the metacarpals.[180] They noted that in 35% of specimens a main artery to the distal epiphysis was absent, making these metacarpal heads dependent on small circumferential pericapsular arterioles.

Distal Fifth Fractures (Boxer's Fracture)

Fractures of the distal fifth metacarpal are relatively common, particularly during adolescence. These injuries may be metaphyseal or physeal injuries (Fig. 17-47). Correction of the angular deformity may be necessary, as remodeling may not correct malunion, particularly in the patient close to skeletal maturity. Infrequently, open reduction, pin stabilization, or both are indicated. Premature epiphysiodesis may occur (Fig. 17-48).

Thurston described closed osteotomy for correction of nonunion of metacarpal neck fractures in which there was excessive flexion.[178] It involved removing a small dorsal wedge followed by tension band wire fixation.

Metacarpophalangeal Dislocation

Reports of complex dislocations of the metacarpophalangeal joints (Fig. 17-49) have combined patients of all ages, but a significant number of these patients are skeletally immature.[181-198] Baldwin reported four patients, three of whom were children.[182] Five of the nine patients reported by Green and Terry were 16 years old or younger.[190] Similarly, 8 of 13 patients reported by Becton, 1 by Bohart, 1 by Milch, 8 of 10 by Murphy and Stark, and 11 by Gilbert were all skeletally immature.[185,186,189,196,197] The incidence of this injury in children and adolescents has been underemphasized.

Forced hyperextension of the proximal phalanx of the index finger, usually from a fall on the hand, results in the metacarpal heads being pushed through the palmar capsule. The fibrocartilaginous palmar plate is torn loose at its weakest point of attachment, the membranous attachment to the metacarpal. The metacarpal head is displaced toward the palm, and the palmar plate remains attached to the phalanx and is folded into the joint, where it becomes

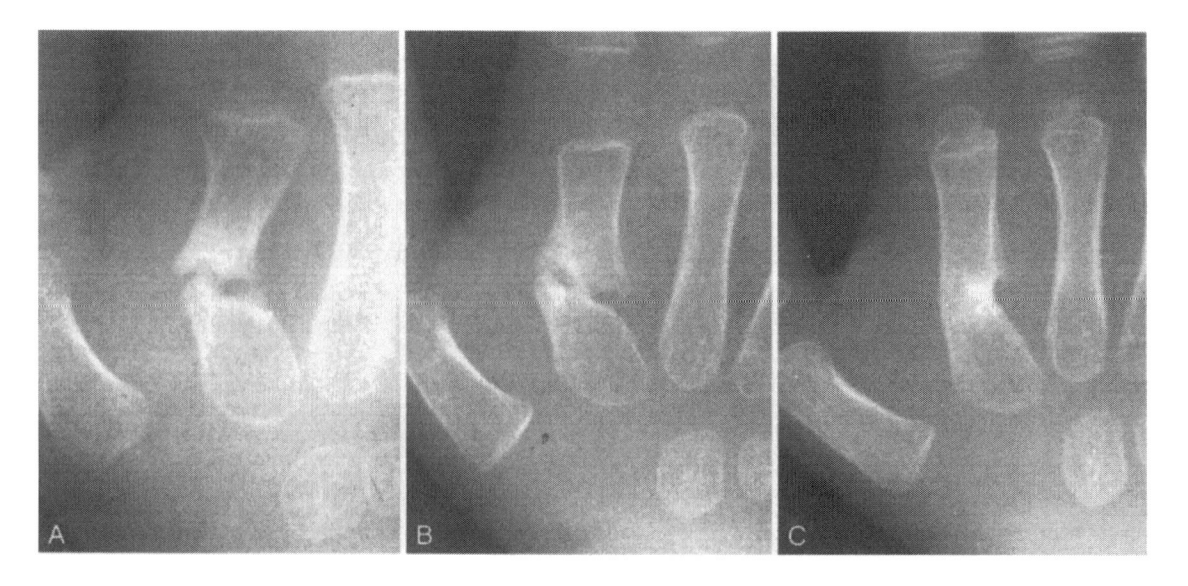

FIGURE 17-40. (A) Delayed union. (B) Progressive healing with continued immobilization. (C) Healed fracture.

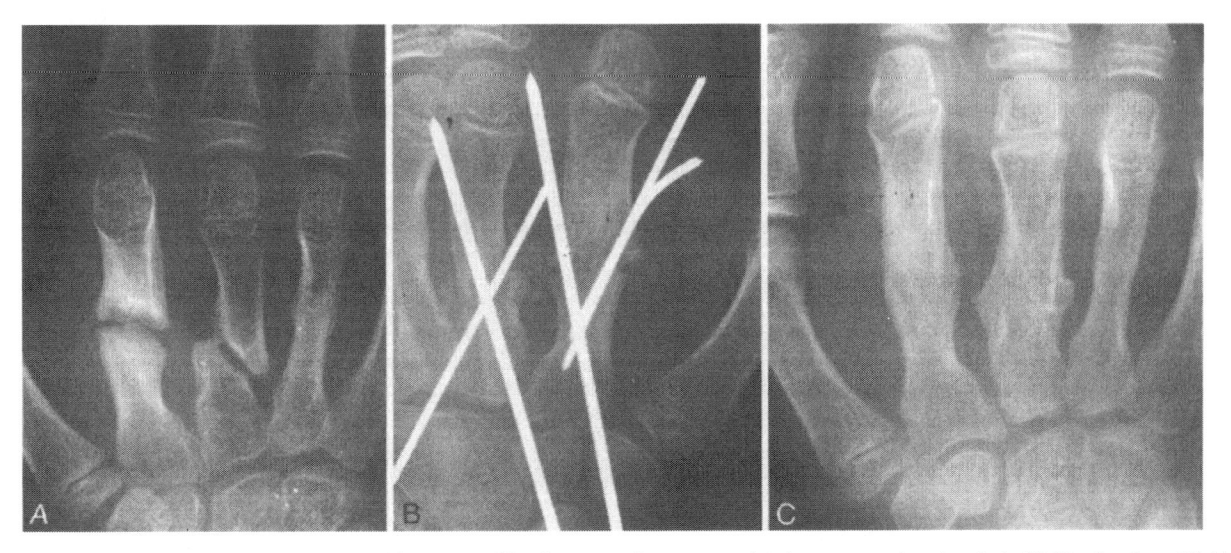

FIGURE 17-41. (A) Nonunion of metacarpal fractures. The fracture of metacarpal 4, in contrast, has healed. (B) Pin fixation. (C) Healing.

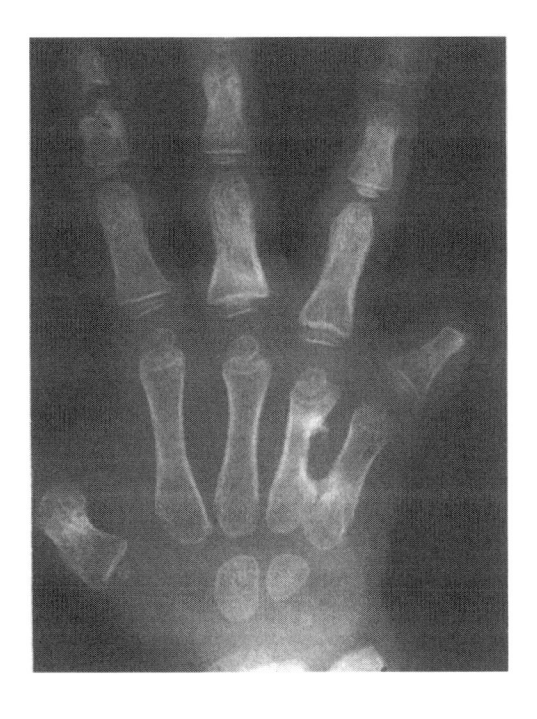

FIGURE 17-42. Synostosis of the fourth and fifth metacarpals after a blast injury to the hand.

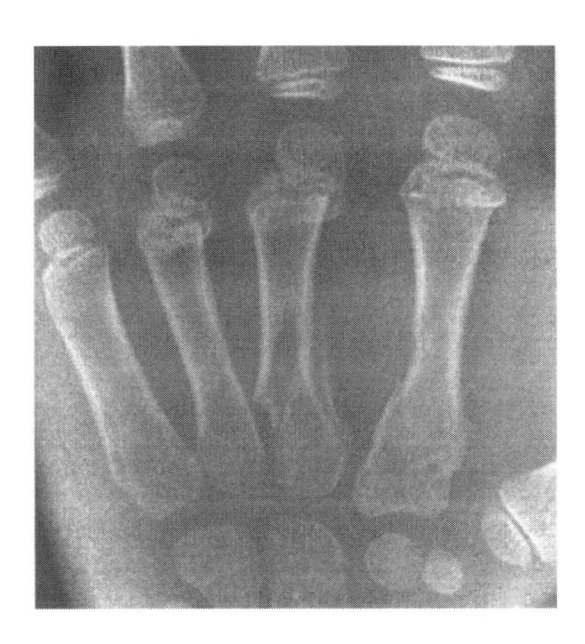

FIGURE 17-43. Distal second, third, and fourth physeal metacarpal fractures associated with fractures of the second and third metacarpal at the diaphyseal/proximal metaphyseal transition.

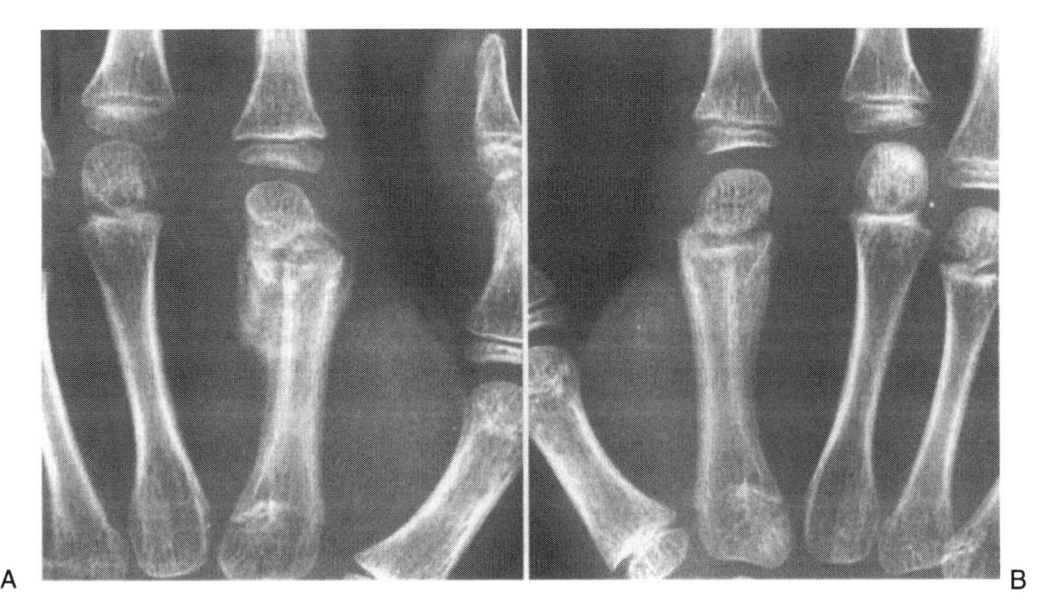

FIGURE 17-44. (A) Fracture of the second metacarpal 4 weeks after injury. (B) Remodeling 10 weeks after injury.

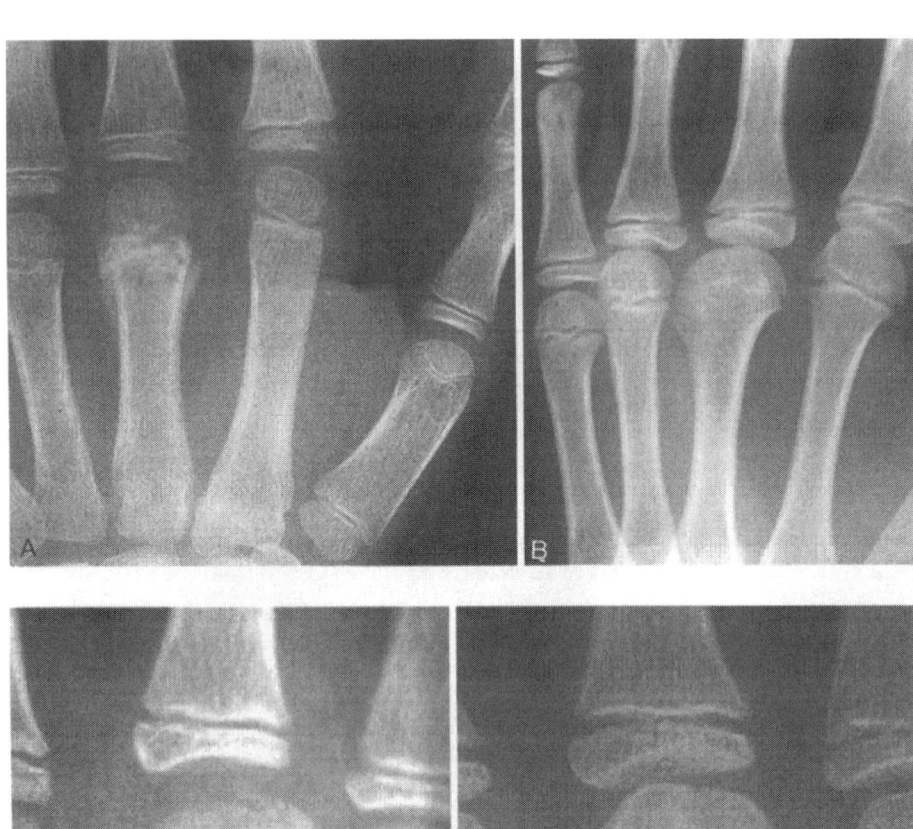

FIGURE 17-45. (A) Type 2 fracture of the third metacarpal head. (B) Three years later the head is large (probably because of hypervascularity following the injury), but the physis has closed; it is leading to shortening.

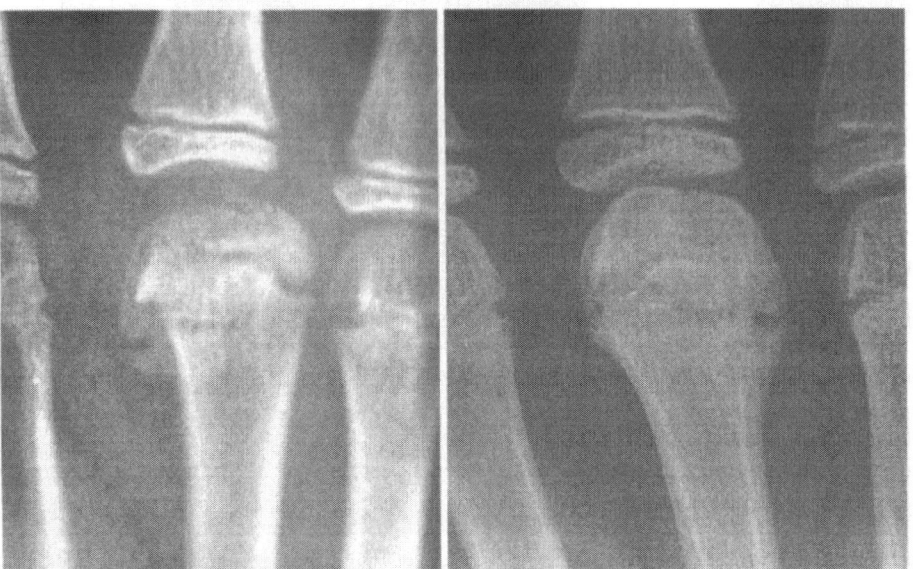

FIGURE 17-46. (A) Type 3 fracture after being hit by a baseball bat. (B) Three months later.

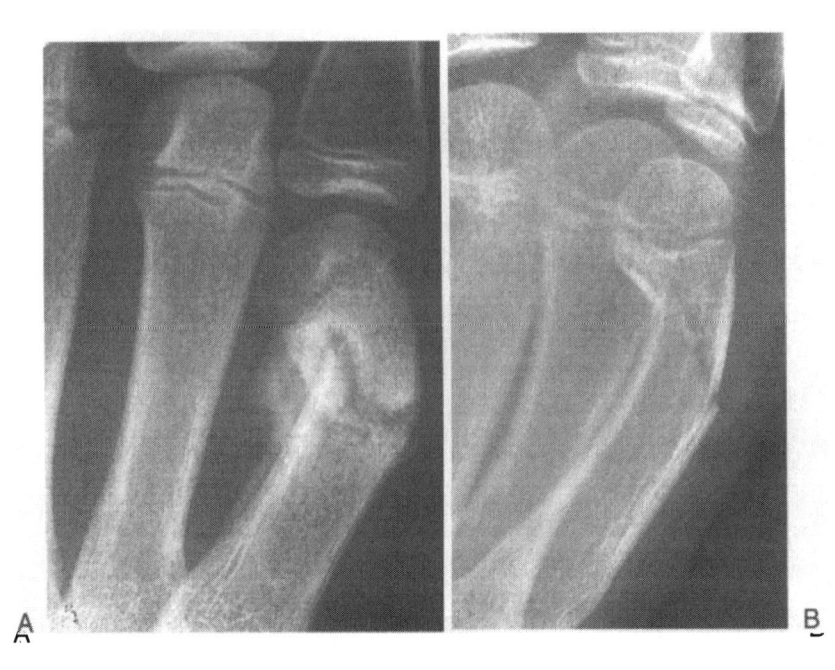

FIGURE 17-47. (A) Metaphyseal fracture of the fifth metacarpal. Angulation was not corrected and has led to malunion. (B) Moderate angulation.

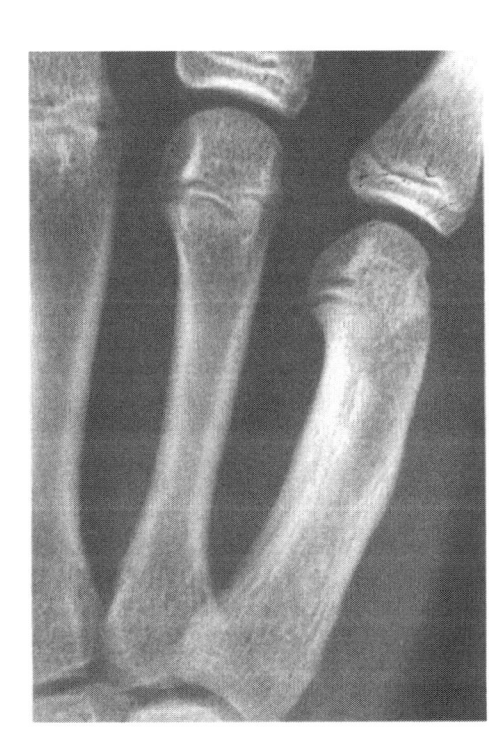

FIGURE 17-48. Premature epiphysiodesis 4 months after a teenage boxer's fracture.

wedged between the metacarpal head and the base of the proximal phalanx. The phalanx is dislocated dorsally on the metacarpal head, which is forced through the transverse metacarpal ligament to become fixed between the ligament and the longitudinal portion of the superficial palmar fascia. The flexor tendons are displaced ulnarward and the lumbrical tendons radialward, with both lying dorsal to the displaced metacarpal head (Fig. 17-50). Gilbert found that the lumbrical and flexor tendons were displaced ulnarward together in eight cases, whereas in two cases the lumbrical was displaced separately to the radial side.[189]

When the fifth finger is involved, because of the more distal course of the long flexor tendons to the little finger, these tendons are displaced radially and trap the metacarpal head on that side; the tendon of the abductor digiti quinti is the lateral trapping element. The fibrocartilaginous plate and superficial transverse ligament, as in the index finger, respectively form the floor and roof of the trap.

Widening or lateralization of the joint space on the anteroposterior radiograph suggests complex dislocation with interposition of the palmar plate within the joint. However, *the anteroposterior radiograph may be deceptive*, not readily showing complete joint disruption (Fig. 17-51). Usually the metacarpal head is directed radially (relative to the proximal phalanx). Lateral films of the hand clearly demonstrate the dorsal dislocation of the proximal phalanx, if care is taken to visualize each of the overlapping proximal phalanges. Lateral tomography through the involved finger removes superimposition of the other metacarpophalangeal joints.

The term "complex metacarpophalangeal dislocation" primarily acknowledges the difficulties of management. The principal impediment to reduction is entrapment of the palmar plate. The treating physician should not undertake multiple attempts at closed reduction before concluding that the dislocation is irreducible because definite clinical and radiographic clues exist. First, displacement of the phalanx on the metacarpal is not at 90° (as it generally is with a simple interphalangeal dislocation) but is more nearly parallel,

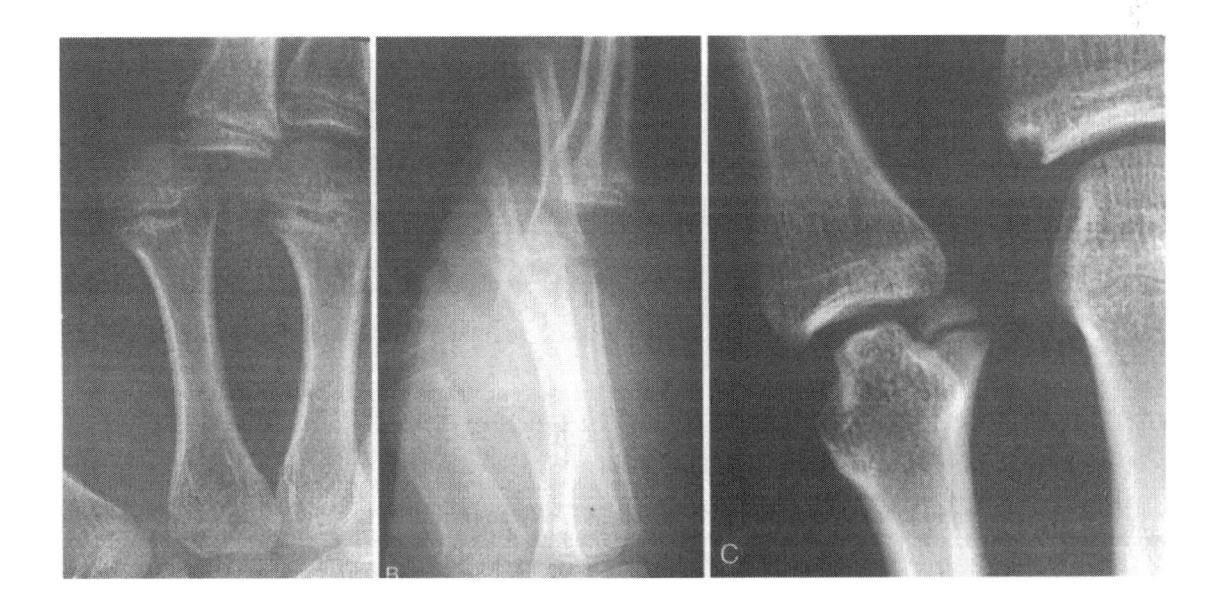

FIGURE 17-49. (A, B) Complex MCP dislocation in a 10-year-old boy following a fall from a tree. It was an open injury but unfortunately was "cleaned, closed, and reduced" (no postreduction roentgenogram) in an emergency ward. When the boy returned to the hospital 1 day later with acute sepsis from clostridial infection, roentgenograms showed that the dislocation was still present. Open reduction was successful, and the infection was controlled with débridement, with the wound kept open, and administration of parenteral antibiotics. (C) Three years later there has been some "regeneration" of the ulnar side of the epiphysis.

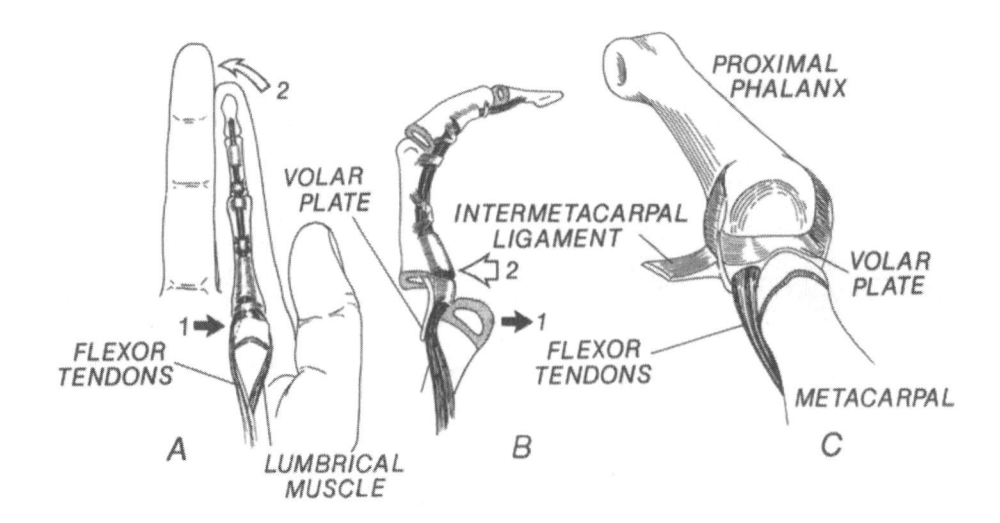

FIGURE 17-50. Structures involved in complex MCP dislocations of the index and little fingers.

often with only slight displacement and minimal angulation. Second, there often is dimpling of the palmar skin (see the engraving at the beginning of this chapter). In the index finger (the most common site of complex dislocation) the dimple may be difficult to visualize because it lies within the proximal palmar crease. Finally, widening or lateralization of the joint space on radiography suggests a complex dislocation because of interposition of the palmar plate within the joint.

Reduction usually can be attained through a palmar approach once the fibrocartilaginous plate has been partially incised, although an attempt should be made to reduce it prior to plate incision. Excessive transection of the palmar plate is not usually necessary in the child because of normally increased laxity of ligamentous structures.[192,194] Only enough fibrocartilaginous plate or ligament to effect a reduction should be incised. If the diagnosis has been delayed longer than 3–4 weeks, the ulnar collateral ligament of the metacarpophalangeal joint must sometimes be incised through a separate dorsal incision before reduction can be accomplished.[183,188]

Early, protected mobilization of the joint with a dorsal splint preventing full extension is the postoperative preference. The reduction is stable so long as hyperextension is avoided the first few weeks after surgery. Internal fixation is usually unnecessary. In fact, K-wires crossing the physis may be harmful in skeletally immature patients; a 10-year-old boy had a deformed metacarpal head and articular surface and a distorted physis.[182]

Concomitant osteochondral fracture (Fig. 17-52) from the ulnar side of the metacarpal epiphysis may occur.[185,189] These chondro-osseous injuries represent the analogue of ligamentous injury in the skeletally immature patient and may involve peripheral physeal injury. It is also important that this fragment not be confused with a sesamoid displaced into the joint.[199] The sesamoid usually remains unossified until mid- to late adolescence.

Gilbert reported concomitant proximal phalangeal physeal injury.[189] This injury mechanism would be similar to the physeal disruption of the radial head that occurs while an elbow dislocation is being reduced (see Chapter 15).

The possibility of vascular damage must be considered in the skeletally immature patient, as the epiphyseal and physeal circulation may be compromised by the dislocation or exposure for the reduction. Irregularity of the metacarpal head has been described after injury and open reduction.[186,198] However, these reports did not discuss vascular compromise as a possible cause, nor did they address any "significant" growth deformities following reduction. Ischemic necrosis and growth damage involving the metacarpal physis and epiphysis have certainly not been recognized in the literature as specific complications of index finger metacarpophalangeal dislocations.

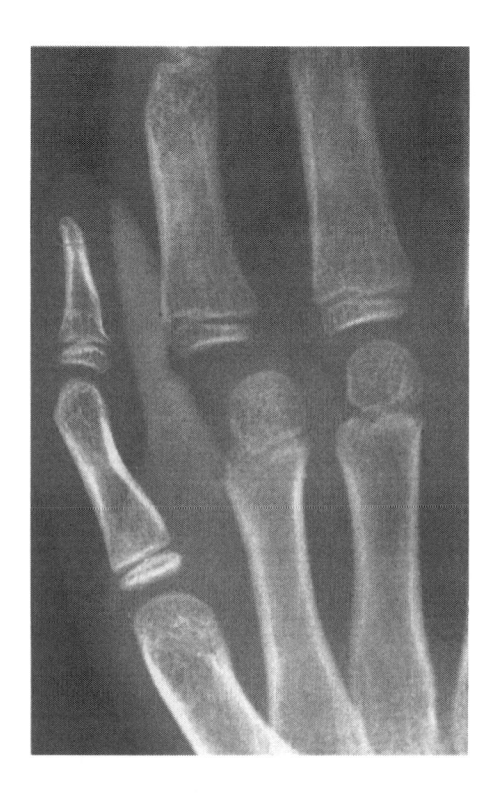

FIGURE 17-51. Subtle second MCP dislocation.

FIGURE 17-52. (A) Osteochondral fragment (arrow) often found in a complex MCP dislocation. (B) Type 3 epiphyseal fracture is evident following reduction of an MCP dislocation.

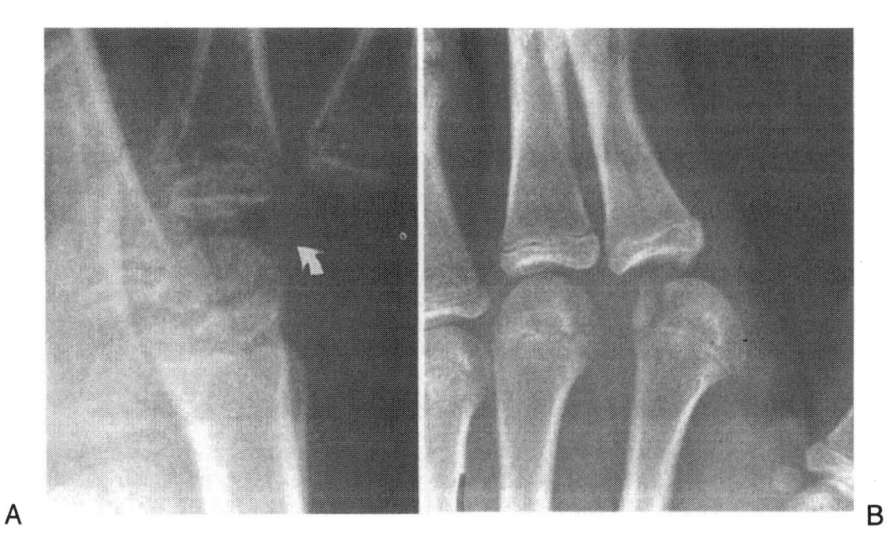

Phalanges

Interphalangeal Dislocation

Dislocations involve the proximal interphalangeal joint (PIP) more than the distal interphalangeal joint (DIP) (Figs. 17-53 to 17-55). These hinge joints allow only flexion and extension. The accessory fibers of the palmar plate and the paired quadrilateral collateral ligaments form three sides of each joint. The thickest portion of the collateral ligament reinforces the insertion of the palmar plate into the base of the middle phalanx. With a dislocation, generally two of the three sides are disrupted. Following relocation, a collateral ligament in a child usually heals with little difficulty.[227] Even in children, however, a collateral ligament may be avulsed and does not become reaffixed to the chondro-osseous structures. Callus may create a mass on the side of the finger. If it occurs, it may be necessary to remove it surgically.

Ligaments and capsular structures around the joints in the child are strong in comparison to the physis, and injuries that would frequently cause a dislocation in an adult more often result in an epiphyseal fracture in the finger of a child or adolescent (Fig. 17-5).[218,235,242] For this reason it is important to obtain roentgenograms of any joint injury prior to and after reduction (Figs. 17-53, 17-55). Concomitant fractures may be more evident after reduction.

As with a slipped capital femoral epiphysis complicating reduction of an acute hip dislocation, a phalangeal epiphyseal-physeal unit may be acutely fractured and left displaced when the rest of the phalanx is "reduced" (Fig. 17-55).[218,235,242]

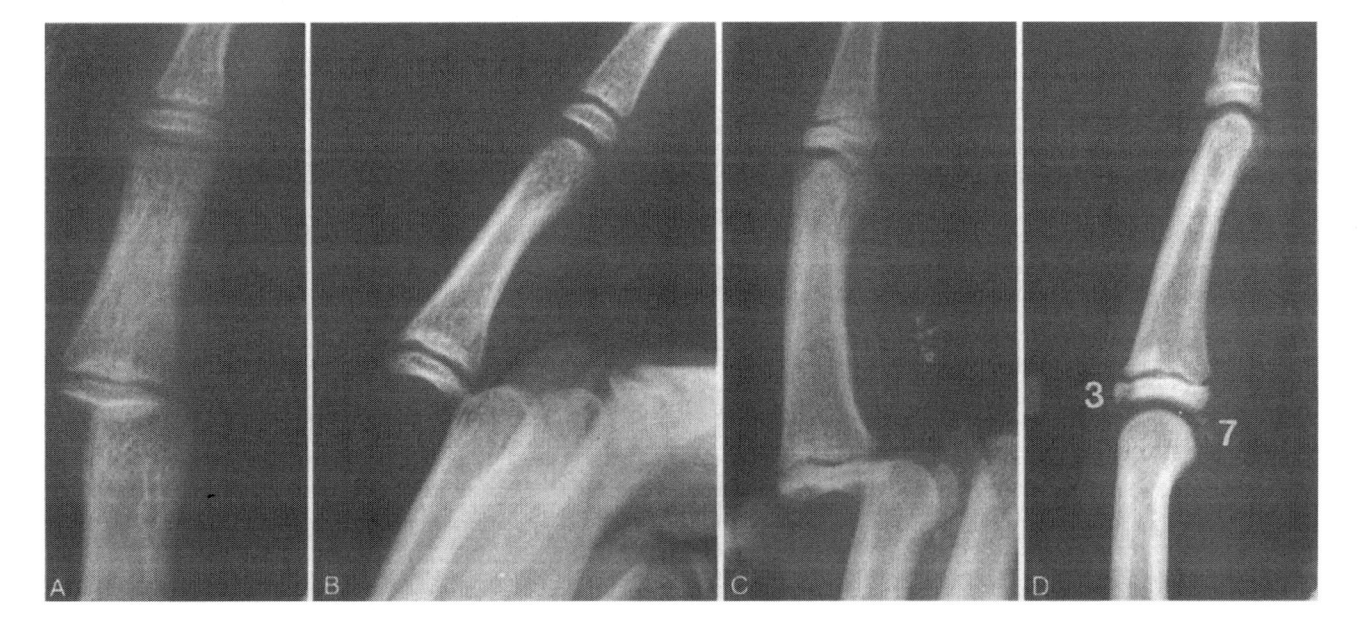

FIGURE 17-53. (A, B) Anteroposterior and lateral views of dislocation of the proximal interphalangeal (PIP) joint. (C) Seemingly simple PIP dislocation. (D) Postreduction films of the fracture shown in (C) demonstrated type 3 dorsal (3) and type 7 palmar (7) epiphyseal ossification center fractures.

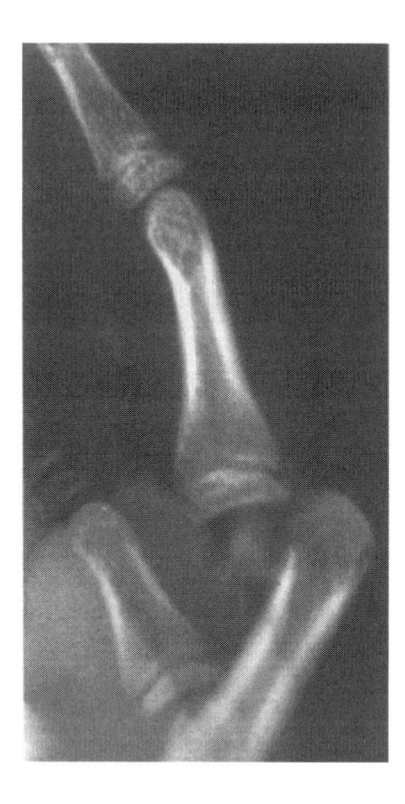

FIGURE 17-54. (A) "Dislocation" of the PIP joint. It is actually a displaced unicondylar fracture-dislocation.

With most interphalangeal dislocations, reduction is easily accomplished by closed manipulation. The correct technique for closed reduction is to hyperextend the joint and then push the distal bone over into the reduced position in a dorsal to palmar direction.[228] One should not apply traction to a dislocated finger joint and attempt to pull the distal bone back into position, as it may entrap soft tissue within the joint and prevent reduction.[219,241] After reduction it is imperative to check the stability of the collateral ligaments, as they may be torn at the time of initial displacement. However, it must be remembered that joint laxity is common in children. The motion should be compared with that of the contralateral digit. If the joint is stable after reduction, which it usually is, immediate protected motion of the finger should be allowed by taping it to an adjacent normal digit (dynamic splinting). An acceptable alternative is to immobilize the finger for 10–14 days in the aforementioned functional position (position of safety).

Crick et al. described dislocation of the proximal interphalangeal joint with an avulsion fracture of the phalangeal head that was locked through a tear in the central slip that required open reduction.[205] Irreducibility of a dorsal dislocation of the distal interphalangeal joint may also be due to the interposition of the volar plate.[217,227,234]

Simultaneous dislocations of the distal and proximal interphalangeal joints may occur.[214,215] The mechanism of injury appears to be a longitudinal compressive force along the extended digit. These dislocations should be reduced by closed manipulation. There may be small avulsion fractures of the volar plates.

Fractures of the Phalanges

Leonard and Dubravicik described 263 phalangeal fractures in children: 75% were treated by simple external immobilization; 15% required manipulative reduction with the patient under anesthesia; and 10% required open reduction.[49] Epiphyseal separations or fractures through the metaphysis formed the largest group (41%); seven open reductions were necessary for these injuries. Only 26% were shaft injuries. Eight diaphyseal fractures necessitated open reduction and lateral fixation, the main indication being marked displacement with comminution and instability. When there was sufficient angulation to warrant surgical

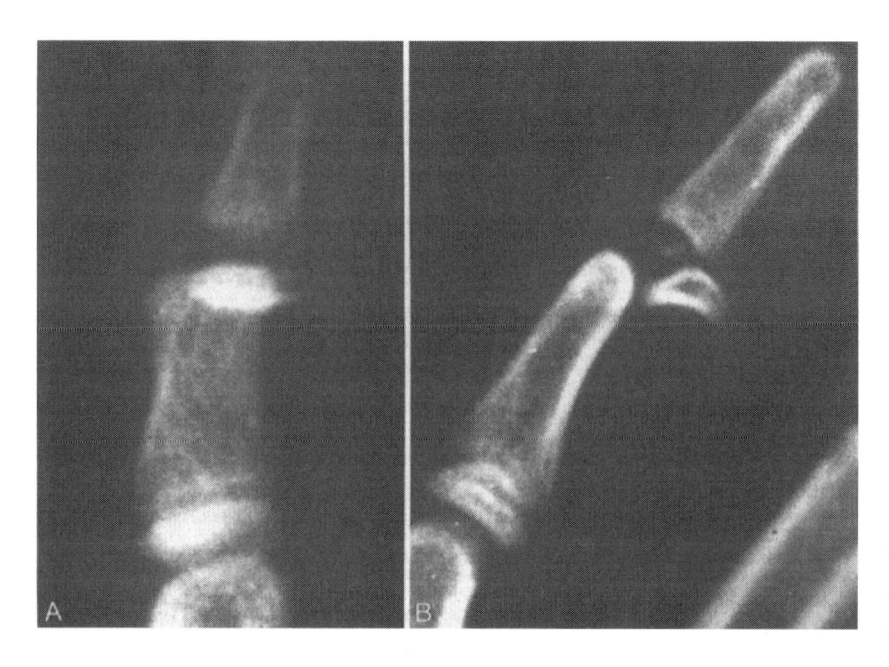

FIGURE 17-55. (A) Apparent dislocation of the distal interphalangeal joint. (B) Lateral view shows a type 2 injury of the distal phalanx. The displaced epiphyseal fragment is also dislocated.

intervention, it was necessary to immobilize the fracture for about 6 weeks, as the distal fragment was relatively avascular and healing was slow. Using small K-wires for internal fixation did not interfere significantly with the ultimate function of the interphalangeal joints or cause degenerative arthritis or epiphyseal arrest in the transfixed joints.[237] DeJonge et al. found that in the 10- to 29-year age group sports injuries and accidental falls were the most common cause of injury of the phalanges.[209] Shewring and Coleman described phalangeal fractures as a complication of finger wrestling.[231]

Some displacement of phalangeal fractures in children may be accepted so long as the fragments are aligned in axial and rotatory planes. Even mild angulation of a fracture in the plane of motion of a hinge joint often disappears, particularly if the apex is toward the flexor side.

Malrotation is the most frequent complication of phalangeal fractures, and must be avoided by careful attention to anatomic detail.[201,233] When the fingers are individually flexed, they do not remain parallel as they do in full extension but, rather, point toward the region of the scaphoid tubercle. However, they do not converge on a single fixed point, as is sometimes depicted (Fig. 17-5). When the finger is only semiflexed, it helps to use the planes of the fingernails as an additional guide. Rotatory malalignment is primarily due to three contributing factors: (1) failure to recognize the rotational deformity; (2) failure to reduce the fracture properly; and (3) failure to immobilize the fracture properly. Malrotation in a finger is especially disabling. The fingers overlap and become entangled when flexed.

A true lateral roentgenogram of the phalanx should show an image of a single condyle if the two are properly superimposed. However, when rotation exists, the shaft may be seen in the lateral position and the head in an oblique position. This arrangement is not easy to assess in children because of the variable degrees of ossification.[220]

Correcting malrotation in an acute fracture is relatively easy. Vandenberk et al. described the use of percutaneous absorbable pins to control rotation of children's finger fractures.[236] If the fracture heals with malrotation, an osteotomy may become necessary to correct the position. Most malrotations occur in the proximal phalanx. If an osteotomy is needed, a useful technique was described by Lewis and Hartman.[223]

Kirner's deformity is a condition of the little finger characterized by palmar and radial curving of the terminal phalanx. Trauma was originally considered a causal factor, but Dykes showed that it probably is congenital (nontraumatic).[211]

Fortens et al. described a fracture through an incomplete preaxial fusion of the phalanges.[212] This type of radiolucency is not unusual when there is failure to form the joint, and probably because of lack of motion it increases susceptibility to injury.

Connelly and Leicester described a 7-year-old boy who underwent pulley reconstruction at the A2 pulley.[202] Two years later he caught the finger in a fence and fractured the proximal phalanx. At surgery it became evident that the reconstructed A2 pulley had become caught between the fracture fragments. Open reduction led to successful healing and resumption of normal motion.

Fracture of the Proximal Portion of the Proximal Phalanx

Fractures of the proximal phalangeal growth region are among the most common finger fractures in children (Figs. 17-56, 17-57). The fracture-failure pattern frequently leaves

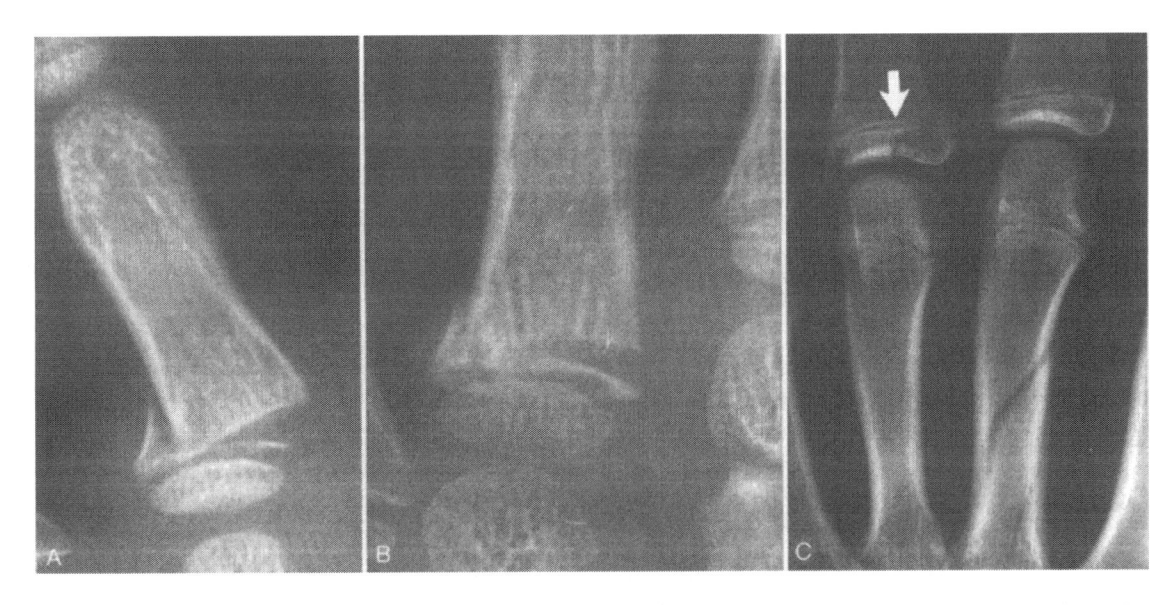

FIGURE 17-56. (A) Angulated (ulnarward) type 2 fracture of the proximal phalanx of the ring finger. As is typical of many of these injuries, there is transverse failure across the entire metaphyseal subchondral plate, rather than just across the physeal cartilage. (B) This fracture was reduced to a more appropriate alignment. (C) Type 3 fracture of the proximal phalanx of the ring finger (arrow), with a concomitant metacarpal fracture in the long finger.

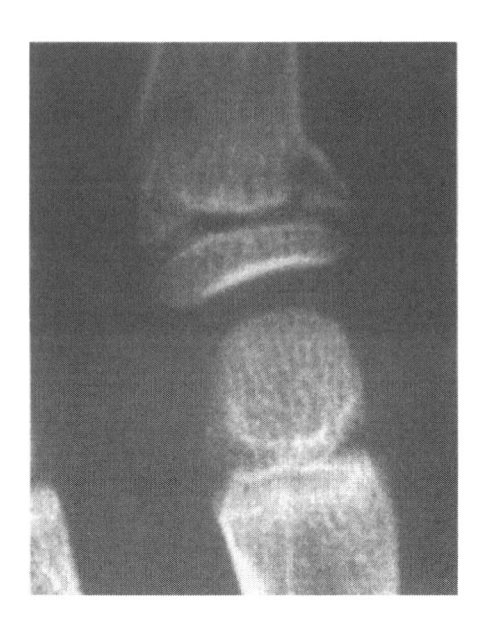

FIGURE 17-57. Variant of a type 2 injury with two peripheral Thurstan Holland fragments.

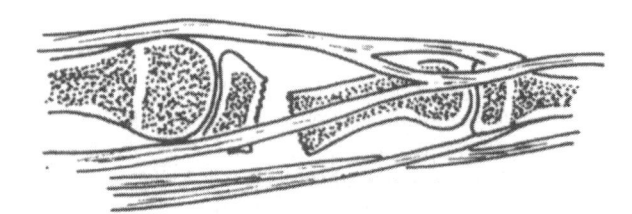

FIGURE 17-58. Proximal phalangeal growth mechanism fracture.

not only the classic Thurstan Holland metaphyseal fragment but also a transverse plate of metaphyseal subchondral bone (the Werenskiöld fragment). Types 3 and 4 growth mechanism fractures may also occur (Fig. 17-56C).

Coonrad and Pohlman focused attention on the poor results obtained in 41 children with impacted fractures of the proximal third of the proximal phalanx of the finger.[203] An impacted fracture of the proximal phalanx in the finger usually angulates toward the palm (Fig. 17-58); and if a significant degree of deformity remains, digital flexion is limited. The fracture angulates toward the palm because the intrinsic muscles flex the proximal fragment, and the long extensor tendon causes shortening by axial pull. If the displaced or impacted fracture is allowed to heal at an angulation of 20° or more, the extensor tendon and its expansion over the proximal phalanx become shortened and exert a tethering effect on the bone.

Closed reduction is usually successful. Open reduction and internal fixation of these proximal phalangeal fractures may be required in the following situations: (1) when closed methods have failed to correct rotation; (2) when open fractures must be reduced; (3) when the articular congruity of small articular fractures must be restored[221]; and (4) when widely displaced fractures are irreducible because of secondary soft tissue interposition. An unusual, irreducible juxtaepiphyseal fracture of the little finger may result from interposition of the flexor tendon.[213,238] Cowen and Dranick reported a badly angulated type 2 injury of the proximal phalanx of the little finger that was irreducible by closed methods because the distal fragment was trapped in a buttonhole rent in the periosteum of the fractured phalanx, and the dorsal hood simulated a "Chinese finger trap."[204]

The most common cause of angular malunion in this type of fracture is immobilization of the digit in insufficient flexion.[202] Extension permits gradual loss of reduction. A true lateral roentgenogram evaluates angulation in these patients both before and after reduction. If the fracture heals in an abnormal position, an opening wedge osteotomy corrects the deformity.

Dameron and Engber described a tension band technique for replacement of adolescent type 3 physeal fractures.[208] The technique is satisfactory if applied with careful surgical technique.

Extra-Octave Fracture

A frequent fracture of the proximal phalanx involves the fifth digit (Fig. 17-59) and is often referred to as the "extra-octave" fracture because of the extreme ulnar angulation (Fig. 17-60). The mechanism of injury and the age of the patient may result in a greenstick fracture of the ulnar cortex. Treatment should correct rotational and angular malalignment.

As with most type 2 epiphyseal fractures, closed reduction usually gives a satisfactory result, although it may be difficult to gain adequate purchase of the proximal fragment while manipulating the distal fragment into anatomic alignment. A pencil placed in the web space may serve as an effective fulcrum to bring the digit radialward (Fig. 17-61). Another method is to flex the metacarpophalangeal joint to 90° (or more), which tightens the collateral ligaments and provides purchase on the proximal (epiphyseal) fragment. Reduction is then accomplished by pushing the distal fragment across the palm and toward the thumb.

If the ulnar cortex is incompletely fractured (greenstick), overcorrection and completion of the cortical fracture may be necessary. The intact periosteal sleeve on the ulnar side of the bone generally prevents overreduction and provides stability in the reduced position. If the ulnar cortex is not completely fractured, the residual plastic deformation may cause gradual recurrence of some, if not all, of the angular deformity.

These fractures may be difficult to control; and once the fracture is reduced, the little finger must be splinted to the adjacent uninjured finger. Protection of the reduction for 3 weeks in an ulnar gutter splint incorporating the adjacent ring finger is advisable. Because of the pull of the abductor digiti quinti muscle, these fractures tend to drift and become redisplaced. Rarely, open reduction with pin fixation is required.

With a severe fracture the epiphysis may remain in place while the remainder of the phalanx is totally dislocated palmarward. Open reduction may be necessary in this fracture pattern.[241]

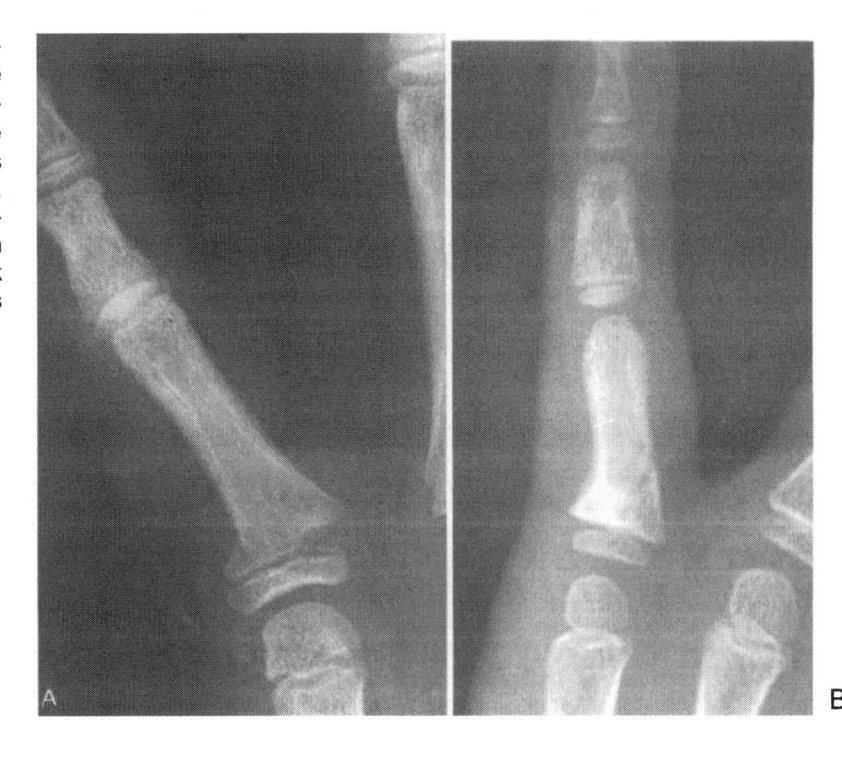

FIGURE 17-59. (A) Type 2 fracture of the fifth proximal phalanx, with concomitant ulnar deviation. Note the transverse metaphyseal fragment, which is characteristic of this type of injury when it occurs in the small longitudinal bones. This greenstick injury is often referred to as the "extra- octave" fracture. Reduction must overcorrect and complete this fracture, or recurrent angular deformity may occur even while the fracture is immobilized. (B) The greenstick component was not completed in this patient. Thus the fracture drifted back and healed in a malunion.

Fractures of the diaphysis of the proximal phalanx (Fig. 17-62) may angulate as well as rotate. Some degree of overriding (shortening) may be accepted. However, malrotation must be corrected. Percutaneous fixation may be used to control rotation. Open reduction is usually unnecessary.

Fractures of the Phalangeal Neck

Phalangeal neck fractures, whether involving the proximal or middle phalanges (Fig. 17-63), are common.[200,206,210,225] Such injuries may be treacherous. It is a classic "booby-trap" fracture in the hand that is transverse through the neck of

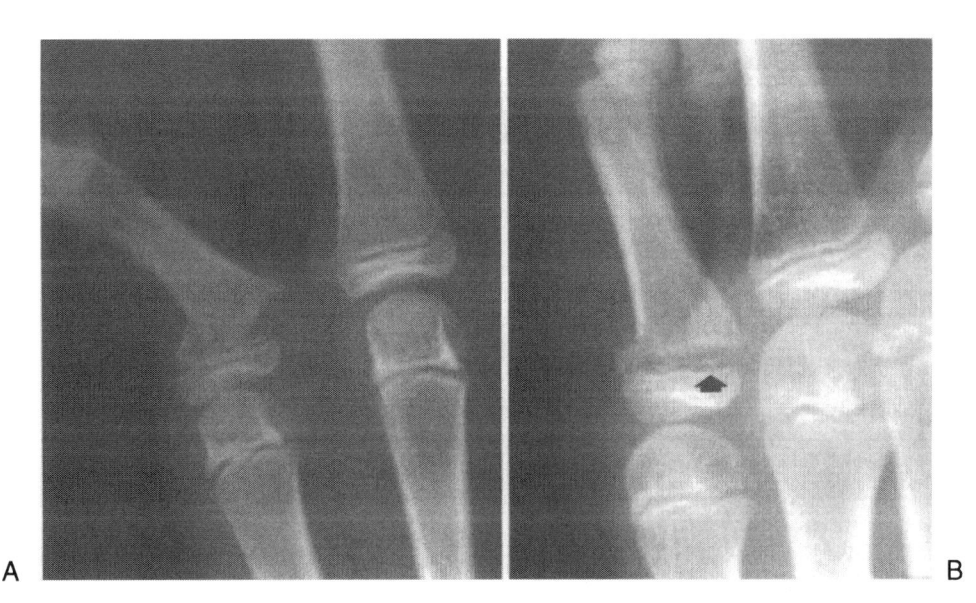

FIGURE 17-60. (A) Stress view showing the extent of angulation probably present at maximum acute deformity. (B) Postreduction film showing a thin linear juxtaphyseal fragment (arrow).

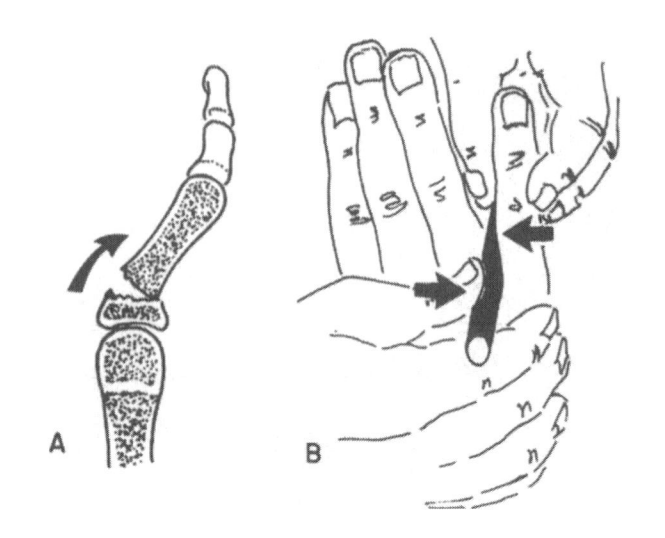

FIGURE 17-61. (A) Extra-octave fracture. (B) Method of reduction utilizing a pencil in the web space.

either the proximal or the middle phalanx, with dorsal displacement of the distal fragment (Fig. 17-63D). In children the palmar plate may roll on itself, causing 90° rotation of the condylar fragment, which is then entrapped by the capsule and collateral ligaments (Fig. 17-64).[226]

The problem of adequate visualization of the fracture in the splint may be overcome by using a tomographic cut (lateral view) coinciding with the long axis of the injured finger. The 90° (or more) rotation of the supracondylar phalangeal fracture can easily be missed. It is essential that an adequate lateral roentgenogram or tomogram be obtained to delineate it thoroughly.

Reduction may be easy, but redisplacement after closed reduction can readily occur. The problem in recognizing this complication is that it is difficult to visualize the bone clearly on the postreduction lateral views because of superimposition of the other fingers in the splint. The resulting loss of reduction may cause an unacceptable deformity (Fig. 17-65), and late treatment of the healed, displaced fracture (even as early as 3 weeks after injury) is difficult. Early open reduction or closed reduction and percutaneous pinning (Fig. 17-66) of the fracture generally yield better results than later attempts to correct the malunion.[222,226]

In the series reported by Leonard and Dubravicik, 9 of 38 phalangeal neck fractures necessitated surgery.[49] Dixon and Moon reported treating five cases of phalangeal fracture through the neck of the proximal phalanx of the finger or thumb with 90° of rotation of the condylar fragment and entrapment by the capsule and collateral ligaments.[210] These fractures could not be reduced by closed methods because the condylar fragment had rotated 90° and was restrained and trapped by the capsule and collateral ligaments. They did not describe any associated injuries of the epiphysis of the middle phalanx. Whipple et al. described an irreducible proximal interphalangeal joint injury in a 6-year-old child and found that the palmar one-half of the articular cartilage of the middle phalanx blocked reduction.[241]

To correct chronic (healed) malunion of fractures of the distal end of the proximal phalanx in children, Simmons and Peters recommended a palmar approach to remove the bony block to flexion.[232]

Complete remodeling of a displaced phalangeal neck fracture may occur.[226] Although this fracture is "removed" from the active proximally located physis, for a few years there is a physis present distally. It ossifies by "pseudoepiphyseal" ossification. The peripheral zone of Ranvier and the temporary presence of a physis explain the remodeling in such cases.

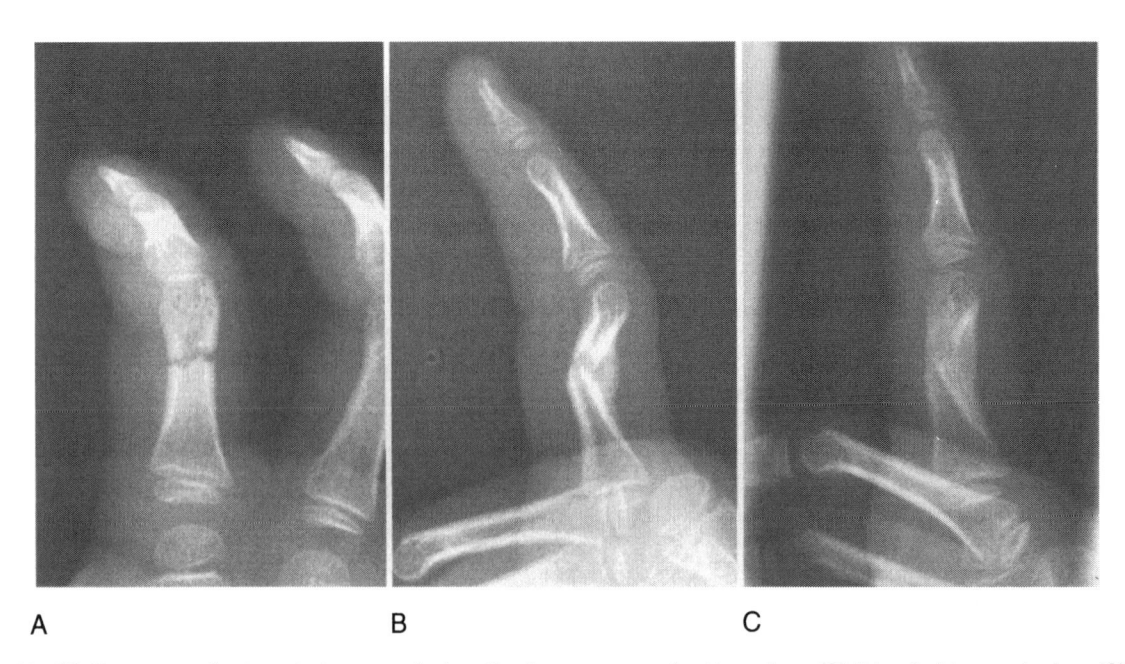

FIGURE 17-62. (A) Transverse fracture that occurred when the finger was crushed in a door. (B) It healed in a malunion. (C) Remodeling and correction of the deformity 7 months later.

Phalanges

FIGURE 17-63. (A) Distal end of a phalanx fracture. (B) Lateral view shows that it is mildly displaced. (C) Fracture of the distal end of the proximal phalanx. (D) Lateral view reveals a major problem: dorsal displacement of the epiphyseal end.

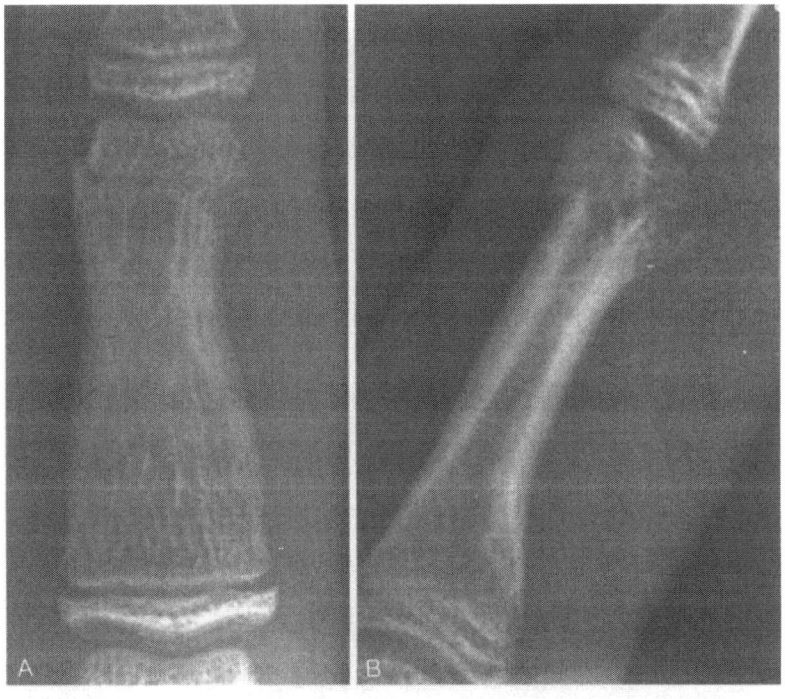

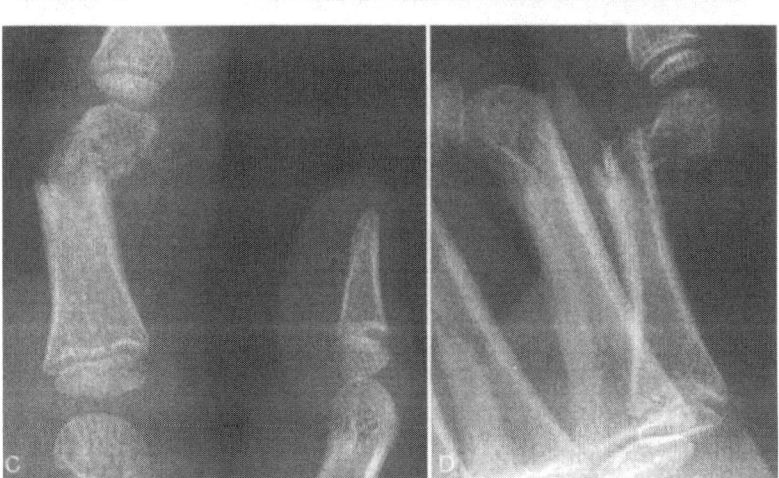

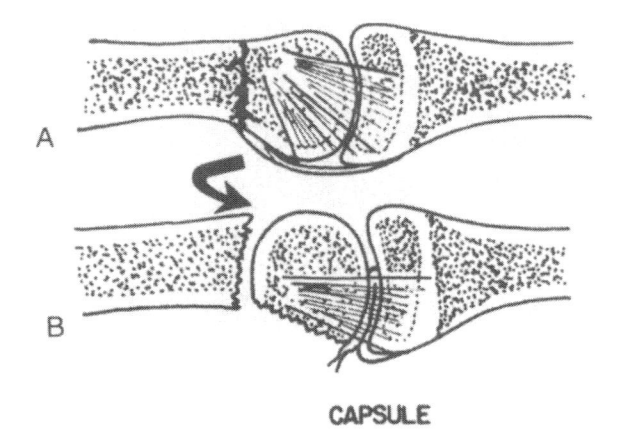

FIGURE 17-64. (A, B) Rotation of the fragment.

A variation of this injury may include both distal phalangeal fracture and adjacent epiphyseal injury.

Intercondylar Fractures

Intercondylar fractures in children should be treated as they are in adults. Displaced T-fractures of the distal end of a phalanx require open reduction and internal fixation with K-wires.[240] When 30% or more of a joint surface is involved or if there is instability of the joint, it should be opened (Figs. 17-67, 17-68).

When pin fixation becomes necessary, healing of the fracture may be delayed. Therefore fixation wires should be left in place for at least 6 weeks. Epiphyseal avascular necrosis has not been described. Stiffness after injury is not as common a problem in children, as they usually regain com-

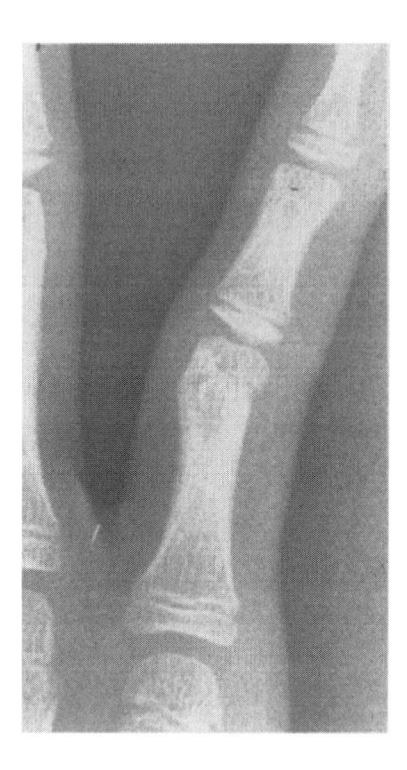

FIGURE 17-65. This distal end fracture healed in malalignment, leaving an ulnar-directed angulation. It will *not* spontaneously correct.

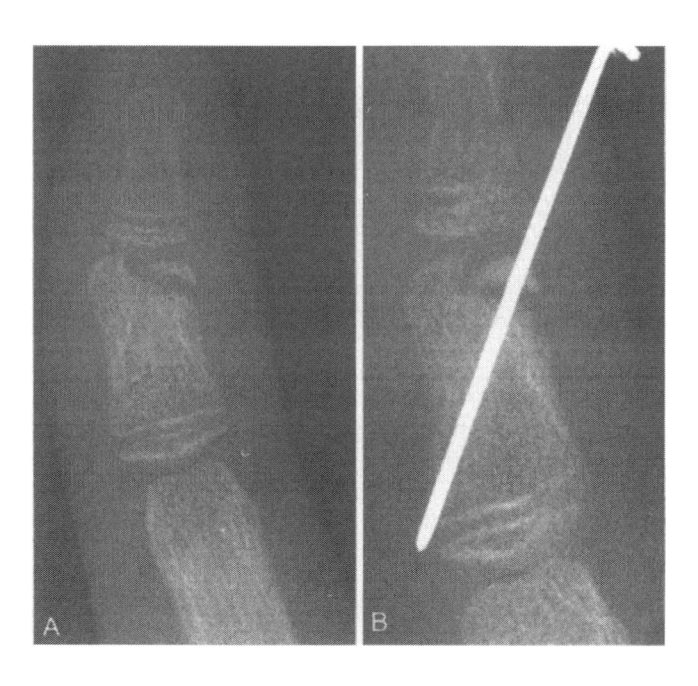

FIGURE 17-67. (A) Displacing unicondylar fracture 4 weeks after injury. (B) Percutaneous fixation. The fragment was left displaced because of concern that open reduction would jeopardize the blood supply.

plete mobility. Stiffness may occur, however, especially in older children; and an extended period (months to years) may be required for motion to return to normal. Arthrodesis may also occur.

Fractures of the Middle Phalanx

Fractures of the epiphysis are common (Figs. 17-69, 17-70). They are ligament injury analogues and are associated with

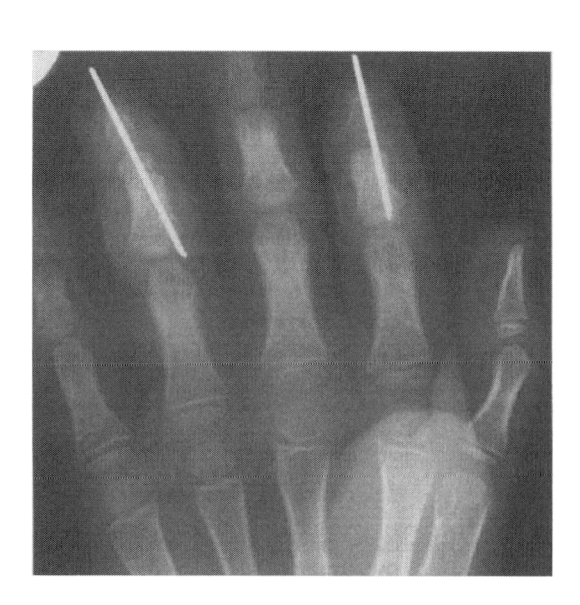

FIGURE 17-66. Open reduction of rotated distal condylar fractures sustained when the fingers were caught in a door.

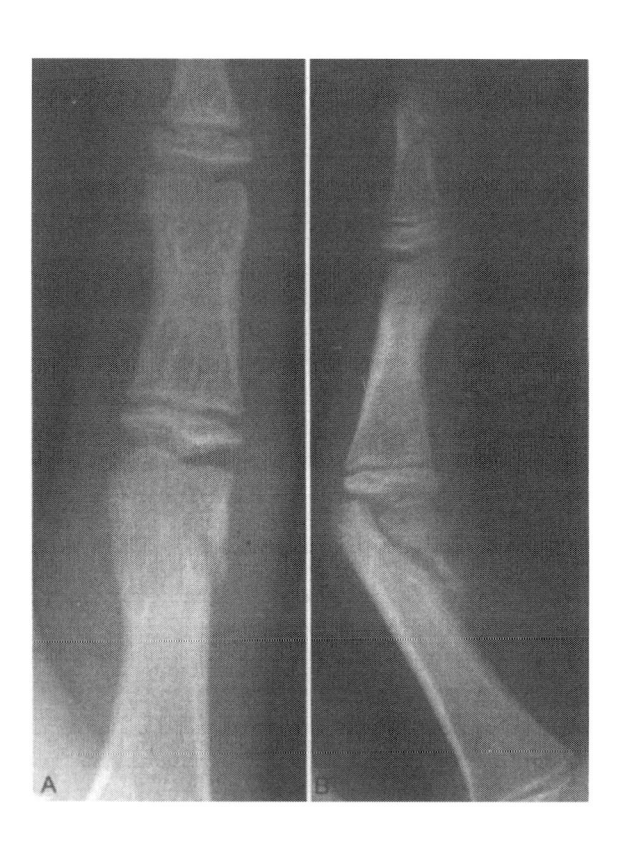

FIGURE 17-68. (A) Undisplaced unicondylar fracture in an adolescent. (B) The patient removed the cast-splint to play basketball, losing the position. The obliquity of the fracture line enhances this complication.

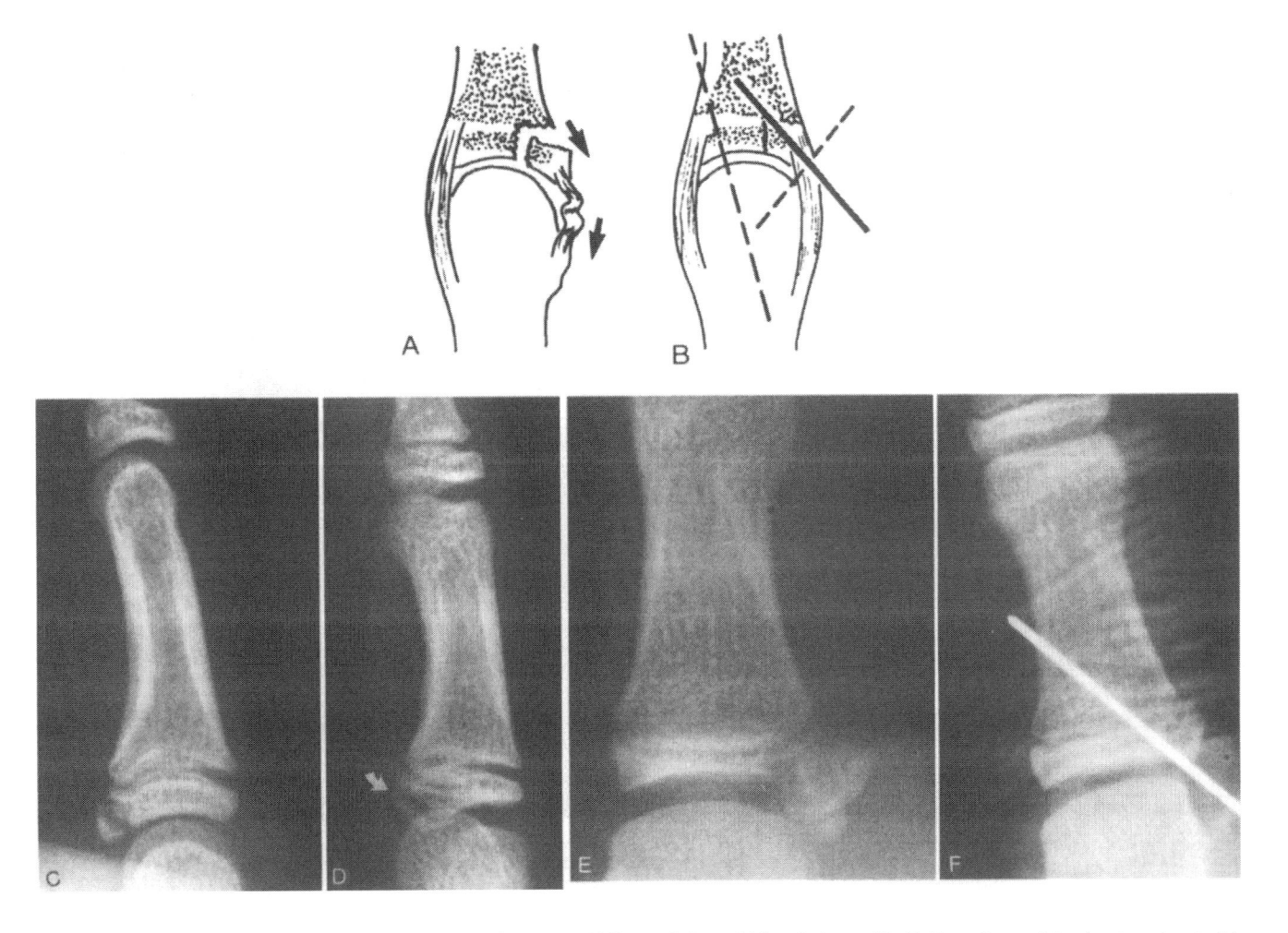

FIGURE 17-69. (A, B) Physeal fracture of the proximal or middle phalanx and method of pinning. Dashed lines represent potential courses for buttress pins. (C, D) Types 3 and 7 condylar fractures of the middle phalanx. (E, F) Type 3 condylar fracture treated by open reduction.

articular surface displacement. They often require open reduction and pin fixation to avoid malunion.

The middle phalangeal shaft injury has specific deforming musculotendinous forces (Fig. 17-71). The important forces are insertion of the central slip onto the dorsal aspect of the proximal middle phalanx and insertion of the flexor digitorum sublimis along the palmar shaft. The central slip extends the proximal phalanx, particularly if it is a more proximal or epiphyseal type of injury. If the fracture is proximal to the sublimis, the distal fragment tends to be flexed. If the fracture is distal to the sublimis tendon, the proximal fragment is flexed and the distal fragment hyperextended.

Fractures of the middle phalanx may be undisplaced or angulated. If the fracture site is distal to the insertion of the flexor superficialis tendon, it can usually be treated by manual traction and flexion of the distal fragment. The extensor tendon pulls the distal fragment into extension, and the flexor superficialis causes flexion of the fragment, producing an overall palmar angulation. Fracture of the middle phalanx proximal to the insertion of the flexor superficialis tendon may also be treated in a closed manner.

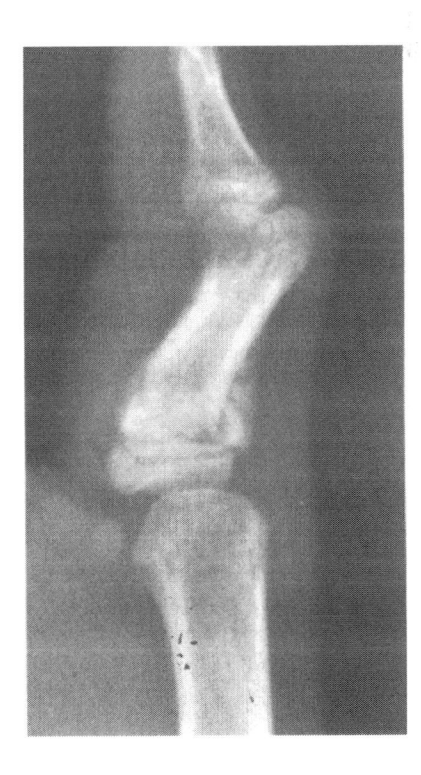

FIGURE 17-70. Malunion of a type 2 injury of the middle phalanx.

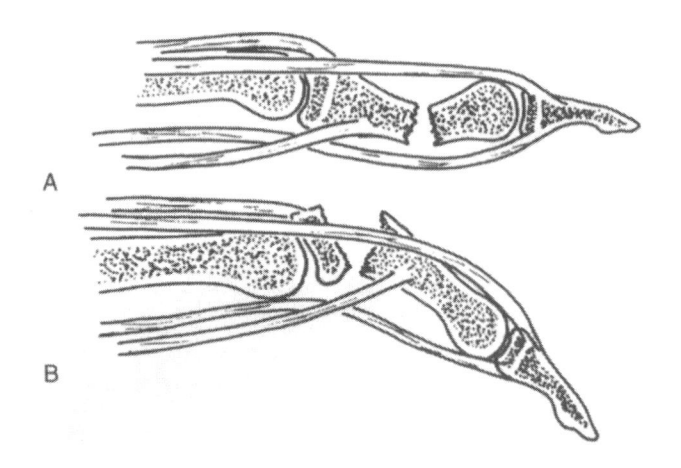

FIGURE 17-71. (A, B) Variable effects of tendons on deformation of fracture fragments in a middle phalangeal injury.

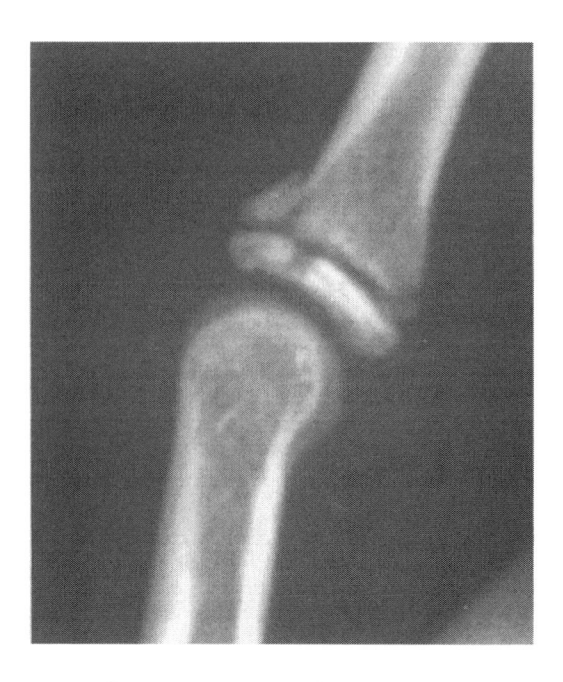

FIGURE 17-72. Complex epiphyseal/physeal fracture due to a crushing injury.

The central slip of the extensor tendon extends the proximal phalanx. The flexor superficialis flexes the distal fragment, producing dorsal angulation of the fragments. Therefore these fractures should be reduced and held in extension. These injuries are often due to the finger being caught in a door. Such crushing injuries may cause severely comminuted epiphyseal fractures (Fig. 17-72).

Fractures of the shaft of the middle phalanx heal correctly so long as the position of immobilization is recognized and maintained. Immobilization for up to 7 weeks may be required, even in a child.

On rare occasions, the proximal epiphysis is displaced (Fig. 17-73).[219] Open reduction is often required in such a situation.

Premature partial physeal growth arrest subsequent to a fracture in the hand of a child appears to be unusual (Fig. 17-74). Culp and Osgood reported a child with a fracture of the middle phalanx that went on to a physeal bar formation.[207] Malunion may fail to remodel (Fig. 17-75).

Mallet Finger

Mallet finger deformities in children are anatomically different from those in adults, but the treatment is similar. In children it is an epiphyseal injury with avulsion of a portion of the epiphysis.[232] In the small child, the deformity is usually a displaced type 1 or 2 epiphyseal fracture at the base of the

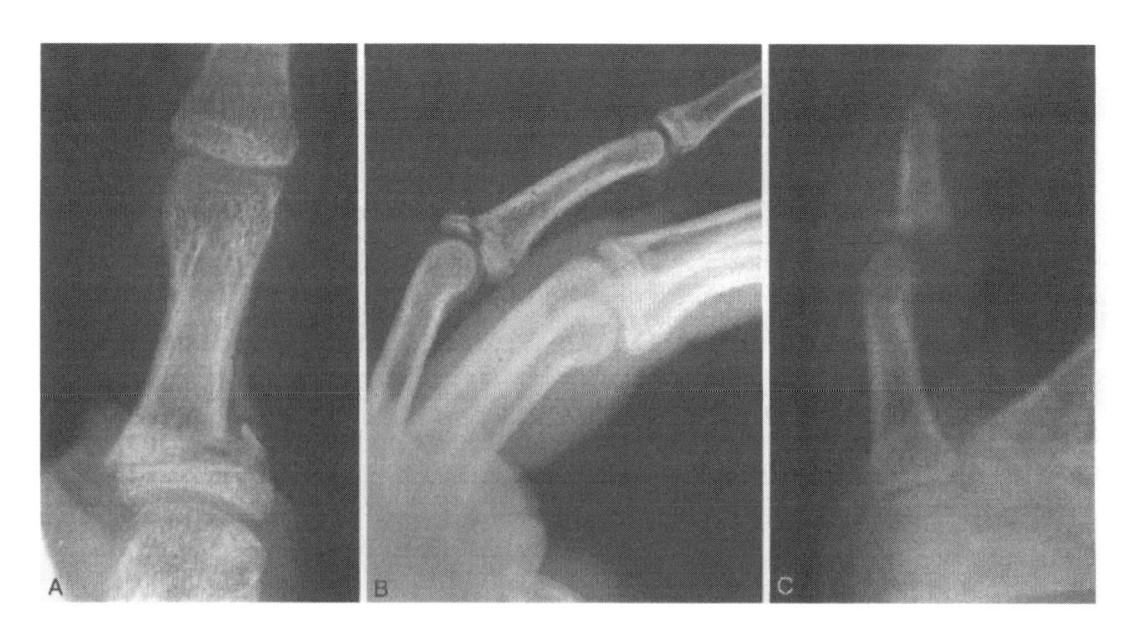

FIGURE 17-73. (A) Displaced type 2 injury of the middle phalanx. (B) Displaced type 3 injury. (C) Displaced type 1 injury (B) and (C) are comparable to a mallet finger injury of the distal phalanx.

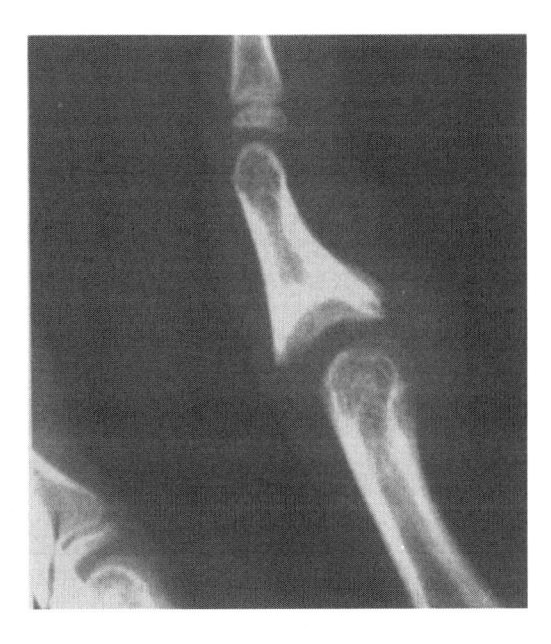

FIGURE 17-74. Lateral view of growth arrest. The physeal fracture was caused by a crushing injury.

distal phalanx (Fig. 17-76). In the adolescent, however, the injury is likely to be a type 3 or type 7 growth mechanism injury, which splits the epiphysis. The deformity ordinarily results from forcible flexion of the end of the finger while the extensor tendon is taut, as when catching a ball or striking an object with the finger extended.

The epiphysis of the terminal phalanx may completely displace, being pulled by the extensor tendon to a position dorsal to the middle phalanx.[224,239] Savage showed that when the distal phalanx epiphysis is displaced it may detach completely from the extensor digitorum communis and flip onto the volar side of the middle phalanx.[229] These injuries require open reduction.

The lateral radiograph is important because rupture of the extensor tendon is uncommon during childhood. The flexor digitorum profundus tendon flexes the metaphysis, into which it is inserted; and the extensor tendon, which inserts into the epiphysis, maintains the epiphysis in the extended position. The proximal epiphysis may be rotated significantly. Sometimes the proximal epiphysis is not ossified, a finding that may lead to diagnostic difficulties and delay in treatment.

Methods of treatment should be directed at joint hyperextension, which may be accomplished with small splints (aluminum) to provide three-point fixation (Fig. 17-77). Commercially available plastic splints are also reasonable. If anatomic reduction cannot be achieved with closed reduction, open reduction and internal fixation may be required. In many children this condition is an intraarticular or intraepiphyseal type 3 injury and warrants open reduction as the initial treatment. Failure to reduce the fragments may result in significant malunion with exostosis formation and joint dysfunction (Fig. 17-78). Partial or complete growth arrest may occur (Fig. 17-79).

Inoue et al. described 14 patients with mallet fingers with a large displaced fracture.[216] They were treated using an extension block Kirschner wire technique.

Because mallet finger injuries are often due to crushing, which causes extensive soft tissue damage, the possibility of infection is high (Fig. 17-80). Any type of fixation should be used judiciously.

Open mallet-type fractures of the distal phalanx pose a significant treatment problem. They are frequently associated with osteomyelitis and poor results. The major problem is that the nail is not elevated sufficiently to expose the open fracture site. This situation may leave the fracture unreduced and inappropriately irrigated, as any open fracture should be. Ideally, the nail is removed, the fracture site properly irrigated and débrided, the fracture reduced, the nail matrix meticulously repaired with 5-0 or 6-0 chromic suture, and the nail replaced as a stent (splint) after having been perforated to allow drainage of any subungual hematoma. Internal fixation of the fracture with K-wires is usually unnecessary.

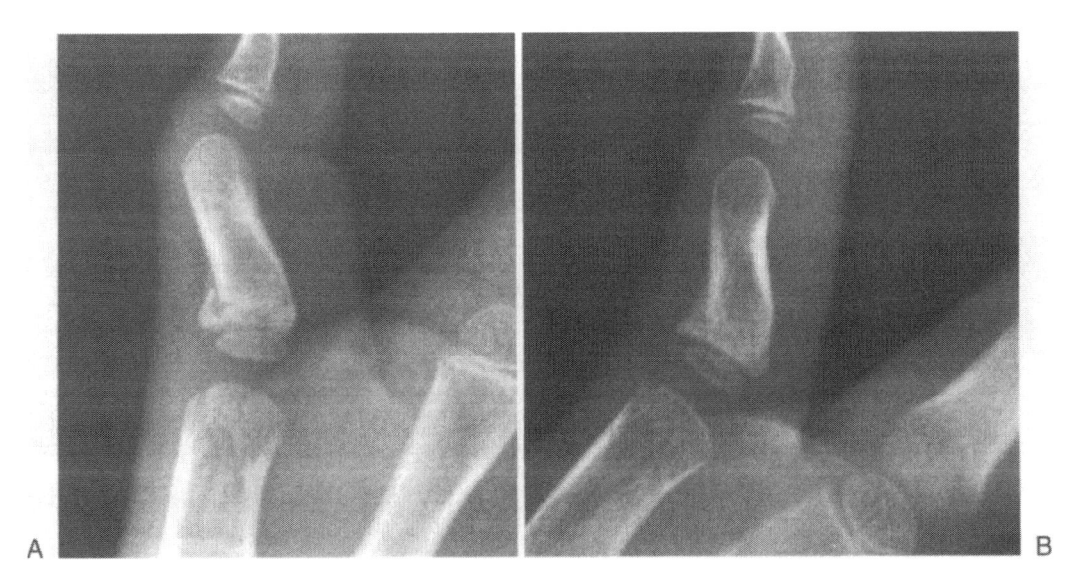

FIGURE 17-75. (A) Crush injury to the metaphysis. Angulation was not sufficiently corrected. (B) The malunion did not remodel.

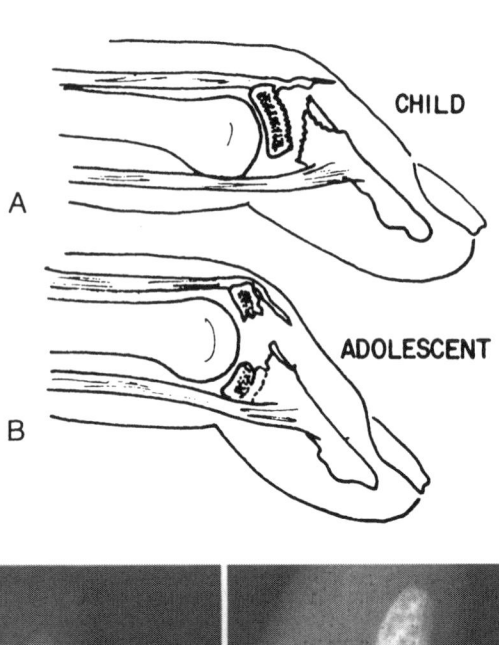

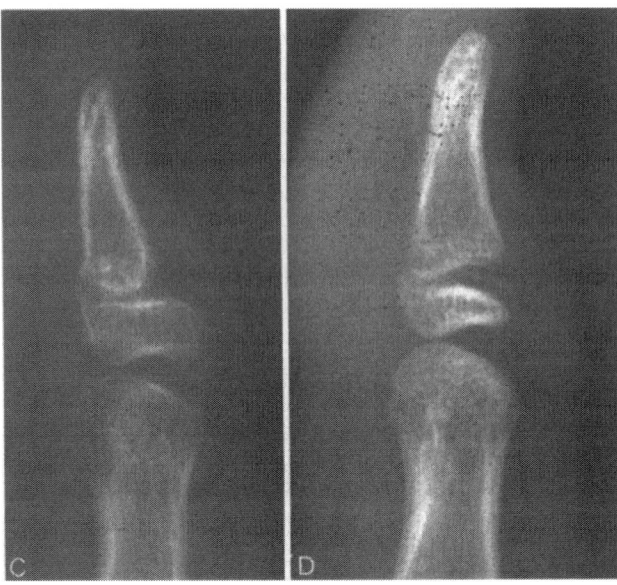

FIGURE 17-76. (A, B) Two types of mallet finger epiphyseal injury in the child and adolescent. (C) Typical appearance of type 1 injury in a 5-year-old. (D) Type 2 injury.

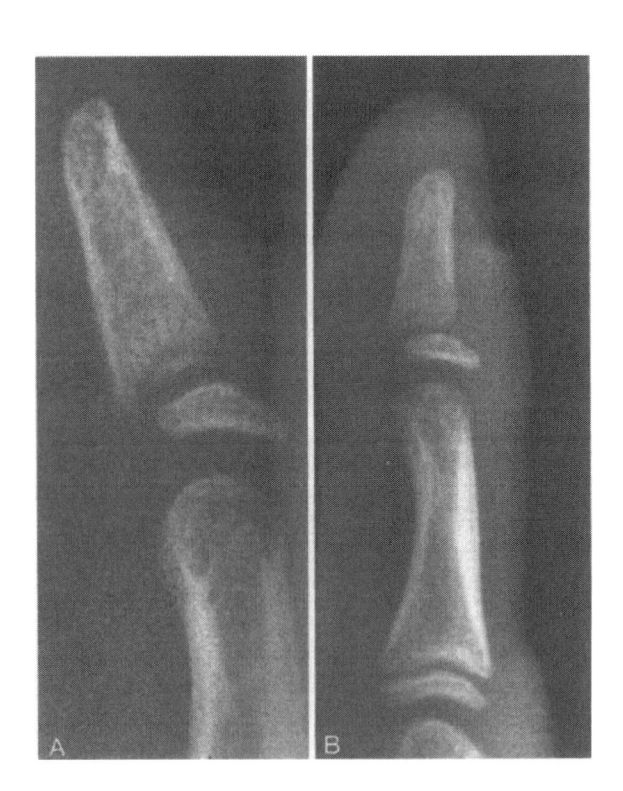

FIGURE 17-77. Mallet finger. (A) Displaced. (B) Acceptable but incomplete reduction with hyperextension.

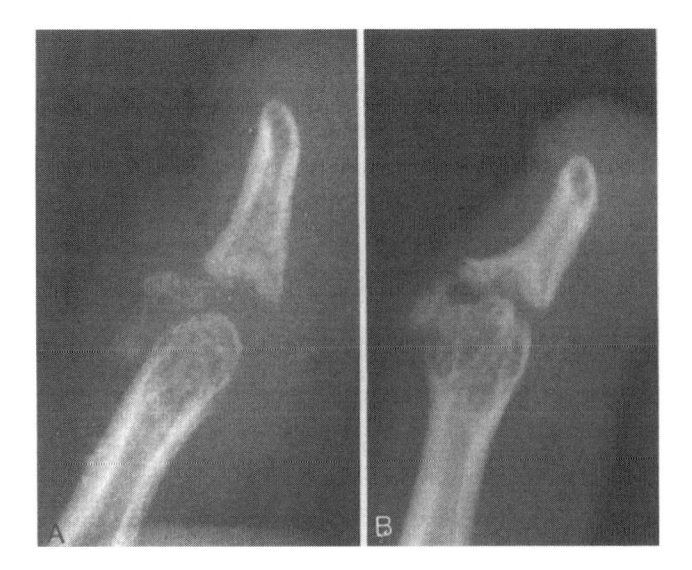

FIGURE 17-78. (A) Fragmented injury of the entire epiphysis in an adolescent. (B) Exostosis formation following nonoperative treatment. It has caused a flexion deformity and impaired joint function.

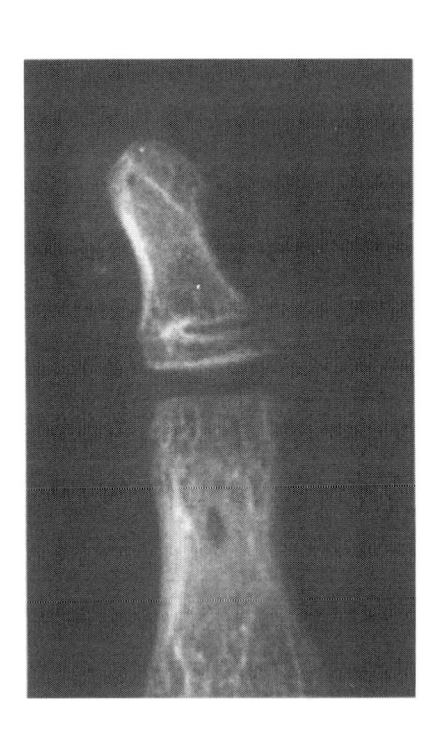

FIGURE 17-79. Partial growth arrest after a mallet finger injury.

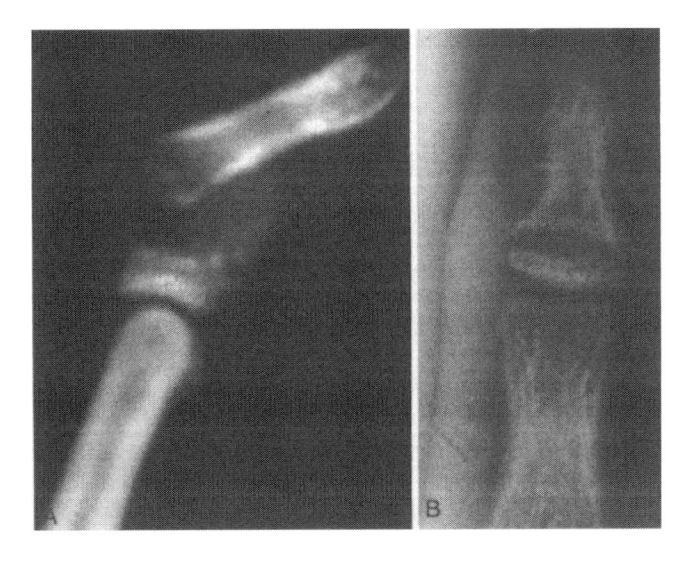

FIGURE 17-80. Mallet finger. (A) Open injury. (B) Widening of the physis due to osteomyelitis in an open injury.

Dameron and Engber described a tension band technique for replacement of adolescent type 3 physeal fractures.[208] The technique is satisfactory if applied with careful surgical technique.

Fractures of the Distal Phalanx

Fractures of the distal phalanx are common. Radiating fibrous septa form a dense meshwork and probably stabilize these fractures, effectively preventing significant displacement (Fig. 17-81). Most of these injuries result from crushing and therefore are usually accompanied by extensive soft tissue damage and subungual hematoma.

The terminal periosteum may be separated from the end of the phalanx, which may or may not be accompanied by a thin sleeve of bone. If fibrous tissue intervenes during the reparative process, nonunion may develop, creating a U-shaped piece of bone (Fig. 17-81C).

Avulsion of the nail and frequently associated lacerations of the nail bed are probably produced by protrusions of the phalangeal fragment. The presence of fracture of the epiphyseal plate in association with avulsion of the nail and laceration of the nail bed has important therapeutic implications because it becomes an open fracture. Simple reduction must also be accompanied with a strong appreciation for the open injury. Engber and Glancy described osteomyelitis and premature closure of the distal phalangeal epiphysis.[249]

Banerjee described two patients with physeal fractures of the distal phalanx in which reduction was prevented by a bridge of nail fold that had herniated into the gap.[244] They noted that Seymour[230] was the first to describe open distal phalangeal epiphyseal injuries with this complication.

Nail Bed

Probably one of the most frequent injuries in children involves the nail bed, usually a crushing injury. About 50% of nail bed injuries have an associated fracture of the distal phalanx. Nail growth occurs at the rate of 0.1 mm per day. If the nail is removed entirely, a delay of 21 days occurs prior to significant evidence of nail growth.

Traumatic avulsion of the fingernail in skeletally immature patients should arouse the physician's suspicion of associated bone injury. Lateral roentgenograms frequently reveal fracture of the distal phalangeal epiphyseal plate.

Inadequate initial treatment may result in permanent residual deformity.[243,250] Lacerations of the nail bed should be sutured as carefully as lacerations of the skin. Although not all late deformity is preventable owing to the crushing nature of the injury, it probably can be minimized by meticulous operative repair of the lacerated nail bed with fine absorbable material.

Meticulous primary repair of the nail bed increases the likelihood of normal growth.[252,253,258,263] The nail plate is completely removed. Incisions are made at the lateral corners of the eponychium to allow evaluation of the nail bed. Any incision required in the eponychium should be made at 90°

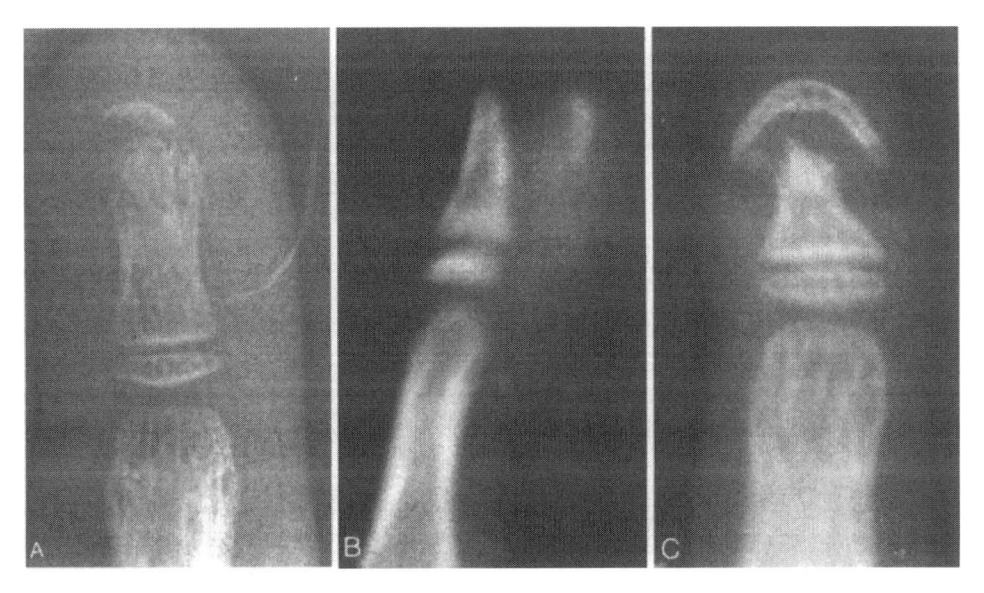

FIGURE 17-81. (A) Closed tip injury. (B) Displaced tip injury. (C) Reactive bone.

angles to minimize the risk of deformity. Copious irrigation is undertaken. The bed is repaired using 7-0 chromic catgut. The avulsed matrix is placed under the eponychial fold with a suture tied over a bolster, and the nail plate may be replaced as a stent. Accompanying fractures should be reduced and stabilized.

Zook et al. found that 90% of repaired nail beds could be graded good to excellent. The poor results generally were due to crush or avulsion injuries to both nail bed and nail fold, usually with an associated infection.[264,265]

In an attempt to determine the most likely contaminating organisms in crushing fingertip injuries in children, Rayan and Flournoy assessed nontraumatized human fingernails. They found that 95% of the subjects had a moderate to heavy growth of *Staphylococcus epidermidis* and that most of these isolates were highly susceptible to antibiotics.[259] It is interesting that 13 of the 20 subjects also had fungi. These organisms, however, do not routinely cause infection in children.

The following treatment protocol is recommended for nailbed injuries. When the fingernail attachment is nearly completely avulsed, the nail should be removed. If only the proximal portion is avulsed, a small proximal portion should be removed, leaving the remainder of the nail to act as a splint. After meticulous débridement and irrigation, a small drain is inserted through the lacerated nail bed, and the epiphyseal separation is reduced and maintained by splinting.[245] Oral antibiotics are given for at least 2 weeks. Because a high percentage of infections of the hand are due to staphylococci resistant to penicillin, appropriate synthetic penicillins (e.g., dicloxacillin) should be used. Cephalosporins may also be given, as they have been shown to decrease the infection rate after open fractures.[257] Consultation with an infectious disease specialist and consideration of other antibiotics are appropriate. The drain is removed after several days, and splinting is maintained for 4–6 weeks.

Subungual Hematoma

Any blood in the nail fold indicates disruption of the nail bed and an open fracture. Bleeding underneath the fingernail may be painful, and significant relief of pain may be attained by draining the blood through the nail. A paper clip may be heated until it glows red. A match does not ordinarily get the tip hot enough to melt painlessly through the nail without having to apply any pressure. Although this technique may be somewhat frightening to the small patient, it is usually less painful than boring a hole in the nail with a sharp instrument. The lunula must not be damaged by the heat or hole. Otherwise, a permanent nail deformity may ensue.

Fingertip

Fingertip injuries in children are generally easier to treat than similar injuries in adults because the regenerative capacity of local tissues in children is greater.[246] Loss of skin only, with intact underlying subcutaneous tissue, is usually managed best by careful neglect (i.e., by allowing the wound to heal by secondary intention). All that is usually required is initial débridement and cleansing of the wound, applying a bulky, compressive dressing for the first 24 hours to control bleeding and then small dressings to keep the wound clean (a small adhesive strip with a gauze pad usually suffices after the first few days). The finger may be soaked daily when the child is bathed, and the wound may then be redressed. Good results with maximal preservation of length and good sensibility may be achieved using this technique, even for injuries in which there is a rather sizable loss of skin. If the tip of the distal phalanx is protruding slightly, the same plan of management may be carried out if the bone is cut with a rongeur at a level underneath the soft tissue at the time of initial débridement. As much bone as possible should be maintained.

The injuries cause exessive parental concern. When an open fracture includes portions of skin and fat that are only partially attached, the tissue should not be removed. Bits of tissue that one suspects would not heal in an adult may completely heal in a child. The regenerative potential in the child is remarkable. Even when the injury has caused complete amputation and the pieces are missing, regeneration occurs and the tip of the stump becomes covered with surprisingly good tissue.[251,255,260,261] In general, one should save as much tissue as possible. However, even when soft tissue healing occurs, the damaged bone ends may not "regenerate."

Duthie and Adams described the use of meshed adhesive tape to treat crushed fingers in children.[247] They believed that this method was better than multiple suturing.

Mennen and Wiese used a semipermeable dressing to cover the avulsed fingertip once a week.[254] The dressing provided a temporary skin, making the finger painless and allowing an appropriate healing environment that actively promoted granulation tissue formation and epithelialization. They found that within an average of 20 days more than 200 fingertip injuries were successfully treated by this methodology. Certainly, it is one to consider in children.

Partial amputations of the fingertip in which the tip is dangling from a narrow bridge of skin should not be removed in the child. Even when the chances of survival of the tip are poor, the tissues should be loosely approximated and given an opportunity to heal. Little has been lost if the tip does not survive. If the tip does become necrotic, it is best to allow it to demarcate spontaneously, so long as it is clean and free of drainage.

The completely amputated fingertip that is picked up at the scene of the accident and brought in separately with the child in some instances warrants replantation. Replacement of the tip with skin sutures is often surprisingly successful.

Moiemen and Elliot found that 11 of 18 amputated digital tips replaced within 5 hours survived completely.[256] In contrast, none of 32 digital tips replaced more than 5 hours after injury survived completely. The mean delay between injury and replacement for the successful group was 3.9 hours. In the unsuccessful group it was 7.2 hours.

Thompson and Sorokolit advocated using the cross-finger flap for treating avulsions of the fingertip.[262] Several authors have recommended using the cross-finger flap in all fingertip injuries in children 7–8 years of age or older but do not advise it in younger children because immobilization is "more difficult in the younger age group." Thompson and Sorokolit arrived at the following conclusions based on 75 children who had undergone 79 operative procedures: (1)

Following cross-finger pedicle grafts the lack of tactile sense, osteogenesis, and disability due to altered sensation is not as common in children as in adults. (2) From the cosmetic standpoint, the pedicle flap and its donor site were not entirely satisfactory. (3) The contour and color of the graft tip were less than ideal. (4) Neglect of the index finger was encountered in 20% of the children, but the middle finger was trained to compensate for this disability. (5) There was no postoperative joint stiffness. (6) Spread scars and interrupted suture scars were noted on the abdomen at the donor site of full-thickness free grafts. (7) The accepted indications for a cross-finger pedicle flap should be modified in children to include all age groups. The procedure has been associated with better clinical results in children than in adults.

Thenar flaps are also useful for these injuries in children. The finger is flexed toward the palm and a flap is elevated from the thenar region to resurface the fingertip pulp deficit. This type of flap often leads to proximal interphalangeal joint stiffness in adults because of the necessary position of immobilization. In contrast, the position is well tolerated by children. The donor site may be closed primarily, so donor site morbidity becomes less than that experienced with cross-finger flaps. This procedure works best for the index and middle fingers, which naturally reach to the thenar region. It may be possible to use it for the ring finger. The little finger, however, cannot be easily brought across and should not be treated with this type of flap.

Elliot and Jigjinni described a lateral pulp flap evolved from the volar tissue.[248] This method, though applicable in the child, should be used as a secondary closure method. The wound is dressed and cleaned with an attempt at covering it to allow primary tissue healing, which is more likely for such a defect in a child.

Amputations at more proximal levels through the distal phalanx or distal interphalangeal joint may require more sophisticated treatment in the operating room, and many techniques for closure and coverage of these amputations have been described.

Partial amputations of the fingertip in which the tip is dangling from a narrow bridge of skin should not be removed in the child. Even when the chances of survival of the tip are poor, the tissues should be loosely approximated and given an opportunity to heal. Little has been lost if the tip does not survive. If the tip becomes necrotic, it is best to allow it to demarcate spontaneously, so long as it is clean and free of drainage.

Bite Injuries

The child's hand often sustains a bite injury or penetration by a sharp organic object. Common household pets (dog, cat) normally have *Eikenella corrodens* or *Pasturella multocida* in their mouth.[271] Wiggins et al. described severe hand infection in a 15-month-old infant bitten by a dog.[273] The wound was initially sutured and the child given oral antibiotics. These lesions should be considered contaminated crush-avulsion injuries requiring aggressive irrigation and débridement; they should never be closed primarily.

Infection of a metacarpophalangeal (MCP) joint resulting from a tooth wound sustained in a fist fight was described in 1911.[268] The injury pattern has been referred to as a "fight bite" and occurs when a clenched fist strikes the opponent's tooth.[267,270] Given the natural tendency of some children to fight, particularly during adolescence, this pattern of injury is likely to occur in all age groups. Because of the flexion of the MCP joint, the impact usually results in a subchondral fracture of the articular and epiphyseal cartilage of the metacarpal epiphysis. The injury also violates the soft tissue dorsal to the joint, allowing bacteria to be implanted directly in the joint, bone, cartilage, and overlying extensor tendons and their sheaths. As the fingers extend after the impact, the soft tissues retract proximally, often sealing the contaminated wound and impeding the search for implanted organisms.

The significance of the fight-bite injury is often overlooked in children. Anyone with a history of such a wound, no matter what size, over a metacarpal head should be treated with suspicion, particularly as children are often poor historians and when involved in fights are reluctant to give a history of the nature of the injury.

Eyres and Allen described a skyline view in which the MCP joint is fully flexed as is the proximal interphalangeal (PIP).[266] The x-ray beam is then directed along the axis of the proximal phalanx. This allows visualization of the metacarpal head and may reveal intraarticular lesions. In the child, with increasing amounts of cartilage involving the epiphysis, such fight-bite lesions may still be difficult to detect. However, it is important to look for these intraarticular fractures, which represent type 3, 4, and 7 growth plate injuries in any child who has a history of hitting an object or person with a hand in a clenched fist position.

Characteristically, roentgenography shows a wedge-shaped defect in the dorsal articular surface subchondral bone of the metacarpal head. It represents a subchondral fracture.

Phair and Quinton studied human bite injuries involving the MCP and PIP joints.[269] All were treated by surgical exploration within 24 hours. In 62% the wound had entered the joint, and in 58% the bone or cartilage was injured. The authors emphasized the concept of "chondral divot fractures," which might increase the likelihood of septic complications. They recommended a combination of surgery and broad-spectrum antibiotics. Bacteriologic culture showed mixed coliforms in eight, *Staphylococcus aureus* in three, *Staphylococcus albus* in one, and anaerobes in 1. In 8 patients the injury was confined to the depths of the skin, whereas in 21 patients the depth of the bite extended to tendon, joint capsule, or chondro-osseous tissue. Seventeen patients had injury to the bone, with eleven osteochondral fragments, four metacarpal head indentations, and two indentations of the metacarpal shaft.

The most important factor governing the final outcome of human fight-bite injuries to the hand is the time elapsed between injury and the commencement of treatment. If left untreated for 24–48 hours, the injury may lead to serious septic arthritis, osteomyelitis, and extension of the soft tissue infection to the deeper spaces of the hand or proximally into the forearm within days to weeks. The two most common organisms usually described for fight-bite injuries include *Staphylococcus* and *Streptococcus* species, although anaerobic organisms may also be encountered.

Seiler et al. reported that venomous snake bites are a relatively common occurrence in the southeastern and southwestern United States.[272] They most commonly involve the pit viper family (Crotalidae). Almost 50% of bites occur on the fingers, and 30% involve children under 13 years. Because of their small size children exhibit the most severe manifestations of envenomation, including coagulopathy, renal failure, compartment syndrome, cardiopulmonary arrest, and even death. There should be judicious use of antibiotics, tetanus, immunization, and antivenom. The use of the latter is preceded by skin testing because of anaphylactic reactions. Compartment syndrome is common and requires appropriate treatment (see Chapters 9, 10).

Open Injuries

The hand is often the site of multiple open injuries (Fig. 17-82). Power tools and machines (especially lawn mowers), explosives (e.g., firecrackers), and firearms may cause not only the obvious acute injuries (Fig. 17-83) but also long-term growth problems (Fig. 17-84).[274,275] The basic treatment of such open wounds is discussed in Chapter 9.

The presence of foreign bodies in open wounds should be suspected in children. Roentgenograms cannot be relied on to visualize foreign bodies, as wood splinters, glass, and other foreign materials, especially biologic ones, may not be radiopaque.

Russell et al. assessed the detection of foreign bodies in the hand.[279,282] Using fresh cadaver hands, they implanted glass, gravel, plastic, and wood in the soft tissues. The methods of assessment were routine radiographs, xeroradiography, CT, and MRI. All types of glass were usually seen by all imaging methods. Gravel was visible with all methods except MRI; usually ferromagnetic streak artifacts obscured visualization. Plastic was not readily seen by routine radiography or xeroradiography, was faintly seen by CT, and was

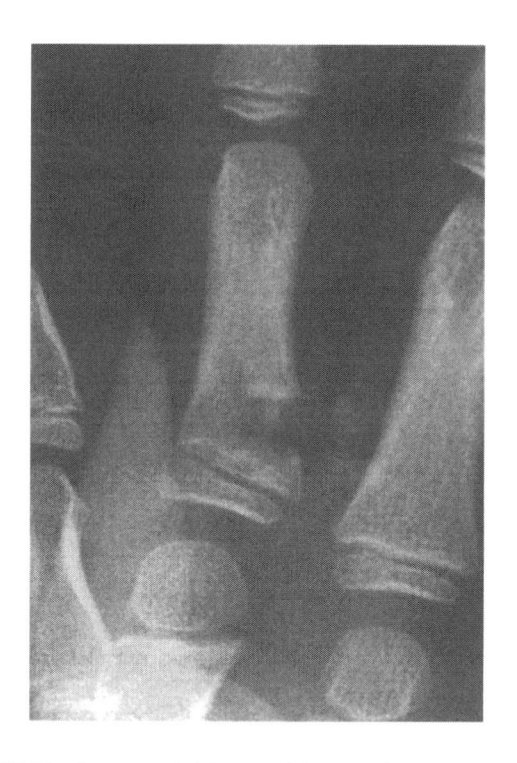

FIGURE 17-82. Open crush injury and fracture from entrapment in a car door.

usually detected by MRI. Wooden foreign bodies, especially when wet, were seen only by CT and MRI. Xeroradiography exhibited no benefit over plain films in identifying foreign bodies and should be discarded in favor of CT or MRI when plain films were unrevealing.

Fackler and Burkhalter emphasized the importance of minimizing excision of uninjured or questionable tissue in the hand and going back to look for further tissue necrosis 24–48 hours later to try to save as much tissue as possible.[277] The intricate anatomy of the hand requires more careful

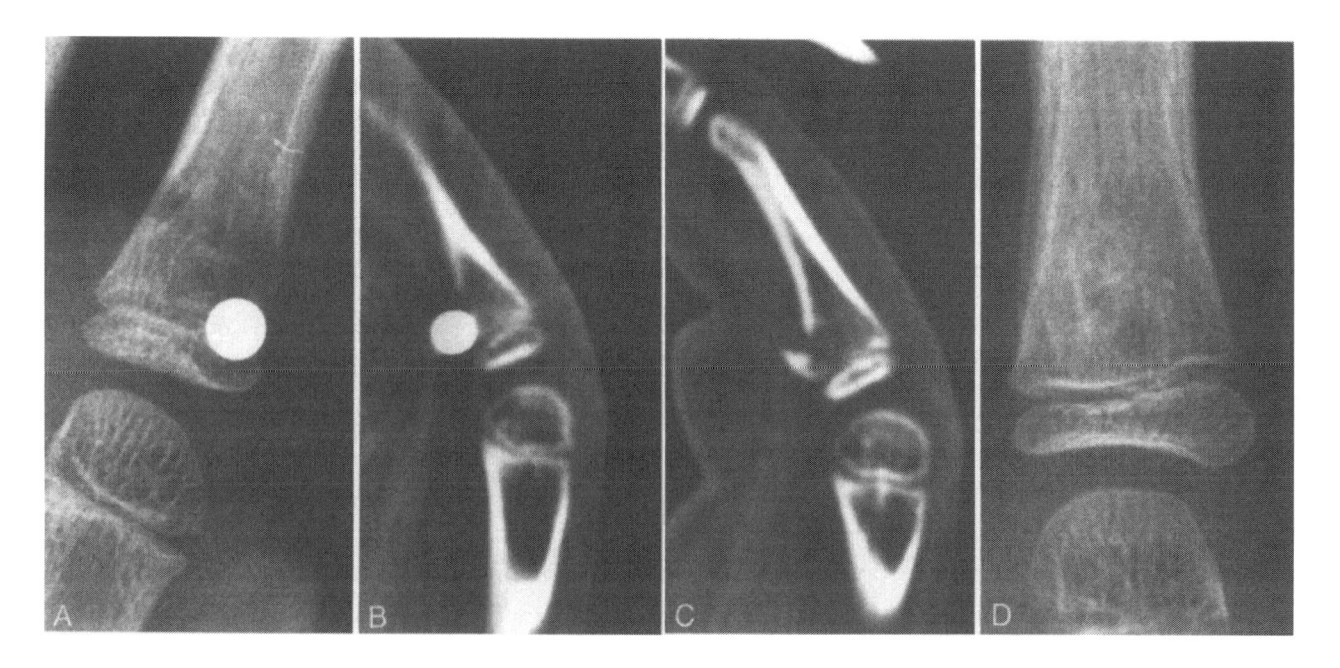

FIGURE 17-83. (A) BB gun injury apparently impinging on the physis. (B, C) Tomographic cuts. (D) Six months after removal.

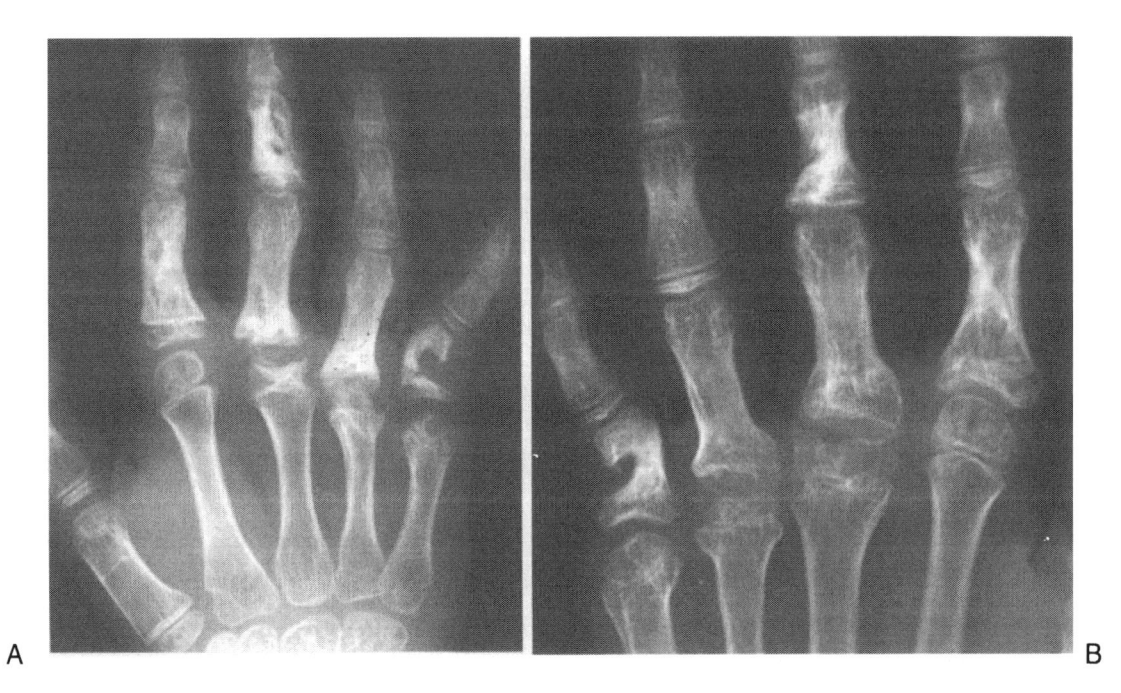

FIGURE 17-84. (A) Lawn mower injury with multiple areas of growth damage. (B) One year later.

attention to tissue excision. Any penetrating projectile must crush sufficient tissue to form a hole, referred to as the permanent cavity. Surrounding tissue is pushed aside by radial stretching. This larger area is referred to as the temporary cavity. The amount of damage caused to such tissue by displacement is dependent on the tissue's elasticity and the extent of displacement.

Fackler and Burkhalter evaluated the ballistics of various penetrating injuries involving bullets and shotgun buckshot.[277] Wound profiles for even the highest velocity military bullets might cause minimal disruption in the initial 12 cm of tissue penetration. Thus when the hand is involved the total tissue path is much less (<12 cm), and the projectile's potential for increased tissue disruption is unlikely to be reached. Accordingly, wounds from high velocity bullets do not differ much from wounds produced by bullets of much lower velocity. However, a bullet striking bone increases the likelihood of more severe tissue disruption. Only necrotic or severely ischemic muscle is excised in the hand and even in the forearm and wrist, as aggressive, potentially unnecessary, excision of questionably viable tissue may increase the ultimate disability by removing tissue that may prove functional so long as it does not become infected. They recommended additional débridement with a "second look" at 1–3 days.

Ada et al. described problems of machinery rolling belt injuries in children in a rural agricultural population.[274] They described 16 children, most of whom were under 4 years of age, whose hands had been caught in the rolling belts of agricultural machinery. Injuries included friction burns; injuries to flexor tendons, digital nerves and arteries, and skin; and fractures. They also had a number of patients who sustained amputations. Their study concentrated on finger injuries. Ten fingers in four patients had total amputations; replantation was attempted in three, with only one patient doing well.

The problems of closure in children who sustain major explosive-type injuries or degloving is the availability of contiguous healthy tissue. Dap et al. described a posterior interosseous flap that they used successfully in 23 cases.[276] The youngest patient was 15 years old.

Reconstruction of these mutilating hand injuries is challenging. Various rotation and free flaps are used for soft tissue loss.[224,226] Phalangeal and metacarpal shortening due to bone loss or growth arrest may be treated by bone graft interposition or gradual lengthening.[278,280,281,283]

Amputations

Amputations at more proximal levels through the distal phalanx or distal interphalangeal joint usually require sophisticated treatment in the operating room. Many techniques for closure and coverage of these amputations have been described.

Replantations and Transplantation

Basic principles of replantation are discussed in Chapter 9. The specific problem of replanted or transplanted epiphyses and their subsequent capacity for growth are discussed in Chapters 6 and 7.

Yamano has recommended replantation of the amputated distal part of the fingers in zones I and II.[304] The normal techniques of microsurgery sometimes have to be modified, especially when there are no veins to anastomose. This modification may require leaving a fishmouth incision and using heparin irrigation. The procedure was done in children as young as 14 months of age.

Significant advances in microvascular surgical techniques have made replantation of entire digits of the hand a clinical reality (Figs. 17-85, 17-86).[284-304] *Not all amputations are suitable for replantation.* If the primary care physician sees a patient with a completely amputated digit, referral should be made as soon as possible to a surgeon experienced in micro-

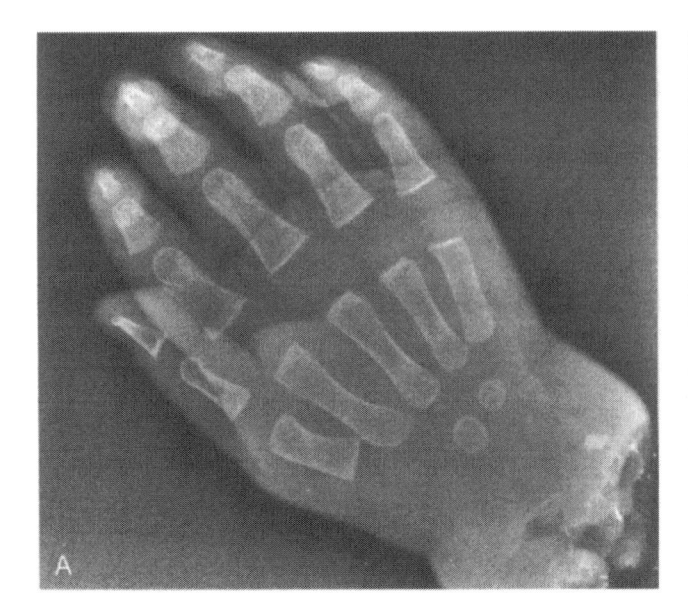

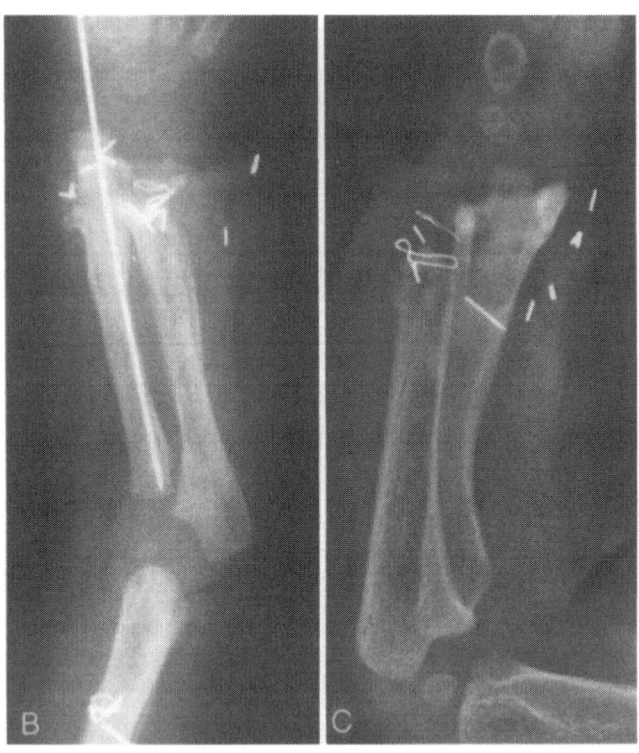

FIGURE 17-85. Replantation of an amputated hand. (A) Radiograph shows the hand to be intact, but fragmentation of the distal radius is present. (B) Four months later. (C) Eight months later.

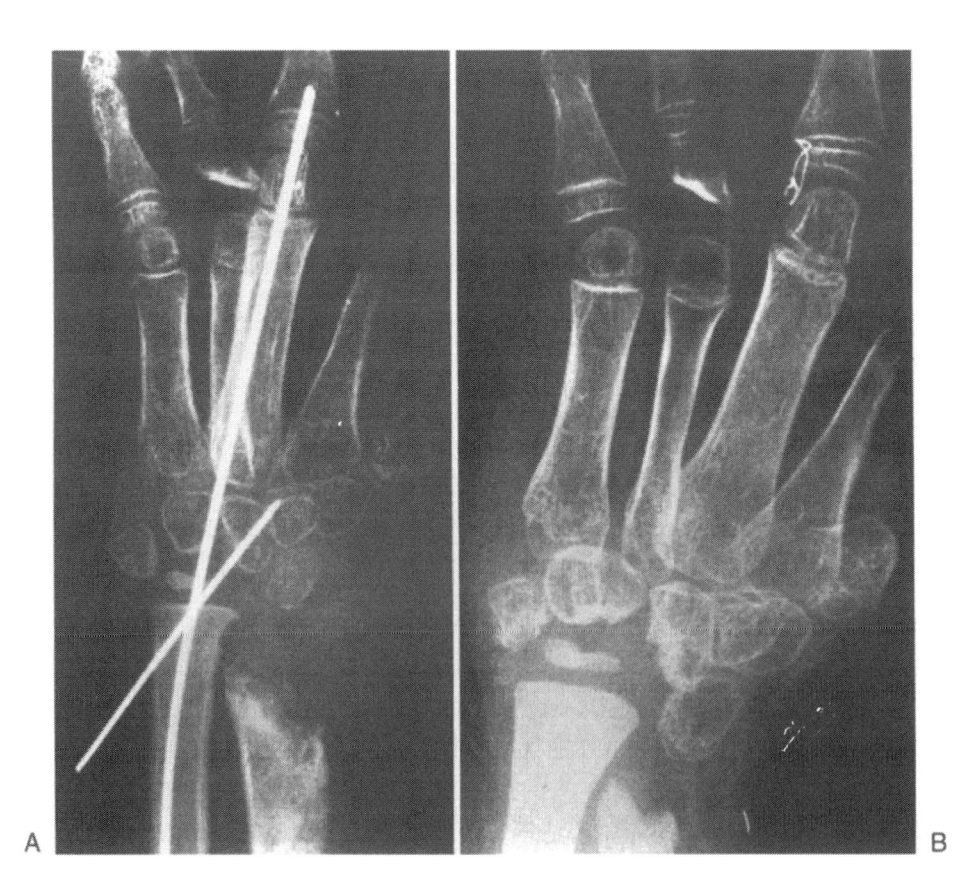

FIGURE 17-86. (A) Centralization of replanted hand on the ulna. (B) One year later.

surgical techniques. The digit should be wrapped in a sterile gauze pad soaked in Ringer's lactate, placed in a plastic bag, and cooled in ice. It should not be frozen, nor should the vessels be cannulated or irrigated.

To be considered thoroughly successful, digital replantation in children after trauma must allow for physeal growth to skeletal maturity, continued finger joint motion, stability of the digit, and viability of the digit. With new techniques for microvascular anastomosis, the survival of replanted digits is becoming more and more frequent. Digital replantation in children has not generally attained the same success achieved with adult replantation, with reported viability rates being no more than 67% compared with 80% in adults. In children undergoing digital replantation with microsurgical repair of digital nerve and flexor tendon, the immediate functional results have generally surpassed results attained in adults. If there is to be normal function of the hand at skeletal maturity, the physis must also continue to grow longitudinally. The hand in a normal child doubles in size between 2 years of age and skeletal maturity.

Saies et al. described the results following 73 replantations and 89 revascularizations of the upper extremity in 120 children.[299] The rate of survival of the amputated part was significantly higher after revascularization (88%) than after replantation (63%). They also found that there was a significantly higher rate of survival after replantation in children who were less than 9 years old (77%) compared to those who were 9-16 years (52%). The one significant factor was the lack of radiographic follow-up to see what the effects were on growth plates and whether compromise of growth plate function similar to frostbite was evident in any of these extremities.

Continuing longitudinal epiphyseal growth has always been a major concern following surgical reconstruction for congenitally defective or traumatically amputated digits in children. Epiphyseal transfers with and without microvascular anastomosis have yielded varying and unpredictable results.[302,303] In general, epiphyses transferred without microvascular anastomosis have rarely grown in a normal manner postoperatively.

Kröpfl et al. stated that only three of their patients had normal growth.[294] Fifteen patients attained 88% of normal growth, and one patient had overgrowth (118%). Four patients developed deviation of the replanted finger in the frontal plane. The cause of deviation in each case was an incorrect primary reposition and not a disturbance of growth of the replanted epiphysis. Demiri et al. reported that the average longitudinal growth in the injured bone was 94.5% in the phalanges of the amputated distal part.[289] Ninkovic et al. described development of an arteriovenous fistula after free flap surgery in a replanted hand.[296]

Phalangeal Lengthening

The lengthening of metacarpals and phalanges after severe hand injuries with loss of bone substance has been used in adults. It has been reported more recently in children.[278,280,281,283] Microfixators should be considered as a means of maintaining length in children who have lost a segment of the phalanx and offer an opportunity for bone grafting when the wound is clean.

Autoamputation

Children with sensory neuropathy syndromes often have severe hand involvement because of self-mutilation. Lack of sensation may result in injuries, especially thermal injuries, which cause skin breakdown and exposure of the chondro-osseous elements. Many of these children have mild mental retardation and may chew their fingers, further exposing bone.

Treatment must always be directed at obtaining soft tissue healing without a complicating infection. Because of the "chewing" mechanism, cellulitis from microorganisms such as *Streptococcus* is just as significant a possibility as staphylococcal osteomyelitis. These wounds should never be closed; granulation and spontaneous epithelialization should be allowed.

Repetitive infection of the bone (chronic osteomyelitis) may require amputation. In a child, amputations are best done at a joint, although this principle is applied less rigidly to a child's hand. Only as much bone as necessary to control infection and assist in soft tissue coverage is removed.

Repetitive trauma may lead to chronic epiphysiolysis or crushing injury to the physis. Either increases the functional loss of the hand and wrist. Because these children cannot perceive pain, the parents should be taught to look for signs of swelling or erythema, especially about the wrist, so roentgenograms may be taken to evaluate the presence of a fracture. Treatment (immobilization) lessens the likelihood of repetitive epiphysiolysis, which is associated with a much higher incidence of premature growth arrest.

Thermal Injuries

The hand is often the site of major thermal injury, which may involve either cold (frostbite) or heat (burn).[305-316] Primary management is generally directed toward obvious soft tissue damage, although long-term effects on the chondro-osseous elements may occur and should be of sufficient concern to warrant serial roentgenograms. The middle phalangeal physes seem particularly susceptible to premature growth arrest, whether the thermal injury is excessive heat or cold.[309,311]

Burns

The appropriate management of a burn injury of the hand is dictated largely by the depth of tissue damage. Superficial epidermal burns are easily diagnosed, and they heal without intervention.[310] On the other hand, partial-thickness (dermal) burns may be superficial or deep, requiring different courses of therapy. Superficial partial-thickness burns also heal by themselves, generally within 3 weeks and without scarring.

In contrast, deep partial-thickness burns, if left alone, heal primarily by wound contracture aided by epidermal proliferation from the few surviving skin appendages. The process takes more than 3 weeks and, if it involves the hand, often results in serious impairment of function.[305,308] As a result, nearly all burn surgeons now recommend early excision and grafting of these wounds. Early wound closure allows early mobilization and prevents joint stiffness and contractures, particularly of the proximal interphalangeal joints. Early wound closure avoids the need for continuous splinting and elevation of the injured extremity. Early wound closure lessens the possibility of wound infection with its attendant risks of further damage to the hand. For all of these reasons, early wound closure reduces the total length of hospitalization of the patient. Finally, the ultimate cosmetic and functional outcome is also improved.

Children with contact burns of the hand that result in more than epidermal injury should be managed in a conservative manner. They should be hospitalized when first seen and consultation arranged. Local wound care and physical therapy can be maximized while providing the opportunity for intensive observation. Given 2–3 days for the burn to declare its own ability to heal, more competent decisions regarding appropriate therapy may be made.

For burns that demonstrate an ability to heal without significant scarring or functional impairment, the brief hospitalization is a justifiable expense. During this time parents may be instructed about the techniques of proper burn care, simplifying outpatient management. An added advantage to hospitalization is the opportunity to provide optimal pain management during the acute stage.

Stern and colleagues reviewed 264 surgically treated proximal interphalangeal joint flexion contractures following burns in children.[312] Contracture severity was determined from preoperative radiographs and physical examination. Eighty per cent of the digits were successfully treated when the postoperative contractures were less than 20°. Unsatisfactory results were present in 12% of the digits, and they were directly proportional to the severity of the contracture and tended to occur in older children with large total body surface burns. The time interval between burn and contracture release did not correlate with contracture severity or therapeutic failure. The most common cause of an unsatisfactory result was failure to release the contracture fully. Generally, simple releases with or without scar excision were performed for type I contractures, with coverage being achieved by skin grafting or Z-plasty. The type I contracture has skin involvement only and does not require joint release. Type II deformities often required a capsular release in addition to the dermal release. Coverage was achieved by skin grafting, Z-plasty, or cross-finger flap. There were only 14 type III contractures; 8 were treated by release and autograft, 5 by arthrodesis, and 1 by cross-finger flap. All fusions were performed through the dorsal approach. Bone shortening was necessary to gain extension and to accommodate the palmar soft tissue contracture.

Graham et al. reviewed 278 postburn MCP joint extension contractures and devised a classification system.[307] Type 1 (47%) had more than 30° of MCP flexion with the wrist fully extended. Scarring was generally limited to the dorsal skin. Type 2 (34%) showed less than 30° of MCP flexion with the wrist maximally extended and scarring typically involved skin, dorsal apparatus, and MCP capsule. Type 3 (19%) exhibited more than 30° of MCP hyperextension and often demonstrated incongruity or dorsal subluxation of the MCP. Improvement after reconstruction was evident in 95% of type 1, 73% of type 2, and 47% of type 3. Failure to improve functionally was related to the adequacy of the scar release. The ring and small fingers accounted for 65% of the digits in this study, 68% of the failures, and all 7 amputations. The authors did not address whether there were areas of thermal injury to the underlying distal metacarpal physes and epiphyses. They did note that an "abnormal radiographic appearance of the MCP joint" often precluded a satisfactory result. They did not stipulate exactly what they meant by "abnormal." The ulnar side of the hand appears particularly vulnerable to the development of extension contractures and accounts for a disproportionally high percentage of unsatisfactory results.

Frostbite

Long-term sequelae of frostbite include premature fusion and abnormal growth of the physes,[314–316] which lead to shortening and deformity of the affected metacarpals and proximal and middle phalanges. There may also be irregular involvement of the physis. The articular surfaces may also have premature degenerative arthritis. Frostbite in children typically affects the forefingers while sparing the thumb, probably because the thumb is protected by being clasped in the palm when the child is outside. The pathologic theories include extracellular ice crystal formation causing chondrocyte damage, ionic shock in chondrocytes owing to abnormal movement of intracellular fluid, and microvascular damage, with the latter being the most likely. A detailed description of this injury pattern and its complications is found in Chapter 6.

Tendon Injuries

Tendon injuries are relatively common in children. They often result from grasping sharp objects. As such, the tendon ends are likely to retract. Treatment of tendon injuries in children is similar to that in adults.[314–346]

In one study glass was the most common cause of injury, involving 30 of 38 patients.[327] Five patients were cut by a knife, and three sustained their injuries by other means. As mentioned previously, the little finger was most commonly injured, followed, in order, by the ring finger, middle finger, and index finger. The most frequent accompanying injury was injury to the digital nerve, which occurred in 20 patients (almost half). There were three fractures of either a carpal or a phalangeal bone.[327]

Levine and Leslie described the use of ultrasonography to detect a radiolucent foreign body in the hand.[279] It was a small piece of glass from a laboratory instrument that was not evident on radiographs. The authors were able to show that the glass was embedded in the deep synovial surface of the flexor pollicis longus, facilitating surgical exposure and removal of a foreign body. They noted that ultrasonography for the detection of small foreign bodies in the hand required slow, meticulous scanning where there are many complex echogenic structures. They also emphasized the importance of studying the extremity from multiple orientations.

Recognizing tendon lacerations is more difficult in the small child than in the adult because of problems of accurate physical examination. Precise testing of specific tendon function in a small child requires considerable skill and patience. It may be virtually impossible to carry out in the painful hand of a frightened, injured child. In such situations the best information is usually gleaned from careful, almost surreptitious observations, specifically looking for a digit that is held in an atypical position or one that does not move in normal synchrony with the other digits. Sometimes the absence of specific muscles is seen by the lack of normal retraction response to gentle pinprick examination.

Passive observation is just as important as active testing of function. Observe whether the child at rest holds all the fingers in the same position. If one finger seems slightly out of position with the rest of the fingers, a tendon injury is suspected. If there is a flexor tendon injury, the involved finger usually lies in more extension than the rest of the digits. In contrast, if a finger lags in flexion when the child extends the fingers, an injury of an extensor tendon should be suspected. Squeezing the forearm may create some motion that aids in diagnosis. Passive motion of the wrist may also be used to look for disparate motion of one finger relative to the rest. Both of the aforementioned tests are suggestive only and do not help diagnose an incomplete injury. In children, nerve injuries frequently occur in association with tendon injuries.

Interestingly, although all children are susceptible to tendon injuries, the incidence appears to be slightly higher during the first 3 years of life. This obviously has a significant effect on the ability to make a diagnosis because of the poor history and the variability of the child to cooperate during a detailed if not complex physical examination. Routine tests for sensation and function may create adverse responses. For instance, a child is more likely to withdraw from pinprick than to be willing to allow repetitive stimulation to delineate a neurologic deficit. The concept of two-point discrimination may not be part of the child's thought processes.

The suspicion of tendon laceration requires thorough exploration with the patient under tourniquet control and adequate anesthesia because it is the only sure way to identify specific tendon injury. Exploration is done in an operating room, where proper equipment is available for tendon repair.

Although concepts regarding the repair of some tendon injuries are often controversial, the current thinking is that the best results in children are likely to be achieved with the primary repair of all lacerated tendons in clean wounds. This includes lacerated flexor tendons in the region often referred to as a "no-man's-land"—that portion of the flexor apparatus between the proximal palmar crease and the proximal interphalangeal joint. Aggressive postoperative therapy is essential to avoid loss of function (Fig. 17-87).

The absence of any part of the total mechanical force, such as the flexor tendons, may be responsible for retardation of bone growth during a child's growth phase.[322] A disturbance in digital growth after an unrepaired tendon injury in the child is a phenomenon that has received little attention. Gaisford and Fleegler reported unrepaired flexor tendon injuries in children that were associated with disturbances of digital growth.[326] No such findings were reported in another study of flexor tendon injuries.[319]

Some studies have documented growth retardation of the finger in which repairs of flexor tendon injuries were significantly delayed.[322,326] The actions of appropriate

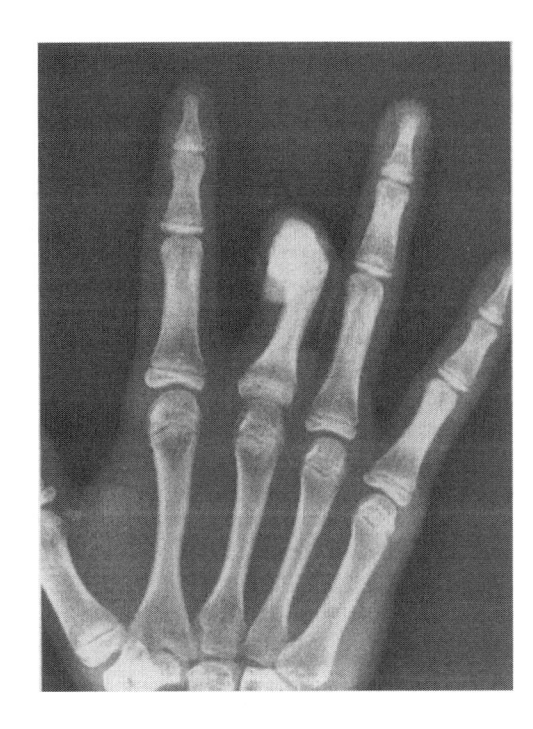

FIGURE 17-87. Tendon injury followed by contracture of the digit.

mechanical forces resulting from tendon lacerations causes the growth disturbance. Again, this complication of delayed repair may be potentially avoided by primary repair. Maintaining normal tension may be the most important factor in longitudinal tendon growth.[340]

There must be concern for whether the tendon will grow. Maintaining normal tension may be the most important factor in longitudinal tendon growth.[340] A study by Hage and Dupuis suggested that the graft elongates with growth of the child,[328] but the elongation may have been growth at either end of the original tendon rather than within the graft itself. Interestingly, they noted that the fingers requiring tendon grafts were smaller and thinner than those of the contralateral hand. There is virtually no published material on the behavior of grafted tendon tissue with growth.

Flexor Tendons

O'Connell et al. reviewed 78 patients younger than 16 years who had 95 flexor tendon lacerations and repairs in zone I or II.[341] The average postrepair follow-up interval was 24 months. They divided their patient groups into 0–5 years, 6–10 years, and 11–15 years of age. All repairs in zone I returned to excellent function. The repairs in zone II achieved comparable results when managed with an early *passive* motion program following immobilization for 3–4 weeks. Immobilization for longer than 4 weeks resulted in appreciable deterioration of function. In many digits, noticeably improved digital motion was found when the patients returned after several years of continued growth.

Lacerations of the flexor tendons in the carpal canal region (zone IV) should be repaired primarily. Some of the carpal ligaments are left intact to prevent bowstring displacement. Primary repairs are indicated for all lacerations in the palm of the hand (zone III). To minimize scarring, the palmar fascia over the tendon juncture is excised. Results of the primary repair of flexor tendons in the digital sheaths (zone II) have been unpredictable. Repair of the profundus tendon and excision of the subliminus tendon are recommended with repair of the sheath when both are injured in children under 4 years of age. If the sheath cannot be repaired, the surgeon should consider a fascia graft, although there is no evidence in children that this practice improves the repair results.

Stahl et al. compared 17 partially lacerated flexor tendons (less than 75% of the cross-sectional area) in children treated by surgical repair to that of 19 tendons treated nonoperatively.[344] The outcome of the two groups was comparably favorable. There were no complications, such as triggering or furthering of the tear in either group. The authors advocated early mobilization for partial tear and exploration for complete tear.

Bell et al. have advocated using tendon grafts for injuries within the digital sheath in children.[319] The proximal superficialis flexor tendon is the preferred source of graft when both tendons have been lacerated. Other sources of tendon grafts include the palmaris longus, a toe extensor, or the plantaris tendon. In children the superficial and deep tendons tend to be the same size, in contrast to those in adults.

Satisfactory results may be obtained by primary repair of tendon lacerations in the distal portions (zone I). It is important in children to repair the tendon laceration rather than advancing the profundus, so suture lines do not cross the epiphyseal plate of the distal phalanx. The flexor pollicis longus may be repaired primarily at any level in children with consistently good results.[327] Two-stage tendon grafts are rarely necessary in children. The advantages of primary repair include a shortened period of disability, lack of stiffness, and decreased incidence of joint contractures. Secondary procedures are not usually necessary.

Postoperatively, it is essential to protect the surgical repair, which is made difficult by the inability or unwillingness of the young child to cooperate or understand the importance of total postoperative immobilization as part of the rehabilitation. Children under 5 years of age should be immobilized, which may involve an enveloping cast that does not allow any type of finger motion. Children over 5 years, particularly over 7 years, are probably more mature and better able to understand the concept of immobilization. It is also important to immobilize the elbow in a cast because the child will move the muscle masses of the extensor and flexor tendons. Immobilization is maintained for 3–4 weeks. Following cast removal use of the hand and wrist is encouraged. The parents are instructed in passive range of motion, and the child is encouraged to play. Aggressive, defined occupational therapy is probably unnecesary in most children.

Tenolysis, the surgical release of nongliding adhesions after tendon repair, may be used in children. The same attention to detail necessary in an adult must be applied to the child. Significant improvement in active flexion after tenolysis is more likely to occur in children over 11 years of age.[320]

Grobbelaar and Hudson studied tendon injuries in 38 children with a mean age of 6.7 years.[327] All were treated by primary suture and controlled remobilization. There were 53 tendon injuries with an average of 1.5 digits per patient; most commonly the little finger was injured (23 of 38 patients). Sixty percent of the injuries occurred in zone II. These authors found that repair of both the flexor digitorum superficialis (FDS) and the flexor digitorum profundus (FDP) was better than repair of the FDP alone, even in zone II. Eighty-two percent achieved excellent or good results. There were three tendon ruptures, and all were classified as poor results. Other poor results occurred with a zone II injury with an associated ulnar nerve palsy. Grobbelaar and Hudson believed that the outcome of flexor tendon repair in children was much better than that in adults because of rapid healing of the tendons. No child in their series required subsequent tenolysis due to adhesions. They strongly emphasized that both flexor tendons should be repaired, irrespective of the zone of injury.

Woods and Sicilia reviewed congenital trigger digits, emphasizing that they sometimes present following an apparent injury with the parent having been unaware of the lesion before.[346] The tendency in the child is for involvement with the thumb. Surgical treatment is simple and effective. The diagnosing physician should be aware of the fact that these injuries are more likely to be congenital than a consequence of trauma.

Miura et al. showed that among 62 patients with camptodactyly of the little finger, only 5 failed to respond to conservative treatment.[339] Ogino and Kato showed that in five of six cases of camptodactyly, the FDS tendon was hypoplastic and there was no continuity of the normal tendon between the muscle belly and the osseous insertion.[342]

Extensor Tendons

Extensor tendon injuries are just as important as flexor tendon injuries (Fig. 17-88) but do not usually receive the same emphasis in the literature. Primary repair in the child is currently the treatment of choice at all levels of injury. Attention must be paid particularly to the various types of mallet finger equivalents at the distal phalanx in which some or all of the epiphysis is displaced, effectively shortening the extensor tendon and leaving the nonrepaired finger with a permanent flexion deformity. Primary repair allows adequate exploration of the wound in an otherwise apprehensive individual. Unrecognized injuries may require tendon grafts or transfers. In either case, postoperative immobilization is paramount. The recommendation of 30° of wrist extension and 15° of MCP flexion should not be approached as rigidly in a child because of the rapidity with which they overcome contractures. These tendons are much thinner and more ribbon-like than the flexor tendon and must be protected for a longer period of time, usually up to 6 weeks.

Posner and McMahon described congenital radial subluxation of the extensor tendons in a boy who complained of increasing pain and snapping at the MCP joints with active finger flexion.[343] It was surgically repaired with an excellent result. They noted that the tightness of the radial, sagittal, and transverse bands of the dorsal hood was the cause of the

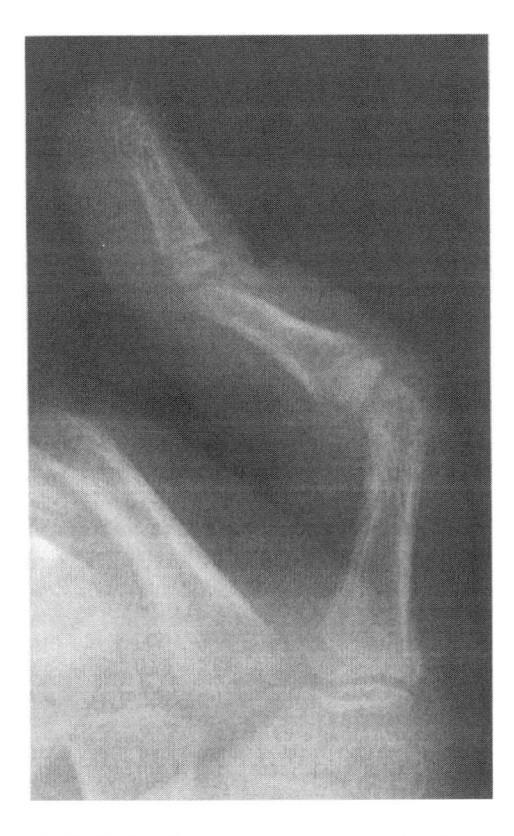

FIGURE 17-88. Deformity after an unrepaired extensor tendon laceration.

radial shift. They also noted that there were at least two similiar cases in the literature that had resulted from trauma involving a single finger.

Calcification

Acute calcific tendinitis has been described in a child.[338] It was found in a 10-year-old boy who had had a week of progressive pain and swelling. It was initially diagnosed as a finger infection. The patient denied trauma. There was calcification in the flexor tendon region adjacent to the proximal phalangeal metaphysis. The patient was splinted, and within 1 month the calcification disappeared.

Nerve Injuries

Recognizing nerve injuries in children is even more difficult than recognizing tendon injuries. A lacerated digital nerve in the small child is almost impossible to diagnose by physical examination alone, and even injury to the major nerves in the forearm may be difficult to demonstrate objectively.

Severance of a peripheral nerve includes sensory and motor function and sympathetic intervention. Simply touching the fingertips may indicate a difference in moistness in a child, which helps with the diagnosis. The diagnosis may be ascertained with little patient cooperation. A smooth piece of plastic, such as the barrel of a pen, may be drawn across the surface of the fingertips. In the presence of sweating, there is adhesion between the plastic and the fingertip; in fact, a plastic device may squeak against dry skin.[353]

Instead of using pinprick, scratch the fingertip with a fingernail and then stroke it with the pulp of the examiner's finger.[350] If the patient can feel the difference, the nerve is probably intact. If the patient cannot discriminate, it is likely that nerve function has been damaged. Furthermore, if the child cannot discriminate between fingernail scratch and simple touch, he probably cannot feel a pin stick. The child may also respond to actual or anticipated poking in a reactive way (i.e., anticipating pain from a sharp object) rather than as a response to the invoked pain. Another trick is to immerse the hand in water. Finger skin with intact sensation wrinkles after being submerged in lukewarm water after about 5 minutes, whereas denervated areas remain smooth.

The size and location of the skin laceration aid little in the diagnosis, as a penetrating wound may extend a great distance from the point of injury, and a small, benign-appearing skin laceration often masks rather extensive underlying soft tissue injuries. A tiny puncture wound in the palm is often overlooked as the point of injury that could result in a digital nerve laceration.

Because primary repair of lacerated nerves in clean wounds is likely to give the best results, recognizing these injuries when the child is first seen is important. It is imperative that all penetrating wounds with any possibility of nerve laceration be examined under appropriate conditions, including adequate anesthesia and tourniquet control. A lacerated nerve should be repaired in the operating room under appropriate magnification.

Primary nerve repair utilizes the operating microscope and may or may not necessitate someone specifically skilled in techniques of nerve repair. Because children in general have better regeneration after repair of peripheral nerves, most surgeons do an epineural suture for divided nerves in the child's hand. Fascicular nerve repairs and suturing are probably not necessary in a child unless there are nontransverse lacerations.

Most articles dealing with peripheral nerve suture conclude that children regenerate sensation better than adults with similar injuries. However, the mechanism of improved functional recovery is still in question. Almquist et al. studied nerve conduction velocities and microscopically evaluated median nerves in baby and adult monkeys.[347] Three years after laceration and repair, nerve conduction velocities were essentially identical. The only difference was that the infants had slightly more accidents than the adults. This study suggested that there is no difference in axon regeneration at any age; rather, the improved sensory recovery is most likely related to the intrinsic elasticity of the central nervous system in children.

Although some surgeons advocate sensory reeducation after suture of peripheral nerves, children probably experience spontaneous postoperative sensory reeducation with the activities of daily living. Children have an intrinsic mechanism that encourages the use of an extremity or a digit if it has sufficient sensation and motion to be of any function.

Return of muscle function following nerve repair usually lags behind return of sensibility. A minimum of a year is required to assess return of motor function, especially in the hand. When motor deficits persist after peripheral nerve injury, standard tendon transfers that apply to adult radial, medial, and ulnar nerve palsies may also be useful in children. The few transfers that require bony insertions must be modified to ensure that open physes are not damaged.

Poilvache et al. described carpal tunnel syndrome (CTS) during childhood.[354] One of their cases was posttraumatic. This boy had sustained a palmar wound in his right hand at the age of 2 years. Surgical exploration had revealed a partial laceration of the transverse carpal ligament. From age 2 to 9 he was asymptomatic, after which pain gradually developed. Surgical release at age 10 years led to complete subsidence of symptoms. Most cases of CTS in children are usually associated with space-occupying lesions (e.g., congenital abnormalities such as neurofibroma or angioma).[349,351,352] CTS may appear after fractures of the distal end of the radius or burns.[348]

Hair Strangulation

Because of the propensity of small children to take hands and fingers they have been sucking and to then twirl them in their hair or to play with clothing that may be frayed may lead to digital constriction.[355–361] According to Abel and McFarland, this was first reported in 1832 and involved a constricting band around the penis.[355] Since then, approximately 70 additional cases have been reported involving the toes, fingers, and genitals. In the various reviews, the incidence of involvement was the toes in 44%, the genitals in 32%, and the fingers in 24%. The mean age for patients with involvement of the toes is 4 months. Finger involvement, interestingly, tends to present within the first month of life, averaging 3 weeks of age.

Abel and McFarland stated that the exact pathologic sequence was not known.[355] Infants have a tendency to twirl objects such as hair, causing it to become encircled around the involved region; and continued movements and growth may result in tightening of the hairs with resultant initial lymphatic obstruction. As swelling and growth continue, the hairs may cut into the skin, causing more inflammation and making a diagnosis more difficult.

These children may present a diagnostic dilemma to a primary care physician or pediatrician who initially confronts a swollen digit in a child, especially in the office or emergency room. The constricting agents are often difficult to see, particularly when it involves blond hair or a light fabric. Successful treatment obviously depends on prompt recognition of the problem and alleviation of the constriction, which usually involves isolating the constriction material, which then may be cut to remove it. The use of magnifying loupes enhances the ability to visualize the material. In rare instances partial resection of some tissue may be necessary. Of the reported cases, approximately 50% were successfully managed with specific removal of the hairs or threads in the emergency room. Operative exploration with sharp dissection was done to release the constrictions in all of the remaining patients, except two who required amputation.[356]

References

Anatomy

1. Ames EL, Bissonnette M, Acland R, Lister G, Firrell J. Arterial anatomy of the thumb. J Hand Surg [Br] 1993;18:427–436.
2. Berger RA, Landsmeer JMF. The palmar radiocarpal ligaments: a study of adult and fetal human wrist joints. J Hand Surg [Am] 1990;15:847–854.
3. Bogumill GP. A morphologic study of the relationship of collateral ligaments to growth plates in the digits. J Hand Surg [Am] 1983;8:74–79.
4. Caffey J. Pediatric X-ray Diagnosis, 8th ed. Chicago: Year Book, 1985.
5. Compson JP, Waterman JK, Heatley FW. The radiological anatomy of the scaphoid. J Hand Surg [Br] 1994;19:183–187.
6. Flake J, Light TR, Ogden JA. Postnatal growth of the flexor tendon pulley system. J Pediatr Orthop 1990;10:612–617.
7. Garn SM, Burdi AR, Babler WJ. Prenatal origins of carpal fusions. Am J Phys Anthropol 1976;45:203–208.
8. Gelberman RH, Menonn J. The vascularity of the scaphoid bone. J Hand Surg [Am] 1980;5:508–513.
9. Haines RW. The pseudoepiphysis of the first metacarpal in man. J Anat 1974;117:145–158.
10. Handley RC, Pooley J. The venous anatomy of the scaphoid. J Anat 1991;178:115–118.
11. Hankin F, Janda D. Tendon and ligament attachments in relationship to growth plates in a child's hand. J Hand Surg [Br] 1989;14:315–318.
12. Kobayashi H, Kosakai Y, Usui M, Ishii S. Bilateral deficiency of ossification of the lunate bone. J Bone Joint Surg Am 1991;73:1255–1256.
13. Kuczynski K. The proximal interphalangeal joint: anatomy and causes of stiffness in the fingers. J Bone Joint Surg Br 1968;50:656–663.
14. Ogden JA, Conlogue GJ, Light TR. Correlative roentgenography and morphology of the longitudinal epiphyseal bracket. Skeletal Radiol 1981;6:107–117.
15. Ogden JA, Ganey TM, Light TR, Belsole RJ, Greene TL. Ossification and pseudoepiphysis formation in the "nonepiphyseal" end of bones of the hands and feet. Skeletal Radiol 1994;23:3–13.
16. Ogden JA, Ganey TM, Light TR, Greene TL, Belsole RJ. Nonepiphyseal ossification and pseudoepiphysis formation. J Pediatr Orthop 1994;14:78–82.
17. Simmons P, Coleridge Smith P, Lees WR, McGrouther DA. Venous pumps of the hand: their clinical importance. J Hand Surg [Br] 1996;21:595–599.
18. Stuart HC, Pyle SI, Cornoni J, Reed RB. Onsets, completions, and spans of ossifications in the 29 bone-growth centers of the hand and wrist. Pediatrics 1962;29:237–249.
19. Watson HK, Light TR, Johnson RT. Checkrein resection for flexion contracture of the middle joint. J Hand Surg [Am] 1979;4:67–71.

General

20. Almquist EE. Hand injuries in children. Pediatr Clin North Am 1986;33:1511–1522.
21. Aufaure PM, Bendjeddou M, Gilbert A. Fractures du poignet et de la main chez l'enfant. Ann Chir 1982;36:499–506.
22. Beaton AA, Williams L, Moseley LG. Handedness and hand injuries. J Hand Surg [Br] 1994;19:158–161.
23. Beaty E, Light TR, Belsole RJ, Ogden JA. Wrist and hand skeletal injuries in children. Hand Clin North Am 1990;6:723–738.

24. Bhende MS, Dandrea LA, Davis HW. Hand injuries in children presenting to a pediatric emergency department. Ann Emerg Med 1993;22:1519–1523.
25. Bora FW Jr, Nissenbaum M, Ignatius P. The treatment of epiphyseal fractures of the hand. Orthop Dig 1976;5:11–13.
26. Borde J, Dayot P. Fractures des metacarpiens et des phalanges chez l'enfant. Ann Orthop Ouest 1972;4:92–110.
27. Borde J, Lefort J. Injuries of the wrist and hand in children. In: Tubiana R (ed) The Hand, vol II. Philadelphia: Saunders, 1985.
28. Campbell RM Jr. Operative treatment of fractures and dislocations of the hand and wrist region in children. Orthop Clin North Am 1990;21:217–243.
29. Carroll RE, Seitz WH Jr, Putnam MD. Acute calcium deposit in the hand of an 11-year-old girl. J Pediatr Orthop 1985;5:468–470.
30. Danilov AA, Schitov VS, Panasink VA, Pokopishin AL. Osteointez pri perelomakh kostei kisti u detei. [Osteosynthesis in hand bone fractures in children]. Orthop Traumatol Protez 1991;4:18–12.
31. Davis TRC, Stothard J. Why all finger fractures should be referred to a hand surgery service: a prospective study of primary management. J Hand Surg [Br] 1990;15:299–302.
32. Eaton RG. Hand problems in children. Pediatr Clin North Am 1967;14:643–658.
33. Ehalt W. Über die Bruche des ersten Mittelhandknochens und ihre Behandlung. Arch Orthop Unfallchir 1929;27:515–520.
34. Fischer MD, McElfresh EC. Physeal and periphyseal injuries of the hand. Hand Clin 1994;10:287–301.
35. Freilinger G. Zur Handchirurgie beim Kleinkind. Z Klin Med 1964;11:212–217.
36. Grad JB. Children's skeletal injuries. Orthop Clin North Am 1986;17:437–449.
37. Green DP. Hand injuries in children. Pediatr Clin North Am 1977;24:903–918.
38. Greene TL, Noellert RC, Belsole RJ, Simpson LA. Composite wiring of metacarpal and phalangeal fractures. J Hand Surg [Am] 1989;14:665–669.
39. Griffin PA, Robinson DN. Paediatric hand injuries and the galvanized-iron fence. Med J Aust 1985;150:644–645.
40. Hager DL. Hand injuries in children. Contemp Orthop 1982;4:631–655.
41. Hastings H II, Simmons BP. Hand fractures in children. Clin Orthop 1984;188:120–130.
42. Herndon JH. Hand injuries: special considerations in children. Emerg Med Clin North Am 1985;3:405–413.
43. Innis PC. Office evaluation and treatment of finger and hand injuries in children. Curr Opin Pediatr 1995;7:83–87.
44. Johnson CF, Kaufman KL, Callendar C. The hand as a target organ in child abuse. Clin Pediatr 1990;29:66–72.
45. Knorr P. Entwicklungsstörungen nach Hand- und Fingerfrakturen im Kindesalter. PhD dissertation, University of Leipzig, 1969.
46. Komarertsev VD, Blandinskii VF. [Closed injuries of finger bones in children] (in Russian). Vestn Khirurg Grekova 1990;145:76–78.
47. Landin LA. Fracture patterns in children: analysis of 8682 fractures with special reference to incidence, etiology and secular changes in a Swedish urban population 1950–1979. Acta Orthop Scand 1983;54(suppl 202):1–109.
48. Larsen CF, Brondum V, Wienholtz G, Abrahamsen J, Beyer J. An algorithm for acute wrist trauma. J Hand Surg [Br] 1993;18:207–212.
49. Leonard MH, Dubravicik P. Management of fractured fingers in the child. Clin Orthop 1970;73:160–168.
50. Lindsay WK. Hand injuries in children. Clin Plast Surg 1976;3:65–75.
51. Lindsay WK. Hand injuries in children. Pediatr Clin North Am 1986;33:1911–1923.
52. Lucas GL. Internal fixation in the hand: a review of indications and methods. Orthopaedics 1980;3:1083–1089.
53. Malek R. Hand surgery in children. In: Tubiana R (ed) The Hand, vol II. Philadelphia: Saunders, 1985.
54. Montgomery MT, Waters PM. Management of acute fractures and late sequelae in pediatric wrist trauma. Curr Opin Orthop 1995;6:11–17.
55. Parsons SW, Fitzgerald JA, Shearer JR. External fixation of unstable metacarpal and phalangeal fractures. J Hand Surg [Br] 1992;17:151–155.
56. Rankin EA, Jabaley ME, Blair SJ, Fraser KE. Acquired rotational digital deformity in children as a result of finger sucking. J Hand Surg [Am] 1988;13:535–539.
57. Rayan GM, Turner WT. Hand complications in children from digital sucking. J Hand Surg [Am] 1989;14:933–936.
58. Reid DA, Price AH. Digital deformities and dental malocclusion due to finger sucking. Br J Plast Surg 1984;37:445–452.
59. Ruggeri S, Osterman AL, Bora FW. Stabilization of metacarpal and phalangeal fractures in the hand. Orthop Rev 1980;9:107–110.
60. Samuel AW. Epiphyseal injuries in the hand. Injury 1981;12:503–505.
61. Sandzen SC. Growth plate injuries of the wrist and hand. Am Fam Physician 1984;29:153–168.
62. Sandzen SC. Physeal (epiphyseal growth plate) injuries. In: Atlas of Wrist and Hand Fractures, 2nd ed. Littleton, MA: PSG Publishing, 1986.
63. Scharli AF. Osteosynthese kindlicher hand- und fussfrakturen nach dem Zuggurtungsprinzip. Unfallchirurgie 1980;6:24–27.
64. Simmons BP. Injuries to and developmental deformities of the wrist and carpus. In: Bora FW (ed) The Pediatric Upper Extremity. Philadelphia: Saunders, 1986.
65. Simmons BP, Hastings H. Hand fractures in children: a statistical analysis. In: Tubiana R (ed) The Hand, vol II. Philadelphia: Saunders, 1985.
66. Simmons BP, Lovallo JL. Hand and wrist injuries in children. Clin Sports Med 1988;7:495–512.
67. Stalter K, Smoot EC, Osler T. Method for elevating the pediatric hand. Plast Reconstr Surg 1988;81:788.
68. Stone OJ, Mullins JF. Chronic paronychia in children. Clin Pediatr 1976;2:104–108.
69. Strickland JW. Bone, nerve and tendon injuries of the hand in children. Pediatr Clin North Am 1975;22:451–463.
70. Wakefield AR. Hand injuries in children. J Bone Joint Surg Am 1964;46:1226–1234.
71. Wavak P. The use of antibiotics in acute hand injuries. Orthop Rev 1981;10:141–143.
72. Williams GS. Hand injuries in children: late problems. Clin Plast Surg 1977;4:503–511.
73. Wood VE. Fractures of the hand in children. Orthop Clin North Am 1976;7:527–542.
74. Worlock PH, Stower MJ. The incidence and pattern of hand fractures in children. J Hand Surg [Br] 1986;11:198–200.
75. Wynn SK, Wiviott W. Hand injuries in children. Int Surg 1966;46:283.

Carpus

76. Abbitt PL, Riddervold HO. The carpal tunnel view: helpful adjuvant for unrecognized fractures of the carpus. Skeletal Radiol 1987;16:45–47.

77. Albert MC, Barre PS. A scaphoid fracture in association with a displaced distal radial fracture in a child. Clin Orthop 1989;240:232–235.
78. Anderson WJ. Simultaneous fracture of the scaphoid and capitate in a child. J Hand Surg [Am] 1987;12:271–273.
79. Aufaure P, Bendjeddou M, Gilbert A. Fracture du poignet et de la main chez l'enfant. Ann Chir 1982;36:499–506.
80. Barrick WT, Terrin A, Mewberg AH. Refracture of a proximal pole scaphoid fracture: a case report. J Hand Surg [Am] 1994;19:241–242.
81. Bloem JJA. Fractures of the carpal scaphoid in a child aged 4. Arch Chir Neerl 1971;23:91–93.
82. Caputo AE, Watson HK, Hissen C. Scaphoid non-union in a child: a case report. J Hand Surg [Am] 1995;20:243–245.
83. Christodoulou AG, Colton CL. Scaphoid fractures in children. J Pediatr Orthop 1986;6:37–39.
84. Compson JP. Transcarpal injuries associated with distal radial fractures in children: a series of three cases. J Hand Surg [Br] 1992;17:311–314.
85. Cooney WP, Linscheid RL, Dobyns JH. Triangular fibrocartilage tears. J Hand Surg [Am] 1994;19:143–154.
86. Craigen MAC. Recurrent locking of the wrist due to dorsal midcarpal subluxation. J Bone Joint Surg [Br] 1996;78:664–666.
87. Cristiani G, Cerojokni E, Squarzina PB, et al. Evaluation of ischaemic necrosis of carpal bones by magnetic resonance imaging. J Hand Surg [Br] 1990;15:249–255.
88. Dautel G, Goudot B, Merle M. Arthroscopic diagnosis of scapho-lunate instability in the absence of x-ray abnormalities. J Hand Surg [Br] 1993;18:213–218.
89. DeBoeck H, Van Wellen P, Haentjens P. Nonunion of a carpal scaphoid fracture in a child. J Orthop Trauma 1991;5:370–372.
90. DeCoster TA, Faherty S, Morris AL. Pediatric carpal fracture dislocation. J Orthop Trauma 1994;8:76–78.
91. De Smet L, Fabry G, Stoffelen D, Broos P. Displaced fracture of the lunate in a child. Acta Orthop Belg 1993;59:137–139.
92. Doman AN, Marcus NW. Congenital bipartite scaphoid. J Hand Surg [Am] 1990;15:869–873.
93. Finkenberg JG, Hoffer E, Kelly C, Zinar DM. Diagnosis of occult scaphoid fractures by ultrasound vibration. J Hand Surg [Am] 1993;18:4–7.
94. Gamble JG, Simmons SC. Bilateral scaphoid fractures in a child. Clin Orthop 1982;162:125–128.
95. Gerard RM. Post-traumatic carpal instability in a young child. J Bone Joint Surg [Am] 1980;62:131–133.
96. Gibbons WW, Jackson A. An isolated capitate fracture in a 9-year-old boy. Br J Radiol 1989;62:487–488.
97. Giddin GEB, Shaw DG. Lunate subluxation associated with a Salter-Harris type 2 fracture of the distal radius. J Hand Surg [Br] 1994;19:193–194.
98. Gilula LA. Carpal injuries: analytic approach and case exercises. AJR 1979;133:503–517.
99. Gilula LA, Weeks PM. Post-traumatic ligamentous instabilities of the wrist. Radiology 1978;129:641–651.
100. Gouldesbrough C. A case of fracture scaphoid and os magnum in a boy ten years old. Lancet 1916;2:792–793.
101. Green WB, Anderson WJ. Simultaneous fracture of the scaphoid and radius in a child. J Pediatr Orthop 1982;2:191–194.
102. Greene MH, Hadied AM, LaMont RL. Scaphoid fractures in children. J Hand Surg [Am] 1984;9:536–541.
103. Gruber W. Os navicular carpi bipartitum. Arch Pathol Anat 1877;69:391–396.
104. Grundy M. Fractures of the carpal scaphoid in children. Br J Surg 1969;56:523–524.
105. Horii E, Nakamura R, Watanabe K, Tsunoda K. Scaphoid fractures as a "puncher's fracture." J Orthop Trauma 1994;8:107–110.
106. Kerlinke L, McCabe SJ. Nonunion of the scaphoid: a critical analysis of recent natural history studies. J Hand Surg [Am] 1993;18:1–3.
107. Kleinman WB, Grantham SA. Multiple volar carpometacarpal joint dislocation. J Hand Surg [Am] 1978;3:377–382.
108. Kohler Z, Zimmer EA. Borderlands of the Normal and Early Pathologic in Skeletal Roentgenology, 10th ed. Orlando: Grune & Stratton, 1956.
109. Lahoti O, Wong J, Regan B, Fogarty EE, Dowling FE. Fracture of the scaphoid associated with volar displacement of a lower radial epiphyseal fracture. Scand J Plast Reconstr Hand Surg 1993;27:195–196.
110. Larson B, Light TR, Ogden JA. Fracture and ischemic necrosis of the immature scaphoid. J Hand Surg [Am] 1987;12:122–127.
111. Letts M, Esser D. Fractures of the triquetrum in children. J Pediatr Orthop 1993;13:228–231.
112. Light TR. Injury to the immature carpus. Hand Clin 1988;4:415–424.
113. Lindström G, Nyström Å. Natural history of scaphoid nonunion, with special reference to "asymptomatic" cases. J Hand Surg [Br] 1992;17:697–700.
114. Littlefield WG, Friedman RL, Urbaniak JR. Bilateral nonunion of the carpal scaphoid in a child. J Bone Joint Surg Am 1995;77:124–126.
115. London PS. The broken scaphoid bone. J Bone Joint Surg Br 1961;43:237–244.
116. Louis DS, Calhoun TP, Garn SM. Congenital bipartite scaphoid: fact or fiction? J Bone Joint Surg Am 1976;58:1108–1112.
117. Mack GR, Bosse JJ, Gelberman RH, Yu E. The natural history of scaphoid nonunion. J Bone Joint Surg Am 1984;66:504–509.
118. Macrosson KI. Sprain fracture of the carpal scaphoid in children. Lancet 1946;1:341–342.
119. Masquelet A-C, Gilbert A. Traumatismes de la main chez l'enfant. Traum Enfant 1986;36:33–41.
120. Maxted MJ, Owen R. Two cases of non-union of carpal scaphoid fractures in children. Injury 1982;12:441–443.
121. Mazet R Jr, Hohl M. Fractures of the carpal navicular. J Bone Joint Surg Am 1963;45:82–112.
122. McClain EJ, Boyer JH. Missed fractures of the greater multangular. J Bone Joint Surg Am 1966;48:1525–1528.
123. McCoy GF, Graham HK, Piggot J. Nonunion of fractures of the carpal scaphoid in a child. Ulster Med J 1956;56:66–67.
124. Minami M, Yamazaki J, Chisaka N, et al. Nonunion of the capitate. J Hand Surg [Am] 1987;12:1089–1091.
125. Mintzer C, Waters PM. Acute open reduction of a displaced scaphoid fracture in a child. J Hand Surg [Am] 1994;19:760–761.
126. Mussbichler H. Injuries of the carpal scaphoid in children. Acta Radiol [Diagn] (Stockh) 1961;56:361–368.
127. Nafie SA. Fractures of the carpal bones in children. Injury 1987;18:117–119.
128. Nakamura R, Imaeda T, Miura T. Scaphoid malunion. J Bone Joint Surg Br 1991;73:134–137.
129. Onuba O, Ireland J. Two cases of nonunion of fractures of the scaphoid in children. Injury 1984;15:109–112.
130. Peiro A, Martos F, Mut T, Aracil J. Trans-scaphoid perilunate dislocation in a child. Acta Orthop Scand 1981;52:31–34.
131. Pennes DR, Braunstein EM, Shirazi KK. Carpal ligamentous laxity with bilateral perilunate dislocation in Marfan syndrome. Skeletal Radiol 1985;13:62–64.

132. Peyton RS, Moore JR. Fracture through a congenital carpal coalition. J Hand Surg [Am] 1994;19:369–371.
133. Pick RY, Segal D. Carpal scaphoid fracture and nonunion in an eight-year-old child. J Bone Joint Surg Am 1983;65:1188–1189.
134. Protas JM, Jackson WT. Evaluating carpal instabilities with fluoroscopy. AJR 1980;135:137–140.
135. Rand JA, Lindscheid RL, Dobyns JH. Capitate fractures: a long-term follow-up. Clin Orthop 1982;165:209–216.
136. Rasmussen F, Schantz K. Lunatomalacia in a child. Acta Orthop Scand 1986;57:82–84.
137. Reider B, Yurkofsky J, Mass D. Scaphoid wrist fracture in a weight lifter. Am J Sports Med 1993;21:329–331.
138. Riegels-Nielsen P. Pseudarthrosis ossis scaphoidei spontan heling hos et barn. Ugeskr Laeger 1980;142:1935.
139. Ruster VD, Napieralski K. Zur Pathogenese von Navikularefrakturen unter Beruchsichtigung der Kombination mit Brucken am distalen Unterarmende. Beitr Orthop Traumatol 1972;19:155–160.
140. Sherwin JM, Nagel DA, Southwick WO. Bipartite carpal navicular and the diagnostic problem of bone partition: a case report. J Trauma 1967;11:440–443.
141. Smith KL, Harvey FJ, Stalley PD. Nonunion of a pathologic juvenile scaphoid fracture after osteomyelitis. J Hand Surg [Am] 1991;16:493–494.
142. Southcott R, Rosman MA. Non-union of carpal scaphoid fractures in children. J Bone Joint Surg Br 1977;59:20–23.
143. Stark HH, Jobe FW, Bayes JH, Ashworth CR. Fracture of the hook of the hamate in athletes. J Bone Joint Surg Am 1977;59:575–582.
144. Stewart MJ. Fractures of the carpal navicular (scaphoid). J Bone Joint Surg Am 1954;36:998–1006.
145. Suzuki K, Herbert TJ. Spontaneous correction of dorsal intercalated segment instability deformity with scaphoid malunion in the skeletally immature. J Hand Surg [Am] 1993;18:403–406.
146. Taleisnik J, Kelly PJ. The extraosseous and intraosseous blood supply of the scaphoid bone. J Bone Joint Surg Am 1966;48:1125–1137.
147. Tiel-Van Buul MMC, Van Beek EJ, et al. The value of radiographs and bone scintigraphy in suspected scaphoid fracture. J Hand Surg [Am] 1990;15:879–884.
148. Trumble TE, Benirschke SK, Vedder NB. Ipsilateral fractures of the scaphoid and radius. J Hand Surg [Am] 1993;18:8–14.
149. Trumble TE, Irving J. Histologic and magnetic resonance imagery correlation in Kienböck's disease. J Hand Surg [Am] 1990;15:879–884.
150. Vahvanen V, Westerlund U. Fracture of the carpal scaphoid in children. Acta Orthop Scand 1980;51:909–913.
151. Viegas SF, Ampar E. Magnetic resonance imaging in the assessment of revascularization in Kienböck's disease. Orthop Rev 1989;18:1285–1288.
152. Whalen JL, Bishop AT, Lindscheid RL. Nonoperative treatment of acute hamate hook fractures. J Hand Surg [Am] 1992;17:507–511.
153. Whitson RO. Carpometacarpal dislocation. Clin Orthop 1955;6:189–195.
154. Wilson-MacDonald J. Delayed union of the distal scaphoid in a child. J Hand Surg [Am] 1987;12:520–522.
155. Young TB. Isolated fracture of the capitate in a ten-year-old boy. Injury 1986;17:133–134.
156. Zimmerman NB, Weiland AJ. Scapholunate dissociation in the skeletally immature carpus. J Hand Surg [Am] 1990;15:701–705.

Thumb

157. Gabuzda G, Mara J. Bone gamekeeper's thumb in a skeletally immature girl. Orthopedics 1991;14:792–793.
158. Griffiths JC. Bennett's fracture in childhood. Br J Clin Pract 1967;20:582–583.
159. Mintzer CM, Waters PM. Late presentation of a ligamentous ulnar collateral ligament injury in a child. J Hand Surg [Am] 1994;19:1048–1049.
160. Patel MR, Moradia VJ. Correction of an angular deformity of the thumb in a juvenile by epiphyseal distraction. J Hand Surg [Am] 1995;20:258–260.
161. Rath S, Kotwal PP. Loss of proximal phalanx of thumb following a closed injury. J Hand Surg [Br] 1990;15:378.
162. Ryba W. Die Bennettfraktur bei Jungendlichen. Z Kinderchir 1967;38(suppl 3):394–397.
163. Shibu MM, Gault D. Post-traumatic digital overgrowth. J Hand Surg [Br] 1996;21:283–285.
164. Smith MA. The mechanism of acute ulnar instability of the metacarpophalangeal joint of the thumb. Hand 1980;12:225–230.
165. Wallace DA, Carr AJ. Rupture of the ulnar collateral ligament of the thumb in a 5-year-old girl. J Hand Surg [Br] 1993;18:501.
166. White GM. Ligamentous avulsion of the ulnar collateral ligament of the thumb of a child. J Hand Surg [Am] 1986;11:669–672.
167. Winslet MC, Clarke NMP, Mulligan PJ. Breakdancer's thumb—partial rupture of the ulnar collateral ligament with a fracture of the proximal phalanx of the thumb. Injury 1986;17:201–202.

Metacarpals

168. Brown JE. Epiphyseal growth arrest in a fractured metacarpal. J Bone Joint Surg Am 1959;41:494–296.
169. Ireland ML, Taleisnik J. Nonunion of metacarpal extraarticular fractures in children: report of two cases and review of the literature. J Pediatr Orthop 1986;6:352–355.
170. Lane CS. Detecting occult fractures of the metacarpal head: the Brewerton view. J Hand Surg 1977;2:131–133.
171. Lang CJ, Ogden JA. Palmar (volar) fracture of the proximal index metacarpal. J Orthop Trauma 1999;13:149–150.
172. Light TR, Ogden JA. Metacarpal epiphyseal fractures. J Hand Surg [Am] 1987;12:460–464.
173. McElfresh EC, Dobyns JH. Intra-articular metacarpal head fractures. J Hand Surg [Am] 1983;8:383–393.
174. Menon J. Correction of rotary malunion of the fingers by metacarpal rotational osteotomy. Orthopedics 1990;13:197–200.
175. Royle SG. Rotational deformity following metacarpal fracture. J Hand Surg [Br] 1990;15:124–125.
176. Schiund F. Locked metacarpophalangeal joint due to an intraarticular fracture of the metacarpal head. J Hand Surg [Br] 1992;17:148–150.
177. Steinert V, Knorr P. Mittelhand und Fingerfrakturen im Kindesalter. Zentralbl Chir 1971;96:113–124.
178. Thurston AJ. Pivot osteotomy for the correction of malunion of metacarpal neck fractures. J Hand Surg [Br] 1992;17:580–582.
179. Waninger KN, Lombardo JA. Stress fracture of index metacarpal in an adolescent tennis player. Clin J Sports Med 1995;5:63–66.
180. Wright TC, Dell PC. Avascular necrosis and vascular anatomy of the metacarpals. J Hand Surg [Am] 1991;16:540–544.

Metacarpophalangeal Joint

181. Adler GA, Light TR. Simultaneous complex dislocation of the metacarpophalangeal joints of the long and index fingers. J Bone Joint Surg Am 1981;63:1007–1009.
182. Baldwin LW. Metacarpophalangeal joint dislocations of the fingers. J Bone Joint Surg Am 1967;49:1587–1590.
183. Barnard HL. Dorsal dislocation of the first phalanx of the little finger: reduction by Farabeuf's dorsal incision. Lancet 1901; 1:88–90.
184. Barry K, McGee H, Curtin J. Complex dislocation of the metacarpophalangeal joint of the index finger: a comparison of the surgical approaches. J Hand Surg [Br] 1988;13:466–468.
185. Becton JL. A simplified technique for treating the complex dislocation of the index metacarpophalangeal joint. J Bone Joint Surg Am 1975;57:698–700.
186. Bohart PG. Complex dislocations of the metacarpophalangeal joint: operative reduction by Farabeuf's dorsal incision. Clin Orthop 1982;164:208–210.
187. Burman M. Irreducible hyperextension dislocation of the metacarpophalangeal joint of a finger. Bull Hosp Joint Dis 1953;14:290–291.
188. Farabeuf LHF. De la luxation du ponce en arriere. Bull Soc Chir 1876;11:21–62.
189. Gilbert A. Dislocation of the metacarpophalangeal joint in children. In: Tubiana R (ed) The Hand, vol II. Philadelphia: Saunders, 1985.
190. Green DP, Terry GC. Complex dislocation of the metacarpophalangeal joint: correlative pathological anatomy. J Bone Joint Surg Am 1973;55:1480–1486.
191. Imbriglia JE, Sciulli R. Open complex metacarpophalangeal joint dislocation: two cases: index finger and long finger. J Hand Surg [Am] 1979;4:72–75.
192. Kaplan EB. Dorsal dislocation of the metacarpophalangeal joint of the index finger. J Bone Joint Surg Am 1957; 39:1081–1086.
193. LeClerc R. Luxations de le index sur son metacarpien. Rev Orthop 1911;2:227–242.
194. Light TR, Ogden JA. Complex dislocation of the index metacarpophalangeal joint in children. J Pediatr Orthop 1988;8:300–305.
195. McLaughlin HL. Complex "locked" dislocation of the metacarpophalangeal joints. J Trauma 1965;5:683–688.
196. Milch H. Subluxation of the index metacarpophalangeal joint. J Bone Joint Surg Am 1965;47:522–523.
197. Murphy AF, Stark HH. Closed dislocation of the metacarpophalangeal joint of the index finger. J Bone Joint Surg Am 1967;49:1579–1586.
198. Ridge EM. Dorsal dislocation of the first phalanx of the little finger. Lancet 1901;1:781.
199. Sweterlitsch PR, Torg JS, Pollack H. Entrapment of a sesamoid in the index metacarpal joint: report of two cases. J Bone Joint Surg Am 1969;51:995–998.

Phalanges

200. Barton NJ. Fractures of the phalanges of the hand in children. Hand 1979;11:134–143.
201. Bora FW, Ignatius P, Nissenbaum M. The treatment of epiphyseal fractures in the hand. J Bone Joint Surg Am 1976; 58:286.
202. Connolly WB, Leicester AW. Fracture of the proximal phalanx: an unusual complication of pulley reconstruction in a child. J Hand Surg [Br] 1992;17:420–421.
203. Coonrad RW, Pohlman MH. Impacted fractures in the proximal portion of the proximal phalanx of the finger. J Bone Joint Surg Am 1969;51:1291–1296.
204. Cowen JJ, Dranick AD. An irreducible juxtaepiphyseal fracture of the proximal phalanx. Clin Orthop 1975;110: 42–44.
205. Crick JC, Conners JJ, Franco RS. Irreducible palmar dislocation of the proximal interphalangeal joint with bilateral avulsion fractures. J Hand Surg [Am] 1990;15:460–463.
206. Crick JC, Franco RS, Conners JJ. Fracture about the interphalangeal joints in children. J Orthop Trauma 1988; 1:318–325.
207. Culp RW, Osgood JC. Posttraumatic physeal bar formation in the digit of a child: a case report. J Hand Surg [Am] 1993;18:322–324.
208. Dameron TA, Engber WD. Surgical treatment of mallet finger fractures by tension band technique. Clin Orthop 1994; 300:133–140.
209. DeJonge JJ, Kingma J, Van der Lei B, Klasen HJ. Phalangeal fractures of the hand: an analysis of gender and age-related incidence and aetiology. J Hand Surg [Br] 1994;19: 168–170.
210. Dixon GL, Moon NF. Rotational supracondylar fractures of the proximal phalanx in children. Clin Orthop 1972;83: 151–156.
211. Dykes RG. Kirner's deformity of the little finger. J Bone Joint Surg Br 1978;60:58–60.
212. Fortens Y, DeSmet L, Stanley JK. Fracture with non-union through an incomplete preaxial distal symphalangism. J Hand Surg [Br] 1994;19:371–372.
213. Harryman DT, Jordan TF. Physeal phalangeal fracture with flexor tendon entrapment. Clin Orthop 1990;250:194–196.
214. Hutchinson JD, Hooper G, Robb JE. Double dislocations of digits. J Hand Surg [Br] 1991;16:114–115.
215. Inoue G. Closed reduction of mallet fractures using extension-block Kirschner wire. J Orthop Trauma 1992;6:413–415.
216. Inoue G, Kino Y, Kondo K. Simultaneous dorsal dislocation of both interphalangeal joints in a finger. Am J Sports Med 1993;21:323–325.
217. Johnson FG, Green MH. Another cause of irreducible dislocation of the proximal interphalangeal joint: a case report. J Bone Joint Surg Am 1966;48:542–544.
218. Jones NF, Jupiter JB. Irreducible palmar dislocation of the proximal interphalangeal joint associated with an epiphyseal fracture of the middle phalanx. J Hand Surg [Am] 1985; 10:261–264.
219. Keene JS, Engber WD, Stromberg WB. An irreducible phalangeal epiphyseal fracture-dislocation. Clin Orthop 1985; 186:212–215.
220. Kojima T, Yanagawa H, Tomonari H. Solitary osteochondroma limiting flexion of the proximal interphalangeal joint in an infant: a case report. J Hand Surg [Am] 1992;17: 1057–1059.
221. Lee MLH. Intra-articular and peri-articular fractures of the phalanges. J Bone Joint Surg Br 1963;45:103–109.
222. Leonard MH. Open reduction of fractures of the neck of the proximal phalanx in children. Clin Orthop 1976;116:176–179.
223. Lewis RC, Hartman JT. Controlled osteotomy for correction of rotation in proximal phalanx fractures. Orthop Rev 1973; 2:11–14.
224. Michelinakis E, Vourexaki H. Displaced epiphyseal plate of the terminal phalanx in a child. Hand 1980;12:51–53.
225. Mintzer CM, Waters PM, Brown DJ. Remodelling of a displaced phalangeal neck fracture. J Hand Surg [Br] 1994; 19:5:594–596.

226. Newington DP, Craigen MA, Bennet GC. Children's proximal phalangeal neck fracture with 180° rotational deformity. J Hand Surg [Br] 1995;20:353–356.
227. Palmer AK, Linscheid RL. Irreducible dorsal dislocation of the distal interphalangeal joint of the finger. J Hand Surg [Am] 1977;2:406–408.
228. Patel MR. Tranverse bayonet dislocation of proximal interphalangeal joint. Clin Orthop 1978;133:219–226.
229. Savage R. Complete detachment of the epiphysis of the distal phalanx. J Hand Surg [Br] 1990;15:126–128.
230. Seymour N. Juxta-epiphyseal fracture of the terminal phalanx of the finger. J Bone Joint Surg Br 1966;48:347–349.
231. Shewring DJ, Coleman MG. Phalangeal fractures resulting from finger wrestling. J Hand Surg [Br] 1992;17:579.
232. Simmons BP, Peters TT. Subcondylar fossa reconstruction for malunion of fractures of the proximal phalanx in children. J Hand Surg [Am] 1987;12:1079–1082.
233. Steinert VV, Knorr P. Mittelhand und Fingerfrakturen im Kindesalter. Zentralbl Chir 1971;4:113–124.
234. Stripling WD. Displaced intra-articular osteochondral fracture: cause for irreducible dislocation of the distal interphalangeal joint. J Hand Surg [Am] 1982;7:77–78.
235. Torre B. Epiphyseal injuries in the small joints of the hand. Hand Clin 1988;4:113–120.
236. Vandenberk P, DeSmet L, Fabry G. Finger fractures in children treated with absorbable pins. J Pediatr Orthop Part B 1996;5:27–30.
237. Viegas SF. Extension block pinning for proximal interphalangeal joint fracture dislocations: preliminary report of a new technique. J Hand Surg [Am] 1992;17:896–901.
238. Von Raffler W. Irreducible juxta-epiphyseal fracture of a finger. J Bone Joint Surg Br 1964;46:229–231.
239. Waters PM, Benson LS. Dislocation of the distal phalanx epiphysis in toddlers. J Hand Surg [Am] 1993;18:581–589.
240. Weiss A-PC, Hastings H III. Distal unicondylar fractures of the proximal phalanx. J Hand Surg [Am] 1993;18:594–599.
241. Whipple TL, Evans JP, Urbaniak JR. Irreducible dislocation of a finger joint in a child. J Bone Joint Surg Am 1980;62:832–833.
242. Zielinski C. Irreducible fracture-dislocation of the distal interphalangeal joint. J Bone Joint Surg Am 1983;65:109–110.

Fingertip and Nail Bed

243. Ashbell TS, Kleinert HW, Putcha SM. The deformed fingernail: a frequent result of failure to repair nailbed injuries. J Trauma 1967;7:177–189.
244. Banerjee A. Irreducible distal phalangeal epiphyseal injuries. J Hand Surg [Br] 1992;17:337–338.
245. Cohen MS, Hennrikus WL, Botte MJ. A dressing for repair of acute nail bed injury. Orthop Rev 1990;19:882–884.
246. Das SK, Brown HG. Management of lost finger tips in children. Hand 1978;10:16–27.
247. Duthie G, Adams J. Meshed adhesive tape for the treatment of crushed fingers in children. J Hand Surg [Br] 1984;9:41.
248. Elliot D, Jigjinni VS. The lateral pulp flap. J Hand Surg [Br] 1993;18:423–426.
249. Engber WD, Glancy WG. Traumatic avulsion of the fingernail associated with injury to the phalangeal epiphyseal plate. J Bone Joint Surg Am 1978;60:713–714.
250. Hoddinott C, Matthews JP. Deformation of the nail following elastic band traction: a case report. J Hand Surg [Br] 1989;14:23–24.
251. Illingworth CM. Trapped fingers and amputated fingertips in children. J Pediatr Surg 1974;9:853–858.
252. Inglefield CJ, D'Arcangelo M, Kolhe PS. Injuries to the nail bed in childhood. J Hand Surg [Br] 1995;208:258–261.
253. Kasdan ML, Stutts JT. One-stage reconstruction of the nail fold. Orthopedics 1993;16:887–889.
254. Mennen U, Wiese A. Fingertip injuries. Management with semiocclusive dressing. J Hand Surg [Br] 1993;18:416–422.
255. Metcalf W, Whalen WP. Salvage of the injured distal phalanx. Clin Orthop 1959;13:114–123.
256. Moiemen NS, Elliot D. Composite graft replacement of digital tips. 2. A study in children. J Hand Surg [Br] 1997;22:346–352.
257. Patzakis M, Harvey J, Ivler D. The role of antibiotics in the management of open fractures. J Bone Joint Surg Am 1974;56:532–541.
258. Pessa JE, Tsai T-M, Li Y, Kleinert HE. The repair of nail deformities with the nonvascularized nail bed graft: indications and results. J Hand Surg [Am] 1990;15:466–470.
259. Rayan GM, Flournoy DJ. Microbiologic flora of human fingernails. J Hand Surg [Am] 1987;12:605–607.
260. Sandzen SC. Management of the acute fingertip injury in the child. Hand 1974;6:190–197.
261. Shrewsbury M, Johnson RK. The fascia of the distal phalanx. J Bone Joint Surg Am 1975;57:784–788.
262. Thompson HG, Sorokolit WT. The cross-finger flap in children: a follow-up study. Plast Reconstr Surg 1967;39:487–492.
263. Usal H, Beattie TF. An audit of hand injuries in a pediatric accident and emergency department. Health Bull 1992;50:289–287.
264. Zook EG. Nail bed injuries. Hand Clin 1985;1:701–716.
265. Zook EG, Guy RJ, Russell RC. A study of nail bed injuries: causes, treatment and prognosis. J Hand Surg [Am] 1984;9:247–252.

Bite Injury

266. Eyres KS, Allen TR. Skyline view of the metacarpal head in the assessment of human fight-bite injuries. J Hand Surg [Br] 1993;18:43–44.
267. Mennen U, Howells CJ. Human fight-bite injuries of the hand: a study of 100 cases within 18 months. J Hand Surg [Br] 1991;16:431–435.
268. Peters LOH. Hand infection apparently due to Bacillus fusiformis. J Infect Dis 1993;8:455–462.
269. Phair IC, Quinton DN. Clenched fist human bite injuries. J Hand Surg [Br] 1989;14:86–87.
270. Resnick D, Pinoda CJ, Weisman MH, Kerr R. Osteomyelitis and septic arthritis following human bites. Skeletal Radiol 1985;14:263–266.
271. Schmidt DR, Heckman JD. Eikenella carrodens in human bite infections of the hand. J Trauma 1983;23:478–482.
272. Seiler JG, Sagerman SD, Geller RJ, et al. Venomous snake bite: current concepts of treatment. Orthopedics 1994;17:707–714.
273. Wiggins ME, Akelman E, Weiss APC. The management of dog bites and dog bite infections to the hand. Orthopedics 1994;17:617–623.

Open Injury

274. Ada S, Bora A, Özerkan F, Kaplan I, Arikan G. Rolling belt injuries in children. J Hand Surg [Br] 1994;19:601–603.
275. Berger LR, Kalishman S, Rivara FP. Injuries from fireworks. Pediatrics 1985;75:877–882.
276. Dap F, Dautel G, Voche P, Thomas C, Merle M. The posterior interosseous flap in primary repair of hand injuries. J Hand Surg [Br] 1993;18:437–445.
277. Fackler ML, Burkhalter WE. Hand and forearm injuries from penetrating projectiles. J Hand Surg [Am] 1992;17:971–975.
278. Kessler I, Hecht O, Baruch A. Distraction lengthening of digital rays in the management of the injured hand. J Bone Joint Surg Am 1979;61:83–87.

279. Levine WN, Leslie BM. The use of ultrasonography to detect a radiolucent foreign body in the hand: a case report. J Hand Surg [Am] 1993;18:218–220.
280. Lundborg G, Sollerman C. A case of phalangeal lengthening. Acta Orthop Scand 1987;58:423–425.
281. Matev IB. Thumb reconstruction in children through metacarpal lengthening. Plast Reconstr Surg 1979;64:665–669.
282. Russell RC, Williamson DA, Sullivan JW, Sucky H, Suliman O. Detection of foreign bodies in the hand. J Hand Surg [Am] 1991;16:2–11.
283. Upton J, Boyajian M, Mulliken JB, Glowacki J. The use of demineralized xenogeneic bone implants to correct phalangeal defects: a case report. J Hand Surg [Am] 1984;9:388–391.

Replantation/Revascularization

284. Baker GL, Leinert JM. Digit replantation in infants and young children: determinants of survival. Plast Reconstr Surg 1994;94:139–145.
285. Balfour W. Two cases, with observations, demonstrative of the powers of nature to reunite parts which have been, by accident, totally separated from the animal system. Edinb Med Surg J 1814;10:421–430.
286. Black EB III. Microsurgery and replantation of tissues in children. Pediatr Ann 1992;11:918–920.
287. Cheng GL, Pan DD, Yang ZX, Fang GR, Gong XS. Digital replantation in children. Ann Plast Surg 1955;15:325–331.
288. Chicarelli ZN. Pediatric microsurgery: revascularization and replantation. J Pediatr Surg 1986;21:706–710.
289. Demiri E, Bakhach J, Tsakoniatis N, et al. Bone growth after replantation in children. J Reconstr Microsurg 1995;11:113–123.
290. Gaul JS, Nunley JA. Microvascular replantation in a seven-month-old girl: a case report. Microsurgery 1988;9:204–207.
291. Jackson A, Reilly M, Watson S. Radiologic appearances following limb replantation: a report of 5 cases. Skeletal Radiol 1992;21:155–159.
292. Jaeger SH, Tsai TM, Kleinert HE. Upper extremity replantation in children. Orthop Clin North Am 1981;12:897–907.
293. Jubi T, Ikitay K, Watari S, et al. The smallest digital replant yet? A case report. Br J Plast Surg 1976;29:313–315.
294. Kröpfl A, Gasperschitz F, Niederwiesser L, et al. Epiphysenwachstum nach Replantation im Kindersalter. Handchir Mikrochir Plast Chir 1994;26:194–199.
295. Nettleblad H, Randolph MA, Weiland AJ. Free microvascular epiphyseal-plate transplantation. J Bone Joint Surg Am 1984;66:1421–1430.
296. Ninkovic M, Sucur D, Starovic B, Markovic S. Arteriovenous fistulae after free flap surgery in a replanted hand. J Hand Surg [Br] 1992;17:657–659.
297. Nunley JA, Spiegel PV, Goldner RD, Urbaniak JR. Longitudinal epiphyseal growth after replantation and transplantation in children. J Hand Surg [Am] 1987;12:274–279.
298. O'Brien BM, Franklin JD, Morrison WA, MacLeod AM. Replantation and revascularization surgery in children. Hand 1980;12:12–24.
299. Saies AD, Urbaniak JR, Nunley JA, et al. Results after replantation and revascularization in the upper extremity in children. J Bone Joint Surg Am 1994;76:1766–1776.
300. Sekiguchi J, Ohmori K. Youngest replantation with microsurgical anastomoses. Hand 1979;11:64–66.
301. Tamai S, Hori Y, Tatsumi Y, et al. Little finger replantation in a 20-month-old child: a case report. Br J Plast Surg 1974;27:1–3.
302. Urbaniak JR. Digital and hand replantation: current status. Neurosurgery 1979;4:551–558.
303. Urbaniak JR, Bright DS. Replantation of amputated digits in hands in children. Interclin Inform Bull 1975;14:1–4.
304. Yamano Y. Replantation of the amputated distal part of the fingers. J Hand Surg [Am] 1985;10:211–218.

Burns

305. Alexander JW, MacMillan BG, Martel L, Krummel R. Surgical correction of postburn flexion contractures of the fingers in children. Plast Reconstr Surg 1981;68:218–226.
306. Clarke HM, Whittpen GP, McLeod AME, et al. Acute management of pediatric hand burns. Hand Clin 1990;6:221–232.
307. Graham TJ, Stern PJ, True MS. Classification and treatment of postburn metacarpophalangeal joint extension contractures in children. J Hand Surg [Am] 1990;15:450–456.
308. Gunn AL. Late complications of burns of the hand in children and their treatment. Guys Hosp Rep 1970;119:71–80.
309. Hoffer M, Lankenan J, Wellisz T. Proximal interphalangeal joint autofusions after extensive burns. J Orthop Trauma 1994;8:249–251.
310. Shugerman R, Rivara F, Parish RA, Heimbach D. Contact burns of the hand. Pediatrics 1987;80:18–21.
311. Stern PJ. Postburn PIP joint contracture in children. J Hand Surg [Am] 1987;12:450–457.
312. Stern PJ, Neale HW, Graham TJ, Warden GD. Classification and treatment of postburn proximal interphalangeal joint flexion contractures in children. J Hand Surg [Am] 1987;12:450–457.
313. Trippi D, Pastacaldi P, Camerini E, Giorgetti M. Effetto dei traumi elettrici sulle strutture osteo-cartilaginee delle mani nell'infanzia. Radiol Med 1990;79:384–386.

Frostbite

314. Crouch C, Smith WL. Long-term sequelae of frostbite. Pediatr Radiol 1990;20:365–366.
315. Nakazato T, Ogino T. Epiphyseal destruction of children's hands after frostbite: a report of two cases. J Hand Surg [Am] 1986;11:289–292.
316. Reed MH. Growth disturbances in the hands following thermal injuries in children: frostbite. J Can Assoc Radiol 1988;39:95–99.

Tendon Injury

317. Al-Qattan MM, Posnick TC, Lin KY. The in vivo response of foetal tendons to sutures. J Hand Surg [Br] 1995;20:314–318.
318. Arons MS. Purposeful delay of the primary repair of cut flexor tendons in "some man's land" in children. Plast Reconstr Surg 1974;53:638–642.
319. Bell JL, Mason ML, Koch SL, Stromberg WB. Injuries to the flexor tendons of the hand in children. J Bone Joint Surg Am 1958;40:1220–1230.
320. Birnie RH, Idler RS. Flexor tenolysis in children. J Hand Surg [Am] 1995;20:254–257.
321. Bora FW. Profundus tendon grafting with unimpaired sublimis function in children. Clin Orthop 1970;71:118–123.
322. Cunningham MW, Yousif NJ, Matloub HS, Sanger JR, Gingrass RP, Valiulis JP. Retardation of finger growth after injury to the flexor tendons. J Hand Surg [Am] 1985;10:115–117.
323. Ejeskar A. Flexor tendon repair in no-man's land. Scand J Plast Reconstr Surg 1980;14:279–286.
324. Entin MA. Flexor tendon repair and grafting in children. Am J Surg 1965;109:287–293.
325. Fetrow KO. Tenolysis in the hand and wrist: a clinical evaluation of 220 flexor and extensor tenolyses. J Bone Joint Surg Am 1967;49:667–685.

326. Gaisford JD, Fleegler EJ. Alterations in finger growth following flexor tendon injuries. Plast Reconstr Surg 1973;51:164–168.
327. Grobbelaar AO, Hudson DA. Flexor tendon injuries in children. J Hand Surg [Br] 1994;19:696–698.
328. Hage J, Dupuis CC. The intriguing fate of tendon grafts in small children's hands and their results. Br J Plast Surg 1965;18:341–349.
329. Herndon JH. Tendon injuries. In: Carter PR (ed) Reconstruction of the Child's Hand. Philadelphia: Lea & Febiger, 1991.
330. Herndon JH. Treatment of tendon injuries in children. Orthop Clin North Am 1976;7:717–731.
331. Herndon JH. Tendon injuries: extensor surface. Emerg Clin North Am 1985;3:333–340.
332. Hunter JM, Salisbury RE. Use of gliding artificial implants to produce tendon sheaths: techniques and results in children. Plast Reconstr Surg 1970;45:564–572.
333. Joseph KN, Kalus AM, Sutherland AB. Glass injuries of the hand in children. Hand 1981;13:113–119.
334. Jozsa L, Reffy A, Demel S, Balint JB. Foreign bodies in tendons. J Hand Surg [Br] 1989;14:84–85.
335. Leddy JP, Packer JW. Avulsion of the profundus tendon insertion in athletes. J Hand Surg 1977;2:66–69.
336. Masquelet AC, Gilbert A. Plaies récentes des tendons fléchisseurs des doigts chez l'enfant. Rev Chir Orthop 1985;71:587–593.
337. McFarlane RM, Hampole MK. Treatment of extensor tendon injuries of the hand. Can J Surg 1973;16:366–375.
338. Millon SJ, Bush DC, Harrington LP. Acute calcific tendinitis in a child: a case report. J Hand Surg [Am] 1993;18:592–593.
339. Miura T, Nakamura R, Tamura Y. Long-standing extended dynamic splintage and release of an abnormal restraining structure in a camptodactyly. J Hand Surg [Br] 1992;17:665–672.
340. Nishijima N, Fujio K, Hamamuro T. Growth of severed flexor tendons in chickens. J Orthop Res 1995;13:138–142.
341. O'Connell SJ, Moore MM, Strickland JW, Frazier GT, Dell PD. Results of zone I and zone II flexor tendon repairs in children. J Hand Surg [Am] 1994;19:48–52.
342. Ogino T, Kato H. Operative findings in camptodactyly of the little finger. J Hand Surg [Br] 1992;17:661–664.
343. Posner MA, McMahon MS. Congenital radial subluxation of the extensor tendons over the metacarpophalangeal joints: a case report. J Hand Surg [Am] 1994;19:659–662.
344. Stahl S, Kaufman T, Bialik V. Partial lacerations of flexor tendons in children: primary repair versus conservative treatment. J Hand Surg [Br] 1997;22:377–380.
345. Vahvanen V, Gripenberg L, Nuntinen P. Flexor tendon injury of the hand in children: a long-term follow-up of 84 patients. Scand J Plast Reconstr Surg 1981;15:43–48.
346. Woods VE, Sicilia M. Congenital trigger digit. Clin Orthop 1992;285:205–209.

Nerve

347. Almquist EE, Smith OA, Fry L. Nerve conduction velocity, microscopic and electron microscopy studies comparing repaired adult and baby monkey median nerves. J Hand Surg [Am] 1983;8:406–410.
348. Fissette J, Onkelinx A, Fandi N. Carpal and Guyon tunnel syndrome in burns at the wrist. J Hand Surg [Am] 1981;6:13–15.
349. Gibson CT, Manske PR. Carpal tunnel syndrome in the adolescent. J Hand Surg [Am] 1987;12:279–281.
350. Harrison SH. The tactile adherence test estimating loss of sensation after nerve injury. Hand 1974;6:148–149.
351. Lettin AW. Carpal tunnel syndrome in childhood. J Bone Joint Surg Br 1965;47:556–559.
352. Lettin AW. Carpal tunnel syndrome in childhood. Proc R Soc Med 1966;59:40–43.
353. McCarroll HR Jr. Nerve injury. In: Carter PR (ed) Reconstruction of the Child's Hand. Philadelphia: Lea & Febiger, 1991.
354. Poilvache P, Carher A, Rombouts JJ, Partoune E, Lejeune G. Carpal tunnel syndrome in childhood: report of five new cases. J Pediatr Orthop 1989;9:687–690.

Hair Constriction

355. Abel MF, McFarland R. Hair and thread constriction of the digits in infants. J Bone Joint Surg Am 1993;75:915–916.
356. Alpert JJ, Filler R, Glaser HH. Strangulation of an appendage by hair wrapping. N Engl J Med 1965;273:866–867.
357. Barton DJ, Sloan GM, Nichter LS, Reinisch JF. Hair-thread tourniquet syndrome. Pediatrics 1988;82:925–928.
358. Beck AR, Wesser DR. Constrictive digital injuries in infants caused by human hair. Plast Reconstr Surg 1972;49:420–422.
359. Kerry RL, Chapman DD. Strangulation of appendages by hair and thread. J Pediatr Surg 1973;8:23–27.
360. Mann TP. Finger-tip necrosis in the newly born: a hazard of wearing mittens. BMJ 1961;2:1755–1796.
361. Miller PR, Levi JH. Hair strangulation. J Bone Joint Surg Am 1977;59:132.

18

Spine

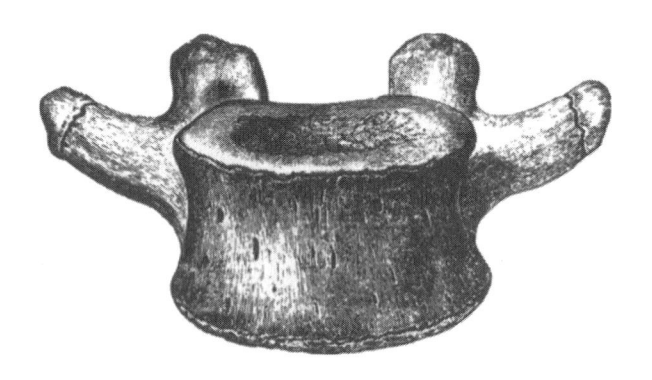

Engraving of an adolescent lumbar vertebra showing the ring apophyses and secondary centers of the transverse processes. (From Poland J. Traumatic Separation of the Epiphyses. *London: Smith, Elder, 1898)*

The morphologic and histologic patterns of spine and spinal cord injury in children and adolescents, especially in the cervical region, relate to the changing anatomy and particularly to the various cartilaginous growth regions of the neurocentral synchondroses, physeal end-plates, and facet growth regions.[3,28] The skull is relatively large at birth when compared to the rest of the body. With subsequent postnatal development, this ratio gradually lessens, such that a decreasing mass (potential angular momentum) is presented to the cervical spine during any traumatic incident. The skull, through the occipital condyles, articulates horizontally with the atlas. The occipitoatlantal joints are relatively tightly constrained, allowing flexion and extension but minimal rotation. Rotation principally occurs between C1 and C2, although some rotation also occurs between each of the other cervical vertebra.

Anatomy

The dens is attached to the anterior arch of the atlas by several ligaments: (1) alar or check ligaments; (2) apical dental ligament; (3) tectorial membrane; and (4) cruciate ligament. The transverse portion of the cruciate ligament is probably the *most important* mechanically, no matter what the age of the patient. The atlantoaxial joints have a contiguous synovial lining between the anterior arch of the atlas and dens, between the transverse ligament and dens, and between the lateral masses (Fig. 18-1).

The atlantoaxial relations permit mobility and rotation combined with intrinsic stability.[5,16,28,29] The possible movements are extension, forward flexion, and rotation. Rotation is limited to approximately 45°, although the usual range is 20°–60°. The atlantoaxial joints may be disrupted in children, in part because the normal ligamentous laxity characteristic of this age group allows significant motion in these joints during rotation. Such disruption, which is most likely to occur at the facet joints rather than at the dens–C1 joint, is likely to be a subluxation rather than a dislocation.

Separate primary ossification centers are present in the lateral masses of the atlas. A third primary center for the anterior arch is ossified in only about 20% of neonates and may not be seen until the child is 1 year of age (Figs. 18-2, 18-3). This particular ossification center may be bifid but is not always symmetric.[13,21,25] Posterior ossification may be incomplete, resulting in a variable ossific spina bifida. (In contrast, the cartilaginous ring may be complete.) These ossification variations and synchondroses should *not* be confused with traumatic disruption of the rings. The diameters of the C1 canal reach "adult" size by the time a child is 4–5 years of age, at which point little further canal growth occurs in C1, although the bone does continue to enlarge by appositional (periosteal) growth.

In the axis the usual primary ossification pattern pertains in the centrum and neural arches. In addition, ossification of the dens begins prenatally with two longitudinal primary ossification centers, which are usually fused by birth.[8,13,26,28] In rare instances one may not form, creating a thin dens.

The dens is separated from the body of the axis by a region of growth cartilage termed the dentocentral synchondrosis (Figs. 18-4, 18-5). This cartilage progressively disappears when the child is 5–7 years old. It is important to realize that this *is* a bipolar growth zone responsible for longitudinal growth of the upper part of the C2 centrum

708

Anatomy

FIGURE 18-1. Relation of C1 and C2 in the immature spine. There are joints anterior and posterior to the dens, as well as the horizontal joints (arrows). The asterisk marks the transverse ligament, a major stabilizer of this joint.

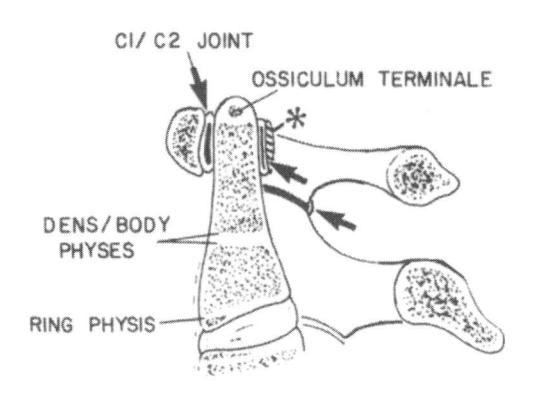

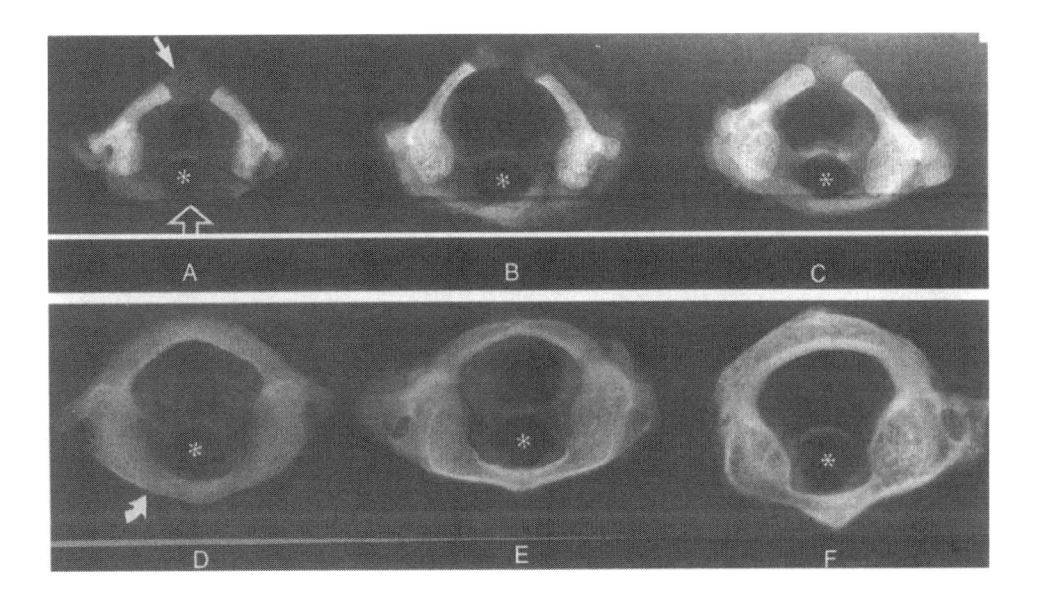

FIGURE 18-2. Early development of C1. (A) At birth. (B) Three months. (C) Seven months. (A) Solid arrow points to the posterior synchondrosis; the open arrow points to the unossified anterior arch. The asterisk (*) marks the locations of the dens, with the transverse ligament intact. Subsequent maturation of C1 is shown in three specimens from cadavers aged 7(D), 9(E), and 12 (F) years. All show comparable shapes and cervical canal size. The arrow in (D) shows the anterior closing synchondrosis.

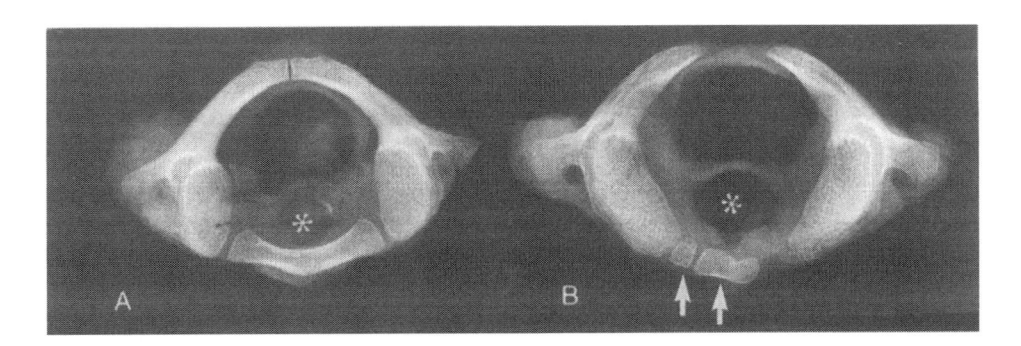

FIGURE 18-3. Variations in the anterior development of C1 at 3 years. (A) Normal development with a posterior synchondrosis and an anterior arch with two synchondroses. (B) Widened posterior region and irregular ossification centers in the arch (arrows). Asterisks mark the location of the dens, with the transverse ligament intact.

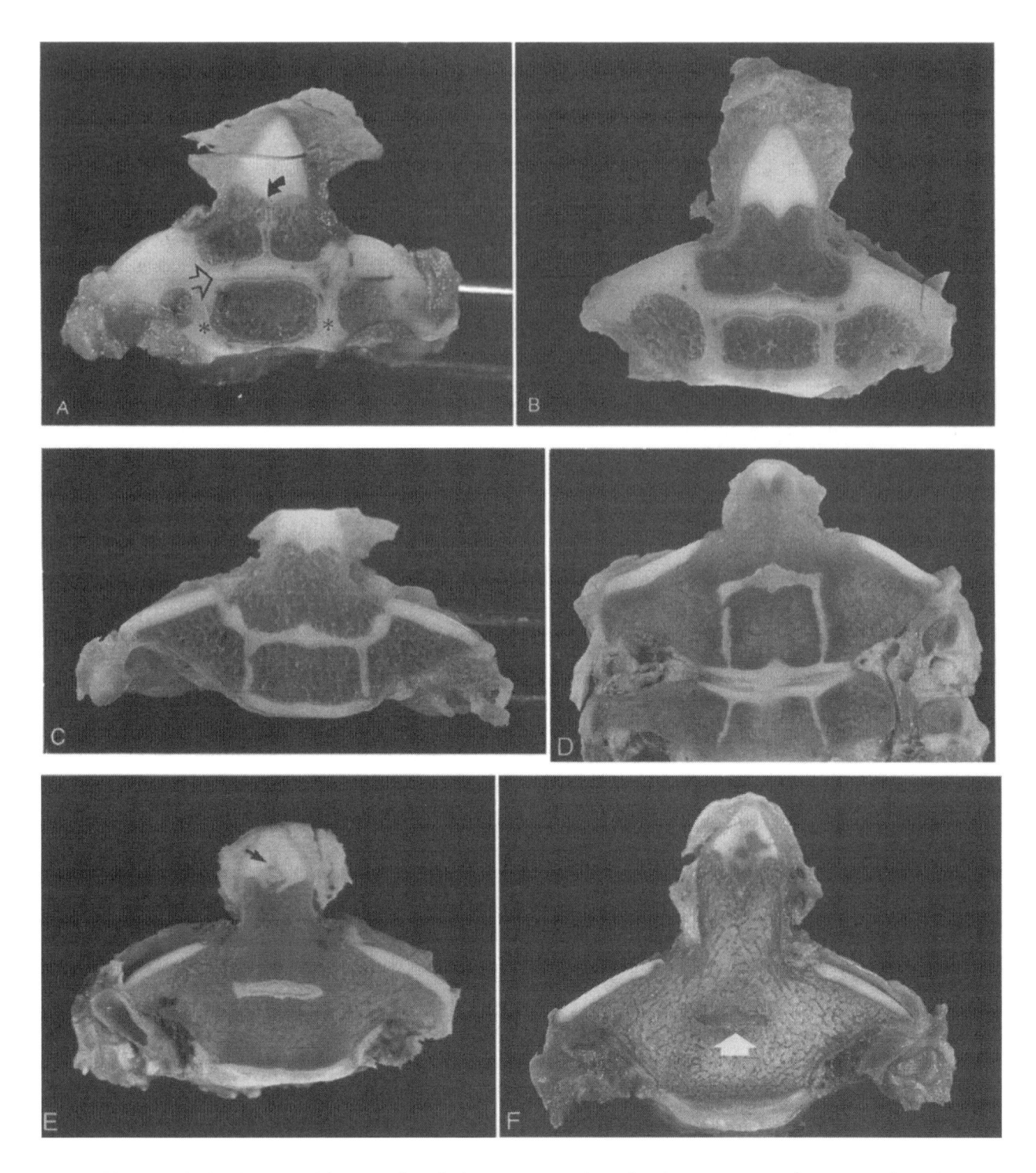

FIGURE 18-4. Morphologic development of the second cervical vertebra. (A) Neonate. The bifid ossification of the dens is evident (solid arrow). There is considerable cartilaginous continuity throughout the centrum, posterior elements, and dens (open arrow). The asterisks indicate the neurocentral synchondroses between the centrum and the posterolateral elements. (B) At 3 months the dens ossification centers have coalesced and the neurocentral synchondroses separate the centrum from the posterolateral elements. (C) At 1 year. (D) At 3 years the dens has fused to the lateral elements. (E) At 7 years the ossiculum terminale is beginning to form (arrow). (F) At 9 years the ossiculum terminale is more evident. (E, F) Note the remnant of the growth cartilage between the dens and centrum (arrow in F). It creates a radiolucent cleft that may be mistaken for a fracture.

Anatomy

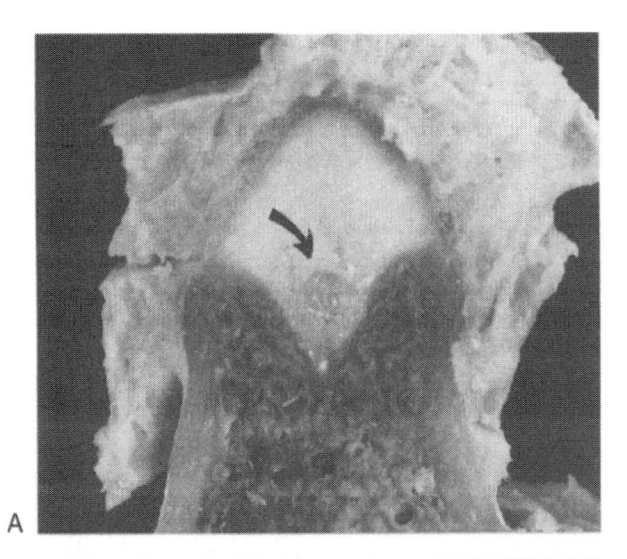

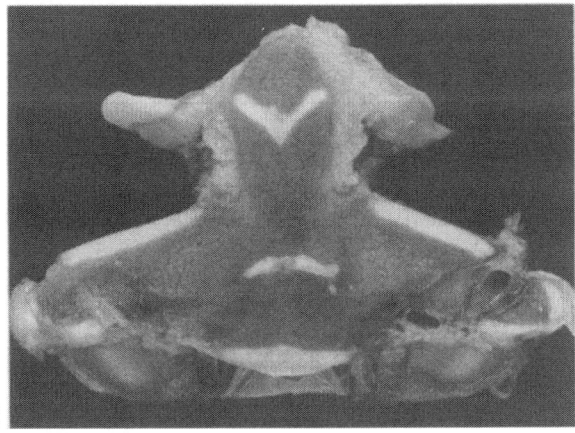

FIGURE 18-5. (A) Chevron-shaped upper dens with early secondary ossification (arrow) at 8 years. (B) Well-formed terminal ossification center at the tip of the dens at 10 years. Some of the dentocentral cartilage remains within the "body" of C2.

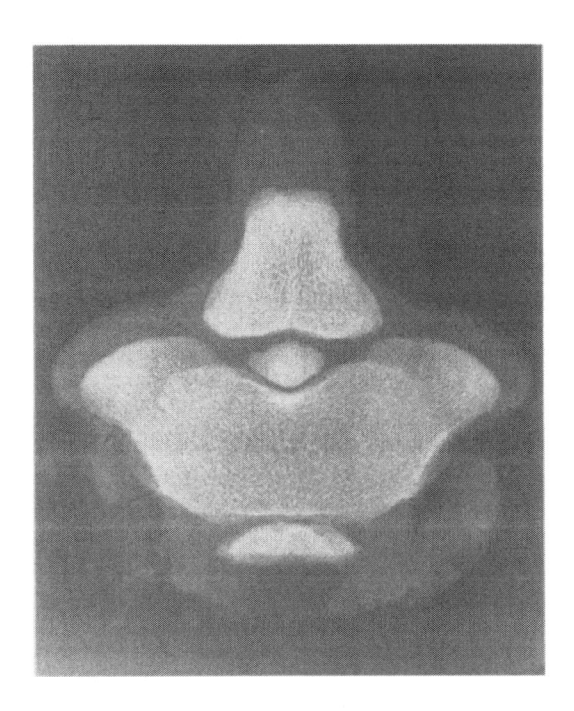

FIGURE 18-6. Comparable C2 ossification in a skeletally immature 3-month-old seal. Secondary ossification is present in the dentocentral synchondrosis. This would be expected, as the area is a developmental fusion of epiphyseal equivalents and thus is comparable to secondary ossification in the human triradiate cartilage (see Chapter 19).

and lower part of the dens. In most animals a secondary ossification center appears within the dentocentral synchondrosis, similar to ossification within the triradiate cartilage (Fig. 18-6).

The dentocentral cartilage is located below the level of the articular facets, within the eventual C2 vertebral body (Fig. 18-4). It is histologically continuous with the neurocentral synchondroses of the centrum and the posterior elements of C2 in the infant and young child. A "ghost" of this structure may remain for several years and should not be confused with a fracture (Fig. 18-4). In children, dens fractures extend along this growth mechanism and thus are partially within the body of C2, a factor that significantly enhances healing. In contrast, the fracture level in the adolescent and adult is usually several millimeters higher, at the articular facet level (Fig. 18-7).

The dentocentral synchondrosis effectively prevents vascularization of the dens by direct extension of vessels from the centrum.[1,22,35] This separation of circulations probably remains, to some degree, after closure of the synchondrosis, similar to the physiologic separation of the metaphyseal and epiphyseal circulations for years after growth plate closure in long bones. The circulation enters the dens from two areas. At the upper end, near the ossiculum terminale, there are soft tissue attachments that allow penetration of vessels. However, the distal end is supplied by vessels entering medial to the facet joints. These go toward the dentocentral synchondrosis and into the main portion of the dens, which is almost totally free of soft tissue attachments. The latter circulation is usually undamaged by childhood fractures but may be cut off by adult fractures because of the aforementioned difference in the fracture patterns.

The tip of the dens usually has a chevron shape in the anteroposterior view (Fig. 18-5). This variation, sometimes termed a bicornuate dens, represents a normal pattern of

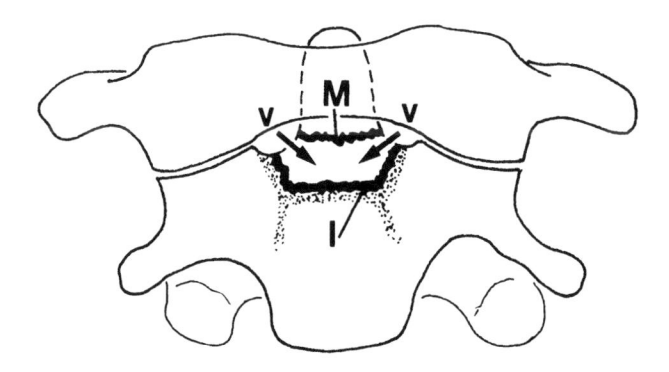

FIGURE 18-7. Dens fracture patterns in the mature (M) and immature (I) dens. Note the vascular entrance points (V) and how the childhood fracture pattern (I) does not interfere with the dental blood supply, whereas the adult fracture pattern (M) does. The neurocentral and dentocentral synchondroses are stippled.

fusion of the two lateral ossification centers that extend superiorly to enclose the normal ossiculum terminale. It should be considered normal. Within this chevron, a separate secondary ossification for the tip of the dens occurs, but not until the child is about 6–7 years old. This ossiculum terminale fuses with the rest of the dens around 12 years of age.[26,28] Although these centers usually fuse completely in the adult, the lines of fusion may be demarcated by clefts in different stages of skeletal maturation. There may also be failure of osseous union of a normal ossiculum terminale with the dens.

Injury theoretically could avulse the terminal epiphysis from the rest of the odontoid. It may enlarge to contribute to the formation of an os odontoideum. In the lateral view, the posteriorly tilted slope of the anterior surface allows normal flexion-extension between C1 and C2.

The lymphatic drainage of the cervical spine region is primarily into the retropharyngeal glands and ultimately into the deep cervical glands. Both sets of glands also drain the nasopharynx. This fact is significant in cervical pseudosubluxation secondary to pharyngitis and lymphadenopathy (Grisel syndrome).

The third through seventh cervical vertebrae and all of the thoracic and lumbar vertebrae exhibit a common ossification pattern.[28,37] One ossification center develops in each of the two neural arch cartilage centers, and one ossification center generally forms in the vertebral centrum (Fig. 18-8). The position of the two neural arches and single vertebral centrum ossification center is such that the cartilage separating them, the neurocentral synchondrosis, is slightly anterior to the anatomic base of the pedicles. This synchondrosis disappears when the child is between the ages of 3 and 6 years. The ossified portions of each neural arch fuse with each other posteriorly by 2–4 years of age. Prior to this time, they produce radiolucent lines on the frontal projection of the spine (Fig. 18-8) and should not be confused with congenital abnormalities (e.g., spina bifida) or trauma.[13] Thus, posterior cervical spinal canal diameters reach maturity long before longitudinal growth (height) of the anterior centrum ceases during mid- to late adolescence.

The normal planes of the articular surfaces change angulation with growth. The lower cervical spine facets change from 55° to 70°, whereas the upper cervical spine (i.e., C2–C4) may have initial angles as low as 30°, which gradually increase to approximately 60°–70° (Fig. 18-9).[27] This angulation variation is a major factor in the pseudosubluxation of the upper cervical spine of infants and young children.[28]

Similarly, development of the upward curve of the lateral margins of the cervical vertebral centra varies considerably with age. This region, referred to as the joint of Luschka or uncinate process, does not exist as a rigid (osseous) structure in the infant and young child, although it is anatomically present as a cartilaginous structure.[27] By 7–10 years of age, the marginal ossification has progressed sufficiently into the antecedent cartilage to begin radiologically detectable formation of this structure. This is another developmental

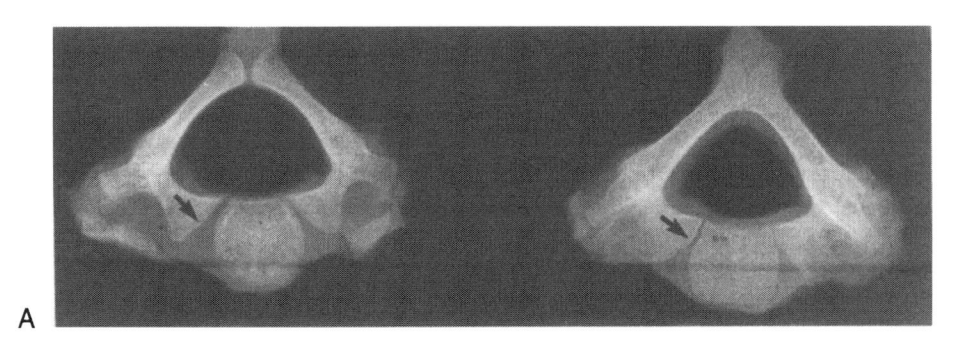

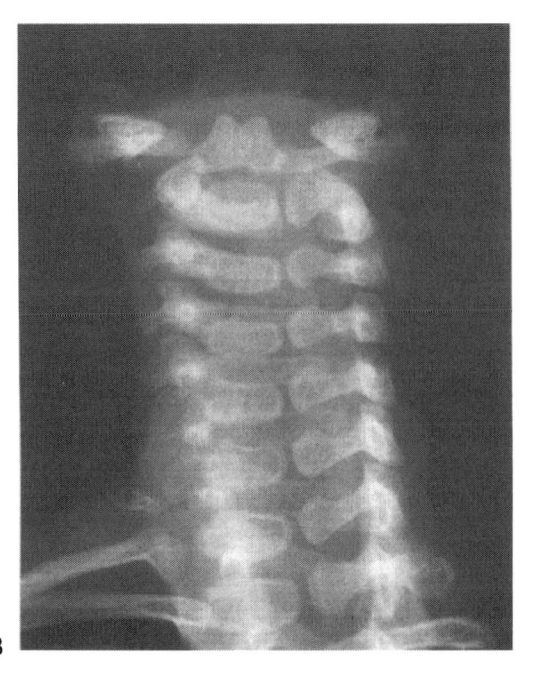

FIGURE 18-8. (A) Representative cervical vertebrae (C4) at 7 months (left) and 15 months (right), showing the location of the three growth regions: the posterior one at the spinous process and two anterior ones at the neurocentral synchondroses (arrows). These growth regions allow diametric increase in spinal canal diameter. (B) Oblique specimen radiograph of the cervical spine from a 7-month-old baby shows the radiolucent appearance of the neurocentral synchondroses.

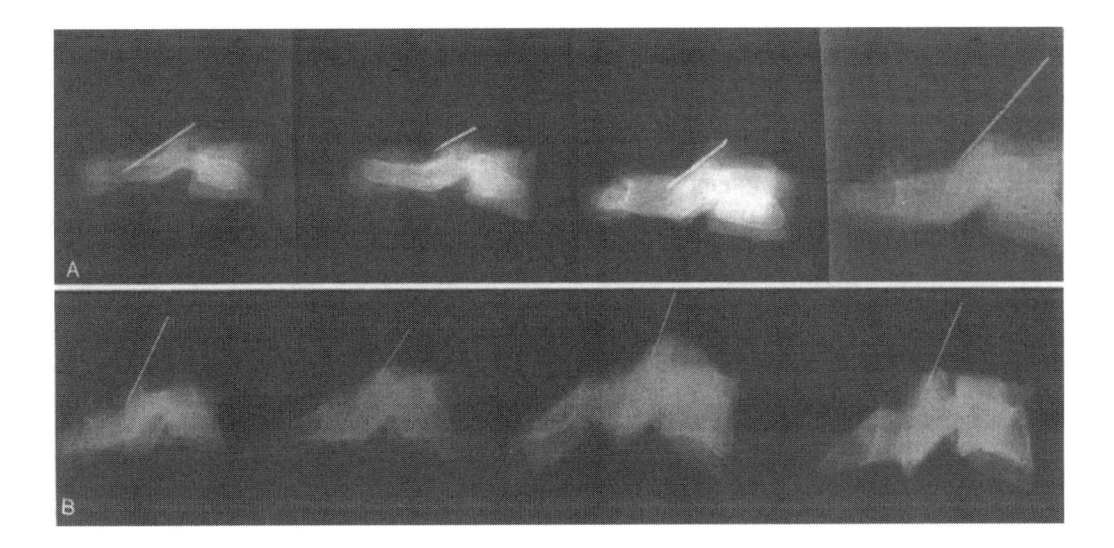

FIGURE 18-9. Changes in angulation of the articular facet plane in the cervical spine from birth to 10 years. The pins follow the articular plane. (A) C3 vertebra, which has a less acute angle than C7, which is shown in (B). This progressive angular change may be a major factor in allowing subluxation of the second, third, and fourth cervical vertebrae in young children compared to adolescents.

anatomic factor affecting mobility and fracture pattern susceptibility in the immature cervical spine.

Development of the thoracic vertebra is comparable to the lower cervical spine,[18,27,28] but this development is integrated with the ribs (Fig. 18-10), which tend to protect the thoracic vertebra from injury. These interrelations also explain some of the patterns of costovertebral injury in child abuse (see Chapter 11).

The neurocentral and posterior synchondroses are usually evident in thoracic spines removed from neonates. Within 2–3 months of postnatal development the posterior synchondroses close, except for an infrequent occurrence in the upper thoracic region. In contrast, the neurocentral synchondroses remain open until 5–6 years of age and begin patterns of closure similar to those of the cervical spine. Closure occurs in the upper region before closure in the middle region, which occurred before closure in the lower region. There may be considerable variation in the overall shape of the canal from spine to spine and among individual thoracic vertebrae of a single spine.

The transverse process develops a progressive posterior angulation during development. When viewed from the anterior projection, there is progressive downward angulation. A similar progressive angulation increase occurs in the aforementioned directions when the upper, middle, and lower thoracic spines are compared. Specifically, there is much greater posterior angulation in the lower thoracic spine than in the upper region.[18,27]

The facet joints maintain a relatively constant alignment along a given spine and throughout development. Significant changes in angulation comparable to those seen in the cervical spine were not evident, but there was a mild angulation of the facets from initially perpendicular to the spinous processes during development. This was more evident in the lower thoracic spine than in the upper thoracic spine.[18,27] The ligaments of the facet joints are relatively lax in the child, similar to joint laxity in the extremities. The amount of longitudinal or angular displacement allowed by such laxity, especially in the cervical spine, may exceed the intrinsic elasticity of the cord.[15]

The relative contributions of the anterior versus the posterior portions of the thoracic spine to the overall sagittal dimensions vary at different levels and ages. The centrum contributes the larger proportion of growth in the latter stages, particularly after the synchondroses have closed. The rate of growth of the vertebral body markedly increases in the lower thoracic levels. The spinous process elongates threefold to fourfold and shows a mild increase in its angulation relative to the longitudinal axis when spines were compared throughout development.[18,27]

Ossification with the vertebral body occurs in a systematic way, beginning as a hemispheric type of expansion during the prenatal stage and continuing with this type of expansion pattern during the postnatal phase to create the bulk of the vertebral body. Expansion occurs much more quickly toward the superior and inferior surfaces than toward the

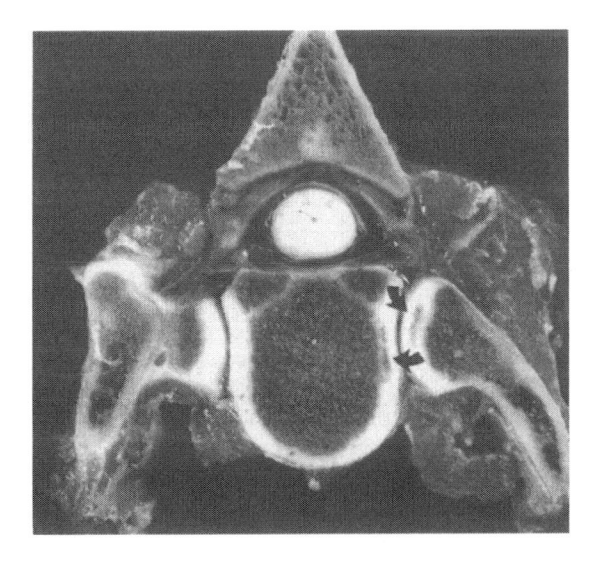

FIGURE 18-10. Juxtaposition of various growth regions of a thoracic vertebra and the ribs in an "adolescent" cape water buffalo. Apposed secondary ossification centers are evident (arrows).

peripheral surfaces around the sides of the vertebra. Similar expansion occurs relatively rapidly toward the posterior portion of the vertebral body, where the junction with the spinal canal is present. Once these factors are established, at approximately 2 years of age, the bulk of expansion of the vertebral body occurs in anterior and latitudinal directions rather than posteriorly.[18,27]

Vascular foramina are evident thoughout the peripheral margins and end-plates superiorly and inferiorly. Expansion of the peripheral margins of the ossification center is undulating. Within the indentations around the peripheral margins, a layer of cartilage is evident. A ring-like secondary ossification center, the ring apophysis, eventually develops in this region. Radial or spoke-like interdigitation of the physis (ring apophysis) with the expanding ossification center is evident by 6–7 years. This pattern is variable and often asymmetric (right half versus left half) within a single vertebra.[18,27]

The first thoracic vertebra has an uncinate process, not unlike the lower cervical vertebra. However, proceeding in a distal direction, this upturned lateral portion shifts to a more posterior position; and by the mid-thoracic region, any vestige of an "uncinate-like" process is no longer evident.[18,27]

The thoracic spinous processes elongate three to four times, depending on the region, and show a mild increase in angulation relative to the longitudinal axis when neonatal and mature spines are compared for any given level. The rates of increase in angulation of the spinous processes of the upper and lower regions are greater than the rate for the middle region. The angulation changes appear necessary to allow close overlap of spinous processes while the vertebral body increases in height.

Lumbar spine development follows the same basic pattern of three primary ossification centers. These vertebra have significant height growth during adolescence through growth plate analogues. This epiphyseal equivalency is more evident in other mammals, including most primates. The posterior synchondrosis of L5 often remains as a fibrous radiolucent defect referred to as spina bifida occulta, which may be present in as many as 20% of the population.[13,36]

The initial ossification centrum of all vertebra is spherical in utero[30] and progressively enlarges after birth to conform to the cartilaginous contours of the vertebral anlage. Because this expansion process is similar to that of the ossification center of a long bone, there may be similar reactions to trauma or illness. Specifically, the chondro-osseous transformation may stop temporarily and then resume, with a thin shell of sclerotic bone the result. It appears as a vertebra within a vertebra (Fig. 18-11).[24] As the ossification center approaches and conforms to the edges of the vertebra and remodels to conform to biologic demands, the vertebral body becomes increasingly responsive to trauma in a manner similar to the adult spine.[11]

The spinal canal, at any level, enlarges so long as the two neurocentral and single posterior synchondroses remain open.[17,20,28] They close first in the cervical region at about 6–7 years of age,[28] followed by thoracic closure (7–9 years) and lumbar closure (9–10 years).[17,28,30] Early closure due to a dysplasia (e.g., achondroplasia), infection, metabolic disease, or trauma may lead to canal stenosis.[3,28]

The thoracolumbar junction is comparable to a "stress riser" because of the motion change between the relatively rigid thoracic spine and the mobile lumbar spine, which increases the risk of injury at this level. Seat belt usage, especially if the chest strap is not adapted to the child, increases the risk of Chance fractures.

Secondary ossification centers variably appear at the tips of the spinous, transverse, and other processes during adolescence (Fig. 18-12). Avulsion or undisplaced chondro-osseous disruptions in these areas could be interpreted as ligamentous injuries because they are so difficult to visualize radiographically. Secondary ossification also appears at the same time in the cartilaginous "ring" apophysis within the vertebral end-plate (Fig. 18-13). This area is involved in the vertical growth (i.e., height) of the vertebral body.

Each of the facets has an epiphyseal analogue, with growth plate, undifferentiated hyaline cartilage, and articular cartilage. These areas are hypothetically susceptible to injuries analogous to physeal fractures in long bones.

The individual vertebral bodies enlarge circumferentially by the process of perichondrial and periosteal apposition

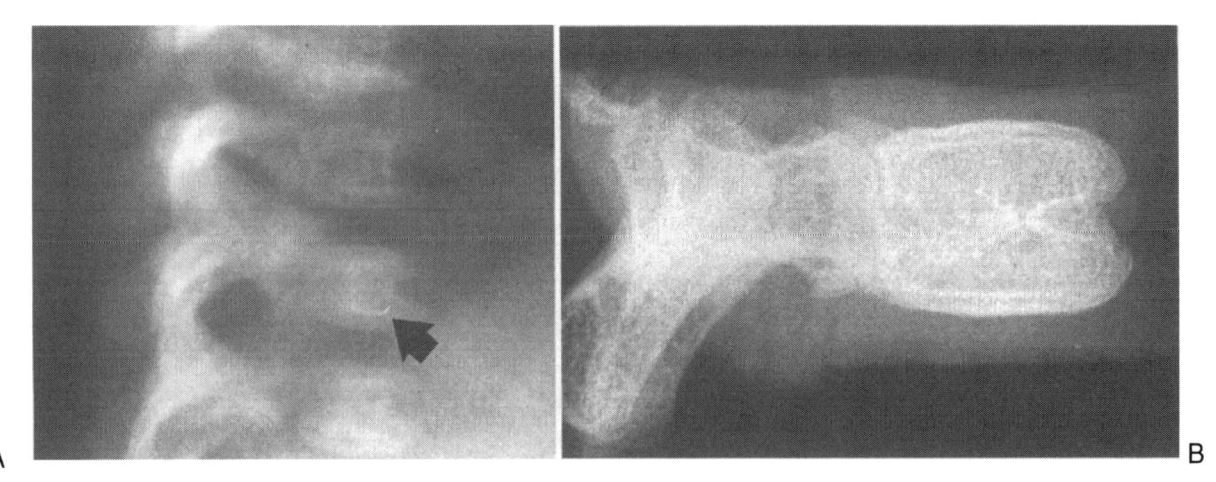

FIGURE 18-11. (A) Vertebra within a vertebra (arrow). This process is the spinal analogue of the Harris growth slowdown line. (B) Anatomic specimen of a thoracic vertebra from a 2-year-old boy showing the vertebra within a vertebra.

Anatomy

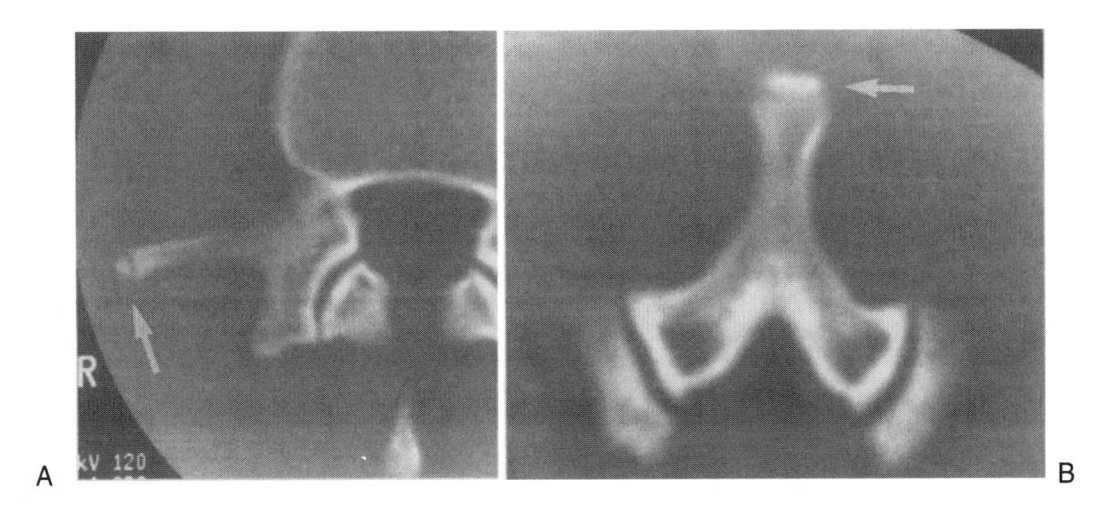

FIGURE 18-12. Secondary ossification in the developing spine. (A) Transverse process (arrow). (B) Spinous process (arrow).

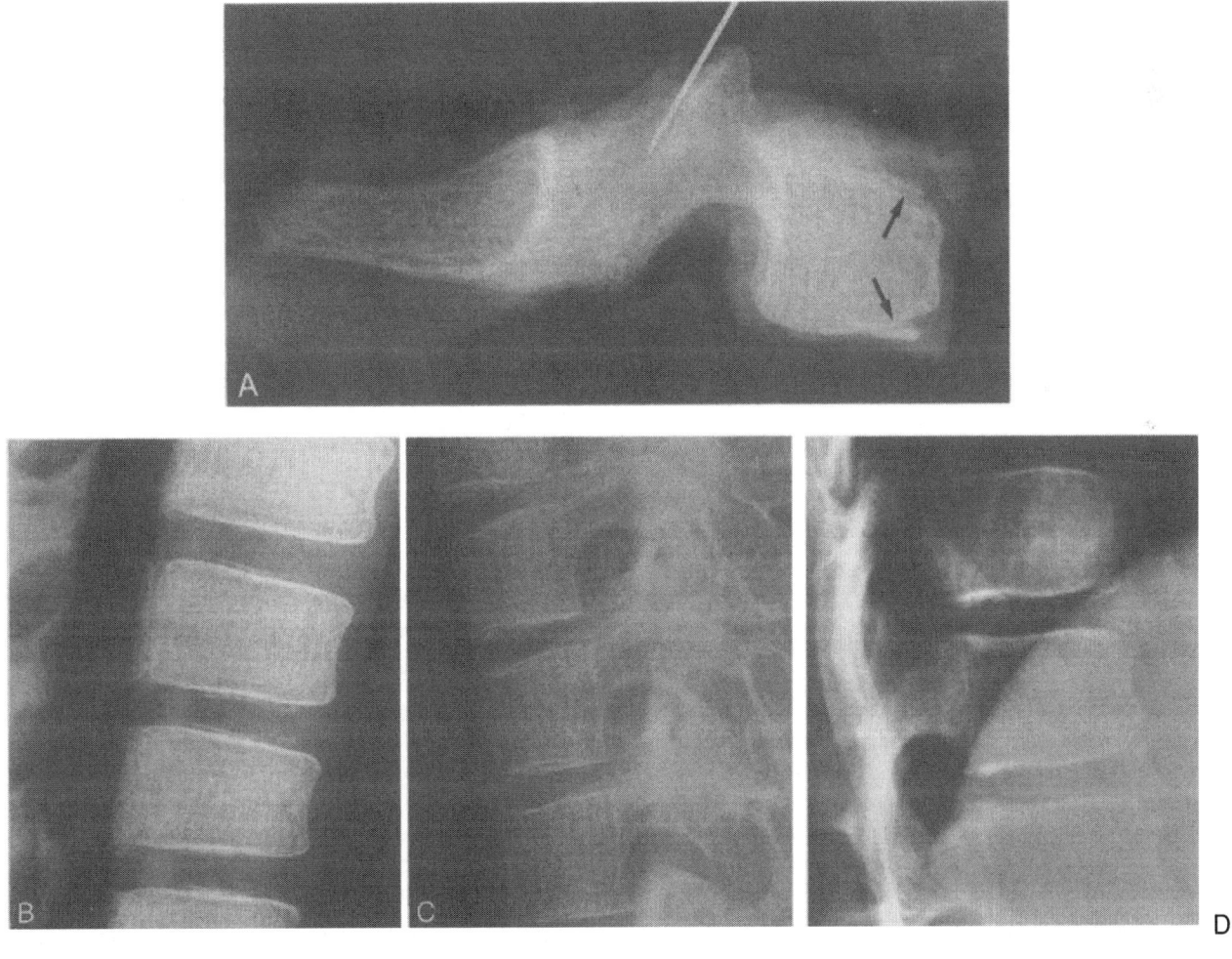

FIGURE 18-13. (A) Superior and inferior ring apophyses of C7 in a 12-year-old child (arrows). (B, C) Thoracolumbar development. (B) At 7 years. Note the greater degree of ring apophyseal maturation in the upper thoracic spine. (C), At 14 years. Note the extensive development of ring ossification. (D) Anterior ring apophyseal ossification in the lumbar vertebra. Abnormal development may lead to Scheuermann's kyphosis in a manner similar to Blount's disease (response to increased pressure).

those with early quadriplegia secondary to spinal cord trauma, the vertebral body may grow disproportionately in height, with the result that the vertebral bodies become relatively tall and thin, with biconvex end-plates and decreased disk spaces.[2,32]

The sacral vertebra, which are fused as a composite bone, have ossification patterns comparable to those of the other

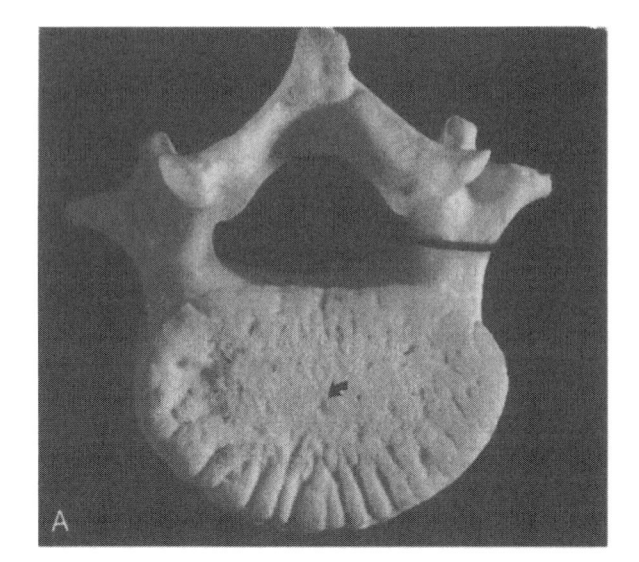

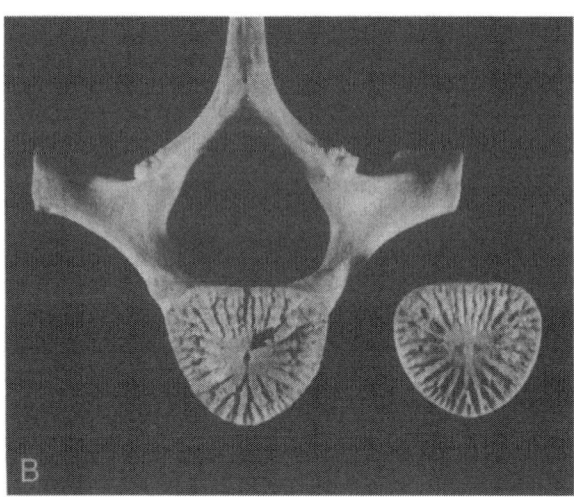

FIGURE 18-14. Comparison of metaphyseal undulations in the thoracic vertebrae of a 7-year-old human (A) and an adolescent dolphin (B). The latter species forms a complete end-plate, whereas the former species forms an incomplete marginal plate (ring). Asymmetric undulation in the human may be a factor in the development of scoliosis. (B) The matching complete end-plate (secondary, or epiphyseal, ossification center) is adjacent to the centrum. Also note the central remnant (ghost) of the notochord (arrow).

and grow vertically by endochondral ossification, with the vertebral end-plates functioning similarly to other physes. It has been said that the "ring" apophysis does not contribute to vertical growth of the vertebral body; it is true, as this particular structure represents a secondary ossification center like that in a long bone (Figs. 18-14 to 18-16). However, it is contiguous with a slow-growing physis covering the superior and inferior surfaces of each vertebral body.[38]

Normal values for the vertebral body height/sagittal diameter ratio and the vertebral height/disk space height ratio have been developed.[2] Such values assume significance only with full maturation of the osseous vertebra. Normal weight-bearing appears to affect vertical growth and keeps it in a normal relation to the anteroposterior diameter. In patients who do not have normal upright or walking posture, such as

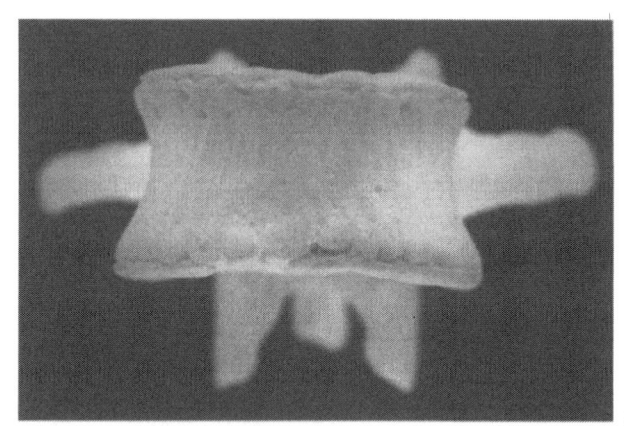

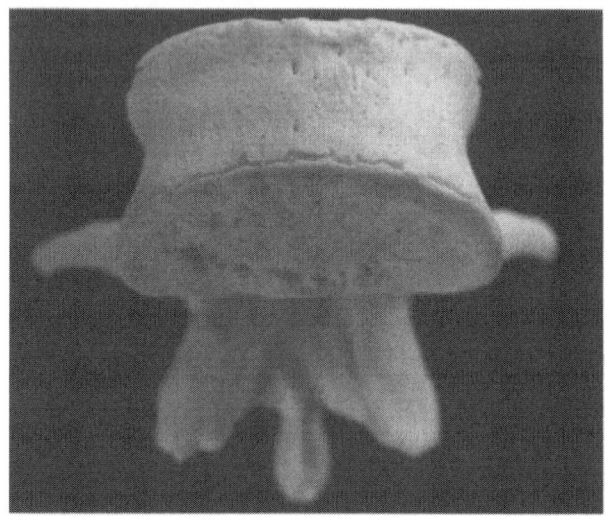

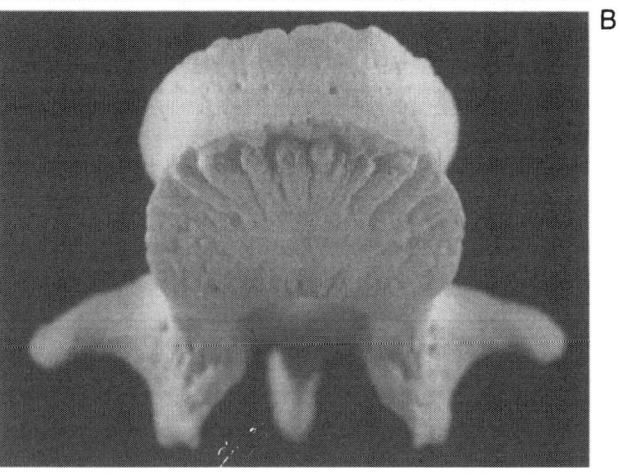

FIGURE 18-15. Ring apophyses in an 11-year-old boy. (A) Anterior view. (B) Oblique view. (C) Appearance of radial undulations after removal of ring apophysis. These undulations are probably adaptations to rotational stresses.

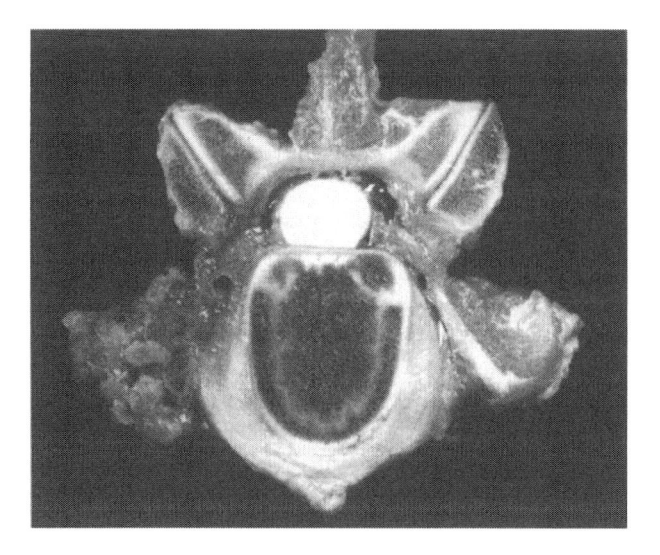

FIGURE 18-16. Transverse section of a thoracic vertebra of a cape water buffalo. The "ring apophysis" extends posteriorly, where it meets the neurocentral synchondroses.

vertebra. Cartilage runs along the margins apposed to the sacroiliac joint. Growth cartilage is part of this structure, which allows the possibility of chondro-osseous separation similar to a growth plate fracture in a long bone.

The basic pattern of blood supply to the spinal cord is established at birth.[4,7,12,23] Segmental arteries supply relatively discrete sections of the cord.[6] These vessels may supply anterior or posterior sections without a great deal of anastomotic communication.[6] The cervical and lumbar cord enlargements receive relatively greater numbers of blood vessels and may be more sensitive to temporary hemodynamic disruption. The lumbar enlargement is often referred to as a watershed region because of its dependence on the artery of Adamkiewicz.[7,9,19,33] Disruption of this specific artery has extreme consequences (especially paralysis).

These penetrating vessels also send branches to the vertebra. The supply of the posterior elements and anterior bodies are essentially separate and remain so even after closure of the neurocentral synchondroses.[10,14,31] Central arteries usually enter the vertebral body both anteriorly and posteriorly.[28] A significant venous supply leaves the vertebral body posteriorly, creating venous plexi (Fig. 18-17) that may be disrupted, causing an extradural hematoma, which may cause cord compression.

The intervertebral disk (Fig. 18-18) is supplied by encircling vessels that enter the periphery of the disk. Vessels also penetrate the enlarging vertebral end-plate.[38] Venous return from the disk tends to go into the vertebral body.[34]

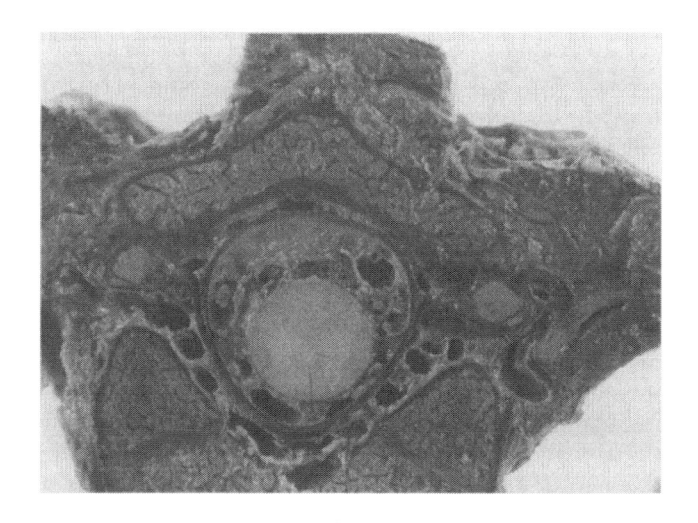

FIGURE 18-17. Extradural and intradural venous circulation in the thoracic vertebra of a 2-year-old child. Disruption of these vessels may play a role in compressive hematoma formation.

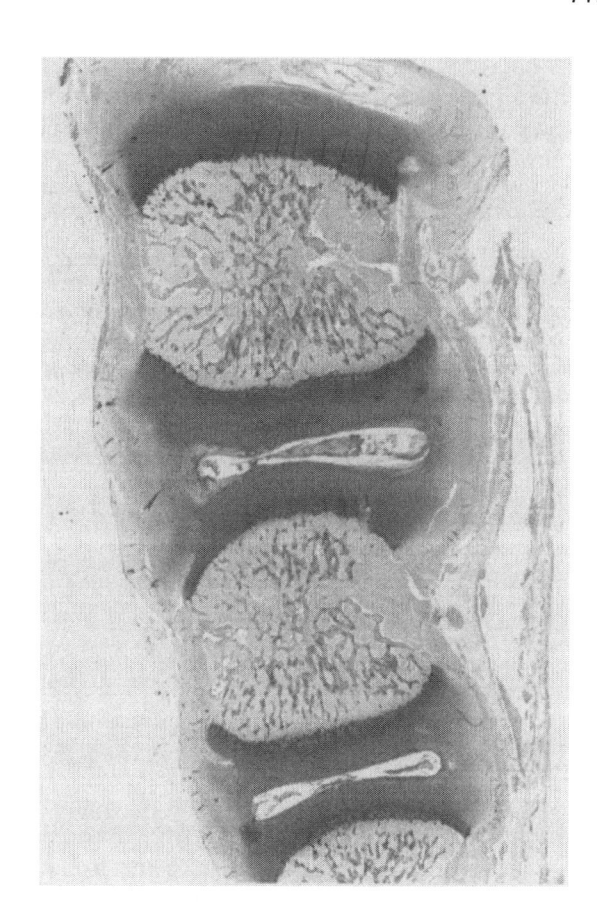

FIGURE 18-18. Appearance of vertebral primary ossification, cartilaginous end-plates, and disk material of the lumbar vertebra at full term.

Response of the Developing Spine to Trauma

Spinal fractures in children have distinct differences from those in adults. Such differences result from the child's inherent resilience to trauma and the potential for altered growth and development subsequent to a discrete injury, a major factor that may dramatically improve or worsen the initial postinjury result. The principal differences observed in children are the relatively benign clinical course, the potential for some gradual restoration of the vertebral body height when anteriorly wedged, and the development of progressive spinal deformity when there is end-plate (physeal) injury, facet physeal injury, or paralysis.[39,41,42,44,46,47,49-52,54-58,60-66,68,70-72,74-76,78] Fractures, dislocations, and fracture-dislocations of the spine in infants and children are relatively uncommon compared to their occurrence in adolescents and adults, who are more likely to be exposed to the major trauma mechanisms that usually cause spinal fractures. Knowledge about spinal and spinal cord injuries has been obtained primarily from experience with the adult population. There are far fewer reports concerning comparable injuries in children. A significant number of the reports pertain to the cervical spine, which in children is injured much more frequently than other regions of the spine. Fractures of the lower cervical and thoracolumbar spine and spinal cord injuries are less common in children than in adults.

Henrys and colleagues reviewed 1299 vertebral traumatic lesions; among them were 631 cervical lesions, of which only 12 were in children under 15 years of age (1.9%).[57] The progressive incidence of osseous injuries in the 6- to 15-year age group reflects the gradual acquisition of adult features of reduced flexibility and increasing exposure to more severe injury mechanisms.

Fracture-dislocations, which usually result from severe violence, account for the most severe neurologic complications. Of the six children with fracture-dislocations reported by Henrys and colleagues, five had significant neurologic complications, and one died.[57]

Hubbard reviewed 42 cases of spinal injury in children ranging in age from 17 months to 17 years; two-thirds were stable, and one-third were unstable.[62,63] None of the patients with stable injuries had neurologic trauma. Of the 14 patients with unstable lesions, however, eight had neurologic damage (six to the spinal cord and two to a nerve root). The neurologic injuries were of immediate onset, with the exception of one patient who sustained injury to the nerve roots 2 days after the initial trauma owing to a redislocation. Of the eight who suffered neurologic damage, there was cervical injury in four, thoracolumbar injury in three, and lumbar injury in one. Radiographs obtained 6 months after injury revealed scoliosis following *stable* thoracic, thoracolumbar, or lumbar injuries associated with hyperflexion force. However, the scoliosis was only slightly progressive and measured less than 10°, eventually becoming balanced with time. With *unstable* injuries, abnormal alignment was often present on the initial radiograph and progressed unless early surgical fusion was undertaken.

Dislocation of spinal segments is rare in children because the ligaments are generally stronger than the bone. However, displacement may occur *without* spinal cord injury; and in fact, in some cases there is no radiographic evidence of fracture. Separation of the centrum from an end-plate may be evident only as apparent widening of a disk space. Similarly, unilateral or bilateral facet disruption may occur in regions such as the thoracolumbar junction because of intrinsic ligamentous laxity. Again, such disruption may be free of concomitant spinal cord injury.[61]

Children have a growth plate and cartilage similar to an epiphysis associated with each of the four facet joints. Injury can theoretically involve these regions and certainly has been seen by me during open reductions of thoracic and lumbar fractures. Morphologic and histologic studies are lacking, however, even in Aufdermaur's classic pathologic study.[40] We have had the opportunity to assess some of these injuries in skeletally immature large zoo animals.

Normal anteroposterior and lateral alignments of the spine are contingent on the chondro-osseous anatomy, ligaments, truncal musculature, and effect of gravity.[3,16] The extent of disruption of perichondrium and periosteum into which these soft tissues components attach also affects stability. Because of the possibility of radiolucent injury, the spine must be immobilized until actual or occult injuries are appropriately evaluated. The large size of the child's head may cause excessive flexion on a flat immobilization board (Fig. 18-19).[45,59]

At any specific level of a motion segment where injury occurs, stability depends primarily on the interrelation between the anterior, middle, and posterior chondroosseous and ligamentous columns. In a traumatized spine, the extent of damage to these columns determines the overall stability during the acute and chronic phases. It is often difficult to assess accurately the amount of stability in the adult spine. It is even more difficult to assess the degree of intrinsic or remaining stability of the cartilaginous portions of the immature spine. The goal of treatment, whether operative or nonoperative, is still the same: spinal stability. Failure to achieve this goal may result in progressive deformity.

In adults spinal deformity is considered a preventable complication of fractures and fracture-dislocations of the axial skeleton provided there is judicious use of bracing or instrumentation and fusion. In the child, however, a different situation arises, as damage to end-plate growth mechanisms may not be obvious and may slowly lead to subsequent deformity during the various periods of growth (especially adolescence). Whether dealing with acute injury or progressive secondary changes due to growth deformity, associated morbidity may significantly limit the ultimate physical and neurologic rehabilitation of the spine and spinal cord-injured child and adolescent months or even years following the original injury. The complex reconstructive surgery that is often required to correct deformities and relieve symptoms is not without potentially serious risk to the child or adolescent. These risks must be considered before choosing surgical approaches, especially in skeletally immature children. Some methods of stabilization may be difficult or inappropriate in the young child.

The clinical picture for patients with stable injury is characteristically benign and not usually associated with long-term problems, strongly suggesting that initial treatment for more than a few months may not be required.[62] However, long-term follow-up to skeletal maturity may help identify the patient who is likely to develop a growth abnormality. Such studies must be encouraged in centers caring for these children. The absence of spontaneous interbody fusion or disk narrowing probably relates to a healthy intervertebral disk and its inherent ability to withstand stress in the child.

There may be variable, incomplete restoration of vertebral body height in thoracolumbar fractures, but it is less likely following cervical compression fractures.[62] There is a difference in the ultimate growth (height) capacity of the cervical spine versus the thoracolumbar spine during growth spurts that may be a major factor in this potential tendency of one region, but not the other, to restore height. The cervical vertebrae approximate adult height sooner than the thoracic and lumbar vertebrae. It is important to realize that complete restoration of vertebral height does *not* always occur in any

FIGURE 18-19. Concept of large head causing spine flexion (top). The support for the body should be higher (middle, bottom).

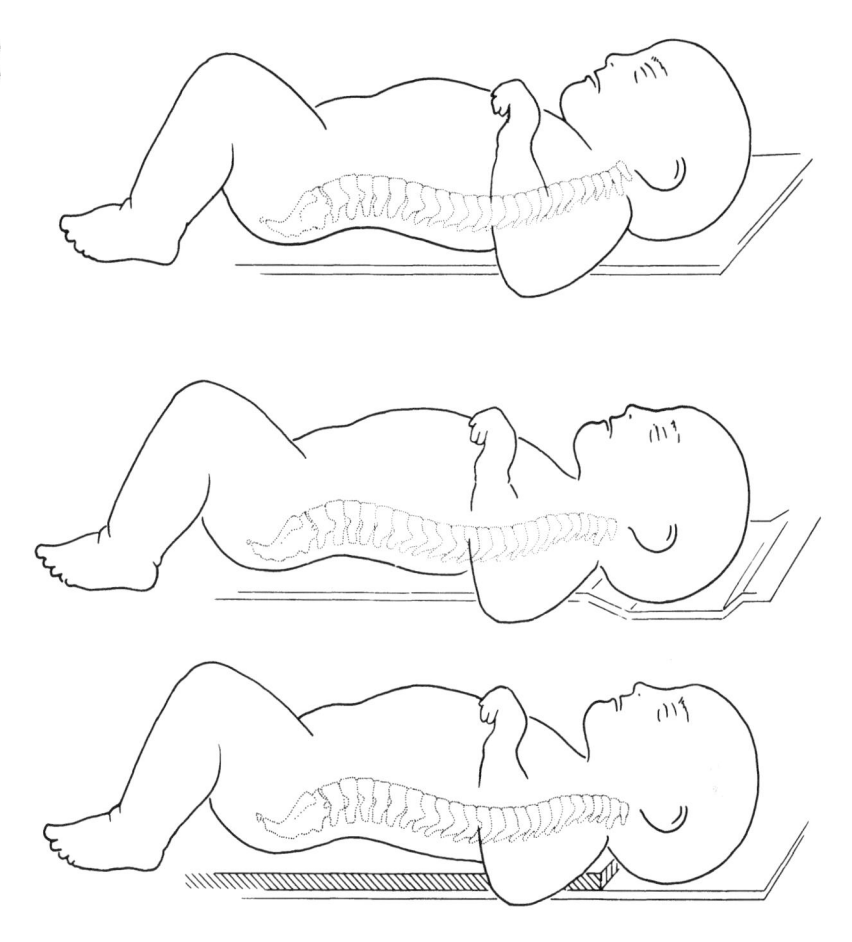

segment of the developing spine, in contrast to generalizations that such complete recovery of height usually occurs.

Gunshot Injury

Spinal and spinal cord injuries consequent to gunshots are becoming increasingly prevalent, particularly among urban children.[43,69,79] These injuries are approached similarly to those in adults and are described in more detail in Chapter 9. The most serious consequence in a child is that dissolution of lead by the cerebrospinal fluid may lead to toxic levels of lead systemically, with subsequent neurodevelopmental consequences.[48,53,77]

Preexisting Disease/Deformity

There are many congenital malformations of the craniovertebral junction that should not be confused with traumatic lesions.[80–116] Anomalies characterized by single or multiple ossification centers must be differentiated from traumatic fragmentation. Well-marginated, distinct ossification centers may be seen anterior to the dens above or below the arch of the atlas. There may be unilateral or bilateral clefts in the ring of the atlas, usually in the posterior arch but rarely in the anterior arch. These clefts vary from small defects (spina bifida occulta) to agenesis of half or even the entire posterior ring.

There are a number of congenital and acquired orthopedic vertebral problems, especially those involving the various skeletal dysplasias. In addition, due consideration should be given to evaluating these children, just as much as a child with Down syndrome, before they participate in various types of athletic activities. Underdevelopment of the dens (hypoplasia) and C1–C2 instability are relatively common.[80,83,103,105] Children with severe osteogenesis imperfecta may also develop micro- and macrofractures, leading to severe deformity (see Chapter 11).

Evaluation for an acute injury to the neck or back may be the first indication of a congenital spinal deformity.[112] In the illustrated case of a child sustaining a hyperflexion injury (Fig. 18-20), there was concern that the wedging was traumatic. However, a bifid, congenitally deformed vertebral body was found on computed tomographic (CT) scan, with no evidence of posterior disruption. Children and adolescents with congenital deformities such as Klippel-Feil syndrome (Fig. 18-21) may develop neck or back pain during sports, which may lead to the initial diagnosis of congenital spine deformity. Once such deformities are diagnosed they may affect the appropriateness of continuation in a given sports activity.[99,108] Sherk and Nicholson reported a fatal injury in an abnormal cervical spine.[158]

Children with Klippel-Feil syndrome and other congenital deformities may be at significantly increased risk for spinal cord injury.[88] Elster reported a case of quadriplegia following minor trauma in a patient with preexisting Klippel-Feil syndrome.[94] Strax and Baran also reported cases of traumatic quadriplegia on an acute basis.[112] Many of these children do not present for diagnosis until they are engaged in some sporting activity that makes them develop neck pain or subtle to obvious neurologic findings, at which point evaluation reveals the abnormality. Most neurologic problems develop slowly. Any patient with a diagnosis of Klippel-Feil syndrome should

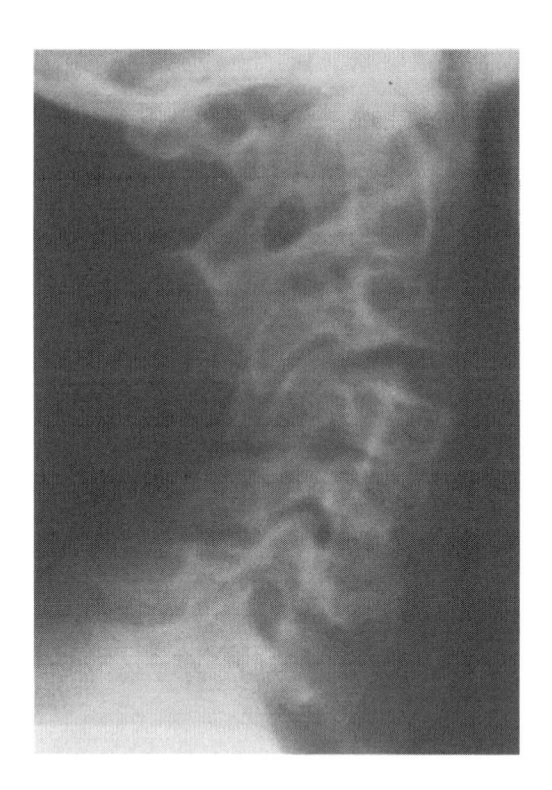

FIGURE 18-21. This 9-year-old patient presented with neck pain while playing soccer. Her only motion segment was C3–C4.

create an increased moment arm at C7–T1, leading to facet displacement (Fig. 18-22).

Down Syndrome

Over the past 20 years there has been increasing recognition of actual and potential cervical instability in children with Down syndrome.[117–167] Much of it has come about because of increased assimilation of these individuals into family units and the rise of activities such as the Special Olympics.

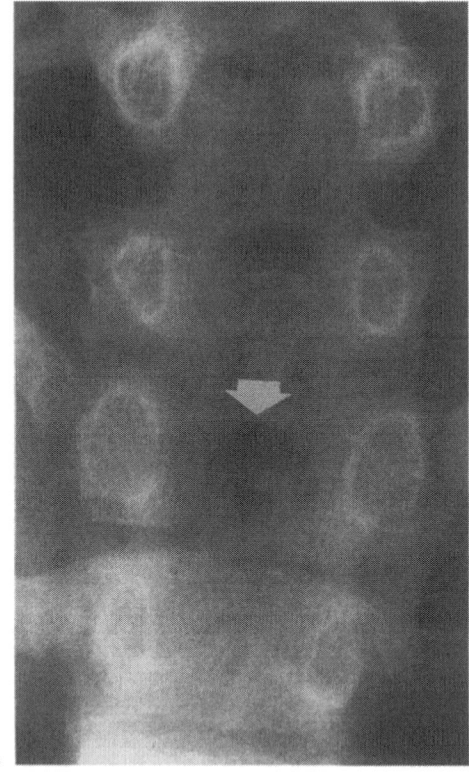

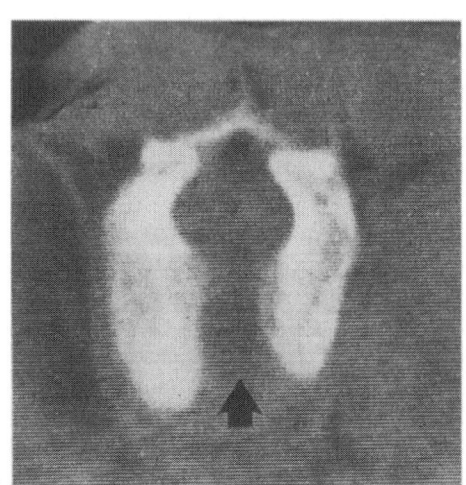

FIGURE 18-20. A 10-year-old boy with back pain after hyperflexion injury. Lateral view showed apparent wedging, which suggested a compression fracture. (A) Anteroposterior view shows widening of the pedicles and a central lucency (arrow). (B) Computed tomographic scan showed a bifid vertebral body (arrow). The ligaments had been strained, but no fractures occurred. The "compression" was part of the congenital deformity.

be thoroughly screened for potential instability through hypermobile segments that develop to accommodate lack of motion in the fused segments.

Scoliosis

Children who have had fusion and instrumentation for scoliosis may be at increased risk for spinal trauma following an accident.[89,114,116] Particularly, a high thoracic fusion may

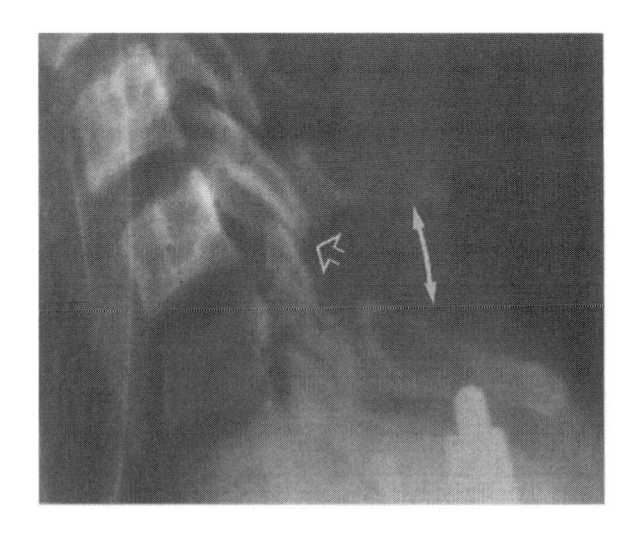

FIGURE 18-22. C6–C7 disruption in an automobile accident victim who had undergone previous Harrington instrumentation to T1 for scoliosis. Closed arrows show widening of spinous processes; open arrow shows facet joint disruption.

Pathobiology

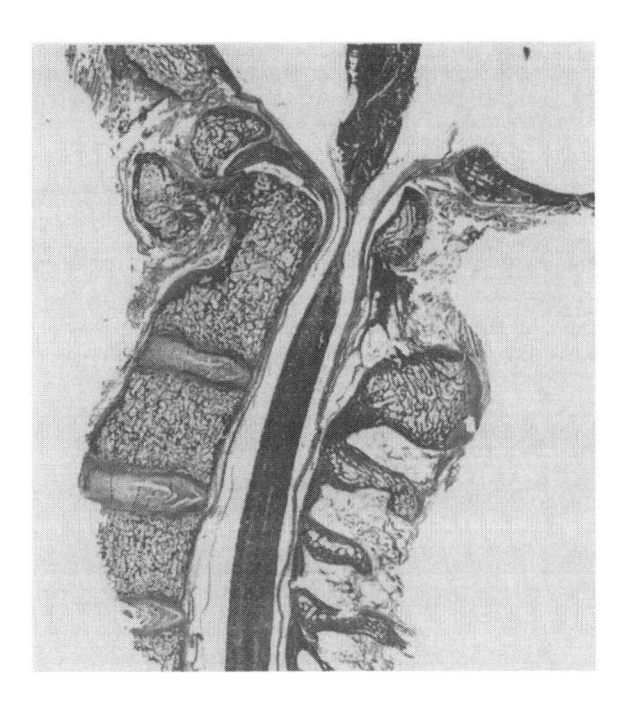

FIGURE 18-23. Histologic section of the occiput to C4 in a patient with Down syndrome. A progressively waddling gait had been evident for more than 2 years. Stabilization was refused by the family. Severe upper cord/medulla attenuation is evident.

The most potentially serious problem is intervertebral instability that leads to acute or progressive compression of the spinal cord (Fig. 18-23). It may occur at the occipitoatlantal joint, the altlantoaxial joint, or both. This instability is probably a consequence of abnormal collagen, rather than acute ligament failure. Children with various types of dysplasia and who are involved in accidents obviously deserve close evaluation of their cervical spine. Great care should be taken when evaluating what represents a preexistent anatomic variant or abnormality versus trauma-related disease.

The consensus is that if an atlas-dens interval (ADI) of 4.5 mm or more is present or if significant odontoid hypoplasia exists, at-risk sports should be avoided. When significant myelopathic signs accompany an increased ADI, C1–C2 fusion should be undertaken. These children seem to be at greater risk to resorb any grafted bone.[156] Postoperative halo-vest immobilization is also recommended because of the hyperactive nature of these children. There is an excellent overview of screening indications and frequency in the AAOS monograph.[885]

Pathologic Fractures

Children may have acute onset of neck pain that is attributed to some activity. The (treating) physician must be aware of the possibility of unusual conditions such as an eosinophilic granuloma or a spinal cord tumor.

Patients with chronic conditions, such as juvenile rheumatoid arthritis (Fig. 18-24), leukemia, or renal osteodystrophy, may develop back pain. It is usually due to pathologic fractures in the osteoporotic/osteopenic bone. Treatment is generally symptomatic (medication, orthotics). Successful treatment of the predisposing cause also obviously affects the continuation or recurrence of these pathologic fractures.

Pathobiology

Aufdermaur presented a detailed morphologic investigation of spinal injuries in 12 children under 18 years of age who were examined after accidental deaths.[40] Each of the spines was completely dissected for evaluation. He also removed 20 intact spines from juveniles of similar age groups who had died from nontraumatic causes (e.g., cancer, drowning) and subjected them to similar mechanical stress testing. A frequent finding was the tendency for the injuries to have occurred through the region of the subcondylar (end) plate and hypertrophic cartilage, creating a physeal injury analogue (Fig. 18-25). Aufdermaur believed that because there was a high likelihood of such growth mechanism injury the most likely radiographic sign, if any, would be widening of the intervertebral space.[40] Such widening may not be readily apparent on routine radiography, as these injuries often reduce spontaneously after deforming forces are dissipated. Stress views might elicit the instability, but this procedure could be dangerous to the spinal cord. Magnetic resonance imaging (MRI) would be more likely to detect areas of altered signal intensity associated with hemorrhage and edema near the vertebral end-plate. This technique has been used to detect occult physeal injuries in the limbs (see Chapters 5–7).

Aufdermaur's cases involved injuries to the following areas: cervical spine (seven cases), thoracic spine (four cases), and lumbar spine (one case).[40] In 10 instances the injury was due to a traffic accident, and in two instances the spine was hyperextended during childbirth. Clinically,

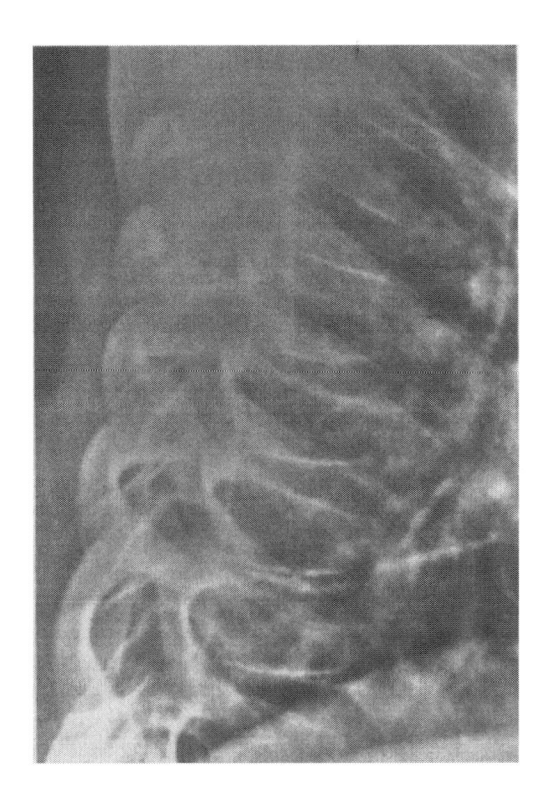

FIGURE 18-24. Multiple compression fractures in a 9-year-old boy with systemic juvenile rheumatoid arthritis on high dose steroids.

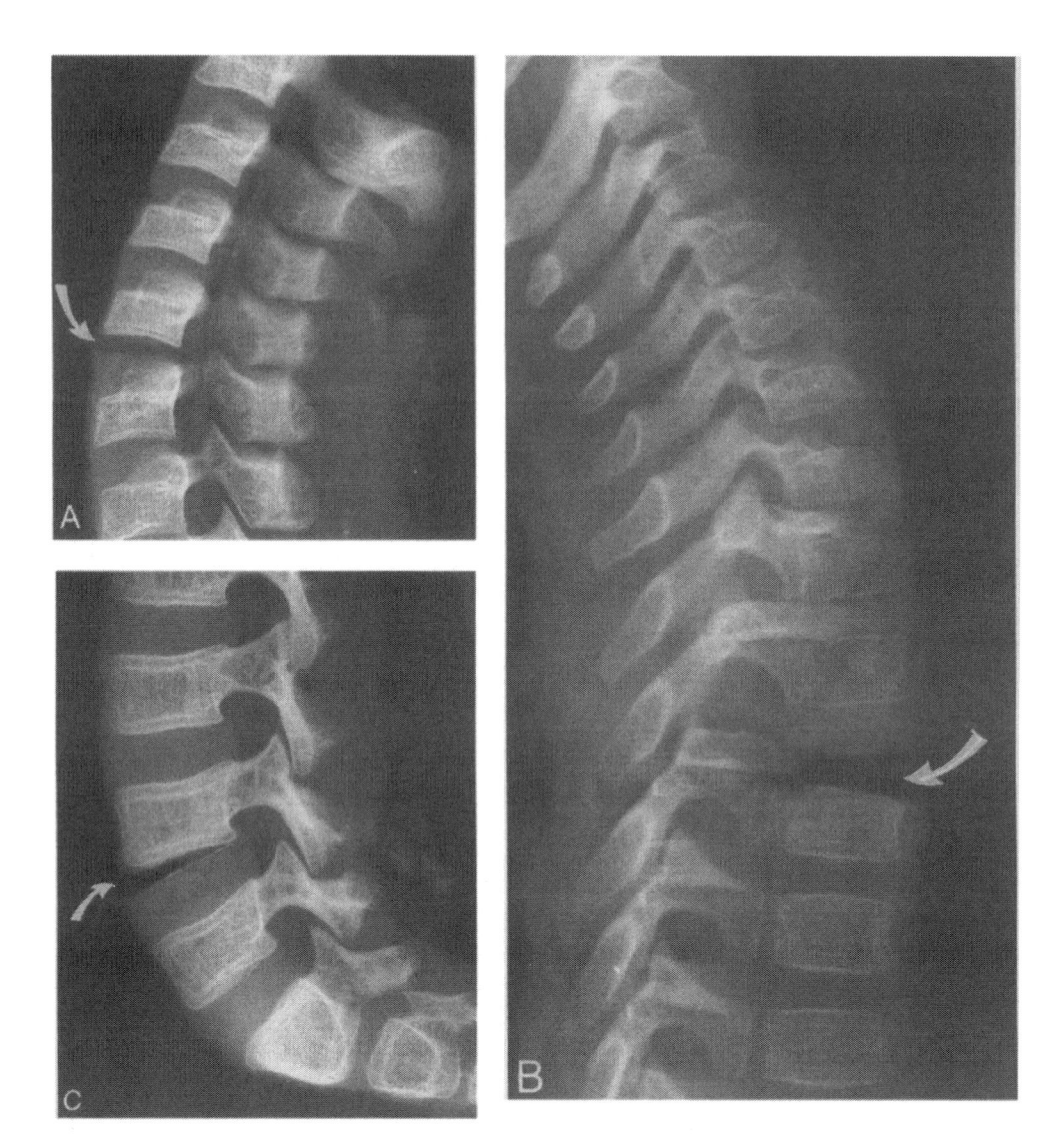

FIGURE 18-25. Injuries of the immature spine found during autopsy following traumatic deaths (usually vehicular versus pedestrian). (A) Cervical (arrow). (B) Thoracic; this is a Chance injury equivalent (arrow). (C) Lumbar (arrow). Each is a separation through the end-plate.

however, a spinal fracture was suspected *only once*. In the other 11 cases, the spinal injury was not diagnosed until autopsy. In all cases, death occurred within 1.0–1.5 days of the accident. In nine of the cases the spinal injuries did *not* contribute to death; in three cases, however, there were significant cervical, epidural, and subdural hematomas and associated brain injury that probably were related to the cause of death. In two cases the anterior longitudinal ligament was ruptured; and in three cases the supraspinous and intraspinous ligaments, ligamentum flavum, and capsules of the posterolateral joints were ruptured, as were the cartilaginous end-plate and the longitudinal ligaments. Histologically, the fracture lines involved the growth zone almost exclusively. Four patients had multiple-level cartilage plate injuries. The top end-plate was injured in 12 patients and the bottom end-plate in 6. Histologic findings were similar for cervical, thoracic, and lumbar vertebrae.

This study by Aufdermaur introduced the anatomic concept of occult injury to the developing spine. He emphasized that separation of an end-plate from the incompletely ossified vertebral body could occur, leading to considerable angular displacement when injurious forces were maximal. As such displacing forces dissipated, the angulation accordingly reversed, effectively (spontaneously) closing the fracture gap. With the maximum morphologic deformity, traction or compression injury to the spinal cord could occur. This phenomenon has become accepted in the pediatric orthopaedic and spinal literature as *s*pinal *c*ord *i*njury *w*ithout *o*bvious *r*adiologic *a*bnormality (SCIWORA).

Animal Fractures

Animal models of spontaneous fractures of the immature spine offer another method of understanding the pathoanatomy of these injuries and the occurrence of SCIWORA. We have studied a number of such physeal fracture analogues.[73]

Pathobiology

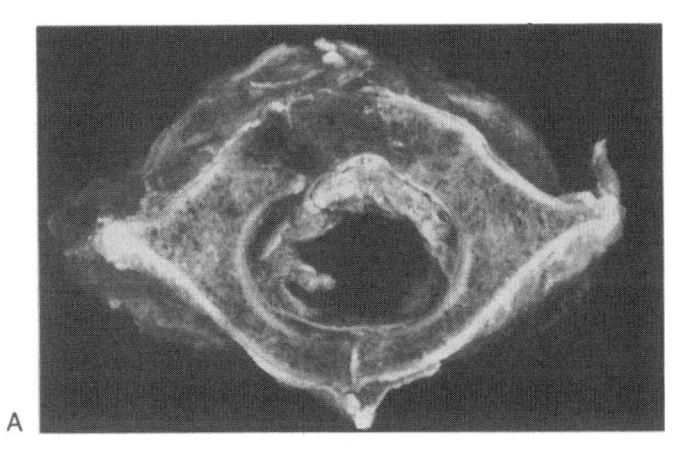

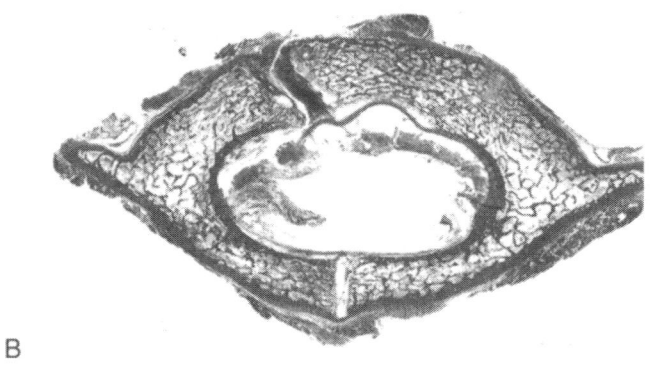

FIGURE 18-26. C1 fracture in an immature giraffe. (A) Transverse section shows anterior injury and intraosseous hemorrhage. (B) Histologic section shows the anterior fracture through the synchondrosis.

As in the skeletally immature human, the most commonly injured regions in the specimens were the cervical spine (five fractures) and lumbar spine (five fractures), followed by the thoracic spine (four fractures).[73] All fractures in these skeletally immature specimens propagated along chondro-osseous growth regions. The atlas and axis were disrupted through their synchondroses, whereas the other vertebrae usually were fractured along the end-plate physes. These end-plate physeal fractures also propagated variably into the neurocentral synchondroses when the mechanism of injury was extension-distraction. Distinct spinal cord injury was noted in four animals.

A "Jefferson fracture" injury was noted in a 2-month-old giraffe (Fig. 18-26). The animal became progressively ataxic following a traumatic delivery and was killed several weeks after the observed injury when no recovery was evident. Dissection revealed organized hematoma anterior to the ring of C1. Radiographs of the atlas demonstrated a thin subchondral separation in the posterior synchondrosis, a closed left anterior synchondrosis, and a normal right anterior synchondrosis. Morphologic examination of the atlas revealed hemorrhage in the right anterior synchondrosis and subperiosteal hemorrhage extending along the spinal canal to the posterior synchondrosis with resulting cord compression. Histology demonstrated hemorrhage and chondro-osseous separation in the right synchondrosis, providing evidence that it was an analogue of a "Jefferson fracture" that had broken through the atlas not only at the posterior synchondrosis but also at the right anterior synchondrosis.

A 3-day-old Thompson's gazelle ran head first into an abutment. The animal developed progressive paralysis over the ensuing hours and as a result was killed. Initial radiographs of the cervical spine showed a C2 fracture of the dens. Dissection revealed hemorrhage in the upper cervical paravertebral tissues and an additional fracture involving the superior articular facet of C2 (Fig. 18-27). The facet fracture appeared nondisplaced on the radiograph, and there was no disruption of the articular surface morphologically. This discrepancy was attributable to the fracture traversing a region of subarticular cartilage. The facet joint was minimally displaced, hinging apart so the displacement was not readily evident on the radiograph.

A 5-month-old giraffe was acutely paralyzed after running into a fence. Radiographs revealed a type 2 physeal fracture traversing the dentocentral synchondrosis with a right articular facet Thurstan Holland fragment. This fragment was partially separated from the physis (Fig. 18-28).

In another injured giraffe the spinal cord was completely severed at the level of a dens fracture and was additionally compressed by a hematoma distally at the C2–C3 junction. Interestingly, most of the hematoma was on the dorsal side of the cord, whereas the fractures were on the ventral side (Fig. 18-29).

A colobus monkey was the victim of physical abuse by another colony member, sustaining a fracture-dislocation at the thoracolumbar junction. This fracture propagated through the posterior elements and exited in two directions: (1) through the vertebral body T12, along the neurocentral

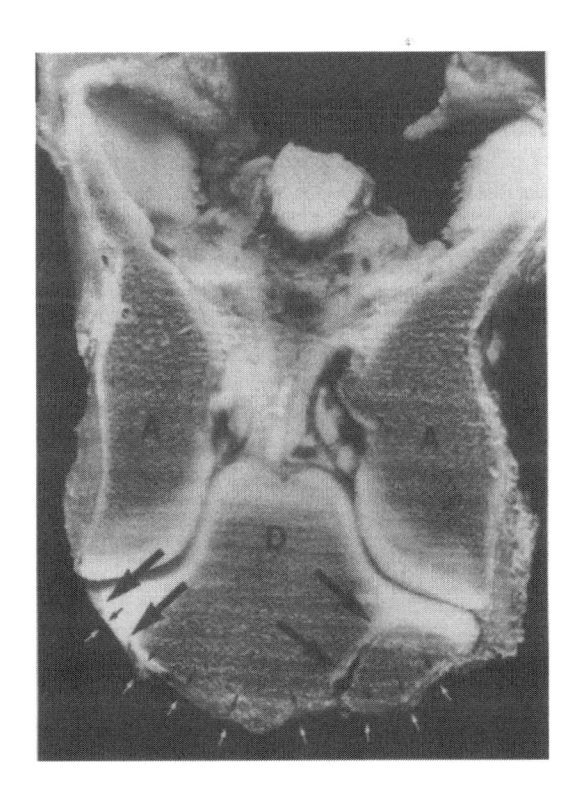

FIGURE 18-27. C2 fracture in a gazelle. As in the child, the dens fracture line followed the dentocentral synchondrosis (arrows).

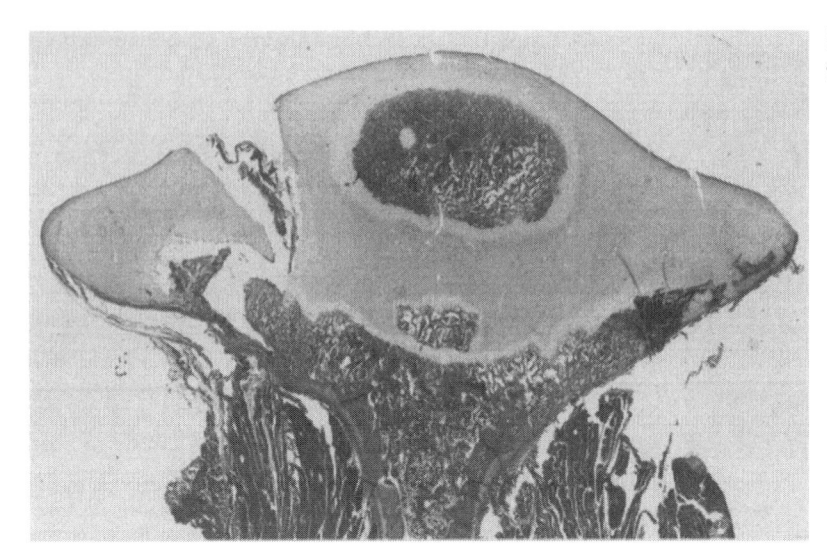

FIGURE 18-28. Facet fracture of C2 in a 5-month-old giraffe that was a chondro-osseous separation.

synchondroses, across the inferior end-plate and intervertebral disk, exiting anteriorly along the superior end-plate of L1; and (2) through the inferior end-plate of T11 (Fig. 18-30). Although these fractures appeared to traverse only the superior end-plates, further inspection revealed that these fractures also propagated along the neuro-central synchondroses toward the inferior end-plates. This pattern has recently been described in a case of child abuse.[677]

Type 3 inferior end-plate fractures of the lumbar spine were sustained by a camel and a zebra (Fig. 18-31). Dissection revealed hemorrhage extending into the intervertebral disk. Histologic examination revealed that the fracture traversed the primary spongiosa of the body, technically making it a type 4 growth mechanism fracture. The injury also propagated across a portion of the intervertebral disk.

Diagnosis

Diagnosis includes accurate evaluation of the level and extent of injury to chondro-osseous and nervous system tissues and the contiguous muscular and vascular structures. Early assessment is essential, as it is the baseline against which the effectiveness of any therapeutic manipulation or development of complications is evaluated. Early assessment comprises inspection and palpation, *accurate determination of neurologic function or dysfunction*, and radiographic examination. The initial neurologic examination should be completed before the patient undergoes radiologic evaluation. Radiographs or other types of diagnostic imaging should be obtained progressively in accordance with neurologic findings and with appropriate protection.

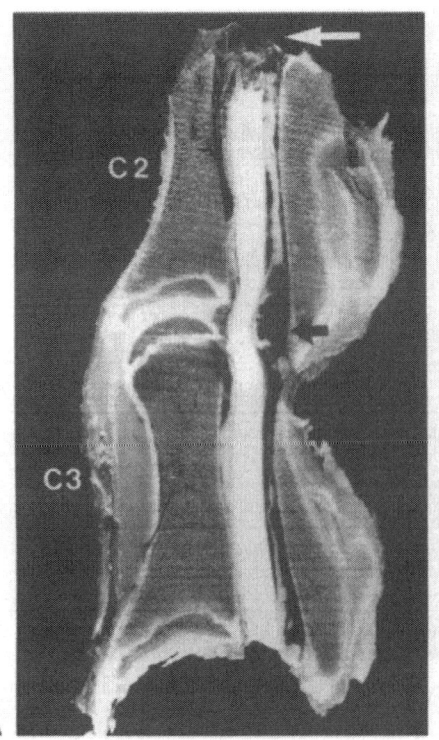

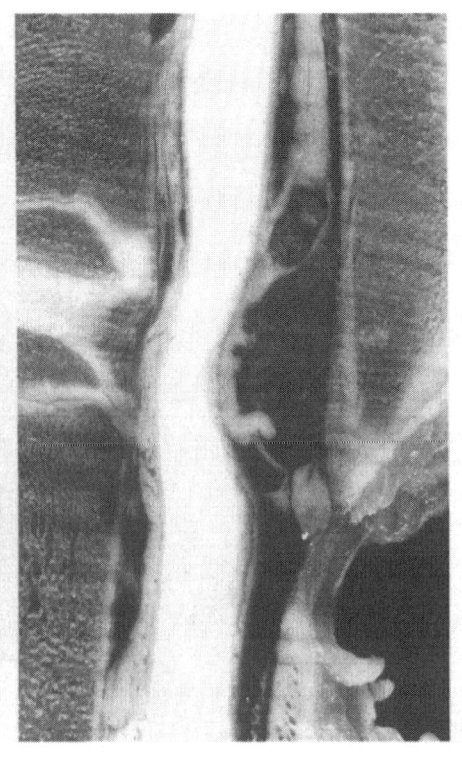

FIGURE 18-29. SCIWORA in a giraffe. A fracture is evident at the top of C2 (arrow), but no obvious osseous injury is seen at C3. (A) Slab section showing a hematoma posterior to the spinal cord. (B) Higher power view showing cord deformity and a smaller area of hemorrhage anterior to the cord. The intraosseous hematoma of the C3 proximal metaphysis suggests occult injury (bone bruising) with incomplete fracture.

Diagnosis

Inspection may reveal associated soft tissue injury. Abrasion of the face suggests cervical hyperextension injury, possibly with a rotatory component; and abrasion of the upper neck suggests hyperflexion of the dorsal spine. Scalp contusion or laceration may indicate an axial loading component in addition to the aforementioned angular, shear, and rotatory components. Palpation may reveal a local area of tenderness. The presence of a palpable gap may indicate disruption of the posterior ligaments and a potentially high degree of instability. Neurologic evaluation is of primary importance, as damage to the spinal cord is the main complication. Of the 18 patients reported by Henrys and colleagues, seven had neurologic injuries.[57] Of subluxations of C1 and C2, two resulted in decerebration; and one patient with subluxation of C1–C2 presented with a transient paresthesia of the left arm, secondary to a football injury.

Detailed neurologic examination should be *repeated frequently*, since changing, especially worsening neurologic patterns may require aggressive action, and improvements may encourage waiting. Motor function in the awake, cooperative patient should be described so subsequent observers are able to assess the improvement or gradual loss of neurologic patterns or function. Loss of deep tendon reflexes generally parallels loss of motor function. In the unconscious patient, facial grimacing when in pain, in the absence of withdrawal of the extremities and loss of deep tendon reflexes, suggests cord injury. In the cervicodorsal region, the spinous process lies about two segments above the corresponding spinal segment (i.e., the spinous process of C5 overlies the C7 cord level). In the dorsolumbar region, as many as 11 spinal segments may lie between the spinous processes of T10 and L1.

Complete loss of motor and reflex function immediately following injury and associated with sensory loss is generally consistent with similar motor level loss and involves all sensory modalities, including deep pain. In the Brown-Sequard syndrome, loss of touch and proprioception occurs on the same side as the motor loss; in contrast, analgesia

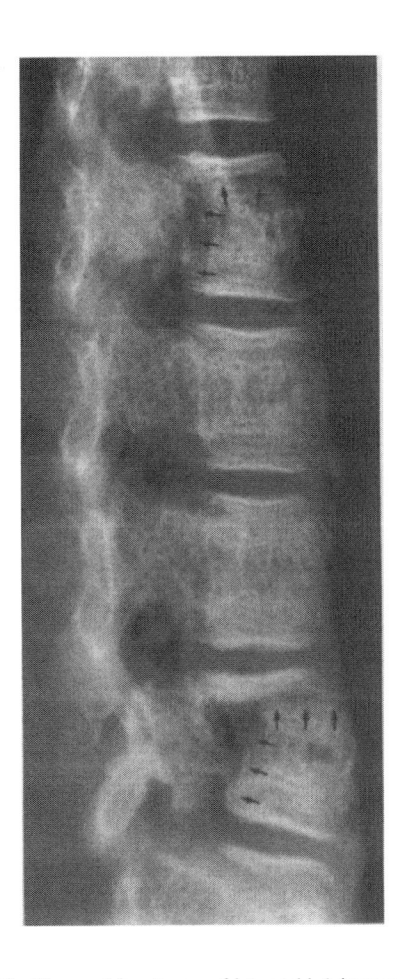

FIGURE 18-30. Physeal fractures of L1 and L4 (arrows) in an infant monkey. These fractures propagated along the superior end-plate physis and turned to follow the neurocentral synchondroses. Although a rare injury in children, it has been reported and may be more common because of lack of familiarity with the pattern of injury.

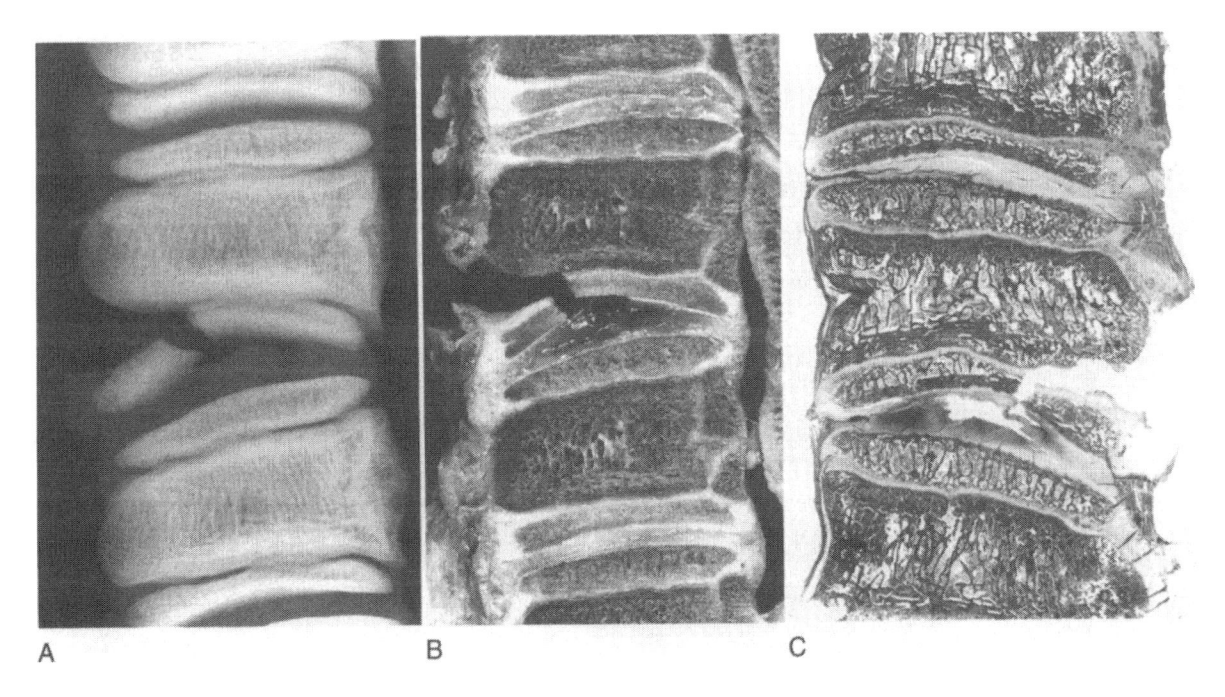

FIGURE 18-31. End-plate physeal fracture (type 3) in an adolescent zebra. (A) Radiograph. (B) Slab section. (C) Histologic section.

occurs on the contralateral side and, because of the manner in which pain fibers cross the sensory level for pain, usually two to three levels below the motor level.

In the anterior spinal artery syndrome, touch and proprioception may be preserved but there is loss of other long tract functions. This situation occurs because the posterior cord (i.e., dorsal and dorsolateral columns) may be supplied by relatively separate branches of the posterior spinal artery. Preservation of touch and proprioception has no predictive value for motor recovery, especially in the young child.

Preservation of sacral sensation is seen occasionally in central cord injuries because of the peripheral location of the sacral portion of the spinothalamic tract. Its predictive value is questionable in children, in whom the recovery potential is often remarkable compared with similarly injured adults.

In contrast, preservation of patchy areas of sensation or appreciation of deep pain indicates that motor loss may be secondary to spinal shock. Spinal shock remains a misunderstood phenomenon. Deep tendon reflexes cannot be elicited, and there is flaccid paralysis below the level of the lesion. Sphincter tone generally is minimally affected, and there is urinary retention. If the injury is not severe, reflexes gradually return, voluntary micturition is reestablished, and motor recovery begins within hours or days of injury. If the cord injury is severe, recovery of reflexes is accompanied by reflex facilitation that may occur within hours or days, unaccompanied by any evidence of sensation or voluntary motor activity. In infants, the reflex activity of the isolated cord may be almost indistinguishable from normal motor function.

Pain in a root distribution, often accompanied by sensory dysfunction, reflex loss, and motor weakness, is generally a reliable indicator of the level of injury. However, preciseness may not be as possible in the frightened, traumatized child as in the adult. Because recovery of function is more likely following decompression, early diagnosis of root entrapment is essential. The value of functional recovery in any of the roots of the brachial plexus cannot be overemphasized, especially in the child.

A common situation in which spinal injury may be overlooked or the extent of damage not appreciated is the polytraumatized child with head or major thoracoabdominal injury. Any severe head trauma caused by a rotation, flexion, or extension force directed against the head is capable of causing injury to the cervical spine, cervical spinal cord, or both. Failure to immobilize the unconscious child adequately can lead to irreversible spinal cord damage.

Unconscious patients with facial injuries or patients who are vomiting may have to be transported on their side to prevent aspiration of blood or vomitus. These patients often require support of the cervical area by manual or halter traction, which is applied to the head. A neutral spine position generally is adequate; and in the case of a suspected cervical spine injury, the head should be supported laterally to prevent rotation or sideways motion. With lower spine injury, a small support under the affected area or lumbar lordotic curve may be required to support the spine in a neutral position without applying stress to the injury.

The position of the relatively large, posteriorly directed head of a young child must be considered to prevent cervical hyperflexion when the child is transported on a flat immobilization board (Fig. 18-19).[67]

Diagnostic Imaging

Radiographic evaluation must be accomplished with regard for potentially severe and unstable injuries and must include prior adequate immobilization of the spine.[173,175,177] Radiographs should show the exact nature of the lesion. The area of involvement, as suspected or defined by neurologic examination, must be included in the films. One of the most frequent errors when evaluating suspected injury of the cervical spine is failure to obtain good visualization of the C7 and T1 vertebral bodies (Fig. 18-32). Anteroposterior and lateral

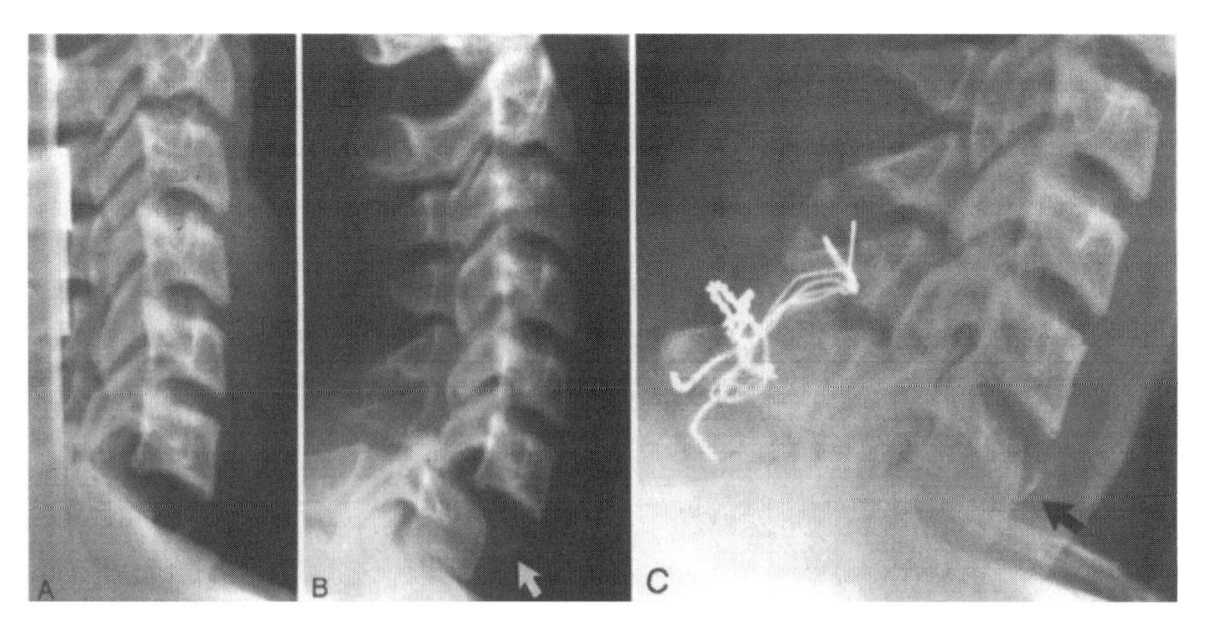

FIGURE 18-32. (A) Spine injury evaluation in an adolescent does not adequately show C7. (B) Better view of C6–C7 shows anterior displacement of C6 and superior end-plate fracture of C7 (arrow). (C) Reduction and posterior fixation. Note the end-plate fracture (arrow). This small fragment is the vertebral equivalent of a Thurstan Holland metaphyseal sign.

tomograms may be helpful; and oblique views may be necessary. A CT scan, MRI, or three-dimensional reconstruction of either may also be indicated.[172,183,202]

The radiology of the developing spine of children differs considerably from that in adults, especially in the cervical region. Lack of awareness of the normal, variant, and traumatically altered roentgenographic appearances may lead to misdiagnoses in pediatric patients.[168,170,171,176,178,180,182,185-187,189,191,193,196,197,203] Common transient developmental features and more unusual normal variants may be mistaken for spinal trauma in children. The multiple primary and secondary ossification centers and their intervening synchondroses are often mistaken for evidence of fracture, avulsion, or fragmentation.

Naik measured the sagittal and interpedicular diameters of the cervical spinal canal on radiographs of normal infants.[187] He assessed the difficulty obtaining accurate measurements and mentioned a new method for measuring the sagittal diameter. Naik's values may be consulted for the interpretation of trauma, even though his main purpose was to assess possible congenital defects.

In young children the lateral thoracic or lumbar spinal radiograph occasionally shows a vertically oriented, lucent cleft. This cleft may represent the more anteriorly placed neurocentral synchondrosis (Fig. 18-8). A similar cleft may also represent a bifid vertebrae (Fig. 18-20). Morphologic variations in the lumbosacral region are common. Lumbarization of the first sacral segment to form a sixth lumbar vertebrae or bilateral or unilateral fusion of L5 to the sacrum is often seen. Incomplete osseous fusion of the neural arch of L5 or S1 (or both) is common in children, with a 50% incidence in some populations. A gradual decrease in incidence occurs throughout childhood, but remains relatively high, even in adolescence.

Certain anatomic regions are of significant concern:

1. *Variations resembling subluxation due to displacement of vertebrae.*[179] Anterior displacement of the second or third cervical vertebrae, resembling a true subluxation, is relatively common in children less than 7 years of age. Less frequently, similar displacement is seen between the third and fourth cervical vertebrae. On lateral roentgenograms, overriding of the atlas on the dens and apparent widening of the space between these two structures is seen in about 20% of normal children. There is apparent subluxation of C2 and C3 in 20% of normal children and absence of lordosis in the cervical spine in about 15%.[59] Absence of uniform angulation, absence of cervical lordosis, and absence of flexion curves have also been reported in a high percentage of normal, asymptomatic children. All of these signs are suggestive of, but do not necessarily specifically indicate, ligamentous or other soft tissue injury.

2. *Variations resembling spasm and ligamentous injury due to curvature of the cervical spine.* An absence of uniform angulation between adjacent vertebrae and an absence of a flexion curvature of the spine between the second and seventh cervical vertebrae are seen on lateral roentgenograms obtained with the cervical spine in flexion.

3. *Variations resembling fractures related to skeletal growth centers.*[169] The cartilaginous plate of the dens (dentocentral synchondrosis) frequently persists beyond the age of 5 years and may resemble an undisplaced fracture (Fig. 18-4). Normal anterior "wedging" of an immature vertebral body (especially in the cervical region) may seem to be a compression fracture. Spinous process secondary centers may be confused with avulsion fractures during adolescence.

An evaluation of clinical observations and findings that might increase the reliability of obtaining diagnostically significant films in children with potential cervical spine injury found that no single clinical predictor had a sensitivity of 100% when considered in isolation.[189] A clinical assessment consisting of a complaint of neck pain or involvement in a vehicular accident with head trauma would have correctly identified all cases of cervical spine injury. If this information had been used prospectively in this study, the number of cervical spine radiographs could have been reduced by approximately one-third.[189]

Hyperextension injuries often reduce spontaneously, especially in the resilient spine of a child. Swelling of the prevertebral fat stripe may be the only indication of this occult injury (Fig. 18-33).[129,188,198,201] Another indication of such an injury is a small piece of bone pulled away from the anteroinferior edge of the ossifying vertebral centrum at the point of separation of the end-plate, anterior longitudinal ligament, and annulus.

In the young child, radiologic diagnosis is further complicated by the relative elasticity of the cartilaginous spine and supporting ligamentous structures, which may deform sufficiently to allow severe cord damage at impact, but with subsequent absence of radiographic evidence of fracture or dislocation when the child is evaluated posttraumatically.

Evaluation by CT has increased in frequency. The method is obviously useful for defining the complete morphology of the fracture and to assess fragments compromising the spinal canal. However, because of the nature of the developing skeleton, significant fracture components may not be readily visible (i.e., a fracture involving the cartilage). Summers and Galli showed that CT scans required a cut interval of 3 mm or less to detect occult fractures of the cervical spine during screening.[196]

Wojcik and associates presented preliminary studies on three-dimensional CT analysis of acute cervical spine trauma and thought that computer-integrated three-dimensional images obtained from CT data were considerably superior to observer mental integration of individual CT images.[202] They did not give the ages of their patients, but at least one of the cases involving a child showed an excellent reconstruction. However, such reconstruction must be put in proper perspective. The decreased visualization of incompletely ossified skeletal elements in young children must be considered during any process of interpretation.

The MRI technique has obviously become increasingly important for detailed evaluation of children with obvious fracture and evidence of cord or root damage.[181,184,199] As when diagnosing chondro-osseous injuries, the interpreting physician should have some familiarity with the normal anatomy of the developing spinal cord.[190] MRI can show noncontiguous cord injury, especially in the cervical spine.[195] These studies are also useful for delineating posttraumatic changes in the spinal cord over time.[174,192,194] Perhaps the most important use of MRI acutely is to define the cord injury and an occult fracture in SCIWORA.[192]

Weng and Haynes assessed flexion-extension MRI in children.[200] Patients with instability also had neurologic mani-

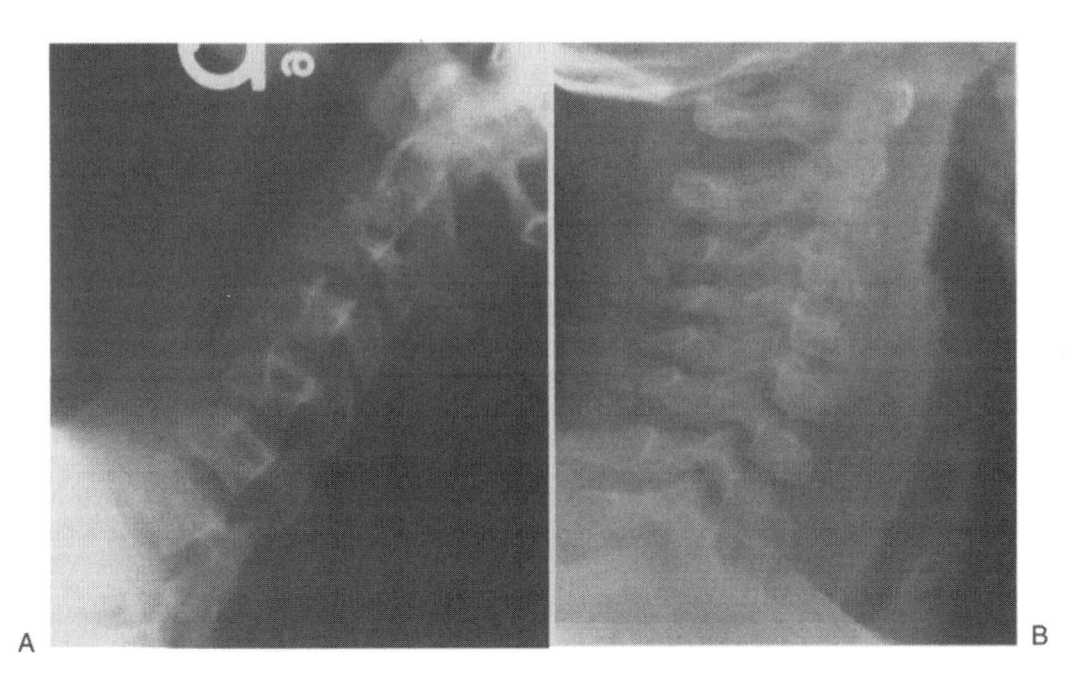

FIGURE 18-33. (A) Subluxation of the upper cervical spine. The prevertebral fat stripe, however, is normal. (B) Four-year-old child who sustained a head and neck injury. The prevertebral fat stripe is markedly widened. No radiologically evident vertebral injuries were noted.

festations and underwent surgery. Patients without spinal cord compression on MRI did not demonstrate neurologic compromise.

Subluxation

The fulcrum of motion of the normal cervical spine in children under the age of 8 years is C2–C3, rather than the more distal C5–C6 fulcrum of the adult.[212,216] A flexion film of the cervical spine frequently seemingly shows the second segment "misaligned" relative to the third. This condition is usually termed pseudosubluxation and is generally a normal finding in children (Fig. 18-34). Failure to recognize this frequent (common) normal variation is responsible for many erroneous concepts and dictated reports regarding the relation of subluxation of the cervical spine; it causes a major diagnostic problem when the finding is noted in children who have sustained actual or perceived neck trauma.[206,209,211,218] Communication between the radiologist and treating

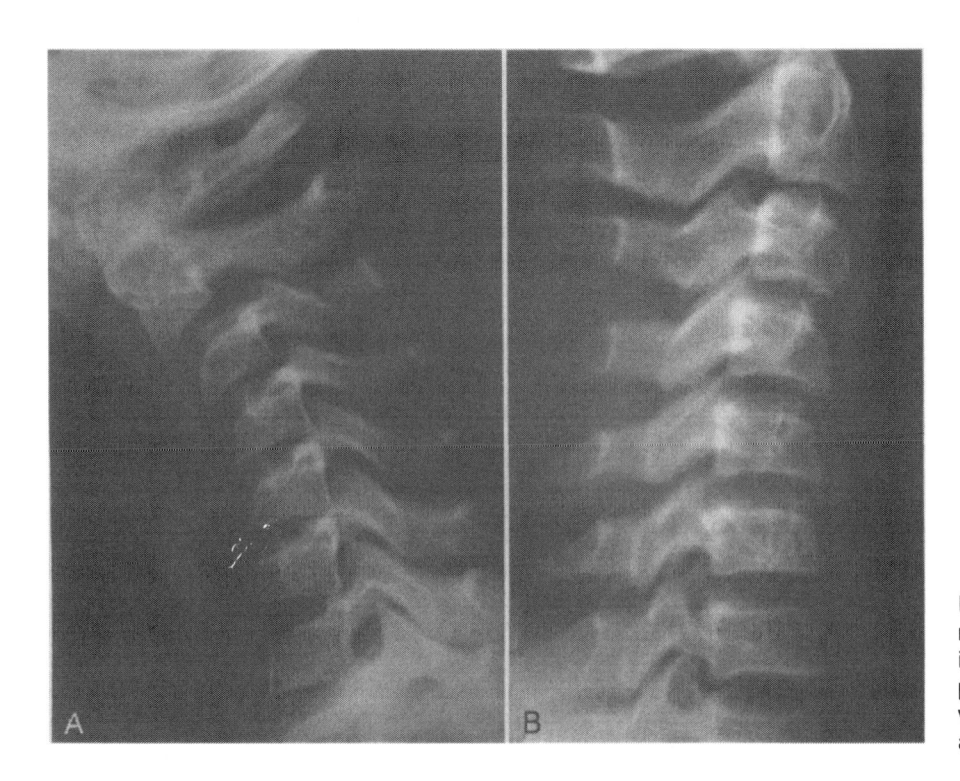

FIGURE 18-34. (A) Pseudosubluxation in a normal child. The C2–C3 joint is most involved. Note the differences in the planes of the facet joint surfaces of C3–C4 versus C6–C7. (B) Anterior pseudosubluxation of the upper cervical spine.

physician is extremely important for the diagnosis of variation versus injury.

Subluxation of the cervical vertebrae *without* associated fracture or spinal cord injury occurs frequently in children.[204,205,208] Anterior displacement (especially rotatory) of the atlas on the axis is a common pattern. Many of these cases occur spontaneously; and although local infection has been cited as a predisposing factor, the high incidence of upper respiratory infection in the age group most frequently encountered (6–12 years) makes this relation statistically difficult to establish.[214]

The facet joints of the upper cervical vertebrae are more horizontal than those of the lower cervical vertebrae, with this variation being more pronounced in the young child (Fig. 18-9). This angulation changes to a more oblique orientation as the cervical spine matures. Some laxity of the transverse ligament must occur for the atlas to slide forward on the axis. Although asymptomatic cases in children have been reported in which the distance between the anterior arch and dens is in excess of 3.5 mm, most authors agree that 3.0 mm is the upper limit of normal for children.[204]

Bailey noted that infants and children should show a normal step-off of as much as 2–3 mm at the level of the second and third cervical vertebrae.[168] Similarly, the gap between the posterior portion of the anterior arch of the adolescent and the anterior portion of the dens may increase with motion. In normal adults it does not usually move more than 2 mm, but in normal children even a 5 mm excursion in flexion may be normal. Furthermore, when the neck is in extension, the arch may appear to move posteriorly and may seem to lie on top of the dens. This may occur because of a combination of ligamentous laxity and the curvilinear angulation of the anterior portion of the dens.

Hypermobility of the cervical spine in young children may be noted at the C2–C3 and C3–C4 levels on lateral roentgenograms obtained with the neck in full flexion.[214] Anterior subluxation of up to 4 mm may be normal. The diagnosis of abnormal motion should be made only when the radiographic finding of subluxation is accompanied by clinical evidence of muscular spasm and pain, generally with limitation of lateral extension of the neck. Evidence of soft tissue swelling with anterior tracheal displacement is sometimes present. Tomography may be helpful for demonstrating fractures not readily apparent on the plain films.

Children who have normal pseudosubluxation and normal vertebral epiphyses do not require extensive and aggressive treatment. An awareness of the normal anatomy of the pediatric cervical spine should prevent overtreatment. Seemingly abnormal radiographic findings should be accompanied by appropriate physical signs to warrant prolonged traction, casting, or surgery under the misconception that serious (actual) injury exists. Dunlap and colleagues reported 12 children between the ages of 3 and 8, only one of whom had a well-documented traumatic injury.[286] Altogether they reviewed 47 children and found 8 with marked subluxation of C2–C3. They believed that children with these normal variations should *not* be subjected to extensive orthopaedic treatment unless there is a supporting history of sufficient injury to the neck and clinical examination bears out the significant probability that these variations are traumatic subluxations.

Intervertebral (disk space) calcification may be found during the evaluation of acute trauma or pain in children.[207,210,215,217] It is usually an asymptomatic, fortuitous finding that should direct the physician to look closely for other etiologies of the pain. Diskitis, which is really vertebral osteomyelitis in children, may also present as relatively acute pain sometimes associated (seemingly) with an injury.[213]

Grisel Syndrome

Differentiation of a traumatic subluxation from an inflammatory subluxation constitutes a major diagnostic problem.[219-244] Grisel syndrome (torticollis and atlantoaxial subluxation in children) infrequently follows a major injury. More often it is associated with the hyperemia and local edema that follow pharyngitis, otitis, tonsillar abscesses, osteomyelitis, tuberculosis, and tumors, which may permit stretching of ligaments, so even normal neck motion produces atlantoaxial displacement.

SCIWORA

As alluded to several times in this chapter the child often presents to the emergency room with obvious neurologic injury, but screening, if not detailed imaging studies, fail to reveal an obvious fracture that could be associated with the neurologic injury. This has been termed *spinal cord injury without obvious radiologic abnormality* (SCIWORA).[245,246,251,252,254,260-268] MRI may show occult intraosseous edema (bone bruising) compatible with a spontaneously reduced end-plate fracture. Another possible mechanism is hypermobility, causing a traction cord injury. This mechanism may be significant in the cervical spine or thoracolumbar junction. Others have suggested some type of vascular injury as an etiologic factor.[247-250,253,255-259]

In sequential MRI studies (Fig. 18-35) in patients with cervical cord injury without bony injury (SCIWORA), 70% of the patients had a major cord injury detected by MRI at the C3–C4 level. Three patterns of signal changes were observed. Enhancement of the damaged cord was observed on gadolinium-enhanced MRI, and the palsy in these patients was more severe than that of those without enhancement. This probably represents necrosis, absorption, and reorganization of the spinal cord and suggests that the injury is permanent. Another imaging finding was a high-intensity signal in the dorsal column that appeared 2–3 months after injury and then disappeared by 6 months. This probably represents wallerian degeneration of the corticospinal tract.

An analysis of 71 patients with cervicothoracic trauma found 7 (10%) patients with clinical or MRI evidence of noncontiguous spinal cord injury and either more than one neurologic level or a cord lesion remote from the suspected or actual major imaging abnormality.[299] The second lesion was probably due to cord stretching after local tethering at the first level. Three of the patients had a small extramedullary hematoma at the distant cord lesion.

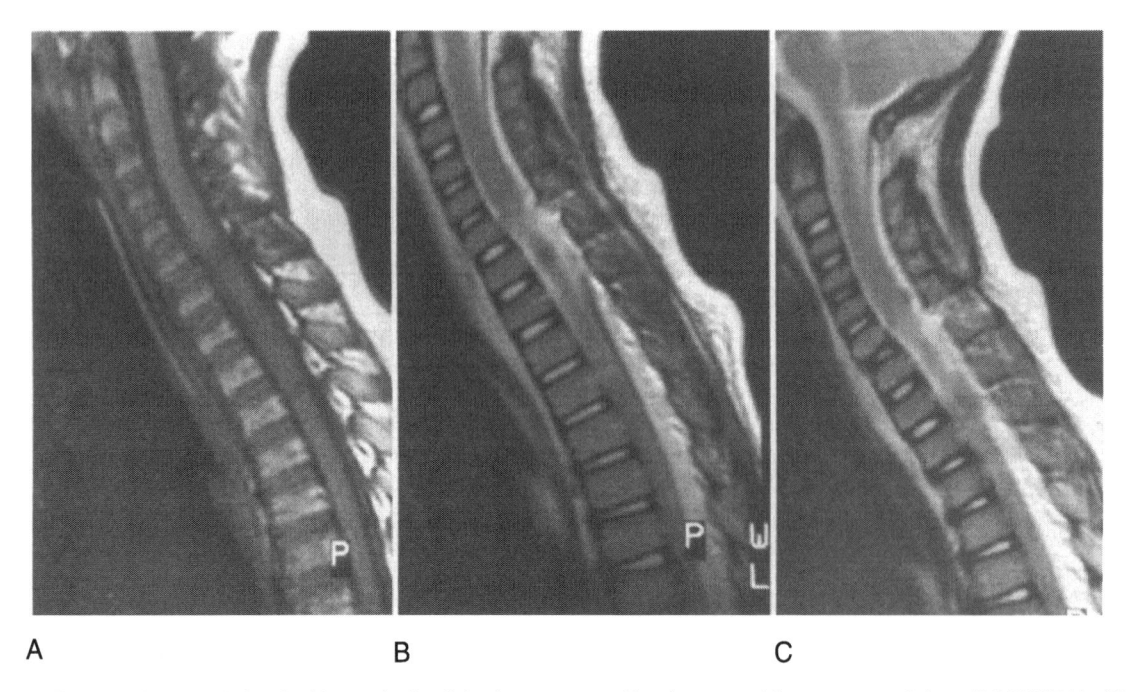

FIGURE 18-35. This child was admitted with paralysis of the lower extremities but no evident osseous injury (SCIWORA). (A) Magnetic resonance imaging (MRI) scan shortly after admission showed a focal cord lesion. (B) Three weeks later. (C) Four months later.

Basic Treatment Guidelines

A number of unique problems are encountered during treatment of infants, children, and adolescents with major spine and spinal cord injuries. With any closed, nonoperative treatment regimen, the spinal osseous deformity should be reduced and adequately protected from redisplacement or increasing deformity during the period of physiologic reaction, repair, and consolidation of the anterior, middle, or posterior columns. Surgical techniques used in adults for external stabilization, operative stabilization, and anatomic reduction may be inapplicable in children because of the differences in skull and spine morphology and the biomechanical resistance, musculature, and ligamentous stability, all of which must be considered when treating significant spinal chondro-osseous injury.

Unstable fractures should be treated with traction and, if necessary, internal fixation. As with the long bones, ligamentous rupture is probably infrequent. Most fractures, including obvious or occult end-plate injuries, stabilize by osseous healing. With thoracic and lumbar injuries, fusion may be needed for subsequent growth displacements. Instability complicating superimposed congenital anomalies may require fusion.

Laminectomy has been used frequently but often indiscriminantly. In general, it is not usually indicated in children. Laminectomy may be appropriate if there is a discrete block on myelography, CT scan, or MRI and especially if it is associated with worsening neurologic signs. For removal of important posterior elements, extensive laminectomy may become a major factor in posttraumatic kyphotic deformity. If laminectomy is indicated, every effort should be made to keep the facet joints and capsules intact. This operation, as an isolated procedure, has limited use for early management of closed spinal injuries in children.

Specific aspects of treatment are discussed in the ensuing sections on anatomic regions. Acute and chronic injuries and posttraumatic consequences are also discussed.

Halo Fixation

The use of a halo may present distinct problems in the child.[269-278,280-282] Halo fixation pins should be placed anterolaterally and posterolaterally, where the bones are usually the thickest. Insertion of halo pins in the temporal fossa region is not recommended because: (1) it is relatively thin; (2) there is a cranial suture; and (3) the temporal muscles may be penetrated, resulting in pain with mastication and during episodes of exaggerated facial expressions (which occur with regularity in children). The anterior portion of the skull should be avoided because of thin bone dimensions and the underlying frontal sinus. The thickest location is directly posterior, but this is not an ideal location for pin placement because patients may lie on this pin when supine.

A limited CT scan may be used to select the best bone to accommodate the pins. Often one has already been obtained as part of the trauma evaluation. Another suggestion for decreasing the risk of pin complications is to use a larger number of pins (eight) instead of the usual four.

As with application of head-halter or cranial traction in children, overdistraction may occur when the halo-vest is used.[279] Adequate positioning of the cervical vertebra must be checked carefully after the device is applied.

Dormans et al. reviewed complications in children immobilized in a halo vest.[272] The halo was not used in conjunction with operative arthrodesis of the cervical spine in 24 patients (65%). The other 13 patients (35%) were being treated for trauma. Complications occurred in 68% of the patients. The most common problem was pin-site infection

(22/25). Grade II infections (purulent drainage) developed more frequently in patients over 11 years of age. Children younger than 10 years tended to have nonpurulent drainage at the pin sites and pin loosening. Additional complications included dural penetration, transient injury to the supraorbital nerve, and three disfiguring pin site scars.

Goodman and Nelson reported a 15-year-old boy who developed a brain abscess while being immobilized in a halo orthosis for a neck fracture.[276] Their case and at least one other may have been due to tightening of a halo pin several weeks after placement.

Specific Injuries

As mentioned previously, the cervical spine appears to be the most commonly involved spinal component injured in the skeletally immature patient, especially the child under 10 years of age.[283–309] Fractures and dislocations of the upper cervical spine, in particular, occur with a greater incidence in children than in adults. Lesions of the atlas and axis were noted in 16% of cervical spine injuries in adults, whereas they constitute almost 70% of cervical spine injuries in children. Locked facets, which are common in adults, are infrequent in children. Facet physeal fracture, however, may occur as the analogue, similar to tibial spine/anterior cruciate ligament in the knee. It is probably associated with ligament laxity. An underlying congenital abnormality (e.g., Klippel-Feil syndrome) may be a predisposing cause of injury. Fuch et al. reported several cases of high cervical spine injuries in children restrained in forward-facing car seats.[288]

Abuse

Abuse during infancy may also cause significant spinal injury.[310–317] The upper cervical spine is not resistant to major torsional stresses under these circumstances, and injury may occur proximal to the tethering of the large brachial nerve roots. The relatively heavy infantile head is poorly supported by cervical musculature. Accordingly, the upper cervical spine is highly vulnerable to repeated shaking, especially in the battered child syndrome. These infants probably have a higher risk of SCIWORA, especially in the shaken baby syndrome. Firmly gripping the infant around the thorax may lead to costotransverse injury that is difficult to diagnose (see Chapter 11), and it may be accompanied by canal hemorrhage or disruption of cord vascularity.

Birth Injury

The youngest patients with upper spine lesions have been newborns in whom autopsy has revealed atlantooccipital and atlantoaxial disruption, fracture of the dens, and transection of the cord. These injuries can occur as anticipated obstetric complications of difficult deliveries. Obviously, efforts should be made to minimize the risk of occurrence.

Birth trauma probably is a common cause of spinal cord injury in infants.[318–376] Most injuries involve breech extraction and sustained laceration of the spinal cord without a roentgenographically evident injury to the spine (i.e., another cause of SCIWORA).[318,322,333,349,351,367,370–373] Spinal cord injury may also result from an accident to the neonate or infant (e.g., child abuse). In the young infant the vertebral column is extremely elastic, certainly more so than the spinal cord, which is tethered by nerve ends and blood vessels. During delivery it is possible to prolong longitudinal traction sufficiently to distract the neck without producing permanent or evident injury to the chondro-osseous structures or dura, yet go beyond the tensile resilience of the spinal cord, which can tear within the intact dura and spinal column.

Yates showed that trauma to the cervical spine at birth could result in damage to the cervical portions of the vertebral artery.[375] There was evidence of distortional trauma but no evidence of major fracture or dislocation to the cervical spine. The lesions could be classified into four main groups: (1) extradural, dural, subdural, and subarachnoid hemorrhage; (2) tears and hemorrhages in the nerve roots and spinal ganglia; (3) evidence of hemorrhage around one or both of the vertebral arteries in the form of a crescentic, adventitial hematoma or massive hemorrhage encircling the vessel; and (4) spinal cord lesions that consisted of contusion and bilateral necrosis of the lateral columns. Vertebral artery hemorrhage may be an important cause of perinatal mortality and morbidity. Many cases of cerebral palsy alleged to be caused by anoxic spells may be explicable on the basis of vertebral artery trauma and ischemic cerebral, cerebellar, and cord damage at birth.

Ligamentous laxity permits a longitudinal force to separate adjacent vertebral bodies sufficiently that breech deliveries may cause total anatomic transection of the cervical cord without apparent fracture-dislocation of the spine. The cervical musculature, so important to the stability and alignment of the adult cervical spine, is still not fully developed in the infant. Thus, distracting and displacing forces at the time of injury are less likely to be checked by the patient. After injury, protective muscular splinting is less effective.

These infants have difficult diagnostic patterns. Presenting symptoms may be a fever of unknown origin due to loss of temperature-regulating mechanisms. Reflex movements may be mistaken for voluntary movements. These infants may have respiratory distress resulting from paralyzed intercostal muscles. Typically, if the child has had a cord transection, painful stimuli above the level of the transection do not induce movement in the limbs affected below the cord transection. Stimulation below the sensory level elicits reflex withdrawal but does not usually produce any irritable response in the infant.

Clinically, there are two primary neurologic syndromes seen in infants who sustain major cervical cord injury at birth. The first type is secondary to complete disruption of the spinal cord, and the clinical picture seen immediately after birth is that of a completely flaccid, areflexic infant with spinal shock. Within a few weeks to several months, the infant loses the flaccidity and areflexia and becomes hyperreflexic and hypertonic. The second type of neurologic syndrome is seen in the infant who remains flaccid, rather than becoming spastic or hyperreflexic. This syndrome probably results from further damage to the lower cord by the disruption of the vascular supply, which leads to anoxia and infarction.

Occipital Fracture

Cottalorda et al. described an occipital condylar fracture in a 15-year-old girl.[379] They found only 36 cases reported since Bell first described the injury in 1817. Occipital fractures are unusual in young children.[377,379-382] When they occur the potential for growth damage must be considered, as there are chondro-osseous growth regions in the occipital bone and occipital condyles.[27] In contrast, most of the cranial and facial bones enlarge by membranous ossification and are less susceptible to disruption of normal growth dynamics.

Nonoperative treatment is the usual method. Care must be taken to assess the extent of bleeding, as a contiguous subdural hematoma may have to be evacuated.[378]

Occipitoatlantal Dislocation

In adults the anatomy of the atlantooccipital joint provides considerable stability.[399] However, the relatively small size of the occipital condyles, the large space of the atlantooccipital joints, and the relatively horizontal plane of these joints in infants and young children make the relation between the atlas and occiput less stable, particularly in extension injuries.[399] Congenital defects also may predispose to injury.[383,390,393] A progressive inclination of the occipitoatlantal joint develops with skeletal maturation. Therefore dislocation without fracture is possible in children.[394,398,400,404,407] Spontaneous, nontraumatic occipitoatlantal subluxations may also be due to various inflammatory diseases (see Grisel Syndrome, above).

In children the (sagittal or coronal) diameter of the cervical portion of the spinal canal is approximately 22 mm at the first cervical vertebrae.[397] Hypermobility in this joint may be confusing.[412] The major changes of growth occur in the surrounding bones. The susceptible areas of neurologic dysfunction associated with occipitoatlantal injury are the caudal cranial nerves, brain stem, proximal portion of the spinal cord, and upper three cervical nerves.

Total dislocation of the atlantooccipital articulation is a rare, usually fatal injury often associated with transection of the medulla oblongata or the spinal medullary junction.[386,387,405,410,411] The vertebral artery may also be damaged.[384] There is displacement of the occipital condyles from the superior facets of the atlas along with retropharyngeal swelling (Fig. 18-36). The relation of the dens to the basiocciput and that of the posterior arch of the atlas to the posterior rim of the foramen magnum are distorted.

There is little information available regarding patients who sustain and, particularly, survive this injury,[388,391,398,403,406] although young children appear most likely to do so.[398,401,402] The clinical and neurologic manifestations vary and include cardiorespiratory arrest, motor weakness, quadriplegia, torticollis, pain in the neck, vertigo, and projectile vomiting.[443] A 6-year-old child demonstrated significant irregularities in pulse and respiration. When the head was extended, they disappeared. After recovery there were no neurologic sequelae.[392] Gabrielson and Maxwell reported a partial dislocation in which the patient initially demonstrated cranial nerve dysfunction and long tract signs, but the only residual neurologic deficit was anesthesia over the distribution of the greater occipital nerve.[391] Evarts described traumatic occipi-

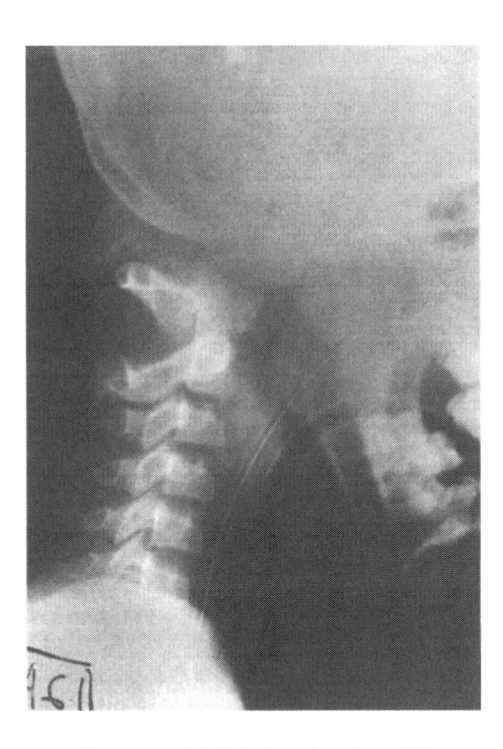

FIGURE 18-36. Atlantooccipital dislocation in a 14-year-old. This case was fatal owing to lack of spontaneous respiration.

toatlantal dislocation in an 11-year-old boy who had acute respiratory distress, stridor, palsy of the sixth left cranial nerve and both twelfth cranial nerves, and a left hemiparesis.[389] The patient had both brain stem and cord involvement initially, but only a partial left lateral rectus paresis and a positive left Babinski reflex persisted.[440] It is evident that a wide spectrum of neurologic abnormalities may be encountered with occipitoatlantal dislocation, from minimal involvement of the brain stem or proximal spinal cord to sufficient dysfunction to result in immediate death.

Sponseller and Cass reported two children who survived atlantooccipital dislocation.[408] In both children (4 and 11 years of age) an occiput to C2 fusion was successfully undertaken. Others have also reported survival of this injury.[384,385,389,409,413,494,497,499]

Conservative management (with a halo) has succeeded in some young children, although surgical fusion may be required in older children and adolescents because of the difficulty obtaining and maintaining reduction.[389,392,395,408] The initial treatment of this dislocation is to relieve any respiratory distress by endotracheal intubation, tracheostomy, or cervical traction. Care must be taken not to increase any displacement with cervical traction, a phenomenon more likely in the child than the adult. Monitoring the occipitoatlantal relation with lateral roentgenograms is essential.

Atlas Fractures

Atlas fractures in children are infrequent.[416,417,420,421,423-425,427-430,432-434,436,438,480,486,495] Birth injury and congenital defects may be associated with C1 injury.[416] In fact, congenital abnormalities may be misdiagnosed as atlas fractures.[414,415,418,419,422,426,431,435,]

Specific Injuries

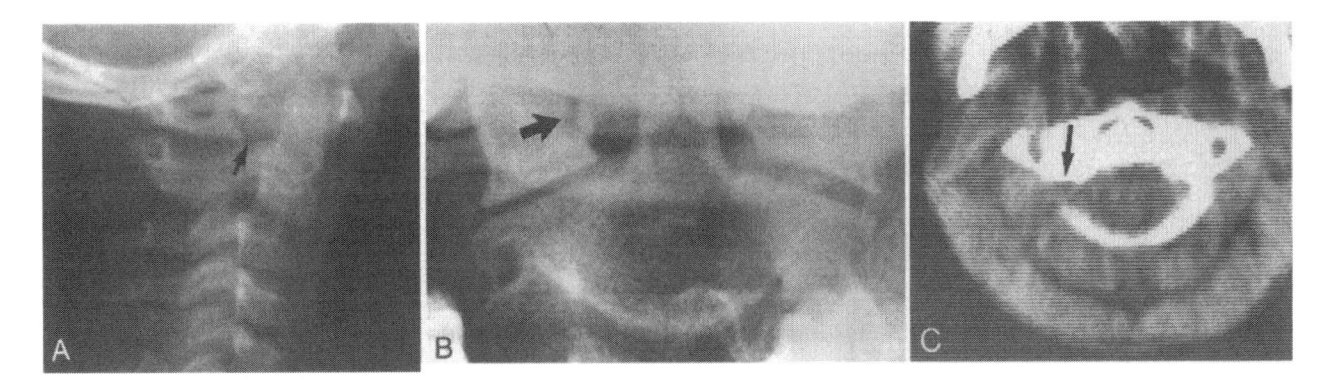

FIGURE 18-37. C1 fracture. (A, B) Lateral mass fracture (arrows) is evident on lateral and open mouth views. (C) Computed tomography (CT) scan shows the fracture clearly (arrow).

Indirect trauma usually causes these injuries.[437] The occiput and multiple muscle layers protect the immature atlas. Fractures ordinarily require reasonably direct axial transmission force through the skull to concentrate stresses on the atlantal components. Direct blows on the head, accordingly, may produce axial compression of the atlas by forcing the occipital condyles downward into the lateral masses of the atlas. If the lower cervical spine remains sufficiently rigid, the lateral masses are displaced centrifugally, albeit minimally (Fig. 18-37). The force may also comminute the lateral masses and rupture the transverse ligament. Axial compression of the skull and cervical spine with hyperextension of the head may also shear the posterior arch of the atlas at its weakest point, through the groove of the vertebral arteries. Detachment of the posterior arch of the atlas leaves it subjected to upward displacement by the posteroinferior oblique muscles, but the lateral masses are not displaced because they generally remain securely attached to the anterior arch.

Usually there is both anterior and posterior injury of the ring. In young children this disruption is usually through the neurocentral synchondroses (Fig. 18-38).[425] If the force is applied eccentrically, there may be only a single fracture. However, if one synchondrosis is involved, it is likely the other is also involved as an occult (microscopic) injury that is not readily evident radiologically (Fig. 18-26). A fracture may occur within the anterior ossification center (Fig. 18-39).

Patients usually complain of a sensation of instability, severe suboccipital discomfort, and pain. Pharyngeal soft tissue swelling and fat pad displacement are not usually prominent features. Spinal cord damage may occur.

Because of the difficulty visualizing this region with routine roentgenographic projections, other imaging methods become essential. CT scanning, in particular, allows excellent visualization of the entire ring and is probably the best method for demonstrating the pattern of injury and degree of fragment displacement. It is also helpful for determining the extent of healing during follow-up evaluation.

Treatment consists of a (Minerva) cast or rigid orthosis (e.g., Somi) for approximately 6–8 weeks followed by a removable cervical orthosis for the child with minimal dis-

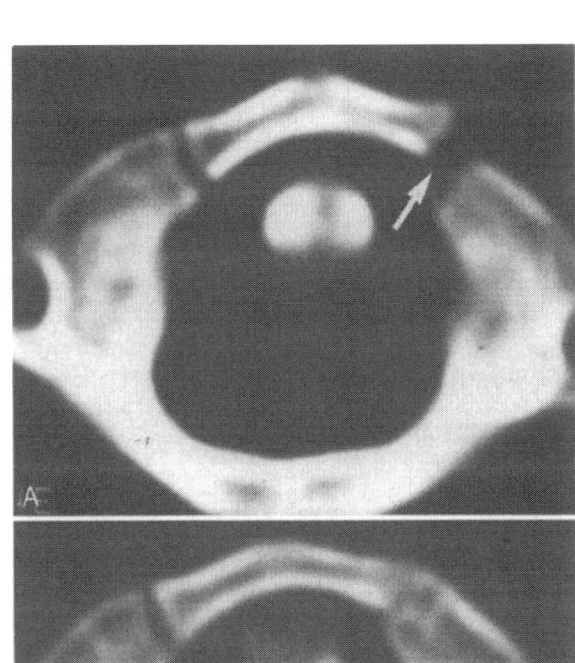

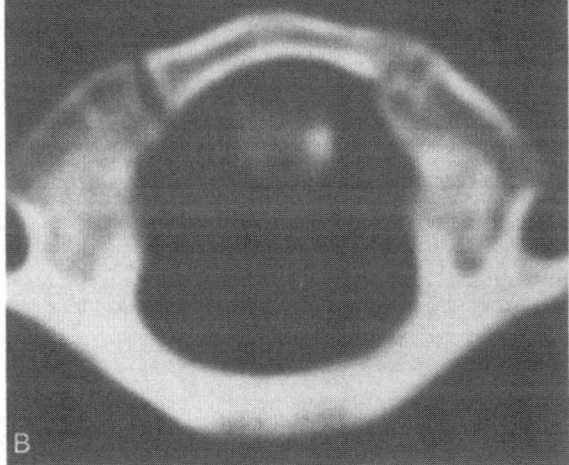

FIGURE 18-38. (A) Fracture (arrow) through one of the neurocentral synchondroses. (B) Several months later healing has closed the disrupted facet, although the other facet remains open. Note that this is anteriorly displaced and probably "hinged" at the other synchondrosis.

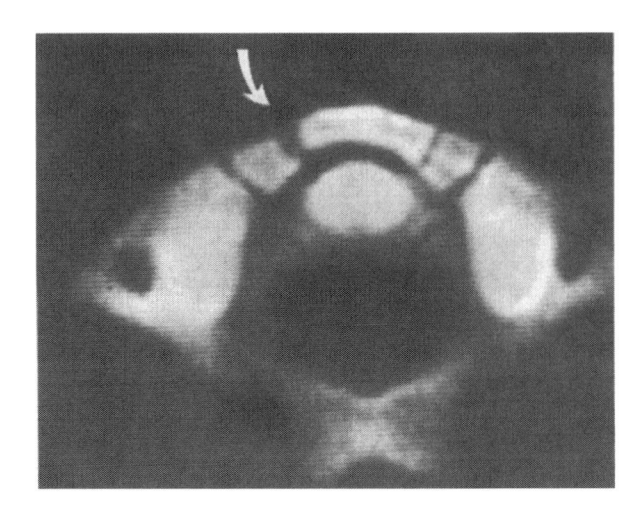

FIGURE 18-39. Fracture within the anterior ossification center (arrow), rather than the synchondrosis.

placement (in whom facet capsules/ligaments and atlantoaxial ligaments are probably intact). Serial CT scans allow assessment of progressive healing of the injury. The older child or adolescent may require application of a halo vest. Infrequently, surgical fusion is necessary.[427]

Rotatory Subluxation of the Atlantoaxial Joint

Rotatory subluxation or dislocation, rather than fracture of the atlantoaxial articulation (Figs. 18-40, 18-41), is one of the more common lesions in children with injuries to the atlas and axis.[439–486] The injury mechanism may seem relatively innocuous in small children.

Isolated atlantoaxial subluxation or dislocation may be secondary to rupture of the transverse ligament (Fig. 18-42), skeletal dysplasia, Down syndrome, inflammation (tonsillitis), pharyngitis, or juvenile rheumatoid arthritis (see previous sections). However, traumatic rupture of the transverse ligament is rare, as the more mechanically vulnerable dens usually fails at the neurocentral synchondrosis before the ligaments do.[446] More importantly, the normal ligamentous laxity may allow displacement without necessarily incompletely or completely tearing the ligament.

With atlantoaxial displacement, the atlas moves anteriorly, which increases the distance between the anterior arch of the atlas and dens and decreases the canal space. Such displacement may significantly damage the spinal cord or medulla.[449] The maximal normal distance in flexion or neutral position in children is 3–4 mm, decreasing to 2 mm at skeletal maturation.[466] Pathologic inflammation may produce increased laxity of the ligaments (e.g., in Grisel syndrome), and there may be rotatory and anterior displacement.

The presenting symptom of patients with atraumatic subluxation is usually an isolated complaint of torticollis.[445] Radiographic studies should be obtained for any child whose cervical spasm and pain do not respond rapidly with conventional therapy. With the most common type, anterior unilateral displacement, the head may be turned away from the affected side, and neck movements are limited. Signs and symptoms of cord compression are infrequent. Underlying disorders such as a syrinx or cord tumor must be sought as part of the differential diagnosis.

On rotation of the head, instead of the atlas moving on the axis, the two moved together. Fielding and Hawkins described 17 cases of irreducible atlantoaxial subluxation.[455] The striking features were delayed diagnosis and persistent

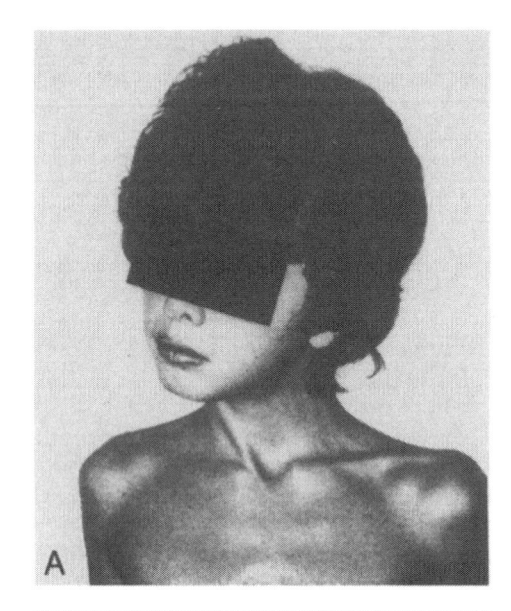

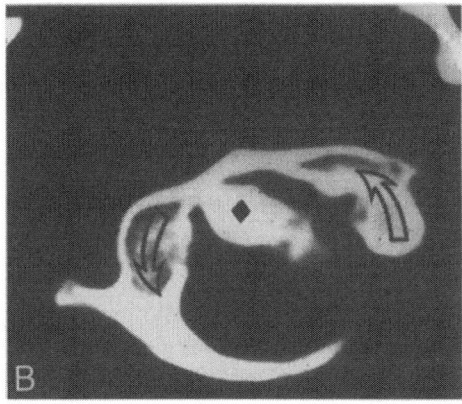

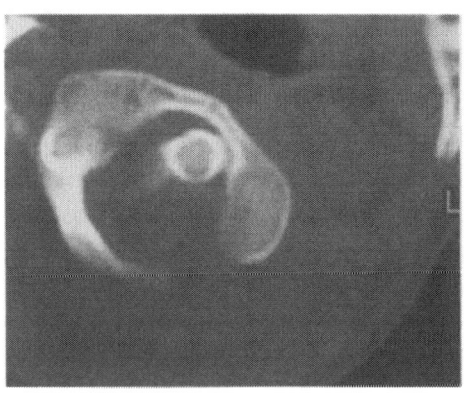

FIGURE 18-40. (A) Torticollis associated with a locked rotatory subluxation. (B) CT scan of counterclockwise (arrows) locked rotatory subluxation of C1 on C2 (= dens). (C) CT scan of clockwise locked rotatory subluxation of C1 on C2. The transverse ligament may be strained, but most likely it is intact.

Specific Injuries

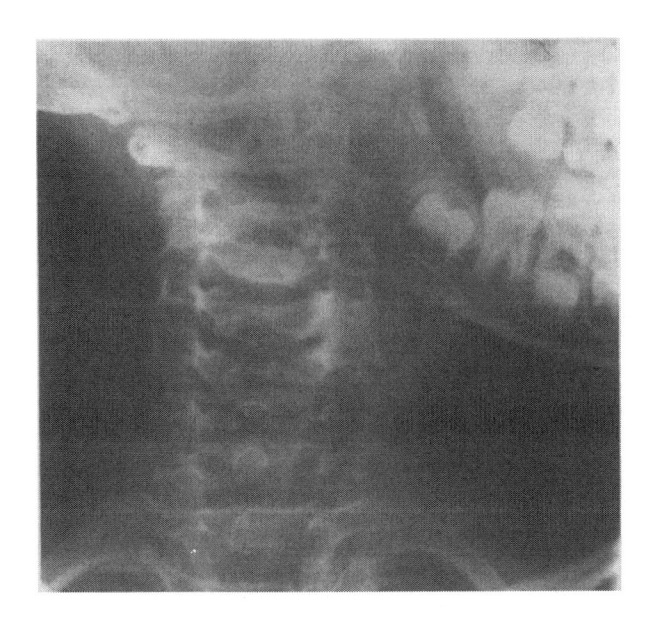

FIGURE 18-41. Torticollis and rotatory subluxation of C1 on C2 in a 7-year-old child. It was gently "unlocked" by controlled traction with the patient awake. The anteroposterior view of the spine contrasts with the lateral view of the skull.

clinical and roentgenographic deformities. All patients presented with torticollis and restricted, often painful neck motion. Seven young patients had long-standing deformity and flattening of one side of the face. These investigators thought that cineroentgenography was particularly helpful for making the diagnosis. Real-time fluoroscopy should also be considered.

Excessive mobility of the atlas and axis has been reported.[441,455,480] This mobility may exist as an independent abnormality or with other regional malformations, such as Klippel-Feil syndrome. The abnormally mobile atlantoaxial joint associated with a hypoplastic dens does not necessarily give rise to symptoms in the upper part of the cervical spine. Because of the absence of the dens, this excessive mobility may be compatible with minimal if any risk, with the exception of acute trauma.

Rotatory subluxation of the atlantoaxial joint is a relatively common problem in a child with an upper respiratory infection and differs from the fixed pattern. Associated hyperemia affects ligaments that support the upper cervical spine and makes the atlantoaxial joint temporarily unstable. Subluxation is produced by twisting the neck suddenly or rotating it beyond its normal range. The child presents with painful torticollis accompanied by marked spasm of the sternocleidomastoid muscle. The child may support the head with the hands or may prefer to be recumbent. There is local tenderness of the atlantoaxial joint when the posterior aspect of the neck is palpated. Neurologic examination is done to rule out spinal lesions.

Rotatory fixation of the atlantoaxial joint may occur with a minor accident, such as a blow to the head or an automobile collision. The child complains of pain and stiffness in the neck and may have occipital neuralgia and torticollis (Fig. 18-40). Patients with atlantoaxial rotatory fixation may also develop a compensatory counterclockwise occipitoatlantal subluxation.[448]

Open-mouth anteroposterior roentgenograms show that the dens is asymmetrically placed between the lateral articular masses of the atlas. The diagnosis is confirmed by additional open-mouth views obtained in various degrees of rotation. It cannot be emphasized too strongly that correct diagnosis of traumatic displacement depends on the analysis of a pair of true right-angle films of the atlas. The crucial observation on the lateral film is the distance of the dens from the anterior arch of the atlas. Overriding of the articular surfaces of the atlas is not significant, as it may be produced by changing the angulation of the roentgenographic beam. If the subluxation is minimally evident on routine radiographs, CT views may be used to demonstrate the altered C1/C2 relations and whether one or both facet joints are disrupted (one is more likely if the transverse ligament is intact).

Ebraheim et al. studied the effect of atlantoaxial rotation on canal size.[452] Anterior translations of the atlas of 3, 4, and 5 mm led, respectively, to canal decreases of 85%, 80%, and 75% of normal. If rotation was then added to the deformity, more significant changes occurred. A 40° degree rotation coupled with an 8-mm anterior displacement resulted in the canal area being only one-fourth normal.

Most rotatory deformities of the atlantoaxial joint are usually temporary and correctable.[544,556] Treatment consists of continuous traction with a head halter. The subluxation may spontaneously reduce within a few days, as the muscle spasm subsides. In some cases gentle reduction is attempted with the patient awake but adequately sedated. One should try to avoid attempting to reduce this lesion with the patient under general anesthesia. Evoked potential monitoring is done whenever possible. After reduction the patient is supported with a cervical collar, orthosis, cast, or halo, depending on the etiology and severity of the injury.

For more severe injuries, treatment may include skull or halter traction followed by atlantoaxial arthrodesis (Fig. 18-43), as necessary.[521,522] Of 13 patients so treated in one study, 11 showed good results, 1 showed fair results, and there was insufficient follow-up of the other patient. One other patient died while in traction as the result of cord transection that was produced by further rotation of the atlas and the axis

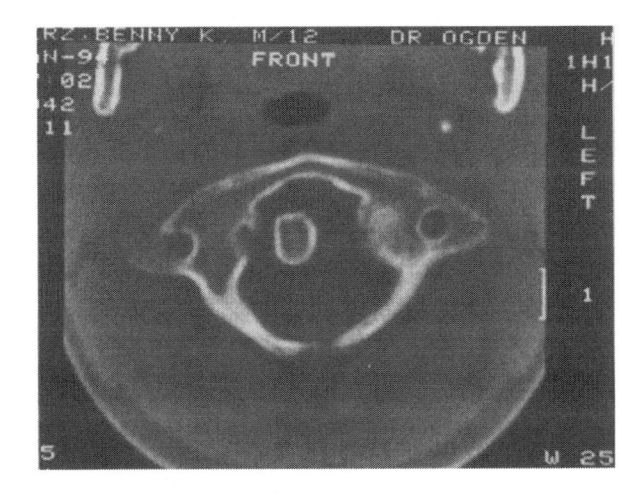

FIGURE 18-42. (A) Anterior subluxation of C1 on C2. The transverse ligament has to be disrupted.

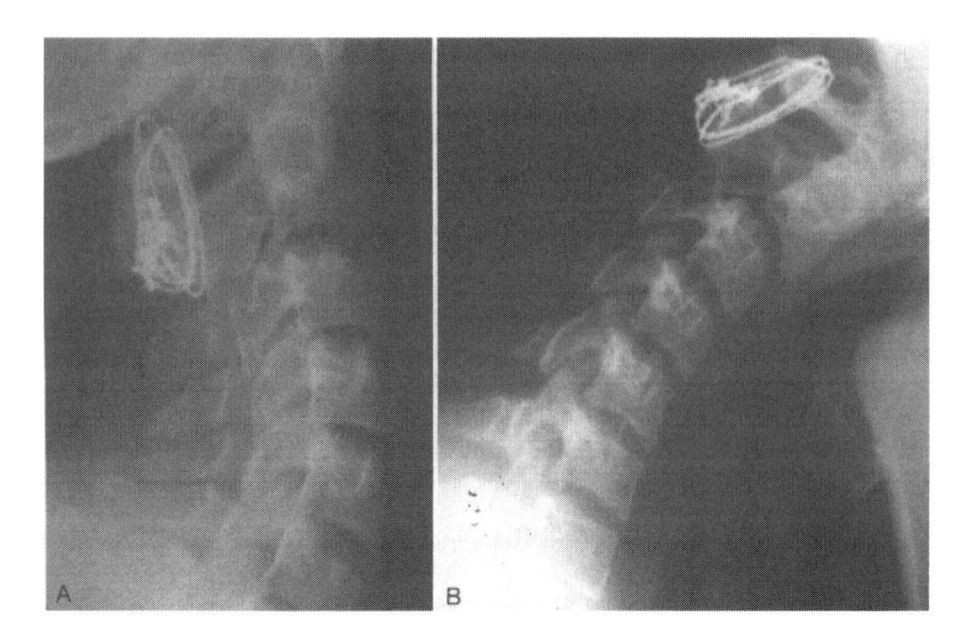

FIGURE 18-43. (A) C1–2 fusion for chronic, painful rotatory subluxation. (B) Postoperative subluxation of C1–C2 on C3. It is probably due to attenuation of facet capsules and the interspinous ligament.

(despite traction). After fusion, other segments may exhibit increased mobility.

The most challenging problem is the chronic, essentially fixed subluxation that does not reduce in traction or following gentle manipulation. It may be necessary to consider an atlantoaxial fusion in situ in the displaced position, accepting the extent of deformity. Alternatively, removal of some of the displaced facet may allow rotational correction, which should be followed by fusion.

Dens Fracture

Fracture of the dens is infrequent in children who are less than 7 years old and especially infrequent in those who are less than 3 years of age.[487,489,490,495,496,499,503,504,512,514,523,527,529,531–533,535,536,539,540,544] In a large series of dens fractures (60 patients), only five were between the ages of 3 and 6 years.[536]

In most recognized instances of dens fracture in children, there is major trauma. Most of these fractures are diagnosed readily on the basis of early roentgenograms (Fig. 18-44), although swelling or widening of the retropharyngeal soft tissue space may be the only diagnostic sign in some young children. Furthermore, the injury mechanism may be relatively "benign" and the radiographs seemingly normal, a factor that may explain an initially missed diagnosis and the subsequent origin of the os odontoideum.

There is a difference in the levels at which the axis fractures in the adult and the young child (Fig. 18-7).[537,539] The lateral radiograph in adults shows that the fracture line usually lies at or above the level of the articular facets, whereas in the young child the fracture line is generally below these facets, within the body of the bone (vertebral centrum). Displacement of the dens may be recognized on the lateral film. The fracture line propagates along the region of the physeal plate, although it may involve bone

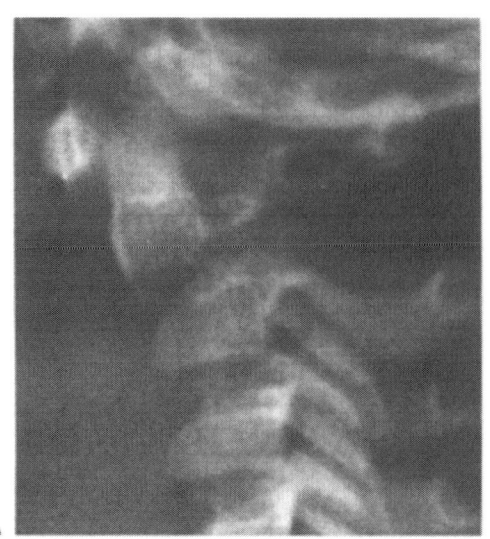

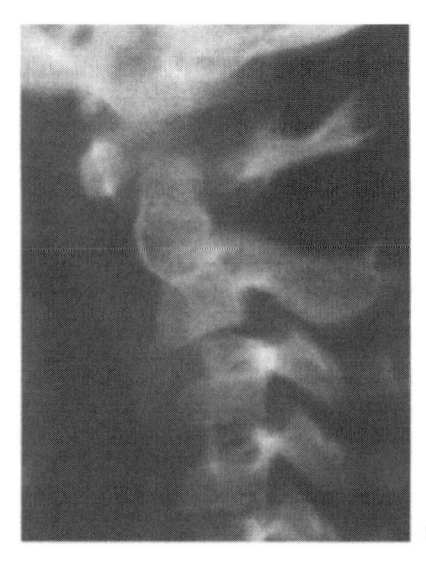

FIGURE 18-44. (A) Dens fracture in a 5-year-old boy. (B) Healing after 7 weeks in a Minerva jacket.

Specific Injuries

FIGURE 18-45. (A) Dens fracture in a 6-year-old child. (B) MRI shows cord injury, but in the lower cervical cord several segments distal to the fracture. This may be a cord traction phenomenon, rather than SCIWORA, at the level of cord injury.

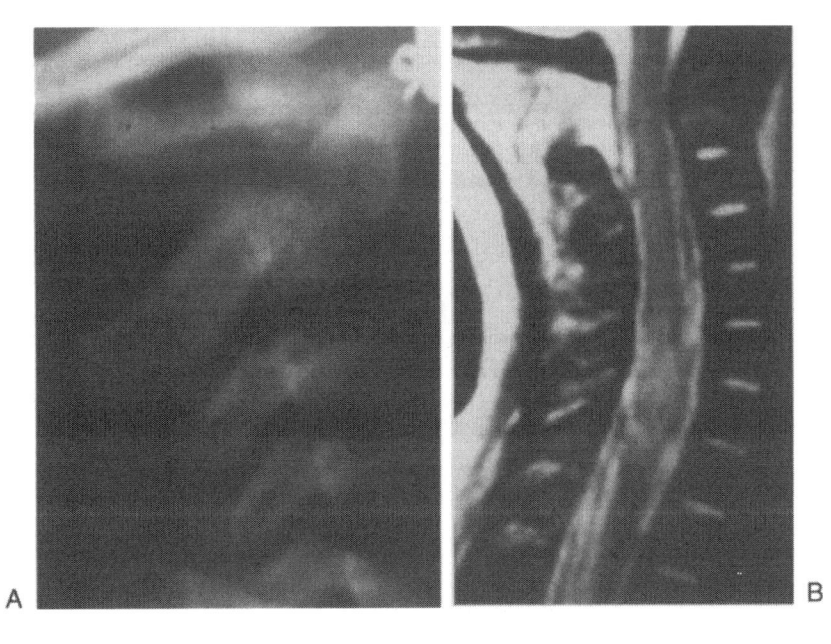

on the dens side compatible with a type 1 or 2 growth mechanism fracture.[527] Blockey and Purser believed that the dens fracture in young children was always an epiphyseal separation.[490]

There is no diagnostic clinical syndrome for a dens fracture. The symptoms and signs may be few and so indefinite that the diagnosis is missed. There may be little pain, but usually there is some stiffness in the neck. The immediate pain may be severe and often is referred to the occipital region. It may be accentuated with any attempt to move the head. Classically, the child supports the head with the hands to prevent any movement and often describes a feeling of the head "falling off." The neck may be held twisted (acute torticollis).

Seimon presented children with dens fractures and described what he considered an important diagnostic clinical sign.[535] In each, injury to the cervical spine was suspected from the description of the trauma mechanics, but initial roentgenograms failed to reveal any fracture. The patients were comfortable when lying supine or when fully erect, and each child strongly resisted any attempt to hyperextend the neck. With extension, the anterior arch of C1 courses along the anterior dens, which would cause micromotion at the fracture site. This symptom is a valuable clinical sign when injury to the dens is suspected, as these fractures usually occur with a flexion mechanism. The radiograph may or may not demonstrate forward displacement of the dens relative to the C2 vertebral centrum.

The most common minor neurologic complication is damage to the greater occipital nerve, with referred pain to the occiput.[490] Obviously, the most serious complication is the immediate damage, followed by the potential for chronic damage to the spinal cord or medulla oblongata.[514,541] The level of neurologic (spinal cord) injury may not be at the same level as the dens fracture (Fig. 18-45). One child had pyramidal signs with absence of the abdominal reflexes and extensor plantar responses.[490] None of these cases was associated with delayed-onset paraplegia, although this is reportedly a potential complication in the adult. Delayed myelopathy may be due to a long-term instability.[488,493]

Open-mouth views may be significant, but lateral and anteroposterior tomographic views are also helpful. Care must be taken not to misinterpret the closing dentocentral synchondrosis as a fracture (Fig. 18-46). Displacement is usually minimal, making the diagnosis more difficult.

In most cases, with minimal or no displacement, treatment is conservative with strict bed rest, initial cervical traction for comfort, and a subsequent rigid collar (e.g., Somi brace). With displaced lesions, with or without neural deficit, treatment may have to be modified.[496] Manipulation and a Minerva cast have been used, as has skeletal traction followed by a halo cast. The ease of reduction, stability with traction or cast support, early callus formation, and prompt

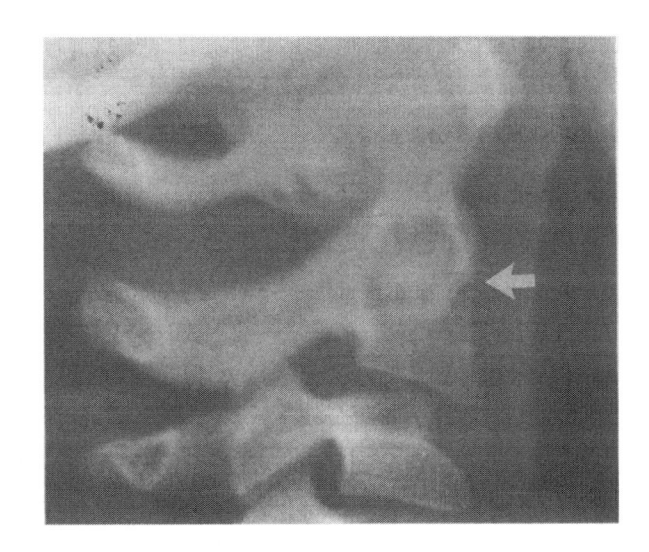

FIGURE 18-46. Apparent fracture of the dens (arrow) that is actually the dentocentral synchondrosis remnant. The absence of contiguous retropharyngeal swelling should lead one to suspect a structural variation, rather than trauma.

healing in most cases offer a good prognosis in these patients. Surgical (manipulative) reduction or fusion rarely is necessary. In older children and teenagers, the synchondrosis at the base of the dens is fused with the body of the axis, and injuries are essentially the same as those of an adult. In general, basilar and apical fractures heal well when reduced and stabilized, whereas fractures of the dens above the level of the atlantoaxial articular facets tend to remain unstable and often require posterior C1–C2 fusion.[521] Remodeling in children after C1–C2 fusion has a tendency to form kyphosis but to gradually remodel. Surgery is rarely necessary in a young child.[521] In rare instances an anterior approach is used.[492]

Like epiphyseal separations in other parts of the body, the separated dens is purported to unite readily. In the two cases reported by Blockey and Purser, union occurred in 7 and 13 weeks, respectively; and at the end of 3 years the clinical and radiologic appearances were normal.[490] Dens fractures in children older than 7 years closely resemble those in adults, especially regarding the likelihood of delayed healing.

Although there is a high incidence of pseudarthrosis or avascular (ischemic) necrosis in adults, these conditions do not seem to be serious complications in skeletally immature patients.[524] Undisplaced fractures at the base of the dens within the substance of the body of the axis have a satisfactory potential for healing. Fractures higher in the dens and displaced fractures, particularly those displaced posteriorly, have a much higher pseudarthrosis rate and usually require some type of fusion after reduction.

Late atlantoaxial instability may complicate even a minimally displaced dens fracture. Follow-up must be accurate and maintained until the child stops growing (Fig. 18-47).

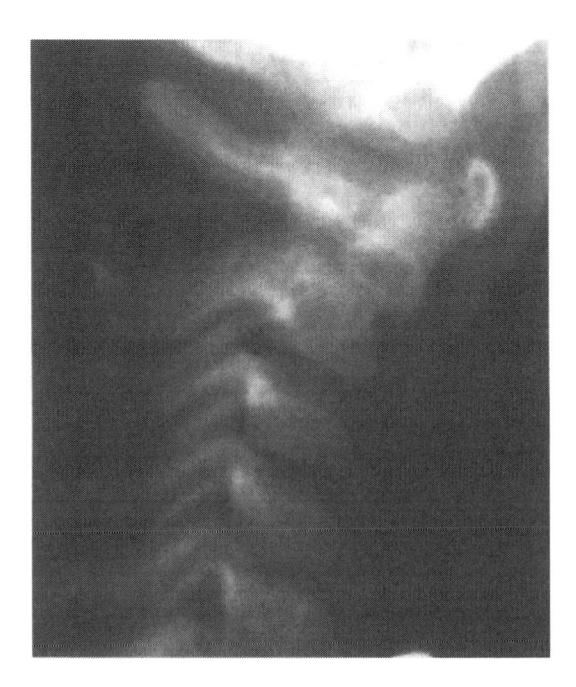

FIGURE 18-47. This 5-year-old child was being evaluated for a "fall." Screening of the cervical spine revealed an old odontoid fracture that had healed in a displaced position. A detailed interview showed a similar presentation after a "fall" 2 years previously. Child abuse was eventually diagnosed as the cause.

Os Odontoideum

Several anomalies are associated with abnormal flexion/extension motion between C1 and C2: hypoplasia of the dens, hypoplasia with an os odontoideum, simple shortening of the dens resulting from failure of the terminal ossification center to develop, and total agenesis of the dens.[498,507,509,513,516,517,522,526] Pizzutillo et al. reported an interesting case in which one of the paired primary ossification centers failed to develop.[530]

In the past, os odontoideum was thought to represent a deformed dens that failed to unite with the body of C2. This theory neglects the fact that the base of the normal dens is lower than the plane of the C1–C2 joints, although the os odontoideum complex may have a protrusion extending above the articular facets. The os odontoideum has also been considered a hypertrophic remnant of the proatlas associated with hypoplasia of the dens in the absence of the distal ossification center.

Trauma, often unrecognized, undoubtedly plays a significant role in the eventual development of an os odontoideum in the child and the adult (Figs. 18-48, 18-49).[491,497,500,502,506,518,519,524,525,534,545] Cases of apparent congenital absence of the dens have been reported frequently, although in some cases there were reports of definite trauma prior to definitive diagnosis.[501,510,515,536,538] Other reports describe the disappearance of the central portion of the dens in the child.[535] In these cases roentgenograms obtained shortly after injury revealed no fracture, whereas abnormalities were found when the patients were reevaluated. Seimon's patients were 22 and 35 months old at the time of their injuries.[535]

Gwinn and Smith reported 27 cases of acquired and congenital absence of the dens.[513] In more than half of these patients there had been antecedent trauma. Associated abnormalities of the cervical spine were present in five cases. Gillman described a case of congenital absence of the dens that was discovered after the patient sustained a head injury.[509] Freiberger and colleagues suggested that although some cases of an absent dens were congenital, some may be due to unsuspected trauma.[504]

Verska and Anderson described an identical twin with an os odontoideum after trauma, with the other twin having a normal cervical spine and no history of trauma.[543] Another report found an os odontoideum in *both* twins.[520]

Resorption of the basilar portion of the dens occurred in three reported cases in which injury of the dens was not recognized and treated. It produced the appearance of complete absence in one patient and the appearance of an os odontoideum in the other two patients.[500]

It seems that the disappearance of the lower portion of the dens is an example of nonunion and fibrous replacement of the bone, not unlike the traumatic acquisition of lumbar spondylolysis (L5) in gymnasts. A similar situation is chondro-osseous fracture of the carpal navicular (scaphoid) leading to a radiologically bipartite scaphoid (see Chapter 17). Certainly, an untreated fracture through a cartilaginous growth plate in a mobile area of the body such as the dens may go on to nonunion, especially if it is inadequately immobilized or not immobilized at all. If the dens is not seen radiographically, it does not necessarily mean there is a loss of all

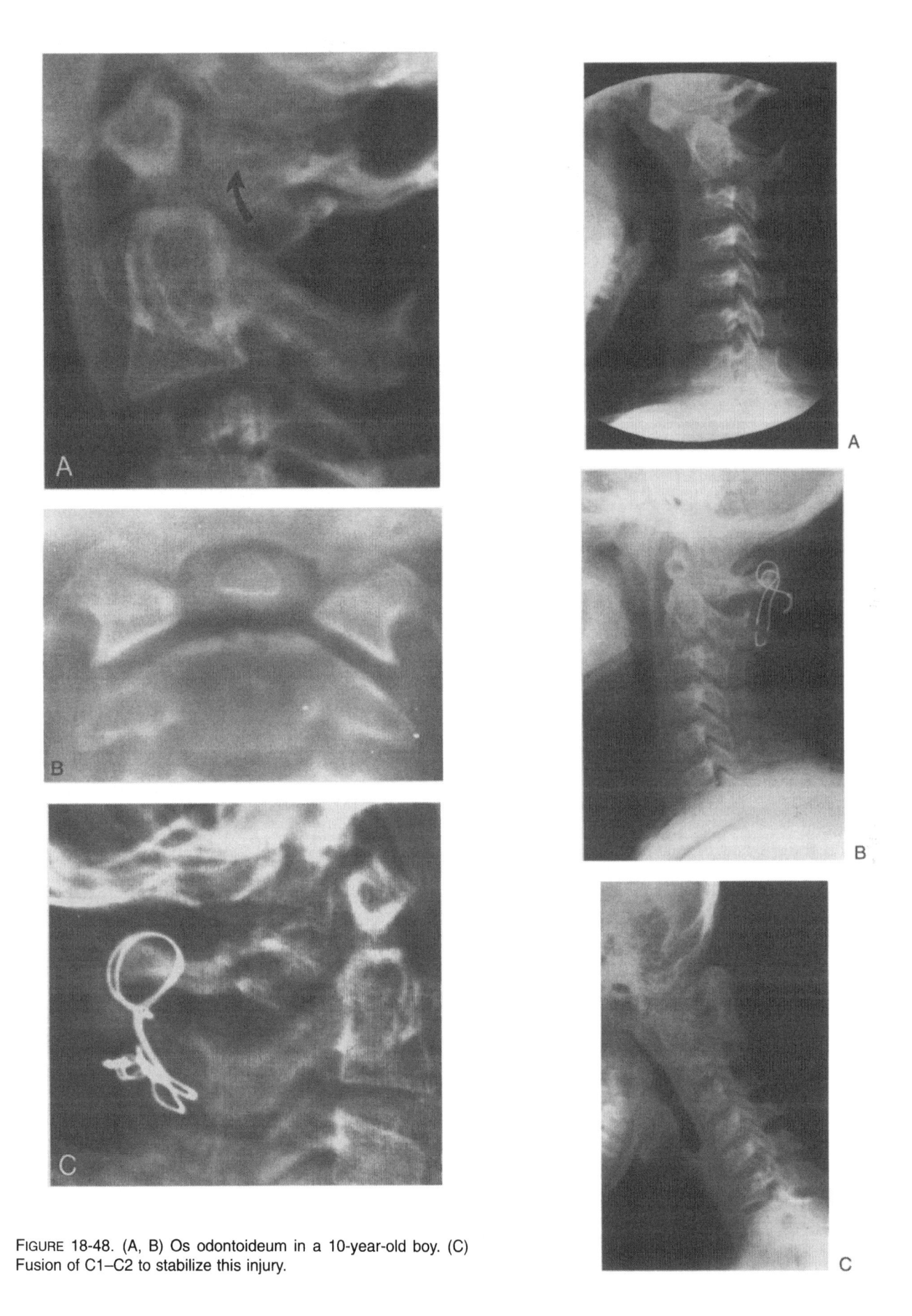

FIGURE 18-48. (A, B) Os odontoideum in a 10-year-old boy. (C) Fusion of C1–C2 to stabilize this injury.

FIGURE 18-49. (A) Unstable C1–C2 relation due to nonunion (os odontoideum) of a dens fracture in a 12-year-old boy. (B) It was treated by posterior fusion and wiring. The latter broke owing to delayed union. (C) Final result after augmentation of the bone graft and removal of the broken wire.

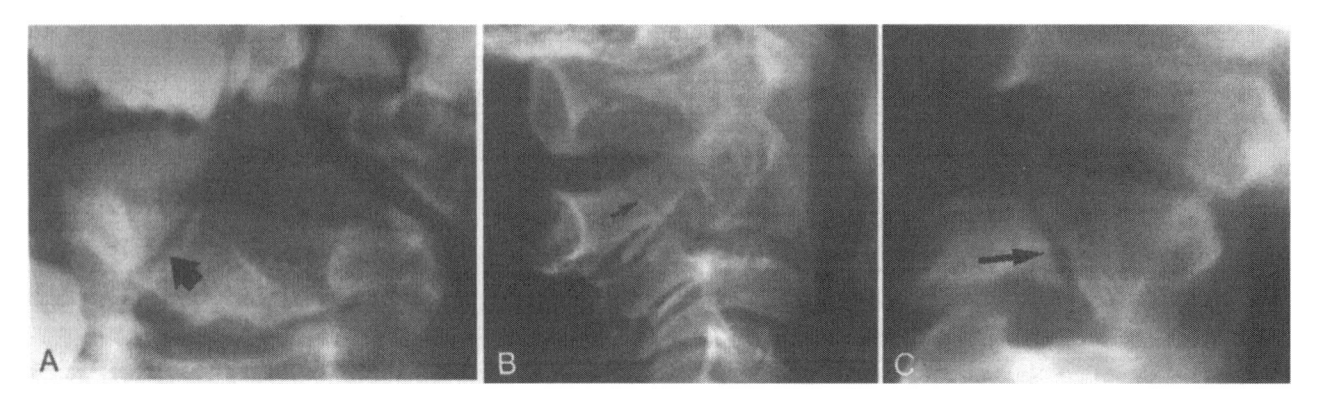

FIGURE 18-50. (A, B) Fracture of pedicle and lateral mass (arrow) of C2. (C) Seemingly comparable case. However, this linear defect was present bilaterally and probably represented a congenital defect (arrow).

tissue with a cystic defect. In a child, roentgenograms are obtained after suspected or definitive dens fracture to demonstrate whether union has occurred or unforeseen problems have arisen (3–4 weeks and 3–4 months after any suspicious injury).

When an os odontoideum is found, the first treatment step is a detailed evaluation of cord function, intrinsic stability, and the potential for cord compression acutely or chronically. This assessment may be done by assessing lateral MRI images in flexion and extension. If there is abnormal mobility or evidence of actual or potential cord damage, C1–C2 fusion should be considered (see Fig. 18-48 below).[497,511,521]

Fractures of the Body and Neural Arch of the Axis (C2)

Fractures of the body and neural arch of the axis, compared with dens or atlas fractures, are infrequent and generally heal satisfactorily with nonoperative treatment.[494,505,508] Congenital pseudarthroses, however, may complicate (confuse) the diagnosis (Figs. 18-50, 18-51).[522,528,542] Nordstrom and associates reported a 9-year-old girl with *familial* spondylolisthesis of C2 and C3.[528] Her father had similar vertebral abnormalities. Her condition was not discovered until she presented with a complaint of mild, localized neck pain after having fallen.

The posterior portion of the spinous process may be fractured through bone (Fig. 18-52) or as a chondro-osseous fracture of the tip (which has a cap of epiphyseal cartilage). The osseous fracture may extend to one or both laminae. The latter situation may lead to partial instability.

Upper Cervical Fracture-Dislocation

As previously mentioned, the focus of flexion-extension in the young child is at C2–C3. It does not shift to the lower cervical spine until after 7–8 years of age if not the second decade of life. The laxity of ligaments may allow facet displacement without fracture (Fig. 18-53). Displacement may be enough to cause a jumped (locked) facet. End-plate (apophyseal)

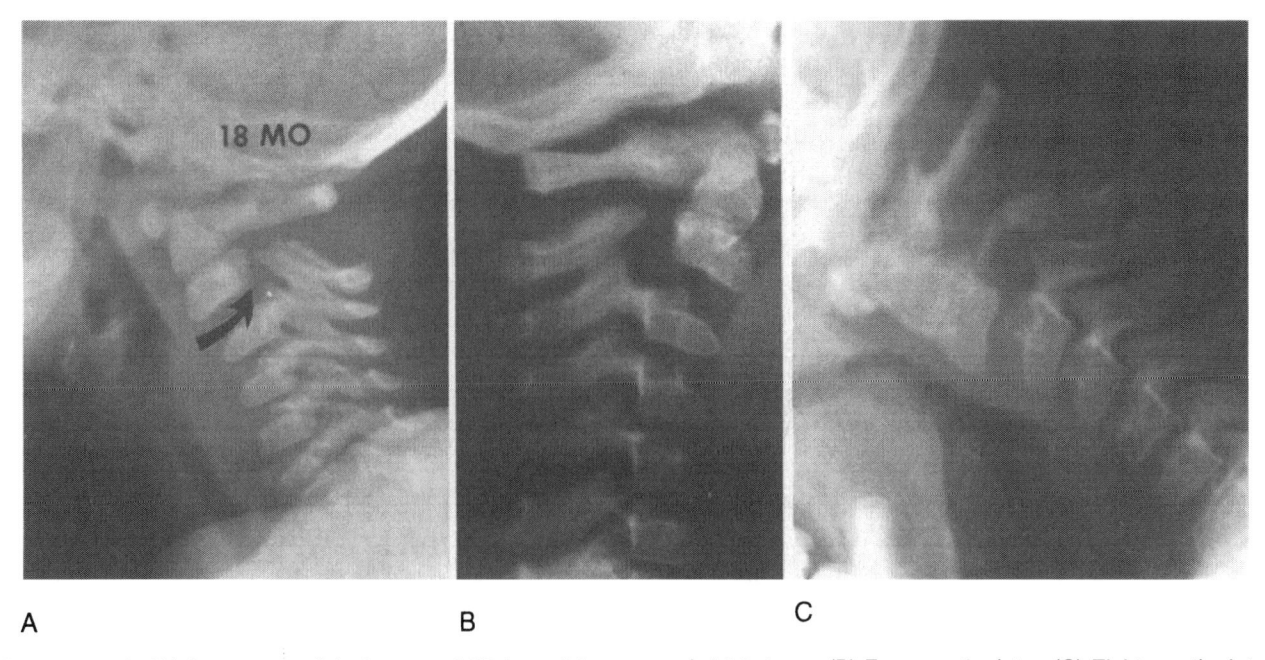

FIGURE 18-51. (A) Apparent pedicle fracture of C2 (arrow) in a case of child abuse. (B) Four months later. (C) Eight months later.

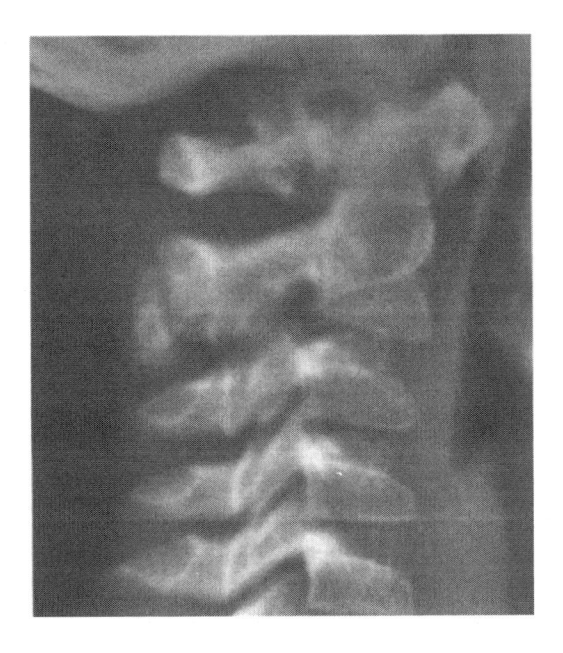

Specific Injuries

FIGURE 18-52. Fracture of the spinous process of C2.

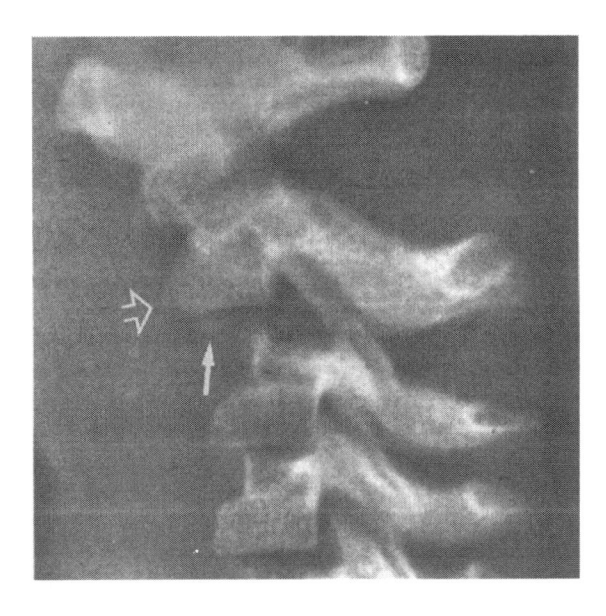

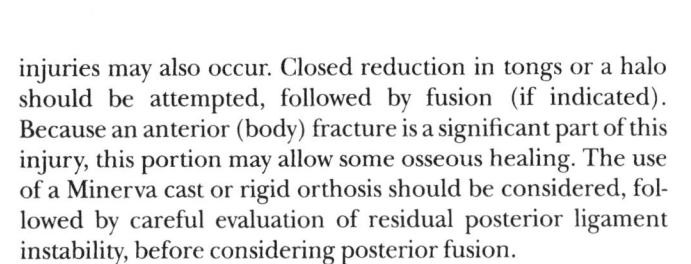

FIGURE 18-53. C2–C3 fracture-dislocation with locked facets. A small fragment (solid white arrow) is probably from the anteroinferior body (open white arrow) of C2.

injuries may also occur. Closed reduction in tongs or a halo should be attempted, followed by fusion (if indicated). Because an anterior (body) fracture is a significant part of this injury, this portion may allow some osseous healing. The use of a Minerva cast or rigid orthosis should be considered, followed by careful evaluation of residual posterior ligament instability, before considering posterior fusion.

Lower Cervical Fracture-Dislocation

The remainder of the cervical spine, with the exception of pseudosubluxation, is less frequently involved after trauma in children under 10 years.[546–554,556,558–560,562,564,566,570,571,573,576,578–581,584,586,588,590,595–600,602,604,637,660,688] Compression fractures of the cervical spine vertebral centra are unusual in children.[577] Congenital deformity may also predispose to injury.[568,574,582,593,594]

There is usually associated disruption of the posterior ligaments that allows vertebral body (anterior) displacement (Fig. 18-54). Posterior ligament disruption is often recognized preoperatively with a lateral roentgenogram that demonstrates widening of the spaces between the posterior spinous processes. This widening may be evident only with application of longitudinal traction. Therefore a lateral roentgenogram made with the patient in traction may be necessary to diagnose accurately whether the posterior ligaments are intact after injury to the immature cervical spine. Loss and lordosis are variable radiologic findings.[561] If

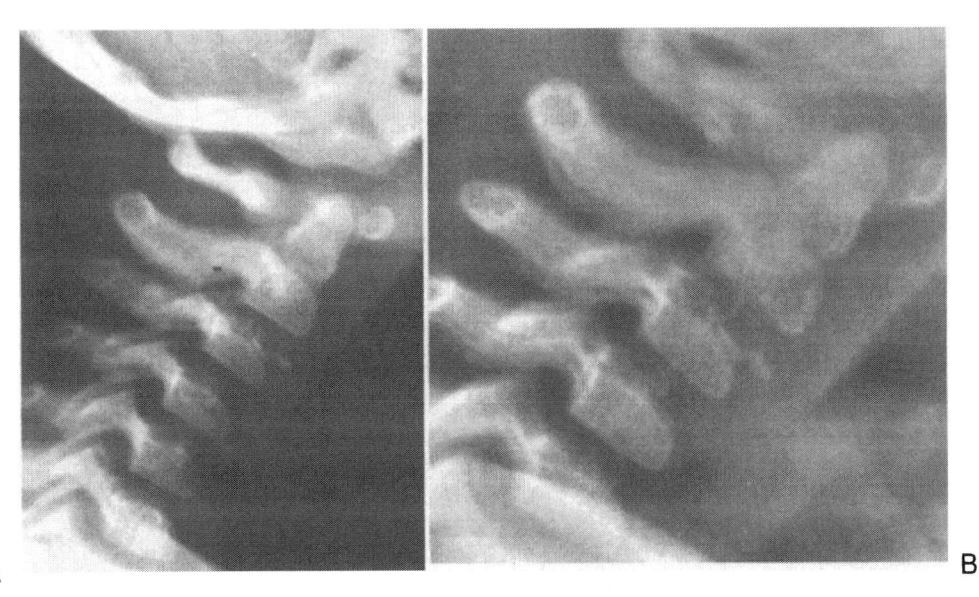

FIGURE 18-54. (A) Traumatic subluxation of C2 on C3. An anterior fragment is evident. (B) Ossification is progressing toward C2 several weeks later.

flexion-stress continues, the superior portion of the vertebral body may be additionally compacted to create a wedged vertebra (Fig. 18-55).

In infants and younger children, reduction of a cervical fracture-dislocation with halter or skeletal traction usually suffices, and surgical stabilization is not always necessary. This treatment generally takes 6–12 weeks in skeletal traction or a halo and another 6–8 weeks in a rigid orthosis or cast.[563] Skeletal traction by any one of several devices is often difficult to maintain in young children because of the thin outer table of their skulls.[592] Tantalum wire, threaded between burr holes, may be effective for treating children under 3 years of age. The halo cast in small children has the advantage of rigid external fixation coupled with ease of application and ample surgical approach. Its use in children appears to be without significant complication.

With tongs or a halo cast, meticulous attention to the sites of pin insertion is necessary to prevent superficial infection. Periodic roentgenograms of the skull are necessary for early detection of penetration of the inner table or osteomyelitis. Complaints of local pain, especially if severe, always suggest penetration of the inner table.

Stability is restored by ligamentous and chondro-osseous healing if the neck is held in a reduced position. If subsequent roentgenographic examination suggests a recurrent displacement, a limited two- to three-level posterior fusion with wires and autogenous bone grafts secures fixation in most instances (Fig. 18-56). Spontaneous fusion at the fracture site is less likely in adolescents, and fusion may be needed as often as it is used in adults. Disturbance of the growth of the anterior centrum, coupled with the disruption of the posterior ligaments, may cause these injuries to remain unstable. Without fusion, these patients may develop kyphotic deformities.

Techniques of anterior interbody fusion were originally developed to treat degenerative cervical spine disease.[583] These techniques are generally contraindicated in young children, as they may damage the superior and inferior endplates (Fig. 18-57).[587,601]

Limited posterior fusions are more appropriate in skeletally immature patients.[565,572] When undertaking posterior fusion of the cervical spine in children, it should be noted

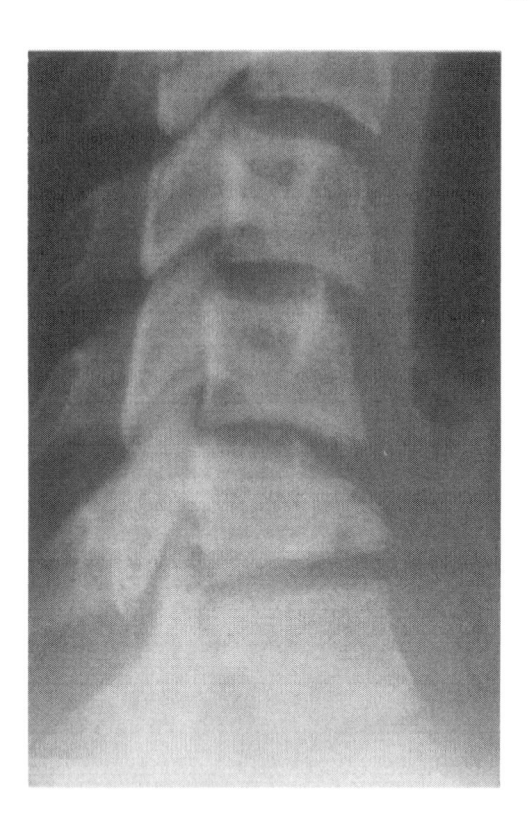

FIGURE 18-55. Wedging of C6 in flexion due to a hyperflexion injury in a 12-year-old boy. Note the appearance of the superior and inferior ring apophyses despite the retained wedging, which has *not* remodeled 18 months after injury.

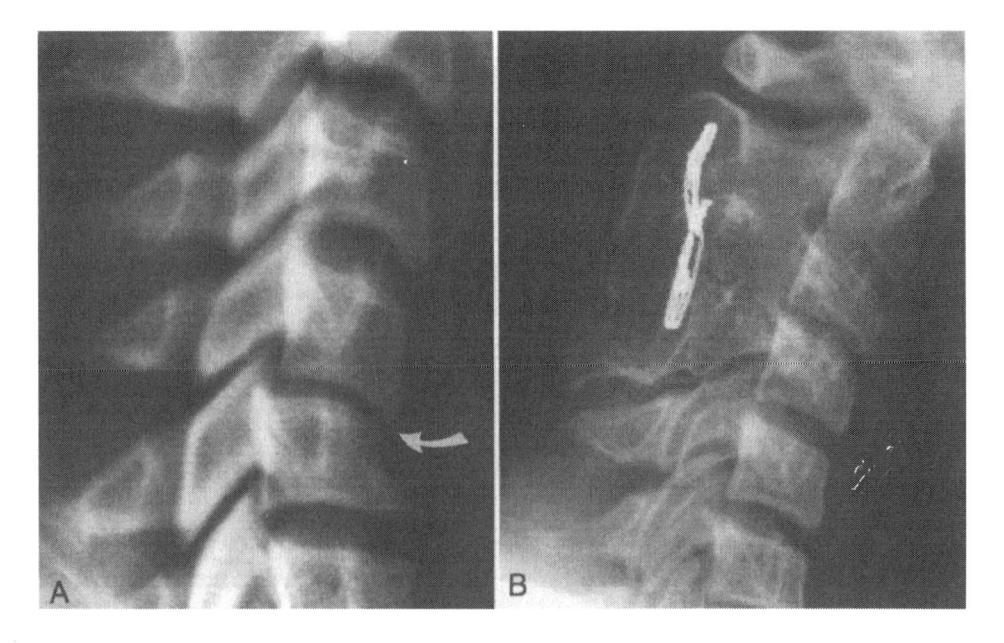

FIGURE 18-56. (A) Instability of C4 on C5. Note the narrowing of the interspace (arrow). (B) Similar case with involvement of two intervertebral levels was treated by wiring three spinous processes.

FIGURE 18-57. (A) Compression fracture of C5 (open arrow). Note the posterior widening (solid arrow), suggesting both anterior and posterior injury. (B) Initial treatment in a brace failed to correct the deformity. (C) It was then correctly stabilized by posterior interspinous wiring. (D) It was thought that anterior fusion was also indicated, a procedure *not* appropriate in such a skeletally immature individual. Surgical elevation of the anterior longitudinal ligament and the anterior vertebral cartilage to expose the incompletely developed central ossification caused fusion not only of C4–C6 (solid arrow) but also of C2 and C3 (open arrow), leading to a major growth abnormality.

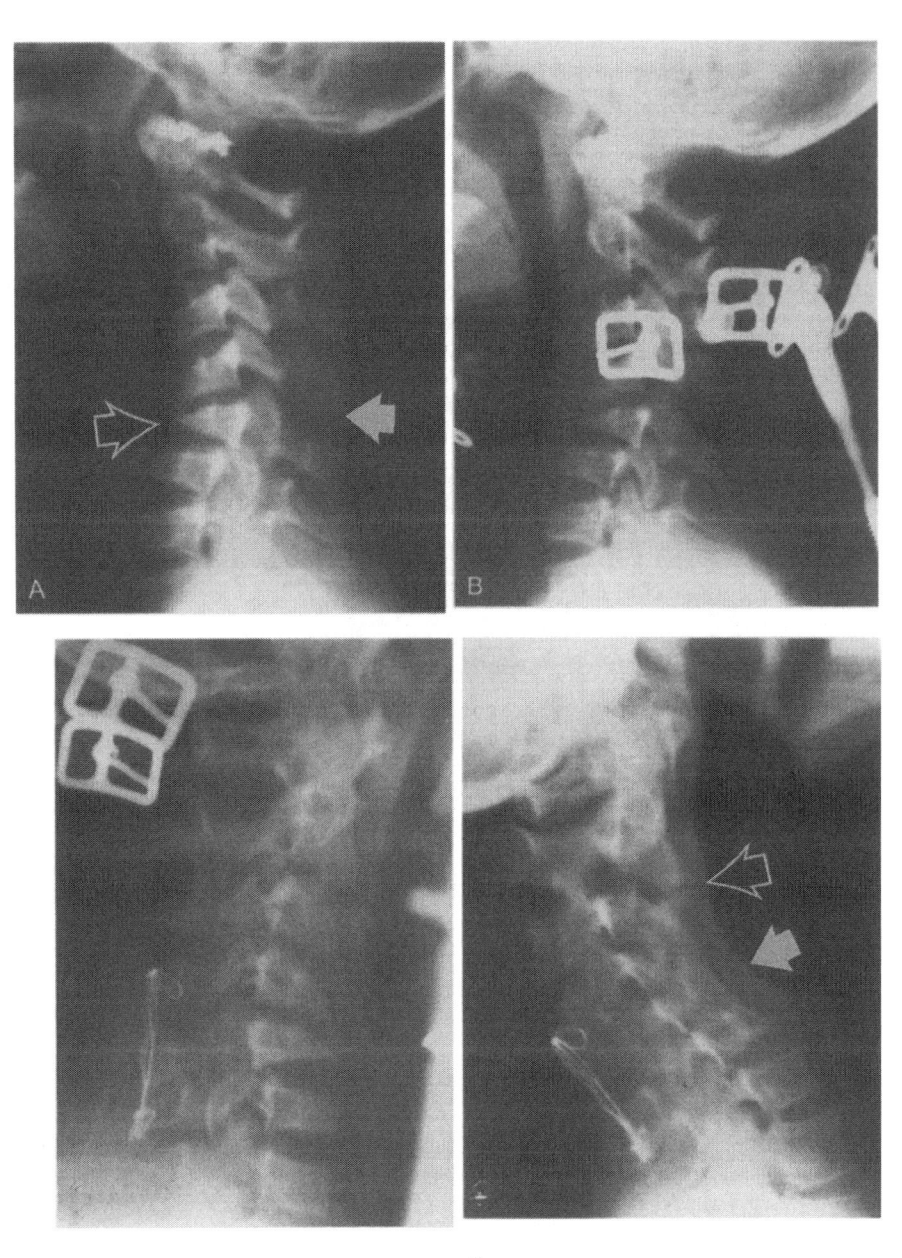

that cadaveric bone grafts in children are less likely to result in posterior cervical fusion.[591] Autogenous iliac bone graft is significantly superior for use in children, athough even it may be resorbed. Furthermore, young children have limited amounts of such bone for grafting.

Combined anterior and posterior fusion has also been advocated in adults. However, when the injury is primarily posterior, the anterior longitudinal ligament usually is intact in the young child, in whom it is a thick structure. It probably is unwise to remove this ligament because it is the final stabilizing structure in a posterior to anterior disruption. Anterior approaches should be minimized in children because of these significant anatomic differences.

Treatment for a fracture or fracture-dislocation of the cervical spine below the axis in children usually does not necessitate laminectomy. Progression of a neurologic deficit while the child is under direct observation is a relative indication for evaluation with MRI or CT. A child who presents with a nonprogressive deficit is unlikely to benefit from decompression. The addition of posterior decompressive laminectomy, allegedly done to relieve pressure in the damaged spinal cord, may involve removal of posterior ligaments, and it increases the degree of instability that may have been caused initially by the osseous injury. Because spinal cord injury frequently extends over several levels, decompression of only one or two segments is inadequate unless there is active progression of the neurologic deficit. In addition, the multiple-level laminectomy has adverse consequences from the standpoint of cervical spine stability in children, resulting in a severe swan-neck deformity (Fig. 18-58).[555,557,575,589,603] If laminectomy has been undertaken, the facet joints usually are stabilized with wiring and bone graft.

Occasionally, a child or adolescent sustains trauma to the cervical spine that produces little or no osseous damage and has no neurologic consequence. Ligamentous injury may render the cervical spine unstable, though, an event that is undetected initially and then is either untreated or undertreated. Because of the lack of obvious osseous damage, treat-

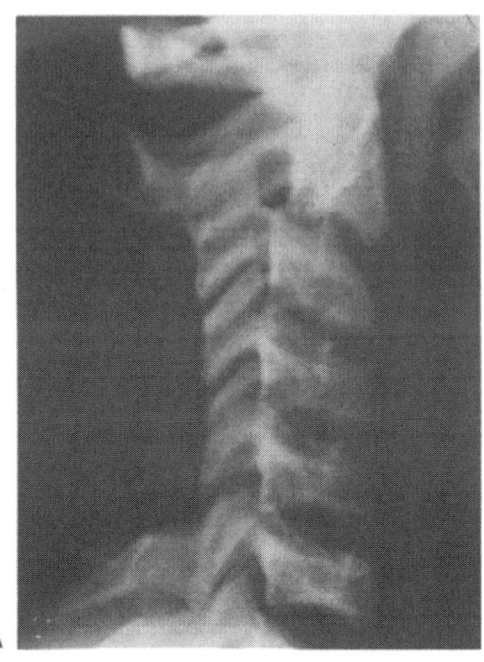

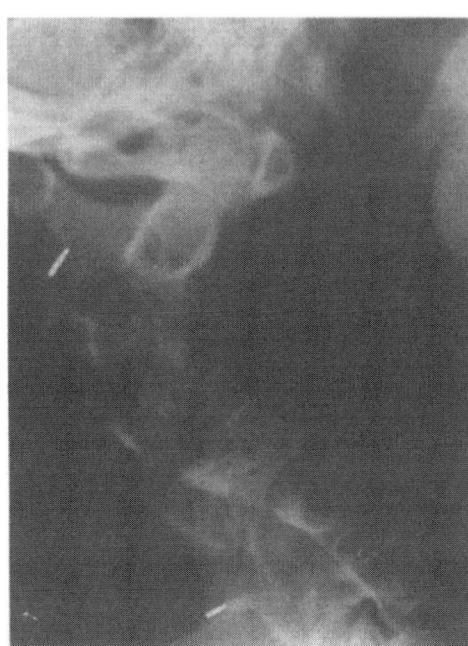

FIGURE 18-58. Resection of stabilizing fulcrum elements may lead to major deformity. (A) Appearance after performance of a multiple laminectomy. (B) Swan-neck deformity 4 years later.

ment may be minimized, and the instability persists or even progresses.

Spinous Processes

Hyperflexion injuries may lead to avulsion of the cartilaginous tips that are responsible for elongation of the spinous processes. Whether initially recognized at the time of injury or later, these particular injuries have a high rate of delayed and nonunion (Fig. 18-59). If they become painful, resection may be necessary.

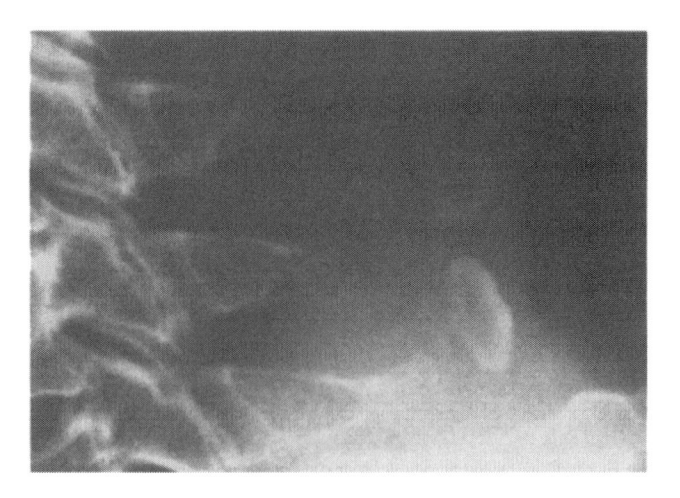

FIGURE 18-59. Multiple avulsions of the spinous processes of C6, C7, and T1. Only the latter (T1) healed. The other two were painful nonunions.

Cervical End-Plate Injury

Physeal injuries of the cervical spine (Figs. 18-60, 18-61) are uncommon injuries usually caused by hyperextension of the cervical spine.[567,569] Significant violence is the usual mechanism, most often due to an automobile accident or diving into shallow water. In infants, child abuse involving severe shaking may completely disrupt an interspace through one of the end-plates.

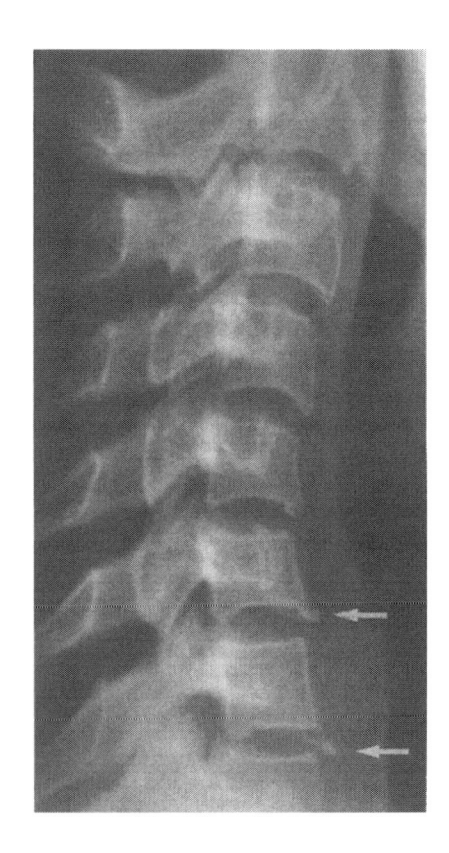

FIGURE 18-60. Double-level end-plate fractures (arrows). Note the subluxations in the upper cervical regions.

Specific Injuries

FIGURE 18-61. (A) Inferior end-plate fracture of C2 (arrow). (B) Healing.

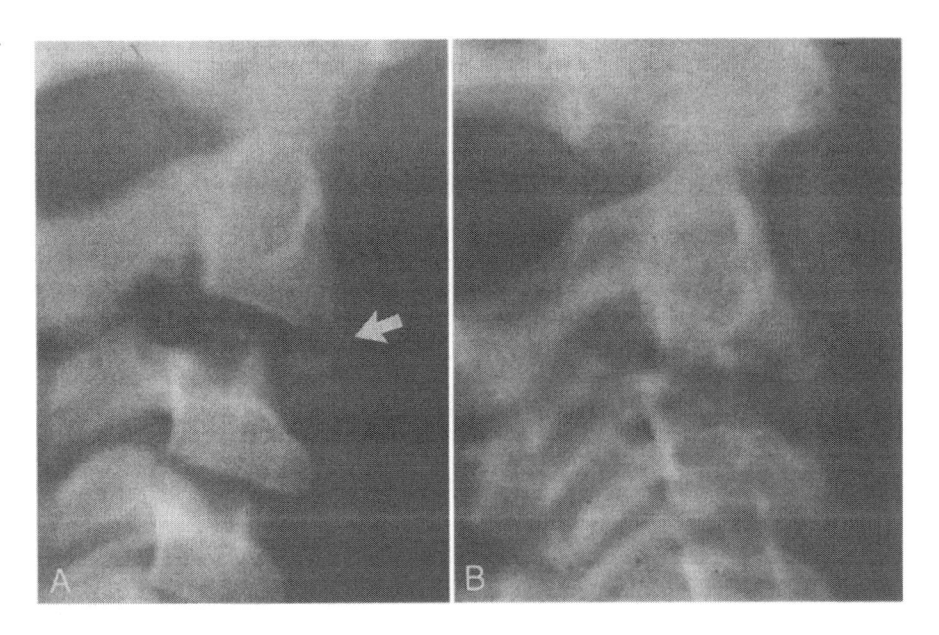

The injury usually involves the inferior growth region (end-plate).[567,569] The uncinate processes may biomechanically protect the superior region, making the inferior end-plate the weaker link relative to fracture susceptibility. Histologic examination (Fig. 18-62) of a case showed concomitant microscopic disruption of the superior end-plate of C3.[569] Stanley et al. described two examples of superior end-plate injury.[592]

With some of these injuries it is difficult to imagine, when the anterior borders of the vertebra above and below the avulsed ossification center maintain their normal anatomic alignment, that the entire growth plate and epiphysis have been involved, as would be expected with a classic type 1 physeal injury. Accordingly, it is possible that a type 3 injury (Fig. 18-63) affecting only the anterior portion of the growth plate and epiphysis may be an appropriate concept for some of the "adolescent" injuries. In animals these anterior end-plate injuries certainly are type 3 growth mechanism injuries (Fig. 18-31), sometimes with an additional type 1 extension. Furthermore, when the posteroinferior "ring apophysis" is

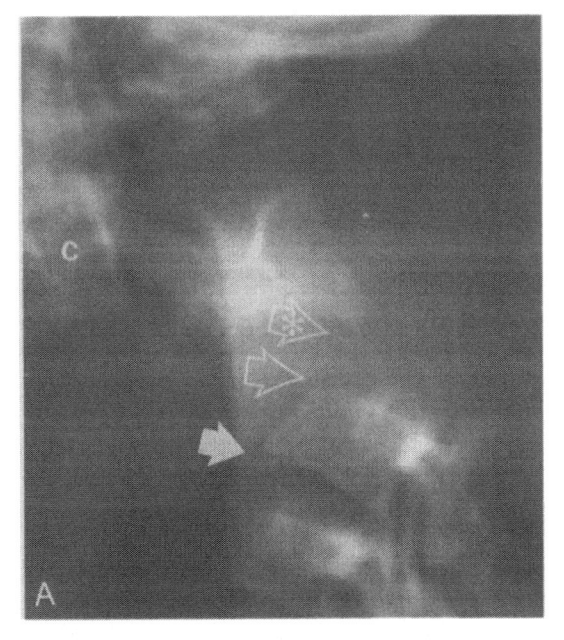

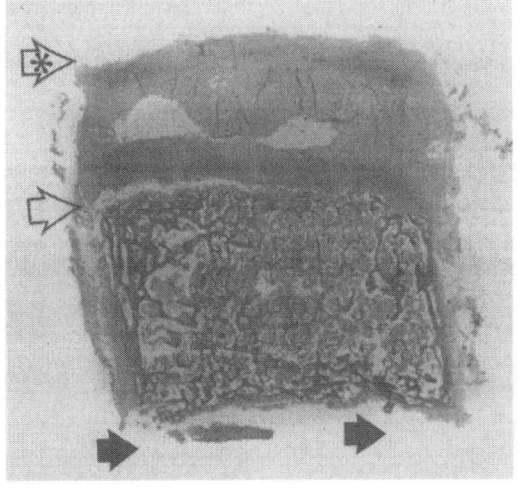

FIGURE 18-62. (A) Epiphyseal fractures of the cervical spine. The arrow with the asterisk points to the C2 end-plate, which has separated from the centrum (C). The intervertebral disk, demarcated by the two open arrows, is intact. However, the interspace of C3–C4 (solid arrow) is probably partially disrupted by hyperextension. (B) Histologic specimen. The arrow with the asterisk points to the C2 end-plate, which has separated from the centrum. Note that the intervertebral-apophyseal region is beginning to separate (open arrow) from the C3 centrum, as it did above at C2. There is also disruption of the inferior subchondral plate of C3 (solid arrows).

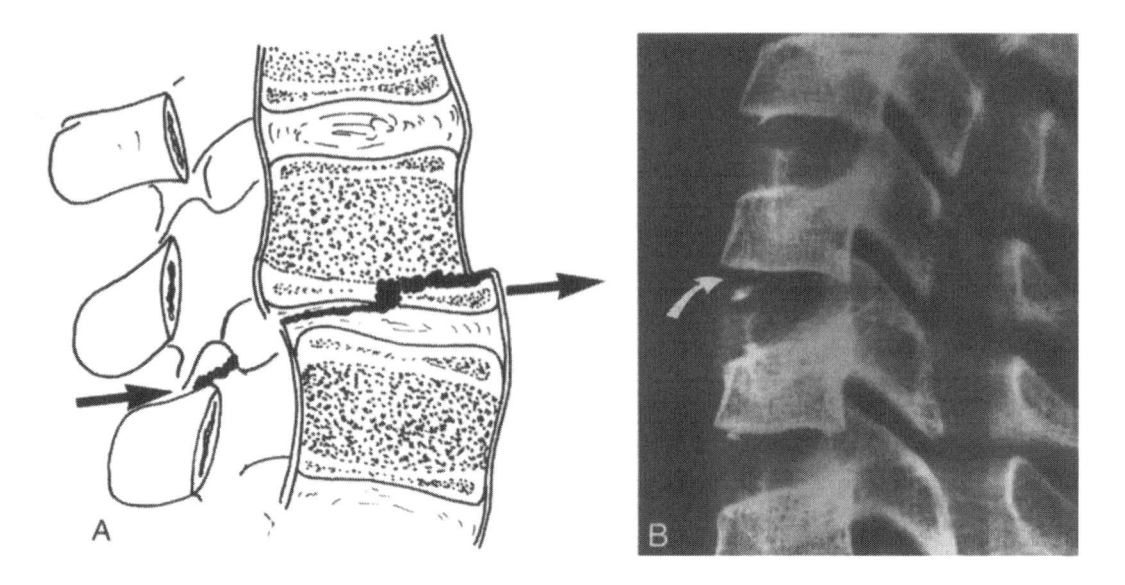

FIGURE 18-63. (A) Type 3 growth mechanism end-plate injury in an adolescent. (B) Traumatic end-plate separation (arrow) in an adolescent cadaver.

injured in adolescent lumbar spines, CT scanning shows a type 3 fracture, rather than involvement of the entire endplate. The type 1 injury (Figs. 18-64, 18-65) more characteristically involves the infant or young child. Such an age-related difference in injury response patterns is certainly consistent with the variability of comparable physeal injuries in the long bones.

Most of the reported patients are adolescents, an observation suggesting age-related susceptibility during the stages of physeal maturation and closure.[567,569] However, Aufdermaur, during postmortem examinations, found cervical endplate fractures in children from birth through adolescence, implying that the injury pattern is not so much related to the extent of chondro-osseous maturation as it is to our inability to diagnose the undisplaced injury radiographically in young patients.[40]

The secondary ossification center of a cervical vertebra appears relatively late. Evaluation and diagnosis of the injury thus may be difficult, if not impossible, before its appearance. The infrequent secondary ossification center of a cervical spine vertebra may be mistaken for a fracture fragment by an inexperienced observer. In contrast, diagnosis of a displaced ring apophysis is relatively easy on the lateral roentgenogram. The secondary ossification center is anteriorly displaced, and there is usually contiguous soft tissue swelling. Although secondary ossification centers are present in children 6–10 years of age, these centers most often first appear in the cervical spine when children are 10–12 years

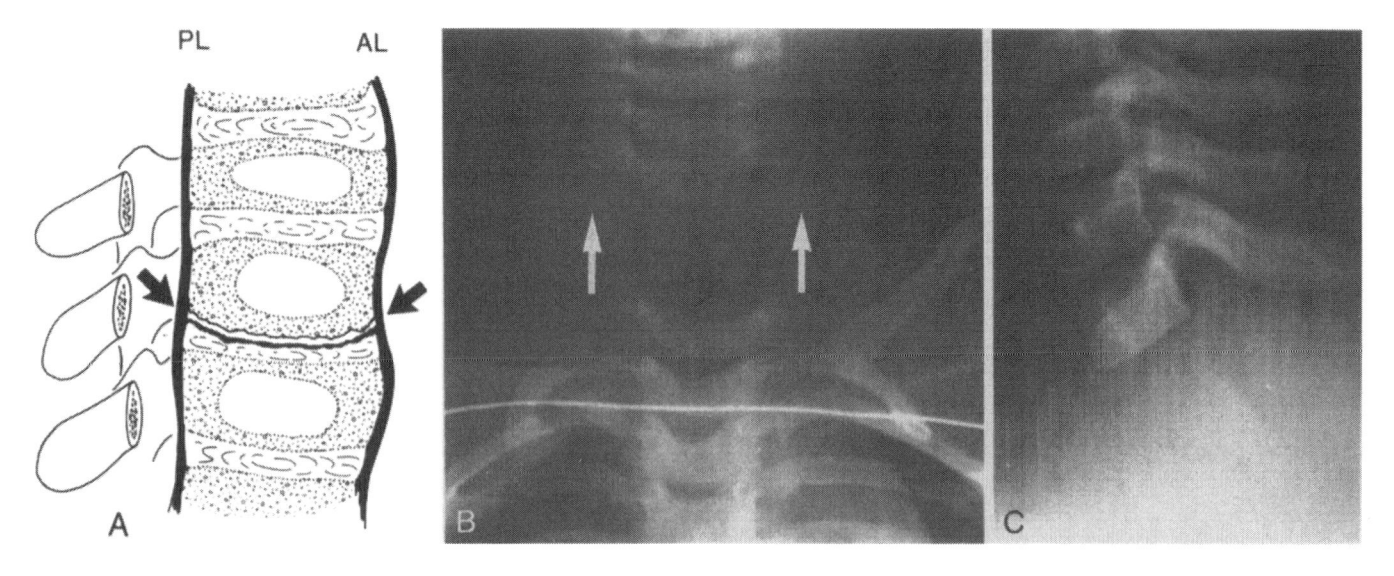

FIGURE 18-64. (A) Type 1 end-plate growth mechanism injury in an infant. PL = Posterior longitudinal ligament; AL = Anterior longitudinal ligament. Anteroposterior (B) and lateral (C) views of such an injury following an automobile accident, showing complete separation of C6 from C7 (arrows).

Specific Injuries

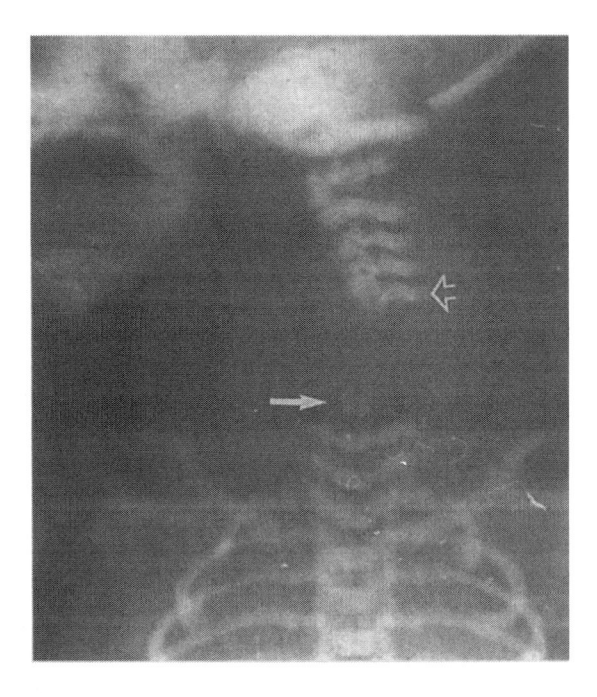

FIGURE 18-65. Traumatic separation of the centrum of C5 (solid arrow) from the posterior element (open arrow). This injury had to occur through the neurocentral synchondroses.

of age. Accordingly, if this injury were to occur before such secondary ossification, the diagnosis would have to be deduced from soft tissue swelling anterior to the vertebral body; and treatment would be rendered empirically on the basis of neck pain following significant trauma. MRI may offer an alternative diagnostic modality in the affected young patient. The separation involves angular displacement and is difficult to diagnose radiographically. Moreover, it probably reduces spontaneously. As in older patients, when C7–T1 lesions are evaluated, it is imperative that the radiographic views adequately visualize the lower margin of C7 and the C7–T1 interspace.

The injury may occur at various levels in the cervical spine. The four patients studied by Keller had C2 or C3 inferior end-plate involvement.[567] In contrast, two of our patients had more caudal involvement of the inferior end-plates (C6 and C7), and a third patient had involvement of the inferior end-plate of C3.[567] In two of Keller's patients the avulsion occurred at a single level, and in the other two it occurred at two levels. Multiple-level involvement was evident radiographically in one of my cases and histologically in another.[569]

Type 3 injuries heal rapidly within a few weeks. The periosteum, which is integrally related to the anterior longitudinal ligament, is pulled away from the inferior portion of the vertebrae associated with the fracture. During childhood this structure is osteogenic, and if it is surgically elevated it may lead to rapid fusion of the cervical vertebrae anteriorly. Such a response lessens with increasing spinal maturity. Keller described uneventful healing with anterior "osteophytes" in three patients and incomplete bridging of the interspace (Fig. 18-66) in a fourth patient.[567] The bridging occurred within the anterior longitudinal ligament. Premature closure of the growth plate may lead to deformity or interspace narrowing (Fig. 18-67).

Keller did not describe flexion-extension lateral views, so it is difficult to say if there was any long-term injury to the contiguous soft tissues in those patients.[567] In our patients, there was definite loss of normal cervical flexion at the injured levels. However, the long-term consequences of these motion losses—particularly whether they eventually predispose to spondylytic changes or disk space narrowing—are currently unknown owing to the lack of a sufficient number of patients followed for extended times after such injuries.

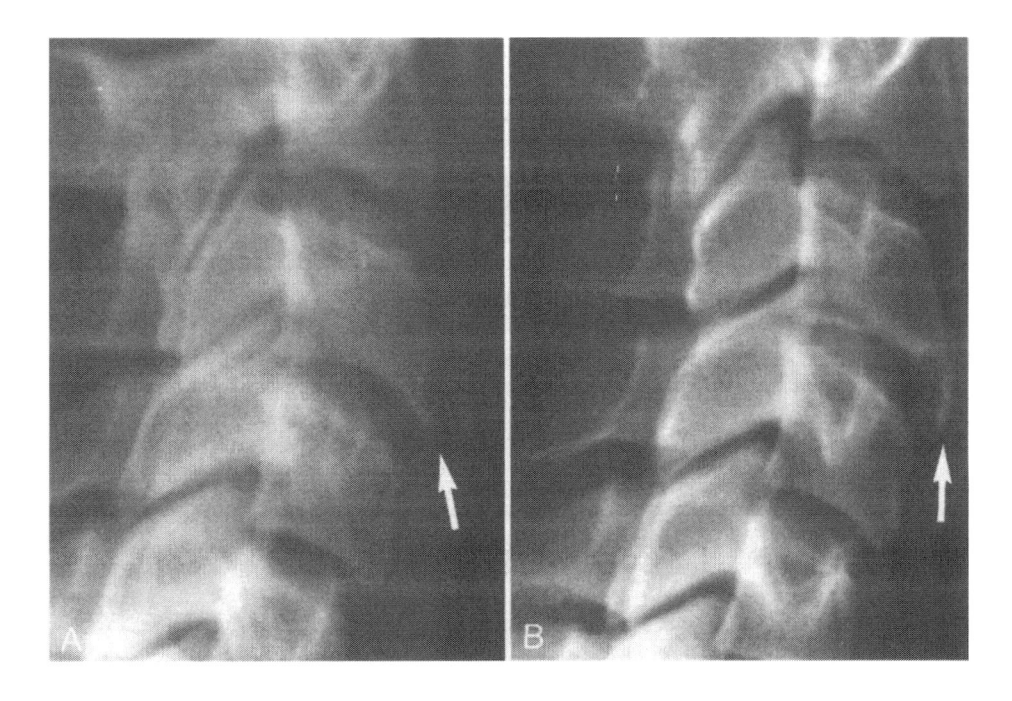

FIGURE 18-66. (A) End-plate fracture (arrow). (B) Subsequent ossification of the annulus (arrow).

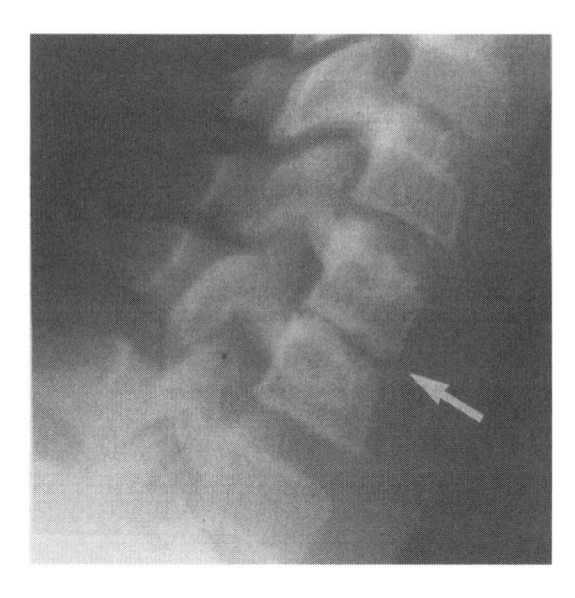

FIGURE 18-67. Narrowing of the posterior part of the C5–C6 interspace with anterior ring apophysis formation (arrow). This child had been a victim of child abuse 7 years before this film was obtained to evaluate neck pain following a football injury.

Type 1 growth mechanism injuries may be fatal, although not necessarily acutely. Small children may be easily overdistracted because the end-plate, ligaments, *and* spinal cord are often all transected, leading to quadriplegia (Fig. 18-65). Cervical traction must be closely monitored. If the infant or small child survives, fusion of the disrupted vertebrae is essential.

Injury to the Thoracic Spine

Injury to the vertebral elements of the developing thoracic spine is relatively infrequent compared to other, more mobile regions.[608,610] Most of these injuries result from vehicular accidents. Falls from a height and sporting accidents are less common causes. Child abuse is a common mechanism. Congenital lesions may also mimic thoracic spine trauma.[612]

Because these fractures are often subtle or reduce spontaneously, additional diagnostic clues should be sought. Widening of the mediastinum, similar to the prevertebral fat stripe seen with a cervical injury, may be a good indicator of possible thoracic spine injury.[605]

Inspection of the back frequently reveals abrasions and contusions, which give a clue to the mechanism of injury. Palpation may elicit tenderness of the paravertebral musculature and spinous processes, but palpable widening of the interspinous distance does not usually occur. Neurologic symptoms and objective neuromuscular findings are typically absent. Traumatic ileus may accompany even a minor injury. Excluding rib fractures, associated skeletal injuries are not particularly helpful for the diagnosis and may often contribute to a delay in appropriate treatment.

The intrinsic elasticity of the region, coupled with the protective effect of the rib cage to prevent excessive translational movements of the thoracic spinal components, maximizes the abnormal stresses necessary to cause fracture or dislocation. In the thoracic region, especially in young children, injury to the spinal cord occurs more often *without* associated vertebral fracture, although significant translation may occur without cord damage.[611] The thoracic cord appears to be susceptible to injury because of its relatively narrow canal and tenuous blood supply (artery of Adamkiewicz).

A relatively rare cause of thoracic spinal cord dysfunction in a child is blunt trauma to the abdomen. This injury usually relates to interference with the abdominal aorta and its branches, particularly the artery of Adamkiewicz, which arises at T11 and is a particularly important feeder to the spinal cord. Most patients with this condition have complete, permanent interruption of cord function.

Ruckstuhl et al. described 26 children and adolescents with 65 vertebral fractures.[610] Most of the fractures occurred in the mid-thoracic spine. Fractures of the vertebral body with sagittal wedge deformity alone had a better prognosis than those with concomitant sagittal *and* frontal wedge deformities. Those in the first group self-corrected partially or completely during subsequent growth, but improvement in the wedge deformity was present in only about one-third of the patients in the second group. When the end-plates were fractured, there was *no* correction, and there was a distinct lack of vertebral growth. Severe destruction of the cartilaginous end-plates and intervertebral disk led to fusion of the corresponding segments. An increase in wedge deformity was observed twice. Slight axial deviations of the intervertebral disks following vertebral body fractures were compensated during growth in most cases. Unstable fractures may be difficult to control, even with a thoracolumbosacral orthosis.[712]

Wedge fractures of the thoracic vertebral bodies, usually of minor degree, are relatively common (Figs. 18-68, 18-69). The intrinsic elasticity in children, in contrast to that in adults, allows these injuries to occur without major damage to the posterior elements, thus causing an intrinsically more stable injury.[607] The posterior and anterior longitudinal ligaments are usually intact, although some posterior damage may allow subluxation (Fig. 18-70). Wedge fractures occur in the thoracolumbar junction more commonly than fractures localized to only the thoracic or lumbar spine. Compression of two or more vertebrae occurs frequently in children.

The presence of a healthy intervertebral disk, in combination with well-mineralized bone, is likely to be responsible for the finding of multiple anterior compression fractures. When a normal disk is present, the injurious force applied to the spine may be transmitted from one vertebral body to an adjacent one. The "normal" intervertebral disk might also explain the infrequency of disk space narrowing and the absence of spontaneous interbody fusion in this group of children, although disk space injury may still occur.

Instability of the thoracic spine after injury depends on the degree of damage to the posterior elements: chondroosseous, ligamentous, or both.[607] If these posterior structures remain intact, the fracture is probably stable. When a fracture of the articular processes or rupture of the posterior ligaments occurs, the injury is potentially unstable. A fracture is grossly unstable when the posterior elements are completely disrupted and vertebral body displacement and dislocations are present on roentgenographic examination.

Simple bed rest is generally indicated, as most children with hyperflexion thoracic compression fractures are asymp-

Specific Injuries

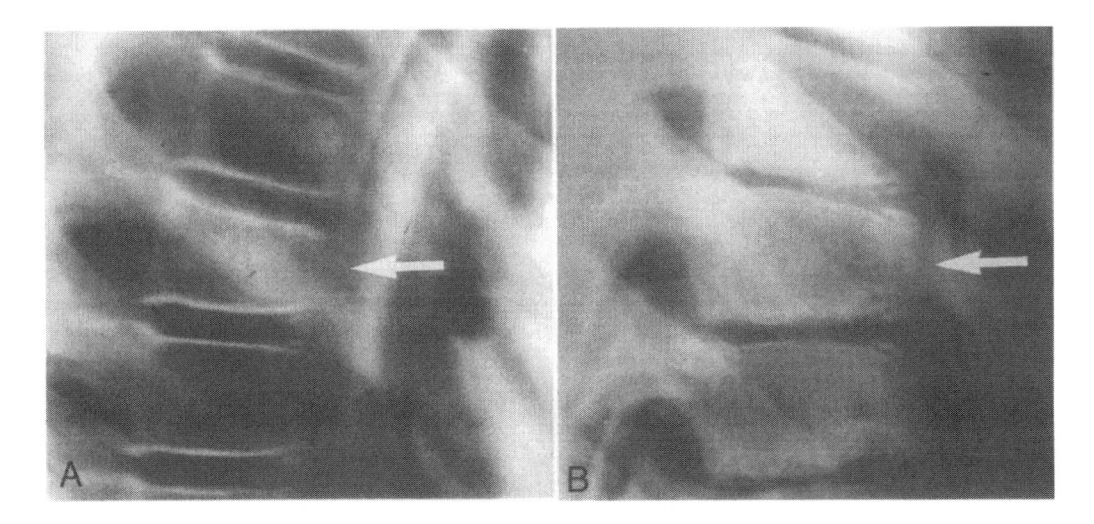

FIGURE 18-68. (A) Mild compression fracture (arrow) of a thoracic vertebra. (B) Appearance 1 year later, with some reconstitution of the anterior height (arrow).

tomatic within a few weeks. External support is appropriate. Activity is gradually increased, depending on the patient's symptoms. Spinal fusion or internal stabilization is rarely necessary in this region in a child but should be considered in patients, especially older ones, with residual instability.[609]

Follow-up through spinal skeletal maturity is warranted to assess potential delayed development of scoliosis or kyphosis due to end-plate damage. An acquired "bar" may form and lead to a situation similar to an uncompensated congenital scoliosis. Pseudomeningocele has also been reported.[606]

Follow-up radiographs after compression fractures of the immature spine show varying degrees of restoration of vertebral body height (Figs. 18-68, 18-69). The extent of restoration is directly related to the severity of the fracture and the age of the patient at the time of injury. In children under 10 years of age with moderate compression injuries, some reconstitution of the vertebral body may occur. Children with severe fractures or those injured when older usually show some permanent asymmetric wedging of the vertebral bodies with concave end-plates and deformity of the anterior contour of the bodies.

In a review of 59 patients who had sustained thoracic fractures during childhood, most of which were localized to the mid-thoracic area, more than 50% had no evidence of posttraumatic growth or response changes during their follow-up examinations. The number of posttraumatically altered

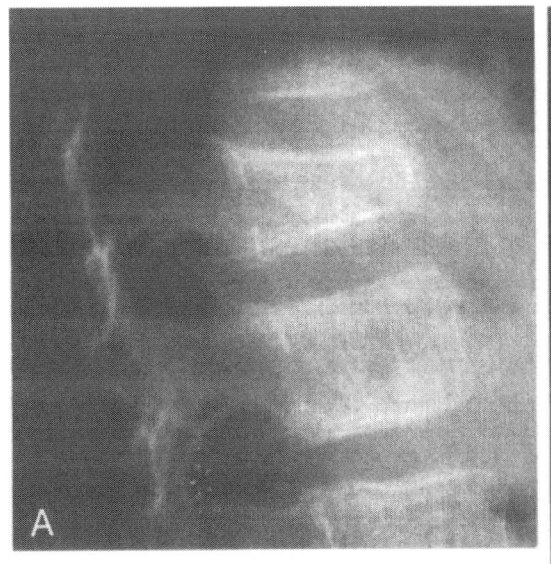

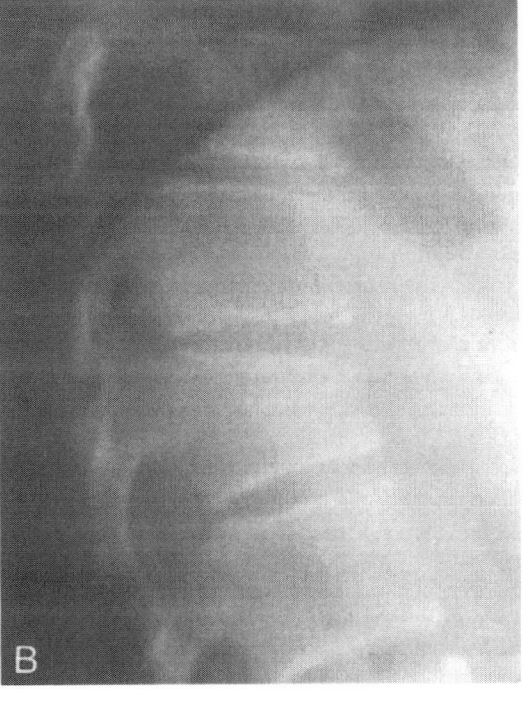

FIGURE 18-69. (A) Crush fracture of T12. (B) Incomplete growth recovery 3 years later.

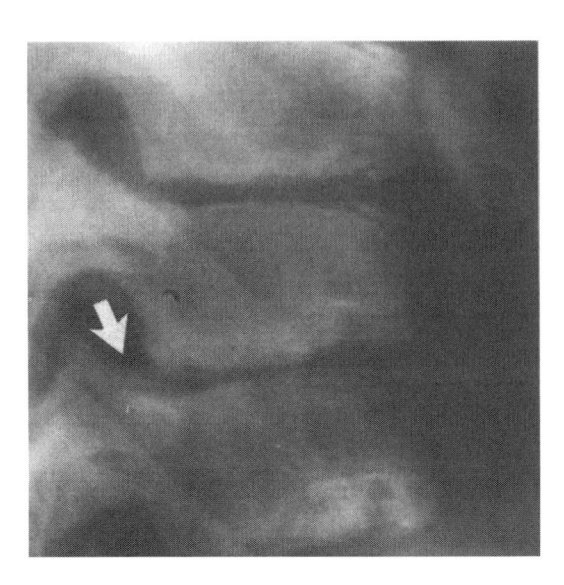

FIGURE 18-70. Anterior subluxation of T11 on T12 (arrow) with mild wedging of T12.

vertebral bodies was significantly lower than the number of those primarily injured.[60]

Anteroposterior radiographs often reveal scoliosis following a hyperflexion thoracic injury. Typically, the scoliosis is a balanced thoracolumbar curve apically centered at the fractured area. From a prognostic standpoint, the deformity is less than 10° and only slightly progressive.

In patients with unstable injuries, with or without paralysis, this same potential for growth and development, combined with the instability of the fracture, may lead to a progressive spinal deformity.

Facet Fractures

The facets not only are comprised of an articular cartilage surface, they also have a variable amount of epiphyseal and physeal cartilage. These regions are initially integrated with the neurocentral synchondroses but gradually become separate, not unlike the gradual separation of the capital femoral, greater trochanteric, and lesser trochanteric regions of the proximal femur. These regions are capable of sustaining an injury pattern similar to a long-bone physeal fracture. Such facet injuries may involve any region of the spine: cervical, thoracic, lumbar, or sacral. This pattern has been documented in animal specimens (Figs. 18-27, 18-28) but is not well documented in children. That it is a separation of the cartilaginous facet away from the metaphyseal bone equivalent makes radiographic demonstration difficult if not impossible.

Because there are growth plates associated with each of the four facets present in each vertebra, involvement leading to physeal damage would affect symmetric growth and could contribute to a scoliotic deformity.

Scheuermann's Disease

The combination of fixed kyphosis of the thoracic spine with radiographic changes of vertebral wedging, end-plate irregularity, and narrowing of the intervertebral disk space with or without intervertebral disk herniation is commonly referred to as Scheuermann's disease.[613–619,621,622,626,629,632,633] Although less common, lumbar and thoracolumbar forms of Scheuermann's juvenile kyphosis have been described (Fig. 18-71)[622] and characteristically produce more pain than the thoracic type.[618,620,624,627,635]

The exact etiology of this "disease" is unknown.[619,621,623,625,630,634] Alexander proposed that it is a traumatic stress spondylodystrophy that is sequential upon traumatic growth arrest and end-plate fractures (perhaps single and microscopic) that occurs during the heightened vulnerability of the adolescent growth spurt.[613] Once one fracture has occurred, an insidious compounding of the deformity may ensue, with adjacent vertebrae being affected by abnormally applied static loads that increasingly cause pathologic stress failure in the anterior region.

In specimens of juvenile Scheuermann's osteochondrosis, Aufdermaur showed that there were foci of various sizes in the cartilaginous end-plates that displayed disruption of the collagen fibers.[614–617] These findings, coupled with an alteration and occasional absence of the growth zone, were thought to result in the typical deformation of the vertebral bodies through a disturbance of collagen or ground substance biosynthesis.

The role of strenuous physical activity or repetitive injury in the pathogenesis of these lesions has been suggested.[625,629–631] I have seen it in adolescents engaged in rigorous overhead (e.g., military press) body building. Several of these patients had a significant kyphotic deformity.

Greene et al. presented 19 adolescent patients with mechanical-type back pain and vertebral changes consisting of intervertebral disk herniation, disk space narrowing, and minimal wedge deformity.[624] Most of the symptoms and signs were located at the thoracolumbar junction, and a specific strenuous activity or traumatic event was clearly associated with the onset of symptoms in 16 of the 19 patients. Despite the thoracic involvement, none of these patients had a progressive kyphotic deformity. A number of authors have noted that juvenile kyphosis was more often associated with hard physical labor or weight lifting before 16 years of age, similar to that initially reported by Scheuermann.[620,622,632,633] Micheli found similar lumbar changes in young rowers and suggested that the etiology was stress injury to the vertebral growth plates, which is a more realistic etiology.[627] Others have supported this concept.[623,626,635]

The concomitant presence of spondylolysis and spondylolisthesis in many patients supports the contention that abnormal stresses were applied to the spine (thoracolumbar and lumbar) in Scheuermann's disease.[624] Further support for this being a stress-related, potentially reversible phenomenon is the reconstitution of vertebral height following the initiation of treatment.

Treatment should be symptomatic for mild deformity. A hyperextension brace should be used for more severe deformation.[628] Surgery is sometimes necessary.

Injury to the Thoracolumbar Junction (T12–L1)

The thoracolumbar junction is a major motion segment during flexion and extension. The ligamentous laxity of the child increases susceptibility to facet displacement

Specific Injuries

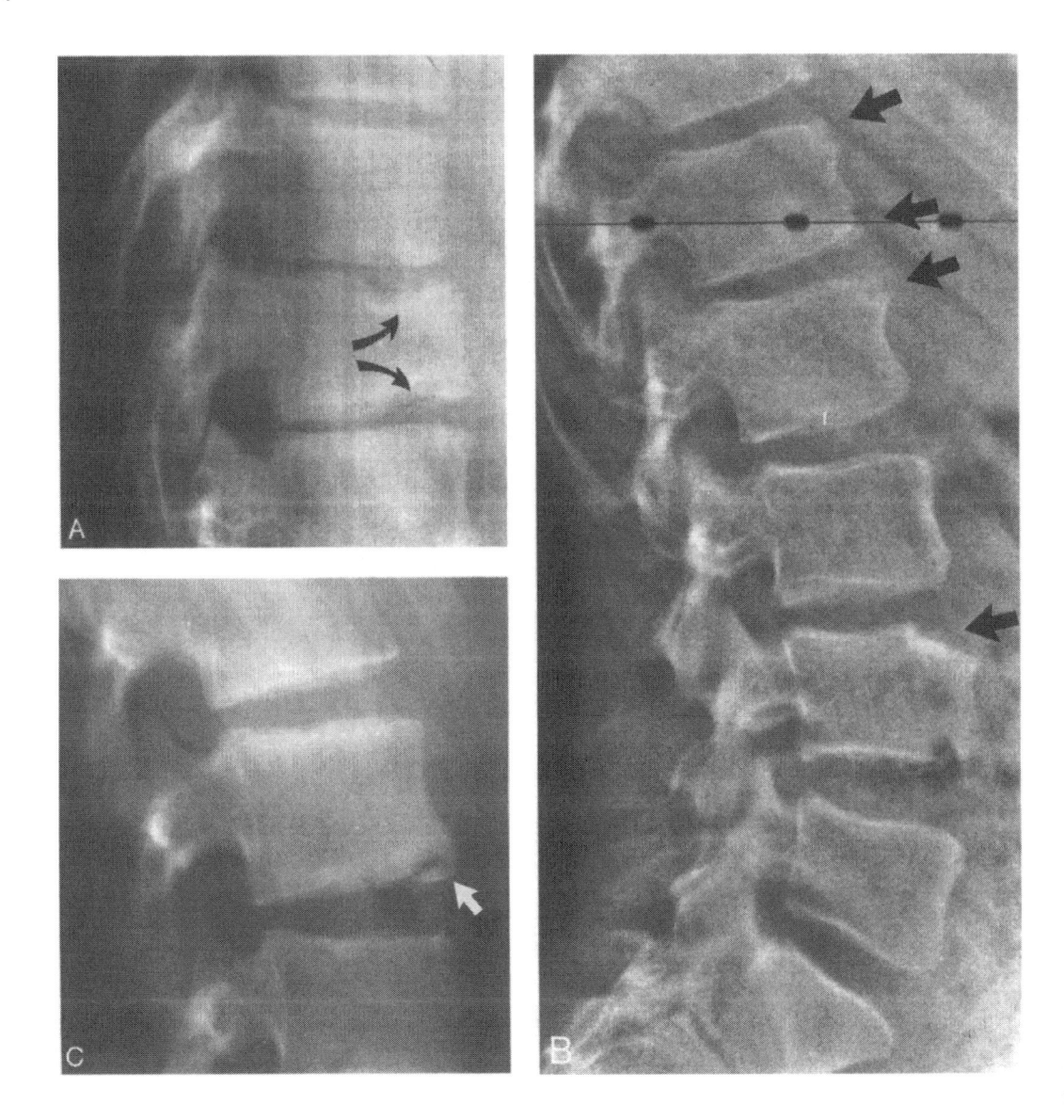

FIGURE 18-71. (A) Scheuermann's disease of vertebral end-plates (arrows). (B) Deformity of multiple levels (arrows), especially L3. (C) Healing Scheuermann's lesion (arrow) during hyperextension brace treatment.

(Figs. 18-72, 18-73), which may occur in the absence of fracture or spinal cord injury. These children should be carefully assessed for stability and then treated with spica cast immobilization. If there is cord damage, early posterior fusion may be indicated.

Injuries secondary to flexion-rotation result in classic fracture-dislocations of the thoracolumbar spine. Anteroposterior and lateral roentgenograms reveal fractures of the articular processes (i.e., facet injuries), a lateral shift of the spinous process, increased interspinous distance, and forward displacement of the superior vertebral fragment. Fusion is usually necessary.

Careful neurologic evaluation determines the presence of spinal cord or nerve root injury. Because the end of the spinal cord lies opposite the lower border of the first lumbar vertebra; fractures below this level may cause only nerve root, rather than specific cord, injury. With fractures at the thoracolumbar region, however, special attention is needed to determine whether complete or incomplete division of the spinal cord, with or without nerve root involvement, has occurred. Complete loss of voluntary power and loss of sensation in all areas supplied by the sacral segments, in association with a bulbocavernosus or anal skin reflex, usually indicates a complete injury of the spinal cord.

Fracture-dislocations at the thoracolumbar junction are frequently unstable. Early fusion is the treatment of choice in these cases. Whether early operative decompression has any role in the treatment of spinal cord or nerve root injuries believed to be complete at impact remains controversial. Operative decompression is indicated when there is a progressive neurologic deficit associated with partial spinal cord or nerve root injury.

Chance Fracture

Chance described a horizontal shearing fracture, principally in adults, in which a relative anterior displacement of the superior vertebral fragment is common.[641] Typically, the

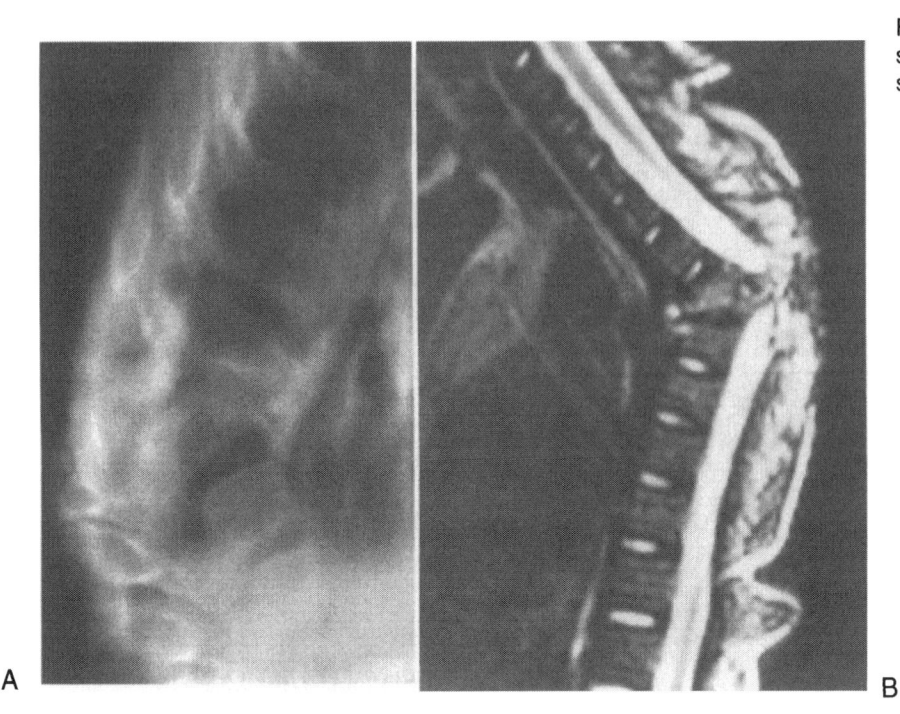

FIGURE 18-72. (A) Flexion injury of the thoracic spine in a 10-year-old boy. (B) Complete transection of the spinal cord.

injury in children involves the twelfth thoracic and first to third lumbar vertebrae (Figs. 18-74 to 18-76).[636,637,644,646,659,664]

The history and physical examination do not vary significantly from those of patients with flexion-rotation injuries, with one exception: abdominal contusion caused by a seat belt, which may lead to a temporary paralytic ileus or other intraabdominal injuries.[640,647,649,650,654,655,658,660,662,668] These particular lumbar injuries may be associated with lap seat belts,[639,642,643,645,648,650,651,653,656–658,660,665–667,669–672] with tension stress primarily responsible for the injury. Because the fractures are characterized by disruption of the posterior and anterior elements, they are potentially unstable. Injuries secondary to tension result in longitudinal separation of the posterior elements. Minimal if any anterior compression of the involved vertebral body may occur in children. Voss et al. reported three children with Chance fractures from the same accident.[671] All three had a different anatomic variant. One was rendered paraplegic.

Neurologic injury appears to be infrequent in children with this injury. Winter and Jani reported a child who presented with total paraplegia after a hyperflexion injury due to a seat belt.[672] The child subsequently had a complete return of neurologic function.

Of 33 reported cases of Chance fracture in one study, only 8 occurred in adolescents and 1 in a young child.[638] The child, a 6-year-old, was treated with a body cast; at 7 months after

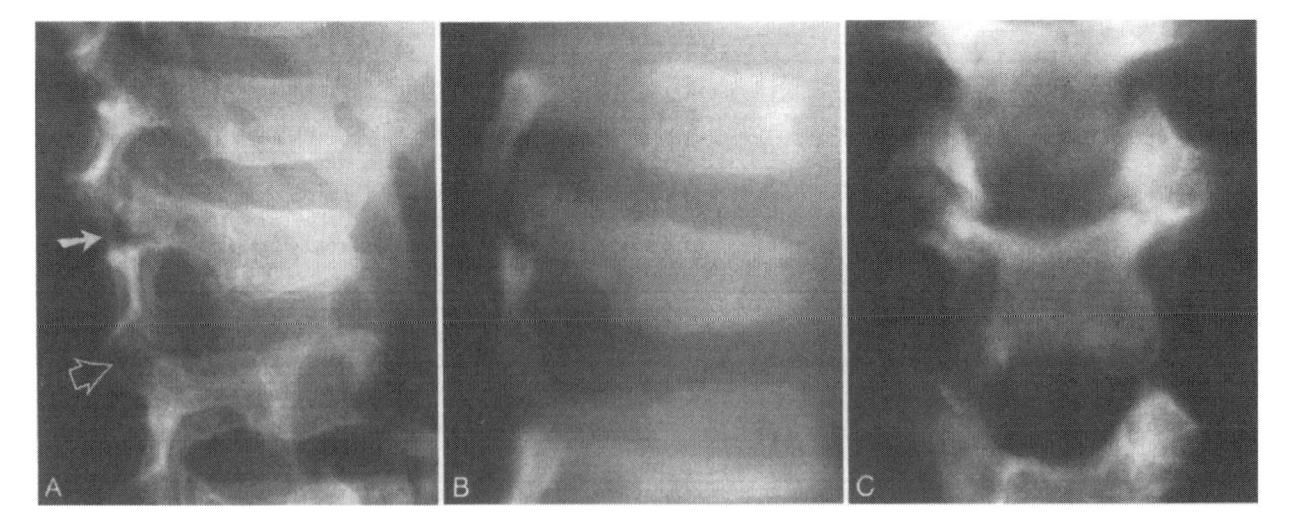

FIGURE 18-73. (A) Hyperflexion injury in a 4-year-old. T12 is anteriorly crushed; but more important, it has a posterior (pedicle) fracture as well as facet disruption and probable fracture. (B) Lateral tomogram shows the fracture and dislocation. (C) Anterior tomogram accentuates the disruption of both facet joints.

Specific Injuries

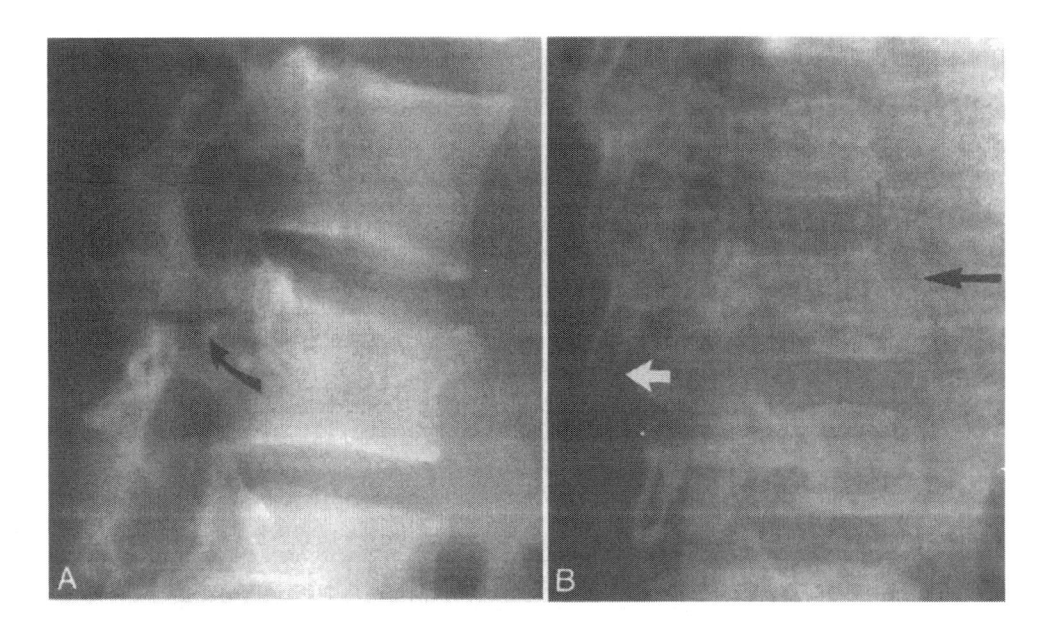

FIGURE 18-74. (A) Moderate crush of L3, with posterior extension (arrow). It is a variation of a Chance fracture. (B) Posteriorly displaced Chance fracture (arrows) in a 5-year-old child.

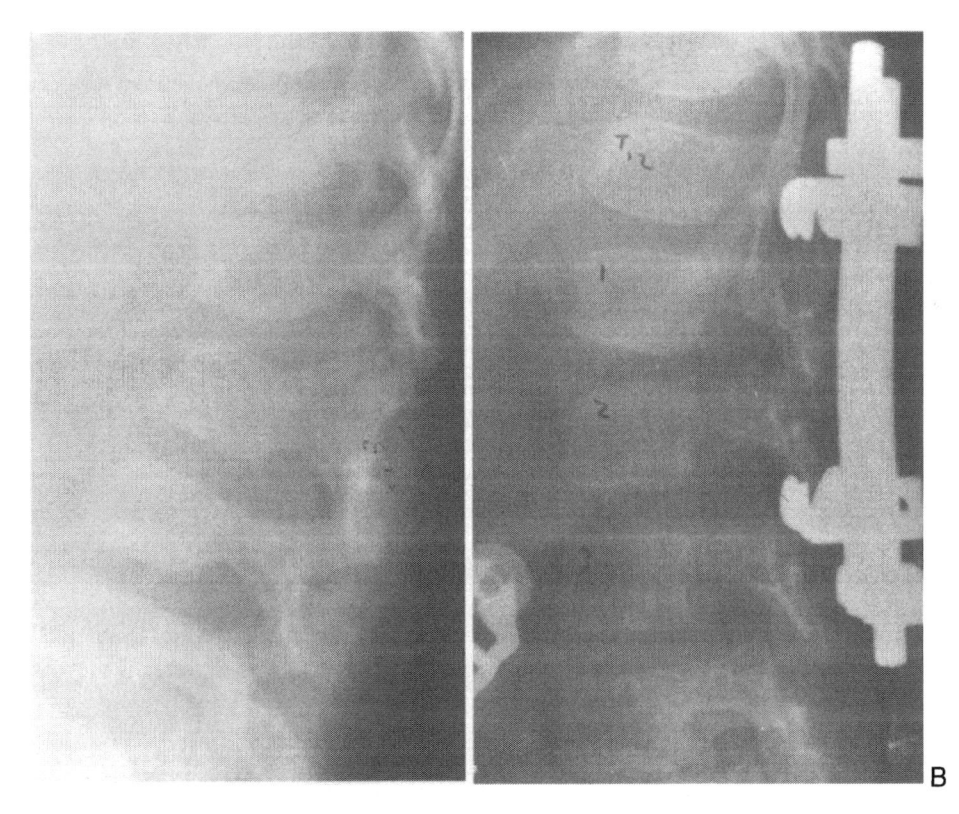

FIGURE 18-75. (A) This lateral film showing a Chance fracture variant (T12–L1) was not obtained until 5 days after injury. The child had already undergone laparoscopy and laparotomy. He was neurologically intact. (B) Limited fusion and stabilization was undertaken.

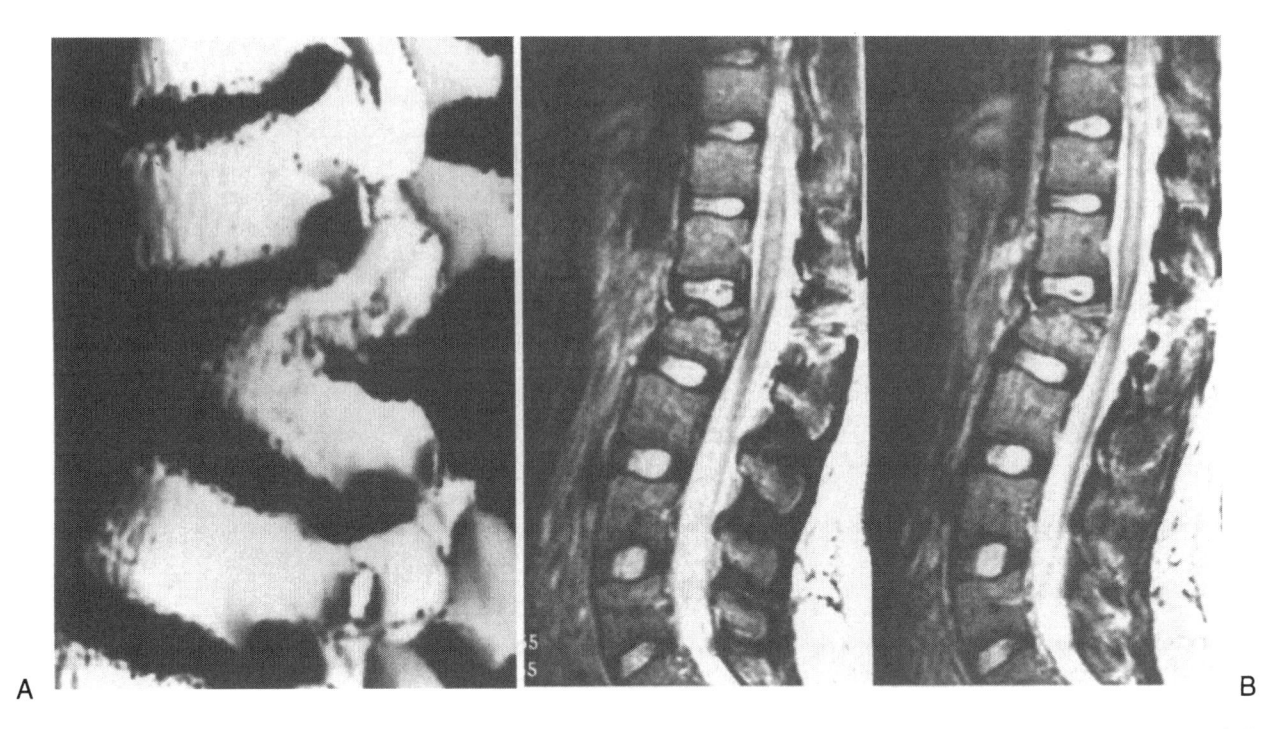

FIGURE 18-76. (A) CT three-dimensional reconstruction of a Chance fracture in a 13-year-old girl. (B) MRI showing posterior soft tissue disruption.

injury there was complete healing of the lumbar spine, full range of motion, no evidence of instability in flexion or extension, and no neurologic problems. It is interesting that this case involved L4, whereas all other reported Chance fractures involved L3 or above.[768] Only Ritchie and colleagues[661] and Rogers et al.[663] have reported other young patients, between 10 and 14 years of age. An analogue of the Chance fracture is a perched facet injury (see Fig. 18-73).

When the vertebral end-plate and growth mechanism are involved, a progressive kyphotic deformity may ensue. It may require surgical stabilization (Fig. 18-77).[652]

Injury to the Lumbar Spine

The lumbar region is infrequently involved in significant injury until the adolescent period, when the maturing spine assumes more of the biomechanical characteristics of the adult spine.[673,678,680,681] Minor and moderate wedge fractures may be seen at all levels (Figs. 18-78 to 18-80). The region is capable of significant translation with a fracture-dislocation, thus increasing the likelihood of spinal cord or, especially, nerve root injury.[691] Physeal (end-plate) fractures may involve the lumbar spine during adolescence. Such injuries may lead to disruption of the interspace with progressive fusion of the vertebrae (Fig. 18-81). Multiple lumbar fractures are not uncommon, and MRI may be required to detect occult lesions.[686]

Glass et al. assessed 35 children with lumbar spine injuries.[684] Most of them (27 of 35, 77%) were restrained by a lap-style safety belt. Abnormalities were not detected with thick-section CT scans in 20 (57%) of the cases. Lumbar spine radiographs must also be obtained in such cases.

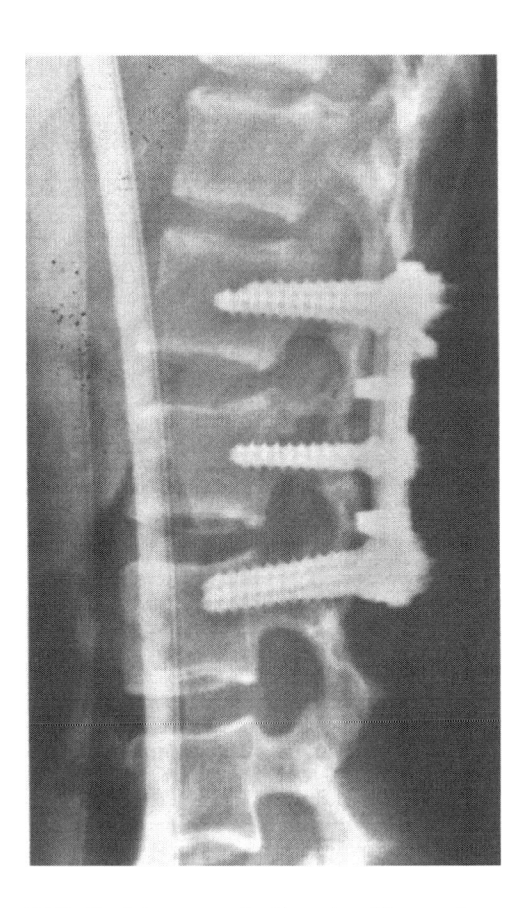

FIGURE 18-77. Pedicle screw fixation of a Chance fracture in a 14-year-old boy.

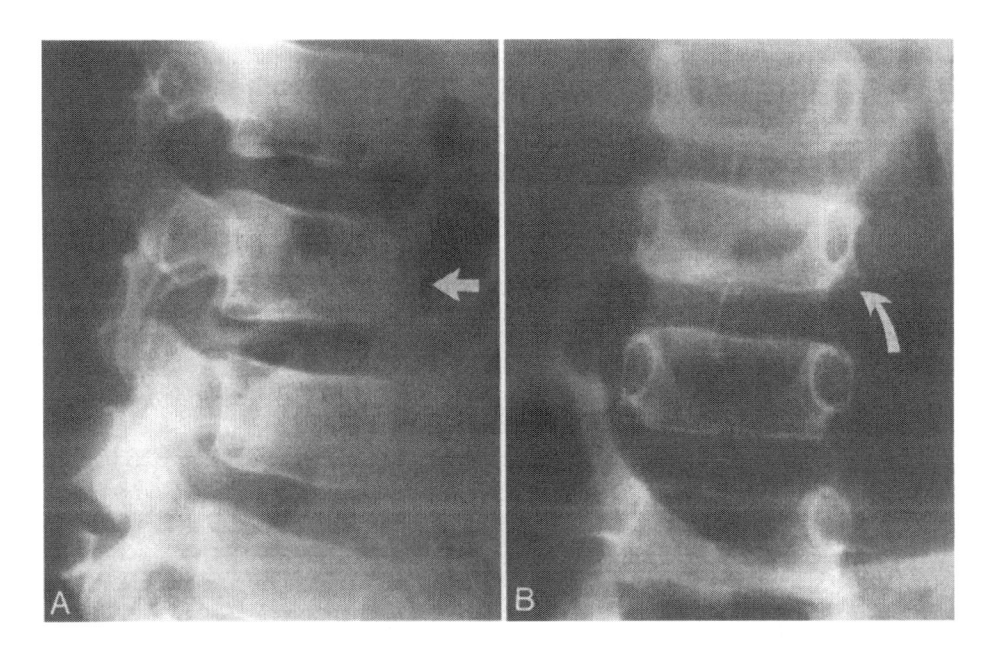

FIGURE 18-78. (A) Lateral view of a mild compression fracture of L2 (arrow). (B) Anteroposterior view showing asymmetric crush (arrow). This injury may lead to asymmetric growth and scoliosis.

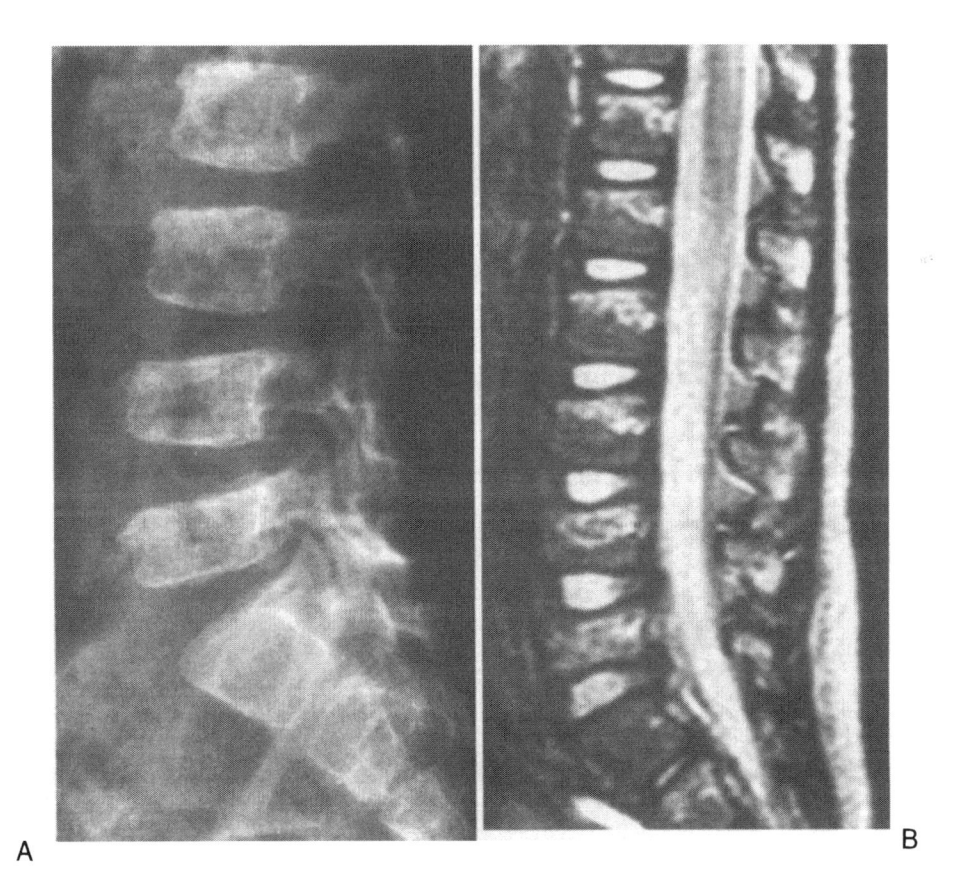

FIGURE 18-79. This 3-year-old girl climbed on the front of a family entertainment center, which fell forward, causing a hyperflexion injury. (A) Multiple lumbar fractures are evident. (B) Focal edema on the T2-weighted MRI scan suggested multiple vertebral involvement. Four years later she has had virtually no change in the shapes of L4 and L5 vertebral bodies.

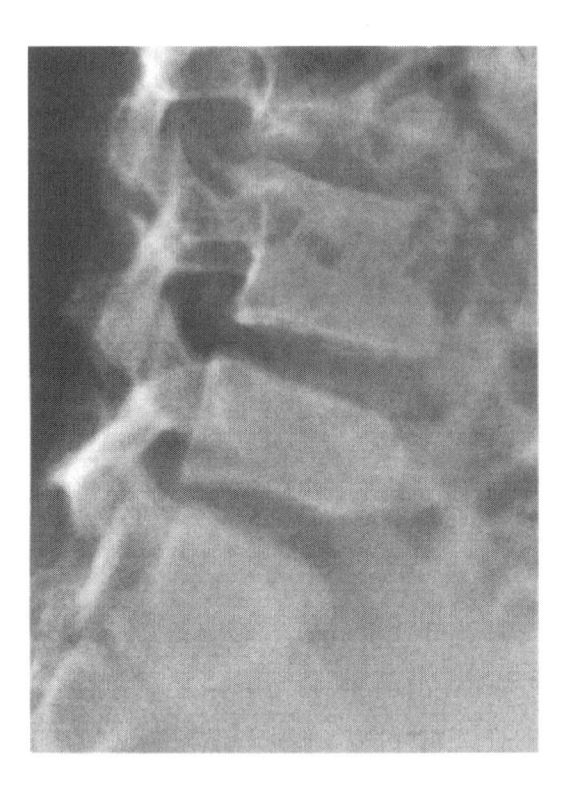

FIGURE 18-80. Compression fracture of L5 in a lap seat-belted 8-year-old girl. Her aorta was also transected. This seemingly innocuous fracture was associatd with complete paraplegia.

Burst fractures may occur in the lumbar area (Figs. 18-82, 18-83). The mechanism of injury is a compression force transmitted directly along the line of the vertebral bodies. One of the end-plates ruptures, and the disk is forced into the body of the vertebrae, causing it to burst. The posterior elements often remain intact. A fragment of the vertebral body or disk extending posteriorly, compromising the spinal canal, may cause neurologic damage.

Children who sustain burst fractures at or before puberty tend to develop mild progressive angular deformity at the site of the fracture if not surgically stabilized. Operative treatment achieves and maintains correction of the deformity, Nonoperative treatment of a burst fracture is a viable option in neurologically intact children, but bony deformity (scoliosis, kyphosis and body collapse) may occur. Residual deformity following operative and nonoperative management does not correlate with symptoms or function at follow-up.

Chatani et al. described a 16-year-old boy who had been in a motor vehicle accident.[679] The vertebral body of L4 was displaced anteriorly in front of L5; and the posterior elements of L3 and L4 were split away from their respective vertebral bodies and remained posteriorly.

Variations in developmental anatomy of the lumbosacral junction may predispose to soft tissue and osseous injury that may be associated with severe back pain.[674,675,682,692,695,696] Some of the pain may be due to disk herniation at the level of the radiologic variant or just above it.[675,696]

Acute pedicle fractures may occur[685,690,694] They are usually chronic in nature and represent stress fractures due to repetitive athletic activities.

Isolated fractures that involve the neural arch, facet, or transverse process account for the remainder of stable injuries.[689,690,693] The most common mechanism of injury is a direct blow. Facet and neural arch fractures are treated best with an external support until evidence of healing is obtained by clinical and radiographic evaluation. With fractures of the transverse process, external support may or may not be used, depending on the patient's discomfort with activity.

Postural reduction is the best initial treatment. Pillows, sandbags, pelvic slings, and various traction techniques may be used, depending on the availability of equipment and the type of fracture.

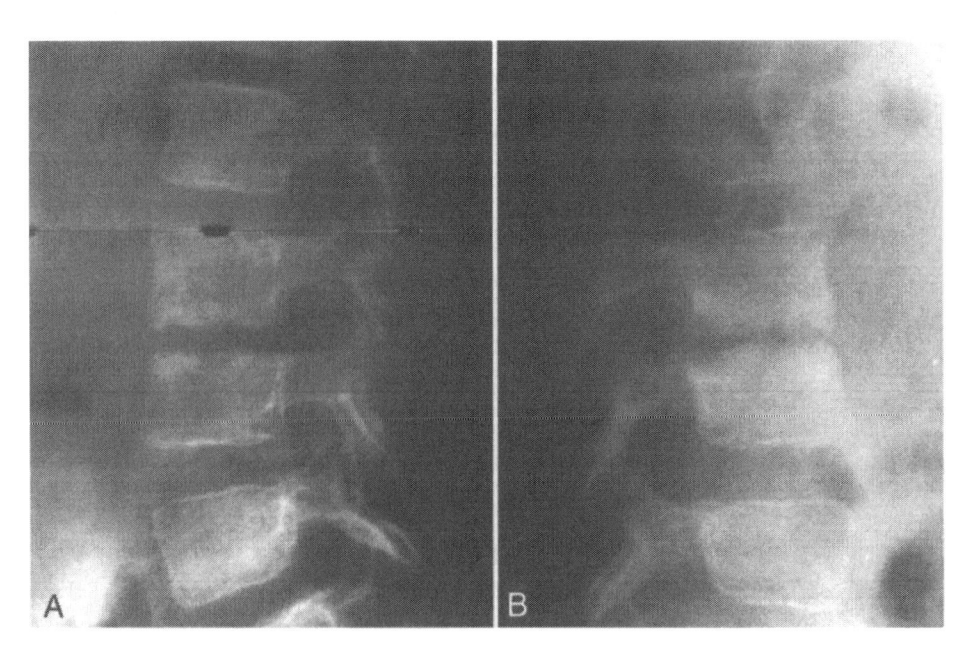

FIGURE 18-81. (A) Irregular end-plates 7 months after hyperflexion injury. (B) Progressive narrowing 18 months after the injury. It should not be confused with diskitis.

Specific Injuries

manipulation with or without the administration of anesthesia is indicated. If the fracture remains unreduced following manipulation, open reduction should be considered.

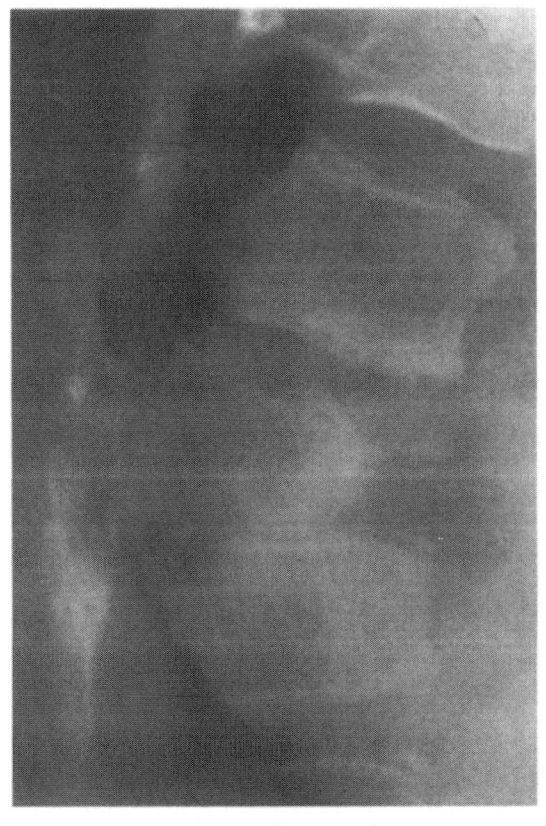

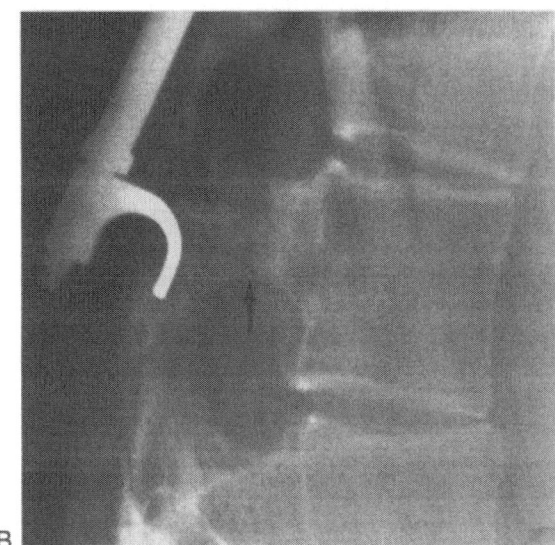

FIGURE 18-82. (A) Burst fracture with retropulsion of T12. (B) During placement of the inferior hook and reduction a pedicle fracture became evident. It may have been partial failure of the bone due to the accident that was worsened by the procedure. The hook was inserted at a lower level.

The effect of this initial treatment on the injury must be carefully and frequently assessed by neurologic and radiographic examination. The CT scan may be helpful for predicting neurologic deficits.[683] Changes are made in the patient's posture until reduction is achieved. If reduction of the fracture is not adequate by postural methods, gentle

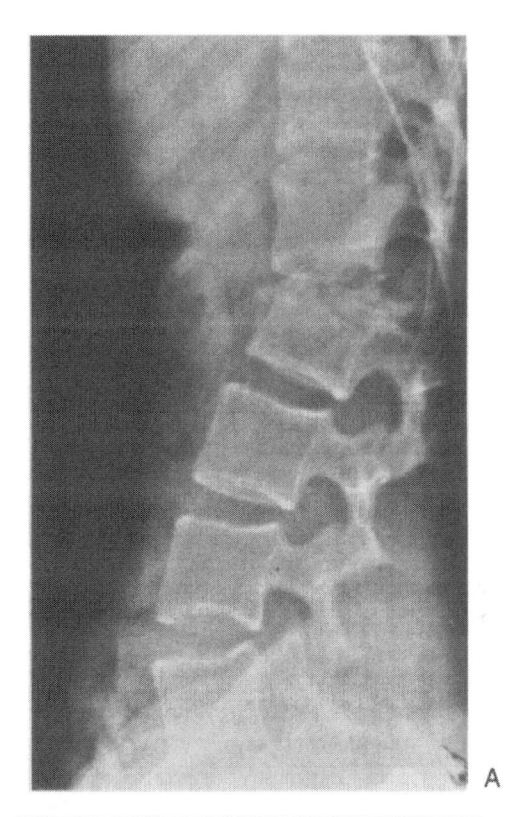

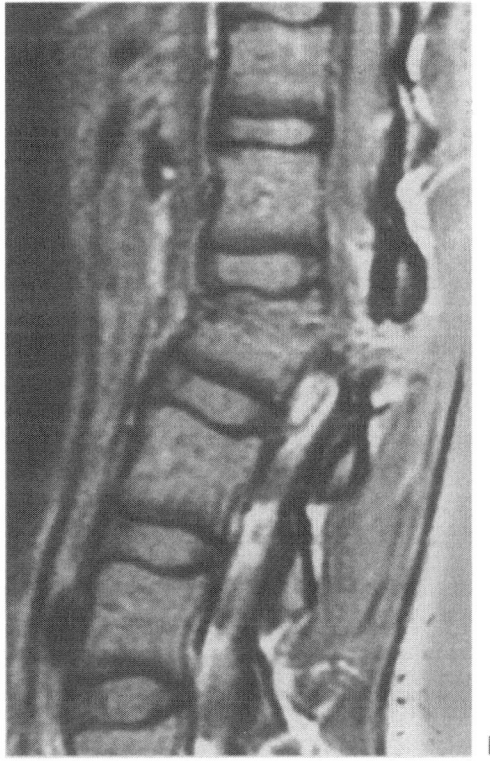

FIGURE 18-83. (A) Flexion injury of L1 in a 14-year-old girl. (B) MRI showing retropulsion and cord/root injury.

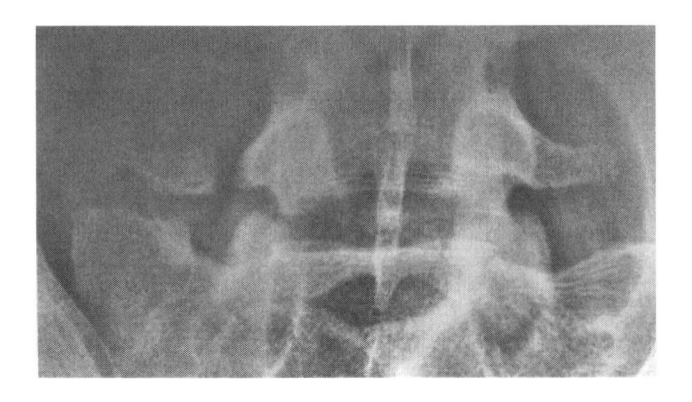

FIGURE 18-84. Nonunion of a lumbar transverse process fracture.

Patients with minimal or no neurologic injury can usually be fitted with external supports and allowed to ambulate if acceptable reduction has been maintained for a period of 3–6 weeks. Paravertebral callus, when seen on roentgenographic examination, is helpful for determining the stability of the fracture and the time when external supports may be discontinued. Most fractures become intrinsically stable by 12 weeks; flexion and extension films should be obtained at such time to determine soft tissue stability and any motion within the fracture itself.

In prepubertal children, supports should be well padded, removable, and utilized until most of the spinal growth has occurred (14 years in girls and 16 years in boys). This approach usually prevents progressive spinal deformity.

If nonoperative treatment fails because of instability or progressive spinal deformity, operative fusion is indicated.[676,687] The surgical procedure (anterior, posterior, or combined) and the type of internal fixation utilized, if any, is best determined on an individual basis. Any nerve root impingement must be decompressed at the neuroforamina. Postoperative immobilization in a spica cast that includes at least one leg is often essential. Close follow-up of possible growth deformity is necessary, particularly if the child is just entering the adolescent growth spurt.

Patients with significant residual neurologic deficit, with or without severe spinal deformity, continue to require special care to obtain maximal independence in the community. Physical findings of decreased mobility and neuromuscular abnormalities are directly proportional to the extent of the residual structural and neurologic damage.

Transverse and Spinous Process

Peripheral areas of the lumbar vertebrae may be injured. The mechanism may be a direct blow or tensile avulsion. Either may occur as an isolated injury or as part of a more extensive fracture. The spinous process has a cartilaginous cap that may be avulsed, or a fracture may occur through the osseous portion of the spine. Similarly, the transverse process may sustain an osseous or chondrosseous fracture. In either instance the injury may progress to nonunion (Fig. 18-84). Fragment excision is indicated only for severe pain.

Spondylosis

A somewhat controversial topic is whether spondylolysis has a traumatic etiology.[696,701,703,708,710,711,713,716–722,724,725,730,733,735,739–745,748] Wiltse and Jackson believe that most, if not all, patients with spondylolysis (Figs. 18-85, 18-86) have a stress fracture through the pars interarticularis.[720–723,745,748] I agree with this concept. Not every symptomatic patient has complete bilateral spondylolysis. The pars may be attenuated (plastic deformation) leading to a thin structure (Fig. 18-87). Only one side may have a defect. Sclerosis (without fracture) may occur that is probably reactive bone to subcortical failure or stress in the pars.

In one study patients with unilateral spondylolysis had reactive sclerosis and hypertrophy of the contralateral pedicle.[740] This study pointed out the importance of differ-

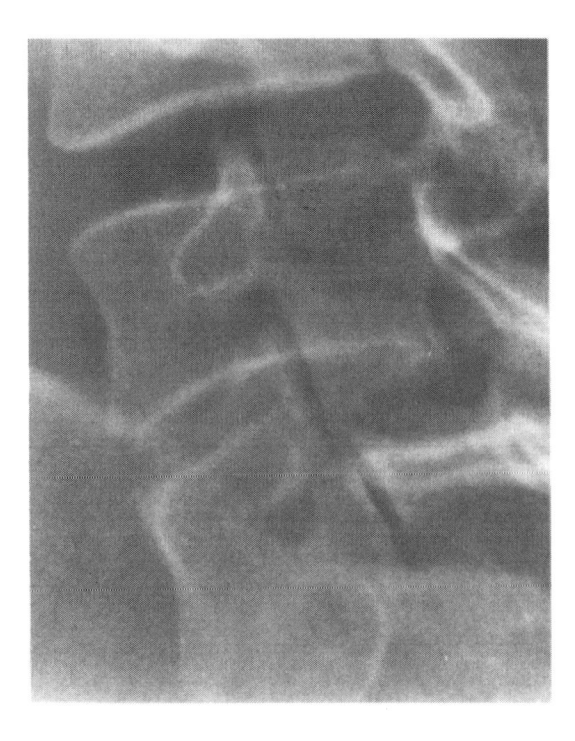

FIGURE 18-85. Spondylolysis of L5 in a gymnast.

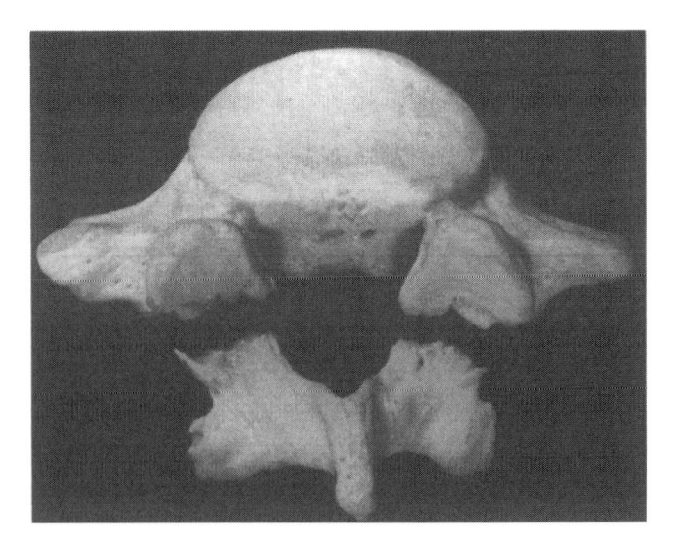

FIGURE 18-86. Bilateral spondylolysis in an anatomic specimen.

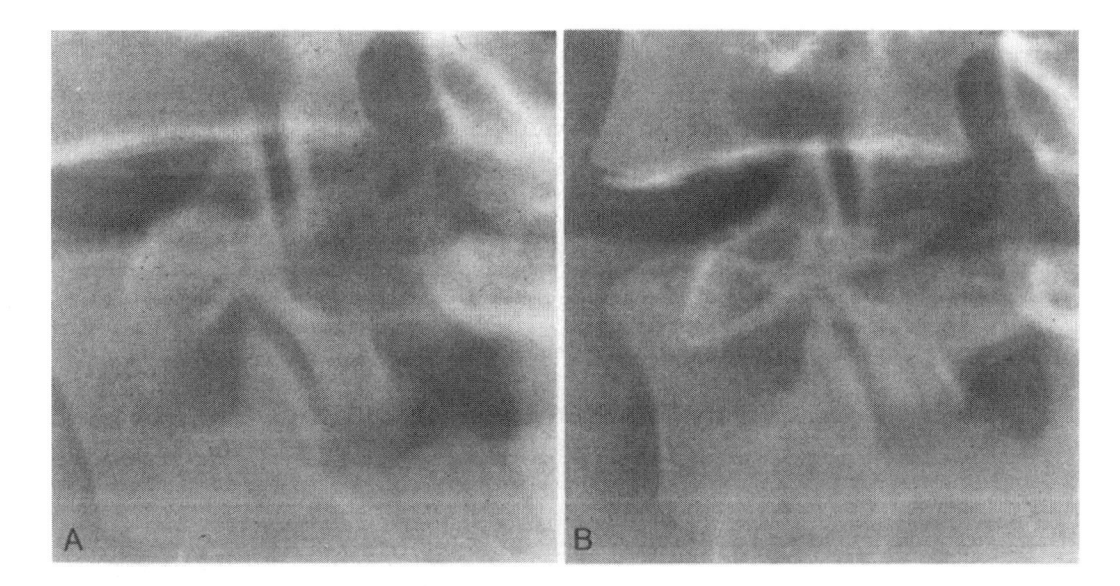

FIGURE 18-87. (A) Attenuated pars. (B) Contralateral spondylolysis.

entiating pars injuries from osteoid osteoma and, furthermore, that the unilateral hypertrophy was probably a physiologic reaction to stress from the contralateral unstable neural arch. The increased sclerosis may make this region susceptible to subsequent failure if the evocative forces continue.[704–706,712,727,738]

Miyake et al. analyzed facet orientation in the lumbar spine in 144 boys without pars defects and 104 boys with pars defects.[732] They found no difference in growth in the two groups up to 13 years of age. After that age, however, the growth of the facet joints in patients with a pars defect was significantly retarded. Miyake et al. thought that the facet changes were due to altered development as the defect developed and were *not* the cause of the defect.

There is a potential inability of the posterior elements of the lower lumbosacral vertebrae to respond appropriately to stress, leading to fracture of the pars interarticularis in adolescent athletes.[714,723,726,728] Repetitive training and competition exercises involving flexion-extension of the lumbar spine stress this region. In vitro cyclic stress loading easily produced fractures of the pars interarticularis after approximately 1500 cycles of applied force involving a vertebral column taken from a 14-year-old child.[716,717]

Jackson et al. described the condition in young athletes (adolescents).[721] In a study of 100 female gymnasts, 11 had radiologically evident spondylolysis, 6 of whom also had at least a grade 1 spondylolisthesis (Fig. 18-88).[702] Of the 89 without radiologic disease, 19 had episodic lumbar pain. Low back pain in any young athlete should be a warning sign.[697,698,707,737]

A routine lumbosacral spine series, which should include oblique views, does not necessarily rule out a developing pars defect. A technetium bone scan is a valuable tool for diagnosing these lesions.[736] In unusual circumstances of chronic pain and a negative bone scan, a single-photon emission computed tomography (SPECT) scan may delineate the presence and level of injury.[697,699] CT scans may also be beneficial.[729]

Restriction of vigorous athletic activity is essential until the lesion has healed.[707,715,746] Use of a brace may alleviate symptoms.[723,731] In the study by Letts and colleagues, the lesion was bilateral in 4 patients and unilateral in 10.[730] Five of the unilateral lesions healed with immobilization in a thoracolumbar orthosis. In none of the patients with bilateral lesions or the other five unilateral lesions did healing take place, despite 3 months of similar immobilization.

Spondylolisthesis

When failure (spondylolysis) has involved both sides, the risk of a progressive spondylolisthesis then arises (Figs. 18-89,

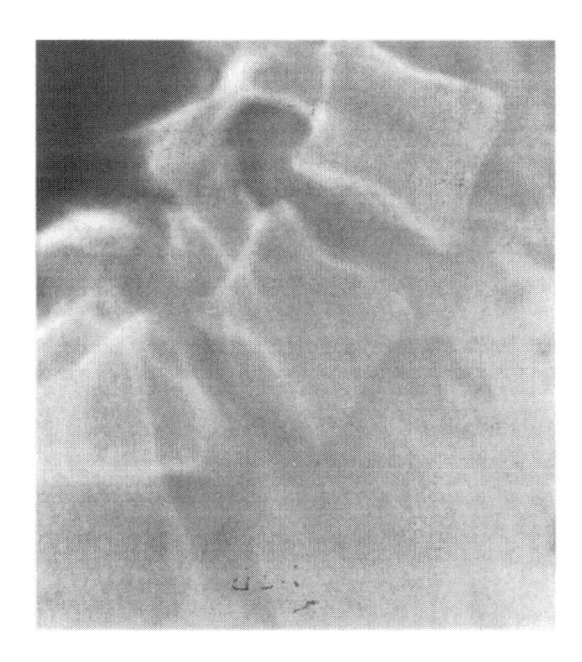

FIGURE 18-88. Traumatic spondylolisthesis in an adolescent gymnast. Bilateral spondylolysis is also present.

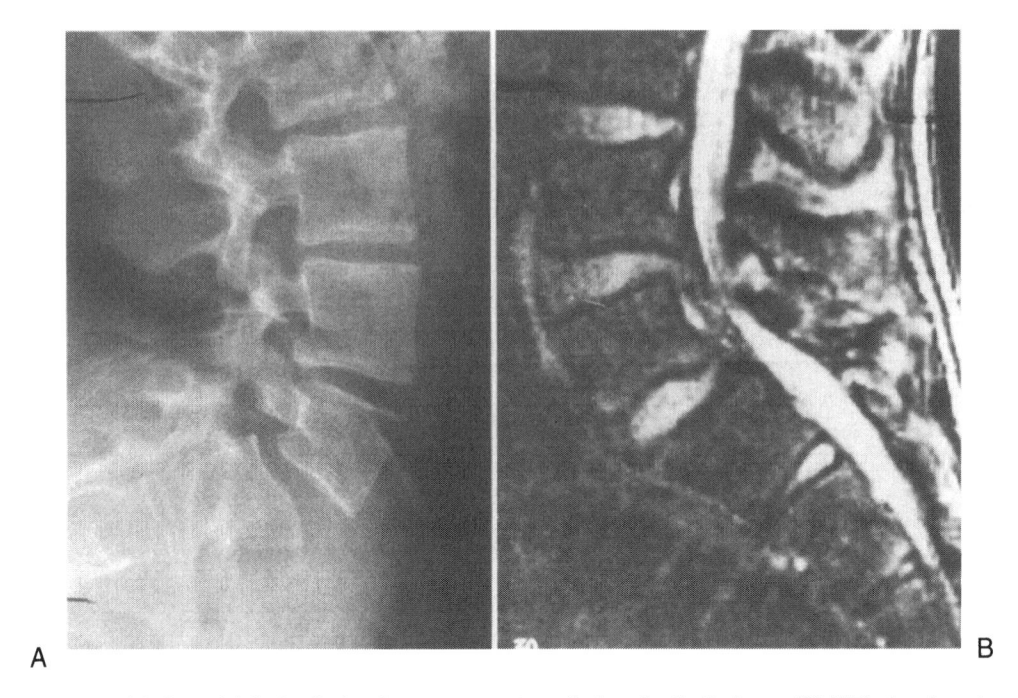

FIGURE 18-89. (A) Spondylolisthesis that became symptomatic in a football player. (B) MRI showing stenosis.

18-90), especially if the evocative activity (e.g., gymnastics) is continued.[702,709,734,747] This posttraumatic spondylolysis/spondylolisthesis progression tends to be painful, in contrast to congenital spondylolisthesis. Spondylolisthesis has also been reported on the newborn, although a difficult delivery could not have been considered the cause.[700]

Stress Fractures

Other areas may sustain stress fractures without developing spondylolysis. Unilateral stress fracture may occur in the pedicle (Fig. 18-91). Another variation is a stress fracture in the pedicle with a laminar fracture on the opposite side.

Lumbar Apophyseal Injury

Avulsion of the posterior portion of the lumbar end-plate (apophysis) is being increasingly recognized as a cause of low back pain in adolescents (Figs. 18-92 to 18-96).[749–795] The apophyseal lesion represents a type 3 or type 4 growth mechanism injury in which a portion of the disk and ring apophysis, with or without an accompanying "metaphyseal" fragment, is displaced posteriorly into the spinal canal (Fig. 18-95). This fragment then variably impinges on the lumbosacral roots.

Because of the association of the injury with sports such as gymnastics and weight lifting, attention is often directed

FIGURE 18-90. Traumatic spondylolisthesis in a 10-year-old following a tobogganing injury.

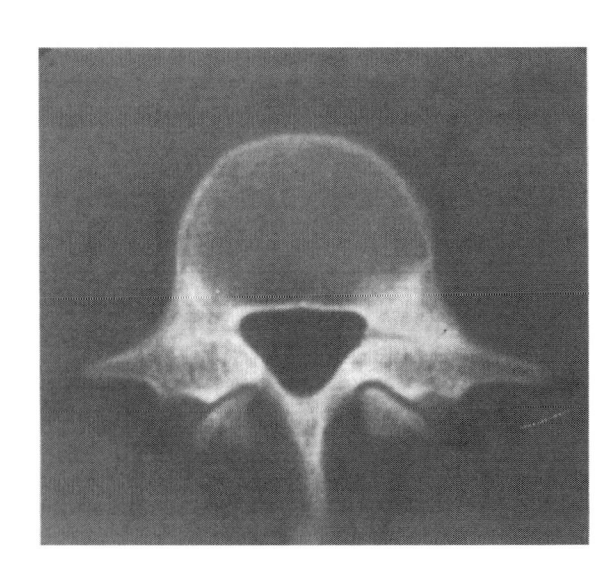

FIGURE 18-91. Pedicle stress fracture.

FIGURE 18-92. (A) Posterior epiphyseal injury that may mimic disk herniation. It is a type 3 or type 4 growth mechanism injury of the inferior end-plate. (B) Appearance of undisplaced posteroinferior ossification (arrow).

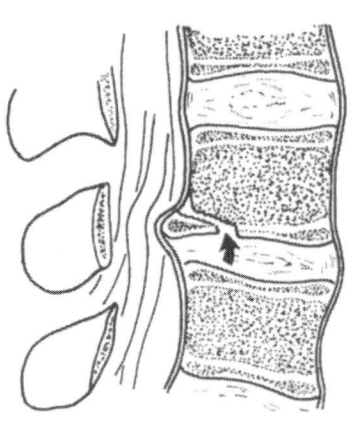

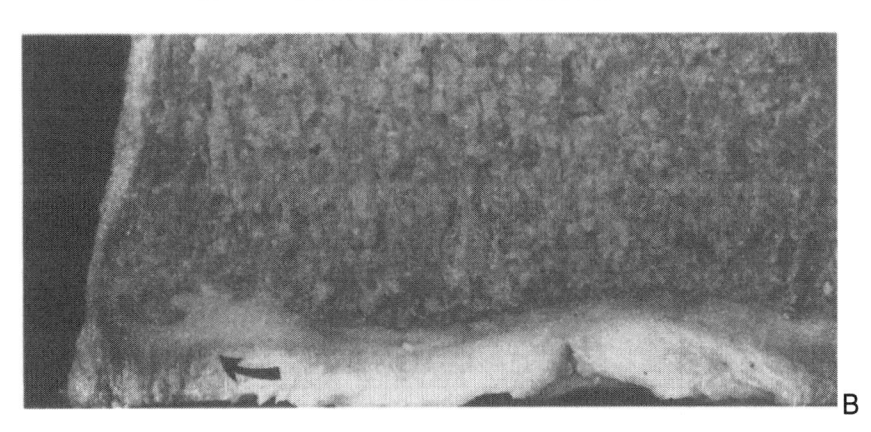

to more common causes of pain (e.g., Scheuermann's disease), which may precede or coexist with an avulsed fragment (Fig. 18-93). The uniform complaint is back pain. It is rarely accompanied by associated sensory or motor loss.

Ikata et al. reviewed 37 patients under 18 years of age who had lesions of the lumbar posterior end-plate.[767] All but one were active in sports, and most were seen for back pain. Abnormalities were most frequent at the inferior rim of L4 and the superior rim of the sacrum. Adjacent intervertebral disks showed a decrease in signal intensity. Ikata et al. thought that the posterior end-plate lesion should be regarded as a vertebral nonarticular osteochondrosis.

When there is a fracture of the lumbar vertebral apophysis, CT scanning is the ideal diagnostic test (Fig. 18-94), as it is sometimes difficult to see the osseous portion on a lateral film. The CT scan shows the size of the fragment and the extent of canal compromise. Experimental end-plate fractures are extremely difficult to visualize.

Surgical excision is recommended. Otherwise, the displaced lesion may heal to the vertebral body, effectively narrowing the spinal canal by causing spinal stenosis (Fig. 18-96).

A usual version of an apophyseal/synchondrosis injury is shown in Figure 18-97. The vertebral centrum may be rotated away from the superior end-plate and the neurocentral synchondroses.[73,677] This is also illustrated in a primate "child abuse" case (Fig. 18-30), and a cervical injury (Fig. 18-65). This injury pattern may be more frequent than we realize because of the diagnostic difficulty.

Disk Herniation

Acutely herniated disks are unusual in children under 16 years of age (Fig. 18-98). Fewer than 200 disk protrusions have been reported in patients 16 years of age or younger.[796-838] Trauma appears to play an important etiologic role in lumbar disk herniation in the child or adolescent. Such trauma may result from contact sports, a fall, or an automobile-related injury. Noncontact sports such as weight lifting have also been implicated. There may be an accompanying fracture of a portion of the vertebral end-plate because of the dense attachments of the annulus, and this structure (rather than the disk) may be the cause of any block.

It is uncommon for children with lumbar disk (or end-plate) protrusions to have the usual signs and symptoms associated with comparable adult disk herniation. Low back pain, limitation of motion on forward flexion, a peculiar gait, and limitation of straight-leg raising are common signs. Pain is not a prominent complaint. Neurologic findings are rare. The physician should be aware of congenital deformities of the posterior elements.

A delay in diagnosis often occurs because many of these patients have pain in the lower limb, rather than in the back. In one study discrete clinical neurologic changes were found in only 19 of 55 patients.[823] This low incidence of nerve root compression is in agreement with the findings of other reports and probably represents (1) significant resistance of maturing neurologic tissue to nerve root compression and (2) the lack of chronic impingement through osteophyte

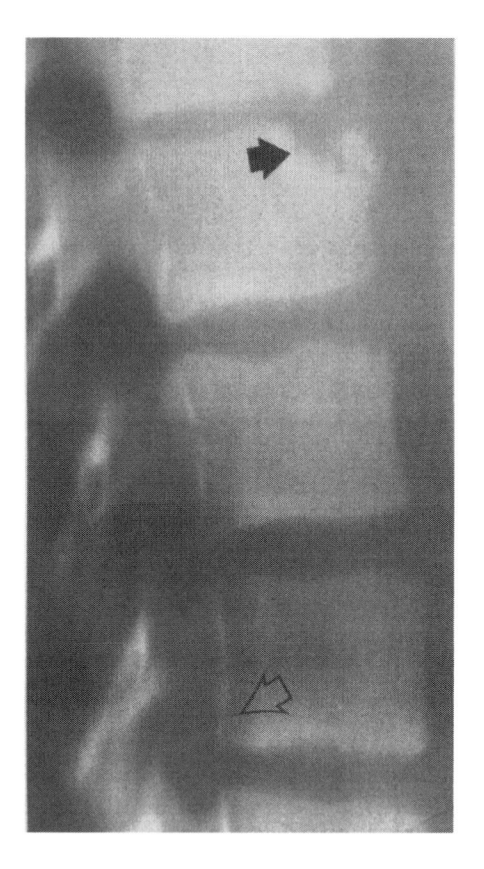

FIGURE 18-93. Attention to a Scheuermann's lesion (solid arrow) led to the diagnosis of this lesion as the cause of back pain. The real cause was a displaced end-plate fracture (open arrow) in this teenage weight lifter.

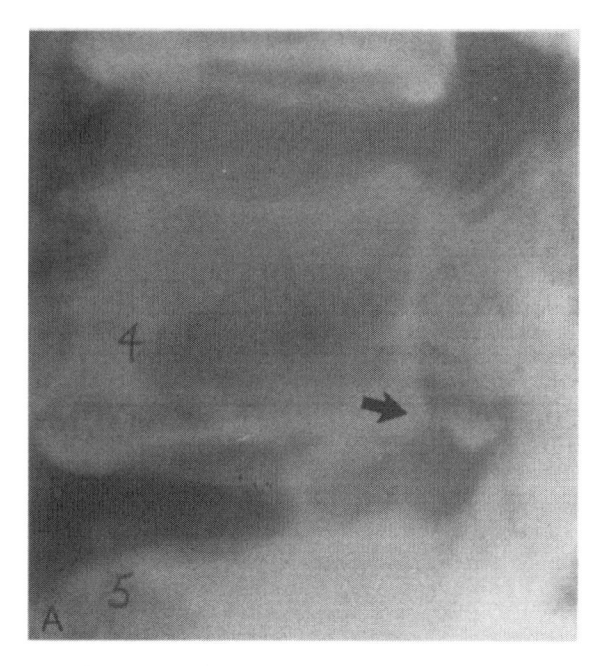

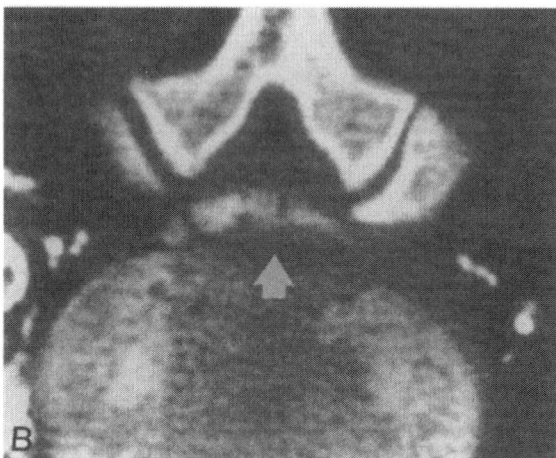

FIGURE 18-94. (A) Displaced end-plate fragment (arrow). (B) CT scan of the injury (arrow).

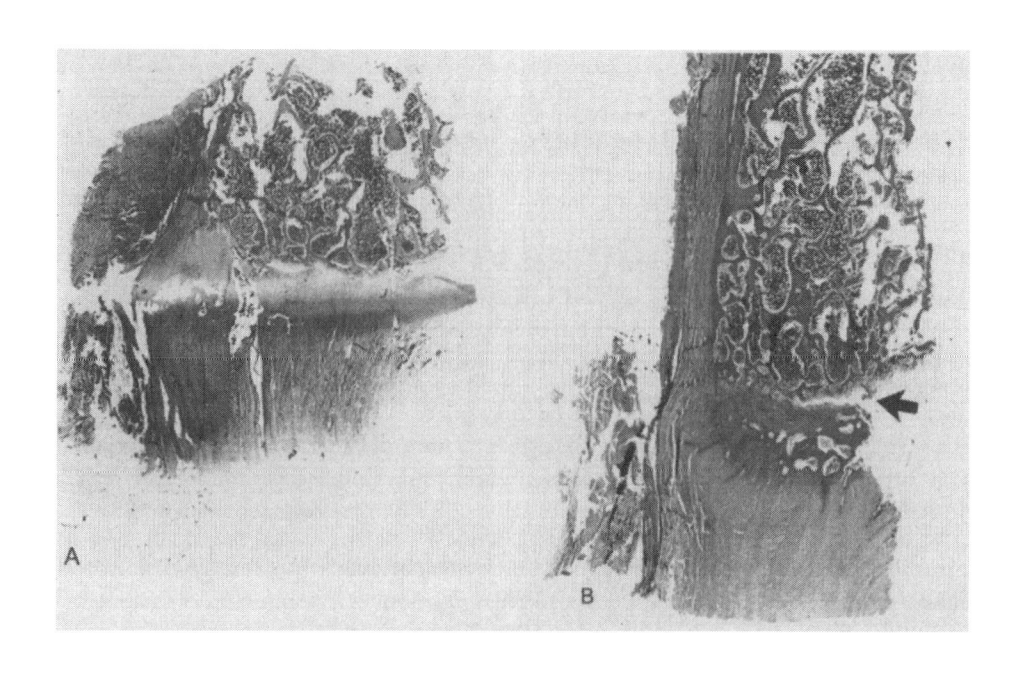

FIGURE 18-95. (A, B) Histopathology of end-plate avulsions surgically excised. (B) Note that the physeal separation (arrow) extends into the fragment.

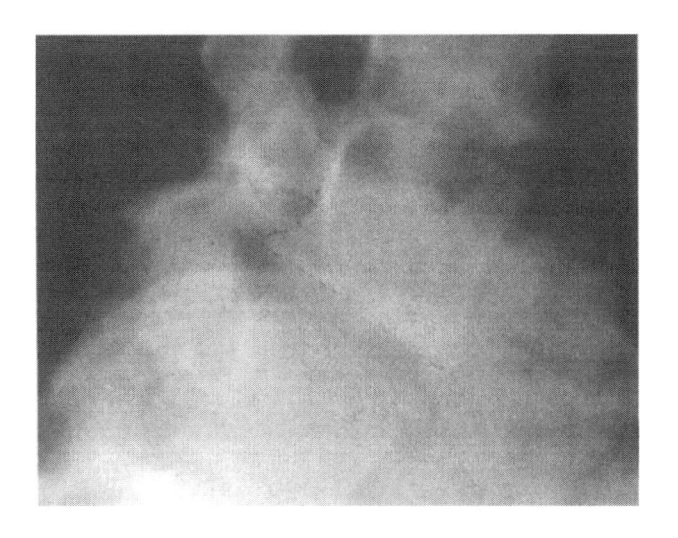

FIGURE 18-96. Lateral view of 24-year-old football player/weight lifter with chronic back pain since adolescence. The posteriorly displaced end-plate healed in its canal position, causing stenosis.

formation in addition to the disk material. Secondary changes in the nerve, over time, may predispose it to greater reaction to acute injury.

Magnetic resonance imaging may be utilized to evaluate adolescent disk herniation (Fig. 18-98). Gibson and associates noted that 15 of their 20 patients had multiple disk abnormalities, which suggested that there was an underlying diasthesis in those patients who developed disk herniation, a finding that is certainly compatible with progressive multiple-level involvement in adults.[811]

Lorenz and McCulloch reported the use of chemonucleolysis for herniated nucleus pulposus in adolescents, utilizing the procedure in 55 patients between the ages of 13 and 19 years.[823] The procedure was considered an alternative to diskectomy and was performed only after the patient failed to respond to previous conservative management. One patient had an anaphylactic reaction. Chemonucleolysis did *not* relieve the symptoms in 11 of the 55 patients, all of whom subsequently required surgical excision of the disk. Of the remaining 44 patients, 27 had no subsequent back pain. The other 17 had occasional backaches but did not require any specific or prolonged treatment.

Injury to the Lumbosacral Region

The regions of major motion capacity change (i.e., the thoracolumbar and lumbosacral junction) may be sites of increased susceptibility to injury, often seemingly innocuous at the onset. This is especially true at the lumbosacral junction, where anatomic variations may predispose to debilitating pain (Figs. 18-99, 18-100).

A rare injury involves facet dislocation at the L5–S1 junction.[847,853] This trauma pattern is usually associated with cervical injury but may also occur in the thoracolumbar junction and lumbar vertebrae. The cervical facet obliquity predisposes to subluxation, but the lumbar facets are more vertical. Disruption of part of the facet joints by fracture probably contributes to the injury mechanism.

Berguiristain et al. described a 5-year-old boy with a traumatic L5–S1 dislocation (traumatic spondylolisthesis).[839] No fracture was evident. Eight years later no significant deformity was evident.

Injury to the Sacrum and Coccyx

Injuries to the sacrum and coccyx are infrequent (Figs. 18-101, 18-102) and are usually produced by direct violence.[840–842,844,846,849,852] They may be difficult to recognize radiographically because of the patterns of ossification in the region.[843] Neurologic damage must be assessed carefully.[850] Treatment should be symptomatic, even if displaced.

Involvement of the sacroiliac joint is covered in detail in Chapter 19. Sacral injuries (Fig. 18-103) often accompany pelvic fractures. Regular CT views are best for visualizing them.

Stress fractures of the sacrum may also occur (Fig. 18-104).[844,845,848,851]

Spinal Cord Injury

Injury to the Spinal Cord

Injury without fracture or open injury may result in concussion, contusion, infarction of the cord, or anterior spinal cord damage.[868,870,873,874] This condition is often referred to as SCIWORA: *s*pinal *c*ord *i*njury *w*ithout *o*bvious *r*adiologic *a*bnormality.[860,867] The mechanism of injury is a matter of conjecture. Most likely a displaced type 1 injury of a cartilaginous end-plate springs back into position and heals with no or few radiographic signs (Fig. 18-105). Another possible mechanism for this particular injury of the young spine is that the excessive mobility may stretch the spinal cord over a hyperextended or hyperflexed region (even fractured but spontaneously reduced) and contuse the anterior portion of the cord (Fig. 18-106), similar to the mechanism in the more rigid spine of an adult. Children with complete paraplegia who have no radiographic signs of injuries may have associated rib fractures or a fractured spinal transverse process. Paraplegia may be spastic or flaccid. Spinal cord injury has been reported in the newborn following umbilical artery catheterization.[859]

Fewer than 5% of patients with traumatic paraplegia are children.[854–857,863,866,872,875,879,882,908,918,923] The decreased frequency of concomitant spinal cord injuries does not mean that childhood back injuries should not be taken seriously. The child's spine is more mobile than that of the adult, so force is more easily dissipated over a greater number of segments. It is interesting that cord injury without evident fracture, which is rare in adults, represents about one-fourth of all injuries in children with neurologic damage. This observation is especially evident with cord injury in the neonate and with that caused by child abuse. The efficacy of steroids in lessening the extent of injury has not been adequately assessed in children.[858] Similarly, acute laminectomy may not be particularly helpful in the child.[865]

Because of the lack of radiologic findings, it is imperative to proceed with further evaluation. MRI offers the best method for detecting occult fractures, cord injury, and hematoma.[861,869,876] MRI evaluation is also important in brain-

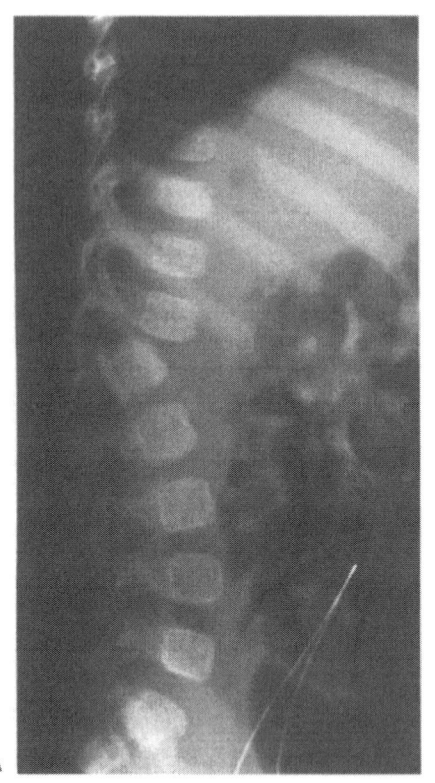

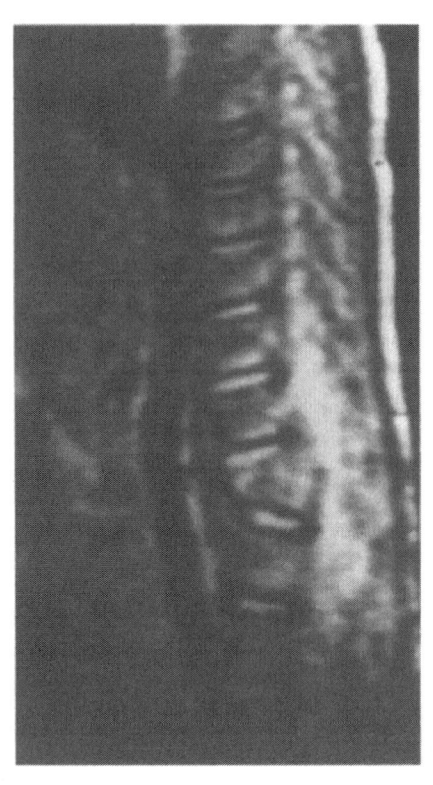

FIGURE 18-97. (A) Apparent posterior displacement of T12 posterior to T11. (B) MRI suggests an apophyseal separation. (C) CT scan shows fracturing through the neurocentral synchondroses.

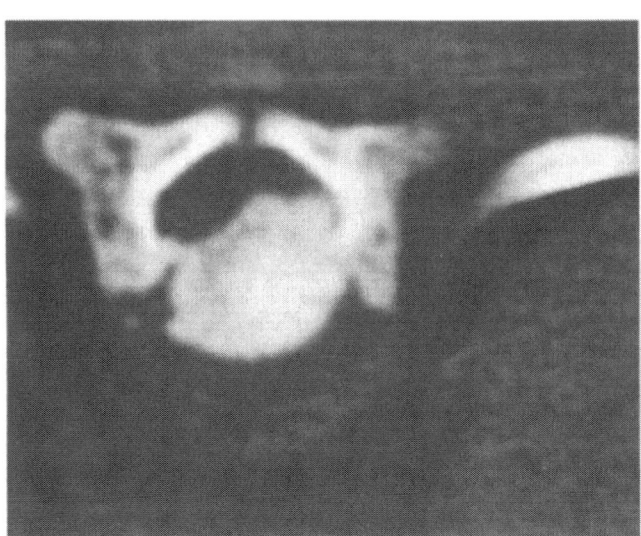

injured children.[871] Children with head trauma may also have an injured cord. The diagnosis may be difficult if not impossible by routine methods. MRI is also useful for detecting posttraumatic lesions such as spinal cord cysts.[862]

Vertebral or spinal cord damage should be suspected in any unconscious child with an injury that is likely to cause flexion or rotation of the spine, in the awake child who complains of loss of sensation or motor power below a transverse level of the body, and in any injured child who complains of localized vertebral pain or tenderness or of pain radiating along radicular distributions. Examination must be done *without* moving the possible areas of spinal column instability. Intubation in a child with a cervical spine injury is best accomplished via the nasotracheal route, and tracheostomy may be indicated if intubation cannot be accomplished without extending or manipulating the neck.

Spinal shock and the resulting loss of sympathetic vasomotor tone may complicate a general evaluation and mimic the symptoms of shock from internal bleeding.[877] Rapid restoration of normal blood pressure is essential to preserve cord function and may be accomplished by vasoconstrictors or blood volume expanders. A subsequent drop in blood pressure suggests blood loss rather than loss of vasomotor tone, and the source should be sought in the abdominal cavity, thoracic cavity, pelvis, or fracture in an extremity. Abdominal reflexes may be absent, and guarding or complaints of abdominal pain may not occur in the patient with a high cord lesion.

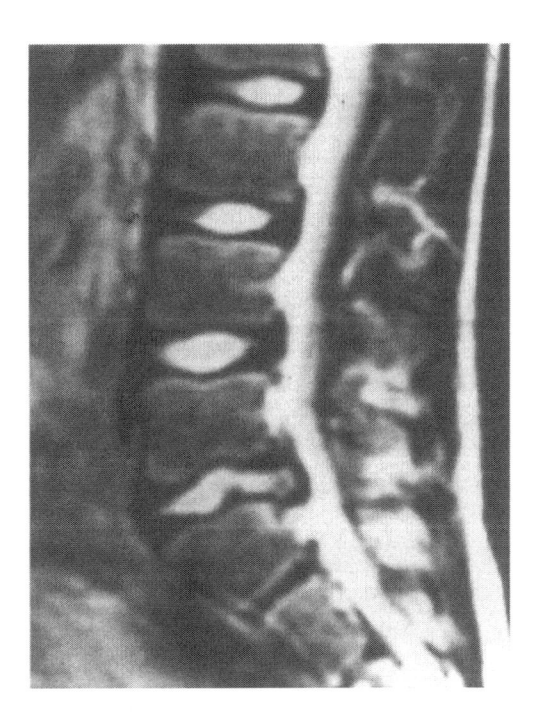

FIGURE 18-98. MRI of a herniated nucleus pulposus in a 12-year old gymnast.

Spinal cord injury associated with spinal shock may produce urinary retention and overdistension of the bladder, which may be avoided by using an indwelling catheter.[899,902] Recovery from spinal shock is usually accompanied by the development of autonomic micturition. If urinary tract infection has been avoided and sphincter tone remains intact (i.e., the level of injury is above S2), intermittent catheterization has proved to be a reasonable means of achieving socially acceptable continence. The older paraplegic child may be instructed in the technique of self-catheterization. For the quadriplegic and younger paraplegic child, instruction of a family member, usually the mother, may be accomplished with relative ease. The low rate of urinary tract infection associated with intermittent catheterization has been well documented. Pharmacologic and surgical methods that increase bladder capacity without causing loss of external sphincter tone are available but not necessarily applicable in each involved child.[906,909] Such procedures may enable the child to attend a full day of school without undue concern. Bowel control is relatively easy to accomplish by means of diet and the use of suppositories. All the complications of flexor spasm frequently seen in patients with high cord injury are due to facilitation of local reflexes. Overflow into visceral channels may also produce a "mass reflex" phenomenon. This reflex phenomenon remains one of the least understood areas of spinal cord injury management. Dorsal myelotomy and sectioning anterior roots have *not* been consistently useful for this condition.[907,917] No available pharmacologic agent has proved useful in the more difficult cases. Variable success has been reported with a variety of agents in the less severe forms of the disorder.

Merriam and associates reviewed 77 patients with traumatic central cord syndrome and found that atypical variations were more common than the existing literature suggested, but that the general outcome was good, with a favorable prognosis most likely when admission evaluation showed good hand function, hyperesthesia, Lhermitte's sign, and normal perianal sensation.[864] Lhermitte's sign is a sudden, shooting paresthesia or paresthesia-like electric shocks spreading down the body or into the limbs on flexion of the neck.

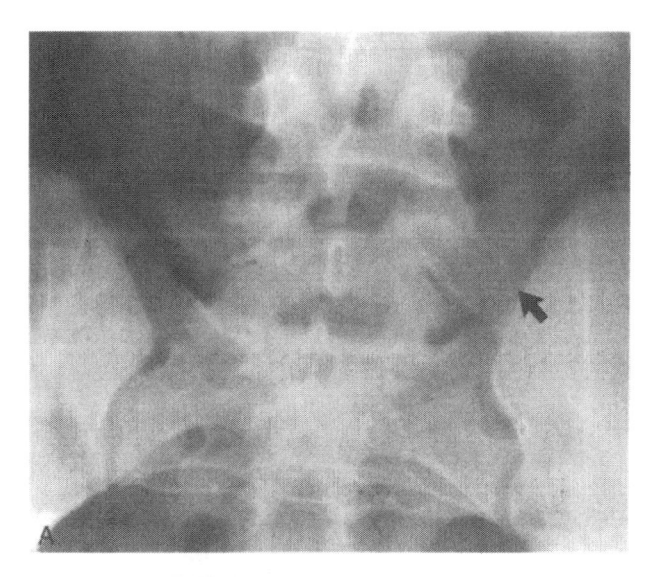

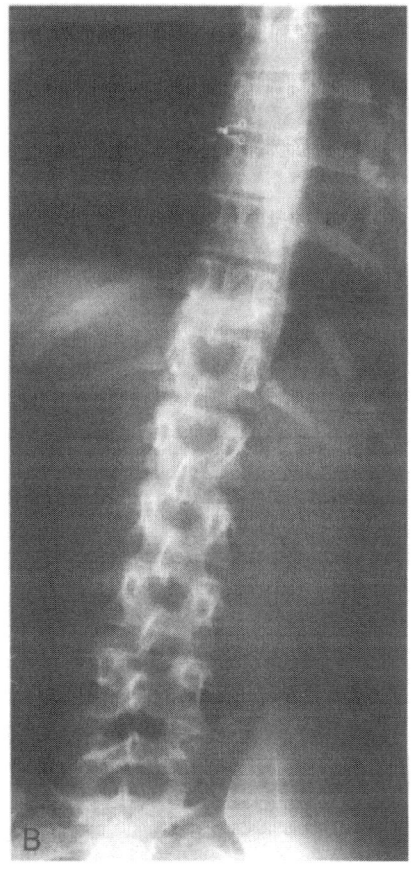

FIGURE 18-99. (A) Partial sacralization of L5 (arrow). (B) This girl fell a few months later during a gymnastics routine, developing severe pain, spasm, and scoliosis.

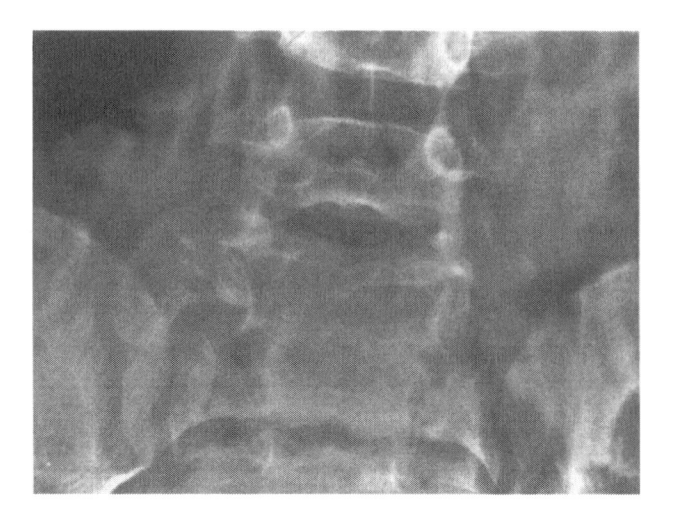

FIGURE 18-100. Painful partial sacralization of the right side of L5 in a 15-year-old female softball pitcher.

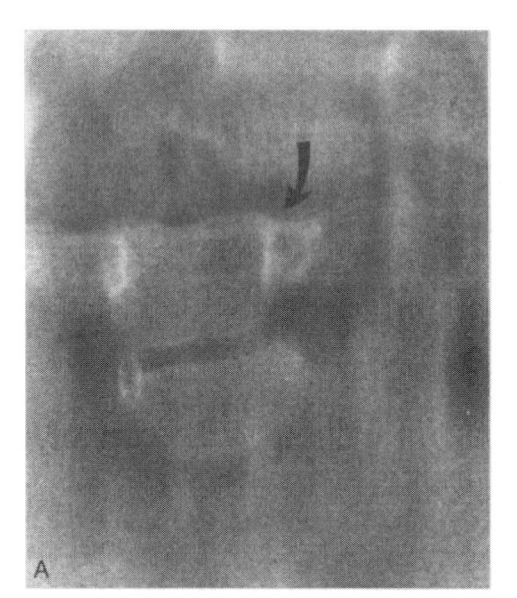

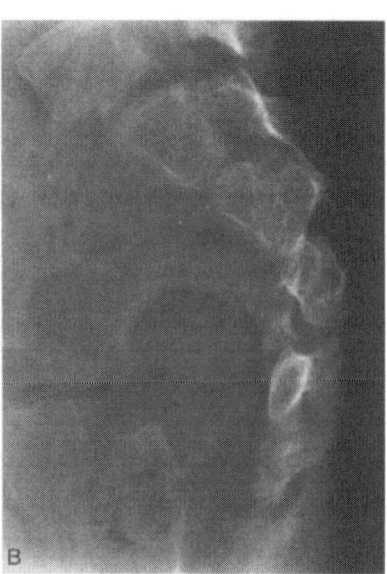

FIGURE 18-101. Anteroposterior (A) and lateral (B) views of a displaced sacral fracture (arrow).

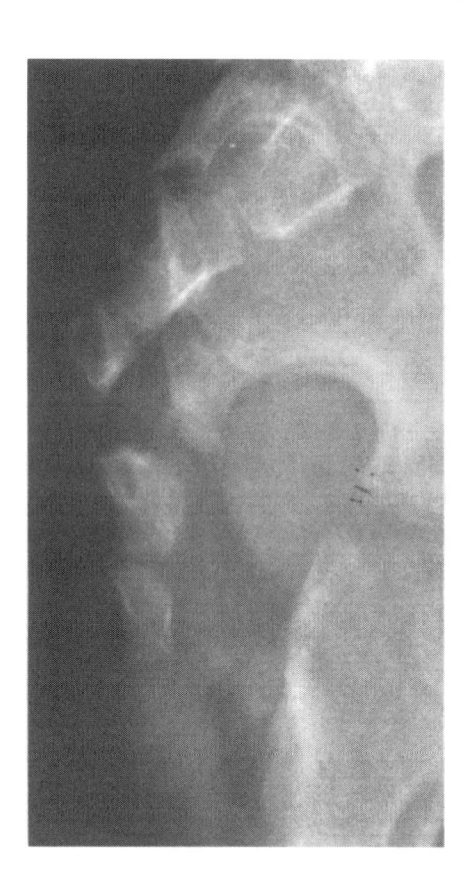

FIGURE 18-102. Displaced sacral fracture in a 10-year-old girl who fell from a ski lift.

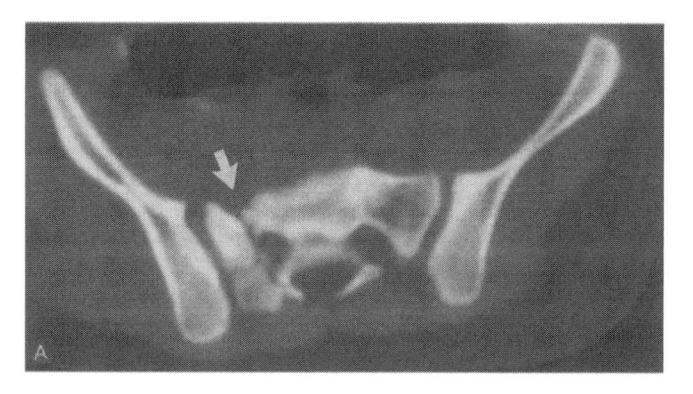

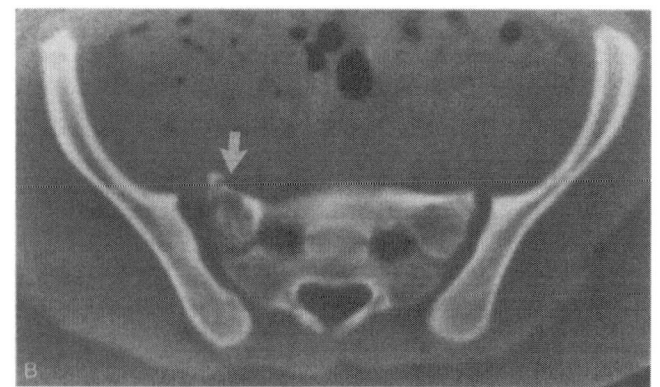

FIGURE 18-103. (A, B) CT views of sacral fractures (arrows) complicating pelvic injuries.

siderable variation in the extent of initial damage. One study reported 31 such children, 18 of whom died. Most of the patients survived long enough to be admitted to the hospital, presenting with symptoms of incomplete hemiplegia (almost 50%).

With complete cord lesions, with or without fracture, the incidence of spinal deformity, lordosis, kyphosis, or scoliosis is higher when the lesion involves the upper thoracic or cervical regions. There is muscle imbalance, the onset of paraplegia is early in life, and laminectomy is often performed. Bracing is difficult, and spinal fusion is usually required. Because progressive angular kyphosis may damage cord functions in partial lesions, early fusion is usually indicated. With extensive thoracic and lumbar lesions, it may be necessary to use appropriate instrumentation.

Autonomic dysreflexia is a syndrome that occurs in patients with spinal cord lesions at or above the sixth thoracic level. It is characterized by exaggerated autonomic responses to stimuli that are usually innocuous in unaffected persons. The spinal cord lesion is above the sympathetic splanchnic visceral outflow. The stimuli that may initiate the reflex include bladder or bowel distension, visceral inflammation, skin irritation, and pain. The initiating afferent stimuli travel to the spinal cord and trigger a gross sympathetic reflex in the caudal stump. Sympathetic efferent motor fibers complete the reflex and cause arteriolar spasm of skin and splanchnic vessels, resulting in severe paroxysmal hypertension. Vasomotor and sudomotor activity below the level of the cord lesion are caused by other efferent sympathetic fibers. Marked hypertension may be associated with a sudden rise in intracranial pressure and may lead to severe

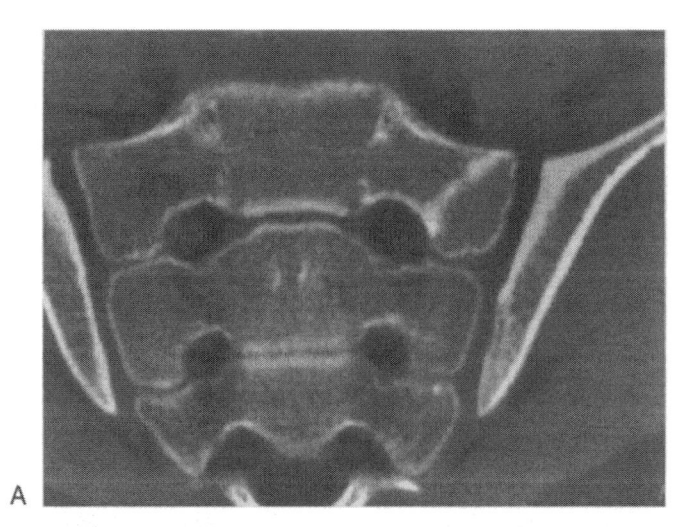

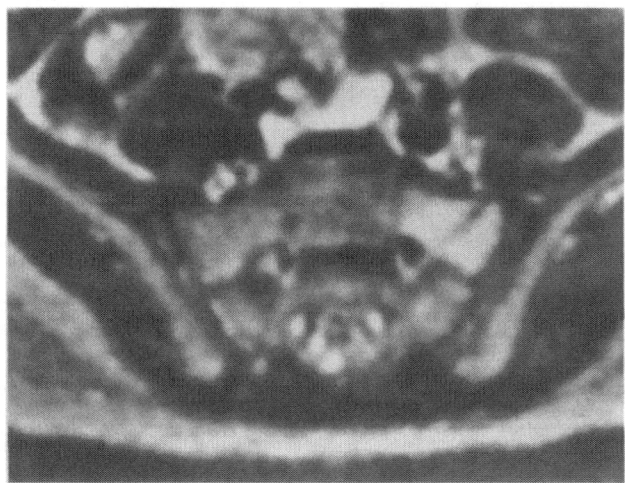

FIGURE 18-104. Stress fracture of sacrum. (A) CT scan showing a stress fracture. (B) MRI showing extensive changes of altered signal intensity due to interosseous edema.

It seems to be widely assumed, in classic central cord syndrome, that the anatomy and neurophysiology of the human spinal cord are accurately known. This is far from true in children who are still in variable stages of neurologic development, maturation, and acquisition of various reflex pathways. The extent of a given central cord injury cannot always be anatomically deduced, and the degree of permanent neurologic deficit varies considerably.

Infarction results in complete, permanent, flaccid paraplegia below the mid-thoracic level.[870,877] The blood supply of the thoracic cord depends significantly on the artery of Adamkiewicz. Anastomosis of the spinal vessels between the first and eleventh intercostal arteries is highly variable and may result in infarction of a major portion of the cord (Fig. 18-106). Because the whole cord is malfunctioning the paraplegia is flaccid, in contrast to spastic paraplegia, which is produced by a segmental lesion.

With thoracic injuries the prognosis for recovery is essentially nonexistent. Most of these injuries are fracture-dislocations. It may be assumed that the cord is severely damaged or transected initially. Cervical injuries show con-

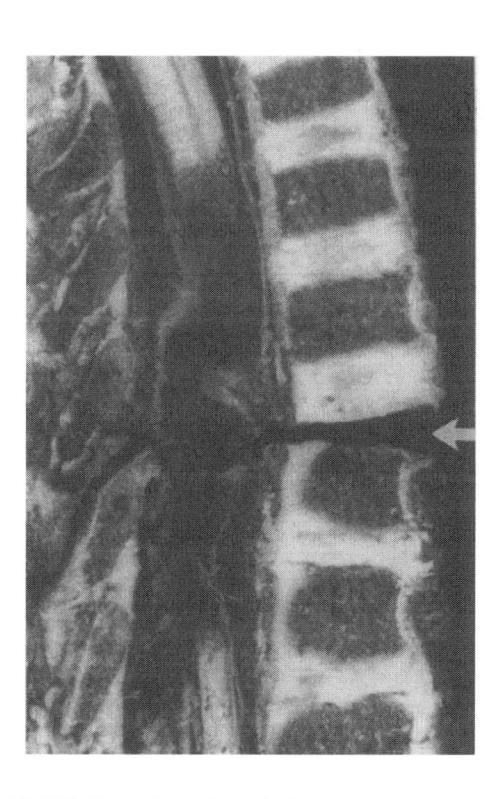

FIGURE 18-105. Fatal thoracic end-plate injury (arrow). Note that the hemorrhage in the spinal cord extends several levels above and below the fracture.

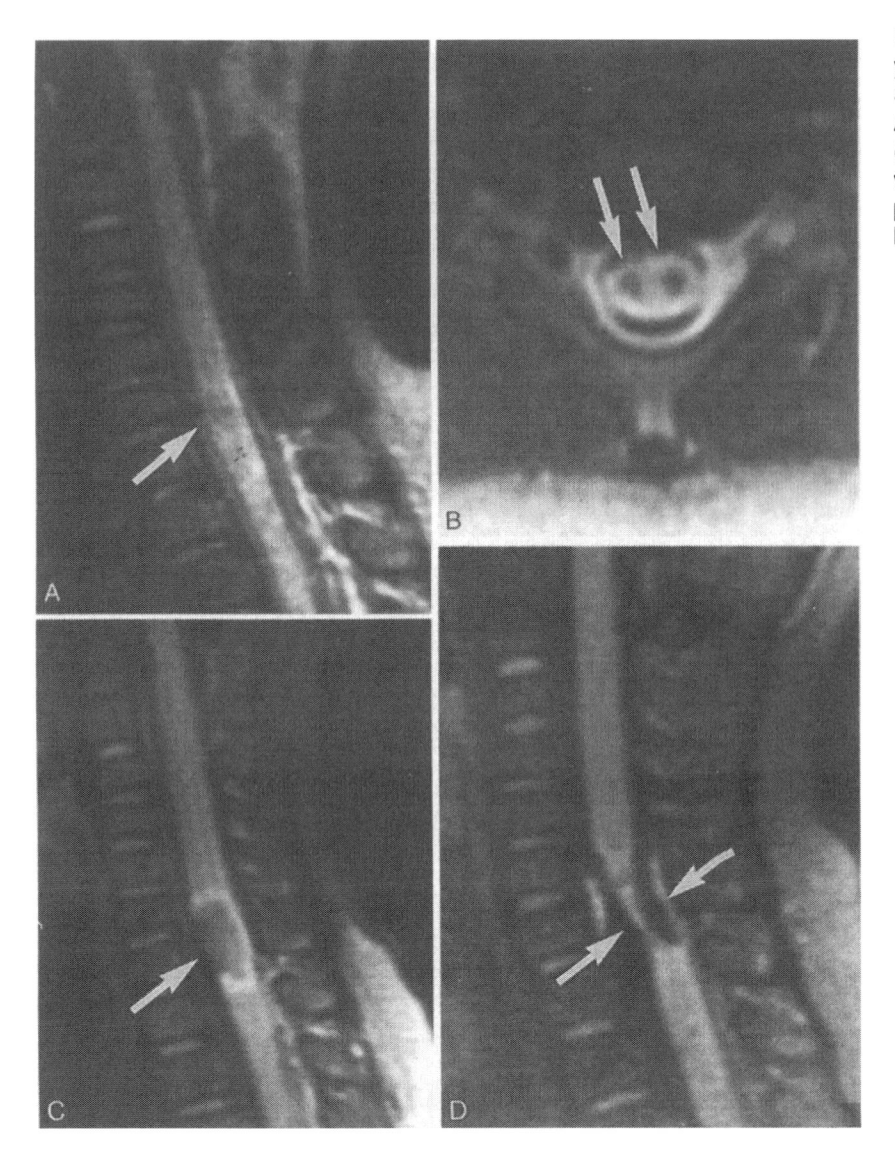

FIGURE 18-106. MRI of the cervical cord of a 2-year-old child injured in a vehicular accident. (A) Spinal cord hemorrhage (arrow) at 48 hours. (B) Axial view of hemorrhage (arrows) at 48 hours. (C) Appearance at 5 days (arrow). (D) At 5 weeks. Resolution of hemorrhage reveals partial cord transection (arrows). The little girl is left with a complete C5 paralysis.

headaches. The vasodilatation above the cord lesion also leads to hyperhidrosis, most often on the forehead, and vasodilatation of the nasal mucous membranes, resulting in nasal congestion. Infants and toddlers, if not older children with relatively early onset of SCIWORA, may be predisposed to develop latex allergy similar to children with myelodysplasia.

Late Sequelae

Spinal injury prior to the completion of vertebral growth may lead to unequal growth and progressive deformity.[880,883,886,888,989,892,894,896,898,904,905,910–912,919–922] Theoretically, premature asymmetric epiphyseal (end-plate) closure comparable to epiphyseal injuries in the appendicular skeleton is responsible for the unequal growth. With lateral wedge compression fractures in children, mild scoliosis is the rule and significant nerve damage and progression are the exceptions. In one study, any residual of anterior wedge compression fractures incurred by adolescents was difficult to find radiographically at follow-up averaging 16 years, leading to the conclusion that unequal growth from an epiphyseal injury was rare.[60] However, other studies and my own experience show that vertebral height is not always completely restored. Osseous bridging may also occur.

Although injury to the vertebral column that results in cord damage is not common in the young child or adolescent, when it does occur the effect of continuing growth on subsequent behavior of the fractured vertebral column must be considered. The normal growth rate slows to a steady rate after the age of 3 years until the growth spurt of puberty. Griffiths followed a boy who initially had a cervical injury at the age of 8 years, with an incomplete Brown-Sequard lesion.[897] His initial injury was a flexion type, with fractures through the vertebral bodies of C3, C4, and C5. Approximately 2 years later he began to show evidence of a kyphotic deformity. Four years after the injury his gait pattern was deteriorating, and both of his legs showed increasing spasm. Again, a further degree of kyphosis was noted. Surgery was refused. Postmortem examination showed well-preserved disk spaces without evidence of anterior callus formation compatible with an attempt at spontaneous fusion. On the basis of the experience in this case, Griffiths subsequently treated fractures with an anterior cervical fusion when he found them in the young adolescent. I disagree. Posterior fusion is probably a more appropriate approach in the skeletally immature individual. The posterior elements are relatively mature in mid-childhood, whereas the anterior end-plates may grow until late adolescence.

Deformation of a vertebral body may result in angular deformity. The most frequent deformities are kyphosis, scoliosis, and kyphoscoliosis. More than a 30% loss in anterior height has the potential for an increasing late deformity, as there may be unrecognized disruption of the posterior elements (i.e., the interspinous ligaments) and unrecognized (occult) end-plate injury similar to that described in long-bone physeal injuries. Alterations in vertebral body shape and deformities below the site of injury are probably the result of unequal pressure that results from neuromuscular imbalance during normal epiphyseal growth.

The late onset of progressive neurologic deficit is usually associated with the extension of a posttraumatic syringomyelia (Fig. 18-107) or the development of a kyphosis or scoliosis with associated cord injury.[881,887] Because both lesions are potentially surgically correctable, early diagnosis is indicated to avoid further extension of an already disabling injury.

The effects of acquired neuromyogenic disorders are determined by the level and degree of spinal cord injury and the age of the patient at the time of injury. The relentless progression of spinal deformity in the untreated pediatric patient with acquired paraplegia exemplifies the effects of asymmetric muscle tension and spasm, fascial contraction, chronic posturing, and gravity on the unsupported growing spine. Almost any combination of deformities is possible. Pelvic obliquity, which may result from contracture above and below the pelvis, makes treatment even more difficult.[893,922]

After management of the acute episode of spinal cord injury, an orthopaedist's primary concern is prevention of subsequent spinal deformation. In a detailed review of 64 juvenile patients who were followed for more than 6 months after injury, spinal deformity, scoliosis, kyphosis, or lordosis were noted in approximately 91%. Girls up to 12 years and boys up to 14 years who had cervical or thoracic injuries developed significant spinal deformity with pelvic obliquity, which may lead to a loss of sitting balance that requires the use of the upper extremities for trunk support, pressure sores on the ischium, and subluxation or dislocation of the hip on the "high" side of the pelvis.[893,922] Children with lumbar lesions are less apt to develop significant spinal deformity, especially one requiring surgical intervention. Most patients with scoliosis had complete lesions, and almost all of those with incomplete lesions had minimal return of function. Scoliosis was the most frequent primary spinal deformity noted. Kyphosis was generally thoracolumbar, and lordosis was either thoracolumbar or lumbar. Pelvic obliquity did not accompany primary kyphosis or lordosis. When it occurred with the scoliosis, it frequently impaired sitting balance. Nonoperative treatment of spinal deformity, employing external support, should be initiated when the potential for spinal deformity exists. In young children it should be prior to radiologic evidence of fixed deformity.

Spinal deformity per se is not an indication for surgery except in an immature patient with a progressive posttraumatic deformity despite bracing or a deformity of more than 40°.[902] The goals of surgical treatment are to prevent increasing deformity and its sequelae, relieve the symptoms of mechanical instability, improve spinal alignment through correction of the deformity, and reverse (or at least halt) increasing neurologic dysfunction.

Scoliosis following hyperflexion injury is probably also due to open epiphyses. The development of scoliosis is

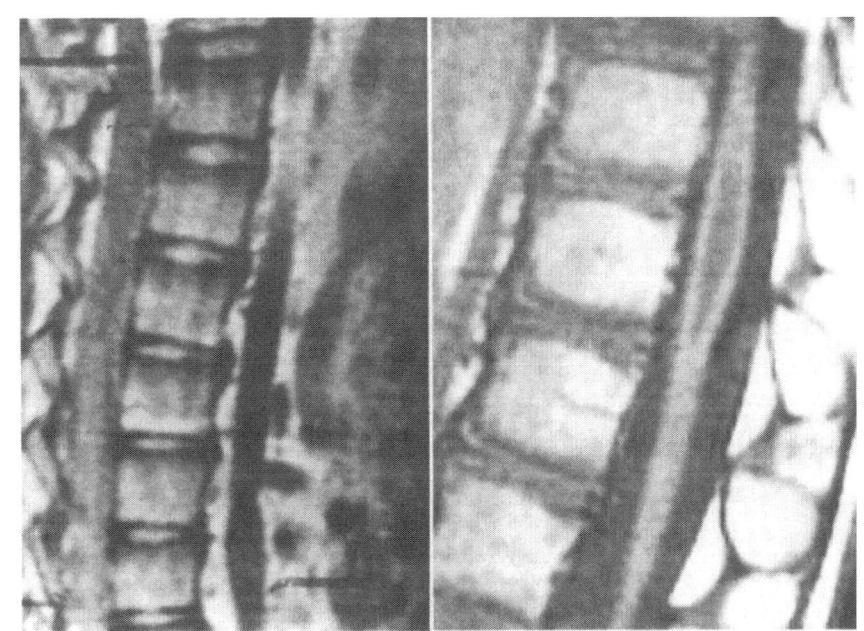

FIGURE 18-107. (A) Edema 36 hours after injury. (B) Four months later a syrinx is evident.

most likely related to unequal compression of the vertebral end-plates. This condition probably causes an incomplete cessation of longitudinal growth or asymmetric stimulation of epiphyseal growth. These processes may continue. This slowing or stimulation of osseous development in the patient who has a stable spinal fracture without neuromuscular deficit also explains why the scoliosis is only mildly progressive.

With scoliosis due to acquired paraplegia, the currently used principles and techniques of instrumentation are applicable. If there is also pelvic obliquity and lumbar kyphosis or lordosis, the fusion mass must extend proximally at least two levels above the injury and distally as an intertransverse process fusion of the sacrum. Cotrel-Dubousset, TSRH, or unit rod instrumentation, as well as a number of other instrumentation systems, offer a stable fixation method. It may be necessary to release the lumbodorsal fascia, iliotibial band, or periarticular hip joint contractures preoperatively.

When there is radiologic evidence of progressive spinal deformity in the growing child receiving nonoperative treatment, surgery should be considered. Posterior spinal fusion was the surgical procedure of choice for scoliosis. The fusion should extend to the sacrum to prevent pelvic obliquity, which is a consistent finding in those patients with fixed scoliosis. Instrumentation of the lumbosacral joint with either the transsacral bar or an enlarged sacral alar hook is desirable. Pseudarthroses may be common, indicating the need for extensive lateral exposure and decortication to the ends of the transverse processes.

With progressive kyphosis, when the deformity exceeds 60° and appears rigid, Kilfoyle and colleagues recommended anterior spinal fusion at the apex of the deformity, followed by a posterior spinal fusion with compression rods.[906] This decision was based on the frequent observation of loss of correction or pseudarthrosis formation at the apex of the kyphotic deformity when only one procedure was used. Progressive lordotic deformity, which generally includes the lumbosacral joint, may be satisfactorily corrected and stabilized by posterior spinal fusion. However, when lordosis is severe or more than 100°, rigid anterior spinal fusion is probably a better approach, but it must be appended with a posterior fusion, as anterior extension to the sacrum is not possible.

In addition to treating the deformity, bracing improves function by restoring sitting balance and freeing the upper extremities for activities other than trunk support. Any orthoses must be well padded to protect the anesthetic skin, easily removable to allow frequent skin checks, and easily adjustable to allow for growth. A thoracolumbosacral orthosis brace is best here and should be used in all patients with spinal lesions above T10. For the levels below T10 a removable axillary-level, high-body jacket is used. Nonoperative treatment is more apt to be successful in the older child with a scoliotic deformity than in the patient with kyphosis alone. Failure usually is seen in the uncooperative patient and in those with moderate or severe spasticity.

The paraplegic and less often the quadriplegic patient is at risk of developing pathologic fractures in the osteoporotic bone.[901] These fractures may be difficult to detect because of loss of symptoms such as pain. The increased emphasis on sports for the disabled (e.g., wheelchair sports) may increase the likelihood of extremity injury in the involved child or adolescent. Fractures may heal with significant amounts of heterotopic bone, particularly if spasticity is present.[895,913,914,924]

Patients with a spinal cord injury have lower bone densities (compared to their nondisabled peers) ranging from 56% to 65% of normal.[878,885,891,900,903,915] Those with a history of fractures have significantly lower bone density.

Great care must be taken to observe the hips carefully so subluxation or dislocation does not occur.[922] Growth abnormalities are more subtle in their presentation. Myelotomy or rhizotomy may relieve some of the spasticity that contributes to these structural contractures.[907] Botox or baclofen may be effective in the young patient and the adult.

The patient with loss of sensation following cord injury is uniquely vulnerable to the development of decubiti. Irreversible local necrosis may be seen after only 3–4 hours. The use of mattresses designed to distribute pressure areas is helpful for preventing decubiti, but the most important factors are frequent turning and good skin care.

Development of a decubitus ulcer may delay rehabilitation weeks or months. The injury frequently occurs during the first few hours after admission, when the attention of the medical and nursing staff is directed to other matters. Early and continued attention to this important parameter of nursing care provides incalculable benefit for long-term management of these patients.

Chao and Mayo followed 40 children with spinal cord injury with an average age at presentation of 9 years and a mean follow-up of 4 years.[890] There were 2 cervical, 13 thoracic, and 5 lumbar injuries. Bladder management included 11 patients with reflex voiding and 29 patients given combined anticholinergic medication with intermittent catheterization. Video-urodynamics showed good function and preservation of the urinary tract in 25 of 28 patients. Failure was equated with noncompliance to the recommended voiding regimens. The authors recommended annual renal ultrasonography and video-urodynamic studies every 1–2 years.

Physical therapy should be directed at maximizing function by preventing contractures and by the use of braces and assistive devices. In general, physical therapy should be combined with a program of occupational therapy aimed at making the child independent in the activities of daily life. Early enrollment in a rehabilitation program is instrumental in a child's rapid return to family and community.

Triolo et al. have applied functional neuromuscular stimulation to children with spinal cord injuries.[925] They found that the procedure required a major commitment from the patient and family but when used selectively improved the patient's standing, walking, and hand grasp.[884]

Obvious causes of treatment failure include (1) incomplete reduction; (2) incorrect assessment of stability with resultant insufficient quality and duration of spinal orthotic protection; and (3) neglect of patients with skeletally stable injuries but a cord deficit.

Assimilation back into the family and school is not easy. A team effort and counseling are often appropriate. The willingness to return to school varies remarkably.[916]

References

Anatomy

1. Althoff B, Goldie IF. The arterial supply of the odontoid process of the axis. Acta Orthop Scand 1977;48:622–629.
2. Carpenter EB. Normal and abnormal growth of the spine. Clin Orthop 1961;21:49–55.
3. Clark CA, Panjabi MM, Wetzel FT. Can infant malnutrition cause adult vertebral stenosis? Spine 1985;10:165–170.
4. Di Chiro G, Harrington T, Fried LC. Microangiography of human fetal spinal cord. AJR 1973;118:193–199.
5. Dickman CA, Crawford NR, Tominaga T, et al. Morphology and kinetics of the baboon upper cervical spine. Spine 1994;19:2518–2523.
6. Dommisse GF. The blood supply of the spinal cord: a critical vascular zone in spinal surgery. J Bone Joint Surg Br 1974;56:225–235.
7. Dommisse GF. The Arteries and Veins of the Human Spinal Cord from Birth. Churchill Livingstone: Edinburgh, 1975.
8. Faborowski Z. Extrafetal development of the axis on the basis of roentgen anthropometric measurements. Folia Morphol (Warsz) 1978;37:167–177.
9. Faure C, Debrun G, Djindjian R. Normal and pathological arterial vascularisation of the lumbar enlargement of the spinal cord in the child: Adamkiewicz's artery. Ann Radiol (Paris) 1967;10:129–140.
10. Fischer LP, Gonon GP, Carret JP, Sayfi Y. Arterial vascularization of the lumbar vertebrae. Bull Assoc Anat (Nancy) 1976;60:347–355.
11. Fyhrie DP, Schaffler MB. Failure mechanisms in human vertebral cancellous bone. Bone 1994;15:105–109.
12. Gillilan LA. The arterial blood supply of the human spinal cord. J Comp Neurol 1958;110:75–86.
13. Girdany BR, Golden R. Centers of ossification of the skeleton. AJR 1952;68:922–924.
14. Guida G, Cigala F, Riccio V. The vascularization of the vertebral body in the human fetus at term. Clin Orthop 1979;65:229–234.
15. Jarzem PF, Kostnik JP, Filaggi M, Doyle DJ, Ethier R, Tator CN. Spinal cord distraction: an in vitro study of length, tension and tissue pressure. J Spinal Disord 1991;4:177–182.
16. Johnson RM. Some new observations on the functional anatomy of the lower cervical spine. Clin Orthop 1975;111:192–200.
17. Larsen JL, Smith D. The lumbar spinal canal in children. Eur J Radiol 1981;1:163–170.
18. Lord MJ, Ogden JA, Ganey TM. Postnatal development of the thoracic spine. Spine 1995;20:1692–1698.
19. Luyendijk W, Cohn B, Rejger V, Vielvoye GJ. The great radicular artery of Adamkiewicz in man: demonstration of a possibility to predict its functional territory. Acta Neurochir (Wien) 1988;95:143–146.
20. Maat GJR, Matricali B, van Mearten EL. Postnatal development and structure of the neurocentral junction: its relevance for spinal surgery. Spine 1996;21:661–666.
21. Macalister A. Notes on the development and variations of the atlas. J Anat Physiol 1892;27:519–942.
22. Menck J, Lierse W. The arterial supply of the cervical vertebral body in newborns. Acta Anat (Basel) 1990;137:165–169.
23. Minami K, Kikkawa F. Anatomical studies of the spinal rami of lumbar arteries in Japanese fetuses. Okajima Folia Anat Jpn 1982;58:1211–1230.
24. O'Brien JP. The manifestations of arrested bone growth: the appearance of a vertebra within a vertebra. J Bone Joint Surg Am 1969;51:1376–1378.
25. Ogden JA. Radiology of postnatal skeletal development. XI. The first cervical vertebra. Skeletal Radiol 1984;12:12–20.
26. Ogden JA. Radiology of postnatal skeletal development. XII. The second cervical vertebra. Skeletal Radiol 1984;12:169–177.
27. Ogden JA, Ganey TM, Sasse J, Neame PJ, Hilbelink DR. Development and maturation of the axial skeleton. In: Weinstein S (ed) The Pediatric Spine: Principles and Practice. New York: Raven, 1994, pp 3–69.
28. Ogden JA, Grogan DP, Light TR. Prenatal and postnatal development of the chondro-osseous skeleton. In: Albright JA, Brand RA (eds) The Scientific Basis of Orthopedics, 2nd ed. Norwalk, CT: Appleton-Century-Crofts, 1988.
29. Ogden JA, Murphy MJ, Southwick WO, Ogden DA. Radiology of postnatal skeletal development. XIII. C1/C2 interrelationships. Skeletal Radiol 1986;15:433–438.
30. Papp T, Porter TW, Aspden RM. The growth of the lumbar vertebral canal. Spine 1994;19:2770–2773.
31. Ratcliffe JF. The arterial anatomy of the developing human dorsal and lumbar vertebral body: a microarteriographic study. J Anat 1981;133:625–628.
32. Roaf R. Vertebral growth and its mechanical control. J Bone Joint Surg Br 1960;42:40–59.
33. Rodriguez Baeza A, Muset Lara A, Rodriguez Pazos M, Domenech Mateu JM. The arterial supply of the human spinal cord: a new approach to the arteria radicularis magna of Adamkiewicz. Acta Neurochir (Wien) 1991;109:57–62.
34. Saywell WR, Crock HV, England JP, Steiner RE. Demonstration of vertebral body endplate veins by magnetic resonance imaging. Br J Radiol 1989;62:290–292.
35. Schiff DCM, Parke WW. The arterial supply of the odontoid process. J Bone Joint Surg Am 1973;55:1450–1456.
36. Sutow WW, Pryde AW. Incidence of spina bifida occulta in relation to age. Am J Dis Child 1956;91:211–217.
37. Tondury G. The cervical spine: its development and changes during life. Acta Orthop Belg 1959;25:602–607.
38. Whalen JL, Parke WW, Mazur JM, Stauffer ES. The intrinsic vasculature of developing vertebral endplates and its nutritive significance to the intervertebral disc. J Pediatr Orthop 1985;5:403–410.

General

39. Anderson JM, Schutt AH. Spinal injury in children: a review of 156 cases seen from 1950 through 1978. Mayo Clin Proc 1980;55:99–104.
40. Aufdermaur M. Spinal injuries in juveniles: Necropsy findings in twelve cases. J Bone Joint Surg Br 1974;56:513–519.
41. Babcocke JL. Spinal injuries in children. Pediatr Clin North Am 1975;22:487–500.
42. Bohlman HH, Rekate HL, Thompson GH. Problem fractures of the cervical spine in children. In: Houghton GR, Thompson GH (eds) Problematic Musculoskeletal Injuries in Children. London: Butterworths, 1985.
43. Conway JE, Crofford TW, Terry AF, Protzman RR. Cauda equina syndrome occurring nine years after a gunshot injury to the spine. J Bone Joint Surg Am 1993;75:760–763.
44. Crawford AH. Operative treatment of spine fractures in children. Orthop Clin North Am 1990;21:325–339.
45. Curran C, Dietrich AM, Bowman MJ, et al. Pediatric cervical-spine immobilization: achieving neutral position? J Trauma 1995;39:729–732.
46. Desgrippes Y, Bensahel H. Les fractures du rachis de l'enfant sans lesions neurologiques definitives. J Chir (Paris) 1976;112:329–334.

47. Dickman CA, Rekate HL, Sonntag VKH, Fadramski JM. Pediatric spinal trauma: vertebral column and spinal cord injuries in children. Pediatr Neurosci 1989;15:237–256.
48. Dwornik JJ, O'Neal ML, Ganey TM, Slater-Hause AS, Ogden JA, Wagner CE. Metallic dissolution of a Civil War bullet embedded in a sternum. Am J Forensic Med Pathol 1996;17:130–135.
49. Forni I. Le fratture del rachide nel bambino. Chir Organi Mov 1947;31:347–361.
50. Funk FJ, Wells RE. Injuries to the cervical spine in football. Clin Orthop 1975;109:50–58.
51. Gelehrter G. Die Wirbelkorperbruche im Kindes und Jugendalter. Arch Orthop Unfallchir 1957;49:253–263.
52. Gorovaia TP. Closed fractures of the spine in children. Chirurgia 1962;38:112–118.
53. Grogan DP, Bucholz RW. Acute lead intoxication from a bullet in an intervertebral disc space: a case report. J Bone Joint Surg Am 1981;63:1180–1182.
54. Hachen HJ. Spinal cord injury in children and adolescents: diagnostic pitfalls and therapeutic consideration in the acute stage. Paraplegia 1977;15:55–64.
55. Hadley MN, Fadramski JM, Browner CM, Rekate H, Sonntsej VKH. Pediatric spinal trauma: review of 122 cases of spinal cord and vertebral column injuries. J Neurosurg 1988;68:18–24.
56. Hemmer R. Versteifungsoperationen an der Halswirbelsaule im Kindesalter. Dtsch Med Wochenschr 1970;44:2218–2220.
57. Henrys P, Lyne ED, Lifton C, Salciccioli G. Clinical review of cervical spine injuries in children. Clin Orthop 1977;129:172–176.
58. Herkowitz HN, Sanberg LC. Vertebral column injuries associated with tobogganing. J Trauma 1978;18:806–810.
59. Herzenberg JE, Hensinger RN, Dedrick DK, Phillips WA. Emergency transport and positioning of young children who have an injury to the cervical spine. J Bone Joint Surg Am 1989;71:15–22.
60. Horal J, Nachemson A, Scheller S. Clinical and radiological long-term follow-up of vertebral fractures in children. Acta Orthop Scand 1972;43:491–503.
61. Horne, J, Cockshott WP, Shannon HS. Spinal column damage from water ski jumping. Skeletal Radiol 1987;16:612–616.
62. Hubbard DD. Injuries of the spine in children and adolescents. Clin Orthop 1974;100:56–65.
63. Hubbard DD. Injuries of the spine in children and adolescents. Orthop Clin North Am 1976;17:605–614.
64. Kewalramani LS, Kraus JF, Sterling HM. Acute spinal cord lesions in a pediatric population: epidemiologic and clinical features. Paraplegia 1980;18:206–219.
65. Leoin F, Kabbaj K, Dhellemmes P, et al. Spinal fractures in children: diagnostic and therapeutic problems; apropos of 67 cases. Neurochirurgie 1984;30:289–294.
66. Letts M, Macdonald P. Sports injuries to the pediatric spine. State Art Rev 1990;4:49–83.
67. Majernick TC, Bieniek R, Houston JB, et al. Cervical spine movement during oro-tracheal intubation. Ann Emerg Med 1986;15:417–420.
68. Mann DC, Dodds JA. Spinal injuries in 57 patients 17 years or younger. Orthopedics 1993;16:159–164.
69. Mann DC, Tall R, Brodkey JS. Bullet within the spinal cord. Orthop Rev 1989;18:453–457.
70. McPhee IB. Spinal fractures and dislocations in children and adolescents. Spine 1981;6:533–537.
71. Micheli LJ, Hall JE, Miller ME. Use of modified Boston brace for back injuries in athletes. Am J Sports Med 1980;8:351–356.
72. Möllenhoff G, Walz M, Muhr G. Korrekturverhalten nach Frakturen der Brust- und Lendenwirbelsäule bei Kindern und Jugendlichen. Chirurg 1993;64:948–952.
73. O'Neal ML, Lord MJ, Ganey TM, Ogden JA. Spontaneously occurring fractures of the spine in skeletally immature animals. Spine 1994;19:1230–1236.
74. Pizzutillo PD. Spinal considerations in the young athlete. AAOS Instr Course Lect 1993;42:463–472.
75. Povacz F. Behandlungsergebnisse und Prognose von Wirbelbrüchen bei Kindern. Chirurg 1969;40:30–33.
76. Ruge JR, Sinson GP, McLane DG, Cerullo LJ. Pediatric spinal injury: the very young. J Neurosurg 1988;68:25–30.
77. Senturia HR. The roentgen findings in increased lead absorption due to retained projectiles. AJR 1942;47:381–391.
78. Vinz H. Vertebral body fractures in children: results of a follow-up study. Zentralbl Chir 1965;90:626–636.
79. Wu WQ. Delayed effects from retained foreign bodies in the spine and spinal cord. Surg Neurol 1986;25:214–218.

Congenital Predisposition

80. Afshani E, Girdany BR. Atlanto-axial dislocation in chondrodysplasia punctata. Radiology 1972;102:399–401.
81. Archer E, Batnitaki S, Franken EA, Muller J, Hale B. Congenital dysplasia of C2–6. Pediatr Radiol 1977;6:121–122
82. Aronson DD, Kahn RH, Canady A, Bollinger RO, Towlin R. Instability of the cervical spine after decompression in patients who have Arnold-Chiari malformation: J Bone Joint Surg Am 1991;73:898–906.
83. Beighton P, Craig J. Atlanto-axial subluxation in the Morquio syndrome. J Bone Joint Surg Br 1973;56:478–481.
84. Bernini FP, Eletante R, Smatino F, Tedeschi G. Angiographic study on the vertebral artery in cases of deformities of the occipito-cervical joint. AJR 1969;107:526–529.
85. Bethem D, Winter RB, Lutter L, et al. Spinal disorders of dwarfism: review of the literature and report of eighty cases. J Bone Joint Surg Am 1981;63:1412–1425.
86. Black KS, Gorey MT, Seideman B, Scuderi DM, Cinnsuron J, Hyoran PA. Congenital spondylisthesis of the 6th cervical vertebra: CT findings. J Comput Assist Tomogr 1991;15:335–337.
87. Blaw ME, Langer LO. Spinal cord compression in Morquio Brailsford's disease. J Pediatr 1969;74:593–600.
88. Born CT, Camden MP, Freed M, DeLong WG. Cerebrovascular accident complicating Klippel-Feil syndrome. J Bone Joint Surg Am 1988;70:1412–1415.
89. Bradford D, King H. Fracture-dislocation of the spine after spinal fusion and Harrington instrumentation for idiopathic scoliosis. J Bone Joint Surg Am 1987;62:1374–1376.
90. Cattell HS, Clark BL. Cervical kyphosis and instability following multiple laminectomies in children. J Bone Joint Surg Am 1967;49:713–720.
91. Dawley JA. Spondylolisthesis of the cervical spine. J Neurosurg 1971;34:99–101.
92. Dawson EG, Smith L. Atlanto-axial subluxation in children due to vertebral anomalies. J Bone Joint Surg Am 1979;61:582–587.
93. Dubousset J. Torticollis in children caused by congenital anomalies of the atlas. J Bone Joint Surg Am 1986;68:178–188.
94. Elster AD. Quadriplegia after minor trauma in the Klippel-Feil syndrome: a case report and review of the literature. J Bone Joint Surg Am 1984;66:1473–1474.
95. Gangeni M, Renier D, Danssarge J, Hirsch JF, Rigault P. Children's cervical spine instability after posterior fossa surgery. Acta Neurol 1982;4:39–43.
96. Goldberg MJ. Orthopaedic aspects of bone dysplasias. Orthop Clin North Am 1976;7:445–456
97. Grant T, Puffer J. Cervical stenosis: a developmental anomaly with quadriparesis during football. Am J Sports Med 1976;4:219–221.

References

98. Guillaume J, Roulleau J, Fardou H, Treil J, Manelfe C. Congenital spondylolysis of cervical vertebrae with spondylolisthesis and frontal narrowing of the spinal canal. Neuroradiology 1976;11:159–163.
99. Hall K, Simmons ED, Daryl Cheek K, Barnes PD. Instability of the cervical spine and neurological involvement in Klippel-Feil syndrome. J Bone Joint Surg Am 1990;72:460–462.
100. Hammerschlag W, Ziv I, Wald U, et al. Cervical instability in an achondroplastic infant. J Pediatr Orthop 1988;8:481–484.
101. Heggeness MH. Charcot arthropathy of the spine with resulting paraparesis developing during pregnancy in a patient with congenital insensitivity to pain. Spine 1994;19:95–98.
102. Kessler JT. Congenital narrowing of the cervical spinal canal. J Neurol Neurosurg Psychiatry 1975;38:1218–1224.
103. Kopits SE. Orthopedic complications in dwarfism. Clin Orthop 1976;114:153–179.
104. Ladd AL, Suranton PE. Congenital cervical stenosis presenting as transient quadriplegia in athletes. J Bone Joint Surg Am 1986;68:1371–1374.
105. Lyson SJ. Dysplasia of odontoid process in Morquio's syndrome causing quadriparesis. J Bone Joint Surg Am 1977;59:340–344.
106. Mopel RH, Raso E, Waltz TA. Central cord syndrome resulting from congenital narrowness of the cevical spinal cord. J Trauma 1989;29:694–664.
107. Moseley I. Neural arch dysplasia of the sixth cervical vertebra: congenital cervical spondylolisthesis. Br J Radiol 1976;49:81–83.
108. Nagib MG, Maxwell RE, Chou SN. Identification and management of high risk patients with Klippel-Feil syndrome. J Neurosurg 1984;61:523–530.
109. Prioleau BR, Wilson CB. Cervical spondylolysis with spondylolisthesis: case report. J Neurosurg 1975;43:750–793.
110. Shapiro J, Herring J. Congenital vertebral displacement. J Bone Joint Surg Am 1993;75:656–662.
111. Sherk HH, Nicholson J. Cervico-oculoacusticus syndrome: case report of death caused by injury to abnormal cervical spine. J Bone Joint Surg Am 1972;54:1776–1778.
112. Strax TE, Baran E. Traumatic quadriplegia associated with Klippel-Feil syndrome: discussion and case reports. Arch Phys Med Rehabil 1975;56:363–365.
113. Svensson O, Aaro S. Cervical instability in skeletal dysplasia: report of 6 surgically fused cases. Acta Orthop Scand 1988;59:66–70.
114. Thomas R, Carl D, Moskowitz A. Multiple spinal fractures after scoliosis fusion with Harrington rods. Spine 1989;14:539–941.
115. Tokgözolu AM, Alpaslan AM. Congenital spondylolisthesis in the upper spinal column. Spine 1994;19:99–102.
116. Tuffley DJ, McPhee IB. Fracture of the spine after spinal fusion for idiopathic scoliosis. Spine 1984;9:538–539.

Down Syndrome

117. Akiyama T, Marius S, Naito M, et al. Treatment of atlanto-axial luxation in Down's syndrome. J Central Jpn J Orthop Trauma 1992;25:871–883.
118. American Academy of Pediatrics, Committee on Sports Medicine. Atlantoaxial instability in Down syndrome. Pediatrics 1984;74:152–154.
119. Arlet V, Rigault P, Padovani JP, Janklevicz P, Tonzet P, Finiidon G. Atlanto-axial instability in children with trisomy 21: atlanto-axial or occipito-axial fusion. J Orthop Surg 1992;6:244–251.
120. Aung MH. Atlanto-axial dislocation in Down's syndrome: report of a case with spinal cord compression and review of the literature. Bull Los Angeles Neurol Soc 1973;38:197–201.
121. Braakhekke JP, Gabreels FJ, Renier WO, et al. Craniovertebral pathology in Down syndrome. Clin Neurol Neurosurg 1985;87:173–179.
122. Brooke DC, Brinkens JK, Benson DR. Asymptomatic occipito-atlantal instability in Down syndrome (trisomy 21). J Bone Joint Surg Am 1987;49:293–295.
123. Brooke DC, Burkus JK, Benson DR. Asymptomatic occipito-atlantal instability in Down syndrome. J Bone Joint Surg Am 1987;69:293–295.
124. Burke SW, Franch HG, Roberts JM, et al. Chronic atlanto-axial instability in Down syndrome. J Bone Joint Surg Am 1985;67:1356–1360.
125. Coria F, Quintana F, Villallis M, Reboths M, Berciano J. Craniocervical abnormalities in Down's syndrome. Dev Med Child Neurol 1983;25:252–255.
126. Curtis BH, Blank S, Fisher RL. Atlanto-axial dislocation in Down's syndrome: report of two patients requiring surgical correction. JAMA 1968;205:464–465.
127. Davidson RG. Atlanto-axial instability in individuals with Down syndrome: a fresh look at the evidence. Pediatrics 1988;81:857–865.
128. Diamond LS, Lynne D, Sigman D. Orthopedic disorders in patients with Down's syndrome. Orthop Clin North Am 1981;12:57–71.
129. Dzentis AJ. Spontaneous atlanto-axial dislocation in a mongoloid child with spinal cord compression: case report. J Neurosurg 1966;25:458–460.
130. El-Khoury GY, Clark CR, Dietz FR, Harre RG, Tozzi JE, Kathal MH. Posterior atlanto-occipital subluxation in Down syndrome. Radiology 1986;159:507–509.
131. Elliott S, Morton RE, Whitelaw RA. Atlanto-axial instability and abnormalities of the odontoid in Down's syndrome. Arch Dis Child 1988;63:1484–1489.
132. Evans DL, Bethem D. Cervical spine injuries in children. J Pediatr Orthop 1989;9:563–568.
133. Fielding JW, Herring JA. Cervical instability in Down's syndrome and juvenile rheumatoid arthritis. J Pediatr Orthop 1982;2:205–207.
134. Finerman GAM, Sakai D, Weingarten S. Atlanto-axial dislocation with spinal cord compression in a mongoloid child: a case report. J Bone Joint Surg Am 1976;58:408–409.
135. French HG, Burke SW, Roberts JM, et al. Upper cervical ossicles in Down syndrome. J Pediatr Orthop 1987;7:69–71.
136. Gabriel KR, Madson DC, Carango P. Occipito-atlantal instability in Down's syndrome. Spine 1990;15:997–1002.
137. Gerard Y, Segal P, Bedochs JS. Instabilité de l'atlas sur l'axis dan le mongolisme. Presse Med 1971;79:573–576.
138. Giblin PE, Micheli LJ. The management of atlanto-axial subluxation with neurologic involvement in Down's syndrome: a review of two cases and a review of the literature. Chir Orthop 1979;140:66–71.
139. Hreidarsson S, Magram G, Singer H. Symptomatic atlanto-axial dislocation in Down syndrome. Pediatrics 1982;69:568–571.
140. Hungerford GD, Akkaraju V, Rawe SE, Young FG. Atlanto-occipital and atlanto-axial dislocations with spinal cord compression in Down's syndrome: a case report and review of the literature. Br J Radiol 1981;54:758–761.
141. Kobori M, Takahashi H, Mikawa Y. Atlanto-axial dislocation in Down's syndrome: report of two cases requiring surgical correction. Spine 1986;11:195–200.
142. Martel W, Tishler JM. Observations on the spine in mongoloidism. AJR 1968;97:630–638.
143. Martel W, Uyham R, Stinson CW. Subluxation of the atlas causing spinal cord compression in a case of Down's syndrome with a manifestation of "occipital vertebra." Radiology 1969;93:839–840.

144. Mautner H, Barnes A, Curtis G. Abnormal findings of the spine in mongoloids. Am J Ment Defic 1950;55:105–107.
145. Michejda M, Menolascino FJ. Skull base abnormalities in Down's syndrome. Ment Retard 1975;13:24–26.
146. Moore RA, McNicholas KW, Warren SP. Atlanto-axial subluxation with symptomatic spinal cord compression in a child with Down's syndrome. Anesth Analg 1987;66:89–90.
147. Nordt JC, Stauffer ES. Sequelae of atlanto-axial stabilization in two patients with Down's syndrome. Spine 1981;6:437–440.
148. Onari K, Ifawa T, Kurski Y. Clinical and radiological evaluation of atlanto-axial instability in children with Down's syndrome. J Orthop Traumatol Surg 1981;24:619–624.
149. Parfenchuck TA, Bertrand SL, Powers MJH, et al. Posterior occipito-atlantal hyperinstability in Down syndrome: an analysis of 199 patients. J Pediatr Orthop 1994;14:304–308.
150. Pueschel SM. Atlantoaxial instability in individuals with Down syndrome: commentaries. Pediatrics 1988;81:879–880.
151. Pueschel SM, Findley FW, Furia J, et al. Atlanto-axial instability in Down's syndrome: roentgenographic, neurologic and somatosensory evoked potential studies. J Pediatr 1987;110:515–521.
152. Pueschel SM, Herndon JH, Gelch MM, Senet KE, Scola FH, Goldberg MJ. Symptomatic atlanto-axial subluxation in persons with Down syndrome. J Pediatr Orthop 1984;6:682–688.
153. Pueschel SM, Scola FH, Perry CD, Pezzuleo JC. Atlanto-axial instability in children with Down's syndrome. Pediatr Radiol 1981;10:129–132.
154. Rosenbaum DM, Blumhagen JD, King HA. Atlanto-occipital instability in Down syndrome. AJR 1986;149:1269–1272.
155. Schaffer TE, Dyment PG, Luckstead EF, Murray JJ, Smith NJ. AAP Committee on Sports Medicine: atlanto-axial instability in Down syndrome. Pediatrics 1984;74:152–154.
156. Segal LS, Drummond DS, Zanotti RM, Ecter ML, Mubarek SJ. Complications of posterior arthrodesis of the cervical spine in patients who have Down syndrome. J Bone Joint Surg Am 1981;73:1547–1554.
157. Semine AA, Erthl AN, Goldberg MJ, Bull MJ. Cervical spine instability in children with Down syndrome (trisomy 21). J Bone Joint Surg Am 1968;60:649–652.
158. Sherk HH, Nicholson JT. Rotary atlanto-axial dislocation associated with ossiculum terminale and Down's syndrome. J Bone Joint Surg Am 1969;51:957–964.
159. Sherk HH, Pasquariello PS, Walters WC. Multiple dislocations of the cervical spine in a patient with juvenile rheumatoid arthritis and Down's syndrome. Clin Orthop 1982;162:37–40.
160. Shikita J, Mikawa Y, Ikeda T, Yamamuro T. Atlanto-axial subluxation with spondyloschisis in Down syndrome. J Bone Joint Surg Am 1985;67:1414–1417.
161. Shikita J, Yamamuro T, Mikawa Y, Lida H, Kobori M. Atlantoaxial subluxation in Down's syndrome. Int Orthop 1989;13:187–192.
162. Stein SM, Kirchner SG, Horev G, Hernanz-Schulman M. Atlanto-occipital subluxation in Down syndrome. Pediatr Radiol 1991;21:121–124.
163. Thalman H, Scholl H, Tonz O. Spontane atlas Dislokation bei einem Kind mit Trisomie 21 an rheumatoider Arthritis. Helv Paediatr Acta 1972;27:391–403.
164. Tischler J, Martel W. Dislocation of the atlas in mongolism: preliminary report. Radiology 1965;84:904–906.
165. Tredwell SJ, Newman DE, Lockitch G. Instability of the upper cervical spine in Down syndrome. J Pediatr Orthop 1990;10:602–606.
166. Van Dyke DC, Gahogan CA. Down syndrome: cervical spine abnormalities and problems. Clin Pediatr 1986;27:362–365.
167. Whaley WJ, Gray WD. Atlanto-axial dislocation and Down's syndrome. Can Med Assoc J 1980;123:35–37.

Diagnostic Imaging

168. Bailey DK. The normal cervical spine in infants and children. Radiology 1952;59:712–719.
169. Brandner ME. Normal values of the vertebral body and intervertebral disk index during growth. AJR 1970;110:618–627.
170. Cadoux CG, White JD. High-yield radiograph considerations for cervical spine injuries. Ann Emerg Med 1986;15:236–239.
171. Clark WM, Gehweiler JA, Laib R. Twelve significant signs of cervical spine trauma. Skeletal Radiol 1979;3:201–205.
172. Colter HB, Kulkarni MV, Bondurant FJ. Magnetic resonance imaging of acute spinal cord trauma: preliminary report. J Orthop Trauma 1988;2:1–4.
173. Daffner RH, Deeb ZL, Rothfus WE. "Fingerprints" of vertebral trauma—a unifying concept based on mechanisms. Skeletal Radiol 1986;15:518–525.
174. Gabriel KR, Crawford AH. Identification of acute posttraumatic spinal cord cyst by magnetic resonance imaging: a case report and review of the literature. J Pediatric Orthop 1988;8:710–714.
175. Hegenbarth R, Ebel K-D. Roentgen findings in fractures of the vertebral column in childhood. Pediatr Radiol 1976;5:34–39.
176. Hinck BC, Hopkins CE, Savara CS. Sagittal diameter of the cervical spinal canal in children. Radiology 1962;79:97–108.
177. Keene JS, Goletz TH, Lilleas F, et al. Diagnosis of vertebral fractures. J Bone Joint Surg Am 1982;64:586–594.
178. Kim KS, Rogers LF, Regenbogen V. Pitfalls in plain film diagnosis of cervical spine injuries: false positive interpretation. Surg Neurol 1986;25:381–392.
179. Locke GR, Gardner JI, Van Epps EF. Atlas-dens interval (ADI) in children's survey based on two hundred normal cervical spines. AJR 1966;97:135–140.
180. Markuske H. Sagittal diameter measurement of the bony cervical spinal canal in children. Pediatr Radiol 1977;6:129–131.
181. Mathis JM, Wilson JT, Barnard JW, Zelenck ME. MR imaging of spinal cord avulsion. AJNR 1988;9:1232–1233.
182. Mazur JM, Stauffer ES. Unrecognized spinal instability associated with seemingly "simple" cervical compression fractures. Spine 1983;8:687–692.
183. McAfee OC, Yuan HA, Frederickson BE, Lubicky JP. The value of computed tomography in thoracolumbar fractures. J Bone Joint Surg Am 1983;65:461–473.
184. Mendelsohn DB, Zollars L, Weatherall PT, Gerison M. MR of cord transection. J Comput Assist Tomogr 1990;14:909–911.
185. Miller DL. Radiology of the cervical spine in trauma patients. AJR 1991;156:638–639.
186. Mirvis SE, Diaconis JN, Chirico PA, et al. Protocol driven radiologic evaluation of suspected cervical spine injury. Radiology 1989;170:831–834.
187. Naik DR. Cervical spinal canal in normal infants. Clin Radiol 1970;21:323–326.
188. Penning L. Prevertebral hematomas in cervical spine injury: incidence and etiologic significance. AJR 1981;136:553–561.
189. Rachesky I, Boyce WT, Duncan B, et al. Clinical prediction of cervical spine injuries in children: radiographic abnormalities. Am J Dis Child 1987;141:199–201.
190. Resio IM, Harwood-Nash DC, Fitz CR, Chuang S. Normal cord in infants and children examined with computed metrizamide myelography. Radiology 1979;130:691–696.
191. Ross SE, Schwab CCO, David ET, et al. Clearing the cervical spine: initial radiological evaluation. J Trauma 1987;27:1055–1060.
192. Schmada K, Tokioka T. Sequential MRI studies in patients with cervical cord injury but without bony injury. Paraplegia 1995;33:573–578.

193. Shaffer MA, Doris PE. Limitations of the cross-table lateral view in detecting spinal injuries. Ann Emerg Med 1981;10:508–513.
194. Shen WC, Lee SK, Ho YJ, Lee KR, Mar SC, Chi CS. MRI of sequela of transverse myelitis. Pediatr Radiol 1992;22:382–383.
195. Silberstein M, McLean K. Non-contiguous spinal injury: clinical and imaging features, and postulated mechanism. Paraplegia 1994;32:817–823.
196. Summers RL, Galli RL. Determining the probability of detecting cervical spine fractures with computed tomographic scans using the visible human database. Emerg Radiol 1997;26:7–9.
197. Swischuk LE. The cervical spine in childhood. Curr Probl Diagn Radiol 1984;13:1–26.
198. Templeton PA, Young JWR, Mirvis SE, Buddemeyer EU. The value of retropharyngeal soft tissue measurements in trauma of the adult cervical spine. Skeletal Radiol 1987;16:98–104.
199. Tracy PT, Wright RM, Hanigan WC. Magnetic resonance imaging of spinal injury. Spine 1989;14:292–301.
200. Weng MS, Haynes RJ. Flexion and extension cervical MRI in a pediatric population. J Pediatr Orthop 1996;16:359–363.
201. Whalen JP, Woodruff CL. The cervical prevertebral fat stripe: a new aid in evaluating the cervical prevertebral soft tissue space. AJR 1970;109:445–451.
202. Wojcik WG, Edeiken-Monroe BS, Harris JH Jr. Three-dimensional computed tomography in acute cervical spine trauma: a preliminary report. Skeletal Radiol 1987;16:261–269.
203. Woodring JH, Lee C. Limitation of cervical radiography in the evaluation of acute cervical trauma. J Trauma 1993;34:32–39.

Cervical Subluxation

204. Cattell HS, Filtzer DL. Pseudosubluxation and other normal variations in the cervical spine in children. J Bone Joint Surg Am 1965;47:1295–1309.
205. Czynski A. Excessive physiological mobility of the cervical spine in children as a cause of diagnostic difficulties. Chir Nrzadow Ruchu Ortop Pol 1963;28:809–814.
206. Donaldson JS. Acquired torticollis in children and young adults. JAMA 1956;160:458–461.
207. Ginalski JM, Landry M, Gudinchet F, Schnyder P. Is tomography of intervertebral disc calcification useful in children? Pediatr Radiol 1992;22:59–61
208. Jacobson G, Bleeker HH. Pseudosubluxation of the axis in children. AJR 1959;82:472–477.
209. Jones ET, Hensinger RN. C2–C3 dislocation in a child. J Pediatr Orthop 1981;1:419–422.
210. Pasquier J. Calcification du disque intervertebral de l'enfant. Ann Chir 1975;16:249–253.
211. Pennecot GF, Leonard P, Peyrot DGS, et al. Traumatic ligamentous instability of the cervical spine in children. J Pediatr Orthop 1984;4:339–345.
212. Penning L. Normal movements of the cervical spine. AJR 1978;130:317–326.
213. Song K, Ogden JA, Ganey T, Guidera KJ. Contiguous discitis and osteomyelitis in children. J Pediatr Orthop 1997;17:470–477.
214. Sullivan CR, Bruwer AJ, Harris LE. Hypermobility of the cervical spine in children: a pitfall in the diagnosis of cervical dislocation. Am J Surg 1958;95:636–640.
215. Swischuk LE, Stansberry SD. Calcific discitis: MRI changes in discs without visible calcification. Pediatr Radiol 1991;21:365–366.
216. Townsend EH Jr, Rowe ML. Mobility of the upper cervical spine in health and disease. Pediatrics 1952;10:567–573.
217. Ventura N, Huguet R, Salvador A, Terricabras L, Cabrera AM. Intervertebral disc calcification in childhood. Int Orthop 1995;19:291–294.
218. Vinz H. Subluxation in the region of the cervical spine in children: causes and differential diagnosis. Arch Orthop Unfallchir 1964;56:531–542.

Grisel Syndrome

219. Berkheiser EJ. Post infectious non-traumatic dislocation of the atlanto-axial joint. AAOS Instr Course Lect 1949;6:248–252.
220. Blunck C. Über die Atlasluxation. Beitr Z Klin Chir 1955;162:285–289.
221. Boiten J, Hageman G, deGraaff R. The conservative treatment of patients presenting with Grisel's syndrome. Clin Neurol Neurosurg 1986;88:95–99.
222. Desfosses P. Un cas de maladie de Grisel: torticollis nasopharyngien par subluxation de l'atlas. Presse Med 1930;38:1179–1180.
223. Finsni-Gallotta G, Luzzatti G. Sublussazione laterale sublussazione rotatorie dell'atlante. Arch Orthop 1957;70:467–484.
224. Fitzwilliams DCL. Inflammatory dislocation of the atlas. BMJ 1934;2:107–109.
225. Grisel P. Enucleation de l'atlas et torticolis naso-pharyngien. Presse Med 1930;38:50–53.
226. Grobman LR, Stricker S. Grisel's syndrome. Ear Nose Throat J 1990;69:799–801.
227. Hanson A, Kraft JP, Adcock DW. Subluxation of the cervical vertebra due to pharyngitis. South Med J 1973;66:427–429.
228. Hess JH, Bronstein IP, Abelson SM. Atlanto-axial dislocations: unassociated with trauma and secondary to inflammatory foci in the neck. Am J Dis Child 1935;49:1137–1140.
229. Keuter EJW. Non-traumatic atlanto-axial dislocation associated with naso-pharyngeal infections (Grisel's disease). Acta Neurochir (Wien) 1969;21:11–22.
230. Marar BC, Balachandrian N. Non-traumatic atlanto-axial dislocation in children. Clin Orthop 1973;92:220–226.
231. Mathern GW, Batzdoof U. Grisel's syndrome. Clin Orthop 1989;244:131–146.
232. Moyson R, Wattiez R. Le faux torticolis aigu. Acta Paediatr Belg 1966;20:259–263.
233. Parke WW, Rothman RH, Brown MD. The pharyngovertebral veins: an anatomic rationale for Grisel's syndrome. J Bone Joint Surg Am 1984;66:560–574.
234. Pinckney LE, Currarino G, Higenbothem L. Osteomyelitis of the cervical spine following dental extraction. Radiology 1980;135:335–337.
235. Pinkham JR. Inflammatory subluxation of the atlanto-axial joint. South Med J 1976;69:1507–1509.
236. Rintala AE. Cervical spondylitis as a complication of secondary cleft palate surgery—a rare variety of the "maladie de Grisel." Scand J Plastic Recontr Surg 1984;18:253–255.
237. Sanner G, Bergstrom B. Benign paroxysmal torticollis in infancy. Acta Paediatr Scand 1979;58:219–223.
238. Sullivan AW. Subluxation of the atlanto-axial joint: sequel to inflammatory processes of the neck. J Pediatr 1949;35:451–464.
239. Washington ER. Non-traumatic atlanto-occipital and atlanto-axial dislocation: a case report. J Bone Joint Surg Am 1959;41:341–344.
240. Watson-Jones R. Spontaneous hyperaemic dislocation of the atlas. Proc R Soc Med 1931;25:586–590.
241. Watson-Jones R. Spontaneous dislocation of the atlas. Proc R Soc Med 1932;25:785–787.
242. Wetzel FT, Rocca HL. Grisel's syndrome: a review. Clin Orthop 1989;240:141–152.
243. Wittek A. Ein fall von distensionluxation im atlantoepistropheal gelenke. Munch Med Wochenschr 1908;55:1936–1939.

244. Wongsiriamnuey S. Grisel's syndrome: a case report. J Med Assoc Thailand 1991;74:292–294.

SCIWORA

245. Ahmann PA, Smith SA, Schwartz JF, Clark DB. Spinal cord infarction due to minor trauma in children. Neurology 1975;25:301–307.
246. Chesire DJE. The paediatric syndrome of traumatic myelopathy without demonstrable vertebral injury. Paraplegia 1971;15:74–85.
247. Choi J-U, Hoffman HJ, Hendrick EB, Humphreys RP, Keith WS. Traumatic infarction of the spinal cord in children. J Neurosurg 1986;65:608–610.
248. Di Chiro G, Grilles FH. Blood flow currents in spinal cord arteries. Neurology 1971;21:1088–1094.
249. Di Chiro G, Wener L. Angiography of the spinal cord. J Neurosurg 1973;39:1–29.
250. Gellan S, Talov IM. Differential vulnerability of spinal cord structure to anoxia. J Neurophysiol 1955;18:170–174.
251. Hachen HJ. Spinal cord injury in children and adolescents: diagnostic pitfalls and therapeutic considerations in the acute stage. Paraplegia 1977;15:55–64.
252. Hardy AG. Cervical spinal cord injury without bony injury. Paraplegia 1977;14:296–305.
253. Hassler O. Blood supply to human spinal cord. Arch Neurol 1966;15:301–307.
254. Hegenbarth R, Ebel KD. Roentgen findings in fractures of the vertebral column in childhood: examination of 35 patients and its results. Pediatr Radiol 1976;5:34–39.
255. Henson RA, Parsons M. Ischaemic lesions of the spinal cord. Q J Med 1967;36:205–222.
256. Hughes JT. Venous infarction of the spinal cord. Neurology 1971;21:794–800.
257. Krogh E. The effect of acute hypoxia on the motor cells of the spinal cord. Acta Physiol Scand 1950;20:263–292.
258. Laguna J, Craviolo H. Spinal cord infarction secondary to occlusion of the anterior spinal artery. Arch Neurol 1973;28:134–136.
259. Lazorthes G. Arterial vascularization of the spinal cord: recent studies of the anastomotic substitution pathways. J Neurosurg 1971;35:253–262.
260. Le Blanc HJ, Nadel J. Spinal cord injuries in children. Surg Neurol 1974;2:411–414.
261. Osenbach RK, Menezes AH. Spinal cord injury without radiographic abnormality in children. Pediatr Neurosci 1989;15:128–174.
262. Pang D, Wilberger JE Jr. Spinal cord injury without radiographic abnormalities in children. J Neurosurg 1982;97:114–129.
263. Puller AR. The mechanism of injury to the spinal cord in the neck without damage to the vertebral column. J Bone Joint Surg [Am] 1951;33:543–550.
264. Scher AT. Trauma of the spinal cord in children. South Afr Med J 1976;50:2023–2025.
265. Taylor AR. The mechanism of injury to the spinal cord in the neck without damage to the vertebral column. J Bone Joint Surg Br 1951;33:543–547.
266. Vines FS. The significance of "occult" fractures of the cervical spine. AJR 1969;107:93–504.
267. Walsh JW, Stevens DB, Young AB. Traumatic paraplegia in children without contiguous spinal fracure or dislocation. Neurosurgery 1983;12:439–445.
268. Yngve DA, Harris WP, Herndon WA, et al. Spinal cord injury without osseous fracture. J Pediatr Orthop 1988;2:153–159.

Halo Fixation

269. Baum JS, Hanley EN Jr, Pullehines J. Comparison of halo complications in infants and children. Spine 1989;14:251–252.
270. Bottle MJ, Byrne TP, Garfin SR. Use of skin incisions in the application of halo skeletal fixator pins. Clin Orthop 1989;246:100–101.
271. Dorfmüller G, Höllerhage H-G. Severe intracranial injury from a fall in the halo external fixator. J Orthop Trauma 1992;6:366–369.
272. Dormans JP, Criscitiello AA, Drummond DS, Davidson RS. Complications in children managed with immobilization in a halo vest. J Bone Joint Surg Am 1995;77:1370–1373.
273. Ebraheim NA, Lu J, Biyani A, Brown JA. Anatomic considerations of halo pin placement. Am J Orthop 1996;22:754–756.
274. Garfin SR, Bottle MJ, Waters RL, Nickel VL. Complications in the use of the halo fixation device. J Bone Joint Surg Am 1986;68:320–325.
275. Garfin SR, Roux R, Bottle MJ, et al. Skull osteology as it affects halo pin placement in children. J Pediatr Orthop 1986;6:434–436.
276. Goodman ML, Nelson PB. Brain abscess complicating the use of a halo orthosis. Neurosurgery 1987;20:27–30.
277. Graziano GP, Hensinger RN. The halo-Ilizarov distraction cast for correction of cervical deformity. J Bone Joint Surg Am 1993;75:996–1003.
278. Haas LL. Roentgenological skull measurements and their diagnostic application. AJR 1952;67:197–209.
279. Jeanneret B, Magerl F, Ward JC. Over distraction: a hazard of skull traction in the management of acute injuries of the cervical spine. Arch Orthop Trauma Surg 1991;110:242–245.
280. Kopits SE, Sterngass M. Experience with the "halo-cast" in small children. Surg Clin North Am 1970;50:935–943.
281. Letts M, Kaylor K, Gouw G. A biomechanical analysis of halo fixation in children. J Bone Joint Surg Br 1988;70:277–279.
282. Mubarek SJ, Camp JF, Vuletich W, Wenger DR, Garfin SR. Halo application in the infant. J Pediatr Orthop 1989;9:612–614.

Cervical Injury (General)

283. Apple JS, Kirks DR, Merten DF, Martinez S. Cervical spine fractures and dislocations in children. Pediatr Radiol 1987;17:45–49.
284. Barcat E, Rigault P, Padovani JP, Martin P. Fractures et luxations du rachis cervical chez l'enfant. Ann Chir Infant 1976;17:197–206.
285. Bensahel H. Luxations et fractures du rachis cervical chez l'enfant. Rev Chir Orthop 1968;54:765–773.
286. Dunlap JP, Morris M, Thompson RG. Cervical spine injuries in children. J Bone Joint Surg Am 1958;40:681–686.
287. Ehara S, El-Khoury GY, Sato Y. Cervical spine injury in children: radiological manifestations. AJR 1988;151:1175–1178.
288. Fuch S, Barthel MJ, Flannery AM, Christoffel KK. Cervical spine fractures sustained by young children in forward-facing car seats. Pediatrics 1989;84:348–354.
289. Gaufin LM, Goodman SJ. Cervical spine injuries in infants: problems in management. J Neurosurg 1975;42:179–184.
290. Hasue M, Hoshino R, Omata S, et al. Cervical spine injuries in children. Fukushima J Med Sci 1974;20:115–121.
291. Hill SA, Miller CA, Kosnik EJ, Hunt WE. Pediatric neck injuries. J Neurosurg 1984;60:700–706.
292. Holmes JC, Hall JE. Fusion for instability and potential instability of the cervical spine in children and adolescents. Orthop Clin North Am 1976;9:923–943.

293. Huerta C, Griffin R, Joyce SM. Cervical spine stabilization in pediatric patients: evaluation of current techniques. Ann Emerg Med 1987;16:1121–1126.
294. Jaffe DM, Binns H, Radkowski MA, et al. Developing a clinical algorithm for early management of cervical spine injury in child injuries. Ann Emerg Med 1987;16:270–276.
295. Mahale YJ, Silver JR, Henderson NJ. Neurological complications of the reduction of cervical spine dislocations. J Bone Joint Surg Br 1993;75:403–409.
296. McCabe JB, Angelos MG. Injury to the head and face in patients with cervical spine injury. Am J Emerg Med 1984;13:512–515.
297. McCoy GF, Piggot J, Macafee AL, Adair IV. Injuries of the cervical spine in schoolboy rugby football. J Bone Joint Surg Br 1984;66:500–503.
298. McGrory BJ, Klassen RA. Arthrodesis of the cervical spine for fractures and dislocations in children and adolescents. J Bone Joint Surg Am 1994;76:1606–1616.
299. McGrory BJ, Klassen RA, Chao EY, Staheli JW, Weaver AL. Acute fractures and dislocations of the cervical spine in children and adolescents. J Bone Joint Surg Am 1993;75:988–995.
300. Murphy MJ, Ogden JA, Bucholz RW. Cervical spine injury in the child. Contemp Orthop 1981;3:615–624.
301. Nitecki S, Moir CR. Predictive factors of the outcome of traumatic cervical spine fracture in children. J Pediatr Surg 1994;29:1409–1411.
302. Rachesky I, Boyce WT, Duncan B, et al. Clinical prediction of cervical spine injuries in children: radiographic abnormalities. Am J Dis Child 1987;141:199–201.
303. Sherk HH, Schut L, Lane JM. Fractures and dislocations of the cervical spine in children. Orthop Clin North Am 1976;17:593–601.
304. Stauffer ES, Mazur JM. Cervical spine injuries in children. Pediatr Ann 1982;11:502–511.
305. Swanepoel HC, Mennen U. Neck injuries in children. S Afr Med J 1983;63:152–157.
306. Taylor AS. Fracture-dislocation of the cervical spine. Ann Surg 1929;90:321–327.
307. Toyama Y, Matsumoto M, Chilz K, et al. Realignment of postoperative cervical kyphosis in children by vertebral remodeling. Spine 1994;22:2565–2570.
308. Vigouroux RP, Baurand C, Choux M, Pellet W, Guillerman P. Les traumatismes du rachis cervical chez l'enfant. Neurochirurgie 1968;14:689–702.
309. Wagner A. Traumatic luxation of cervical vertebra in children. Wiad Lek 1965;18:65–69.

Abuse

310. Babcock JL. Spinal injuries in children. Pediatr Clin North Am 1979;22:487–500.
311. Caffey J. The whiplash shaken infant syndrome. Pediatrics 1974;54:396–403.
312. Cullen JC. Spinal lesions in battered babies. J Bone Joint Surg Br 1975;57:364–366.
313. Kleinman PK, Zito JL. Avulsion of the spinous processes caused by infant abuse. Radiology 1984;151:389–391.
314. Kogutt MS, Swischuk LE, Fagan CJ. Patterns in injury and significance of uncommon fractures in the battered child syndrome. AJR 1974;121:143–149.
315. McGrory BE, Fenichel GM. Hangman's fracture subsequent to shaking in an infant. Ann Neurol 1977;2:82–84.
316. Romer KH, Wolff F. On spinal injuries due to mistreatment in very small children. Arch Orthop Unfallchir 1963;55:203–211.
317. Sumchai AP, Sternbach GL. Hangman's fracture in a 7 week old infant. Ann Emerg Med 1991;20:119–122.

Birth Injury

318. Abroms IF, Bresnan MJ, Zuckerman JE, et al. Cervical cord injuries secondary to hyperextension of the head in breech presentation. Obstet Gynecol 1973;41:369–378.
319. Adams C, Babyn PS, Logan WJ. Spinal cord birth injury: value of computed tomographic myelography. Pediatr Neurol 1988;4:105–109.
320. Alexander E, Masland R, Harris C. Anterior dislocation of first cervical vertebra simulating cerebral birth injury in infancy. Am J Dis Child 1953:85:173–181.
321. Allen JP, Birth injury to the spinal cord. Northwest Med 1920;69:323–326.
322. Allen JP, Myers GG, Condon VR. Laceration of the spinal cord related to breech delivery. JAMA 1969;208:1019–1022.
323. Behrman SJ. Fetal cervical hyperextension. Clin Obstet Gynecol 1962;5:1018–1030.
324. Bell HT, Dykstra DD. Somatosensory evoked potentials as an adjunct to diagnosis of neonatal spinal cord injury. J Pediatr 1985;106:298–301.
325. Biemond A. Birth injury of the spinal cord. Ned Tijdschr Geneeskd 1962;106:105–108.
326. Brans YW, Cassady G. Neonatal spinal cord injuries. Am J Obstet Gynecol 1975;123:918–919.
327. Bresnan MJ, Abroms IF. Neonatal spinal cord transection secondary to intrauterine hyperextension of the neck in breech presentation. J Pediatr 1974;5:734–737.
328. Bucher HV, Boltshauser E, Friderich J, Isler W. Birth injury to the spinal cord. Helv Pediatr Acta 1979;34:517–527.
329. Burr CW. Hemorrhage into the spinal cord at birth. Am J Dis Child 1920;19:473–478.
330. Byers RK. Transection of the spinal cord in the newborn: a case with autopsy and comparison with a normal cord at the same age. Arch Neurol Psychiatry 1932;27:585–592.
331. Byers RK. Spinal cord injuries during birth. Dev Med Child Neurol 1975;17:103–110.
332. Crothers B. Injury of the spinal cord in breech extraction as an important cause of fetal death and of paraplegia in childhood. Am J Med Sci 1923;165:94–102.
333. Crothers B, Putnam MC. Obstetrical injuries of the spinal cord. Medicine 1927;6:41–46.
334. Daw E. Hyperextension of the head in breech presentation. Br J Clin Pract 1970;24:485–487.
335. Deacon AL. Hyperextension of the head in a breech presentation. J Obstet Gynecol 1951;58:300–301.
336. De Souza SW, Davis JA. Spinal cord damage in a new-born infant. Arch Dis Child 1974;49:70–71.
337. Duncan JM. Laboratory note: On the tensile strength of the fresh adult foetus. BMJ 1874;2:763–765.
338. Ehrenfest H. Injuries of the vertebral column and spinal cord in birth injuries in the child. In: Ehrenfest H (ed) Birth Injuries. New York: Appleton, 1931.
339. Enriquez G, Also C, Lucaya J, Creixell S, Fernandez E. Traumatic cord lesions in the newborn infant. Ann Radiol (Paris) 1976;19:179–186.
340. Evrard JR, Hilrich N. Hyperextension of the fetal head in breech presentations. Obstet Gynecol 1955;5:789–792.
341. Falls FH. Opisthotonus foetus. Surg Gynecol Obstet 1917;24:65–67.
342. Foderl V. Die halsmarkquetschung, eine unter art der geburtstraumatischen Schädigung des Zentralnervensystems. Arch Gynaekol 1930;143:598–634.
343. Ford FR. Breech delivery and its possible relations to injury of the spinal cord. Arch Neurol Psychiatry 1925;14:742–747.
344. Franken EA Jr. Spinal cord injury in the newborn infant. Pediatr Radiol 1975;3:101–104.

345. Gilles FH, Bina M, Setrel A. Infantile atlantooccipital instability: the potential danger of extreme extension. Am J Dis Child 1979;133:30–37.
346. Glasauer FE, Cares HL. Traumatic paraplegia in infancy. JAMA 1972;219:38–41.
347. Glasauer FE, Cares HL. Biomechanical features of traumatic paraplegia in infancy. J Trauma 1973;13:166–170.
348. Guilhem P, Pontonnier A, Baux R. Deux cas de presentation du siege avec hyperextension du cou. Bull Fed Soc Gynecol Obstet Lang Fr 1951;3:706–707.
349. Hellstrom B, Sallmander V. Prevention of spinal cord injury in hyperextension of the fetal head. JAMA 1968;204:1041–1044.
350. Hillman JW, Sprofkin BE, Parrish TF. Birth injury of the cervical spine producing a "cerebral palsy" syndrome. Am Surg 1954;20:900–906.
351. Hoffmeister HP. Beitrag zur Wirbelsaulenverletzung beim Neugebornen. Geb Frauenheilkd 1964;24:1085–1090.
352. Hoffmeister HP. Contribution to spinal injury in newborn infants. Fortschr Rontgenstr 1964;101:190–195.
353. Jellinger K, Schwingshackl A. Birth injury of the spinal cord. Neuropaediatrics 1973;4:111–123.
354. Jones EL. Birth trauma and the cervical spine. Arch Dis Child 1970;45:147–156.
355. Koch BM, Eng GM. Neonatal spinal cord injury. Arch Phys Med Rehabil 1979;60:378–381.
356. Lacoste A. Sur le développements de l'écaille occipitale étudie comparative chez le mouton et chez l'homme. Arch Anat Histol Embryol 1930;12:1–47.
357. Laffont A. Un cas de presentation du siege avec foetus en hyperextension: rupture de sac dure merien pendant l'extraction. Bull Fed Soc Obstet Gynecol Lang Fr 1919;18:50–54.
358. Lanska MJ, Roessmann U, Wiznitzer M. Magnetic resonance imaging in cervical cord birth injury. Pediatrics 1990;85:760–764.
359. Lazar MR, Salvaggio AT. Hyperextension of the fetal head in breech presentation. Obstet Gynecol 1959;14:198–199.
360. Leventhal HR. Birth injuries of the spinal cord. J Pediatr 1960;56:447–453.
361. Longley JD, Trueman GE. Fetal cervical hyperextension. J Can Assoc Radiol 1961;12:96–98.
362. Marion J, Daudet M, Carron JJ, et al. Luxation obstetricale de la colonne cervicale. Ann Chir Infant 1969;10:193–201.
363. Norman MG, Wedderburn LC. Fetal spinal cord injury with cephalic delivery. Obstet Gynecol 1973;42:355–358.
364. Pierson RN. Spinal and cranial injuries of the baby in breech deliveries. Surg Gynecol Obstet 1923;37:802–806.
365. Ross P. Neonatal spinal cord injury. Orthop Rev 1980;9:95–97.
366. Sabouraud O, Coutel Y, Pecker J. 2 cas de lesions spinales d'origine obstetricale. Rev Neurol (Paris) 1959;101:766–769.
367. Shulman ST, Madden JD, Esterly JR, Shanklin DR. Transection of spinal cord: a rare obstetrical complication of cephalic delivery. Arch Dis Child 1971;46:291–294.
368. Stern WE, Rand RW. Birth injuries to the spinal cord. Am J Obstet Gynecol 1959;78:498–512.
369. Stoltzenberg F. Zerreissungen der intervertebralen Gelenkkapseln der Halswirbelsaule: eine typische Geburtsverletzung. Berl Klin Wochenschr 1911;2:1741–1745.
370. Towbin A. Spinal cord and brain stem injury at birth. Arch Pathol 1964;77:620–632.
371. Towbin A. Spinal injury related to the syndrome of sudden death ("crib death") in infants. Am J Clin Pathol 1968;49:562–567.
372. Towbin A. Latent spinal cord and brain stem injury in newborn infants. Dev Med Child Neurol 1969;11:54–68.
373. Towbin A. Central nervous system damage in the human fetus and newborn infant. Am J Dis Child 1970;119:529–542.
374. Warwick M. Necropsy findings in newborn infants. Am J Dis Child 1921;21:488–496.
375. Yates PO. Birth trauma to vertebral arteries. Arch Dis Child 1959;34:436–441.
376. Zellweger H. Über geburtstraumatische Bruckenmarksläsionen. Helv Paediatr Acta 1945;1:13–30.

Occipital Injury

377. Anderson PA, Montesano PX. Morphology and treatment of occipital condyle fractures. Spine 1988;13:731–736.
378. Ashkenszi E, Carmon M, Pasternak D, Israel F, Beni L, Pomeranz S. Conservative treatment of a traumatic subdural hematoma of the posterior fossa in a child: case report. J Trauma 1994;36:406–407.
379. Cottalorda J, Allard D, Dutour N. Fracture of the occipital condyle: case report. J Pediatr Orthop Part B 1996;5:61–63.
380. Leventhal MR, Boydstron WR, Sebeg JI, Pinstein ML, Lostridge CB, Lowery R. The diagnosis and treatment of fractures of the occipital condyle. Orthopedics 1992;15:944–947.
381. Stroobants J, Seynaeve P, Fidlers L, et al. Occipital condyle fracture must be considered in the pediatric population: case report. J Trauma 1994;36:440–441.
382. Wessels LS. Fracture of the occipital condyle: a report of 3 cases. S Afr J Surg 1990;28:155–156.

Occipital-Atlantal Injury

383. Badelon O, Bensahel H. Fracture separation du massif articulaire du rachis cervical chez l'enfant. Rev Chir Orthop 1984;70:83–85.
384. Bernini FP, Elefante R, Smatrino F, Tedeschi G. Angiographic study on the vertebral artery in cases of deformities of the occipitovertebral joint. AJR 1969;107:526–529.
385. Bools JC, Rose BS. Traumatic atlanto-occipital dislocation: two cases with survival. AJNR 1986;7:901–904.
386. Bucholz RW, Burkhead WZ. The pathologic anatomy of fatal atlantooccipital dislocations. J Bone Joint Surg Am 1979;61:248–250.
387. Collalto PM, DeMuth WW, Schwentker EP, Boal DK. Traumatic atlantooccipital dislocation. J Bone Joint Surg Am 1986;68:1106–1109.
388. Dublin AB, Marks WM, Weinstock D, Newton TH. Traumatic dislocation of the atlanto-occipital articulation (AOA) with short-term survival. J Neurosurg 1980;52:541–546.
389. Evarts CM. Traumatic occipito-atlantal dislocation: report of a case with survival. J Bone Joint Surg Am 1970;52:1653–1660.
390. Farley FA, Graziano GP, Hensinger RN. Traumatic atlanto-occipital dislocation in a child. Spine 1992;17:1539–1541.
391. Gabrielsen O, Maxwell JA. Traumatic atlanto-occipital dislocation. AJR 1966;97:624–629.
392. Georgopoulos G, Pizzutillo PD, Lee MS. Occipito-atlantal instability in children. J Bone Joint Surg Am 1987;69:429–436.
393. Gilles FH, Bina M, Sotrel A. Infantile atlanto-occipital instability: the potential danger of extreme extension. Am J Dis Child 1979;133:30–37.
394. Hosono N, Yonenobu K, Kawagoe K, Hirayamanan, Ono K. Traumatic anterior atlanto-occipital dislocation: a case report with survival. Spine 1993;18:786–790.
395. Jovtich V. Traumatic lateral atlanto-occipital dislocation with spontaneous bony fusion. Spine 1989;14:123–124.
396. Kaufman RA, Carroll CD, Buncher CR. Atlanto-occipital junction: standards for measurement in normal children. AJNR 1987;8:995–999.

397. Kaufman RA, Dunbar JS, Botford JA, McLaurin RL. Traumatic longitudinal atlanto-occipital distraction injuries in children. AJNR 1982;3:415–419.
398. Kawabe N, Hirotani H, Tanoka O. Pathomechanism of atlanto-axial rotatory fixation in children. J Pediatr Orthop 1989;9:569–574.
399. Lee C, Woodring JH, Goldstein SJ, et al. Evaluation of traumatic atlanto-occipital dislocations. AJNR 1987;8:19–26.
400. Matava MJ, Whitesides TE Jr, Davis PC. Traumatic atlanto-occipital dislocation with survival serial computerized tomography as an aid to diagnosis and reduction. Spine 1993;18:1897–1903.
401. Maves CK, Souza A, Prenger EC, Kirks DR. Traumatic atlanto-occipital disruption in children. Pediatr Radiol 1991;21:504–507.
402. Page CP, Stoory JL, Wissinger JP, Branch CL. Traumatic atlanto-occipital dislocation: case report. J Neurosurg 1973;39:394–397.
403. Nischal K, Chumas P, Sparrow O. Prolonged survival after atlanto-occipital dislocation: two case reports and review. Br J Neurol 1993;7:677–682.
404. Pang D, Wilberger JE. Traumatic atlanto-occipital dislocation with survival: case report and a review. Neurosurgery 1987;7:503–508.
405. Parrot J. Note sur un case de rupture de la moelle chez un nouveau: ne par suite des manoevres pendant l'accouchement. Bull Mem Soc Med Paris 1869;6:38–40.
406. Powers B, Miller MD, Kramer RS, Martinez S, Gehwerler JA. Traumatic anterior atlanto-occipital dislocation. Neurosurgery 1979;4:12–17.
407. Ramsey AH, Waxman BP, O'Brien JF. A case of traumatic atlanto-occipital dislocation with survival. Injury 1986;17:412–420.
408. Sponseller PD, Cass JR. Atlanto-occipital fusion for dislocation in children with neurologic preservation. Spine 1997;22:344–347.
409. Traynelis VC, Marano GD, Dunbar RO, Kaufman HA. Traumatic atlanto-occipital dislocation: a case report. J Neurosurg 1986;65:863–870.
410. Van Don Bout AA, Domisse GF. Traumatic atlanto-occipital dislocation. Spine 1986;11:174–176.
411. Werne S. Studies in spontaneous atlas dislocation. Acta Orthop Scand 1957;28(suppl 23):11–83.
412. Wiesel S, Kraus D, Rothman RH. Atlanto-occipital hypermobility. Orthop Clin North Am 1978;9:969–972.
413. Woodring JM, Selke AC Jr, Duff DE. Traumatic atlanto-occipital dislocation with survival. AJR 1981;137:21–24.

C1 Injury

414. Budin E, Sondheimer F. Lateral spread of the atlas without fracture. Radiology 1952;59:713–719.
415. Dalinka MK, Rosenbaum AE, Van Houten F. Congenital absence of the posterior arch of the atlas. Radiology 1972;103:581–583.
416. Galindo MJ, Francis WR. Atlantal fracture in a child through congenital anterior and posterior arch defects. Clin Orthop 1983;178:220–222.
417. Garber JN. Abnormalities of the atlas and axis vertebrae: congenital and traumatic. J Bone Joint Surg Am 1964;46:1782–1791.
418. Gehweiler JA Jr, Daffner RH, Robert L Jr. Malformations of the atlas vertebra simulating the Jefferson fracture. AJR 1983;140:1083–1086.
419. Haakonsen M, Gudmundsen TE, Histøl O. Midline anterior and posterior atlas clefts may simulate a Jefferson fracture. Acta Orthop Scand 1995;66:369–371.
420. Jefferson G. Fractures of the atlas vertebra. Br J Surg 1920;7:407–412.
421. Landell SCD, VanPeteghem PK. Fractures of the atlas: classification, treatment and immobility. Spine 1988;13:450–492.
422. Logan WW, Stuard ID. Absent posterior arch of the atlas. AJR 1973;18:431–434.
423. Lui TN, Lee ST, Wong CW, et al. C1–C2 fracture-dislocations in children and adolescents. J Trauma 1996;40:408–411.
424. Marlin AE, Gayle RW, Lee JF. Jefferson fractures in children. J Neurosurg 1983;58:277–279.
425. Mikawa Y, Watanabe R, Yamano Y, Ishii K. Fracture through a synchondrosis of the anterior arch of the atlas. J Bone Joint Surg Br 1987;69:483.
426. Motateanu N, Gudinchet F, Sarraj H, Schnyder P. Case report 665: congenital absence of the posterior arch of the atlas. Skeletal Radiol 1991;20:231–232.
427. Nicholson JT. Surgical fixation of dislocation of the first cervical vertebra in children. NY State J Med 1956;56:3839–3843.
428. Ogden JA, Ganey TM, Olsen JH. Fractures of C1 and C2 in an infant gazelle. J Pediatr Orthop 1993;13:572–576.
429. Plant HF. Fracture of the atlas or development abnormality? Radiology 1937;29:227–229.
430. Richards PG. Stable fractures of the atlas and axis in children. J Neurol Neurosurg Psychiatry 1984;47:781–783.
431. Richardson EG, Boone SC, Reid RL. Intermittent quadriparesis associated with a congenital anomaly of the posterior arch of the atlas. J Bone Joint Surg Am 1975;57:853–854.
432. Routt ML Jr, Green NE. Case report: Jefferson fracture in a 2 year old child. J Trauma 1989;29:1710–1712.
433. Segal LS, Grimm JO, Stauffer ES. Nonunion of fracture of the atlas. J Bone Joint Surg Am 1987;69:1423–1434.
434. Sherk HH, Nicholson JT. Fractures of the atlas. J Bone Joint Surg Am 1970;52:1017–1024.
435. Suss RA, Zimmerman RD, Leeds NE. Pseudospread of the atlas: false sign of Jefferson fracture in young children. AJNR 1983;4:183–186.
436. Tippett GO. Atlanto-axial fracture dislocation: report of a case. J Bone Joint Surg Br 1951;33:108–109.
437. Tolo VT, Weiland AJ. Unsuspected atlas fracture and instability associated with oropharyngeal injury: case report. J Trauma 1979;19:278–280.
438. Wirth RL, Zatz LM, Parker BR. CT detection of a Jefferson fracture in a child. AJR 1987;149:1001–1002.

Atlantoaxial Instability

439. Allington NJ, Zembo M, Nadell J, Bowen JR. C1–C2 posterior soft-tissue injuries with neurologic impairment in children. J Pediatr Orthop 1990;10:596–601.
440. Altongy JF, Fielding JW. Combined atlanto-axial and occipito-atlantal rotatory subluxation. J Bone Joint Surg Am 1990;72:923–926.
441. Balau J, Hupfauer W. The differential diagnosis of injuries of the atlanto-axial joint in childhood. Arch Orthop Unfallchir 1974;78:343–355.
442. Barros TEP, Olivera RP, Rodriques NR, Greve JM, Basile R Jr. Atlanto-axial dislocation in children. Rev Paul Med 1992;110:11–13.
443. Bhatnagar M, Sponseller PD, Carroll C IV, Tolo VT. Pediatric atlanto-axial instability presenting as cerebral and cerebellar infarcts. J Pediatr Orthop 1991;11:103–107.
444. Bondarenkons ML, Kazitskii VM, Dougam BL. Dislocations and subluxation of the atlas in children. Ortop Travmatol Protez 1988;2:51–55.
445. Burkus JK, Deponte RJ. Chronic atlantoaxial rotatory fixation: correction by cervical traction, manipulation and bracing. J Pediatr Orthop 1986;6:631–635.

446. Carlioz H, Dubossett J. Les instabilites entre l'atlas et l'axis chez l'enfant. Rev Chir Orthop 1973;59:291–294.
447. Casey ATH, O'Brien M, Kumar V, Hayward RD, Crockard HA. Don't twist my child's head off: iatrogenic cervical dislocation. BMJ 1995;311:1212–1213.
448. Clark CR, Kathol MH, Walsh T, El-Khoury GY. Atlanto-axial rotatory fixation with compensatory counter occipito-atlantal subluxation: a case report. Spine 1986;11:1048–1050.
449. Dastur DK, Wadia NH, Desai AD, Sing G. Medullospinal compression due to atlanto-axial dislocation and sudden haematomyelia during decompression: pathology, pathogenesis and clinical correlations. Brain 1965;88:897–924.
450. De Beer J, Hoffman EB, Kieck CF. Traumatic atlanto-axial subluxation in children. J Pediatr Orthop 1990;10:397–400.
451. Dvorak J, Panjabi M, Gerger M, Wichmann R. CT functional diagnostics of the rotatory instability of upper cervical spine: an experimental study on cadavers. Spine 1987;12:197–206.
452. Ebraheim NA, Xu R, Ahmad M, Heck B. The effect of atlas anterior translation and rotation on axis canal size: a computer-assisted anatomic study. Am J Orthop 1998;27:29–33.
453. El-Khoury GY, Clark CR, Gravett AW. Acute traumatic rotatory atlanto-axial dislocation in children: a report of three cases. J Bone Joint Surg Am 1984;66:774–777.
454. Fielding JW, Cochran G, Lawsing JF, Hohl M. Tears of the transverse ligament of the atlas. J Bone Joint Surg Am 1984;56:1683–1691.
455. Fielding JW, Hawkins RJ. Atlanto-axial rotatory fixation. J Bone Joint Surg Am 1977;59:37–44.
456. Fielding JW, Hawkins RJ, Hensinger RN, Francis WR. Atlanto-axial rotary deformities. Orthop Clin North Am 1978;9:955–967.
457. Fielding JW, Hawkins RJ, Ratzan SA. Spine fusion for atlanto-axial instability. J Bone Joint Surg Am 1976;58:400–407.
458. Filipe G, Berges O, Lebard JP, Carlioz H. Post-traumatic instability between the atlas and the axis in children: apropos of 5 cases. Rev Chir Orthop 1982;68:461–469.
459. Floman Y, Kaplan L, Elidon J, Umansky F. Transverse ligament rupture and atlanto-axial subluxation in children. J Bone Joint Surg Br 1991;73:640–643.
460. Gonzalez Lopex DL, Forte G-T Martin JS, Durantez JAR, Yalverde SL. Chronic atlanto-axial rotatory fixation. J Pediatr Orthop 1991;28:99–101.
461. Greely RW. Bilateral (ninety degrees) rotatory dislocation of the atlas upon the axis. J Bone Joint Surg 1930;12:953–962.
462. Grogaard B, Dullend R, Magnaes B. Acute torticollis in children due to atlanto-axial rotatory fixation. Arch Orthop Trauma Surg 1993;112:185–186.
463. Hardy J, Poutiques JC, Livernaux P. Lusations traumatiques C1–C2 chez l'enfant: etude pronstiquet indications therapeutiques. Rev Chir Orthop 1990;76:17–22.
464. Harouchi A, Padovani JP, Andaloussi ME, Refass A. Des dislocations atlanto-axisiennes chez l'enfant. Chir Pediatr 1984;25:136–144.
465. Highland TR, Aronson DD. Traumatic rupture of the cranial ligament in a child with a normal odontoid process. Spine 1986;11:73–75.
466. Hohl M, Baker HR. The atlanto-axial joint: roentgenographic and anatomical study of normal and abnormal motion. J Bone Joint Surg Am 1954;46:1739–1752.
467. Jacobson G, Adler DC. Examination of the atlanto-axial joint following injury, with particular emphasis on rotational subluxation. AJR 1956;76:1081–1094.
468. Kawabe N, Hirotani H, Tanoka O. Pathomechansim of atlanto-axial rotatory fixation in children. J Pediatr Orthop 1989;9:569–574.
469. Mazzara JT, Fielding JW. Effect of C1–C2 rotation on canal size. Clin Orthop 1988;237:115–119.
470. Morani BC, Balanchandrian N. Non-traumatic atlanto-axial dislocation in children. Clin Orthop 1973;92:220–226.
471. Nagashimo C. Surgical treatment of irreducible atlanto-axial dislocation with spinal cord compression. J Neurosurg 1973;38:374–378.
472. Nerubay J, Lin E, Weiss J, et al. Posttraumatic atlanto-axial rotatory fixation. J Pediatr Orthop 1985;5:734–736.
473. Ono K, Yonenobu K, Fuji T, Okada R. Atlanto-axial rotatory fixation: radiographic study of its mechanism. Spine 1985;10:602–608.
474. Phillips WA, Hensinger RN. The management of rotatory atlanto-axial subluxation in children. J Bone Joint Surg Am 1989;71:664–668.
475. Rinaldi J, Mullins WJ Jr, Delaney WF, Filzer PM, Toonberg DN. Computerized tomographic demonstration of rotational atlanto-axial fixation: a case report. J Neurosurg 1979;50:115–119.
476. Roach JW, Duncan D, Wenger DR, Maraoilla A, Maravilla K. Atlanto-axial instability and spinal cord compression in children: diagnosis by computerized tomography. J Bone Joint Surg Am 1984;66:708–714.
477. Scapinelli R. Three-dimensional computed tomography in infantile atlanto-axial rotatory fixation. J Bone Joint Surg Br 1994;76:367–370.
478. Schwartz N. Die vertebrate rotations subluxation der Halswirbelsäule. Unfallchirurg 1992;95:367–374.
479. Shammiganothan K, Mirvis SE, Levine AM. Rotational injury of cervical facets: CT analysis of fracture patterns with implications for management and neurologic outcome. AJR 1994;163:1165–1169.
480. Sherk HH. Lesions of the atlas and axis. Clin Orthop 1975;109:33–41.
481. Swischuk LE. Anterior displacement of C2 in children: physiologic or pathologic. Radiology 1977;122:759–763.
482. Teng P, Papatheodorou C. Traumatic subluxation of C2 in young children. Bull Los Angeles Neurol Soc 1967;32:197–202.
483. Van Holsbeeck EMA, MacKay NNS. Diagnosis of acute atlanto-axial rotatory fixation. J Bone Joint Surg Br 1989;71:90–91.
484. Washington ER. Non-traumatic atlanto-occipital and atlanto-axial dislocation: a case report. J Bone Joint Surg Am 1959;41:341–344.
485. Wittek A. Ein fälle von distensionluxation in atlanto-epiphyseal gelenke. Munch Med Wochenschr 1908;55:1836–1837.
486. Wortzman G, Dewar FP. Rotatory fixation of the atlanto-axial joint: rotational atlanto-axial subluxation. Radiology 1968;90:479–487.

C2 Injury

487. Alp MS, Crockard HA. Late complication of undetected odontoid fracture in children. BMJ 1990;300:319–320.
488. Bachs A, Barraquer-Bodas L, Barraquer-Ferre L, et al. Delayed myelopathy following atlanto-axial dislocation by separated odontoid process. Brain 1955;78:537–553.
489. Bhattacharyya SK. Fracture and displacement of the odontoid process in a child. J Bone Joint Surg Am 1974;56:1071–1072.
490. Blockey NJ, Purser DW. Fractures of the odontoid process of the axis. J Bone Joint Surg Br 1956;38:794–817.
491. Buirski G, Booth A, Watt I. Case report 419: os odontoideum with an ossified pedicle lying between the os and the body of C2. Skeletal Radiol 1987;16:240–245.
492. Crockard HA. Anterior approaches to lesions of the upper cervical spine. Clin Neurosurg 1988;34:389–416.

493. Crockard HA, Heilman AE, Stevens JM. Progressive myelopathy secondary to odontoid fractures: clinical, radiological and surgical features. J Neurosurg 1993;78:579–586.
494. Currarino G. Primary spondylolysis of the axis vertebra (C2) in three children, including one with pyknodysostosis. Pediatr Radiol 1989;19:535–538.
495. Diekema DS, Allen D. Odontoid fracture in a child occupying a child restraint seat. Pediatrics 1988;82:117–119.
496. Dunn ME, Seljeskog EL. Experience in the management of odontoid process injuries: an analysis of 128 cases. Neurosurgery 1986;18:306–310.
497. Dyck P. Os odontoideum in children: neurological manifestations and surgical management. Neurosurgery 1978;2:93–99.
498. Evarts CM, Lonsdale D. Ossiculum terminale: an anomaly of the odontoid process; report of a case of atlanto-axial dislocation with cord compression. Cleve Clin Q 1970;37:73–76.
499. Ewald FC. Fracture of the odontoid process in a seventeen month old infant treated with a halo. J Bone Joint Surg Am 1971;53:1636–1640.
500. Fielding JW. Disappearance of the central portion of the odontoid process. J Bone Joint Surg Am 1965;47:1228–1230.
501. Fielding JW, Griffin PP. Os odontoideum: an acquired lesion. J Bone Joint Surg Am 1974;56:187–190.
502. Fielding JW, Hensinger RN, Hawkins RJ. Os odontoideum. J Bone Joint Surg Am 1980;62:376–383.
503. Finnegan MA, McDonald H. Hangman's fracture in an infant. Can Med Assoc J 1982;127:1001–1002.
504. Freiberger RH, Wilson PO, Nicholas JA. The odontoid process. J Bone Joint Surg Am 1965;47:1231–1236.
505. Gehweiler JA Jr, Martinez S, Clarke WM Miller MD, Stewart GC. Spondylolisthesis of the axis vertebrae. AJR 1977;128:682–686.
506. Giacomini C. Sull esistenza a dé "os odontoideum" nell' uomo. G R Acad Med Torino 1886;49:24–38.
507. Giannestras NJ, Mayfield FH, Provencis FP, Maurer J. Congenital absence of the odontoid process: case report. J Bone Joint Surg Am 1964;46:839–843.
508. Gille P, Bonneville JF, Francois JY, et al. Fracture des pedicules de l'axis chez hourrisson battu. Chir Pediatr 1980;21:343–344.
509. Gillman EL. Congenital absence of the odontoid process of the axis. J Bone Joint Surg Am 1959;41:345–348.
510. Granger DK, Rechtine GR. Os odontoideum: a review. Orthop Rev 1987;16:909–916.
511. Grosse L, Bohly J, Taglang G, Dosch JC, Kempf I. Osteosynthese par vissage des fractures de l'apophyse odontoide. Rev Chir Orthop 1991;77:425–431.
512. Griffiths SC. Fracture and displacement of the odontoid process in child. J Pediatr Surg 1972;7:680–683.
513. Gwinn JL, Smith JL. Acquired and congenital absence of the odontoid process. AJR 1962;88:424–431.
514. Handyside PS. On a remarkable dimunition of the medulla oblongata and adjacent portion of the spinal marrow, consequent upon spontaneous dislocation of the processus dentatus and ankylosis of the upper part of the spine—yet unattended with any signs of paralysis. Edinb Med Surg J 1840;53:376–379.
515. Hawkins RJ, Fielding JW, Thompson WJ. Os odontoideum: congenital or acquired. J Bone Joint Surg Am 1976;58:413–414.
516. Hensinger RN. Osseous abnormalities of the craniovertebral junction. Spine 1986;11:323–333.
517. Hensinger RN, Fielding JW, Hawkins RJ. Congenital anomalies of the odontoid process. Orthop Clin North Am 1978;9:901–912.
518. Hukuda S, Ota H, Okabe N, Tazima K. Traumatic atlanto-axial dislocation causing os odontoideum in infants. Spine 1980;5:207.
519. Jubl M, Seerip KK. Os odontoideum: a cause of atlanto-axial instability. Acta Orthop Scand 1983;54:113–118.
520. Kirlew KA, Hathout GM, Reiter SD, Gold RH. Os odontoideum in identical twins: perspectives on etiology. Skeletal Radiol 1993;22:525–527.
521. Koop SE, Winter RB, Lonstein JE. The surgical treatment of instability of the upper part of the cervical spine in children and adolescents. J Bone Joint Surg Am 1984;66:403–411.
522. Matthews LS, Vetter WL, Tolo VT. Cervical anomaly simulating hangman's fracture in a child. J Bone Joint Surg Am 1982;64:299–300.
523. McGrory Be, Fenichel GM. Hangman's fracture subsequent to spanking an infant. Ann Neurol 1977;2:82–83.
524. Michaels L, Prevost MJ, Crang DF. Pathological changes in a case of os odontoideum (separate odontoid process). J Bone Joint Surg Am 1969;51:965–972.
525. Minderhoud JM, Braakman, Penning L. Os odontoideum: clinical radiological and therapeutic aspects. J Neurol Sci 1969;8:521–544.
526. Miyakawa G. Congenital absence of the odontoid process: a case report. J Bone Joint Surg Am 1952;34:676–677.
527. Mouradian WH. Fractures of the odontoid: a laboratory and clinical study of mechanisms. Orthop Clin North Am 1978;9:985–1001.
528. Nordstrom RE, Lahdenranta TV, Kaitila II, Laasonen EM. Familial spondylolisthesis of the axis vertebra. J Bone Joint Surg Br 1986;68:704–706.
529. Parisi M, Lieberson R, Shatsky S. Hangman's fracture or primary spondylolysis: 1 patient and a brief review. Pediatr Radiol 1991;21:367–368.
530. Pizzutillo PD, Rocha EF, D'Astous J, et al. Bilateral fracture of the pedicle of the second cervical vertebra in the young child. J Bone Joint Surg Am 1986;68:892–896.
531. Richards PG. Stable fractures of the atlas and axis in children. J Neurol Neurosurg Psychiatry 1984;47:781–783.
532. Ries MD, Ray S. Posterior displacement of an odontoid fracture in a child. Spine 1986;11:1043–1044.
533. Ruff SJ, Taylor TKF. Hangman's fracture in an infant. J Bone Joint Surg Br 1986;68:702–703.
534. Schuler TC, Kurz L, Thompson DE, et al. Natural history of os odontoideum: case report. J Pediatr Orthop 1991;11:222–225.
535. Seimon LP. Fracture of the odontoid process in young children. J Bone Joint Surg Am 1977;59:943–948.
536. Sherk HH, Nicholson J, Chung SMK. Fractures of the odontoid process in young chldren. J Bone Joint Surg Am 1978;60:921–924.
537. Smith JT, Skinner SR, Shonnard NH. Persistent synchondrosis of the second cervical vertebra simulating a hangman's fracture in a child. J Bone Joint Surg Am 1994;75:1228–1230.
538. Stillwell W, Fielding JW. Acquired os odontoideum. Clin Orthop 1978;135:71–73.
539. Swischuk LE, Hayden CK Jr, Sarwar M. The dens-arch synchondrosis versus the hangman's fracture. Pediatr Radiol 1979;8:100–102.
540. Teng P, Papatheodorou C. Traumatic subluxation of C2 in young children. Bull Los Angeles Neurol Soc 1967;32:197–202.
541. Thompson W. Morbid changes of the spinal cord: a case of spontaneous luxation of the vertebra dentata. Edinb Med Surg J 1834;42:711–714.
542. Togozoglu AM, Alpaslan AM. Congenital spondylolisthesis in the upper spinal column. Spine 1994;19:99–102.
543. Verska JM, Anderson PA. Os odontoideum: a case report of one identical twin. Spine 1997;22:706–709.
544. Weiss MH, Kaufman B. Hangman's fracture in an infant. Am J Dis Child 1973;126:268–269.

545. Wokin DG. The os odontoideum: a separate odontoid process. J Bone Joint Surg Am 1963;45:1459–1471.

Lower Cervical Spine

546. Badelon O, Bensahel H. Fracture séparation du massif articulaire du rachis cervical chez l'enfant. Rev Chir Orthop 1984;70:83–85.
547. Bayless P, Ray VG. Incidence of cervical spine injuries in association with blunt head trauma. Am J Emerg Med 1989;7:139–142.
548. Birney TJ, Hanley EN Jr. Traumatic cervical spine injuries in childhood and adolescence. Spine 1989;14:1277–1282.
549. Black BE, An HS, Simpson JM. Cervical spine injury in the skeletally immature patient. In: An HS, Simpson JM (eds) Surgery of the Cervical Spine. Baltimore: Williams & Wilkins, 1991.
550. Bohn D, Armstrong D, Becher L, Humphreys R. Cervical spine injuries in children. J Trauma 1990;30:463–469.
551. Bollini G. Fracture du rachis de l'enfant et croissance. Ann Chir 1990;44:189–192.
552. Bollini G, Choux M, Tallet JM, Clement JL, Jacquemier M, Bouyala JN. Fractures, entorses graves et lesions médullaires du rachis de l'enfant. Rev Chir Orthop 1986;72(suppl II):48–50.
553. Braakman R, Vinden PJ. Unilateral facet interlocking in the lower cervical spine. J Bone Joint Surg Br 1967;42:249–257.
554. Budrick TE, Anderson PA, Rivara FP, Cohen W. Flexion-distraction fractures of the cervical spine. J Bone Joint Surg Am 1991;73:1097–1100.
555. Cattell HS, Clark GL. Cervical kyphosis and instability following multiple laminectomy in children. J Bone Joint Surg Am 1967;49:713–720.
556. Conroy BG, Hall CM. Cervical spine fractures and rear seat restraints. Arch Dis Child 1987;62:1267–1268.
557. Daussange J, Rigault P, Renier D, et al. Les instabilites et cyphoses apres laminectomie cervicale et craniectomie occipitale chez l'enfant et l'adolescent. Rev Chir Orthop 1980;66:423–440.
558. Dietrich AM, Ginn-Pesse ME, Barthrowski HM, King DR. Pediatric fractures: predominantly subtle presentation. J Pediatr Surg 1991;26:995–1000.
559. Evans DL, Bethem D. Cervical spine injuries in children. J Pediatr Orthop 1989;9:563–568.
560. Farley FA, Hensinger RN, Herzenberg JE. Cervical spinal cord injury in children. J Spinal Disord 1992;5:410–416.
561. Fineman S, Bortelli FJ, Rubenstein BM, Epstein H, Jacobson HG. The cervical spine: transformation of the normal lordotic pattern into a linear pattern in the neutral posture. J Bone Joint Surg Am 1963;45:1179–1183.
562. Forsyth HF. Neck injuries in children. N C Med J 1961;22:122–125.
563. Gaskill SJ, Marlin AE. Custom fitted thermoplastic Minerva jackets in the treatment of cervical spine instability in preschool age children. Pediatr Neurosurg 1990;16:35–39.
564. Gourand D. Étude radiologique de la stabilité du rachis cervical chez l'enfant. Thése Médicine. Université de Paris, 1981.
565. Hardy JR, Puliquen JC, Pennecot FG. Posterior arthrodeses of the upper cervical spine in children and adolescents: apropos of 19 cases. Rev Chir Orthop 1985;71:153–166.
566. Jones ET, Hensinger RN. C2–C3 dislocation in a child. J Pediatr Orthop 1981;1:419–422.
567. Keller RH. Traumatic displacement of the cartilaginous vertebral rim: a sign of intervertebral disk prolapse. Radiology 1974;110:21–24.
568. Ladd AL, Scranton PE. Congenital cervical stenosis presenting as transient quadriplegia in athletes. J Bone Joint Surg Am 1986;68:1371–1374.
569. Lawson JP, Ogden JA, Bucholz RW, Hughes SA. Physeal (endplate) injuries of the cervical spine. J Pediatr Orthop 1987;7:428–435.
570. Lebwohl NH, Eismont FJ. Cervical spine injuries in children. In: Weinstein SL (ed) The Pediatric Spine: Principles and Practice. New York: Raven, 1994.
571. McKee TR, Tinkoff G, Rhodes M. Asymptomatic occult cervical spine fracture: case report and review of the literature. J Trauma 1990;30:623–626.
572. McWhorter JM, Alexander E Jr, Davis CH, Kelly DL Jr. Posterior cervical fusion in children. J Neurosurg 1976;45:211–215.
573. Merle P, Georget AM, Viallet JF. Etude radiologique dynamique des rapports de l'atlas et l'axis chez l'enfant. J Radiol 1970;51:373–377.
574. Meyer SA, Schulte KR, Callaghson JJ, et al. Cervical spinal stenosis and stingers in collegiate football players. Am J Sports Med 1994;22:158–166.
575. Mikawa Y, Shikata J, Yamamuro T. Spinal deformity and instability after multilevel cervical laminectomy. Spine 1987;12:6–11.
576. Neville BG. Hyperflexion cervical cord injury in a children's car seat. Lancet 1981;2:103–104.
577. Norton WL. Fractures and dislocations of the cervical spine. J Bone Joint Surg Am 1962;44:115–139.
578. Olerud C, Karlstrom G. Cervical spine fracture caused by high jump: case report. J Orthop Trauma 1990;4:179–182.
579. Orenstein JB, Klein BL, Ochsenschlager DW. Delayed diagnosis of pediatric cervical spine injury. Pediatrics 1992;89:1185–1188.
580. Papavasiliou V. Traumatic subluxation of the cervical spine during childhood. Orthop Clin North Am 1978;9:945–954.
581. Reynen PD, Clancy WG Jr. Cervical spine injury, hockey helmets and face masks. Am J Sports Med 1994;22:167–170.
582. Robinson MD, Northrup B, Sabo R. Cervical spinal canal plasticity in children as determined by the vertebral body ratio technique. Spine 1990;15:1003–1005.
583. Roy L, Gibson DA. Cervical spine fusions in children. Clin Orthop 1970;73:146–151.
584. Saleh J, Rayerof TJF. Hyperextension injury of cervical spine and central cord syndrome in a child. Spine 1992;17:234–237.
585. Scher AT. Diving injuries to the cervical spinal canal. S Afr Med J 1981;59:603–605.
586. Schneider RC, Cherry G, Pantek H. The syndrome of acute central cervical spinal cord injury: special reference to the mechanisms involved in hyperextension injuries of cervical spine. J Neurosurg 1954;11:546–577.
587. Shacked I, Ram Z, Hadam M. The anterior cervical approach for traumatic injuries to the cervical spine in children. Clin Orthop 1993;292:144–150.
588. Silver JR, Silver DD, Godfrey JJ. Injuries of the spine sustained during gymnastic activities. BMJ 1986;293:861–863.
589. Sim FH, Svien HJ, Bickel WH, et al. Swan-neck deformity following extensive cervical laminectomy. J Bone Joint Surg Am 1974;56:564–580.
590. Sneed RC, Stover SL. Undiagnosed spinal cord injuries in brain-injured children. Am J Dis Child 1988;142:965–967.
591. Stabler CL, Eismont FJ, Brown MD, et al. Failure of posterior cervical fusions using cadaveric bone graft in children. J Bone Joint Surg Am 1985;67:370–375.
592. Stanley P, Duncan AW, Isaacson J, Isaacson AS. Radiology of fracture-dislocation of the cervical spine during delivery. AJR 1985;145:621–625.

593. Sullivan CR, Bruwer AJ, Harris LE. Hyperinstability of the cervical spine in children: a pitfall in the diagnosis of cervical dislocation. Am J Surg 1958;95:636–640.
594. Swischuk LE. Anterior displacement of C2 in children: physiologic or pathologic? Radiology 1977;122:759–763.
595. Taylor TKF, Nade S, Bannister JH. Seat belt fractures of the cervical spine. J Bone Joint Surg Br 1976;58:328–331.
596. Torg JS, Glasgon CG. Criteria for return to contact activities following cervical spine injury. Clin J Sport Med 1991;1:12–26.
597. Torg JS, Sennett B, Pavlov H, Liventhal MR, Glasgon SG. Spear tackler's spine: an entity precluding participation in tackle football and collision activities that expose the cervical spine to axial energy inputs. Am J Sports Med 1993;21:640–649.
598. Vines FS. The significance of "occult" fractures of the cervical spine. AJR 1969;107:493–504.
599. Webb JK, Broughton RBK, McSweeney T, Park WM. Hidden flexion injury of the cervical spine. J Bone Joint Surg Br 1976;58:322–327.
600. Weston WJ. Clay shoveler's disease in adolescents (Schmitt's disease): a report of two cases. Br J Radiol 1957;30:378–380.
601. Wickboldt J, Sorenson N. Anterior cervical fusion after traumatic dislocation of the cervical spine in childhood and adolescence. Childs Brain 1978;4:120–128.
602. Woodring JH, Lee C. The role and limitations of computed tomographic scanning in the evaluation of cervical trauma. J Trauma 1992;33:698–708.
603. Yasuoko S, Peterson H, MacCarty C. Incidence of spinal column deformity after multilevel laminectomy in children and adults. J Neurosurg 1982;57:441–445.
604. Zike K. Delayed neuropathy after injury to the cervical spine in children. Pediatrics 1959;24:413–417.

Thoracic Spine

605. Bolesta MJ, Bohlman HH. Mediastinal widening associated with fractures of the upper thoracic spine. J Bone Joint Surg Am 1991;73:447–450.
606. Cook DA, Heiner JP, Breed AL. Pseudomeningocele following spinal fracture. Clin Orthop 1989;274:74–79.
607. Denis F. The three column spine and its significance in the classification of acute thoracolumbar spinal injuries. Spine 1983;8:817–831.
608. Denis F, Burkus JK. Shear fracture-dislocations of the thoracic and lumbar spine associated with forceful hyperextension (lumber jack paraplegia). Spine 1992;17:156–161.
609. Murphy MJ, Ogden JA, Southwick WO. Spinal stabilization in acute spine injuries. Surg Clin North Am 1980;60:1035–1047.
610. Ruckstuhl J, Morscher E, Jani L. Behandlung und prognose von Wirbelfrakturen im kindes und jugendalter. Chirurg 1987;47:458–467.
611. Simpson AHRW, Williamson DM, Golding SJ, Houghton QR. Thoracic spine translocation without cord injury. J Bone Joint Surg Br 1990;71:80–83.
612. Swichieff J. Torsion spasms and abnormal postures in children with hiatus hernia: Sandifer's syndrome. Prog Pediatr Radiol 1969;2:190–197.

Scheuermann's Disease

613. Alexander CJ. Scheuermann's disease: a traumatic spondylodystrophy? Skeletal Radiol 1977;1:209–221.
614. Aufdermaur M. Zur pathologischen Anatomie der Scheuermannschen Krankheit. Schweiz Med Wochenschr 1965;95:264–268.
615. Aufdermaur M. Zur Pathogenese der Scheuermannschen Krankheit. Dtsch Med Wochenschr 1974;89:73–79.
616. Aufdermaur M. Juvenile kyphosis (Scheuermann's disease): radiology, histology, and pathogenesis. Clin Orthop 1981;154:166–174.
617. Aufdermauer M, Spycher M. Pathogenesis of osteochondrosis juvenilis Scheuermann. J Orthop Res 1986;4:452–457.
618. Bradford DS. Juvenile kyphosis. Clin Orthop 1977;128:45–55.
619. Butler RW. The nature and significance of vertebra osteochondritis. Proc R Soc Med 1955;48:895–902.
620. Cannon SR, James SE. Back pain in athletes. Br J Sports Med 1984;18:159–164.
621. Cleveland RH, Delong GR. The relationship of juvenile lumbar disk disease and Scheuermann's disease. Pediatr Radiol 1981;10:161–164.
622. Edgren W, Vainio S. Osteochondrosis juvenilis lumbalis. Acta Chir Scand Suppl 1957;227:1–47.
623. Ferguson AB. The etiology of pre-adolescent kyphosis. J Bone Joint Surg Am 1956;38:149–157.
624. Greene TL, Hensinger RN, Hunter LY. Back pain and vertebral changes simulating Scheuermann's disease. J Pediatr Orthop 1985;5:1–7.
625. Hilton RC, Ball J, Benn R. Vertebral end-plate lesions (Schmorl's nodes) in the dorsolumbar spine. Ann Rheum Dis 1976;35:127–132.
626. Lowe TG. Current concepts review: Scheuermann disease. J Bone Joint Surg Am 1990;72:940–945.
627. Micheli LJ. Low back pain in the adolescent: differential diagnosis. Am J Sports Med 1977;7:362–364.
628. Montgomery SP, Erwin WE. Scheuermann's kyphosis: long-term results of Milwaukee brace treatment. Spine 1981;6:5–8.
629. Nathan L, Kuhns JG. Epiphysitis of the spine. J Bone Joint Surg 1940;22:55–58.
630. Resnick D, Niwayama G. Intravertebral disk herniations: cartilaginous (Schmorl's) nodes. Radiology 1978;126:57–65.
631. Revel M, Andre-Deshays C, Roudier R, et al. Effects of repetitive strains on vertebral end plates in young rats. Clin Orthop 1992;279:303–309.
632. Scheuermann VH. Kyphosis dorsalis juvenilis. Z Orthop Chir 1921;41:305–326.
633. Scheuermann VH. Kyphosis juvenilis (Scheuermann's Krankheit). Fortschr Rontgenstr 1936;53:1–23.
634. Schmorl G, Junghanns H. The Human Spine in Health and Disease. Orlando: Grune & Stratton, 1959.
635. Swärd L, Hellström M, Jacobsson B, Peterson L. Back pain and radiologic changes in the thoraco-lumbar spine of athletes. Spine 1990;15:124–129.

Chance Fracture

636. Agran PV, Winn D, Dunkle D. Injuries among 4 to 9 year old restrained motor vehicle occupants by seat location and crash impact site. Am J Dis Child 1989;143:1317–1321.
637. Anderson PA, Henley MB, Rivara FP, Maier RV. Flexion distraction and Chance injuries to the thoraco-lumbar spine. J Orthop Trauma 1991;5:153–160.
638. Blasier RD, LaMont RL. Chance fracture in a child: a case report with nonoperative treatment. J Pediatr Orthop 1985;5:92–93.
639. Burdi AR, Huella DF. Infants and children in the adult world of automobile safety design: pediatric and anatomical consideration for design of child restraints. Biomechanics 1969;2:267–280.
640. Carragher AM, Cranley B. Seat belt stomach transection in association with a Chance vertebral fracture. Br J Surg 1987;74:397.
641. Chance GQ. Note on a type of flexion fracture of the spine. Br J Radiol 1948;21:452–453.

642. Ebraheim NA, Savolaine ER, Southworth SR, et al. Pediatric lumbar seat belt injuries. Orthopedics 1991;14:1010–1013.
643. Fish J, Wright WH. The seat belt syndrome: does it exist? J Trauma 1965;5:746–750.
644. Gallagher DJ, Heinrich SD. Pediatric Chance fracture. J Orthop Trauma 1990;4:183–187.
645. Glassman SD, Johnson JR, Holt RT. Seat belt injuries in children. J Trauma 1992;33:882–886.
646. Hall HE, Robertson WW. Another Chance: a non-seat belt related fracture of the lumbar spine. J Trauma 1985;25:1163–1166.
647. Hardacre JM II, West KW, Rescorla FR, et al. Delayed onset of intestinal obstruction in children after recognized seat belt injury. J Pediatr Surg 1990;25:967–969.
648. Hoffman MA, Spence LJ, Wesson DE, et al. The pediatric passenger: trends in seat belt use and injury patterns. J Trauma 1987;27:974–976.
649. Holgersen LO, Bishop HC. Non-operative treatment of duodenal hematomata in childhood. J Pediatr Surg 1977;12:11–17.
650. Hope PG, Houghton GR. Spinal and abdominal injury in an infant due to the incorrect use of a car seat belt. Injury 1986;17:368–369.
651. Huelke DF, Kaufer H. Vertebral column injuries and seat belts. J Trauma 1975;15:304–318.
652. Jodoin A, Gillet P, Dupuis PR, Maurals G. Surgical treatment of post traumatic kyphosis: a report of 16 cases. Can J Surg 1989;32:36–42.
653. Johnson DC, Falci S. The diagnosis and treatment of pediatric lumbar spine injuries caused by rear seat lap belts. Neurosurgery 1990;26:434–441.
654. Massot P. Occlusion du jéjunam au cours d'une fracture du rachis chez un enfant. Ann Chir Orthop 1965;6:141–144.
655. Metaizeau JP, Prevot J, Schmitt M, Bretogne MC. Intestinal strangulation between two vertebra following an axial dislocation of L1/L2. J Pediatr Surg 1980;15:193–194.
656. Miller JA, Smith TH. Seat belt induced Chance fracture in an infant. Pediatr Radiol 1991;21:575–577.
657. Moskowitz A. Lumbar seat belt injury in a child: case report. J Trauma 1989;29:1279–1282.
658. Newman KD, Bowman LM, Eichelberger MR, et al. The lap belt complex; intestinal and lumbar spine injury in children. J Trauma 1990;30:1133–1138.
659. Raney EM, Bennett JT. Pediatric Chance fracture. Spine 1992;17:1522–1524.
660. Reid AB, Lelts RM, Black GB. Pediatric Chance fractures: association with intra-abdominal injuries and seat belt use. J Trauma 1990;30:384–391.
661. Ritchie WP Jr, Ersek RA, Bunch WL, Simmons RL. Combined visceral and vertebral injuries from lap-type seat belts. Surg Gynecol Obstet 1970;131:431–435.
662. Roger RM, Missiuna P, Ein S. Bowel entrapment within spinal fracture. J Pediatr Orthop 1991;11:783–785.
663. Rogers LF. The roentgenographic appearance of transverse or Chance fractures of the spine: the seat belt fracture. AJR 1971;111:844–849.
664. Rolander SD, Blair WE. Deformation and fracture of the lumbar vertebral end plate. Orthop Clin North Am 1975;6:75–81.
665. Rumball K, Jarvis J. Seat belt injuries of the spine in young children. J Bone Joint Surg 1992;74:571–574.
666. Sivit CJ, Taylor GA, Newman KD, et al. Safety-belt injuries in children with lap-belt ecchymosis: CT findings in 61 patients. AJR 1991;157:111–115.
667. Smith WS, Kaufer H. Patterns and mechanisms of lumbar injuries associated with lap seat belts. J Bone Joint Surg Am 1969;51:239–254.
668. Statter MB, Coran AG. Appendiceal transection in a child associated with a lap belt restraint: case report. J Trauma 1992;33:765–766.
669. Taylor GA, Eggli KD. Lap belt injuries of the lumbar spine in children: a pitfall in CT diagnosis. AJR 1988;150:1355–1358.
670. Vandershirs R, O'Connor HMC. The seat belt syndrome. Can Med Assoc J 1987;137:1023–1024.
671. Voss L, Cole PA, D'Amato C. Pediatric Chance fractures from lapbelts: unique case report of three in one accident. J Orthop Trauma 1996;10:421–428.
672. Winter M, Jani L. Seat belt injury with total paraplegia and recovery in a child. J Pediatr Orthop 1993;18:162–164.

Lumbar Spine

673. Abel MS. Jogger's fracture and other stress fractures of the lumbo-sacral spine. Skeletal Radiol 1985;13:221–227.
674. Avrahami E, Cohn DF, Yaron M. Computerized tomography, clinical and x-ray correlations in the hemi-sacralized 5th lumbar vertebra. Clin Rheumatol 1986;5:332–338.
675. Bertolotti M. Contributo allo conoscenza dei vizi, differenzazione regionale del rachid con speciale reguardo all' assimilazione sacrale della v lombare. Radiol Med 1977;4:113–144.
676. Brenner B, Moid R, Dickson J, Harrington P. Instrumentation of the spine from fracture-dislocations in children. Childs Brain 1977;3:249–255.
677. Carrion WV, Dormans JP, Drummond DS, Christofersen MR. Circumferential growth plate fracture of the thoracolumbar spine from child abuse. J Pediatr Orthop 1996;16:210–214.
678. Chambers HG, Akbarnia BA. Thoracic, lumbar and sacral spine fractures and dislocations. In: Weinstein SL (ed) The Pediatric Spine: Principles and Practice. New York: Raven, 1994.
679. Chatiani K, Yoshioka M, Hase H, Hirasawa Y. Complete anterior fracture-dislocation of the fourth lumbar vertebra. Spine 1994;7:726–729.
680. Chiroff RT, Sachs BL. Discontinuity of the spinous processes on standard roentgenograms as an aid in the diagnosis of unstable fractures of the spine. J Trauma 1976;16:313–316.
681. Denis F, Burkus JK. Lateral distraction injuries to the thoracic and lumbar spine. J Bone Joint Surg Am 1991;73:1049–1053.
682. Epstein BS, Epstein JA, Lavine L. The effects of anatomic variations in the lumbar vertebrae and spinal canal on cauda equina and nerve root syndrome. AJR 1964;91:1055–1063.
683. Fontijne WPJ, deKlerk LWL, Braakman R, et al. CT scan prediction of neurological deficit in thoracolumbar burst fractures. J Bone Joint Surg Br 1992;74:683–685.
684. Glass RBJ, Sivit CJ, Sturm PF, Bulas DI, Eichelberger MR. Lumbar spine injury in a pediatric population: difficulties with computed tomographic diagnosis. J Trauma 1994;37:815–819.
685. Gunzberg R, Fraser RD. Stress fracture of the lumbar pedicle: case reports of pediculolysis and review of the literature. Spine 1991;16:185–189.
686. Kaplan FS, Scheol JD, Wisneski R, Chestle M, Haddad JO. The cluster phenomenon in patients who have multiple vertebral compression fractures. Clin Orthop 1993;297:161–167.
687. Keene JS, Lash EG, Kling TF Jr. Undetected post-traumatic instability of "stable" thoracolumbar fractures. J Orthop Trauma 1988;2:202–211.
688. Keenen TL, Antony J, Benson DR. Dural tears associated with lumbar burst fractures. J Orthop Trauma 1990;4:243–245.
689. Mandell GA, Harcke HT. Scintigraphy of persistent vertebral transverse process epiphysis. Clin Nucl Med 1987;12:359–362.
690. Maxwell KM, Newcomb CE. Bilateral traumatic L4 pedicular fractures in a healthy male athlete: a case report. Spine 1993;18:407–409.

691. Nykamp PW. Computed tomography for a bursting fracture of the lumbar spine. J Bone Joint Surg Am 1978;60:1108–1109.
692. Postacchini F, Massobrio M, Ferro L. Familial lumbar stenosis. J Bone Joint Surg Am 1985;67:321–323.
693. Shore RM, Cain GP, Lloyd TV. Secondary ossification centre of the transverse process: a bone scan normal variant. Eur J Nucl Med 1985;10:88–89.
694. Traughber PD, Havlina JM Jr. Bilateral pedicle stress fractures: SPECT and CT features. J Comput Assist Tomogr 1991;15:338–340.
695. Wigh RE. The thoraco-lumbar and lumbo-sacral transitional junctions. Spine 1980;5:215–222.

Spondylolysis/Spondylolisthesis

696. Beeler JW. Further evidence on the acquired nature of spondylolisthesis. AJR 1970;108:796–798.
697. Bellah RD, Summerville DA, Treves ST, Micheli LJ. Low back pain in adolescent athletes: detection of stress injury to the pars interarticularis with SPECT. Radiology 1991;180:509–511.
698. Blanda J, Bethem D, Moats W, Lew M. Defects of pars interarticularis in athletes: a protocol for non-operative treatment. J Spinal Disord 1993;6:496–411.
699. Bodner RJ, Heyman S, Drummond DS, Gregg JR. The use of single photon emission computed tomography (SPECT) in the diagnosis of low-back pain in young patients. Spine 1988;13:1155–1160.
700. Borkow SE, Kleiger B. Spondylolisthesis in the newborn. Clin Orthop 1971;81:73–76.
701. Ciullo Jr, Jackson DW. Pars interarticularis stress reaction, spondylolysis and spondylolisthesis in gymnasts. Clin Sports Med 1985;4:95–110.
702. Commandre FA, Taillan B, Gagerie F, et al. Spondylolysis and spondylolisthesis in young athletes: 28 cases. J Sports Med Phys Fitness 1988;28:104–107.
703. Cope R. Acute traumatic spondylolysis: report of a case and review of the literature. Clin Orthop 1988;230:162–165.
704. Cyron BM, Hutton WC. The fatigue strength of the lumbar neural arch in spondylolysis. J Bone Joint Surg Br 1978;60:234–238.
705. Dietrich M, Kurowski P. The importance of mechanical factors in the etiology of spondylolysis. Spine 1985;10:532–542.
706. Farfan HF, Osteria V, Lamy C. The mechanical etiology of spondylolysis and spondylolisthesis. Clin Orthop 1976;117:40–55.
707. Ferguson RJ, McMaster JH, Stanitski CL. Low back pain in college football linemen. J Sports Med 1975;2:63–69.
708. Frederickson BE, Balcer DR, McHolick WJ, Yuan HA, Lubicky J. The natural history of spondylolysis and spondylolisthesis. J Bone Joint Surg Am 1984;66:699–707.
709. Frennered AK, Danielson BI, Nachemsom AL. Natural history of symptomatic isthmic low-grade spondylolisthesis in children and adolescents: a seven-year follow-up study. J Pediatr Orthop 1994;11:209–214.
710. Gainor BJ, Hagen RJ, Allen WC. Biomechanics of the spine in the pole vaulter as related to spondylolysis. Am J Sports Med 1983;11:53–57.
711. Galakoff C, Kalifa G, Dubousset J, Bennet J. Lyse isthmique et spondylolisthesis. Arch Fr Pediatr 1985;42:437–440.
712. Garber GE, Wright AM. Unilateral spondylolysis and contralateral pedicle fracture. Spine 1986;11:63–66.
713. Goldberg MA. Gymnastic injuries. Orthop Clin North Am 1980;11:717–724.
714. Green TP, Allvey JC, Adams MA. Spondylolysis: bending of the inferior articular process of lumbar vertebrae during simulated spinal movements. Spine 1994;19:2683–2692.
715. Hardcastle PH. Repair of spondylolysis in young fast bowlers. J Bone Joint Surg Br 1993;75:398–402.
716. Hutton WC, Cyron BM. Spondylolysis. Acta Orthop Scand 1978;49:604–609.
717. Hutton WC, Stott JR, Cyron BM. Is spondylolysis a fatigue fracture? Spine 1977;2:202–209.
718. Jackson DW. Low back pain in young athletes: evaluation of stress reaction and discogenic problems. Am J Sports Med 1979;7:364–366.
719. Jackson DW, Wiltse LL. Low back pain in young athletes. Phys Sports Med 1974;2:53–58.
720. Jackson DW, Wiltse LL, Cirinclone RJ. Spondylolysis in the female gymnast. Clin Orthop 1976;117:68–73.
721. Jackson DW, Wiltse LL, Dingeman RD, Hays M. Stress reactions involving the pars interarticularis in young athletes. Am J Sports Med 1981;9:304–312.
722. Kälebo P, Kadziolka R, Sward L, Zachrisson BE. Stress views in the comparative assessment of spondylolytic spondylolisthesis. Skeletal Radiol 989;17:570–575.
723. Kip PC, Esses SI, Doherty BI, Alexander JW, Crawford MJ. Biomechanical testing of pars defect repairs. Spine 1994;19:2692–2697.
724. Klinghoffer L, Murdock MG. Spondylolysis following trauma. Clin Orthop 1982;166:72–74.
725. Kotani PT, Ichikawa MD, Wakabiayashi MD, Yoshii T, Koshiimune M. Studies of spondylolysis found among weight lifters. Br J Sports Med 1971;6:4–8.
726. Kraus H. Effect of lordosis on the stress in the lumbar spine. Clin Orthop 1976;117:56–58.
727. Krenz J, Troup JDG. The structure of the pars interarticularis of the lower lumbar vertebrae and its relation to the etiology of spondylolysis with a report of a healing fracture in the neural arch of a fourth lumbar vertebra. J Bone Joint Surg Am 1977;59:154–198.
728. Lafferty JR, Winter WG, Gambaro SA. Fatigue characteristics of posterior elements of vertebrae. J Bone Joint Surg Am 1977;59:154–158.
729. Langston JW, Gravant ML. "Incomplete ring" sign: a simple method for CT detection of spondylolysis. J Comput Assist Tomogr 1985;9:728–729.
730. Letts M, Smallman T, Afanasiev R, Gouw G. Fracture of the pars interarticularis in adolescent athletes: a clinical-biomechanical analysis. J Pediatr Orthop 1986;6:40–46.
731. Micheli LJ, Hall JE, Miller ME. Use of the modified Boston brace for back injuries in athletes. Am J Sports Med 1980;8:351–356.
732. Miyake R, Ikata T, Katoh S, Morita T. Morphologic analysis of the facet joint in the immature lumbosacral spine with special reference to spondylolysis. Spine 1996;21:783–789.
733. Newell RL. Historical perspective: spondylolysis. Spine 1995;20:1950–1956.
734. Oakley RH, Carty H. Review of spondylolisthesis and spondylolysis in pediatric practice. Br J Radiol 1984;57:877–895.
735. O'Neill DB, Micheli LJ. Post-operative radiographic evidence for fatique fracture as the etiology in spondylolysis. Spine 1989;14:1342–1355.
736. Papanicolau N, Wilkinson RH, Romans JB, Treves S, Micheli LJ. Bone scintigraphy and radiography in young athletes with low back pain. AJR 1985;145:1039–1044.
737. Schneiderman GA, McLain RF, Hambly MF, Nielson SL. The pars defect as a pain source: a histologic study. Spine 1995;20:1761–1764.
738. Sherman FC, Wilkenson RH, Hall JE. Reactive sclerosis of a pedicle and spondylolisthesis in the lumbar spine. J Bone Joint Surg Am 1977;59:49–54.

739. Szot F, Boron Z, Galaj Z. Overloading changes in the motor system occurring in elite gymnasts. Int J Sports Med 1985;6:36–40.
740. Taillard WF. Etiology of spondylolisthesis. Clin Orthop 1976;117:30–39.
741. Troup JG. The rise of weight training and weight lifting in young people: functional anatomy of the spine. Br J Sports Med 1970;5:27–33.
742. Troup JG. Mechanical factors in spondylolisthesis and spondylolysis. Clin Orthop 1976;117:59–67.
743. Weir MR, Smith DS. Stress reaction of the pars interarticularis leading to spondylolysis: a cause of adolescent back pain. J Adolesc Health Care 1989;10:573–577.
744. Wertzberger KL, Peterson HA. Acquired spondylolysis and spondylolisthesis in the young child. Spine 1980;5:437–442.
745. Wiltse LL. The etiology of spondylolisthesis. J Bone Joint Surg Am 1962;44:539–560.
746. Wiltse LL, Jackson DW. Treatment of spondylolisthesis and spondylolysis in children. Clin Orthop 1976;117:92–100.
747. Wiltse LL, Newman PH, MacNab I. Classification of spondylolysis and spondylolisthesis. Clin Orthop 1976;117:23–29.
748. Wiltse LL, Widdell EH, Jackson DW. Fatigue fracture: the basic lesion in spondylolisthesis. J Bone Joint Surg Am 1975;57:17–22.

Lumbar Physis

749. Albeck MJ, Madisen FF, Wagner A, Gjerris F. Fracture of the lumbar vertebral ring apophysis imitating disc herniation. Acta Neurochir (Wien) 1991;113:52–56.
750. Bailey W. Persistent vertebral process epiphyses. AJR 1939;42:85–89.
751. Bick EM, Copel JW. The ring apophysis of the human vertebra. J Bone Joint Surg Am 1951;33:783–789.
752. Clark JE. Apophyseal fracture of the lumbar spine in adolescence. Orthop Rev 1991;20:512–516.
753. Dake MD, Jacobs RP, Margolin FR. Computed tomography of posterior lumbar apophyseal ring fracture. J Comput Assist Tomogr 1985;9:730–732.
754. Dieterman JL, Runge M, Badoz A, et al. Radiology of posterior lumbar apophyseal ring fractures: report of 13 cases. Neuroradiology 1988;30:337–344.
755. Edelson JG, Nathan H. Stages in the natural history of the vertebral end-plates. Spine 1988;13:21–26.
756. Ehni C. Schneider SJ. Posterior lumbar vertebral rim fracture and associated disc protrusion in adolescence. J Neurosurg 1988;68:912–916.
757. Epstein NE, Epstein JA. Limbus lumbar vertebral fractures in 27 adolescents and adults. Spine 1991;16:962–966.
758. Epstein NE, Epstein JA, Mauri T. Treatment of fractures of the vertebral limbus and spinal stenosis in five adolescents and five adults. Neurosurgery 1989;24:595–604.
759. Ghelman B, Freiberger RH. The limbus vertebra: an anterior disk herniation demonstrated by discography. AJR 1976;127:854–855.
760. Goldman AB, Ghelman B, Doherty J. Posterior lumbar vertebrae: a cause of radiating back pain in adolescents and young adults. Skeletal Radiol 1990;19:501–507.
761. Gooding CA, Hurwitz ME. Avulsed vertebral rim apophysis in a child. Pediatr Radiol 1974;2:269–268.
762. Handel SF, Twiford TW Jr, Reisel DH, Kaufman HH. Posterior lumbar apophyseal fractures. Radiology 1979;130:629–633.
763. Hellmer H. Röntgenologische Beobachtungen über Ossifikations Störungen im limbus vertebrae. Acta Radiol 1932;13:183–187.
764. Hellstadius A. A contribution to the question of the origin of anterior paradiscal defects and so-called persisting apophyses on the vertebral bodies. Acta Orthop Scand 1948;18:377–386.
765. Henales V, Hervas JA, Lopez P, Martinez JM, Ramos R, Herrera M. Intervertebral disc herniations (limbus vertebrae) in pediatric patients: report of 15 cases. Pediatr Radiol 1993;23:608–610.
766. Hirayama Y, Mitsuhashi T, Shiojima K, et al. Five cases of disk herniation in young adults associated with avulsion fracture of the ring apophysis. Orthop Trauma Surg 1982;25:857–862.
767. Ikata T, Morita T, Katoh S, Tachibana K, Maoka H. Lesions of the lumbar posterior end-plate in children and adolescents. J Bone Joint Surg Br 1995;77:991–995.
768. Ishida K, Otani A, Matsumura T, Furuta M. A case of juvenile lumbar disk herniation with a slipped ring apophysis. Seikei Geka 1974;25:841–843.
769. Joisten C. Über persistirende Apophysen an der Lenden wirbelsaule. Arch Orthop Unfallchir 1930;28:622–625.
770. Kubo T, Koyama K, Murakami K. Two cases of posterior apophysis in adolescent children. Chubu Seisai 1974;17:160–162.
771. Laredo J-D, Bard M, Chretien J, Kahn M-F. Lumbar posterior marginal intra-osseous cartilaginous node. Skeletal Radiol 1986;15:201–208.
772. Lippitt AB. Fracture of a vertebral body end-plate and disk protrusion causing subarachnoid block in adolescents. Clin Orthop 1976;116:112–115.
773. Lowrey JJ. Dislocated lumbar vertebral apophysis in adolescent children. J Neurosurg 1973;38:232–234.
774. Lyon E, Marum G. Krankheiten der wirbelkorperepiphysen. Fortschr Geb Roentgen 1931;44:498–501.
775. Mahaisavariya B, Wittayakom T. Lumbar vertebral growth plate displaced into the vertebral canal: a case report of a 15 year old boy. Acta Orthop Scand 1993;64:103–104.
776. Mardersteig K. Zur Frage der persistierrenden wirbelkorperepiphysen. Fortschr Geb Roentgen 1932;46:441–445.
777. Martel W, Seeger JF, Wicks JD, Washburn RL. Traumatic lesions of the discovertebral junction in the lumbar spine. AJR 1976;127:457–464.
778. Momma M, Honda Y, Takasu K, et al. A case report of the lower extremity paralysis due to the fragment of the posterior lower margin of the lumbar vertebra. Kanto Seisai 1972;3:311–312.
779. Munetaka M, Kataoka O, Ito T, et al. Lumbar disc herniation with a traumatic fracture-dislocation of the end-plate: report of two cases. Orthop Trauma Surg 1984;27:129–133.
780. Nishijima M, Tatezaki S, Yamada H, et al. Lumbar disk herniation with a traumatic fracture-dislocation of the end-plate: report of two cases. Orthop Trauma Surg 1984;27:129–132.
781. Petterson H, Harwood-Nash DC, Fitz CR, Chung S, Armstrong E. The CT appearance of avulsion of the posterior vertebral apophysis. Neuroradiology 1981;21:145–147.
782. Reigel NH. Slipped lumbar apophyseal ring. Concepts Pediatr Neurosurg 1985;5:34–40.
783. Rothfus WE, Goldberg AL, Deeb FL, Daaffnea RH. MR recognition of posterior lumbar vertebral rim fracture. J Comput Assist Tomogr 1990;14:790–794.
784. Sovio OM, Bell HM, Beauchamp RD, Tredwell SJ. Fracture of the lumbar vertebral apophysis. J Pediatr Orthop 1985;5:550–552.
785. Swärd L, Hellström M, Jacobsson B, Peterson L. Acute injury of the vertebral ring apophysis and intervertebral disc in adolescent gymnasts. Spine 1990;15:144–148.
786. Swärd L, Holstrom M, Jacobsson B, Karlsson L. Vertebral ring apophysis injury in athletes: is the etiology different in the thoracic and lumbar spine? Am J Sports Med 1993;21:841–845.

787. Takata K, Inoue SI, Takahashi K, Ohtsuka Y. Fracture of the posterior margin of a lumbar vertebral body. J Bone Joint Surg Am 1988;70:589–594.
788. Techakapuch S. Rupture of the lumbar cartilage plate into the spinal canal in an adolescent: a case report. J Bone Joint Surg Am 1981;63:481–482.
789. Teramoto K, Nosaka K, Yasuda K, et al. Four cases of juvenile lumbar disk herniation and slipped ring apophysis. Chubu Seisai 1983;26:1788–1793.
790. Tsubuku M. Posterior "kantenabtrennung." Rinsho Seikei Geka 1968;3:79–82.
791. Tsukada T, Shiba T. Traumatic displacement of the posterior ring apophysis: a case report. Kanto Seisai 1975;6:386–388.
792. Wagner A, Albeck MN, Madsen FF. Diagnostic imaging in fracture of lumbar vertebral ring apophysis. Acta Radiol 1990;33:72–75.
793. Yagan R. CT diagnosis of limbus vertebra. J Comput Assist Tomogr 1984;8:149–151.
794. Yoh K, Marumo S, Matsumoto M, et al. A case of upper lumbar disk herniation associated with displaced ring apophysis in adolescent. Seikei Geka 1982;33:1183–1184.
795. Yoshihati H, et al. Five cases of disc herniation in young adults associated with avulsion fracture of the ring apophysis. Orthop Trauma Surg 1982;25:897–860.

Disk Herniation

796. Billot C, Desgrippes Y, Bensahel H. La hernie discale lombaire chez l'enfant. Rev Chir Orthop 1980;66:43–46.
797. Borgesen SE, Vang PS. Herniation of the lumbar intervertebral disk in children and adolescents. Acta Orthop Scand 1974;45:540–549.
798. Bradford DS, Garcia A. Herniations of the lumbar intervertebral disk in children and adolescents: a review of 30 surgically treated cases. JAMA 1969;210:2045–2051.
799. Bulos S. Herniated intervertebral lumbar disk in the teenager. J Bone Joint Surg Br 1973;55:273–278.
800. Bunnell WP. Back pain in children. Orthop Clin North Am 1982;13:587–604.
801. Callahan DJ, Pack LL, Bream RC, Heisinger RN. Intervertebral disk impingement syndrome in a child: report of a case and suggested pathology. Spine 1986;11:402–404.
802. Carcassonne G. Sciatique de l'enfant. In: Entretien de Chirurgie Infantile. Paris: Expansion Scientifique Francaise, 1977, pp 151–173.
803. Clark NMP, Cleak DK. Intervertebral disc prolapse in children and adolescents. J Pediatr Orthop 1983;3:202–206.
804. Day PL. The teenage disk syndrome. South Med J 1967;60:247–250.
805. DeLuca PF, Mason DE, Weiand R, Howard R, Bassett GS. Excision of herniated nucleus pulposus in children and adolescents. J Pediatr Orthop 1994;14:318–322.
806. DeOrio JK, Bianco AJ Jr. Lumbar disk excision in children and adolescents. J Bone Joint Surg Am 1982;64:991–996.
807. DeSeze S, Levernieux J. La sciatique des adolescents: étude sur 52 observations. Rev Rhum Mal Osteoartic 1957;24:270–276.
808. Epstein JA, Lavine LS. Herniated lumbar intervertebral disks in teen-age children. J Neurosurg 1964;21:1070–1075.
809. Fernstrom U. Protruded lumbar intervertebral disk in children. Acta Chir Scand 1956;111:71–79.
810. Garrido E, Humphreys RP, Hendrick EB, Hoffman HJK. Lumbar disc disease in children. Neurosurgery 1978;2:22–26.
811. Gibson MJ, Szypryt EP, Buckley JH, et al. Magnetic resonance imaging of adolescent disk herniation. J Bone Joint Surg Br 1987;69:699–703.
812. Girodias J-B, Azonz EM, Marton D. Intervertebral disk space calcification: a report of 51 children with a review of the literature. Pediatr Radiol 1991;21:541–546.
813. Giroux JC, Leclerq TA. Lumbar disk excision in the second decade. Spine 1982;7:168–170.
814. Grobler LJ, Simmons EH, Barrington TW. Intervertebral disk herniation in the adolescent. Spine 1979;4:267–278.
815. Hashimoto K, Fujita K, Kojimoto H, Shimomura Y. Lumbar disc herniation in children. J Pediatr Orthop 1990;10:394–396.
816. Herring JA, Asher MA. Intervertebral disc herniation in a teenager. J Pediatr Orthop 1989;9:615–617.
817. Kamel M, Rosman M. Disc protrusion in the growing child. Clin Orthop 1984;185:46–52.
818. Key JA. Intervertebral disk lesions in children and adolescents. J Bone Joint Surg Am 1950;32:97–102.
819. Kimura Y, Fujimaki E, Miyaoka H, et al. Operated cases of lumbar disk herniation in children under fifteen years old. Kanto Seisai 1984;16:187–191.
820. King AB. Surgical removal of a ruptured intervertebral disk in early childhood. J Pediatr 1959;55:57–62.
821. Kozlowski K. Anterior intervertebral disk herniations in children. Pediatr Radiol 1977;6:32–35.
822. Kurihara A, Kataoka O. Lumbar disk herniation in children and adolescents: a review of 70 operated cases and their minimum 5-year follow-up studies. Spine 1980;5:443–451.
823. Lorenz M, McCulloch J. Chemonucleolysis for herniated nucleus pulposus in adolescents. J Bone Joint Surg Am 1985;67:1402–1404.
824. MacGee EE. Protruded lumbar disk in a 9 year old boy. J Pediatr 1968;73:418–419.
825. Mainzer F. Herniation of the nucleus pulposus: a rare complication of intervertebral disk calcification in children. Radiology 1973;107:167–170.
826. Mandell AJ. Lumbosacral intervertebral disk disease in children. Calif Med 1960;93:307–308.
827. Mori T, Tajima T, Yui S. Herniated lumbar intervertebral disk in teenage children. Chubu Seisai 1966;9:206–209.
828. Nelson CL, Janecki CJ, Gildenber PL, Sava G. Disk protrusion in the young. Clin Orthop 1972;88:142–190.
829. O'Connell JE. Intervertebral disk protrusions in childhood and adolescence. Br J Surg 1960;47:611–616.
830. Pasquier J. Calcification du disque intervértebral de l'enfant Ann Chir Inf 1975;16:249–253.
831. Rugtveit A. Juvenile lumbar disk herniations. Acta Orthop Scand 1966;37:348–356.
832. Russwurm H, Bjeakreim I, Ronglan E. Lumbar intervertebreal disc in children and adolescents. Acta Orthop Scand 1971;45:940–944.
833. Sutton TJ, Turcotte B. Posterior herniation of calcified intervertebral discs in children. J Can Assoc Radiol 1973;24:131–136.
834. Tsuji H, Ito T, Toyoda A, et al. Lumbar disk herniation in teenage children. Rinsho Seikei Geka 1977;12:945–949.
835. Wahren H. Herniated nucleus pulposus in a child of twelve years. Acta Orthop Scand 1945;16:40–42.
836. Webb JH, Svien HJ, Kennedy RL. Protruded lumbar intervertebral disks in children. JAMA 1954;227:1153–1154.
837. Wigh RE. The transitional lumbo-sacral discs: probability of herniation. Spine 1981;6:168–171.
838. Zamani MH, MacEwan GD. Herniation of the lumbar disk in children and adolescents. J Pediatr Orthop 1982;2:528–533.

Sacrum

839. Beguiristain J, Schweitzer J, Mora G, Pombo V. Traumatic lumbosacral dislocation in a 5 year old boy with eight year follow-up. Spine 1995;20:362–366.

840. Bonnin JG. Sacral fractures and injuries to the cauda equina. J Bone Joint Surg 1945;27:113–127.
841. Day DL, Letouornay JG, Grass JR, Goldberg ME, Drake DG. Musculoskeletal case of the day. AJR 1987;148:1048–1052.
842. Denis F, Davis S, Comfort T. Sacral fractures: an important problem; retrospective analysis of 236 cases. Clin Orthop 1988;227:67–81.
843. Fujita K, Sinmei M, Hashimoto K, Shimomura Y. Posterior dislocation of the sacral apophyseal ring. Am J Sports Med 1986;14:243–245.
844. Grier D, Wardell S, Sarwak J, Poznanski AK. Fatigue fractures of the sacrum in children: two case reports and a review of the literature. Skeletal Radiol 1993;22:215–218.
845. Haasbeek JF, Green NE. Adolescent stress fractures of the sacrum: two case reports. J Pediatr Orthop 1994;14:336–338.
846. Heckman JD, Keats PK. Fracture of the sacrum in a child: a case report. J Bone Joint Surg Am 1978;60:404–409.
847. Kramer KE, Levine AM. Unilateral facet dislocation of the lumbosacral junction: a case report and review of the literature. J Bone Joint Surg Am 1989;71:1258–1261.
848. Phelan ST, Jones D, Bishay M. Conservative management of transverse fractures of the sacrum with neurological features: a report of four cases. J Bone Joint Surg Br 1991;73:969–971.
849. Pohlemann T, Gängglen A, Tscherne H. Die Problematik der Sakrumfraktur: klinische Analyse von 377 Fällen. Orthopade 1992;21:400–412.
850. Rai SK, Far RF, Ghovanlon B. Neurologic deficits associated with sacral wing fractures. Orthopedics 1990;13:1363–1366.
851. Rajah R, Davies AM, Carter SR. Fatigue fracture of the sacrum in a child. Pediatr Radiol 1993;23:145–146.
852. Rodriquez-Fuentes AE. Traumatic sacrolisthesis S1–S2: report of a case. Spine 1993;18:768–771.
853. Zoltan D, Gilula LA, Murphy WA. Unilateral facet dislocation between the fifth lumbar and first sacral vertebrae: case report. J Bone Joint Surg Am 1979;61:767–769.

Acute Injury

854. Anderson JM, Schutt AH. Spinal injury in children: a review of 156 cases seen from 1950 through 1978. Mayo Clin Proc 1980;55:499–504.
855. Andrews LG, Jung SK. Spinal cord injuries in children in British Columbia. Paraplegia 1979;17:442–451.
856. Arlington NJ, Zembo M, Nadell J, Bowen JR. C1–C2 posterior soft-tissue injuries with neurologic impairment in children. J Pediatr Orthop 1990;10:596–601.
857. Babcock JL. Spinal injuries in children. Pediatr Clin North Am 1975;22:487–500.
858. Bracken MB, Shepard MJ, Collins WF, et al. A randomized controlled trial of methylprednisolone or naloxone in the treatment of acute spinal cord injury: results of the second national acute spinal cord injury study. N Engl J Med 1990;322:1405–1411.
859. Brown MS, Phibbs RH. Spinal cord injury in newborns from use of umbilical artery catheters. J Perinatol 1988;8:105–110.
860. Cheshire DJ. The paediatric syndrome of traumatic myelopathy without demonstrable vertebral injury. Paraplegia 1977;15:74–85.
861. Cotler HB, Kulkarni MV, Bondurant FJ. Magnetic resonance imaging of acute spinal cord trauma: preliminary report. J Orthop Trauma 1988;12:1–4.
862. Gabriel KR, Crawford AH. Identification of acute post-traumatic spinal cord cyst by magnetic resonance imaging: a case report and review of the literature. J Pediatr Orthop 1988;8:710–714.
863. Hadley MN, Zabramski JM, Browner CM, Rekate H, Sonntag VK. Pediatric spinal trauma: review of 122 cases of spinal cord and vertebral injuries. J Neurosurg 1988;68:18–24.
864. Merriam WF, Taylor TKF, Ruff SJ, McPhail MJ. A reappraisal of acute traumatic central cord syndrome. J Bone Joint Surg Br 1986;68:708–713.
865. Morgan R, Brown JC, Bonnett C. The effect of laminectomy on the pediatric spinal cord-injured patient. J Bone Joint Surg Am 1974;56:1767–1772.
866. Posnikoff J. Spontaneous spinal epidural hematoma of childhood. J Pediatr 1968;73:178–183.
867. Rathbone D, Johnson G, Letts M. Spinal cord concussion in pediatric athletes. J Pediatr Orthop 1992;12:616–620.
868. Renard M, Tridon P, Kuhna ST, et al. Three unusual cases of spinal cord injury in childhood. Paraplegia 1978;16:130–134.
869. Schwartz A. Spinal cord infarction: MRI and MEP findings in these cases. J Spinal Disord 1992;5:212–216.
870. Silwa JA, MacLean IC. Ischaemic myelopathy: a review of the spinal vasculature and related clinical syndromes. Arch Phys Med Rehabil 1980;39:1–8.
871. Sneed RC, Stover SL. Undiagnosed spinal cord injuries in brain injured children. Am J Dis Child 1988;142:965–967.
872. Sneed RC, Stover SL, Fine PR. Spinal cord injury associated with all-terrain vehicle accidents. Pediatrics 1986;77:271–274.
873. Tator CH. Review of experimental spinal cord injury with emphasis on the local and systemic circulatory effects. Neurochirurgie 1991;37:291–302.
874. Tator CH, Fehlings MG. Review of the secondary injury theory of acute spinal cord trauma with emphasis on vascular mechanisms. J Neurosurg 1991;75:15–26.
875. Wilberger JE Jr. Spinal Cord Injuries in Children. Mount Kisco, NY: Futura, 1986.
876. Wittenberg RH, Boetel U, Boyer HK. Magnetic resonance imaging and computer tomography of acute spinal cord trauma. Clin Orthop 1990;260:176–185.
877. Wohman L. The neuropathology of traumatic paraplegia. Paraplegia 1964;1:233–251.

Spinal Cord Injury (Chronic)

878. Abramson AS. Bone disturbances in injuries to the spinal cord and cauda equina (paraplegia): their prevention by ambulation. J Bone Joint Surg Am 1948;30:982–987.
879. Audic B. Paraplegies traumatiques: problemes specifiques des enfants. Rev Prat 1971;21:456–461.
880. Audic B, Maury M. Secondary vertebral deformities in childhood and adolescence. Paraplegia 1969;7:10–16.
881. Backe HA, Betz RR, Mezgarzadeh M, Beck T, Clancy M. Post-traumatic spinal cord cysts evaluated by magnetic resonance imaging. Paraplegia 1991;29:607–612.
882. Banta JV. Rehabilitation of pediatric spinal cord injury: the Newington Children's Hospital experience. Conn Med 1984;48:14–18.
883. Bedbook CM. Correction of scoliosis due to paraplegia sustained in pediatric age group. Paraplegia 1977;15:90–96.
884. Betz RR, Mulcahey MJ. Spinal cord injury rehabilitation. In: Weinstein SL (ed) The Pediatric Spine. Principles and Practice. New York: Raven, 1994.
885. Betz RR, Mulcahey MJ. The Child with a Spinal Cord Injury. Rosemont, IL: AAOS, 1996.
886. Boltshauser E, Isler W, Bucher HM, Friderich H. Permanent flaccid paraplegia in children with thoracic spinal cord injury. Paraplegia 1981;19:227–234.
887. Bradway JK, Kavanagh BF, Houser OW. Post-traumatic spinal-cord cyst. J Bone Joint Surg Am 1986;68:932–933.

888. Brown JC, Swank SM, Matta J, Barras DM. Late spinal deformity in quadriplegic children and adolescents. J Pediatr Orthop 1984;4:456–461.
889. Bucher HM, Boltshauser E, Forderich J, Isler W. Traumatische quer-Schmitts' lähmungen im Kindesalter. Schweiz Med Wochenschr 1980;110:331–337.
890. Chao R, Mayo ME. Long-term urodynamic follow-up in pediatric spinal cord injury. Paraplegia 1994;32:806–809.
891. Cristofaro RL, Brink JD. Hypercalcemia of immobilization in neurologically injured children: a prospective study. Orthopedics 1979;2:486–491.
892. Dearolf WW III, Betz RR, Vogel LC, Levin J, Clancy M, Steel HH. Scolosis in pediatric spinal cord injured patients. J Pediatr Orthop 1990;10:214–216.
893. Drummond DK. A study of pressure distribution measured during balanced and unbalanced sitting. J Bone Joint Surg Am 1982;64:1034–1039.
894. Gangloff S, Onimus M. Post-traumatic scoliosis. J Pediatr Orthop Part B 1996;5:216–219.
895. Garland DE, Shimoyama ST, Lugo C, Barra SD, Gilgoff I. Spinal cord insults and heterotopic ossification in the pediatric population. Clin Orthop 1989;245:303–310.
896. Garrett AL, Perry J, Nickel VL. Paralytic scoliosis. Clin Orthop 1961;21:117–124.
897. Griffiths GR. Growth problems in cervical injuries. Paraplegia 1974;12:277–289.
898. Haffner DL, Hoffer MM, Wiedbusch R. Etiology of children's spinal injuries at Rancho Los Amigos. Spine 1993;18:679–684.
899. Head H, Riddoch G. The automatic bladder, excessive sweating and some other reflex conditions in gross injuries of the spinal cord. Brain 1917;40:188–193.
900. Hill EL, Martin RB, Gunther E, Morey-Holton E, Holets VR. Changes in bone in a model of spinal cord injury. J Orthop Res 1993;11:537–547.
901. Hyre HM, Stelling CB. Radiographic appearance of healed extremity fractures in children with spinal cord lesions. Skeletal Radiol 1989;18:189–192.
902. Jane MJ, Freehafer AA, Hazel C, et al. Autonomic dysreflexia. Clin Orthop 1982;169:151–154.
903. Jeannopolous CL. Bone changes in children with lesions of the spinal cord or roots. NY State Med 1954;54-II:3219–3224.
904. Kewalramani LS, Kraus JF, Sterling HM. Acute spinal cord lesions in a pediatric population: epidemiological and clinical features. Paraplegia 1990;18:206–219.
905. Kewalramani LS, Tori JA. Spinal cord trauma in children: neurologic patterns, radiologic features, and pathomechanics of injury. Spine 1980;5:11–18.
906. Kilfoyle RM, Foley JJ, Norton PL. Spine and pelvic deformity in childhood and adolescent paraplegia: a study of 104 cases. J Bone Joint Surg Am 1965;47:659–682.
907. Laitinen L, Singounas E. Longitudinal myelotomy in the treatment of spasticity of the legs. J Neurosurg 1971;35:536–540.
908. Lancourt JE, Dickson JH, Carter RE. Paralytic spinal deformity following traumatic spinal-cord injury in children and adolescents. J Bone Joint Surg Am 1981;63:47–53.
909. Lapides JL. Neurogenic bladder: principles of treatment. Urol Clin North Am 1974;1:81–97.
910. Mayfield JK, Erkkila JC, Winter RB. Spine deformity subsequent to acquired childhood spinal cord injury. J Bone Joint Surg Am 1981;63:1401–1411.
911. McCall IW, Galvin E, O'Brien JP, Park WM. Alterations in vertebral growth following prolonged plaster immobilization. Acta Orthop Scand 1981;52:327–330.
912. McSweeney T. Spinal deformity after spinal cord injury. Paraplegia 1969;6:212–221.
913. Melzak J. Paraplegia among children. Lancet 1969;2:45–48.
914. Mital MA, Garber JE, Stinson JT. Ectopic bone formation in children and adolescents with head injuries: its management. J Pediatr Orthop 1987;7:83–90.
915. Moynahan M, Betz RR, Triolo RJ, Maurer AH. Characterization of the bone mineral density of children with spinal cord injury. J Spinal Cord Med 1997;19:249–254
916. Mulcahey MJ. Returning to school following spinal cord injury: perspectives of four adolescents. Am J Occup Ther 1992;46:395–413.
917. Munro D. The rehabilitation of patients totally paralyzed below the waist: anterior rhizotomy for spastic paraplegia. N Engl J Med 1945;233:453–461.
918. Norton PL, Foley JJ. Paraplegia in children. J Bone Joint Surg Am 1959;41:1291–1309.
919. Odom JA, Brown CLO, Jackson RR, Hahn HR, Cade TV. Scoliosis in paraplegia. Paraplegia 1970;8:42–47.
920. Pouliquen JC, Pennecot GF. Progressive spinal deformity after spinal injury in children. In: Houghton GR, Thompson GH (eds) Problematic Musculoskeletal Injuries in Childen. London: Butterworths, 1985.
921. Renshaw TS. Spinal cord injury and post traumatic deformities. In: Weinstein SL (ed) The Pediatric Spine: Principles and Practice. New York: Raven, 1994.
922. Rink P, Miller F. Hip instability in spinal cord injury patients. J Pediatr Orthop 1990;10:583–587.
923. Sterling HM. Physical rehabilitation of young children with spinal cord lesions. JAMA 1961;175:584–587.
924. Stover SL, Hahn HR, Miller JM III. Disodium etidronate in the prevention of heterotopic ossification following spinal cord injury. Paraplegia 1976;14:146–156.
925. Triolo RJ, Betz RR, Mulcahey MJ, Gardner ER. Application of functional neuromuscular stimulation to children with spinal cord injuries: candidate selection for upper and lower extremity research. Paraplegia 1994;32:824–843.

19
Pelvis

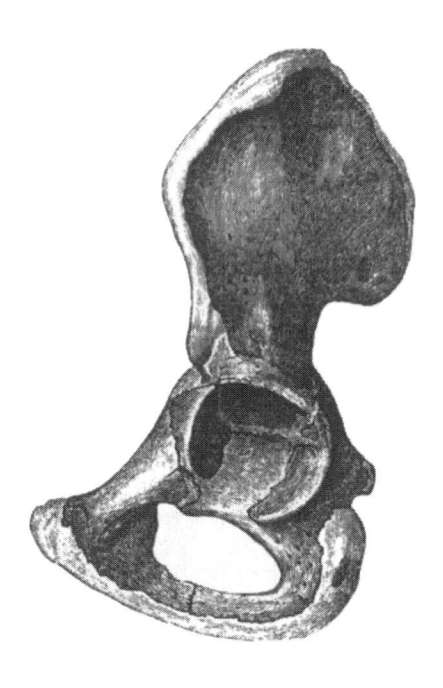

Engraving of immature hemipelvis. (From Poland J. Traumatic Separation of the Epiphyses. London: Smith, Elder, 1898)

The child's pelvis is a complex structure that includes the termination of the spine (sacrum and coccyx). Multiple growth regions are present throughout the developing pelvis. These regions are the equivalents of the epiphyses of the long bones. Secondary ossification within these epiphyses and apophyses may be confusing when evaluating the possibility of fracture. These regions certainly may be fractured at the chondro-osseous interface to create a physeal injury.

The developing pelvic bone, especially the ilium, may be quite flexible, a factor that allows considerable deformation without obvious fracture. Rebound following deformation may create a false sense of security when evaluating the extent of injury. Such deformation also puts contained soft tissue structures at risk for injury. The potential for urethral, gynecologic, bladder and rectal injuries must be assessed carefully, even when the radiologic appearance of the pelvis does not suggest severe injury.

Anatomy

Each hemipelvis initially forms from three primary centers of ossification located within the chondral anlagen of the ischium, pubis, and ilium. The primary ossification centers of these anlagen converge within the acetabulum to delineate the triradiate cartilage (Fig. 19-1). The triradiate cartilage is a composite of the epiphyses of three contributing anatomic (embryologic) structures that comprise each hemipelvis.[5,6] The particular chondro-osseous interrelations allow continual integrated growth and hemispheric expansion of the acetabulum commensurate with the progressive spherical growth of the capital femoral epiphysis. During adolescence secondary centers of ossification develop within the "arms" of the triradiate cartilage (Figs. 19-2, 19-3). These arms should not be misconstrued as fracture fragments during the evaluation of a pelvic injury during childhood or adolescence (Fig. 19-4). This modified growth region (triradiate cartilage) normally undergoes physiologic epiphysiodesis at approximately 12–14 years in girls and 14–16 years in boys. Damage to the triradiate growth mechanism may lead to deformity of the acetabulum (e.g., a shallow acetabulum), especially if such an injury occurs in a young child (under 10 years of age).

Within each arm of the triradiate cartilage the physeal cartilage is bipolar, being directed toward two of the three component pelvic bones. The germinal zone runs along the central portion of each arm. Small blood vessels are also present within this central region of the cartilage. Extending from the central germinal zone toward each metaphysis are the dividing and hypertrophic zones. These zones are not as wide as they are in longitudinal bones, reflecting the less rapid rates of endochondral ossification occurring within the triradiate physes. The capacity for continued growth and endochondral ossification within this structure may be damaged by certain fracture patterns.

The intrapelvic side of the triradiate cartilage is covered by perichondrium and a thick layer of fibrous tissue.[6]

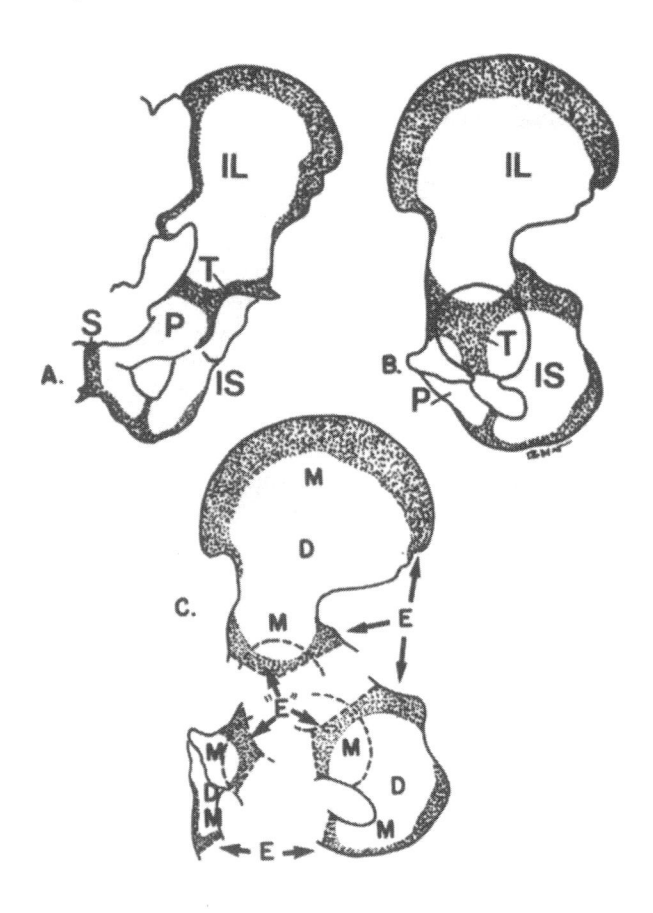

FIGURE 19-1. Anterior (A) and lateral (B) developing pelvis, showing relative areas of bone (white) and cartilage (stippled). IL = ilium; IS = ischium; P = pubis; S = symphysis pubis; T = triradiate cartilage. (C) Exploded view to emphasize analogy of each component bone to a long bone and how several "epiphyses" fuse to form the triradiate cartilage. Similar "epiphyseal" fusions form the ischiopubic junctions and the symphysis pubis. E = epiphysis; M = metaphysis; D = diaphysis.

Traumatic stripping of the periosteal attachments in this region may result in abundant formation of callus and can contribute to the intrinsic stability. Because of such periosteal tissue this region may rapidly form a small or large osseous bridge if injured.

The composite radiolucency of the two superior arms of the triradiate cartilage is usually visualized on the standard anteroposterior roentgenogram of the pelvis. However, the appearance of the triradiate cartilage is shown best by a direct roentgenogram through the acetabulum (Figs. 19-2, 19-3). In the clinical setting, such a roentgenogram is difficult to obtain because of the obliquity of the acetabulum and the superimposed presence of the capital femoral ossification center. Routine internal and external oblique roentgenograms (e.g., Judet views[105]) may assist in visualizing different portions of the triradiate cartilage, allowing reconstruction of the entire unit for diagnostic or follow-up purposes. Computed tomography (CT) may also offer improved three-dimensional reconstruction of the region. It is important to understand the anatomy of this cartilage, as it represents the "epiphyseal" ends of the iliac, pubic, and ischial rami and may be variably disrupted when these bones are also fractured in other anatomic regions. The seeming absence of a concomitant fracture in a childhood single-ramus injury, in contrast to the double-ramus concept in adults, may be explained by the fact that a physeal injury (separation) may also be present at the triradiate cartilage, the cartilage of the pubic symphysis, or the ischiopubic synchondrosis. If displacement is minimal (or even occult), such an injury pattern may be virtually impossible to detect by routine radiography.

The anatomic os acetabuli (i.e., the equivalent of secondary epiphyseal ossification centers) appear within the triradiate cartilage when the child is 12–14 years of age and fuse by 16 years. These secondary centers coalesce with the peripheral radiographic os acetabulum

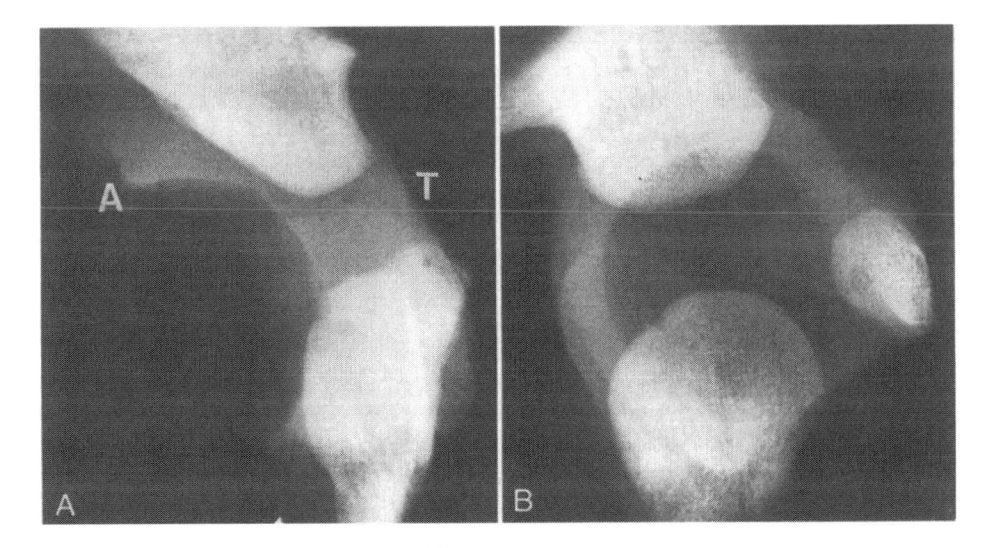

FIGURE 19-2. Early developmental patterns of the triradiate cartilage. (A) Duplication of the standard anterior view of the acetabular segment and composite bones from the pelvis of a stillborn neonate. Note the extent of the acetabular, A, and triradiate, T, cartilage. (B) Direct view of acetabulum to show the true appearance of the triradiate cartilage.

(Figs. 19-4, 19-5), which is a normal secondary ossification center located along the margins of the acetabulum.[5,7,8] The peripheral os acetabulum may be avulsed traumatically, especially with posteriorly directed hip dislocations (see Chapter 20). During late adolescence the triradiate ossification centers fuse with the peripheral center.

The ischium and pubis also have an additional ongoing interposed bipolar growth cartilage within the inferior ramus. Fusion of this particular region normally occurs between the ages of 4 and 7 years. Fusiform enlargement of this ischiopubic junction during physiologic closure is often evident radiographically.[1,2,4] Caffey and Ross reported that fusion could occur any time between 4 and 12 years of age and was often preceded by irregularity of ossification. The latter is most frequent between the ages of 5 and 8 years and may be asymmetric in 22% of normal patients.[1]

Kloiber et al. noted that the bone adjacent to the unfused ischiopubic synchondrosis has a structure and vascular anatomy comparable to that of the metaphysis of long bones of children and thus is a potential site of injury or osteomyelitis.[4] Normal variability in the radiographic and scintigraphic appearance of the synchondrosis may make the evaluation of images difficult. Just prior to fusion the normal synchondrosis may show a combination of expansion and irregular ossification. The age of fusion varies and, in the same patient, often proceeds asymmetrically, negating or minimizing the value of comparison with the opposite side. Correspondingly, increased asymmetric activity has also been described in bone scintigraphy in normal patients.

Enlargement of the ischiopubic junction has been variably described as normal, an osteochondrosis, a stress fracture, infection, or malignancy. In children in the 6- to 10-year range irregularity of this area should be considered a

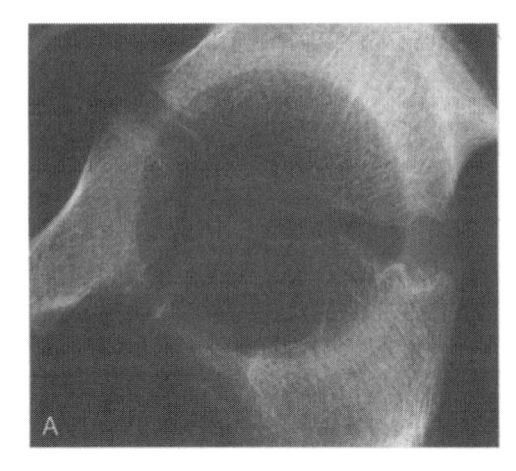

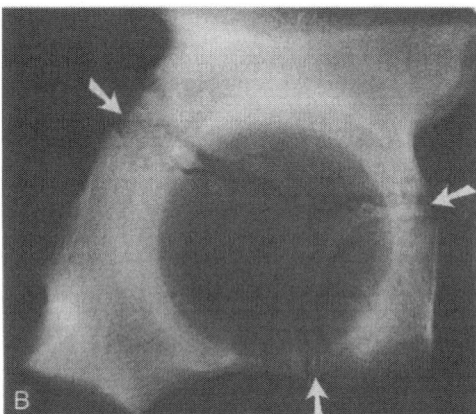

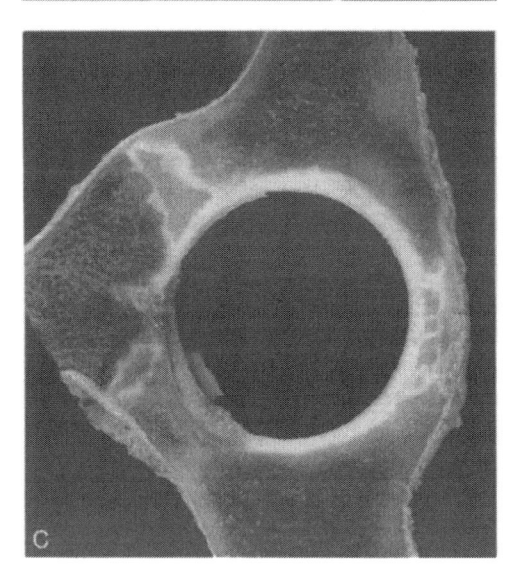

FIGURE 19-3. Later development of the triradiate cartilage. (A) At 12 years, prior to the development of secondary ossification. (B) At 14 years, with development of secondary ossification centers in the arms of the triradiate cartilage (arrows). Serial sectioning shows the morphology (C) of these centers.

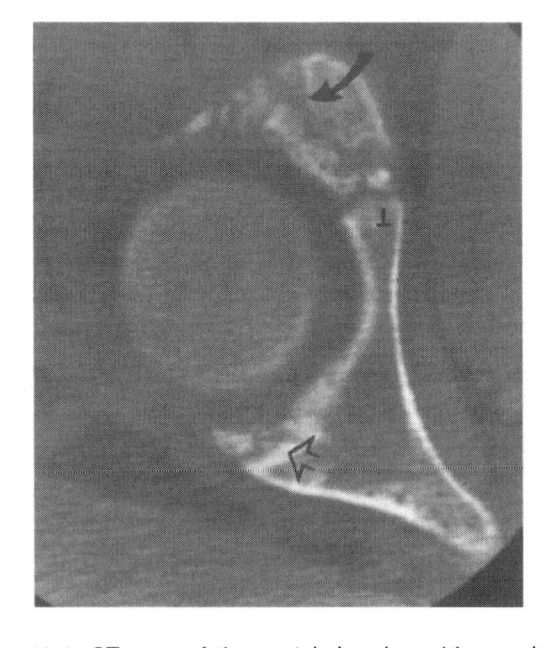

FIGURE 19-4. CT scan of the acetabulum in a 14-year-old boy being evaluated for pelvic trauma following a motor vehicle accident. Secondary ossification centers are present within the triradiate cartilage and the anterior (open arrow) and posterior (solid arrow) rims.

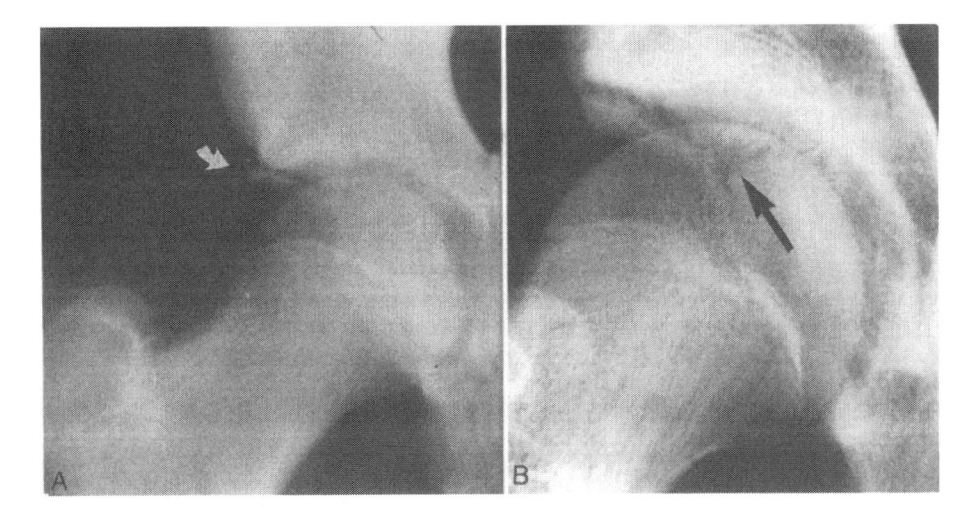

FIGURE 19-5. Normal peripheral acetabular ossification characteristic of adolescence. (A) Beginning formation along the superior rim (arrow), which should not be confused with an avulsion fracture of the adjacent anteroinferior spine. (B) Complete rim ossification with posterosuperior continuity with the triradiate ossification (arrow).

normal variation of skeletal maturation. It should *not* be misinterpreted as a healing fracture, even though the radiographic appearance may be suggestive of callus formation or reactive new bone caused by osteomyelitis or neoplasia.[4] However, in the older child, particularly one with pain in the groin region, any apparent increased bone formation in the ischiopubic junction should be considered a possible stress fracture, infection, or neoplasia. A bone scan showing asymmetric radionuclide uptake may help make a specific diagnosis. Chondro-osseous fractures may occur through this region or the symphysis when there is a triradiate fracture and a rotational displacement of the pubis, ischium, or both.

The normal, maturing ischial tuberosity may appear irregular and may be mistaken for a fracture, infection, or tumor, especially if the patient presents with excessive reactive bone formation several weeks after injury. Because secondary ossification is often not present until midadolescence, the only indication of a traction injury, with or without displacement, may be cystic change in the metaphyseal-equivalent region.

The iliac crest and spines are cartilaginous until adolescence (Fig. 19-6). Secondary centers of ossification appear along the anterolateral iliac crest when the child is approximately 13–15 years old. Posterior advancement continues until the posterior iliac spine is reached. Fusion of crest ossification to the rest of the ilium occurs by 15–17 years, although complete fusion may be delayed until 25 years. Alternatively, after the ossification center first appears, separate ossification may proceed from a posterior center, with the central portion being ossified at a later date as the two centers grow toward each other.

The anterosuperior iliac spine develops from the anterior apophysis of the iliac crest. This area ossifies at about age 15 years and unites completely with the ilium between 20 and 25 years. Several muscles originate or insert on the anterosuperior iliac spine, including the sartorius, tensor fasciae lata, and gluteus medius.

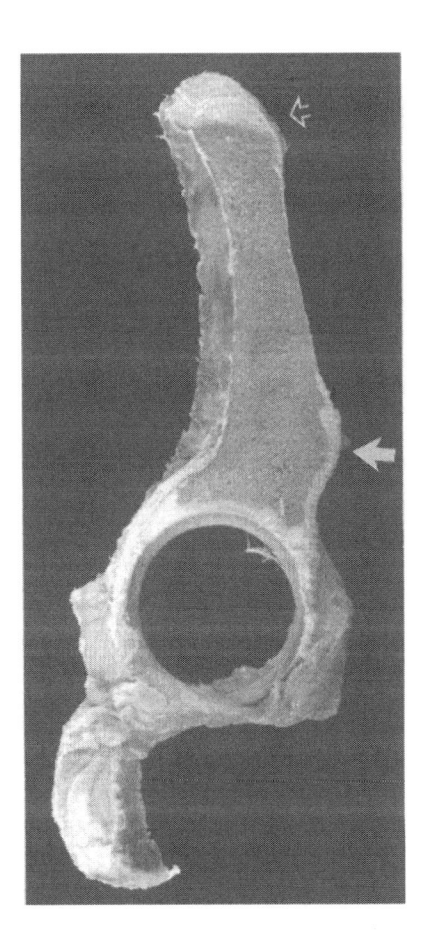

FIGURE 19-6. Slab section of the pelvis showing the anterosuperior iliac spine (open arrow) and the anteroinferior iliac spine (solid arrow) above the acetabulum. A portion of the ischial synchondrosis is evident below the acetabulum.

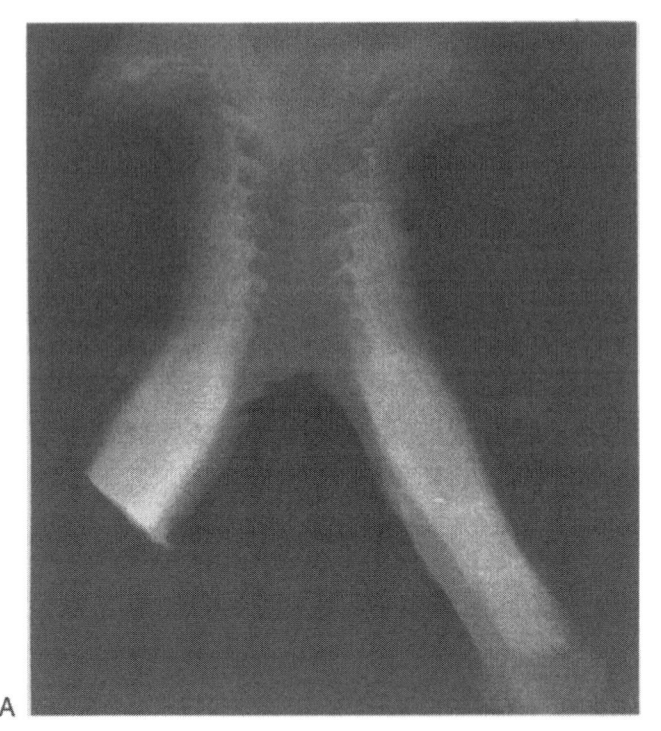

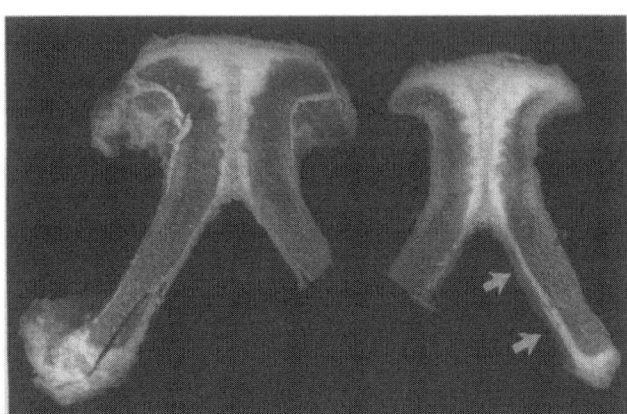

FIGURE 19-7. Development of the symphysis pubis. (A) Radiograph of a slab specimen from a 14-year-old, showing the normal undulated appearance that progressively develops. It should not be misinterpreted as an inflammatory process. (B) Morphologic slab sections of the immature pubic symphysis showing undulated epiphyseal cartilage on either side of central fibrocartilage (which remains in adults) and extension of the epiphyseal cartilage along the ramus to the ischiopubic synchondrosis (arrows).

There may be a secondary center of ossification at the anteroinferior iliac spine, appearing at 13–15 years and fusing at 16–18 years. This is evident more commonly in boys than girls and may be contiguous with secondary ossification extending from the acetabular margin.

The symphysis pubis is a growth region connecting the two hemipelves anteriorly. As an epiphyseal analogue it may be injured, comparable to epiphyseal fractures of the long bones. The normal endochondral ossification process may be associated with an irregular, undulated appearance that should not be confused with that due to trauma (Fig. 19-7). "Widening" of the symphyseal region is highly variable and depends on the degree of maturation of chondral into osseous tissue.[3]

General Considerations

The pelvis of the child differs from that of the adult in that the bone, cartilage, and joints (sacroiliac, symphysis pubis, triradiate, ischiopubic) are more pliant (Fig. 19-8) and susceptible to separation (fractures) at the chondro-osseous interfaces. This greater volume of cartilage and the less brittle bone provide a significant buffer for energy absorption, much like the developing skull and its sutures. Accordingly, pelvic osseous fractures are less common than in adults.[9–45] When fractures do occur, the contiguous radiolucent cartilage may be damaged (often occultly) at the time of injury or later, particularly if the fracture heals in such a way that abnormal forces result in altered growth. As an example, the triradiate cartilage may be damaged microscopically (i.e., not radiologically evident), leading to acetabular maldevelopment and a morphologic situation similar to developmental hip dysplasia. A displaced fracture of the ischiopubic ring (essentially reversing an innominate or similar pelvic osteotomy) may lead to uncovering of the femoral head with subsequent capital femoral subluxation. The presence of growth cartilage along several pelvic margins allows avulsion fractures to occur (type 3, 4, and 7 growth mechanism injuries, as described in Chapter 6). These fractures are comparable to epiphyseal-physeal injuries in a long bone and are subject to all the potential acute and long-term complications. Leg length discrepancy may be a problem when a hemipelvis is shifted superiorly and may lead to scoliosis during the adolescent period owing to the posttraumatic pelvic obliquity and the relative leg length discrepancy.

The developing chondro-osseous pelvis is more resilient than that in an adult and therefore affords less rigid protection to the contained viscera, which because of immature fibrous capsules and stroma may be damaged more easily than comparable adult organs. The juvenile pelvis may undergo considerable elastic and plastic distortion without actual fracture. Therefore organ damage may occur with little subsequent roentgenographic evidence of the severity of the maximum degree of chondro-osseous trauma.

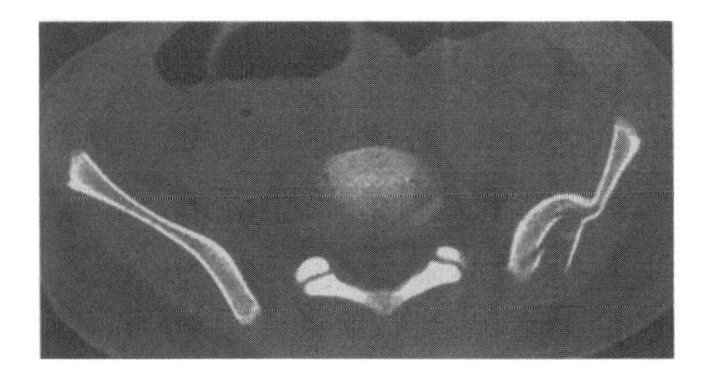

FIGURE 19-8. Plastic deformation of the ilium following direct pelvic trauma in a 7-year-old boy. The anterior cortex is deformed but intact, whereas the posterior cortex is plastically deformed and cortically disrupted.

General Considerations

The identification of a pelvic fracture in a child, particularly if displaced, thus assumes even more clinical significance. The array of injuries, including genitourinary ones, is roughly proportional to the severity of the pelvic fracture pattern.

Reed reviewed 84 cases of pelvic fractures in children, more than 80% of which were due to vehicular accidents[33]; 39% were unstable. The most frequent type was the diametric fracture, in which there was a fracture of the ilium or sacrum or sacroiliac separation, combined with a pubic fracture anteriorly on either the same or the opposite side. However, many diametric fractures in children are stable, because the posterior fractures are often undisplaced or incomplete epiphyseal separations through the sacroiliac region with a considerable degree of retained soft tissue (periosteal and ligamentous) continuity and stability. The other injuries, most of which were isolated pubic fractures, were stable. Sixteen patients had associated visceral injuries. Eighteen had transient microhematuria, but none had significant injuries to the genitourinary tract. Eleven had gross hematuria, and all had major injuries to the lower urinary tract or the kidney. Two patients had severe intracranial injuries. One-third of the patients sustained fractures of other bones, the most common being the femur and the skull. Four children had acetabular fractures through the triradiate cartilage, a pattern that must be closely sought as it is easy to overlook.

Fractures of the pelvic components must be placed in proper perspective. During the initial phase the orthopaedist must be acutely aware of potential injury to the intrapelvic and intraabdominal visceral and vascular contents, rather than the obvious osseous injuries.[55-102] Osseous damage often assumes secondary importance until internal tissue injuries are completely evaluated and treated as necessary. Massive retroperitoneal bleeding following pelvic fracture produces high morbidity and mortality in victims of blunt trauma, no matter what their age. Although less common in children, hemorrhage still represents a significant potential complication.[46-54]

Quinby reported 20 pediatric patients with fractures of the pelvis,[32] 19 of whom were involved in vehicular accidents. The patients were divided into three treatment groups. Group 1 (six patients) did not require laparotomy; the pelvic fractures were relatively mild and essentially undisplaced (including one mild separation of the sacroiliac joint); and none showed clinical shock or required blood transfusion. Group 2 (nine patients) all underwent laparotomy for visceral injuries accompanying the pelvic fractures. All but one of the patients with organ lacerations were in this group. One of the children died. Group 3 (five patients) all had massive retroperitoneal and pelvic hemorrhage with severe pelvic fractures. All group 3 patients had extensive disruption of the sacroiliac joint. All were in clinical shock, with one of the patients dying while control of hemorrhage was attempted during laparotomy. Two others died within 24 hours of surgery, and another died 36 hours postoperatively. The amount of blood replacement from admission to either death or recovery was 3500–8000ml, which represented 175–400% of the estimated volumes. Vascular injuries were combined arterial and venous and were both specific and diffuse. Four of these children had no femoral pulse. In all cases there was injury to the primary branches of the iliac artery near the disrupted sacroiliac joint. There was also diffuse bleeding from injured muscle and bone. Thus among 20 patients there were five deaths: one due to associated brain injury, three to uncontrolled major vascular lacerations, and 1 to a mixture of possible causes but primarily hemorrhage.

Bond et al. studied children consecutively admitted to a regional pediatric trauma center with blunt trauma.[56] Fifty-four of the children (2.4% of 2248 injured children) had an injury to the pelvis. Only 13 of these 54 children had a concomitant abdominal or genitourinary injury. Nine of the children required transfusion, and nine required exploratory or reparative surgery. Six children died. The location of the fracture was strongly associated with the probability of abdominal injury; 80% of children with multiple pelvic fractures had a concomitant abdominal or genitourinary injury, compared with only 33% involvement when there was an isolated fracture of the ilium or pelvic rim, and 6% with isolated pubic fractures. According to their study, the probability of abdominal injury and associated pelvic injury was less than 1% for isolated pubic fractures, 15% for iliac or sacral fractures, and 60% for multiple fractures of the pelvic ring. They noted that in adults the two major conditions leading to death from severe pelvic fracture were hemorrhage and subsequent infection of the intrapelvic hematoma. In contrast, children with pelvic fractures usually died from complications of an associated head injury.

Garvin et al. reviewed 36 pediatric patients who were classified using Torode and Zieg's system.[14,41] They also classified the severity of injury using the Modified Injury Severity Score (MISS). Associated injuries occurred in 67% of the patients, with a long-term morbidity or mortality in 30%. They stressed the high probability of minimal bony injury being associated with life-threatening visceral injuries and morbidity. The most common concomitant organ system involved was musculoskeletal, with 18 long bone fractures in 11 patients. The abdomen was the second most common site of injury (11 patients). Six injuries involved the prostatic urethra ($n = 3$) and spine ($n = 3$). Two patients with prostatic urethral injuries were still incontinent. The third patient died of sepsis. Two of the spinal injury patients had permanent neurologic sequelae. One was monoplegic secondary to lumbosacral plexus injury. The second patient eventually underwent a hemipelvectomy after a sacral plexus injury, femoral neurovascular disruption, and subsequent fungal fasciitis that eventually necessitated the procedure. There were lacerations or severe contusions in two livers, two kidneys, two vaginas, two rectums, and one spleen. However, a partial splenectomy was the only major abdominal surgery required. Three patients sustained closed head injuries. None of them had permanent damage from the associated injury. None of the eight patients had involvement of the sacroiliac joint. None underwent surgery. They found that all patients with long-term morbidity had a fracture classified as ring disruption. However, the morbidity was never attributed to the pelvic bone injury but, rather, to the other nonosseous injuries the patient sustained.

Lacheretz and Herbaux questioned whether unstable ring fractures in children should ever be treated surgically.[19] They reviewed 126 cases, 10 of whom had acetabular involvement. They classified the other 116 cases according to Tile.[40] There were 80 stable fractures (type A), 29 unstable transverse fractures (type B), and seven unstable transverse and vertical fractures (type C). They found that all type A and B fractures healed by conservative means. Only in type C fractures was there a need to consider closed reduction with external fixation or surgical intervention.

McLaren et al. studied long-term pain and disability after displaced pelvic ring fractures.[25] All patients were adults. They found that in 43 patients with high-energy pelvic fractures 5 years or more earlier, the occurrence of chronic pain and the functional outcome was related to residual deformity of the pelvic ring. Among the patients with no residual deformity (i.e., a displacement of less than 1 cm), 88% had no serious pain and 82% had normal function. However, among the patients with residual deformity, with the displacement being more than 1 cm posteriorly, 70% had serious pain and only 70% had normal function. They recommended definitive reduction and stabilization as early after the injury as possible. Schwartz et al. found that near-anatomic reduction in children gave the best functional/pain results 2–25 years after pelvic fracture.[37] Remodeling in children, however, makes mandatory anatomic reduction of the pelvis and sacroiliac joints less necessary. Remodeling does *not* correct upward displacement of a hemipelvis at the sacroiliac junction.

Having treated many pelvic disruptions in children, I have observed that the patients with hemipelvic displacements of more than 1–2 cm may have minimal problems as a child but frequently develop pain and discomfort during adolescence and their early adult years when they are followed for an extended period of time. The leg length inequality often requires treatment. Back pain becomes a significant problem with further growth and increasing physical demands.

Diagnosis

The accurate diagnosis of pelvic injuries is difficult only on the basis of clinical findings. Children tend to be at the extremes, with either a relatively simple pelvic injury or multiple trauma. Variable levels of consciousness may limit the response to pain. Physical examination should include pelvic compression, which may elicit pain. The absence of pain, however, does not effectively rule out injury because of possible lumbosacral plexus and spinal cord injury. Posterior subluxation of the ilium on the sacrum at the sacroiliac joint is generally missed because the patient is usually supine, especially if severely injured. The region may not be examined with sufficient care, particularly when there are multiple injuries. Soft tissue injury—abrasions, lacerations, ecchymoses—should increase the index of suspicion. The perineum should be examined carefully.

As reasonable a neurologic examination as possible should be undertaken, depending on the level of consciousness of the patient. In particular, sacral sensation should be tested. Many nerve injuries are missed because detailed initial neurologic examination is neglected or cursory, especially in the child with life-threatening injury. The lumbosacral plexus is closely related to the sacroiliac joint; there may be some neural damage when the "joint" is dislocated or separated. The lumbosacral trunk, the superior gluteal nerve, and the obturator nerve may be stretched or even disrupted. Intrathecal rupture of the roots of the cauda equina may be produced by traction. Chondro-osseous distortion or displacement may be greater at the time of the accident than when the child presents for treatment. The actual extent of tissue deformity may cause stretch (traction) nerve injuries.

Adequate radiographic examination is critical. However, always remember that this static radiographic appearance may not indicate the maximum deformity that was attained when the injury was actually occurring. A gonad shield should *not* be used during the initial screening, as it may obliterate areas that need to be critically evaluated. The anteroposterior view of the pelvis that adequately demonstrates the pelvic ring is not always acceptable for determining fracture details because of the normal lumbar lordosis. The best view in the anteroposterior position may be oblique, depending on how much curvature there is in the spine.[80] An inlet or downshot view is obtained 30° off the vertical, with the cone aimed distally to demonstrate bursting of the ring. Other projections (e.g., Judet's views) may provide important information about fragment displacement, especially in the adolescent.[105]

Computed tomography (Figs. 19-9 to 19-11) offers the best method for detecting subtle injuries and defining the specific fracture anatomy more precisely.[30] For example, apparent sacroiliac disruption was actually a chondro-osseous disruption comparable to a type 1 or 2 growth mechanism injury of a long bone. CT scanning is also useful for detecting inward or outward winging hinged at the sacroiliac joint (Fig. 19-10), as well as the diagnosis of posterior displacement of an ilium (Fig. 19-11).

Magid et al. discussed the role of two- and three-dimensional CT imaging in the evaluation of acetabular and pelvic fractures in pediatric patients.[23] Using standard technology, the acquired images may be rotated through multiple positions in any 360° sequence until the best view is obtained. This capability is important, as conventional films may not provide the optimum view or because the injured young patient may be unable or unwilling to comply with positioning maneuvers. Furthermore, colonic air and solid contents may obscure the posterior pelvic ring. Magid et al. noted that much of the recent trend toward more conservative, less invasive management of patients with abdominal or thoracic trauma is related to the ability to document adequately the extent of injury by CT rather than resorting to exploratory laparotomy or laparoscopy.

Magid et al. found that three-dimensional CT reconstruction was useful in 50% of the cases in terms of better fracture definition, 56% in terms of deciding between conservative or operative management, 46% in terms of selecting the ideal operative approach, and 30% in terms of selecting the hardware to be used for the operation.[23] CT also provides a convenient, noninvasive method for follow-up of a complex pelvic fracture.

Although CT imaging provides additional information for evaluating traumatized patients, not every pediatric patient with pelvic trauma requires such a study. Particularly, patients with simple, stable injuries to the symphysis or anterior ring that were readily evident on routine films did not

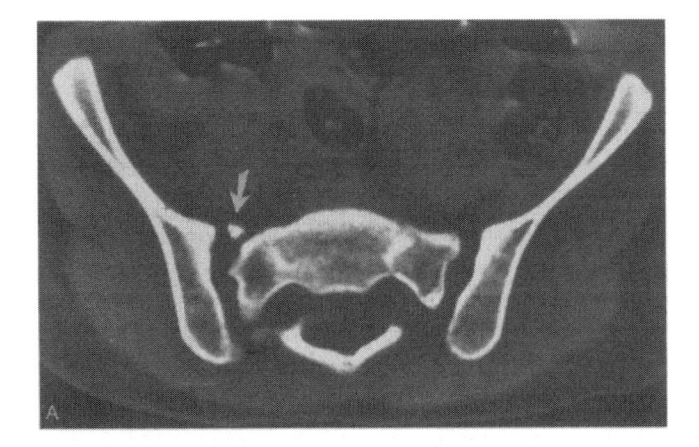

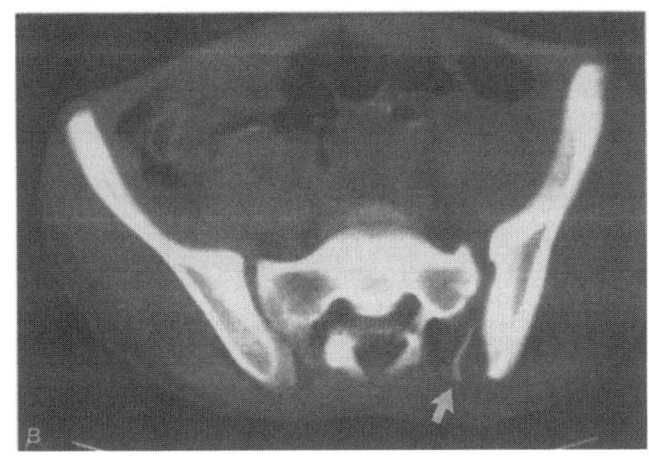

FIGURE 19-9. (A) CT scan shows that the apparent sacroiliac separation seen on the routine anteroposterior film was really a type 2 growth mechanism with separation at the chondro-osseous interface, leaving a small Thurstan Holland fragment (arrow) from the ilium. (B) Similar case but with a posterior Thurstan Holland fragment (arrow). This hemipelvis had been internally rotated by direct impact from an automobile bumper.

Types of Pelvic Fracture

Adult pelvic fractures may be simply classified according to the direction of the impact force: anteroposterior compression, lateral compression, vertical shear, or a combination of these forces. Such classification correlates well with the presence or lack of pelvic stability and the appropriate treatment requirements. This classification, however, is not as easily applied to children as it is to adults because of the presence of multiple regions of physeal and epiphyseal-equivalent cartilage, all of which have additional injury failure patterns.

Fractures of the immature pelvis may be classified into four basic groups: (1) stable fractures with continuity of the pelvic ring; (2) unstable fractures with disruption of the pelvic ring anteriorly, posteriorly, or both; (3) fractures of the acetabulum especially involving the triradiate cartilage; and (4) avulsion (apophyseal) fractures, often resulting from muscular avulsion rather than direct violence. The most common pelvic osseous fracture in children, constituting almost 50%, is a ramus fracture, with most being unilateral and primarily involving the superior (pubic) ramus. The basic fracture types are shown in Figures 19-12 to 19-15.

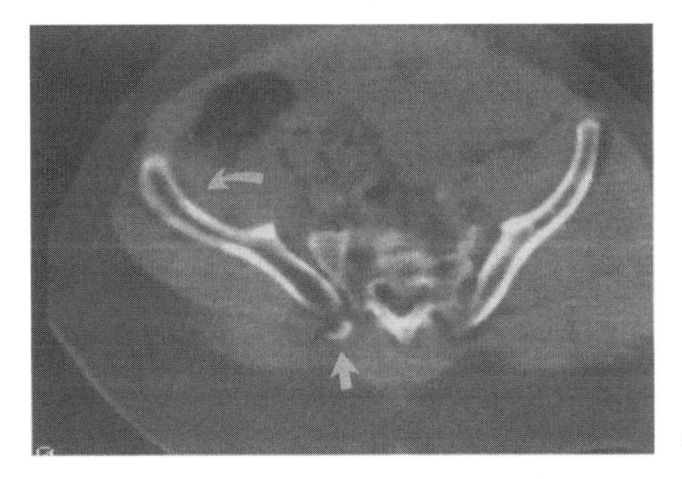

require scanning. The two- and three-dimensional CT images are most useful in pediatric patients with complex injuries in whom the full definition of injury is essential to determine whether external fixation or operation was necessary. Contrast in the bladder or intravenous pyelography does not interfere with the CT scan and usually delineates any extravasation.

Scanning by CT is also useful for follow-up of disruptive pelvic injuries (Fig. 19-10). It allows evaluation of the extent of healing and residual anatomic deformity. Magnetic resonance imaging (MRI) probably has limited use in pelvic fractures, as osseous detail is better visualized in a CT scan. However, intraabdominal and intrapelvic soft tissue injury, hematoma accumulation, and so on may be discerned and documented. Furthermore, cartilaginous damage (e.g., avulsion of an unossified anteroinferior iliac spine) may become evident.

Because of the increased amount of trauma often incurred during adolescence, multiple injuries may occur. In particular, a hip dislocation may also occur with pelvic fractures.

FIGURE 19-10. (A) Outward winging of left ilium (curved arrow) due to a chondro-osseous disruption of the sacroiliac joint. A small posterior iliac fragment is evident (straight arrow). (B) CT scan 3 months after right hinging injury. Remodeling of the iliac side of the sacroiliac joint is evident.

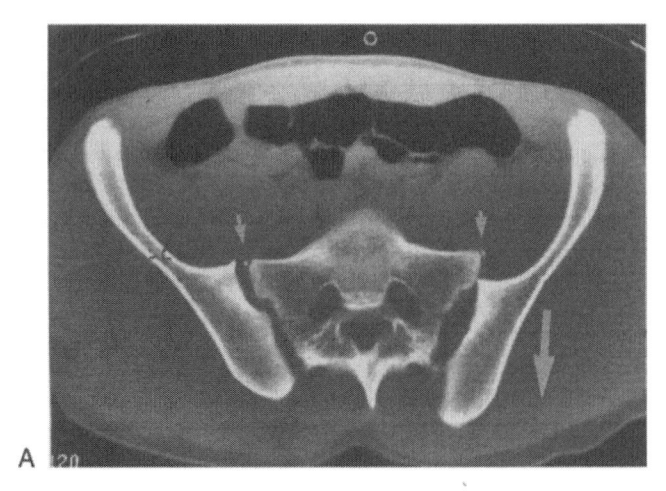

FIGURE 19-11. (A) Posterior displacement of the ilium (large arrow) in a 12-year-old girl. Small anterior accessory ossifications of the sacrum (small arrows) are normal and should not be construed as fractures. (B) Posterior shift of the left hemipelvis. Note the posterior accessory ossification centers of the sacrum (arrows). The shift of this accessory center on the left implies a chondro-osseous separation, rather than a sacroiliac dislocation.

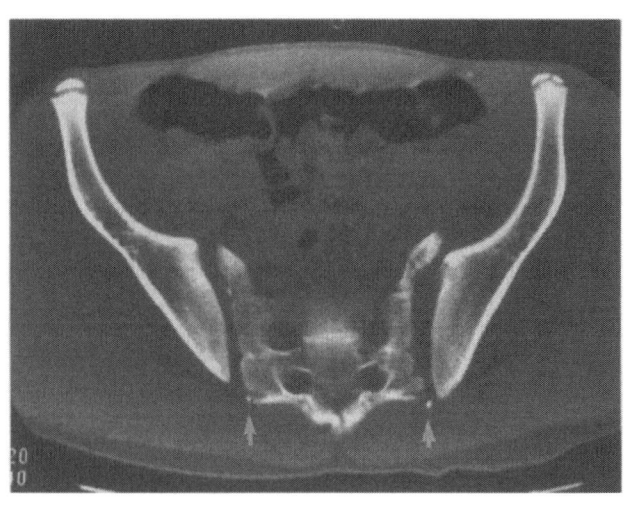

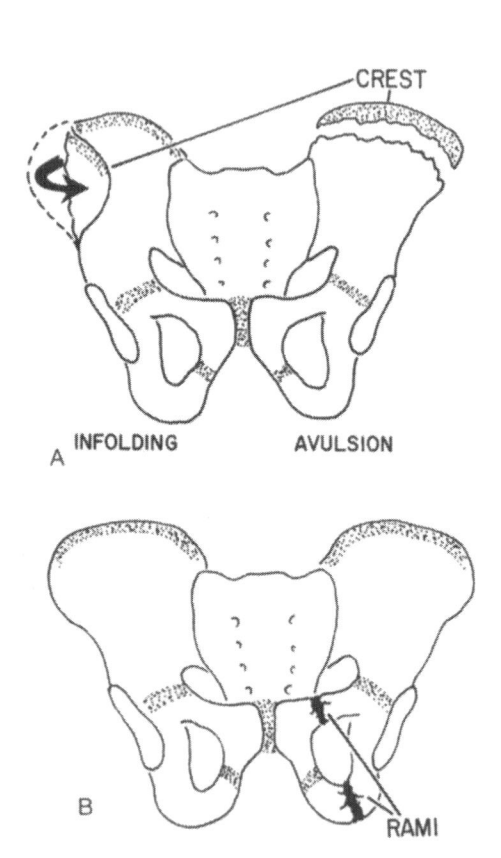

FIGURE 19-12. Stable fracture patterns. (A) Infolding of the iliac wing, which is analogous to a type 4 growth mechanism injury and may cause irregularity of crest development. Type 1 or 2 growth mechanism injuries of the iliac crest may occur, although such avulsion patterns are unusual. Direct contusion (type 5 growth mechanism injury) may also occur. (B) Fractures of the ischiopubic rami are rarely displaced significantly in a child because of extensive cartilage and strong periosteum. In fact, the chondro-osseous fracture response in a child may allow fracture of only one ramus, a highly unusual injury in adults. The examiner should always look for accompanying disruption of the sacroiliac joint, symphysis pubis, or triradiate cartilage.

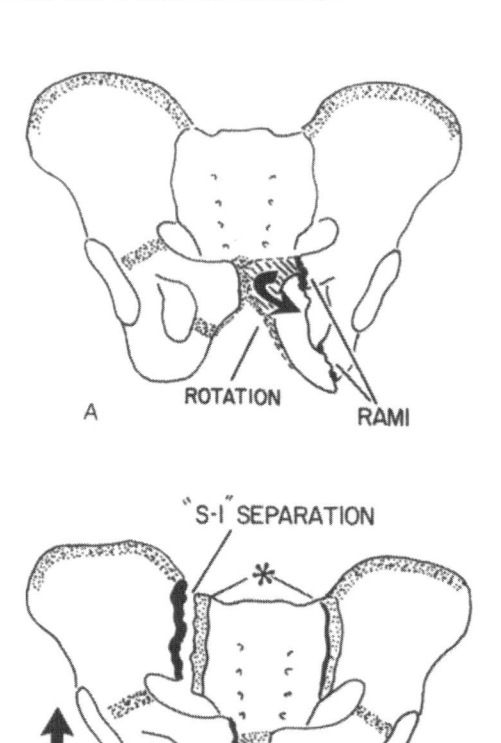

FIGURE 19-13. Unstable fracture patterns. (A) Rami fractures may be accompanied by displacement of the medial ischiopubic fragment from the symphysis (stippled areas) and periosteum (lined area). The fragment is externally rotated, hinging at the fracture site. This is a type 1 growth mechanism fracture. If the fragment is not reduced, the relatively intact periosteal tube makes bone (membranous and some endochondral) to fill the defect. Alternatively, the ramus fracture may extend to the triradiate cartilage and allow inward hinging of the ramus. (B) "Malgaigne" fracture of the immature pelvis. The true sacroiliac joint (*) is intact, but a chondro-osseous separation occurs on the iliac side, mimicking a sacroiliac disruption radiographically (see Figure 19-12). The inferior disruption may be a type 1 symphysis-ischiopubic separation or fracture of the rami. The relatively free hemipelvis is then displaced superiorly, but soft tissue (periosteal) constraints generally limit the degree of displacement.

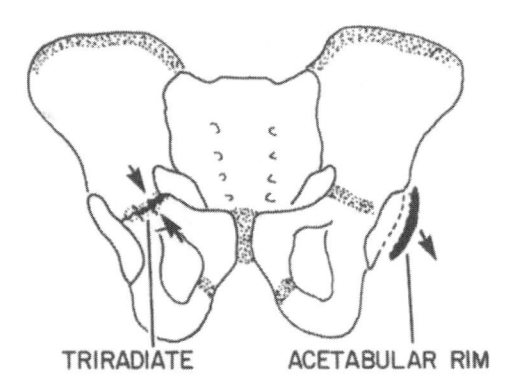

FIGURE 19-14. (Left) Crush injury to the triradiate cartilage (arrows) Translation may also occur. (Right) Ossifying region of the acetabular rim may be avulsed. This injury may occur prior to ossification, as an accompaniment to hip dislocation. The diagnosis is extremely difficult in such a situation and should not be confused with normal ossification patterns (see Chapter 20).

In contrast to adult pelvic disruption, pelvic fractures in children are less likely to be significantly displaced; most are stable, including diametric fractures in which the posterior fractures tend to be incomplete. This stability is the result of the relatively thick periosteum and the frequent involvement of chondro-osseous regions with partial zone of Ranvier disruption in children. Many of these injuries are analogous to physeal-metaphyseal injuries. They have intrinsic stability because some of the periosteal sleeve is intact. Fractures are also likely to be incomplete (i.e., greenstick) due to the resilient nature of the immature bone.

Stable Pelvic Ring Fractures

Wing of the Ilium

The wing of the ilium may be displaced outward, inward, upward, or downward (Fig. 19-16). The pull of muscles on this fragment may be reduced by abduction and flexion. This type of fracture, which is not common in children, is a result of direct force against the pelvis, causing disruption of the iliac apophysis or an infolding of the pliable wing of the ilium. Altered iliac crest development may occur.

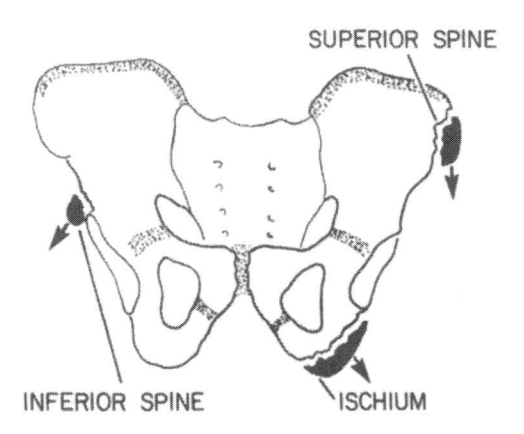

FIGURE 19-15. Avulsion fracture patterns of iliac and ischial regions in which secondary ossification centers normally develop.

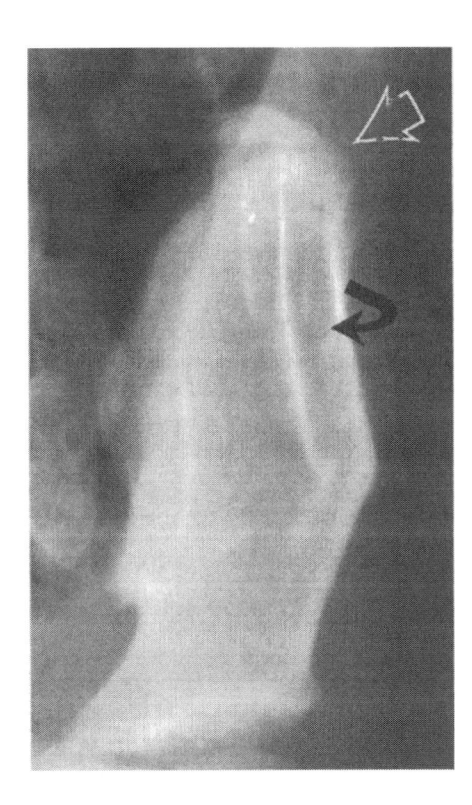

FIGURE 19-16. Fracture of the iliac wing, with infolding of the anterior portion (solid arrow) and some comminution of the superior metaphyseal region (open arrow).

The infolding may cause a splitting injury of the iliac crest apophysis along the rim or at the iliac spines. Such disruption may lead to subsequent growth distortion of the iliac wing or elongation (prominence of an iliac spine).

Ischiopubic Rami

If one ramus is fractured, or both rami on the same side (Figs. 19-17 to 19-21), the patient usually may be treated symptomatically. If only one ramus is fractured, the physician must always remember to look carefully for concomitant injury completing the fracture somewhere within the pelvic ring. Particularly, the possibility of a "physeal" fracture at the junction of the involved ramus with the triradiate or symphyseal cartilage should be assessed. Confirmation of a concomitant chondro-osseous injury may not adversely affect the intrinsic fracture stability. However, separation that allows angulation renders the ramus fracture unstable (see ensuing section). These injuries are relatively stable, as a portion of the periosteal sleeve is intact. Significant displacement may require manipulative (closed) or operative reduction. The intact periosteal tube allows new bone formation, which fills the "displacement" gap, again lessening the need for reduction. Evaluation is also particularly important at the sacroiliac joint. However, because the pelvic components are resilient in the child, a solitary ramus fracture is possible, whereas in the adult a fracture is invariably completed through contraposed portions of the ring. Even multiple fractures of three or four

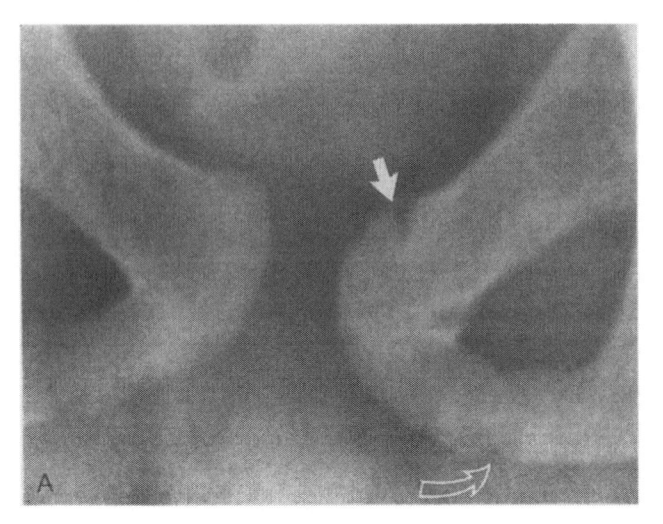

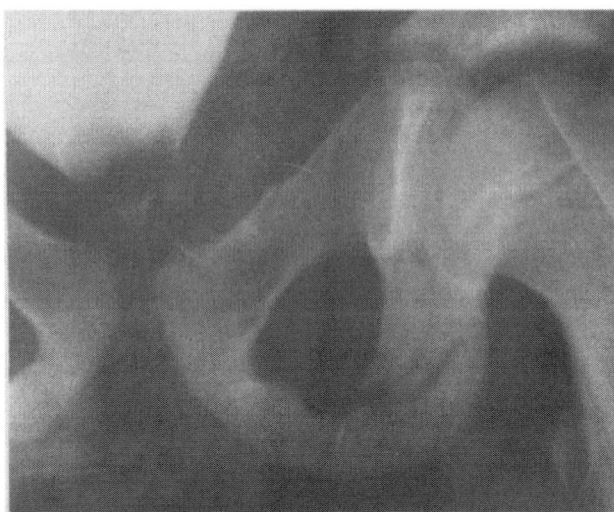

FIGURE 19-17. (A) Minimally disrupted pubic ramus fracture (solid arrow). The ischial radiolucency (open arrow) is the normal synchondrosis, not a fracture. (B) Multiple fractures of both rami.

rami (see Fig. 19-23, below) may be reasonably stable in a child because of the dense ligamentous, periosteal, and cartilaginous continuities.

Separation of the Symphysis

The changing size and irregular undulation of the symphysis region during growth must always be borne in mind. Frequently, an injury to this area must be diagnosed by physical examination (e.g., pain, overlying ecchymosis), as there may be little radiographic evidence. These separations are physeal injuries with separation of the ramus metaphysis from the epiphyseal and fibrocartilage of the symphysis (Figs. 19-22 to 19-25). In children, diastasis of the pubic symphysis is by separation of the bone–cartilage junction on one or both sides, rather than by disruption of the fibrous joint, as in the adult.

Radiographic diastasis of the pubic symphysis may occur in children without resultant instability of the sacroiliac joints posteriorly, presumably because of the elasticity of the bony pelvis, partial disruption of the anterior sacroiliac joint, or triradiate fracture. The sacroiliac joint in the young child may split anteriorly at the bone–cartilage interface of either the posterior ilium or sacrum.

More importantly, a displaced ramus with separation at the pubic symphysis is more likely to fail additionally within the triradiate cartilage (i.e., the other end of this bone), rather than posteriorly at the sacroiliac joint. This difference between ramus fractures in adults and children is extremely important.

Webb et al. described use of a two-hole fixation plate for traumatic diastasis of the symphysis pubis.[44] All of their patients were skeletally mature. The need to use such fixation in a child is unlikely, particularly as the symphysis per se is not disrupted but, rather, is a "physeal fracture analogue." However, early application of plate fixation restored the disrupted anterior pelvic ring, contributed to early immobilization of the patients, and made reduction of the

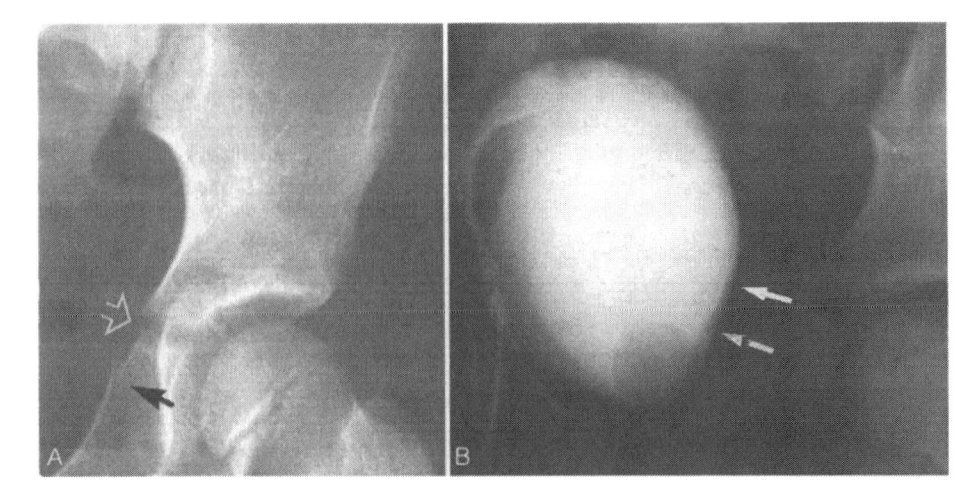

FIGURE 19-18. (A) Fracture of the superior pubic ramus (solid arrow). There also was concern for the triradiate region (open arrow), as it appeared offset, but it was a variation due to the projection. Three years later there was no evidence of triradiate growth injury. (B) A catheter was inserted, dye was injected, and displacement of the bladder (arrows) by retropubic hematoma was evident.

Types of Pelvic Fracture

FIGURE 19-19. (A) Fractures of all four rami. (B) CT scan showed that the right pubic ramus fracture (arrow) did not involve the triradiate cartilage.

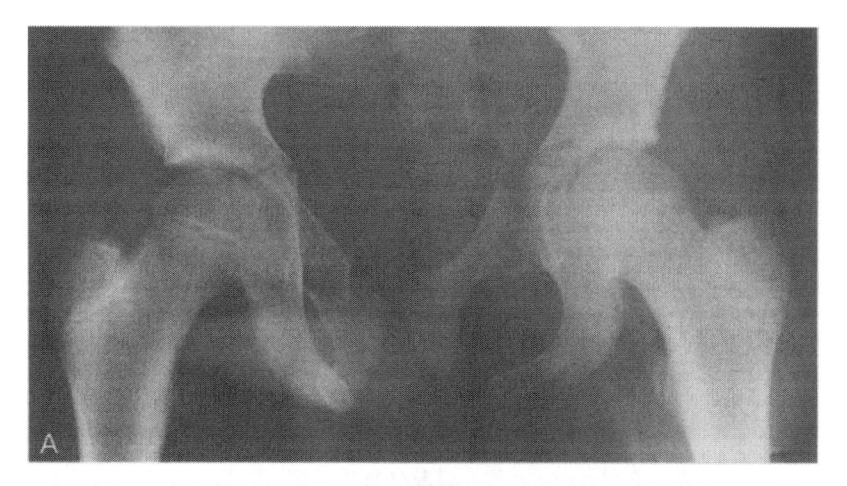

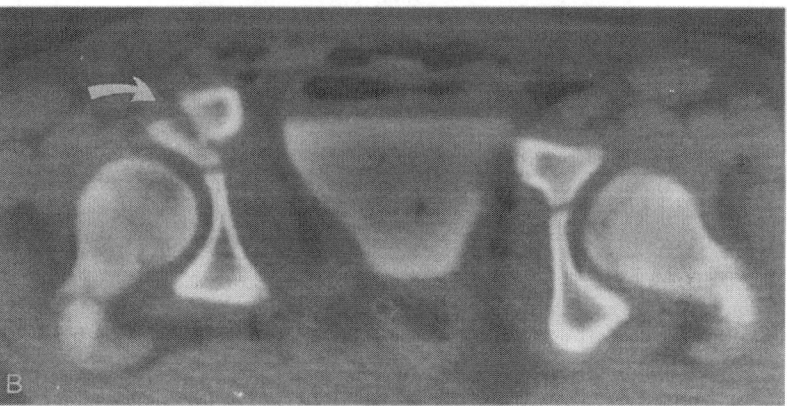

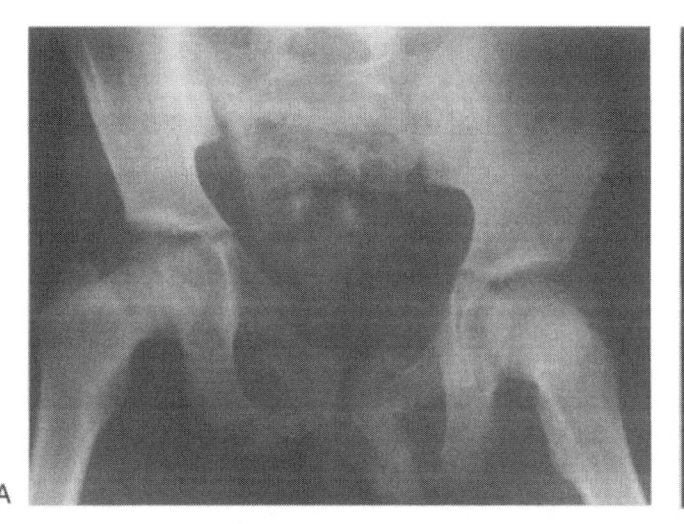

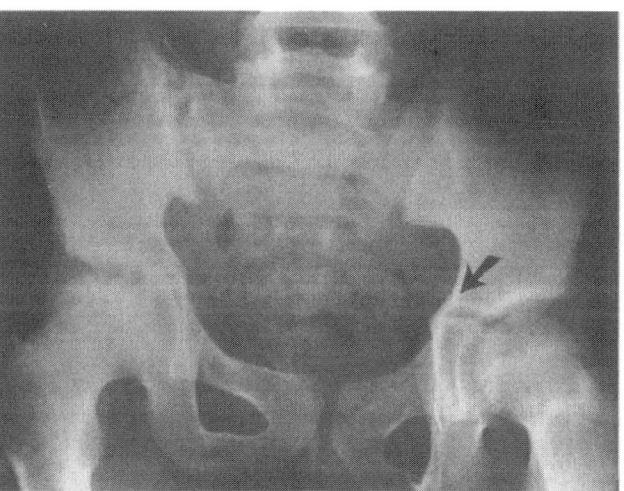

FIGURE 19-20. (A) Four ramus fracture, with hinging of the left rami at the triradiate cartilage. (B) Appearance 1 year later. Note the remodeling of the ramus fractures. The left triradiate cartilage has a medial osseous bridge (arrow).

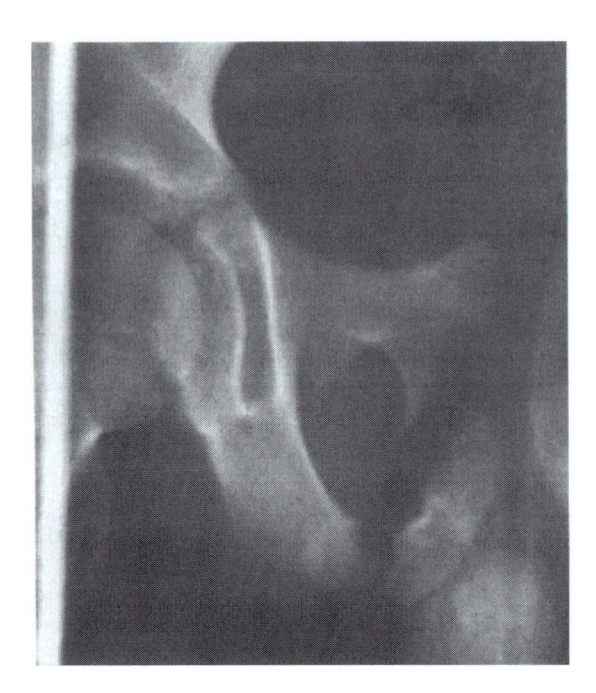

FIGURE 19-21. Fracture at the junction of pubic and ischial rami at the symphysis. The other end of the fracture is a chondro-osseous separation at the ischial synchondrosis.

concomitantly disrupted sacroiliac joint easier. A child is more likely to have a concomitant injury at the triradiate cartilage than at the sacroiliac joint. Open reduction back into the periosteal sleeve, with repair of periosteum, with or without temporary pin fixation, may be considered. The pin should be percutaneous, bent at 90° and removed at 2–3 weeks to avoid the risk of breakage or migration. An external fixator applied to the ilia can close the anterior chondro-osseous fracture (not diastasis) as effectively as a plate. Because the fracture is a growth mechanism injury it usually stabilizes within a few weeks.

Unstable Pelvic Ring Fractures

Separation of the Symphysis Pubis, Accompanied by Partial Disruption at the Sacroiliac Joint
(Figs. 19-24, 19-25)

With separation of the symphysis pubis, the ring is disrupted and opened anteriorly at the symphysis. The posterior separation at the sacroiliac joint may be due to disruption of the anterior capsule of the joint or an epiphyseal iliac fracture. Comparable epiphyseal separation at the sacrum may occur but is less likely because of developmental patterns of the sacrum.

The supine position aggravates the deformity, and the child may be more comfortable lying on his or her side. Frequently, placement of a pelvic sling relieves symptoms. This sling may allow some control of the pelvic diastasis, as the straps may be crossed to increase compression. Compression immobilization with a sling or a spica should be maintained for 6–8 weeks, depending on the age of the child, to ensure adequate ligamentous or chondro-osseous union at the symphysis and to prevent late spreading.

Fractures of the Anterior Arch (Fig. 19-26)

Crush injuries in the anteroposterior direction may cause fractures of both rami bilaterally to give a floating segment. In the child, a variation of this injury is fractures of both rami but with an ipsilateral separation of the bone from the symphyseal cartilage or the triradiate cartilage. The fragment may be displaced posteriorly to cause bladder displacement or damage. Disruption of the symphysis pubis is usually associated with separation of the bone (i.e., metaphysis) away

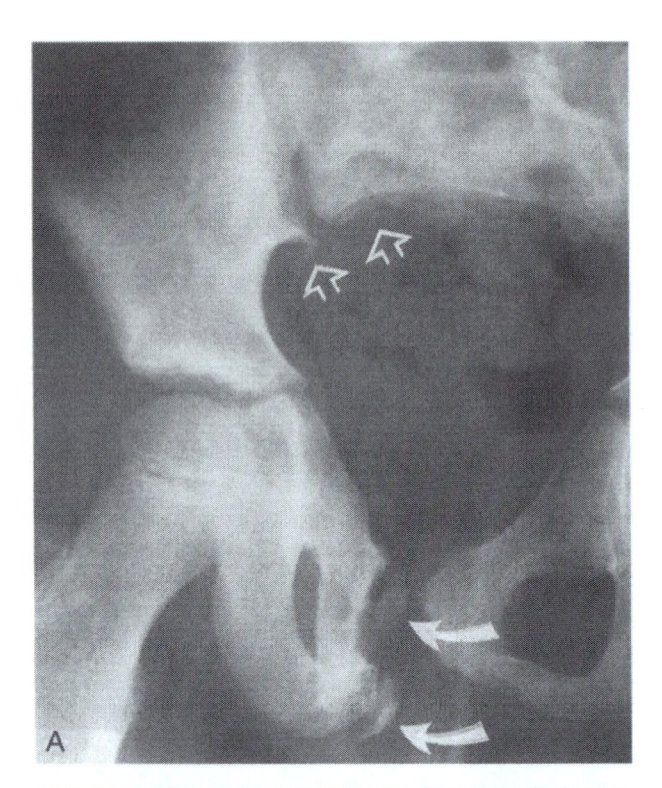

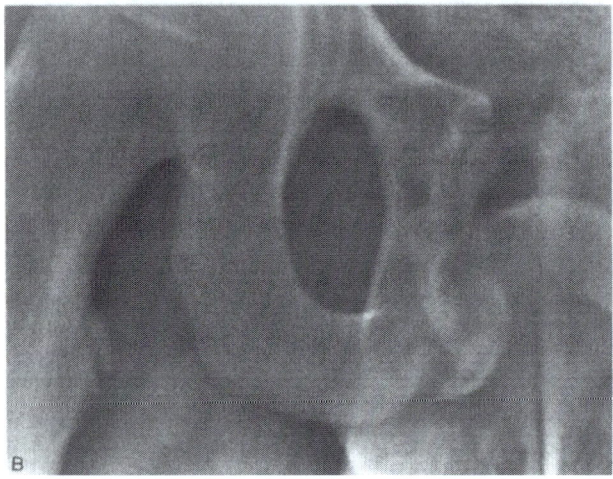

FIGURE 19-22. (A) Stable separation of the right sacroiliac region (open arrows) and ipsilateral separation of the symphysis (solid arrows). This roentgenogram was obtained 2 months after injury and shows subperiosteal new bone at the sacroiliac joint and subperiosteal and endosteal bone at the symphysis. (B) At 6 months more bone is evident adjacent to the symphysis.

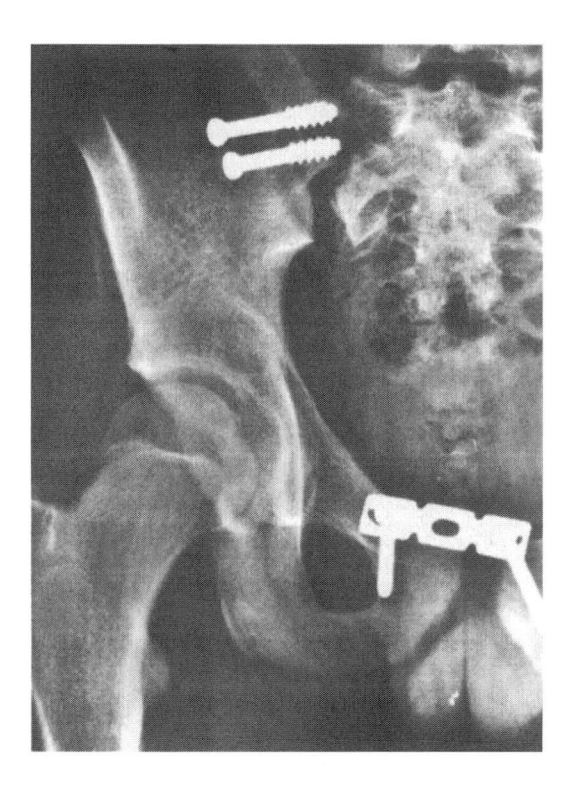

FIGURE 19-23. Reduction of a symphyseal diastasis with a small plate. The posterior screws are not sufficiently across the sacroiliac separation.

from the cartilage and thick periosteal sleeve. The separation gap may subsequently be filled in by endochondral bone formation. The segment may be displaced posteriorly (usually by impact), superiorly because of the rectus abdominis muscles, or inferiorly because of the adductors and hamstrings.

A pelvic sling should not be used in this situation, as it may cause inward compression of an unstable ramus. Children with this injury should be rested supine and placed in a semi-Fowler's position to relax the abdominal and adductor muscles. Treatment is maintained for 3 weeks, depending on the degree of displacement. Disruption of this region must be carefully assessed, particularly with regard to urethral and bladder injuries (Fig. 19-27). Thickened periosteum may not be damaged completely, so major fragment displacement is not common in children. External fixation may be considered. If the fragment is displaced into the pelvis, injuring or potentially injuring the bladder, consider using some type of stabilization.

Vertical Shear

With vertical shear the ring is broken in front and in back, and the free hemipelvis is shifted upward, inward, or outward (Fig. 19-28). The free pelvic segment is displaced by spasm of the muscles whose origin is fixed to the floating piece (e.g., the psoas, adductors, gluteus maximus, lateral abdominal muscles). If upward displacement is sufficient, leg length discrepancy may result.

Such fractures may be treated by skeletal traction using a pin through the distal femoral metaphysis. However, multiple system injury may preclude use of this method, as rigorous attempts at reduction may precipitate further retroperitoneal hemorrhage or nerve damage (traction or avulsion) and are thus contraindicated. Traction with 10–15 pounds, usually requiring a skeletal pin, may be necessary to reduce the fracture. After reduction is achieved, which is usually

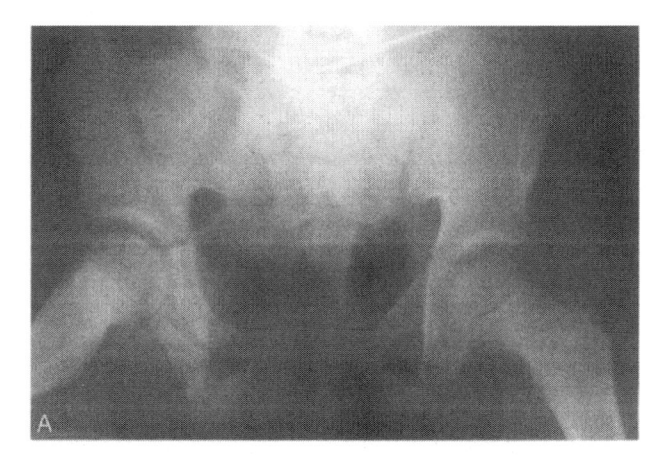

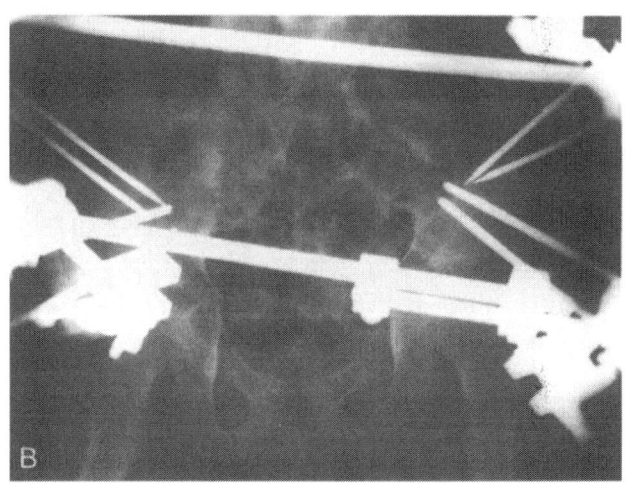

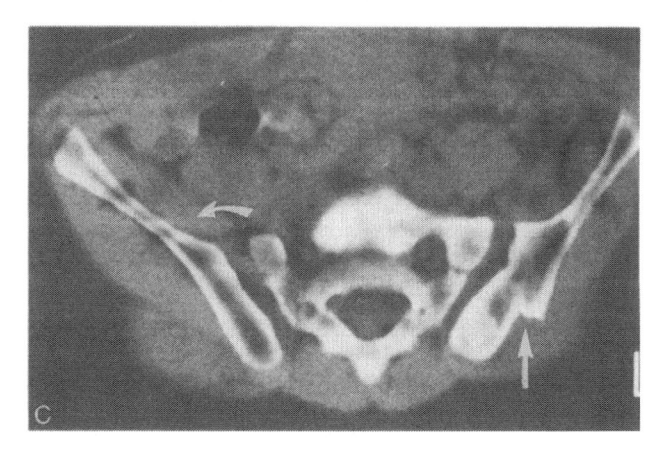

FIGURE 19-24. (A) Externally rotated right hemipelvis with a greenstick iliac fracture of the left side. Note the marked widening of the symphysis. (B) Treatment with pelvic external fixation. (C) The right hemipelvis had been externally rotated through the sacroiliac joint (curved arrow). The left hemipelvis had a fracture near the sacroiliac joint (straight arrow).

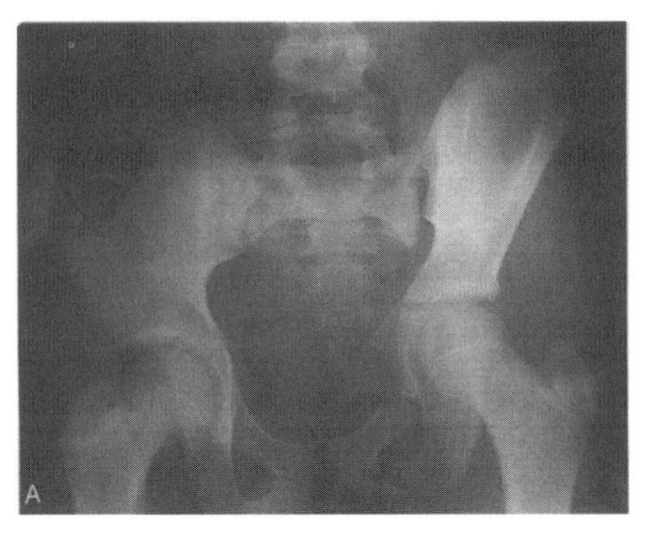

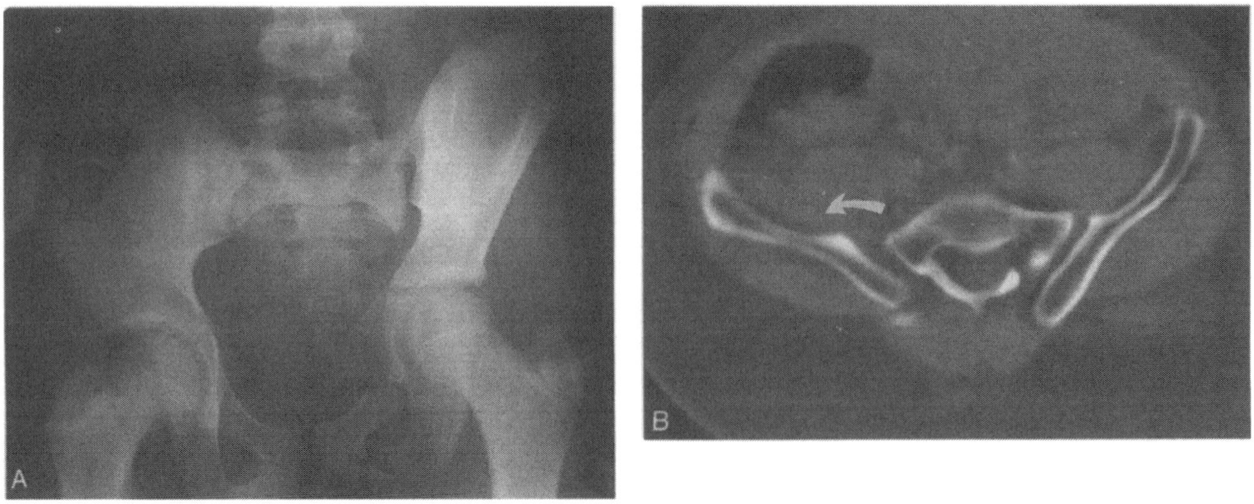

FIGURE 19-25. (A) Marked eversion of the right hemipelvis with a posterior fracture and sacroiliac "disruption." The left hemipelvis has an upward shift through the sacroiliac joint and ramus fractures. (B) CT scan shows external rotation (arrow) of the hemipelvis through the sacroiliac joint.

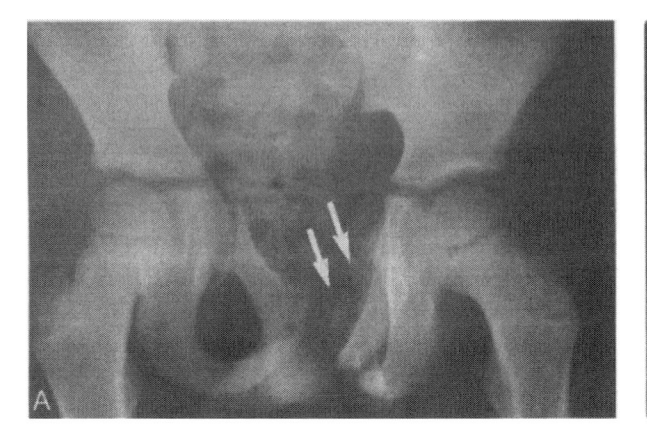

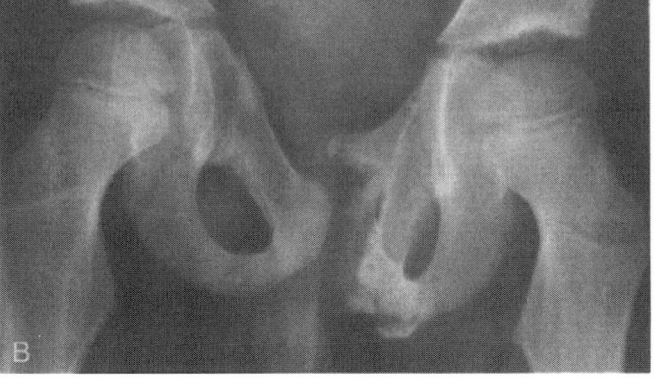

FIGURE 19-26. (A) Four weeks after multiple trauma, causing a right-sided Malgaigne injury and subperiosteal rotational displacement of the contralateral rami, there is new bone formation (arrows). (B) Two months later, significant membranous bone is filling the intact periosteal tube along the ramus displacement.

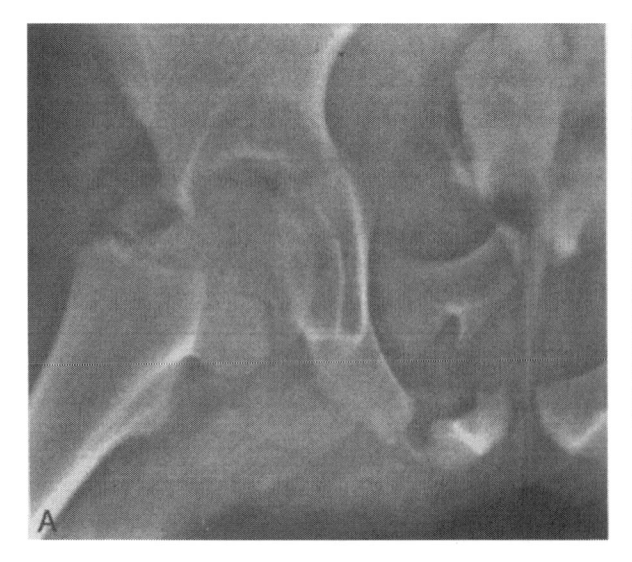

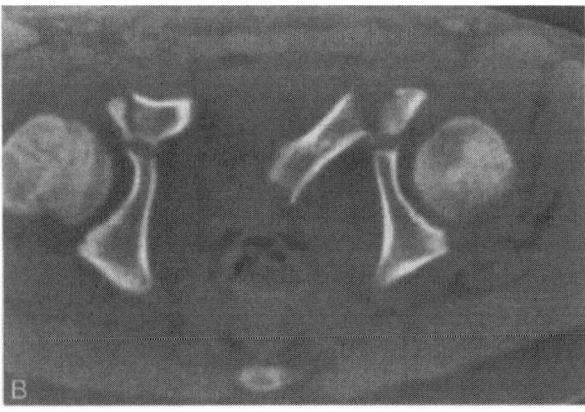

FIGURE 19-27. (A) Severely damaged pubic ramus is separated from the symphysis and hinging at the triradiate cartilage. (B) CT scan showed that this fragment was directed into the pelvic cavity and was injuring the bladder. Open reduction was done during bladder repair.

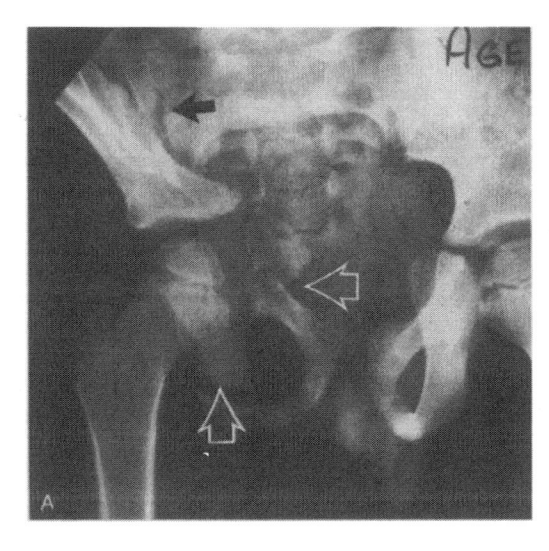

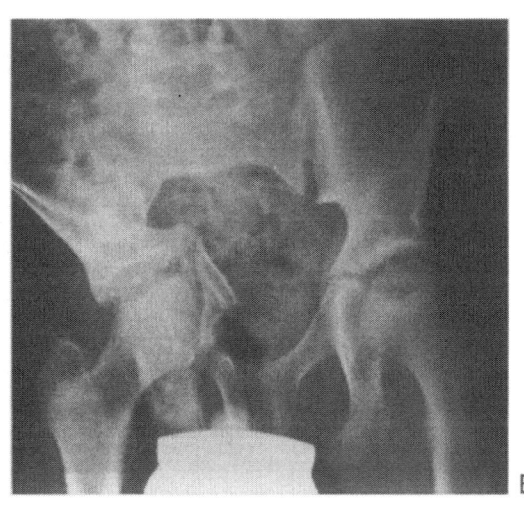

FIGURE 19-28. (A) Vertical shear fracture with probable involvement of the triradiate cartilage. The iliac fracture (open arrows), combined with pubic and ischial fractures (closed arrow), allowed rotation of the "free" fragment. (B) Four years later there is obvious altered growth of the acetabulum.

within a week, the position should be held. Countertraction should be maintained to prevent the child from inadvertently placing the injured leg in relative abduction. Open reduction is rarely indicated.

Bucket Handle Injury

With a bucket handle injury the pelvic ring is broken in front and back, and the floating pieces are rotated so the iliac crest is displaced medially and the ischial tuberosity laterally. This condition may be combined with some vertical shear. This type of injury, in effect, causes the reverse of an innominate osteotomy and thereby "uncovers" the femoral head. Again, this injury should be treated by skeletal traction or an external fixator whenever possible. It is important to reduce this deformity, as uncovering the femoral head, particularly in the young child up to 8–9 years of age, may cause relative or actual dysplasia of the acetabulum by the time growth is finished.

Lateral Compression

Lateral crushing injury folds the wing of the pelvis, hinged posteriorly on the sacroiliac joint or hinged anteriorly at the pubis. However, the free edge of the fragment may be displaced centrally. When a child is run over, one ilium may be rotated externally at the sacroiliac joint and the other hemipelvis rotated internally.

Traction may be applied through the hip joint and proximal femur in an attempt to reduce it over time. Such reduction takes approximately 1 week and should be followed by maintenance of bed rest. Open reduction may be indicated, particularly in the small child in whom skeletal traction is not readily applicable. External fixation with a pelvic frame may also be used. Using the "lengthening" attachments, winging of a hemipelvis may be gradually reduced to a normal (or near-normal) anatomic position.

General Management Guidelines

Osseous Injuries

Pelvic fractures may be accompanied by other skeletal injuries. Because many pelvic injuries are caused by direct blows and vehicular trauma, fractures of the proximal femur, hip dislocation, and spinal fractures may occur. Such injuries should not be overlooked during the initial evaluation. Associated injuries may require much more treatment than the pelvic fracture itself.

With stable injuries, function is minimally impaired. Usually the basic pelvic ring is undisplaced or minimally displaced. Comfort, the primary treatment goal, is attained most effectively by bed rest (frequently mandated by accompanying injuries). Reduction, either closed or open, is rarely necessary, particularly in the young child, because of the extent of remodeling that will occur and the possibility of damaging intrapelvic structures.

However, given the inherent instability of posterior disruption of the pelvis, closed reduction and minimal external fixation are recommended when displacement is evident (Fig. 19-29). Fixation frames allow easier nursing care and access to management of soft tissue damage and catheters.[27,35] However, external fixation must be used carefully in the young child, as placement of threaded pins or screws through apophyseal regions (e.g., iliac crest) may cause localized physeal damage. Because the chondroosseous nature of these fractures allows relatively rapid healing, fixators do not have to remain in place in a child as long as they would in an adult. It may be necessary to use limited internal fixation (Fig. 19-30).

One of the most common complications is leg length inequality secondary to a shifted hemipelvis (Fig. 19-31). Vigorous manipulation in the child to reduce the superior shift anatomically may not be appropriate and may cause recurrent bleeding or genitourinary damage. Remodeling,

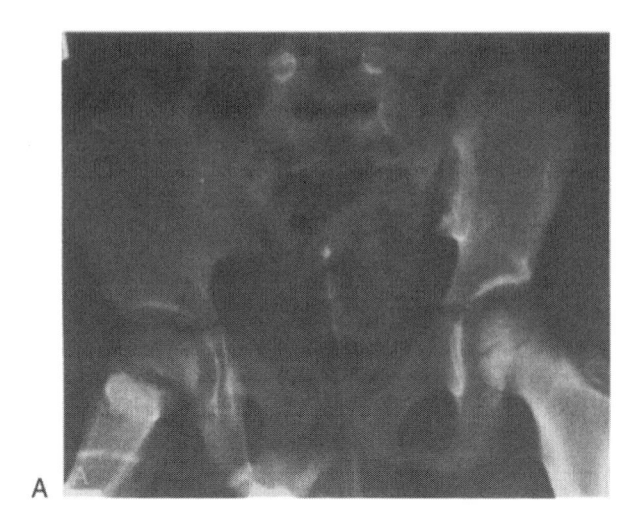

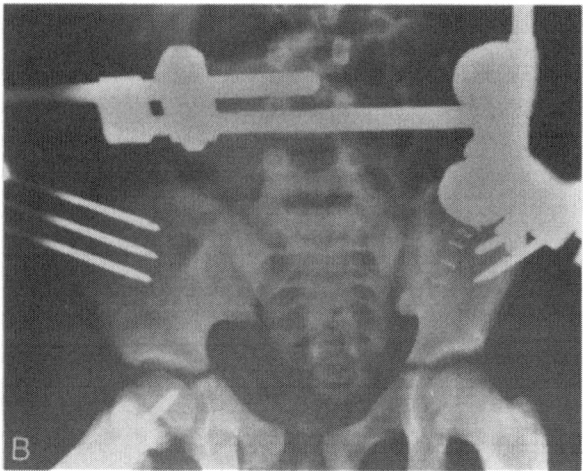

FIGURE 19-29. (A) Unstable fracture of the pelvis. (B) It was stabilized with external pelvic fixation.

as in long bones, may alter such relations in a positive way. Nonunion and delayed union are uncommon complications of childhood pelvic injuries.[35] Limb lengthening may be corrected at a later date. Because the discrepancy is usually less than 2 cm most children may be treated effectively with a lift and, if indicated, an appropriately timed contralateral epiphysiodesis.

Vascular Injuries

Despite having a distribution of pelvic fractures sites similar to that of adults, only 5 of 372 children in four separate investigations died as a result of hemorrhage.[14,20] Possible explanations for reduced bleeding from pelvic fractures in children have anatomic bases. First, the periosteal tissues appear to be more adherent to the underlying bone in the child, which may limit the displacement and thus lessen the likelihood of disruption of major vessels that course over and around the pelvis. Second, children's vessels are much more vasoconstrictive, which potentially helps limit hemorrhage from smaller vessels.

McIntyre et al.[52] reviewed 57 pelvic fractures in children. Eighteen required blood transfusion within 48 hours (i.e., one-third of patients). Skeletal fixation was applied in ten of these patients and was believed to control bleeding in six. Pelvic arteriography was used to identify arterial hemorrhage in three patients, all of whom underwent successful embolization to control the bleeding.

Shock may accompany severe pelvic fractures and is usually hemorrhagic rather than neurogenic (see Chapter 10). Appropriate volume replacement, transfusion, and temporary postponement of laparotomy or laparoscopy until the

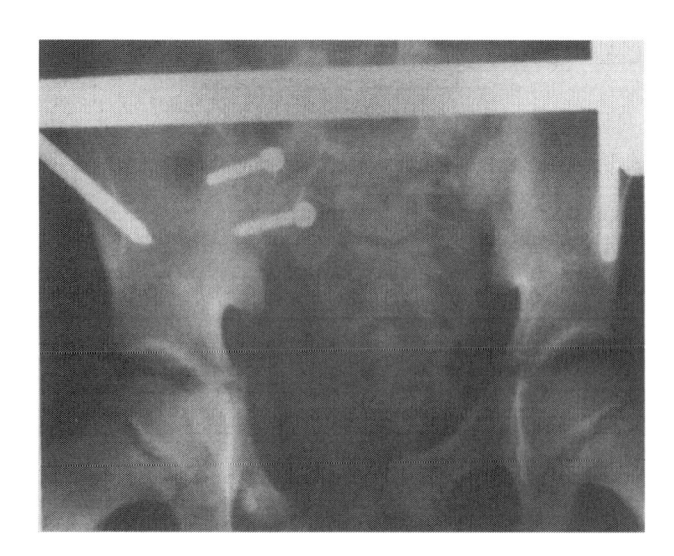

FIGURE 19-30. Combined use of an external pelvic fixation device with internal stabilization of a fracture-separation of the sacroiliac region.

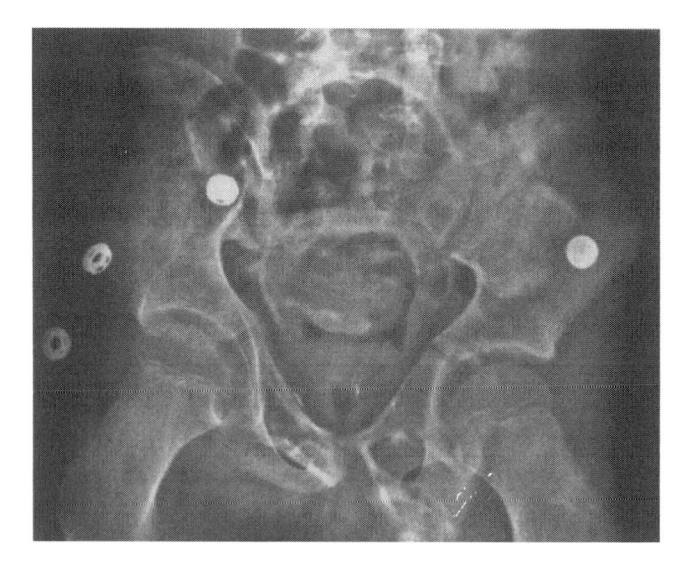

FIGURE 19-31. Five years after a severe pelvic fracture in a head-injured patient with multitrauma, there is a permanent upward shift of the right hemipelvis and clinically evident leg length inequality.

circulatory and volume status are stable are strongly recommended. A delay in the repair of visceral or arterial injuries is probably less serious than the crisis of cardiac arrest during an exploratory operation performed while the general circulation is in a tenuous state. The sacroiliac region of the child and adolescent seems to be the point where the vessels and nerves are most susceptible to significant injury. If this area is disrupted, there should be concern for laceration of vessels up to the size of the iliac artery. Shock poorly responsive to volume replacement and pressor agents in the presence of a rapidly enlarging abdomen, with absence of one or both femoral pulses, should be cause for immediate surgical exploration (e.g., laparoscopy), rather than delay. It is a good surgical principle *not* to disturb stable retroperitoneal hematomas, regardless of their size but, rather, to control the specific visceral or vascular lacerations. CT and MRI scans may be more efficacious than abdominal taps for identifying large hematomas. In addition to being a method of repair, limited laparoscopy may be helpful for diagnosis.

Certain fractures have been correlated with specific vascular injuries. Lacerations or avulsions of the common external iliac vessels are associated with disruption of the ilium or separation of the sacroiliac joint. In children, disruption of the posterior pelvis has been associated with avulsion of the superior gluteal artery.[32]

Sources of external hemorrhage should be sought around the urethral meatus, vagina, and anus. Abdominal and rectal examinations are essential. Pulses in the lower extremities must be assessed carefully by palpation. Doppler studies should be obtained if a pulse cannot be felt.

When the sacroiliac joint is separated and pulses in one leg are diminished or absent, a major branch of the internal iliac artery has probably been disrupted.[49] The child generally is in profound shock and requires rapid transfusion of blood in massive quantities. This type of injury is associated with high mortality, even in children. The importance of concealed hemorrhage due to fractures of the pelvis cannot be overstated. In one case, a 7-year-old child lost more than half of his blood volume into such a hematoma.[53] The possible consequences of allowing continued rapid retroperitoneal blood loss, such as intraperitoneal rupture with exsanguination, prolonged jaundice, renal failure, coagulopathy, and prolonged ileus, should be avoided.

Autopsy studies of 200 consecutive fatally injured pedestrians showed that 45% had pelvic fractures, and all had significant retroperitoneal bleeding.[47] The hemorrhage accompanying pelvic fracture was the direct cause of death or contributed substantially to the fatal outcome. In contrast, in a similar study of 500 pedestrians who did *not* succumb to their injuries, only 4% sustained pelvic fractures.

Hemorrhage may be intraperitoneal or extraperitoneal. Intraperitoneal bleeding often necessitates control by laparotomy or laparoscopy. Extraperitoneal bleeding is much more difficult to control, and explorative surgery and attempts to ligate vessels may be difficult. The bleeding often originates from branches of the obturator artery that supply the pubic rami.[51]

The magnitude of blood loss may go unrecognized. Operative attempts at stemming hemorrhage are frequently unsuccessful because identification of the primary bleeding site is difficult. Opening the peritoneum when tamponade has occurred may increase blood loss substantially. In addition, if the hemorrhage is eventually controlled, the risk of later sepsis within the hematoma is enhanced (especially if there has been accompanying urethral or bladder injury). Success with internal iliac artery ligation has been variable. In fact, the morbidity associated with retroperitoneal exploration and arterial ligation may outweigh the risk of nonoperative management with continued blood replacement.

Angiographic evaluation of bleeding associated with pelvic fracture and treatment by selective embolization of clotted blood to sites in the vicinity of the fractures (usually branches from the obturator artery along the pubic rami) have been described in adults and more recently in children.[46,48,50,51] This technique may be considered a nonoperative approach to massive pelvic hematomas,[54] when contrasted with the hazards of surgical exploration. The technique involves arterial catheterization on the side opposite the trauma. A flush aortogram is performed with the catheter at the level of the renal arteries, with the urinary tract visualized as well. Selective celiac axis arteriography then follows to evaluate the liver and spleen. For embolization, the catheter is advanced proximally to the obturator artery, and pieces of Gelfoam (mixed with contrast material) or autologous clot may be injected into the obturator artery under fluoroscopic control.

For detecting occult vascular problems MRI angiography may help.[31] New spin echo sequences may allow visualization of regional anatomic structures contiguous to metallic devices.

Abdominal Organs

Injury to the bowel is an uncommon complication of childhood pelvic fracture and probably occurs in fewer than 3% of cases.[56,62] In contrast, a reactive ileus and gastric dilatation (air swallowing) are common, especially in children. A nasogastric tube may be used if such complications are present. Children have a propensity to swallow air when injured. Accordingly, gastric dilatation per se does not indicate a definite bowel injury.

Entrapment of bowel between osseous fragments of the pelvis has been reported.[55,57,62,63] Everett described a 5-year-old boy who sustained a fractured pelvis with dislocation of the left sacroiliac joint.[61] Small bowel obstruction subsequently developed. At exploration, the apparent fracture-separation of the sacroiliac joint was a type 1 growth mechanism injury in which the cartilage at the sacroiliac joint had retained normal continuity, whereas the osseous portion of the ilium had hinged away, allowing small bowel to herniate into this area. The bowel became entrapped when the fracture spontaneously reduced after the injurious forces dissipated.

Nimityongskul et al. reported an 8-year-old who had small bowel incarceration associated with a central fracture dislocation of the hip.[64] Again, the bowel was entrapped when the temporarily widened fracture spontaneously reduced, progressively leading to perforation of the bowel, infection of the hip joint, separation of the capital femoral epiphysis, and osteomyelitis of the femoral shaft (Fig. 19-32).

In the long term, if there is severe disruption of the anterior ring, especially when it is rotated and disrupted by a symphysis pubis diastasis, the inguinal ligament may be dis-

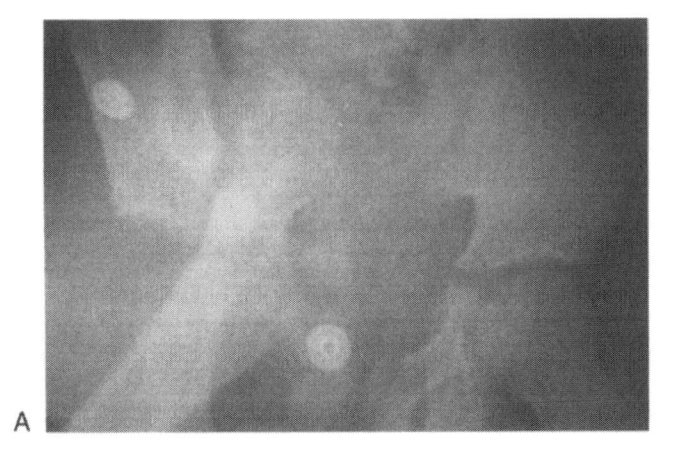

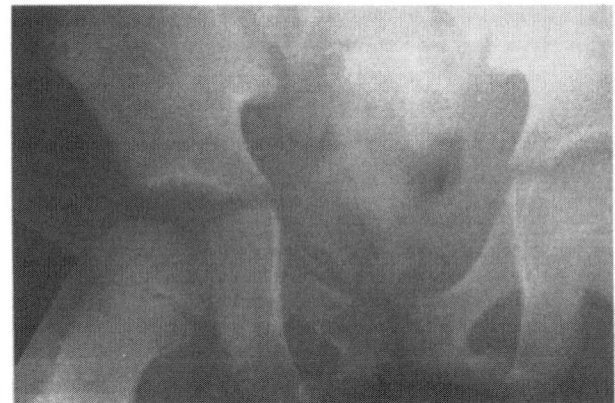

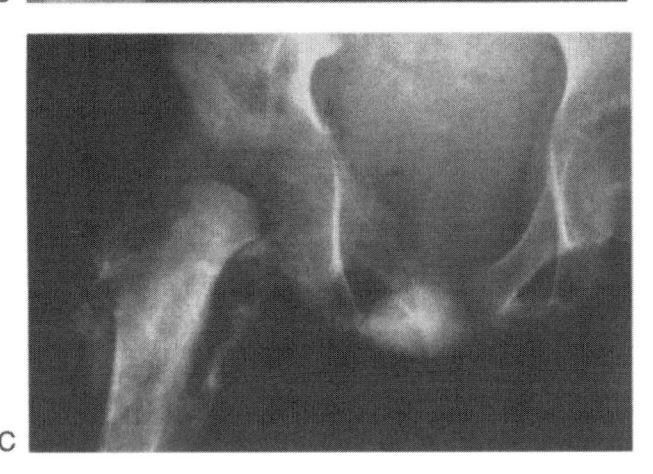

FIGURE 19-32. (A) Central fracture dislocation. (B) Closed reduction. The widening of the joint space was due to entrapped bowel. (C) Result after infection supervened (coliform bacteria).

rupted and a hernia may ensue. Similarly, disruption along the region of the iliac crest may lead to a lumbar or abdominal hernia.

The liver is the second most commonly injured intraabdominal organ in pediatric patients.[58,59] The need for operative therapy for liver lacerations in children is controversial. Further discussion of liver and spleen injury may be found in Chapter 13, as these organs are also frequently injured with rib and thoracic trauma.

Perineal avulsion may be associated with genitourinary and rectal injury.[60] Stabilization of the pelvic injury may contribute substantially to the necessary reconstruction of these tissues and organs. Perineal trauma is associated with mortality rates of 32–58%, which are improved by control of hemorrhage and sepsis.

Neurologic Injuries

Neurologic injury may occur at several levels, particularly when the sacroiliac region is disrupted.[65,66] The nerve roots may be stretched or avulsed at the spinal foramina. Injury to the sciatic nerve as it courses past the acetabulum is unusual, primarily because these injuries usually leave an intact periosteum that protects the nerve. If the sciatic nerve is injured, some degree of function may be permanently lost.

Children with residual nerve damage, no matter what the final level, may have major problems with recurrent fractures, Charcot-like joints, soft tissue contractures, and decubiti. Relative osteoporosis may significantly weaken the metaphyseal areas, predisposing to growth mechanism and metaphyseal fractures (see Chapters 6, 10, 11).

Incomplete injuries to the lumbosacral plexus, especially stretch injuries, are relatively easy to overlook when evaluating more life-threatening aspects of a traumatized child. Lesions around the areas of the sacral roots are often painless. Because of overlap of sensory fields it may not be easy to detect discrete sensory loss, and there may be subtle motor damage that results in problems around the hip region and distally.

Urologic Injuries

Disruption of the symphysis or displaced fractures of the pubic rami may cause injury to the bladder and urethra.[68,77,83,87] Complete urologic evaluation with urethrography, cystography, and an intravenous pyelogram may be required (Figs. 19-33, 19-34).

Hendren and Peters noted that with multiple trauma the urinary tract is second only to the central nervous system in terms of the frequency of injury.[80] Injuries to the lower genitourinary tract and perineum account for about 1% of pediatric trauma center admissions. In one study 10% had urethral injuries and one-third had head injuries.[21]

About 10–25% of bladder injuries are due to penetrating trauma, especially when the bladder is full at the time of injury.[70,72,82] Allison reported that 17% of pelvic fractures are associated with rupture of the bladder or urethra.[67] The latter injury is potentially serious (Fig. 19-33B). The degree of bladder trauma may be classified into four groups: (1) contusion; (2) extraperitoneal rupture; (3) intraperitoneal rupture; and (4) combined extraperitoneal and intraperitoneal rupture.

Suprapubic tenderness may be associated with a contusion or tear of the bladder wall. A catheter should be placed through the urethra; if it proves difficult, a tear of the urethra should be suspected. Should the catheter enter the bladder without difficulty, a major urethral injury can usually be excluded. If the urine is blood-stained, cystography may be performed by injecting dye into the bladder through the catheter and looking for extravasation of the dye beyond the bladder outline. Detailed management of major urinary tract injuries—bladder or urethral tears—should be left to the discretion of the urologic surgeon. If it is necessary to make a suprapubic approach to the urethra to place a stent, it may be possible to perform, concomitantly, a better reduc-

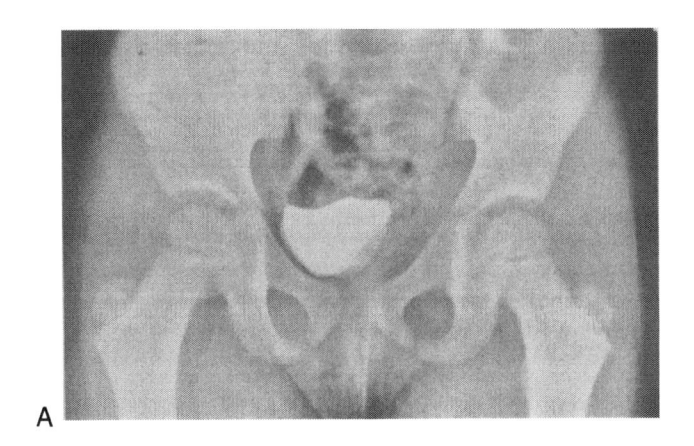

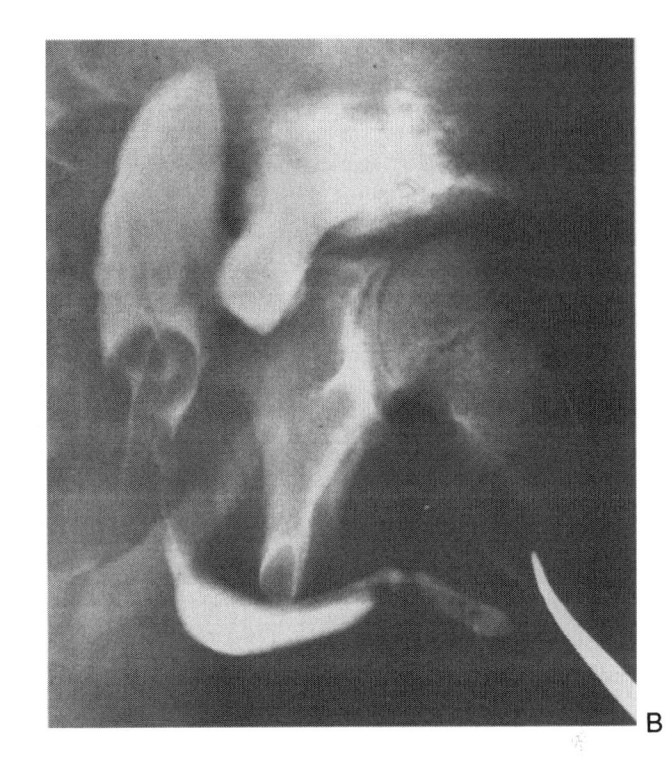

FIGURE 19-33. (A) There is no obvious pelvic fracture. Intrapelvic bleeding has displaced the bladder. (B) Extravasation of dye from a bladder tear.

tion of the fracture fragment.[69] However, metallic internal or external fixation should be used cautiously, as there is a risk of bladder infection during the early postinjury course. Osteomyelitis by hematogenous or direct spread is a complication to be avoided.

Cystography is one of the best methods for revealing damage. With contusion, the bladder is generally elevated, deviated from the midline, teardrop-shaped, and there is no dye extravasation. With extraperitoneal injury, the cystogram shows that the base of the bladder is obscured, and there are small to extensive lines of contrast within the fascial planes. With intraperitoneal rupture, there is contrast around the bowel and an hourglass-shaped bladder; there may also be contrast in and around the abdominal organs. It is important to evaluate the ureters and kidneys as well.[73] Retrograde cystourethrography permits this type of study. Excretory urography is also beneficial. Intravenous pyclography is an easy way to obtain basic information.

Urethral trauma is infrequent in children but may be caused by blunt or penetrating trauma. Boys are more likely to be injured than girls.[86,88] Tears are more common than complete severance of the urethra.[74] The most significant injury is disruption of the urethra close to the apex of the prostate.[77,78,81,84] The puboprostatic ligament is ruptured, and the bladder is displaced upward and posteriorly. In a rupture below the urogenital diaphragm, the extravasation of dye is often contained within Buck's fascia.[79] Urethral injury should always be suspected and ruled out in any child with a pelvic fracture. There is usually an inability to void, and frequently blood is seen at the urethral meatus. A retrograde

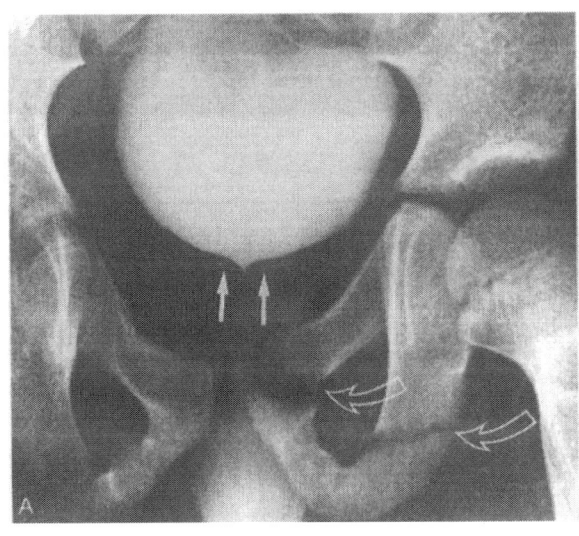

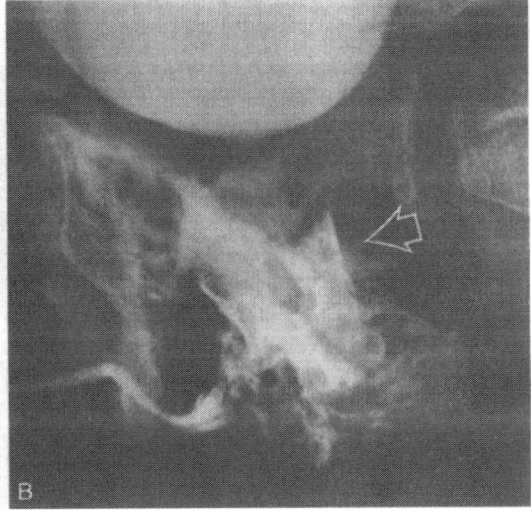

FIGURE 19-34. Multiple rami injuries (curved open arrows) were associated with bladder injury (A, straight arrows) and urethral injury (B, arrow).

urethrogram should be obtained, as it can demonstrate the area of tear or severance with extravasation of contrast. Multiple projections may be required.

Impotence may complicate urethral injury in the male patient.[85] Gibson reported impotence in 37% of their patients with urethral injury, the largest percentage occurring in patients with rupture of the membranous prostatic portion.[76] These studies were done in adults, however, and there are *no* long-term studies of young children who have had comparable pelvic fractures to determine whether they eventually exhibit similar problems once they reach sexual and physical maturity. Gibson further noted that fertility was frequently impaired, and that only 14% of the adult patients had subsequently fathered children.[75] I sent questionnaires to male patients who had sustained significant anterior pelvic injury, with 11 responses. None had difficulty with erection or ejaculation. Four were married, but only one patient had been unable to have a child. Evaluation in this instance showed extensive scarring.

Dhubuwala et al. found impotence following pelvic fracture in 26 patients including a 7-year-old boy.[71] They believed the impotence was caused not by disruption of the prostatic membranous urethra but, rather, by disruption of the neurovascular supply to the penis.

Obstetric/Gynecologic Injuries

There is a possibility of future obstetric problems if the pelvic outlet is significantly narrowed or distorted owing to a displaced fracture. Again, long-term studies in immature girls who sustain pelvic fractures have not been conducted to ascertain whether there is a significant risk of such a complication and increased need for cesarean section. Heinrich et al. noted the association of an open pelvic fracture coupled with vaginal laceration and pelvic diaphragmatic rupture in a 4-year-old.[89]

Acetabular Fractures

Treatment of a pediatric patient with a fractured acetabulum is determined by the general condition and associated injuries. Most authors have advised conservative treatment, especially in the child. In contrast, Judet and colleagues recommended greater emphasis on surgical repair, but their series included only skeletally mature patients.[105] From this series, it appeared that conservative treatment was better for inner wall or posterior acetabular fractures. Superior fractures had poor results whether treatment was nonoperative or operative. The most important factor seemed to be reestablishment of the superior dome and extraction of any loose fragments of bone, cartilage, or muscle that might be herniated into the defects, thereby reconstituting a normal relation between the femoral head and acetabulum. The future of the hip depends primarily on the condition of the weight-bearing portions of the acetabulum and femoral head, the potential for the development of ischemic necrosis in either the acetabulum or femoral head, an accurate femoral-acetabular relation, and intrinsic stability of the joint.

Heeg and coworkers reviewed 23 acetabular fractures in patients younger than 17 years of age.[102-104] Good or excellent functional results were achieved in 21 patients, and radiographic healing was good or excellent in 16. Conservative treatment gave consistently good results with fractures with minimal initial displacement, stable posterior fracture dislocations, and type 1 and 2 triradiate physeal cartilage fractures. Less favorable results were seen with type 5 triradiate fractures and comminuted fractures, but no operation was better than any other. Unstable posterior fracture-dislocations and irreducible central fracture-dislocations usually require operative treatment, but the results may still be unsatisfactory.

Peripheral Fractures

Peripheral acetabular fractures are often associated with dislocations of the hip in the adult. However, because of the structure of the child's acetabulum—particularly the pliable cartilaginous components such as the labrum—dislocations of the hip often occur without concomitant acetabular fracture or at least a radiologically evident (i.e., osseous) one (see Chapter 20). In the older child, posterior dislocation is more likely to displace an osseous acetabular fragment than is the less common anterior dislocation (Fig. 19-35). The chance for displacement of an acetabular fragment is also influenced by the relative extent of ossification of the posterior and anterior walls. Any acetabular fracture that accompanies a hip dislocation should be reduced as accurately as possible, as it is an intracapsular injury in the child. Whether there are fragments within the joint is not always easy to determine, as portions of radiolucent cartilage may be displaced into the joint, particularly when there is separation of the fibrocartilaginous acetabular labrum away from the main hyaline cartilage. Any suggestion of limitation of motion or failure to attain complete, concentric reduction (widening of the radiolucent cartilage or joint space) should make one suspicious of this possibility. An arthrogram is

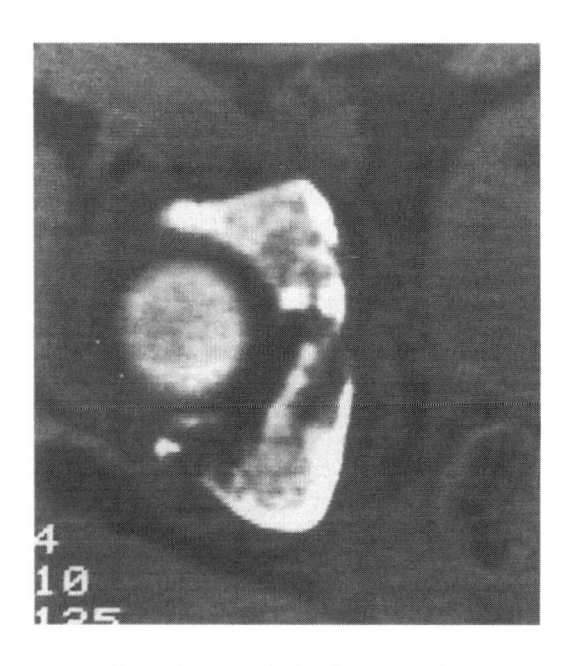

FIGURE 19-35. Posterior acetabular fracture, along with some central propagation just posterior to the triradiate cartilage.

often of benefit diagnostically. Oblique radiographs with the pelvis rotated 45° (both right and left oblique views) must be obtained to reveal the posterior acetabulum in profile. Depending on the age of the patient, the os acetabulum must be considered a source of roentgenographic "fracture" (Fig. 19-5). Large superior fragments should be viewed with caution and must be followed carefully through skeletal maturity in case they lead to subsequent acetabular dysplasia and hip subluxation. CT evaluation is often definitive.

The problem of concomitant hip dislocation and peripheral acetabular fracture, especially with displacement of the osseous or cartilaginous fragment into the joint, is discussed in Chapter 20.

Central Injuries

The femoral head is infrequently driven centrally into the pelvis in children prior to adolescence, probably because of the resilience of this area compared to other portions of the pelvis (Fig. 19-36). Watts described total dislocation of the acetabulum through the triradiate cartilage anteriorly and the sacroiliac joint posteriorly in a 12-year-old child; it was

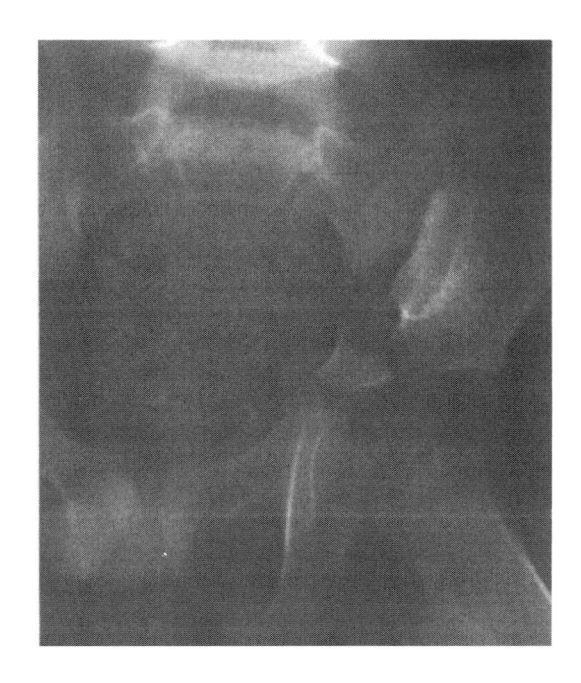

FIGURE 19-37. Superior acetabular fracture (nontriradiate).

successfully treated by open reduction and internal fixation.[43] The fracture may involve the weight-bearing superior portion lateral to the triradiate cartilage (Fig. 19-37).

Triradiate Injuries

Traumatic disruption of the acetabular triradiate physeal cartilage is an infrequent injury.[91,92,95,97,100–104,106,110,111,114–117,119,121] Ljubosic described 13 patients with premature closure of the triradiate cartilage consequent to injury to the acetabulum.[109] Jurkovskj found 2 epiphyseal injuries of the acetabulum among 237 fractures of the pelvis in children.[106] Bryan and Tullos reported 3 cases in 52 pelvic fractures; only one patient demonstrated significant growth disturbance.[10] Of the 84 pelvic fractures in children reviewed by Reed, 4 had evidence of acetabular triradiate involvement.[33]

It is my experience that triradiate fracture is often overlooked in many children with seemingly solitary ramus fractures. If a ramus fracture is displaced, there must be another injury that allows such hinging to occur. It is often due to an unrecognized chrondro-osseous separation at one or more arms of the triradiate cartilage. Such displacement, which may be subtle, is better detected by CT scans than routine radiography of the pelvis.

If one of the pelvic bones (pubis or ischium) in a child is displaced and rotated at the symphysis pubis, it must hinge. In adults the hinging is usually through the sacroiliac joint; in the skeletally immature patient, however, rather than injury to the entire hemipelvis, the forces may be summated at the triradiate cartilage, disrupting a portion (or all) of the triradiate end and the symphyseal end. Lateral compression forces in an adult may produce a hemipelvic disruption, whereas the child may sustain a quadrant disruption with rotatory disruption of the ischiopubic and triradiate units.

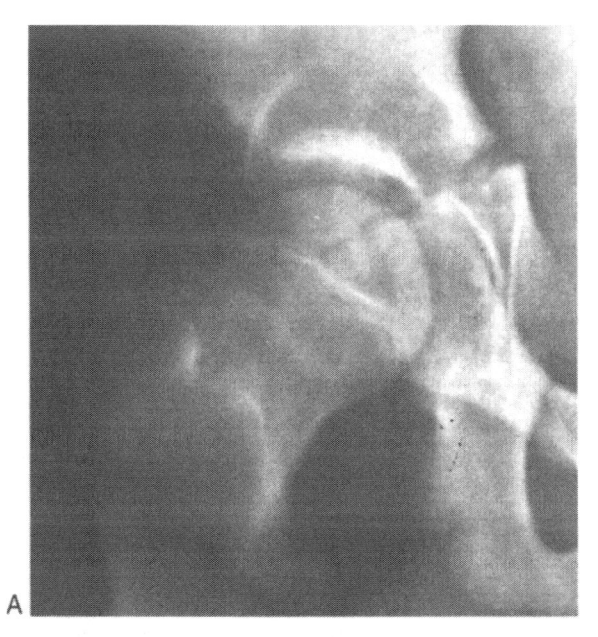

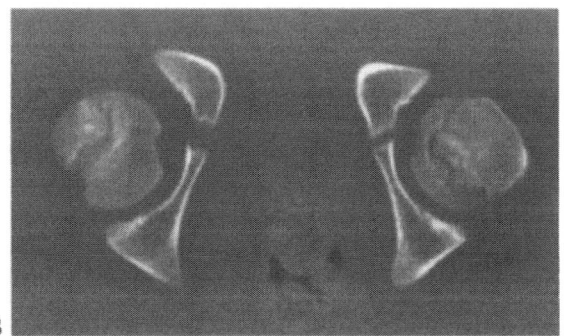

FIGURE 19-36. (A) Central fracture with a split through the closing or recently closed triradiate cartilage. (B) CT scan.

These fractures are usually undisplaced and infrequently require open reduction. However, when a displaced type 2 growth mechanism is observed and CT scan shows joint disruption, open reduction may be indicated.

Injuries to the triradiate cartilage constitute physeal trauma comparable to fractures involving the physes of longitudinal bones. The potential for this injury should always be assessed whenever a single ramus fracture is noted. However, the bipolar anatomy of the triradiate cartilage and the lack of ossified epiphyses until late adolescence may make classification of these injuries difficult. During adolescence the appearance of multiple secondary ossification centers may make diagnosis confusing. Three basic patterns occur that are similar to physeal fractures elsewhere in the developing appendicular skeleton.

The first pattern is a shearing-type injury due to a blow to the ilium or the proximal end of the femur that causes a type 1 or 2 injury at the interface of the two superior arms of the triradiate cartilage and the metaphyseal spongiosa of the ilium (Figs. 19-38 to 19-42). A triangular medial metaphyseal fragment (Thurstan Holland sign) may be present. This fragment effectively splits the acetabulum into a superior (main weight-bearing) one-third and an inferior (minimally weight-bearing) two-thirds. The germinal zones contained within the bipolar physes would be unaffected by such a fracture mechanism, and so continued growth would be expected. Comparable disruption between the triradiate arms and the metaphysis of either the ischial or the pubic ramus is theoretically possible. Type 1 and type 2 injuries appear to carry a favorable prognosis for continued (relatively) normal growth.

The second pattern is a displaced ramus fracture (more often involving the pubic ramus) in either the diaphyseal (analogous) segment or the metaphysis at the symphysis. The fulcrum of rotation becomes the inferior arm of the triradiate cartilage along with the anterior or posterior portion of the superior arm (contingent on whether the pubic or ischial ramus is involved). This rotational component at the physeal–metaphyseal interface of the triradiate cartilage is analogous to a displaced growth plate fracture in a long bone. Furthermore, there has to be subchondral separation from the contiguous articular cartilage (Fig. 19-41). They are usually type 1 or 2 growth mechanism injuries.

The third pattern of disruption causes a type 5 injury pattern, either as a primary injury (Fig. 19-43) or as part of the aforementioned type 1 or type 2 pattern. Such a type 5 injury may be difficult if not impossible to detect on the initial roentgenogram, although narrowing of the triradiate space suggests the possibility. The variability of the radiographic appearance of the triradiate cartilage makes assessment of "width" changes difficult (even with a CT scan). Accordingly, one must look for osseous bridging several months after the injury. Premature closure of the triradiate cartilage appears to be the usual outcome of a type 5 injury; and, depending on the age of the patient at the time of initial injury, it may cause progressive acetabular dysplasia

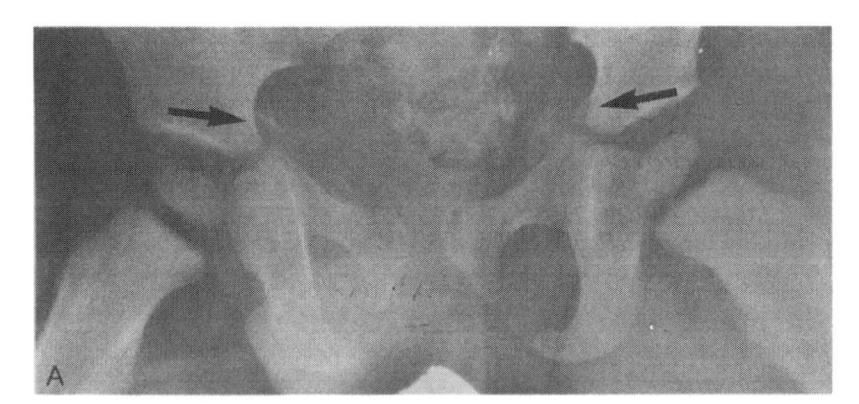

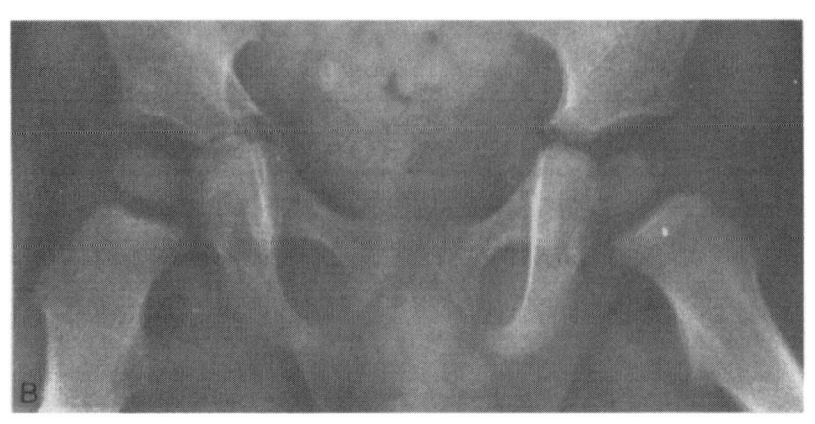

FIGURE 19-38. (A) Bilateral type 2 growth mechanism injuries (arrows) of the triradiate cartilage. (B) Extent of healing 2 months later.

Acetabular Fractures

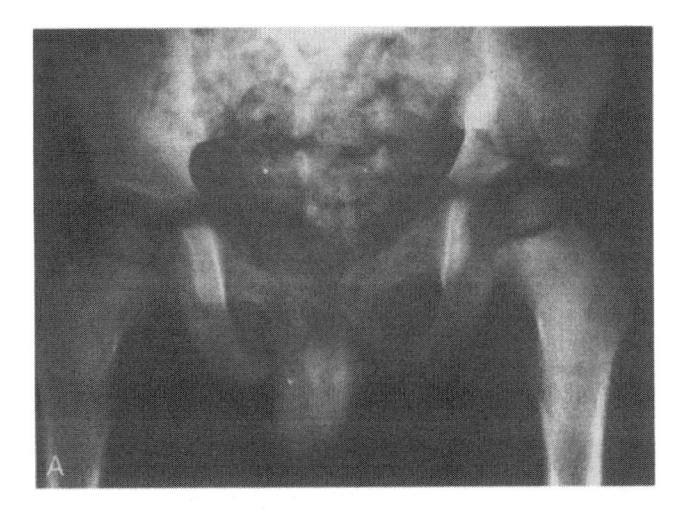

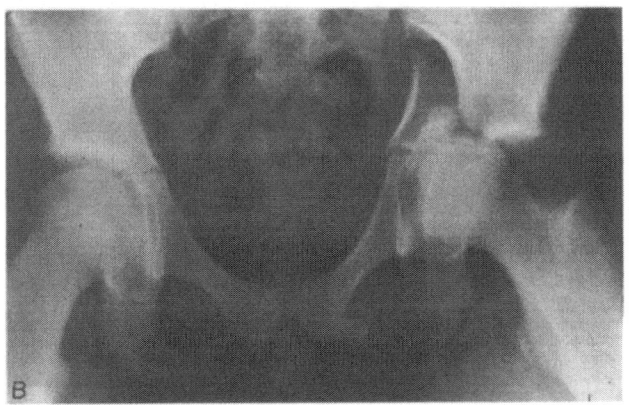

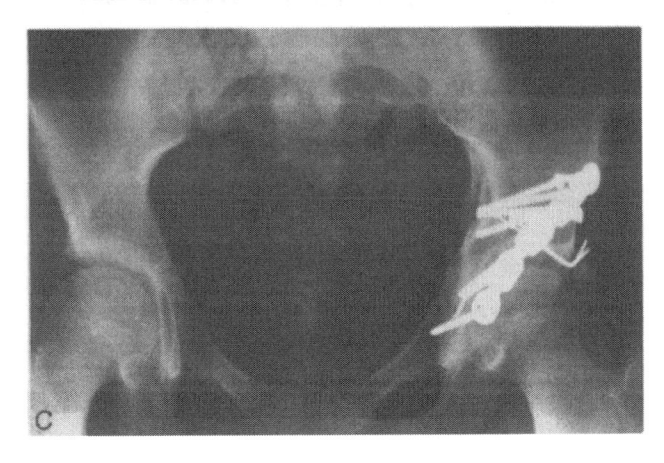

FIGURE 19-39. (A) Type 2 injury of the left acetabulum in a 2-year-old child. (B) Similar injury in a 13-year-old. (C) Internal fixation.

(Fig. 19-44). The earlier in life any premature closure occurs, the greater is the potential for change in acetabular morphology with subluxation and lateralization of the less affected or unaffected femoral head.

Growth mechanisms about the pelvis are dependent on an adequate vascular supply. It is feasible that trauma disrupts significant portions of the blood supply to the central germinal zone of the bipolar physis, further contributing to permanent disruption of growth. This region, like other epiphyses, is penetrated by cartilage canals that supply the germinal zones necessary for continued growth. A vascular injury may be the real cause of premature closure (variation of a type 5 injury), rather than crushing of germinal cells. Furthermore, microscopic type 4 shear fractures and comminution (see Chapter 6) may be factors.

During the final normal stages of closure of the triradiate cartilage, severe trauma to the pelvis may result in a fracture through one or more of the regions of the arms of the triradiate cartilage (Fig. 19-42). This pattern during late adolescence is analogous to the Tillaux fracture of the distal tibia, with the remodeling bone plate creating a region of temporary susceptibility to fracture until osseous remodeling across the physeal region is well under way. During this stage secondary (epiphyseal analogue) centers occur within the triradiate cartilage (Figs. 19-3 to 19-5). These ossification regions should not be confused with a fracture or comminution in an adolescent being evaluated for acute pelvic trauma.

Pina-Medina and Pardo-Montaner reported an unusual combination of triradiate cartilage fracture associated with transphyseal separation of the femoral head.[113]

Figure 19-50 (below) shows a representative patient who sustained growth injury to the triradiate cartilage. Potential injury may only be suggested contingent on the degree of trauma and possible limitation of movement. The diagnosis may have to be made retrospectively.[120] Narrowing of the triradiate cartilage and displacement are difficult to detect roentgenographically, especially when other pelvic components are damaged.

These fractures are usually undisplaced and infrequently require open reduction. However, when a displaced type 2 growth mechanism is observed and CT scan shows joint disruption, open reduction may be indicated.

The major subsequent problem is disparate growth of the acetabulum and the femoral head (Fig. 19-44). The femoral head continues to grow, whereas the normal mechanism of concomitant hemispheric expansion of the acetabulum cannot occur responsively. Growth may occur only at the periphery. Such growth at the periphery becomes increas-

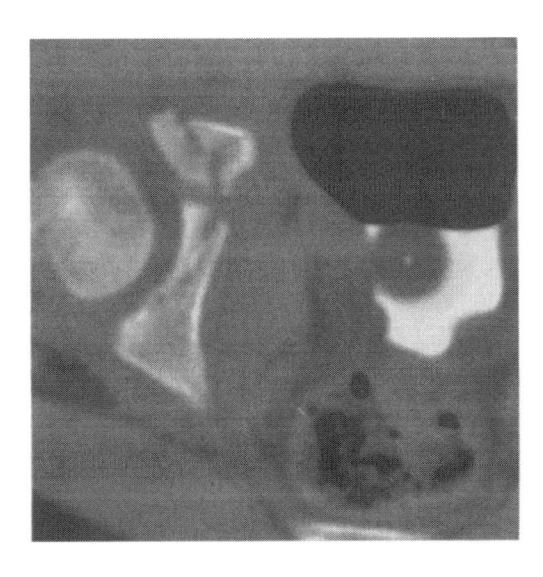

FIGURE 19-40. Pubic ramus fracture extending to the triradiate cartilage. Note the anterior greenstick fracture of the opposite side.

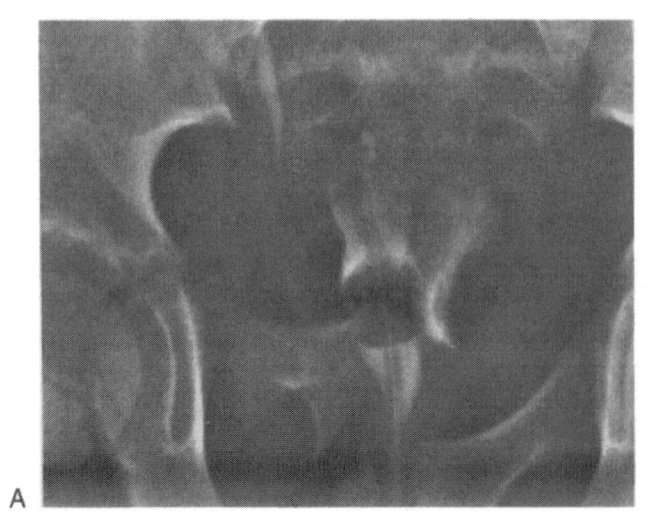

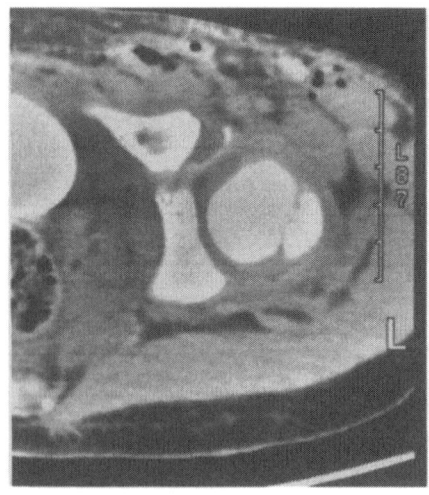

FIGURE 19-41. (A) Apparent type 1 injury of the triradiate (pubic-ischial arm) with rotation of the fragment toward the bladder. (B) Posteriorly displaced fracture of the pubic ramus leaving a subchondral shell at the anterior acetabular wall. The ramus is hinged at the triradiate cartilage.

ingly subjected to pathologic pressure from the femoral head, causing eversional deformation, not unlike that seen in developmental hip disease. When the fracture occurs during adolescence, subsequent growth-related changes in acetabular morphology and congruency of the hip joint are unlikely. However, in young children, especially those who are less than 10 years old, acetabular growth abnormalities are a complication of this injury and may result in a shallow acetabulum similar to that seen in patients with developmental dysplasia of the hip.

Trousdale and Ganz thought that the radiographic appearance of posttraumatic acetabular dysplasia was distinctly different from developmental dysplasia.[120] The acetabular teardrop width and inner wall of the acetabulum were significantly enlarged, with lateralization of the femoral head.

By the end of skeletal maturity, disparate growth increases the incongruence of the hip joint and may lead to progressively more severe subluxation of the proximal femur. Acetabular reconstruction may be necessary to correct the gradual subluxation of the femoral head. Variable irregularities of growth at the proximal end of the femur may also occur. Whatever the etiology, once the bridge is formed it acts as a bone graft across the acetabular physis. Experi-

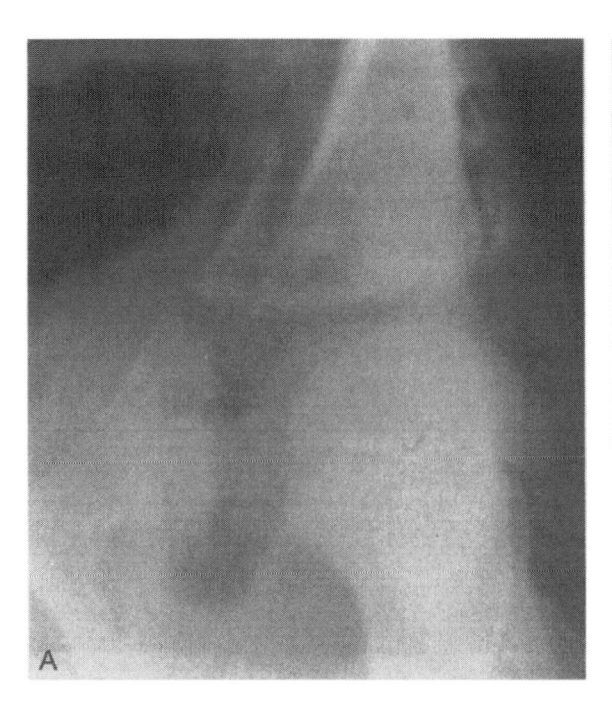

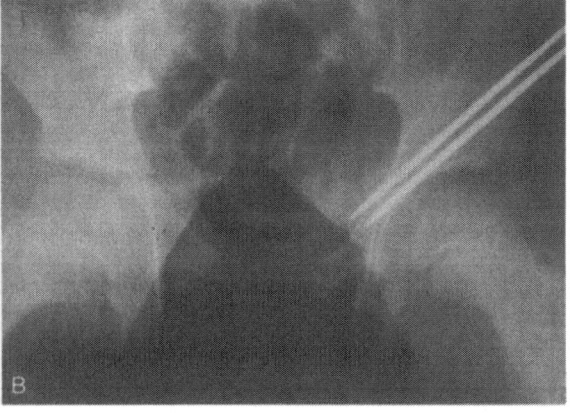

FIGURE 19-42. (A) Thurstan Holland fragment evident only on the Judet view. (B) Internal fixation.

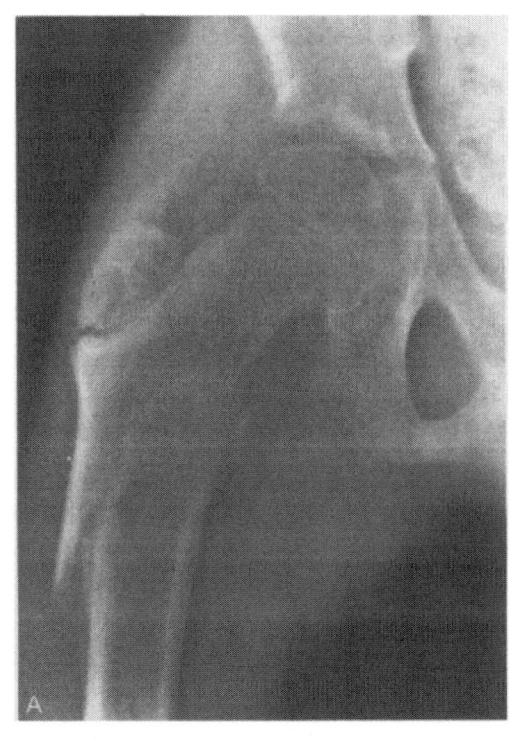

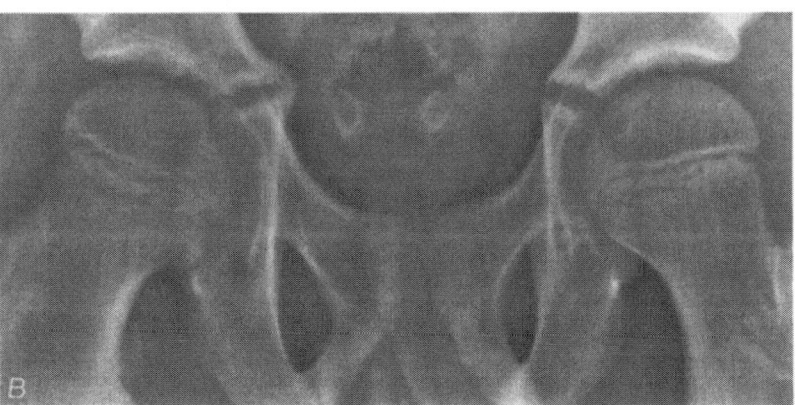

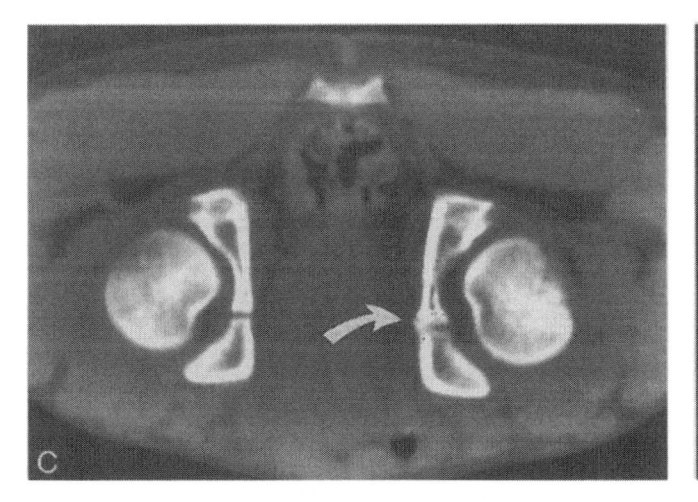

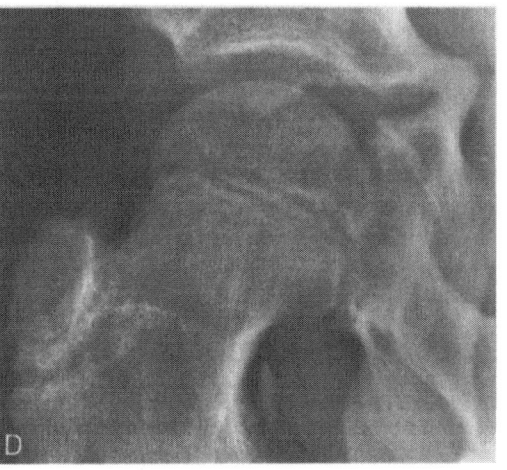

FIGURE 19-43. (A) Attention to a subtrochanteric fracture led to failure to assess a triradiate injury. (B) Three months later a bridge is forming. (C) CT view of the osseous bridge (arrow). (D) Fourteen months later. The parents refused bridge resection.

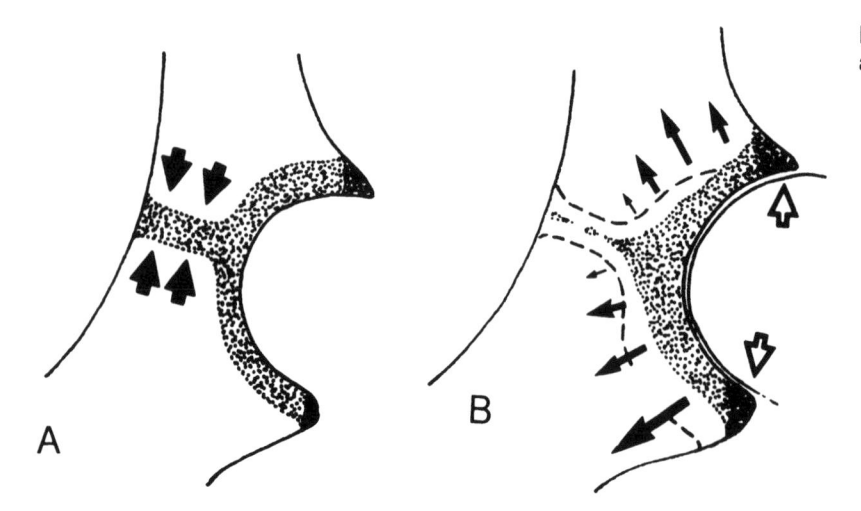

FIGURE 19-44. Growth arrest leading to a shallow acetabulum.

mentally, a bone graft across a physis may cause distortion or arrest of growth that ceases only when the graft (progressively) breaks, is resorbed, or is replaced by nonosteogenic material.[101] Theoretically, if the osseous bridge were removed surgically, growth would resume and the normal shape of the acetabulum might be preserved. However, the rapid development of the osseous bridge and progression to closure of the triradiate cartilage suggest that resection of the bridge and implantation of fat or some other interpositional material, as recommended for injuries to long bone physes, may not have much success in this particular anatomic region. Presumably, there are different degrees of damage to the triradiate cartilage, so variable inhibition of growth may occur. Peterson and Robertson reported the first resection of a triradiate growth arrest.[112]

The growth physes of the three pelvic bones extend continuously from the triradiate cartilage laterally into the discrete acetabular peripheral physis. Fusion of the triradiate cartilage may still leave the peripheral physis intact. Depending on the age of the child at the time of injury, this acetabular growth plate continues to grow, effectively enlarging the acetabulum laterally (i.e., circumferentially and posteriorly). The medial wall of the acetabulum becomes thicker and the acetabulum more shallow. Concomitantly, as the femoral head expands and is displaced laterally and superiorly (subluxates), it exerts increased pressure against the superior part of the acetabulum, impairing normal endochondral ossification and increasing the acetabular index, similar to the mechanism of developmental dysplasia of the hip.

Reconstructive surgery may be necessary in some of these children and must be individualized to the specific injury, concomitant pelvic deformation from other fractures, and the degree of anticipated growth. Shelf augmentation procedures offers a solution in many of these cases.

None of the reported patients with triradiate fracture had significant pain in the hip at skeletal maturation, although one did have some pain with exertion at extremes of motion during the physical examination. Blair and Hanson reported a patient who was originally injured at the age of 4 years when he sustained a fracture of the left femur, right pubis, and diastases of the pubic symphysis, right sacroiliac joint, and left triradiate cartilage.[91] Premature bridging was present in the triradiate cartilage 2 months after the injury. At 14 years he was having significant pain in the hip, and evaluation showed subluxation of the hip. By the age of 16 the pain required a Chiari osteotomy. Rodrigues noted growth arrest following injury to the triradiate cartilage, causing a miniacetabulum.[115] Similar growth arrest has been reported by Hallel and Salvati.[101]

Experimental closure of the triradiate cartilage, with gradual acetabular dysplasia, has been reported.[90,93,94,96,98,99,101,107,108,118] Gepstein and associates found no significant difference in acetabular dysplasia or hip displacement resulting from fusion of all three limbs versus selective fusion of the ilioischial limb.[98] Delgado-Baeza and coworkers have shown that experimental traumatic lesions of the iliac and pubic regions of the triradiate cartilage of the acetabulum in rats produced interference with the pubic growth plate that eventually caused acetabular dysplasia and dislocation of the hip.[93,94,99] Although their primary emphasis was to look at damage that could lead to some of the changes seen with developmental dysplasia of the hip, obviously the traumatic nature is germane for evaluating the results from injury to this region during trauma. With severe disruption of growth, a shallow acetabulum results, with progressive subluxation if not dislocation of the hip.

Avulsion Fractures

Avulsions are the most common type of pelvic chondro-osseous injury in the child and especially in the adolescent athlete. Most may be treated by rest, relief from weight-bearing with crutches, muscle relaxants, and cessation of the evocative athletic activity for several weeks. These regions may be avulsed prior to the appearance of secondary ossification (which frequently does not appear until late adolescence). In such absence of definitive radiologic diagnosis, the injury must be strongly suspected clinically, and treatment should be directed toward the presumptive injury. Several weeks later the diagnosis may be confirmed by the appearance of "metaphyseal" callus (Fig. 19-45). Because of the thick periosteum and perichondrium, these fractures are not usually significantly displaced. Postinjury muscle function is generally not impaired by eventual healing in a mildly

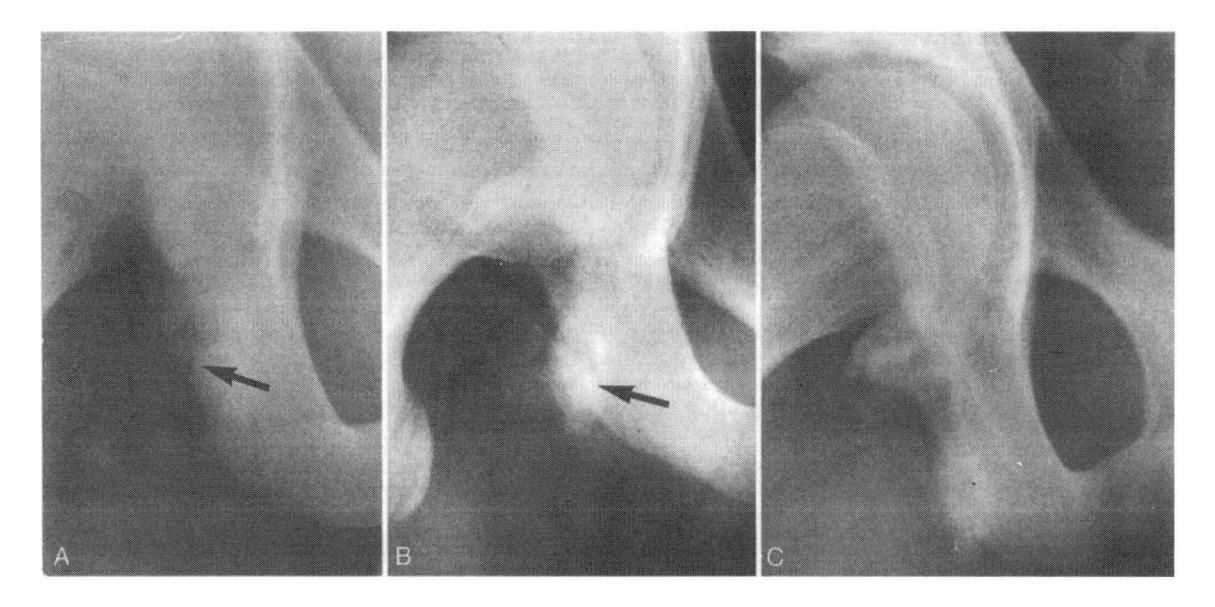

FIGURE 19-45. (A) Appearance of the ischial tuberosity following a "split" injury during water skiing. Note a small linear crack suggestive of fracture (arrow). (B) Three weeks later some reactive bone (arrow) confirms the diagnosis. (C) Four months later the area is beginning to remodel.

displaced position, even if a fibrous, rather than osseous, union results owing to the persistent tensile forces. However, significant displacement, which is much less common, may cause functional insufficiency (inefficiency) of the involved muscles and may require open reduction or reconstruction (i.e., shortening) for optimal muscle function. Complications are unusual, as these fractures are ordinarily associated with minor athletic stress, rather than major trauma.

When a musculotendinous unit is subjected to excess stress, whether an acute overload or a less forceful but repetitive application, the contraction or contractions may be transmitted to the apophysis. This may result in a fracture at either the chondro-osseous interface or through a segment of the subchondral bone. The excessive, invariably repetitive demands of adolescent athletics make this age group especially susceptible to avulsion fractures.

Various studies suggest that iliac spine avulsions are the most common, whereas others list ischial injuries as more frequent.[159] Frequency is not as important as suspicion and recognition by the clinician.

The basic treatment protocol is to stop the evocative activity, prescribe rest (including bed rest), prescribe nonsteroidal drugs, recommend appropriate positioning of the leg, and gradual resumption of activity. There should be protected weight-bearing with crutches. Most avulsion fractures may be managed nonoperatively, with attention directed at minimizing tension in the musculotendinous insertion.

Confusion with neoplasia or even osteomyelitis may be likely when there is irregular radiodensity and radiolucency. If a biopsy is done, the callus may be misinterpreted as an osteosarcoma.[161] Such a mistake may lead to unnecessary and costly evaluation and to inappropriate, even ablative surgery.

For competitive adolescent athletes conservative treatment of pelvic avulsion injuries may cause difficulties, despite good functional results. The disadvantages include a relatively long period of immobilization, use of crutches, risk of reinjury, alteration of functional length of involved muscles, disruption of normal training regimens, and the risk of missing a significant part of a sport season.

Iliac Crest

Butler and Eggert reported a fracture of the iliac crest as a variation of "hip pointer," which is usually defined as an iliac crest contusion.[122] Their patient sustained a direct blow to the crest from a football helmet. Clancy and Foltz reviewed iliac crest apophysitis and thought that it was a significant cause of disability in the adolescent athlete.[123] They reported 13 cases of anterior iliac crest apophysitis and 3 cases of stress fractures of the anterior iliac apophysis in adolescent runners.

Godshall and Hansen reported a case of incomplete avulsion fracture of the iliac epiphysis resulting from a sudden, severe contraction of the abdominal muscle associated with abrupt directional changes while running.[124] They were unable to find any comparable cases, although they subsequently saw a 16-year-old boy with a similar injury. They thought this particular condition in adolescent athletes could be confused with the "hip pointer," or a contusion of the iliac crest.

Symptoms may occur acutely or, at the other end of the spectrum, may persist for months following questionable injury. Some adolescent athletes have a posterior iliac crest apophysitis with pain localized at the posterior iliac crest (Fig. 19-46). This condition may be duplicated by resistance to abduction with the hip flexed and the patient lying on the unaffected side.

Roentgenograms are frequently unremarkable. One often must seek subtle differences in contour or physeal width. Variable radiolucencies within the iliac crest apophyseal ossification center are common, just as they are in the calcaneal apophysis (see Chapter 24); they are not indicative per se of

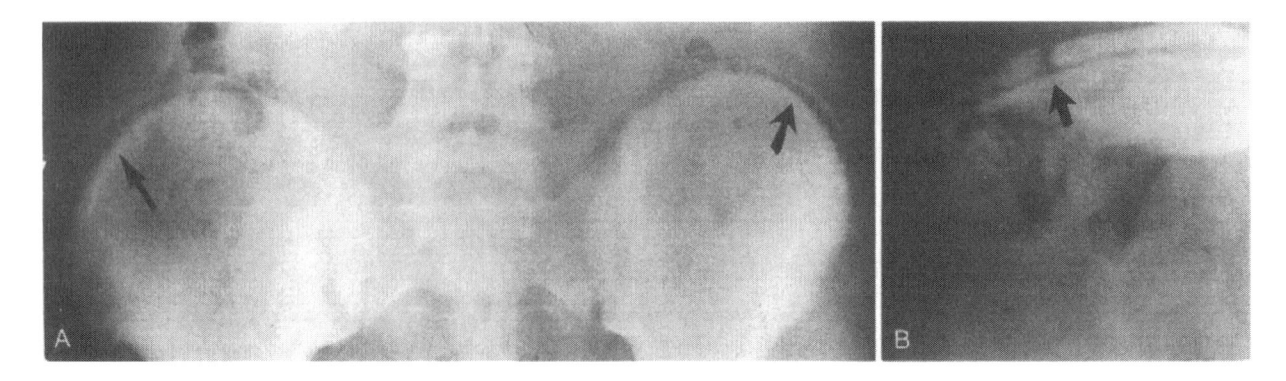

FIGURE 19-46. Adolescent complaining of "hip pointer" after a football tackle. (A) There is mild separation (arrow) of the iliac ossification center on the right. (B) Fracture through crest ossification (arrow) following a direct blow to the pelvic rim.

either an avulsion fracture or a fracture within the ossification center.

To avoid the risk of further avulsion and more serious damage, crutches should be used for 5–7 days, followed by limited physical activity for approximately 4 weeks. Patients treated by rest and discontinuation of their usual athletic activity generally have complete relief of symptoms within 4–6 weeks and are able to resume training programs at that point.

More significant trauma may avulse significant portions of the iliac crest (Fig. 19-47). The more violent the trauma, the greater is the risk of damage to growth potential, creating underdevelopment of the iliac wing. McDonald showed that growth disturbance of the ilium may be associated with premature fusion of the sacroiliac joint.[24]

Physeal avulsion of a nonossified iliac crest may result in intestinal obstruction because of a lumbar hernia or entrapment of bowel segments.[55,61] Damage to the iliac crest physis during early childhood may lead to growth discrepancy (Fig. 19-48). Olney et al. found that experimental splitting of the rabbit iliac apophysis significantly affected growth of the ilium.[125] Altered iliac growth, development, and attainment of a normal shape and orientation might negatively affect the origin and vector efficiency of the adductor muscles, which could, over time, affect the biomechanics of the hip.

Iliac Spines

The anterosuperior iliac spine (ASIS) serves as the attachment of the sartorius muscle and some of the tensor fascia lata; and the anteroinferior iliac spine (AIIS) is the attachment for the rectus femoris muscle. The muscles arising from either spine cross two mobile joints, both of which are major hip flexors and may be under extreme force during vigorous athletic activity or during an accident. Either iliac spine may be avulsed.[126–169] The anterosuperior spine is probably injured more often than the anteroinferior spine. The classic presentation is an adolescent sprinter who feels a sudden, sharp pain in the groin upon leaving the starting blocks. Less commonly repetitive stress of training may lead to insidious prodromal microfailure that can go on to complete avulsion (similar to the patterns of slipped capital femoral epiphysis and Osgood-Schlatter's lesion).

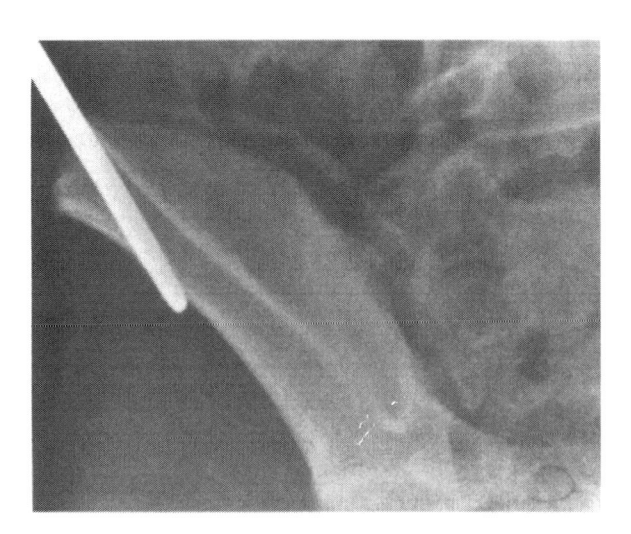

FIGURE 19-47. Subchondral equivalent of an iliac apophysis avulsion. This 4-year-old boy was severely injured when pinned under the tire of a large truck.

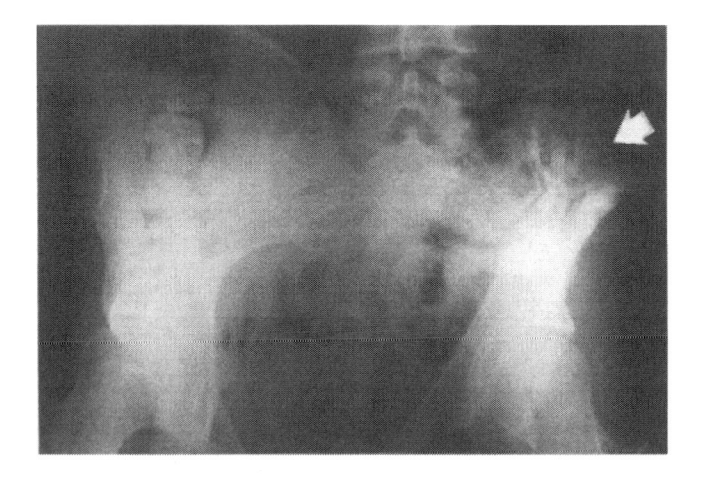

FIGURE 19-48. Adolescent who as an infant had sustained an injury to the left pelvis when thrown from a car during an accident. The left hemipelvis is hypoplastic; and the entire pelvis is rotated, with displacement of the symphysis. The injury appeared to involve only a portion of the iliac crest (arrow), as the acetabulum formed in a reasonably normal manner.

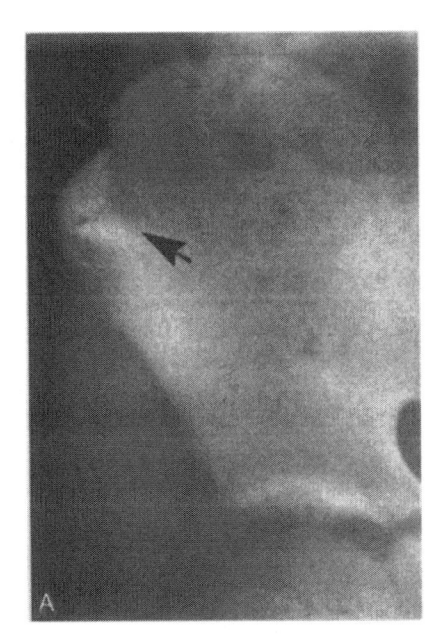

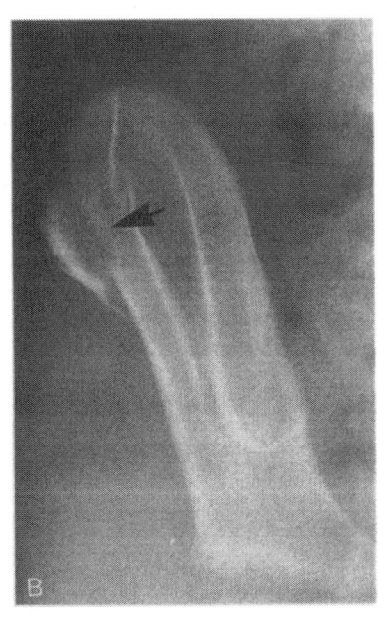

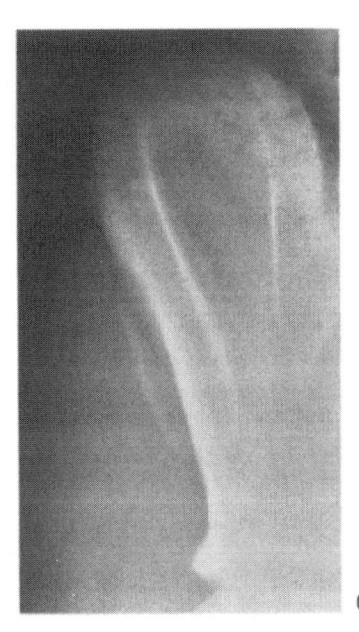

FIGURE 19-49. Fractures of the superior iliac spine. (A) Direct blow, with mild displacement. (B) Avulsion following a direct blow. (C) Injury of the anterosuperior iliac spine with downward displacement.

Two mechanisms of injury have been proposed. The first is a forceful contraction of the sartorius and tensor fasciae lata muscles against a hyperextended trunk (e.g., while running, playing soccer), such as at the start of a race or while slipping. The second is the sudden, repetitive movements of short sprints. This injury pattern most frequently affects adolescent runners. Essentially the two joints are moving in opposite directions simultaneously.

Most patients complain of acute pain, which is usually severe enough to cause them to stop the activity. Pain is increased during active movement of the hip. A snap was felt by the patients in 45% of cases. Swelling and tenderness are often present.

Diagnosis may be difficult. In a young child the spine may be cartilaginous, and thus impossible to detect with routine radiography. The adolescent usually has a fracture through the equivalent of metaphyseal bone, pulling off the cartilage and enough osseous tissue to be detected radiographically. Rarely, a secondary ossification center is evident in a cartilaginous disruption in the adolescent.

Usually these fractures do not separate significantly, although in rare instances they may be displaced several centimeters, especially when the trauma is repetitive (Figs. 19-49, 19-50). Hamsa described a displaced superior iliac spine that had led to formation of an osseous bar extending down from the pelvis.[190] Chronic, repetitive avulsion may

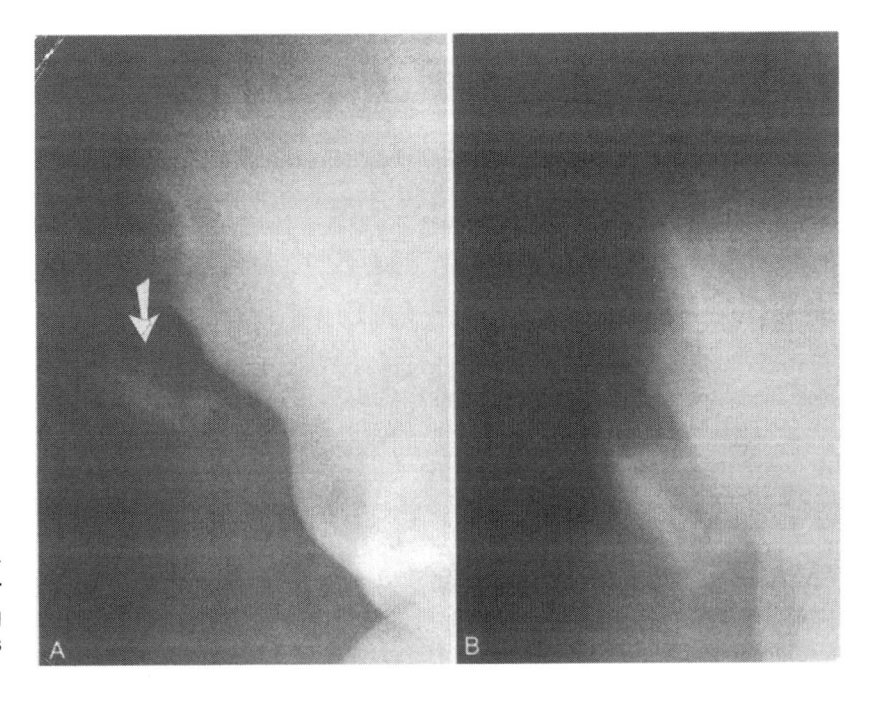

FIGURE 19-50. (A) Avulsion injury of the superior iliac spine (arrow) in a 14-year-old sprinter who sustained a tear coming out of the starting blocks. (B) Appearance 7 weeks later with callus formation.

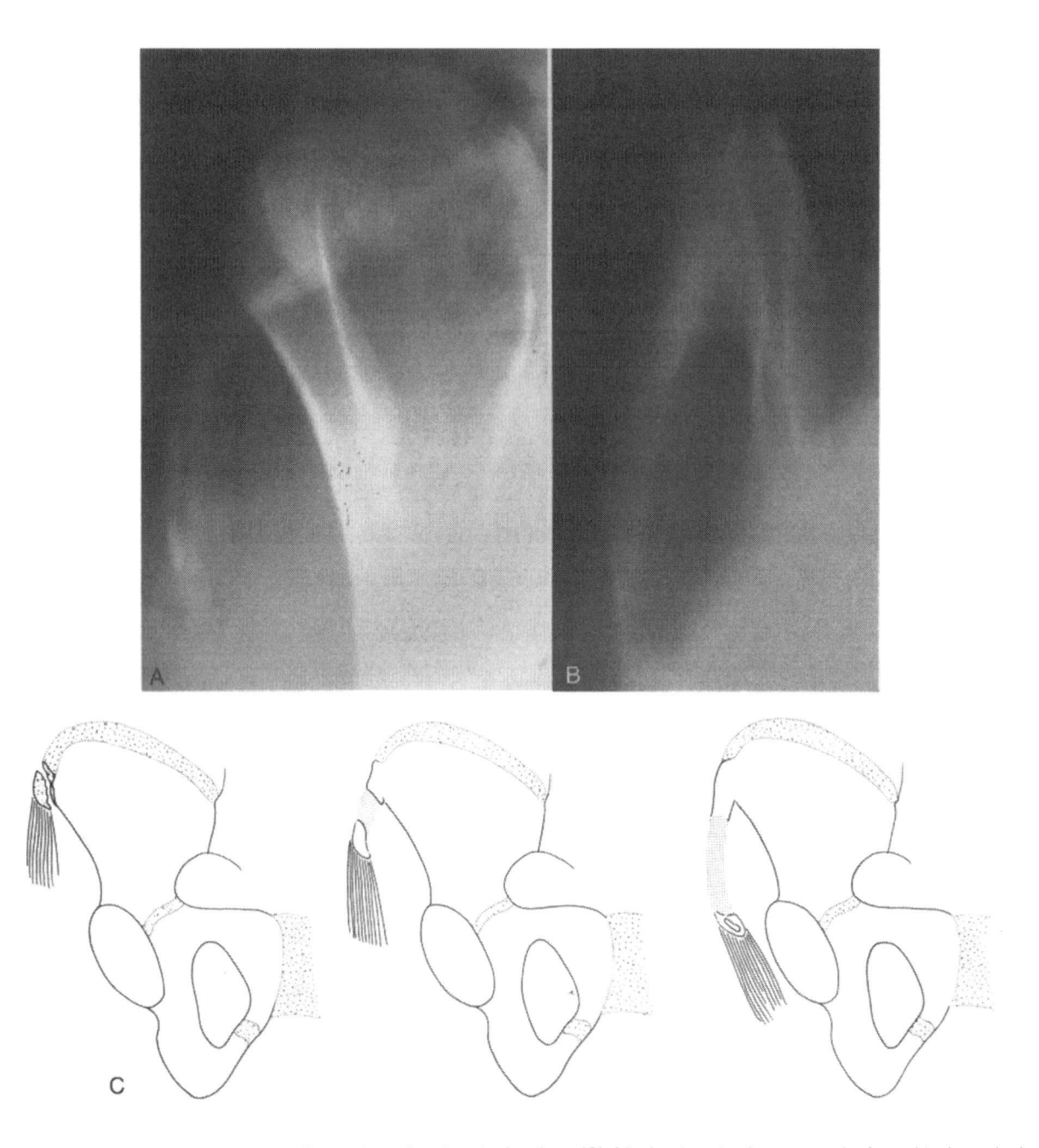

FIGURE 19-51. (A,B) Elongated superior iliac spine after break dancing. (C) Mechanism is the traumatic (repetitive) equivalent of surgical bone lengthening by chondrodiatasis.

lead to formation of an extensively elongated superior spine (Fig. 19-51).[138,154]

Treatment includes rest, minimal weight-bearing with the use of crutches, and discontinuation of athletic activities for 4–6 weeks. If a significant separation has occurred, open reduction may be indicated. However, open reduction and internal fixation are rarely needed (Fig. 19-52).

Walking on crutches for 1–2 weeks and abstaining from vigorous activities yield the best results. The average duration of disability is approximately 20 days. Pain should be absent before evocative athletic activities are resumed.

Irving reported two cases of exostosis formation after traumatic avulsion of the AIIS.[144] This particular injury (Figs. 19-53, 19-54) is much less common than other avulsion fractures around the pelvis and should not be considered myositis ossificans. This enlarged reactive bone must be interpreted carefully.

Exostosis formation of either the ASIS or AIIS is due to acute or chronic traction avulsion of the cartilaginous apophysis. The intervening gap is filled in with endochondral bone (chronic traction) or a combination of membranous and endochondral bone (acute avulsion). In the chronic situation the repetitive minimal avulsion/traction duplicates the same phenomenon as with limb lengthening through the growth plate (i.e., chondrodiatasis).

Avulsion Fractures 821

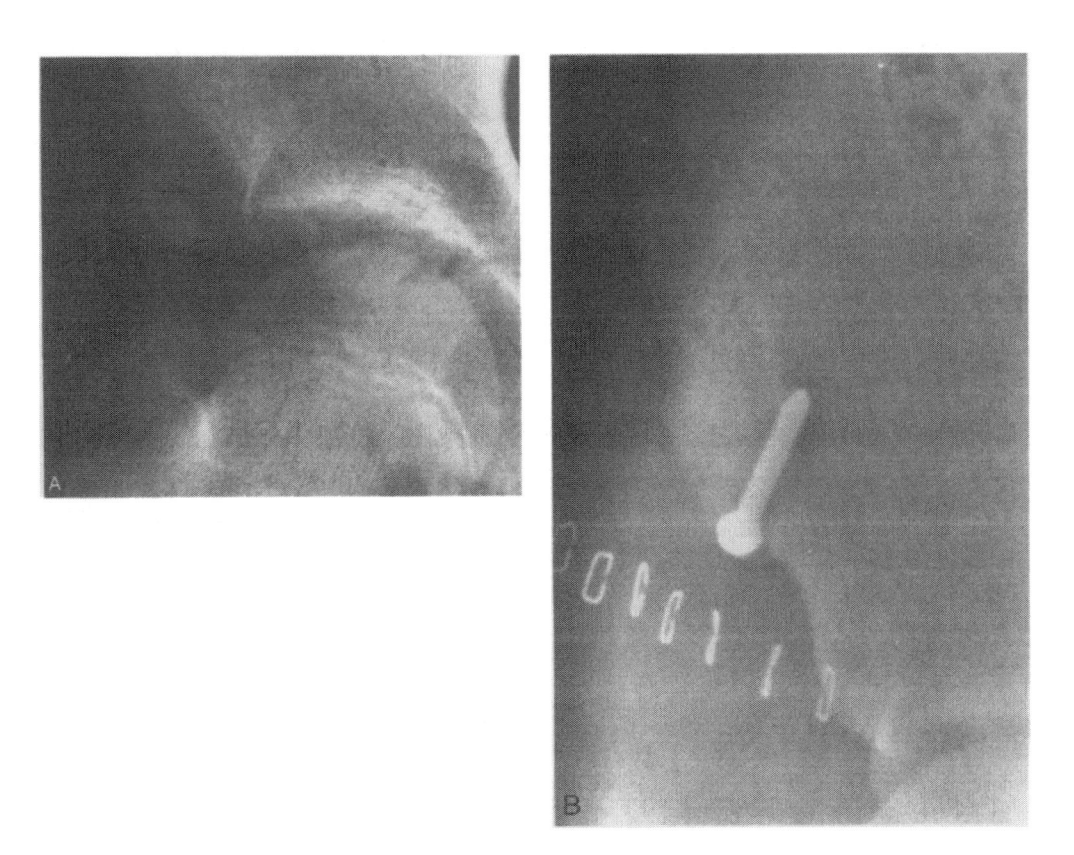

FIGURE 19-52. (A) Avulsion of the anteroinferior spine. (B) Internal fixation.

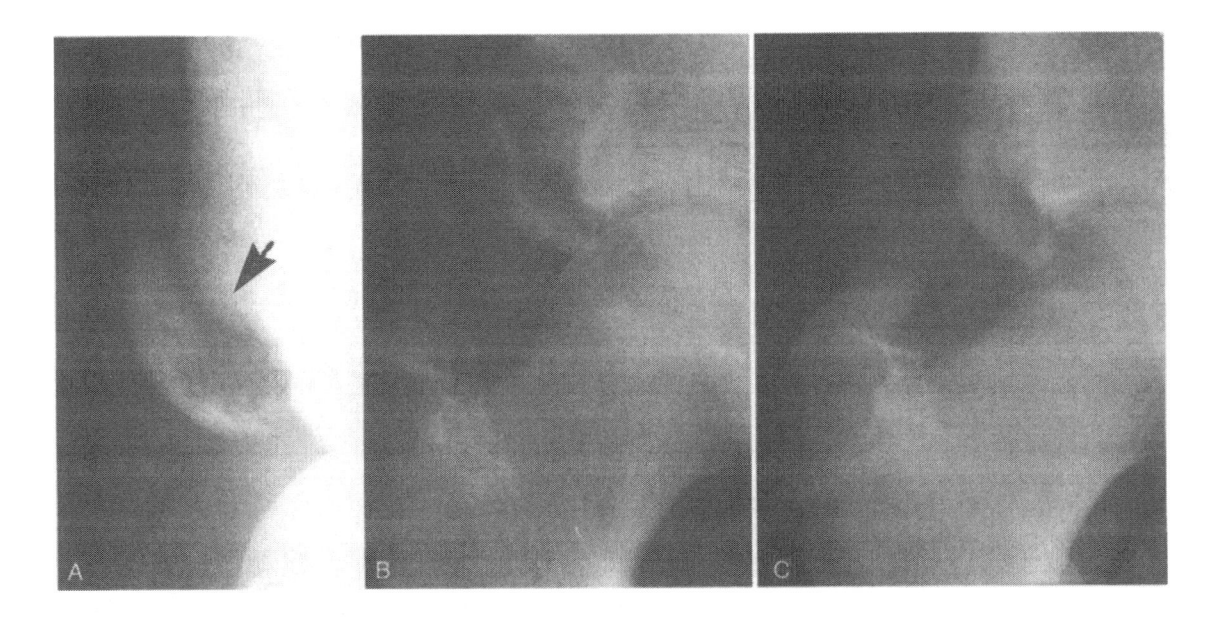

FIGURE 19-53. (A) Avulsion of the inferior iliac spine (arrow). (B) Avulsion of the combined inferior spine and acetabular rim ossification center. (C) Four months later extensive healing is evident.

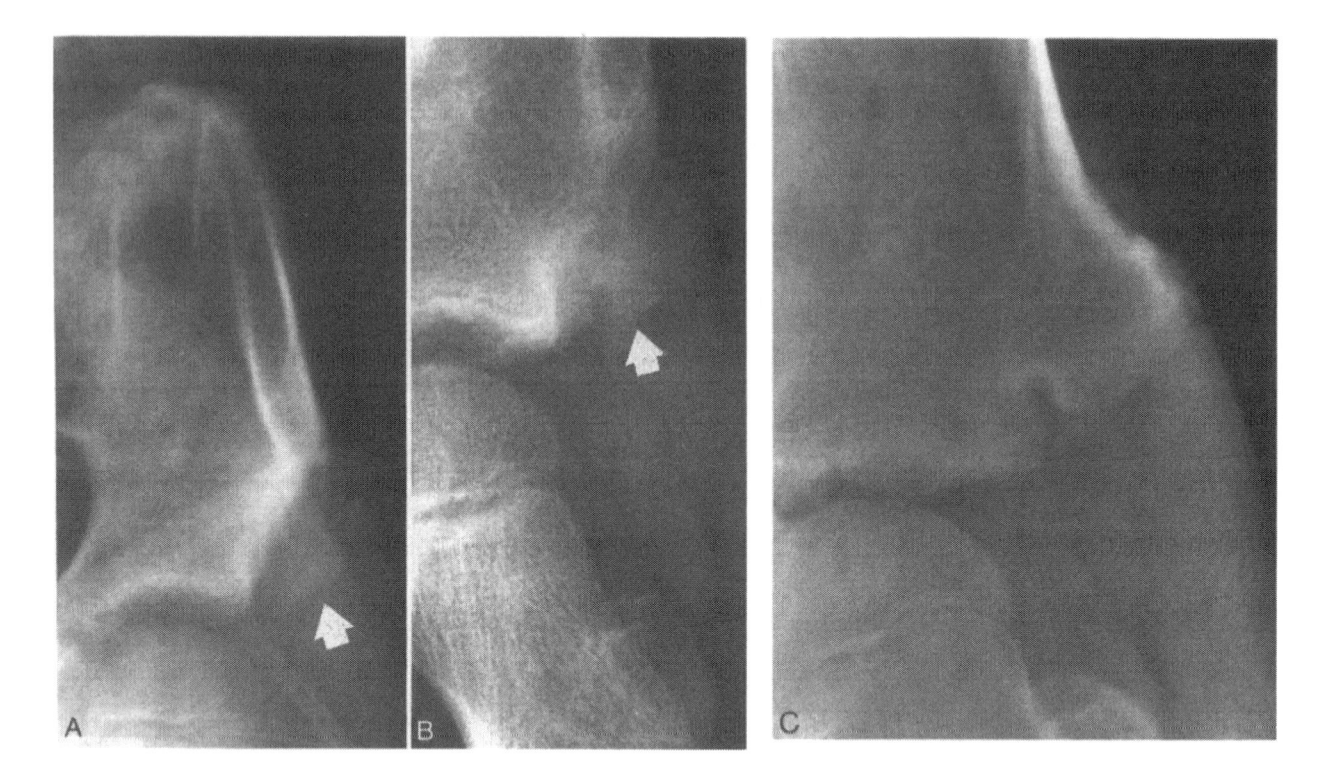

FIGURE 19-54. Exostosis formation following anteroinferior spine injury in a 6-year-old child. There was no evidence of osseous spine injury during initial major pelvic trauma. In retrospect, the cartilaginous inferior spine had avulsed. New bone formation (arrow) is evident 3 weeks after injury (A) and 8 months later (arrow) (B). (C) Five years later.

Ischial Tuberosity

Injury to the ischial tuberosity has been discussed frequently,[170–232] and Hamada and Rida presented an excellent review.[189] Irregularity of the apophysis of the ischial tuberosity is termed Kremser's disease. The typical patient is a young adolescent athlete. This area may be avulsed (Fig. 19-55), which may lead to nonunion although not necessarily a symptomatic one (Fig. 19-56).[200,206]

Ischial apophysiolysis is often diagnosed only after considerable time. In these delayed cases, commonly the precipitating injury is not considered significant by either the patient or the physician.

The mechanism of injury appears to be the action of the hip flexors on the pelvis, transmitted across the femoral head as a fulcrum, which tends to elevate the ischium. This elevation is counteracted by the hamstring muscle, which pulls downward and laterally, a force neutralized by the sacrosciatic ligaments.

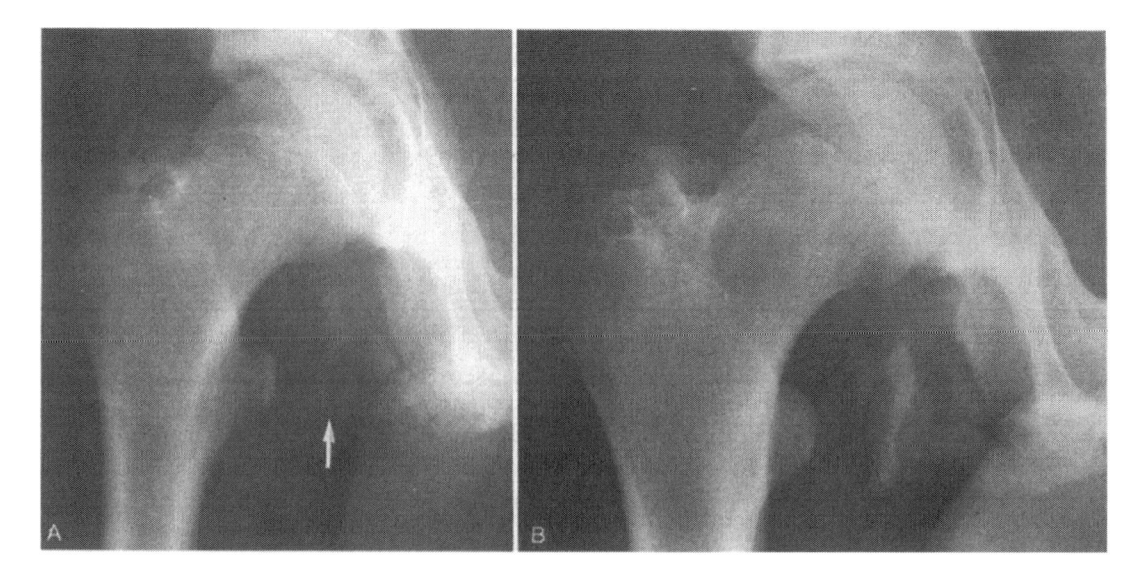

FIGURE 19-55. (A) Avulsion of the ischial tuberosity with early bone formation (arrow). (B) At 7 weeks extensive bone formation is evident.

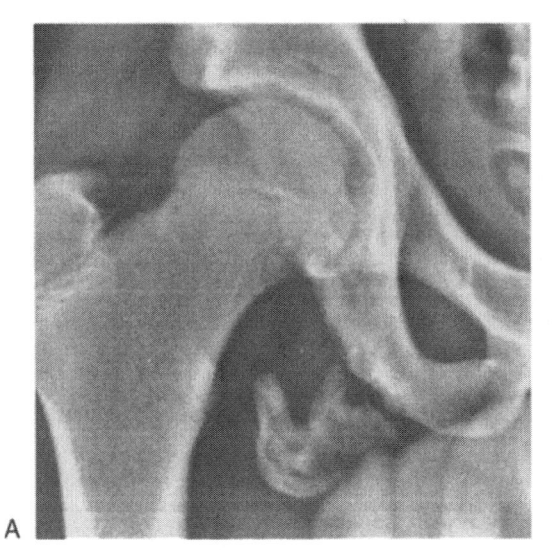

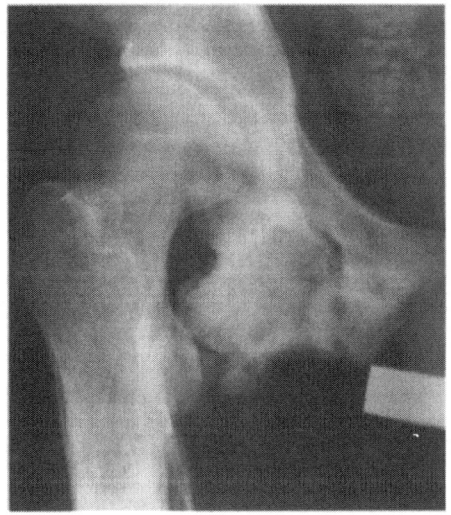

FIGURE 19-56. (A) Avulsion of the ischial tuberosity 10 months after injury. (B) Three years later. Sitting was painful. This fragment was subsequently excised.

Therefore the degree of displacement of the ischial apophysis depends on the specific role of these ligaments. The most likely conditions for the injury are attained when a powerful muscle contraction takes place in the hamstrings with the pelvis fixed in flexion and the knee in extension. These conditions commonly occur with hurdling and gymnastics, although many other sports are associated with the injury. For example, in the boy shown in Figure 19-45, the injury was acquired during water skiing when he did an inadvertent split while both skis were in contact with the water.

From an anatomic standpoint, an avulsion is likely to be partial (incomplete). The ischial tuberosity is roughly divisible into two portions, one for insertion of the hamstrings and the other for insertion of the adductor magnus. Thus the pattern of injury in a high hurdler could be different from that in a dancer doing a split.

Diagnosis often is difficult in these children. Figure 19-45 shows an absence of any significant area, although the small crack, coupled with the history, should make one suspicious. Yet later, with formation of new bone, the diagnosis became obvious. Watanabe and Chigira described a detailed study with serial CT scans showing avulsion of small bone fragments that subsequently enlarged (in the unossified cartilaginous apophysis, similar to the Osgood-Schlatter injury pattern).[228] They also found that MRI studies strongly supported the concept of an avulsion fracture.[229]

Treatment may vary. Most patients with ischial apophysiolysis do well with rest and a protective program. Ideally, osseous union is demonstrable by roentgenography before strenuous exercises are again permitted. Milch's study indicated it may require up to 2–4 years in the younger age groups.[209] Failure to follow a protective program could result in avulsion fracture of the apophysis from a subsequent undisplaced injury. The possibility of contralateral involvement should always be kept in mind.

Avulsion fractures with significant separation (1 cm or more) probably should be reduced anatomically by closed or open reduction (Fig. 19-57). An attempt at closed reduction

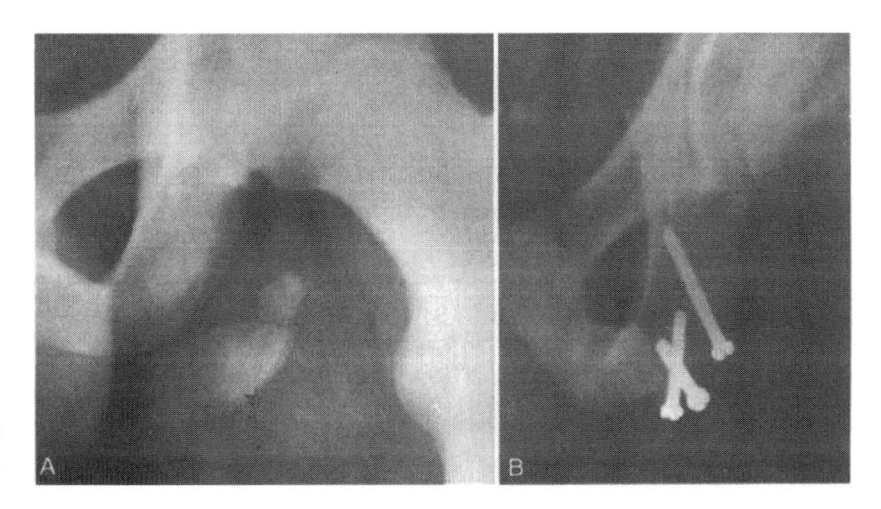

FIGURE 19-57. Open reduction of an avulsion of the ischial tuberosity. (A) Original injury. (B) Postoperative appearance.

probably is worthwhile and may be possible with direct pressure over the tuberosity. Open reduction of an avulsion fracture is a relatively straightforward procedure. Attachment may be made with cancellous screws. Pruner and Johnston discussed the use of fixation of the ischial tuberosity when it was displaced.[215] Wootton et al. also recommended open reduction and internal fixation for significantly displaced fractures.[231] Their cases were associated with marked chronic disability after delay in diagnosis and nonunion of the fracture. Howard and Piha suggested that avulsions with more than 2 cm displacement needed operative reduction and fixation.[194]

An untreated avulsion fracture may unite spontaneously or may form a fibrous union with subsequent enlargement of the tuberosity.[219] The symptoms include inability to sit comfortably on the enlarged, nonunited tuberosity and pain, with associated discomfort in the back or limb especially while involved in excessive activity.[21,214,221] The subsequent enlargement of the tuberosity may be irregular enough to suggest a tumor, and a diagnosis of osteogenic sarcoma or Ewing's sarcoma has been rendered in some cases. Sciatic-type pain is not a general feature of the older, chronic lesions; and if this symptom is encountered, one should rule out a coexistent herniated intervertebral disk before attributing neurologic symptomatology to this lesion.

Chronic injuries, when symptomatic, may be treated by excision of the ununited fragment and repair of the tendinous origin of the hamstrings or by fixation and bone graft. I prefer resection and musculotendinous reattachment.

Other Pelvic Injuries

Stress Fracture

The increased emphasis on competitive sports not only puts skeletally immature individuals at risk for the previously described avulsion injuries, it also may lead to unusual avulsions and stress fractures. As discussed in the section on anatomy, the pubic symphysis and ischiopubic synchondrosis are areas of progressive chondro-osseous growth and maturation. Repetitive use may cause strain and lead to chronic

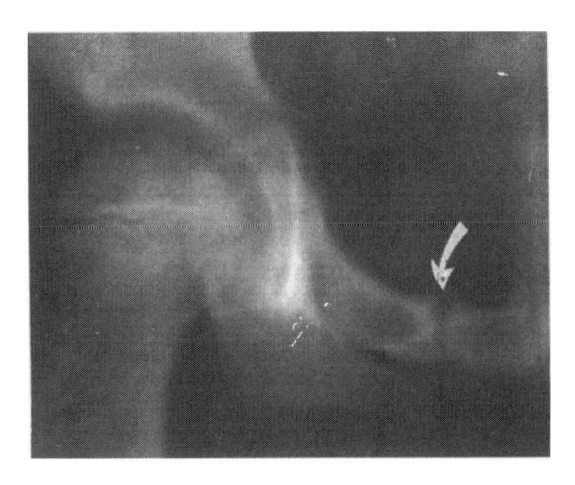

FIGURE 19-58. Stress fracture (arrow) of the pubic ramus.

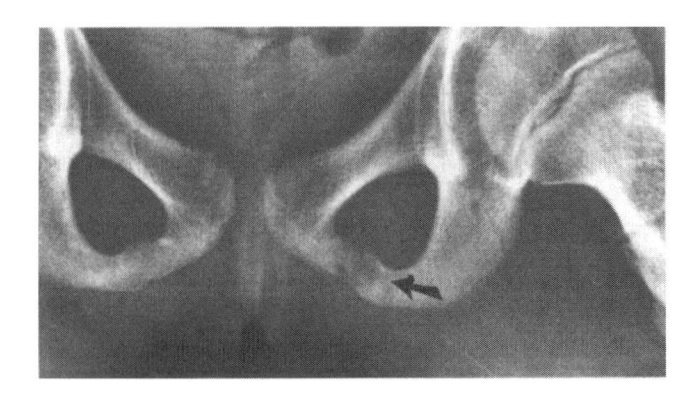

FIGURE 19-59. Stress fracture of the left ischial synchondrosis (arrow). The right ischial synchondrosis is physiologically closed although still slightly enlarged.

fatigue manifesting as pain (i.e., an incomplete or microscopic fracture of the evolving chondro-osseous interface). These stress fractures (Fig. 19-58) should be treated symptomatically, with the emphasis on decreasing or stopping the evocative activity.

Ischiopubic Osteochondrosis

The ischiopubic osteochondrosis region may be the site of stress fractures in young joggers and runners (Fig. 19-59). Such fractures are nondisplaced.[213] These injuries are more frequent in females, which may be due to differences in pelvic anatomy and running styles. The increased participation of young individuals in these sports leads to similar symptoms (groin/thigh pain) but with radiolucency/radiodensity or enlargement of the synchondrosis.

Treatment is symptomatic. Temporary cessation of the physical activity for 2–3 weeks usually alleviates the pain. Preactivity stretching may lessen muscle pull at the pelvic attachment.

Pubic Symphysis

In the adolescent the onset of midline pain at the symphysis may be due to a fatigue (tension) failure of the chondro-osseous origin of the gracilis muscle.[237] Changes (radiographic) usually involve only one side of the symphysis. It is referred to by several names: osteitis pubis, pubic symphysitis, osteochondritis of the symphysis pubis, adductor injury, and gracilis syndrome.

Pain may be in the groin, perineum, or medial thigh and is usually gradually insidious in its onset. On examination there may be discrete tenderness at the symphysis. Radiographic proof is contingent on a cartilaginous avulsion (radiolucent) or a piece of subchondral bone along with a cartilage fragment. Fragment displacement is not significant. Reactive bone may form in the gap (similar to other apophyseal pelvic avulsions), sometimes leading to a small "exostosis." Chronic motion may also cause erosive irregularities in the bone margin, akin to gymnast's wrist (see Chapters 12, 16). In Wiley's case the bone fragment was excised.[237] Histology was compatible with chronic avulsion failure. Others have reported similar cases in adolescent athletes.[233–236]

Meralgia Paresthetica

Edelson and Stevens[239] and MacNichol and Thompson[240] reviewed children and adolescents with meralgia paresthetica. It was usually associated with injury during sports activities. Bilateral involvement is common. The average duration of symptoms was 24 months. In about half of the cases the diagnosis was missed initially. Predisposing factors appeared to include previous pelvic osteotomy and pelvic fracture. The usual pain was over the anterior or lateral thigh.

Pain reproduced by direct palpation of the nerve (inferior to the ASIS) and a trial injection of lidocaine (Xylocaine) usually produced transient relief of symptoms. Pain decreased normal activities, including sports. Several were eventually treated with decompression of the lateral cutaneous nerve. Surgery revealed thickened fascial constrictive bands. Previously unrecognized repetitive (stress) avulsion of the ASIS may present with chronic pain attributed to meralgia paresthetica.[238,241]

References

Anatomy

1. Caffey J, Ross SE. The ischiopubic synchondrosis in healthy children: some normal roentgenologic findings. AJR 1956;76:488–494.
2. Cawley KA, Dvorak AD, Wilmot MD. Normal anatomic variant: Scintigraphy of the ischiopubic synchondrosis. J Nucl Med 1982;24:14–16.
3. Gamble JG, Simmons SC, Freedman M. The symphysis pubis: anatomic and pathologic considerations. Clin Orthop 1986;203:261–272.
4. Kloiber R, Udjus K, McIntyre W, Jarvis J. The scintigraphic and radiographic appearance of the ischiopubic synchondroses in normal children and in osteomyelitis. Pediatr Radiol 1988;18:57–61.
5. Ogden JA. Hip development and vascularity: relationship to chondro-osseous trauma in the growing child. In: The Hip, vol 9. St Louis: Mosby, 1981.
6. Ponseti IV. Growth and development of the acetabulum in the normal child: anatomical, histological, and roentgenographic studies. J Bone Joint Surg Am 1978;60:575–585.
7. Schinz HR. Altes und neues zur Beckenossifikation: Zugleich ein Beitrag zur Kenntnis des Os acetabuli. Fortschr Röntgenstr 1922;30:66–73.
8. Zander G. Os acetabuli and other bony periarticular calcifications at the hip joint. Acta Radiol [Diagn] (Stockh) 1943;24:317–322.

General Considerations

9. Allouis M, Bracq H, Catier P, Babut JM. Traumatismes pelviens graves de l'enfant. Chir Pediatr 1981;22:43–50.
10. Bryan WJ, Tullos HS. Pediatric pelvic fractures: review of 52 patients. J Trauma 1979;19:799–805.
11. Carlioz H, Michelutti D. Traumatismes du bassin et de la hanche chez l'enfant. Ann Chir 1982;36:50–56.
12. Craig CL. Hip injuries in children and adolescents. Orthop Clin North Am 1980;11:743–754.
13. Engelhardt P. Die Malgaigne-Becken ring verletzung in Kindesalter. Orthopade 1992;21:422–426.
14. Garvin KL, McCarthy RE, Barnes CL, Dodye BM. Pediatric pelvic ring fractures. J Pediatr Orthop 1990;10:577–582.
15. Habacker TA, Heinrich SD, Dehne R. Fracture of the superior pelvic quadrant in a child. J Pediatr Orthop 1995;15:69–72.
16. Harder JA, Bobechko WP, Sullivan RS, Daneman A. Computerized axial tomography to demonstrate occult fractures of the acetabulum in children. Can J Surg 1981;24:409–411.
17. Heiss W, Daum R, Fischer H. Beckenfrakturen bei Kindern und Jugendlichen. Hefte Unfallheilkd 1975;124:283–286.
18. Keshishayan RA, Rozinov VM, Malakhovoa et al. Pelvic polyfractures in children. Clin Orthop 1995;320:28–33 [contains a number of references from the Russian literature].
19. Lacheretz M, Herbaux B. Faut-il opérer les fractures instables du bassin chez l'enfant. Chirurgie 1988;114:510–515.
20. Lacheretz M, Noel JL, Fontaine C, Hodin B. Les lesions associées et les complications propres aux fractures du bassin chez l'enfant. Chirurgie 1988;106:541–545.
21. Lane-O'Kelly A, Fogarty E, Dowling F. The pelvic fracture in childhood: a report supporting nonoperative management. Injury 1995;26:327–329.
22. Lim EVA, Abrahan LM Jr, Altre TL, Songco RS. External pelvic fixation in an infant. J Trauma 1995;38:820–821.
23. Magid D, Fishman EK, Ney NR, et al. Acetabular and pelvic fractures in the pediatric patient: value of two- and three-dimensional imaging. J Pediatr Orthop 1992;12:621–625.
24. McDonald GA. Pelvic disruptions in children. Clin Orthop 1980;151:130–134.
25. McLaren AC, Rorabeck CH, Halpenny J. Long-term pain and disability in relation to residual deformity after displaced pelvic ring fractures. Can J Surg 1990;33:492–494.
26. Mears DC, Fu F. External fixation in pelvic fractures. Orthop Clin North Am 1980;11:465–479.
27. Metzmaker JN, Pappas AM. Fractures of the pelvis. Am J Sports Med 1985;13:349–358.
28. Morden ML. Pelvic fractures in children. In: Houghton GR, Thompson GH (eds) Orthopaedics. London: Butterworths, 1983.
29. Musemeche CA, Fischer RP, Cotler HB, Andrassy RJ. Selective management of pediatric pelvic fractures: a conservative approach. J Pediatr Surg 1987;22:538–540.
30. Nierenberg G, Volpin G, Bialik V, Stein H. Pelvic fractures in children: a follow-up in 20 children treated conservatively. J Pediatr Orthop Part B 1993;1:140–142.
31. Potter HG, Mongomery KD, Padgett DE, Salvati EA, Helfet DL. Magnetic resonance imaging of the pelvis. Clin Orthop 1995;319:223–231.
32. Quinby WC. Fractures of the pelvis and other associated injuries in children. J Pediatr Surg 1966;1:353–361.
33. Reed MH. Pelvic fractures in children. J Can Assoc Radiol 1976;27:255–261.
34. Reichard SA, Helikson MA, Shorter N, et al. Pelvic fractures in children: review of 120 patients with a new look at general management. J Pediatr Surg 1980;15:727–734.
35. Sahlstrand T. Disruption of the pelvic ring treated by external skeletal fixation. J Bone Joint Surg Am 1979;61:433–434.
36. Schmidt HD, Hofmann S. Die Problematik schwerer Beckenfrakturen im Wachstumsalter. Hefte Unfallheilkd 1975;124:286–288.
37. Schwarz N, Mayr J, Fischmeister FM, Schwartz AF, Posch E, Öhner T. 2-Jahres-Ergebnisse der conservatiren Therape instabiler Beckenringfrakturen bei Kindern. Unfallchirurgie 1994;97:439–444.
38. St. Pierre RK, Oliver T, Somoygi J, et al. Computerized tomography in the evaluation and classification of fractures of the acetabulum. Clin Orthop 1984;188:234–237.

39. Stewart MJ, Milford LW. Fracture-dislocation of the hip. J Bone Joint Surg Am 1954;36:315–342.
40. Tile M. Pelvic fractures: operative versus nonoperative treatment. Orthop Clin North Am 1980;11:423–464.
41. Torode I, Zieg D. Pelvic fractures in children. J Pediatr Orthop 1985;5:76–84.
42. Ward RE, Clark DG. Management of pelvic fractures. Radiol Clin North Am 1981;19:167–170.
43. Watts H. Fractures of the pelvis in children. Orthop Clin North Am 1976;7:615–624.
44. Webb LX, Gristina AG, Wilson JR, Rhyne JR, Meredith JH, Hansen SV Jr. Two-hole plate fixation for traumatic symphysis pubis diastasis. J Trauma 1988;28:813–817.
45. Young JW, Burgess AR, Brumback RJ, Poka A. Lateral compression fractures of the pelvis: the importance of plain radiographs in the diagnosis and surgical management. Skeletal Radiol 1986;15:103–109.

Vascular Injuries

46. Barlow B, Rottenberg RW, Santulli TV. Angiographic diagnosis and treatment of bleeding by selective embolization following pelvic fracture in children. J Pediatr Surg 1975; 10:939–942.
47. Braunstein PW, Skudder PA, McCarroll JR, et al. Concealed hemorrhage due to pelvic fracture. J Trauma 1964;4:832–838.
48. Canarelli JP, Collet LM, Ricard J, Boboyon JM. Complications vasculaires des traumatismes pelviens chez l'enfant. Chir Pediatr 1988;28:233–241.
49. Ger R, Condrea H, Steichen FM. Traumatic intrapelvic retroperitoneal hemorrhage: an experimental study. J Surg Res 1969;9:31–34.
50. Lacheretz M, Herbaux B. Traitement des hématomes souspéritoneaux des fracture du pelvis chez l'enfant: intérêt de l'hémostase par embolisation. Chirurgie 1986;112: 541–545.
51. Margolies MN, Ring EJ, Waltman AC, et al. Arteriography in the management of hemorrhage from pelvic fractures. N Engl J Med 1972;287:317–321.
52. McIntyre RC, Bensard DD, Moore EE, Chambers J, Moore FA. Pelvic fracture geometry predicts risk of life-threatening hemorrhage in children. J Trauma 1993;35:423–429.
53. Moreno C, Moore EE, Rosenberger A, Cleveland HC. Hemorrhage associated with major pelvic fracture: a multispecialty challenge. J Trauma 1986;26:987–994.
54. Ring EJ, Waltman AC, Athanasoulis C, et al. Angiography in pelvic trauma. Surg Gynecol Obstet 1974;139:375–380.

Abdominal Injuries

55. Arnold GT. A case of fracture of the pelvis with nipping of the small intestine between the fragments. Lancet 1907; 1:1157–1158.
56. Bond SJ, Gotschall CS, Eichelberger MR. Predictors of abdominal injury in children with pelvic fracture. J Trauma 1991;31:1169–1173.
57. Buchanan JR. Bowel entrapment by pelvic fracture fragments: a case report and review of the literature. Clin Orthop 1980;147:164–166.
58. Cooney DR, Billmire DF. Abdomen: hepatic, biliary tree and pancreatic injury. In: Touloukian RJ (ed) Pediatric Trauma, 2nd ed. St. Louis: Mosby, 1990.
59. Cywes S, Rode H, Millar AJW. Blunt liver trauma in children: non-operative management. J Pediatr Surg 1985;20: 14–18.
60. Davidson BS, Simmons GT, Williamson PR, Bueok CA. Pelvic fractures associated with open perineal wounds: a survivable injury. J Trauma 1993;35:36–39.
61. Everett WG. Traumatic lumbar hernia. Injury 1972;4:354–356.
62. Levine JI, Crampton RS. Major abdominal injuries associated with pelvic fractures. Surg Gynecol Obstet 1963;62:223–226.
63. Lunt HRW. Entrapment of bowel within fractures of the pelvis. Injury 1970;2:121–126.
64. Nimityongskul P, Anderson LD, Powell RW. Small bowel incarceration associated with a central fracture-dislocation of the hip in a child: case report. Contemp Orthop 1989;18:607–609.

Neurologic Injuries

65. Harris WR, Rathbun JB, Wortzman G, Humphrey JG. Avulsion of lumbar roots complicating fracture of the pelvis. J Bone Joint Surg Am 1973;55:1436–1442.
66. Lam CR. Nerve injury in fractures of the pelvis. Ann Surg 1936;104:945–950.

Urologic Injuries

67. Allison R. Urethrography in pelvic trauma. J Urol 1974;111: 778–779.
68. Brereton RJ, Philip N, Buyukpamukcu N. Rupture of the urinary bladder in children: the importance of the double lesion. Br J Urol 1980;52:15–20.
69. Brock WA, Kaplan GW. Use of the transpubic approach for urethroplasty in children. J Urol 1981;125:496–501.
70. Coffield KS, Weems WL. Experience with management of posterior urethral injury associated with pelvic fractures. J Urol 1974;117:722–724.
71. Dhabuwala CB, Hamid S, Katsikas DM, Pierce JM Jr. Impotence following delayed repair of prostatomembranous urethral disruption. J Urol 1990;144:677–678.
72. Donohue JP. Ureteral and bladder injuries in children. Pediatr Clin North Am 1975;22:393–399.
73. Emanuel B, Weiss H, Gollin P. Renal trauma in children. J Trauma 1977;17:275–278.
74. Garret RA. Pediatric urethral and perineal injuries. Pediatr Clin North Am 1975;22:401–406.
75. Gibson GR. Impotence following fractured pelvis and ruptured urethra. Br J Urol 1970;42:86–88.
76. Gibson GR. Urological management and complications of fractured pelvis and ruptured urethra. J Urol 1974;111: 353–355.
77. Glassberg KI, Tolete-Velcek F, Ashley R, Waterhouse K, et al. Partial tears of prostatomembranous urethra in children. Urology 1979;13:500–504.
78. Glassberg KI, Kassner EG, Haller JO, Waterhouse K. The radiographic approach to injuries of the prostatomembranous urethra in children. J Urol 1979;122:678–683.
79. Goswami AK, Indudhara R, Sharama SK. Case report: traumatic loss of the entire urethra and bladder neck in a girl: reconstruction by modified Flocks bladder tube. J Trauma 1992;32:545–546.
80. Hendren WH, Peters CA. Lower urinary tract and perineal injuries. In: Touloukian RJ (ed) Pediatric Trauma, 2nd ed. St. Louis: Mosby, 1990:371–398.
81. Kaiser TF, Farrow FC. Injury of the bladder and prostatomembranous urethra associated with fracture of the boy pelvis. Surg Gynecol Obstet 1965;120:99–112.
82. Kaufman JJ, Brosman SA. Blunt injuries of the genitourinary tract. Surg Clin North Am 1972;52:747–760.

83. Livne PM, Gonzalez ET Jr. Genitourinary trauma in children. Urol Clin North Am 1985;12:53–65.
84. Malek RS, O'Dea MJ, Kelalis PP. Management of ruptured posterior urethra in childhood. J Urol 1977;117:105–109.
85. Mark SD, Kesne TE, Vandemark RM, Webster GD. Impotence following pelvic fracture urethral injury: incidence, aetiology and management. Br J Urol 1995;75:62–64.
86. Merchant WC III, Gibbons MD, Gonzales ET Jr. Trauma to the bladder neck, trigone and vagina in children. J Urol 1984;131:747–750.
87. Reda EF, Lobowitz RL. Traumatic ureteropelvic disruption in the child. Pediatr Radiol 1986;16:164–167.
88. Williams DI. Rupture of the female urethra in childhood. Eur Urol 1975;1:129–130.

Obstetric-Gynecologic Injuries

89. Heinrich SD, Sharps CH, Cardea JA, Gervin AS. Open pelvic fracture with vaginal laceration and diaphragmatic rupture in a child. J Orthop Trauma 1988;2:257–261.

Acetabular (Triradiate) Fracture

90. Akbas A, Ünsaldi T, Körüklü O, Göze F. The effect of physeal traction applied to the triradiate cartilage on acetabular growth. Int Orthop 1995;19:122–126.
91. Blair W, Hanson C. Traumatic closure of the triradiate cartilage: report of a case. J Bone Joint Surg Am 1979;61:144–145.
92. Bucholz RW, Ezaki M, Ogden JA. Injury to the acetabular triradiate physeal cartilage. J Bone Joint Surg Am 1982;64:600–609.
93. Delgado-Baeza E, Gil E, Serrada A, Davidson WM, Miralles C. Acetabular dysplasia associated with a lesion of iliopubic limb of the triradiate cartilage. Clin Orthop 1988;234:75–81.
94. Delgado-Baeza E, Sanz-Laguna A, Miralles-Flores C. Experimental trauma of the triradiate epiphysis of the acetabulum and hip dysplasia. Int Orthop 1991;15:335–339.
95. Dias L, Tachdjian MO, Schroeder KE. Premature closure of the triradiate cartilage. J Bone Joint Surg Br 1980;62:46–48.
96. Garay EG, Baeza ED, Hierro AS. Acetabular dysplasia in the rat induced by injury to the triradiate growth cartilage. Acta Orthop Scand 1988;59:516–519.
97. Geleherter G. Pelvis. In: Ehalt W (ed) Traumatologia de la Infancia y Adolescencia. Madrid: Labor, 1965.
98. Gepstein R, Weiss RE, Hallel T. Acetabular dysplasia and hip dislocation after selective fusion of the triradiate cartilage: an experimental study in rabbits. J Bone Joint Surg Br 1984;66:334–336.
99. Gervin KL, McCarthy RE, Barnes CL, Dodge BM. Pediatric pelvic fractures. J Pediatr Orthop 1990;10:577–582.
100. Guingard O, Rigault P, Padovani JP, et al. Luxations traumatiques et fractures du cotyle chez l'enfant. Rev Chir Orthop 1985;71:575–579.
101. Hallel T, Salvati EA. Premature closure of the triradiate cartilage: a case report and animal experiment. Clin Orthop 1977;124:278–281.
102. Heeg M. Fractures of the acetabulum. Thesis, Rihksunwersitent Groningen, 1990.
103. Heeg M, Klasen HJ, Visser JD. Acetabular fractures in children and adolescents. J Bone Joint Surg Br 1989;71:418–421.
104. Heeg M, Visser JD, Oostvogel HJM. Injuries of the acetabular triradiate cartilage and sacroiliac joint. J Bone Joint Surg Br 1988;70:34–37.
105. Judet R, Judet J, Letournel E. Fractures of the acetabulum: classification and surgical approaches for open reduction. J Bone Joint Surg Am 1964;46:1615–1646.
106. Jurkovskj II. Perdelomy taza u detej. Diss Kand Med, Czechoslovakia, 1945.
107. Laguna AS. Lesiones traumaticas del cartilago triradiado estudio experimental. Thesis, Univ Autonoma Madrid, 1988.
108. Lansinger O. Fractures of the acetabulum: a clinical and experimental study. Acta Orthop Scand Suppl 1977;165:1–125.
109. Ljubosic NA. Poraneni jamky kycelniho kloubu u deti. Acta Chir Orthop Traumatol Cech 1967;34:393–400.
110. Mesquita J, Vieira MJ, Lino AP, Corte Real A. Lesao traumatica rara da anca infantil. Rev Orthop Trauma 1982;8:163–165.
111. Nerubay J, Glancz G, Katznelson A. Fractures of the acetabulum. J Trauma 1973;13:1050–1062.
112. Peterson HA, Robertson RC. Premature partial closure of the triradiate cartilage treated with excision of a physeal osseous bar. J Bone Joint Surg Am 1997;79:767–770.
113. Pina-Medina A, Pardo-Montaner J. Triradiate cartilage fracture associated with a transepiphyseal separation of the femoral head. J Orthop Trauma 1996;10:575–585.
114. Rigault S, Hannouche D, Judet J. Luxations traumatiques de hanche et fractures du cotyle chez l'enfant. Rev Chir Orthop 1968;54:361–382.
115. Rodrigues KF. Injury of the acetabular epiphysis. Injury 1972;4:258–260.
116. Rowe CR, Lowell JD. Prognosis of fractures of the acetabulum. J Bone Joint Surg Am 1961;43:30–59.
117. Scuderi G, Bronson MJ. Triradiate cartilage injury: report of two cases and review of the literature. Clin Orthop 1987;217:179–189.
118. Soini J, Ritsila V. Experimentally produced growth disturbance of the acetabulum in young rats. Acta Orthop Scand 1984;55:14–17.
119. Sprenger TR. Fracture of the acetabulum in a 14-year-old patient. Orthop Rev 1984;13:709–716.
120. Trousdale RT, Ganz R. Post traumatic acetabular dysplasia. Clin Orthop 1994;305:124–232.
121. Weisel A, Hecht HL. Occult fracture through the triradiate cartilage of the acetabulum. AJR 1980;134:1262–1264.

Ilium-Wing and Crest

122. Butler JE, Eggert AW. Fracture of the iliac crest apophysis: an unusual hip pointer. J Sports Med 1975;3:192–193.
123. Clancy WG, Foltz AS. Iliac apophysitis and stress fractures in adolescent runners. Am J Sports Med 1976;4:214–218.
124. Godshall RW, Hansen CA. Incomplete avulsion of a portion of the iliac epiphysis: an injury of young athletes. J Bone Joint Surg Am 1973;55:1301–1302.
125. Olney BW, Schler FJ, Asher MA. Effects of splitting the iliac apophysis on subsequent growth of the ilium: a rabbit study. J Pediatr Orthop 1993;13:365–367.

Ilium-Spines

126. Ahmadi A, Kreusch-Brinker R, Mellerowicz H, Wolff R. Apophysenausriss am Becken und der unteren Extremität durch Sport. Sportverletzung Sportschaden 1987;3:113–115.
127. Albrecht LUD, Pollahne W. Partielle und Komplete post traumatische desinsertion mit appositionellen Verkalkungen und Röntgenbild des Becken Skeletts der fügendlichen sportlern. Radiol Diagn 1975;16:849–856.

128. Bachmann W. Un cas d'arrachement bilateral de l'epine iliaque anteroinferieure. Schweiz Med Wochenschr 1941;22:721–722.
129. Boccanera L. La frattura isolata della spina iliaca anteriore inferiore. Minerva Orthop 1960;11:171–173.
130. Bousseau A. Disj. epiphysaire traumatique de la tete du femur et des epines iliaques ant. Bull Soc Anat Paris 1867;42:283–284.
131. Burghardt I. Abriss der Spinaca iliaca Anterior inferior beim Fussball spiel. Sportzartz Sportmed 1994;25:32–33.
132. Cords H. Frakturen durch muskelzug beim sport. Arch Orthop Unfallchir 1935;35:563–567.
133. Cotta H, Krahl H. Apophysenverletzungen jugendlicher Fussballspieler. Sportzartz Sportmed 1971;26:266–268.
134. Crespi M. La frattura isolata della spina iliaca anteriore inferiore. Arch Ortop (Milan) 1961;74:348–352.
135. De Cuveland E, Heuck F. Osteochondropathie der Spina iliaca ant. inf. unter Beruchsichtigung der Oss. Fortschr Rontgenstr 1951;75:430–431.
136. Deeham DJ, Beattie TF, Knight D, Jongschaaph LO. Avulsion fracture of the straight and reflected heads of rectus femoris. Arch Emerg Med 1992;9:310–313.
137. Draper DO, Dustmen AJ. Avulsion fracture of anterior superior iliac spine in a collegiate distance runner. Arch Phys Med Rehabil 1992;73:881–882.
138. Duclover P, Fillipe G. Les avulsions apophysaires du bassin chez l'enfant. Chir Pediatr 1988;29:91–92.
139. Fernbach SK, Wilkinson RH. Avulsion injuries of the pelvis and proximal femur. AJR 1981;137:581–584.
140. Gallagher JR. Fracture of the anterior inferior spine of the ilium: "sprinter's fracture." Ann Surg 1935;102:86–89.
141. Ghetti PL. A proposito della interpretazione della immagine radiografica nelle fratture delle spine iliache anteriori. Arch Putti Chir Organi Mov 1965;20:261–264.
142. Goodwin MA. Myositis ossificans in the region of the hip-joint. Br J Surg 1959;46:547–549.
143. Hanson PG. Bilateral avulsion fracture of the anterior superior iliac spine. Acta Chir Scand 1970;136:85–86.
144. Irving MH. Exostosis formation after traumatic avulsion of the anterior inferior iliac spine. J Bone Joint Surg Br 1964;46:720–722.
145. Khoury MB, Kirks DR, Martinez S, Apple J. Bilateral avulsion fractures of the anterior superior iliac spines in sprinters. Skeletal Radiol 1985;13:65–67.
146. Klose HH, Schuchardt E. Die beckennahen Apophysenabrisse. Orthopade 1980;9:229–236.
147. Lagier R, Jarret G. Apophysiolysis of the anterior inferior iliac spine. Arch Orthop Unfallchir 1975;83:81–89.
148. Lehnhardt K, Dietschi C. Abriss frakturen der Becken apophysen. Z Orthop 1974;112:1218–1225.
149. Lombardo SJ, Retting AC, Kerlan RK. Radiographic abnormalities of the iliac apophysis in adolescent athletes. J Bone Joint Surg Am 1983;65:444–446.
150. Mader TJ. Avulsion of the rectus femoris tendon: an unusual type of pelvic fracture. Pediatr Emerg Care 1990;6:198–199.
151. Metges PJ, Delahaye RP, Mine PJ, Kleitz CR, Prigent M. Décollements apophysaires des épines iliaques antérieures. J Radiol 1979;60:251–254.
152. Resniche JM, Carrasco CH, Edeiken J, Hasko AW, Ro JY, Ayala AG. Avulsion fracture of the anterior inferior iliac spine and abundant reactive ossification in the soft tissue. Skeletal Radiol 1996;25:580–584.
153. Rinonapoli E. Distacchi apofisari da trauma sportivo. Clin Orthop (Padova) 1955;7:337–340.
154. Rosenberg N, Noiman M, Edelson G. Avulsion fractures of the anterior superior iliac spine in adolescents. J Orthop Trauma 1996;10:440–443.
155. Rothbart L. Abrissfraktur der Spina iliaca ant. inf. Zentralbl Chir 1932;59:781–782.
156. Schwobel MG. Apophysenfrakturen bei jugendlichen. Chirurg 1985;56:699–704.
157. Stanislajevic S. Fracture of the anterior inferior spine of the ilium. Arch Orthop (Milan) 1958;71:626–630.
158. Stewart MJ. Unusual athletic injuries. AAOS Instruct Course Lect 1960;17:377–391.
159. Sundar M, Carty H. Avulsion fractures of the pelvis in children: a report of 32 fractures and their outcome. Skeletal Radiol 1994;23:85–90.
160. Taillard W. L'epiphysiolyse de la hanche. Triangle 1968;8:217–224.
161. Tehranzadeh J. The spectrum of avulsion and avulsion-like injuries of the musculoskeletal system. Radiographics 1987;7:945–974.
162. Vacirca M. Fratture de strappamento a sede rara in adolescenti sportivi. Minerva Chir 1954;9:89–90.
163. Valdiserri L. Distacco apofisario traumatico della spine iliaca anteriore inferiore. Osped Ital Chir 1966;15:411–415.
164. Veselko M, Smrkolj V. Avulsion of the anterior-superior iliac spine in athletes: case reports. J Trauma 1994;36:444–446.
165. Waters PM, Millis MB. Hip and pelvic injuries in the young athelete. Clin Sports Med 1988;7:513–526.
166. Weitzner I. Fractures of the anterior superior spine of the ilium in one case and anterior inferior in another. AJR 1935;33:39–40.
167. Winkler AR, Barnes JC, Ogden JA. Break dance hip: chronic avulsion of the anterior superior iliac spine. Pediatr Radiol 1987;17:501–502.
168. Wuensch K. Die Apophysenlosung der spinaca Iliaca anterior inferior. Z Orthop 1959;91:119–131.
169. Zilkens KW, Defrain KW. Apophysen-Abrissfrakturen beim Jugendlichen. Akt Traumatol 1985;15:260–263.

Ischial Tuberosity

170. Abbate CC. Avulsion fracture of the ischial tuberosity. J Bone Joint Surg 1945;27:716–717.
171. Barnes ST, Hinds RB. Pseudotumor of the ischium. J Bone Joint Surg Am 1972;54:645–647.
172. Berry JM. Fracture of the tuberosity of the ischium due to muscular action. JAMA 1912;59:1450–1451.
173. Cappelli B, Garosi G. La necrosi asettica della tuberosita ischiatica. Riv Radiol 1962;2:153–155.
174. Carnevale V. Apofisiolysis del isquion (avulsion del isquion). Bol Soc Argent Orthop Traumatol 1951;16:234–235.
175. Castellana A. Les apophysiolyses de l'ischion. Rev Orthop 1948;34:145–146.
176. Castellana A. Su di un caso di apofisiolisi dell'ischio. Arch Orthop 1950;63:417–419.
177. Christini V, Marangoni L. Osteocondropatia delle tuberosita ischiatiche: variante tuberositaria della mala. Radiol Med 1955;41:451–452.
178. Cohen H. Avulsion fracture of the ischial tuberosity. J Bone Joint Surg 1937;19:1138–1139.
179. Cossi CG, Cossi A, Colawita S, Bairle L. Apophyseolysis and osteochondrosis of the ischial tuberosity: criteria of differential diagnosis. Ital J Orthop Traumatol 1986;12:515–524.
180. DeLucchi G. Distacco epifisario della tuberosita ischiatica. Clin Orthop (Padova) 1954;6:245–247.

181. DePalma AF, Silberstein CE. Avulsion fracture of the ischial tuberosity in siblings. Clin Orthop 1965;38:120–122.
182. Ellis R, Greene AG. Ischial apophyseolysis. Radiology 1966;87:646–648.
183. Fernbach SK, Wilkinson RH. Avulsion injuries of the pelvis and proximal femur. AJR 1981;137:581–584.
184. Ferrand J, Barsotti J. Avulsion apophysaire de l'ischion. Rev Chir Orthop 1961;47:241–244.
185. Finby N, Begg CF. Traumatic avulsion of ischial epiphysis simulating neoplasm. New York J Med 1967;67:2488–2490.
186. Franciosi A. Raro caso di distacco del nucleo di oss. della tuberosita ischiatica. Ann Radiol Diagn 1947;20:63–64.
187. Graziati G. Il distacco della tuberosita ischiatica. Clin Orthop (Padova) 1960;12:79–81.
188. Gutschalk A. Doppelseitige Abrissfraktur des Tuber ossis ischii. Arch Orthop Unfallchir 1933;33:256–257.
189. Hamada G, Rida A. Ischial apophysiolysis (IAL). Clin Orthop 1963;31:117–119.
190. Hamsa WR. Epiphyseal injuries about the hip joint. Clin Orthop 1957;10:119–124.
191. Hellmer H. Ein Fall von traumatischer Ablösung der Epiphyse des Os ischii. Arch Orthop Unfallchir 1934;34:45–47.
192. Holereiter F. Fur Atió-Pathogenese der Sitzbeintuber-Osteochondropathie und Apophyseolyse. Radiol Diagn 1968;9:621–631.
193. Hösli P, Vilaer L. Traumatische Apophysenlösungen in Berich des Beckens und des koxalen Femurendes. Orthopade 1995;24:429–435.
194. Howard FM, Piha RJ. Fractures of the apophysis in adolescent athletes. JAMA 1929;92:1597–1598.
195. Karfiol G. Abrissfraktur des Tuber Ischiadicum. Zentralbl Chir 1930;57:2466–2467.
196. Kelly J. Ischial epiphysitis. J Bone Joint Surg Am 1963;45:435.
197. Kozlowski K, Campbell JB, Azouz EM. Traumatised ischial apophysis. Australas Radiol 1989;33:140–143.
198. Krahl H. Sliding of the ischial apophysis. Z Orthop 1973;111:210–216.
199. Kressin W. Apophysenlösung nach tumor am Os ischii in der Differential diagnose der Keugexxerung an der Oberschenkel rükseite. Med Sport 1968;8:93–96.
200. Labuz EF. Avulsion of the ischial tuberosity: report of a case. J Bone Joint Surg 1946;28:388–389.
201. Lindner HO, Winkeltau G, Kalemba J. Apophyseal rupture of ischial bone tuberosity. Zentrabl Chir 1987;112:109–114.
202. Lorenc S. Isolierter Bruch der Sitzbeinknorrens: klinischer Beitrag. Areiv Orthop Unfallchir 1958;49:514–515.
203. MacLeod SB, Levin P. Avulsion of the epiphysis of the tuberosity of the ischium. JAMA 1929;92:1597–1598.
204. Major S, Lakos J. Traumatic epiphyseolysis of the os ischii. Magyar Traumatol Orthop 1968;11:296–297.
205. Martin TA, Pipkin G. Treatment of avulsion of the ischial tuberosity. Clin Orthop 1957;10:108–118.
206. McMaster PE. Epiphysitis of the ischial tuberosity: a case report. J Bone Joint Surg 1945;27:493–495.
207. Metzmaker JN, Pappas AM. Avulsion fractures of the pelvis. Am J Sports Med 1985;13:349–358.
208. Milch H. Avulsion fracture of the tuberosity of the ischium. J Bone Joint Surg 1926;8:832–833.
209. Milch H. Ischial apophysiolysis: a new syndrome. Clin Orthop 1953;2:184–193.
210. Miller A, Stedman GH, Beisaw NE, Gross PT. Sciatica caused by an avulsion fracture of the ischial tuberosity. J Bone Joint Surg Am 1987;69:143–145.
211. Mooney V. Avulsion fracture of the tuberosity of the ischium. Penn Med J 1947;50:1072–1074.
212. Munich B, Boros Z, Endes J, Barath E. Tuber ossis ischii apophyseolysise. Magyar Traumatol 1990;33:63–66.
213. Pavlov H. Roentgen examination of groin and hip pain in the athlete. Clin Sports Med 1987;6:829–843.
214. Poulsen TK, Enggaard TP. Afrivningsfraktur af tuber ischiadicum. Ugeskr Leger 1995;157:6140–6141.
215. Pruner RA, Johnston CE II. Avulsion fracture of the ischial tuberosity. Orthopedics 1990;13:357–358.
216. Raspe R. Über eine seltene Veranderung am Tuber ischi durch Sport. Rontgenpraxis 1937;9:124–126.
217. Rogge E, Romano R. Avulsion of the ischial apophysis. J Bone Joint Surg Am 1956;38:442.
218. Rogge E, Romano R. Avulsion of the ischial apophysis. Clin Orthop 1957;9:239–243.
219. Saenz L, Mottram M. Avulsion of ischial apophysis. Calif Med 1972;116:64–68.
220. Scheggi S. Frattura da strappamento della tuberosita ischiatica per trauma sportivo. Chir Organi Mov 1950;35:736–737.
221. Schlonsky J, Olix ML. Functional disability following avulsion fracture of the ischial epiphysis. J Bone Joint Surg Am 1972;54:641–644.
222. Schneider G. Uber isolierter Frakturen des Sitzbeines und Apophysenlosungen am Tuber ossisisakii. Arch Orthop Unfallchir 1956;48:326–339.
223. Scott W. Non-union of the ischial tuberosity associated with epiphysitis vertebrae. J Bone Joint Surg 1946;28:862–864.
224. Stayton CA. Ischial epiphysiolysis. AJR 1965;76:1161–1163.
225. Stulz E, Jenny G. A propos d'un nouveau cas de decollement apophysaire traumatique de la tuberosite. Lyon Chir 1961;57:840–843.
226. Vostal O. Odtrzeni hrbolu kosti sedaci u atletu. Acta Chir Orthop Cesk 1957;24:38–42.
227. Wardle EN. Epiphysitis of the tuber ischii. Br J Surg 1952;40:180–181.
228. Watanabe H, Chigira M. Irregularity of the apophysis of the ischial tuberosity. Int Orthop 1993;17:248–253–255.
229. Watanabe H, Shinozakit, Arita S, Chigira M. Irregularity of the apophysis of the ischial tuberosity evaluated by magnetic resonance imaging. Can Assoc Radiol J 1995;46:380–385.
230. Winkler H, Rapp IH. Ununited epiphysis of the ischium: report of a case. J Bone Joint Surg 1947;29:234–236.
231. Wooton JR, Cross MJ, Holt KW. Avulsion of the ischial apophysis: the case for open reduction and internal fixation. J Bone Joint Surg Br 1990;72:625–627.
232. Young LW, Tan KM. Radiological case of the month: traumatic ischial apophyseolysis. Am J Dis Child 1980;134:885–886.

Symphysis Pubis

233. Adams RJ, Chandler FA. Osteitis pubis of traumatic etiology. J Bone Joint Surg Am 1953;35:685–696.
234. Burman M, Weinkle IN, Langsam MJ. Adolescent osteochondritis of the symphysis pubis. J Bone Joint Surg 1934;16:649–657.
235. Klinefelter EW. Osteitis pubis: review of literature and report of a case. AJR 1950;63:368–371.
236. Schneider R, Kaye JJ, Ghelman B. Adductor avulsion injuries near the symphysis pubis. Radiology 1976;120:567–569.
237. Wiley JJ. Traumatic osteitis pubis: the gracilis syndrome. Am J Sports Med 1983;11:360–363.

Meralgia Paresthetica

238. Buch KA, Campbell J. Acute onset meralgia paresthetic after fracture of the anterior superior iliac spine. Injury 1993; 24:569–570.
239. Edelson R, Stevens P. Meralgia paresthetica in children. J Bone Joint Surg Am 1994;76:993–999.
240. MacNichol MF, Thompson WJ. Idiopathic meralgia paresthetica. Clin Orthop 1990;254:270–274.
241. Thanikachalam M, Petros JG, O'Donnell S. Avulsion fracture of the anterior superior iliac spine presenting as acute-onset meralgia paresthetica. Ann Emerg Med 1995;26: 515–517.

20

Hip

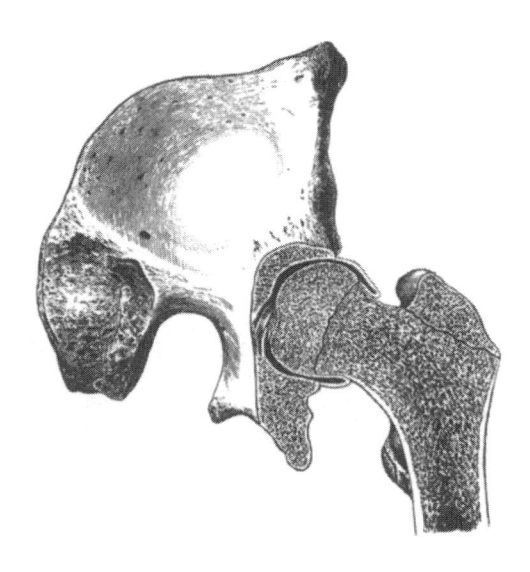

Engraving of the adolescent hip. (From Poland J. Traumatic Separation of the Epiphyses. *London: Elder, Smith, 1898)*

The relevant anatomy of the acetabulum is presented in Chapter 19, and aspects of proximal femoral development are presented in Chapter 21. However, certain morphologic structures relate directly to the hip joint and the specific problems encountered during traumatic dislocation of the hip joint in the skeletally immature individual.

Anatomy

The capsule inserts along the chondro-osseous junction of the pelvis, making the cartilaginous acetabular labrum intracapsular.[1] This is evident as the "rose thorn" in arthrographic studies. The femoral capsular insertion along the intertrochanteric margins totally encapsulates the developing capital femur and femoral neck, creating an enveloping "spherical" structure comprised of synovium, capsule, and dense ligamentous condensations (Fig. 20-1). The capsule has intrinsic laxity that allows considerable displacement of the joint components if the suction effect is disrupted. The allowable displacement may be significant (Fig. 20-2). Joint effusion following trauma, similar to pus in septic arthritis, may accumulate rapidly, break the suction effect, and hydraulically stretch the capsule.

The iliofemoral ligament (ligament of Bigelow), which may be an obstacle to reduction, resembles an inverted Y. The ligament is often referred to as the Y-ligament. The apex of the ligament is the thickened longitudinal fibers of the capsule originating from the anterior inferior iliac spine and traversing the anterior aspect of the hip joint to attach to the anterior intertrochanteric line (Fig. 20-3). Distally, this fibrous band broadens and separates into two relatively distinct bands. The iliofemoral ligament normally limits hyperextension and lateral rotation of the hip joint. The ligament is under maximum tension in extension, which also may increase intracapsular pressure, especially when a posttraumatic hemarthrosis is present.[2,3] The capsular confinement is used as a rationale for the need to perform capsulotomy for hip dislocation or femoral neck fracture to decompress a posttraumatic hematoma. Placing the hip in flexion, however, either in bed in balanced suspension or in a cast may alleviate much of such pressure without having to release the fluid operatively or percutaneously. Furthermore, the capsule is usually torn with traumatic hip dislocation, allowing extracapsular extravasation of blood into the contiguous soft tissues.

Tears may involve the midcourse of the ligament because the ligamentous attachments into the cartilage and bone are dense. Buttonhole displacement through a capsular tear may impose constricting restraints to closed reduction and necessitate open reduction (Fig. 20-4). The Y-ligament may become taut during dislocation and thus become a significant impediment to closed reduction.

When the capsule is torn, it is likely that the tear is closer to the pelvic attachment than to the thicker femoral attachments. Such avulsion may include marginal bone (Fig. 20-5) and cartilaginous labrum from the acetabulum. In young children only cartilage may be involved, making routine radiographic diagnosis difficult. Such avulsions are analogous to growth mechanism injuries in the long bones.

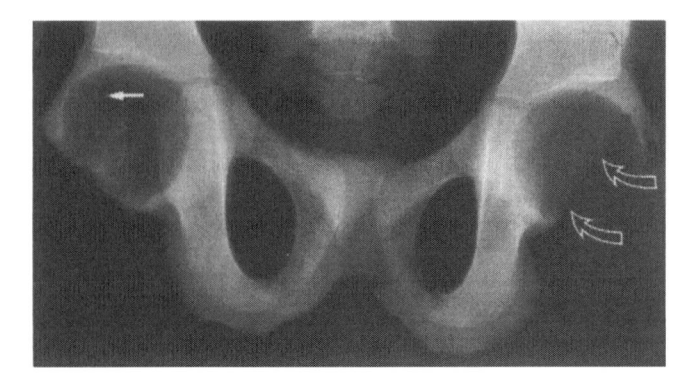

FIGURE 20-1. Appearance of the hip joints in a 7-year-old child. The right hip capsule has been cut along the femoral insertion to emphasize the contour and anterior extent of this structure. The solid arrow depicts the demarcation between the labrum and capsule. Essentially, the capsule extends the hemispheric acetabulum to create an enveloping structure that is approximately three-fourths of a sphere. The left hip capsule has been cut to emphasize the posterior intertrochanteric line (open arrows). This portion does not extend as far along the femoral neck as the anterior portion.

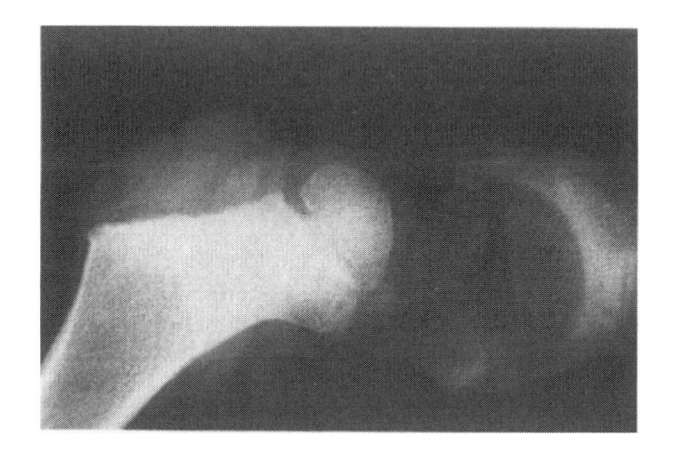

FIGURE 20-2. Once the suction effect is broken, the proximal femur may be displaced from the acetabulum. The capsule allows considerable displacement before constraining the femoral head.

The iliopsoas tendon may be displaced behind the dislocated femoral head and may indent the capsule, as with developmental hip dislocation (Fig. 20-4). Such displacement may present a major obstacle to closed reduction. Other muscles in the direct path of the dislocating femoral head may be stretched or partially torn. The external rotator muscle group (obturator externus and internus, piriformis, and quadratus femoris) is either partially or completely torn, along with the posterior part of the capsule. The femoral head occasionally pushes between the short external rotators without tearing them. The gluteus maximus, medius, and minimus muscles are stretched and pushed backward by the femoral head, which usually lies deep to these muscles, similar to the distortion caused by developmental hip dislocation. These muscles and tendons may, by a buttonhole effect, prevent or impede reduction.

The ligamentum capitum femoris may limit the extent of displacement of the femoral head, no matter what the age of the patient,[3,4] but it has to rupture to allow complete acute anterior or posterior dislocation. Accordingly, any blood supply from the ligament into the femoral head is disrupted. The significance of this particular blood vessel system to the overall hemodynamics within the femoral head is unknown, although it does not appear to be a major supply.[1-3]

Incidence

Hip dislocation in children has been frequently reported, although a large number of the reports are case studies.[5-82] Epstein reported 75 dislocations in 74 skeletally immature patients over a practice span of 48 years.[19,21] They represented 9% of an overall series of 830 hip dislocations in patients of all ages. Approximately 75% of the young patients were boys and 25% were girls. The right and left hips were almost equally involved. There were 11 dislocations in the 2- to 4-year age group, 13 in the 5- to 7-year age group, 18 in the 8- to 12-year age group, and 33 in the 13- to 15-year age group. Of these dislocations, 67 were posterior, 8 were anterior, 4 were accompanied by ipsilateral femoral fractures, and 1 was not recognized for 2.5 months.

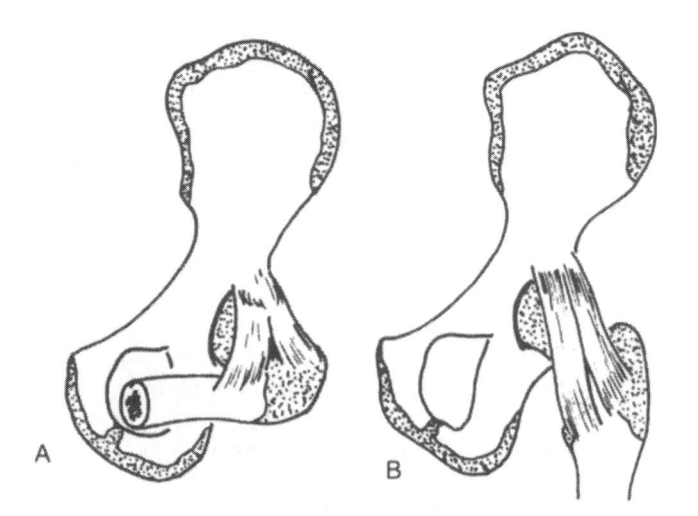

FIGURE 20-3. Y-Ligament of Bigelow. (A) In flexion, the ligament relaxes. (B) In extension, the ligament is taut.

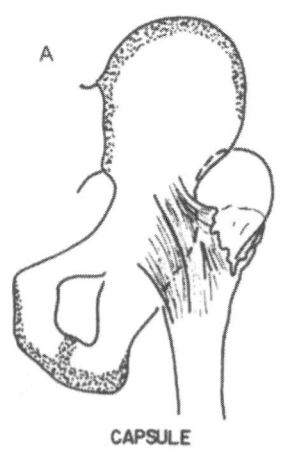

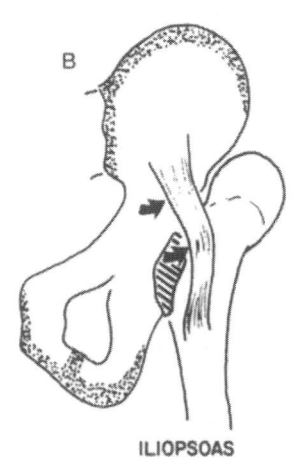

FIGURE 20-4. (A) Effect of buttonholing through the capsule. (B) Effect of a displaced iliopsoas tendon on preventing reduction. The structure marked by lines is the acetabulum.

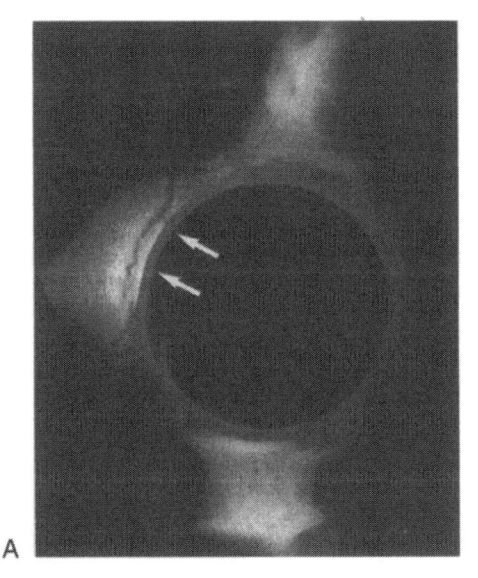

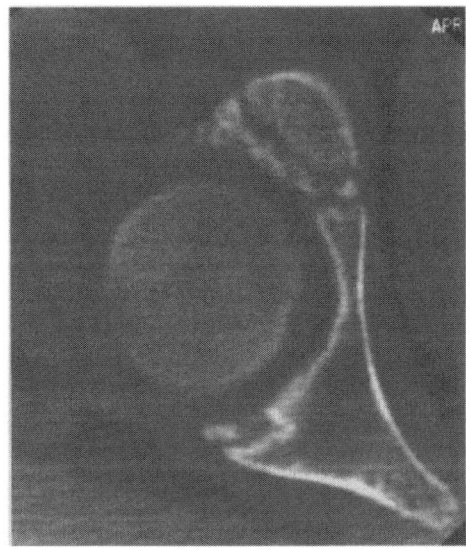

FIGURE 20-5. (A) Peripheral secondary ossification (arrows). It may be fractured as an equivalent of a physeal fracture when the hip dislocates. (B) Computed tomography (CT) scan shows the continuity of the secondary ossification of the anterior rim and the triradiate cartilage. A seemingly separate posterior osssification center is also evident. These ossification variations must be distinguished from a peripheral fracture complicating a hip dislocation.

The Pennsylvania Orthopaedic Society collected 51 cases of hip dislocation in skeletally immature patients: 41 were posterior, 8 were anterior, and 2 were central.[63,64] Nine patients had associated fractures of the acetabulum, femoral head, or greater trochanter. These particular concomitant injuries strongly influenced the prognosis. Five additional patients had associated ipsilateral tibial or femoral shaft fractures; these injuries did not influence the final results in four instances but did delay diagnosis and treatment of the hip injury.

Using multivariate analysis to assess reported cases of hip dislocation in patients under 16 years of age, 87% were posterior, and the male/female ratio was 4:1. Minimum trauma is more likely to cause dislocation in those 8 years old or younger. The young child has increased susceptibility to minimal injury because of relative ligamentous laxity and the biologic plasticity of the fibrocartilaginous acetabular margin. After 8 years of age, hip dislocation is associated with increasingly forceful mechanisms. Overall, approximately 15% of children have a concomitant fracture, with the femoral diaphysis or greater trochanter being the most common.

Types of Dislocation

Traumatic dislocation of the hip may be classified according to the position of the displaced femoral head relative to the acetabulum. They are depicted in Figure 20-6 and are subsequently illustrated with patient radiographs.

Posterior iliac. The femoral head lies posterosuperiorly along the lateral aspect of the ilium, usually with a significant portion of the femoral head above the acetabular roof and lateral edge (Figs. 20-7 to 20-9).

Posterior ischial. The femoral head is displaced posteroinferiorly and lies adjacent to the greater sciatic notch (Figs. 20-10, 20-11).

Anterior obturator (anterior-inferior). The femoral head lies near the obturator foramen. The perineal type is an extremely inferiorly displaced form of anterior dislocation.

Anterior pubic (anterior-superior). The femoral head is displaced anterosuperiorly along the superior (pubic) ramus.

Central. There is a comminuted fracture of the central or superior portion of the acetabulum with displacement of the femoral head and acetabular fragments into the pelvis. This injury is unusual in a child and often involves disruption of the triradiate cartilage Alternatively, the acetabular roof is split superiorly, at a variable distance from the superior arms of the triradiate cartilage. These patterns are discussed in detail in Chapter 19.

Inferior. There is a dislocation with the femoral head lying directly inferior to the acetabulum (Fig. 20-12). It may be referred to as luxatio erecta when the head is directed completely inferior and the femoral shaft is longitudinally aligned with the spine (Fig. 20-13).

Medial. A medial segment of the femoral head may remain. This type of comminution is rare in children. In the adult it is classified as a type 4 injury (see Chapter 21).

Slipped capital femoral epiphysis (SCFE). With dislocation of the hip in association with separation of the capital femoral epiphysis, the capital femur may remain in the joint while the femoral neck "dislocates"; or the capital femur may be totally extracapsular but is displaced at the time of dislocation or with reduction.

Posterior Dislocation

Mechanism of Injury

The trauma sustained with a posterior dislocation varies considerably. One of the most striking observations is the frequently benign nature of the injury that causes hip dislocation in an infant or young child. In contrast to the

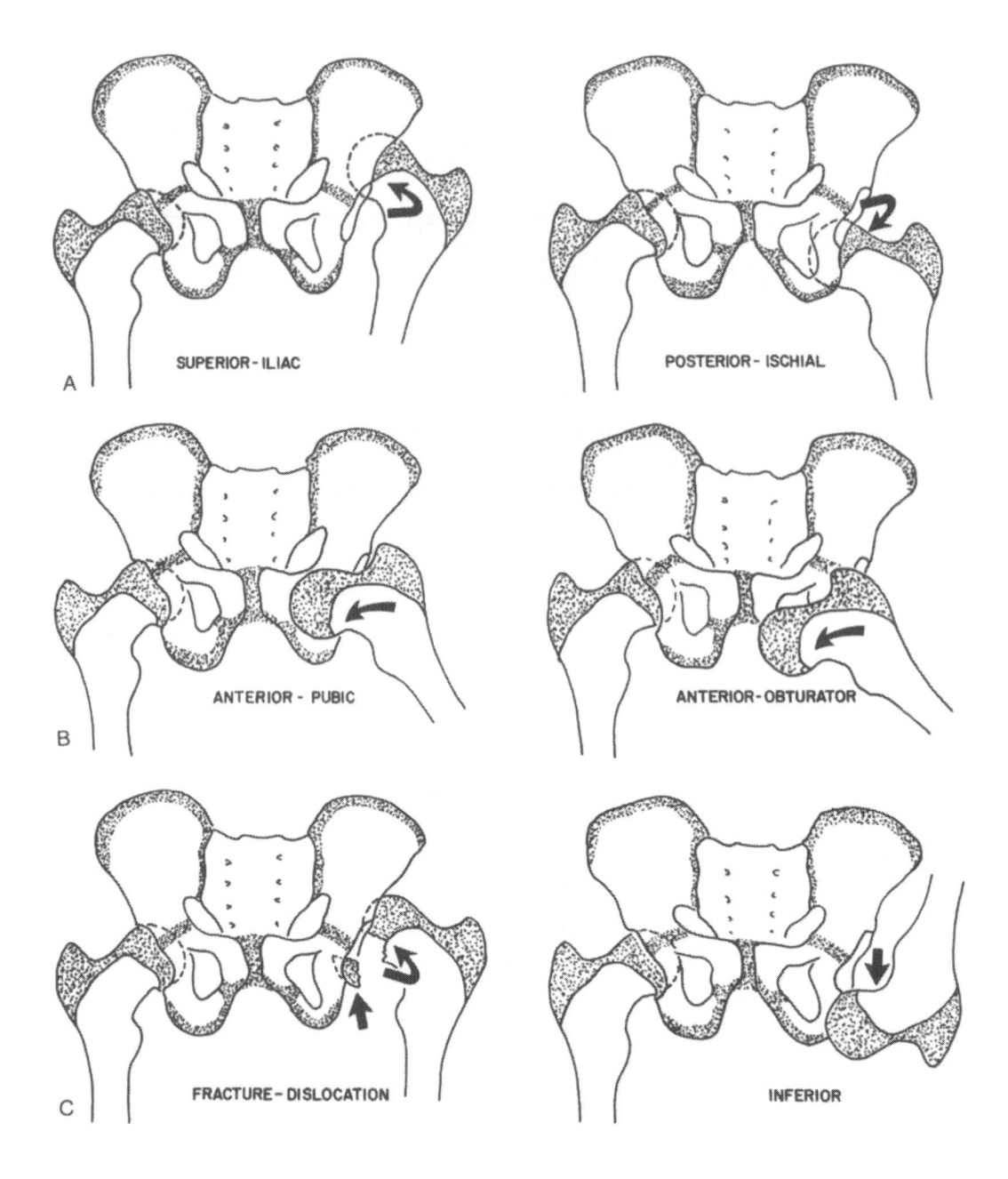

FIGURE 20-6. Types of dislocation.

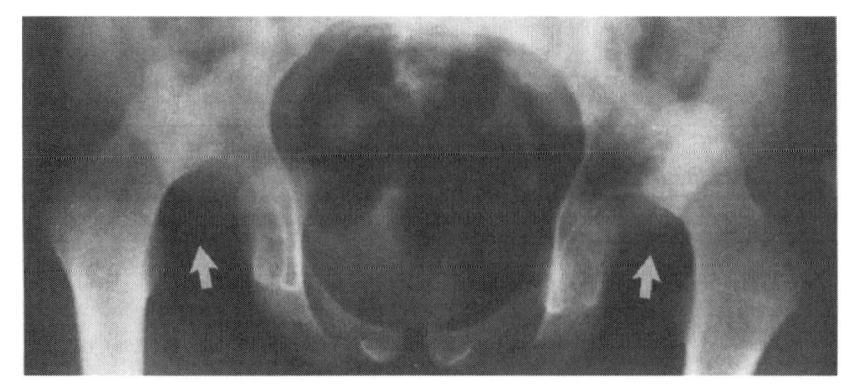

FIGURE 20-7. Bilateral traumatic dislocation (arrows).

Posterior Dislocation

FIGURE 20-8. (A) Posterior iliac dislocation in a 6-month-old infant. This injury is rare but may be distinguished from a developmental hip dislocation by the history (an accident) and normal acetabulum. With trauma a fracture of the proximal femur is more likely. Often such dislocations in this age group are due to a septic process. (B) Posterior iliac dislocation in a 3-year-old child.

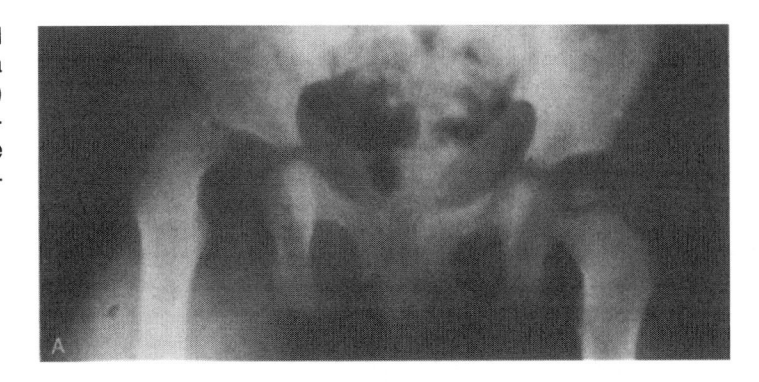

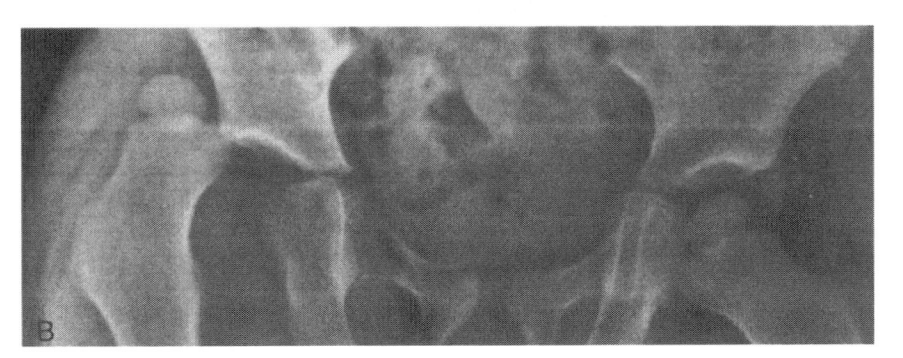

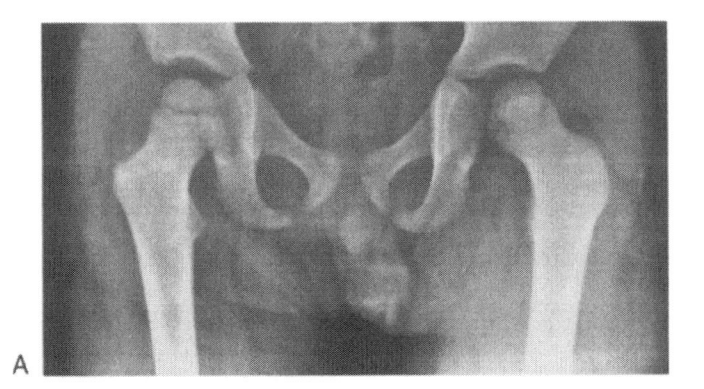

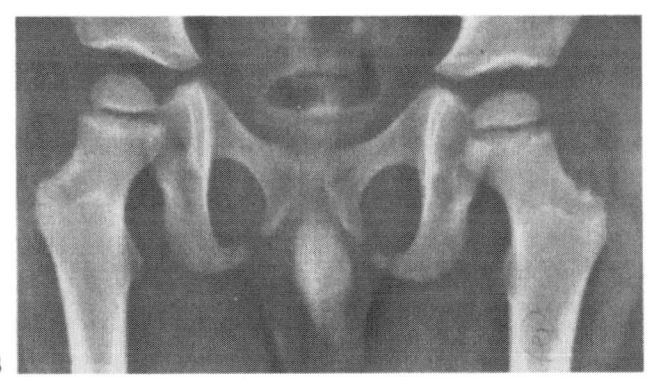

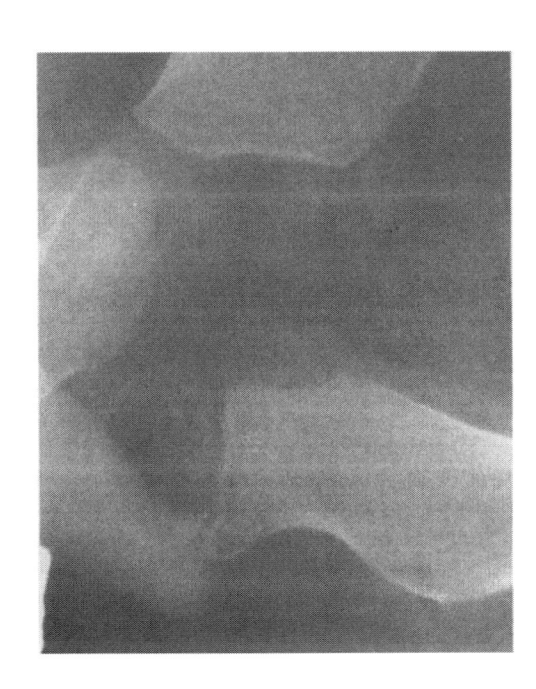

FIGURE 20-10. Posterior ischial dislocation in a 3-year-old child.

FIGURE 20-9. (A) Direct posterior dislocation of the left hip in a 4-year-old boy. Note the widening of the cartilage space medially and "rotation" of the femoral head. (B) After closed reduction.

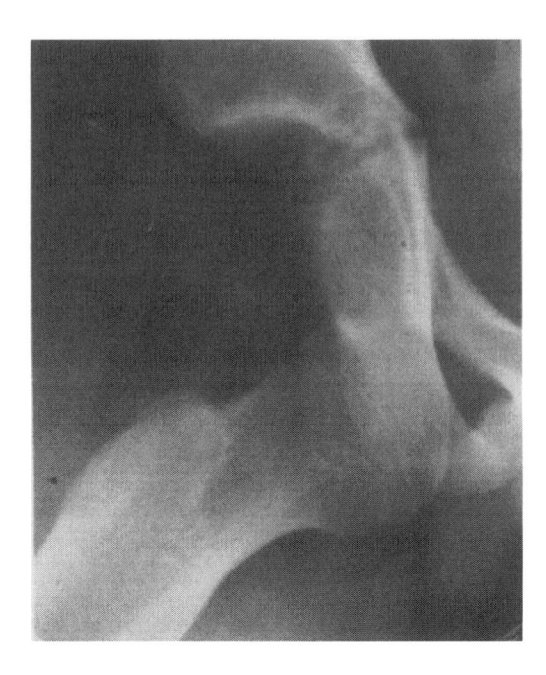

FIGURE 20-11. Posteroinferior dislocation in a 7-year-old child.

significant force usually required to dislocate the adult hip, seemingly trivial injuries may have the same result in younger age groups.

Because minor injuries can cause traumatic dislocation of the hip in children under 5 years of age, the dislocation may be missed because of a lack of suspicion of the possibility of such injury. These injured children may present with a complaint of knee pain through referred pain from the hip disorder. This is a well-known stumbling block in the diagnosis of *any* hip disorder in children and certainly can occur even with an acute hip dislocation.

The immature acetabulum has much pliable cartilage. Joint laxity is also common in young children. Often minimal force is required to subluxate the proximal femur to the acetabular rim, while little additional applied force is required to subsequently dislocate the femoral head completely from the acetabulum. As age increases, greater portions of the acetabulum progressively ossify, and there is a gradual lessening of joint laxity, so more violent trauma is necessary to produce the same type of injury and is more likely to create associated osseous damage at the acetabular periphery.

In Epstein's series, however, most of the hip dislocations were due to relatively severe trauma. About 60% involved vehicular accidents, 5% occurred during football, and 30% involved less severe trauma, such as falling down stairs or tripping.[21]

Diagnosis

Most posterior dislocations are of the iliac type, with the femur positioned between the sciatic notch and the acetabulum. High iliac and ischial posterior luxations are less common in children. On rare occasions, bilateral traumatic dislocation of the hips (Fig. 20-8) occur.[9,21,72]

With posterior iliac dislocations, the deformity has a typical appearance. The involved lower limb is held in flexion, adduction, and internal rotation. There is shortening of the limb. The femoral head may be palpable in the gluteal region. The child generally is in severe pain and unable to stand or walk. Motion of the hip is usually painful and guarded by muscle spasm. The motions of extension, abduction, and external rotation are markedly restricted and painful. Flexion and internal rotation posturing of the hip are primarily produced by tension in the Y-ligament of Bigelow.

Because this injury is often sustained while the child is sitting in a car with the hip flexed, the femur, patella, and upper end of the tibia must also be evaluated for concomitant injury. Dislocation of the hip, even in children, may be missed if there is an ipsilateral femoral fracture. These are, however, comparatively infrequent concomitant injuries in children relative to those in adults.

Knee pain may be present as a consequence of pain radiating down the obturator nerve. The nerve may be stretched in either anterior or posterior dislocations. Sciatic nerve injury may arise because of impact, attenuation, or displacement by the posteriorly dislocated femoral head. Because the anterior portion of the nerve is usually affected, dysfunction (sensory, motor, or both) is most likely evident in the distribution of the perineal nerve. Nerve function, or lack of it, must be carefully documented before and after reduction. Neurologic injury, which usually resolves spontaneously, occurs in 3% of children.[30,75,80] A thorough neurologic examination of the sciatic nerve is an integral part of both pre- and postreduction testing.

Delayed Diagnosis

If a dislocated hip is found more than 24 hours after injury, a bone scan or magnetic resonance imaging (MRI) should

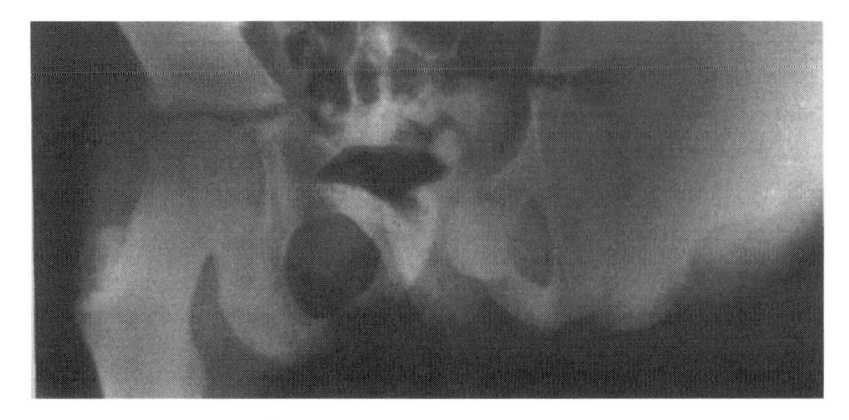

FIGURE 20-12. Inferior dislocation in a 10-year-old child.

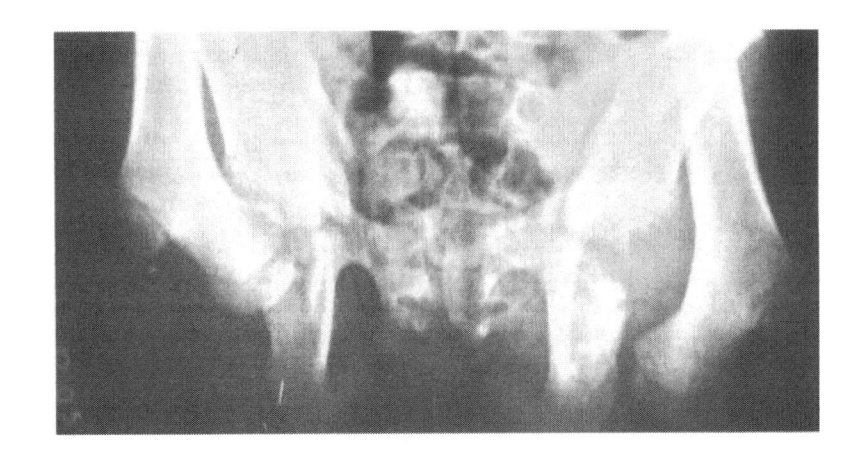

FIGURE 20-13. Luxatio erecta of the left hip.

be done to assess potential femoral (ossification center and physis) head viability. General anesthesia and muscle relaxation should be used, as soft tissue contraction begins early and may preclude reduction by the usual closed methods without medications.

If the traumatic dislocation has been present for more than a few weeks, adequate prereduction evaluation is essential. It should include a detailed neurologic examination, as the sciatic nerve may be under chronic stretch. Arthrography may determine whether fibrotic tissues are filling the acetabulum, and dye may flow through a residual capsular tear to delineate the shape of the femoral head. MRI may afford the same anatomic information. Open reduction is usually necessary to remove soft tissues within the acetabulum. Any capsular rent should be repaired to prevent recurrent dislocation.

Delayed diagnosis is more likely to occur in underdeveloped countries[57] or in association with ipsilateral diaphyseal femoral fracture. Skeletal traction followed by closed or open reduction was the most frequent method of treatment. However, the incidence of osteonecrosis was high. A reduction probably should be attempted as long as 6–9 months after the traumatic incident, especially if the apparent cause was relatively benign. There probably should be *no* arbitrary time limit between injury and possible reduction.

Even a poor result from closed or open delayed reduction may be acceptable. It prevents proximal migration, may lessen soft tissue contractures, and decreases the amount of muscle atrophy. The restored anatomy, even if osteonecrosis and collapse develop, still makes total hip replacement a viable possibility and technically easier if soft tissues are stretched to normal length rather than being contracted from chronic displacement.

Roentgenography

Roentgenography usually discloses the specific pattern of dislocation. It is imperative that adequate films be obtained to rule out associated fractures, especially of the triradiate cartilage or the acetabular margin (see Chapter 19). The entire hip region must be roentgenographed when *any* fracture of the femur is present to rule out concomitant hip dislocation, femoral shaft fracture, or both.

Barquet reported six retroacetabular dislocations.[6] He stressed the difficulty of diagnosing this particular dislocation pattern in children, as standard frontal roentgenograms may show a seemingly normal "concentric" projection of the capital femoral physis and acetabulum. Other authors have also described this problem.[15,123] A true cross-table lateral view of the pelvis should demonstrate any posterior or anterior displacement. Computed tomographic (CT) scanning also usually shows this displacement pattern. CT scanning is useful for revealing small rim fragments, whether in or out of the joint, before *and* after reduction. Completely cartilaginous fragments may be difficult to identify on CT scanning but should be suspected if there is asymmetry of the cartilage space width ("joint" width).

Improved imaging techniques have become available. The definition of CT scans is of much better quality. The method allows good definition of posterior acetabular rim fractures and intraarticular loose bodies. Three-dimensional CT is being used increasingly for the evaluation of pelvic trauma, although its use in young children may be misleading because of the "irregularities" of the immature ossification center.[22]

Although MRI does not provide significant further information regarding the basic anatomy of the hip dislocation, it may reveal the status of altered hemodynamics and allow better prediction of the likelihood of subsequent ischemic changes. It is more useful in the postreduction patient with joint space widening to assess interposed capsule or cartilage. Bone scans may show immediate changes, but there may also be a delayed reaction. Similarly, the use of MRI to detect acute vascular compromise may be limited—even though of benefit several weeks to months later.

Treatment

Early reduction, preferably within 8–12 hours, is important to lessen the risk of potential sequelae such as ischemic necrosis. Closed reduction of uncomplicated, acute posterior dislocations is almost always possible, leaving open reduction for only a small number of neglected cases and those irreducible, acute dislocations that are usually due to some type of capsular or musculotendinous interposition. The chief obstacle to reduction of a posterior hip dislocation is usually the iliofemoral ligament. Other possible impediments to closed reduction are the piriformis tendon, an inverted labrum, or an osteocartilaginous fragment.

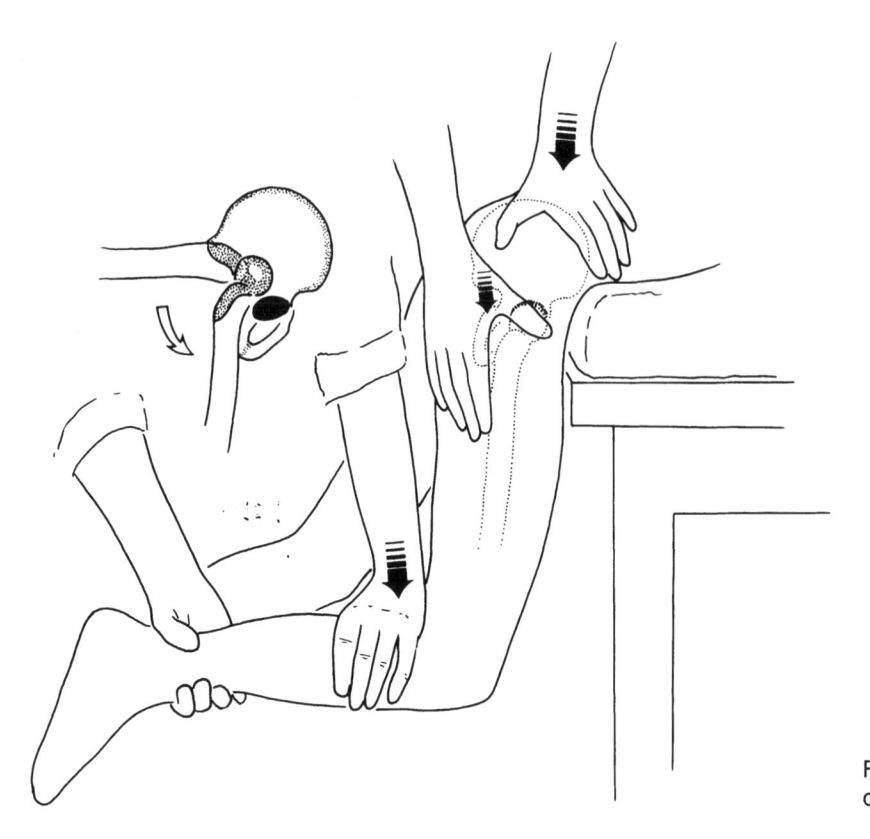

FIGURE 20-14. Closed reduction using the method of Stimson.

The following common methods for closed reduction of posterior dislocations utilize the principle of hip flexion, which should cause the Y-ligament to relax and bring the femoral head adjacent to the acetabular margin near the capsular rent.

Method of Stimson

Using the method of Stimson (Fig. 20-14), the patient is placed prone, with the lower limb hanging free from the end of the table. The pelvis is immobilized by pressing down on the sacrum. The knee is then flexed to 90°, and pressure is applied just below the bent knee. Gentle rocking, rotatory motions of the limb, and direct pressure on the femoral head and trochanter assist in the reduction. This method is not forceful and utilizes the weight of the limb to help in the reduction. If necessary, a sandbag may be strapped to the leg to relax tight muscles gradually. If this procedure is done with the patient under adequate anesthesia with appropriate muscle-relaxing agents, excessive force is not usually necessary and should be avoided to prevent complications such as iatrogenic slipped capital femoral epiphysis.

Method of Allis

Using the method of Allis (Fig. 20-15), the patient is placed in a supine position, and the pelvis is immobilized by pressing on the anterosuperior spine. The hip and knee are both flexed to 90°, with the thigh maintained in slight adduction and medial rotation. Direct vertical traction is applied with the forearm behind the knee, lifting the femoral head over the posterior rim of the acetabulum and through the rent in the capsule into the acetabular socket. The hip and knee are then gradually extended. Soft tissue resistance is encountered occasionally and may be relaxed by increasing the degree of hip adduction and internal rotation. If the hip cannot be extended easily after the reduction, there probably is soft tissue interposition, and another attempt at closed reduction should be undertaken before resorting to open reduction.

Method of Bigelow

Using the method of Bigelow (Fig. 20-16), the patient is placed supine, and countertraction is applied. The thigh is adducted and internally rotated, the hip is flexed to 90° or more, and longitudinal traction is applied in the line of the deformity. These motions convert an iliac displacement to an ischial displacement by running the femoral head along the posterior margin of the acetabulum and relaxing the Y-ligament. The femoral head is freed from the short external rotators by gently rotating and rocking while distally directed traction is maintained. This maneuver allows levering the femoral head into the acetabulum.

It may be wise to use general anesthesia or a muscle relaxant with any of these methods, particularly in the older child. Attempts to reduce an acute hip dislocation with the patient under analgesia, or a combination of analgesia and a drug such as diazepam, may not allow sufficient muscle relaxation for a mechanically easy reduction. Because most dislocations are posterior, attempts to reduce the hip without adequate relaxation could result in the femoral head being pushed backward against the posterior acetabular rim, comparable to the mechanism in chronic SCFE. Because of morphologic constraints, reduction of an anterior dislocation would not be as likely to cause such a complicating displacement of the femoral head.

Posterior Dislocation

FIGURE 20-15. Closed reduction using the method of Allis.

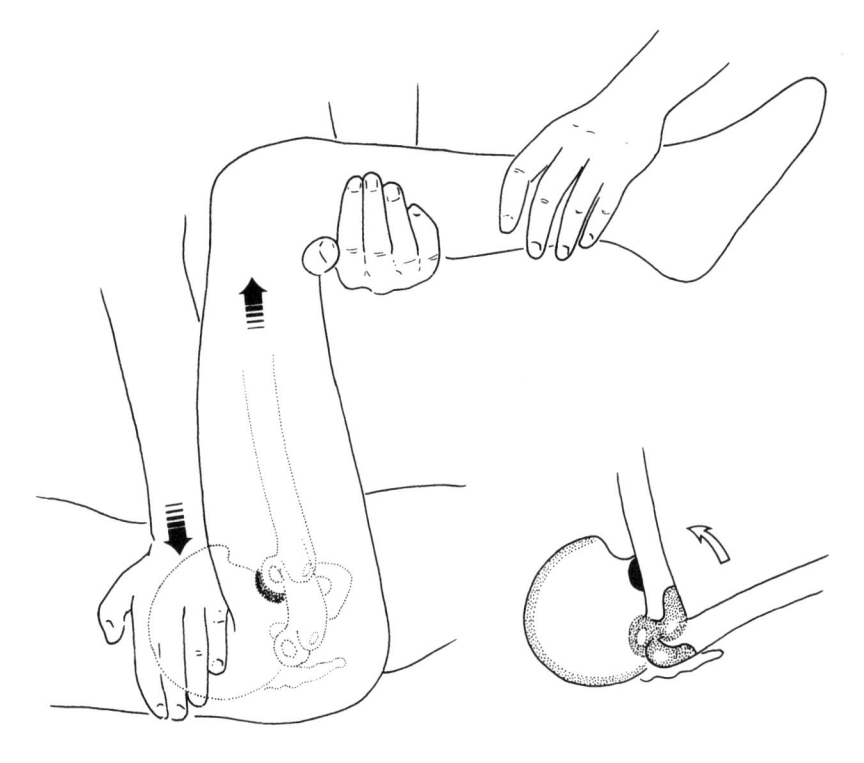

If two or three attempts at closed reduction (with adequate muscle relaxtion) are unsuccessful, an open reduction should be considered. An associated acetabular fracture with displacement of the fragment lessens the likelihood of a satisfactorily closed reduction. Either the fragment mechanically impairs the reduction, or the reduction is unstable. Thus if a significant fracture fragment is present, open reduction and fracture stabilization are often indicated.

Following closed reduction my preference is 2–3 days in traction (balanced suspension) with the hip flexed 30° or more. The stability is verified by active push–pull testing under fluoroscopy. If the hip is stable, non-weight-bearing ambulation is continued for a month.

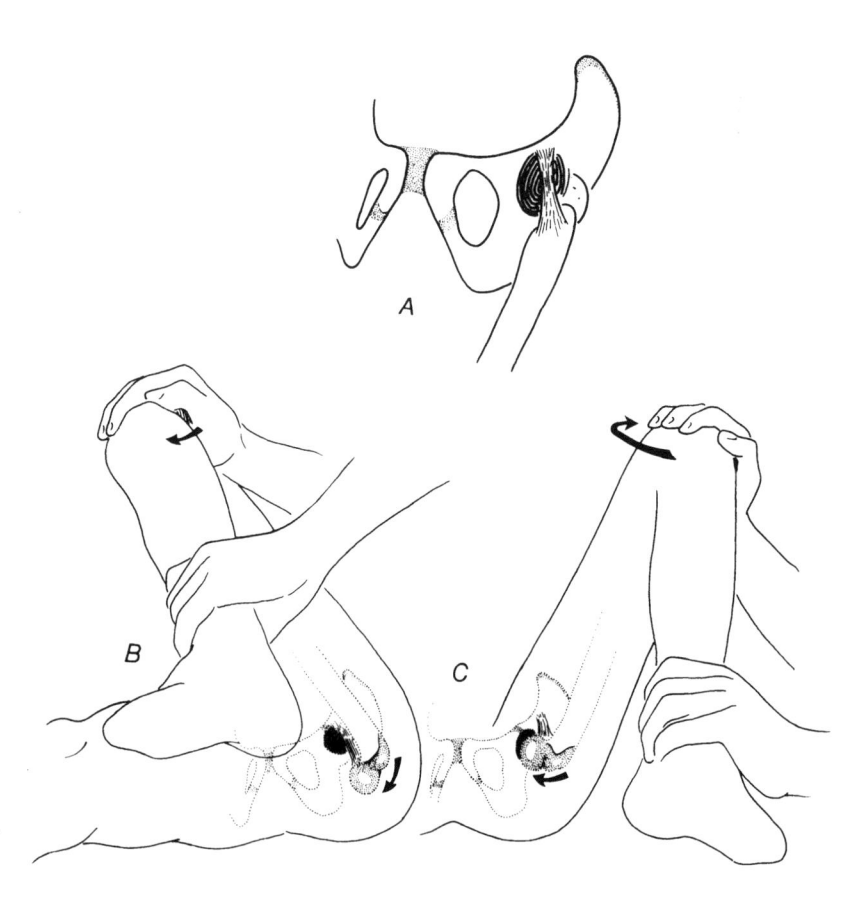

FIGURE 20-16. Closed reduction using the circumduction method of Bigelow.

If there is an accompanying fracture, the relative stability may be assessed fluoroscopically while confirming the reduction. Traction, with or without a skeletal pin, is instituted for 2–3 weeks. The stability is reassessed fluoroscopically.

Some authors have recommended hip joint aspiration under image intensification.[68] The concept is to decrease the volume of intracapsular hematoma that might lead to vascular occlusion. Although theoretically this concept is sound, the dislocation more often than not causes a capsular tear that allows decompression of contained fluids. I do *not* routinely aspirate the hip in a patient with a traumatic hip dislocation.

Postreduction Care

It is imperative that a satisfactory, anatomic reduction be confirmed by fluoroscopy or routine radiography. It verifies the concentric reduction or delineates any widening of the radiolucent cartilage space (compared to the opposite side) that should make one suspect an interposed cartilaginous or chondro-osseous fragment. It can also demonstrate complications such as a postreduction SCFE. The acetabular rim should also be reassessed for any injuries. My preference is to obtain a CT scan as well to assess any acetabular fracture or fragment interposition.

There is little agreement on immediate postreduction treatment. Most surgeons use some sort of immobilization that lasts a few weeks to about 2 months. This immobilization may be achieved by bed rest or spica cast. I use traction for approximately 3–10 days in balanced suspension, with the hip flexed about 30° to relax the capsule and Y-ligament. A period of about 3 weeks of subsequent immobilization is probably sufficient to allow initial healing of capsular and soft tissue structures. It may be accomplished by use of a hip spica cast or an orthosis that restricts certain ranges of motion, especially flexion. Small children may be treated with abduction orthoses (e.g., Scottish Rite orthosis).

The presence of synovial irritation should be one of the guidelines to determine when the child is allowed out of balanced suspension or protected weight-bearing activity. So long as acute synovial irritation or pain is present, the child should probably be in traction and suspension, not in a cast. If symptoms of synovial irritation recur after the resumption of progressive weight-bearing, the patient is again placed in traction, balanced suspension, or at least restrained from weight-bearing; and diagnostic studies are undertaken to determine the cause of the recurrent pain.

It is difficult to assess the importance of the duration of the non-weight-bearing period; recommendations range from a few days to 3 months. A correlation between the period of non-weight-bearing and the frequency of ischemic necrosis was proposed by Funk,[27] but according to other authors there is absolutely no correlation.[26] Hammelbo[174] recommended that weight-bearing should be avoided for 2–3 months, although most patients start weight-bearing 2–3 weeks after release from traction or casting. *Children are invariably noncompliant* about the status of anything other than full weight-bearing.

In children under the age of 6 years, despite their excellent prognosis, it is probably advisable to attempt to discourage weight-bearing for at least a month, after which gradual resumption of activity may be permitted. Children over the age of 6 years should not bear weight for an additional period of several more weeks but should engage in muscle range of movement and strengthening programs. When persistent symptoms (e.g., synovitis) are present, this period should be further prolonged. However, it should be noted that almost all children resume full activities and full weight-bearing *promptly* after removal of any restrictive device, regardless of advice to the contrary.

Results

Epstein described the results in 44 posterior dislocations with an average follow-up of 78 months. Of these children, 24 had excellent results, 11 had good results, and 9 had fair to poor results. Invariably, these patients were severely injured and usually had concomitant chondral or chondro-osseous injury that complicated the dislocation.[19]

The final results in the Pennsylvania series showed 43 normal hips and 8 abnormal hips. However, the predictive value was tentative, as only 18 of the 51 patients had attained skeletal maturity. After reviewing the literature, as well as their series, these investigators thought that one-third of the children had, or would have, abnormal hips or poor results by the time they reached skeletal maturity.[64]

Any child who has sustained a traumatic hip dislocation should be followed regularly, both clinically and radiographically, to anticipate and document complications as early as possible. Ischemic necrosis may not become radiologically evident until 6 months or more following the dislocation. An MRI or bone scan 2–3 months following the hip injury may allow early diagnosis of osteonecrosis. Prior to this time, reactive changes to the dislocation may create "false" findings.

Patterns of ischemic necrosis complicating the closed treatment of developmental hip dysplasia may not cause significant morphologic deformity until the adolescent growth spurt. Similarly, follow-up of traumatic hip dislocation patients should be considered complete only when the patients are skeletally mature.

Anterior Dislocation

Traumatic anterior dislocation constitutes roughly 10% of all pediatric hip dislocations.[83-104] Barquet reviewed 111 traumatic anterior dislocations of the hip in children.[84] The incidence of traumatic anterior hip dislocation, unlike that of posterior dislocation, is no different between children and adults. Anterior hip dislocations are usually extrusions of the femoral head through the joint capsule, often terminating as a large bulge in the inguinal region.

The most important causal factor is forced abduction and external rotation. Anterior and central dislocations may also be caused by a direct blow to the greater trochanter. Anterior dislocation is often sustained in a fall from a height, with the impact being a direct blow on the posterior aspect of the abducted and externally rotated thigh.

Anterior hip dislocations may be classified as pubic (superior) or obturator (inferior) (Fig. 20-17). An avulsion fracture of the greater trochanter may accompany an anterior dislocation. Direct anterior dislocation may be difficult to diagnose (Fig. 20-18).

Anterior Dislocation

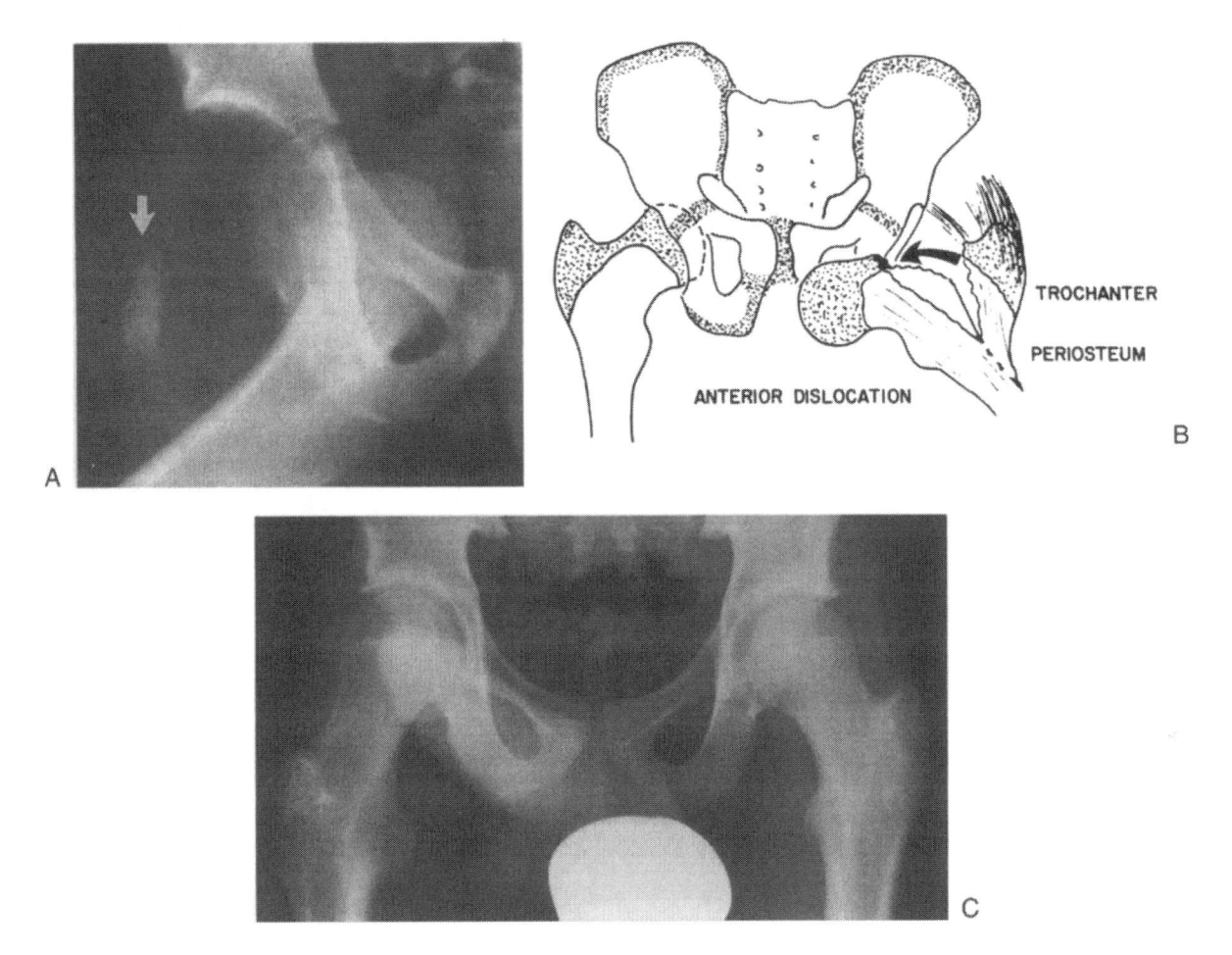

FIGURE 20-17. Anterior pubic dislocation. (A) Acute injury, with a greater trochanteric fragment (arrow). (B) Greater trochanter remained attached to the periosteal sleeve and gluteal musculature. (C) Greater trochanter underwent premature epiphysiodesis, leading to an elongated femoral neck and valgus at skeletal maturity (6 years later). Most likely, the medial displacement of the main fragment disrupted the normal medial and lateral circumflex circulation to the greater trochanter. The capital femur exhibited no evidence of ischemic necrosis.

With anterior dislocations, the hip is usually held in abduction, external rotation, and some flexion. There is fullness in the region of the obturator foramen, where the femoral head may be palpable. The motion of the hip is markedly restricted, with almost no adduction and external rotation. It is often difficult to palpate the greater trochanter.

The nerve most likely to be damaged is the femoral nerve. Careful evaluation of its function is essential before and after reduction.

With an uncomplicated anterior dislocation, prompt closed reduction generally gives a good result. Unlike posterior dislocations, there is not a good osseous fulcrum available to assist in the reduction. The iliofemoral ligament lies

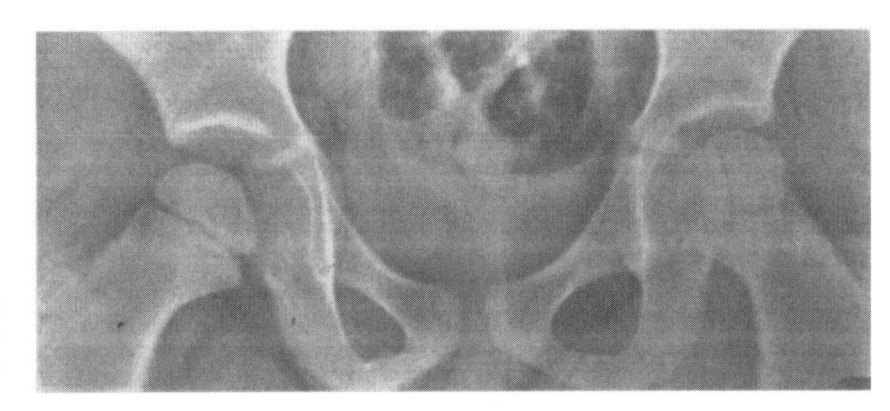

FIGURE 20-18. Direct anterior dislocation. It was initially missed, despite the obviously widened space between the teardrop and the femoral head in the right hip.

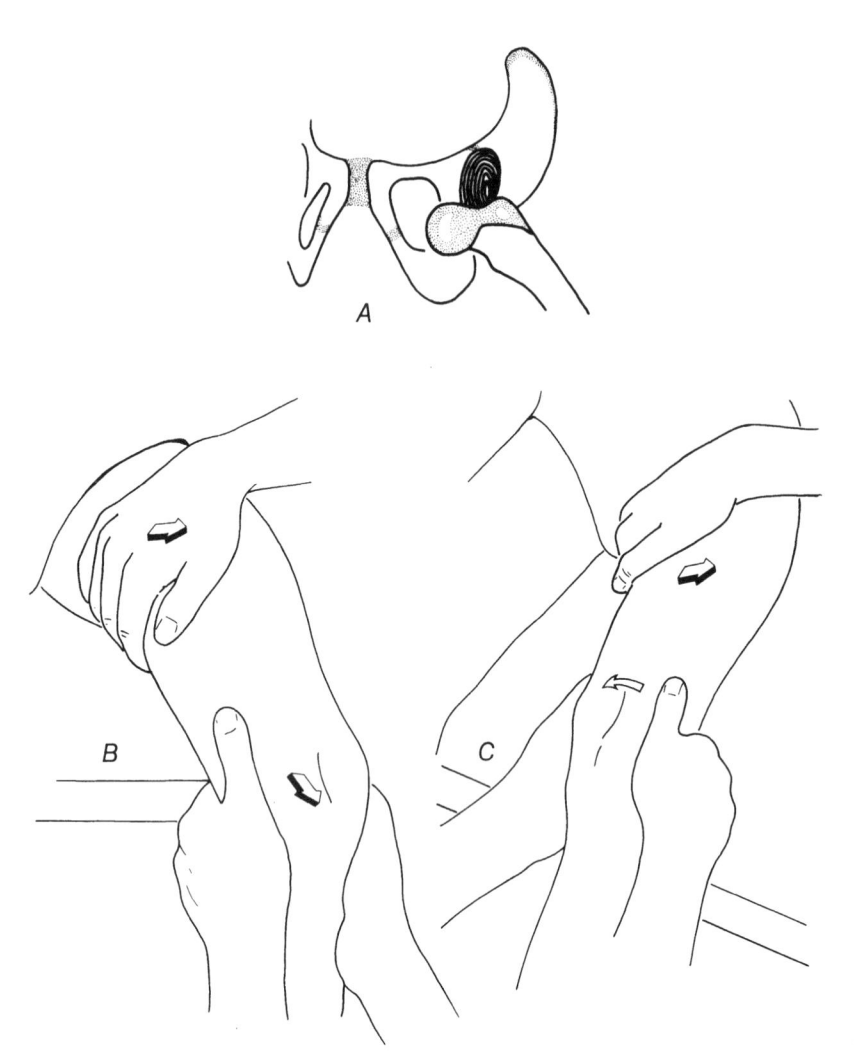

FIGURE 20-19. Method for closed reduction of an anterior dislocation.

across the displaced femoral neck. The patient is placed supine, the knee flexed to relax the hamstrings, and the hip adducted and brought into increasing flexion (Fig. 20-19). The femoral head is gradually brought opposite the tear in the capsule, through which it is levered into the acetabular socket. Longitudinal traction is then applied in the line of the axis of the femur, and lateral traction is applied concomitantly at the level of the femoral head. The hip may be rotated internally as it is adducted to try to achieve reduction.

Failure of initial closed manipulation, which is unusual, may be due to interposition of the torn capsule, a buttonhole lesion of the capsule, or iliopsoas interposition behind the femoral head.[93–95] Open reduction may be necessary in such situations.

Younge and Lifeso described a 16-year-old boy who had sustained an anterior dislocation of the hip when he was 10 years old. An open reduction was attempted but led to a poor result. He eventually underwent hip fusion.[104] Four other examples of anterior hip dislocations occurring 5 months to 12 years before definitive diagnosis are in the literature.[91,96]

When the greater trochanter is avulsed concomitantly (see Fig. 20-22, below), open reduction may be essential to restore chondro-osseous morphology. Such an avulsion pattern represents a type 3 or 4 growth mechanism injury to the trochanteric region. Internal fixation of the trochanter should be used and may be removed once healing occurs.

Acute occlusion or damage of the femoral artery, vein, or both may occur.[85,87,92,102] Nerubay reported a 15-year-old boy who sustained an anterior dislocation of the hip, bilateral fractures of the pubic rami, and a fracture of the ischium.[97] At surgery the femoral head was found to be compressing the femoral artery against the inguinal ligament, completely occluding flow. The patient developed severe ischemic necrosis 2 years after his injury. Bonnemaison and Henderson[85] and Hampson[92] observed cases of venous obstruction.

Inferior Dislocation

Inferior dislocation, sometimes referred to as luxatio erecta (Fig. 20-13), is rare in children.[105–110] The mechanism of injury probably consists of a combination of flexion, abduction, and internal rotation. All reported cases have been reduced closed. Recurrent dislocation and osteonecrosis have occurred.[108]

Central Dislocation

Central dislocations are discussed in Chapter 19. They are most often associated with disruption of the triradiate cartilage in the skeletally immature patient.

Associated Injuries

Femoral Fracture (Diaphysis)

Concomitant dislocation of the hip and fracture of the femoral shaft may not be diagnosed acutely. The simultaneous occurrence of hip dislocation and femoral shaft fracture has also been reported in children.[111–113,115–123] Missing such a concurrence is as inappropriate as missing a Monteggia injury in the forearm (see Chapter 16). In 42 cases of dislocation of the hip with ipsilateral fracture of the femur, the dislocation was recognized at initial examination in only 15 cases. In most cases the diagnosis was not made until 4–6 weeks later.[111]

Vialas used open reduction of the hip dislocation followed by traction for both the hip dislocation and femoral fracture in a 5-year-old girl.[122] The outcome was satisfactory.

Fracture of the Femoral Head

Kelly and Yarbrough described posterior dislocation of the hip with a portion of the femoral head remaining within the acetabulum.[114] This remaining fragment possessed attachments of the ligamentum (capitis) femoris. They described 27 patients, the youngest being a 20-year-old. This injury is not generally associated with the immature skeleton, although it certainly may occur (Fig. 20-20). Like the fracture of Tillaux (see Chapter 23), it is most likely to occur when the capital femoral physis is undergoing closure.

Open reduction, particularly with excision of the medial head fragment (even though it is relatively non-weight-bearing), produced inferior results compared with those obtained with either open reduction with internal fixation or closed reduction. Epstein described a 6-year-old girl who underwent closed reduction.[21] At follow-up 13 years later the fragment had reattached to the neck to form an exostosis that blocked full flexion and adduction.

A variation of segmental femoral head fracture occurs when the attachment of the ligamentum teres detaches.[144] This is analogous to a tibial spine avulsion of the anterior cruciate ligament in the knee. The stability of the hip should be assessed fluoroscopically. If necessary, the avulsed ligament is excised (including the avulsed fragment).

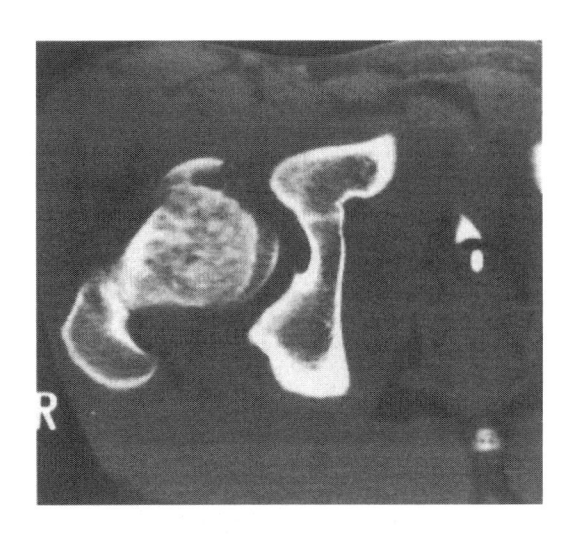

FIGURE 20-20. Split femoral head in a 15-year-old boy. It is a variant of the adult type 4 injury.

Traumatic Separation of the Capital Femoral Epiphysis

The capital femur may be injured during a hip dislocation,[124–143] and the injury may involve a partial physeal separation that is easy to overlook when there is a seemingly more obvious hip dislocation (Fig. 20-21). The femoral head may remain within the confines of the acetabulum, with the femoral neck and greater trochanter being displaced laterally (Fig. 20-22). The capital femur may be displaced from the acetabulum and significantly separated from the femoral neck.

The capital femur may also be displaced during reduction of a posterior dislocation (Fig. 20-23). Fiddian and Grace

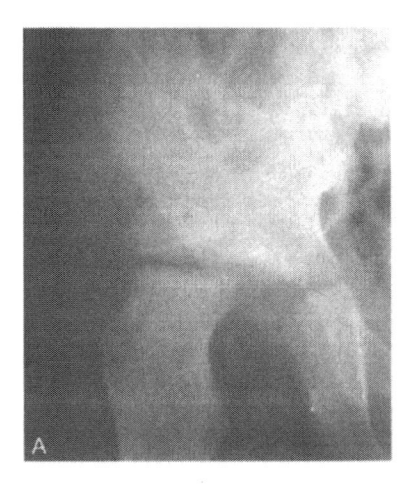

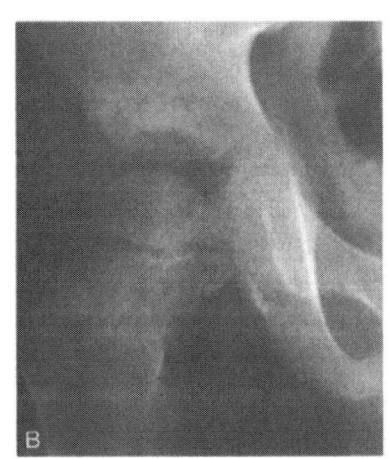

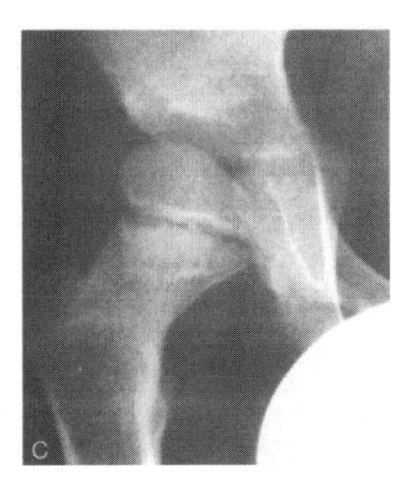

FIGURE 20-21. (A) Hip dislocation associated with type 1 physeal fracture in a 2-year-old. (B) Follow-up at 6 months shows physeal narrowing. (C) Mild coxa magna 11 months later.

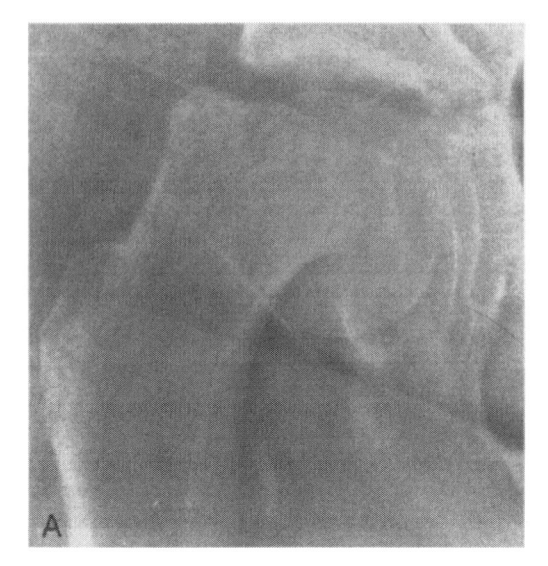

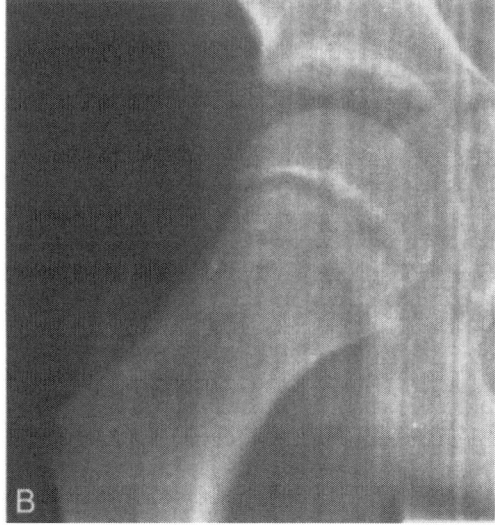

FIGURE 20-22. (A) Anteriorly dislocated femoral neck with located femoral head. (B) Open reduction.

reported two patients in whom there was a traumatic dislocation of the hip with separation of the capital epiphysis.[132] In both cases the slip occurred *during* the subsequent attempted closed reduction of the traumatic hip dislocation. However, the capital femoral physis may have been microscopically damaged during the dislocation (occult physeal injury), rendering it more mechanically susceptible to macro-injury from relatively minor forces than it would have otherwise been.

Open reduction is virtually always necessary. It is difficult to consider how closed reduction might be possible. In fact, several reported cases occurred while attempting closed reduction. In these instances the femoral neck reduced into the acetabulum, leaving the femoral head behind (extracapsular).

The importance of gentle manipulative reduction of a hip dislocation, with the patient under general anesthesia and with adequate muscle relaxation, must be emphasized to avoid such an unusual complication. Capital femoral displacement, whether part of the original injury or a complication of the reduction, requires gentle restoration of anatomy and (under anesthesia) fixation.

Barquet and Vécsei reported a case of traumatic dislocation of the hip with accompanying dislocation of the capital femoral epiphysis. Because of severe fat embolism, the patient's dislocated femoral head was not reduced into the hip until approximately 4 weeks after injury. The result 11 years later was poor.[125]

Osteonecrosis has developed in *all* reported cases of this combined injury, with the exception of one case that became

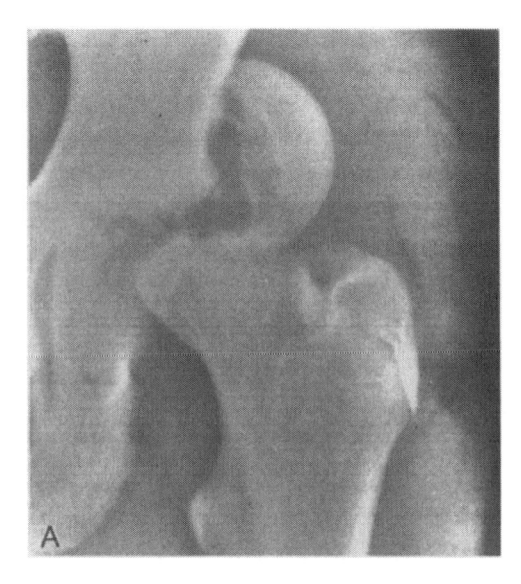

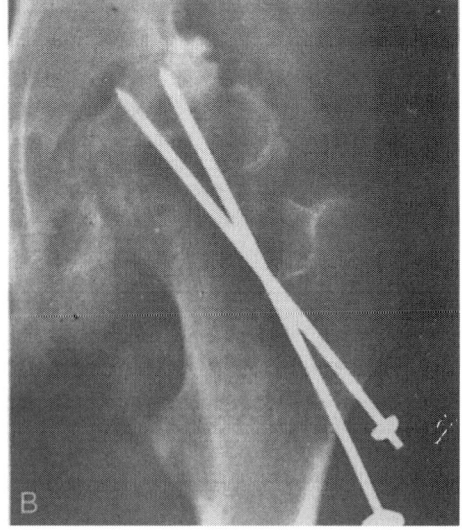

FIGURE 20-23. (A) Slipped capital femoral epiphysis complicating attempted reduction of a hip dislocation. (B) Ischemic damage and collapse 11 months later.

Associated Injuries

infected and required removal of the femoral head. According to Mass and colleagues, *none* of the patients with this injury have had a good result.[138]

Fifteen reported patients with at least 2 years of follow-up all developed osteonecrosis. In one case the dislocated capital epiphysis was never successfully reduced. Interestingly, this capital femoral epiphysis developed osteonecrosis while the capital femur was in its unreduced extracapsular position.

Pedina-Medina and Pardo-Montaner reported a variation in which a traumatic SCFE, with displacement of the femoral head from the acetabulum, was associated with a fracture of the triradiate cartilage.[139] Barquet and Vécsei divided the condition into (1) dislocation with complete separation and displacement of the epiphysis and (2) dislocation with incomplete separation of the epiphysis.[125]

Acetabular Fragments

The chondro-osseous periphery of the acetabulum may be fractured during the hip dislocation or subsequently during attempted reduction (Figs. 20-24, 20-25). Following any reduction, roentgenograms should be obtained to confirm the completeness of the reduction of both the hip dislocation and the acetabular fragment.

Sometimes associated fractures of the margin of the acetabulum are not readily evident on prereduction films but become evident after reduction.[144-164] Shea and associates described two cases illustrating problems of displaced unossified and ossified acetabular margins.[162] Any widening of the cartilage ("joint") space relative to the contralateral hip should arouse a suspicion of soft tissue or cartilage interposition (Figs. 20-26, 20-27) and the need for exploratory arthrotomy and excision of interposed tissue. Kaelin reported a 7-year-old boy who had locking of the hip after a minor fall.[154] The major finding was marked widening of the radiolucent space.

Bennett and Cash encountered a nonconcentric reduction of the hip in a 7-year-old boy 6 days after closed reduc-

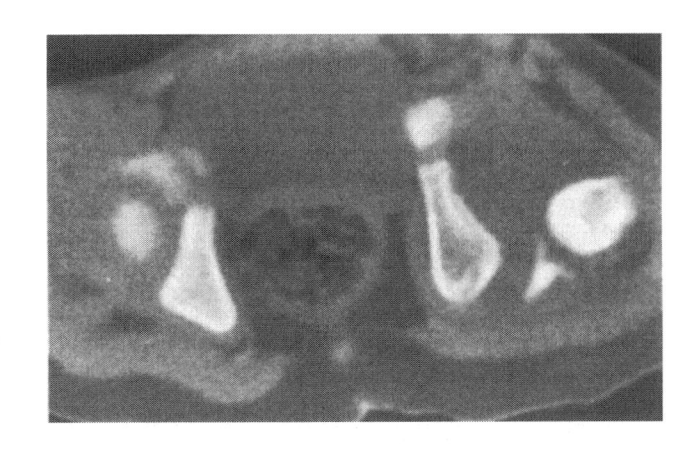

FIGURE 20-25. Posterior acetabular fracture with separation. This was treated with open reduction and internal fixation.

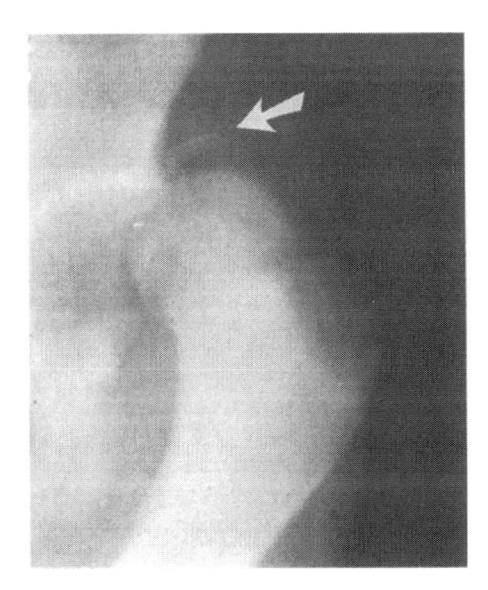

FIGURE 20-24. Acetabular rim fracture (arrow) in a teenager.

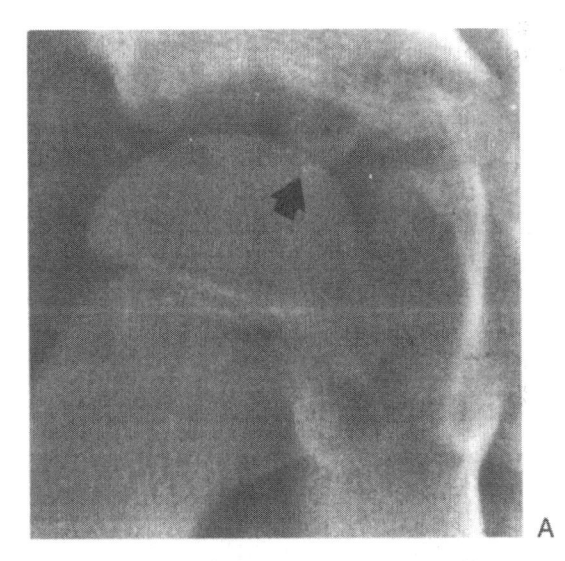

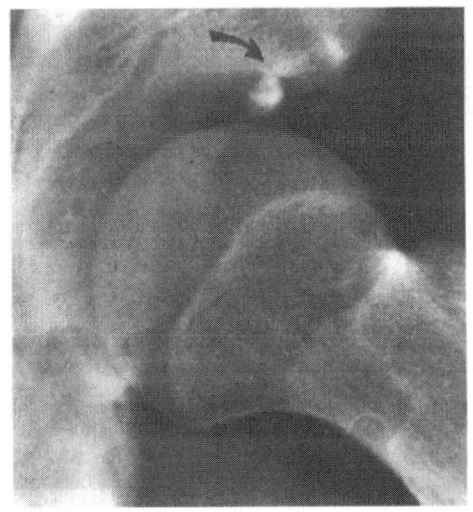

FIGURE 20-26. Retained chondro-osseous fragments (arrows).

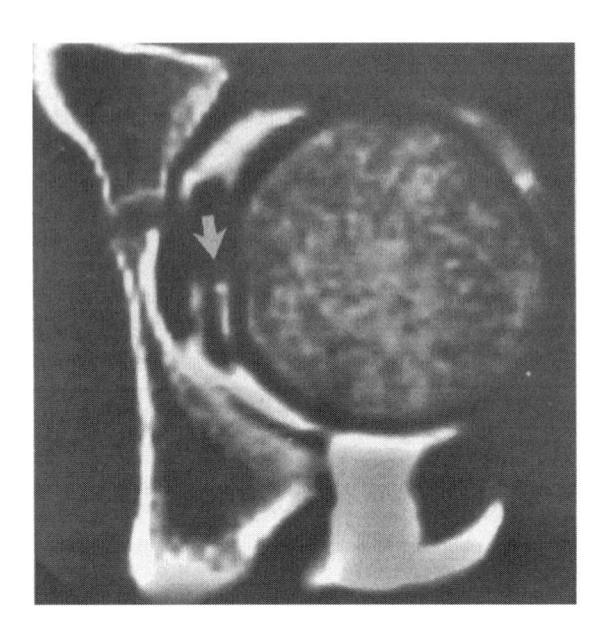

FIGURE 20-27. Interposed fragment (arrow). This injury was an avulsion of the ligamentum capitum femoris (ligamentum teres).

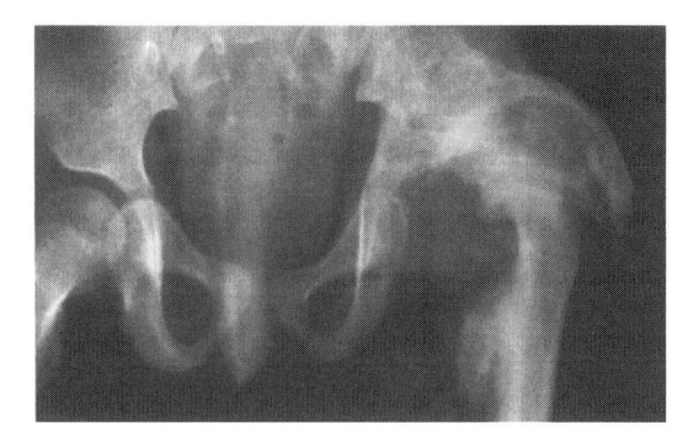

FIGURE 20-28. Untreated hip dislocation with acetabular injury. This patient also had a lumbosacral plexus nerve injury, with permanent muscular impairment and a Charcot joint at the hip.

tion and casting.[145] CT scans suggested posterior soft tissue interposition. During injection of contrast for an arthrogram a spontaneous concentric reduction occurred abruptly, along with outflow of dye from the inferior aspect of the capsule.

If closed (i.e., concentric) reduction is unsuccessful or if there are unstable chondro-osseous acetabular fractures, open reduction may be necessary. A posterior or lateral approach is best for visualizing the damaged areas. Large acetabular fragments are secured, but fixation pins or screws should not damage the triradiate cartilage. Any capsular rent is repaired.

An intraarticular fragment may not be recognized until after the reduction. Care is taken to ensure that the intraarticular distances (cartilage space widths) are bilaterally equal after reduction, as this may give an early indication that soft tissue or cartilaginous interposition is present, possibly indicating a need for open reduction and removal of the continued tissue. An arthrogram may show the interposed tissue. Demonstration of this interposed tissue may not be easy in the child whose injury has been acutely reduced, as tears in the capsule may allow extravasation of dye, which makes interpretation of the arthrogram difficult.

Relocation of the femoral head may disrupt the peripheral acetabular epiphysis or labrum and displace either tissue into the acetabulum, comparable to the way the femoral head may also be displaced from the neck. The size and consistency (cartilage or partially ossified tissue) of the epiphyseal fragment vary and make radiographic diagnosis difficult. Persistent widening of the medial cartilage space and continued pain and limitation of motion should alert the physician to the need for further studies. CT scans may be useful for delineating interposed cartilage fragments, even after reduction. If one has to resort to MRI, arthrotomy is probably justifiable instead.

Frich and coworkers found that arthroscopy was useful for diagnosing and removing intraarticular fragments and labral tears.[149] However, the application of arthroscopy to the hip is still controversial.

Santora et al. described six adolescents with intraarticular loose bodies diagnosed 2 months to 2 years after hip trauma. All were treated with excision. Four were symptom-free, and two had occasional pain.[161]

Failure to stabilize a peripheral acetabular injury may lead to chronic instability and severe, destructive joint changes (Fig. 20-28). Using CT scanning, Rashleigh-Belcher and Cannon described a lesion of the posterior acetabulum due to a posterior dislocation with no associated fracture.[160] Exploration of the hip, because of recurrent dislocation, revealed disruption of the posterosuperior acetabular labrum with formation of a pouch between the posterior acetabular wall and the external rotator muscles. They thought that it resembled a Bankart-type lesion of the shoulder. Repair was done using a bone block.

Tears of the acetabular labrum, which certainly can occur with a dislocation, are usually accompanied by a small fragment or involve the secondary ossification marginal process. These small fragment/labral tears may be detected by CT scan. Pure labral tears are more difficult to diagnose. Nishii et al. used contrast-enchanced MRI, with continuous leg traction to delineate such tears successfully.[158]

In all the reported cases, the chronic labral injury was associated with subsequent acetabular dysplasia. A constant early radiologic sign was a cyst above the lateral aspect of the acetabulum. The cysts occurred as a consequence of abnormal stresses imposed by the uncovered lateral portion of the femoral head.

Complications

Ischemic Necrosis (Osteonecrosis)

A significant long-term complication is vascular compromise eventuating in ischemic osseous and physeal/epiphyseal

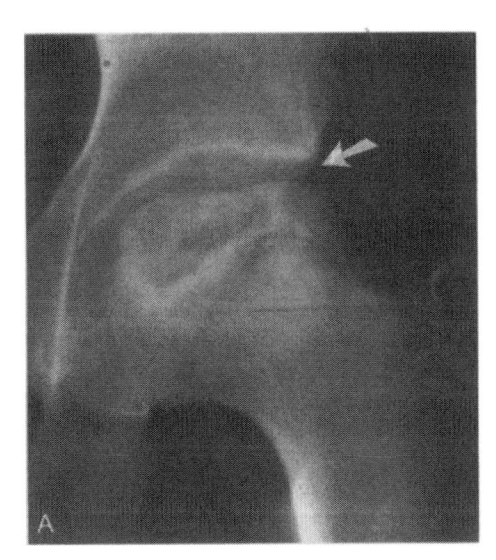

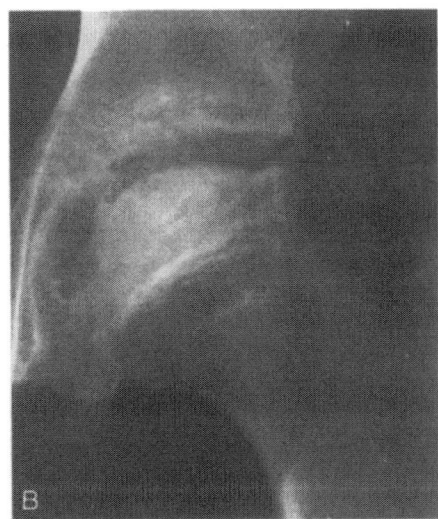

FIGURE 20-29. (A) Ischemic necrosis (arrow) with central collapse of the femoral head following previous dislocation. (B) Recovery 7 months later.

changes (Figs. 20-29 to 20-32).[165–187] Fineschi reviewed approximately 150 cases and found 16 complicated by ischemic necrosis.[23] This figure concurs with that of the Pennsylvania Orthopaedic Society; their reported incidence of ischemic necrosis was only 4%.[63,64] Epstein reported a 6% incidence.[19] Robertson and Peterson thought that if ischemic necrosis was not evident by 15 months after the injury it probably would not develop.[72]

Elmslie described ischemic necrosis of the femoral head secondary to traumatic dislocation and termed it coxa plana.[169,170] Goldenberg described "Perthes" disease following hip dislocation; it most likely was ischemic necrosis.[172] Undoubtedly, comparisons with the Legg-Calvé-Perthes (LCP) lesion are not appropriate because one is a more chronic kind of condition. However, the roentgenographic patterns and delayed presentation are often similar in comparable age groups.

Glass and Powell presented a study of 47 children who sustained posterior traumatic hip dislocations.[30] Their incidence of ischemic necrosis was approximately 20%. The average follow-up was 28 months. Of 26 children under the age of 10 years, 1 developed ischemic necrosis. Of the 21 children aged 10 years or over, 5 were so affected. There was premature epiphyseal fusion in only one child.

There seems to be an age variation with regard to susceptibility to posttraumatic ischemic necrosis. This complication appears to be infrequent in children under 6 years of age, whereas in older children the frequency is probably about 10%. The observation is sometimes made that the young patient has some protection against the complication of ischemic necrosis. This protection is probably due to the anatomic particularities of the circulation and continuity of the proximal femoral epiphysis, the greater amount of epiphyseal cartilage, and the relative positions of capsular

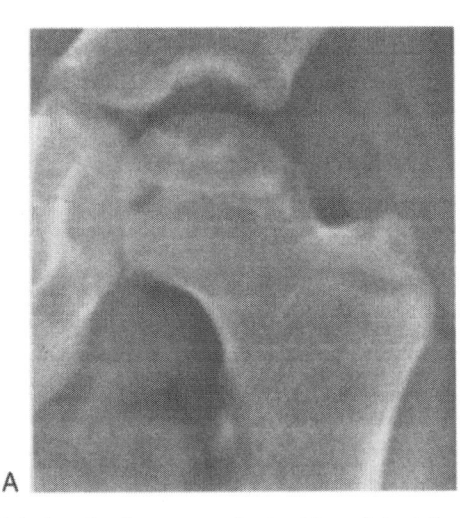

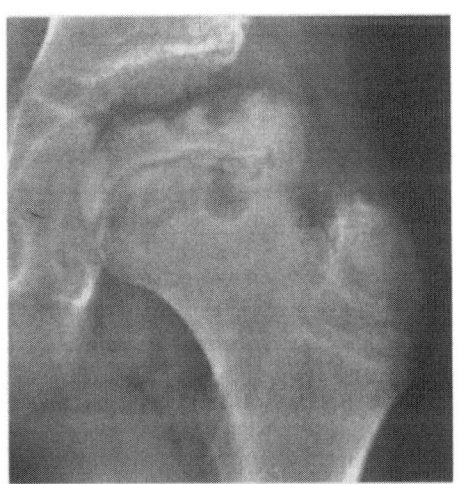

FIGURE 20-30. (A) Ischemic changes on both sides of the joint 11 months after hip dislocation. (B) Ten months after a hip dislocation there is ischemic involvement of the physis and ossification center.

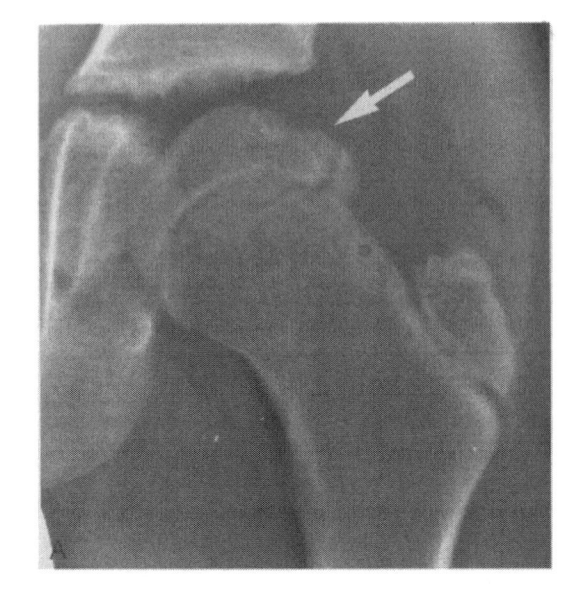

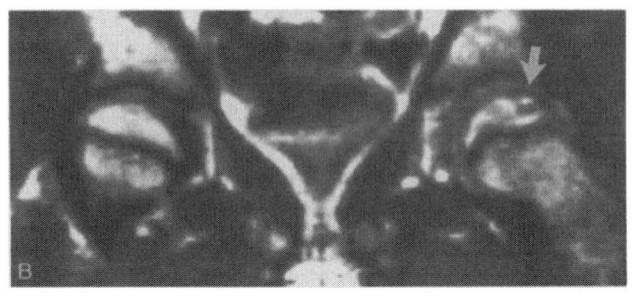

FIGURE 20-31. (A) Mild ischemic change (arrow). (B) MRI localizes the lesion (arrow).

not appear until adolescence, even though the vascular insult may have been rendered within the first few months of life.[167]

Once the patient has gotten over the acute healing phase, usually 2–3 months after the injury, a baseline bone scan may insertion to blood vessels in the various age groups. This complication has also been attributed to changes in the function of the artery of the ligamentum capitis femoris, which is usually completely disrupted. It seems more likely that the age-related differences relate to the volume of ossification within the capital femoral epiphyseal cartilage. The developing osseous centrum is a more vascularly dependent structure than is the surrounding unossified cartilage.[180,181,187] The greater the mass of epiphyseal bone at the time of injury, the more is the normal vascular demand, so the bone is less likely to withstand prolonged ischemia. Macrovascular and microvascular patterns also change significantly with age.

The patient who sustains a posterior dislocation usually tears the capsule in the direction of the longitudinal fibers and does not usually destroy the area where the blood supply courses. The capsular rent allows decompression; therefore there usually is no buildup of hematoma under pressure within the joint. Furthermore, the intracapsular course of vessels should not be seriously compromised by this type of dislocation.

Of all the reported cases of ischemic necrosis, only two were first diagnosed more than 2 years after the injury.[173] The final prognosis should be reserved until the patient reaches skeletal maturity, as unanticipated changes may occur during the adolescent growth spurt. Some of the subtle changes of ischemic necrosis that complicate the developmental hip do

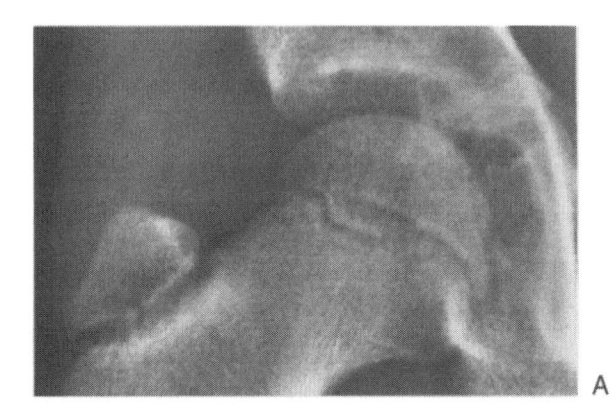

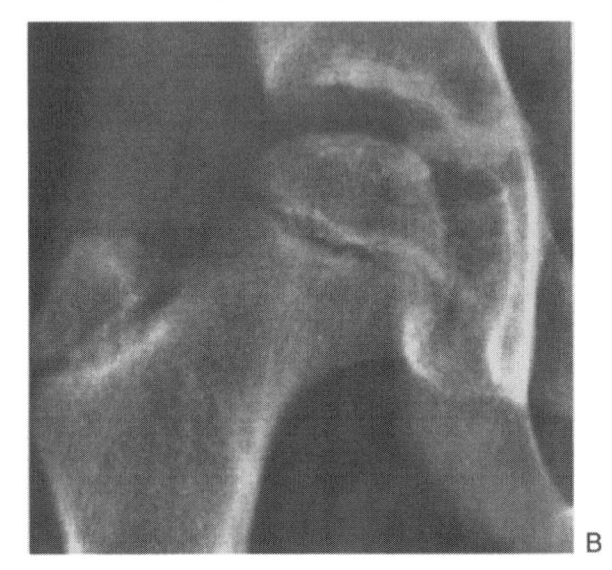

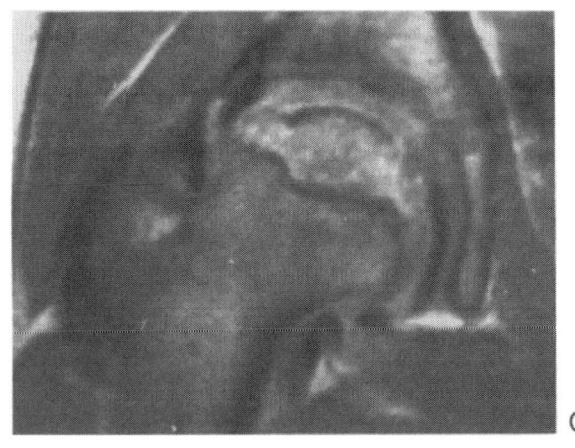

FIGURE 20-32. Appearance 4 months after traumatic hip dislocation. (A) The hip appears normal, although the child has intermittent complaints of hip and groin pain. (B) One year later a subchondral fracture is evident. (C) MRI shows evidence of osteonecrosis.

be obtained to see if there is any decrease in the blood supply to the affected femoral head. Serial radiographic review should continue until skeletal maturity to detect any developing problems, particularly long-term changes in the femoral head, as some changes do not manifest until the growth spurt.

Magnetic resonance imaging may also help delineate the extent of vascular damage. Poggi et al. reviewed 14 patients who had an MRI evaluation after hip dislocation (only one was under 18 years).[183] Eight of the hips had abnormal marrow within 6 weeks after injury, but progression to radiologically evident damage occurred in only three patients. Repeat MRI studies in the other five patients showed resolution of the process. They did not differentiate between bone bruising (contusion) and osteonecrosis. They also noted the MRI was not reliable during the first week after injury, nor was it useful for predicting which patients would progress to osteoarthritic change. In some cases MRI may be detecting contusion and hemorrhage similar to the bone bruise of the distal femur (see Chapter 22).

Li and Hiette used a specialized technique of contrast-enhanced fat saturation MRI to study the pathophysiology of osteonecrosis (nontraumatic).[176] They believed that early nontraumatic osteonecrosis was associated with hyperemia, an increase in capillary permeability rather than acute devascularization, or both, and that diffuse marrow edema was the initial finding. Trauma could easily cause comparable changes.

If ischemic necrosis should occur, the first step is prohibition of or protected weight-bearing to try to prevent osseous collapse during the revascularization period. Osteotomy may also be beneficial, as it may align the head in a more effective weight-bearing position and enhance revascularization and venous outflow.

A complication that is not stressed in the literature is the development of coxa magna, which is probably caused by injury-induced hyperemia to the capital femur. If this complication causes acetabular-femoral incongruity, there may be a predisposition to subsequent osteoarthritis.

Chronic vascular complications of anterior dislocation are rare. The incidence of ischemic necrosis of the femoral head after anterior dislocation was reported by Brav as 9% in 62 cases, although these patients were primarily adolescents and adults.[86] Litton believed that ischemic necrosis was a rarity with anterior dislocation because the main vessels supplying blood to the femoral head were posterior.[95] Although damage to the posterior capsule is less likely with this injury, the fact that the femoral head is often buttonholed through a piece of tight anterior capsule may cause direct pressure from the capsular rent and the displaced iliopsoas tendon on some of the vessels. This condition can predispose to a greater risk of vascular injury if urgent reduction of the dislocation is not carried out.

Recurrent Dislocation

A less frequent complication is recurrent dislocation.[188–202] Choyce described five cases of recurrent dislocation.[168] Mauck and Anderson reported a 6-year-old boy who had a subsequent dislocation 13 months after the initial injury.[51] Morton cited five cases of recurrent dislocation.[53] The reports of the Pennsylvania Orthopaedic Society mentioned only one case.[63,64] With few exceptions, all children suffering the complication of recurrent dislocation appeared to be under 8 years of age at the time of initial injury. One child developed ischemic necrosis following the recurrent dislocation.

The longest interval between recurrent dislocations was 7 years, with a 1.5-year follow-up after the second dislocation.[199] The average time between the initial and final dislocation was 2 years, and the shortest interval between successive dislocations was 1 month. Based on these findings, Simmons and Elder suggested that a minimal period of follow-up is 2 years.[199]

An important causal factor of recurrent dislocation may be inadequate immobilization of the hip after reduction, with consequent incomplete healing of the capsular damage (Fig. 20-33). Liebenberg and Dommisse thought that the mechanism was incomplete healing of a posterior capsular defect, particularly if the reduction was delayed.[196] If there is incomplete healing, a false cavity with synovial lining may develop and communicate with the true joint. Synovial fluid may then flow freely between the two regions.

Treatment, following definitive diagnosis, consists of excision of the pouch and repair of the capsular defect. The hip is immobilized for 4–6 weeks with a hip spica cast to allow complete healing.

Simmons and Elder reported a case of a 5-year-old child who sustained a posterior dislocation of the hip. On subsequent occasions 5, 7, and 9 months afterward, the femur redislocated as a result of minimal trauma.[199] Exploration revealed a large herniation of the posterior joint capsule, laxity, and a large capsular tear deep to the quadratus femoris muscle. This tear was successfully closed without significant problems or subsequent recurrent dislocation.

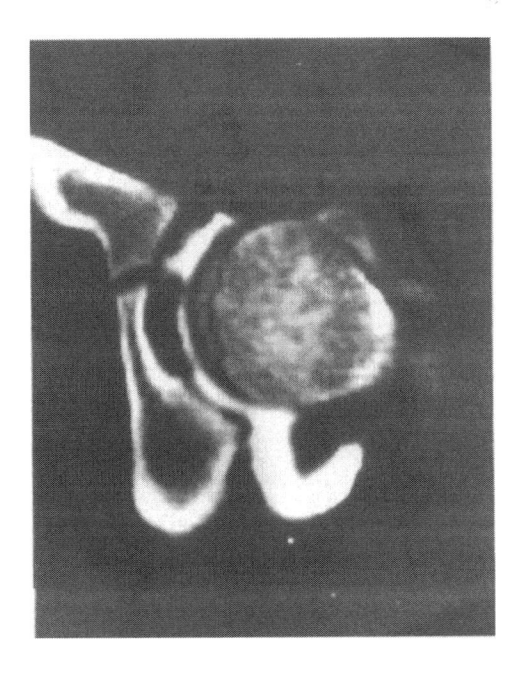

FIGURE 20-33. Recurrent dislocation in a 12-year-old boy. CT arthrogram shows extravasation of dye through a large posterior capsule defect.

Dall and colleagues[87] and Scudese[103] reported cases of recurrent anterior dislocation. The complication appears less prevalent with anterior dislocations than following posterior dislocations.

Routine hip arthrography after the initial dislocation in a child has not been advocated, but it may have some merit for detecting hips that might redislocate by localizing a large defect in the joint capsule. If the results of arthrography suggest a capsular defect, repair should be considered. The operation is done in such a way that the capsular tear or stretch is demonstrated and specifically repaired.

Osteochondrosis

An 8-year-old boy developed osteochondrosis of the upper femoral epiphysis 3.5 years after his original posterior dislocation.[203] This condition may represent a focal variation of ischemic necrosis.

Myositis Ossificans

Myositis ossificans is a rare complication in the normal child. It is more likely in the patient with concomitant head injury. When it does occur, the process must be allowed to mature completely before resection is attempted.

Periarticular calcification was present in Nerubay's[97] case and was previously reported by Aggarwall and Singh in all six of their reported unreduced anterior hip dislocations.[83] Brav found an incidence of 11% among 228 posterior dislocations but none with anterior dislocations.[86]

Neurologic Deficits

Neurologic deficiency was the most frequent complication in the series by Pearson and Mann.[62] Although all experienced some degree of functional recovery, only one patient had complete recovery of nerve function. Epstein reported three cases of neurologic deficiency: two patients with full recovery, although one still had weakness in the great toe extensor 21 years after the injury.[21] These deficits all accompanied posterior dislocation and involved variable sensory or motor deficiency of the sciatic nerve. Injury accompanying posterior dislocations may be due to the marked internal rotation of the hip that occurs at the time of dislocation. Sciatic injury may cause serious long-term consequences (Fig. 20-28).[204]

Osteoarthritis

It is essential to follow hip-injured children beyond skeletal maturity. Long-term changes not evident during the early posttraumatic period may subsequently become significant osteoarthritis. Epstein reported six such cases.[21] Severe injuries in young children may lead to this complication even before skeletal maturity is attained.

Chronic Hip Pain

The choice of treatment for the patient with disabling hip pain consequent to complications of childhood hip dislocation is difficult, especially as some available treatment modalities involve major risks and compromises for a young patient. Certainly, total joint replacement, a bipolar prosthesis, and an endoprosthesis are not reasonable initial alternatives in a skeletally immature patient who is otherwise healthy. For the child sufficiently disabled to warrant surgical relief of hip pain, the essential options available (other than acceptance of the pain) are pelvic or femoral osteotomy or hip fusion.[205-210]

Fulkerson presented a comprehensive long-term follow-up of hip fusions done for disabling hip pain in children.[206] One of the significant findings was that following hip fusion there was a tendency for the fused hip to progressively adduct. This observation was true of each and every hip fused in skeletally immature patients. The average increase of adduction was 10°, usually occurring within 2 years after the initial fusion. The reasons for this postoperative increase in adduction have not been identified, but certainly growth at the trochanteric epiphysis and lateral capital epiphysis can contribute. The hips were fused in 20°–40° of flexion, which is allowable in a more active child.[206] Rotational alignment was not a problem, and fusion near neutral rotation was generally accepted.

The results of adolescent hip fusions are satisfactory. Many of these children returned to vigorous physical activities and normal life styles. Fusion of the hip certainly does not negate the possibility of subsequent conversion to a total hip arthroplasty.[210]

Obstetric "Dislocation"

All presumed *acute* dislocations of the hip in the newborn have been found to be fractures across the entire proximal femoral metaphysis and physis. This type of injury was produced easily when attempting acute dislocation of the hip in stillborns and infants (see Chapter 21). Traumatic dislocation of the femoral head in the newborn is essentially nonexistent because the ligaments that reinforce the capsule are strong (although they may be hyperlax during the perinatal period because of the influence of maternal hormones). In cases of excessive trauma, as from energetic traction during delivery, epiphysiolysis or fracture of the femoral metaphysis may be produced. Elizalde reported two cases he believed were true dislocations of the hip, but the roentgenograms indicated that the most likely diagnosis was a fracture through the transepiphyseal region.[211] In contrast to developmental hip dysplasia, these injuries are painful if the leg is manipulated. They are discussed in detail in Chapter 21.

Any neonate who returns to the hospital and is found to have a traumatic "hip dislocation" deserves careful evaluation. First, the true diagnosis is probably a fracture-separation of the entire proximal femoral epiphysis. Second, and much more important, a skeletal survey and detailed physical examination must be done. This infant is most likely the victim of child abuse, not unrecognized obstetric trauma.

Snapping Hip Syndrome

Many children and adolescents who pursue athletics or dance (e.g., ballet) on a highly competitive basis develop repetitive, painful snapping in the hip.[212–215] One of two syndromes may be present. The most common is the external variant, caused by the posterior border of the iliotibial band or the outer border of the gluteus maximus impinging on the greater trochanter with hip rotation. The less common internal variant is usually attributed to the iliopsoas tendon temporarily impinging on the femoral head, anterior hip capsule, or iliopectineal eminence.[212,214]

Symptoms with the external variation are a snapping sensation and lateral thigh pain. The internal variant exhibits palpable or audible snapping in association with anterior inguinal pain.

Vaccaro et al. used contrast imaging of the iliopsoas bursa (an anatomic extension of the hip joint) to pinpoint the impingement during fluoroscopy.[215] Therapeutic injection into the iliopsoas bursa was found to alleviate pain in a significant number of patients.

Voluntary Habitual Dislocation

Recurrent voluntary or habitual dislocation of the hip in children, in the absence of a well-defined antecedent dislocation, is unusual.[216–227] There may be predisposing factors such as paralysis or collagen disorders (see Chapter 11). In the latter situation the repetitive displacement continues because of capsular distortion (attenuation) and loss of support of surrounding tissues.

Children with voluntary dislocation probably have an intact capsule and reasonable contiguous soft tissue support. These factors cause decreased intracapsular pressure as the femur displaces from the acetabulum, causing liberation of gas into the joint.[225] It typically produces what is referred to as a "vacuum arthrogram" and is due to the physics principle of cavitation (release of dissolved gas with a change in applied pressure). This phenomenon is pathognomonic of habitual dislocation.

These children also have clinical "clunks." However, this sign may occur with recurrent dislocation due to other causes or the snapping hip syndrome.

As with nursemaid's elbow the phenomenon decreases over time. Expectant treatment and parental education are ususally sufficient. An intertrochanteric derotation osteotomy was used in one patient.[224]

References

Anatomy

1. Diméglio A, Kaelin A, Bonnel F, DeRosa V, Couture A. The growing hip: specifications and requirements. J Pediatr Orthop Part B 1994;3:135–147.
2. Ganey TM, Ogden JA. Pre- and post-natal development of the hip. In: Callaghan JJ, Rosenberg AG, Rubash HE (eds) The Adult Hip. Philadelphia: Lippincott, 1998:3–19.
3. Ogden JA. Hip development and vascularity: relationship to chondro-osseous trauma in the growing child. In: The Hip, vol 9. St. Louis: Mosby, 1981:139–137.
4. Ponseti IV. Growth and development of the acetabulum in the normal child: anatomical, histological, and roentgenographic studies. J Bone Joint Surg Am 1978;60:575–585.

General

5. Barcat J, Testas P. A propos des luxations traumatiques recentes de la hanche chez l'enfant. Mem Acad Chir 1958;84:659–664.
6. Barquet A. Traumatic hip dislocation in children. Acta Orthop Scand 1979;50:549–553.
7. Barquet A. Luxations irreductibles de la hanche chez l'enfant. Lyon Chir 1980;76:329–334.
8. Barquet A. Traumatic Hip Dislocation in Childhood. New York: Springer, 1987. [This monograph contains 524 references to this injury in children.]
9. Bernhang AM. Simultaneous bilateral traumatic dislocation of the hip in a child. J Bone Joint Surg Am 1970;52:365–366.
10. Brug E, Ziegelmuller F. Die traumatischen Huftgelenksluxation im Kindesalter. Munch Med Wochenschr 1974;116:315–320.
11. Brunner C, Gysler R, Morger R. Traumatische Hüftluxation beim kind. Z Kinderchir 1988;43:174–175.
12. Bunnell WP, Webster DA. Late reduction of bilateral traumatic hip dislocations in a child. Clin Orthop 1980;147:160–163.
13. Canale ST, Manugian AH. Irreducible traumatic dislocation of the hip. J Bone Joint Surg Am 1979;61:7.
14. Carlioz H, Michelutti D. Traumatisme du bassin et de la hanche chez l'enfant. Ann Chir 1982;36:50–56.
15. Chavette J. Luxation traumatique de la hanche chez l'enfant. Thesis, University of Lyon, 1968.
16. Chorney GS, Forese LL. Late diagnosis of traumatic dislocation of the hip in a child. Surg Rounds Orthop 1989;3:44–46.
17. Clarke HO. Traumatic dislocation of the hip joint in a child. Br J Surg 1929;16:690–691.
18. Endo S, Yamada Y, Fejii, et al. Bilateral traumatic hip dislocation in a child. Arch Orthop Trauma Surg 1993;112:155–156.
19. Epstein HC. Traumatic anterior and simple posterior dislocations of the hip in adults and children. AAOS Instr Course Lect 1973;22:115–1145.
20. Epstein HC. Traumatic dislocations of the hip. Clin Orthop 1973;92:116–142.
21. Epstein HC. Traumatic Dislocation of the Hip. Baltimore: Williams & Wilkins, 1980.
22. Ferran JL, Diméglio A, Lebonco N, Couture A, DeRosa V. Three-dimensional computed tomography of the infantile hip. J Pediatr Orthop Part B 1994;3:131–134.
23. Fineschi G. Die traumatische Huftverrenkung bei Kindern. Literaturubersicht und statistischer Beitrag von 7 Fallen. Arch Orthop Unfallchir 1956;48:225–236.
24. Fischer L, Venouil J, Baulieux J. Luxations traumatiques de la hanche chez l'enfant. Cah Med Lyon 1971;47:3325–3331.
25. Fordyce AJW. Open reduction of traumatic dislocation of the hip in a child. Br J Surg 1971;l58:705–707.
26. Freeman GE Jr. Traumatic dislocation of the hip in children. J Bone Joint Surg Am 1961;43:401–406.
27. Funk FJ. Traumatic dislocation of the hip in children: factors influencing prognosis and treatment. J Bone Joint Surg Am 1962;44:1135–1145.
28. Germaneau J, Vital JM, Bucco P, et al. Luxations traumatiques de la hanche de l'enfant de moins de 6 ans: a propos de 10 observations. Chir Pediatr 1980;21:239–244.
29. Giraud D. Contribution a l'etude de la luxation traumatique de la hanche chez l'enfant. Thesis Bordeaux, 1927.
30. Glass A, Powell HDW. Traumatic dislocation of the hip in children. J Bone Joint Surg Br 1961;43:29–37.
31. Glynn P. Two cases of traumatic dislocation of the hip in children. Lancet 1932;1:1093–1094.
32. Godley DR, Williams RA. Traumatic dislocation of the hip in a child: usefulness of MRI. Orthopedics 1993;16:1145–1147.

33. Gouin JL. A propos des luxations traumatiques chez l'enfant. Mem Acad Chir 1961;87:612–615.
34. Grobelski M. Die traumatischen Huftverrenkungen im kindesalter. Arch Orthop Unfallchir 1957;48:691–697.
35. Guingand O, Rigault P, Padovani JP, Finidori G, Touzet P, Depatter J. Luxations traumatiques de la hanche et fractures du cotyle chez l'enfant. Rev Chir Orthop 1985;71:575–585.
36. Gupta RC, Shravat BP. Traumatic dislocation of the hip in children. Indian J Orthop 1978;12:17–24.
37. Haines C. Traumatic dislocation of the head of the femur in a child. J Bone Joint Surg 1937;19:1126–1127.
38. Hougaaod K, Thomsen PB. Traumatic hip dislocation in children: follow-up of 13 cases. Orthopedics 1989;12:375–378.
39. Hovelius L. Traumatic dislocation of the hip in children. Acta Orthop Scand 1974;45:746–751.
40. Huckstep RL. Neglected traumatic dislocation of the hip in children. J Bone Joint Surg Br 1971;53:355.
41. Hunter GA. Posterior dislocation of fracture dislocation of the hip. J Bone Joint Surg Br 1969;51:38–44.
42. Ingram A, Bachynski B. Fractures of the hip in children. J Bone Joint Surg Am 1953;35:867–887.
43. Klasen HJ. Traumatic dislocation of the hip in children. Reconstr Surg Traumatol 1979;17:119–129.
44. Libri R, Calberson E, Capelli A, Soncini G. Traumatic dislocation of the hip in children and adolescents. Ital J Orthop Traumatol 1986;l12:61–67.
45. Londonberry P. Traumatic dislocation of the hip in childhood. J Bone Joint Surg Br 1961;43:29–37.
46. Lugger LJ. Traumatische Huftverrenkung und gleichzeitiger Oberschenkelschaftbruch im Kindesalter. Zentralbl Chir 1974;99:340–342.
47. Mabit C, Robert M, Moulies D, Alain JL. Les luxations traumatiques de la hanche chez l'enfant. Acta Orthop Belg 1985;51:905–913.
48. MacFarlane L, King D. Traumatic dislocation of the hip joint in children. Aust NZ J Surg 1976;46:227–231.
49. MacGoff JP, Ramoska EA. Traumatic hip dislocation in a child. Ann Emerg Med 1987;16:108–110.
50. Mason ML. Traumatic dislocation of the hip in childhood. J Bone Joint Surg Br 1954;36:630–632.
51. Mauck HP, Anderson RL. Infracotyloid dislocation of the hip. J Bone Joint Surg 1935;17:1011–1013.
52. Meng CI. Traumatic dislocation of the hip in childhood. Chin Med J 1954;48:736–741.
53. Morton KS. Traumatic dislocation of the hip in children. Br J Surg 1959;47:233–237.
54. Moseley CF. Fractures and dislocations of the hip. AAOS Instr Course Lect 1992;41:397–401.
55. Murphy DP. Traumatic luxation of the hip in childhood. JAMA 1923;80:549–551.
56. Nagi ON, Dhillon MS. Neglected hip dislocations in young children. Contemp Orthop 1995;30:407–412.
57. Nagi ON, Dhillon MS, Gill SS. Chronically unreduced traumatic anterior dislocation of the hip: a report of four cases. J Orthop Trauma 1992;6:433–436.
58. Offierski CM. Traumatic dislocation of the hip in childhood. J Bone Joint Surg Br 1981;63:194–197.
59. Pai VS. The management of unreduced traumatic dislocation of the hip in developing countries. Int Orthop 1992;16:136–139.
60. Pai VS, Kumar B. Management of unreduced traumatic dislocation of the hip: heavy traction and abduction method. Injury 1990;21:225–227.
61. Paus B. Traumatic dislocations of the hip. Acta Orthop Scand 1951;21:99–112.
62. Pearson DE, Mann RJ. Traumatic hip dislocation in children. Clin Orthop 1975;92:189–194.
63. Pennyslvania Orthopaedic Society. Traumatic dislocations of the hip joint in children: final report by the scientific research committee. J Bone Joint Surg Am 1960;42:705–710.
64. Pennyslvania Orthopaedic Society. Traumatic dislocations of the hip joint in children: a report by the scientific research committee. J Bone Joint Surg Am 1968;50:79–88.
65. Petrie SG, Harris MB, Willis RB. Traumatic hip dislocation during childhood: a case report and review of the literature. Am J Orthop 1996;25:645–649.
66. Piggott J. Traumatic dislocation of the hip in childhood. J Bone Joint Surg Br 1959;41:20–29.
67. Platt H. Traumatic dislocation of the hip joint in a child. Lancet 1916;1:80–81.
68. Rieger H, Pennig D, Klein LO, Grumert J. Traumatic dislocation of the hip in young children. Acta Orthop Trauma Surg 1991;110:114–117.
69. Rigault P, Hannouche D, Judet J. Luxations traumatiques de la hanche et fractures du cotyle chez l'enfant. Rev Chir Orthop 1958;44:361–367.
70. Rigault P, Moreau J, Iselin F, Judet J. Fractures de col du femur chez l'enfant (25 cas). Rev Chir Orthop 1966;52:325–336.
71. Ritter G, Höllwarth M, Hausbrandt D, Linhart W. Die traumatische Hüftluxation in Kindesalter. Unfallheilkunde 1984;87:24–26.
72. Robertson RC, Peterson HA. Traumatic dislocation of the hip in children: review of Mayo Clinic series. In: The Hip, vol 2. St. Louis: Mosby, 1974.
73. Rocher HL, Rocher C, Cuzard M. Luxation traumatique de la hanche chez l'enfant. Bordeaux Chir 1937;8:255–256.
74. Sankarankutty M. Traumatic inferior dislocation of the hip (luxatio erecta) in a child. J Bone Joint Surg Br 1967;49:145.
75. Schlonsky J, Miller PR. Traumatic hip dislocations in children. J Bone Joint Surg Am 1973;55:1057–1063.
76. Schonbauer H. Begleitverletzungen am Oberschenkel Bei Huftverrenkungen. Klin Med 1961;16:39–43.
77. Swiontkowski MF. Fractures and dislocations about the hip and pelvis. In: Green NE, Swiontkowski MF (eds) Skeletal Trauma in Children. Philadelphia: Saunders, 1994.
78. Tronzo RG. Traumatic dislocation of the hip in children: a problem in anesthetic management. JAMA 1961;176:526–527.
79. Von zlrt L. Traumatische Hüftverletzungen in Wachstumsalter. Z Orthop 1990;128:415–417.
80. Wilchinsky MS, Pappas AM. Unusual complications in traumatic dislocation of the hip in children. J Pediatr Orthop 1995;5:534–539.
81. Wilson DW. Traumatic dislocation of the hip in children: a report of four cases. J Trauma 1966;6:739–743.
82. Yang RS, Tsuang YH, Hang LS, Lyu TK. Traumatic dislocation of the hip. Clin Orthop 1991;265:218–227.

Anterior Dislocation

83. Aggarwall ND, Singh H. Unreduced anterior dislocation of the hip. J Bone Joint Surg Br 1967;49:288–292.
84. Barquet A. Traumatic anterior dislocation of the hip in childhood. Injury 1982;13:435–440.
85. Bonnemaison MFE, Henderson EDD. Traumatic anterior dislocation of the hip with acute common femoral occlusion in a child. J Bone Joint Surg Am 1978;50:753–756.
86. Brav EM. Traumatic dislocation of the hip. J Bone Joint Surg Am 1962;44:1115–1134.
87. Dall D, MacNab I, Gross A. Recurrent anterior dislocation of the hip. J Bone Joint Surg Am 1970;52:574–576.

88. Erb RE, Steele JR, Nance EP Jr, Edwards JR. Traumatic anterior dislocation of the hip: spectrum of plain film and CT findings. AJR 1995;165:1215–1219.
89. Fernandez-Herrera E. Luxacion traumatica anterior de la cadera en la infancia. Bol Med Hosp Infant Mex 1965;22:95–98.
90. Gaul RW. Recurrent traumatic dislocation of the hip in children. Clin Orthop 1973;90:107–109.
91. Hamada G. Unreduced anterior dislocation of the hip. J Bone Joint Surg Br 1957;39:471–476.
92. Hampson WGJ. Venous obstruction by anterior dislocation of the hip joint. Injury 1972;4:69–73.
93. Henderson RS. Traumatic anterior dislocation of the hip. J Bone Joint Surg Br 1951;33:602–603.
94. Katznelson AM. Traumatic dislocation of the hip. J Bone Joint Surg Br 1962;44:129–130.
95. Litton LO. Traumatic anterior dislocation of the hip in children. J Bone Joint Surg Br 1958;40:1419–1422.
96. Mikhail IK. Unreduced traumatic dislocation at the hip. J Bone Joint Surg Br 1956;38:899–901.
97. Nerubay J. Traumatic anterior dislocation of the hip joint with vascular damage. Clin Orthop 1976;116:129–132.
98. Niloff P, Petrie J. Traumatic anterior dislocation of the hip. Can Med Assoc J 1950;62:574–576.
99. Pries P, Gayet LE, Bonnet L, Clarac JP. A case of traumatic obdurator luxation of the hip in a 4 year old child. Rev Chir Orthop 1991;77:94–97.
100. Renato L. Open anterior dislocation of the hip in a child. Acta Orthop Scand 1987;58:669–670.
101. Scadden WJ, Dennyson WG. Unreduced obdurator dislocation of the hip: a case report. S Afr Med J 1978;53:601–602.
102. Schwartz D, Haller J. Open anterior hip dislocation with femoral vessel transection in a child. J Trauma 1974;14:1054–1059.
103. Scudese VA. Traumatic anterior hip redislocation. Clin Orthop 1972;88:60–63.
104. Younge D, Lifeso R. Unreduced anterior dislocation of the hip in a child. J Pediatr Orthop 1988;8:478–480.

Inferior Dislocation

105. Abad Rico JI, Barquet A. Luxatio erecta of the hip: a case report and review of the literature. Arch Orthop Trauma Surg 1982;99:227–229.
106. Beauchesne R, Kruse R, Stanton RP. Inferior dislocation (luxatio erecta) of the hip. Orthopedics 1994;17:72–75.
107. Mauck H, Anderson R. Infracotyloid dislocation of the hip. J Bone Joint Surg 1935;17:1011–1013.
108. Rao JP, Read RB. Luxatio erecta of the hip: an interesting case report. Clin Orthop 1975;110:137–138.
109. Sankarankutty M. Traumatic inferior dislocation of the hip (luxatio erecta) in a child. J Bone Joint Surg Br 1967;49:145.
110. Wendel W. Die luxatio femoris infracotyloiden. Dtsch Z Chir 1904;72:193–195.

Associated Femoral Fracture

111. Dehne E, Immermann EW. Dislocation of the hip combined with fracture of the shaft of the femur on the same side. J Bone Joint Surg Am 1954;33:731–745.
112. Fardon D. Femoral shaft fracture with ipsilateral hip dislocation in a child. J Am College of Emerg Physic 1978;7:159–161.
113. Fina CP, Kelly PJ. Dislocations of the hip with fractures of the proximal femur. J Trauma 1970;10:77–87.
114. Kelly RP, Yarbrough SH III. Posterior fracture-dislocation of the femoral head with retained head fragment. J Trauma 1971;11:97–108.
115. Lugger L. Traumatische Hüftverrenkung und gleichseitiger Ober-Schenkelschaftbruch im Kindesalter. Zentralbl Chir 1974;99:340–342.
116. Lyddon DW, Hartman JT. Traumatic dislocation of the hip with ipsilateral femoral fracture. J Bone Joint Surg Am 1971;53:1012–1016.
117. Malkawi H. Traumatic anterior dislocation of the hip with fracture of the shaft of the ipsilateral femur in children: case report and review of the literature. J Pediatr Orthop 1982;2:307–311.
118. Rinke W, Protze J. Offene traumatische Hüftgelenksluxation und gleichseitige Oberschenkelschaftfraktur im Kindesalter. Zentrabl Chir 1976;101:177–179.
119. Schoenecker P, Manske P, Sertle G. Traumatic hip dislocation with femoral shaft fractures. Clin Orthop 1978;130:233–238.
120. Slater RNS, Allen PR. Traumatic hip dislocation with ipsilateral femoral shaft fracture in a child: an open and closed case. Injury 1992;23:60–61.
121. Trillat A, Ringot A. Erreurs d'interpretation radiographique dans les fractures du cotyle avec luxation de la tete femorale. Lyon Chir 1951;46P:472–475.
122. Vialas M. Luxation traumatique de la hanche avec fracture diaphysaire du fémur chez une enfant de cinq ans. Rev Chir Orthop 1986;72:81–84.
123. Wadsworth TG. Traumatic dislocation of the hip with fracture of the shaft of the ipsilateral femur in a 3 year old. J Bone Joint Surg Br 1961;43:47–49.

SCFE Complicating Reduction

124. Barbieri M. Distacco-lussazione dell'epifisi femorale prossimale. Chir Organi Mov 1955;41:338–339.
125. Barquet A, Vécsei V. Traumatic dislocation of the hip with separation of the proximal femoral epiphysis: report of two cases and review of the literature. Arch Orthop Trauma Surg 1984;103:219–223.
126. Bonvallet JM. Sur un cas exceptional de luxation traumatique de la hanche de l'enfant, associe an un decallement epiphysaire complet et a une fracture du noyau cephalique. Rev Chir Orthop 1965;51:723–728.
127. Cady RB. Posterior dislocation of the hip associated with separation of the capital epiphysis. Clin Orthop 1987;222:186–189.
128. Calderon M. Décollement et luxation traumatique de l'épiphyse supérieure du fémur. Cir App Locomotor 1950;7:393–398.
129. Collado JR, Vivas J, Sesma P. Asociacion de luxación posterior de cadera y epifisiolisis traumática femoral superior. Rev Ortop Trauma 1984;28:233–236.
130. Drevermann P. Isolierte luxatio iliaca des Schenkelkopfes bei traumatischer Epiphysenlösung. Dtsch Z Chir 1924;185:422–424.
131. Economou T, Gavrilita N, Nastase N. Formes rares de luxation traumatique de la hanche chez des enfants. Lyon Chir 1958;54:203–211.
132. Fiddian NJ, Grace DL. Traumatic dislocation of the hip in adolescence with separation of the capital epiphysis. J Bone Joint Surg Br 1983;65:148–149.
133. Fina CP, Kelly PJ. Dislocation of the hip with fractures of the proximal femur. J Trauma 1970;10:77–87.
134. Herring JA. Fracture dislocation of the capital femoral epiphysis. J Pediatr Orthop 1986;6:112–114.

135. Hougaard K, Thomsen PB. Traumatic posterior dislocation of the hip associated with separation of the capital epiphysis. Orthopedics 1990;13:891–894.
136. Langan P, Fontanetta AP. Reduction of dislocated hip with transepiphyseal fracture. Orthop Rev 1986;15:586–589.
137. Lesourd G. Luxation traumatique de la hanche droite, avec decallement epiphysaire de la tete femorale et fracture du sourcil cotyloidien posterieur chez un enfant de 15 ans. Rev Chir Orthop 1969;55:61–64.
138. Mass DP, Spiegel PG, Laros GS. Dislocation of the hip with traumatic separation of the capital femoral epiphysis. Clin Orthop 1980;146:184–187.
139. Pina-Medina A, Pardo-Montaner J. Triradiate cartilage fracture associated with a transepiphyseal separation of the femoral head: a case report. J Orthop Trauma 1996;10:575–585.
140. Poilleux-Edelman A. Fracture partielle de la tête fémoral associée a une luxation traumatique de la hanche. Rev Orthop 1949;35:3–4.
141. Ruffoni R. Su un raro caso di lussazione traumatica bilaterale d'anca associato a distacco epifisario prossimale del femore sinistro. Arch Orthop 1962;75:325–333.
142. Schiele E. Traumatische huftgelenksluxation mit femurkopf-epiphysenlösung und ihre behandlung durch kopfresektion und fascientransplantation. Chirurg 1947;17:703–707.
143. Walls JP. Hip-fracture dislocation with transepiphyseal separation: case report and literature review. Clin Orthop 1991;284:170–175.

Acetabular Fragment

144. Barrett IR, Goldberg JA. Avulsion fracture of the ligamentum teres in a child. J Bone Joint Surg Am 1989;71:438–439.
145. Bennett JT, Cash JD. Reduction of a nonconcentrically relocated hip dislocation in a seven year old boy. Clin Orthop 1992;280:208–213.
146. Cinats JG, Noreau MJ, Swersky JF. Traumatic dislocation of the hip caused by capsular interposition in a child. J Bone Joint Surg Am 1988;70:130–133.
147. Dameron TB. Bucket-handle tear of acetabulum accompanying posterior dislocation of the hip. J Bone Joint Surg Am 1959;41:131–134.
148. Dorrell JH, Catterall A. The torn acetabular labrum. J Bone Joint Surg Br 1986;69:400–403.
149. Frich LH, Lauritzen J, Juhl M. Arthroscopy in diagnosis and treatment of hip disorders. Orthopaedics 1989;12:389–392.
150. Hall RL, Scott A, Oakes JE, Urbaniak JR, Callaghan JJ. Posterior labral tear as a block to reduction in an anterior hip dislocation. J Orthop Trauma 1990;4:204–207.
151. Harder JA, Bobechko WP, Sullivan R, Daneman A. Computerized axial tomography to demonstrate occult fractures of the acetabulum in children. Can J Surg 1981;24:409–411.
152. Huo MA, Root L, Baly RL, Mauri TM. Traumatic fracture-dislocation of the hip in a 2 year old child. Orthopedics 1992;15:1430–1433.
153. Judet J, Judet R, Letournel E, Vacher D. L'incarceration fragmentaire au cours des fractures du cotyle. Presse Med 1968;76:411–414.
154. Kaelin A. Une cause rare de blocage traumatique de la hanche chez l'enfant. Int Orthop 1984;8:9–12.
155. Lachertz M, Noel JL, Fontaine C, Hodin B. Les lesions associées et les complications propres aux fractures du bassin chez l'enfant. Chirurgie 1980;106:541–545.
156. Lesourd G. Luxation traumatique de la hanche avec decollement epiphysaire de la tete femorale et fracture du sourcil cotyloidien posterieur. Rev Chir Orthop 1969;55:55–59.
157. Lieberman JR, Altchek DW, Salvati EA. Recurrent dislocation of a hip with a labral lesion: treatment with a modified Bankart-type repair. J Bone Joint Surg Am 1993;75:1524–1527.
158. Nishii T, Nakanishi K, Sugano N, Naito H, Tamura S, Ochi T. Acetabular labral tears: contrast-enhanced MR imaging under continuous leg traction. Skeletal Radiol 1996;25:349–356.
159. Paterson I. The torn acetabular labrum: a block to reduction of a dislocated hip. J Bone Joint Surg Br 1957;39:306–309.
160. Rashleigh-Belcher HJC, Cannon SR. Recurrent dislocation of the hip with a "Bankart-type" lesion. J Bone Joint Surg Br 1986;68:398–399.
161. Santora SD, Stevens PM, Coleman SS. Intraarticular loose bodies in the adolescent hip: results of treatment of those recognized late. J Pediatr Orthop 1990;10:261–264.
162. Shea KP, Kalamchi A, Thompson GH. Acetabular epiphysis-labrum entrapment following traumatic anterior dislocation of the hip in children. J Pediatr Orthop 1986;6:215–219.
163. Sprenger TR. Fracture of the acetabulum in a 14 year old patient. Orthop Rev 1984;13:709–716.
164. Wilchinsky ME, Pappas AM. Unusual complications in traumatic dislocation of the hip in children. J Pediatr Orthop 1985;5:534–539.

Ischemic Necrosis

165. Barquet A. Avascular necrosis following traumatic hip dislocation in childhood. Acta Orthop Scand 1982;53:809–813.
166. Barquet A. Natural history of avascular necrosis following traumatic hip dislocation in childhood. Acta Orthop Scand 1982;53:815–820.
167. Bucholz RW, Ogden JA. Patterns of ischemic necrosis of the proximal femur in nonoperatively treated congenital hip disease. In: The Hip, vol 6. St. Louis: Mosby, 1978.
168. Choyce CC. Traumatic dislocation of the hip in childhood and relation of trauma to pseudocoxalgia. Br J Surg 1924;12:52–55.
169. Elmslie RC. Pseudocoxalgia following traumatic dislocation of the hip in a boy aged four years. J Orthop Surg 1919;1:109–110.
170. Elmslie RC. Traumatic dislocation of the hip in the child age seven with subsequent development of coxa plana. Proc R Soc Med 1932;25:1100–1102.
171. Fairbank HAT. Case of pseudo-coxalgia following traumatic dislocation in a boy. Proc R Soc Med (Sect Orthop) 1924;17:40.
172. Goldenberg R. Traumatic dislocation of the hip followed by Perthes disease. J Bone Joint Surg 1938;20:770–772.
173. Haliburton RA, Brockenshire FA, Barber JR. Avascular necrosis of the femoral capital epiphysis after traumatic dislocation of the hip in children. J Bone Joint Surg Br 1961;43:43–47.
174. Hammelbo T. Traumatic hip dislocation in childhood. Acta Orthop Scand 1976;47:546–551.
175. Kleinberg S. Aseptic necrosis of the femoral head following traumatic dislocation: report of two cases. Arch Surg 1939;39:637–639.
176. Li KCP, Hiette P. Contrast-enhanced fat saturation magnetic resonance imaging for studying the pathophysiology of osteonecrosis of the hips. Skeletal Radiol 1992;21:375–379.
177. Maffei F. Contribute alla studio della lussazione traumatica dell' anca nell infanzia. Chir Organi Mov 1922;6:604–607.
178. McCue SF. Bliven FE, Shaker IJ, Hall LH. An unusual vascular injury in the region of the hip in a child. J Bone Joint Surg Am 1994;76:1717–1719.
179. Mutschler HM. Sekundare Oberschenkelkopf-necrose nach traumatischer Ausrenkung des Huftgelenkes bei einem 14 Jahrigen. MMW 1939;86:258–261.

180. Ogden JA. Anatomic and histologic study of factors affecting development and evolution of avascular necrosis in congenital dislocation of the hip. In: The Hip, vol 2. St. Louis: Mosby, 1974.
181. Ogden JA. Changing patterns of proximal femoral vascularity. J Bone Joint Surg Am 1974;56:941–945.
182. Petrini A, Grassi G. Long-term results in traumatic dislocation of the hip in children. Ital Orthop Traumatol 1983;9: 225–230.
183. Poggi JJ, Callaghan JJ, Spritzer CE, Roark T, Goldner RD. Changes on magnetic resonance images after traumatic hip dislocation. Clin Orthop 1995;319:249–259.
184. Quist-Hanssen S. Caput necrosis after traumatic dislocation of the hip in a 4-year-old boy. Acta Chir Scand 1945;92: 393–402.
185. Scholder-Dumur C. Necrose de la tete femorale a la situe d'une luxation traumatique de la hanche chez l'enfant. Rev Chir Orthop 1959;45:504–505.
186. Shim SS. Circulatory and vascular changes in the hip following traumatic hip dislocation. Clin Orthop 1979;140:255–261.
187. Trueta J. The normal vascular anatomy of the human femoral head during growth. J Bone Joint Surg Br 1957;39:358–394.

Recurrent Dislocation

188. Aufranc OE, Jones WN, Harris HH. Recurrent traumatic dislocation of the hip in a child. JAMA 1964;190:291–294.
189. Body J. Luxation recidivante de la hanche chez un garcon de 7 ans. Rev Chir Orthop 1969;55:65–68.
190. Duytjes F. Recurrent dislocation of the hip joint in a boy. J Bone Joint Surg Br 1963;45:432.
191. Gaul RW. Recurrent traumatic dislocation of the hip in children. Clin Orthop 1973;90:107–109.
192. Gula D. Recurrent traumatic dislocation of the hip in children. J Am Osteopath Assoc 1972;72:32–39.
193. Hensley CD, Schofield GW. Recurrent dislocation of the hip. J Bone Joint Surg Am 1969;51:573–577.
194. Hohmann D. Recidivierende traumatische Huftluxation beim Kind nach fehlerhafter Gipsfixation. Monatsschr Unfallheikd 1964;67:352–355.
195. Klein A, Sumner TE, Volberg FM, Orbon RJ. Combined CT-arthrography in recurrent traumatic hip dislocation. AJR 1982;138:963–964.
196. Liebenberg F, Dommisse GF. Recurrent post-traumatic dislocation of the hip. J Bone Joint Surg Br 1969;51:632–637.
197. Llagone B, Sandra J, de Miscault G, David S. A propos d'une luxation traumatique de hanche mal réduite chez l'enfant. J Chir (Paris) 1987;124:57–58.
198. Niloff R, Petrie JG. Traumatic recurrent dislocation of the hip: report of a case. Can Med Assoc J 1950;62:574–576.
199. Simmons RL, Elder JD. Recurrent post-traumatic dislocation of the hip in children. South Med J 1972;65:1463–1466.
200. Slavik M, Dungl P, Spindorich J, Stedry V. Recurrent traumatic dislocation of the hip in a child: significance of early hip arthrography. Arch Orthop Traum 1986;104:385–388.
201. Sullivan CR, Bickel WH, Lipscomb PR. Recurrent dislocation of the hip. J Bone Joint Surg Am 1955;37:1266–1270.
202. Townsend RG, Edwards GE, Bazant FJ. Post traumatic recurrent dislocation of the hip without fracture. J Bone Joint Surg Br 1969;51:194.

Osteochondrosis

203. Cros A. Osteochondrosis of the upper femoral epiphysis following traumatic dislocation of the hip joint. J Bone Joint Surg Am 1959;41:1335–1338.

Nerve Injury

204. Kleiman SG, Stevens J, Kolb L, Pankovich A. Late sciatic nerve palsy following posterior fracture-dislocation of the hip. J Bone Joint Surg Am 1971;53:781–782.

Hip Fusion

205. Choyce CC. Traumatic dislocation of the hip in childhood and relation of trauma to pseudocoxalgia. Br Surg 1924/1925;12: 52–59.
206. Fulkerson JP. Arthrodesis for disabling hip pain in children and adolescents. Clin Orthop 1977;128:296–301.
207. Mowery CA, Houkom JA, Roach JW, Sutherland DH. A simple method of hip arthrodesis. J Pediatr Orthop 1986;6:7–10.
208. Murrell GAC, Fitch RD. Hip fusion in young adults: using a medial displacement osteotomy and cobra plate. Clin Orthop 1994;300:147–154.
209. Price CT, Lovell WW. Thompson arthrodesis of the hip in children. J Bone Joint Surg Am 1980;62:1118–1123.
210. Sponseller PD, McBeath AA, Perpich M. Hip arthrodesis in young patients: a long-term follow-up study. J Bone Joint Surg Am 1984;66:853–859.

Obstetric Injuries

211. Elizalde EA. Obstetrical dislocation of the hip associated with fracture of the femur. J Bone Joint Surg Am 1946;28:838–841.

Snapping Hip Syndrome

212. Lyonds JC. The snapping iliopsoas tendon. Mayo Clin Proc 1984;59:327–332.
213. Schaberg JE, Harper MC, Allen W. The snapping hip syndrome. Am J Sports Med 1984;12:361–365.
214. Staple TW. Arthrographic demonstration of iliopsoas bursa extension of the hip joint. Radiology 1972;102:515–516.
215. Vaccaro JP, Sauser DD, Beals RK. Iliopsoas bursa imaging: efficacy in depicting abnormal iliopsoas tendon motion in patients with internal snapping hip syndrome. Radiology 1995;197:853–856.

Voluntary Dislocation

216. Ahmadi B, Harrkes MB. Habitual dislocation of the hip. Clin Orthop 1983;175:209–212.
217. Broudy AS, Scott AD. Voluntary posterior hip dislocation in children. J Bone Joint Surg Am 1975;57:716–717.
218. Chan YL, Cheng JCY, Tang APY. Voluntary habitual dislocation of the hip: sonographic diagnosis. Pediatr Radiol 1193;23:147–148.
219. Goldberg L, Rousso I. Voluntary habitual dislocation of the hip. J Bone Joint Surg Am 1984;66:1117–1119.
220. Hikkinen ES, Sulama M. Recurrent dislocation of the hip: a case report. Acta Orthop Scand 1971;42:58–62.
221. Iwamoto Y, Katsuki I, Eguchi M, Oishi T, Sugioka Y, Saski K. Voluntary dislocation of both hips in a child. Int Orthop 1989;13:283–285.
222. Keret D, Reis ND. Voluntary habitual dislocation of the hip joint in a child: case report. J Pediatr Orthop 1986;6:222–223.
223. Mastromario R, Impagliazzo A. Voluntary dislocation of the hip (case report). Ital J Orthop Trauma 1979;5:219–224.

224. Moon M-S, Sun DH, Moon Y-W. Habitual voluntary dislocation of the hip in a child: a case report. Int Orthop 1996;20:330–332.
225. Petterson H, Theander G, Danielsson L. Voluntary habitual dislocation of the hip in children. Acta Radiol Diagn 1980;21:303–307.
226. Stuart PR, Epstein HP. Habitual hip dislocation. J Pediatr Orthop 1991;11:541–543.
227. Takekowa Y, Okulo K, Nagafuchi T, Murata K, Moriyama M. Voluntary dislocation of the hip in a child (in Japanese). Orthop Surg 1987;38:1592–1595.

21
Femur

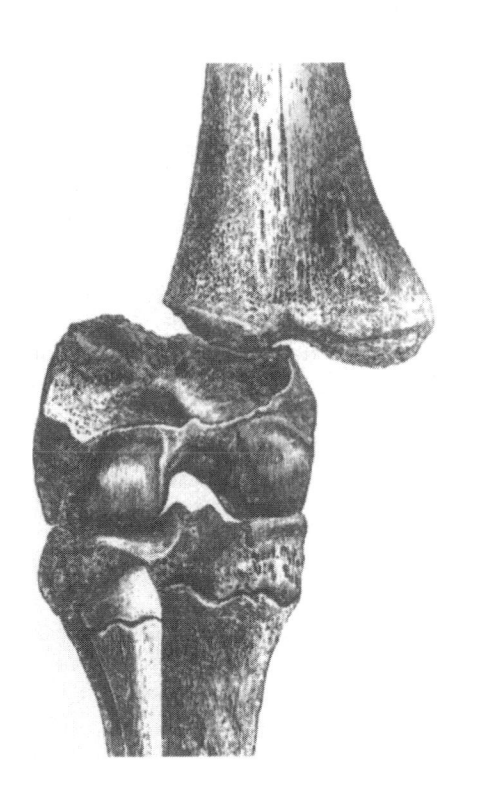

Engraving of a specimen of type 1 growth mechanism fracture of the distal femur. (From Poland J. Traumatic Separation of the Epiphyses. *London: Smith, Elder, 1898)*

The femur is the longest bone in the human body. It must develop appropriately at both the proximal and distal ends to allow coordinated musculoskeletal activity at the hip and knee. Subtle as well as major alterations of development consequent to trauma may alter normal bone and joint morphology and adversely affect the biomechanics of a specific joint if not the entire leg.

Anatomy

Proximal Femur

Development of the proximal femoral chondro-osseous epiphysis and physis is probably the most complex of all the appendicular skeletal growth regions.[12] Figure 21-1 illustrates several stages in the development of the proximal femur. Perhaps the two most important features are (1) the continuity of epiphyseal and physeal cartilage along the posterosuperior neck throughout much of postnatal development and (2) the intracapsular course of the limited capital femoral blood vessels. Fortunately, significant growth mechanism injury secondary to direct trauma or selective vascular damage to the area is infrequent. When it does occur, however, complications assume great importance for subsequent morphology and hip and leg biomechanics.

Secondary ossification usually begins in the capital femur by 4–6 months postnatally (range 2–10 months). This process is a centrally located sphere of ossification that expands centrifugally, eventually conforming to the hemispheric shape of the articular surface by the time the child is 6–8 years old and forming a discrete subchondral plate that follows the capital femoral physeal contour. The ossification center is dependent on an intact vascular supply; and any temporary or permanent decrease in blood flow, as might be sustained with a femoral neck fracture, has variable effects on the ability of capital femoral ossification to continue normal maturation and chondro-osseous transformation.

Femoral Neck

Throughout most of the development the capital femoral and trochanteric epiphyses have a cartilaginous continuity along the posterior and superior portions of the femoral neck (Fig. 21-2).[12] Although this region gradually thins as the child grows, it is essential for the normal latitudinal growth of the femoral neck (Fig. 21-2) and, in part, the normal decrease in anteversion. Damage, as with a femoral neck fracture, may seriously impair the capacity of these cartilaginous neck regions to develop normally. This posterosuperior

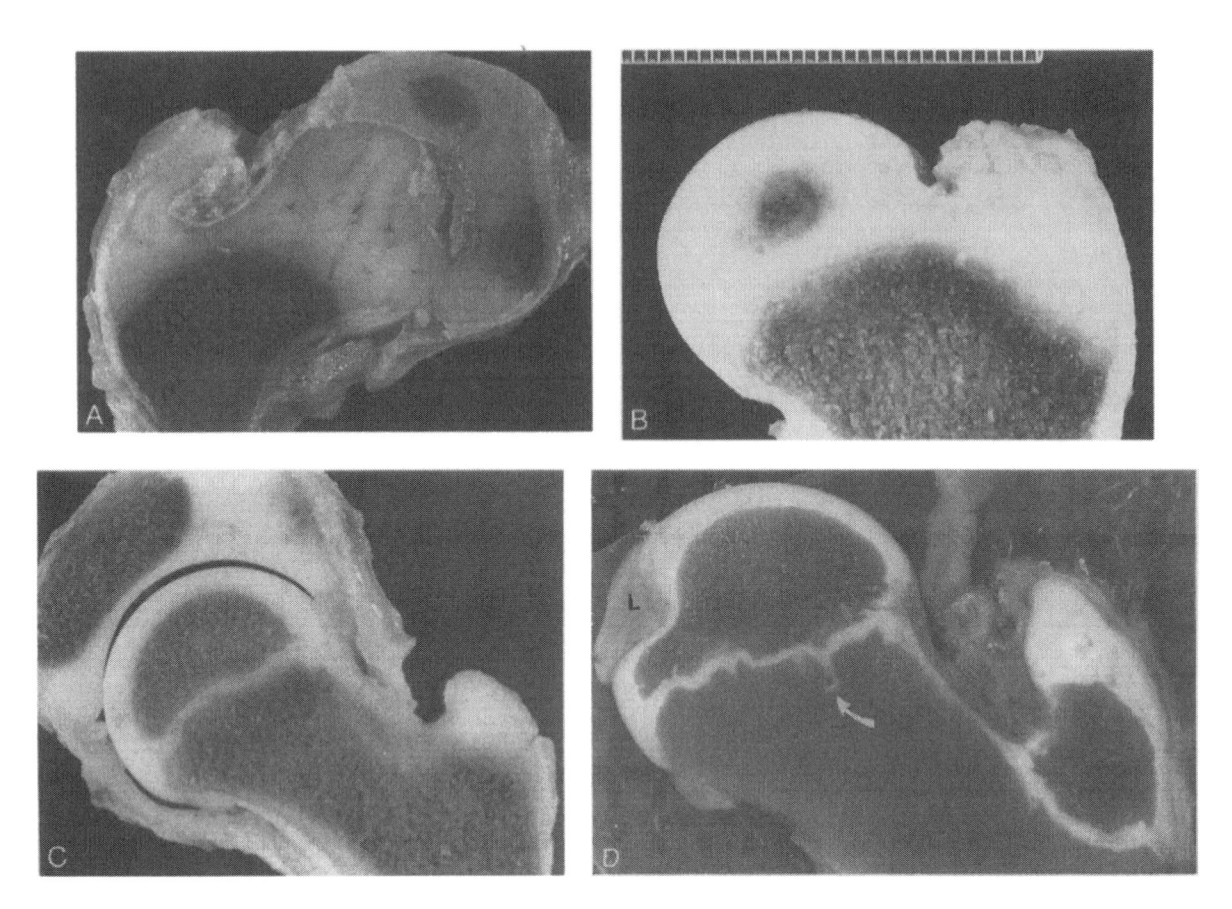

FIGURE 21-1. Slab sections showing proximal femoral development. (A) At 2 months a contiguous epiphysis encompasses the capital femur and greater trochanter. The intrinsic vascularity of the capital femoral cartilage is evident. (B) At 8 months the capital femoral ossification center is developing, and the femoral neck (metaphysis) is forming. (C) At 8 years undulations are developing in the capital femoral physis. (D) At 12 years there is a normal indentation of the ossification center at the site of attachment of the capital femoral ligament (L); the capital femoral physis is extensively undulated, and a mammillary process (arrow) is evident.

femoral neck cartilage is radiolucent. Hence the true extent of a femoral neck fracture may be underdiagnosed if only the osseous fracture line is considered. The blood vessels course along the posterosuperior femoral neck. However, they have a variable intracartilaginous course, which makes them more susceptible to fracture if the injury to the subcapital or neck region propagates into or through this cartilage.

Selective growth along the capital femorointertrochanteric physis establishes a discrete femoral neck. The primary spongiosa initially formed during neck development is not completely oriented to biologic forces across the hip joint. The more responsive secondary spongiosa begins to form the typical trabecular patterns oriented to compression and tension forces. This process becomes more prominent during the second decade of life. The area between these major osseous patterns is often referred to as Ward's triangle.

The development of the femoral neck brings about changes in the contour of the capital femoral physis. Initially, the femoral neck is transversely directed (Fig. 21-1); but during the first year there is preferential growth in the medial, and middle sections. As these regions develop, the capital femoral physis becomes more medially (varus) and posteriorly oriented, which eventually may predispose to slipped capital femoral epiphysis. Lappet formation, undulations, and mammillary processes develop in the physis (Fig. 21-1), again becoming more evident after 10 years of age. These processes and contours serve to "anchor," or stabilize, the capital femoral epiphysis to prevent displacement due to biologic shear stresses.

Greater Trochanter

Ossification begins in the greater trochanter at 5–7 years (Fig. 21-3) and is initially present directly above the trochanteric physis. With further development, ossification proceeds cephalad into the remainder of the epiphysis. This cartilaginous portion may be injured without obvious roentgenographic evidence. Epiphysiodesis of the greater trochanter occurs at 14–16 years (usually later than in the capital femoral physis).

The greater trochanter typically is considered a "traction apophysis," but this is a simplistic misconception. The biomechanical forces are usually schematically depicted as traction applied at the tip of the trochanter. In reality, there are multiple muscle attachments and forces on the entire surface, including attachments of the quadriceps (vastus

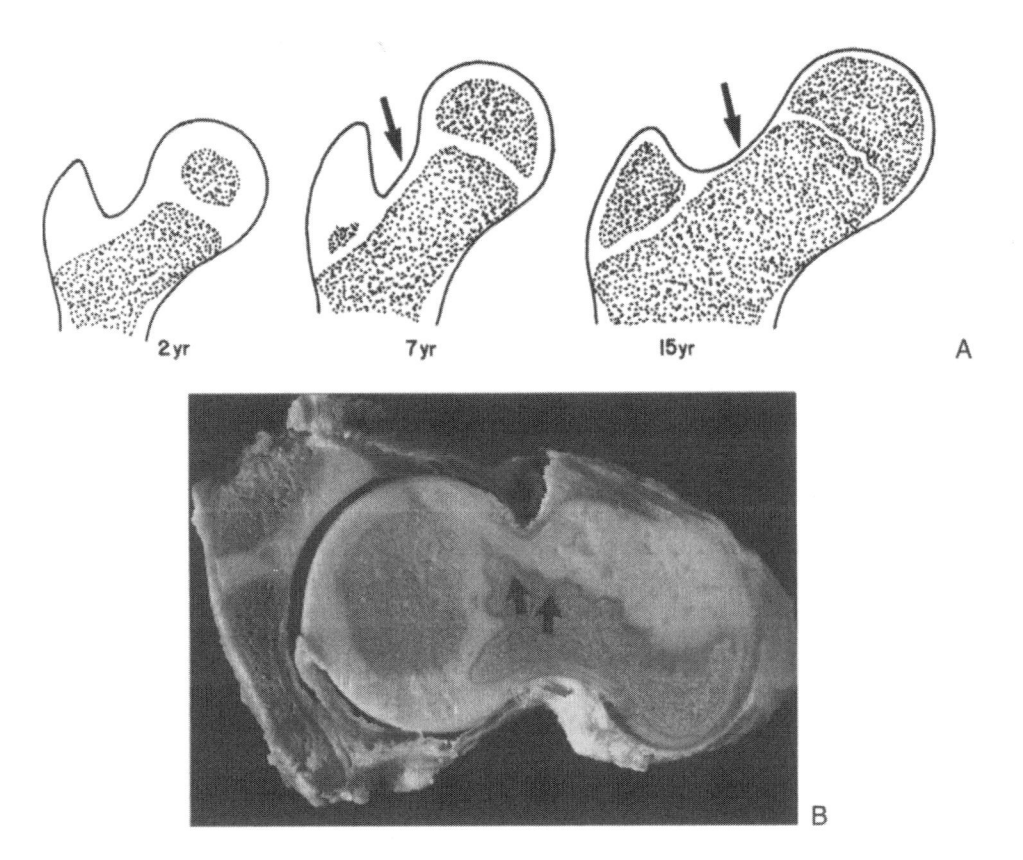

FIGURE 21-2. (A) Progressive proximal femoral development. A segment of physeal cartilage (arrows) is present along the posterosuperior femoral neck throughout most of development. It is necessary for widening of the femoral neck and posteriorly directed growth of the femoral neck to spontaneously decrease the amount of anteversion. (B) Transverse section through the proximal femur showing the capital femoral epiphysis and the posterior cartilaginous continuity (arrows) with the unossified greater trochanter.

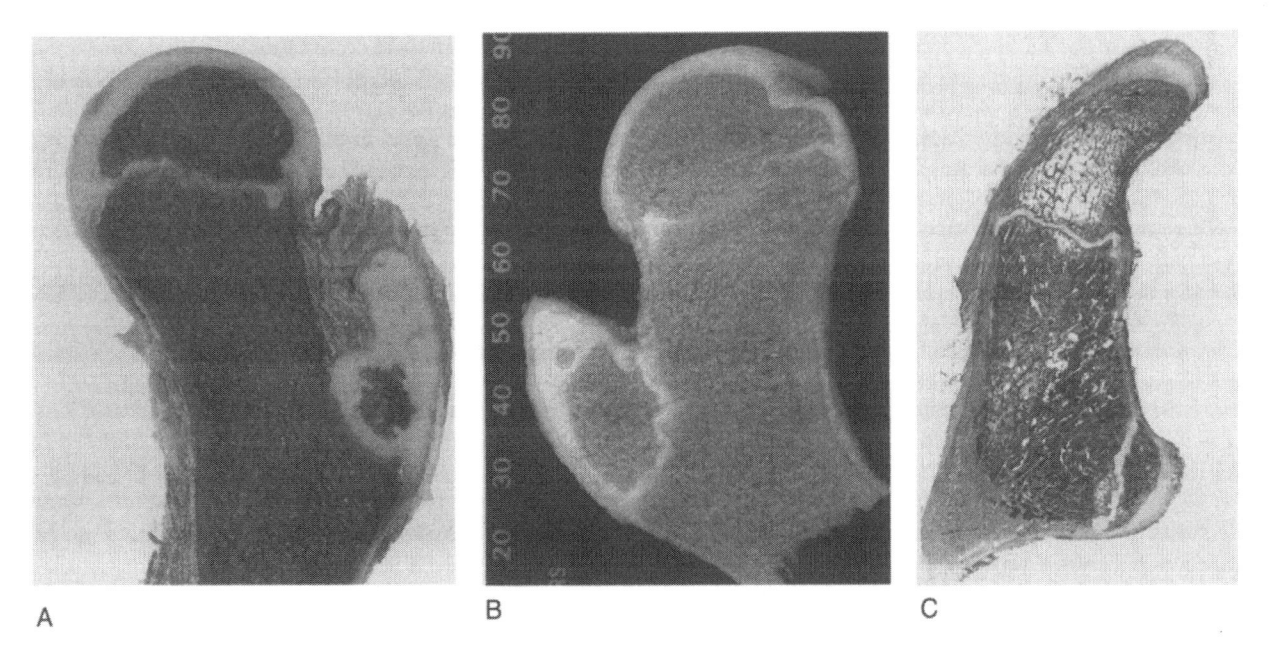

FIGURE 21-3. (A) Development of trochanteric ossification in an 8-year-old child, showing the irregular margins of secondary ossification and the extensive cartilaginous nature of the trochanteric epiphysis, especially proximally at the tip. (B) Later stage (12 years) showing an accessory (tertiary) ossification center. (C) Histologic section through the greater and lesser trochanters in a 15-year-old boy.

lateralis) and the posteriorly located external rotators (gemelli, piriformis). There is also overlying compression from the tensor fascia and muscle. The summated vector force is compression, which is reflected in the histologic appearance of the greater trochanteric physis.

Growth occurs through the trochanteric physis and interstitial expansion. True growth does not occur proximally, as some have suggested. Rather, this presumed proximal growth is, in reality, an expansion of ossification into the already formed cartilage. Magnetic resonance imaging (MRI) readily shows such unossified, but well-formed, trochanteric cartilaginous morphology.

Lesser Trochanter

The lesser trochanter does not usually ossify until adolescence (Fig. 21-3). Fusion occurs between 15 and 19 years. This region is subject to high tensile stresses from the attached iliopsoas tendon and represents a traction apophysis. Overgrowth may occur owing to chronic stress, as with cerebral palsy.

Proximal Vascularity

The blood supply to the proximal femur varies with the extent of skeletal maturation.[6,7,8,10,11,18,19] A vascular loop circles the capsular insertion at the base of the femoral neck, adjacent to the greater trochanter. A limited number of vessels cross the capsule and extend toward the capital femur. Their course is defined by morphology. A short femoral neck is present in the infant, whereas the teenager has an elongated neck. Essentially, a small group of vessels traverses the inferior femoral neck to a retinacular reflection, entering the medial side of the capital femoral epiphysis. Another group of vessels courses along the superoposterior portion of the developing femoral neck. Some of these vessels may become encased in the cartilage along the femoral neck. This posterosuperior vascular grouping enters the lateral side of the capital femoral epiphysis and becomes the dominant blood supply. Unfortunately, because of the close proximity to, or even incorporation into, the femoral neck cartilage, these vessels are at risk for disruption whenever the femoral neck or capital femur sustains a fracture.

The greater trochanteric blood supply is derived from the aforementioned extracapsular loop and other vascular systems. It is not particularly susceptible to traumatically induced vascular damage. Accordingly, trauma that affects capital femoral circulation creates a situation comparable to the ischemic necrosis seen with developmental hip dysplasia, namely, disruption of capital femoral growth and maturation coupled with normal growth and maturation of the greater trochanter. This causes variable morphologic change to the proximal femur, contingent on the age of the patient and the extent of vascular disruption.

Femoral Diaphysis

The diaphysis is a long cylinder of heavy, compact bone composed of progressively modeled and remodeled osteon structure. The femoral diaphysis is the only region to have significant osteon conversion of woven (fetal) bone during the perinatal period. The lack of well-defined osteons probably is a factor in the rapid healing associated with perinatal and infantile femoral fractures. The diaphyseal bone normally is bowed anteriorly and laterally. Treatment methods for femoral shaft fractures should be directed at some restoration of this anterolateral bowing, even when the fragments are left overriding. The linea aspera is a sturdy, elevated ridge that extends along the posteromedial surface of the femoral shaft. This ridge acts as a thickened buttress, providing strength and serving as a longitudinal musculofascial attachment.

The circulation of the diaphysis and the proximal and distal metaphyses is derived from the nutrient artery and from a peripheral circulation around each metaphysis. Vessels derived from the nutrient artery course toward each end of the bone, supplying small vessels to the marrow and endosteal circulation. At each end the vessels ramify to create a more retiform network within the metaphysis. These vessels end as vascular loops that abut the hypertrophic cells of the growth plate, and they contribute to the chondroosseous transformation of these cells.

Distal Femur

The epiphyseal ossification center of the distal femur is usually present at birth if the infant is full term. Expansion occurs relatively rapidly to fill both condylar regions (Fig. 21-4).[5,13] This area is the largest and most actively growing epiphyseal-physeal unit in the body, contributing almost 70% of the length of the femur and 40% of the entire leg. It fuses with the metaphysis at 14–16 years of age in girls and 16–18 years in boys. The distal epiphysis, which includes the entire articular surface of the lower end of the femur, serves as the origin of part of the gastrocnemius muscle.

The distal femoral physis is essentially a transverse plane at birth. As the infant commences walking and places increased weight-bearing and shearing forces across the knee, the distal femoral physis develops macroscopic undulations. Viewed from the anteroposterior projection, there appear to be two convexities directed toward the epiphyseal ossification center (Fig. 21-5). There is a central peak or apex directed toward the metaphysis. In the lateral view a similar binodal contour is evident. In three-dimensional terms there are four convex protuberances of the metaphysis and physis extending toward the epiphyseal ossification center. These extensions are directed at dissipating shearing and rotatory stress within the physis. In large animals that run and leap, the extension of these cones may be dramatic (see Chapter 1). The physis also exhibits microscopic undulations and mammillary processes, which represent further biomechanical adaptation to applied loads. Peripherally, physeal/epiphyseal lappet formation is evident and is most pronounced anteriorly in the patellofemoral groove.[4]

The distal femoral metaphysis is the site of numerous developmental (maturational) variations (Figs. 21-6 to 21-8) that should not be misconstrued as due to trauma. Fibrous cortical defects have been recognized as normal variants (Figs. 21-7, 21-8), although small pathologic fractures sometimes occur in these defects. Another relatively common lesion is the avulsive cortical irregularity. Although usually

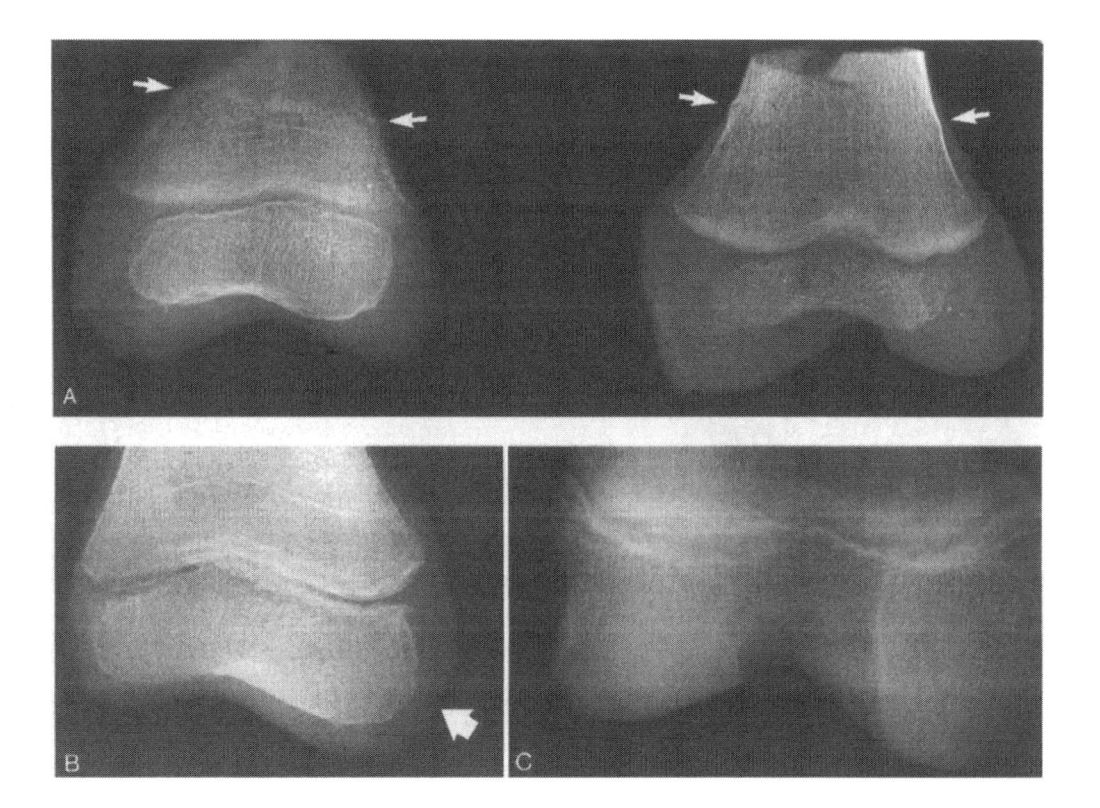

FIGURE 21-4. Roentgenographic development of the distal femur. (A) Serial sections from a 3-year-old child (accident victim). Note the differences in the physeal/metaphyseal contours. There is a torus fracture in the distal metaphysis (arrows). (B) Irregular medial ossification (arrow) is evident in this specimen from a 7-year-old. (C) Femur from a 15-year-old showing early stages of physiologic epiphysiodesis.

benign in appearance, these radiologically apparent cortical erosions are sometimes suggestive of destructive or infiltrative lesions such as osteomyelitis or osteogenic sarcoma.[1-3,14,15,17,20] The distal femoral metaphyseal "lesion" is almost exclusively located on the posteromedial aspect of the femoral condyle, above the adductor tubercle (Fig. 21-7). This portion of the medial ridge is the site of insertion of a portion of the transverse fibers of the adductor magnus aponeurosis. Intense bone remodeling usually occurs continuously in this region during periods of rapid skeletal growth. The cortex of the bone may be affected by this constant remodeling, so excessive mechanical stress produces microavulsions of the relatively porous cortical bone. These microavulsions may elicit a hypervascular, fibroblastic response, which in turn stimulates osteoclastic activity and bone resorption. In this way, a cycle of microfracture–resorption–microfracture is established. The rapid appearance and subsequent regression of the lesion and its common occurrence in active, adolescent boys suggest a mechanically induced lesion that may be a tension stress failure.

The circulation of the distal femur is multifocal.[4,9,16] Small vessels enter the epiphysis medially, laterally, and posteriorly. The main circulatory input/output is through the posterior femoral notch. As in the capital femoral epiphysis and spinal cord, there are "watershed" areas in the condyles (especially medially) that have limited circulation, and they may be susceptible to ischemic changes eventuating in osteochondritic lesions.

Proximal Femoral Injuries

Although proximal femoral fractures are infrequent injuries in the immature skeleton, they have received considerable attention in the literature.[21-244] These fractures are more common in boys, with the male/female ratio approximately 3:2. Fractures may occur at any age, with the highest incidence being at 11–12 years. Proximal femoral fractures may occur at birth and must be isolated diagnostically from developmental hip dysplasia. The injury may also occur in an abused infant (Fig. 21-9). Because considerable violence is required to fracture the proximal femur in older children and adolescents, there are often accompanying injuries. During adolescence an acute injury represents one segment of the spectrum of slipped capital femoral epiphysis. Pathologic fractures (see Chapter 11) may occur in many diseased states, including renal osteodystrophy, fibrous dysplasia, bone cysts, hypothyroidism, juvenile rheumatoid arthritis, septic arthritis, and malignancies.

There are several important differences between proximal femoral fractures in adults and those in children. Because the combined periosteal-perichondrial region is much

862

21. Femur

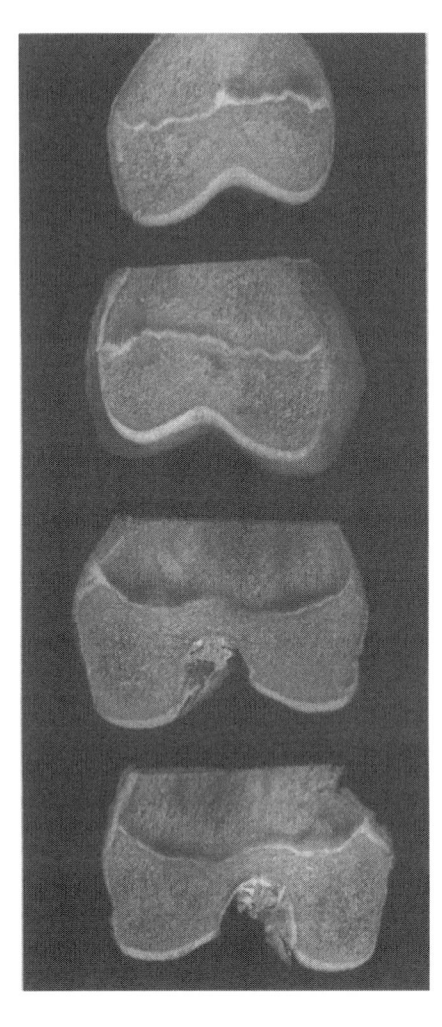

FIGURE 21-5. Undulating nature of the distal femoral physis. These are 5-mm serial slab sections of the same specimen. The contour variability affects physeal fracture patterns.

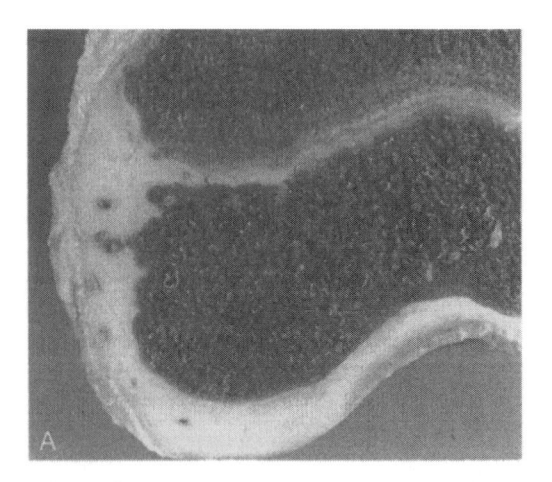

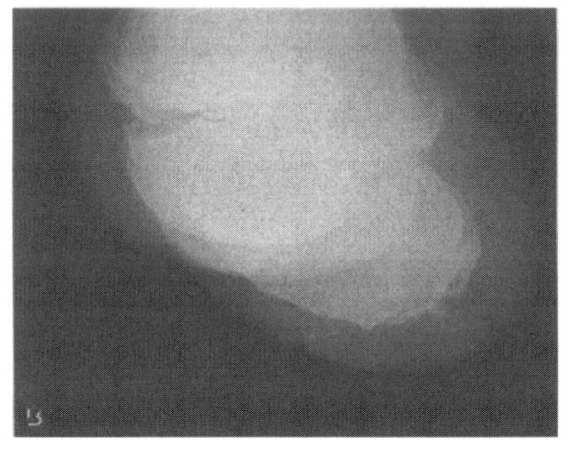

FIGURE 21-6. (A) Slab section showing irregularity of development of the medial side of a secondary ossification center. (B) Roentgenogram showing similar irregularity along the inferior region. These variations are normal.

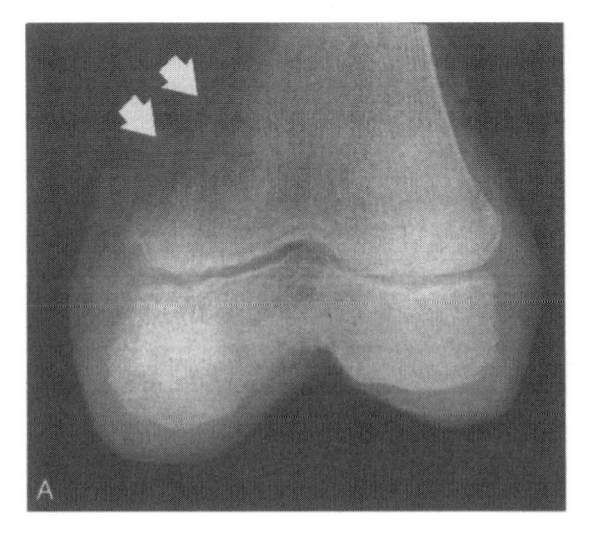

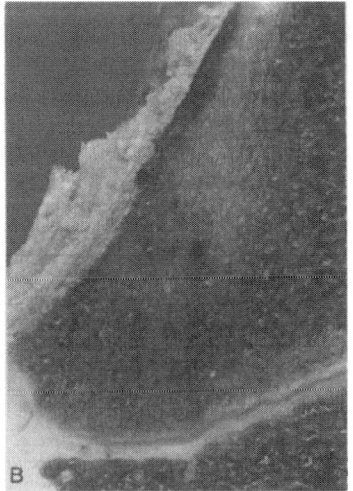

FIGURE 21-7. (A) Roentgenogram of 6-year-old child showing irregularity of the distal femoral metaphysis medially at the adductor insertion (arrows). Compare this cortex with the lateral cortex. (B) Sclerotic and porotic bone characteristic of this region.

Proximal Femoral Injuries

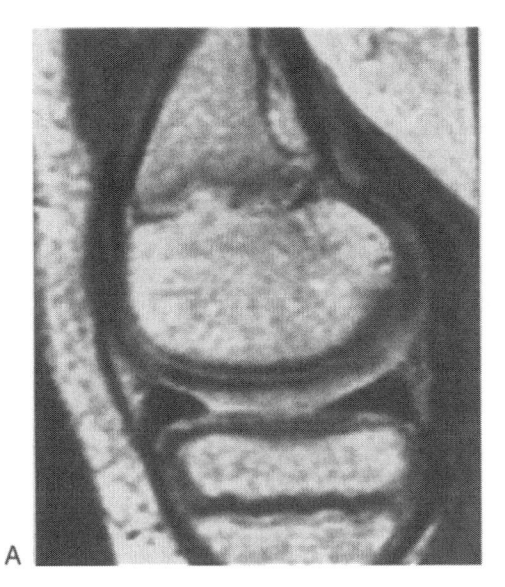

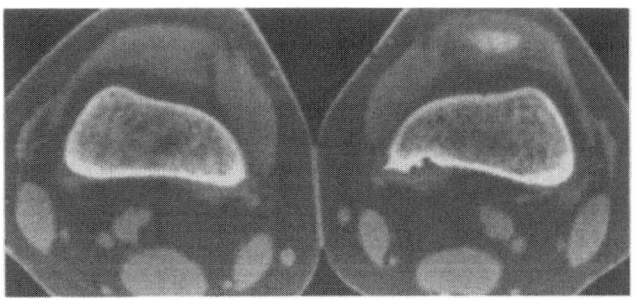

FIGURE 21-8. Typical posterior fibrous cortical defect. (A) MRI shows the osseous demarcation and continuous fibrous tissue. (B) CT shows indentation of the posteromedial cortex.

stronger in children, fractures are not always significantly displaced. In addition, the presence of the cartilaginous intraepiphyseal bridge along the superior and posterior aspect of the neck tends to prevent displacement of the physis unless this cartilage is also significantly disrupted, a factor that is impossible to discern with standard roentgenographic techniques. Damage to this region of cartilage may affect development of the femoral neck. A potential complication, ischemic necrosis, may affect, specifically or in combination, the epiphysis, the metaphysis, and the physis. The violence of the initial injury is generally blamed for the high incidence of ischemic necrosis in children (as high as 80–90% in some series, with an average of 40%). Direct damage to the vessels coursing along or within the intraepiphyseal cartilage may also be a factor.

Children generally readily tolerate the duration of cast immobilization necessary to attain acceptable union with an undisplaced or reduced fracture. However, malunion of the developing femoral neck is a real hazard if only casting is used. Like the lateral condylar fracture of the distal humerus, the femoral neck fracture has a reasonable risk of loss of reduction or nonunion in a young child because of the relatively constant micromotion even while in a cast. When a displaced or potentially unstable fracture is reduced and held in a cast, insidious, progressive coxa vara may still occur. The hardness of a child's bone and the small size of the femoral neck often limit the choice of fixation devices. Pins or screws of small caliber should be used. If transphyseal pins are necessary (as they often are), they must be smooth in the region that crosses the physis. Threaded fixation devices should not cross the physis. When fracture healing problems arise in a child, endoprosthetic replacement is usually *not* an available solution. Accordingly, avoidance of complications, especially ischemic necrosis, becomes paramount.

Classification

Proximal femoral fractures in children may occur at different levels along the femoral neck (Fig. 21-10). However, because the femoral neck is actively elongating and maturing, certain types cannot occur at young ages, and any given type may vary morphologically with age.

The type I injury can assume several patterns contingent on the age of the patient and the presence of predisposing disease conditions, such as a tumor or rickets. During the neonatal period and the first year of life, the entire proximal femoral chondroepiphysis, including the capital femur, the

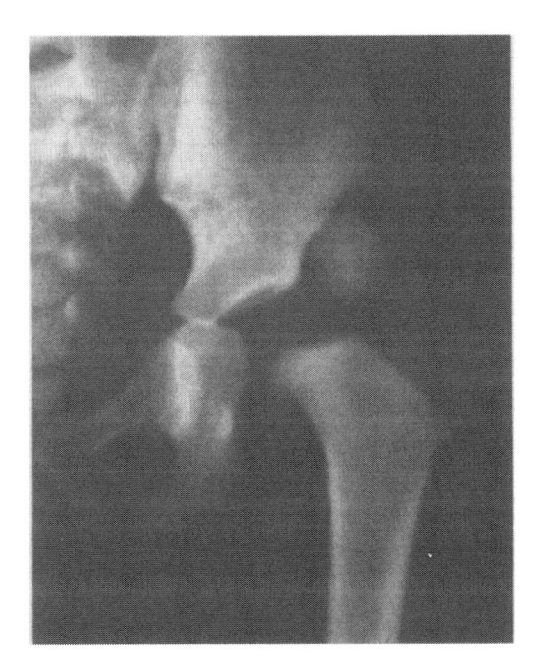

FIGURE 21-9. Type 1 injury of the capital femur in a 10-month-old victim of child abuse. The capital femur was completely dislocated.

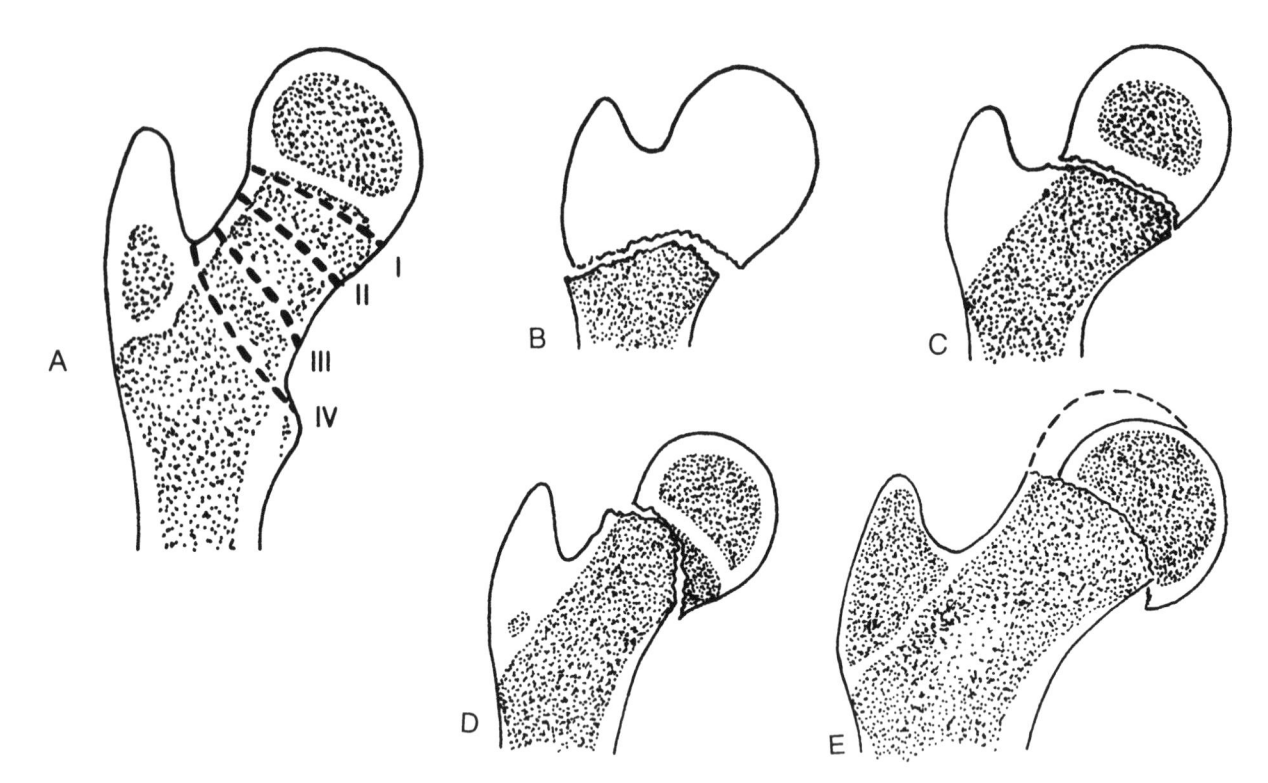

FIGURE 21-10. (A) Types of fracture of the femoral neck: type I, transphyseal injury; type II, transcervical injury; type III, cervicotrochanteric injury; type IV, peritrochanteric injury. A type I injury is transphyseal during infancy, but in the older child and adolescent the fracture splits the capital femoral and intraepiphyseal segments so a type 3 growth mechanism injury occurs. In pathologic conditions (e.g., renal rickets) the presence of the metaphyseal fragment indicates a type 4 growth mechanism injury. (B–E) Age-related variations of type I fractures. (B) Type I growth mechanism injury in an infant. (C) Type 3 growth mechanism injury in a 4-year-old child. (D) Type 3 growth mechanism injury in an adolescent (acute slipped capital femoral epiphysis). (E) Type 4 growth mechanism injury in a 7-year-old.

intraepiphyseal region, and the greater trochanter, traumatically separates as a contiguous, complete unit. The lesser trochanter may or may not be included depending on the patient's age and the mechanism of injury. As is discussed later, increased medial disruption may cause localized type 5 injury with the potential for temporary or permanent growth arrest and a progressive traumatic coxa vara. As the anatomic femoral neck develops, the type I fracture pattern changes and increasingly localizes only to the capital femoral region. The fracture line may extend across the intraepiphyseal cartilage and along the capital femoral physis or partially along the capital femoral physis and into the metaphysis of the femoral neck. During adolescence the type I fracture involves the capital femoral physeal–metaphyseal interface, crossing the remnants of the intraepiphyseal region; this is an acute slipped capital femoral epiphysis.

Type II (transcervical) is a fracture through the midportion of the femoral neck. Type III is cervicotrochanteric, through the base of the femoral neck. Type IV is peritrochanteric, between the base of the femoral neck and lesser trochanter. The latter injury essentially follows the capsular insertions. Obviously, the length of the femoral neck affects which pattern is present at any given age.

A more realistic classification in children, because of the changing length of the neck, would be: I, physeal fracture; II, intracapsular neck fracture; and III, intertrochanteric fracture (at the capsular insertion or extracapsular). The distinction between transcervical and cervicotrochanteric is difficult to distinguish until adult morphology is reached at skeletal maturity.

Although limited development of the length of the neck affects the pattern of fracture, at least from the standpoint of defining types II, III, and IV, treatment is essentially the same; and the risks of complications such as ischemic necrosis and coxa vara are reasonably similar for all patterns. It is important to remember that there is a variably thick cartilaginous continuity along the posterosuperior neck (Fig. 21-2), and that most femoral neck fractures undoubtedly propagate into and through this area, essentially making types II, III, and IV each a type 4 growth mechanism injury, which requires reasonably accurate anatomic reduction to prevent or minimize subsequent growth deformity.

Transphyseal Injury (Type I)

A transphyseal fracture of the proximal femur of a young child is infrequent.* Such fractures occur insidiously in patients with myelomeningocele.[142] With the exception of birth trauma, these children often sustain multiple trauma. Transepiphyseal fractures infrequently are associated with dislocation of the capital femoral epiphysis from the acetabulum (see Chapter 20).

---

*Refs. 37–39,83,107,117,173,180,184,186,193,233,237.

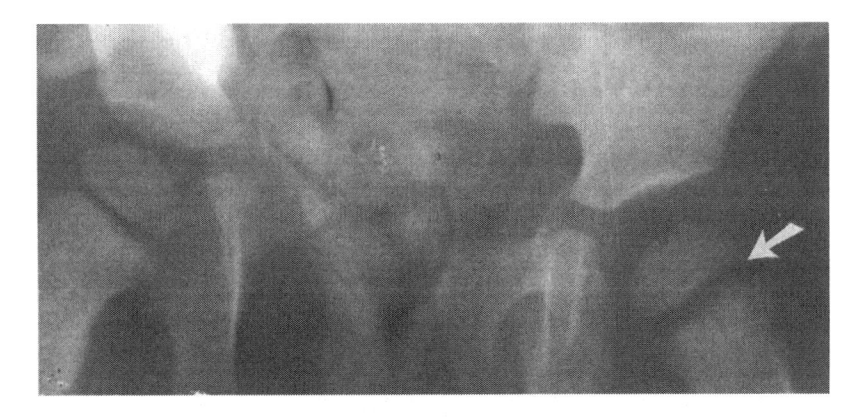

FIGURE 21-11. Type 1 injury with widening of the physis of the left capital femur (arrow).

This injury pattern may be difficult to diagnose in the young child (Fig. 21-11). The diagnosis must often be made as a clinical assumption, as roentgenographic corroboration may be lacking or difficult to visualize. The distinction from developmental hip dislocation may be difficult when the child is first seen, as a roentgenogram may show only upward and lateral displacement of the femoral shaft. A septic hip may also be difficult to distinguish from a traumatic lesion due to child abuse, particularly because both conditions can cause fever (blood in a joint may cause a temporary febrile response).

Milgram and Lyne obtained postmortem specimens from children who died of disease without osseous involvement.[142] Manipulative epiphyseal separation was produced by simultaneously rotating and bending the specimens. Microscopically, the zone of disruption was variably through the hypertrophic cell layer.

Radiographically, the separation occurs at the physis and may or may not be associated with displacement from the neck (Fig. 21-12). Because of anatomic constraints there may be only widening of the physis (Fig. 21-11). In the lateral view, the neck of the femur may be displaced forward in relation to the epiphysis, comparable to the type of external rotation that occurs with slipped capital femoral epiphysis. In some patients only widening of the physis is seen, without significant displacement. Wide displacement is uncommon because the periosteal and perichondrial attachments are usually intact. Displacement may occur only in certain ways because of the epiphyseal continuity along the posterosuperior surface of the neck. Displacement of the proximal fragment is most likely to be posterior.

Treatment must be individualized. Many of these fractures are minimally displaced (if at all) and clinically stable, which may be determined by ranging the hip under fluoroscopy. Thus whenever possible, conservative, nonoperative treatment is instituted, with resultant growth deformities corrected at a later date. If the fracture line is undisplaced or minimally displaced, the hip may be immobilized in a spica

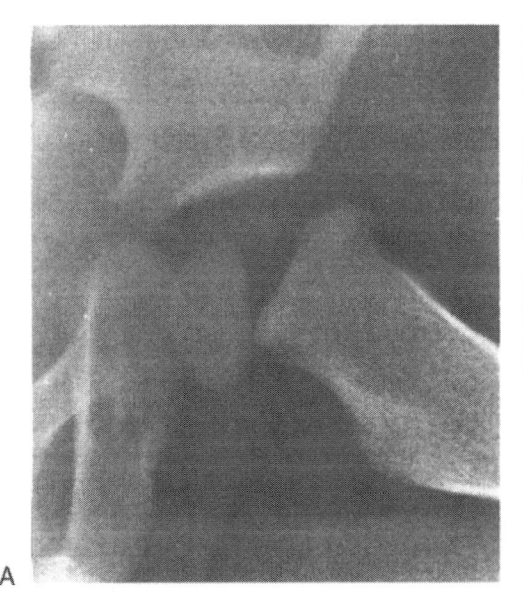

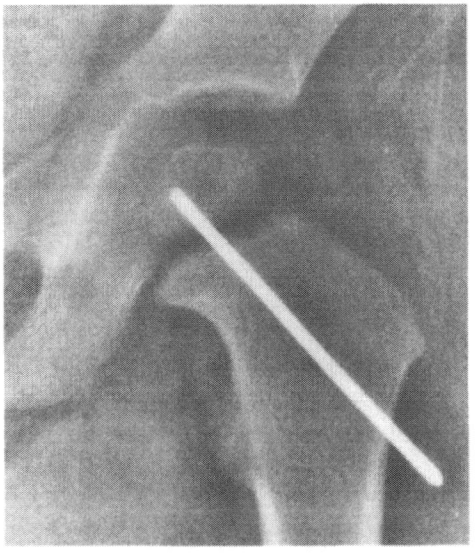

FIGURE 21-12. (A) Transphyseal fracture in an 11-month-old infant (unrestrained passenger in a motor vehicle accident). (B) Fracture was reduced under anesthesia, proved to be unstable, and was treated with a single smooth percutaneous pin, which was removed 6 weeks later. There was no subsequent growth arrest 3 years after the injury.

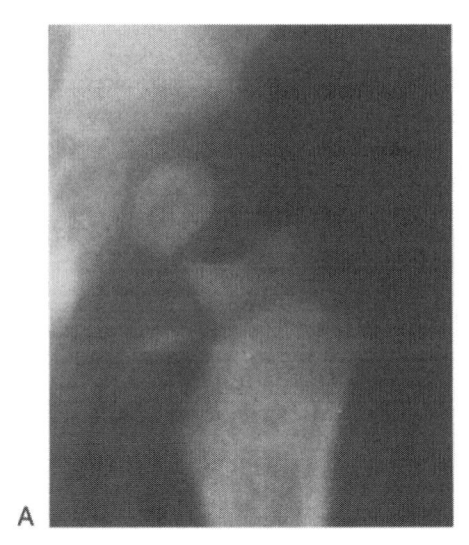

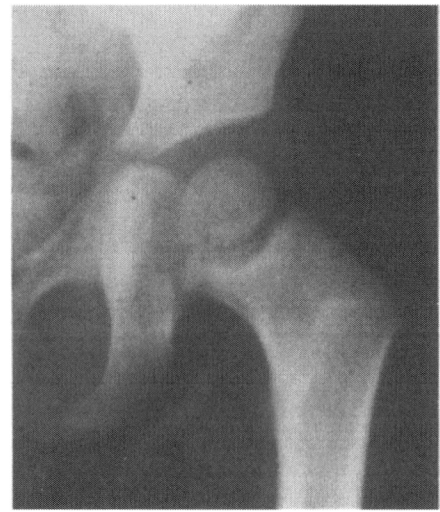

FIGURE 21-13. (A) Child abuse led to fracture of the proximal femur in this 7-month-old baby. (B) Mild deformity and concavity of the physeal metaphyseal interface at age 1 year.

cast, with the affected side in moderate abduction, neutral extension, and mild internal rotation. If displaced more than one-fourth of the physeal length, a gentle closed reduction with the patient under general anesthesia may be considered. In the older child, if displacement is significant and a manipulative reduction has to be undertaken, or if the fracture appears unstable to fluoroscopic examination, it may be necessary to fix the fracture internally with *smooth* pins that penetrate the epiphysis and then immobilize the hip in a spica cast. Four to six weeks is usually required to achieve osseous union sufficient to allow discontinuation of the casting. The pins should be left outside the skin or in the subcutaneous tissues so they can be removed within 4–8 weeks, at which time the physeal injury should be mechanically stable (although not necessarily stable for active, normal weight-bearing).

The potentially poor prognosis of these lesions must be emphasized to the parents. The prognosis may be guarded because of damage to the physis at the time of the injury, which may represent a localized type 5 injury, or because of vascular injury that eventually leads to radiographic evidence of ischemic necrosis (Fig. 21-13). Each patient must be carefully followed by periodic roentgenograms for the possible development of the complications of ischemic necrosis, coxa vara, or premature fusion of the physis. Premature fusion may occur even though there is no ossification center in the epiphysis at the time of the injury. Early treatment of complications by appropriate osteotomy may salvage the hip. Using fat interposition after resection of the osseous bridge in this particular region would not be easy and has not been reported.

Neonatal Injury (Type I)

Although infrequent, fractures involving the proximal femur in the neonate must be diagnostically differentiated from developmental hip dysplasia or infection (septic hip or proximal femoral osteomyelitis). Numerous authors have reported one or more cases of this injury.[39,142,162,163,189,228,245–289] The injury involves the entire proximal femoral epiphysis, which at birth is comprised of the capital femur, greater trochanter, and lesser trochanter. These regions do not become anatomically separate until several months after birth.

These particular proximal femoral fractures usually occur during a difficult delivery (Fig. 21-14), such as those involving breech or footling presentations. Michail and colleagues described obstetric separation of the upper femoral epiphysis and the appearance of the ossification center of the femoral head 15 days after birth; it was believed to be a consequence of the injury. They emphasized that "the existence of an obstetric (traumatic) dislocation of the hip has never been demonstrated,"[266] a concept with which I completely agree.

Prevot et al. reported obstetric disruption of the upper femoral epiphysis.[275] They noted that the fracture occurred even though the delivery was by cesarean section. Three patients were treated with traction followed by a hip spica cast, and one patient had a pin osteosynthesis. Two patients had an excellent result, but two patients had increased external rotation of the leg.

Fairhurst opened the hip of a 10-day-old baby who was the product of a difficult delivery and breech extraction.[257] They directly observed a severely displaced fracture between the cartilaginous head and neck and the osseous metaphysis. It was reduced and percutaneously pinned. There was normal development of the hip.

Meier reported two cases of children with epiphysiolysis consequent to birth trauma.[265] One of these children died several weeks later. An autopsy showed marked callus formation around the shaft with a fracture through the region just below the common growth plate. Pfeiffer[272] and Truesdell[287] described similar autopsy findings. Harrenstein manipulated hips of newborn cadavers and found that "the

Proximal Femoral Injuries

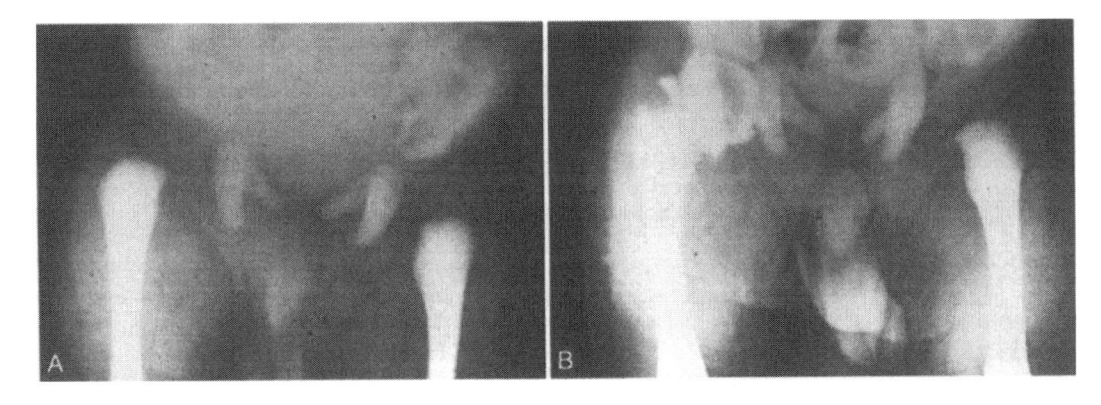

FIGURE 21-14. (A) This injury to the proximal femur occurred during birth. The hip appears to be dislocated. (B) Arthrogram shows an intact hip joint, and the hip eventually developed normally. The injury was a fracture, not a dislocation.

line of cleavage passed below the cartilage of the femoral head."[258]

Duplication of the lesion in stillborn cadavers shows that the fracture is usually a type 1 growth mechanism injury traversing the entire physis underneath both the capital femur and the greater trochanter (Fig. 21-15).[269,270] The periosteal sleeve is intact posteriorly and still attached to the proximal physis. There may be comminution (rather than crushing) of the epiphysis, physis, and metaphysis medially. Such longitudinal splitting and separation along cell columns, with these separations extending through the germinal zone and into the epiphysis, creates multiple, microscopic type 3 and 4 physeal injuries. Such findings of cellular microdisruption afford a more plausible explanation of premature growth arrest than the previously hypothesized type 5 mechanism of cellular crush injury within the terminal zone. Animal models have shown similar histologic damage.[270]

Acute traumatic dislocation of the femoral head in the newborn is essentially *nonexistent* because the ligaments and capsule, although they may be lax during the perinatal period owing to the influence of selective maternal hormones, are still biomechanically stronger than the proximal femoral physis. Any unstable (i.e., subluxating or dislocating) hip found during examination is invariably the result of *chronic*, progressive intrauterine deformation, and cartilaginous, ligamentous, and capsular distortion and stretching.

The clinical symptoms are characteristic. Swelling is reasonably constant in the inguinal crease, gluteal area, and proximal thigh. The newborn holds the leg in external rotation, flexion, and adduction, usually avoiding and resisting movements of the leg. Irritability during diaper changing is usually evident. Considerable pain, often with crepitation, is elicited, an important finding when distinguishing a fracture from developmental hip dysplasia, which is invariably pain-free. An almost constant feature appears to be pseudoparalysis of the affected limb. However, the "paralysis" rapidly disappears as the fracture becomes nonpainful through early healing and callus stabilization.

Roentgenograms usually show lateral displacement of the proximal femoral metaphysis (Fig. 21-14). The displacement may be slight and difficult to interpret. If the metaphysis appears to be displaced laterally, in the presence of a normal-appearing acetabulum, one should be suspicious of a fracture. Developmental hip dysplasia may be considered because of the superolateral displacement of the femur. However, the acetabulum usually has a normal acetabular index in a neonate with a proximal femoral fracture.

Whenever possible, the diagnosis should be made before fracture callus is evident (Fig. 21-16), as any anatomic deformity is undoubtedly irreducible at that stage. Subperiosteal ossification around the proximal metaphysis gives irrefutable evidence of the injury. Usually, such callus formation is evident within 8–14 days. This callus may be considerable, depending on both the extent of periosteal stripping at

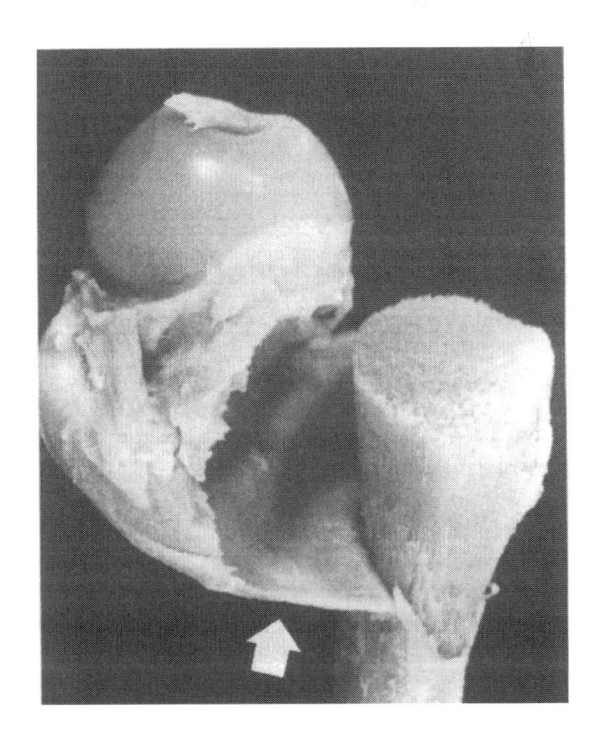

FIGURE 21-15. Experimental proximal femoral fracture. Posterior displacement associated with stripping of the posterior periosteum (arrow).

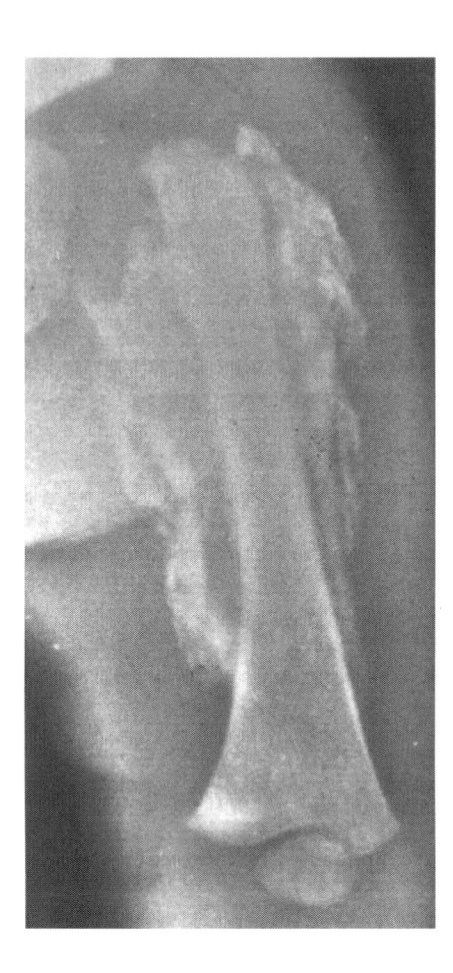

FIGURE 21-16. Extensive subperiosteal new bone. Note that the shaft is laterally displaced. The radiolucent proximal (capital) femur is still in the acetabulum.

the time of injury and how much continued motion the injury was subjected to until and after the diagnosis was made. Stripping and subperiosteal bleeding that further elevate the periosteum are present because the injury invariably occurs prior to the neonate receiving a prophylactic vitamin K injection.

Because the diagnosis is difficult when the clinical and routine radiographic findings are minimal, other diagnostic studies may be indicated. Arthrography may define the injury (Fig. 21-14). Injected dye should outline the anatomically located capital femur, although there may be extravasation of dye beyond the capsule, especially medially, where some of the metaphysis is normally within the capsular boundaries. Any joint fluid removed at the time of arthrography should be cultured to rule out an infectious process. Ultrasonography may be used to make the diagnosis. Diaz and Hedlund described the use of sonography to diagnosis traumatic separation of the proximal femoral epiphysis in a patient with myelomeningocele.[251]

Experimental observations regarding the periosteal sleeve are important. This structure is intact posteriorly and disrupted anteriorly, allowing the proximal metaphysis to "buttonhole" through the tear. The posterior attachment of the periosteum to the physeal periphery may be used to advantage during traction and reduction to introduce intrinsic stability, similar to the soft tissue continuity used in other areas (e.g., dorsally displaced fracture of the distal radius fracture). This practice contributes to fracture stability and prevents overreduction.

Traction seems to be the easiest method for controlling the fracture and is certainly the reasonable choice for initial management. The child is carefully placed in Bryant's traction with the hips flexed to 90° and the knees flexed 15°–20°. Skin traction straps should extend to the upper thigh. Only 1 pound (or less) may be necessary for *gentle suspension* of the legs in this position. This position usually corrects varus displacement and takes advantage of the *posteriorly intact* periosteal tissue. Once the child is pain-free (usually only a few days), an abduction pillow splint or Pavlik's harness may be used. Casting is used if the aforementioned methods are unsuccessful. The abduction device usually may be discontinued 4–6 weeks later. The rapid rate of healing supports conservative therapy. The long-term results are usually excellent, with a low incidence of growth complications.

Subsequent coxa vara has been described by a few authors.[247,258,260,261,265,267] Some degree of coxa vara was usually evident early in the healing phase because of the anatomy of the displacement. Usually such a varus deformity corrects itself within a few months and is followed by normal proximal growth, although it may persist as long as 4 years after the injury.[259,267] Some cases of congenital and infantile coxa vara are actually missed cases of neonatal epiphysiolysis or even intrauterine disruption.[261,267]

Cases of ischemic necrosis have been described following this specific neonatal fracture in the literature, but the anatomy of the fracture relative to the blood supply makes it unlikely. The fracture line is primarily extracapsular (subtrochanteric) and away from the main blood supply, which is proximal to the injury and should be relatively undisturbed.[270,280] In fact, the capital femoral ossification center may appear earlier than normal owing to a hyperemic, not ischemic, vascular response to the injury.[266]

Acute Slipped Capital Femoral Epiphyseal Injury (Type I)

Slipped epiphysis of the capital femur (SCFE) may occur with traumatic hip injury or dislocation.[290–318] These injuries are serious and are associated with a high incidence of complications. SCFE may also occur acutely without a concomitant dislocation. The distinction between acute and chronic cases of SCFE may be difficult. By definition, only slips seen within 3 weeks of the onset of symptoms and particularly after definable trauma are considered acute.[291]

This injury may occur in children with preexistent mild (chronic) slips or beginning (prodromal) symptoms. The femur undergoing physiologic and biomechanical changes that predispose it to eventual slipping may be acutely stressed, causing more significant displacement (Fig. 21-17). Acute slips of the proximal femoral epiphysis are usually characterized by abrupt onset of severe pain, limitation of motion, external rotation deformity, and the inability to bear

Proximal Femoral Injuries

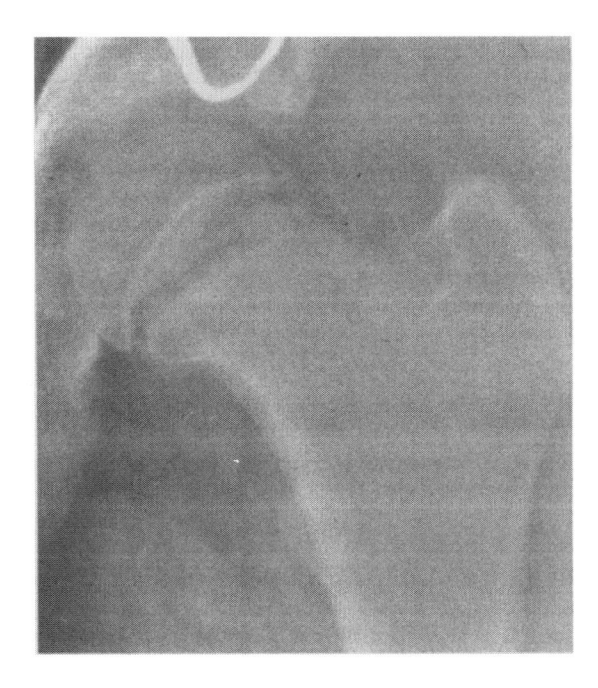

FIGURE 21-17. Acute-on-chronic slipped capital femoral epiphysis (SCFE). This patient had intermittent thigh pain for a month, followed by an acute increase in pain when he misjudged the height of a school bus step.

weight on the affected limb in association with a specific traumatic event (Fig. 21-18).

The acute cases do not differ significantly from the more common chronic type with regard to age, sex, or body build, except for the patients having concomitant hip dislocation. Prodromal symptoms of a dull ache or pain during the affected or ipsilateral knee may be present for extended periods, suggesting that acute slips do not necessarily occur only during the early phase of epiphysiolysis. In fact, Barash and associates showed a roentgenogram obtained 10 months prior to an acute slip, demonstrating early epiphysiolysis that had not been treated with prophylactic pinning.[291]

When symptoms have been present prior to the acute slipping or earlier roentgenograms showed mild slipping, there is little doubt that trauma only acutely precipitates further displacement. Prodromal symptoms were recorded in all patients reported by Fahey and O'Brien and in 60 of 89 acute cases reported in the literature.[299] Lack of complaints, however, does not exclude the possibility of mild asymptomatic slipping. It may be difficult to ascertain the relative importance of trauma in an adolescent without previous symptoms, especially when acute displacement of the capital femoral epiphysis is seen after a moderate to severe injury. Fahey and O'Brien believed that in only 17 cases from the literature was trauma the exclusive causal factor, and most of these cases occurred in the younger age group rather than in the group for which slip was characteristic.[299] The trauma sustained was usually severe, and associated injuries were frequently present. Of the reported cases, there were eight with complete dislocations of the capital femur from the acetabulum (see Chapter 20).

Several authors have described lateral slipping of the capital femoral epiphysis (epiphyseal coxa valga).[298,299,301,307,310,315,318] It seems likely that this direction of slipping occurs in the older child in whom there is a thin remnant of cartilage along the posterior femoral neck that allows the capital femur to be pushed laterally as it is slipping posteriorly. Rothermel also thought that the slip tended to occur more frequently in patients with a horizontally oriented growth plate.[310]

Some form of gentle closed reduction may be attempted for acute slipping, but closed reduction is not uniformly successful for repositioning. In general, most cases may be treated with balanced suspension, an internal rotation strap, and bed rest. Operative manipulation should be used cautiously. Fahey and O'Brien thought that the results of their 10 cases supported the observation that gentle manipulation was the preferred method of reduction, believing that the earlier closed reduction is attempted, the more likely it is to succeed in repositioning the femoral head, with minimal risk of vascular damage.[299] Traction is usually carried out with the hip in extension, which is a position that may increase joint pressure and predispose to vascular problems in an acutely injured and possibly effused joint. When traction or balanced suspension is used, with or without derotation straps, I believe that the hip should be flexed at least 30°. Gentle reduction attempts in the operating room should have the hip flexed 90°.

Dietz noted that gentle reduction of acute or acute on chronic severe SCFE was generally recommended.[297] Dietz attempted to study gentle reduction using longitudinal traction with medial rotation. Only 5 of 13 hips had discernible reduction with this method, and one developed ischemic necrosis. In review, however, this hip had been distracted from the acetabulum by excessive longitudinal traction. Casey et al. also described a similar technique and noted that longitudinal traction with medial rotation was an acceptable approach.[295]

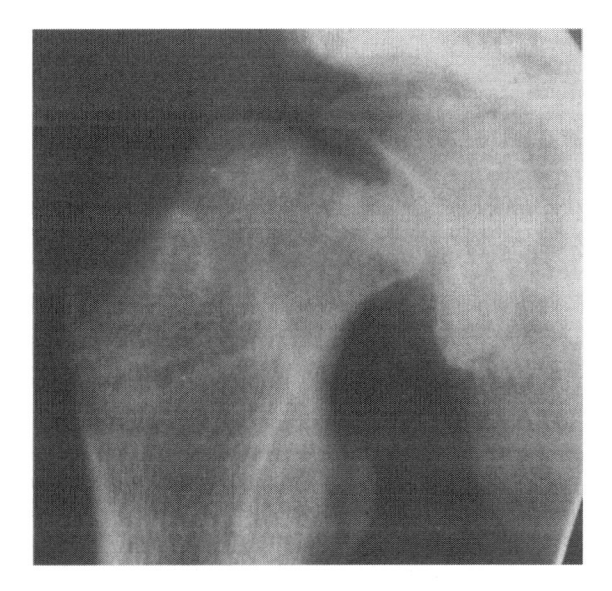

FIGURE 21-18. Acute SCFE following a fall. The patient had had no prodromal symptoms. It was reduced over 2 days in traction (split Russell's with derotation strap) and subsequently pinned.

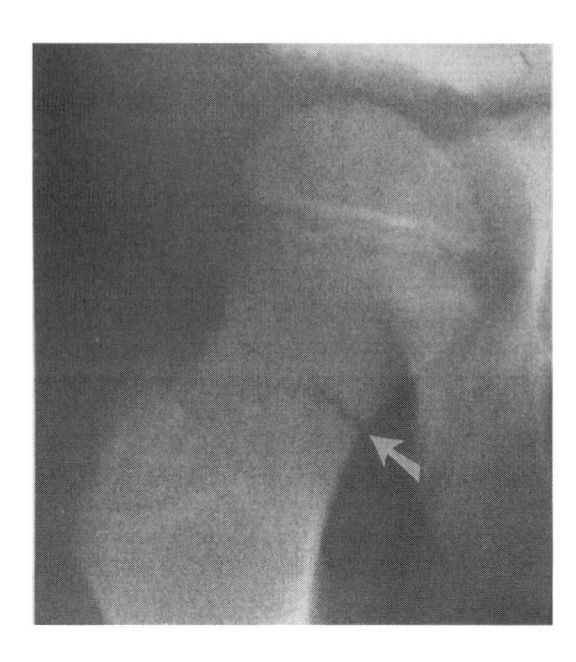

FIGURE 21-19. Femoral neck fracture, type III injury pattern (arrow). The fracture was undisplaced, and the child was treated with immobilization in a cast. The fracture did not appear to extend completely across the neck (metaphysis), thereby decreasing the likelihood of intraepiphyseal cartilage injury.

Aadalen et al.[290] and Casey et al.[295] reported the ability to obtain reduction in acute-on-chronic SCFE. Jerre, in contrast, found successful manipulative reduction present in only 19 of 26 patients (73%).[304] Schein successfully reduced three acute hips with traction and internal rotation.[313] Based on the literature, ischemic necrosis probably occurs in 10–20% of cases with acute slips no matter what the treatment, and traction and reduction appear safe so long as excessive weight is not used that might result in hip joint distraction.

Closed reduction should probably not be attempted if a period of more than 1 week has elapsed since the probable acute episode. In situ extraarticular fixation with threaded pins or screws is indicated. The postoperative management consists of avoiding weight-bearing for 3–4 weeks, followed by a gradual increase in weight-bearing. The main complication, other than ischemic necrosis, is subtrochanteric fracture after pin removal, especially if they were in the lateral cortex. Pins are usually removed to avoid future difficulties. Titanium pins are avoided, as they may be difficult to remove. Biomechanical studies suggest that internal fixation devices reach peak efficacy at 6 months and that surrounding bone begins to weaken progressively after that while the bone "incorporates" the plate, pins, or screws into "normal" stress patterns. Pin removal is controversial and not without complications, but I usually remove them within a year of insertion. Other methods of stabilizing the hip, such as the use of a transphyseal bone peg, may be considered to avoid the necessity of removing the pins at a later date.

Baynhamn et al. described two patients who developed femoral neck fractures as a complication of in situ pinning for an SCFE.[292] The first patient developed pain postoperatively. The pins were removed 14 months following surgery, at which time there was an area of lucency at the base of the right femoral neck, and the patient had coxa vara with a neck shaft angle of 100°. Tomograms showed a fracture, and it was treated conservatively. The second patient developed a left femoral neck fracture and coxa vara, despite having a pin in place. She subsequently required a vascularized pedicle bone graft. The authors studied heat production during reaming for cannulated screws and postulated that the fractures probably developed through areas of osteonecrosis secondary to thermal injury.

Acute slip may occur as a complication of a hip dislocation or its attempted reduction (see Chapter 20).[293,294,300,302,306,311,312] An SCFE may also complicate a fracture of the femoral neck or diaphysis that has been left in nonanatomic alignment.[308]

Femoral Neck Fractures

In children, femoral neck and intertrochanteric fractures are the most frequent levels of injury (Figs. 21-19 to 21-22). Ratliff reviewed 71 cases of femoral neck fractures of patients under 17 years of age.[182,184,186] The highest incidence of the injury appeared to be in the 11- to 13-year range. There were 2 physeal fractures, 39 cervical fractures, 26 basal fractures, and 4 intertrochanteric fractures; 22 were undisplaced and 49 were displaced fractures.

Pathomechanics

Various muscle forces may lead to varus or valgus deformation of the fragments relative to each other (Fig. 21-23). The iliopsoas tends to move the greater trochanter proximally, medially, and anteriorly and rotates it externally. The gluteus maximus moves the femur proximally, medially, and posteriorly and rotates it externally. The external rotators rotate

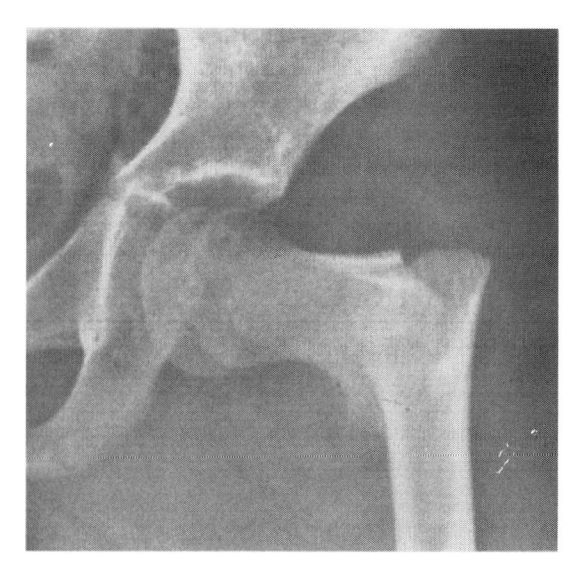

FIGURE 21-20. Femoral neck fracture with a varus tilt. The severity of injury and displacement place this patient at high risk for ischemic necrosis.

Proximal Femoral Injuries

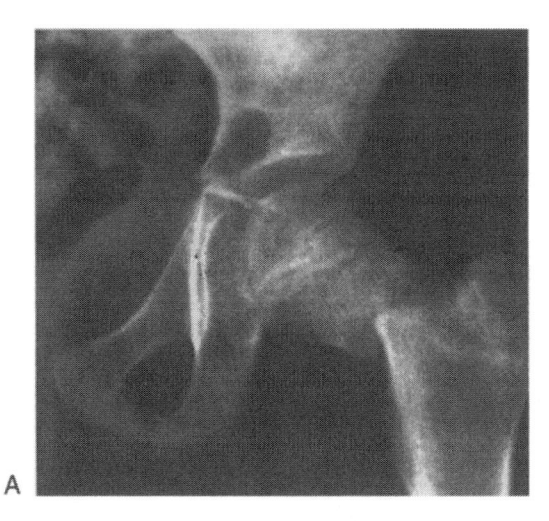

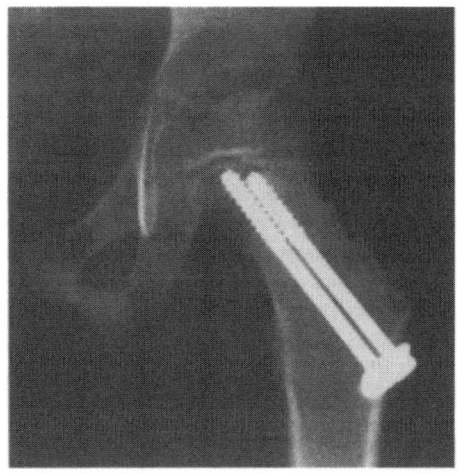

FIGURE 21-21. (A) Femoral neck fracture in a 9-year-old boy. (B) It was reduced and the fracture stabilized by percutaneous screws (and a hip spica).

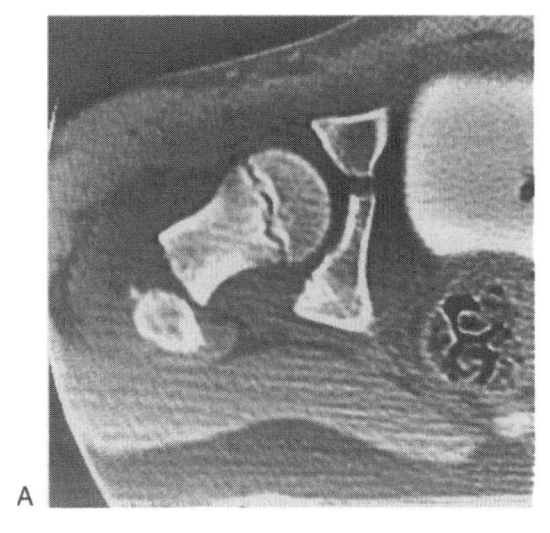

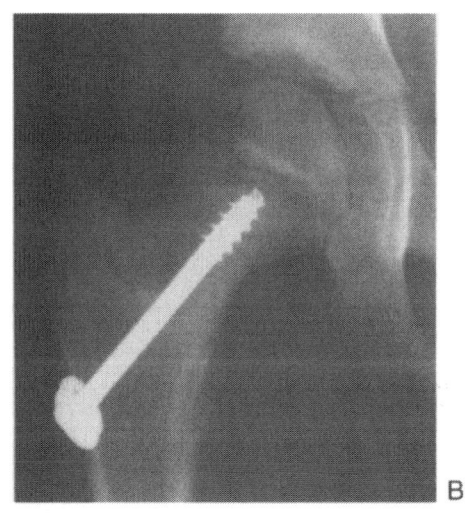

FIGURE 21-22. This 8-year-old girl was involved in a bicycle–car accident. She sustained bilateral femoral diaphyseal, unilateral femoral neck and proximal tibial physeal fractures. (A) CT of the femoral neck fracture. (B) The femoral neck fracture was reduced and stabilized with a cannulated screw that stopped short of the physis.

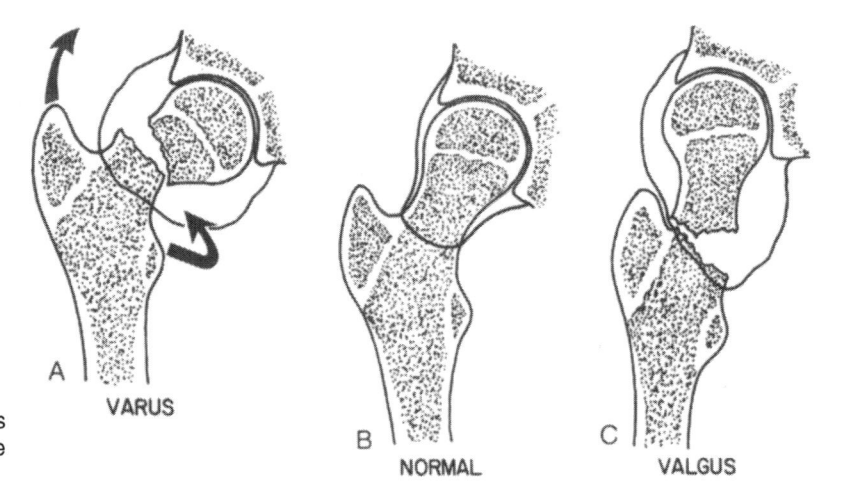

FIGURE 21-23. Varus and valgus neck deformities in femoral neck fractures. Arrows in (A) show the major vectors of the deforming forces.

the femur and shift it medially. Thus, in theory, four muscular forces contribute to the medial shift and three to external rotation. However, the iliopsoas basically neutralizes the opposite action of the gluteus maximus and external rotators. Therefore after most fractures the greater trochanter is pulled upward, rotated externally, and shifted medially. This displacement tends to take place regardless of the exact anatomic position of the fracture line.

Diagnosis

The diagnosis is generally not difficult. There is a history of a severe injury, following which the patient complains of sudden pain in the hip and usually cannot stand or walk. However, greenstick or impacted fractures and stress fractures may allow some weight-bearing. The injured limb is usually held rigidly and in varying degrees of external rotation and slight adduction, and it may be flexed to allow some relief of capsular distension by hematoma. When the fracture is displaced, the patient is generally unable to move the hip actively. Shortening of 1–2 cm may be present. Generally, there is marked restriction of passive motion of the hip, particularly flexion, abduction, and internal rotation. The diagnosis is confirmed by roentgenograms, which should be obtained in both anteroposterior and lateral views. The direction of the fracture line, the degree of traumatic coxa vara, and the amount of posterior tilt should be noted, as well as whether the femoral head is retained in the acetabulum in its normal location (the distal fragment is usually displaced upward and anteriorly or into slight external rotation).

It is important to remember that the fracture is evident only through the osseous portion of the neck. The fracture may propagate further through the intraepiphyseal cartilage, extending across the rest of the superoposterior femoral neck (Fig. 21-2).

Treatment

Excellent results are generally, although not universally, achieved with undisplaced fractures, no matter how they are treated. Undisplaced fractures in children have some inherent stability, possibly because the contiguous cartilage of the pertense or prior femoral neck is not completely disrupted. The safest way to treat them is by a hip spica with the leg held in internal rotation flexion and abduction for 8–12 weeks. This practice is usually sufficient, especially in the young child. The stability may be assessed fluoroscopically prior to applying the cast; and it is imperative that the fracture be radiographed regularly (at 1, 3, and 6 weeks) to assess it for insidious displacement. After 6 weeks the likelihood of displacement is minimal provided healing is progressing and there is no progressive varus deformation. A spica cast cannot maintain hip stability in most instances when the fracture is not intrinsically stable.

Anatomic alignment may be progressively (insidiously, nonpainfully) lost and may lead to displacement and a greater incidence of complications, particularly coxa vara. As a general rule, if Pauwel's angle (fracture line) is less than 40°, such fractures may be treated by a spica cast without weight-bearing. Inclusion of both legs may be necessary for a particularly active child. Frequent roentgenograms are essential. If there is significant loss of anatomic position, the fracture probably should be fixed internally (percutaneous pinning).

For displaced fractures, the eventual risks of coxa vara and ischemic necrosis increase significantly. Manipulation with the patient under anesthesia generally corrects the displacement, but it may be easily lost once the traction has been released. Initial reduction of a fracture may be obtained by counteracting muscle forces acting in the trochanteric area. A condition as close to anatomic reduction as possible should be attained.

Anatomic alignment, achieved closed reduction, may be maintained by internal fixation with percutaneous small, threaded or nonthreaded pins, which should stop short of the physis. Again, a hip spica cast is also applied to provide additional immobilization. The importance of internal fixation in maintaining reduction when Pauwel's angle is greater than 40° cannot be overemphasized.

Although it has been stated that pinning in a young child may enhance the risk of ischemic change, there is *no* reason for the blood vessels to be damaged so long as the pins are kept within the femoral neck. Should ischemic changes occur, they are most likely caused by the original injury (damage to vessels coursing along the femoral neck), rather than by the surgical intervention.

The relatively short neck of the femur in a young child sometimes makes fixation difficult. The best type of internal fixation relates to the differing anatomy. Large-diameter nails may cause distraction of the fragments, are often difficult to drive into the dense bone (compared with adult bone), and may lead to fragmentation and propagation of the fracture or to premature epiphysiodesis. I prefer threaded fixation pins or screws that stop short of the capital femoral physis. It is rarely necessary to cross the growth plate, except with fractures less than 1 cm from the physis. In such cases smooth pins should be used, with the pins being removed as soon as possible to avoid interfering with subsequent growth. However, continued growth in the capital femur may occur, such that the epiphysis progressively grows away from the pin ends, leaving them in the metaphysis. Threaded pins that cross the growth plate may enhance the risk of premature epiphysiodesis. A lag-screw through a predrilled and tapped hole also offers a good fixation method, but it requires placing a relatively large device and displacing much bone, and the lag-screw should not cross the physis.

Displaced femoral neck fractures should be treated by gentle closed reduction under fluoroscopy followed by internal fixation with two or three threaded pins, with any pin crossing the plate being smooth. Age is not a factor with this suggested treatment modality. This treatment should be followed by the use of a supplementary hip spica cast.

If adequate reduction cannot be achieved or if after reduction Pauwel's angle is still more than 50°–60° with a consequently high shearing stress, a subtrochanteric valgus osteotomy may be considered. In this situation, an anterior approach or extension of the exposure with direct visualization of the fracture may allow adequate reduction. If the capsule is opened, it should be opened anteriorly, and great care should be taken not to place any instruments forcefully through the fracture line into the posterior region or around the neck for exposure, as such placement may damage the major circulatory systems to the femoral head.

Some intertrochanteric fractures in the child may be reduced and held in traction. When callus is present at 2–3 weeks, a hip spica may be applied. An indication for internal fixation is irreducibility or inability to hold the fracture in traction because of concomitant injuries, particularly those involving the central nervous system. Open reduction may be difficult. Ischemic necrosis does not carry the same potential risk as with higher neck fractures, and the tendency toward varus deformity is more easily overcome than with proximal fractures. Fixation should avoid the greater trochanteric physis. Generally, pins should be placed so they parallel the neck cortices. Thus, the entry points on the lateral cortex should be *below* the greater trochanteric physis.

Results

Canale and Bourland reviewed 61 fractures, including 5 transepiphyseal, 27 transcervical, 22 intertrochanteric, and 7 subtrochanteric fractures.[50] Among them, 55% had good results, 20% fair results, and 25% poor results. The use of internal fixation appeared to reduce the complications of nonunion and coxa vara. Ischemic necrosis caused most of the poor results. There were 26 patients who developed necrosis, 13 developed a coxa vara deformity, and 4 had nonunion. Of 54 hips with adequate follow-up, 33 (62%) showed premature capital physeal closure compared to the opposite hip. Canale and Bourland believed that subtrochanteric osteotomy was not indicated as a reparative procedure, as recommended by Ratliff.[182,184,186]

McDougall observed equally good or bad results from conservative or operative methods.[139] However, these statistics were misleading because all the intertrochanteric fractures were treated conservatively by casts or traction, whereas the transcervical fractures were usually treated by internal fixation.

Leung and Lam[129] reassessed some of the patients originally reported by Lam.[123,124] They were able to evaluate 41 of the 92 children between 13 and 23 years after injury. Although the early clinical results reported by Lam 3–5 years after treatment showed excellent clinical results despite a high incidence of complications, the subsequent review showed that 83% of the patients had a radiographic abnormality and 24% had pain, a limp, or leg shortening. This type of study is indicative of what needs to be done following most childhood skeletal injuries, especially those involving an epiphysis or physis. Long-term effects—a decade or more after skeletal maturity is attained—give more realistic results regarding the likelihood that osteoarthritis, joint dysfunction, or other chronic problems may develop.

Complications

There is a high incidence of complications independent of the therapeutic approach. Complications of varying severity develop in about 50% of children with fractures of the femoral neck. Such complications include (1) coxa vara, (2) ischemic necrosis, (3) delayed union, (4) nonunion, (5) leg length inequality, and (6) epiphyseal slip. The incidence of ischemic necrosis has ranged from 16% to 45%. The incidence of coxa vara has ranged from 25% to 55%. Nonunion occurs in approximately 10–33% of cases. Of 189 cases reported in five large series, one or more of these complications developed in 60% of the patients.[72,184,186,189,216] This fracture is one of the more challenging childhood injuries.

Ischemic necrosis is the major complication.[67,111,216] In one series this complication developed in 30 patients (42%); the fragments had been displaced in 26 patients, whereas in 4 patients there was no displacement.[111] Ischemic necrosis is usually apparent within a year after injury, although radiographic signs of necrosis may not be obvious for as long as 2 years after the injury.[139] Earlier diagnosis may be detected with MRI.

The basic cause of necrosis is presumed to be damage to or occlusion (partial, temporary) of the posterosuperior and posteroinferior vessels passing along the neck of the femur. It is not clear whether ischemia results from complete division of all vessels, kinking of those vessels that remain intact, or tamponade by hemarthrosis within the hip capsule (Figs. 21-24, 21-25).

Weber et al. stressed the importance of pressure exerted on the blood vessels by the hematoma formed within the capsule after a proximal femoral fracture and stated that it may be a significant factor in reducing the blood supply.[231] They recommended that the capsule be opened and the pressure thereby alleviated. Kay and Hall have argued that the hip should be aspirated to prevent tamponade of the vessels.[111] This concept remains controversial.

Vegter and Lubsen showed that temporary vascular occlusion for 6 hours resulted in necrosis of trabecular bone in rabbit femoral heads.[229] Only 2 hours of increased intracapsular pressure was necessary to result in a much more complex picture of trabecular osteocyte death. They concluded that transient occlusion due to this type of pressure phenomenon could cause cellular death despite intact perfusion of the bone. Such fractional osteonecrosis was characterized by necrosis of some trabecular osteocytes, whereas the vascular and bone-forming marrow tissue seemed to remain alive. This observation probably can be explained by a difference in susceptibility to ischemia of the various cell types within the epiphysis.

Melberg and colleagues showed that joint pressures in adults were less than 20 mmHg when the hip fracture was unreduced. When the hip was extended and internally rotated, however, the pressure rose to values exceeding the normal arteriolar pressure, with a peak pressure of 135 mmHg. Prolonged reduction maneuvers with the hip joint in extension and internal rotation may create intracapsular pressure increases high enough to temporarily jeopardize the circulation of the femoral head. They believed their findings did *not* support the hypothesis that hip joint tamponade *per se* was the common etiologic factor for the development of femoral head necrosis after femoral neck fracture; rather, the position maintained during the treatment was more likely to be responsible.[141]

There appear to be three basic roentgenographic patterns of ischemic necrosis (Figs. 21-26, 21-27). One is a total involvement of the epiphysis, physis, and metaphysis extending from the level of fracture. The second is anterolateral involvement, comparable to Legg-Calvé-Perthes disease, with

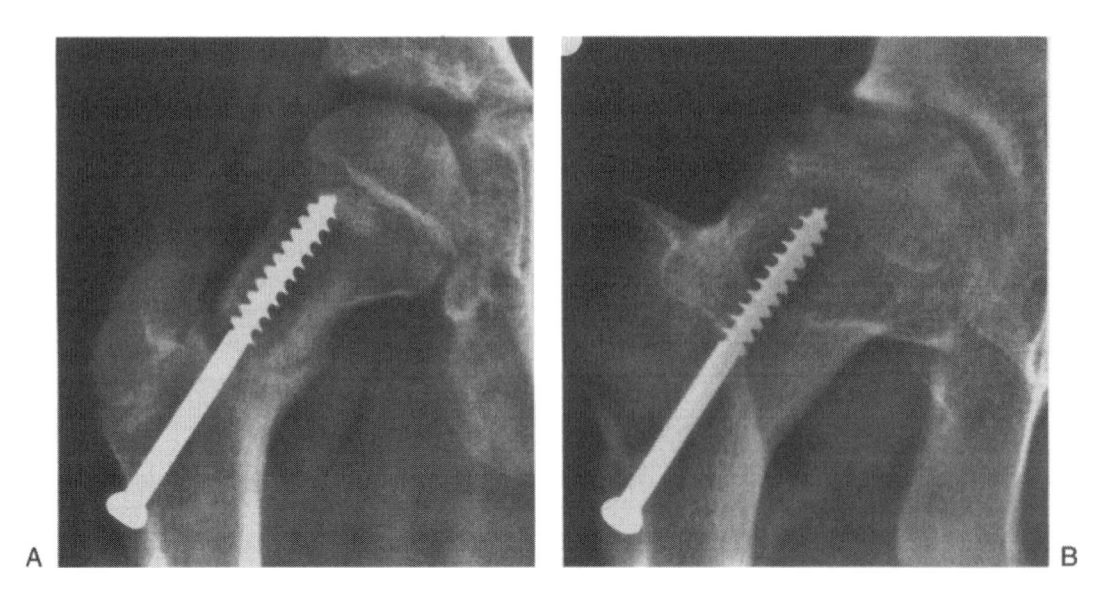

FIGURE 21-24. (A) Femoral neck fracture treated by closed reduction and fluoroscopically directed percutaneous internal fixation. (B) Development of ischemic (avascular) necrosis 11 months after the injury.

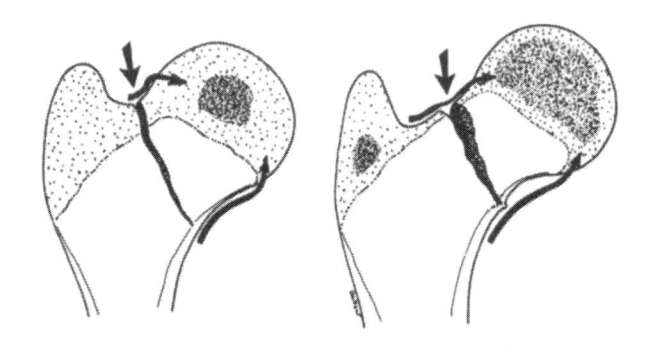

FIGURE 21-25. Femoral neck fractures, showing how the fracture propagates into the intraepiphyseal cartilage. They may attenuate or transect the posterosuperior vessels, especially with varus deformation, yet leave the posteroinferior vessels relatively undamaged.

presumed involvement of only the metaphysis and an intact, uninvolved epiphysis. The third type represents involvement of the anterior vessels from the lateral circumflex artery.

The method of treatment seems to be a factor in the development of ischemic necrosis. Of fractures treated conservatively, 35% were complicated by this problem, in contrast to only 27% of those treated by internal fixation. Extreme abduction of the hip during the treatment of developmental dislocation of the hip certainly decreases circulation, and it is significant that with some of the recommended conservative methods of casting the fractured hip is forced into extreme positions to reduce the fracture. After reduction the affected hip should be brought into 30°–40° of abduction and moderate flexion to lessen mechanical impingement and attenuation of vessels. Similarly, following internal fixation the hip should not be immobilized in extreme positions.

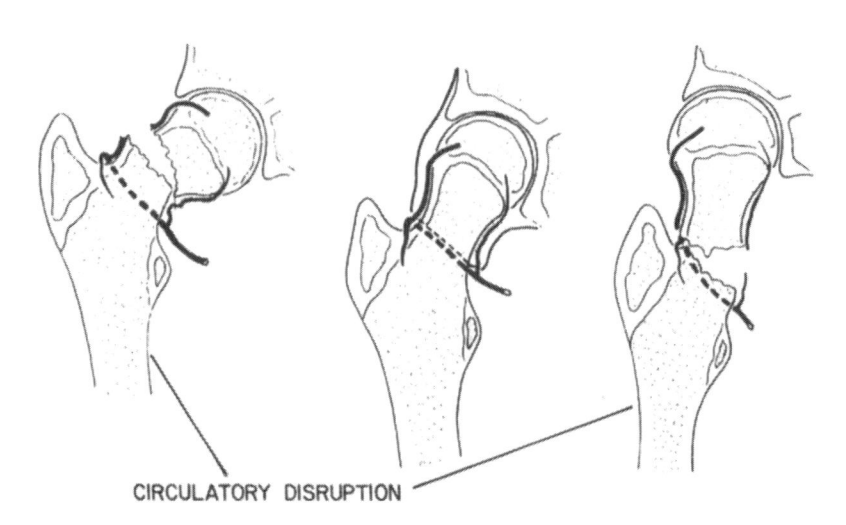

CIRCULATORY DISRUPTION

FIGURE 21-26. Vascular disruption with varus and valgus injuries.

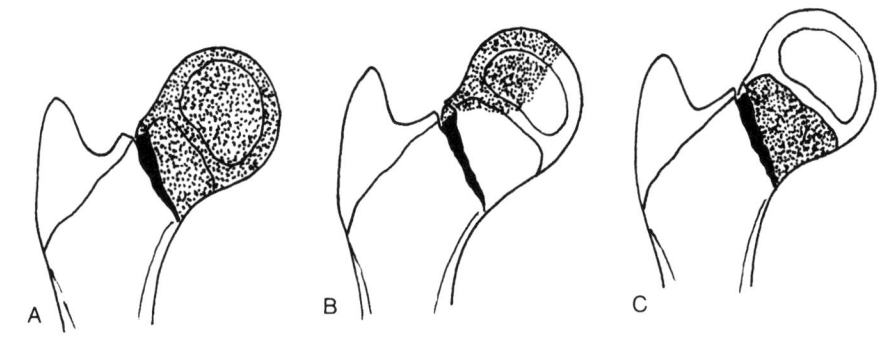

FIGURE 21-27. Ischemic (avascular) necrosis patterns. (A) Total involvement of the capital femoral epiphysis, physis, and metaphysis (all vessels). (B) Anterolateral involvement (probably of only the posterosuperior vessels). (C) Metaphyseal involvement only, with unaffected capital femoral epiphysis and physis.

This complication may occur after undisplaced or displaced fractures of the femoral neck in children. Chong and coworkers believed that the most important prognostic factor was the degree of displacement at the time of injury. They reported an incidence of ischemic necrosis of 50%.[56] I tend to agree with this concept that vascular damage occurs at the time of injury.

Femoral neck fractures appear more likely to undergo necrosis than do intertrochanteric fractures. Displaced transepiphyseal fractures have the poorest prognosis, with development of avascular necrosis in 80% of the involved patients. The incidence of ischemic necrosis in those who are 10 years of age or younger is 21%, whereas in those over 10 years of age it increases to 47%.

These "at risk" children should have a bone scan 3–4 months after the injury, with the scan repeated approximately 1 year after the injury to look for possible delayed vascular damage or compromise. A bone scan may be difficult to interpret because of the new bone formation from the healing fracture and the changes in the femoral head consequent to injury and immobilization. Ischemia is usually detectable on a scan within the first few months and probably always within a year, at which time radiographic changes are also becoming evident. The first signs of ischemic necrosis are that the head does not become osteoporotic and that it does not grow and mature compared with the opposite side. The cartilage space widens. These signs are present long before fragmentation and deformity of the head, comparable to Legg-Calvé-Perthes disease. MRI is of questionable value because of the artifactual changes due to the internal fixation.

If there is any suggestion of ischemic change or if roentgenographic changes seem to be gradually appearing, premature epiphysiodesis of the greater trochanter should be considered to minimize the overgrowth and loss of the normal articulotrochanteric distance.

Premature fusion of the capital femoral physis is sometimes an early sign of ischemic necrosis. Premature fusion may result in shortening of the lower limb and a relative coxa vara. This situation may lead to a short neck and a weak lever arm for the hip abductor muscles, shortened leg, and limitation of abduction resulting from overgrowth of the greater trochanter. It appears reasonable to implicate specific ischemic involvement to selected regions of the physis, along with continued growth in other regions, similar to the avascular necrosis encountered in the various patterns following closed and open treatment of developmental dislocation of the hip.[216]

In contrast, an increase in circulation consequent to the trauma may produce a coxa magna, which is poorly covered if the acetabulum does not also overgrow congruously. This development is a good prognostic sign, as it implies more than adequate circulation, rather than ischemia.

Coxa vara is a common complication.[68] Lam reported 23 instances in 75 fractures.[124] The deformity developed in fractures during the immediate postinjury period in 18 patients and as a late complication in 5. It may be caused by several factors: (1) failure to reduce the fracture; (2) loss of alignment in the hip spica because of inadequate immobilization or delayed union; and (3) ischemic necrosis and premature fusion of the capital femoral physeal plate, in which instance relative discrepancy of growth between the capital femur and greater trochanter may result in a progressive decrease in the neck–shaft angle. The clinical signs of coxa vara are prominence and elevation of the greater trochanter, shortening of the limb, decreased hip abduction, and gluteus medius limp. Treatment usually consists of a subtrochanteric abduction (valgus) osteotomy. If the capital femoral epiphyseal plate is prematurely fused, the relative varus deformity recurs with continued growth of the trochanter. It is reasonable to consider a greater trochanteric epiphysiodesis at the time of the abduction osteotomy. The resultant leg length discrepancy may require arrest of the contralateral distal femoral epiphysis at the appropriate age (or ipsilateral leg lengthening).

Delayed union or nonunion may develop with femoral neck fractures. It occurs in about 85% of the cases with a Pauwel's angle of more than 60° (Fig. 21-28), particularly when treated conservatively by cast immobilization alone. In those treated by internal fixation, the fracture fragments may be separated by the threaded portion of a large pin. Nonunion should be treated by bone grafting and subtrochanteric abduction osteotomy aimed at converting the fracture angle from one of shearing or tensile stress to one of compression. With delayed union, abduction osteotomy is adequate. Usually it is unnecessary to insert a bone graft as well. When evaluating these patients prior to considering surgery, a bone scan is useful for determining if there is ade-

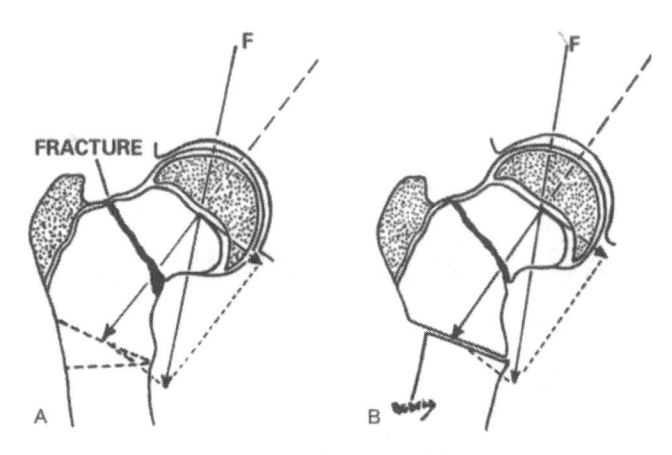

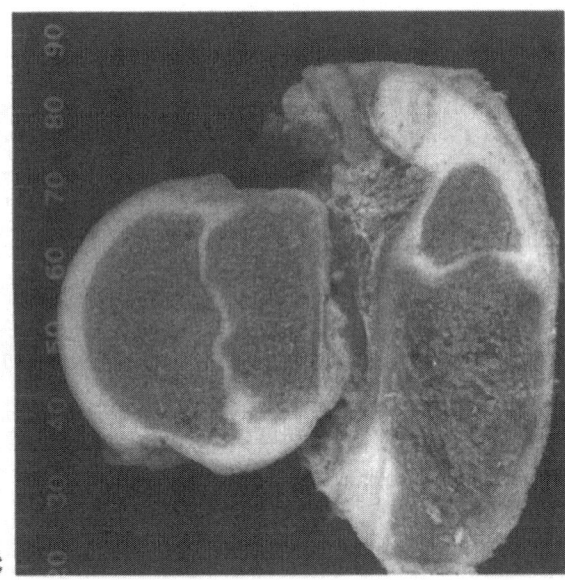

FIGURE 21-28. (A, B) Femoral neck fracture left in varus. (C) Simulation of such nonunion and coxa vara after a femoral neck fracture.

quate blood supply to the proximal portion, particularly in the metaphysis.

A rare complication of coxa vara is the subsequent development of an SCFE during adolescence.[204]

Stress Fractures

Stress fractures of the femoral neck are relatively common in young men in their early twenties but less likely prior to skeletal maturity. Wolfgang described a stress fracture of the femoral neck in a 10-year-old child.[241] There are two types of stress fracture of the femoral neck. The transverse type appears as a small lucency in the superior part of the femoral neck and often becomes displaced. This type is less likely in a child, in whom there is still epiphyseal cartilage along the neck. The second, a compression type that appears as a haze of callus on the inferior aspect of the femoral neck associated with slight varus displacement, is more likely to occur in a young patient.

Ipsilateral Proximal/Diaphyseal Fracture

Double level fractures of the femoral neck and diaphysis are infrequent in the child. The femoral neck fracture has the same potential problems as the isolated injury. It should be stabilized first. The diaphyseal fracture may be treated by closed or open means. However, a cast (immediate), open reduction, and plating or an external fixator are also reasonable alternatives.

Trochanteric Injuries

Greater Trochanter

Injuries to the greater trochanter (Fig. 21-29) generally occur as a result of a direct blow or a hip dislocation.[329,332,338,340,341,346,349–351,358,359,362] The greater trochanter may be avulsed by sudden contraction against resistance in the gluteus medius and minimus muscles. Such a fracture is usually undisplaced or minimally displaced. With more severe injury, the chondro-osseous fragment is retracted proximally, posteriorly, and medially (see Fig. 21-35, below).

Care must be taken not to interpret a small accessory ossification center at the tip of the greater trochanter as an avulsion fracture. This finding usually is a normal variation in the tip of the greater trochanter that appears in children 7–10 years of age (Fig. 21-3).

Depending on the age of the patient at the time of trochanteric injury, part of the fracture most likely occurs through the intraepiphyseal cartilaginous continuity between the capital femur and greater trochanter. This description may cause damage to the blood vessels along the posterosuperior femoral neck and lead to ischemic changes in the femoral head as a consequence of the injury.[346] If the trochanter is avulsed from the lateral femoral metaphysis, an additional complication may be premature fusion of the physis with continued growth of the capital femur to create an elongated femoral neck (see Chapter 20).

Treatment is closed reduction if the fracture is minimally displaced. When significant displacement occurs, tension band wiring or transphyseal fixation may be indicated (Fig. 21-30).

Churchill et al. found that there were few anastomoses between the vessels of the greater trochanter and those of the adjacent cancellous bone of the shaft.[326] They believed that ischemia of the greater trochanter could thus contribute to nonunion following trochanteric osteotomy. The studies by Churchill et al. suggested that even in the adult the greater trochanter has a separate blood supply after bony fusion to the shaft.[326] This is not unexpected. When one analyzes MRI studies in young to middle-aged adults there often is residual independence of the circulation of the metaphyseal and diaphyseal bone from the epiphyseal and apophyseal regions. A relatively avascular plane physiologically separates the two circulatory patterns even well after skeletal maturation.

Linhart et al. described a 12-year-old girl who sustained an apparent isolated fracture of the greater trochanter.[346] The patient was treated conservatively, and approximately 6 months later she was noted to be developing ischemic necro-

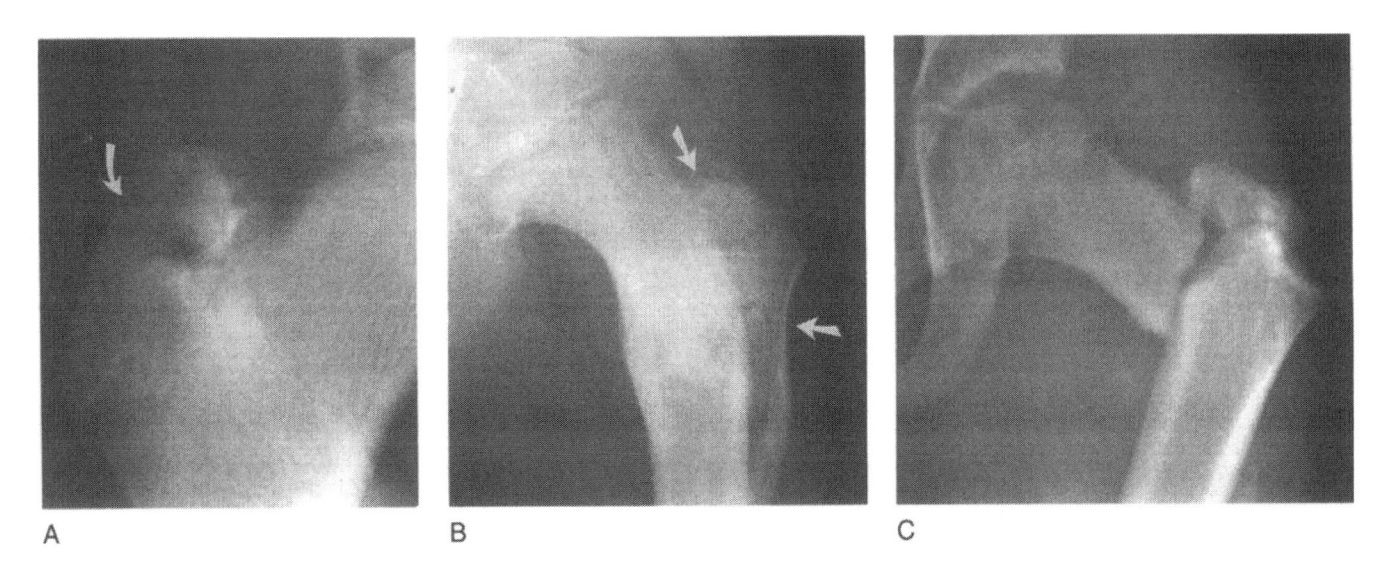

FIGURE 21-29. (A) Greater trochanteric fracture (arrow). (B) Healed avulsion (arrows) of the greater trochanter. (C) Trochanteric injury accompanying a femoral neck fracture.

sis of the capital femur. This is the only reported case of this complication. Probably there was avulsion of the main branch of the lateral retinacular vessels as they coursed along the posterosuperior femoral neck. These vessels or even the main circumflex may have been significantly injured by the pattern of fracture.

Lesser Trochanter

Wilson and colleagues[366] reviewed 78 cases of this injury; 90% occurred in adolescents, usually following the appearance of the secondary ossification center in the lesser trochanter.[319-325,327,328,330,331,333-339,342-345,347-349,352-366] The avulsion of the lesser trochanter usually occurs with hyperextension and abduction of the hip. It often occurs in boys playing running games when they stop suddenly to avoid a fall or collision.

It is also common in hurdlers, and it may occur coming out of starting blocks in a sprint race. There is a sudden snap in the groin, immediate pain, and an inability to stand erect comfortably. Climbing stairs is difficult. Some hip flexion may be retained because the iliacus portion has a broader insertion, and the psoas portion inserts directly into the tip of the lesser trochanter.

There is pain along the inner thigh, a limp, and frequent inability to flex the thigh, with deep-seated tenderness in the region of the lesser femoral trochanter. External rotation is a common finding. These findings are comparable to those of slipped capital femoral epiphysis. Patients usually are able to support the weight of the body on the injured limb, but the inability to bring the leg forward comfortably and the associated pain may interfere with walking or other activities. The inability to flex the hip when in a sitting position is usually diagnostic of the loss of power.[335] It is conceivable that

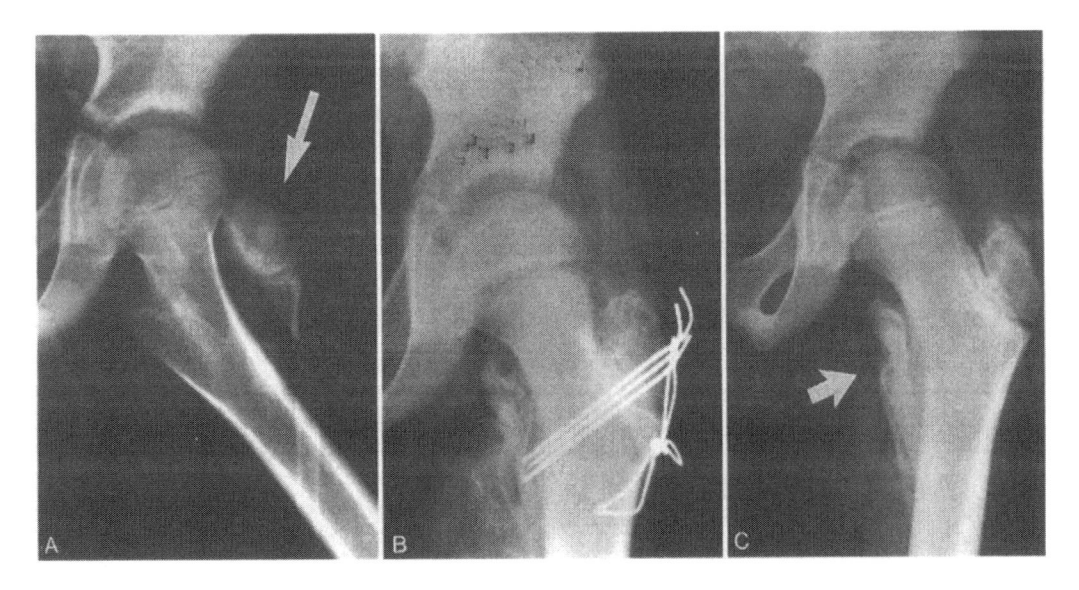

FIGURE 21-30. (A) Avulsion of the greater trochanter (arrow). (B) Reduction with tension band wiring. (C) Follow-up showed that the lesser trochanter was also involved (arrow).

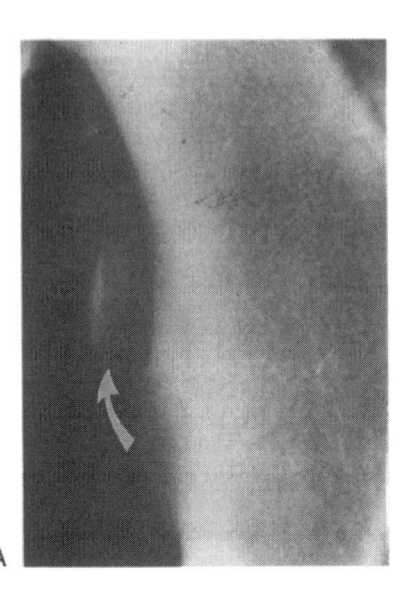

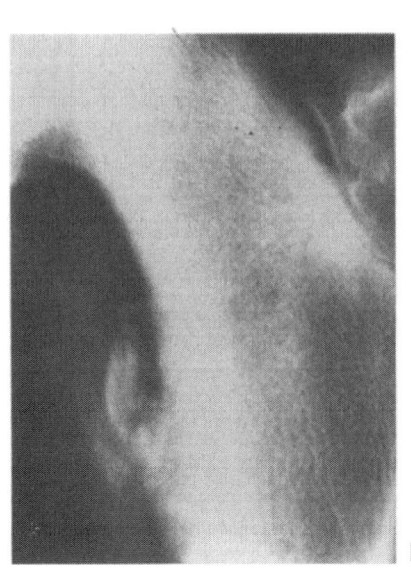

FIGURE 21-31. (A) Avulsion fracture (arrow) of the lesser trochanter in a female gymnast. (B) Follow-up 1 year later showing extensive bone formation.

some degree of flexion is possible if some periosteal attachments of the trochanter remain intact. Good functional results have been obtained by merely immobilizing the limb. There have been no long-term complications, even if an apparent fibrous union developed.

Roentgenograms must be obtained with the thigh in external rotation to rotate the lesser trochanter into an adequate view. Usually the lesser trochanter is avulsed and upwardly displaced, although not necessarily completely separated from the femur (Fig. 21-31). Obviously, the lack of a secondary ossification center makes the radiographic diagnosis difficult.[328,334] MRI may be useful in such situations (Fig. 21-32).

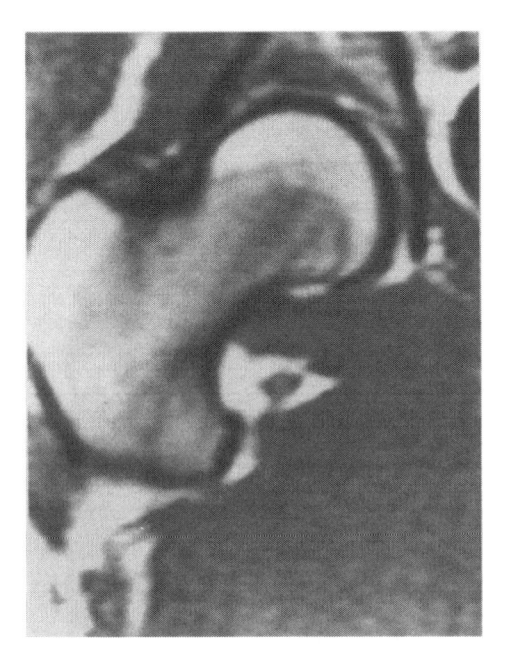

FIGURE 21-32. MRI showing avulsion of the lesser trochanter and surrounding tissue edema (acute injury).

The displaced fracture heals with minimal if any disability. Most of these fractures respond simply to rest and decreased activity. The patient is kept in bed with the hip in flexion until comfortable and then allowed to ambulate with crutches and a three-point partial weight-bearing gait. Immobilization in a cast is rarely necessary. Open reduction is not usually indicated.[328,366]

Parisel reported an avulsion of the lesser trochanter that eventually healed with elongation of the trochanter.[356] Dimon reviewed 30 fractures of the lesser trochanter,[328] 22 of which occurred during vigorous sports. He noted that 26 of the 30 patients were treated symptomatically. Two were treated with a spica cast and two with open reduction. He further found that beginning resumption of athletic activities was possible by 6–8 weeks.

Subtrochanteric Fractures

Little attention has been given to children's subtrochanteric fractures, with these injuries generally grouped with fractures of the proximal third of the femur.[367,368,370–373] These particular fractures are usually the result of a direct blow during an automobile accident or athletic activity. Unlike most children's fractures, many have some degree of comminution, along with overriding and anterior and varus angulation.[367,370,372] Kehr and Starke thought that subtrochanteric fractures in children differed from those in adults in that there was usually a simple fracture line and much less likelihood of comminution of the fragments.[371]

These fractures in children are difficult management problems because of the tendency of the proximal fragment to be displaced into a flexed, abducted, and externally rotated position consequent to muscle forces (Fig. 21-33). Moreover, remodeling is not as extensive in this region, and malalignment may remain as a permanent deformity (Fig. 21-34).

Treatment initially may consist of skeletal traction with a distal femoral (metaphyseal) pin. Skin traction is rarely suf-

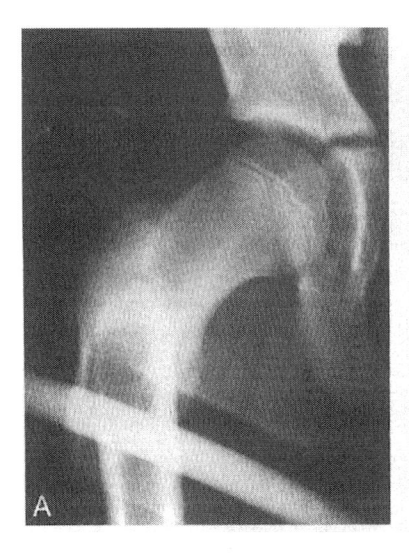

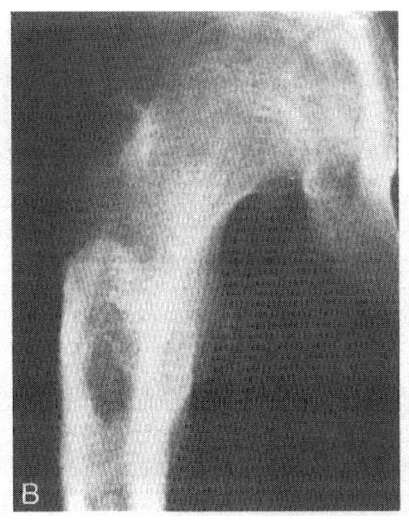

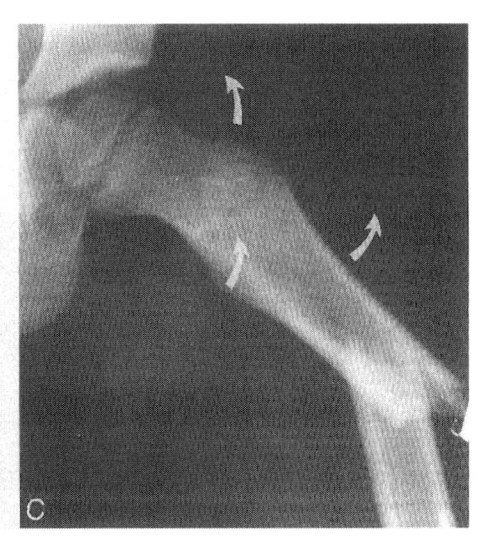

FIGURE 21-33. (A) Subtrochanteric fracture in an 8-year-old child. Overriding has been accentuated by varus and flexion of the proximal fragment. (B) Final healed position. (C) Abduction flexion deformation due to subtrochanteric fracture. Arrows show deforming vectors.

ficient, except in a very young child. The leg is placed in traction with 90° of hip flexion and 90° of knee flexion. This positioning tends to counter both flexion and abduction of the proximal fragment. Use of less than 90° of hip flexion may make alignment difficult. Frequent roentgenograms may be necessary to be certain that adequate alignment is maintained. Traction may be followed by casting or a cast-brace.[368] Frequent radiographs are necessary to determine if the angulation increases in the cast. The average duration of traction and cast immobilization is 9–12 weeks.

Because of instability, costs of traction (i.e., prolonged hospitalization), and frequent verification of position by radiation exposure, alternative methods are gaining popularity. My preference is a uniaxial fixator. Depending on the level of the fracture, one or more fixator pins may have to be placed in the greater trochanteric epiphysis or the femoral neck. The use of a longitudinal rod and locking screws is contraindicated in young patients because of potential damage to the greater trochanteric physis.

Older patients (adolescents) with subtrochanteric fractures that cannot be adequately controlled by traction may be candidates for open or closed reduction and internal fixation. The possibility or necessity of using open reduction is particularly increased if it is difficult to control the fracture because of the associated head injury.[367] The choice of a fixation technique is difficult if the physes of the greater trochanter and capital femur are still functional. An intramedullary nail is contraindicated if it must traverse portions of still functional trochanteric and intraepiphyseal physes. One method is a compression side plate and screw fixation, a method *routinely and effectively* used for elective subtrochanteric osteotomy in children and adolescents. Care must be taken not to damage the trochanteric physis. An alternative is the use of flexible rods, usually inserted retrogradely from the distal femoral metaphysis, across the fracture, and into the femoral neck but not impinging on the capital femoral physis. A uniaxial external fixator is also feasible.

Regardless of the method of treatment, virtually all subtrochanteric fractures in children and adolescents develop adequate osseous union. Mild anterior angulation and some varus or valgus alignment of the fractures may persist. In young children angular deformity may self-correct to a significant extent, whereas in older children little change in

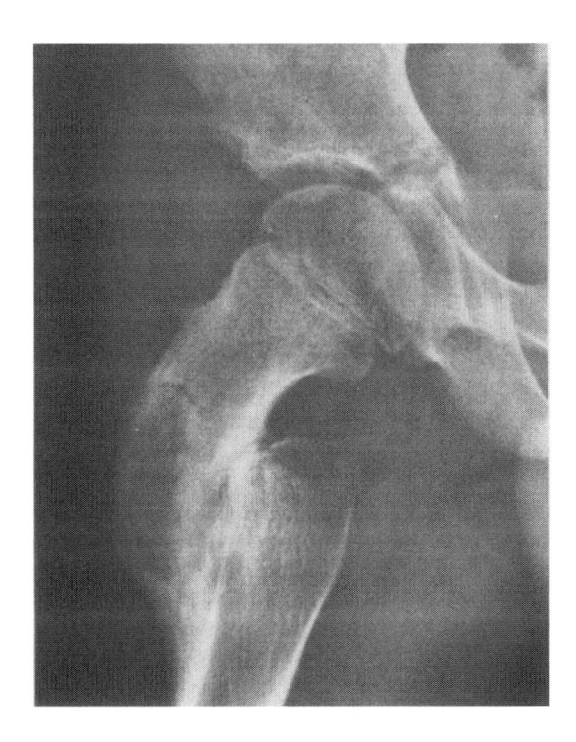

FIGURE 21-34. Malunion of a subtrochanteric fracture.

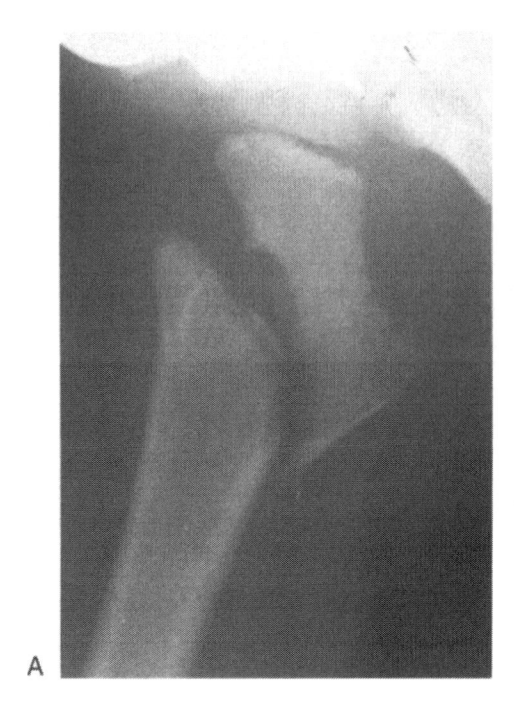

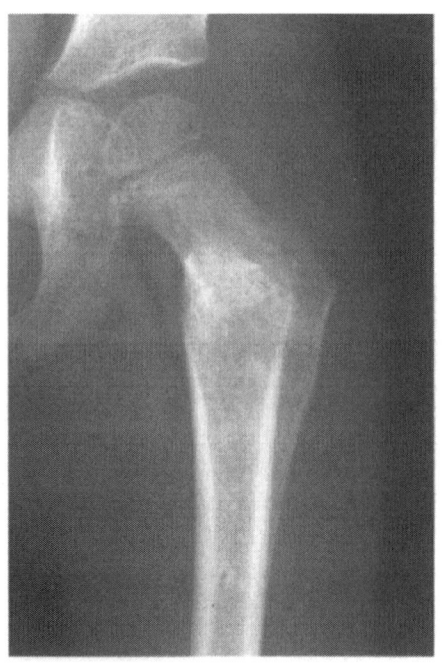

FIGURE 21-35. Cervicopertrochanteric fracture. (A) Injury. (B) Four months later.

alignment occurs with growth. In none of the children was this angulation or rotation at the fracture site a significant functional problem, although there should be some concern for the child with increased varus and posterior direction of the growth plate that might increase susceptibility to slipped capital femoral epiphysis.[205]

The spontaneous correction of leg length inequality by growth stimulation is better in children under 10 years of age, and an overriding of 10–15 mm is acceptable. In contrast, in teenage children there is little remodeling or compensation for shortening after a subtrochanteric fracture.

Gamble et al. described a subtrochanteric fracture variation they classified as a transverse cervicopertrochanteric fracture (Fig. 21-35).[369] The injury was just above the lesser trochanter but below the greater trochanter. It should be considered a variant of the subtrochanteric fracture.

Femoral Shaft Fractures

Diaphyseal fractures of the femur are relatively frequent in children and must be considered serious injuries because of the blood loss and potential shock accompanying the primary trauma. Such fractures often result from violent injuries, especially automobile accidents, and great care must be taken to rule out associated injuries as well as neurologic and vascular complications.[374–731]

Femoral shaft fractures in children may behave differently from similar fractures in adults. The important points to consider are (1) early consolidation, often with considerable callus formation, especially in young children; (2) a reactive increased rate of longitudinal growth of the femur for approximately 1 year (even the tibia may similarly respond); and (3) spontaneous but limited correction of axial deformity without corresponding rotational correction. Because femoral shaft fractures in children generally heal easily and satisfactorily, conservative (i.e., nonoperative) treatment has usually been advocated.

The most frequent site of diaphyseal fracture is the middle third, where normal anterolateral bowing of the diaphysis is at its maximum. This area is most commonly subjected to direct violence; injuries involve the proximal third less commonly and the distal third least frequently. Greenstick fractures may occur but are more frequent in the distal metaphysis. Fractures that result from obstetric trauma usually occur in the middle third of the shaft and ordinarily are transverse. Child abuse femoral diaphyseal fractures tend to be spiral.

Hedlund and Lindgren studied 851 femoral shaft fractures in children and adolescents, reporting that the maximal incidence was in children 2–5 years of age and the total incidence was 2.6 times higher in boys than in girls. The cases were about equally divided between fractures caused by falls and fractures caused by traffic accidents. Falls were the most common cause in children under 3 years of age.[493]

Nafei et al. studied the incidence of femoral shaft fractures in children in a Danish urban population from 1977 to 1986.[585] There were 144 femoral shaft fractures in 138 children less than 15 years of age. The boy/girl ratio was 2.8:1.0. The incidence rate was 28 per 100,000 child-years. Young children less than 3 years of age had the highest incidence per year. The most common etiologies were trauma due to traffic accidents (43.1%) and falls (42.2%).

Proper emergency care, such as initial gentle handling and adequate splinting of the fracture, is extremely important to prevent shock and further injury to soft tissues. Any movement of the acutely injured limb is usually painful. An efficient means of immobilization is the Thomas splint, which must be appropriately sized to the child.

Pathomechanics

The displacement of the fracture fragments depends on the breaking force, the pull of the attached muscles, and the force of gravity acting on the limb. The severity of violence and the strong pull of muscles cause fracture fragments to be completely displaced, leading to variable amounts of overriding. The distal fragment is usually laterally (externally) rotated. With fractures of the upper third of the femoral shaft, the proximal fragment is pulled into flexion by the iliopsoas, abduction by the gluteus medius and minimus, and external rotation by the short external rotators and gluteus maximus. The shorter the proximal fragment, the greater is the degree of displacement. The distal fragment is drawn proximally by the hamstrings and quadriceps femoris muscles and medially by the adductors. Thus the upper end of the distal fragment tends to lie posterior and medial to the proximal fragment, which is in flexion, abduction, and external rotation. Displacement of fragments in a middle third diaphyseal fracture does not follow as regular a pattern. The tendency is for the proximal fragment to be in flexion and the distal fragment to be displaced forward. When the fracture level is in the upper half of the middle third, the proximal half may be abducted. When the break is in the lower half, it tends to abduct. Displacements are not necessarily constant, however; they depend on the relative insertion and the strength of muscles, factors that change considerably as the child grows.

Diagnosis

A history of injury with resultant local pain, tenderness, and swelling, inability or reluctance to move the affected limb, deformity, shortening, abnormal mobility, lateral rotation of the limb, and crepitus render the diagnosis evident. The patient should be examined gently to avoid unnecessary pain. Neurovascular status in the lower limb must be carefully assessed and recorded because injury to the femoral vessels, sciatic nerve, or both may occur, especially from posterior displacement of the distal fragment. Because femoral shaft fractures often result from major violence, it is imperative that the general condition of the patient be evaluated. The patient should be carefully examined to detect any damage to the abdominal, pelvic, and genitourinary area, any cranial injuries, or other fractures or hip dislocation. The last-named injury must be ruled out carefully with a good film of the hip joint. *It is inappropriate to finish treatment of a fracture of the femur and discover that the hip has been dislocated for the entire duration of treatment.* Similarly, the knee should be examined to rule out injury, such as an anterior cruciate ligament avulsion (see Chapter 22).

Roentgenograms are necessary to determine the exact level and nature of the fracture. They should not be done until the patient has been properly examined, subsequently immobilized on a Thomas splint (or similar device), and given adequate medication for relief of pain and muscle spasm.

Khalil described an unusual complication in which there was a comminuted midshaft femoral fracture with the butterfly fragment ending up in the subcutaneous abdominal tissue, having been telescoped into that region at the time of the original fracture.[532]

Treatment

Soft tissue injury inevitably accompanies a femoral shaft fracture. Excessive hemorrhaging with a blood loss of 500 ml or more may occur. The sources of bleeding may be branches of the profunda femoris artery, which course around the posterior and lateral surfaces of the femoral shaft, the vessels of the muscles that envelop the femur, or the medullary vessels of the bone. Occasionally, the femoral artery is damaged. Major damage to the femoral artery, necessitating repair, is one of the situations in which internal fixation is definitely indicated in a child, as it minimizes the tension of the suture line of the vascular repair.

Hypotension is not usually present in children in whom the closed femoral fracture is the only major injury and in whom there is no major vascular injury.[338] Only one-third of the children have a clinically significant change in hematocrit, with most averaging a 4% drop. Children with femoral fractures in whom hypotension or a rapid drop in hematocrit develops should be *promptly* evaluated for an alternative source of significant blood loss (e.g., abdominal, retroperitoneal, intrapelvic).

Ostrum et al. reviewed 100 patients who had either an isolated femoral shaft fracture or a femoral shaft fracture in addition to other non-shock-producing fractures of minor injuries.[600] They found that femoral fractures alone or in combination with other minor injuries should not be considered the cause of hypotensive shock in the traumatized patient. For any traumatized patient who presents with a closed femoral shaft fracture and hypotension, an alternative source of hemorrhage should be sought.

There is no routine treatment for displaced femoral fractures in children. A decision must be made regarding what type of acute reduction, traction, or fixation is indicated for the specific injury complex in a given patient. One must consider the age and weight of the patient; local soft tissue trauma; the type and location of the femoral fracture; other injuries to the head, thorax, and abdomen; and additional fractures of the same or opposite leg.

Several principles should be applied to the treatment of femoral shaft fractures in children: (1) The simplest form of satisfactory treatment usually is the best. (2) If possible, the initial treatment should be maintained. (3) Absolute anatomic reduction may not be essential for adequate long-term function. (4) Restoration of longitudinal and rotational alignment is more important than the positions of the fractured surfaces relative to each other. (5) The more growth remaining in the fractured femur, the more likelihood it is that normal osseous architecture can be restored as the bone remodels. (6) Overtreatment is usually worse than undertreatment. (7) The hope that all deformities in children will correct themselves spontaneously is no excuse for ignoring any deformity that could be corrected by simpler means and manipulation. Shortening of less than 2 cm, angulation of less than 15°, and minimization of rotation are the major goals to achieve with nonoperative treatment.

Traction

Several types of skin and skeletal traction may be used; each has its advantages and advocates. The simplest, safest, most effective method for a child, for a given fracture, and for a particular age group should be the treatment of choice. Bryant's traction, *properly applied and carefully watched*, is appropriate for children weighing less than 18 kg (25 lb) or under 2 years of age. For children weighing more, Russell's traction (or a modification thereof) is probably used most commonly. The increased emphasis on decreasing the time of hospitalization has led to a deemphasis on traction. *However, the methods are safe and are often used in parts of the world where internal or external or fixation are not available.*

The fracture fragments should be longitudinally aligned as near to a normal anatomic relation as possible. Angulation exceeding the normal range by more than 15°–20° should not be accepted. The surgeon should strive for as complete correction of rotational deformity as possible and should try to achieve angulation that does not exceed 10° in the medial or lateral direction, 10° anteriorly, and 5° posteriorly. This objective requires frequent radiographic evaluation of the fracture and adjustment of the traction. The child should not be subjected to frequent manipulations simply to correct minor angulation.

In infants and children up to 2 years of age, Bryant's traction is probably satisfactory, provided there is no spasticity and contracture of the hamstrings and provided that the hips may be easily flexed to 90° with the knees in slight flexion. Traction should be applied to both legs. The legs (knees slightly flexed) should be wrapped from upper thigh to the malleoli, with padding (e.g., lamb's wool or soft cotton) placed over the malleoli to prevent undue pressure. The same amount of weight should be applied to each leg and should be sufficient to lift the infant's pelvis until the sacrum is slightly elevated from the mattress. One must be *cautious* not to overpull a small infant. The position of the fracture must be checked by periodic roentgenograms so distraction of the fragments is avoided. Medial bowing caused by an excessive pull of the hip abductors may be corrected by decreasing the amount of weight on the affected limb and increasing traction on the contralateral normal limb, thereby tilting the pelvis and countering the pull of the hip abductors. The expectation that an osseous deformity during childhood will correct itself spontaneously with growth and remodeling is *not* an acceptable excuse for ignoring it, especially if correction may be obtained by simple traction modification. Callus forms rapidly in young children; at 2–3 weeks after trauma the tenderness disappears and the fracture is probably stable enough to allow removal of the limb from traction and to place it in a hip spica for an additional 6–8 weeks.

Bryant's traction should *not* be used in children over 2 years of age or those weighing over 25 lb. The patient must be monitored closely for the development of vascular and neurologic skin complications. Circulatory problems are the most serious. Bryant's traction is not completely safe in children; tight dressings and abnormal pressure may impair circulation and lead to Volkmann's ischemic contracture, even in the normal limb that is also being treated.[401,426,592] There are three basic patterns of circulatory insufficiency: (1) ischemic fibrosis of the muscles of the lower leg with patches of sensory loss and almost complete paralysis of the muscle distal to the knee, particularly the short toe flexors; (2) involvement characterized both by the aforementioned changes and by circumferential necrosis of the skin and underlying muscles in the calf; and (3) gangrenous changes in the foot and ankle in addition to circumferential necrosis of the calf.

For children older than 2 years of age, there are several types of traction: (1) skin traction with the knee in extension; (2) suspension skeletal traction with the knee in flexion; and (3) 90°–90° skeletal traction with a pin through the distal femur or the proximal tibia.[413,425,515,572,587] I prefer the distal femoral pin, as it avoids risk to the tibial tuberosity with premature growth arrest (Figs. 21-36, 21-37). It also avoids traction across the knee joint, which may have sustained occult soft tissue injury (e.g., to the anterior cruciat ligament). In general, traction is employed to maintain alignment until there is adequate callus for stability (i.e., the callus and fracture site are no longer tender, and the femur moves as a unit on manipulation). The leg may be effectively immobilized in a hip spica cast without loss of the reduction or position.

Because of its effectiveness and simplicity, 90°–90° skeletal traction with a pin through the distal femur is frequently

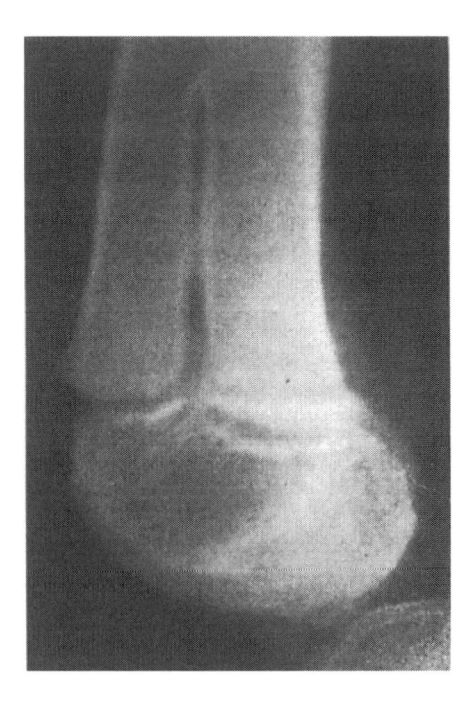

FIGURE 21-36. Effect of a traction pin being too close to the growth plate.

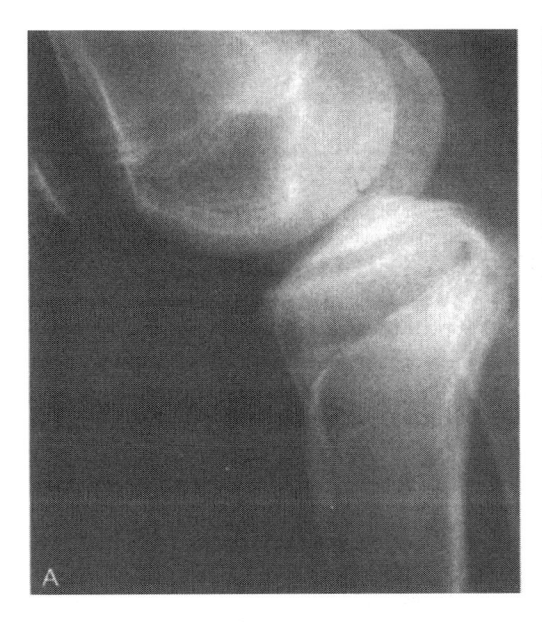

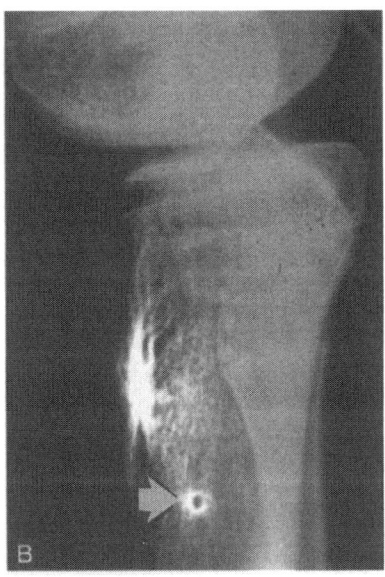

FIGURE 21-37. (A) Recurvatum secondary to pin damage. (B) Recurvatum even with pin (*arrow*) located below and behind the tuberosity.

used (Fig. 21-38). Alignment of the fracture is achieved and maintained, as there is essentially one vector of traction. The pin through the distal femur provides good rotational control of the fracture fragments. The gastrocnemius, hamstring, and iliopsoas muscles are relaxed by the flexed position of the hip and knee, making alignment of the fracture fragments relatively easy.

Other advantages of 90°–90° traction are that it promotes dependent drainage, the thigh is readily accessible for clinical evaluation of alignment with the use of portable roentgenographic equipment, and it facilitates change of dressings and wound inspection in infected or open fractures. A threaded Steinmann pin or large K-wire is inserted 2 cm proximal to the adductor tubercle and distal femoral physis. Injuring the physis must be avoided. Pushing the skin slightly upward while inserting the wire through should prevent undue traction on the skin when the weights are applied. Sterile dressings are placed over the skin incisions, and a traction bow is applied, with the pin under tension. A below-knee cast may be applied, with the ankle in a neutral position. This cast should be well padded in the popliteal area, the dorsum of the foot, and the ankle to prevent pressure sores. Traction ropes suspend the lower leg in a horizontal position, and the knee is in 90° of flexion. The traction forces act vertically, in line with the longitudinal axis of the femoral shaft.

Angulation and rotation may be corrected by shifting the overhead traction in the appropriate direction. If additional external support is necessary in an unstable fracture, coaptation splints may be employed. Slings with 1–2 kg of traction may be applied over the fracture site to control lateral or anteroposterior angulation.

The position and alignment of the fracture fragments must be checked by periodic roentgenograms. Distraction of the fragments should not occur. In children between 2 and 10 years of age, side-to-side (bayonet) apposition, with 0.5–1.0 cm overriding, is an ideal position. Overriding should not exceed 1.5 cm in infants and adolescents. End-to-end apposition is more desirable because of the decreased likelihood of overgrowth.

Traction is continued for 2–4 weeks until the callus is no longer tender and the femur moves as a unit. When adequate callus is evident on the roentgenogram and the patient is comfortable with limb movements, he or she is placed in a hip spica cast. The affected thigh should be in 10° of abduction or in neutral position, with the opposite hip in moderate abduction to facilitate perineal hygiene. The fractured thigh should not be in marked abduction, as the pull of the strong adductors may cause lateral bowing. The pin in the femur may be removed or incorporated into the cast, according to preference.

Humberger and Eyring described a method of 90°–90° skeletal traction with the Kirschner wire inserted through the proximal tibia.[513] *This method is not recommended.* The traction pin may injure the apophysis of the tibial tuberosity. A wire in the proximal tibia does not provide direct control of the femur, as does a wire through the distal femoral metaphysis. Furthermore, patients treated with 90°–90° traction and a proximal tibial traction pin may exhibit knee subluxation or dislocation, genu recurvatum, progressive knee pain, and prolonged rehabilitation.[572]

Bjerkreim and Benum reported seven cases of genu recurvatum after tibial traction for femoral shaft fracture. Six of the patients eventually required corrective osteotomy. The anterior part of the growth plate may be damaged, as may be that part under the tibial tuberosity.[397] Only a small amount of damage need occur to the growth plate to lead to an osseous bridge sufficient to cause angular deformity. Although it is expected that large deformities occur only with large growth slowdowns, it should be realized that even with type 6 injuries a small peripheral osseous bridge may lead to a major angular deformity in this particular region.

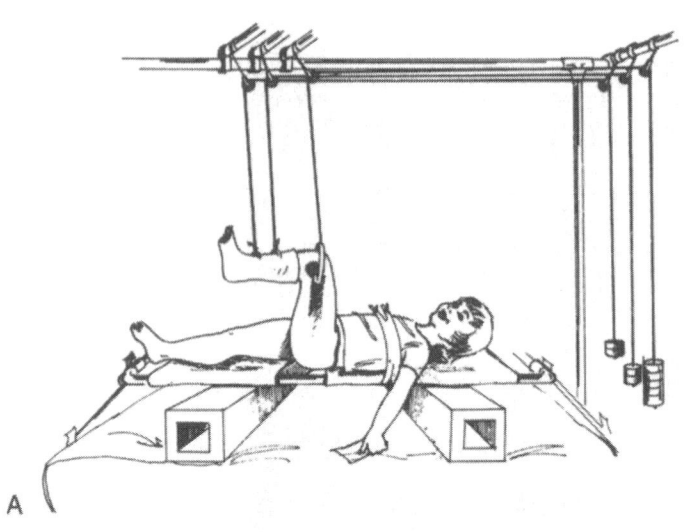

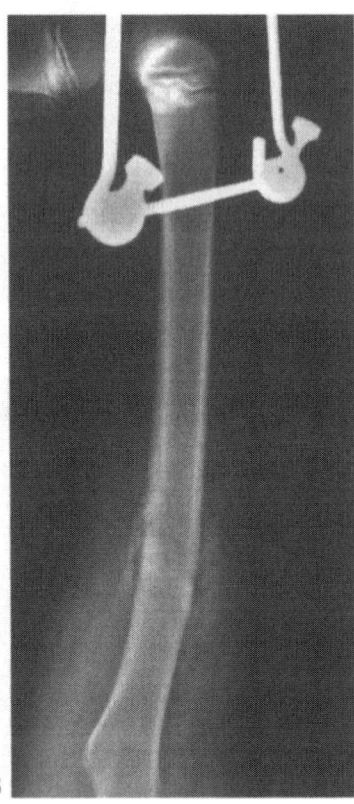

FIGURE 21-38. (A) The 90°–90° skeletal traction positioning with the lower leg in a cast. (B) Early callus formation in a patient in skeletal traction.

Bowler et al. reported two cases of premature closure of the anterior portion of the proximal tibial physis with genu recurvatum in patients who had sustained closed femoral fractures.[406] In *neither* case had a tibial traction pin been used. One patient had been treated with distal femoral pin traction and the other with skin traction and a spica cast.

Havránek et al. used a single screw in the proximal tibia for skeletal traction for femoral shaft fractures.[490] It was inserted into the tibia perpendicular to the surface and well below the tibial tubercle physis. There were no complications such as knee pain, knee joint, subluxation, or growth disturbance.

Suspension traction is preferred by many orthopedic surgeons for older children and adolescents, as skin traction is often unsatisfactory in the older child. Skeletal traction is applied with a K-wire inserted through the distal femur (Fig. 21-39). The thigh and leg are supported on a felt pad covered with a stockinette and are placed on a Thomas splint with a Pearson attachment. With the hip in 35°–40° of flexion, the Thomas splint is placed against the ischial tuberosity and supported by sufficient weight to balance the limb. The traction ropes on the Thomas ring should prevent the splint from sliding distally. The level of the Pearson attachment should be just above the knee joint level so the knee can be flexed approximately 30° to relax the hamstrings. A traction rope with sufficient weight on the distal end of the Pearson attachment supports the weight of the leg. By adjusting the weights the limb may be counterbalanced so it moves comfortably with the patient. The foot of the bed is elevated so the weight of the patient's body acts as countertraction.

With midshaft fractures the tendency is toward posterior angulation. To prevent this and to restore the normal anterior bowing of the femur, the slings under the thigh should be taut and the knee in flexion to relax the gastrocnemius muscle. If there is persistent posterior angulation, a pad may be placed underneath the thigh at the fracture site; alternatively, a sling with direct overhead vertical pull at the appropriate level may be employed. Medial or lateral angulation may be corrected by aligning the distal fragment with the proximal one, which may be accomplished by shifting the position of the ends of the Pearson attachment proximally or distally on the Thomas splint, by changing the direction of the pull, or both. Rotation may be controlled by adjusting the suspension.

Mital and Cashman advocated the use of skeletal traction for 2–3 weeks, followed by cast-brace application and ambulation.[576] They followed 28 children who had been treated with this method. Their ages ranged from 2 to 14 years. The average time for cast-brace application was 20 days after trac-

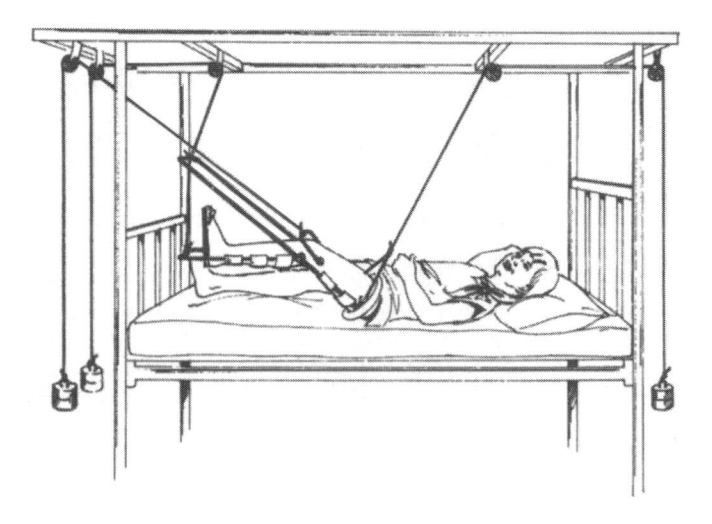

FIGURE 21-39. Skeletal traction combined with splint.

Femoral Shaft Fractures

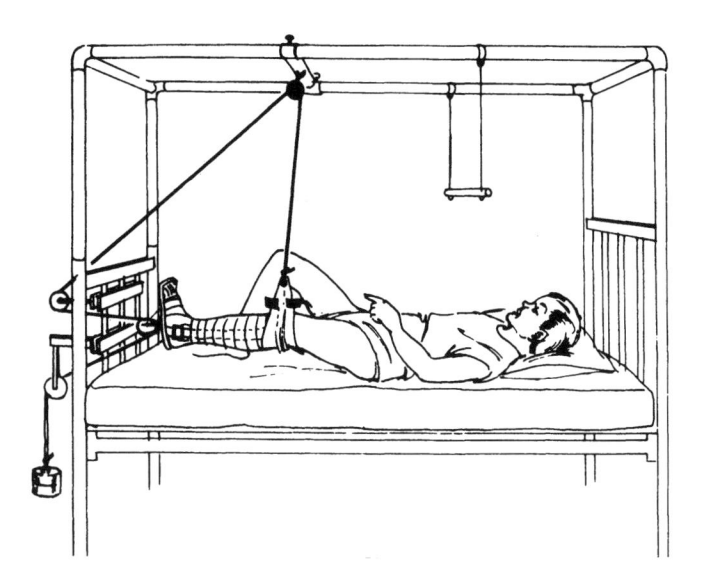

FIGURE 21-40. Variation of Russell's skin traction applicable to femoral fractures in children.

tion, and the average time in the cast-brace was an additional 6.5 weeks.

Russell's skin traction is preferred by some as a method for treating femoral shaft fractures in children (Fig. 21-40). The medial and lateral adhesive traction strips extend from the ankle to a foot plate with a pulley on its inferior surface. There should be two pulleys at the foot of the bed and one overhead. A well-padded sling is placed underneath the knee. The traction rope extends from the sling to the overhead pulley, which is distal to the knee joint, so the rope is directed upward and distally at an angle of 25°, passing over the superior pulley attached to the end of the bed to which the skin traction straps are fixed and back again over the inferior pulley at the foot of the bed, where 2–5 kg of weight is suspended. The lower limb rests on two pillows arranged so the knee is in 30° of flexion, the thigh is supported, and the foot clears the mattress. The foot of the bed is raised to provide countertraction. The vertical traction force is roughly equal to the amount of weight used, whereas the horizontal traction force is equal to approximately twice the amount of weight. The vertical and horizontal forces create a paralellogram of forces, with the resultant force in line with the long axis of the shaft of the femur.

Russell's traction is often preferred because of the ease with which it may be applied, but there are potential problems: (1) peroneal nerve palsy with resultant footdrop due to pressure by the knee sling in the region of the common peroneal nerve; (2) development of posterior bowing at the fracture site due to lack of effective external support under the thigh (often it is necessary to apply an additional sling underneath the thigh with vertical traction to restore the normal anterior bowing of the femur); (3) the difficulty of nursing care and the need for careful vigil to ensure that the correct traction is maintained; and (4) the child's pain, which initially may be greater than that with 90°–90° traction.

Split Russell's traction may be used instead of the original Russell's traction with its 2:1 ratio forces. With split Russell's traction, skin traction is applied in the longitudinal axis of the limb, and a balanced sling with a vertical force is placed under the distal femur or knee and suspended by weights to support the part and supply the necessary resolution of forces. External rotation of the leg is controlled with medial rotation traction straps.

A relatively simple hip flexion-knee extension method may be used for children up to 8 years of age (Fig. 21-41). The leg is placed in a Thomas splint. Skin traction is carefully applied up to the fracture site. The splint is initially placed at 40°–50° but may be adjusted if further flexion deformity is present in the proximal fragment. Up to 7 lb of skin traction may be tolerated by this method. Rotation is initially controlled by allowing the leg to assume a natural, comfortable position. If necessary after a few days, rotation may be controlled by a derotation strap placed across the knee or by restraining the foot. However, the child usually controls rotation spontaneously as he or she begins to move about the bed when swelling and pain subside.

Foy and Colton described four patients with irreducible distal-third femoral shaft fractures.[465] They were irreducible

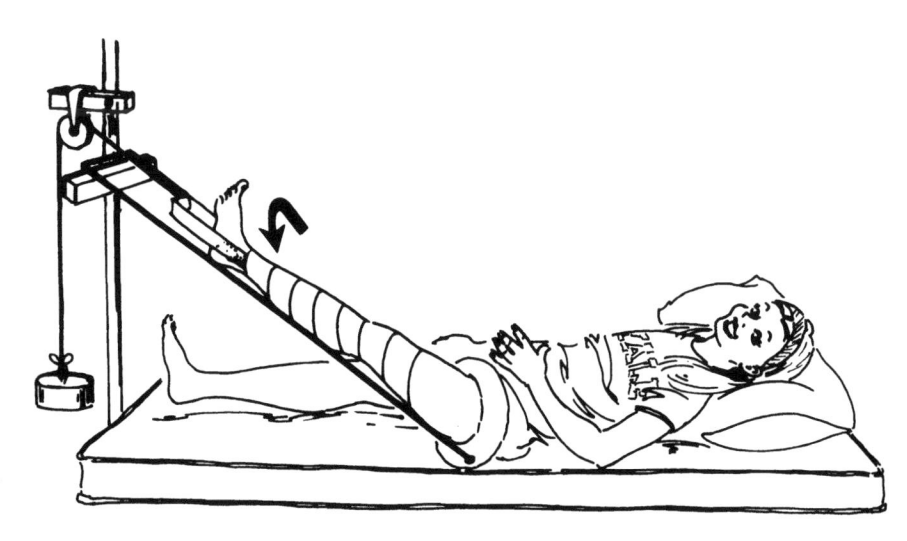

FIGURE 21-41. Straight-leg traction method.

because either the proximal or distal end of the fracture was found to be buttonholed through the lateral intramuscular septum. Continued anatomic separation of the bone ends may indicate entrapped quadriceps muscle. A small exposure allows the bone to be manipulated out of the enveloping muscle and back into the periosteal sleeve. The patient may be placed back in traction, casted, or treated with skeletal fixation.

Rauch et al. described the use of a Weber vertical extension frame for treating femoral fractures in young children to control rotation.[620] They reported good results in eight patients.

Immediate Casting

Because of increasing hospitalization costs, there has been an emphasis on casting femoral fractures in children as soon as possible.[376,432,499,516,566,649,662,663,711,712] This approach may include "immediate" application of a cast, which is probably best for infants and young children. For older children, a brief period of traction or suspension should probably precede casting.

Dameron and Thompson described closed reduction and immediate double hip spica immobilization as a preferred method for treating infants and young children.[438] Their method is as follows. Under aseptic conditions and with the patient under general anesthesia, a K-wire is inserted distal to the proximal tibial epiphysis of the affected side. The foot on the uninjured side is secured by strapping it to the footpiece of the fracture table. Traction is applied to the fractured thigh and normal leg while the pelvis is steadied against the well-padded perineal post. The pull on the distal fragment should be in line with the proximal fragment. Roentgenograms are obtained to determine the alignment of the fracture fragments. If there is any angulation, it is corrected by altering the direction of the traction forces. A well-molded double hip spica cast is then applied to include both feet, incorporating the K-wire in the plaster. The cast is left on for 6–8 weeks. If the method is used for adolescents, an additional 2–4 weeks of immobilization may be necessary for solid bony union. The K-wire placement in the tibia has the same potential risks as when it is used for traction. The use of a K-wire is not essential if the cast is applied with the patient under anesthesia and with adequate muscle relaxation.

The method I prefer is as follows. The small infant or child is casted on the infant spica frame; the fracture table may be used for the older child or adolescent. Adequate cast padding and felt strips are applied. In the young child I also use the Gortex cast liner. A short leg cast is first applied to the injured leg, and then the pelvis and opposite leg are casted. Once these casts are hardening, the assistant puts traction on the injured leg (through the short leg cast); adequate reduction is verified fluoroscopically, and the remainder of the cast is applied to the injured leg. After completion of cast application the position of the fracture fragments is verified by fluoroscopy.

The end results in 53 patients treated by this method, with an average duration of follow-up of 6.9 years, showed no deformity, abnormality of gait, or limitation of hip and knee motion in any of the patients. The fractured leg was, on average, not significantly longer than the normal leg. Complications of malunion, delayed union, nonunion, Volkmann's contracture, and gangrene were not encountered. Dameron and Thompson recommended this method for treating femoral shaft fractures.[438] The chief advantage of this method is that it decreases the duration of the hospital stay, which has obvious financial benefits. However, in the older child, maintenance of reduction is sometimes difficult, requiring close supervision by repeated roentgenograms and wedging of the cast to correct angulation should it occur.

Some studies have concluded that cast-bracing femoral fractures should be restricted to fractures in the distal third of the shaft because of the difficulty of controlling varus and anterior angulation with proximal shaft fractures.[409,432,482,544,567,576,664] In the study by Gross and colleagues, of the 72 femoral fractures treated with immediate cast-bracing, 22 resulted in excessive residual angulation or shortening.[482] These injuries were primarily mid- and proximal shaft fractures. Scott et al. reported that 4 of 14 femoral shaft fractures treated by cast-bracing had excessive angulation or shortening.[649]

Before considering casting, a push-pull evaluation under fluoroscopy may yield important information.[410] The amount of overriding in an emergency room film or in traction may not reflect the extent of soft tissue damage, which may allow further shortening in the cast. Accordingly, prior to casting (but after anesthesia) the distal fragment is pushed proximally. If overriding is less than 3 cm, a cast may be tried. If more than 3 cm of overrriding results, this patient is probably not a good candidate for immediate casting. Other methods (e.g., traction or operative) to reasonably maintain length should be considered.

Hughes et al. assessed the psychosocial aspects when hip spica casts were used to treat femoral fractures.[512] Work interference was identified by families as the major problem. For families with two working parents, a mean of 3 weeks time off work is necessary. None of the children was accepted into schools in spica casts, and home tutoring became necessary. However, none of the children in the study fell behind class permanently (only two temporarily). No child required physical therapy beyond simple instruction in walking, and 12 did not even have this. The mean time to independent walking following cast removal was 5 days and to running 25 days. Skills returned faster in the young children. All aspects of spica treatment were easier for the preschool children.

Weiss et al. reviewed 110 consecutive pediatric femoral shaft fractures treated with early hip spica cast application.[720] Four patients developed peroneal nerve palsy. All palsies resolved with immediate cast removal.

No matter what type of casting is used, immediate removal of the entire cast is not recommended. The child develops contractures and ligament tightness while in the cast. I prefer to remove the uninjured leg side and the injured side to above the knee. This practice allows reattainment of motion in the uninjured leg and knee motion on the injured side. Two to three weeks later the rest of the cast is removed, and hip motion is begun. This regimen decreases the likelihood of refracture.

Pavlik Harness

Stannard et al. detailed the use of the Pavlik harness for treating 16 femur fractures sustained between birth and 18 months of age. Stable union was evident within 5 weeks. The indications included fracture of the proximal and middle thirds of the femur, nonambulatory infants less than 4 months old at the start of treatment or small size of selected patients after 6 months of age, and shortening of less than 2 cm.[668]

Results

No matter what the method of traction or casting, these fractures generally heal well and rapidly in children. Roentgenographically evident callus formation occurs within 2–3 weeks in infants, 4 weeks in children, and 5–6 weeks in adolescents (Figs. 21-42, 21-43). Such callus formation accompanied by subsidence of pain usually indicates that the patient in traction is ready for a spica cast. Casting is necessary inasmuch as the callus is biologically plastic and may still deform if too much muscular activity is allowed, even in a spica cast. Cast removal should be based on clinical and roentgenographic appearance. The absence of pain on compression of the fracture site is an important sign. As a general rule, the amount of time (in weeks) needed for sufficient healing to begin protected activity out of the cast relates to the patient's age. For example, fractures in a 10-year-old child take about 10 weeks for adequate healing; those in a 16-year-old child take about 16 weeks.

Functional recovery to preinjury status is usually more rapid in children than in adults, although they may limp for

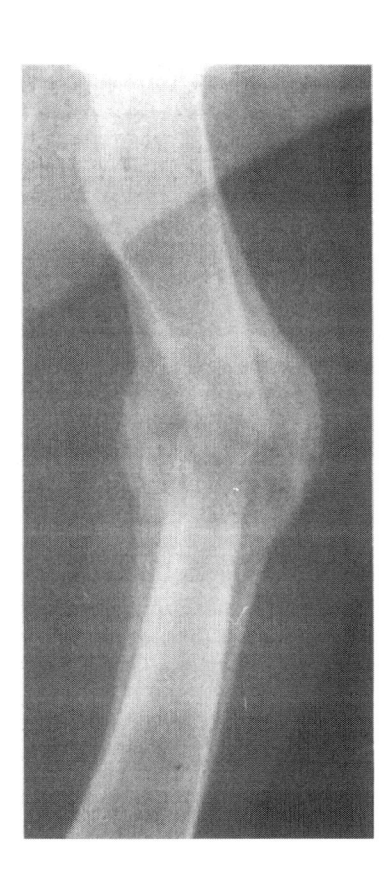

FIGURE 21-42. Typical healing pattern shows subperiosteal new bone confined by a tissue plane, associated with irregular callus around the fracture site, at which much of the periosteum presumably was disrupted.

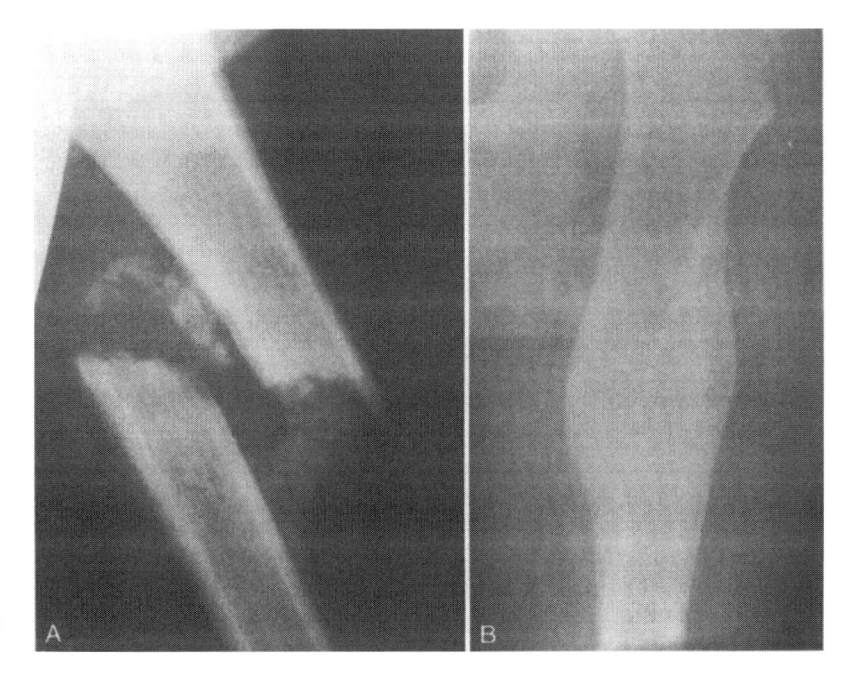

FIGURE 21-43. (A) Early subperiosteal to endosteal healing pattern. (B) Result 16 months later.

a long time afterward owing to leg length inequality and weak thigh musculature. This situation is often disturbing to relatives and parents, but an explanation of the reasons usually allays concerns. Leg length inequality, rotational differences, and muscular weakness may be routinely expected following these injuries.

Operative Methods

The operative treatment of femoral shaft fractures in children generally has been considered unnecessary and to be avoided as much as possible.[538,548,583,618,682,696] Perfect anatomic reduction of fracture fragments is less important in the child than in the adult, as most malunions are corrected with growth and remodeling, union occurs rapidly, pseudarthrosis is rare, and there is a tendency toward spontaneous correction of deformities. There is, however, an increasing advocacy for the use of internal or external skeletal fixation, especially in the older child. Some of this emphasis is due to the desire to decrease the length of hospitalization. However, these methods may allow more rapid rehabilitation of the injured child or adolescent.

Betterman et al. reviewed 270 femoral shaft fractures and thought that surgical intervention or some type of external fixation should be considered after 7 years of age and definitely used after age 12.[395]

Of 191 children in a series reported by Viljanto and associates, 45 (18%) were treated by surgery (18 by intramedullary nailing, 16 by other means of osteosynthesis, and 1 with a crushed extremity by primary amputation).[696] No infections occurred. The mean longitudinal overgrowth of 9.8 mm did not differ significantly from that of 10.7 mm in nonoperatively treated patients. It is interesting that overgrowth was less in those treated by intramedullary nailing than in those treated by other means of osteosynthesis. These investigators preferred intramedullary nailing, recommending it for the following situations or groups of patients: transverse fractures that involved the middle third of the femoral shaft; pathologic fractures; patients in whom primary conservative treatment had not led to an acceptable position; when there were vascular or neural injuries together with shaft fractures and large soft tissue defects; for multiple injuries of the same and other limbs; or the unconscious, neurologically injured patient in whom traction and casting may be difficult due to spasticity.[696] Mohan thought that further indications for open reduction included muscle interposition and gross instability of the fracture.[577]

Some methods of osteosynthesis may be contraindicated in skeletally immature patients, as they may damage the physis along the femoral neck (Fig. 21-44) and may also create distal problems. Ischemic necrosis may also occur (Fig. 21-45). Raisch showed that intramedullary nailing may impinge against the distal epiphyseal plate, resulting in retarded growth of the extremity.[618] This may be avoided by proper choice of nail length and the use of locking screws to prevent migration. In contrast, Griessman[479] and Kuntscher[548] suggested that operative treatment by means of internal fixation did not cause a harmful reaction in children and could therefore be carried out equally well in both children and adults.

When there is an open fracture of the femur, the wound is thoroughly débrided of all foreign material and any damaged tissue excised. After copious irrigation the wound should be left open and the leg placed in 90°–90° skeletal traction to increase spontaneous drainage. Appropriate antibiotics and tetanus antitoxin are administered. There is no justification for immediate internal fixation when the fracture is open. An open fracture does not ordinarily require a longer period to consolidate in a child, but an external fixator should be considered for the open femoral fracture.

Reeves et al. evaluated 90 adolescent patients with 96 femoral fractures.[623] Fifty-two fractures were treated with rigid internal fixation. Forty-four fractures underwent traction and subsequent casting. The traction casting group had

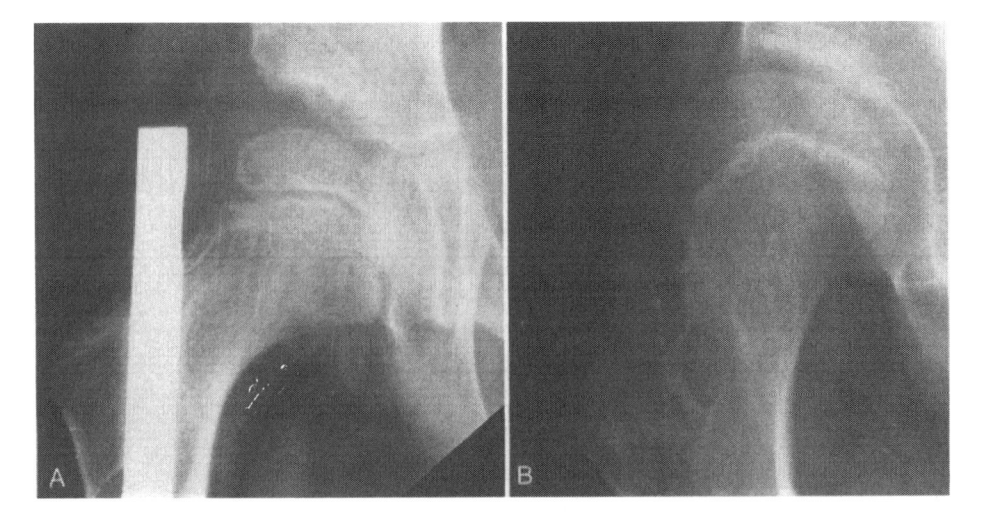

FIGURE 21-44. (A) Intramedullary rodding of a femoral fracture. (B) Subsequent growth deformity of the proximal femoral neck with increased valgus of the capital femur and premature epiphysiodesis of the greater trochanteric physis.

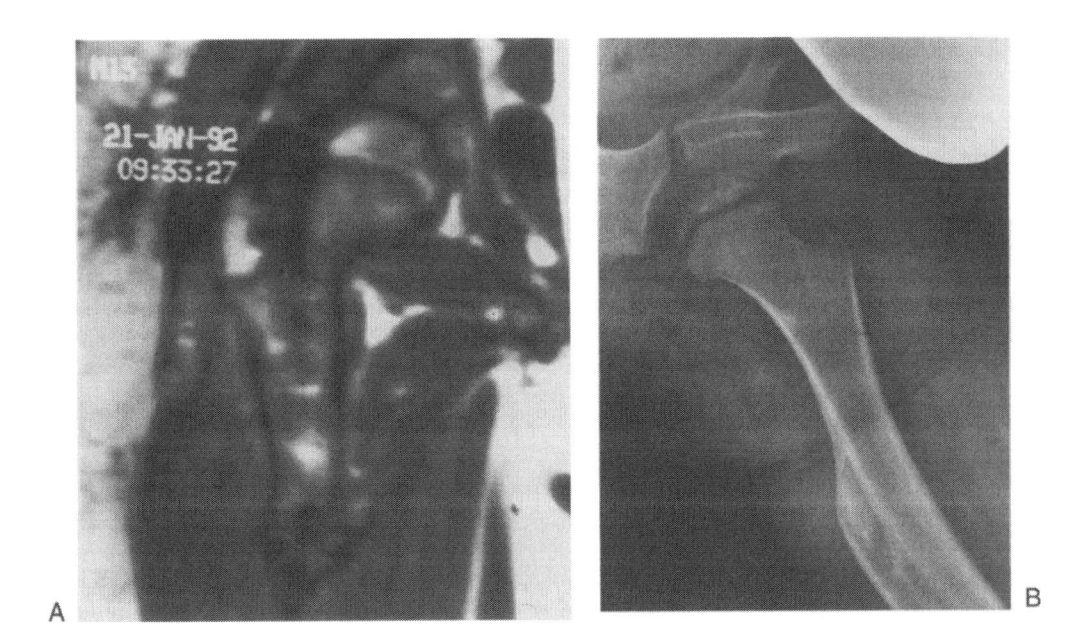

FIGURE 21-45. (A) Ischemic necrosis of the femoral head (partial) after femoral rodding. (B) Ischemic necrosis of the femoral head following *closed* treatment of a femoral fracture.

a mean hospitalization of 26 days. The operative group had a mean stay of 9 days and had fewer complications. The authors concluded that femoral shaft fractures in adolescents could be operatively treated with excellent results and fewer complication.

Intramedullary Rodding

The use of intramedullary rodding, with or without reaming, has been advocated for the treatment of femoral shaft fractures in children during the second decade of life. Part of this advocacy has been based on various statements that premature growth arrest either does not occur, or if it does occur, it does not lead to functional problems. Herndon et al. described 21 fractures in adolescents treated by intramedullary nailing; none of the patients developed premature growth arrest.[502] Reeves et al. treated 33 adolescent patients with intramedullary rods and did not observe any trochanteric growth disturbances.[623] In neither study was it clear whether patients were followed to skeletal maturity.

Valdiserri and colleagues reported that medullary nailing did not cause adverse effects provided it was carried out in children older than 8–9 years of age.[691] If it was done before that time, there were significant problems with trochanteric arrest and a marked valgus deformity. Knittel and Romer reported 47 cases of children who had intramedullary pinning with Rush's rods.[539] They noted that there was a 2- to 20-mm increase in length (average 9.4 mm) compared with the opposite side. In some children there was shortening of 1–15 mm (average 4.6 mm).

Cases of trochanteric apophyseal arrest have been reported.[503,530,729] All reported growth arrests have been asymptomatic. Ziv and coworkers concluded that proximal reaming should be avoided in the growing child and that femoral head necrosis could be a potential complication of reaming, as the area of the circumflex artery might be impaired.[729]

Beaty et al. described the use of interlocking intramedullary nails in 30 patients aged 10–15 years.[392] Two of the patients had an overgrowth of more than 2.5 cm. None had angular or rotational malunions, and there were no trochanteric growth alterations. They noted two important complications: leg length discrepancy and avascular necrosis of the femoral head. The average leg length discrepancy was 0.5 cm. Because of the risk of ischemic necrosis, they recommended that dissection be limited to the base of the femoral neck and into the piriformis fossa–greater trochanter junction; it should not extend into the posterior capsule of the midportion of the femoral neck.

Raney et al. studied skeletally immature patients who developed premature closure of the greater trochanteric physis consequent to placement of an intramedullary rod for primary treatment of the femoral diaphyseal fracture (Fig. 21-44).[619] Each patient developed increased femoral neck valgus when compared to the contralateral hip. None of these patients developed functional disability, although one had a radiographic subluxation. Anatomic specimens demonstrated the likelihood of traversing a portion of the greater trochanteric physis. These authors recommended that other methods of fracture treatment, either operative or nonoperative, be considered in skeletally immature patients who have not entered the final phase of maturation characterized by subchondral sclerosis along the greater trochanteric physis.

The diameter of most rods exceeds the size of the physeal defect that could be associated with a high incidence of premature growth arrest (see Chapter 7). Any defect larger than 0.25 inch generally leads to formation of an osseous bony bridge across the physis.

Extensive analysis of development of the proximal femur shows not only that active growth is present in the greater trochanteric physis, but the physis extends toward the capital femur well into the second decade, with this extension being posterior and superior along the femoral neck. Furthermore, although there is appositional enlargement of the trochanter through its perichondrium, the "growth" that has been attributed to the end of the trochanter was, more properly, proximal (upward) *expansion* of the secondary ossification center into the already formed but still unossified cartilaginous portion of the trochanter.

Premature fusion of the growth plate of the greater trochanter has been used as a method of altering the mechanics of proximal femoral growth for deformities such as coxa plana and vara in patients with Legg-Perthes disease or developmental dysplasia of the hip, and in patients who have developed a deformity secondary to septic arthritis of the hip or proximal femoral osteomyelitis. The stipulated aim of such greater trochanteric epiphysiodesis was "redirection" of growth into a "valgus" pattern.

Operative damage to the greater trochanter during osteotomy for developmental dysplasia of the hip has led to a long valgus femoral neck without significant disturbance of acetabular development. Premature closure of the greater trochanteric epiphysis has also been described as a complication following traumatic avulsion of this structure and led to the development of an elongated valgus femoral neck (see Chapter 20).

Because children enter growth spurts at different stages and skeletal maturity does not always correlate with chronologic age, the use of intramedullary rods that cross the greater trochanteric physis should be used with caution. Certainly, a child who is in the middle or at the end of the growth spurt and who has evidence of thickening of the subchondral plates on either side of the physis of the greater trochanter and capital femur could undergo placement of an intramedullary rod without significant consequence.

An effort should be made to evaluate the skeletal age and extent of maturity in any patient for whom treatment of a femoral shaft fracture with an intramedullary rod is considered. For children who have not yet entered their (pre)adolescent growth spurt, alternative methods of fracture treatment should be considered. It is safer to consider internal fixation with a plate and screws, internal fixation with small rods (e.g., Enders nails) that do not cross a physis, or placement of an external fixator that may be kept in place until the fracture has healed or that may be removed when the fracture is stable and replaced with a cast, cast-brace, or full contact orthosis.

Galpin et al. reported the use of intramedullary nailing in 37 fractures.[469] Twenty-two patients with an average age of 12 years 9 months were treated with reamed nails, whereas fifteen patients at an average age of 6 months were treated with nonreamed nails. Fractures united within 6–12 weeks. None of the patients developed avascular necrosis. One patient required excision of heterotopic bone to restore function. Galpin et al. particularly looked at changes in the articulotrochanteric distance (ATD) and found five patients, two 11-year-olds and three 13-year-olds, at the time of injury and surgery in which the ATD had increased an average of 1.7 cm (range 1.2–2.5 cm); all five had undergone reamed intramedullary (IM) nailing. None of the nonreamed nailings sustained trochanteric growth arrest. When using small rods such as Rush rods, the authors recommended at least two rods to obtain rotational and angular stability. Six patients treated with reamed nailing developed myositis.

Grundes and Reikeras studied the effect on blood flow on healing in rats with closed versus intramedullary nailing of femoral fractures.[483] Reaming had no acute impact on the bone blood flow, whereas reaming combined with a fracture reduced total bone blood flow by half and reduced cortical diaphyseal flow to approximately one-fourth. At 4 weeks the bending strength, rigidity, and fracture energy of the fractures treated by closed medullary nailing were greater than those treated by open nailing; but by 12 weeks there were no differences in the mechanical parameters.

Pape et al. assessed the effect of pulmonary damage after intramedullary femoral nailing in traumatized sheep.[605,606] They found that nailing after severe shock and lung contusion caused further lung damage as a result of polymorphonuclear leukocyte activation and triglyceride embolism. These effects were significantly less if the nailing was performed without prior reaming.

Blitzer and Hamilton monitored oxygen saturation during reaming and intramedullary nailing of 15 femoral fractures.[399] There was no statistically significant drop in oxygen saturation during the procedure.

Kao et al. described 10 pudendal nerve palsies (15%) among 65 intramedullary nailings.[526] All palsies were transient. The authors noted that the patient should be informed preoperatively of this risk.

Nontrochanteric Rodding

Mann and associates described closed reduction and intramedullary Ender's nailing (Figs. 21-46, 21-47) of femoral fractures in children.[562] The average time to independent ambulation was 7.1 days. No patient had an angular deformity of more than 10° in any plane. No patient had clinically evident loss of motion, leg length discrepancy, or radiographic evidence of growth disturbance. It is important, when placing the nails, that the entry point be proximal to the distal physis. An image intensifier should be used to identify the distal physis. For fractures distal to the midshaft, nail insertion is performed in a proximal to distal direction. The proximal portal for Ender's nailing is distal to the greater trochanteric physis on the lateral cortex. Again, the image intensifier is used to identify this insertion point. The distal insertion is used for fractures proximal to the midshaft. Passage of the nail should be stopped at least 1 cm away from the physis at the opposite end.

Bourdelat and coworkers treated children between the ages of 6 and 14 with flexibile medullary nailing, principally through a descending route from the subtrochanteric region.[403–405] They found the results to be satisfactory.

Heinrich et al. described the use of Ender's nails in children 6 years of age or older.[496,497] They found that three points of fixation should be established around the fracture,

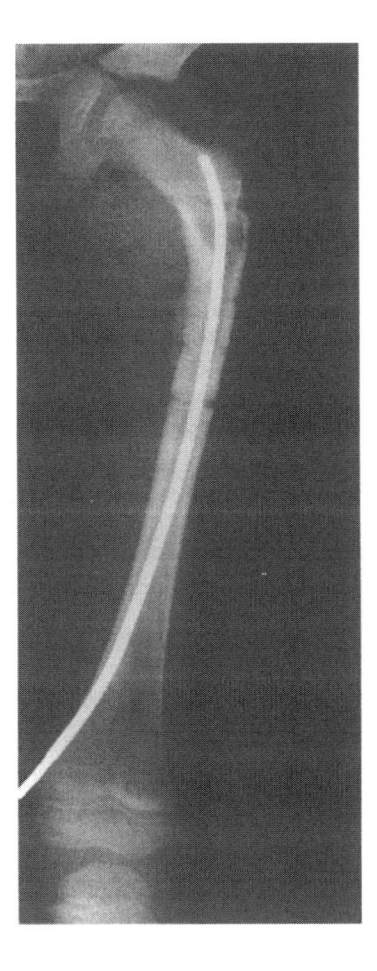

FIGURE 21-46. Single flexible rod used after failure of an external fixator.

common reason for fixation was to simplify nursing care and rehabilitation of children who had associated severe head injury or polytrauma. Twenty-three fractures healed within an average of 11 weeks. Leg length discrepancy was not a clinical problem in any of the patients. Interestingly, when using this rigid fixation method with the AO compression plate, 75% of the fractures healed by periosteal callus formation, not primary bone healing, which reflects the activity (hyperactivity) of the periosteum in the child. Despite instructions of the contrary, many children begin weight-bearing as tolerated as soon as possible after their injury. Although it certainly increases the risk of plate breakage, the stimulus of early weight-bearing probably enhances early periosteal callus formation, despite the use of rigid plates. One 14-year-old boy with unrecognized medial cortex comminution experienced plate breakage 6 weeks after operation. Ward et al. also noted, when reviewing the literature, that there was a plate breakage rate ranging from 3% to 15%, with most series reporting an incidence of 6–7%. They thought that the most important factors contributing to plate breakage in the pediatric/adolescent population were unrecognized medial cortex comminution, early weight bearing, and premature return to full activity. Interestingly, these authors recommended that reamed intramedullary nailing rather than plate fixation be used for adolescents over 12 years of age. One of their patients in whom the plate was removed sustained a stress fracture through the empty

or the intramedullary canal must be stacked with multiple nails to prevent angulation. Any failure to stack the canal or achieve multiple fixation points increased the risk of angular deformity. They thought that subtrochanteric and proximal third fractures should be stabilized retrogradely with insertion through a single site in the distal femoral diaphysis. In general, two divergent C-configuration nails or one standard C- and one S-configuration nail approximately 5 cm distal to the fracture usually provides sufficient fixation. Noncomminuted isthmus fractures should be stabilized through a single approach from either the medial or lateral aspect of the distal femur, with the nail stacked to fill the medullary canal at the site of the fracture. The distal one-third and comminuted middle one-third of femur fractures should be stabilized with at least one retrograde C-configuration nail inserted from the medial metaphysis and one from the lateral. They further thought that children 6–10 years old should be stabilized with 4 mm flexible nails. They noted that 4.5 mm flexible nails were too stiff for use in pediatric patients.

Plate Fixation

Ward et al. reviewed children who underwent compression plate fixation for a diaphyseal femoral fracture.[710] The most

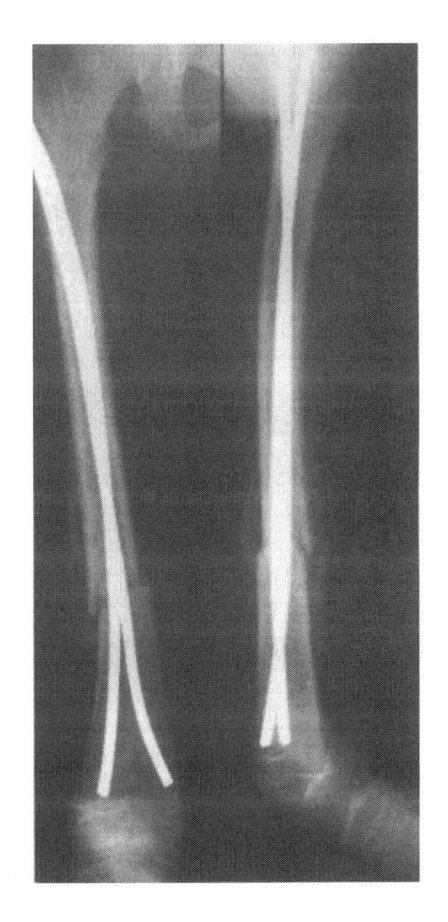

FIGURE 21-47. Double rod fixation of a femoral diaphyseal fracture.

screw hole 2 months after plate removal following blunt trauma from a bicycle accident.

Kregor et al. evaluated plate fixation of femoral shaft fractures in multiply injured children.[542] They reviewed 15 fractures (9 closed, 6 open). There were no infections and were radiographically healed at an average of 8 weeks. The plates were removed at an average of 10 months (range 3–24 months). After the index operation, overgrowth of the injured femur averaged 0.9 cm (range 0.3–1.4 cm).

External Fixator

The external fixator offers a relatively simple, minimally invasive method of stabilizing a femoral shaft fracture (Fig. 21-48). The method is especially useful in the presence of multiple trauma, head injury, and a comatose state or open fractures. Two to three pins are placed proximal and distal to the fracture. Additional pins may be inserted into large comminuted fragments.

The device chosen depends on the preference of the surgeon. Several are available. Their purported biomechanical attributes and differences probably are not a factor in the biologically plastic immature skeleton.

The main potential problems are pin tract inflammation leading to osteomyelitis and refracture after removal of the fixator. To lessen the risk of the latter, the same method used for limb lengthening may be applied. The device is removed, but the pins are left in place for up to a week. If the patient develops pain, the fixator may be readily reapplied. After 5–7 days the radiograph is repeated to see if any stress-induced radiolucency is developing at the fracture site. The pins are then removed.

Other Considerations

Strickland and Wittgen reported a case of pathologic fracture of the femoral shaft 55 years after circumferential banding.[675] The size of the band was only about 50% of the final diameter. There was occlusion of the medullary canal with compact bone. The band probably was responsible for the formed compact bone occluding the area. Occlusion of the medullary cavity may predispose to pathologic fracture in children by increasing the brittleness of the otherwise hollow bone.

Complications

Vascular Problems

Arterial injuries associated with femoral shaft fractures present management problems. A slow arterial leak may not be readily recognized owing to the presence of normal pulse and capillary filling. Dehne and Kriz reported five cases of unrecognized slow arterial leakage.[444] In three patients amputation became necessary because of the delayed diagnosis. Increasing limb girth, absent or diminishing pulse, and progressive neurologic signs in the presence of a closed fracture strongly suggest arterial injury and indicate the need for prompt arteriography. The collateral circulation varies widely in its capacity to maintain viability in the limb. It may be possible to treat young children with skeletal traction following vascular surgery, although internal fixation is usually done. The use of internal fixation has been advocated because a more stable fracture site adds protection to arterial repair.[247] Internal fixation may prolong the surgical procedure and increase the risk of infection; and dissection of soft tissue for insertion of the plate may produce increased venostasis and potential loss of collateral circulation. I prefer an external fixator in these situations.

Because of vascular damage to one or more branches of the deep femoral artery, significant intracompartment bleeding may occur. It may lead to a compartment syndrome that must be assessed and, when necessary, decompressed.

False aneurysm has been described following a closed femoral fracture in a child.[451,593,651]

Bone Length/Overgrowth

Leg length inequality is the most frequent result of femoral shaft fractures during childhood.[375,387,442,450,478,568,688] Staheli studied 84 patients followed for 2–16 years after nonoperative treatment of closed femoral shaft fractures.[665] Tibial length was not affected greatly by the femoral fractures, although some reactive overgrowth may occur even in the tibia. Among the 17 patients sustaining fracture during infancy, no late significant femoral inequality was observed. Among the children 2–8 years of age, 25% showed inequal-

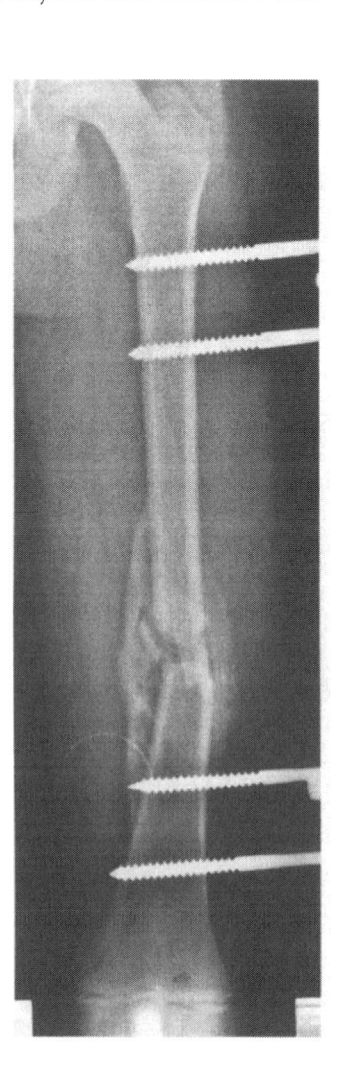

FIGURE 21-48. Uniaxial fixation.

ity. Among children 8–12 years old, significant inequality was observed in 44%. Growth acceleration was less consistent in this age group. Fractures in the proximal third and oblique-comminuted types were also associated with relatively more growth acceleration.

Differences in limb length following femoral shaft fractures may result from excessive overriding or distraction of the fragments or from stimulation of linear growth. These differences usually stabilize within the first year after injury and do not change significantly thereafter. However, in children under 2 years of age and in adolescents, the normal growth stimulation is not as dramatic as in children of the middle childhood years. The infant and young child heal rapidly. During adolescence there are fewer years of growth remaining to correct a deformity. Thus in these two age groups, minimal overriding should be accepted.

The relative tension of the periosteum sleeve is a normal physiologic control factor; it changes with age and becomes more "adult" in character during adolescence. The potential control and interplay between periosteal tension and growth rates at the physis are undoubtedly affected. Periosteal stripping without fracture may promote overgrowth. Furthermore, larger initial fragment displacements may stimulate increased overgrowth through a temporary decrease in periosteal tension.

The extent of overgrowth is not predictable in the individual patient. Since Truesdell's original description, many authors have observed that the relative lengthening of the fractured femur averages approximately 1 cm.[688] This extent of overriding of fracture ends is most commonly accepted as a treatment goal and normal biologic response.

Shapiro documented femoral overgrowth after femoral shaft fractures with sequential orthoroentgenograms in 74 patients followed until skeletal maturity.[652] The femoral overgrowth averaged 0.92 cm (range 0.4–2.7 cm) and was found to be independent of age, level of fracture, or position of the fracture at the time of healing. Ipsilateral tibial overgrowth averaged 0.29 cm (range 0.1–0.5 cm) and added to the length discrepancy. About 78% of the overgrowth had occurred during the first 18 months after fracture. By 18 months after fracture only 12% of the patients had completed the overgrowth, and by 3.5 years after fracture 85% had completed this overgrowth. In 9%, the overgrowth continued throughout the remaining growth period, although at a slower rate than during the first 18 months following fracture.

Overgrowth is a physiologic process associated with both the increased vascularity of the physes of the involved bone produced by healing and changes in tension in the periosteal sleeve. This observation now appears amply confirmed, especially as overgrowth occurs regardless of the position of fracture healing and in virtually all patients, indicating that it is an obligatory phenomenon rather than one compensating for shortening. It also often involves the ipsilateral tibia, which would be related to temporarily increased vascularity, as the periosteum is obviously intact. The phenomenon also occurs with humeral and tibial fractures. Kellernova and associates demonstrated increased vascularity to the entire limb following experimental tibial fracture.[528]

Hehl et al. studied posttraumatic limb shortening after conservative and operative treatment of diaphyseal femoral fractures in children.[495] They treated 120 fractures in 116 children. The treatment of choice was conservative in young patients with overhead traction in the 1- to 3-year-old child and Weber traction in a 3- to 8-year-old child. Operative treatment was usually used in older children. Plate fixation was performed in children 5–16 years of age, and external fixation was used in children 2–14 years of age. Measurements showed a mean limb length increase of 5.5 mm following overhead traction and 7 mm for 90°–90° traction. Following plate fixation it was 5.5 mm and following external fixation 8.5 mm. Their results did not show any statistically significant differences for the various treatment methods regarding the likelihood of overgrowth.

Corry and Nicol studied 50 children roughly 1.9 years after injury.[436] There was a mean 6.9 mm of overgrowth. Age was the only influential variable, with overgrowth being less in children under 4 and 7 years of age. The authors thought that much less shortening should be accepted than is commonly recommended.

Hougaard studied 67 femoral shaft fractures.[509] He could not demonstrate any relation between shortening at the time of healing and the magnitude of overgrowth 2 years later. Nor was he able to demonstrate any relation among sex, age, type of fracture, level of fracture, and magnitude overgrowth. The mean overgrowth was 10.8 mm and the largest 26 mm. Almost all the children who healed with little shortening showed no angulation, whereas almost all of the femoral fractures that healed with considerable shortening had some angulation. The importance of angulation with respect to shortening after femoral shaft fractures in children had not been previously emphasized.

Stephens et al. reviewed 30 skeletally mature patients who had isolated closed femoral shaft fractures during childhood that had been treated conservatively.[671] When the fracture had occurred between the ages of 7 and 13 years, the limb overgrew about 1 cm. These authors found that excessive fracture overlap at the time of injury but not at time of union increased limb overgrowth. Angulation of the fracture remodeled in children injured when they were under 10 years of age. The authors recommended that in the 7- to 13-year-old patient treatment should aim at a 1 cm overlap at union and correction of any angular deformity in children over 10 years of age.

Angulation/Bowing

Restoration of the normal anterolateral bow should also be a goal, no matter what the treatment method. Residual angulation may worsen in a cast. Angular deformities should be minimal. The degree of remodeling and restoration of longitudinal alignment is unpredictable and less likely the closer the fracture is to the middle of the bone (Figs. 21-49, 21-50). The greatest amount of anticipated axial correction was cited by Nonnemann, according to whom axial deviation up to 30° tended to correct spontaneously.[594] Lateral displacement may correct varus deformity on an average of up to 40% and valgus deformity up to 60% of the initial angular defect, whereas antecurvatum and recurvatum may correct nearly 70% of any original deformity over 10°.[697] Viljanto et al. considered the relatively slow and limited correction of varus and valgus deformities the most significant finding.[697]

Wallace and Hoffman studied remodeling of the angular deformity of femoral shaft fractures in children.[708] They

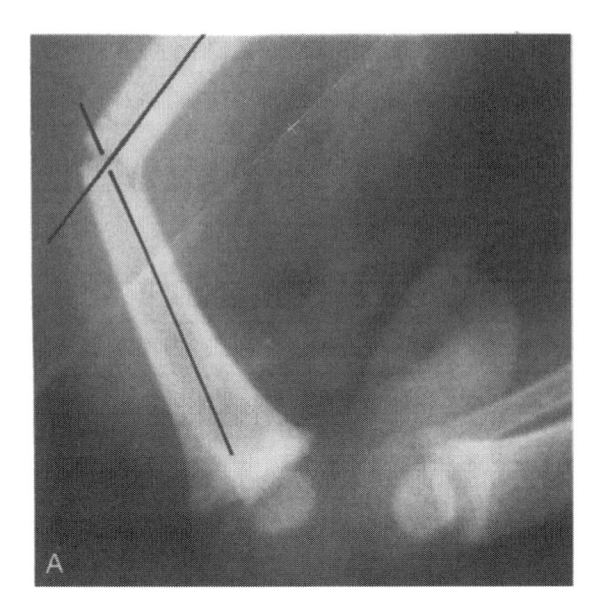

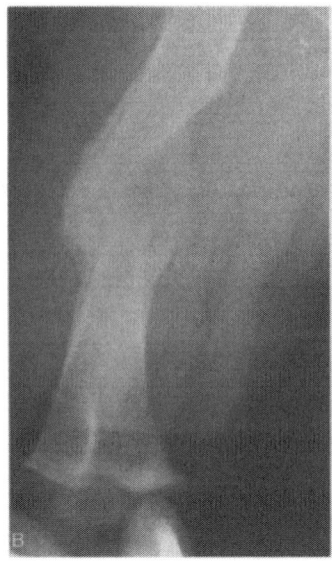

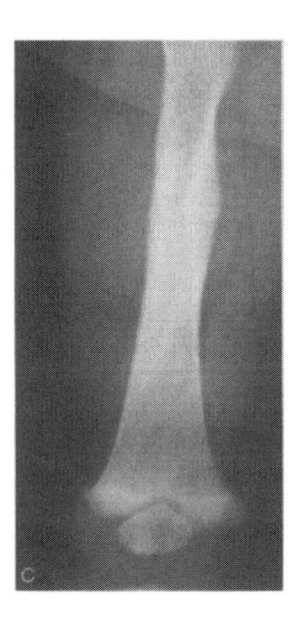

FIGURE 21-49. (A) Excessive malunion in an infant (7 months). (B) It was partially corrected and healed by callus. (C) Eight months later a mild deformity was present. Significant angular deformities are likely to correct themselves only in this young age group.

reviewed 28 children with unilateral middle third fractures who had angular deformities of 10°–26° after union. At an average follow-up of 45 months after the injury, the average correction was 85% of the initial deformity; 74% of the correction occurred at the physes, and only 26% at the fracture site. They concluded that in children under 13 years of age malunion of as much as 25° in any plane can remodel sufficiently to give normal alignment at the joint surfaces, even though the bone per se may continue to appear deformed.

Shaft fractures left with angular deformities have a possibility of long-term complications, such as slipped capital femoral epiphysis.

Rotation

Rotational deformity may occur with any of the traditional methods of treatment.[607,705] A study of rotational deformities 27–32 years after injury found persistent rotational disability in only one case and refuted the established view that

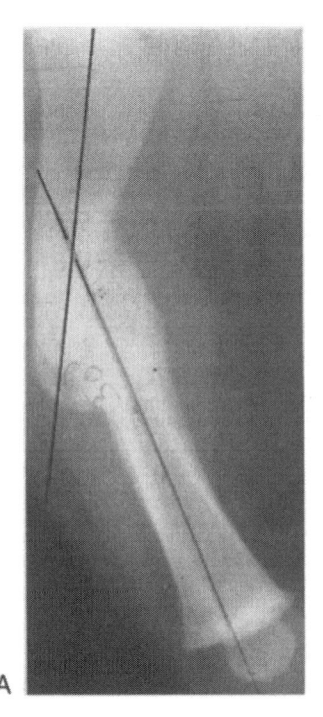

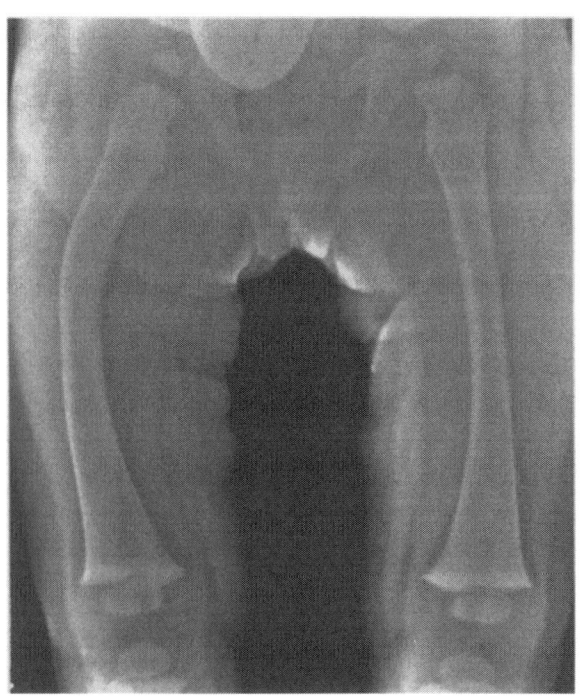

FIGURE 21-50. (A) Angular malunion in a young child (19 months). This degree of deformity should not be accepted in children older than 6–8 years of age. (B) Lack of angular correction, although there is obvious remodeling. It has led to a recurvatum.

rotational displacement is incapable of spontaneously correcting.[408] Hagglund et al. showed that the mean anteversion difference of 9.6° between the fractured and uninvolved sides after femoral shaft fracture decreased to 5.6°, suggesting that children have an ability to correct some rotational deformity by continued growth.[486]

Strong et al. showed that in malrotated femoral fractures created in rabbit models there was 55% improvement of malrotation by 4 weeks.[676] This may not extrapolate to humans because of different biomechanical forces.

Muscle Function

Isometric and dynamic measurements of quadriceps function in children with femoral fractures revealed a significant reduction of strength in the affected leg.[439,500] This function is rarely used as a criterion for assessing the therapeutic results, particularly in children. The status of the muscles after femoral fractures has often been evaluated by measurements of leg circumference, but direct measurements of quadriceps function have not been carried out. There also was a greater reduction of strength the more distally the fracture was located. This factor should be taken into account during the rehabilitation of patients. Miller and associates reported severe loss of muscle function in a child sustaining ischemic fibrosis of the lower leg that was a complication of femoral fracture.[573] Muscle herniation also may complicate healing as well as return of function.

Hennrikus et al. studied muscle strength in the quadriceps muscle following femoral fracture.[500] They examined the patients an average of 33 months after injury; 39% of the patients had a persistent deficit in the strength of the quadriceps on testing with the Cybex machine. Six patients (18%) had a deficit according to the one leg hop for distance test. Forty-two percent had a loss of 10° of flexion. The amount of maximum displacement of the fracture as seen on the initial radiographs appeared to be the only factor that was significant for predicting weakness. Despite the weakness as tested, none of the patients had a clinical problem. A subclinical deficit in the strength of the quadriceps may be related to damage sustained by the muscle at the time of the fracture.

Refracture

Refracture of the shaft of the femur is an infrequent complication. Saimon reviewed 21 patients ranging in age from 7 to 58 years and found that the incidence of refracture was highest in those in the 16- to 20-year range.[635] He thought that excessive emphasis on restoration of knee movement after removal of the cast was a factor because of muscular tightness, particularly in the quadriceps. Rigorous rehabilitation is rarely necessary in children and adolescents. The amount of overriding of the fragments did not seem to be related in any way to the liability to refracture. Careful clinical assessment of the degree of union is important when considering discontinuation of bracing or casting. It is not sufficient only to palpate the callus gently to apply stress to the bone. Firm pressure and strong stresses to the bone should be applied, because if the bone cannot withstand these maneuvers, it almost certainly cannot withstand the vigorous mobilization of the child. Radiologic criteria of "adequate" union are more difficult to define. In some cases refracture occurred despite the presence of a great deal of callus.[635] The radiologic demonstration of "warning" cracks is obviously of great importance and indicates the need for further immobilization.

Nerve Injury

Concomitant injury to the sciatic nerve does not affect the rate of fracture healing. However, the remainder of the bone may become excessively osteoporotic and susceptible to fracture following removal of the cast.

Growth Arrest

Hunter and Hensinger reported an 11-year-old child with a comminuted spiral fracture of the femoral shaft.[514] Growth arrest occurred in all physes of the extremity, with the exception of the distal fibular epiphysis. This instance of multiple premature epiphyseal closure after a seemingly uncomplicated fracture of the femoral shaft appears to be unique, particularly as there was no detectable neurovascular injury to the affected extremity and no history or clinical evidence of direct trauma to the physes. They thought that some generalized vascular or neural disturbance seemed to be the most reasonable explanation for the monomelic growth arrest.

Myositis

Steinberg and Hubbard showed that heterotopic ossification after femoral intramedullary rodding was a significant complication of the procedure.[669] A statistically significant increase of myositis ossificans was found in males when there was an increased delay from injury to surgery and in patients requiring prolonged intubation because of multiple injuries. The heterotopic ossification tended to be present in the dissected tissues for the approach to the intratrochanteric region for insertion of the rod.

Distal Femoral Metaphyseal Injuries

Distal femoral metaphyseal injuries are relatively common. The fracture line is usually transversely oriented. Torus (greenstick) fractures are frequent (Fig. 21-51) and must be treated carefully, as angular deformity (varus or valgus) may be introduced at the time of injury, comparable to supracondylar humeral injuries, and may not be readily recognized during diagnosis or treatment. The fracture may also be complete but undisplaced. Again, the degree of compression deformity of a portion of this fracture must be watched. The fracture may be displaced, but this is an uncommon injury in this region. There may be comminution, with extension (longitudinally) of the fracture from the primary trabecular fracture toward the physis (Fig. 21-52).

The gastrocnemius muscle is the chief deforming force. The muscle arises (by two heads) from the posterior surface of the distal femur and angulates the distal fragment posteriorly toward the popliteal space. Either fragment may

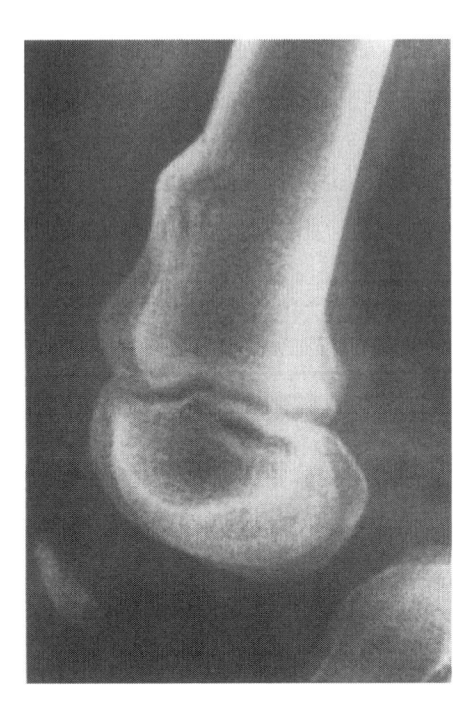

FIGURE 21-51. Torus metaphyseal fracture.

impinge on the popliteal vessels and nerves, partially occluding or compressing them or even causing some degree of laceration. Careful assessment of neurovascular function is essential following injury and during care. The proximal fragment may be driven into the quadriceps femoris muscle and may cause significant damage to the vastus intermedius, with subsequent scarring, restriction of flexion, and fibrosis. The fragment may become entrapped (buttonholed) within the muscle.

For the displaced fracture, treatment should consist of reducing any angular deformity followed by application of a long leg cast with 10°–15° of knee flexion. This cast should be maintained for 3–4 weeks, at which time a cylinder (knee extension) cast or knee immobilizer may be applied to begin protected weight-bearing. Knee stiffness is not a major concern in the young child, although a hinged cast may be used to allow some knee motion in the adolescent who requires longer casting because of the extended time of healing.

For the undisplaced fracture, casting may be used. Frequent checks are necessary to be certain that angular deformation, resulting from the pull of the gastrocnemius, does not occur. Mild knee and ankle flexion should relax the muscle. If the fracture is unstable or there is any neurovascular compromise, the patient should be placed in skin or skeletal traction; alternatively, percutaneous fixation can be used followed by a cast.

If the fracture cannot be controlled effectively, percutaneous pinning or an external fixator should be considered. One of the pins may be placed transversely across the epiphyseal ossification center if there is not enough metaphysis between the fracture and physis to accept more than one pin.

These fractures usually heal rapidly and without major complications. Angular deformity, especially in the varus/valgus plane, does not correct spontaneously and requires correction at the inception of treatment. Residual malunion may require a corrective osteotomy.

Distal Femoral Epiphyseal Injuries

Distal femoral epiphyseal injuries are common, especially in adolescents.[732–802] They were once termed "cartwheel" injuries because the prevalent mechanism of injury involved jumping onto large-wheeled wagons. The literature of the nineteenth and early twentieth centuries called attention to the high incidence of injuries in the distal femoral epiphysis caused principally by horse-drawn vehicles. Boys who attempted to jump on wagons frequently caught one of the lower limbs in the wheel spokes and sustained a hyperextension injury. Automobile, bicycle, skateboard, go-kart, and athletic injuries have superseded the horse-drawn wagon.

Obstetric Injury

Type 1 distal femoral epiphyseal plate separation is an infrequent obstetric injury. Nevertheless, it is an important clinical entity because it may remain undiagnosed or be misdiagnosed as dislocation, septic arthritis, osteomyelitis, or pseudoparalysis. A strong hyperextension force on the knee may produce rupture of the periosteum, causing displacement.[781] An audible snap may be felt. The infant is usually irritable upon examination. Crepitation may be felt during examination.

The radiograph may be interpreted as normal unless careful attention is paid to the position of the distal femoral epiphysis relative to the metaphysis (Fig. 21-53). Otherwise, assess the tibia relative to the femoral axis. This particular

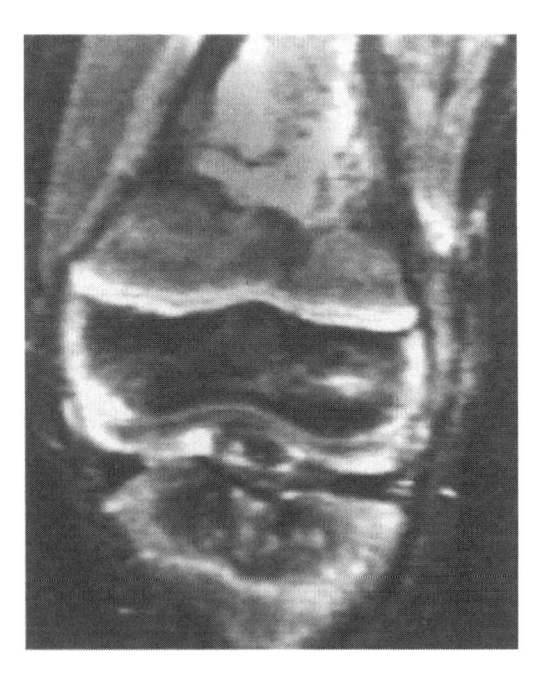

FIGURE 21-52. MRI of a distal femoral metaphyseal fracture. Extensive hemorrhage is evident proximal to the fracture line. There is also a bone bruise in the medial portion of the distal femoral ossification center.

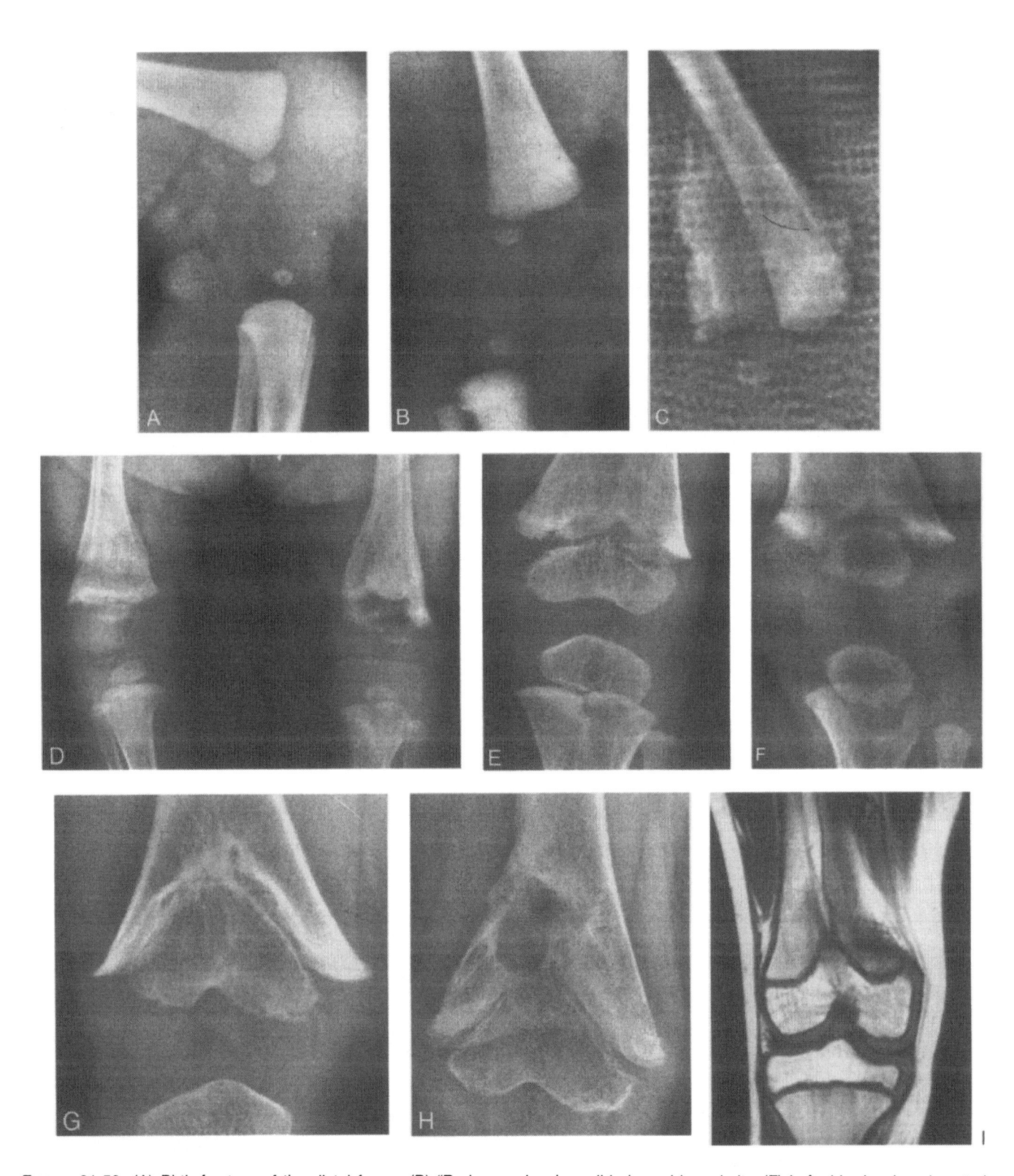

FIGURE 21-53. (A) Birth fracture of the distal femur. (B) "Reduction." (C) Extensive subperiosteal bone. Note the loss of reduction. (D) At 6 months the right side is healing well, but the left side is suggestive of a developing problem. (E) Right side at 18 months showing mild physeal irregularity. (F) Left side developed central arrest. (G) Growth arrest at 2 years. (H) Resection of bridge. (I) MRI 4 years later. The elongated "migration" tract of the resected bridge is readily evident.

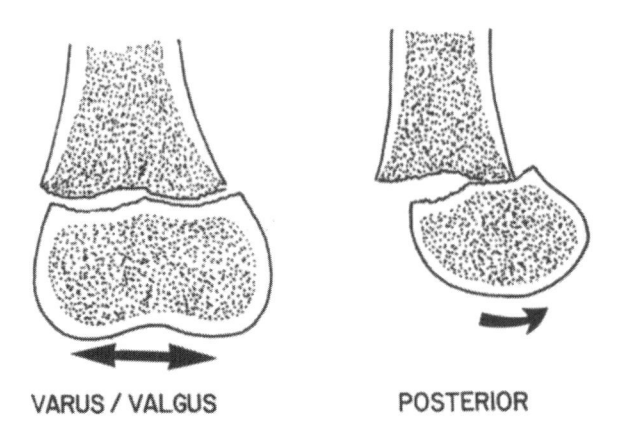

FIGURE 21-54. Type 1 growth mechanism injury patterns.

Classification

Several patterns of growth mechanism injury may affect the distal femoral physis and epiphysis. Certainly, types 1 and 2 are relatively common. Types 3 and 4 may occur with a relatively significant frequency and may be difficult to diagnosis. Types 5 and 6 are infrequent. Type 7 is common as either an acute osteochondral fragment or the more common chronic osteochondritis dissecans (see Chapter 22). Type 7 is also present as a sleeve fracture. Intraepiphyseal fracture or bone bruising is now being described frequently by utilizing MRI to assess painful injuries without obvious radiologic abnormality. These injuries fit the broad category of type 7 growth mechanism injury pattern. Type 8 (Peterson version) may also occur. (see Fig. 21-52.)

Type 1 injuries involve a fracture that traverses the entire physeal–metaphyseal interface (Fig. 21-54). This involvement of the entire physis requires the fracture to follow a contour that becomes increasingly undulated during adolescence. The undulation increases the risk of focal cell damage and subsequent growth impairment.

Because of the major undulations the central "peak" is at risk for focal injury. The direction of epiphyseal displacement varies: anterior, posterior, varus, and valgus. Severe displacement may be associated with vascular injury (Fig. 21-55). However, displacement may be minimal and may be indicated only by slight physeal widening or metaphyseal buckling. With child abuse, the distal femur is frequently injured. The only diagnostic finding may be a small peripheral metaphyseal flake (Fig. 21-56) caused by the curvilinear peripheral extension of the physis over the metaphysis (corner sign).

Type 2 injury is the most common pattern (Fig. 21-57). Hyperextension injuries lead to anterior displacement of the epiphysis underneath the patella (Fig. 21-58). Varus or

injury is much more readily diagnosed because the epiphysis usually undergoes ossification at 38–40 gestational weeks, providing an anatomic marker. Ultrasonic examination of the affected area may demonstrate not only the injury but also the presence of subperiosteal hematoma, which may be extensive.

The treatment of this type of injury during the newborn period is usually relatively simple. When only minimal to moderate displacement of the epiphysis is noted, immobilization with a splint for 2–3 weeks is necessary. When there is marked displacement, gentle reduction should be undertaken. If the reduction is not stable, a spica cast may be applied. Pin fixation may be used. Reparative bone formation is rapid and usually effective for stability (clinical) within about 2–3 weeks. Long-term follow-up is absolutely necessary because of the significant risk of physeal damage.

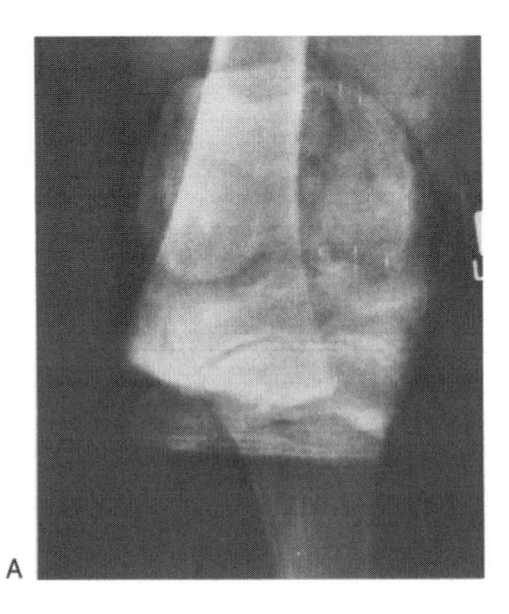

FIGURE 21-55. (A) Complete displacement of a type 1 physeal injury. The epiphyseal fragment was displaced posteriorly. (B) Arteriogram shows complete vascular occlusion. Primary vascular repair was necessary. The physeal fracture was reduced and stabilized by Kirschner wires.

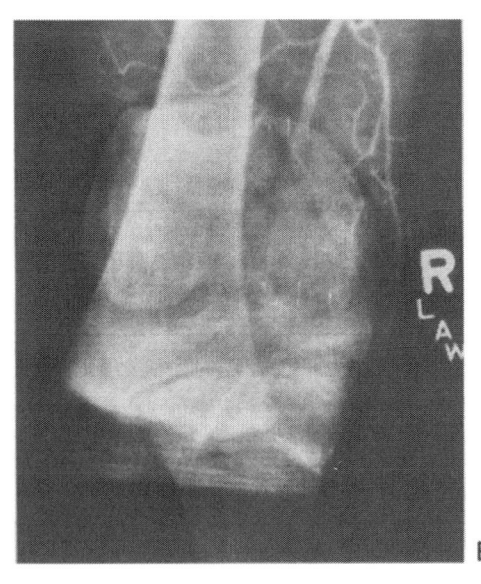

Distal Femoral Epiphyseal Injuries

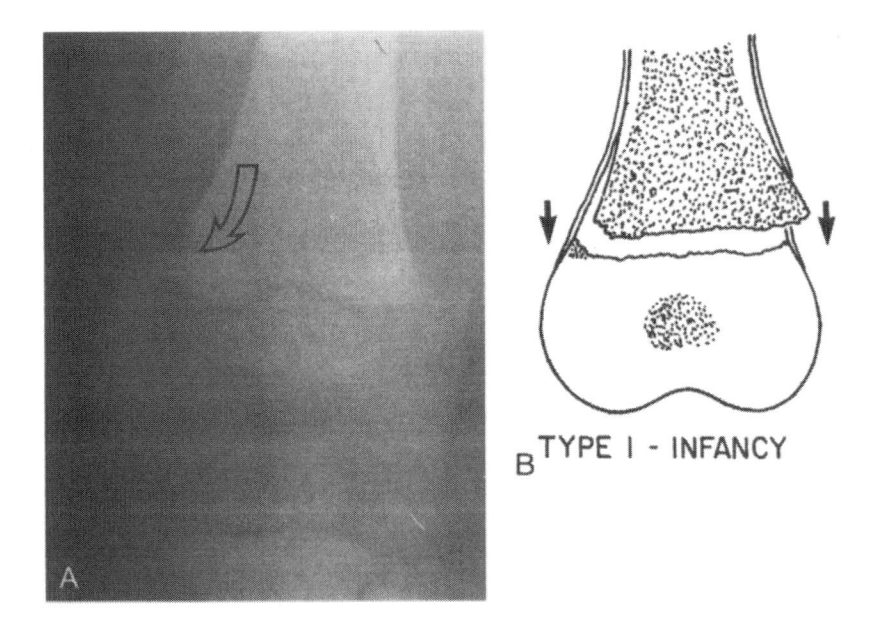

FIGURE 21-56. (A) Metaphyseal "beak" fracture (arrow) characteristic of type 1 physeal injury due to child abuse. (B) Schematic of this injury.

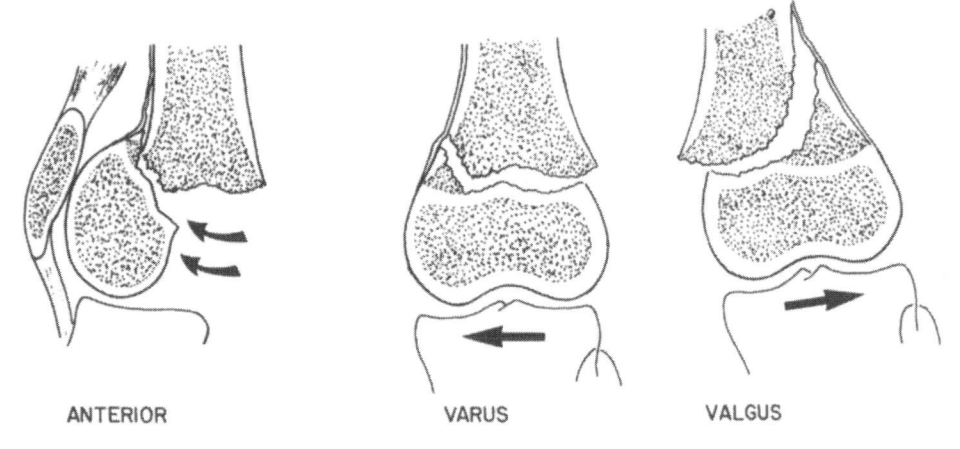

FIGURE 21-57. Type 2 injury.

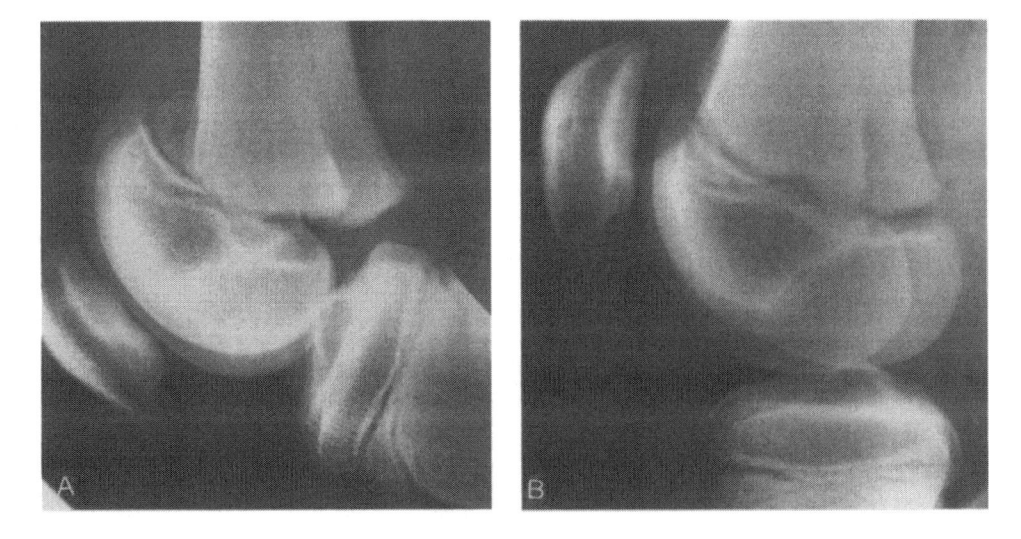

FIGURE 21-58. (A) Type 2 hyperextension injury. (B) Appearance after closed reduction.

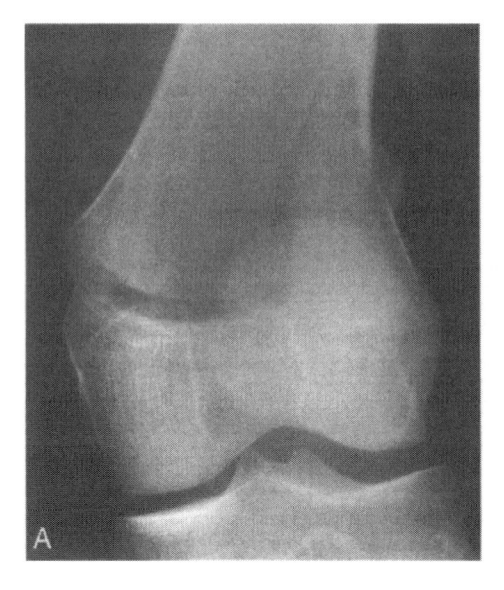

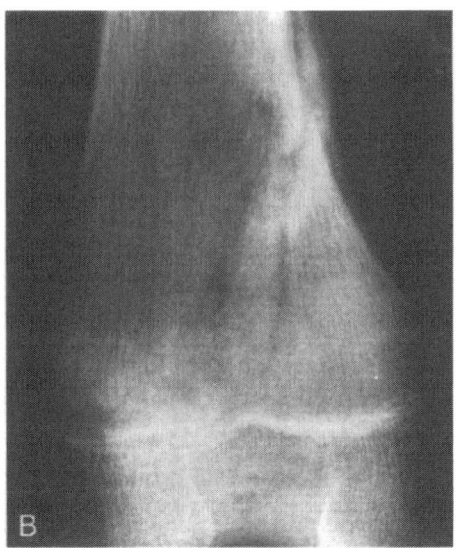

FIGURE 21-59. (A) Type 2 valgus injury with greenstick injury of the lateral metaphyseal component. (B) One year later.

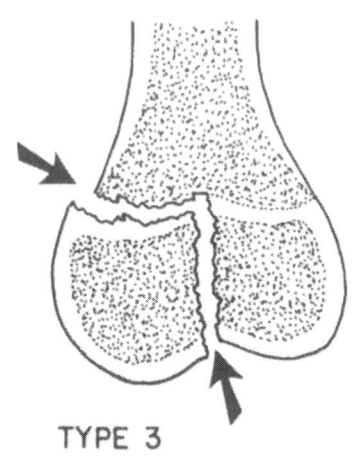

FIGURE 21-60. Type 3 injury.

FIGURE 21-60. Type 3 injury.

valgus displacements are associated with metaphyseal fragments of variable size (Fig. 21-59). Posterior metaphyseal fragment fracture is the least frequent pattern. The central metaphyseal peak probably plays a role in redirecting the propagating fracture proximally into the metaphysis.

Type 3 injuries involve either the medial or the lateral condyle (Figs. 21-60 to 21-62). On rare occasions, a posterior (quadrant) condylar element is involved. These injuries may be difficult to diagnose and may require stress roentgenography (Fig. 21-63). Small pieces of the articular surface and subchondral bone may be fragmented and displaced into the joint.

Type 4 injuries may involve the medial or lateral condyle, or both (Fig. 21-64); or they may occur in conjunction with a type 3 injury (Fig. 21-65). The fragment tends to be dis-

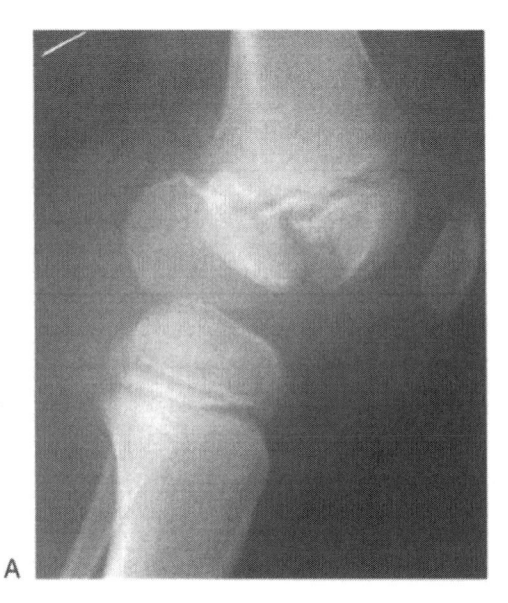

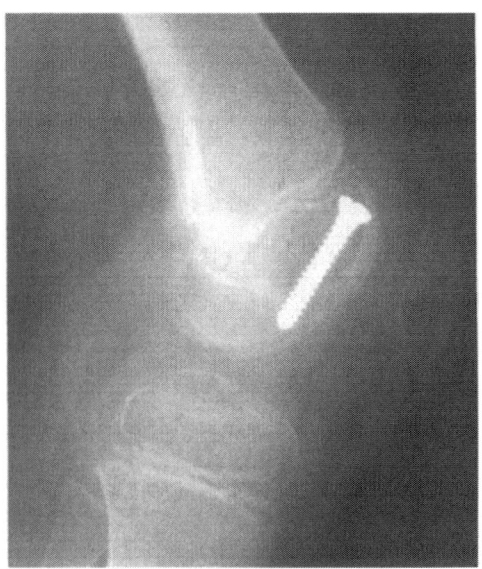

FIGURE 21-61. (A) Type 3 injury of the posteromedial portion of the distal femur. (B) Treatment was open reduction and internal fixation.

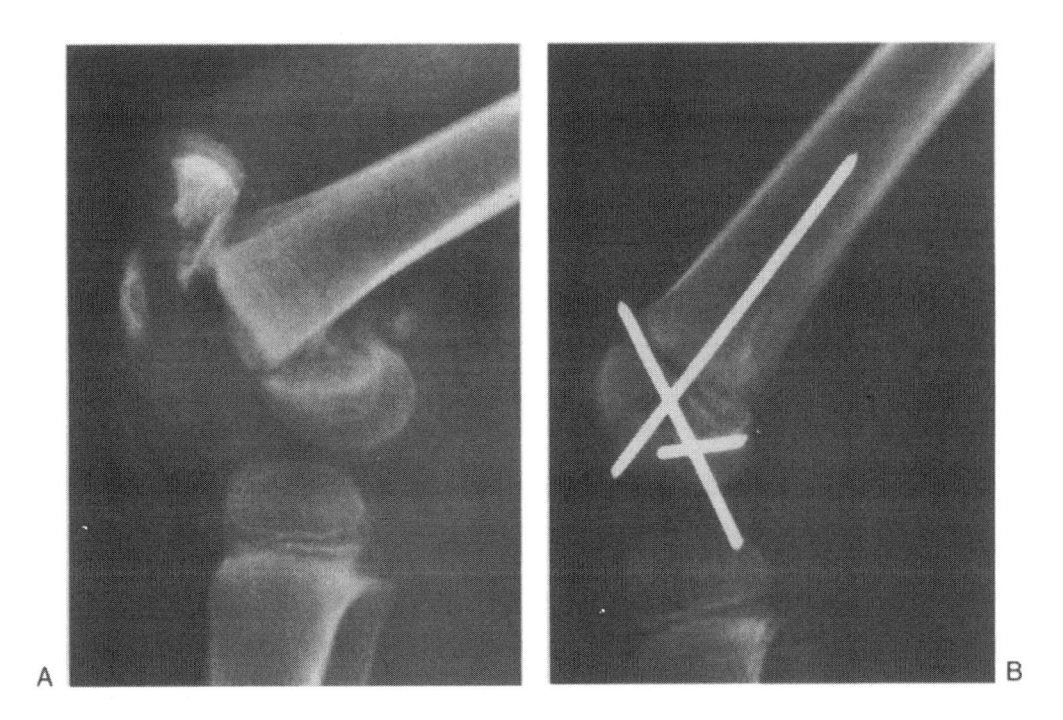

FIGURE 21-62. (A) Severe comminuted type 3 injury with both anterior and posterior fragment displacement. (B) Open reduction was stabilized with internal fixation.

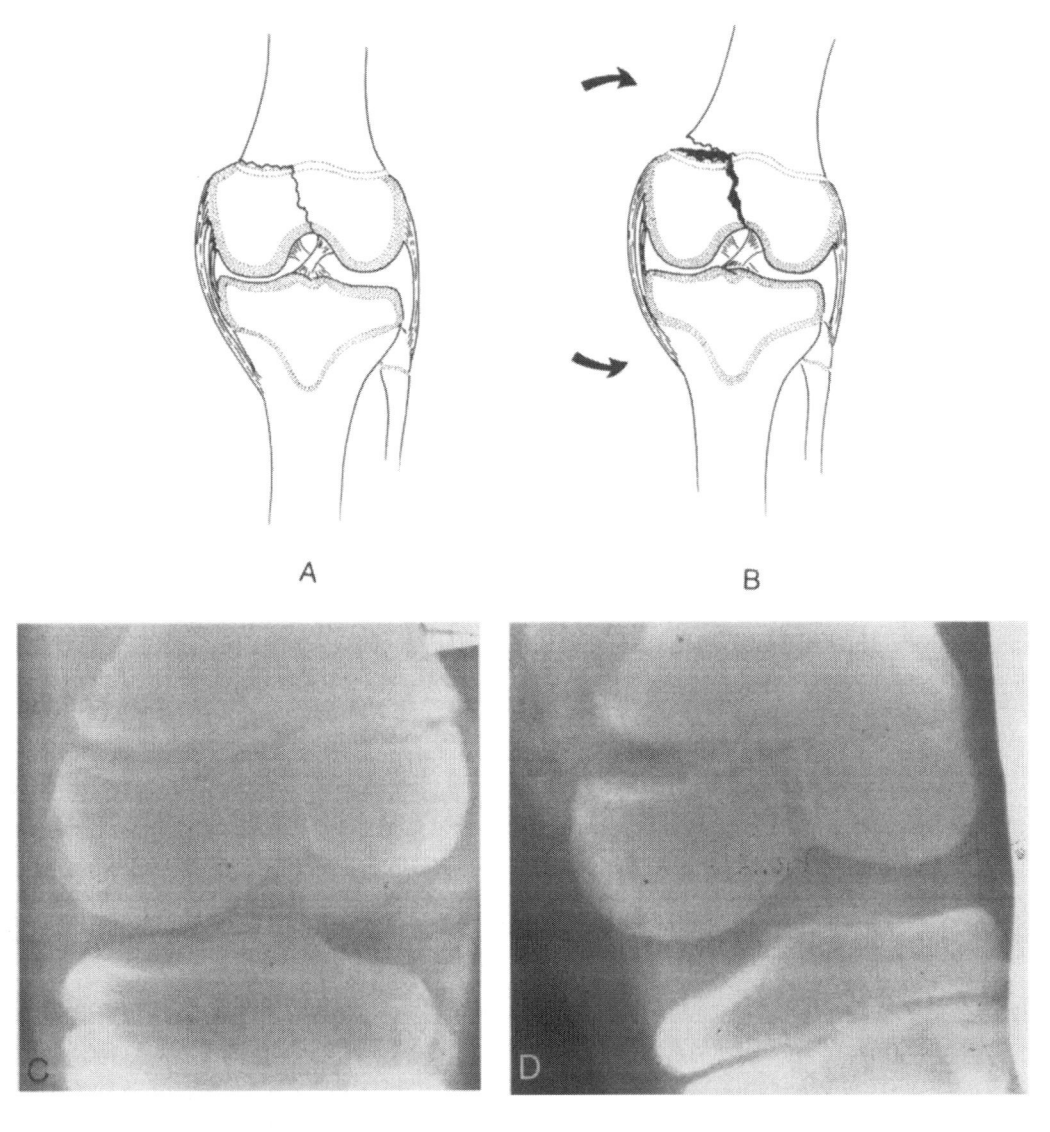

FIGURE 21-63. (A, B) Stress testing. (C, D) Nonstress view (C) and stress view (D).

902

21. Femur

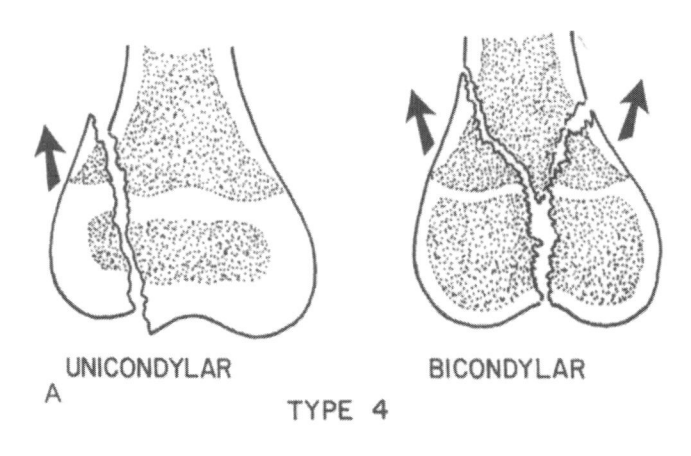

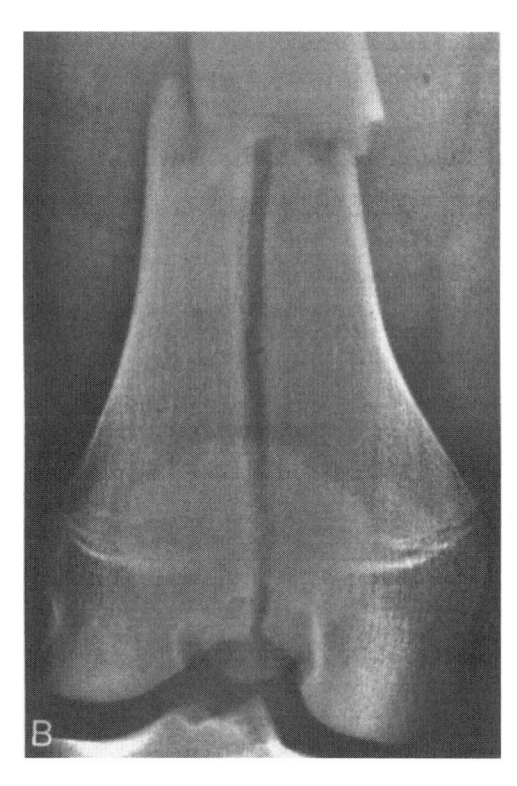

FIGURE 21-64. (A) Unicondylar type 4 injury (left), which can occur medially or laterally. Bicondylar type 4 injury (right). (B) Bicondylar, or T-type injury.

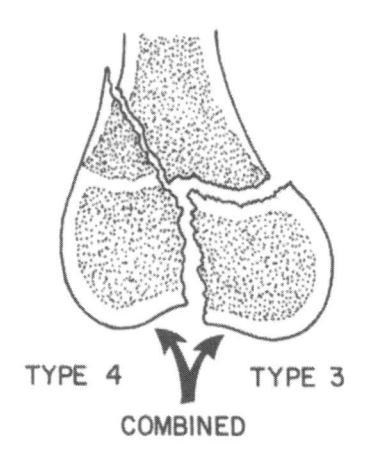

FIGURE 21-65. Combined type 3 and 4 injuries.

placed proximally to a variable degree (Figs. 21-66 to 21-68). When both condyles are involved, the fragments not only are proximally displaced but also split apart. Similarly, types 3 and 4 injuries may occur concomitantly (Fig. 21-69). There is a high incidence of osseous bridge formation, especially in the smaller lesions (Fig. 21-70).

In other cases, there is initial growth slowdown and irregularity in the secondary ossification center. Some of the type 3–4 combinations may constitute the triplane pattern of fracture.

Type 5 injuries are uncommon and more likely to occur in patients with other disorders, such as myelomenginocele. Lombardo and Harvey described a fracture of the proximal tibial metaphysis and diaphysis extending as a type 4 injury into the proximal tibial epiphysis but also leading to an initially unrecognized type 5 injury of the distal femur.[774]

Type 6 injuries may include glancing blows that lead to destruction of a small peripheral segment (Fig. 21-71), which may lead to eventual formation of a physeal bridge. Other mechanisms, such as burns, osteomyelitis, or irradiation, may also contribute to this injury. Hyperextension injury may also damage areas where the capsule, periosteum, and

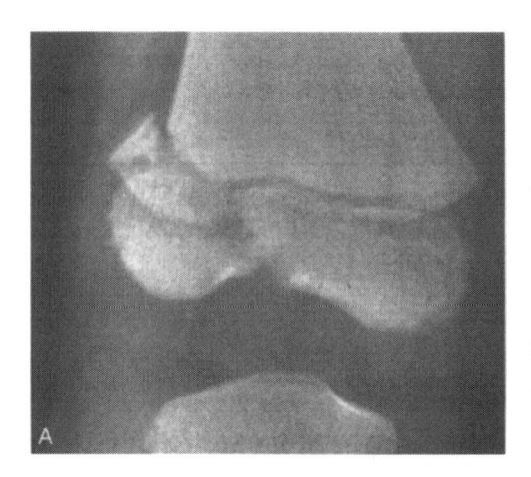

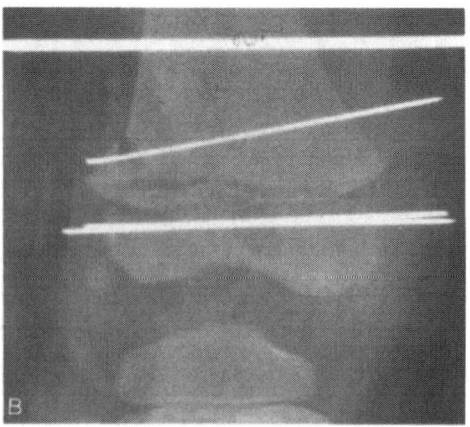

FIGURE 21-66. (A) Type 4 injury. (B) Transverse fixation following open reduction.

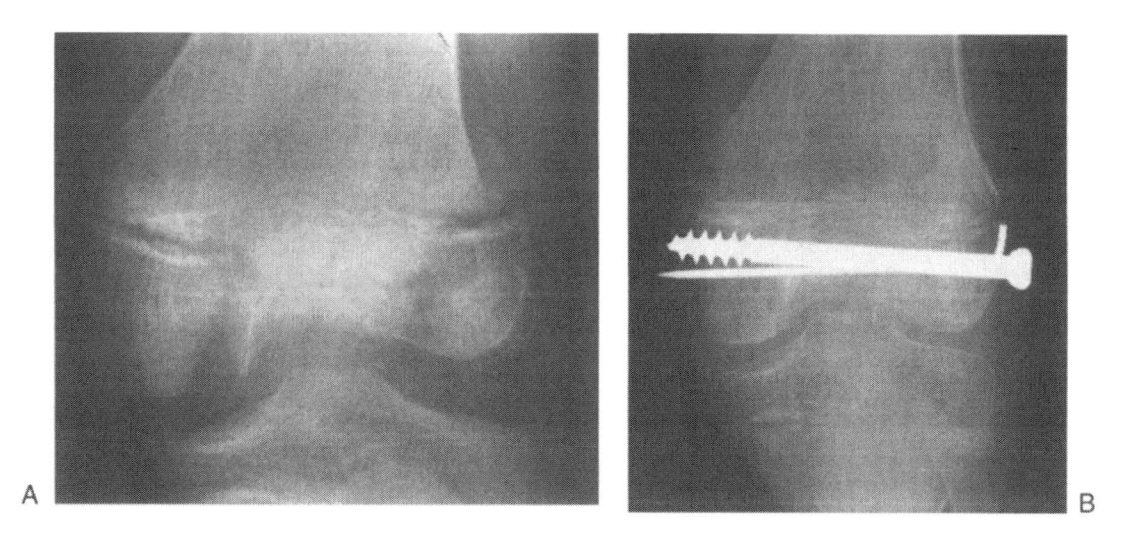

FIGURE 21-67. (A) Lateral type 4 injury. (B) Open reduction and internal fixation.

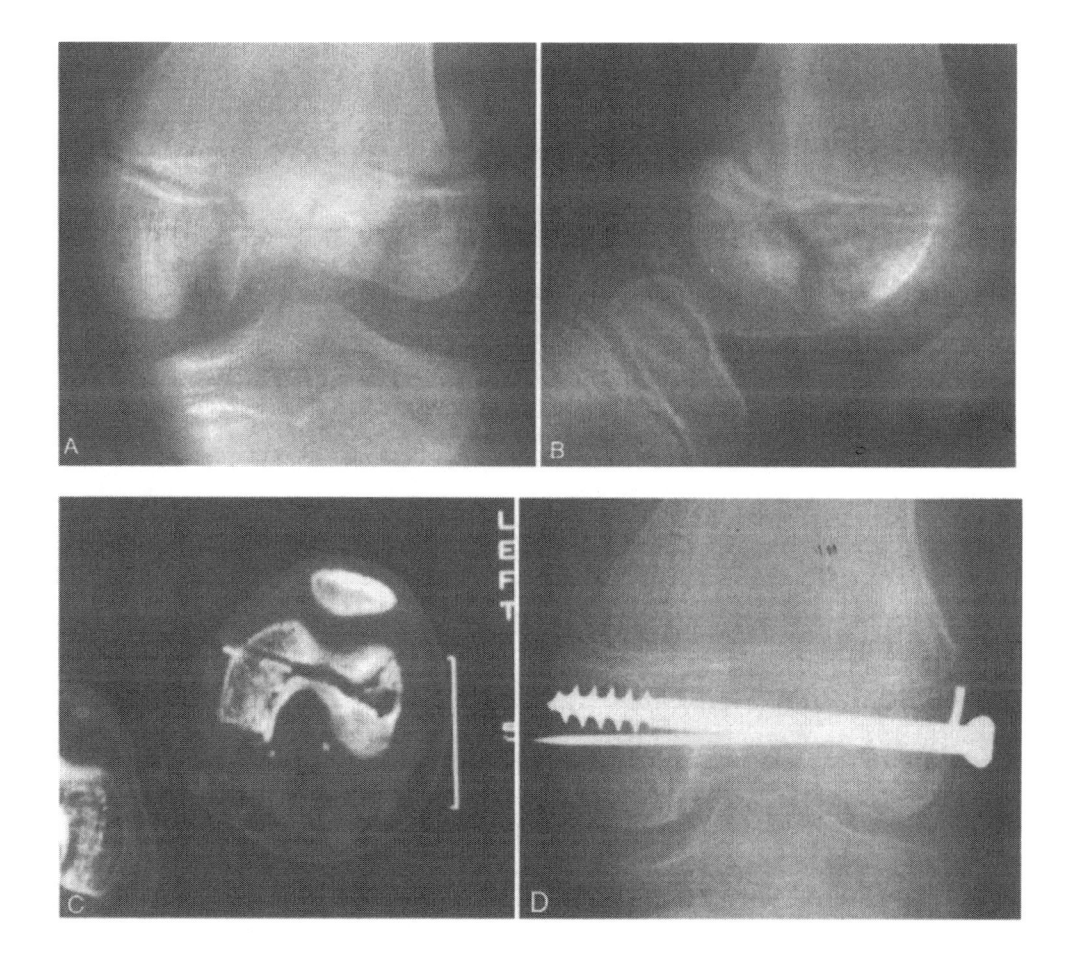

FIGURE 21-68. (A) Anteroposterior view of a type 4 injury. (B) Lateral view. (C) Computed tomographic (CT) scan. (D) Fixation.

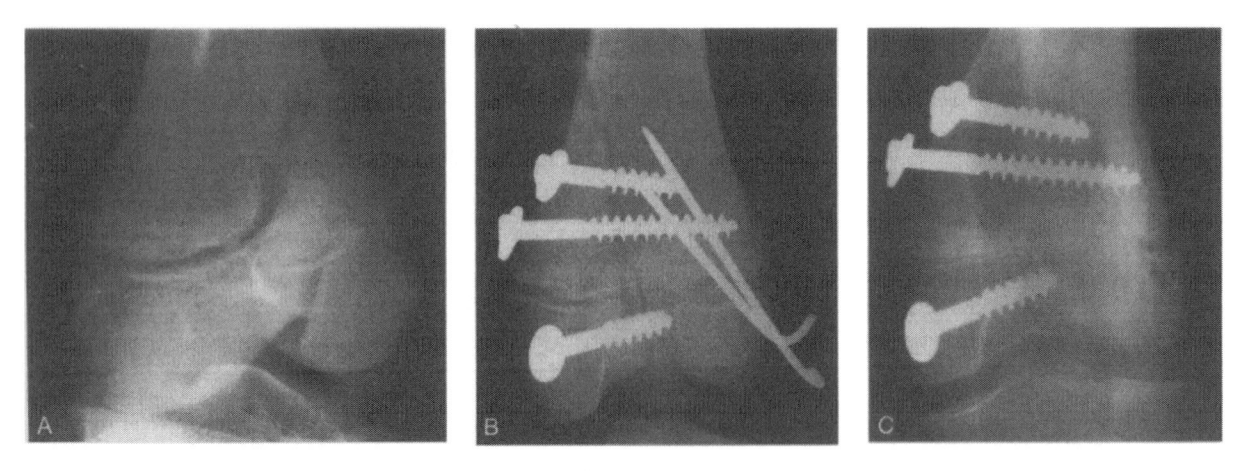

FIGURE 21-69. (A) Type 4 injury of the medial condyle. It proved to be a combined lateral type 3 and medial type 4 injury. (B) Reduction. (C) Growth arrest of the type 3 side.

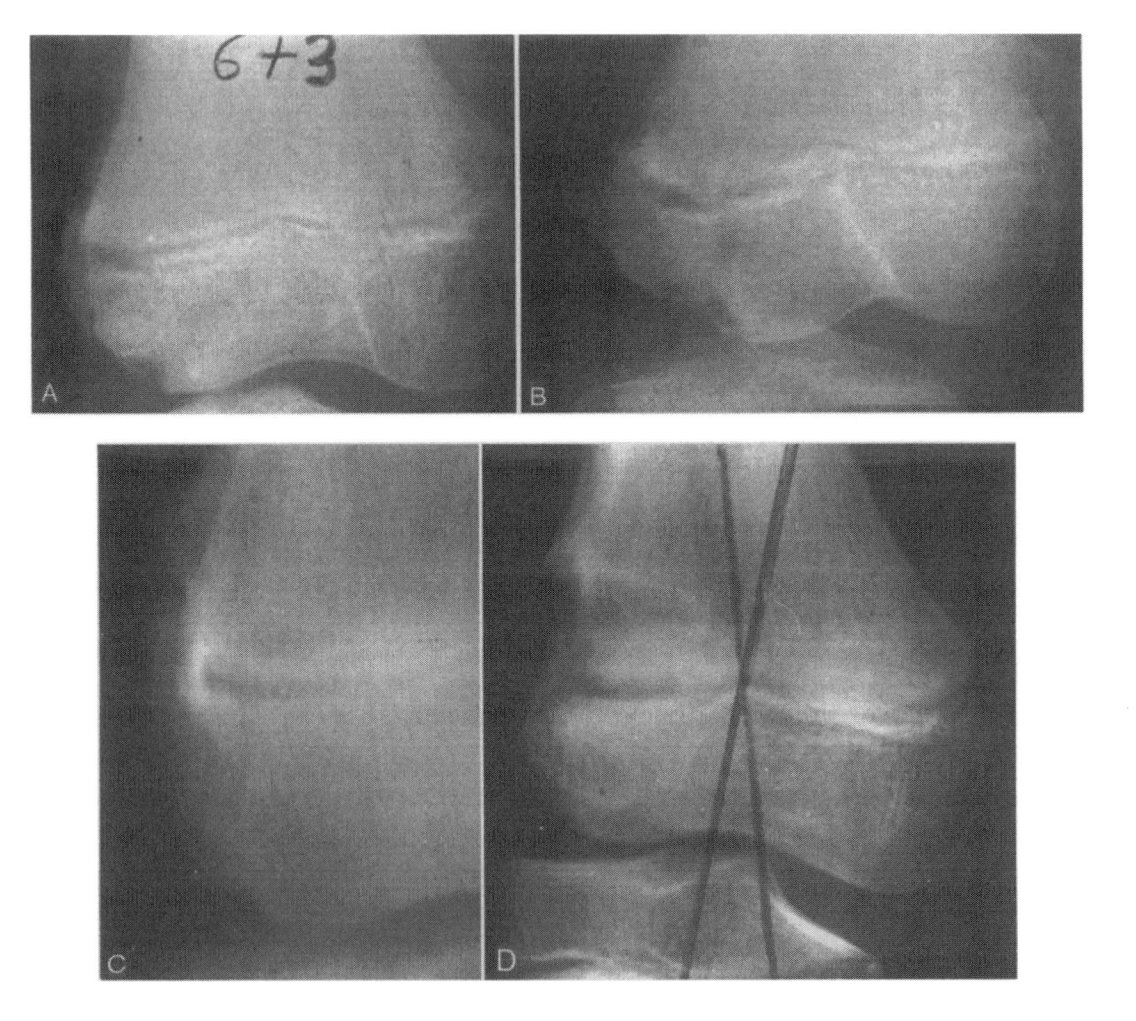

FIGURE 21-70. (A) Early bridge formation in a peripheral type 4 injury. (B) Appearance 6 months later. (C) Tomogram of bridge. (D) Resection and fat transplant.

Distal Femoral Epiphyseal Injuries

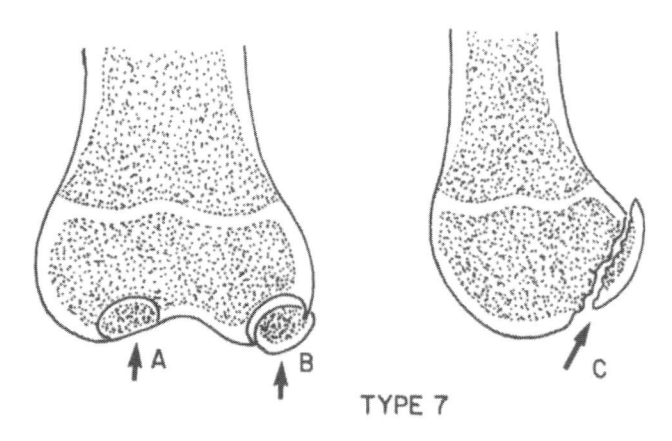

FIGURE 21-72. Type 7 injury: undisplaced (A); displaced (B); and posterior involvement (C).

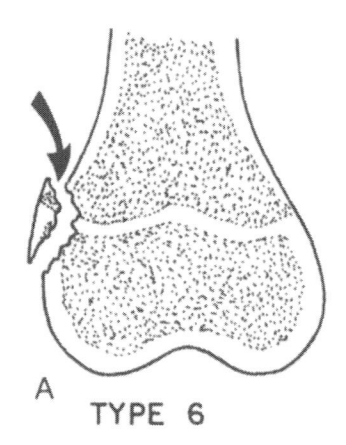

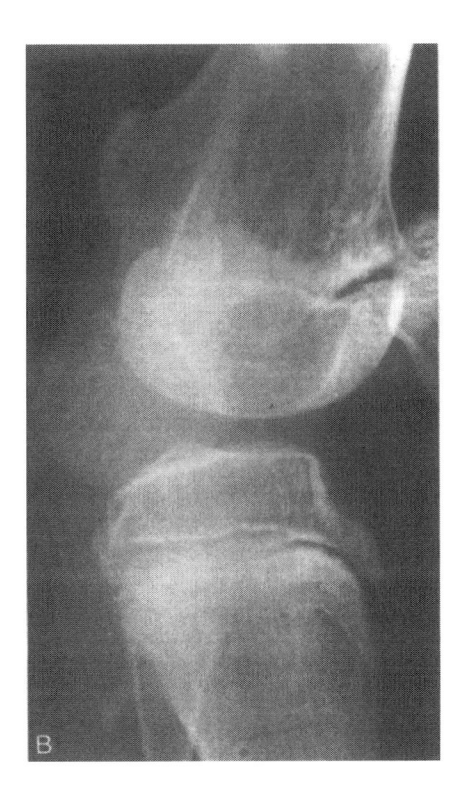

FIGURE 21-71. (A) Type 6 injury to the peripheral zone of Ranvier. (B) Hyperextension type 6 injury of the posterior distal femoral and proximal tibial physes, leading to formation of osteochondromas posteriorly.

perichondrium blend, leading to formation of a solitary osteochondroma.

Type 7 injuries involve fragments of the femoral condyles (Figs. 21-72, 21-73) that vary considerably in size. Alternatively, there may be a sleeve fracture of cartilage and subchondral bone (collateral ligament injury analogue); irregular ossification appears later. Bone bruising (Figs. 21-74, 21-75) occurs within the substance of the epiphyseal trabecular bone. The involvement may be within a condyle, at the periphery (in conjunction with a sleeve injury), or at an articular surface. The latter pattern may be a precursor of an osteochondritis dissecans lesion.

With type 8 injuries the main fracture is a metaphyseal injury. Longitudinal extensions propagate distally toward the physis, where the fracture further extends transversely along the physeal–metaphyseal interface.

Pathomechanism

Distal femoral epiphyseal injuries may be grouped according to the etiologic mechanism: (1) abduction; (2) adduction; (3) hyperextension; and (4) hyperflexion. These four basic

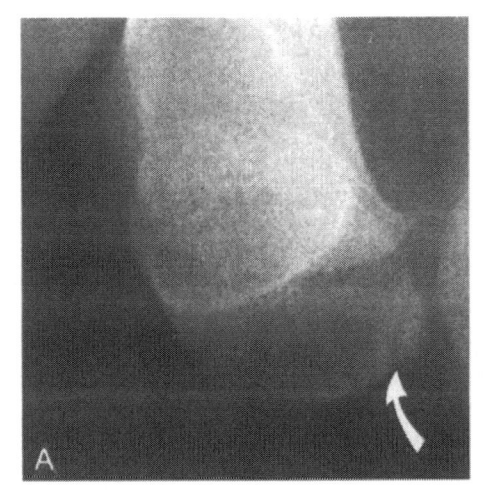

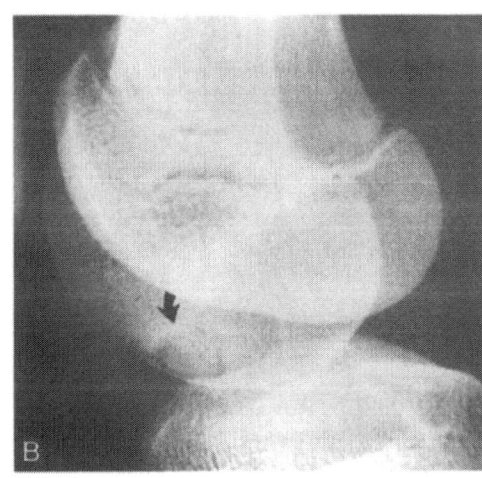

FIGURE 21-73. (A) Acute type 7 fracture of the posterior femoral condyle (arrow). (B) Chronic type 7 injury. Note the osteochondritis dissecans (arrow).

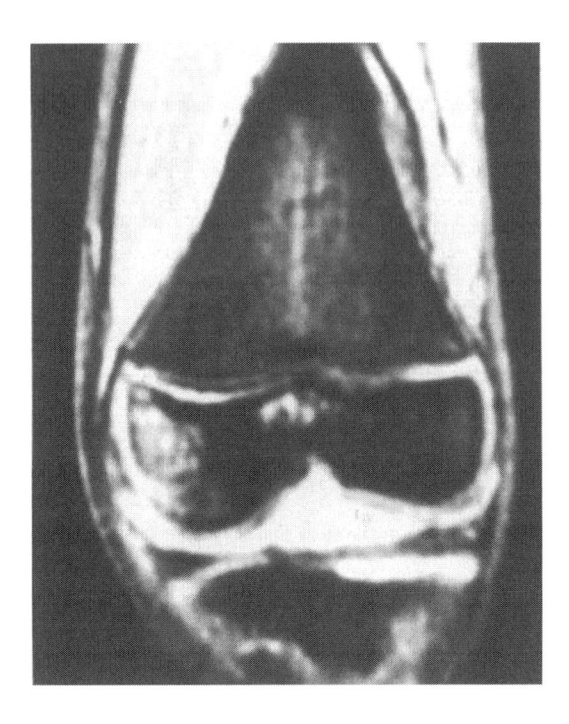

FIGURE 21-74. Type 7 injury of the medial distal femoral epiphysis. There is increased signal intensity within the trabecular bone extending to the subchondral bone medially.

mechanisms are not isolated, often existing in combination, and are accompanied by variable rotation.

Abduction Type

An abduction injury, caused by a blow to the lateral side of the distal femur, frequently occurs in athletes. It is the same type of stress that causes medial soft tissue injuries (especially meniscal and ligamentous) in an older patient. The result is generally a type 2 physeal injury, in which the periosteum is ruptured on the medial side and the distal femoral epiphysis is displaced laterally with a lateral fragment of the metaphysis. It is usually associated with rotation. This fracture may reduce spontaneously and may be missed initially if the triangular piece of metaphyseal bone is small. One should carefully scrutinize the roentgenogram and, if indicated, take additional abduction stress views to detect the lesion. MRI may also delineate the metaphyseal propagation.

Adduction Type

An adduction injury is caused by a medial blow or an indirect injury. The epiphysis is medially displaced as a type 1 or 2 injury pattern. With the addition of a rotational component, a type 3 or 4 injury may occur.

Hyperextension Type

A hyperextension injury was the most common variety in the past because of wagon-wheel injuries, and it is still seen in vehicular accidents. The distal femoral epiphysis is displaced anteriorly by the hyperextension force and by the pull of the quadriceps muscle. The posterior periosteum is torn, and the fibers of the gastrocnemius are stretched or partially torn. The triangular metaphyseal bone fragment and the intact periosteal hinge are anterior, although the latter structure is modified by synovial extension into the suprapatellar pouch. The distal end of the femoral shaft is displaced posteriorly and may injure structures in the popliteal region. Grogan and Bobechko presented an interesting photograph of the mechanism of injury of hyperextension of the knee in a patient with a type 2 fracture of the distal femoral epiphysis.[765] The injury was sustained while landing during a track and field event (long jump).

Hyperflexion Type

Posterior displacement of the distal femoral epiphysis, a hyperflexion injury, is rare. It usually results from a forceful flexion injury caused by a direct blow to the distal femur.

Diagnosis

The usual history is a relatively violent injury with severe pain and inability to bear weight on the leg. The knee is markedly swollen and tense, and the limb is abnormally angulated. There may be a joint effusion, depending on where the fracture line propagates and if there is extension into the joint, either through the intercondylar region or through the suprapatellar extension of the synovium and capsule. Neurovascular function must be examined closely.

These injuries are particularly prone to partial to complete spontaneous reduction following cessation of the evocative force. The diagnosis may be suspected on the basis of a slightly widened growth plate or a fracture extending into the metaphysis. Oblique projections are sometimes as revealing as stress roentgenograms.

Undisplaced type 1 and 2 epiphyseal fractures of the distal femur in the adolescent athlete may mimic injury to the knee ligaments. Roentgenographic examination with the knee under stress often reveals the diagnosis, thereby avoiding

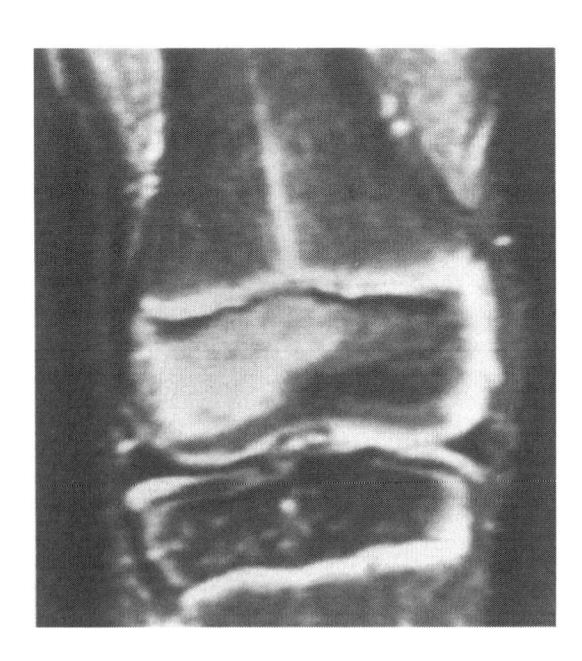

FIGURE 21-75. Medial condylar bone bruise.

unnecessary arthrotomy and indicating appropriate treatment.

Simpson and Fardon reported three cases that initially appeared to be pure ligamentous injuries until stress films were obtained.[797] They noted that one type 3 injury had been misdiagnosed as a ligamentous disruption. Rogers and associates described a "clipping injury" fracture of the epiphysis in the adolescent football player as an occult lesion of the knee.[789] They described seven cases of type 3 and one of type 2, all of which were definitively diagnosed with stress films. It is important to realize that ligament injury may also be present with an epiphyseal injury. MRI should be considered if such concomitant ligamentous injury is suspected.

Treatment

In general, these fractures are variably stable injuries, most of which require some degree of force to effect a reduction. Manipulation in the emergency room may increase the already considerable pain. Accordingly, reductions undertaken in the operating room under more ideal anesthetic conditions are more likely to be anatomic. The following general recommendations should be considered:

1. Displaced distal femoral fractures should be treated with early anatomic reduction under general anesthesia. Stability is then checked fluoroscopically. Unsuccessful or unstable closed reduction should be followed by open reduction with fixation or closed reduction with percutaneous fixation.
2. Following fracture reduction some type of internal fixation is the most effective method of maintaining anatomic reduction. Percutaneous smooth K-wire fixation is traditional. However screw fixation, provided the immature physis is not violated, is acceptable, especially for type 2, 3, and 4 injuries.
3. Long leg cast immobilization is usually inadequate for maintenance of fracture reductions if no internal fixation has been employed. A fracture not internally fixed should be closely followed to allow early intervention if reduction is lost. A hip spica may be more appropriate.
4. Patients and families should be made aware of the high potential for late complications related to physeal damage. It necessitates periodic examination until the child reaches skeletal maturity.

The position for immobilization of type 1 and 2 injuries is usually determined by the characteristics of the original displacement. If there is anterior displacement of the distal fragment, the patient is treated by reduction with traction followed by immobilization in flexion. With posterior displacement, the patient is treated by reduction and immobilization in extension. Any medial or lateral displacement should be corrected by appropriate manipulation. Factors affecting the choice of treatment should include the ease of obtaining and maintaining reduction, the amount of swelling, the body habitus, and the presence of associated injuries.

Treatment may also include skeletal traction, traction followed by cast immobilization, and immediate application of a long leg cast. Percutaneous pin fixation is also effective as an adjunct. As pointed out by Bassett and Goldner, treatment of these injuries must be individualized.[737]

Hyperextension-type fractures present two problems of management: (1) potential injury to the popliteal vessels and nerves; and (2) the difficulty of achieving and maintaining reduction, as the plane of displacement and the plane of the knee joint motion are the same. There is an adequate lever arm to grasp the distal fragment effectively. A closed reduction is attempted first and, if successful, is followed by casting. Flexion may be necessary to maintain anatomic reduction, although swelling in the popliteal region may prevent the use of much flexion.

Recurrence of anterior displacement is usually caused by immobilization with insufficient flexion. If necessary, pins may be used to stabilize the fracture.

The posteriorly displaced distal femur (hyperflexion-type fractures) must be reduced by pulling the distal epiphysis anteriorly. This fracture must be immobilized in extension and should not be immobilized in a position of semiflexion. Immobilization varies, with a mean of 7 weeks (range 3–16 weeks).

Type 3 injuries invariably require open reduction (Fig. 21-76). This procedure includes an arthrotomy or arthroscopy so there is accurate restoration of articular

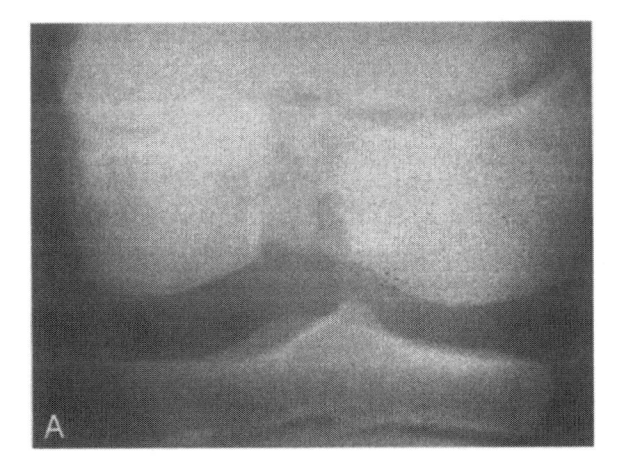

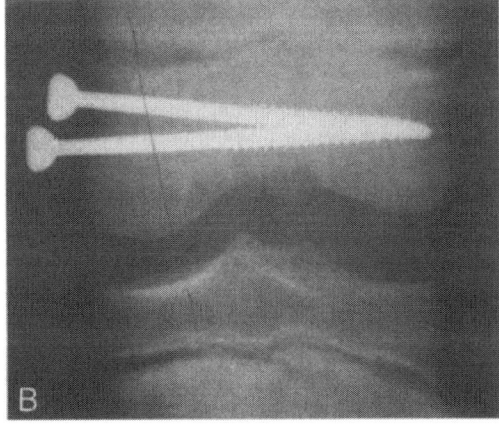

FIGURE 21-76. (A) Type 3 injury. (B) Open reduction and fixation with transcondylar screws.

anatomy. Fixation, as much as possible, should be directed transversely across the epiphyseal ossification center fragments. Smooth pins may be placed across the physis. Alternatively, transversely directed fixation may affix the free fragment to the nonfractured condyle.

Type 4 fractures usually require open reduction and internal fixation with smooth K-wires (if the physis is crossed) or screws directed from the metaphyseal fragment with the uninjured metaphysis. An arthrotomy or arthroscopy is a recommended part of the procedure to gauge restoration of the articular surface and to remove any small fragments that could potentially form loose bodies. Failure to reduce and fix the fragment adequately may result in malunion or nonunion.

Treatment of the type 7 injury is discussed in Chapter 22.

Results

These fractures generally heal rapidly. However, when they involve a child or adolescent with any significant remaining growth potential, this region probably has the highest rate of complications. *Most patients with more than 1 year of development remaining demonstrate some type of a growth disturbance: focal arrest or slowdown of longitudinal growth.* Lee and colleagues emphasized that at least 90% of patients with this type of injury have some degree of shortening.[773] Stephens et al. thought that growth disturbance was an all-or-none phenomenon.[798] Fortunately, many patients are nearing skeletal maturity and do not exhibit major growth deformity as a consequence.

Prognosis based on the growth mechanism classification alone is not reliable. The development of deformity appears to be related to the severity of the injury mechanism, the degree of initial displacement of the fracture, the ease and exactness of the reduction, the type of fracture, and the age of the patient. There undoubtedly are focal areas of physeal damage due to the multiple undulations of this physis. The central "peak" seems particularly susceptible.

Complications

The sequelae of distal femoral physeal fractures include leg length discrepancy, varus or valgus angulation, limitation of knee motion, and quadriceps atrophy. The primary problem is leg length discrepancy, which may occur even in the absence of obvious premature epiphysiodesis because of a generalized slowdown (rather than a complete arrest) of growth relative to the contralateral distal femur. It is imperative to follow these patients to skeletal maturity to document this type of complication adequately, even when the fracture appears to heal satisfactorily.

Neer reported a 42% incidence of leg length discrepancy.[778] Cassebaum and Patterson noted a 25% incidence.[748] The combined series of Nicholson and Neer revealed that 40% of patients had leg length inequality.[778,780] Lombardo and Harvey reviewed 34 fractures of the distal femur and found an average limb length discrepancy of 2 cm in 36% and a varus or valgus deformity of more than 5° in 33%.[774] Twenty percent of the patients required some type of reconstructive procedure, such as an osteotomy, epiphysiodesis, or both. Other complications include limitation of knee motion, ligament laxity, and quadriceps atrophy.

Riseborough and associates, studying 66 distal femoral physeal fractures, found that leg length discrepancies in excess of 2.4 cm or leading to contralateral distal femoral physeal arrest occurred in 37 patients (56%) and that angular deformity requiring corrective osteotomy occurred in 17 patients (26%).[786] Central growth arrest occurred in 13 patients (20%) and was associated primarily with type 1 and 2 growth mechanism injuries. The development of this arrest had an excellent predictive value for progressive limb length discrepancy. Fractures in the juvenile age group (2–11 years) were almost invariably caused by severe trauma and had the poorest prognosis. Of 23 injuries in juveniles, 19 resulted in growth problems. In contrast, fractures in the adolescent age group, those 11 years old or older, were caused by less extensive trauma and were most often associated with sports injuries. *However*, 50% of these individuals also had growth problems.

The distal femoral epiphyseal growth plate contributes 70% of the longitudinal growth of the femur and 40% of the length of the lower extremity. Any injury that completely or partially arrests growth potential may lead to significant shortening or angular deformity of the extremity. The younger the child at the time of injury, the greater the potential for these undesirable complications. If one of these sequelae becomes evident during long-term follow-up, appropriately timed epiphysiodesis or lengthening, as well as osteotomy or even resection of the bridge, may serve to minimize the disability, the deformity, or both.

As noted previously, the undulated contour of the growth plate and the mechanisms of injury—whether varus, valgus, anterior, or posterior—introduce combined shearing–compression forces into the physis as it is displaced. If a large metaphyseal fragment is present, it is less likely that problems will occur than when shearing across the entire "transverse" plane of the epiphysis takes place (Fig. 21-77).

The distal femoral epiphyseal cartilage plate is prone to growth disturbances not generally seen roentgenographically with equivalent injuries at other sites (Figs. 21-78, 21-79). This finding specifically relates to differences in the contour of this particular physis that predispose to certain

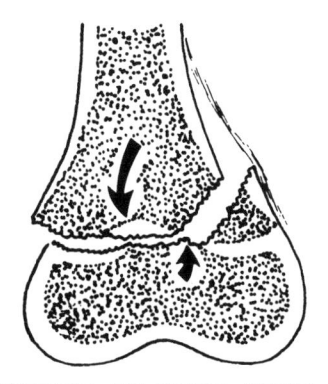

FIGURE 21-77. Effect of undulation. Arrows show the central physeal area with a proximal fragment, which disrupts physeal continuity.

Distal Femoral Epiphyseal Injuries

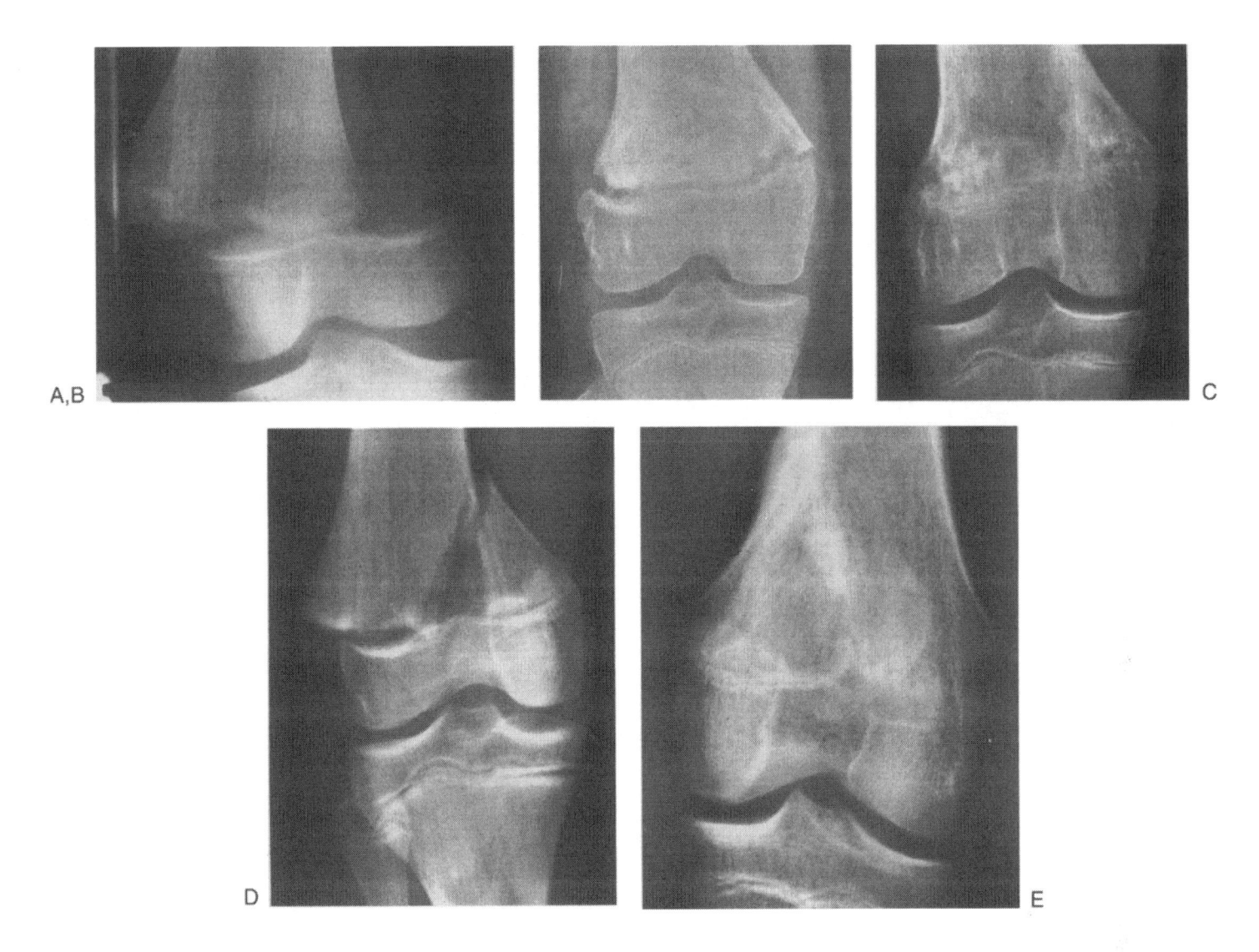

FIGURE 21-78. Effect of grating impingement in type 1 (A–C) and type 2 (D, E) injuries. The microscopic physeal damage leads to premature growth arrest.

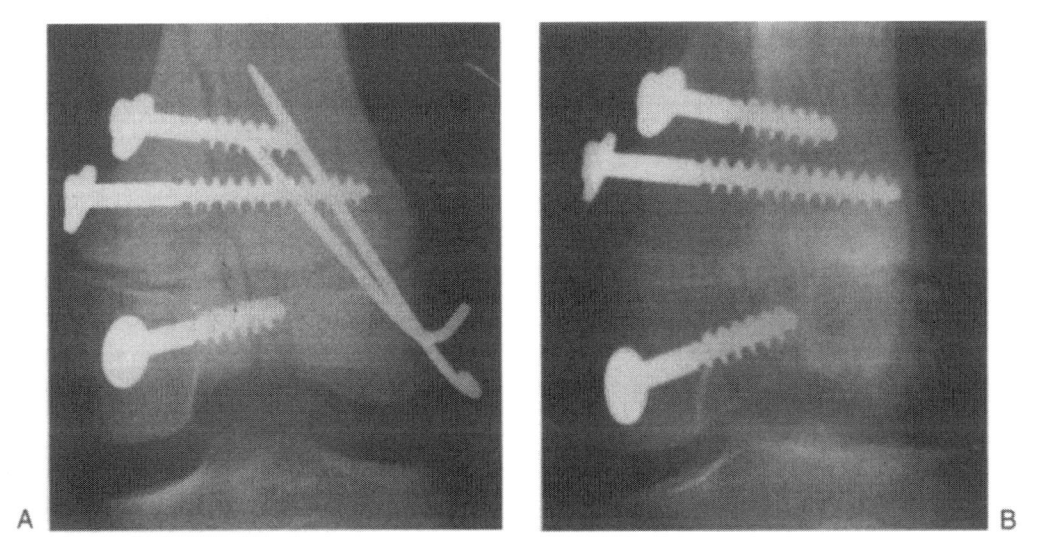

FIGURE 21-79. Growth arrest and osteonecrosis in the type 3 fragment of a type 3/type 4 fracture.

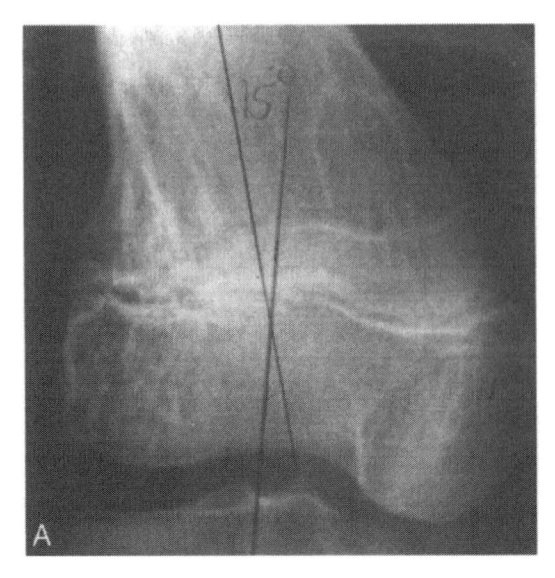

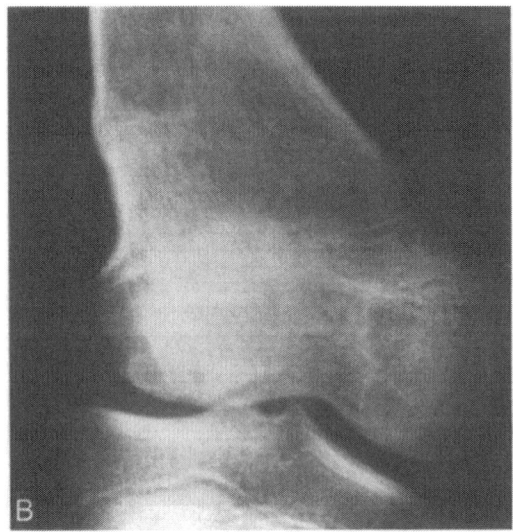

FIGURE 21-80. (A) Angular deformity due to premature closure of the lateral physis. (B) Progressive changes 6 months later.

kinds of injury. Fortunately, many epiphyseal injuries to the distal femur occur at an age when little potential for major longitudinal growth remains. Microscopic disruption of the germinal cartilage cells or blood vessels seems to be the most logical explanation for this cessation of growth. Usually premature epiphysiodesis is evident within 6 months after the injury. The rapidity of the phenomenon indicates both a direct effect of the injury and a gradual growth deceleration process.

Mäkelä et al. studied injury to the distal femoral growth plate. A central drill-hole defect of variable size was used.[775] They found that destruction of 7% of the cross-sectional area of the physis resulted in permanent growth disturbance.

Varus-valgus angular deformities may result from partial or complete unicondylar epiphysiodesis (Fig. 21-80). Treatment is dictated by the anticipated remaining growth. If less than one-third of the area of the physis is involved, bridge resection may be considered. An epiphysiodesis in the other condyle may also be completed. Correction of angular deformity by osteotomy may be necessary.

Thompson and Mahoney reviewed 28 fractures of the distal femoral growth plate and showed that complications were more frequent in displaced than nondisplaced fractures.[682] No fractures treated with internal fixation displaced, whereas 38% of the fractures reduced without fixation subsequently displaced during casting. The authors were unable to demonstrate that gentle reduction under general anesthesia offered any additional protection against subsequent physeal arrest.

Concomitant Ligament Injury

Bertin and Goble reviewed 29 cases of epiphyseal injuries about the knee and found that 50% of the patients had ligament instability at follow-up evaluation an average of 66 months following the original injury.[740] Of the 29 patients, 16 had distal femoral injury; and 6 of the 16 patients also had ligament insufficiency. Proximal tibial physeal fractures were noted in 13 of the patients, and 8 of them had ligament laxity. They concluded that ligament insufficiency was probably a reasonably common concomitant injury to the physeal fracture of the knee. They also reported a complex proximal tibial physeal fracture associated with medial collateral ligament rupture that resulted in genu valgum and early degenerative osteoarthritic changes.

Buess-Watson et al. thought the Salter classification to be of little prognostic value at the knee, as type 2 fractures (in their series) were usually followed by asymmetric growth arrest.[744] They also stressed that associated ligament injuries were not rare (43%) and deserved more attention.

Floating Knee

The floating knee has received little attention in children.[803,804] The injury comprises combined fractures of the ipsilateral femur and tibia (Fig. 21-81). In children, fractures through the growth plates of the distal femur or proximal tibia, along with a similar physeal fracture on the other side of the knee or a metaphyseal or diaphyseal fracture in the contraposed bone, create many analogous situations.

Letts and associates reviewed 15 children with this combined injury pattern. They found that there was a high incidence of floating knee in childhood cyclists, and they proposed a treatment protocol.[804] For a type A injury, in which both the femoral and the tibial fractures are diaphyseal and closed, open reduction and internal fixation of the tibia and balanced skeletal traction for the femur are recommended. For a type B injury, in which one fracture is diaphyseal, one fracture is metaphyseal, and both are closed, open reduction and internal fixation of the diaphyseal fracture and balanced skeletal traction (or casting) for the metaphyseal fracture are recommended. For a type C injury, in which one fracture is diaphyseal and the other is an epiphyseal displacement, it is recommended that the epiphyseal

FIGURE 21-81. Types of floating knee. (A) Diaphyseal injuries. (B) Diaphyseal-metaphyseal pattern. (C) Epiphyseal-diaphyseal pattern.

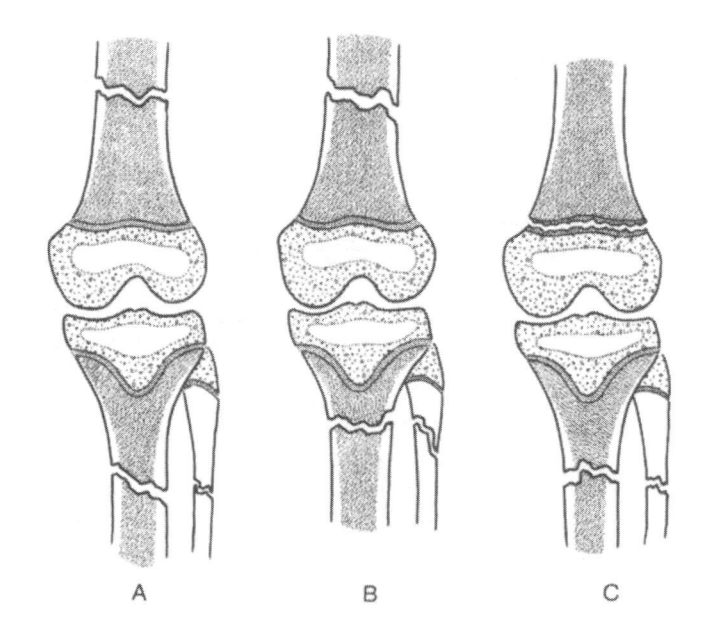

injury be reduced and internally fixed and the other fracture be treated with traction or casting, as indicated. For a type D injury, in which one fracture is open, débridement and external fixation are recommended for the open tibial fracture, with femoral traction for the open or closed fractured femur. For a type E injury in which both fractures are open, external fixation of the tibial fracture and traction or external fixation of the femur are recommended. Results were worst when both fractures were treated nonoperatively.[804]

Any treatment plan has exceptions. If it is essential that the child be mobilized as quickly as possible, internal fixation of both femoral and tibial fractures may be indicated (Fig. 21-82). The type of internal fixation may also depend on the equipment available, the experience of the surgeon, and the age of the child. In older children, intramedullary nailing of the femur or tibia may be more appropriate than plate fixation. In children under 6 years of age, it may be possible to obtain a stable closed reduction of the tibia that may be held with a cast while the femur is treated with traction. Because fractures of the femur in children may be managed safely and effectively by traction, it seems unwarranted to open this fracture, unless necessary, for the well-being of the child.

Lett et al.'s basic premise was that with fractures of the ipsilateral femur and tibia, no matter what the area of involvement, at least one fracture should be stabilized. They thought that such fixation was most appropriate for the tibia. Letts et al. did not believe that routine internal fixation of both fractures should be performed in children, as it may result in overgrowth and is occasionally complicated by osteomyelitis.[804]

Bohn and Durbin reviewed 44 ipsilateral femur and tibial fractures in 42 children and adolescents.[803] One patient died from head injury, and one patient had fat embolism syndrome. The age was found to be the most important variable

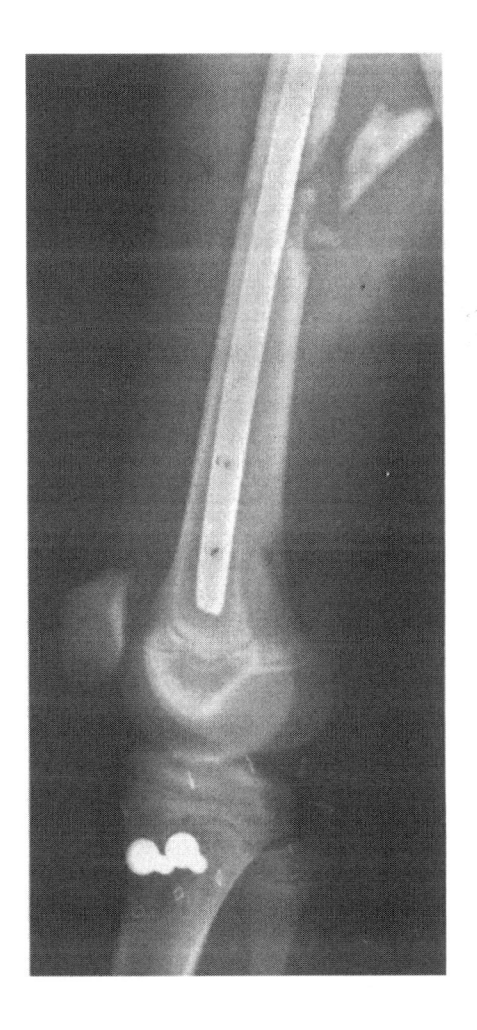

FIGURE 21-82. Adolescent with a femoral diaphyseal fracture associated with a type 2 epiphyseal fracture. Both were treated with open reduction and internal fixation.

related to the clinical course. Of the 15 patients less than 10 years of age, 3 had an early complication. The average time to complete weight-bearing was 13 weeks, and the average combined femoral and tibial overgrowth was 1.8 cm. Of the 15 children who were more than 10 years old, 8 had an early complication. The average time to full weight-bearing was 20 weeks, and there was variable femoral and tibial growth. The juxtaarticular pattern of fracture was associated with the highest incidence of early and late problems. Most children who were younger than 10 years were treated successfully with closed methods, but limb length discrepancy developed. Children older than 10 years were treated successfully with reduction and fixation, but they had a high rate of complications. There is a high incidence of concomitant injuries to the ligaments of the knee resulting in long-term dysfunction. Of 19 patients with long-term follow-up, only 7 had normal function without major problems. The remainder had a compromised result due to limb length discrepancy, angulated deformity, or instability of the knee, particularly ligamentous instability.

References

Anatomy

1. Barnes GR Jr, Gwinn JL. Distal irregularities of the femur simulating malignancy. AJR 1974;122:180–185.
2. Brower AC, Culver JE, Keats RE. Histologic nature of the cortical irregularity of the medial posterior distal femoral metaphysis in children. Radiology 1971;99:389–392.
3. Bufkin WJ. The avulsive cortical irregularity. AJR 1971;112:487–492.
4. Burkus JK, Ogden JA. Development of the distal femoral epiphysis: a microscopic morphological investigation of the zone of Ranvier. J Pediatr Orthop 1984;4:661–668.
5. Caffey J, Madell SH, Royer C, Morales P. Ossification of the distal femoral epiphysis. J Bone Joint Surg Am 1958;40:647–654.
6. Chung SMK. The arterial supply of the developing proximal end of the human femur. J Bone Joint Surg Am 1976;58:961–970.
7. Crock HV. A revision of the anatomy of the arteries supplying the upper end of the human femur. J Anat 1965;99:77–88.
8. Crock HV. An atlas of the arterial supply of the head and neck of the femur in man. Clin Orthop 1980;152:17–27.
9. Crock HV. An Atlas of Vascular Anatomy of the Skeleton and Spinal Cord. St. Louis: Mosby, 1996.
10. Lagrange J, Dunoyer J. La vascularisation de la tête fémorale de l'enfant. Rev Chir Orthop 1962;48:123–137.
11. Ogden JA. Changing patterns of proximal femoral vascularity. J Bone Joint Surg Am 1974;56:941–950.
12. Ogden JA. Development and growth of the hip. In: Katz JE, Siffert RS (eds) Management of Hip Disorders in Children. Philadelphia: Lippincott, 1983.
13. Ogden JA, Ganey TM. Radiology of postnatal skeletal development: the distal femur. Submitted.
14. Ogden JA, Ganey TM. The distal femoral "irregularity." Submitted.
15. Olson SA, Holt BT. Anatomy of the medial distal femur: a study of the adductor hiatus. J Orthop Trauma 1995;9:63–65.
16. Rogers WM, Gladstone H. Vascular foramina and arterial supply of the distal end of the femur. J Bone Joint Surg Am 1950;32:867–874.
17. Simon H. Medial distal metaphyseal femoral irregularity in children. Radiology 1968;90:258–260.
18. Trueta J. The normal vascular anatomy of the human femoral head during growth. J Bone Joint Surg Br 1957;39:358–394.
19. Wertheimer LG, Fernandes Lopes SDL. Arterial supply of the femoral head. J Bone Joint Surg Am 1971;53:545–556.
20. Young DW, Nogrady MB, Dunbar JS, Wigelsworth FW. Benign cortical irregularities in the distal femur of children. J Can Assoc Radiol 1972;23:107–115.

Proximal Femur (Capital and Neck Regions)

21. Allende G, Lezama LG. Fracture of the neck of the femur in children: a clinical study. J Bone Joint Surg Am 1951;33:387–395.
22. Ansorg P, Graner G. Valgisierung des Schenkelhalses nach nagelung kindlicher Oberschenkelschaftfrakturen. Zentralbl Chir 1976;101:968–973.
23. Arel F. Spontannekrose des Schenkelkopfes bei Jugendlichen. Zentrabl Chir 1936;63:617–621.
24. Asrus SE, Gould ES, Bansal M, Rizzo PF, Bullough PG. Magnetic resonance imaging of the hip after displaced femoral neck fractures. Clin Orthop 1994;298:191–198.
25. Aufranc OE, Jones WM, Harris WH. Fracture of the neck of the femur in a child. JAMA 1962;182:348–350.
26. Azouz EM, Karamitsos C, Reed MH, Baker L, Kozlowski K, Hoeffel JC. Types and complications of femoral neck fractures in children. Pediatr Radiol 1993;23:415–420.
27. Badelon O, Ciaudo O, Vie P, Mazda K, Bensahel H. Décollement épiphysaire pour de l'extrémité supérieure du fémur chez le petit enfant: a propos de 2 cas. Chir Pediatr 1986;27:114–117.
28. Barber ET. Fractures of the neck of the femur in a child seven years of age: suit for malpractice. Pacific Med Surg 1871–1872;14:61–64.
29. Bauer J, Andrasina J, Brandebur O, Kovac M. Aussprache über Schenkelhalsbrüche des Wachstumsalters. Monatsschr Unfallheilkd 1968;97:160–169.
30. Berger D. Steinhanslinch: fracture du col fémoral de l'enfant. Ther Umsch 1983;40:960–964.
31. Bester JE. Fracture of the femoral neck in children. J Bone Joint Surg Br 1967;49:200.
32. Bhansali RM. Defunctioning osteotomy for fractures of the femoral neck in children. J Bone Joint Surg Br 1966;48:198.
33. Bloch R. Les fractures de cuisse chez l'enfant. Orthop Rev 1922;9:447–453.
34. Bluemke DA, Petri M, Zerhoumi EA. Femoral head perfusion and composition: MR imaging and spectroscopic evaluation of patients with systemic lupus erythematosus and at risk for avascular necrosis. Radiology 1995;197:433–438.
35. Bohler J. Die Operationsindikation kindlicher Frakturen. Medizinische 1957;35:1207–1214.
36. Bohler J. Fractures of the neck of the femur in children and juveniles. In: Fractures in Children. Stuttgart: Georg Thieme Verlag, 1981:228–233.
37. Bohler J. Hip fracture in children. Clin Orthop 1981;161:339–348.
38. Boitzy A. La Fracture du Col du Femur Chez l'Enfant et l'Adolescent. Paris: Masson, 1971.
39. Bonvallet JM. Sur un cas exceptionnel de luxation traumatique de la hanche de l'enfant, associee a un décollement épiphysaire complet et a une fracture du noyan cephalique. Rev Chir Orthop 1965;51:723–728.
40. Borchard A. Die operative Behandlung der Schenkelhalsbruche, besonders in Jugendlichem alter. Dtsch Z Chir 1909;100:275–279.

References

41. Borgsmiller WK, Whiteside LA, Goldsand EM, Lange DR. The effect of hydrostatic pressure in the hip joint on proximal femoral epiphyseal and metaphyseal blood flow. Trans Orthop Res Soc 1980;5:23.
42. Bouyala JM, Bollini G, Clement JL, et al. Femoral transcervical fractures in children: apropos of 50 cases. Rev Chir Orthop 1986;72:43–49.
43. Bucholz RW, Ogden JA. Patterns of ischemic necrosis of the proximal femur in non-operatively treated congenital hip disease. In: The Hip: Proceedings of the Hip Society, vol 6. St. Louis: Mosby, 1978.
44. Butler JE, Cary JM. Fracture of the femoral neck in a child. JAMA 1971;218:398–400.
45. Cabanela ME, Russell TA, Swiontkowski MF, et al. Fractures of the proximal part of the femur. J Bone Joint Surg Am 1994;76:924–950.
46. Cady RB. Posterior dislocation of the hip associated with separation of the capital epiphysis. Clin Orthop 1987;222:186–189.
47. Calandruccio RA, Anderson WE III. Post-fracture avascular necrosis of the femoral head: correlation of experimental and clinical studies. Clin Orthop 1980;152:49–84.
48. Calvert PT, Kernohan JG, Sayers DCJ, Catterall A. Effects of vascular occlusion on the femoral head in growing rabbits. Acta Orthop Scand 1984;55:526–530.
49. Canale ST. Fractures of the hip in children and adolescents. Orthop Clin North Am 1990;21:341–352.
50. Canale ST, Bourland WL. Fracture of the neck and intertrochanteric region of the femur in children. J Bone Joint Surg Am 1977;59:431–443.
51. Carrell B, Carrell WB. Fracture in the neck of the femur in children with particular reference to aseptic necrosis. J Bone Joint Surg 1941;23:225–239.
52. Catier PH, Bracq H, Allouis M, Babut JM. Décollements épiphysaires traumatiques de la téte fémorale. Chir Pediatr 1981;22:237–241.
53. Cervenansky J, Makai F. Aussprache über Schenkelhalsbrüche des Wachstumsalters. Monatsschr Unfallheilkd 1968;97:161.
54. Chigot PL, Davay A. A propos des fractures du col du femur de l'enfant. Ann Chir 1958;12:1143–1149.
55. Chigot PL, Vialas M. Fractures du col du femur chez l'enfant. Ann Chir Infant 1963;4:209–215.
56. Chong KC, Chacha PB, Lee BT. Fractures of the neck of the femur in childhood and adolescence. Injury 1975;7:111–119.
57. Chrestian P, Bollini G, Jacquemier M, Ramaherison P. Fractures du col du fémur dé l'enfant. Chir Pediatr 1981;22:397–403.
58. Clifford L, Craig MD. Hip injuries in children and adolescents. Orthop Clin North Am 1980;11:743–754.
59. Coldwell D, Gross GW, Boal DK. Stress fracture of the femoral neck in a child. Pediatr Radiol 1981;14:174–176.
60. Colonna PC. Fracture of the neck of the femur in childhood: a report of six cases. Ann Surg 1928;88:902–906.
61. Colonna PC. Fracture of the neck of the femur in childhood. Am J Surg 1929;6:793–797.
62. Cornacchia M. Le frattura del collo del femoro nell'infanzia. Chir Organi Mov 1951;36:1–7.
63. Craig CL. Hip injuries in children and adolescents. Orthop Clin North Am 1980;11:743–754.
64. Cromwell BM. A case of intracapsular fracture of the neck of the femur in a young subject. NC Med J 1885;15:309–310.
65. Davison BL, Weinstein SL. Hip fractures in children: a long-term follow-up study. J Pediatr Orthop 1992;12:355–358.
66. Delbet MP. Fractures du col de fémur. Bull Mem Soc Chir 1909;35:387–389.
67. Delporte J. Les fractures du col du femur chez l'enfant. Thesis, University of Lille, 1966.
68. Deluca FM, Kech CH. Traumatic coxa vara: a case report of spontaneous correction in a child. Clin Orthop 1976;116:125–128.
69. Drake JK, Meyers MH. Intracapsular pressure and hemarthrosis following femoral neck fracture. Clin Orthop 1984;182:172–176.
70. Dromer H, Penndorg K. Oberschenkelbruch im Kindesalter: Ergebnisse einer mehrjahrigen Verlaufsbeobachtung. Chirurg 1967;38:284–290.
71. Duhaime M, Lascombes P. Pronostic des fractures du col du fémur de l'enfant. Chir Pediatr 1984;25:152–160.
72. Durbin FC. Avascular necrosis complicating undisplaced fractures of the neck of femur in children. J Bone Joint Surg Br 1959;41:758–762.
73. Engels M, Lassnig I, Manzl M. Die konservative Behandlung der Oberschenkelfrakturen. Z Kinderchir 1977;20:79–84.
74. Fardon DF. Fracture of the neck and shaft of the same femur. J Bone Joint Surg Am 1970;52:797–799.
75. Fauvy A. Luxation traumatique de la hanche droite avec decollement epiphysaire de la tete fèmorale chez un enfant de 13 ans. Ouest Med 1976;29:1783–1784.
76. Feigenberg Z, Pauker M, Levy M, Seelenfreund M, Fried A. Fractures of the femoral neck in childhood. J Trauma 1977;12:937–942.
77. Flach A, Kudlich H. Schenkelkopfnekrosen nach traumatischen Huftluxationen und Schenkelhalsfrakturen jugendlicher. Zentralbl Chir 1962;20:860–863.
78. Forlin E, Guille JT, Kumar J, Rhee KJ. Complications associated with fracture of the neck of the femur in children. J Pediatr Orthop 1992;12:503–509.
79. Forlin E, Guille JT, Kumar SJ, Rhee KJ. Transepiphyseal fractures of the neck of the femur in very young children. J Pediatr Orthop 1992;12:168–172.
80. Fornaro E, Brunner C, Weber BG. Die Behandlung des Schenkelhalsbruches im Kindesalter: not fall massige Arthrotomie, Reposition und Verschraupung. Hefte Unfallheilkd 1982;158:247–253.
81. Gamble JG, Lettice J, Smith JT, Rinsky LA. Transverse cervicopertrochanteric hip fracture. J Pediatr Orthop 1991;11:779–782.
82. Ganz R, Luthi U, Rahn B, Perren SM. Intraartikulaire Druckerhoheng und epiphysaire Durchblutungsstorung: ein experimentelles Untersuchungsmodell. Orthopade 1981;10:6–8.
83. Gaudinez RF, Heinrich SD. Transphyseal fracture of the capital femoral epiphysis. Orthopaedics 1989;12:1599–1602.
84. Gerber C, Lehmann A, Ganz R. Schenkelhalsfrakturen beim Kind: eine multizentrische Nachkontrollstudie. Z Orthop 1985;123:767–775.
85. Graig CL. Hip injuries in children and adolescents. Orthop Clin North Am 1980;11:743–754.
86. Grassi G, Nigrisoli P. Traumatic separation of the upper femoral epiphysis in a child aged two. Ital J Orthop Traumatol 1976;2:135–139.
87. Greig DM. Fracture of the cervix femoris in children. Edinb Med J 1919;2:75–97.
88. Guilleminent M, Germain D. Aspects radiologiques des fractures traumatiques ou pathologiques du col fémoral chez les jeunes enfants. Lyon Chir 1954;49:351–353.
89. Gupta AK, Chaturvedi SN. Traumatic femoral neck fractures in childhood. Indian J Surg 1973;35:567–572.
90. Gupta AK, Chaturvedi SN, Pruthi KK. Fracture of femoral neck in children. Proc SICOT 1975;4:105–106.
91. Haldenwang O. Über echte Schenkelhalsfrakturen im Kindlichen und Jugendlichem alter. Bruns Beitr Klin Chir 1908;59:81–87.

92. Hamilton CM. Fractures of the neck of the femur in children. JAMA 1961;178:799–801.
93. Havránek P, Staudacherová I, Hájková H. Proximal femoral fractures in children. Acta Univ Carol Med 1989;35:223–242.
94. Heiser JM, Oppenheim WL. Fractures of the hip in children: a review of forty cases. Clin Orthop 1980;149:177–184.
95. Herring JA. Post-traumatic femoral head lesions. J Pediatr Orthop 1982;2:325–328.
96. Hoeksema HD, Olsen C, Rudy R. Fracture of femoral neck and shaft and repeat neck fracture in a child. J Bone Joint Surg Am 1976;57:271–272.
97. Hoekstra HJ, Binnendyk B. Fracture of the neck and shaft of same femur in children: a report of two cases. Arch Orthop Traumatol Surg 1982;100:197–198.
98. Hoffa A. Über Schenkelhalsbruche im Kindlichen und Jugendlichen alter. Z Orthop Chir 1903;11:528–539.
99. Hofmann W. Über Schenkelhalsfrakturen bei Kindern. Beitr Orthop Traumatol 1964;11:412–417.
100. Hughes LO, Beatty JH. Fractures of the head and neck of the femur in children: current concepts review. J Bone Joint Surg Am 1994;76:283–292.
101. Huo MH, Root L, Buly RL, Mauri TM. Traumatic fracture dislocation of the hip in a 2-year-old child. Orthopaedics 1992;15:1430–1433.
102. Imamaliev AS, Zoria VI, Parshikov MV. Treatment of post-traumatic coxa vara in adolescence (in Russian). Ortop Travmatol Protez 1990;2:28–30.
103. Imhauser G. Der Schenkelhalsbruch des Kindes und seine Komplikationen insbesondere die Pseudarthrose. Arch Orthop Unfallchir 1963;55:274–288.
104. Ingelrans P, Lacheretz M, Debeugny P, Vandenbusch F. Les fractures du col du femur chez l'enfant: a propos de huit observations. Acta Orthop Belg 1966;32:809–824.
105. Ingram AJ, Bachynski B. Fractures of the hip in children. J Bone Joint Surg Am 1953;35:867–887.
106. Jacob R, Niemann K. Fractures of the hip in childhood. South Med J 1976;69:629–631.
107. Johansson S. Über Epiphysennekrose bei geheilten Collumfrakturen. Zentralbl Chir 1927;35:2214–2217.
108. Jonasch E. Der eingekeilte Schenkelhalsbruch bei Kindern. Unfallllheilkunde 1981;150:85–92.
109. von Jungbluth KH, Daum R, Metzger E. Schenkelhalsfrakturen im Kindesalter. Z Kinderchir 1968;3:392–403.
110. Katz JF. Spontaneous correction of angulational deformity of the proximal femoral epiphysis after cervical and trochanteric fracture. J Pediatr Orthop 1983;3:231–234.
111. Kay SP, Hall JE. Fractures of the hip in children and its complications. Clin Orthop 1971;80:53–71.
112. Kite JH, Lovell WW, Allman FL. Fracture of the hip in the young. J Bone Joint Surg Am 1962;44:1710–1713.
113. Klasen HJ. Traumatic dislocation of the hip in children. Reconstr Surg Traumatol 1979;17:119–129.
114. Kleinefeld F, Erdwig W. Beidseitige Hüftkopfepiphysenfrakturen beim Kind. Akt Traumatol 1983;13:198–200.
115. Ko J-Y, Meyers MH, Wenger DR. "Trapdoor" procedure for osteonecrosis with segmental collapse of the femoral head in teenagers. J Pediatr Orthop 1995;15:7–15.
116. Kohli SB. Fracture of the neck of the femur in children. J Bone Joint Surg Br 1974;56:776.
117. Korisek G, Schneider H, Breitfuss H. Der kindliche oberschenkelbruch: die konservative therapie und ihre vorzüge. Hefte Unfallheilk 1984;170:336–338.
118. Kotzenberg W. Zwei Fälle von Pseudarthrosen des Schenkelhalses nach Fraktur im Jugendlichen Alter. Langenbeck Arch Clin Chir 1907;82:191–197.
119. Kovac M, Brandebur O. Fractures of the proximal end of the femur in childhood. Acta Chir Orthop Traumatol Cech 1980;47:240–245.
120. Kristensen H, Okholm K. Results after fracture of the neck of the femur in children. Acta Orthop Scand 1974;45:796.
121. Kujat R, Suren EG, Rogge D, Tscherne H. Die Schenkelhalsfraktur in Wachstumsalter. Chirurg 1984;55:43–48.
122. Kurz W, Grumbt H. Die Schenkelhalsfraktur im Kindesalter. Zentalbl Chir 1988;113:881–892.
123. Lam SF. Fractures of the neck of the femur in children. Thesis, University of Hong Kong, 1967.
124. Lam SF. Fractures of the neck of the femur in children. J Bone Joint Surg Am 1976;53:1165–1179.
125. Lange M. Die Gefahr der Pseudoarthrosenbildung und Femurkopfnekrose nach Schenkelhals und Schenkelkopfbruchen jugendlicher. Z Orthop Chir 1932;27:531–542.
126. Lausten GS, Arnoldi CC. Blood perfusion uneven in femoral head osteonecrosis: Doppler flowmetry and intraosseous pressure in 12 cases. Acta Orthop Scand 1993;64:533–536.
127. Leconte PH, Bastien J. Evolution favorable d'un décollement épiphysaire traumatique de l'extremité supérieure du fémur. Rev Chir Orthop 1978;64:695–697.
128. Lee KE, Pelker RR, Rudicel SA, Ogden JA, Panjabi MM. Histologic patterns of capital femoral growth plate fracture in the rabbit: the effect of shear direction. J Pediatr Orthop 1985;5:32–39.
129. Leung PC, Lam SF. Long-term follow-up of children with femoral neck fractures. J Bone Joint Surg Br 1986;68:537–540.
130. Linhart W, Stampfel O, Ritter G. Post-traumatische Femurkopfnekrose nach Trochanterfraktur. Z Orthop 1984;122:766–769.
131. Lombard JLA. Fractures du col du femur chez les enfants. Thesis, University of Nancy, 1910.
132. Lucht U, Bunger C, Krebs B, Hjermind J, Bulow J. Blood flow in the juvenile hip in relation to changes of the intraarticular pressure: an experimental investigation in dogs. Acta Orthop Scand 1983;54:182–187.
133. Maini SP, Moda SK, Singh K. Fracture of the neck of the femur in patients below 17 years of age. Indian J Orthop 1982;16:83–88.
134. Manninger J, Kazar G, Nagy E. Phlebography for fracture of the femoral neck in adolescence. Injury 1974;5:244–254.
135. Manninger J, Zolcer L, Nagy E, et al. The diagnostic role of the intraosseous phlebography in the affections of the hip in childhood. Arch Orthop Trauma Surg 1980;96:203–211.
136. Maroske D, Thon K. Schenkelhalsfrakturen im Kindesalter. Unfallheilkunde 1981;84:186–193.
137. Marsh HO. Intertrochanteric and femoral neck fractures in children. J Bone Joint Surg Am 1967;49:1024.
138. Mattner HR. Schenkelhalsfrakturen im Kindesalter. Arch Orthop Unfallchir 1958;49:473–479.
139. McDougall A. Fracture of the neck of the femur in childhood. J Bone Joint Surg Br 1961;43:16–28.
140. Meaney JFM, Carty H. Femoral stress fractures in children. Skeletal Radiol 1988;16:365–377.
141. Melberg PE, Korner L, Lansinger O. Hip joint pressure after femoral neck fracture. Acta Orthop Scand 1986;57:501–504.
142. Milgram JW, Lyne ED. Epiphysiolysis of the proximal femur in very young children. Clin Orthop 1975;110:146–153.
143. Miller F, Wenger DR. Femoral neck stress fracture in a hyperactive child. J Bone Joint Surg Am 1979;61:435–437.
144. Miller WE. Fracture of the hip in children from birth to adolescence. Clin Orthop 1973;92:155–188.
145. Minikel J, Sty J, Simons G. Sequential radionuclide bone imaging in avascular pediatric hip conditions. Clin Orthop 1983;175:202–208.
146. Mir D, Lustig KA. Femoral neck fractures in children: case report and discussion. Contemp Orthop 1984;9:47–50.
147. Mitchell JI. Fracture of the neck of the femur in children. JAMA 1936;107:1603–1606.

148. Morrissy RT. Hip fractures in children. Clin Orthop 1980;152: 202–210.
149. Morrissy RT. Fractured hip in childhood. AAOS Instr Course Lect 1984;33:229–237.
150. Mortensson W, Rosenberg M, Gretzer H. The role of bone scintigraphy in predicting femoral head collapse following cervical fractures in children. Acta Radiol 1990;31:291–292.
151. Moser H. Zur frage der nagelung jugendlicher Schenkelhalsbruche. Wien Klin Wochenschr 1949;61:55–58.
152. Naerra A. On secondary epiphyseal necrosis after collum femoris fracture in young persons. Acta Chir Scand 1937; 80:238–243.
153. Nagi ON, Dhillon MS, Gill SS. Fibular osteosynthesis for delayed type II and type III femoral neck fractures in children. J Orthop Trauma 1992;6:306–313.
154. Nahoda J, Stryhal F. Otazka spontanni kompenzace prerustu femuru po zlomenine v detstvi. Acta Chir Orthop Traumatol Cech 1969;4:211–215.
155. Naito M, Schoenecker PL, Owen JH, Sugioka Y. Acute effect of traction, compression, and hip joint tamponade on blood flow of the femoral head: an experimental model. J Orthop Res 1992;10:800–806.
156. Nicholson JT, Foster RM, Heath RD. Bryant's traction: a provocative cause of circulatory complications. JAMA 1955; 157:415–418.
157. Nicolas FJM. Traitement des fractures du col du femur de l'enfant. Thesis, University of Nancy, 1922:200.
158. Nielsen B. Om Calve-Perthes sygdom efter fractura colli femoris hos unge of dens betydning for forstaaelsen af de aseptiske epifysenekrosers patogenese. Hospitalstidende 1938;81:773–779.
159. Nielsen PT, Thaarup P. An unusual course of femoral head necrosis complicating an intertrochanteric fracture in a child. Clin Orthop 1984;183:79–81.
160. Niethard FU. Pathophysiologie und Prognose von Schenkelhals frakturen im Kindesalter. Hefte Unfallheilkd 1982; 158:221–232.
161. Noble M. Fractures du col du femur de l'enfant. Thesis, University of Bordeaux, 1907:143.
162. Ogden JA. Hip development and vascularity: relationship to chondro-osseous trauma in the growing child. In: The Hip: Proceedings of the Hip Society, vol 9. St. Louis: Mosby, 1981.
163. Ogden JA. Trauma and the developing hip. In: Tronzo R (ed) Surgery of the Hip, 2nd ed. New York: Springer, 1986.
164. O'Malley DE, Mazur JM, Cummings RJ. Femoral head avascular necrosis associated with intramedullary nailing in an adolescent. J Pediatr Orthop 1995;15:21–23.
165. Oveson O, Arreskov J, Bellstrom T. Hip fractures in children: a long-term follow-up of 17 cases. Orthopaedics 1989; 12:361–367.
166. Papadimitriou DC. Fractures of the neck of the femur in children. Thesis, University of Athens, 1956.
167. Papadimitriou DC. Fractures of the neck of the femur in children. Am J Surg 1958;95:132–137.
168. Parrini L. Le fratture del collo del femore nei bambini. Minerva Ortop 1955;6:293–298.
169. Pathak RH, Saraf ML, Shahana MN, Kamdar BD. Fractures of neck of femur in children. Indian J Surg 1980;42:28–35.
170. Pathi KM. Fracture neck of femur in children. Indian J Orthop 1986;20:132–135.
171. Pazzaglia UE, Finardi E, Pedrotti L, Zatti G. Fracture with loss of the proximal femur in a child. Int Orthop 1991;15:143–144.
172. Peltokallio P, Kurkipaa M. Fractures of the femoral neck in children. Ann Chir Gynaecol Fenn 1959;48:151–163.
173. Pforringer W. Schaden der Femurkopfepiphyse. Z Orthop 1981;119:145–156.
174. Pforringer W, Rosemeyer B. Schenkelhalsfrakturen im Kindesalter. Arch Orthop Unfallchir 1977;88:281–308.
175. Pforringer W. Rosemeyer B. Schenkelhasfrakturen bei Jugendlichen: eine Langzeituntersuchung von 22 Fällen vor und nach Epiphysenschluss. Arch Orthop Unfallchir 1977; 90:169–185.
176. Pforringer W, Rosemeyer B. Fractures of the hip in children and adolescents. Acta Orthop Scand 1980;51:91–108.
177. Pilgaard S. Treatment of fractures of the femoral neck in children. Acta Orthop Scand 1976;45:796.
178. Pistor G, von Hofmann KHS, Batz W. Femoral neck fractures in childhood. Unfallchirurgie 1984;10:293–302.
179. Quinlan WR, Brady PG, Regan BF. Fracture of the neck of the femur in childhood. Injury 1977;11:242–2247.
180. Raju KK, Tepler M, Dharapak C, Pearlman HS. Transepiphyseal fractures of the hip in children. Orthop Rev 1984;13: 65–77.
181. Ratliff AHC. Avascular necrosis of the head of the femur after fracture of the femoral neck in children and Perthes disease. Proc R Soc Med 1962;55:504–505.
182. Ratliff AHC. Fractures of the neck of the femur in children. J Bone Joint Surg Br 1962;44:528–542.
183. Ratliff AHC. Fractures of the neck of the femur in children: a study of 132 cases. Thesis, University of Bristol, 1968.
184. Ratliff AHC. Tramatic separation of the upper femoral epiphysis in young children. J Bone Joint Surg Br 1968;50:757–770.
185. Ratliff AHC. Complications after fracture of the femoral neck in children and their treatment. J Bone Joint Surg Br 1970; 52:175.
186. Ratliff AHC. Traumatic separation of the upper femoral epiphysis in young children. Orthop Clin North Am 1974; 5:925–931.
187. Ratliff AHC. Fractures of the neck of the femur in children. In: Lloyd-Roberts GC, Ratliff AHC (eds) Hip Disorders in Children. London: Butterworths, 1978:165–196.
188. Rehli V, Slongo TH, Gerber CH. Femurkopfnahe Frakturen bei Kindern und Jugendlichen. Helv Chir Acta 1992; 59:547–552.
189. Riedel K. Frakturen im Kindesalter. Dtsch Med Wochenschr 1956;81:32–37.
190. Rigault P, Iselin F, Moreau J, Judet J. Fractures du col du fémur chez l'enfant. Rev Chir Orthop 1966;52:325–336.
191. Rizzo PF, Gould ES, Lyden JP, Asnis SE. Diagnosis of occult fractures about the hip. J Bone Joint Surg Am 1993; 75:395–401.
192. Romer KH, Reppin G. Zur Marknagelung kindlicher Oberschenkelfrakturen. Zentralbl Chir 1973;98:170–171.
193. Rouiller R, Griffe J, Crespy G. Epiphyseolyse femorale superieure apres fracture basicervicale: resultat apres trois ans. Rev Chir Orthop 1971;57:66–67.
194. Rudicel S, Pelker RP, Lee KE, Ogden JA, Panjabi MM. Shear fractures through the capital femoral physis of the skeletally immature rabbit. J Pediatr Orthop 1985;5:27–31.
195. Ruggieri F. La fratture del collo del femore nell'enfanzia. Minerva Ortop 1954;20:276–281.
196. Russell RH. A clinical lecture on fracture of the neck of the femur in childhood. Lancet 1898;1:125–128.
197. Ruter A, Kreuzer U. Schenkelhalsfrakturen beim kind—therapie und ergebnisse. Hefte Unfallheilkd 1982;158:233–240.
198. St. Pierre P, Staheli LT, Smith JB, Green NE. Femoral neck stress fractures in children and adolescents. J Pediatr Orthop 1995;15:470–473.
199. Sanchetti KH, Damle AN, Electrochvala JT. Fractures of the neck of the femur in children. Indian J Orthop 1980;14: 26–31.
200. Sanguinetti C. Le fratture del collo del femore nel bambino. Boll Med Soc Tosco Umbra Chir 1967;28:455–459.
201. Sattel W, Koch A, Stankovic P. Spadergebnisse nach Schenkelhalsfrakturen im Kindesalter. Hefte Unfallheilkd 1982; 158:255–259.

202. Scharli AF, Osterwalder M, Winiker H. Huftnähe Frakturen im Kindesalter. Helv Chir Acta 1992;59:999–1009.
203. Schlachetzki H. Fraktura colli femoris im Kindesalter. Zentralbl Chir 1930;57:549–556.
204. Schlesinger I, Wedge JH. The management of hip fractures in children and adolescents. Techn Orthop 1989;4:48–52.
205. Schwartz E. Was wird aus der Schenkelhalsfraktur des Kindes? Beitr Klin Chir 1913;88:125–128.
206. Schwartz N. Konservative und operative Behandlung der einigekeilten subkapitalen Schenkelhalsfraktur. Unfallheilkunde 1981;84:503–508.
207. Schwartz N, Leixnerung M. Abjuktions frakturen des femurhalses bei Adolesczenten. Akt Traumatol 1988;18:268–270.
208. Schwartz NM, Leixnering M, Frisee H. Aktuelle Therapie und prognose der Femur hals frakturen im Wachstumsalter. Unfallchirurg 1986;89:235–240.
209. Seddon HJ. Necrosis of the head of the femur following fracture of the neck in a child. Proc R Soc Med 1937;30:210–212.
210. Shahane MN, Manelkar KR. Intracapsular fracture of the neck of the femur in children. Clin Orthop (Indian) 1987;1:83–90.
211. Sharma JC, Biyani A, Kalla R, et al. Management of childhood femoral neck fractures. Injury 1992;23:453–457.
212. Shimizu K, Moriya H, Akita T, Sakamoto M, Suguro T. Prediction of collapse with magnetic resonance imaging of avascular necrosis of the femoral head. J Bone Joint Surg Am 1994;76:215–223.
213. Sonheim K. Fracture of the femoral neck in children. Acta Orthop Scand 1972;43:523–531.
214. Sorrel E. Fracture du col du fémur chez un enfant de 7 ans: pseudarthrosis; resultat à longue échéance d'une ostéosynthèse par greffe tibiale. Mem Acad Chir 1951;77:521–523.
215. Soto-Hall R, Johnson LH, Johnson RA. Variations in the intraarticular pressure of the hip joint in injury and disease. J Bone Joint Surg Am 1964;46:509–516.
216. Stougard J. Post-traumatic avascular necrosis of the femoral head in children. J Bone Joint Surg Br 1969;51:354–355.
217. Streicher HJ. Schenkelhalsfrakturend bei Kindern und Jugendlichen. Arch Klin Chir 1957;287:716–722.
218. Swiontkowski MF. Complications of hip fractures in children. Complications Orthop 1989;4:58–64.
219. Swiontkowski MF, Winquist RA. Displaced hip fractures in children and adolescents. J Trauma 1986;26:384–388.
220. Sybrandy S. Correctie van verschil in beenlengte door epiphysiodese, en de betekenis van groeilijnen in het skelet. Ned Tijdschr Geneeskd 1968;112:692–696.
221. Tachdjian MO, Grana L. Response of the hip joint to increased intraarticular hydrostatic pressure. Clin Orthop 1968;61:199–212.
222. Takeuchi T, Shidou T. Impairment of blood supply to the head of the femur after fracture of the neck. Int Orthop 1993;17:325–329.
223. Talwalkar CA. Fracture of the femoral neck in children. ChM thesis, University of Liverpool, 1974.
224. Taylor HL. Fractures of the neck of the femur in children. NY State J Med 1917;17:508–511.
225. Thomas CL, Gage JR, Ogden JA. Treatment concepts for complications of ischemic necrosis complicating congenital hip disease. J Bone Joint Surg Am 1982;64:817–828.
226. Titze A. Vortrag über Schenkelhalsbrüche des Wachstumsalters. Hefte Unfallheilkd 1968;97:157–159.
227. Tondeur G, Bosman J. Fractures spontanées chez l'enfant. Acta Orthop Belg 1966;32:825–838.
228. Touzet P, Rigault P, Padovani JP, Pouliquen JC, Mallet JF, Guyonvarch G. Les fractures du col du fémur chez l'enfant. Rev Chir Orthop 1979;65:341–349.
229. Vegter J, Lubsen CC. Fractional necrosis of the femoral head epiphysis after transient increase in joint pressure. J Bone Joint Surg Br 1987;69:530–535.
230. Wagner H. Orthopedic problems after femoral neck fractures in childhood. Hefte Unfallheilkd 1982;158:141–147.
231. Weber U, Rettig H, Brudet J. Die Schenkelhalsfraktur im Kindesalter. Unfallchirurg 1985;88:512–517.
232. Weiner D, O'Dell HW. Fractures of the hip in children. J Trauma 1969;9:62–76.
233. Werkman DM. The transepiphyseal fracture of the femoral neck. Injury 1980;12:50–52.
234. Whitman R. Fracture of the neck of the femur in a child. Med Rec 1891;39:165–167.
235. Whitman R. Observations on fractures of the neck of the femur in childhood with special reference to treatment and differential diagnosis from separation of the epiphysis. Med Rec 1893;43:227–241.
236. Whitman R. Further observations in the fracture of the neck of the femur in childhood. Ann Surg 1897;25:673–676.
237. Whitman R. Further observations on depression of the neck of the femur in early life; including fracture of the neck of the femur, separation of the epiphysis and simple coxa vara. Ann Surg 1900;31:145–162.
238. Whitman R. Further observations on injuries of the neck of the femur in early life. Med Rec 1909;75:1–9.
239. Wiedman H, Parsch K. Schenkelhalsfraktur bei Kindern. Z Orthop 1990;128:418–421.
240. Wilson JC. Fractures of the neck of the femur in childhood. J Bone Joint Surg 1940;22:531–546.
241. Wolfgang GL. Stress fracture of the femoral neck in a patient with open capital femoral epiphyses. J Bone Joint Surg Am 1977;59:680–681.
242. Worms G, Hamant A. Les fractures du col du femur dans l'enfance et dans l'adolescence. Rev Chir 1912;46:416–422.
243. Zolczer L, Kazar G, Manninger J, Nagy E. Fracture of the femoral neck in adolescents. Injury 1973;4:41–46.
244. ZurVerth M. Sekundäre Nekrose des Schenkelkopfes nach Schenkelhals brüchen Jugendlicher. Zentralbl Chir 1935;62:2549–2553.

Proximal Femur (Neonatal)

245. Azouz EM. Apparent or true neonatal hip dislocation? Radiologic differential diagnosis. Can Med Assoc J 1983;129:595–597.
246. Camera R. Il distacco epifisario ostetrico dell'estremita prossimate del femore. Chir Organi Movi 1929;33:331–334.
247. Camera U. Il distacco epifisario traumatico ostetrico dell'estremita superiore del femore. Arch Orthop 1930;46:1019–1023.
248. Caveric N, Strinovic B. Folgenlös ansgeheilten geburtstraumatischen epiphysenlösungen am proximalen Femur und Humerusende. Akt Traumatol 1977;7:103–108.
250. Define D. Sobre un caso de descollamento epiphysario obstetrico das extremidades femurae. Argent Cir Clin Exp 1938;2:347–349.
251. Diaz MJ, Hedlund GL. Sonographic diagnosis of traumatic separation of the proximal femoral epiphysis in the neonate. Pediatr Radiol 1991;21:238–240.
252. Dimitriou J. Obstetrical injury of the upper femoral epiphysis. Orthopaedics (Oxf) 1971;4:23–25.
253. Ehrenfest H. Birth Injuries of the Child. New York: Appleton, 1931.
254. Ekengren K, Bergdahl S, Ekstrom G. Birth injuries to the epiphyseal cartilage. Acta Radiol 1978;19:197–204.
255. Elizalde EA. Obstetrical dislocation of the hip associated with fracture of the femur. J Bone Joint Surg 1946;28:838–841.

256. Emmeus H, Gerner-Smidt M. Frakturer hos Born. Albertslund, Denmark: Richards Scandinavia, 1979.
257. Fairhurst MJ. Transepiphyseal femoral neck fracture at birth. J Bone Joint Surg Br 1990;72:155–156.
258. Harrenstein RJ. Pseudoluxatio coxae durch abreissen der Femurepiphyse bir der Geburt. Beitr Klin Chir 1929;146:592–595.
259. Kennedy PC. Traumatic separation of the upper femoral epiphysis: a birth injury. AJR 1944;51:707–719.
260. Kleine HO. Zur roentgenologischen differentialdiagnose zwischen Huftgelenksluxation und traumatischer Epiphysenlösung beim Neugeborenen. Arch Kinderheilkd 1933;193:213–217.
261. Lindseth RE, Rosene HA. Traumatic separation of the upper femoral epiphysis in a newborn infant. J Bone Joint Surg Am 1971;53:1641–1644.
262. Lubrano di Diego JG, Chappuis JP, Montsegur P, et al. A propos de 82 traumatismes obstetricaux osteo-articulares du nouveau-ne (paralysies du plexus brachial exceptees). Chir Pediatr 1978;19:219–226.
263. MacKenzie IG, Seddon HJ, Trevor D. Congenital dislocation of the hip. J Bone Joint Surg Am 1960;42:689–705.
264. Madsen ET. Fractures of the extremities in newborn. Acta Obstet Gynecol Scand 1955;34:41–74.
265. Meier A. Geburtstraumatische Epiphysenlösung am proximalen Femurende. Arch Kinderheilkd 1939;116:267–270.
266. Michail JP, Theodorou S, Houliaras K, Siatis N. Two cases of obstetrical separation (epiphysiolysis) of the upper femoral epiphysis: appearance of ossification centre of the femoral head in a fifteen-day-old child. J Bone Joint Surg Br 1958;40:477–482.
267. Mortens J, Christensen P. Traumatic separation of the upper femoral epiphysis as an obstetrical lesion. Acta Orthop Scand 1964;34:238–250.
268. Nathan W. Gerburtstrauma und Huftgelenkverrenkung. Z Orthop Chir 1928;49:383–387.
269. Ogden JA. Birth related injuries to the hip. In: Steinberg M, Hensinger RM, Ogden JA (eds) The Hip and Its Disorders. Philadelphia: Saunders, 1990.
270. Ogden JA, Lee KE, Rudicel SA, Pelker RR. Proximal femoral epiphysiolysis in the neonate. J Pediatr Orthop 1984;4:285–292.
271. Pavlik A. Treatment of obstetrical fractures of the femur. J Bone Joint Surg 1939;21:939–947.
272. Pfeiffer R. Die traumatische Lösung der oberen femurepiphyse, eine typische Gerburtsverletzung. Beitr Klin Chir 1936;164:18–21.
273. Poland J. Traumatic Separation of the Epiphyses. London: Smith, Elder, 1898.
274. Poli A. Quadruplice distacco epifisario ostetrico. Chir Ital 1935;3:212–216.
275. Prevot J, Lascombes P, Blanquart D, Gagneux E. Geburtstraumatische Epiphysenlösung des proximalen Femur: 4 Falle. Z Kinderchir 1989;44:289–292.
276. Puppel E. Die kongenitale huftgelenksluxation als Geburtstrauma. Z Geburtshilfe Perinatol 1930;97:39–43.
277. Rigault P, Iselin R, Moureau J, Judet J. Fractures du col du femur chez l'enfant. Rev Chir Orthop 1966;52:325–336.
278. Robinson WH. Treatment of birth fractures of the femur. J Bone Joint Surg 1938;20:778–780.
279. Ruschenburg E. Die geburtstraumatisene Epiphysenlösung am oberen femurschaft ein typisches Krankheitsbild und ihre abgrenzung zur kongenitalen Huftgelenksverrenkung. Z Orthop 1940;71:81–84.
280. Scott WA. The relationship of fetal birth injuries to obstetric difficulties. Am J Obstet Gynecol 1938;35:491–499.
281. Snedecor ST, Knapp RE, Wilson HB. Traumatic ossifying periostitis of the newborn. Surg Gynecol Obstet 1935;61:385–391.
282. Snedecor ST, Wilson HB. Some obstetrical injuries to the long bones. J Bone Joint Surg Am 1949;31:378–384.
283. Theodorou SD, Ierodiaconou MN, Mitsou A. Obstetrical fracture-separation of the upper femoral epiphysis. Acta Orthop Scand 1982;53:239–243.
284. Thorndike A Jr, Pierce FR. Fractures in the newborn. N Engl J Med 1936;215:1013–1016.
285. Towbin R, Crawford AH. Neonatal traumatic proximal femoral epiphysiolysis. Pediatrics 1979;63:456–459.
286. Truesdell ED. Birth Fractures and Epiphyseal Dislocations. New York: Hoeber, 1917:121–135.
287. Truesdell ED. Further observations upon birth dislocations of the cartilaginous epiphyses. Bull Lying-In Hosp March 1918.
288. Weigel K, Conforty B. Die traumatische Epiphysenablösung am oberen Femurende beim Neugebornen. Z Orthop 1974;112:1286–1289.
289. Wojtowycz M, Starshak RJ, Sty JR. Neonatal proximal femoral epiphysiolysis. Radiology 1980;136:647–648.

Slipped Capital Femoral Epiphysis (Acute)

290. Aadalen RJ, Weiner DS, Hoyt W, Herndon H. Acute slipped capital femoral epiphysis. J Bone Joint Surg Am 1974;56:1473–1487.
291. Barash HL, Galante JO, Ray RD. Acute slipped capital femoral epiphysis. Clin Orthop 1971;79:96–101.
292. Baynham GC, Lucie RS, Cummings RJ. Femoral neck fracture secondary to in situ pinning of slipped capital femoral epiphysis: a previously unreported complication. J Pediatr Orthop 1991;11:187–190.
293. Cady RB. Posterior dislocation of the hip associated with separation of the capital epiphyseal. Clin Orthop 1987;222:186–189.
294. Cannon SR, Pool CJ. Traumatic separation of the proximal femoral epiphysis and fracture of the midshaft of the ipsilateral femur in a child: a case report and review of the literature. Injury 1983;15:156–158.
295. Casey BH, Hamilton HW, Bobechko WP. Reduction of acutely slipped upper femoral epiphysis. J Bone Joint Surg Br 1972;54:607–614.
296. Chung SM, Batterman SC, Brighton CT. Shear strength of the human femoral capital epiphyseal plate. J Bone Joint Surg Am 1976;58:94–103.
297. Dietz FR. Traction reduction of acute and acute-on-chronic slipped capital femoral epiphysis. Clin Orthop 1994;302:101–110.
298. Duncan JW, Lovell WW. Anterior slip of the capital femoral epiphysis. Clin Orthop 1975;110:171–173.
299. Fahey JJ, O'Brien ET. Acute slipped capital femoral epiphysis. J Bone Joint Surg Am 1965;47:1105–1127.
300. Fiddian NJ, Grace DL. Traumatic dislocation of the hip in adolescence with separation of the capital epiphysis: two case reports. J Bone Joint Surg Br 1983;65:148–149.
301. Finch AD, Roberts WM. Epiphyseal coxa valga. J Bone Joint Surg 1946;28:869–872.
302. Herring JA, McCarthy RE. Instructional case: fracture dislocation of the capital femoral epiphysis. J Pediatr Orthop 1986;6:112–114.
303. Imhauser G. Zur Pathogenese und Therapie der jugendlichen Huftkupflösung. Z Orthop 1957;88:3–41.
304. Jerre T. A study in slipped upper femoral epiphysis. Acta Orthop Scand 1950;21(suppl 6):1–146.

305. Kampner SL, Wissinger HA. Anterior slipping of the capital femoral epiphysis. J Bone Joint Surg Am 1972; 54:1531–1536.
306. Mass DP, Spiegel PG, Laros GS. Dislocation of the hip with traumatic separation of the capital femoral epiphysis: report of a case with successful outcome. Clin Orthop 1980;146: 184–187.
307. Meyer LC, Stelling RH, Wise F. Slipped capital femoral epiphysis. South Med J 1957;50:453–459.
308. Ogden JA, Gossling HR, Southwick WO. Slipped capital femoral epiphysis following ipsilateral femoral fracture. Clin Orthop 1975;110:167–172.
309. Rattey T, Wright JG. Acute slipped capital femoral epiphysis. J Bone Joint Surg Am 1996;78:398–402.
310. Rothermel JE. Lateral slipping of the upper femoral epiphysis (epiphyseal coxa valga). Orthop Rev 1979;8:81–83.
311. Rouiller R, Griffe J, Crespy G. Epiphyseolyse femorale superieure apres fracture basicervicale: resultat apres trois ans. Rev Chir Orthop 1971;57:65–69.
312. Savage LJ. Transepiphyseal fracture-dislocation of the femoral neck. Injury 1990;21:187–188.
313. Schein AJ. Acute severe slipped capital femoral epiphysis. Clin Orthop 1967;51:151–155.
314. Schmidt R, Gregg JR. Subtrochanteric fractures complicating pin fixation of slipped capital femoral epiphysis. Orthop Trans 1985;9:497.
315. Skinner SR, Berkheimer GA. Valgus slip of the capital femoral epiphysis. Clin Orthop 1978;135:90–92.
316. Speer DP. Experimental epiphyseolysis: an etiologic model of slipped capital femoral epiphysis. Trans Orthop Res Soc 1978;3:47.
317. Speer DP. Experimental epiphysiolysis: etiologic models of slipped capital femoral epiphysis. In: The Hip. St. Louis: Mosby, 1982:68–88.
318. Wilson PD, Jacobs B, Schecter L. Slipped capital femoral epiphysis: an end result study. J Bone Joint Surg Am 1965; 47:1128–1145.

Trochanters

319. Balensweig I. Traction fracture of the lesser trochanter. J Bone Joint Surg 1924;6:696–703.
320. Basso A. Frattura da strappamento del piccolo trocantere. Chir Organi Mov 1962;50:501–506.
321. Binet H. Les fractures isolées du petit trochanter. Rev Chir 1911;31:5–8.
322. Carl K. Isolierte Abrissfrakturen des Trochanter minor femoris. Dtsch Z Chir 1923;179:266–268.
323. Casacci A. Fratture da strappamento nell' adolescenza. Clin Orthop 1949;1:146–148.
324. Cavicchi L. Su di un caso di frattura del piccolo trocantere. Chir Organi Mov 1953;38:280–285.
325. Chaput P. Fracture par arrachement du petit trochanter. Bull Mem Soc Paris 1910;35:207–210.
326. Churchill MA, Brookes M, Spencer JD. The blood supply of the greater trochanter. J Bone Joint Surg Br 1992;74:272–274.
327. Corsi G. La frattura isolata del piccolo trocantere. Arch Orthop 1950;63:311–314.
328. Dimon JH III. Isolated fractures of the lesser trochanter of the femur. Clin Orthop 1972;82:144–148.
329. Eikenbarry CF. Avulsion or fracture of the trochanter. J Orthop Surg 1921;3:464–468.
330. Ettore E. Su distacco isolato del piccolo trocantere. Osped Maggiore 1927;15:74–76.
331. Fasting OJ. Avulsion of the lesser trochanter. Arch Orthop Trauma Surg 1978;91:81–83.
332. Fernbach SK, Wilkinson RH. Avulsion injuries of the pelvis and proximal femur. AJR 1981;137:581–584.
333. Finzi O. Sulla frattura isolata del piccolo trocantere. Arch Ital Chir 1927;18:669–671.
334. Green JT, Gay FH. Avulsion of the lesser trochanter epiphysis. South Med J 1956;49:1308–1310.
335. Hannamuller J. Des Ludloffische symptom bei der isolierten Abrissfraktur des Trochanter Minor. Beitr Klin Chir 1910; 70:479–482.
336. Herzog K. Zur isolierte Abriss des Trochanter Minor in die Epiphiselinie eine tipische Sportverletzung des Jugendalters. Dtsch Z Chir 1939;251:449–453.
337. Hoch E. Abriss des Trochanter Minor bei einem jugendlichen Individuum. Dtsch Z Chir 1939;251:449–451.
338. Jacobson S. Apofyseavulsioner: baekken og proksimale femur. Ugeskr Laeger 1993;155:2124–2125.
339. Jonasch E. Epiphysenlösung des trochanter minor. Monatsschr Unfallheilkd 1965;58:50–52.
340. Kawelblum M, Lehman WB, Grant AD, Strongwater A. Avascular necrosis of the femoral head as sequela of fracture of the greater trochanter. Clin Orthop 1993;294:193–195.
341. Kehr H, Starke W. Treatment of trochanteric fractures in juvenile and young adult patients. Akt Traumatol 1978;8:413–418.
342. King D. Avulsion of the epiphysis of the small trochanter. Chir Narz Ruchu Ortop Polska 1955;20:225–227.
343. Kuur E. Isoleret afspraengning at trochanter minor. Ugeskr Laeger 1987;149:2981–2982.
344. Lapidus PW. Epiphyseal separation of the lesser femoral trochanter. J Bone Joint Surg 1930;12:548–554.
345. Lasserre C, Lasserre J. Fractures isolée et asolées et associées du petit trochanter. Bordeaux Chir 1952;3:144–147.
346. Linhart W, Stampfel O, Ritter G. Posttraumatische Femurkopfnekrose nach Trochanterfraktur. Z Orthop 1984; 122:766–769.
347. LoDico F, Mandala I. La frattura del piccolo trocantere. Minerva Ortop 1962;13:36–38.
348. Magistroni A, Viscontini GR. Sul distacco isolato del piccolo trocantere. Minerva Ortop 1967;18:219–221.
349. Marty H. Wie lautet ihre Röntgendiagnose? Schweiz Rund Med Prax 1992;81:207–208.
350. Merlino AF, Nixon JE. Isolated fractures of the greater trochanter: report on twelve cases. Int Surg 1969;52:121–120.
351. Milch H. Avulsion fracture of the great trochanter. Arch Surg 1939;38:334–350.
352. Misliborski T. Injury of the femoral nerve associated with avulsion of the lesser trochanter in an athlete. Chir Narz Ruchu Ortop Polska 1952;17:395–397.
353. Morera F. La fratture isolata def piccolo trocantere. Minerva Ortop 1964;15:133–136.
354. Moreau J, Lecouterier M. Fracture isolée du petit trochanter. Arch Francobelg Chir 1923;26:1121–1124.
355. Oudart G. Un cas de fracture isolée du petit trochanter. Rev Orthop 1929;16:237–238.
356. Parisel F. Fracture du petit trochanter chez le grand infant. Acta Orthop Belg 1966;32:423–424.
357. Pugh WTG. Fracture of the small trochanter. Proc R Soc Med 1923;16:14–19.
358. Rinonapoli E. Distacchi epifisari da trauma sportivo. Clin Ortop 1955;7:337–341.
359. Roth L. Des Schenkelhals Brüch und die isolierten Brüch und die isolierten Brüch des Trochanter Major und Minor. Erge Chir Orthop 1913;6:109–113.
360. Ruhl E. Über isolierten abriss des trochanter minor. Beitr Klin Chir 1920;118:676–699.
361. Schlutter SA. Avulsion of the lesser trochanter. J Bone Joint Surg 1926;8:766–768.
362. Schwöbel MG. Apophysenfrakturen bei Jugendlichen. Chirurg 1985;56:699–704.
363. Sweetman RJ. Avulsion fracture of the lesser trochanter. Nier Times 1972;68:122–123.

364. Vorschutz B. Die isolierte Abrissfraktur des Trochanter Minor. Dtsch Z Chir 1912;177:243–245.
365. Walbaum E. Zwei Falle von Abrissbruch des Trochanter Minor. Dtsch Z Chir 1914;128:139–142.
366. Wilson MJ, Michele AA, Jacobson EW. Isolated fracture of the lesser trochanter. J Bone Joint Surg 1939;21:776–777.

Subtrochanteric

367. Daum R, Jungbluth KH, Metzger E, Hecker WC. Subtrochantere und suprakondylare Femurfrakturen im Kindesalter: Behandlung und Ergebnisse. Chirurg 1968;40:217–224.
368. DeLee J, Clanton TO, Rockwood CA Jr. Closed treatment of subtrochanteric fractures of the femur in a modified cast-brace. J Bone Joint Surg Am 1981;63:773–779.
369. Gamble JG, Lettice J, Smith JT, Rinsky LA. Transverse cervicopertrochanteric hip fracture. J Pediatr Orthop 1991;11:779–782.
370. Ireland DCR, Fisher RL. Subtrochanteric fractures of the femur in children. Clin Orthop 1975;110:157–166.
371. Kehr H, Starke W. Zur Behandlung per und subtrochanterer Femurfrakturen in jüngeren Lebensalter. Akt Traumatol 1978;8:413–419.
372. Munson M. Operative treatment of subtrochanteric fractures. Orthopedics 1983;6:874–879.
373. Schwarz N, Leixnerung M, Frisee H. Results of treatment and indications for osteosynthesis in subtrochanteric fractures during growth. Akt Traumatol 1990;20:176–180.

Diaphyseal

374. Aitken AP. Overgrowth of the femoral shaft following fracture in children. Am J Surg 1940;49:147–153.
375. Aitken AP, Blackett CW, Cincotti JJ. Overgrowth of the femoral shaft following fractures in childhood. J Bone Joint Surg 1939;21:334–338.
376. Allen BL, Kant AP, Emery RE. Displaced fractures of the femoral diaphysis in children: definitive treatment in a double spica cast. J Trauma 1977;17:8–19.
377. Allen BL, Schoch EP, Emery FE. Immediate spica cast system for femoral shaft fractures in infants and children. South Med J 1978;71:18–22.
378. Anderson RL. Conservative treatment of fractures of the femur. J Bone Joint Surg Am 1967;49:1371–1375.
379. Anderson WA. The significance of femoral fractures in children. Ann Emerg Med 1982;11:174–177.
380. Ansorg P, Graner G. Valgisierung des Schenkelhalses nach Nagelung Kindlicher Oberschenkelfrakturen. Zentralbl Chir 1976;101:986–993.
381. Aronson DD, Singer RM, Higgins RF. Skeletal traction for fractures of the femoral shaft in children. J Bone Joint Surg Am 1987;69:1435–1439.
382. Aronson J, Tursky EA. External fixation of femur fractures in children. J Pediatr Orthop 1992;12:157–163.
383. Astion DJ, Wilber JH, Scoles PV. Avascular necrosis of the capital femoral epiphysis after intramedullary nailing for a fracture of the femoral shaft. J Bone Joint Surg Am 1995;77:1092–1094.
384. Baccarini G, Gottardi G. Influenza dell'accrescimento osseo delle fratture extra-epiphysairie nelle ossa lunghe del bambino. Chir Organi Mov 1979;65:483–489.
385. Bahuaud C, Benetean M, Dorr M-F. Traitement de la fracture de la diaphyse fémorale chez l'enfant. Soins Chir 1993;150:36–42.
386. Barfield GA, Versfeld GA, Schepers A. Overgrowth following femoral fractures in children. J Bone Joint Surg Br 1979;61:256–257.
387. Barfod B, Christensen J. Fractures of the femoral shaft in children with special reference to subsequent overgrowth. Acta Chir Scand 1958;116:235–252.
388. Barlow B, Niemirska M, Gandhi R, Shelton M. Response to injury in children with closed femur fractures. J Trauma 1987;27:429–430.
389. Barthlet M. Les fractures diaphysaires du fémur chez l'enfant: a propos de 300 cas. Thèse médecine, University of Besançon, 1978.
390. Beals RK, Tufts E. Fractured femur in infancy: the role of child abuse. J Pediatr Orthop 1983;3:583–586.
391. Beaty JH. Femoral-shaft fractures in children and adolescents. J Am Acad Orthop Surg 1995;3:207–217.
392. Beaty JH, Austin SM, Warner WC, Canale ST, Nichols L. Interlocking intramedullary nailing of femoral shaft fractures in adolescents: preliminary results and complications. J Pediatr Orthop 1994;14:178–183.
393. Benum P, Ertesvag K, Hoiseth K. Torsion deformities after traction treatment of femoral fractures in children. Acta Orthop Scand 1979;50:87–91.
394. Best PNB, Verhage CC, Molenaar JC. Torsion deviations after conservative treatment of femoral fractures. Z Kinderchir 1971;11:814–819.
395. Betterman A, Kunze K, van Ackeren V. Oberschenkelschaft frakturen im Wachstumsalter: resultate nach Wachstumabschluss. Unfall Versicherungsmed 1990;83:44–48.
396. Bisgard JD. Longitudinal overgrowth of long bones with special reference to fractures. Surg Gynecol Obstet 1936;62:823–831.
397. Bjerkriem I, Benum P. Genu recurvatum: a late complication of tibial wire traction in fractures of the femur in children. Acta Orthop Scand 1975;46:1012–1019.
398. Blanquard D. L'embrocharge elastique stable des fractures du fémur chez l'enfant. Thése du Médicine, Nancy 1987.
399. Blitzer CM, Hamilton L. Oxygen saturation during reaming and intramedullary nailing of the femur. Orthopaedics 1992;15:1403–1405.
400. Blomquist E, Rudstrom P. Über Femurfrakturen bei Kindern unter besonderer Berucksichtigung des gesteigerten Langenwachstums. Acta Chir Scand 1943;88:267–272.
401. Blount WP, Schaefer AA, Fox GW. Fractures of the femur in children. South Med J 1944;37:481–493.
402. Böstman O, Varjonen L, Vainiopää S, Majola A, Rokkanen P. Incidence of local complications after intramedullary nailing and after plate fixation of femoral shaft fractures. J Trauma 1989;29:639–645.
403. Bourdelat D. Fracture of the femoral shaft in children: advantages of the descending medullary nailing. J Pediatr Orthop Part B 1996;5:110–114.
404. Bourdelat D, Chazel J, Gross PH. Fracture de la diaphyse femorale de l'enfant: traitement par embryochage élastique interne et modifications de cete technique. Chir Pediatr 1989;30:54–57.
405. Bourdelat D, Sanguina M. Fracture de la diaphyse femorale chez l'enfant: embrochage centro-medullaire ascendant ou descendant; un choix de principe ou de necessité? Ann Chir 1991;45:52–57.
406. Bowler JR, Mubarek SJ, Wenger DR. Tibial physeal closure and genu recurvatum after femoral fracture: occurrence without a tibial traction pin. J Pediatr Orthop 1990;10:653–657.
407. Breck LW. Treatment of femoral shaft fractures in children. Clin Orthop 1953;1:109–116.
408. Brouwer KJ, Molenaar J, VanLinge B. Rotational deformities after femoral shaft fractures in children: a retrospective study 27–32 years after the accident. Acta Orthop Scand 1981;52:81–89.
409. Brown PE, Preston ET. Ambulatory treatment of femoral shaft fractures with a cast brace. J Trauma 1975;15:860–868.

410. Buehler KC, Thompson JD, Sponseller PD, Black BE, Buckley SL, Griffin PP. A prospective study of early spica casting outcomes in the treatment of femoral shaft fractures in children. J Pediatr Orthop 1995;15:30–35.
411. Bull MJ, Weber K, DeRosa JP, Stroup KB. Transporting children in body casts. J Pediatr Orthop 1989;9:280–284.
412. Burdick CG, Siris IE. Fractures of the femur in children: treatment and end results in 268 cases. Ann Surg 1923;77:736–751.
413. Burton V, Fordyce A. Immobilization of femoral shaft fractures in children aged 2–10 years. Injury 1973;4:47–53.
414. Burwell HN. Fractures of the femoral shaft in chidren. Postgrad Med J 1969;45:617–621.
415. Bush LF. Treatment of the fractured femur in children. Am J Surg 1944;64:375–378.
416. Calati A, Poli A. Il penomeno dell'iperallungamento osseo consequent a fratture diàfisarie di ossa lunghe reportate nell'infanzia et nell' adolescenza. Minerva Ortop 1959;10:827–846.
417. Campen K. Concerning the treatment of fractures of the femur in children. Arch Orthop Trauma Surg 1980;96:305–308.
418. Canale ST, Beaty JH. Complications of femoral fractures. In: Epps CH, Bowen JR (eds) Complications in Pediatric Orthopaedic Surgery. Philadelphia: J Lippincott, 1995, pp. 155–175.
419. Canale ST, Tolo VT. Fractures of the femur in children. J Bone Joint Surg Am 1995;77:294–315.
420. Carlioz H, Coulon JP. Fracture métaphysaire et diaphysaire de l'enfant. Ann Chir 1980;34:491–500.
421. Catier P, Bracq H, Canciani JP, et al. Indication inhabituelle de l'enclouage de Ender: Le kyste osseux femoral de l'enfant. Rev Chir Orthop 1981;67:147–149.
422. Celiker O, Cetin I, Sahlan S, Pestilci F, Altug M. Femoral shaft fractures in children: technique of immediate treatment with supracondylar Kirschner wires and one-and-a-half spica cast. J Pediatr Orthop 1988;8:580–584.
423. Cheng JCY, Cheng SSC. Modified functional bracing in the ambulatory treatment of femoral shaft fractures in children. J Pediatr Orthop 1989;9:457–462.
424. Cheng JCY, Shih CH, Shih HN, Lee ZL. 90-90 Femoral skeletal traction in the treatment of femoral shaft fracture in children aged 2–10 years. Chang Gung Med J 1988;11:14–22.
425. Childress HM. Distal femoral 90-90 traction for femoral shaft fractures of the femur in children. Orthop Rev 1979;8:45–51.
426. Clark MW, D'Ambrosia RD, Roberts JM. Equinus contracture following Bryant's traction. Orthopedics 1978;1:311–312.
427. Clark WA. Fractures of the femur in children. J Bone Joint Surg 1926;8:273–281.
428. Clarke TA, Edwards DK, Merritt A. Neonatal fracture of the femur: iatrogenic? Am J Dis Child 1982;136:69–70.
429. Clement DA, Colton CL. Overgrowth of the femur after femoral fractures in childhood. J Bone Joint Surg Br 1986;68:534–539.
430. Cole WH. Results of treatment of fractured femurs in children (with special reference to Bryant's overhead traction). Arch Surg 1922;5:702–709.
431. Compere EL, Garrison M, Fahey JJ. Deformities of the femur resulting from arrestment of growth of the capital and greater trochanteric epiphyses. J Bone Joint Surg 1940;22:909–915.
432. Connolly JF, Dehne E, LaFollett B. Closed reduction and early cast brace ambulation in the treatment of femoral shaft fractures. Part II. Results in one hundred and forty-three fractures. J Bone Joint Surg Am 1973;55:1581–1599.
433. Connolly JF, Whittaker D, Williams E. Femoral and tibial fractures combined with injuries to the femoral or popliteal artery: a review of the literature and analysis of fourteen cases. J Bone Joint Surg Am 1971;53:56–68.
434. Conwell HE. Acute fractures of the shaft of the femur in children. J Bone Joint Surg 1929;11:593–647.
435. Corea JR, Ibrahum AW, Hegazi M. The Thomas splint causing urethral injury. Injury 1992;23:340–341.
436. Corry IS, Nicol RO. Limb length following fracture of the femoral shaft in children. J Pediatr Orthop 1995;15:221–219.
437. Curtis JF, Killian JT, Alonso JE. Improved treatment of femoral shaft fractures in children utilizing the portion spica cast: a long-term follow-up. J Pediatr Orthop 1995;15:36–40.
438. Dameron TB, Thompson HA. Femoral-shaft fractures in children. J Bone Joint Surg Am 1959;41:1201–1212.
439. Damholt V, Zdravkovic D. Quadriceps function following fractures of the femoral shaft in children. Acta Orthop Scand 1974;45:756–762.
440. Damsin JP, Videcog P, Filipe G. Traitement des fractures du femur de l'enfant. Chirurgie 1988;42:346–356.
441. Daum R, Metzger E, Kurschner S, et al. Analyse und Spätergebnisse kindlicher Femurschaftfrakturen. Arch Orthop Unfallchir 1969;66:18–29.
442. David VC. Shortening and compensatory overgrowth following fractures in children. Arch Surg 1924;9:438–451.
443. Davids JR. Rotational deformity and remodeling after fracture of the femur in children. Clin Orthop 1994;302:27–35.
444. Dehne E, Kriz FK Jr. Slow arterial leak consequent to unrecognized arterial laceration: report of five cases. J Bone Joint Surg Am 1967;49:372–376.
445. Dencker H. Wire traction complications associated with treatment of femoral shaft fractures. Acta Orthop Scand 1964;35:158–163.
446. DePalma L, Shiavone PA. L'allungamento scheletro negli esiti di fratture diafisarie di femore nel bambino. Chir Organi Mov 1981;67:31–39.
447. Desbrosses J, Rebouillat J, Bosser C, Guilleminet M. Quelques reflexions sur le traitement des fractures des os longs chez l'enfant. Presse Med 1958;66:1929–1230.
448. Deubelle A, Vanneuville G, Tanguy A, Levai JP. Fractures of the femoral shaft in children: apropos of a homogeneous series of 97 fractures. Rev Chir Orthop 1983;69:513–519.
449. Ecke H. Klinische und röntgenologische diagnostik der kindlichen fraktur. Langenbecks Arch Chir 1976;342:277–281.
450. Edvardsen P, Syversen GM. Overgrowth of the femur after fracture of the shaft in childhood. J Bone Joint Surg Br 1976;58:339–344.
451. Esposito PW, Crawford AH. Pediatric update #6: false aneurysm arising from a closed femur fracture in a child. Orthop Rev 1989;18:114–118.
452. Evanoff M, Strong ML, MacIntosh R. External fixation maintained until fracture consolidation in the skeletally immature patient. J Pediatr Orthop 1993;13:98–101.
453. Farkas B, Bak Z, Fazekas I. Femoral fractures in childhood. Beitr Orthop Traumatol 1983;30:143–147.
454. Fass J, Kaufner HK. Follow-up and late results following treatment of childhood femoral shaft fractures. Zentralbl Chir 1985;110:1436–1448.
455. Fein LH, Pankovich AM, Spero CM, Baruch HM. Closed flexible intramedullary nailing of adolescent femoral shaft fractures. J Orthop Trauma 1989;3:133–141.
456. Feldkamp G, Häusler U. Daum R. Verlaufsbeobachtungen kindlicher Unterschenkelschaftbruche. Unfallheilkunde 1977;80:139–146.

457. Feldkamp G, Mitarb U. Welche Frakturen beeinflussen die Wachstumsphanomene nach kindlichen Schaftbruchen. Unfallheilkunde 1978;81:96–102.
458. Fenselau W. Ergebnisse konservativer behandelter Femurschaft frakturen im Kindesalter. Dissertation, Hamburg, 1980.
459. Ferry AM, Edgar MS Jr. Modified Bryant's traction. J Bone Joint Surg Am 1966;48:533–536.
460. Festge OA, Tischer W, Reding R. Operative und konservative Behandlung kindlicher Oberschenkelfrakturen. Zentralbl Chir 1975;100:473–480.
461. Field C, Gotzen L, Hannich T. Die kindliche Femur schaft fraktur in der Altersgruppe 6–14 Jahre: ein retrospectiver Therapie vergleich zwischen konservativer Behandlung, Plattenosteosynthese und externer stabilisurung. Unfallchirurg 1993;96:169–174.
462. Flach A, Geisbe H, Fendel H. Wachstumsstörungen nach Frakturen der Extremitäten im Kindesalter. Z Kinderchir 1967;4:58–71.
463. Flach A, Kudlich H. Das Langenwachstum des Rohrenknochens nach Schaftfrakturen an der unteren Extremität bei Kindern und Jugendlichen. Zentralbl Chir 1962;87:2145–2151.
464. Flach A, Mitarb U. Wachstumsveranderungen nach Frakturen der Extremitäten im Kindesalter. Z Kinderchir 1967;4:58–63.
465. Foy MA, Colton CL. "Button holed" femoral shaft fracture in adolescents: an indication for internal fixation? Injury 1990;21:382–384.
466. Fraser KE. The hammock suspension technique for hip spica cast application in children. J Pediatr Orthop 1995;15:27–29.
467. Fraser RD, Hunter GA, Waddell JP. Ipsilateral fracture of the femur and tibia. J Bone Joint Surg Br 1978;60:510–515.
468. Fry K, Hoffer M, Brink V. Femoral shaft fractures in brain-injured children. J Trauma 1976;16:371–373.
469. Galpin RD, Willis RD, Sabano N. Intramedullary nailing of pediatric femoral fractures. J Pediatr Orthop 1994;14:184–189.
470. Gillquist J, Reiger A, Sjodahl R, Bylund P. Multiple fractures of a single leg. Acta Chir Scand 1973;139:167–172.
471. Glenn J, Miner M, Peltier L. The treatment of fractures of the femur in patients with head injuries. J Trauma 1973;13:958–961.
472. Gonzalez-Herranz P, Burgos-Flores J, Raparie JM, et al. Intramedullary nailing of the femur in children. J Bone Joint Surg Br 1995;77:262–266.
473. Gonzalez-Herranz P, Lopez-Mondejar JA, Burgos-Flores J, et al. Fractures of the femoral shaft in children: a study comparing orthopaedic treatment, intramedullary nailing and monolateral external fixation. Int J Orthop Trauma Suppl 1993;3:64–68.
474. Goodrich A, Ballard A. Posterior cruciate avulsion associated with ipsilateral femur fracture in a ten-year-old. J Trauma 1988;28:1393–1396.
475. Gottschalk E, Ackermann A. Rush-pin und Becken-bein-schiene bei kindlichen Oberschenkelfrakturen. Zentralbl Chir 1977;102:1449–1450.
476. Gregory P, Sullivan JA, Herndon WA. Adolescent femoral shaft fractures: rigid versus flexible nails. Orthopedics 1995;18:645–649.
477. Gregory RJH, Cubison TCS, Pinder IM, Smith SR. External fixation of lower limb fractures in children. J Trauma 1992;33:691–693.
478. Greville NR, Irvins JC. Fractures of the femur in children: an analysis of their effect on the subsequent length of both bones of the lower limb. Am J Surg 1957;93:376–384.
479. Griessman H. Die Besonderheiten in Heilablauf der Frakturen beim Kinde. Med Klin 1941;37:299–311.
480. Griffin PP. Fractures of the femoral diaphysis in children. Orthop Clin North Am 1976;7:633–638.
481. Griffin PP, Anderson M, Green WT. Fractures of the shaft of the femur in children. Orthop Clin North Am 1972;3:213–224.
482. Gross RH, Davidson R, Sullivan J, et al. Cast brace management of the femoral shaft fracture in children and young adults. J Pediatr Orthop 1983;3:572–582.
483. Grundes O, Reikeras O. Closed versus open medullary nailing of femoral fractures: blood flow and healing studied in rats. Acta Orthop Scand 1992;63:492–496.
484. Guttman GG, Simon R. Three-point fixation walking spica cast: an alternative to early or immediate casting of femoral shaft fractures in children. J Pediatr Orthop 1988;8:699–703.
485. Guzzanti V, DiLazzaro A, Falciglia F. L'esito in dismetria delle fratture metafisarie e diaphysarie del femore in bambini fino ai 3 anni di eta. Arch Putti Chir Organi Mov 1991;39:101–113.
486. Hagglund G, Hansson LI, Norman O. Correction by growth of rotational deformity after femoral fracture in children. Acta Orthop Scand 1983;54:858–861.
487. Hammacher ER, Schütte PR. Fixateur externe voor femurschaft fracturen bij kinderen. Ned Tijdschr Geneeskd 1990;134:416–422.
488. Hansen TB. Fractures of the femoral shaft in children treated with an AO-compression plate. Acta Orthop Scand 1992;63:50–52.
489. Havemann D, Schmidt M, Zenker W. Indikation, Zeitpunkt und Verfahrenswahl der Osteosynthese kindlicher Femurschaft frakturen. Hefte Unfallheilkd 1990;212:3512–3517.
490. Havránek P, Westfelt JN, Henrikson B. Proximal tibial skeletal traction for femoral shaft fractures in children. Clin Orthop 1992;283:270–275.
491. Hecker WC, Daum R. Grundsatzliche Indikationsfehler bei kindlichen Frakturen. Langenbecks Arch Chir 1970;327:864–870.
492. Hedberg E. Femoral fractures in children. Acta Chir Scand 1944;90:568–588.
493. Hedlund R, Lindgren U. The incidence of femoral shaft fractures in children and adolescents. J Pediatr Orthop 1986;6:47–50.
494. Hedstrom O. Growth stimulation of long bones after fracture or similar trauma. Acta Orthop Scand 1969;40(suppl 122):12–134.
495. Hehl G, Kiefer H, Bauer G, Völck C. Post traumatische Beinlängendifferenzen nach konservativer und operativer therapie kindlicher oberschenkel schaftfrakturen. Unfallchirurg 1993;96:651–655.
496. Heinrich SD, Drvaric D, Darr K, MacEwen GD. Stabilization of pediatric diaphyseal femur fractures with flexible intramedullary nails. J Orthop Trauma 1993;6:452–459.
497. Heinrich SD, Drvaric DM, Darr K, MacEwen GD. The operative stabilization of pediatric diaphyseal femur fractures with flexible intramedullary nails: a prospective analysis. J Pediatr Orthop 1994;14:501–507.
498. von Heisel J, Kopp K. Spatergebnisse nach Kuntschermarknagelung von Unter- und Oberschenkelbruchen bei noch wachsendeum Knochenskelett. Akt Traumatol 1983;13:5–12.
499. Henderson OL, Morrissy RT, Gerdes MH, McCarthy RE. Early casting of femoral shaft fractures in children. J Pediatr Orthop 1984;4:16–21.
500. Hennrikus WL, Kesser JR, Rand F, Millis MB, Richards KM. The function of the quadriceps muscle after a fracture of the femur in patients who are less than seventeen years old. J Bone Joint Surg Am 1993;75:508–513.
501. Henry AN. Overgrowth after femoral shaft fractures in children. J Bone Joint Surg Br 1963;45:222.

502. Herndon WA, Mahnken RG, Yngve DA, Sullivan JA. Management of femoral shaft fractures in the adolescent. J Pediatr Orthop 1989;9:28–32.
503. Herzog B, Affalter P, Jani L. Spätbefunde nach Marknagelung kindlicher Femurfrakturen. Z Kinderchir 1976;19:74–77.
504. Hildebrandt G. Spätergebnisse konservativ behandelter Oberschenkelfrakturen bei Kindern. Dtsch Ges Wesen 1965;20:1528–1533.
505. Hofmann V, Kapherr S. Vergleich operativer und konservativer Behandlungs: methoden am Beispiel Kindicher Oberschenkel. Z Unfallchir Versicherungsmed 1989;82:236–242.
506. Holmes SJ, Sedgwick DM, Scobie WG. Domiciliary gallows traction for femoral shaft fractures in young children: feasibility, safety and advantages. J Bone Joint Surg Br 1983;65:288–291.
507. Holschneider AM, Vogl D, Dietz HG. Differences in leg length following femoral shaft fractures in childhood. Z Kinderchir 1985;40:341–346.
508. Horeau M, Carlioz H. Fractures de la diaphyse fémorale chez l'enfant. Ann Orthop Ouest 1974;6:110–114.
509. Hougaard K. Femoral shaft fractures in children: a prospective study of the overgrowth phenomenon. Injury 1989;20:170–172.
510. Howes CL, Erickson KL, Heere LM, Henderson RC, DeMasi RA. Isokinetic measurements of knee flexion-extension strength in children. Phys Ther 1991:137–142.
511. Huber RI, Kaller HW, Huber P. Rehm KE. Flexible intramedullary nailing as fracture treatment in children. J Pediatr Orthop 1996;16:602–605.
512. Hughes BF, Sponseller PD, Thompson JD. Pediatric femur fractures: effects of spica cast treatment on family and community. J Pediatr Orthop 1995;15:457–460.
513. Humberger RW, Eyring EJ. Proximal tibial 90-90 traction in treatment of children with femoral shaft fractures. J Bone Joint Surg Am 1969;51:499–504.
514. Hunter LY, Hensinger RN. Premature monomelic growth arrest following fracture of the femoral shaft. J Bone Joint Surg Am 1978;60:850–852.
515. Hupfauer W, Balau J. Die konservative Behandlung kindlicher oberschenkelfrakturen und ihre Ergebnisse. Monatsschr Unfallheilkd 1971;74:441–456.
516. Irani R, Nicholson J, Chung S. Long-term results in treatment of femoral shaft fractures in young children by immediate spica immobilization. J Bone Joint Surg Am 1976;58:945–951.
517. Isaacson J, Louis DS, Costenbader JM. Arterial injury associated with closed femoral-shaft fracture: report of five cases. J Bone Joint Surg Am 1975;57:1147–1150.
518. Izhar UH, Munkonge L. Femoral fracture in children (a prospective study of two hundred and four fractures). Med J Zambia 1982;16:51–53.
519. Jahna H. Conservative treatment of the femoral shaft fracture. Hefte Unfallheilkd 1982;158:106–111.
520. Jani L. Indikation zur osteosynthese der kindlichen Fraktur. Helv Chir Acta 1978;45:623–625.
521. Jawish R, Saikaly J, Ponet M. L'accéleration de croissance dans les fractures diaphysaires du fémur traitées or orthopédiquement chez l'enfant. Chir Pediatr 1990;31:235–239.
522. Jonasch E. Die geschlossene Bruche des Oberschenkelschaftes bei Kindern. Chir Prax 1959;3:421–426.
523. Joost MC. Malrotation after femoral shaft fractures. Arch Chir Neerl 1972;24:101–105.
524. Jungblut KH, Daum R, Metzger E. Schenkelhalsfrakturen im Kindesalter. Kinderchirurg 1968;6:392–397.
525. Kaelin L, Freiburghaus U, von Laer L, Lampert C. Extension oder osteosynthese kindlicher oberschenkelfrakturen: Erfahrungen mit dem Fixateur externe. Z Unfallchir Versicherungsmed 1990;83:30–36.
526. Kao JT, Burton D, Comstock C, McClellan RT, Carrage E. Pudendal nerve palsy after femoral intramedullary nailing. J Orthop Trauma 1993;7:58–63.
527. Kasser JR. Femur fractures in children. AAOS Instr Course Lect 1992;41:403–408.
528. Kellernova E, Delius W, Olerud S, Strom G. Changes in the muscle and skin blood flow following lower leg fracture in man. Acta Orthop Scand 1970;41:249–260.
529. Keret D, Harcke HT, Mandez AA, Bowen JR. Heterotopic ossification in central nervous system injured patients following closed nailing of femoral fractures. Clin Orthop 1990;256:254–259.
530. Kern E, Loch H. Knochenbrache Konservative oder operative Behandlung geschlossener Fraktur. Chirurg 1967;38:437–441.
531. Kettek C, Haas N, Tscherne H. Versorgung der Femurschaftfraktur im Wachstumsalter mit dem Fixateur externe. Akt Traumatol 1989;19:255–261.
532. Khalil SA. An unusual complication of a fractured femur in a child: case report. J Trauma 1994;36:601–602.
533. Kirby R, Winquist R, Hansen S. Femoral shaft fractures in adolescents: a comparison between traction plus cast treatment and closed intramedullary nailing. J Pediatr Orthop 1981;1:193–198.
534. Kirschenbaum D, Albert MC, Robertson WW, Davidson RS. Complex femur fractures in children: treatment with external fixation. J Pediatr Orthop 1990;10:588–591.
535. Kissel IU, Miller ME. Closed intramedullary nailing of femoral fractures in older children. J Trauma 1989;29:1585–1588.
536. Klapp F, Arfeen N, Hertel P, Scheiberer L. Ergebnisse nach konservativer Behandlung der Oberschenkelschaftfraktur im Kindesalter. Akt Traumatol 1974;4:205–210.
537. Klein W, Penning D, Brug D. Die andvendung eines unilateralen fixateur externe bei der kindlichen femurschaftfraktur im rahmen des polytraumas. Unfallchirurg 1989;92:282–286.
538. Klems H, Weigert M. Stable Osteosynthese kindlicher Oberschenkelfrakturen: Indikation und Methode. Chirurg 1973;44:511–513.
539. Knittel G, Romer KH. Erfährungen mit der intramedullaren offenen Rush-pin-Schienung kindlicher Femurschaftfrakturen. Z Kinderchir 1984;39:59–64.
540. Kohan L, Cumming WJ. Femoral shaft fractures in children: the effect of initial shortening on subsequent overgrowth. Aust NZ J Surg 1982;52:141–144.
541. Korisek G, Schneider H, Breitfuss H. Der kindliche oberschenkelbruch: die konservative therapie und ihre vorzüge. Hefte Unfallheilk 1984;170:336–338.
542. Kregor PJ, Song KM, Routt LC Jr, et al. Plate fixation of femoral shaft fractures in multiply injured children. J Bone Joint Surg Am 1993;75:1774–1780.
543. Kettek C, Haas N, Walker J, Tscherne H. Treatment of femoral shaft fractures in children by external fixation. Injury 1991;22:2673–266.
544. Kumar R. Treatment of fracture of the femur in children by a "cast-brace." Int Surg 1982;67:551–552.
545. Kuner EH. Die Osteosynthese bei der kindlichen Fraktur. Langenbecks Arch Chir 1976;342:291–298.
546. Kuner EH. Die Plattenosteosynthese zur Behandlung von Femurschaftfrakturen bei Kindern. Operat Orthop Traumatol 1991;3:227–237.
547. Kuner EH, Weyand F. Indikationen zur operativen Behandlung kindlicher Frakturen. Akt Traumatol 1971;1:63–70.
548. Kuntscher G. Die stabile Osteosynthese bei der Osteotomie. Chirurg 1942;14:161–173.

549. Kunz K, Grohs M. Follow-up study of 124 juvenile femoral shaft fractures. Hefte Unfallheilkd 1982;158:150–153.
550. Kuur E, Hougaard K. Osteosynthesis of femoral shaft fractures in children. Ugeskr Laeger 1988;150:595–596.
551. Lansche WE, Mishkin MR, Stamp WG. The management of complications of femoral shaft fractures in children. South Med J 1963;56:1001–1112.
552. Lascombes P, Prevot J, Bardoux J. Pronostic des fractures de l'extremité inférieure du fémur chez l'enfant et l'adolescent. Rev Chir Orthop 1988;74:438–445.
553. Lauterbach HH, Flintsch K. Extreme axis deviation of the pediatric femur as a cause of spontaneous fracture. Chirurg 1986;57:753–755.
554. Lefort J. Fractures de la diaphyse fémorale chez l'enfant. Ann Chir 1981;35:51–57.
555. Levander G. Über die Behandlung von Bruchen des Oberschenkelschaftes, nebst Beitrag zur Kenntnis des gesteigerten Langenwachstums der Röhrenknochen der unteren Extremitäten nach Bruch derselben. Acta Chir Scand 1929;23(suppl 12):1–193.
556. Levy J, Ward WT. Pediatric femur fractures: an overview of treatment. Orthopaedics 1993;16:183–189.
557. Ligier JN, Metaizeau JP, Brevot J, Lascombes P. Elastic stable intramedullary nailing of femoral shaft fractures in children. J Bone Joint Surg Br 1988;70:74–77.
558. Logie JRC, Garvie WHH. Urethral injury following use of a Thomas splint. Br J Urol 1977;49:522–523.
559. Lorenz GL, Rossi P, Quaglia F, et al. Growth disturbances following fractures of the femur and tibia in children. Ital J Orthop Traumatol 1985;11:133–137.
560. Lüthi UK, Engelhardt P, Weber BG. Femurschaftfrakturen im Kindesalter: 25 Jahre Erfahrung mit dem Webertisch. Z Unfallchir 1990;83:38–43.
561. Malkawi H, Shannak A, Hadidi S. Remodeling after femoral shaft fractures in children treated by the modified Blount method. J Pediatr Orthop 1986;6:421–429.
562. Mann DC, Weddington J, Davenport K. Closed Enders nailing of femoral shaft fractures in adolescents. J Pediatr Orthop 1986;6:651–655.
563. Martin-Ferrero MA, Sanchez-Martin MM. Prediction of overgrowth in femoral shaft fractures in children. Int Orthop 1986;10:89–93.
564. Martinez AG, Carroll NC, Sarwak JF, et al. Femoral shaft fractures in children treated with early spica cast. J Pediatr Orthop 1991;11:412–716.
565. Maruendo-Paulino JI, Sanchia-Alfonso V, Gomar-Sanchio F, et al. Kuntscher nailing of femoral shaft fractures in children and adolescents. Int Orthop 1993;17:158–161.
566. McCarthy RE. A method for early spica cast application in treatment of pediatric femoral shaft fracture. J Pediatr Orthop 1986;6:89–91.
567. McCullough NC, Vinsant J, Sarmiento A. Functional fracture-bracing of long-bone fractures of the lower extremity in children. J Bone Joint Surg Am 1978;60:314–319.
568. Meals RA. Overgrowth of the femur following fractures in children: influences of handedness. J Bone Joint Surg Am 1979;61:381–384.
569. Merki A. Coxa valga nach Femurnagelung Jugendlicher. Helv Chir Acta 1968;35:127–129.
570. Metaizeau JP. L'ostéosynthèse chez l'enfant: techniques et indications. Chir Pediatr 1983;69:495–511.
571. Mileski RL, Garvin KL, Huurman WW. Avascular necrosis of the femoral head after closed intramedullary shortening in an adolescent. J Pediatr Orthop 1995;15:24–26.
572. Miller DS, Martin L, Grossman E. Ischemic fibrosis of the lower extremity in children. Am J Surg 1972;84:317–322.
573. Miller ME, Bramlett KW, Kissell EU, Niemann KMW. Improved treatment of femoral shaft fractures in children. Clin Orthop 1987;219:140–146.
574. Miller PR, Welch MC. The hazards of tibial pin replacement in 90-90 skeletal traction. Clin Orthop 1978;135:97–103.
575. Miller R, Renwick SE, DeCoster TA, Shonnard P, Jabczenski SD. Removal of intramedullary rods after femoral shaft fracture. J Orthop Trauma 1992;6:460–463.
576. Mital MA, Cashman WF. Fresh ambulatory approach to treatment of femoral shaft fractures in children: a comparison with traditional conservative methods. J Bone Joint Surg Am 1976;58:285.
577. Mohan K. Fracture of the shaft of the femur in children. Int Surg 1975;60:282–284.
578. Molnar GE, Alexander J. Objective, quantitative muscle testing in children: a pilot study. Arch Phys Med Rehabil 1973;54:224–228.
579. Molnar GE, Alexander J. Development of quantitative standards for muscle strength in children. Arch Phys Med Rehabil 1974;55:490–493.
580. Mommsen U, Fenselau W, Sauer H, Jungbluth KH. Ergebnisse konservativ behandelter Femurschaftfrakturen im Kindesalter. Z Kinderchir 1978;24:56–62.
581. Montero M. Diametrias postfracturarias de la diafisis del femur en niños. Rev Esp Cir Osteoar 1982;17:34–39.
582. Montgomery SP, Mooney V. Femur fractures: treatment with roller traction and early ambulation. Clin Orthop 1981;156:196–200.
583. Morita S. Surgical treatment of femur shaft fractures in children. Arch Jpn Surg 1967;36:627–636.
584. Muller ME. Zur Einteilung und Reposition der Kinderfrakturen. Unfallheilkunde 1977;80:187–190.
585. Nafei A, Teichert G, Mikkelsen SS, Hvid I. Femoral shaft fractures in children: an epidemiological study in a Danish urban population, 1977–1986. J Pediatr Orthop 1992;12:499–502.
586. Neel AB, Glancy GL. Residual quadriceps weakness following childhood femur fractures. Orthop Trans 1990;14:292.
587. Neer CS II, Cadman EF. Treatment of fractures of the femoral shaft in children. JAMA 1957;163:634–637.
588. Neugebauer R, Becker U, Stinner A. Die Behandlung der Kindlichen oberschenkel frakturen mit dem lateralen klammer fixateur (Technik, Machsorge, Ergebnisse). Hefte Unfallheilkd 1990;212:363–368.
589. Neurath F, van Lessen H. Die unter Verkurzung geheilte kindliche Oberschenkelfraktur. Z Kinderchir 1972;11(suppl):791–808.
590. Newton PO, Mubarek SJ. Financial aspects of femoral shaft fracture treatment in children and adolescents. J Pediatr Orthop 1994;14:508–512.
591. Newton PO, Mubarek SJ. The use of modified Neufeld's skeletal traction in children and adolescents. J Pediatr Orthop 1995;15:467–469.
592. Nicholson JT, Foster RM, Health RD. Bryant's traction: a provocative cause of circulatory complications. JAMA 1955;157:415–418.
593. Nogi J. Nonunion of a closed fracture in a child's femoral shaft. VA Med 1980;107:568–570.
594. Nonnemann HC. Grenzen dur Spontankorrektur fehlgeheilte: Frakturen bei Jugendlichen. Langenbecks Arch Chir 1969;324:78–86.
595. Norbeck DE Jr, Asselmeier M, Pinzur MS. Torsional malunion of a femur fracture. Orthop Rev 1990;19:625–628.
596. Nutz V, Giebel D, Heuser R. Schädelhirntrauma und Femurfraktur beim kindlichen polytrauma. Unfallchirurg 1986;89:539–546.

597. Oelsnitz G. Marknagelung kindlicher Oberschenkelfrakturen. Z Kinderchir 1972;11(suppl):803–815.
598. Ogden JA. Editorial: femoral fractures. J Pediatr Orthop 1995;15:1–2.
599. Osterwalder A, Mitarb U. Langenwachstum an der unteren Extremität nach jugendlichen Schaftfrakturen. Unfallheilkunde 1979;82:451–547.
600. Ostrum RF, Verghese GB, Santner TJ. The lack of association between femoral shaft fractures and hypotonic shock. J Orthop Trauma 1993;7:338–342.
601. Pachucki A, Dremsek JA. Femoral shaft fractures in early childhood. Unfallchirurgie 1984;10:303–308.
602. Pachuki A, Predinger G. Nachuntersuchung ergebnisse von Oberschenkelschaft-brüchen im kindes und Jugendalter unter besonderer Berüchsichtigung des vermehrten Längenwachstums und der Achsenkorrekturpotenz. Hefte Unfallheilkd 1984;206:368.
603. Pankovich AM. Plating of a femoral shaft fracture in a child. Orthopaedics 1985;8:285–287.
604. Pankovich AM, Goldfies ML, Pearson RL. Closed Ender nailing of femoral shaft fractures. J Bone Joint Surg Am 1979;61:222–232.
605. Pape HC, Dwenger A, Regel G, et al. Pulmonary damage after intramedullary femoral nailing in traumatized sheep: is there an effect from different nailing methods. J Trauma 1992;33:574–581.
606. Pape HC, Regel G, Dwenger A, Krettek C, et al. Effekte unterschiedlicher intramedullärer Stabilisierungs vertahren des Femurs auf die Lungenfunktion bei polytrauma. Unfallchirurg 1992;95:634–640.
607. Parvinen T, Viljanto J, Paanenen M, Vilkki P. Torsion deformity after femoral fracture in children. Ann Chir Gynaecol Suppl 1973;62:25–29.
608. Pazolt HJ, Thomas E. Zur operative behandlung der oberschenkel fraktur in kindesalter. Beitr Orthop Traumatol 1974;21:472–477.
609. Pease CN. Fractures of the femur in children. Surg Clin North Am 1957;37:213–221.
610. Pederson HE, Serra JB. Injury to the collateral ligaments of the knee associated with femoral shaft fractures. Clin Orthop 1968;60:119–121.
611. Pelinka H, Schwartz N. Fixateur externe beim kindlichen oberschenkelbruch. Unfallheilkunde 1986;182:348–352.
612. Piroth P, Bliesener JA. Rotationsfehlstellung nach conservativer Behandlung kindlicher Oberschenkelschaftfrakturen. Z Kinderchir 1977;20:172–175.
613. Pollak AN, Cooperman DR, Thompson GH. Spica cast treatment of femoral shaft fractures in children: the prognostic value of the mechnism of injury. J Trauma 1994;37:223–229.
614. Porat S, Milgrom C, Nyska M, et al. Femoral fracture treatment in head-injured children: use of external fixation. J Trauma 1986;26:81–84.
615. Prévot J, Gagneux E, Sessa S. Correction of malunion of the femur in a child by Ilizarov apparatus. Fr J Orthop Surg 1991;5:422–425.
616. Probe R, Lindsey RW, Hadley NA, Barnes DA. Refracture of adolescent femoral shaft fractures: a complication of external fixation. A report of two cases. J Pediatr Orthop 1993;13:102–105.
617. Rahn HD, Kilic M, Tolksdorff G, Schauwecker F. Osteosynthese bei kindlichen oberschenkelfrakturen: konkurrenz zur conservativen Behandlung oder Verfahren der Wahl? Vergleichende Nachuntersuchungsergenrisse in 54 Fällen bei Kindern zwischen 2 und 16 Jahren. Hefte Unfallheilkd 1990;212:361–368.
618. Raisch O. Experimenteller Beitrag zur Frage der Osteosynthese mit besonderer Beruchsichtigung der Marknagelung nach Kuntscher. Beitr Klin Chir 1944;175:548–553.
619. Raney EM, Ogden JA, Grogan DP. Premature greater trochanteric epiphyseodesis secondary to intramedullary femoral rodding. J Pediatr Orthop 1993;13:516–520.
620. Rauch J, Schönitz A, Schramm H, Schmid R. Ergebnisse der Behandlung kindlicher oberschenkelschaftfrakturen mit der Vertikalextension nach Weber mittels Extensiongerät eigener Konstruktion. Zentralbl Chir 1990;115:609–615.
621. Raugstad TS, Alho A, Hvidsten K. Vekstkorreksjon av feilstillinger etter femurshaftfrakturer hos barn. Tidsskr Nor Laegeforen 1979;99:1460–1462.
622. Reding H. Zur Behandlung kindlicher Oberschenkelfrakturen. Dtsch Ges Wesen 1966;21:87–90.
623. Reeves RB, Ballard RI, Hughes JL. Internal fixation versus traction and casting of adolescent femoral shaft fractures. J Pediatr Orthop 1990;10:592–595.
624. Rehbein F, Hofmann S. Knochenverletzungen im Kindesalter. Langenbecks Arch Chir 1963;304:539–562.
625. Rehn J. Zur Toleranzgrenze konservativ behandelter kindlicher Schaftfrakturen. Z Kinderchir 1976;18:305–309.
626. Reisman B. Die Ursachen des Mehrwachstums nack Frakturen im Kindesalter. Z Kinderchir 1979;26:348–364.
627. Resch H, Oberhammer J, Wanitschek P, Seykora P. Der Rotationsfehler nach kindlicher oberschenkelfraktur. Akt Traumatol 1989;19:77–81
628. Reynolds DA. Growth changes in fractured long bones: a study of 126 children. J Bone Joint Surg Br 1981;63:83–88.
629. Ribeyrol JL. Place de l'enclouage centromédullaire a foyer fermé dans le traitement des fractures diaphysaires du femur de l'enfant. These, Bordeaux, 1979.
630. Riew KD, Sturm PF, Rosenbaum D, Robertson WW Jr, Yamaguchi K. Neurologic complications of pediatric femoral nailing. J Pediatr Orthop 1996;16:606–612.
631. Rippstein J. Zur bestimmung der antetorsion des schenkelhalses mittels zweier röntgenaufnahmen. Z Orthop 1955;86:345–360.
632. Romer KH, Reppin G. Zur Marknagelung kindlicher Oberschenkelfrakturen. Zentralbl Chir 1973;98:170–171.
633. Rosenberg NM, Vranesich P, Bottonfield G. Fractured femurs in pediatric patients. Ann Emerg Med 1982;11:84–85.
634. Ryan JR. 90°-90° skeletal femoral traction for femoral shaft fractures in children. J Trauma 1981;21:46–48.
635. Saimon LP. Refracture of the shaft of the femur. J Bone Joint Surg Br 1964;46:32–39.
636. Sasse W, Ellerbrock U. Spontankorrektur fehlgeheilter kindlicher Frakturen. Z Kinderchir 1975;17:154–157.
637. Saxer U. Die Behandlung kindlicher Femurschaftfrakturen mit der Vertikalextension nach Weber. Helv Chir Acta 1974;41:271–275.
638. Schafer JH, Huber C. Unfallursachen, Frakturlokalisation und Behandlung der kindlichen Oberschenkelfrakturen. Bruns Beitr Klin Chir 1974;221:453–460.
639. Schedl R, Fasol P. Spätergebnisse nach der Behandlung von kindlichen oberschenkelschaftbrüchen. Unfallchirurg 1981;7:249–255.
640. Schenk KH. Der Femurschaftbruch beim Kind: Spätergebnisse. Arch Klin Chir 1957;286:144–148.
641. Schenk RK. Besonderheiten des kindlichen Skeletts im Hinblick auf die Frakturheilung. Langenbecks Arch Chir 1976;342:267–276.
642. Schmittenbrecher PP, Dietz HG, Germann C. Spätergebisse nach Unterschenkelfrakturen im Kindesalter. Unfallchirurg 1989;92:79–84.
643. Schoppmeyer K. Die Behandlung kindlicher berschenkelschaftbruche mit dem "Weber-Bock": eine

Moglichkeit, um Drehverschiebungen mit allen daraus Entstenhenden folgen zu vermeiden. Chirurg 1977;48: 348–357.
644. Scott J, Wardlaw D, McLauchlan J. Cast bracing of femoral shaft fractures in children: a preliminary report. J Pediatr Orthop 1981;1:199–201.
645. Schuermans JMR. Femurfracturen bij kinderen. NTVG 1970;114:2145–2152.
646. Schuttemeyer W, Flach A. Die Behandlung kindlicher Frakturen der unteren Extremitäten und ihre Heilunsergebnisse. Monatsschr Unfallheilkd 1950;53:4–11.
647. Schwarz N. Der Fixateure externe als Behandlungsmethode beim Oberschenkelbruch des Kindes. Unfallheilkunde 1983; 86:359–365.
648. Schweiberer L, Hofmeier G, Faust W. Oberschenkelschaftbruche im Kindesalter. Z Kinderchir 1968;5:435–438.
649. Scott J, Wardlaw D, McLauchlan J. Cast bracing of femoral shaft fractures in children: a preliminary report. J Pediatr Orthop 1981;1:199–201.
650. Seyfarth H. Zur Therapie der Frakturen im Kleinekindesalter. Zentralbl Chir 1958;83:72–75.
651. Shah A, Ellis RD. False aneurysm complicating closed femoral shaft fracture in a child. Orthop Rev 1993; 22:1265–1267.
652. Shapiro F. Fractures of the femoral shaft in children. Acta Orthop Scand 1981;52:649–655.
653. Shih H, Chen L, Lee Z, Shih C. Treatment of femoral shaft fractures with the Hoffman external fixator in prepuberty. J Trauma 1989;29:498–501.
654. Shively JL. Genu recurvatum after femoral fracture. Contemp Orthop 1990;21:577–580.
655. Siebenmann R. Die Osteomyelitis aus der Sicht de Pathologen. Z Kinderchir 1970;8:10–16.
656. Siebert HR, Pannike A. Kriterien zur Behandlung von oberschenkelschaft Frakturen im Kindesalter. Unfallchirurgie 1954;10:45–50.
657. Silver D. Treatment by suspension of fracture of femur on young children. Ann Surg 1909;49:105–110.
658. Simonian PT, Chapman JR, Selznicle HS, Benirschke SK, Claudi BF, Swiontkowski MF. Iatrogenic fractures of the femoral neck during closed nailing of the femoral shaft. J Bone Joint Surg Br 1994;76:293–296.
659. Skak SV, Jensen TT. Femoral shaft fracture in 265 children: log-normal correlation of age with speed of healing. Acta Orthop Scand 1988;59:704–707.
660. Skak SV, Overgaard S, Nielson JD, Andersen A, Nielsen ST. Internal fixation of femoral shaft fractures in children and adolescents: a ten to twenty-one-year follow-up of 52 fractures. J Pediatr Orthop Part B 1996;5:195–199.
661. Speed K. Analysis of results of treatment of fracture of femoral diaphysis in children under 12 years of age. Surg Gynecol Obstet 1921;32:527–532.
662. Spinner M, Freundlich BD, Miller IJ. Double-spica technic for primary treatment of fractures of the shaft of the femur in children and adolescents. Clin Orthop 1967; 53:109–114.
663. Splain SH, Denno JJ. Immediate double hip spica immobilization as the treatment for femoral shaft fractures in children. J Trauma 1985;25:994–996.
664. St. Pierre RH, Holmes HE, Fleming LL. Cast bracing of femoral fractures: experience of Emory University Hospitals. Orthopedics 1982;5:739–745.
665. Staheli LT. Femoral and tibial growth following femoral shaft fracture in childhood. Clin Orthop 1967;55:159–163.
666. Staheli LT, Sheridan G. Early spica cast management of femoral shaft fractures in young children. Clin Orthop 1977;126:162–166.
667. Stannard JP, Christensen KP, Wilkins KE. Femur fractures in infants: a new therapeutic approach. J Pediatr Orthop 1995;15:461–466.
668. Steinberg GG, Hubbard C. Heterotopic ossification after femoral intramedullary rodding. J Orthop Trauma 1993; 7:536–542.
669. Stellmann W. Dringliche Osteosynthesen im Kindesalter. Akt Traumatol 1979;9:175–184.
670. Stephens DC, Louis E, Louis DS. Traumatic injury of the distal femur. J Bone Joint Surg Am 1974;56:1383–1390.
671. Stephens MM, Hsu LCS, Leong JCY. Leg length discrepancy after femoral shaft fractures in children. J Bone Joint Surg Br 1989;71:615–618.
672. Stock HJ. Die Marknagelung der kindlichen Oberschenkelschaftfraktur unter Schönung der Wachstumszonen. Zentralbl Chir 1978;103:1072–1075.
673. Stock HJ. Pediatric femoral shaft fractures: evaluation of 504 follow-up studies. Zentralbl Chir 1985;110:969–982.
674. Streissuth AP, Steissguth DM. Planning for the psychological needs of a young child in a double spica cast. Clin Pediatr 1978;17:277–283.
675. Strickland JC, Wittgen EM Jr. An unusual case of pathological femoral shaft fracture fifty-five years after placement of Parham band. Orthopedics 1981;4:287–290.
676. Strong ML, Wong-Chung J, Babikian G, Brody A. Rotational remodeling of malrotated femoral fractures: a model in the rabbit. J Pediatr Orthop 1992;12:173–176.
677. Sturn PF, Alman BA, Christie BL. Femur fractures in institutionalized patients after hip spica immobilization. J Pediatr Orthop 1993;13:246–248.
678. Sugi M, Cole W. Early plaster treatment for fractures of the femoral shaft in childhood. J Bone Joint Surg Br 1987; 69:743–745.
679. Teutsch W. Nachuntersuchungsergebnisse kindlicher Femurschaftfrakturen. Zentralbl Chir 1969;94:1761–1770.
680. Thaer K, Dallek M, Meenan NM, Jungbluth KH. Post traumatische Längendifferenz und muskelatrophie nach oberschenkelfrakturen im Kindesalter. Unfallchirurg 1992;18: 162–167.
681. Thometz JG, Landan R. Osteonecrosis of the femoral head after intramedullary nailing of a fracture of the femoral shaft in an adolescent. J Bone Joint Surg Am 1995;77:1423–1426.
682. Thompson SA, Mahoney LJ. Volkmann's ischemic contracture and its relationship to fracture of the femur. J Bone Joint Surg Br 1951;33:336–347.
683. Timmerman LA, Rab GT. Intramedullary nailing of femoral shaft fractures in adolescents. J Orthop Trauma 1993;7: 331–337.
684. Tischer W. Indikationen und Gefahren der Osteosynthese im Kindesalter. Zentralbl Chir 1975;101:129–140.
685. Tittel K, Tittel M, Schauwecker F. Erfährungen mit der operativen Versurgung von oberschenkel schaftfrakturen bei Kindern. Unfallheilkunde 1986;182:344–349.
686. Tjong Tjin Tai H. Femurschachtfracturen bij kinderen. Thesis, R.C. University Nijmegen, 1974.
687. Träger D, Rode P. Die Behandlung von Femurschaftfrakturen beim kindern Endernägeln. Akt Traumatol 1988;18:173–176.
688. Truesdell ED. Inequality of lower extremities following fracture of the shaft of the femur in children. Ann Surg 1921;74:498–503.
689. Tscherne H, Sükamp N. Offene Frakturen bei kindern. Z Orthop 1985;123:490–497.
690. Turrettini F. Fractures de la diaphyse femorale chez l'enfant. Orthop Rev 1947;33:328–341.
691. Valdiserri L, Marchiodi L, Rubbini L. Kuntscher nailing in the treatment of femoral fractures in children: is it completely contraindicated? Ital J Orthop Traumatol 1983;3:293–296.

692. Van Meter J, Branick R. Bilateral genu recurvatum after skeletal traction. J Bone Joint Surg Am 1980;62:837–839.
693. Van Tets WF, vander Werken C. External fixation for diaphyseal femoral fractures: a benefit to the young child. Injury 1991;23:162–164.
694. Verbeek HOF. Does rotation deformity following femur shaft fracture correct during growth? Reconstr Surg Traumatol 1979;17:75–81.
695. Verbeek HO, Bender J, Sawidis K. Rotational deformities after fracture of the femoral shaft in childhood. Injury 1976;8:43–48.
696. Viljanto J, Kiviluoto H, Paanenen M. Remodeling after femoral shaft fracture in children. Acta Orthop Scand 1971;141:360–369.
697. Viljanto J, Linna MI, Kiviluoto H, Paananen M. Indications and results of operative treatment of femoral shaft fractures in children. Acta Chir Scand 1975;141:366–375.
698. Vinz H. Die festigkeitsmechanischen Grundlägen der typischen Frakturformen des Kindesalters. Zentralbl Chir 1969;94:1509–1514.
699. Vinz H. Die Marknagelung kindlicher Oberschenkelschaftfrakturen. Zentralbl Chir 1972;97:90–95.
700. Vinz H. Operative Behandlung von Knochenbruchen bei Kindern. Zentralbl Chir 1972;97:1377–1384.
701. Vinz H, Grobler B, Wiegand E. Osteitis nach Osteosynthese im Kindesalter. Beitr Orthop Traumatol 1978;25:349–361.
702. Von Laer L. Beinlangendifferenzen und Rotationsfehler nach Oberschenkelschaftfrakturen im Kindesalter. Arch Orthop Unfallchir 1977;89:121–137.
703. Von Laer L. Neue Behandlungskriterien fur die Oberschenkelschaftfraktur im Kindesalter. Z Kinderchir 1978;24:165–172.
704. Von Laer L, Herzog B. Beinlangendifferenzen und Rotationsfehler nach Oberschenkelschaftfrakturen im Kindesalter: therapeutische Beeinflussung und spontant Korrektur. Helv Chir Acta 1978;45:17–23.
705. Vontobel V, Genton N, Schmid R. Die spatergebnisse der kindlichen dislozierten Femurschaftfraktur. Helv Chir Acta 1961;28:655–670.
706. Wagner M, Deisenhammer W, Kutscha-Lissberg E. Indikation zur osteosynthese kindlicher oberschenkelfrakturen. Hefte Unfallheilkd 1984;182:340–346.
707. Walker DM, Kennedy JC. Occult knee ligament injuries associated with femoral shaft fractures. Am J Sports Med 1980;8:172–174.
708. Wallace ME, Hoffman EB. Remodeling of angular deformity after femoral shaft fractures in children. J Bone Joint Surg Br 1992;74:765–769.
709. Walsh MG. Limb lengths following femoral shaft fracture in children. J Ir Med Assoc 1973;66:447–453.
710. Ward WT, Levy J, Kaye A. Compression plating for child and adolescent femur fractures. J Pediatr Orthop 1992;12:626–632.
711. Wardlaw D. Cast brace treatment of femoral shaft fractures. J Bone Joint Surg Br 1977;59:411–416.
712. Wardlaw D. Cast bracing in practice: a two year study in Aberdeen. Injury 1980;12:213–218.
713. Weber BG. Inwieweit sind isolierte extreme Torsionsvariaten der unteren Extremitaten als Deformitäten aufzufassen und welche klinische Bedeutung kommt ihnen zu? Z Orthop 1961;94:287–303.
714. Weber BG. Wie kommt der kindliche einwartsgang zustande, und was hat er zu bedeuten? Helv Paediatr Acta 1961;16:82–89.
715. Weber BG. Zur Behandlung kindlicher Femurschaftbruche. Arch Orthop Unfallchir 1963;54:713–723.
716. Weber BG. Prophylaxe der Achsenfehlstellungen bei der Behandlung kindlicher Frakturen. Unfallmed Berufskr 1966;1:80–95.
717. Weber BG. Indikationen zur operativen Frakturbehandlung bei Kindern. Chirurg 1967;10:441–444.
718. Weber BG. Fractures of the femoral shaft in childhood. Injury 1969;1:65–71.
719. Weber BG. Das besondere bei der Behandlung der Frakturen im Kindesalter. Monatsschr Unfallheilkd 1975;78:193–198.
720. Weiss A-PC, Schenck RC, Sponseller P, Thompson JD. Peroneal palsy after early cast application for femoral fractures in children. J Pediatr Orthop 1992;12:25–28.
721. Weller S. Die konservative Behandlung kindlicher Frakturen. Langenbecks Arch Chir 1976;342:287–290.
722. West WK. Treatment of fractures in children by the use of skeletal traction. South Med J 1933;26:644–646.
723. Whitehouse WM, Coran AG, Stanley B. Pediatric vascular trauma: manifestation, management, sequelae of extremity arterial injury in patients undergoing surgical treatment. Arch Surg 1976;111:1269–1275.
724. Wiesner F, Seyffartn G. Behandlungsergebnisse von Oberschenkelbruchen bei Kindern. Beitr Orthop Traumatol 1980;27:260–266.
725. Wilde CD, Kohler A. Oberschenkelschaftfrakturen im Kindes- und Wachstumsalter. Unfallchirurgie 1978;4:133–138.
726. Yano S, Sawada M. Rotationsfehler nach kindlichen Femurschaftfrakturen. Z Orthop 1975;113:119–129.
727. Zenker W, Buchhammer T, Gottorf T. Spätergebnisse nach conservativer und operativer Therapie kindlicher Femurschaftfrakturen. Hefte Unfallheilkd 1990;212:373–379.
728. Zimmerman R, Stöger A, Golserk, Gabl M, Lyall HA, Benedetto KP. Tibial growth after isolated femoral shaft fractures in children. J Pediatr Orthop 1997;17:421–424.
729. Ziv I, Blackburn N, Rang M. Femoral intramedullary nailing in the growing child. J Trauma 1984;24:432–434.
730. Ziv I, Rang M. Treatment of femoral fracture in the child with head injury. J Bone Joint Surg Br 1983;65:276–278.
731. Zuckerman JD, Veith RG, Johnson KD, et al. Treatment of unstable femoral shaft fractures with closed interlocking intramedullary nailing. J Orthop Trauma 1987;1:209–218.

Distal Femur

732. Abbott LC, Gerald GG. Valgus deformity of the knee resulting from injury to the lower femoral epiphysis. J Bone Joint Surg 1942;24:97–113.
733. Ackerman R. Frakturen und Lysen der distalen Femurepiphyse. In: Rahmanzadeh R, Breyer H-G (eds) Verletzungen der unteren Extremitäten bei Kindern und Jugendlichen. Berlin: Springer, 1990:140–143.
734. Aitken AP, Magill HK. Fractures involving the distal femoral epiphyseal cartilage. J Bone Joint Surg Am 1952;34:96–108.
735. Ansorg P, Graner G. Zur Behandlung distaler Oberschenkelfrakturen im Kindesalter. Beitr Orthop Traumatol 1976;23:359–366.
736. Banagale RC, Kuhns LR. Traumatic separation of the distal femoral epiphysis in the newborn. J Pediatr Orthop 1983;3:396–398.
737. Bassett FJ III, Goldner JL. Fractures involving the distal femoral epiphyseal growth line. South Med J 1962;55:545–547.
738. Bellin H. Traumatic separation of epiphysis of lower end of femur. Am J Surg 1937;37:306–309.
739. Bergenfeldt E. Beitrage fur Kenntnis der traumatischen Epiphysenlösungen an den langen Rohrenknochen der Extremitäten: eine klinisch-Röntgenologische Studie. Acta Chir Scand 1933;27:(suppl 73):1–158.
740. Bertin KC, Goble EM. Ligament injuries associated with physeal fractures about the knee. Clin Orthop 1983;177:188–195.

References

741. Bollini G. Traumatologie et ostésynthèse chez l'enfant. Rev Chir Orthop 1986;72(suppl II):13–17.
742. Bollini G, Christian P, Kohler R, Boulays JM, Carcassone M. La décollement épiphysaire du cartilage conjugal après fracture décollement épiphysaire de l'extrémité inférieure du fémur chez l'adolescent. Marseilles: Chirurg Sud-Est, 1984.
743. Botting TDJ, Serase WH. Premature epiphyseal fusion at the knee complicating prolonged immobilization for congenital dislocation of the hip. J Bone Joint Surg Br 1965;47:280–282.
744. Buess-Watson E, Exner GU, Illi OE. Fractures about the knee: growth disturbances and probems of stability at long-term follow-up. Eur J Pediatr Surg 1994;4:218–224.
745. Burman MS, Langsam MJ. Posterior dislocation of lower femoral epiphysis in breech delivery. Arch Surg 1939;38:250–253.
746. Cage JB, Ivey FM. Intercondylar fracture of the femur in an adolescent athlete. Physician Sportsmed 1983;11:115–118.
747. Cam J. Les traumatismes du cartilage de croissance fémoral inférieur. J Orthop Pediatr Hosp Trousseau Paris 1983;3.
748. Cassebaum WH, Patterson AH. Fractures of the distal femoral epiphysis. Clin Orthop 1965;41:79–91.
749. Coetzee GL. Supracondylar and distal epiphyseal femur fractures in the dog and cat. J S Afr Vet Assoc 1983;54:171–179.
750. Connolly JF, Shindell R, Huurman WW. Growth arrest following minimally displaced distal femoral epiphyseal fracture. Nebr Med 1987;72:341–343.
751. Courtivron B, Bonnard C, Letouze A. Les décollements épiphysaires du genou. Ann Chir 1994;48:46–54.
752. Crawford AH. Fractures about the knee in children. Orthop Clin North Am 1976;7:639–656.
753. Criswell AR, Hand WL, Butler JE. Abduction injuries of the distal femoral epiphysis. Clin Orthop 1976;115:189–194.
754. Czitrom AA, Salter RB, Willis RB. Fractures involving the distal epiphyseal plate of the femur. Int Orthop 1981;4:269–277.
755. Dal Monte A, Manes E, Cammarota U. Post-traumatic genu valgum in children. Ital J Orthop Traumatol 1983;9:5–11.
756. Edmunds I, Wade S. Injuries of the distal femoral growth plate and epiphysis: should open reduction be performed? Aust NZ J Surg 1993;63:195–199.
757. Ehlers PN, Eberlein H. Epiphysenfrakturen: Klinischer Beitrag zur Frage der Spatfolgen. Langenbecks Arch Chir 1963;304:627–632.
758. Ehrlich MG, Strain RE Jr. Epiphyseal injuries about the knee. Orthop Clin North Am 1979;10:91–103.
759. Farine I, Spira E. Décollements épiphysaires traumatiques. Rev Chir Orthop 1968;54:3–23.
760. Feldkam G, Krastel A, Braus T. Welche Faktoren beeinflussen die wachstamsphänomene nach kindlichen Schaftbrüchen? Unfallheilkunde 1978;81:96–102.
761. Ford LT, Key JA. A study of experimental trauma to the distal femoral epiphysis in rabbits. J Bone Joint Surg Am 1956;38:84–102.
762. Gast D, Niethard FU, Cotta H. Fehlverheilte kindliche frakturen im kriegelenkbereich. Orthopäde 1991;20:360–366.
763. Graham JM, Gross RH. Distal femoral physeal problem fractures. Clin Orthop 1990;255:51–53.
764. Griswold AS. Early motion in the treatment of separation of the lower femoral epiphysis: report of a case. J Bone Joint Surg 1928;10:75–78.
765. Grogan DP, Bobechko WP. Pathogenesis of a fracture of the distal femoral epiphysis. J Bone Joint Surg Am 1984;66:621–622.
766. Hubert M, Evrard H. Condylar and supracondylar fractures of the femur in children and adolescents. Acta Orthop Belg 1982;48:749–756.
767. Kaplan JA, Sprague SB, Benjamin HC. Traumatic bilateral separation of the lower femoral epiphyses. J Bone Joint Surg 1942;24:200–201.
768. Kasser JR. Femur fractures in children. AAOS Inst Course Lect 1992;41:403–408.
769. Keller H, Siebler G, Kuner EH. Verletzungen der distalen Femur-epiphyse-Klassifikation, Behandlung: Ergebnisse. In: Rahmanzadeh R, Brayer HG (eds) Verletzungen der unteren Extremitäten bei Kindern und Jugendlichen. Berlin: Springer, 1990:144–145.
770. Kestler PC. Unclassified premature cessation of epiphyseal growth about the knee joint. J Bone Joint Surg 1947;29:788.
771. Knapp DR, Price CT. Correction of distal femoral deformity. Clin Orthop 1990;255:75–80.
772. Lascombes P, Prevot J, Bardoux J. Pronostic des fractures de l'éxtremité inférieure du fémur chez l'enfant et l'adolescent. Rev Chir Orthop 1988;74:438–445.
773. Lee CL, Peterson HE, Lamont RL. Fractures of the distal femoral epiphysis. Presented at the 44th meeting. American Academy of Orthopaedic Surgeons, February 1977.
774. Lombardo SJ, Harvey JP Jr. Fractures of the distal femoral epiphyses. J Bone Joint Surg Am 1977;59:742–751.
775. Mäkelä EA, Vainionpää S, Vihtonen K, Mero M, Rokhanen P. The effect of trauma to the lower femoral epiphyseal plate: an experimental study in rabbits. J Bone Joint Surg Br 1988;70:187–191.
776. Massart R. Decollement epiphysaire de l'éxtremité inférieure des deux femurs consecutif a un traumatisme obstetrical. Bull Soc Anat Paris 1921;18:498–506.
777. Meyers MC, Calvo RD, Sterling JC, Edelstein DW. Delayed treatment of a malreduced distal femoral epiphyseal plate fracture. Med Sci Sports Exerc 1992;24:1311–1315.
778. Neer CS II. Separation of the lower femoral epiphysis. Am J Surg 1960;99:756–761.
779. Nemsadse WP. Die operative Frakturbehandlung der langen Rohrenknochen bei kindesalte. Vestn Chirurg 1965;4:73–84.
780. Nicholson JT. Epiphyseal fractures about the knee. AAOS Instruct Course Lect 1961;18:74–82.
781. Obletz BE, Casagrande PA. Traumatic displacements of the lower femoral epiphyses. NY State J Med 1950;50:2820–2822.
782. Padovani JP, Rigantt P, Raux P, Lignac F, Guyonvarch G. Décollements épiphysaires traumatiques de l'éxtremité inférieure du fémur. Rev Chir Orthop 1976;62:211–230.
783. Patterson WJ. Separation of the lower femoral epiphysis. Can Med Assoc J 1929;21:301–303.
784. Pincherle B. Distacco epifisario inferiori bilaterale del femore da trauma ostetrico. Pediatria 1936;44:816–818.
785. Rhebein F, Joffman S. Knochenverletzungen in Kindesalter. Arch Klin Chir 1963;304:539–544.
786. Riseborough EJ, Barrett IR, Shapiro F. Growth disturbances following distal femoral physeal fracture-separations. J Bone Joint Surg Am 1983;65:885–893.
787. Robert M, Moulies D, Longis B, et al. Décollements épiphysaires traumatiques de l'extrémité inférieure du fémur. Rev Chir Orthop 1988;74:69–78.
788. Roberts JM. Operative treatment of fractures about the knee. Orthop Clin North Am 1990;21:365–379.
789. Rogers L, Jones S, David A. "Clipping injury" fracture of the epiphysis in the adolescent football player: an occult lesion of the knee. AJR 1974;121:69–78.
790. Ross D. Disturbance of longitudinal growth associated with prolonged disability of the lower extremity. J Bone Joint Surg Am 1948;30:103–115.
791. Rumlova E, Vogel E. Dislocated supracondylar femoral fractures, slipped epiphyses and epiphyseal fractures in children. Z Kinderchir 1983;38:48–50.

792. Schneider T. Spatergebnisse der kuntschernagelung am junglichenden Knocher. Arztl Wochenschr 1950;5:846–849.
793. Shulman BH, Terhune CB. Epiphyseal injuries in breech delivery. Pediatrics 1951;8:693–700.
794. Shivley JL. Genu recurvatum after femoral fracture. Contemp Orthop 1990;21:577–580.
795. Sideman S. Traumatic separation of the lower femoral epiphysis. J Bone Joint Surg 1943;25:913–916.
796. Siebler G. Frakturen des distalen Femur. Hefte Unfallheilkd 1988;200:468–470.
797. Simpson WC Jr, Fardon DF. Obscure distal femoral epiphyseal injury. South Med J 1976;69:1338–1340.
798. Stephens DC, Louis E, Louis DS. Traumatic separation of the distal femoral epiphyseal cartilage plate. J Bone Joint Surg Am 1974;56:1383–1390.
799. Tessore A, Pollono F. Il distacco dell'epifisi inferiore del femore. Minerva Ortop 1966;17:35–43.
800. Torg JS, Pavlov H, Morris VB. Salter-Harris type III fracture of the medial femoral condyle occurring in the adolescent athete. J Bone Joint Surg Am 1981;63:586–591.
801. Vogt P. Die traumatische Epiphysenfrennung und deren Einfluss auf des Langenwachstum der Rohrenknochen. Arch Klin Chir 1878;22:343–349.
802. Wajanavisit W, Orapin S. Biplane fracture of distal femoral epiphysis: a case report. J Med Assoc Thai 1994;77:501–504.

Floating Knee

803. Bohn WW, Durbin RA. Ipsilateral fractures of the femur and tibia in children and adolescents. J Bone Joint Surg Am 1991;73:429–439.
804. Letts M, Vincent N, Gouw G. The "floating knee" in children. J Bone Joint Surg Br 1986;68:442–446.

22

Knee

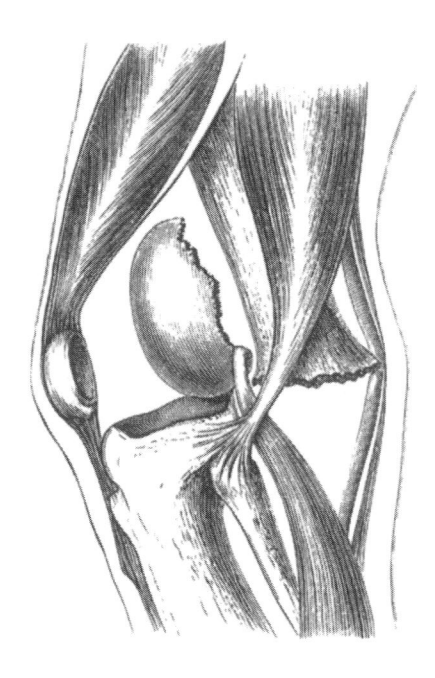

Engraving of a fracture involving the adolescent knee. (From Poland J. Traumatic Separation of the Epiphyses. *London: Smith, Eder, 1898)*

The developmental patterns of the distal femoral and proximal tibial epiphyses are detailed, respectively, in Chapters 21 and 23. The other anatomic structures of the knee joint include the patella, the quadriceps expansion and patellar tendon, the medial and lateral menisci, the component ligaments (collateral and cruciate), and the capsule. These structures are discussed in this chapter.

Anatomy

Patella

The patella is a large sesamoid bone that, with the exception of the articular surface, lies within the tendinous expansion of the quadriceps femoris muscle. The lower third of the patella is covered by a large fat pad and synovial reflection, and it is extra-synovial (Figs. 22-1, 22-2). Synovial recesses extend between the fat pad, patella, and tibia (Fig. 22-2). The patellar tendon is also separated from the synovial joint by this fat pad. The patellar tendon progressively blends into both the inferior patella and tibial tuberosity by fibrous to fibrocartilaginous to cartilaginous tissue. Mature fibers attaching the tendon directly into bone are not present until late adolescence, when both of these structures have finished chondro-osseous transformation and maturation.

Initially the patella is completely cartilaginous and thus radiolucent in the preschool child.[8,14] Primary patellar ossification begins around 5–6 years of age, although small foci may be evident as early as 2–3 years. The initial chondro-osseous transformation is usually typified by multiple small foci that rapidly coalesce (Figs. 22-3, 22-4), similar to secondary ossification in the trochlear region of the distal humerus.[12] Patellar ossification occurs centrifugally within the mass of epiphyseal cartilage that is well vascularized by cartilage canals and is thus comparable to postnatal epiphyseal (secondary) ossification in long bones. Sometimes there is a distinct origin between the inferior and superior portions of the early ossification center, which may be mistaken for a fracture. Similarly, multifocal ossification should not be misconstrued as a comminuted fracture in a young child being evaluated for knee trauma. Ossification progressively expands toward the various margins. Ossification rapidly proceeds to the anterior surface, where periosteum initially forms. In contrast, the posterior, inferior, medial, and lateral margins retain a chondro-osseous interface, with peripheral perichondrium and posterior articular cartilage. During adolescence the anterior, medial, and lateral cortical bone of the expanding ossification center becomes confluent with the fibrous tissue of the quadriceps tendon and progressively creates a dense continuity between tendon and subchondral bone through Sharpey's fibers. Until skeletal maturation, these chondro-osseous interfaces remain as areas mechanically susceptible to tensile forces and thus may incur avulsion fractures.

Developing patellar ossification is usually irregular at the margins, not unlike the expanding distal femoral ossification center.[12] Because of this normal variability of marginal ossification, a diagnosis of osteochondrosis or osteochondritis

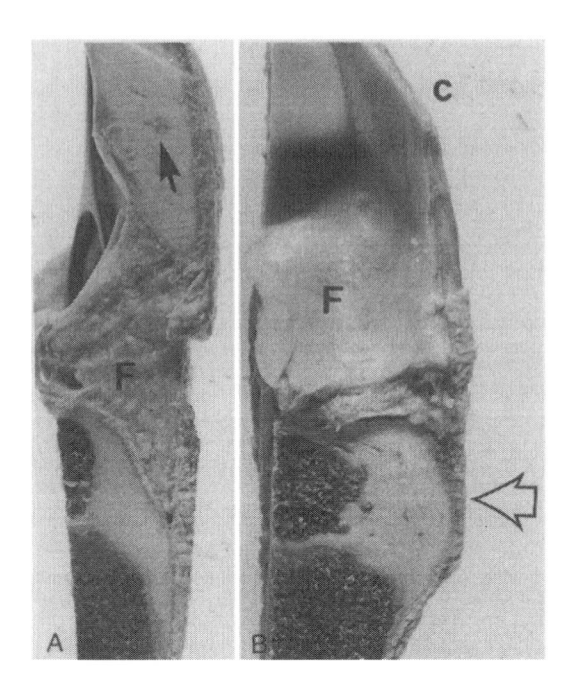

FIGURE 22-1. Coronal (A) and sagittal (B) sections of the patella, capsule, and proximal tibia from a 6-year-old child. Cartilage occupies much of the mass of the patella. A small focus of ossification (solid arrow) is present. The retropatellar fat pad (F) covers much of the lower pole of the patella. The open arrow indicates the medial collateral ligament. Note how it blends into the epiphyseal cartilage and the capsule (c).

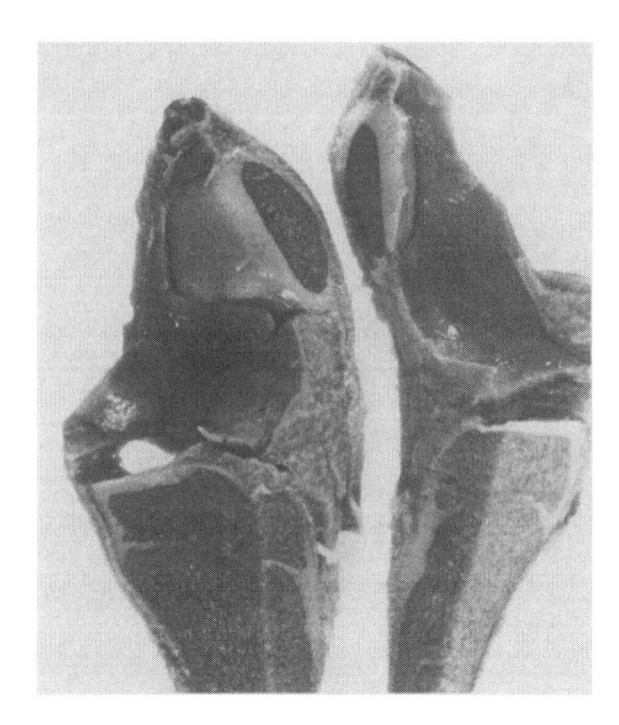

FIGURE 22-2. Coronally split knee from a 10-year-old boy showing a well-ossified patella. Note how the synovium covers the fat pad.

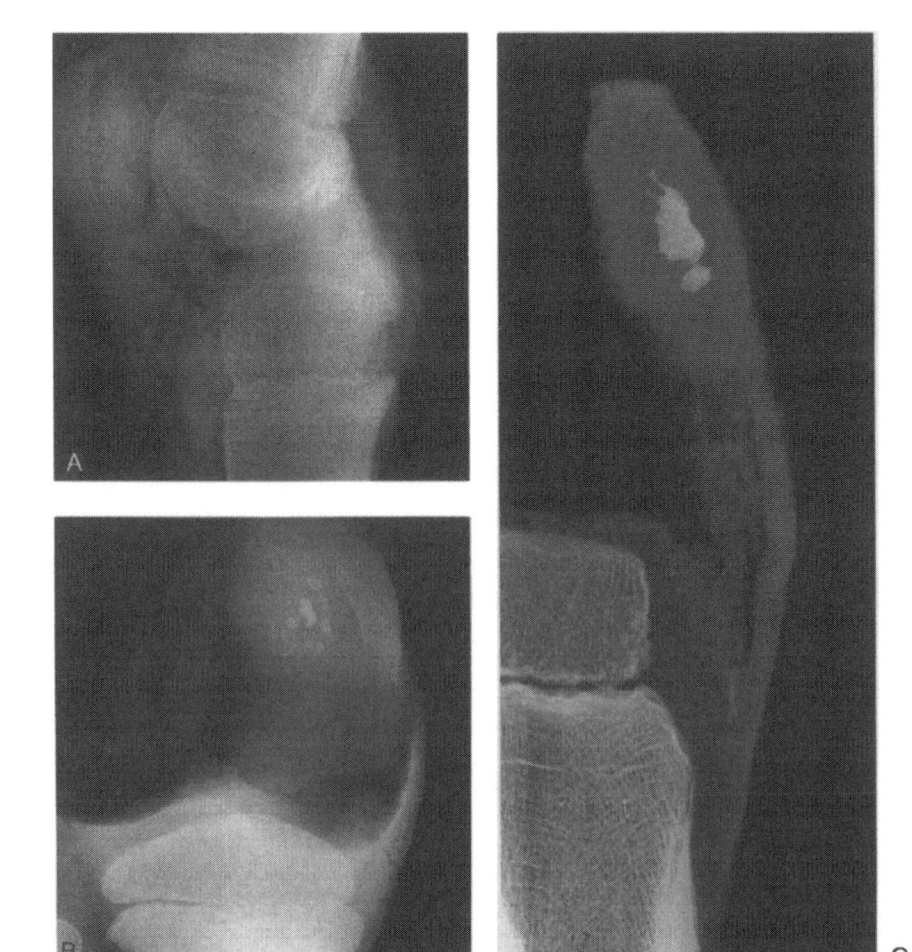

FIGURE 22-3. Cadaver specimens showing progressive patellar development. (A) At 2 years, no ossification is present. However, air/cartilage contrast outlines the patella in the lateral view. (B) Early ossification in a 6-year-old, which is often multifocal. (C) Multifocal ossification then begins to coalesce.

Anatomy

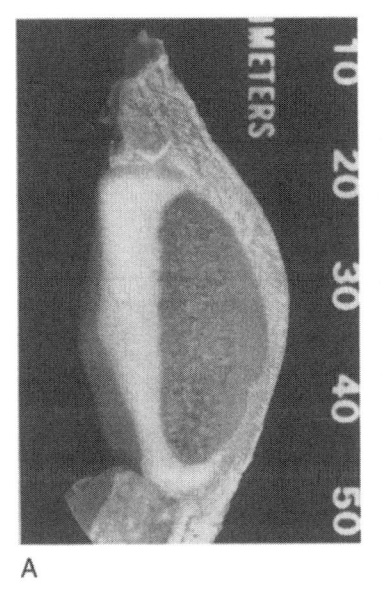

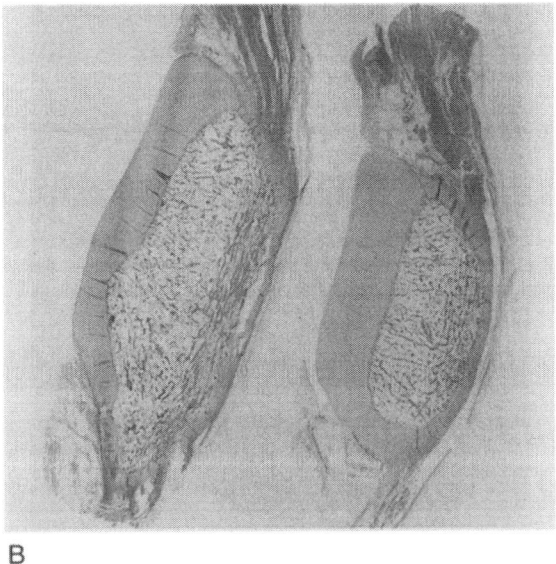

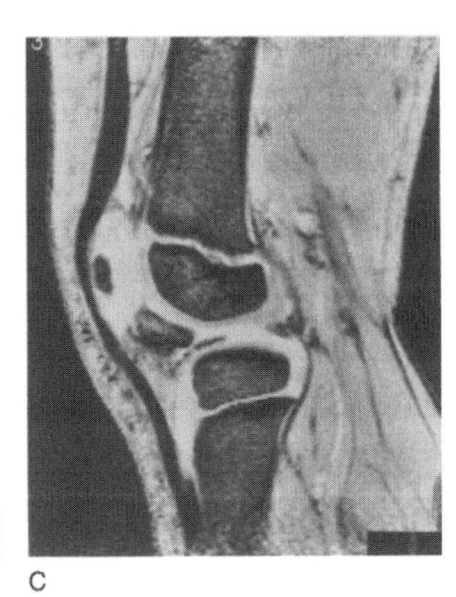

FIGURE 22-4. Ossification rapidly proceeds centrifugally to fill out the cartilaginous patella. Anatomic (A) and serial histologic (B) sections show enlargement of the patellar ossification center. Note how the ossification replaces the anterior cartilage before the posterior cartilage. (C) MRI of patellar ossification in a 6-year-old boy. Note the anterior position of ossification within the cartilaginous patella.

of the patella, or even fracture, solely on the basis of the roentgenographic appearance, must be made with caution. Accessory ossification centers may develop, particularly in the superolateral portion of the bone. A separate ossification center of the inferior pole probably does not exist. Instead, one must consider the diagnosis of a Sinding-Larsen-Johansson lesion, the patellar equivalent of the Osgood-Schlatter lesion. After 10 years of age the patellar subchondral bone becomes more smooth and develops a distinct, shell-like appearance with a thin plate of bone surrounding the patellar trabecular bone.

When a normal, mature patella is sectioned transversely, the medial and lateral articular surfaces are approximately equal and subtend reasonably equivalent angles. However, if the immature patella does not track properly (e.g., subluxates laterally), the cartilage may gradually deform (plastic deformation) and the subsequently appearing ossification center "mirrors" the antecedent, deformed cartilaginous precursor. This eventually leads to the unequal osseous angles characteristic of a chronically maltracking, subluxating, or dislocating patella.

The patella may be situated relatively high or low. Normally, the distance from the lower pole of the patella to the tendinous insertion on the tuberosity should equal the sagittal length of the patella (Fig. 22-5). More than 20% variation probably indicates an abnormal patellar position,[6,10,11]

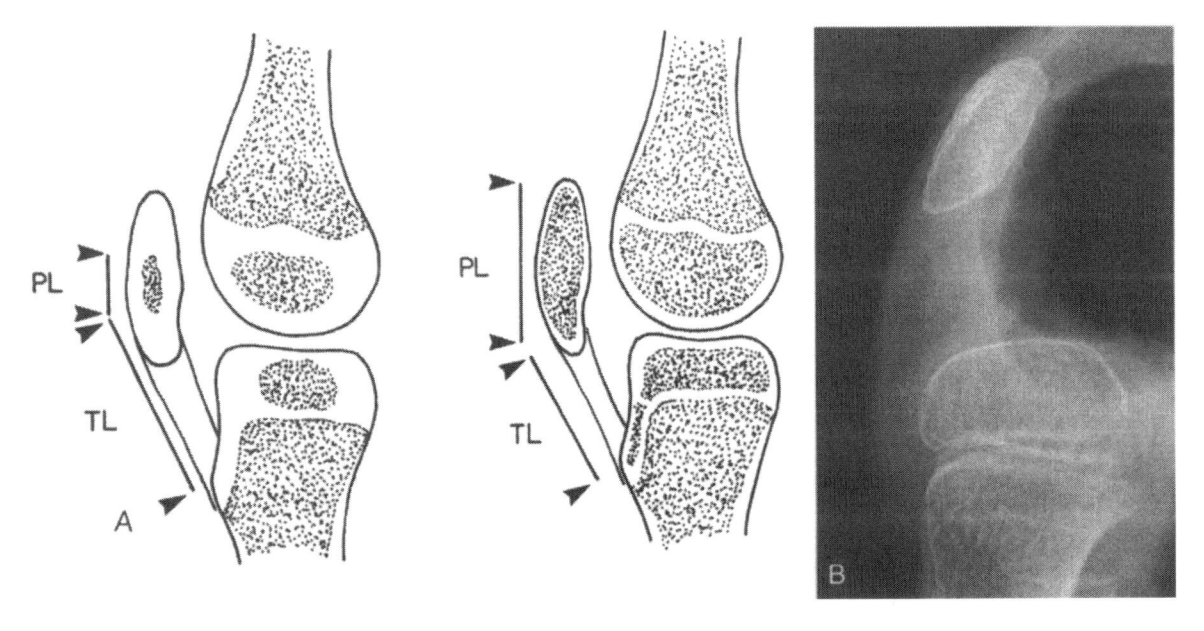

FIGURE 22-5. (A) Normal patella/tendon measurements. Insall's measurement is the ratio of patellar length (PL) to tendon length (TL). (B) Specimen of the knee of an 8-year-old showing problems of such measurement, even in a skeletally immature cadaver. The tuberosity, in particular, is not well defined.

although these measurements and ratios are *not* realistic in the growing child. Depending on the age and extent of chondro-osseous transformation, there are significant amounts of epiphyseal cartilage at both the superior and inferior patellar poles and the tibial tuberosity, such that the sagittal length of the ossified patella and the distance from the patellar ossification center to the tibial tuberosity ossification center may be considerably different from the actual patellar and tendon lengths.

The patella, similar to any epiphysis, is a mass of cartilage interlaced with an intrinsic vascular system within cartilage canals. When ossification expands toward the anterior surface, discrete intraosseous vessels penetrate and supply the ossification. A number of vessels penetrate from around the periphery of the patella.[13]

Meniscus

The menisci assume their characteristic shape during prenatal development.[4,5] The major postnatal changes are progressively decreased vascularity, morphologic growth commensurate with enlargement of the distal femur and proximal tibia, and accommodation of this growth to changing femorotibial contact.[4,5,7] Weight-bearing obviously affects these postnatal changes, which are accompanied by changes at the cellular level and in the extracellular matrix. The progressive decrease in vascularity obviously affects the inflammatory response stage after an injury. The lateral meniscus tends to have more developmental variation, but at *no* time is it normally discoid. Anterior extensions from both menisci to the anterior cruciate ligament and to each other are a residual of their common origin. The transverse anterior (intermeniscal) ligament between the menisci may be a source of some discomfort in children complaining of anterior knee pain. The more fixed medial meniscus possesses important peripheral capsular attachments, including the thickened medial capsular ligament and posteromedial capsular complex. The more mobile lateral meniscus has no attachment posterolaterally at the popliteus tendon recess. There may be a communication to the proximal tibiofibular joint. The meniscofemoral ligaments of Humphrey and Wrisberg are variable, both as to size and presence.

The microscopic structure and collagen fiber alignment of the menisci change over time due to changes in weight-bearing function and applied mechanical loading.[2,3,9] Most of the fibers are arranged in circumferential fashion in the long axis of the meniscus. Other radially directed fibers are located mainly on the surfaces of the meniscus, more on the tibial than the femoral side, and probably act as tie rods resisting longitudinal splitting. A few radial fibers change direction and run in a vertical fashion through the substance of the meniscus. These patterns undergo changing patterns as the child begins ambulation. There are no studies relative to how they change, particularly during adolescence, when there are both significant morphologic (size) changes in the knee and often excessive demands of athletic activity.

The meniscus of the infant is a relatively vascular structure.[4,5] As weight-bearing commences, the more central regions lose their microvascularity. However, peripheral vascularity is retained and allows the likelihood of spontaneous repair of an incomplete tear in the skeletally immature individual.[1,5,7]

Ligaments and Capsule

Throughout most of development the cruciate ligaments blend into the epiphyseal cartilage of the distal femur (intercondylar notch) and proximal tibia (tibial spines). There is a progressive transition of fibrous, fibrocartilaginous, and cartilaginous tissues. Only during late adolescence do the cruciate ligaments insert directly into the maturing ossification centers through the development of Sharpey's fibers. Accordingly, childhood cruciate injuries usually are chondro-osseous failures, rather than intraligamentous ruptures.

It is commonly taught that the medial and lateral collateral ligaments attach primarily into the distal femoral epiphysis and proximal tibial metaphysis, an anatomic configuration that, accordingly, makes the distal femur more susceptible to epiphyseal-physeal injury. The ligaments blend densely into the distal femoral epiphyseal perichondrium. However, dissection of skeletally immature knees shows that the deep collateral ligaments also attach directly into the proximal tibial epiphyseal perichondrium (Fig. 22-6). Some of the more superficial collateral fibers do continue onto the metaphysis, as does the pes anserinus. *The classic concept that the collateral ligaments have no tibial epiphyseal attachments is thus incorrect.* The increased susceptibility to injury is more likely due to the moment arm of any applied deformation force, along with the extent of forceful muscular contracture.

The suprapatellar pouch normally extends under the quadriceps. Developmental variations of the synovium (plicae) in this region may lead to compartmentalization of this pouch (plica syndrome) and chronic knee effusions. The posterior capsule has minimum redundancy. There are no normal communications from the posterior capsule into the popliteal space other than along the popliteal tendon and the communication to the proximal tibiofibular joint. Popliteal cysts in children may develop *without* a discrete communication with the knee joint.

General Examination

Any child or adolescent presenting for the evaluation of an acute or chronic knee injury must be evaluated carefully for possible congenital abnormalities as well as the more typical traumatic lesions that are most often present in young adults.[15–23] Although the injuries commonly afflicting adults, such as a meniscal tear or anterior cruciate ligament injury, are much less frequent in the skeletally immature patient, such lesions do occur. Extensive amounts of cartilage make normal diagnostic methods less likely to be specific. They also increase the likelihood of chondro-osseous disruption, which may or may not be accompanied by a variable layer of subchondral bone. Bleeding within epiphyseal bone (bone bruising) is a real phenomenon that is probably prevalent in children, especially with direct blows to the knee. Magnetic resonance imaging (MRI) is the only way to establish this diagnosis unequivocally. Such studies are indicated when routine imaging fails to indicate

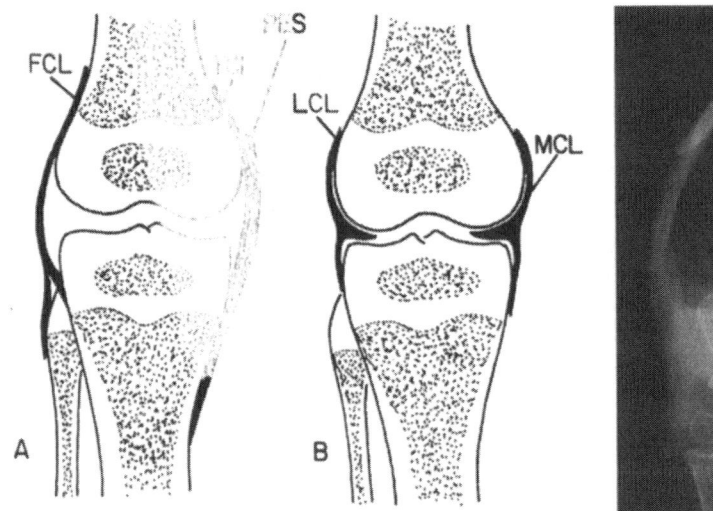

FIGURE 22-6. Superficial (A) and deep (B) collateral ligament attachments. Note the fibular collateral ligament (FCL), pes anserinus (PES), tibial collateral ligament (TCL), the deep medial collateral ligament (MCL), and lateral collateral ligament (LCL). The collateral ligaments attach to the epiphyseal perichondrium of the proximal tibia, *not* the metaphysis. (C) The distal femur has been removed to show the anterior, medial, and lateral capsular reflections and collateral ligaments in an 11-year-old boy.

the cause of acute or persistent symptoms following knee trauma.

Flanagan et al. showed that even minor knee injuries cause pain and functional problems.[18] Rest, ice, and antiinflammatory medications are the usual initial treatment. Range of motion exercises should be started as soon as possible, preferably after an accurate diagnosis has been made. Stretching and strengthening exercises for involved muscle groups provide pain relief and help prevent recurrence. Even minor knee trauma may lead to subluxation due to quadriceps atrophy or tightening of (contracture) of the lateral retinaculum.

Stanitski et al. showed that in 70 children aged 7–18 years with acute traumatic knee hemarthrosis there was a high incidence of intraarticular lesions[22,23]: 47% of preadolescents (age 7–12 years) had meniscal tears and 47% had anterior cruciate ligament tears. Among the adolescents (age 13–18 years), 45% had meniscal tears and 65% had anterior cruciate ligament tears. Osteochondral fractures accounted for 7% of the lesions. Stanitski et al. thought that meniscal and anterior cruciate ligament damage was common in children, especially adolescents. They noted that accurate examination of acute intraarticular injury is arduous. Young patients may be limited historians with regard to the mechanism of injury. Guarding secondary to pain may significantly limit the range of motion and stability testing.

Diagnostic Imaging

When evaluating injury to the knee, the patella is best seen in either the lateral or tangential projections. In the anteroposterior view, because of the normal position of the patella overlying the distal femoral metaphysis and epiphysis, much of the patella is obscured especially when the ossification center is small. However, this anteroposterior view may be the best way to visualize a bipartite patella. Oblique views may also allow adequate visualization of the superolateral region.

Because the epiphyseal regions of the younger child contain more radiolucent cartilage than during the adolescent period, the evaluation of suspected internal derangement of the knee becomes more challenging.[32] Only a thin piece of subchondral bone may be associated with a large cartilaginous fragment in a lesion such as osteochondritis dissecans, an acute osteochondral fracture, or a patellar sleeve fracture. If the knee is placed in the usual diagnostic positions, especially tangential views, portions of the anterior proximal tibia or tibial tuberosity ossification centers may appear to be an osteochondral fragment. The apparent lucency is the physis of the tuberosity, which parallels the roentgenographic beam in this particular view.[28]

Children normally have a greater degree of ligamentous laxity than adults. It enchances the likelihood of phenomena such as "vacuum arthrography," which is due to cavitation of gas from joint fluid when stress is applied. Such cavitation may outline all or part of the joint and should not be misinterpreted as a loose body, chondro-osseous fracture, or open injury.

Arthrography is useful in the child's knee because of the extensive radiolucency.[27,31] Cartilage damage may have little involvement of contiguous subchondral bone, and may be depicted only by single- or double-contrast arthrography. This procedure may be undertaken as a diagnostic study in a child prior to using more invasive procedures such as arthroscopy. However, knee arthrography is rapidly being supplanted by MRI.

Computed tomographic (CT) scanning may be useful to define complex fractures of the distal femur. Such fracture "definition" is important to plan proper reduction and fixation. Certain fractures of the patella and femoral condyles may be visible only with a CT scan. The subluxated, dislo-

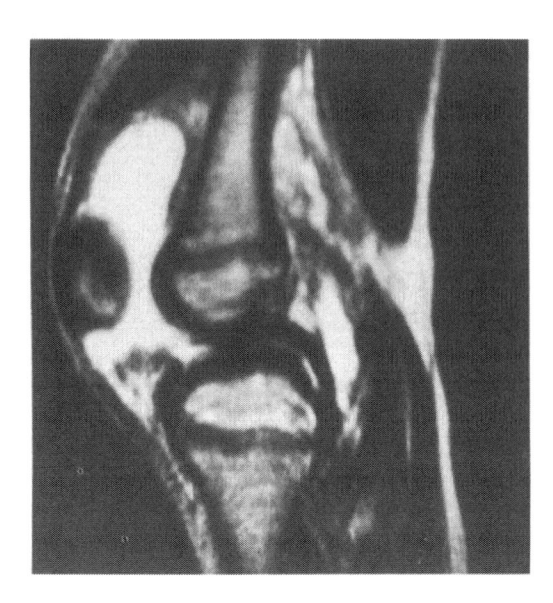

FIGURE 22-7. MRI scan of a 9-year-old demonstrating posttraumatic knee effusion. It fills the suprapatellar pouch and elevates the patella away from the condyles. A bone bruise is evident in the patella.

cating, or dislocated patella may also be assessed with CT scanning.

Magnetic resonance imaging is becoming a more clinically useful tool for evaluating the skeletally immature knee.[24,26,29,30,33] Unfortunately, the younger the child the more likely is sedation or anesthesia necessary to maintain the "stillness" necessary to accomplish a meaningful study.

Because MRI is helpful for diagnosing pathology within the knee, it is important to be familiar with the MRI appearance of normal anatomic variants that might be confused with meniscal tears such as the transverse geniculate ligament, the hiatus of the popliteus tendon, and the meniscofemoral ligaments.[24] Such familiarity must also include variations of chondro-osseous transformation and maturation in the child and adolescent. Meniscal fragments may be difficult to detect on MRI, even though clinically significant, and one of the easier injuries to overlook.[25] MRI may not reliably exclude articular cartilage injury.[30] Evolving sequencing methods may allow such delineation in the future.

There is significant variation in the MRI appearance within the patellar tendon.[29] Many changes may represent subclinical injury. Changes in signal intensity within this tendon may also occur secondary to joint effusions, anterior cruciate ligament tears, or strain (microinjury) within the patellar tendon itself.

The MRI scan is useful for evaluating the presence of effusion or hemarthrosis (Fig. 22-7). The presence of significant distension of the capsule by fluid should make the physician search carefully for an anatomic lesion responsible for such fluid increase. The posterior distension of the joint capsule may cause the patient to complain of posterior knee pain and may even be misdiagnosed as a popliteal cyst.

Perhaps the most important use of MRI is for delineating obscure or occult intraepiphyseal fractures of the knee (Figs. 22-8, 22-9). The knee, like the wrist, is an area of frequent injury in an active child. Competitive, increasingly physically demanding team sports put the knee at risk for direct impact injuries and chondro-osseous interface tensile failure. Children and adolescents often present with a painful knee, with or without joint effusion, only to have a "normal" radiograph. MRI allows a more definitive diagnosis in the enigmatic patient.

The incidence of chondral injury within the femoral condyles may eventually become the most important clinical consequence of the MRI evaluation. The potential role of the initial injury in the development of progressive chondral injury is uncertain. Acute, transarticular load injuries to the calcified cartilage–bone interface generate no initial abnormalities on the surface articular cartilage. The initial concussive blow might exceed some supraphysiologic threshold

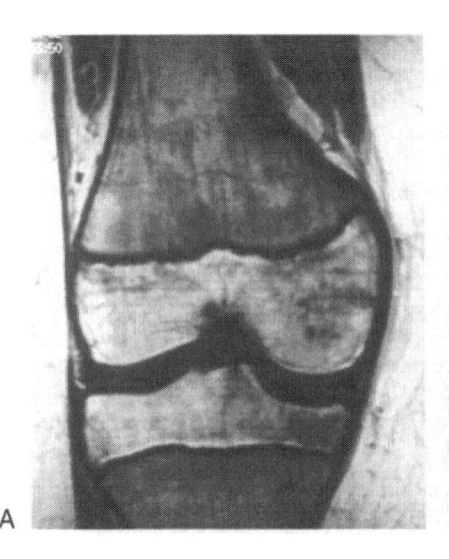

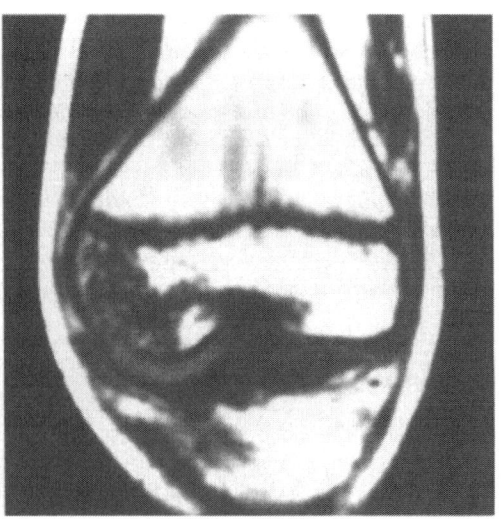

FIGURE 22-8. Bone bruising. (A) Medial femoral and tibial intraepiphyseal involvement after vehicular (bumper) impact to the knee. (B) Medial involvement after being struck by a baseball bat.

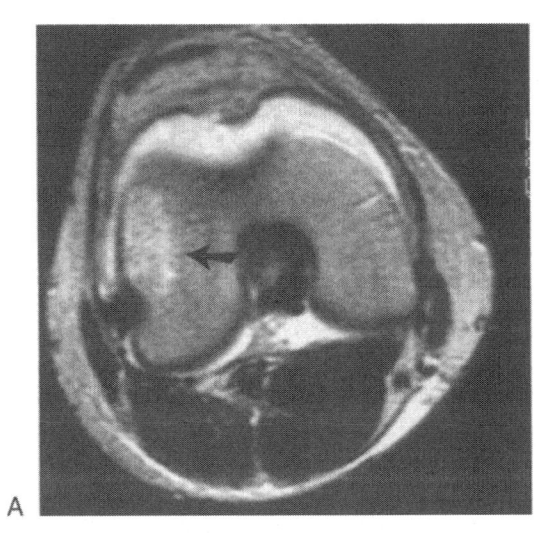

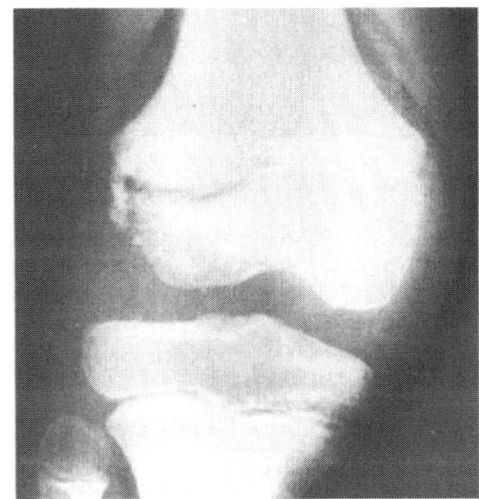

FIGURE 22-9. (A) Transverse MRI scan showing a peripheral bone bruise (arrow) after a shearing injury to the knee. (B) Five months later the lateral chondro-osseous transformation is irregular.

and lead to progressive chondral damage. Another possibility is that the osseous lesion might heal into a stiffer subchondral plate than the previously normal bone. The decreased compliance might then generate greater stiffness in the articular cartilage and predispose to lesions such as osteochondritis dissecans.

Arthroscopy

The diagnosis of traumatic disorders of the knee presents special problems in the pediatric population. The index of suspicion for internal derangement, particularly meniscal or ligament substance tears, is often low. The history of the injury is often inadequate in young children. Physical findings may be nonspecific. Arthroscopy may be advantageous in children, as it provides evidence of significant internal derangements, confirms serious articular damage, and allows the inception of appropriate therapy.[34–57]

Although arthroscopy is not a substitute for a careful history and physical examination, adequate historical and physical findings may be difficult to elicit and are often nonspecific in children. In the preadolescent, provision of historical data often becomes the burden of the parents. With increased sports involvement at earlier ages by larger numbers of children and the increased emphasis on sports participation by girls, a higher incidence of minor to significant knee injuries is expected. In one study group, 31% had a major hemarthrosis.[41]

In preadolescent patients only 55% of the preoperative clinical diagnoses were confirmed at arthroscopy. The younger the patient, the less correlation there was between findings of arthroscopy and the preoperative clinical diagnosis. Even in the adolescent, arthroscopy facilitated a more complete diagnosis. Meniscal injury was frequently overdiagnosed in both children and adolescents. In the preadolescent group with meniscal pathology as the preoperative diagnosis, the knee is often normal at arthroscopy. During adolescence chondromalacia is the most common arthroscopic finding.[38] There was also an "unanticipated" incidence of anterior cruciate ligament structural damage in the preadolescent patient. Even in the child, hemarthrosis is a harbinger of significant intraarticular insult to the knee and is a requisite for an accurate diagnosis so specific treatment may be undertaken.

Ziv and Carroll reviewed 156 arthroscopic examinations in children with knee complaints; 43 of these patients and adolescents were under 12 years of age.[57] In 93% of the cases arthroscopy was useful for preventing unnecessary arthrotomy, providing additional anatomic findings and biopsy material. In only 5% of their cases did the arthroscopy fail to provide additional information. There were no complications from the procedure. Arthroscopy is an effective diagnostic tool for children; it is easier to perform owing to the relative joint laxity, and it allows visualization of the anatomic structures, whether normal or abnormal. Although most initial reports of arthroscopy in children emphasized its diagnostic potential, treatment (arthroscopic surgery) should be done when indicated.

The results of arthroscopy in patients older than 13 years of age were not dissimilar to those reported in adults.[47] However, when patients *under* 13 years of age were analyzed, the presumptive clinical diagnosis was confirmed in only 27% of patients. Some children had significant damage to the articular cartilage that probably had been worsened by the delayed diagnosis of a meniscal tear. Progressive degenerative arthritis of the knee, often seen with undiagnosed meniscal lesions in adults, may be the outcome of similar lesions in the child. The still unossified epiphyseal cartilage is biologically plastic and may readily deform when repetitively exposed to an anatomic abnormality such as a mobile meniscal flap (tear), a joint mouse, or a foreign body. This problem is typically evident during the relatively rapid change from a spherical to a bullet-shaped femoral head in developmental hip dysplasia.

Harvell et al. reviewed 310 knee arthroscopies in 285 children. The preoperative clinical diagnoses were correlated with arthroscopic findings in only 55%;[41] 35% of this group were found to have additional pathology that had not been anticipated preoperatively. In adolescents (13–18 years), 70% of the clinical diagnoses were confirmed arthroscopically; additional pathology was also found in 25% of this group.

Romdane et al. described the formation of a pseudoaneurysm of the popliteal artery following arthroscopic meniscectomy in an 8-year-old boy.[52] They alluded to the fact that popliteal artery injury was rare in children.

Knee Dislocation

Complete dislocation of the knee is infrequent in children and adolescents. It must be clinically and radiographically distinguished from a completely displaced type 1 distal femoral physeal fracture. The trauma usually necessary to produce dislocation is more likely to cause a fracture of the distal femoral or proximal tibial epiphysis.[61,63] Dislocation is usually accompanied by variable disruptions of the unossified epiphyseal cartilage, capsular soft tissues, and ligaments and frequently by neurovascular damage, which must be accurately diagnosed so appropriate repairs may be instituted. The complication of gangrene is usually avoidable, although an incompletely patent popliteal artery may cause ischemia, which may worsen with growth and increasing functional demands. Vascular complications are usually preventable if the initial diagnosis and treatment are adequate.[60,64,65]

Because the clinical appearance of a dislocated knee may be indistinguishable from the appearance of a significantly displaced physeal/epiphyseal fracture, radiographic evaluation is essential. It allows rapid diagnosis that allows intelligent reduction if neurovascular compromise is evident during the antecedent physical examination. MRI may help to accurately define the specific soft tissue injuries.[66]

Dislocation may occur in any direction (Figs. 22-10, 22-11). Particularly, a rotational dislocation may occur, leaving some of the soft tissues intact (Fig. 22-12).[58]

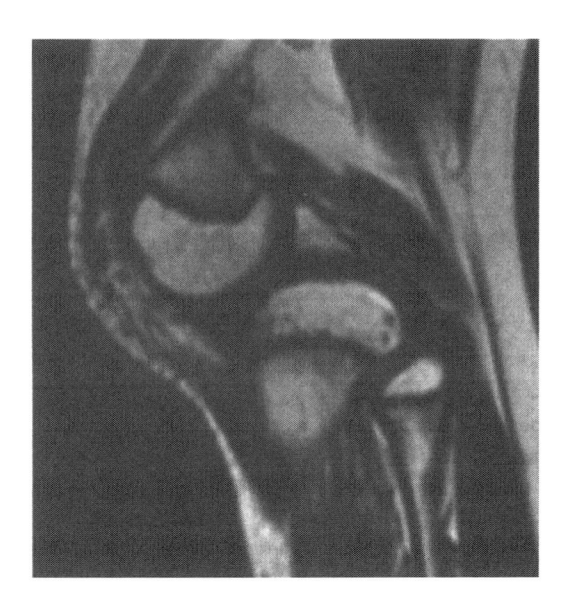

FIGURE 22-10. Dislocation of the knee with anterior femoral displacement in a 12-year-old boy.

The posterior tibialis and dorsalis pedis pulses should be evaluated thoroughly in any child with knee dislocation. If they are not present, the dislocation must be reduced as quickly as possible and the distal circulation immediately reevaluated. If at this point the circulation is still not normal, the popliteal artery should be assessed. Arteriography provides additional information, although the location of the lesion should be obvious. Intimal damage may be more easily diagnosed by arteriography. If performed, arteriography should not prolong the interval between injury and completion of surgical exploration, repair, or anastomosis beyond 6–8 hours. Postoperatively, the patient must be monitored closely for compartment syndrome. Even if no vascular damage occurs, the patient must be monitored closely. Normal circulatory dynamics are disrupted while the knee remains dislocated. The rapid restoration of arterial inflow following reduction may not be accompanied by normal venous/lymphatic outflow. This situation increases capil-

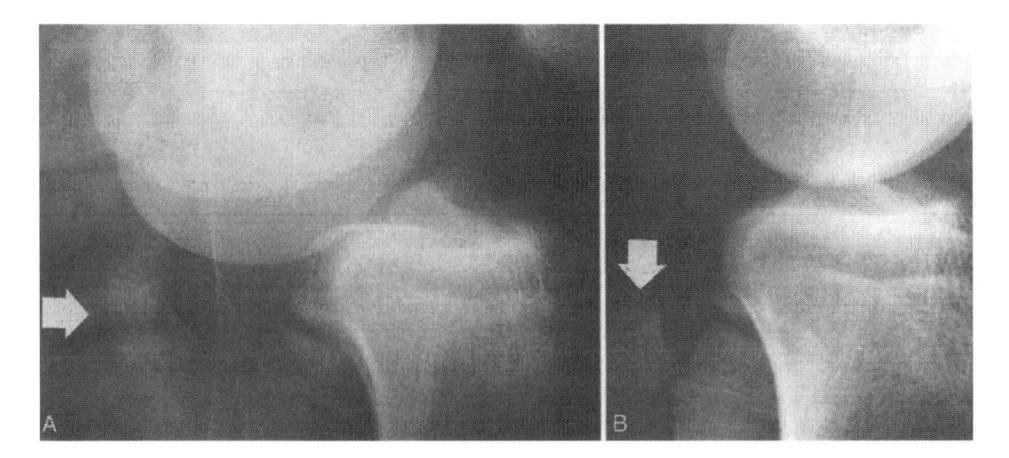

FIGURE 22-11. (A) Knee dislocation with posterior femoral displacement in a 14-year-old boy. The arrow indicates a concomitant type 3 fibular growth mechanism injury. (B) Initial reduction was successful. However, the concomitant type 3 fracture of the proximal fibular epiphysis did not reduce (arrow). Several days later this fracture was reduced surgically, and at the same time the fibular collateral ligament was reattached to the femoral condyle (the ligament avulsed along with a segment of epiphyseal cartilage).

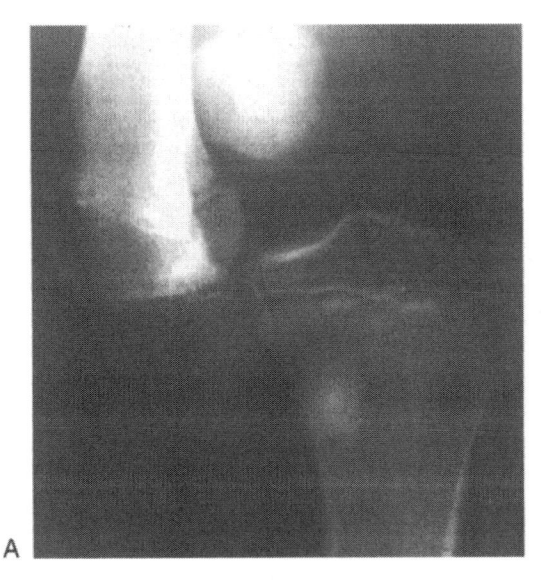

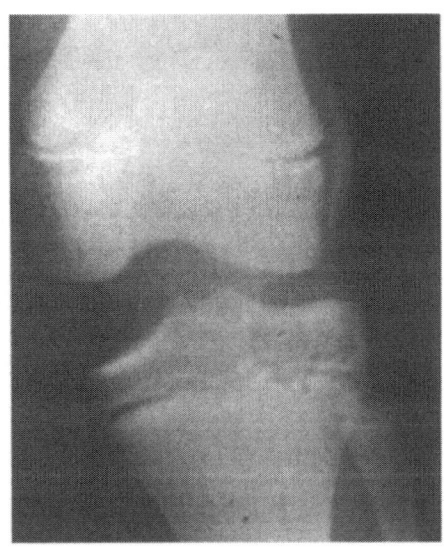

FIGURE 22-12. (A) Dislocation of the knee with medial displacement of the femur. The distal femur is also rotated, whereas the patella still appears attached to the tibia. The tibia, soft tissue, and patella resemble that in Figure 22-6C. It was reduced and treated nonoperatively. (B) Fourteen months later there is medial instability (widening of the joint space during stance). Laterally, it has undergone ossification within the sleeve of lateral cartilage that had been avulsed as a sleeve chondro-osseous fracture when the rest of the epiphysis displaced medially. The lateral collateral ligament was intact, as the original injury was a peripheral fracture rather than a ligament tear.

lary perfusion into the interstitial space with subsequent increased hydrostatic pressure within the myofascial compartments.

The collateral circulation about the knee is variable, especially from the standpoint of being able to sustain completely the rigorous functional activity of the lower leg of an adolescent. The femoral-popliteal artery is variably fixed to the femur at the adductor hiatus and tibia by a fibrous arch. Within the popliteal region, the artery gives rise to the geniculate branches. Although these arteries eventually anastomose with the branches of the anterior tibial recurrent artery, they may not provide adequate blood supply to maintain the *functional* needs of the lower leg musculature of an active child or adolescent, even though the resting circulatory demands may be adequate. An acute popliteal artery injury, particularly one associated with concomitant damage to some of the smaller vessels, hardly allows time for compensatory hypertrophy of collateral circulatory patterns. In some cases the viability of the musculature and skeleton, even at rest, is not adequately provided by an acute circulatory deficiency, which may lead to Volkmann's ischemia in the lower leg.

Vascular repair should be completed within 6–8 hours *from the time of injury* to avoid amputation or the subsequent chronic ischemic problems of *relative functional insufficiency*.[64] Of the patients not treated within that defined time period, 86% went on to amputation and two-thirds of the remaining 14% had chronic ischemic changes. Even if the artery was repaired after 8 hours, many of these patients required eventual amputation of the leg.[64]

Following vascular repair it is essential that the lower leg be closely observed for compartment syndrome. Even if the artery is intact, one must be alert to the appearance of this syndrome as the consequences of muscle infarction and subsequent lower leg and foot dysfunction obviously affect rehabilitation of the reduced knee.

Cummings et al. described an unusual syndrome of popliteal artery entrapment in children.[59] The symptoms of vascular insufficiency were caused by an anomalous course of the popliteal artery or anomalous muscles' impingement on it. Surgical excision of the fibrous band that is often present is the recommended treatment choice. A similar phenomenon could feasibly occur after knee dislocation if extensive posterior scarring occurred.

During vascular repair extensive reconstruction of the knee ligaments usually should not be undertaken, as it would increase the swelling, tissue damage, and potential for further damage to the collateral circulation. At the time of arterial repair, reasonably complete fasciotomies are recommended because of the marked increase in muscular compartment swelling after restoration of the circulation.

Knee dislocation usually heals well if it is reduced immediately (closed reduction). However, adequately documented follow-up of young children less than 10–11 years of age with this injury is rare.[61] Acute surgery should not be undertaken in children except under well-defined circumstances (neurovascular damage, in particular). Reconstructive surgery should be deferred for several months to allow assessment of healing. Cruciate ligament reconstruction must be approached cautiously prior to skeletal maturity. Collateral ligaments may heal well because the failure may be a peripheral sleeve fracture (Fig. 22-12) that heals by fracture healing, not by ligament healing.

Figure 22-11 shows a 14-year-old boy who sustained a knee dislocation and a concomitant fibular epiphyseal fracture. He was treated with a closed reduction. The epiphyseal fracture of the fibula did not reduce commensurate with the reduction of the knee dislocation. Several days later the lateral side of the knee was explored and the fibular fracture reduced. The lateral collateral ligament was repaired where it directly avulsed from the femoral epiphysis. There was no repair of the medial collateral ligament. Follow-up 5 years later showed a knee that was sufficiently functional to allow him to play competitive football.

If there is well-defined abnormal capsular laxity after the child goes through a subsequent period of development, the knee may be explored and a formal repair undertaken. When these procedures are done, care must be taken to restore the normal anatomic relations and not damage cartilage along the epiphyseal margins or physis. The pes anserinus attaches along the medial metaphysis of the proximal tibia; and during reflection for a repair it should be elevated away with the periosteum, with which it is confluent, and reflected proximally. Such a procedure may damage the physeal periphery (zone of Ranvier) and lead to a localized osseous bridge and angular growth deformity of either the main tibial or tuberosity physes.

Cooper et al. noted that complete knee dislocation usually causes disruption of both the anterior and posterior cruciate ligaments.[58] However, they described four cases of complete knee dislocation *without* posterior cruciate ligament disruption. All their patients sustained either anterior or anteromedial dislocation with anterior cruciate ligament disruption and collateral ligament injury. An intact posterior cruciate ligament obviously affects treatment options favorably.[67]

Knee Subluxation

Ferris described a syndrome of congenital snapping knee by habitual anterior subluxation of the tibia in extension.[62] In each instance, the tibia subluxated anteriorly on the femur when the knee was extended and reduced spontaneously during flexion. All patients had dysplastic features in the knee and had different clinical syndromes (e.g., Larson syndrome, congenital short tibia). The authors did not use MRI to look at the morphology of the cruciate ligaments.

Patellar Dislocation

Patellar displacements are relatively common in children and adolescents when the entire spectrum of acute and chronic subluxation and dislocation is considered. However, complete dislocation of the patella is infrequent in a physically normal, skeletally immature individual.[82] In contrast, in children with predisposing factors (e.g., Down syndrome, muscular dystrophy, arthrogryposis), other neuromuscular abnormalities or excessive ligament laxity dislocation may be frequent and repetitive.[80] Chronic or habitual subluxation often mimics dislocation in terms of subjective complaints. Some children with neurologic disorders, such as hyperactivity or attention deficit syndrome, voluntarily dislocate the patella as an attention-getting maneuver.

McManus et al. reviewed 55 cases and thought that most children with acute dislocation of the patella demonstrated roentgenographic signs of patellofemoral dysplasia, suggesting that most of the acute dislocations occurred in the knees of children who had some preexistent anatomic variation or abnormality.[82] Acute dislocations simply add further damage to the dysplasia and result in the knee becoming increasingly symptomatic. The early onset of recurrent dislocation undoubtedly affects development of the cartilaginous patella and femoral condyles. Repetitive displacement leads to lateral tightening and medial attenuation in the retinacular tissues and may impede lateral condylar development of the femur.

Acute lateral dislocation may be caused by a direct blow to the medial side of the patella or twisting, muscular contractions when the knee is placed in valgus stress. The dislocation may be complete or incomplete (Fig. 22-13). Acute lateral displacement must be accompanied by a variable degree of soft tissue injury to the medial patellar retinaculum or avulsion of a portion of the medial chondro-osseous tissue (Figs. 22-14 to 22-16). There is usually hemorrhage within the joint.

The laterally displaced patella often reduces spontaneously, or it may be pushed back inadvertently. The orthopaedic surgeon rarely sees the patella in its dislocated state. The knee is maintained in some flexion with a definite limitation toward full extension. Unless the patient presents with the patella dislocated, the diagnosis must be made on an historical basis; it is often difficult to distinguish from chronic subluxation.

If the patient is seen acutely, the diagnosis should be evident clinically. Radiography of the dislocation may be done to confirm the diagnosis and rule out other fractures, but, radiography is more important after reduction.

Gilbert et al. described medial retinacular tears that also included osteochondral fragments by utilizing MRI.[77] They described bone bruising of the lateral aspect of the distal lateral femoral condyle, probably due to the impingement at the time of the dislocation. Condylar osteochondral injury may also occur.[89,90]

Ordinarily, reduction of an acute dislocation is easy. The hip is flexed to relax the rectus femoris, and the knee is gradually extended and the patella pushed medially into its normal position. General anesthesia is rarely necessary. There is usually effusion in the knee joint, but aspiration is not necessary unless the swelling is painful. Because the patella usually does not redislocate easily, the knee should be radiographed following reduction, with good views to determine if there are any obvious osteochondral fractures from the condyles or patella, and whether they are intra-articular. It may not be possible to obtain a complete roentgenographic examination at the time of acute injury, as a sunrise view may be uncomfortable.

Following reduction, adequate radiographic views should be attained to look for peripheral avulsions, especially medially. The disruption of soft tissues on the medial side, as the patella displaces laterally, may occur within the retinacular tissues. Prior to skeletal maturity there may be a chondro-osseous separation along the edges, especially medially (see Patellar Fractures, Sleeve Fracture, below). If some of the subchondral bone is avulsed, the diagnosis may be made before or after treatment. If the separation is purely cartilaginous, diagnosis of a true patellar fracture, in contrast to a soft tissue injury, may be difficult. In such cases the avulsed

Patellar Dislocation

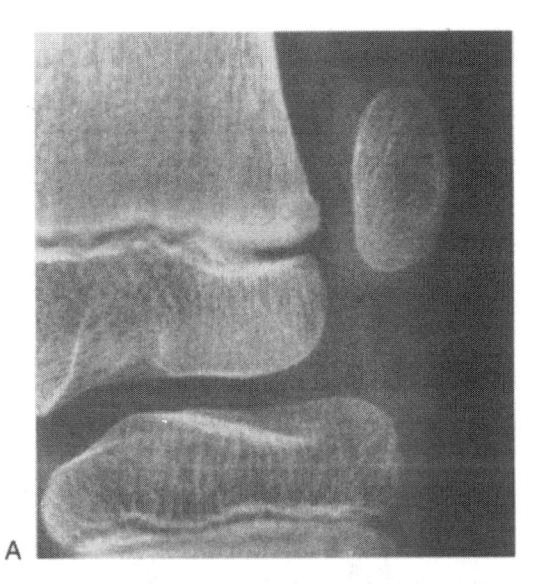

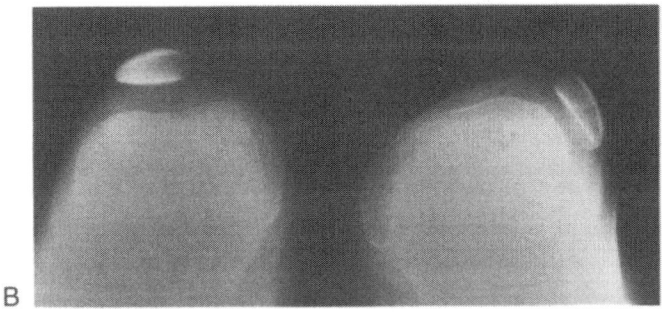

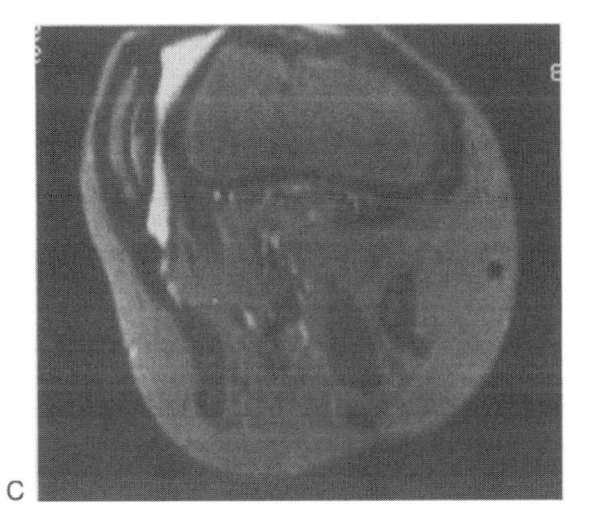

FIGURE 22-13. Complete lateral dislocation of the patella. (A) Oblique. (B) Sunrise. (C) MRI.

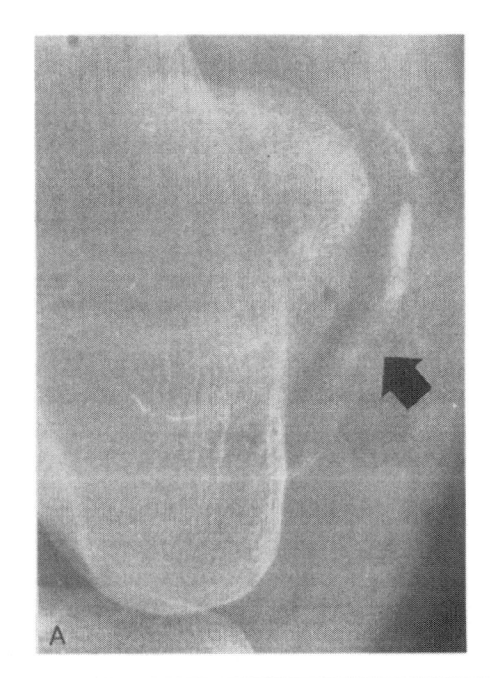

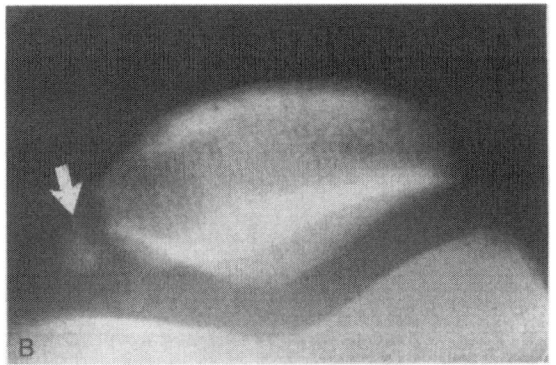

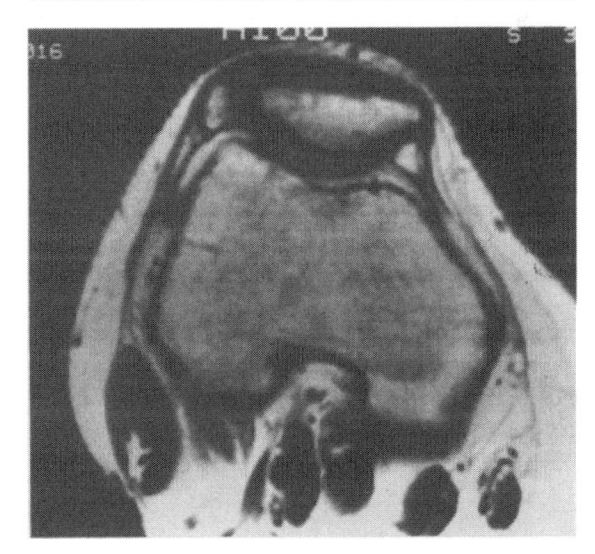

FIGURE 22-14. Anterior (A) and sunrise (B) views of an avulsion fracture of the lateral margin (arrow) of the patella following acute dislocation. (C) MRI of a similiar case involving the medial side.

segment eventually ossifies and may give the appearance of a bipartite patella or peripheral nonunion. If significant separation of such fragments can be detected after the initial reduction, the treating surgeon should consider tension band fixation if a sufficient gap (more than 2–3 mm) persists.

Acute surgical intervention is indicated only in the patient who exhibits significant concomitant soft injury or when

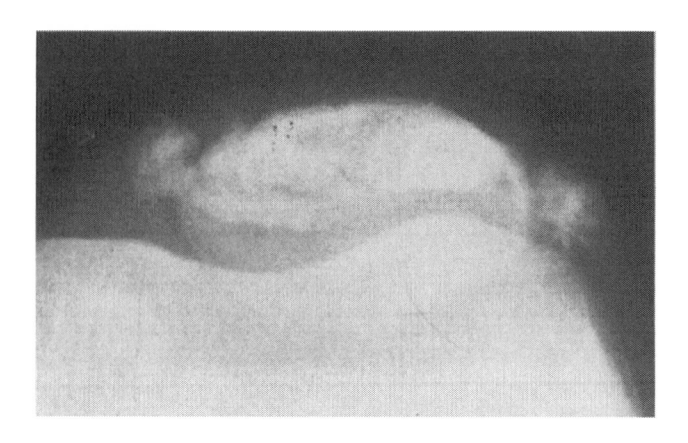

FIGURE 22-15. Medial and lateral sleeve avulsions in a patient who sustained an acute dislocation followed by multiple recurrences of subluxation and dislocation. Note the lateral position of the patella in the intercondylar notch.

there is displacement of the patella or a fragment into the joint, which occurs when the quadriceps muscle contracts strongly after the blow. The failure is usually at the chondroosseous junction.

Roger et al. noted that traumatic lateral dislocations with internal rotation of the patella may be unreducible because they involve locking of the patella on the lateral femoral condyle.[87] These authors believed that reduction could be achieved by applying a downward force to the lateral aspect of the patella, reducing the rotational deformity and unlocking the medial patellar facet. This type of locking and difficulty of reduction is more likely to occur in older patients (adolescent) than in the more loosely ligamentous child.

The limb is placed in a cylinder cast or knee immobilizer for 3–6 weeks. The aforementioned imaging evaluation procedure is repeated during the subsequent recovery phase after return of sufficient motion to allow adequate positioning for roentgenographic examination.

During the reparative (immobilization) phase, a contracture may develop in the iliotibial band and lateral retinaculum, leading to further lateralization. This accentuates the tendency for the patella to then chronically subluxate or dislocate following acute dislocation (Fig. 22-17). In the patient with a chronically subluxating or dislocating patella, surgery

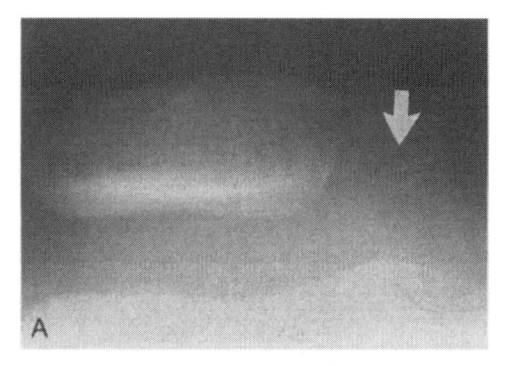

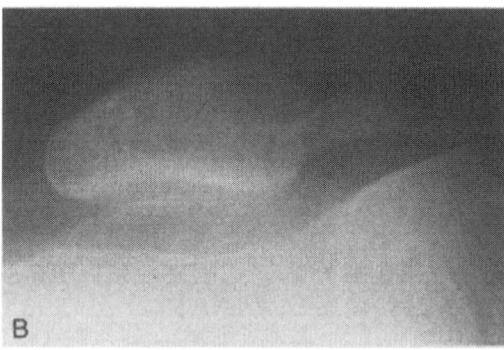

FIGURE 22-16. (A) Appearance of a minimally discernible acute medial avulsion (arrow). (B) One year later the avulsed area has further ossified.

may be more effective if done electively, after the knee has recovered from the acute injury.[70]

Rarely is the patella displaced medially. Miller et al. reported traumatic medial dislocation of the patella in a child.[83] Interestingly, all three of their patients had undergone lateral retinacular release for chronic knee pain or recurrent lateral patellar subluxation.

Intraarticular Dislocation

Intraarticular dislocation of the patella is unusual in children.[69,71–76,78,79,83–86,88] The lesion occurs in skeletally immature individuals because the soft tissue attachments to the patella

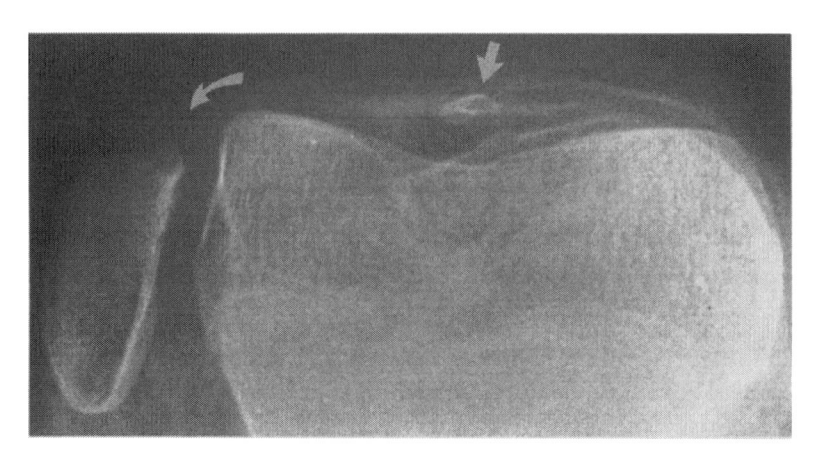

FIGURE 22-17. Sunrise view of repetitive lateral dislocation (curved arrow) of the patella, with a residual medial remnant (straight arrow).

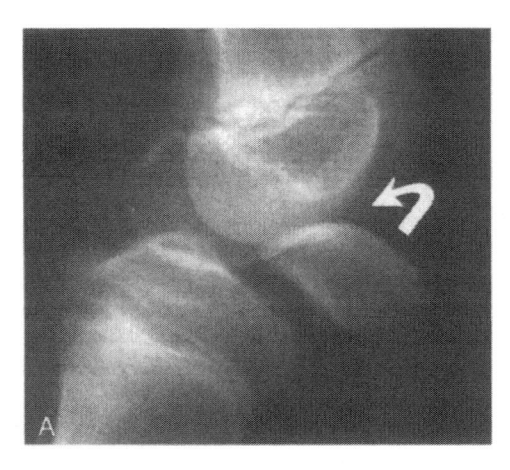

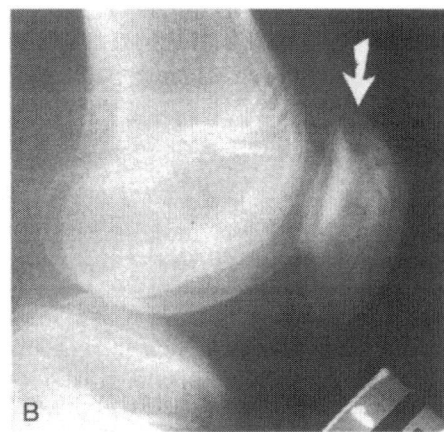

FIGURE 22-18. (A) Lateral roentgenograms of intraarticular dislocation (arrow) of the patella. (B) Postreduction film showing early irregular ossification (arrow) 4 months after the injury.

are more lax, and mobility is greater; with direct trauma to the flexed knee the cartilage and soft tissues may be stripped relatively easily from the osseous patella (i.e., at or near the chondro-osseous interface). In adults a comparable injurious force would most likely cause a fracture.

There are two basic types of intraarticular dislocation. The most common type involves the patella being torn loose from the quadriceps mechanism, with or without the superior cartilage (i.e., a sleeve fracture), so it lodges in the femoral intercondylar notch, with its articular surface directed toward the tibia (Fig. 22-18). With the other type, which is rare, the inferior portion of the patella is separated from the patellar tendon and cartilage (again, a sleeve fracture), and pushed posteriorly into the intercondylar notch. Alioto and Kates[68] and Levin[81] have described a vertical intraarticular dislocation.

The mechanism of injury is probably a direct blow initially displacing the patella into the intercondylar notch; the dissection of the patella from the extensor mechanism undoubtedly occurs when the quadriceps contracts strongly from the blow. The failure is at the chondro-osseous junction.

Additional associated lesions should be sought with both types of intraarticular dislocation. The quadriceps tendon may be ruptured completely, or the patellar tendon may be partially torn from the tibial tuberosity. Tears of the cruciate and collateral ligaments may also occur.

Some authors believe that this type of dislocation is secondary to rupture of the quadriceps tendon. Frangakis described an 11-year-old boy who fell while running, striking his left knee against the edge of a step.[76] In this case the quadriceps tendon was intact and there was associated ligamentous laxity. Frangakis thought that a ruptured quadriceps tendon, although it may occur, was by no means necessary for this type of dislocation to manifest in a child.

Closed reduction is generally not effective. Open reduction should be the primary procedure, if only to inspect the extent of injury and repair both soft tissue and chondro-osseous damage.

Habitual Dislocation

As for the shoulder, certain children become habitual dislocaters of the patella. These children have frequent displacement, sometimes several times a day. Many have underlying personality disorders (e.g., hyperactive behavior, attention deficit syndrome) and may repetitively dislocate the joint to get someone's attention. These patients rarely have soft tissue or chondro-osseous disruption as in the patient who has an acute traumatic dislocation. Instead, they attenuate medial retinacular tissues and contract lateral retinacular tissues.

Treatment may be difficult. Obviously, treatment of any behavioral problem to try to decrease the "need" to demonstrate dislocatibility is necessary. Muscle strengthening and orthotics are minimally effective. In fact, the behavioral problem is likely to make the child inattentive to the therapist's efforts. Lateral retinacular release (arthroscopic) with or without vastus medialis advancement is usually necessary.

Dabezies and Schutte reported a 2-year-old with chronic habitual dislocation of the patella in whom there was a significant contracture of the iliotibial band (probably congenital) that was divided along with advancement of the vastus medialis muscle.[96] I have encountered significant iliotibial band thickening in children with hypoplasia of the femur along with the characteristic lateral condylar hypoplasia. Surgical release was necessary in most cases to correct patellar maltracking that became increasingly problematic during the limb lengthening process.

Chronic Subluxation

Chronic subluxation of the patella is a common knee disorder, especially in adolescent girls.[92,94,99,101,102,110] A significant number of subluxations and recurrent dislocations of the patella in the young child or adolescent are associated with a congenital or developmental deficiency of the extensor mechanism, the femoral condyles, or the shape of the patella and femoral notch (groove).[97,98] Such deficiencies of the extensor mechanism may be divided into three categories: (1) abnormalities of patellofemoral configuration; (2) deficiencies of the supporting muscles or guiding mechanism; and (3) malalignment of the extremity relative to knee mechanics. Often deficiencies in more than one category contribute to patellar instability.[95] Wiberg and Baumgartl have described various types of patella based on relative degrees of sloping of the medial and lateral articular facets in the sunrise view.[114] Such measurements are variably applicable to the incompletely ossified patella. Transverse MRI views may allow such measurement of the unossified cartilage.[111] Weakness of the anteromedial retinaculum, dystrophy or weakness of the vastus medialis obliquus muscle, and hypermobility of the patella due to poor muscle tone also constitute predisposing factors. Genu recurvatum may cause laxity of the extensor mechanism. Patella alta and tightness of the lateral retinaculum also predispose the patella to subluxation or dislocation.

Posttraumatic tightness in the lateral rectinaculum may lead to chronic subluxation following an acute patellar dislocation. This probably occurs because of the medial soft tissue disruption.

Moller et al. induced chondromalacia in rabbits by surgical patellar subluxation.[106] The experiment included 20 immature and 20 mature rabbits. The tibial tuberosity was laterally displaced. At 6 weeks after surgery all the nonoperated knees appeared microscopically normal. Histologically, cartilage degeneration was evident on the experimental side. By 3 months macroscopic changes were evident in 5 of the 10 mature rabbits *but not in the immature rabbits*. Moller et al. thought that this model suggested the importance of malalignment in the development of patellofemoral cartilage degeneration. The initial lesion of the cartilage was primarily a change in the ground substance of the intermittent zones, alone or in association with surface defibrillation. Alteration of glycosaminoglycans may occur in knees during experimental femoral lengthening. Altered mechanics due to subluxation may change joint reaction forces sufficiently to affect the matrix, creating molecular and cellular changes that alter the consistency of the cartilage, beginning the cycle of softening and breakdown consistent with chondromalacia.

Early changes in chondromalacia patella may heal by cartilaginous or fibrous metaplasia, which may account for the resolution of clinical symptoms.[93] In view of findings of the response of cartilage cells to increased pressure with dissolution of cartilage matrix to excessive pressure (see Chapter 1), simple surgical procedures, such as lateral retinacular release to decrease pressure, may be effective prior to skeletal maturity.

Symptoms may be vague. Chronic patellar instability is frequently confused with meniscal injury and certainly should be considered in all patients with relatively nonspecific knee complaints. Limited use of the knee in these painful stages may lead to chondromalacia.

The patella may forcefully reduce if it has been partially displaced onto the lateral condyle and cause injury to the medial patellar articular surface or intercondylar region of the medial femoral condyle. Damage may also be intratrabecular (i.e., bone bruising), which could affect the physiology of the deeper layers of unossified hyaline cartilage.

Thompson et al., in a study of injuries to the patellofemoral joint after acute transarticular loading, found significant changes in the subchondral bone when a fracture was not identifiable on conventional radiographs.[112] They further found that under certain conditions there was a potential for repair of the histopathologic abnormalities and restoration of normality to the articular cartilage and subchondral bone.

Diagnosis is usually by history, as the patella is rarely completely displaced. Maltracking may be evident on physical examination. It is more important, as suggested by Yates and Grana,[32] to base the diagnosis of patellofemoral pain on a precise history and physical examination rather than relying on the radiographic appearance and measurements.

The primary difficulty when treating patellofemoral pain syndrome in children has been the inability to translate distinct problems recognized during the physical examination into a specific clinical classification. Yates and Grana used a classification system based on etiology rather than symptoms and thought it was a better guide for treatment.[32] They believed that most patellofemoral pain in children was caused by trauma or malalignment syndromes (or a combination of the two) and could usually be managed successfully with nonoperative methods. The classification of patellar disorders proposed by Merchant[104] is a clinically relevant system that helps the clinician categorize complaints and physical findings in a manner based on etiology. The chondromalacic lesion seen in a young patient as a result of trauma usually is associated with flaps, chondral separations, or osteochondral fractures, in contrast to the soft fibrillated lesions seen in adults.

Roentgenograms may show patellar deformation and a less prominent lateral femoral condyle (Fig. 22-19). The radiographic diagnosis is sometimes subtle and difficult in young children or adolescents. Anteroposterior views are not particularly remarkable. A lateral view obtained with the knee at 30° to assess certain relations has resulted in the concept of the line of Blumensaat.[114] Insall and Salvati also described the length of patella to length of tendon ratio.[100] However, *these assessments require a completely ossified patella and tibial tuberosity; otherwise they are inaccurate*. Similarly, tangential views such as the Hughston view require almost complete ossification of the femoral condyles and patella to create accurate lines.

Reikeras and Hoiseth measured the relations of the patellofemoral joint with a knee in extension in 43 normal adults.[109] They did not find any significant differences between men and women. They noted that CT scans of the upper and lower halves of the patellofemoral joint showed variations in the sulcus angle, the congruence angle, and the lateral patellar angle. They found that individual variations were great, especially for the congruence angle, and that there were variations apparent in the patellofemoral relations from the proximal to the distal parts of the joint that may be reflected in different degrees of knee flexion. However, it must be remembered that these measurements in still ossifying femoral condyles and patellas in a skeletally immature child or adolescent may be misleading if they are treated as arbitrary measurements. Ando et al. described a method using CT scans to measure the rectus femoris/patellar tendon Q-angle compared with conventional methods.[91]

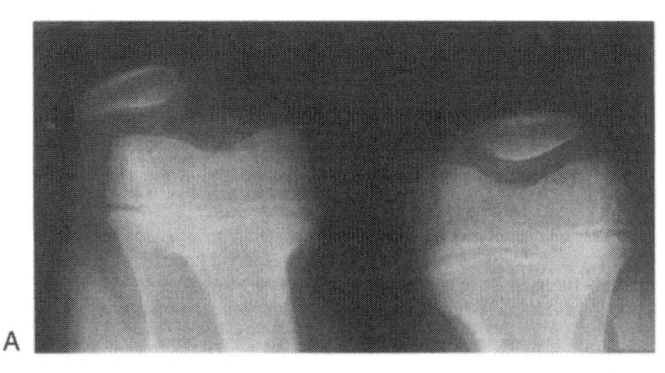

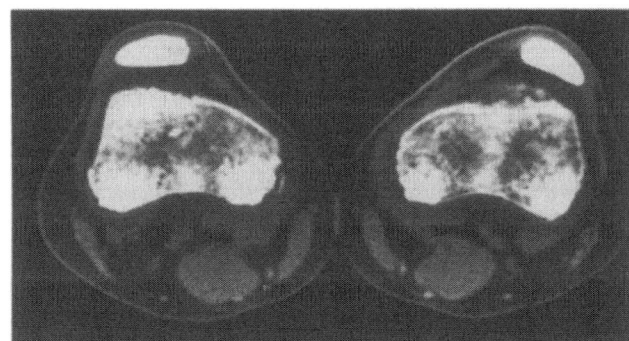

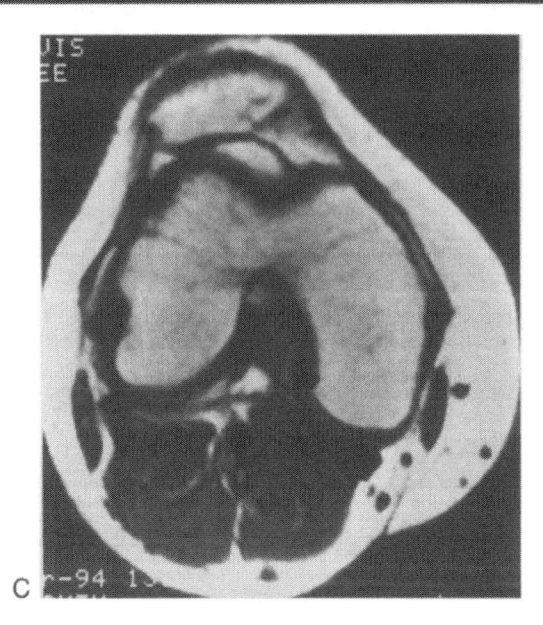

FIGURE 22-19. (A) Sunrise view of patellar subluxation. (B) CT scan. (C) MRI. Note the "short" lateral retinaculum and the attenuated medial tissues.

Nietosvaara and Aalto used ultrasonography to evaluate patellar tracking and found significant changes of maltracking in early flexion as a predisposing factor to patellar subluxation and dislocation, especially when compared with normal knees.[107] The Q-angle was wider and the patellar position more lateral and proximal than in the normal knee.

Initial treatment is immobilization when the patient is acutely symptomatic and a rigorous exercise program subsequently. Failure of conservative therapy should lead to consideration of surgery.[113]

O'Neill et al. studied 30 patients, including 13 skeletally immature patients, in a prospective study designed to evaluate the effect of isometric quadriceps strengthening exercises on the patellofemoral pain syndrome.[108] Each of these patients had an anatomically normal knee with no history of trauma. The authors found that an equal number of skeletally immature patients and adults had a decrease in peripatellar pain. However, 5 of 17 adults had to limit their physical activities, whereas no adolescent patient had to limit activity after the exercise program. Furthermore, eight skeletally immature knees had a more than 5° change in their congruence angles; adults did not exhibit a similar change. O'Neill et al. recommended immediate inception of an isometric progressive resistance quadriceps program with iliotibial band and hamstring stretching exercises to alleviate the patellofemoral pain syndrome. Two of the skeletally immature girls required arthroscopic lateral releases after 6 months of exercise therapy. Patellar bracing and antiinflammatory medications had failed to lessen the pain. One patient did not experience a decrease in the pain after the release. Long-term compliance with an exercise program was the major problem.

Micheli and Stanitski performed 41 lateral retinacular releases in 33 adolescent patients and analyzed 24 of these patients 8–16 months after surgery.[105] None of these patients had undergone surgery until they had had a minimum of 3 months of supervised nonoperative management emphasizing flexibility and static strengthening of the quadriceps and hamstrings. The authors found that lateral knee retinacular release did not interfere with the permanent alignment of the extensor mechanism in the skeletally immature individual and recommended the procedure for patients who do not have evidence of significant patellar malalignment, who are skeletally immature, and who fail a supervised, conscientious preoperative therapeutic program.

Lefort et al. described 93 knees in 74 children and adolescents, ranging in age between 9 and 20 years who were operated on because of patellofemoral instability.[103] In 76 knees there was intractable patellofemoral pain, and in 17 cases there had been one or more episodes of patellar dislocation. All patients had been subjected to rigorous physical therapy that had failed. In 14 instances a vastus medialis advancement was performed coupled with lateral retinacular release; in 71 knees there was transfer of the patellar ligament. Altogether 85 knees were followed for an average of 6 years: 45 were completely free of symptoms; 34 had residual pain; and 6 patellas redislocated. The authors believed that patellar tendon realignment was more effective than vastus medialis transfer.

Bonnard et al. described translation of the medial third of the patellar tendon combined with lateral retinacular release in 16 patients (27 knees).[94] They found that the results were excellent in 60% and good in 20%. There was no evidence of growth disturbance of the tibial tuberosity.

Transposition of the tibial tuberosity medially to effect a better biomechanical axis of the patellofemoral joint is frequently advocated for chronic patellar subluxation. However, its use in children who have not yet attained skeletal maturity may be associated with premature epiphysiodesis of the anterior portion of the proximal tibial physis. Rosenthal and Levine studied the effects of tibial tubercle transplantation in skeletally immature children (16 patients with 20 transplantations).[258] Many of these children had neuromuscular disorders, with cerebral palsy being the most common. Six had recurrent lateral dislocation of the patella. The procedures were performed when the children were under 11 years of age. All were treated by transplanting the tibial tuberosity. Three patients sustained a fracture through the operative site. Growth continued in the contiguous proximal tibial epiphysis in many of these cases, with resultant further distal "migration" of the transplanted tuberosity. In all cases, however, the tibial tuberosity epiphysis failed to develop normally after transplantation.

Ligaments

Ligament injury must be considered in the differential diagnosis of any child sustaining knee trauma, even though fractures, especially physeal injuries, are more likely to occur.[119,126,136,144,148,154,156,162,168,175,183,187] *A physeal fracture may occur in combination with a ligament injury.* Congenital ligament deficiencies may not become evident until the child sustains an acute injury.[124,147] However, such deficiencies are usually associated with other congenital deficiencies (e.g., anterior cruciate ligament absence in a hypoplastic femur or fibular hemimelia). Another factor is the degree of laxity around a joint, which is significant in young children (Fig. 22-20) but becomes progressively less as physeal closure is approached. Injury to the ligaments of the knee in children less than 14 years old is uncommon, presumably because the resilience and strength of the ligaments are greater than those of the chondro-osseous interfaces, physis, and bone. However, utilizing arthroscopy to evaluate acute hemarthrosis reveals that ligamentous tears probably occur more often in children than is currently appreciated.[39]

Baxter assessed normal pediatric knee ligament laxity, examining 464 normal knees in 232 children between the ages of 7 and 14 years.[118] A progressive decrease in the absolute value of both translation and rotation laxity was evident as the age of the child increased. Significant differences between right and left knees of the same patient were not seen, nor did there appear to be any sex-related difference in laxity. Simple clinical testing to evaluate loose jointedness is believed to be of some value for identifying children who might be at greater risk of joint injury during competitive sports.[157] Attempts to predict athletic injury rates in children and adolesents in this fashion have produced conflicting results.[140,142] The absolute value of the measure of translation in the anterior, posterior, and varus-valgus plane decreased progressively from age 7 to 14 years. The translation index showed the same progressive decrease, as did rotational maneuvers. Thus as the child ages, the knee ligament laxity clearly changes. Interestingly, Baxter confirmed the long-standing impression that the ligaments of a child who was large for his or her age appeared to be tighter than those in the small, aesthenic child of the same age.[118] The incidence of disruption of knee ligaments in the older child or adolescent is increasing. Reasons probably relate to more vigorous participation in athletic activities and increased awareness of the possibility of ligamentous lesions in this age group that has led to the increased application of diagnostic modalities such as arthroscopy and MRI. The belief that open physes invariably fail before supporting ligaments is *not* always true. When the child is undergoing physiologic epiphysiodesis during adolescence, the ligaments do increase their relative propensity to failure compared to the physis.

Numerous factors are involved at the site of ligament failure, including the histologic structure, attachment to bone or cartilage, degree of chondro-osseous maturation in the epiphysis, and physeal anatomy.[167,190] The rate of strain and the site and direction of the application of force related to the position of the knee when the strain is applied are important.[128,167] The relation of the attachment of the col-

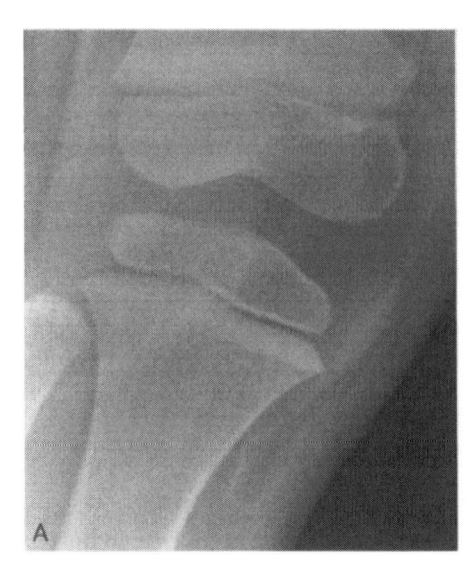

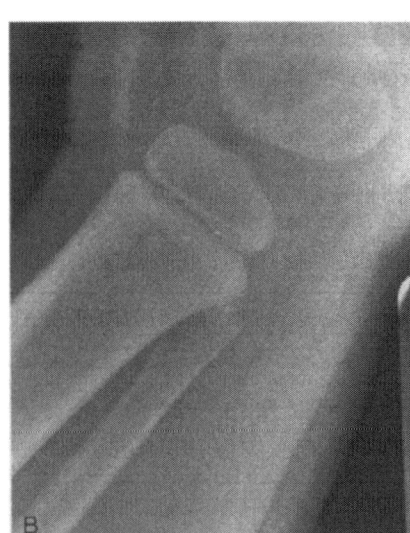

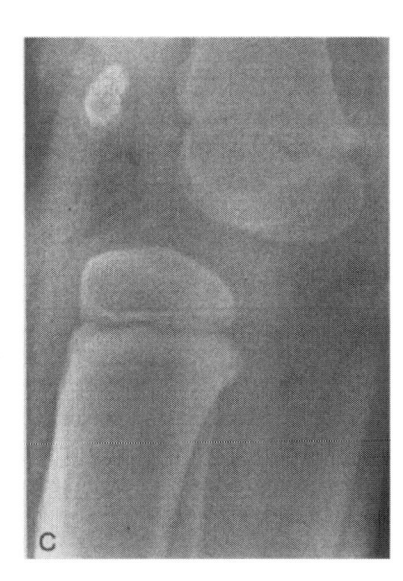

FIGURE 22-20. Ligamentous laxity in a 9-year-old boy. (A) Valgus stress. (B) Accentuated recurvatum. (C) Accentuated drawer test. Some degree of hyperlaxity is not uncommon in children.

FIGURE 22-21. (A) Patient with joint injury and avulsion of the tibial spine. (B) Stress films of both knees showed widening of the medial joint space (arrow) of the right knee due to a medial collateral ligament tear. Comparision should be done because of the normally increased ligament laxity in children.

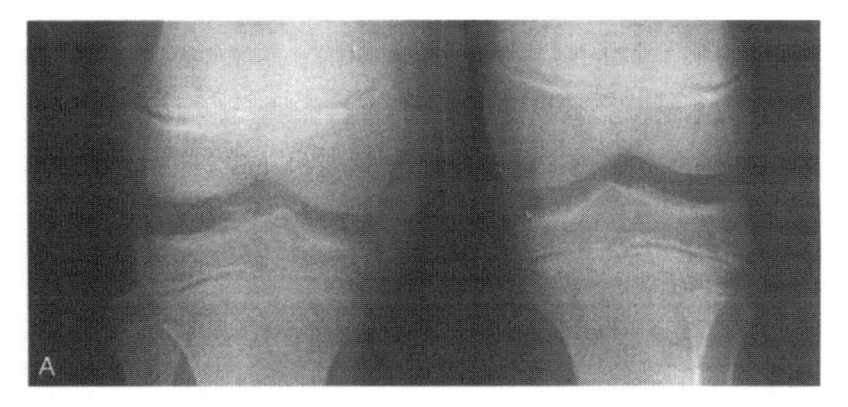

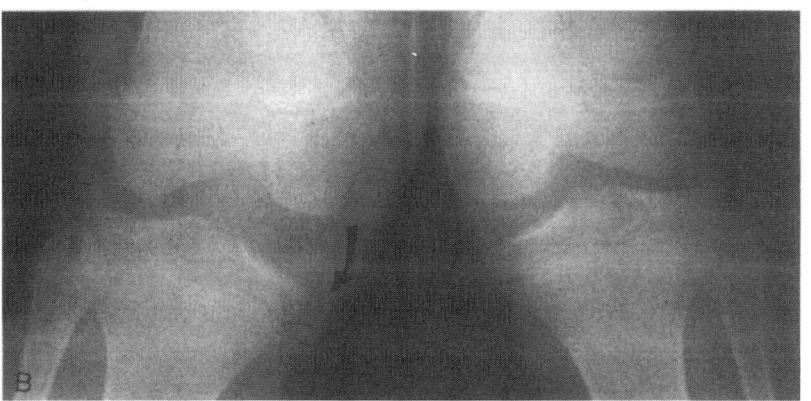

lateral ligaments and joint capsule to the physis influences the site of injury.

Combinations of physeal separation and ligamentous disruption may occur (Fig. 22-21). Kennedy and Grainger reported a 14-year-old who suffered a type 3 physeal injury and avulsion of the anterior cruciate ligament from the tibial spine; reduction of the physeal injury alone would not have controlled the existing instability.[153] When physeal separations are diagnosed in the adolescent, be alert to the fact that ligamentous damage may accompany the chondro-osseous lesion.

Bertin and Goble studied 29 cases of epiphyseal separations and found that 14 of the patients *also* had ligament instability at follow-up an average of 66 months after injury.[119] Of 16 patients with distal femoral fractures, 6 had ligament insufficiency, and 8 of 13 proximal tibial physeal fractures had associated ligamentous injuries. These authors concluded that a physeal fracture about the knee did *not* exclude obvious or occult ligament damage and, in fact, was associated with a high incidence of ligament injury.

Kannus and Jarvinen reviewed 32 patients who sustained a substantial knee ligament injury during adolescence when their knee physes were open.[152] All were treated nonoperatively and reexamined an average of 8 years after the injury. There were 25 partial tears and seven complete tears. After partial tears injuries, the functional results were excellent or good, although static instability had not improved significantly from the initial posttraumatic examination. The long-term results of complete injuries were poor because of chronic functional instability, with continuous symptoms and, in some, posttraumatic osteoarthritis. The poor results from complete injuries suggest that every patient with open physes and a complete tear of one or more ligaments should be treated acutely or subsequently by operation.

Lipscomb and Anderson described a method of reconstruction in adults and used their method for adolescent patients, not noting any disturbances of growth with the graft crossing either the tibial or the femoral physes.[158] Further clinical outcome research in this particular field is needed. In addition, irrespective of the type of injury, it seems that during adolescence the extent of damage to the ligaments is the most important factor for the long-term prognosis and that which of the specific ligaments is involved is only of secondary importance.

In the study of Clanton et al., despite primary surgical repair followed by 6 weeks of immobilization, some degree of ligament laxity persisted, suggesting that such injuries in children are analogous to ligament injuries in adults.[126] Although some degree of objective knee ligament laxity may persist, it may not be associatd with subjective symptoms of instability. Always compare laxity to the opposite side because of the normal laxity in children and adolescents.

Collateral Ligaments

Few patients under 14 years of age with collateral ligament injuries have been reported.[115,122,135,169,170,182] Hyndman and Brown described 15 cases of acute knee ligament injuries in children between the ages of 9 and 15 years.[144] One of the youngest children reported was a 4-year-old boy who sustained an isolated traumatic rupture of the medial collateral ligament; the site of the rupture was the midportion, rather than the origin or insertion of the medial collateral ligament.[150] O'Donoghue described a 6-year-old girl in a series of 82 patients; she was the only patient in his series less than 15 years of age.[169]

The initial examination must be undertaken carefully, as it is probably the evaluation that leads to major decisions for or against surgery. Medication may be appropriate to ensure relaxation.

The medial structures are tested with the knee in extension and at 30° of flexion (Fig. 22-21). The examination includes a thorough check for rotatory instability. The anterior drawer sign must be sought with the knee tested in neutral, internal, and external rotation. This sign is best elicited by having the patient lie supine with the knee flexed to 90°. The foot should be on the table to minimize dependent stretch in the cruciate ligaments, as happens when the knee hangs over the side of the table. Instability of the lateral side is less common but may be more disabling. The lateral compartment tends to be capable of a greater amount of physiologic widening, and comparison should be made with the contralateral uninjured side.

After standard history, physical examination, and roentgenograms, several other diagnostic alternatives are available to delineate the lesion.[196] Aspiration of the knee may allow a more thorough examination, especially when a local anesthetic is instilled. Stress roentgenograms may be obtained. Examination under anesthesia may help. Arthroscopy is another useful tool. MRI may delineate a tear (Fig. 22-22).

Stress roentgenograms of a relaxed patient allow acceptable initial evaluation of potential acute instability (Fig. 22-21). Kennedy and Drainger has published guidelines for limits of medial side widening,[153] but they were for skeletally mature individuals; great care must be taken when using these as guidelines for children inasmuch as the normal cartilage space width is greater owing to incomplete ossification of the entire epiphysis, and the child's knee joint exhibits a certain amount of normal laxity.

If a fracture is obvious, it is less likely that there is concomitant collateral ligament injury. However, if the stress only opens the joint, an isolated ligament injury is more probable. Look for peripheral disruption of the secondary ossification center, which may be an extremely small fragment (Fig. 22-23) that attaches to the ligament (sleeve fracture concept).

Acute treatment should be conservative in the skeletally immature individual, especially as the fragment heals to the rest of the epiphyseal ossification center by osseous union.[149] Conservative treatment consists of immobilization with the knee in approximately 30°–40° of flexion and no weight-bearing for 3–6 weeks. There are no certain indications for surgical repair even in the adolescent patient. Specific surgical treatment of the ligaments depends on the particular pattern of instability.

Pellegrini-Stieda Lesion

In the adolescent a medial collateral ligament avulsion may pull a portion of the femoral epiphysis away from the contiguous ossification center. Such a fragment may be radiolucent. However, the normal chondro-osseous maturation process may lead to formation of a seemingly separate "ossicle," referred to as the Pellegrini-Stieda lesion (Figs. 22-24, 22-25).[173,174,186,193] The lesion may be continuous with the metaphysis or epiphysis through connective tissue. If the lesion is tender, however, a pseudarthrosis is likely and may require surgical exploration, fixation, or removal.

Segond Lesion

The Segond lesion is the analogue of the Pellegrini-Stieda lesion, involving an avulsion from the lateral tibial epiphysis.[120,130,138,145,155] It was originally described by Segond in 1879.[181] The lesion, which may be lateral or medial, is an avulsion of a cartilaginous peripheral fragment, which may or may not contain some of the contiguous subchondral bone (Fig. 22-26).

Felenda and Dittel described a Segond fracture from the lateral tibial condyle in 11 patients.[134] They noted that all patients showed additional major ligamentous damage, and 10 patients had a concomitant injury of the anterior cruciate ligament along with the lateral collateral ligament. They noted that this "harmless" lateral capsular sign should be a warning to undertake further diagnostic measures, particularly arthroscopic or MRI examination.

Cruciate Ligaments

Anterior Cruciate Ligament

Children who have nontraumatic anterior cruciate ligament (ACL) insufficiency fall into two groups. The first group

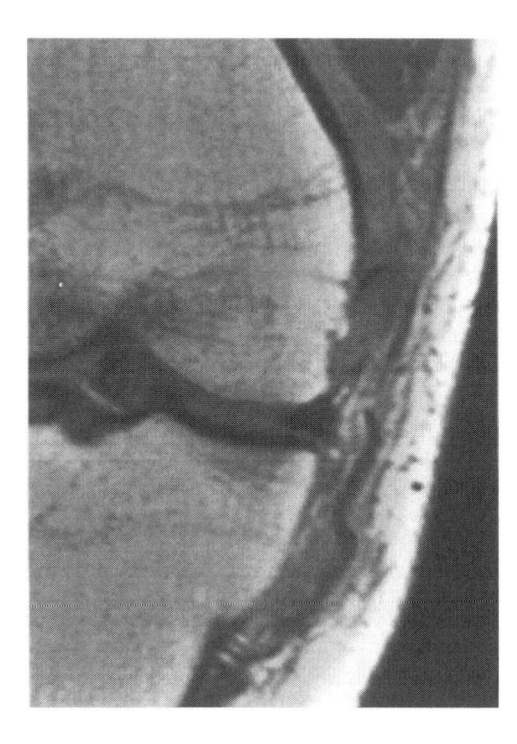

FIGURE 22-22. Tear of the medial collateral ligament in a 15-year-old female gymnast following an uneven bars dismount.

Ligaments

FIGURE 22-23. (A) Avulsion of the deep portion of the lateral collateral ligament has included an osteochondral fragment (arrow) from the tibial epiphysis. This is the site of the collateral ligament attachment. (B) Medial osteochondral fragment (arrow) from the distal femur. (C) These osteochondral fragment fractures, are analogous to ligament disruption in children and adolescents. The tibial lesion is referred to as a Segond fracture, and the femoral lesion is referred to as a Pellegrini-Stieda lesion.

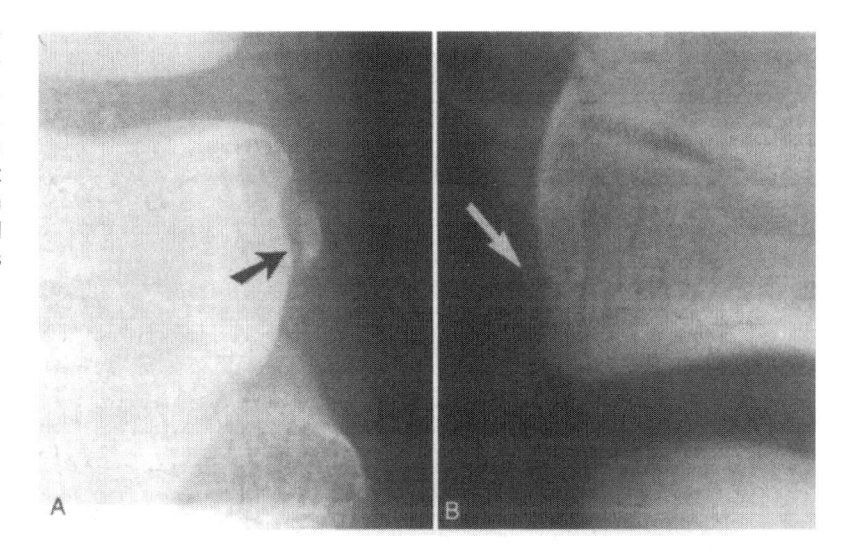

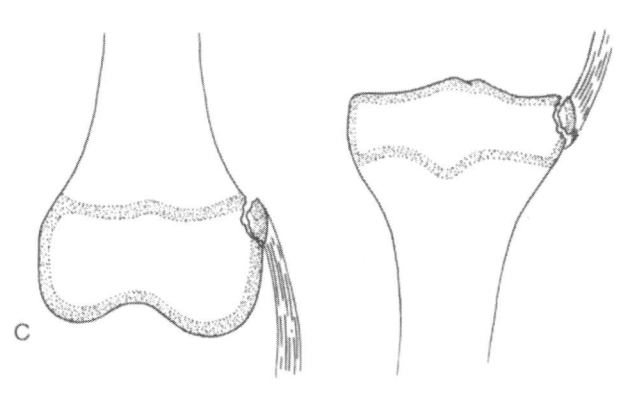

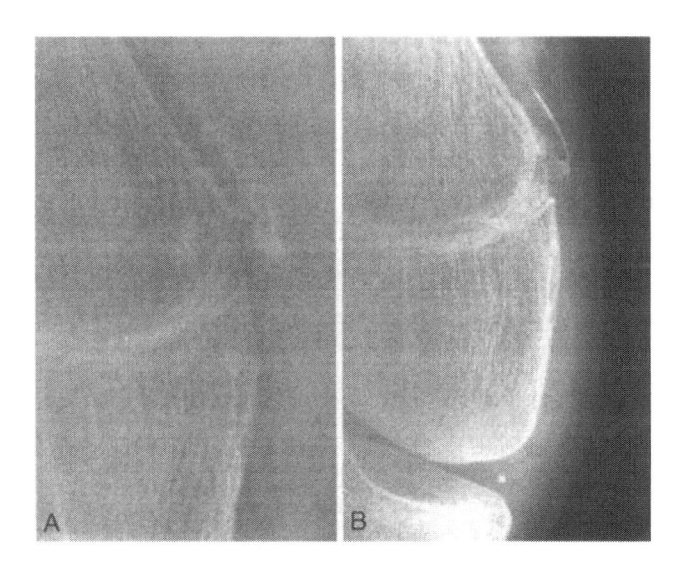

FIGURE 22-24. Early (A) and later (B) stages of Pellegrini-Stieda lesions.

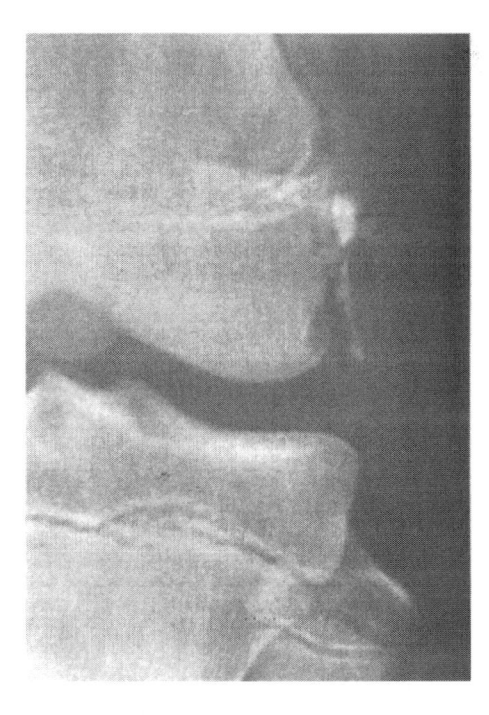

FIGURE 22-25. Tear of the medial collateral ligament and chondro-osseous lateral fracture, creating the equivalent of a lateral collateral ligament tear.

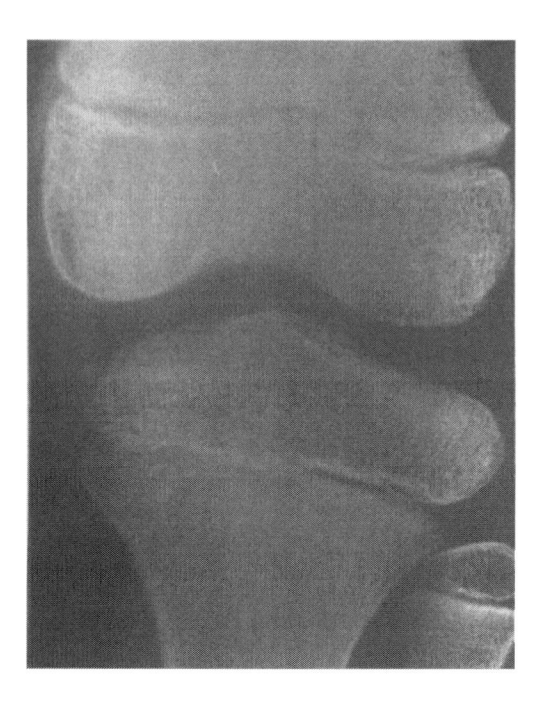

FIGURE 22-26. Medial Segond lesion equivalent. Early development.

has the laxity in conjunction with generalized joint laxity throughout the upper and lower extremities. They usually have a 1+ to 2+ positive anterior drawer sign bilaterally but no associated symptomatology. Such generalized laxity must be considered when evaluating knee injuries in children. Examination of the opposite uninjured knee is essential to establish a baseline for ligamentous laxity in any child. The other group with nontraumatic insufficiency has congenital absence of the anterior cruciate ligament, which is often associated with other congenital abnormalities of the extremity, such as congenital dislocation of the knee, proximal femoral focal deficiency, and fibular hemimelia. Radiographic analysis of the intercondylar eminence often shows aplasia of the intercondylar eminence in congenital absence of the ACL.[137] Eilert reported that most knee problems in children younger than 12 years of age are usually congenital in origin, whereas those in children older than 12 years are more often related to trauma.[38] Similarly, in a series of patients younger than 13 years of age who underwent knee arthroscopy, Morrissy et al. found that only 36% had a history of trauma.[47]

Complete cruciate ligament injuries are infrequent in children.[117,125,131,143,144,146,151,159,163,172,185,189,192,197] Instead, the ligament usually fails at the chondro-osseous transition, which most often affects the tibial spine (see Chapter 23) but may also involve the femoral attachment (Fig. 22-27). Robinson and Driscoll reported a single case in which both femoral and tibial insertions of the ACL were avulsed as fractures.[176]

More recently it has been stressed that there is an association of avulsion of the intercondylar eminence with other ligamentous injuries to the knee in children.[191] For example, Hyndman and Brown reported seven cases of avulsion of the tibial spine, all of which were associated with other ligamentous disruptions of the knee.[144] Bradley et al. reported six cases of medial collateral ligament (MCL) disruption in children younger than 12 years of age; three of the patients had associated ACL injuries.[122] Accordingly, when an anterior tibial spine avulsion is evident radiographically, associated collateral knee ligamentous injuries must be assessed. The ACL also should be assessed, either by arthroscopy if doing a reduction or after healing if closed treatment is used.

Clanton et al. reported nine skeletally immature patients.[126] Despite thorough initial physical and roentgenographic evaluations, the full extent of the lesions was determined only during surgery in seven of the nine patients. The intercondylar eminence of the tibia was avulsed in five patients, four of whom had associated collateral ligament injuries and a positive anterior drawer sign.[126] This association in children must be emphasized. Whereas Meyers and

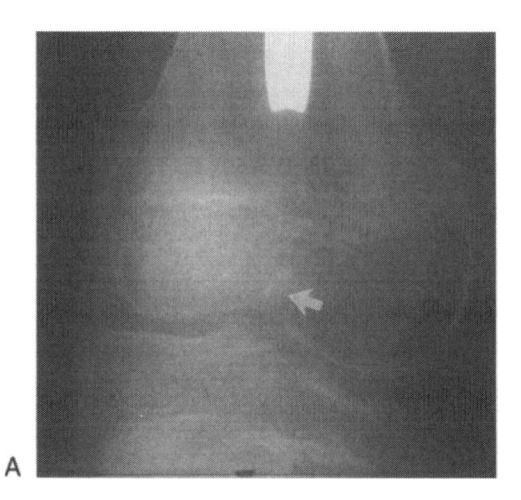

FIGURE 22-27. This 16-year-old boy sustained a femoral fracture in an automobile accident. He was treated with an intramedullary rod. During postoperative rehabilitation he complained of knee pain and intermittent effusion. (A) A fragment is barely evident (arrow) "within" the distal femoral ossification center. (B) MRI delineated the femoral avulsion fragment and the damaged anterior cruciate ligament.

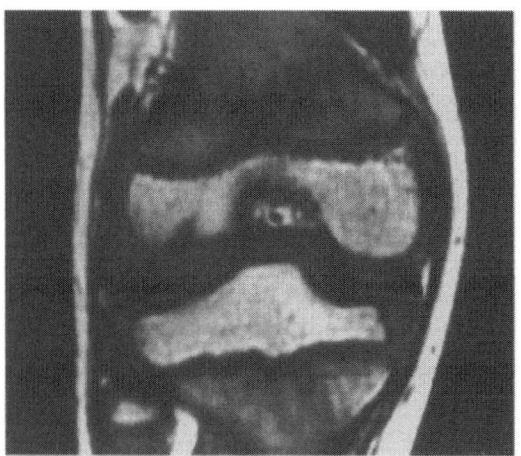

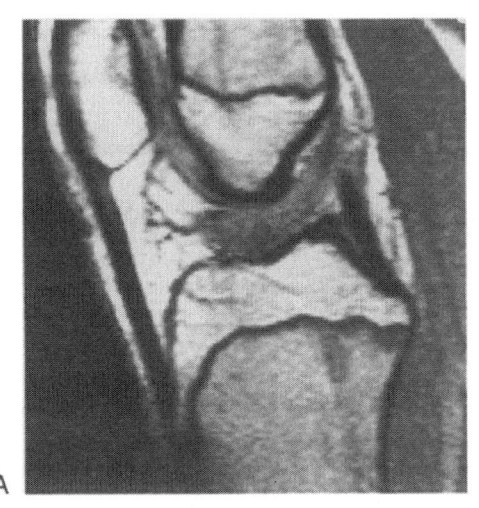

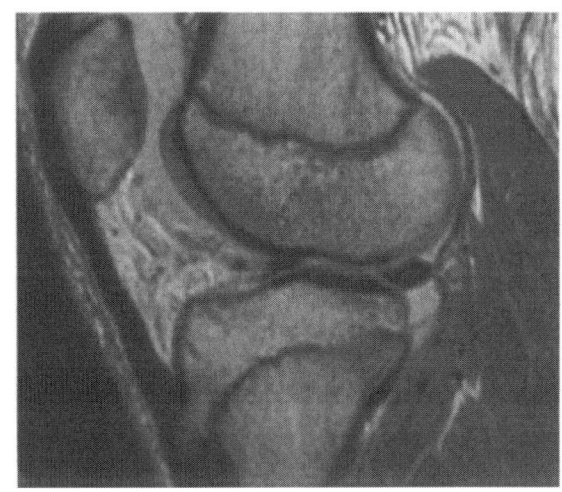

FIGURE 22-28. (A) MRI of an anterior cruciate tear in an adolescent. The tear, at arthroscopy, was in the midportion. (B) Anterior drawer test duplication during an MRI scan.

McKeever[163] noted no associated collateral ligament injuries in children with tibial spine avulsions, Zaricznyj[197] and Hyndman and Brown[144] described concomitant collateral-cruciate damage.

Magnetic resonance imaging (Fig. 22-28) may be used to evaluate presumptive acute ACL injury.[132,177] Among 18 knees 28 osseous lesions were detected by MRI in 15 knees, but none of them had been detected by radiography or arthroscopy.[133] These lesions can best be described as bone bruising of various degrees and particularly were areas of edema or hemorrhage as well as occult (i.e., undisplaced) tibial spine fractures.

Speer et al., using MRI in patients with cruciate ligament injuries, showed accompanying osseous injury associated with acute tears of the ACL.[184] Altogether 83% (45 of 54) of the knees had an osseous contusion directly over the lateral femoral condyle terminal ligament attachment. The lesion was highly variable in size and imaging intensity, although the most intense signal was always contiguous with the subchondral plate. They reported one patient, a 14-year-old, with an open distal femoral physis in which the superior progagation of the abnormal signal was limited by the physes. There is general agreement that a diminished signal on T1-weighted images and an increased signal intensity on T2-weighted images depends on the occurrence of microtrabecular injury and subsequent hemorrhage and fluid transudation at the site of the injury.

Panjabi et al. studied subfailure injury of the rabbit ACL.[171] The overall strength of the ligament, however, did not change. The shape of the load-displacement curve, especially at low loads, was significantly altered.

Aspiration of the hemarthrosis and successful closed reduction by extension of the knee followed by immobilization in extension have produced good results in ACL/tibial spine injuries.[179] Persistent displacement of the tibial eminence following closed reduction may block knee extension and cause knee laxity. The elevated tibial spine effectively shortens the ACL, altering its function and strength. Laxity in the anteroposterior plane increases with time owing to stretching of the secondary capsular restraints.[121] Therefore residual displacement after an attempted closed reduction requires anatomic reduction. Furthermore, there is no evidence to suggest that knee ligaments in children have the potential to heal any better than those in adults.[128]

Injury to the cruciate ligaments in children, excluding avulsion of the tibial spine, may initiate a syndrome of cruciate insufficiency when nonoperative treatment is used. DeLee noted that posttraumatic ACL insufficiency, acute or chronic, was unusual in children younger than 14 years.[129] Details of the treatment of the avulsed tibial spine are covered in Chapter 23.

Wasilewski and Frankl reported an 11-year follow-up of a patient who had an osteochondral avulsion fracture of the femoral insertion of the ACL.[194] It was treated by an open procedure. Follow-up at 11 years showed an asymptomatic patient with a stable knee.

McCarroll et al. described 40 patients under the age of 14 with an open physis who had midsubstance tears of the ACL.[161] Sixteen were treated conservatively with rehabilitation, bracing, and counseling on activity modification, and the remaining 24 underwent arthroscopic examination and an extraarticular or an intraarticular reconstruction based on growth potential. The average follow-up was 26 months. In the conservative group 6 of 16 patients subsequently underwent arthroscopy for meniscal tears, and only 7 patients returned to sports, with all of the patients experiencing recurrent episodes of instability, effusions, and pain. In the surgical group, 12 medial and 6 lateral meniscal tears were found at arthroscopy. All 24 of the patients returned to sports activity, and 22 of 24 were still competing. The two remaining patients suffered reinjury 3 years after their surgery. The authors recommended arthroscopic examination under anesthesia in a young patient with an ACL tear. These authors specifically excluded patients with avulsion of the intercondylar eminence or associated ligamentous damage.

Perhaps the most controversial aspect of repair of an ACL tear prior to skeletal maturity is the potential risk of distal femoral or proximal tibial physeal damage and growth arrest from the tunneling process, the bone plugs, or the interference screw. The size of the usual tunnels exceeds the size of reported experimental physeal defects that are likely to lead to a significant transphyseal bridge. The placement of a soft tissue graft (e.g., hamstring tendon) through the tunnel probably has little effect on preventing such bridging.

Most studies with adequate long-term follow-up show that the results of ACL repair are similar to those attained in young adults and are not accompanied by growth arrest that adversely compromises skeletal maturation.[116,164,195] Most adolescents, especially athletic females, who undergo ACL repairs are close to skeletal maturity, which minimizes the risk of growth abnormality even if a bony bridge or complete epiphysiodesis occurs.

Alternative methods that do not utilize transphyseal drill holes may also be undertaken in skeletally immature patients.[123] However, these may not duplicate knee joint mechanics as well as the tunneled graft.

The problem with any of the aforementioned methods and studies is that very few children under 12 years of age are included in the study cohorts. The risk of transphyseal procedures may increase with the decreasing skeletal maturity of the ACL deficient patients.

Schaefer et al. described a 4-year-old child with an ACL injury who was followed for 11 years.[180] Repair was attempted 4 months after injury. Five years later the surgical repair had failed with evidence of complete disruption, suggesting that these injuries and attempts at surgical repair are neither benign nor successful in every patient.

Mylle et al. used screw fixation for ACL avulsion.[165] This screw crossed the physis and led to an anterior growth arrest with development of recurvatum, leading the authors to suggest a new technique with smaller screws that did not cross the growth plate.

Graf et al. found eight meniscal tears (four medial, four lateral) in six patients with ACL tears.[141] Of the 12 patients in the study, 7 sustained further meniscal damage an average of 15 months (range 7–27 months) after the initial injury.

Posterior Cruciate Ligament

The posterior cruciate ligament (PCL) originates as a broad, flat band from the posterior portion of the proximal tibia just distal to the physeal plate. PCL injury is much less frequent than ACL injury (Fig. 22-29). Sanders et al. reported acute insufficiency of the PCL in two children, noting that it usually detached from the femur along with a chondral fragment, whereas tibial spine/ACL injury is the more classic presentation.[178] Crawford treated two patients with avulsion of the PCL.[127] One underwent surgical repair and did well; the other was treated nonoperatively and had unacceptable instability. Mayer and Micheli also reported an 11-year-old with a similar injury and result.[160]

Suprock and Rogers reported a 4-year-old boy who traumatically avulsed his PCL.[188] The ligament was avulsed from its femoral osseous attachment, along with a piece of cartilage. The posterior horn of the medial meniscus is often avulsed, and there was a tear of the meniscotibial ligament. The PCL was reattached with absorbable sutures placed through a drill hole into the medial femoral epiphysis. It was done fluoroscopically to avoid crossing the physes. The medial meniscus and the meniscotibial ligament injuries were also repaired. Two years later the patient had laxity of the PCL compared to the other side, but he was asymptomatic.

Goodrich and Ballard reported a patient with a closed right distal femoral diaphyseal fracture who also had a PCL avulsion with a bony fragment that was not noted until the patient was placed in traction.[139] They noted that this type of injury had been described previously.[122,126,160] Clanton et al. described two patients with PCL avulsed from the femur.[126] Sanders et al. also added two cases avulsed from the femoral origin.[178]

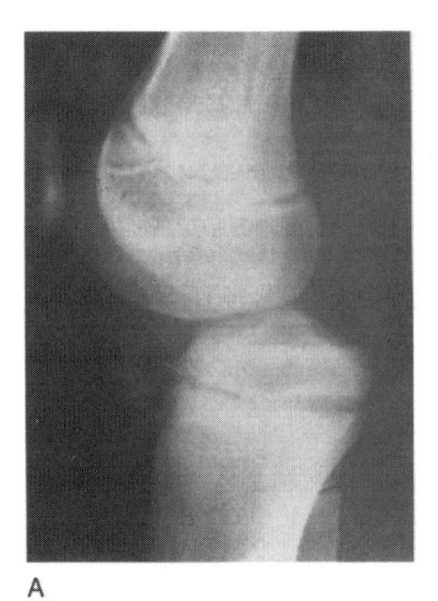

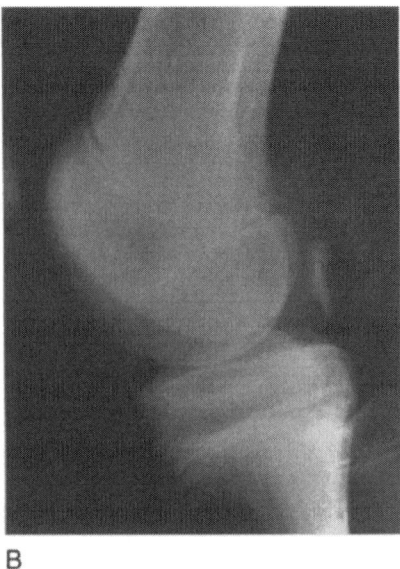

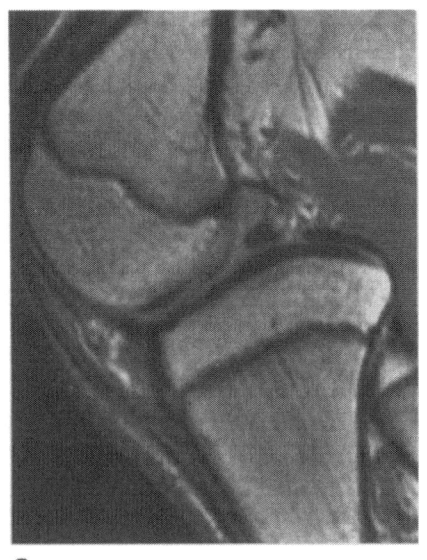

FIGURE 22-29. Posterior cruciate ligament injuries. (A) Posterior subluxation stress film. (B) Avulsed fragment-femoral attachment. (C) MRI showing anterior displacement of the femur.

Patellar Fractures

Fractures may occur when a direct blow is applied to the patella or during displacement or relocation of a patellar dislocation. A direct blow may cause the patella to impact against the femoral condyles and cause a splitting fracture, which is more likely in an adolescent than a younger child, in whom the resilience of the primarily cartilaginous patella usually protects it from major osseous injury. Bone bruising or chondro-osseous separation (sleeve fracture) may occur. A sudden, powerful contraction of the quadriceps mechanism may cause an avulsion fracture through a segment of the chondro-osseous margins. Fractures of the patella must be adequately differentiated from developmental "variations," such as a bipartite patella.[220] Medial and lateral patellar fractures may follow subluxation or, more often, dislocation of the patella. Peterson and Stener reported an interesting case showing that the cause of the ectopic bone around a patella in a 12-year-old boy was due to avulsions of the medial and lateral margins of the patella produced by the medial and lateral longitudinal patellar retinacula.[232] They further showed that not only were these retinacular portions of the tendons of the vastus medialis and lateralis into the patella, they constituted a direct fibrous connection of considerable strength between the patella and the tibia and thus are capable of producing avulsion fractures.

Only 1% of patellar fractures involve patients under 15 years of age.[198,201,207,208,211,214,226,231,234,235,236,238,242] The youngest reported patient is a 2-year-old child. It is common for the diagnosis to be missed or delayed, especially if the patella is not ossified or is minimally ossified. Ronget[235] and Hallopeau[218] both reported cases in which the diagnosis was not made until several months after fracture.

Ray and Hendrix reviewed 185 patients who had defined patellar fractures.[233] Of the 185 there were 12 between 8 and 16 years of age, accounting for a 6.5% incidence in skeletally immature individuals. All the young patients were male, at an average age of 12.7 years. Sleeve fractures were the most common type ($n = 5$) followed by transverse fractures ($n = 4$). Of the 12 cases, 10 required operative management.

Previous injury to the knee with compromised quadriceps mechanism and function may also be a predisposing factor. These fractures often occur in children who take part in activities that require forceful extension of the knee with the quadriceps contracting against resistance. There is an association of this type of injury with high-jumping.[204,239,243] Interestingly, in Houghton and Ackroyd's series, the injury always involved the "take off" leg, with no direct trauma to the knee in any case.[221] Chronic or acute on chronic patellar failure may occur with certain neuromuscular diseases (e.g., cerebral palsy).

Roentgenograms usually define the fracture best in the lateral projection (Figs. 22-30 to 22-33). Because of the thickness of the hyaline cartilage and articular cartilage, there may be an incomplete separation of the articular cartilaginous portion of the patella, even though the patella appears separated within the osseous portion. Elasticity of the cartilage allows hinging, similar to the incomplete fracture of the lateral condyle. In rare instances the patellar tendon may be avulsed from the tibial tuberosity, rather than a fracture of the patella itself. Usually a small osseous fragment is evident.[199,202,209,237]

Treatment of the transversely fractured patella in a child should follow the same principles as in an adult.[205,215,228,241] Undisplaced or minimally displaced fractures should be treated by immobilization of the knee in extension in a cylinder cast. Fractures with significant separation of the fragments require open reduction and repair of the torn quadriceps expansions. Circumferential fixation through the soft tissues, rather than the patella, is less likely to disrupt growth patterns in the patella.

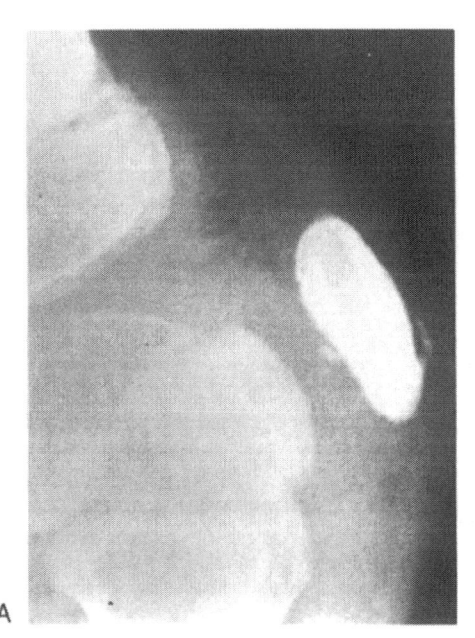

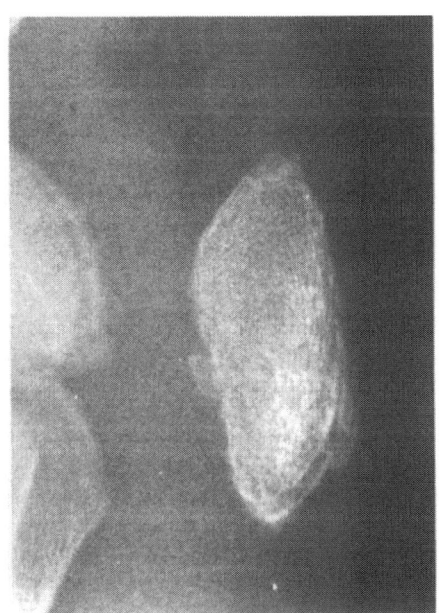

FIGURE 22-30. (A) Anterior and posterior chondro-osseous fractures following direct impact to the knee during a fall. (B) Appearance 8 months later.

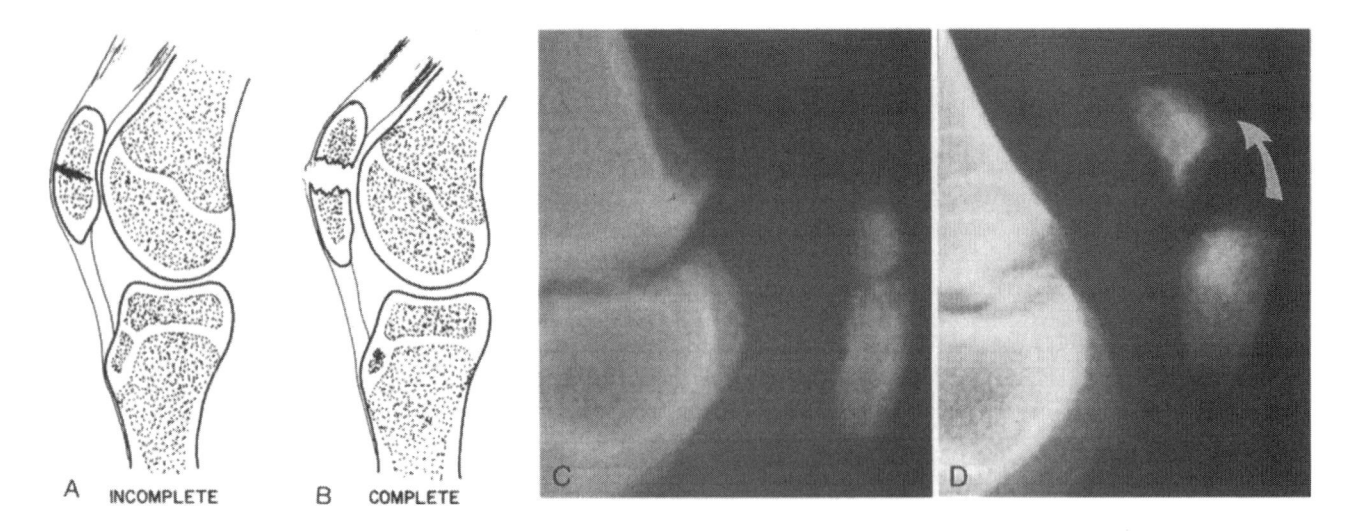

FIGURE 22-31. (A, B) Incomplete and complete fractures of the midportion of the patella. (C) Undisplaced fracture of the patella. (D) Displaced fracture (arrow) that was treated by open reduction.

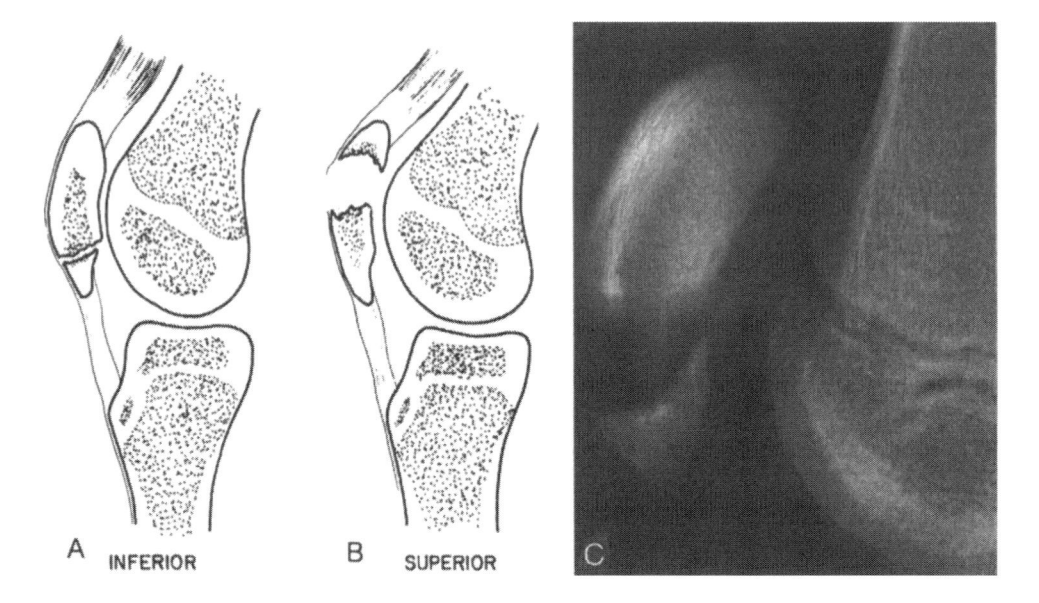

FIGURE 22-32. Patellar fracture showing involvement of the inferior pole (A) and the superior pole (B). (C) Fracture of the inferior pole.

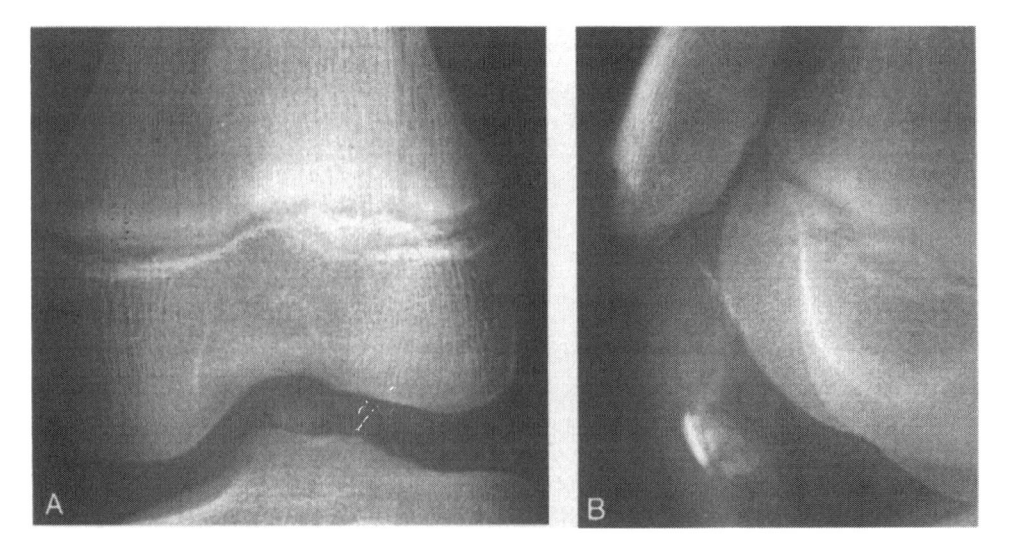

FIGURE 22-33. (A) Anteroposterior view was interpreted as a tibial spine injury. (B) However, the lateral view showed that it was an avulsed inferior pole injury.

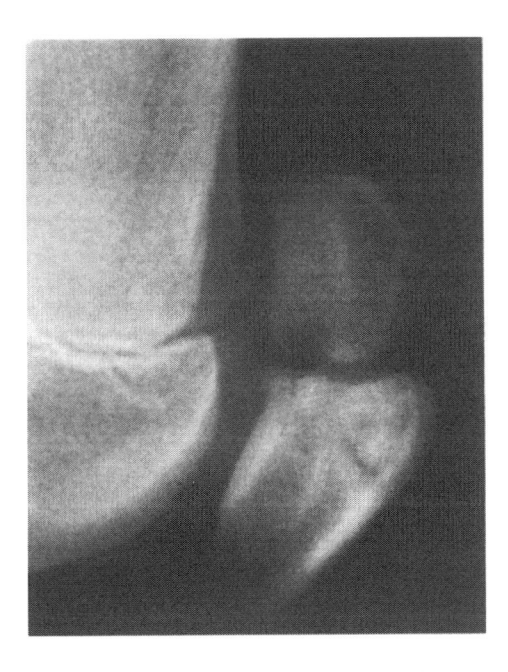

FIGURE 22-34. Radiologic nonunion of a patellar fracture. Quadriceps function was still good because the soft tissues were reasonably intact. The fragments moved as a unit from flexion to extension.

Tension band fixation of the superficial region is often sufficient to restore anatomy and not cause separation at the articular surface.[200]

Failure to diagnose and adequately treat these injuries may result in an established nonunion between the superior and inferior fragments (Fig. 22-34), although there may be sufficient intrinsic healing of the quadriceps expansion to stabilize the extent of separation of the fragments. Nonunion may lead to unusual patellar morphology.[210]

Maguire and Canale described 66 children with patellar fractures.[227] Twenty-four had adequate long-term follow-up with results that were good in 13, fair in 8, and poor in 3. Children with fractures of the ipsilateral femur, tibia, or both and those with comminuted displaced fractures had the poorest results. Altogether 40% of the fractures in their series were incurred in motorcycle or automobile accidents, and 13% were associated with ipsilateral fractures of the tibia, femur, or both. Comminuted fractures were the most common pattern in adolescents. A significant number of the fractures were open. These data are indicative of high-energy trauma. Open reduction and internal fixation produced good results. No growth disturbances were noted after the use of cerclage wires. Absorbable sutures, and/or temporary transfixation pins may be better in a growing child.

Stress Fracture

Dickason and Fox described a transverse stress fracture of the patella in a child athlete.[213] They noted that stress fractures have been described in only three animals: thoroughbred race horses, greyhounds, and humans.[213] Such a condition, also termed overuse syndrome, is defined as a partial or complete fracture of bone due to an inability to withstand nonviolent stress applied in a rhythmic or repeated subthreshold manner.

Devas described three children with stress fractures of the patella; in two there was a crack along the lateral side, and the other case was a transverse fracture.[212] These injuries occurred during vigorous athletic activity. Devas believed that patellar stress fractures in children were seldom severe enough to require operative treatment. However, there may be significant problems associated with the articular surface of the patella that one must look for and evaluate thoroughly before stating that it will be a normal joint. Treatment is discontinuation of the repetitive evocative activity.

Iwaya and Takatori reported three cases of lateral longitudinal stress fractures of the patella.[222] They were in young children, and all healed with discontinuation of athletics. It appears that this injury is due to excessive stress applied through the vastus lateralis.[232]

Teitz and Harrington described two patients with patellar stress fractures due to activities that required prolonged isometric quadriceps contraction and relatively constant knee flexion.[240] They noted that these injuries have been described in patients with cerebral palsy[166] and in adolescent athletes.[207,212,213,219,222,239] The authors concluded that the stress fractures occurred because of repeated bending moments that initiated a fracture on the superficial surface of the patella. Those whose activities require frequent knee flexion and quadriceps use, either isotonically or in sudden bursts, are at risk for these injuries. Children are likely to fail at the lower pole of the patellar or the attachment of the tendon into the tuberosity (Sinding-Larsen-Johansson or Osgood-Schlatter lesions). Such patients presenting with knee pain and superficial patellar tenderness should undergo radiographic examination and possible bone scan to identify early stress fractures of the patella before the injuries become complete fractures.

Sleeve Fracture

A patellar injury pattern unique to children is the sleeve fracture.[206,217,225,234,244] The diagnosis may be missed because the distal osseous fragment may be sufficiently small to be minimally detectable radiographically.[221] An extensive sleeve of cartilage may be pulled from the main body of the osseous patella, with or without an osseous fragment from the distal pole. The small size of the osseous fragment may belie the actual size of the more peripheral radiolucent cartilaginous component.

When the patellar tendon disrupts in children, it usually does so at the upper or lower pole, rather than interstitially.[219,232] Although avulsion of the tibial tuberosity has been reported, avulsion of the lower pole of the patella is more common.[218] These cases tend to occur in children participating in sporting activities that require vigorous extension of the knee, often without proper warm-up or progressive conditioning.

Avulsion fractures may involve any segment of the patellar periphery, with the anatomic extent of the injury not always appreciated on the initial diagnostic film, as minimal bone may be present in the avulsed fragment, especially in young patients.[217] This makes the diagnosis difficult because of

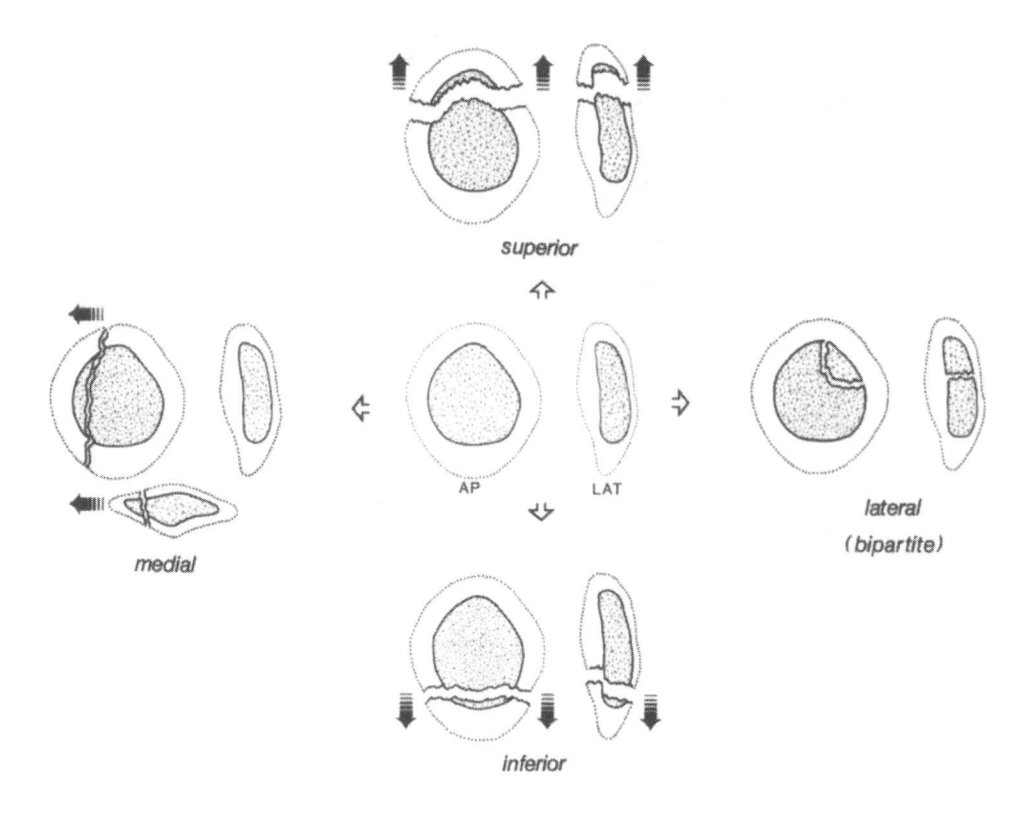

FIGURE 22-35. Various types of patellar sleeve fracture.

the radiolucency of the concomitantly disrupted, unossified peripheral cartilage that comprises the rest of the fragment. These fractures separate at the interface between subchondral bone and nonossified cartilage or involve this layer of the subchondral bone along the biosusceptible margin.

The patterns of avulsion (sleeve) fracture are classified as follows (Fig. 22-35).

Inferior: The fragment involves the lower pole of the patella (Figs. 22-36 to 22-39). It is usually caused by an acute injury. A more chronic injury is the Sinding-Larsen-

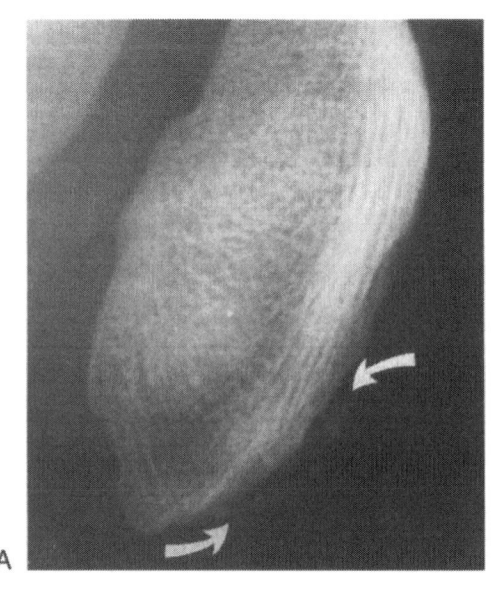

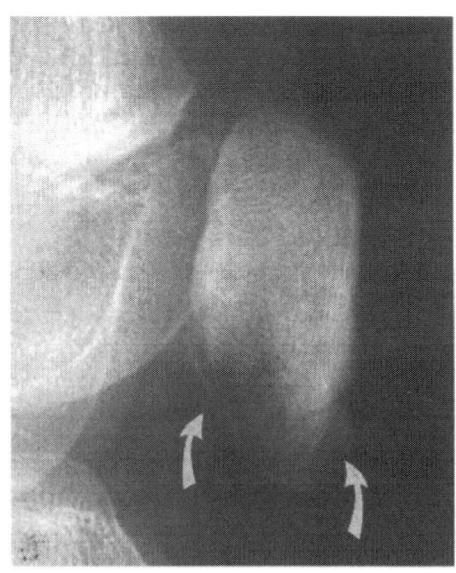

FIGURE 22-36. (A) Sleeve fracture in a 10-year-old. This close-up view shows bone avulsion (arrows) at the chondro-osseous separation interface. (B) Thin linear sleeve fracture (arrows). This segment of the patella is nonarticular and is covered by the retropatellar fat pad.

Patellar Fractures

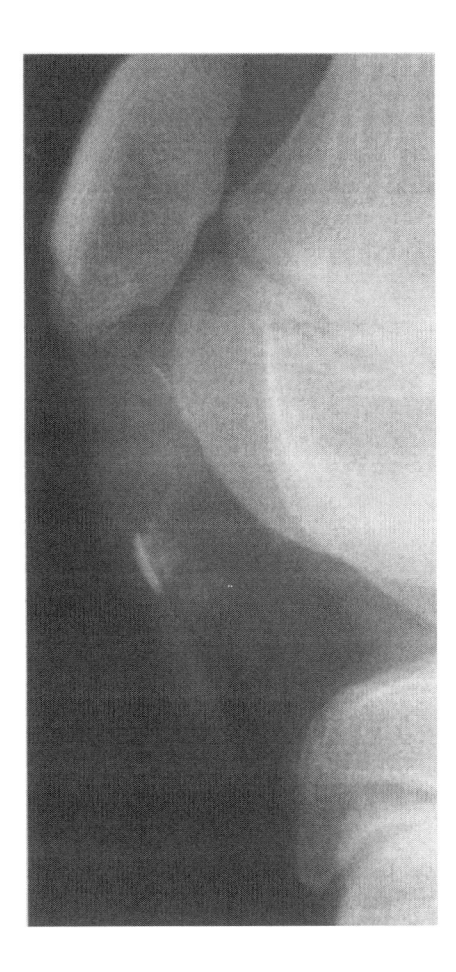

FIGURE 22-37. Sleeve fracture with displacement.

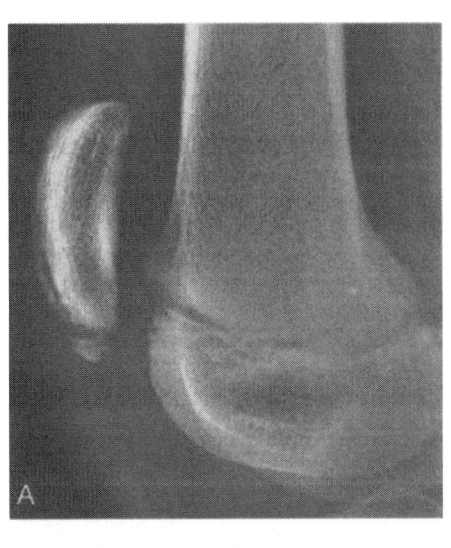

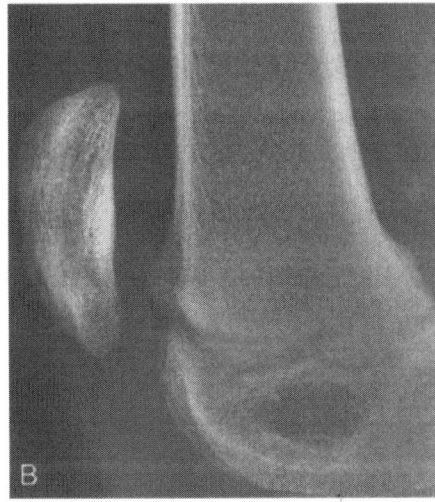

FIGURE 22-38. (A) Acute sleeve fracture. (B) Extent of healing 3 months later.

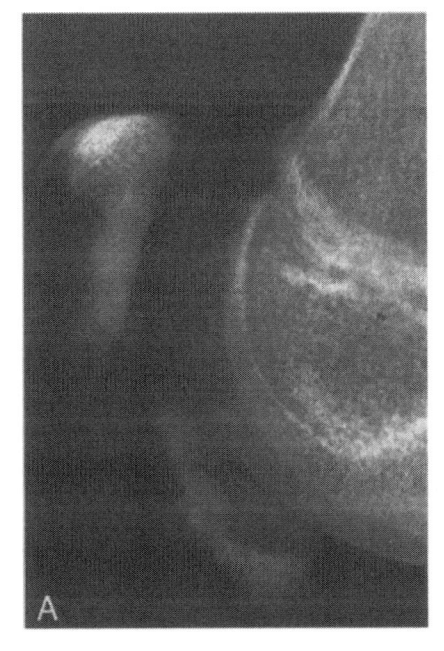

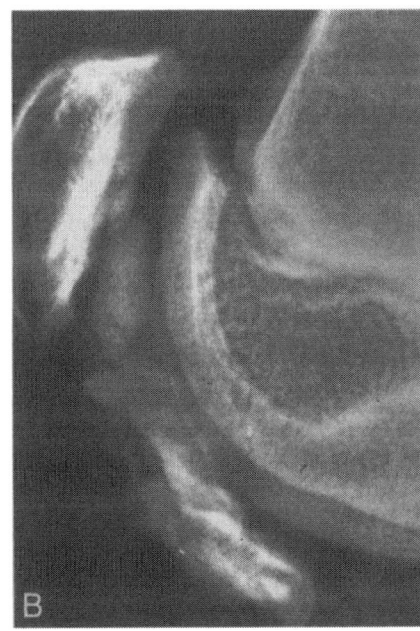

FIGURE 22-39. (A) Several weeks prior to this displaced sleeve fracture, a "normal" radiograph was reported. (B) Five weeks later even more ossification was evident. It was eventually resected.

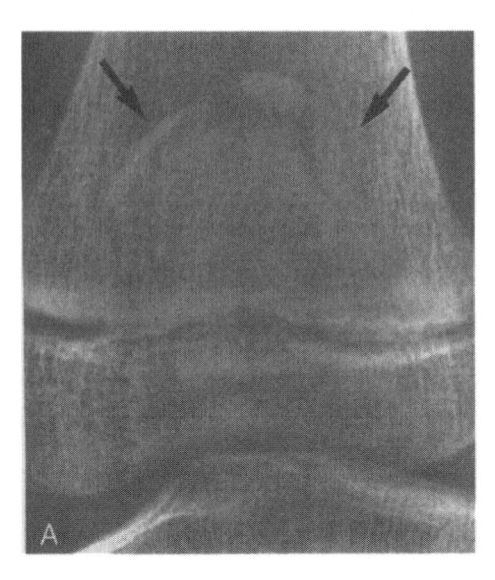

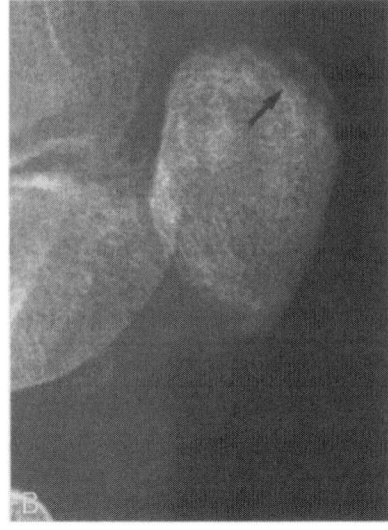

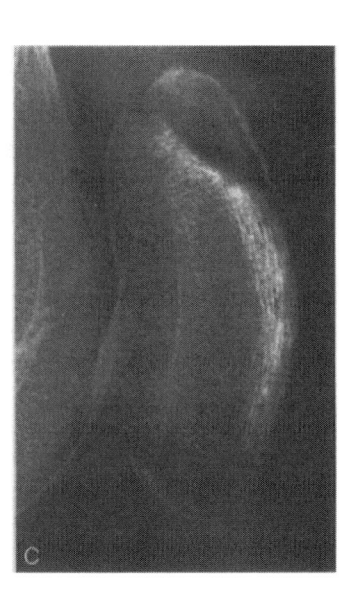

FIGURE 22-40. (A) Superior sleeve fracture (arrow). (B) Superior sleeve fracture (arrow). (C) Displaced superior sleeve fracture. This film was obtained several weeks after the acute onset of symptoms while broad-jumping.

Johansson lesion, although it may be considered an incomplete variation of an insidious avulsion (chronic stress injury) analgous to the Osgood-Schlatter lesion.

Superior: The fragment involves the superior pole of the patella (Figs. 22-40, 22-41). It appears to be the least common pattern.[203]

Medial: The fragment involves most of the medial margin of the patella. The most likely mechanism is that of an acute chondral separation from the ossified patella when the bulk of the patella dislocates laterally. The cartilaginous rim stays medially with the retinaculum. This rim eventually undergoes osseous transformation as a separate ossicle.

Lateral: This lesion is often described as a bipartite patella or dorsal defect of the patella. It may be a chronic stress lesion resulting from repetitive tensile pull from the vastus lateralis muscle during the process of chondro-osseous transformation. As in the accessory navicular (see Chapter 24), a "congenital" bipartite patella may become symptomatic owing to acute or repetitive stress. It is an occult separation along the cartilage separating the ossification centers. However, acute disruption of the entire lateral margin, in conjunction with similar injuries to the medial and inferior margins, has been described.

All the margins (superior, inferior, medial, lateral) are subjected to varying amounts of tensile pull through the quadriceps mechanism, patellar tendon, and retinacular tissues. The peripheral chondro-osseous transformation margin is often radiographically irregular and may have small accessory foci of ossification that are progressively incorporated into the main center. The marginal bone is irregularly formed and not initially mechanically adapted. Accordingly, it is susceptible to fracture along any patellar margin, comparable to a physeal fracture in the metaphyseal primary spongiosa.

The avulsed patellar osseous fragment, which may be only a thin piece of bone, invariably includes an important "sleeve" of cartilage that should be accurately reduced to reestablish the articular surface of the patella. Houghton and Ackroyd recommended the importance of (adequate) fixation.[221] Conservative treatment with extension or hyperextension immobilization may lead to marked deformity of the patella with elongation of the patella and restriction of eventual knee movement. Fixation allows more rapid rehabilitation.

The diagnosis is suggested by the frequent absence of a direct blow, a sudden giving way, severe pain in the knee, and

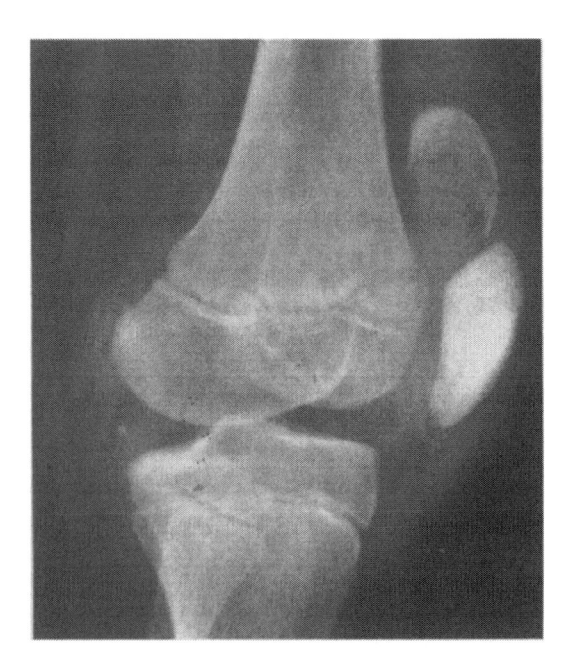

FIGURE 22-41. Superior pole sleeve avulsion with displacement.

difficulty or inability to bear weight. Active extension of the knee may not be possible. Frequently, a gap is palpable at the involved margin of the patella. This gap is a particularly valuable clinical sign, as the peripheral fragment of avulsed bone and cartilage may not be easily detectable radiographically (Fig. 22-39). There may be an effusion. Diagnosis may be delayed, particularly if irregular ossification is interpreted as a developmental variation. The avulsion becomes obvious when progressive ossification occurs, although reactive bone is minimal (as bone is not yet present in one of the fracture fragments), and there is limited periosteum. Flexion/extension lateral films should be obtained. In fact, because much of the peripheral patella is cartilage around a centripetally expanding osseous center, perichondrium is the primary peripheral tissue until adolescence.

No matter which margin is involved, displaced fracture may include partial to complete disruption of the quadriceps mechanism, although the disruption may not be severe enough to compromise function, especially after healing. One of the primary purposes of exploration is to assess the extent of involvement of the articular cartilage. The avulsed patellar fragment may include an important segment (sleeve) of cartilage that must be accurately reduced to establish the articular surface of the patella. The superior and inferior fractures in particular may involve nonarticular cartilage, especially inferiorly where the region is covered by a large retropatellar fat pad.

Closed treatment with the knee extended is used when minimal displacement exists. Conservative treatment with immobilization may lead to deformity. Elongation of the patella and restriction of eventual knee movement may occur if the extent of separation of radiolucent cartilage is not adequately considered. Attenuation of the inferior region on a chronic basis may lead to, or be diagnostically confused with, a Sinding-Larsen-Johansson lesion.

Widening of the fracture gap usually indicates a need for surgical stabilization. Open reduction should be performed when there is fragment displacement to minimize the potential complications of extensor lag and nonunion. Fixation also allows more rapid rehabilitation. Jacquemier et al. reported three patients with sleeve fractures.[223] Surgical repair was undertaken in two; transient ischemic changes developed in both patients (one required secondary patellectomy). In a third patient, not treated operatively, extensive ectopic bone developed within the knee, and function was decreased.

Despite the initial delay in the diagnosis of many of these avulsion fractures, healing often occurs without significant functional disability. Because the patellar ossification center is surrounded by cartilage, much of the outer surface is perichondrium, rather than periosteum. Ossification proceeds peripherally, but only on the anterior surface does it reach the "edge" and become associated with a tissue change to periosteum. Accordingly, the usual childhood osteogenic subperiosteal callus response is minimal in these injuries. Primary healing of trabecular bone is the mechanism of repair. If minimal chondro-osseous transformation exists in the avulsed fragment, this repair process may be delayed.

Sinding-Larsen-Johansson Lesion

The Sinding-Larsen-Johansson (SLJ) lesion is comparable to partial separation of the tibial tuberosity (Osgood-Schlatter lesion), affecting the patella at the attachment of the patellar ligament inferiorly.[216,245–252] The type of trauma is consistent with a chondro-osseous fatigue (stress) fracture with disturbance of normal ossification patterns. The patient is usually an active boy in the 10- to 14-year age group who complains of pain in the knee accompanied by a limp. Bilateral symptoms are relatively common. As with the Osgood-Schlatter lesion, there may be bilateral involvement radiographically but only unilateral symptoms. The lesion may coexist with an Osgood-Schlatter lesion (Fig. 22-42).

Examination shows tenderness and occasional swelling located at the inferior or superior pole of the patella.

Radiographs may reveal fragmentation at the inferior pole, or there may be anteroinferior extension on the patella (Figs. 22-43, 22-44). The inferior pole may develop an overenlarged appearance comparable to the deformity seen in the tibial tuberosity. As with the Osgood-Schlatter lesion, the roentgenographic appearance is not necessarily related to the severity of the symptoms.

Kalebo et al. used ultrasonography to detect partial ruptures in the proximal part of the patellar ligament (jumper's knee).[247] A cone-shaped, poorly echogenic area exceeding 0.5 cm in length in the center of the patellar tendon, in combination with localized thickening, proved to be a reliable indicator of jumper's knee. The site of attachment of the

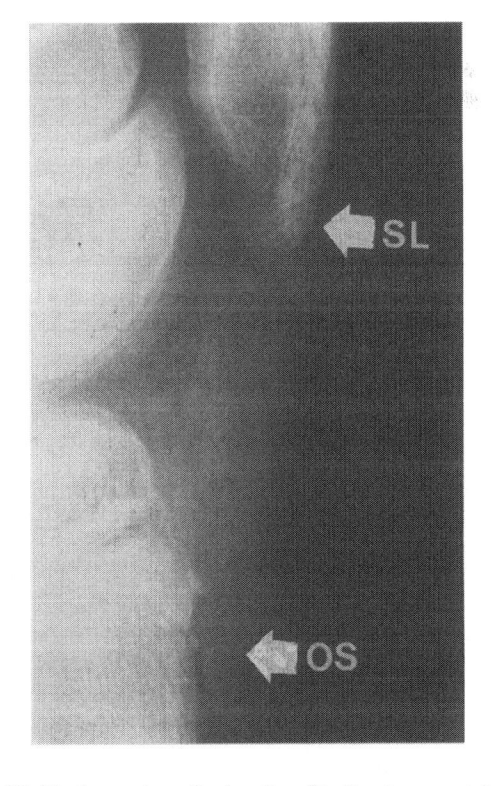

FIGURE 22-42. Asymptomatic, healing Sinding-Larsen-Johansson lesion (SL, arrow) in a child who presented with tibial tuberosity pain compatible with an Osgood-Schlatter lesion (OS, arrow).

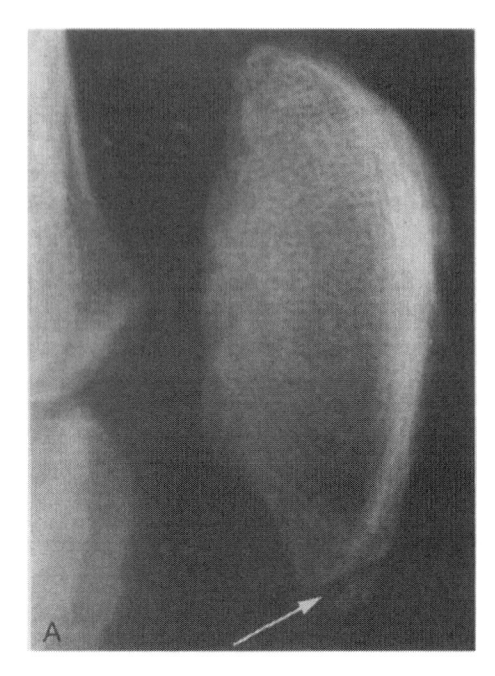

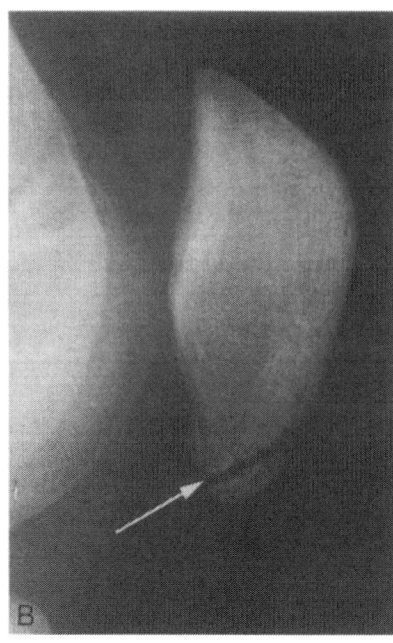

FIGURE 22-43. Sinding-Larsen-Johansson (SLJ) lesions (arrows) in a 9-year-old (A) and a 13-year-old (B).

patellar ligament at the inferior pole of the patella is by far the most common location of jumper's knee, although other sites have been reported. The various entities of patellar tendonitis, jumper's knee, and SLJ probably represent a spectrum of similar pathomechanical processes.[229,230]

Sinding-Larsen-Johansson "disease" is a chronic traction lesion. As with any traction "epiphysitis," treatment is directed at the symptoms and the probable inciting cause. This condition should be treated with rest for a sustained period of 3–6 weeks using extension immobilization, followed by progressive quadriceps mechanism strengthening.

The lesion tends to be self-limited but may remain insidiously active during skeletal growth. Because the involved area is nonarticular and separated from the joint by the fat pad, joint changes other than chondromalacia are unlikely.

Treatment of SLJ is conservative, with the symptoms usually running a course of 2–14 months. A knee immobilizer or cylinder cast is applied for 3–4 weeks in the patient with acute or severe pain. The patient with less severe symptoms is treated with a prescribed rehabilitation protocol and antiinflammatory drugs. These patients often have tight hamstrings and relatively weak hip flexors, such that

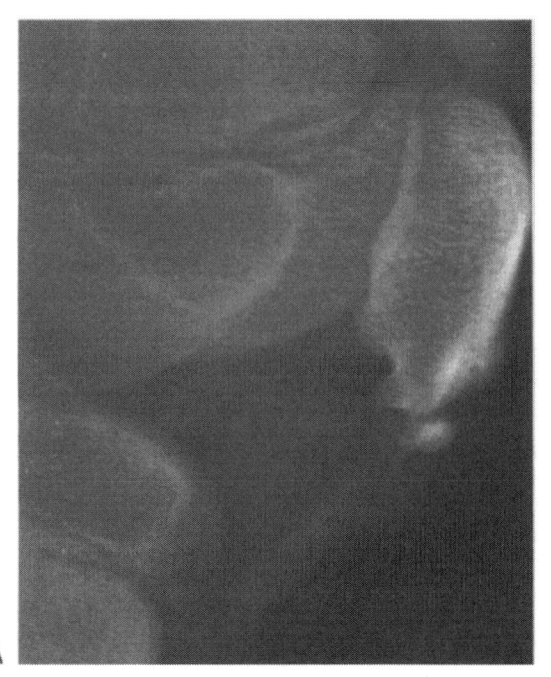

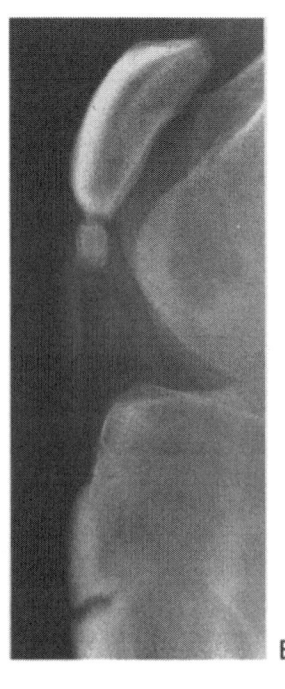

FIGURE 22-44. (A) Delayed healing in a patient who continued to play sports despite pain. (B) Appearance 4 years later.

FIGURE 22-45. (A) Proximal pole SLJ lesion in a 12-year old. (B) Chronic proximal SLJ lesion in a 14-year-old female gymnast.

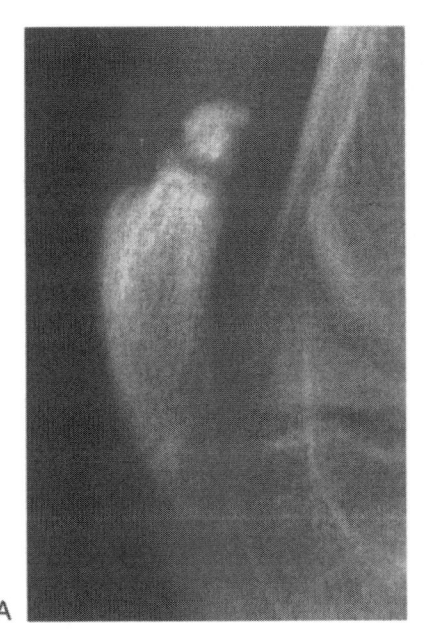

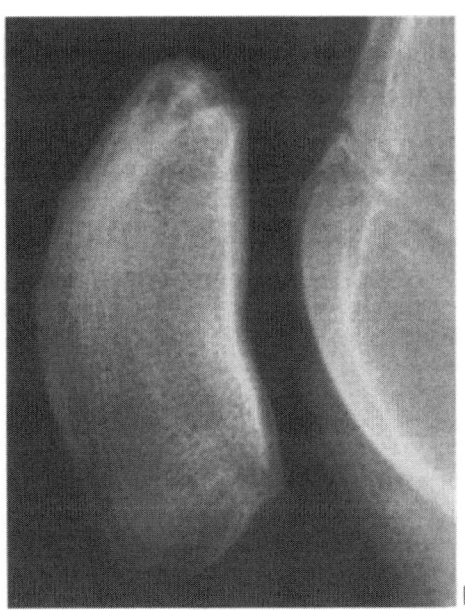

stretching and strengthening of these muscle groups becomes necessary. Cessation of the evocative activity is essential.

Radiographic incorporation of the ossific lesion of the anterior/inferior pole to the rest of the patella is not a prerequisite for activity resumption. Clinical healing with absence of pain and tenderness is a more appropriate endpoint. This is followed by a gradual, progressive, directed strengthening of the quadriceps-patella mechanism. The severity of the lesion must not be underestimated on the basis of a seemingly benign radiographic appearance. Patients treated conservatively may develop prominence of the patella.

The problem may persist to the end of skeletal maturity, may lead to irregular development of the lower end of the patella, and may even be associated with the development of a radiographic "loose body," although there is usually fibrous or fibrocartilaginous continuity.

Proximal Pole Lesion

The SLJ lesion is well recognized in the distal pole of the patella, but similar changes may occur in the proximal pole (Fig. 22-45). The radiographic appearances result from traction exerted through the ligamentous attachments of the quadriceps muscle into the superior edge of the patella.

The patients reported by Batten and Menelaus, ages 10 and 11, presented with anterior knee pain.[245] Batten and Menelaus thought that the lesion represented (1) an abnormality of ossification of the proximal pole of the patella; (2) avascular necrosis related to the poor blood supply of this portion as described by Scapinelli[13]; or (3) the result of traction on the superior pole of the patella or a combination of any of these possibilities.[245] However, the abnormal repetitive traction (overuse) response is the most likely explanation. In one patient who was followed for 2 years there was restoration of the normal trabecular pattern and only minimal alteration in the contour of the bone at the end of the pathologic process.

Association with Neuromuscular Disorders

Rosenthal and Levine reported 88 patients with spastic cerebral palsy and found 10 instances of variable fragmentation of the distal pole of the patella.[258] In addition, 12 knees, including the uninvolved ones, exhibited changes in the tibial tuberosity compatible with an Osgood-Schlatter lesion. Excessive tension in the quadriceps mechanism, usually in the presence of a significant knee flexion contracture, appeared to be the cause of the lesions. Of the fragmented patellas, four healed after hamstring release and correction of the flexion deformity. The association between fragmentation of the distal pole of the patella and cerebral palsy was further emphasized by Kaye and Freiberger, who described fragmentation of the patella in seven patients ranging in age from 7 to 15 years.[253] They thought that the patellar fragmentation was traumatic, with the flexion contractures and spasticity causing chronic, abnormal stresses and *repetitive* microtrauma (to the inferior chondro-osseous interface).

It seems feasible that this lesion is a more extensive version of the SLJ lesion with an osteochondral or sleeve-type fracture pulling away slowly as a chronic separation (Fig. 22-46).

Rosenthal and Levine supported the contention that elongation of the patellar tendon and the secondarily high position of the patella seen in spastic patients represented adaptive changes caused by prolonged increased tension during the phases of rapid growth, particularly in the presence of a knee flexion contracture and crouched-gait ambulation.[258] In their study of the results of surgical advancement of the insertion of the patella tendon in patients with cerebral palsy, Roberts and Adams found one spontaneous fracture of the patella in a patient who had not sustained any

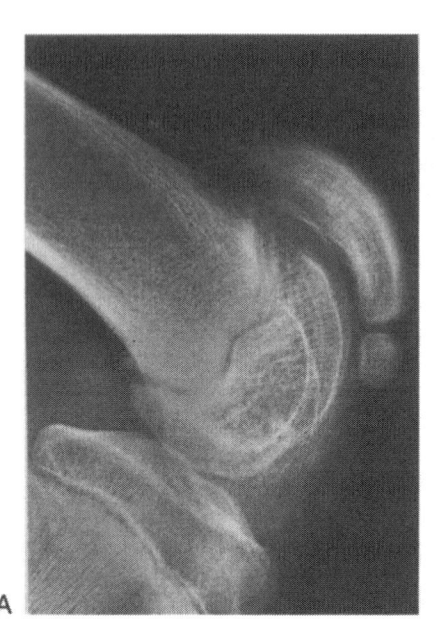

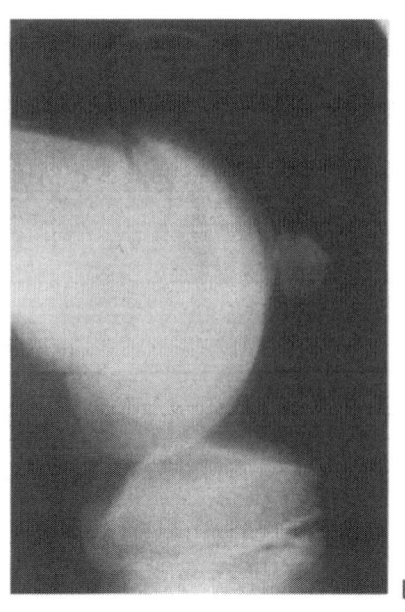

FIGURE 22-46. (A) Attenuated, curvilinear patella with inferior SLJ lesion in a child with cerebral palsy (CP). (B) Similar CP patient with a crouched knee gait and episodic pain. She had an acute onset of pain while walking and was unable to extend the knee. The inferior pole has acutely fractured through an area rendered chronically susceptible.

trauma and proposed that overactivity of the quadriceps had caused the avulsion fracture.[257] If the tension in the extensor mechanism in a growing child is prolonged and of sufficient grade, a high-riding patella or stress fragmentation of the distal pole of the patella or tibial tuberosity may occur, especially in the presence of a knee flexion contracture. Perry and coworkers showed that the quadriceps force required to stabilize the flexed knee during stance in children with cerebral palsy was proportional to the angle of the knee flexion; and that for each degree of flexion, the required force increased an average of 6%.[256] Therefore a flexion contracture of 30° may cause forces of 210% of body weight.[255]

Lloyd-Roberts et al. discussed avulsion of the distal pole of the patella in cerebral palsy as a cause of the crouched-knee gait.[254] It should be emphasized that such avulsion may occur painlessly, although pain may subsequently develop. During long-term follow-up it seems that these individuals are predisposed to develop unusual contours of the patella and an apparent bipartite nature that may become progressively painful with chondromalacia, osteoarthritis, or both. When this lesion affects the individual, there is usually pain in one or both knees. Knee flexion increases, and the child may support the knee with a hand. There may be acute local tenderness at the distal pole. Treatment with bilateral hamstring releases or lengthening and progressive correction of the flexion deformity by serial splints is indicated. Only two of eight patients in the Lloyd-Roberts et al. series required removal of the fragment. Most responded to soft tissue flexion contracture release.

Bipartite Patella

The bipartite patella is a variation of ossification that often must be distinguished from an acute or chronic (stress) fracture,[259–281] which is sometimes difficult. Theoretically, a bipartite patella may be the result of a nonunited avulsion fracture or failure of primary and accessory ossification centers to fuse. Smooth articular cartilage usually covers the area of roentgenographic discontinuity (radiolucency) on the inner (joint) surface.

Bipartite patellas have been anatomically grouped.[276] Class I involves the distal patellar pole, class II the lateral margin, and class III the superolateral pole (Fig. 22-47).[224] Symptomatic cases tend to be class III. Class I appears to be, realistically, the end result of the Sinding-Larsen-Johansson lesion. Class II seems likely to follow traumatic subluxation or dislocation in the child or adolescent (see Sleeve Fracture, above).

The accessory ossification center in bipartite patellae usually appears around 12 years of age, although occasionally it is seen in children as young as 8 years of age. It may persist into adulthood. Ruggles reported an autopsy case of a 63-year-old man with bilateral involvement.[275] It is unilateral in 57% of patients, and it is more common in males than females.[279]

The histologic appearance of surgical and anatomic specimens (Figs. 22-48 to 22-50) is similar to that described in specimens of the Osgood-Schlatter lesion, a factor strongly suggesting a chronic, chondro-osseous, tensile failure in some patients. It is also similar to the histologic changes reported in symptomatic patients with a tarsal accessory navicular (see Chapter 24). One of the weakest areas of the developing skeleton is the margin between an

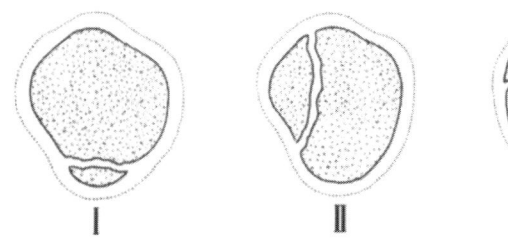

FIGURE 22-47. Anatomic classification of Saupe for bipartite patella. (I) Inferior. (II) Lateral. (III) Superolateral.

Bipartite Patella

FIGURE 22-48. (A) Bipartite patella (arrows) from an 11-year-old. (B) Bipartite patella (arrows) from a 14-year-old. (C) Slab roentgenogram showing multiple accessory ossification in the superolateral region. (D) Slab section of bipartite patella (arrows).

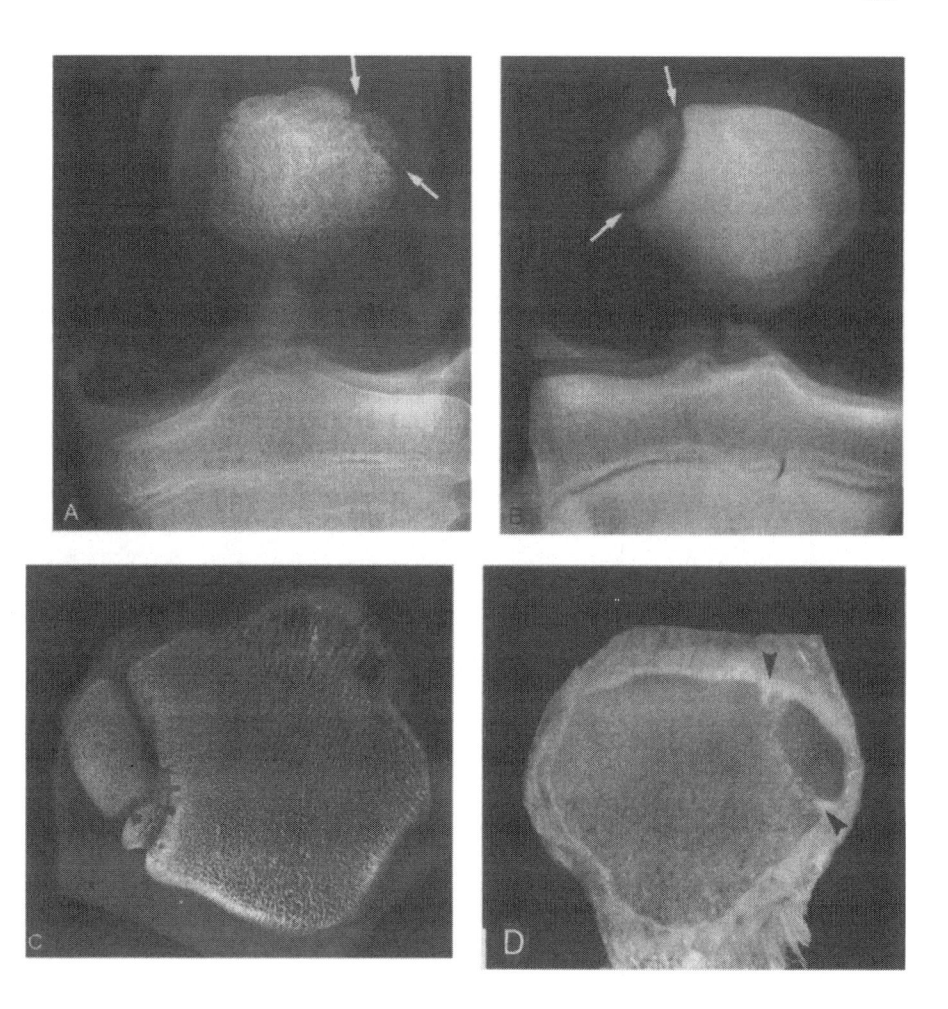

expanding ossification center and the overlying cartilage, similar to the weakness at the physeal–metaphyseal interface. Excessive tensile force, whether applied to the superolateral patellar pole (bipartite patella), inferior patellar pole (Sinding-Larsen-Johansson lesion), or tibial tuberosity (Osgood-Schlatter lesion), may partially separate (avulse) a segment of incompletely developed cartilage that eventually ossifies, thus appearing as an "accessory" or separate region of ossification. Similar postavulsion ossification certainly appears in the avulsed tibial spine in the skeletally immature patient. This bipartite fragment subsequently may fuse to the remainder of the ossifying patella, or it may be separated by an area of irregular cartilage and fibrocartilage.

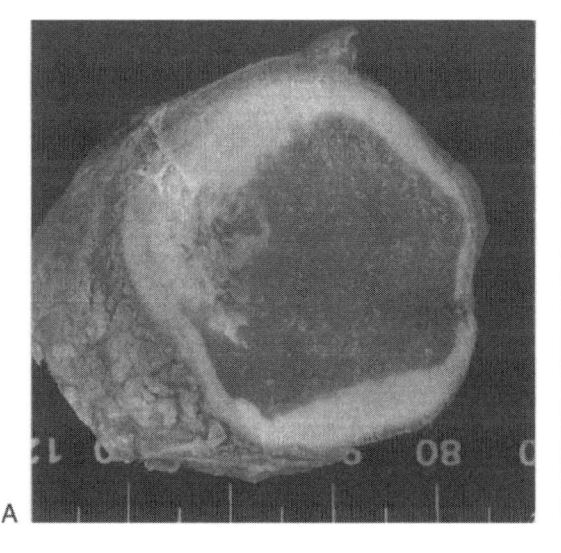

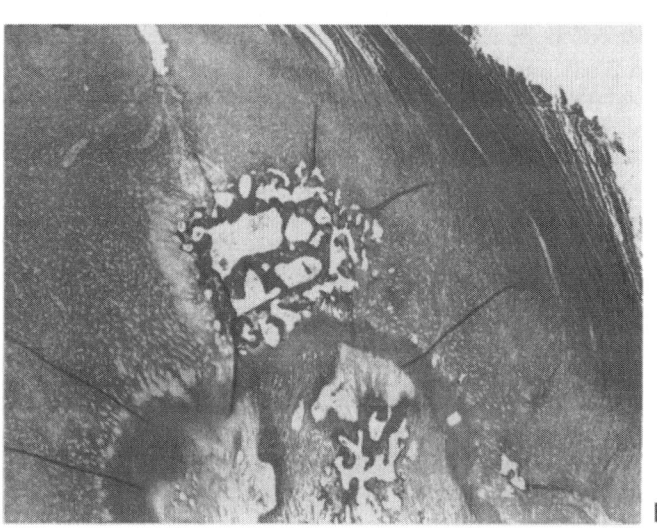

FIGURE 22-49. (A) Irregular ossification of a bipartite patella. Note the superolateral involvement. (B) Histology.

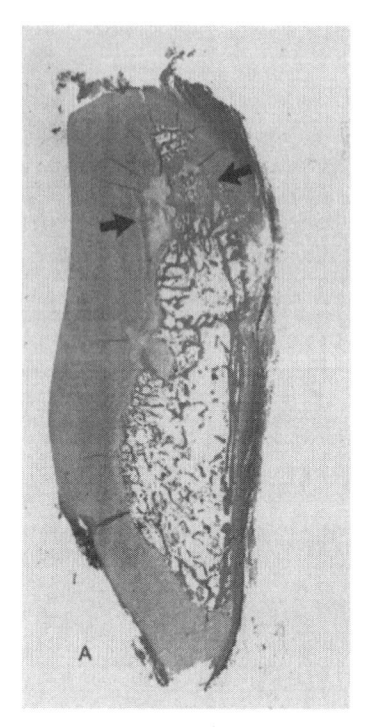

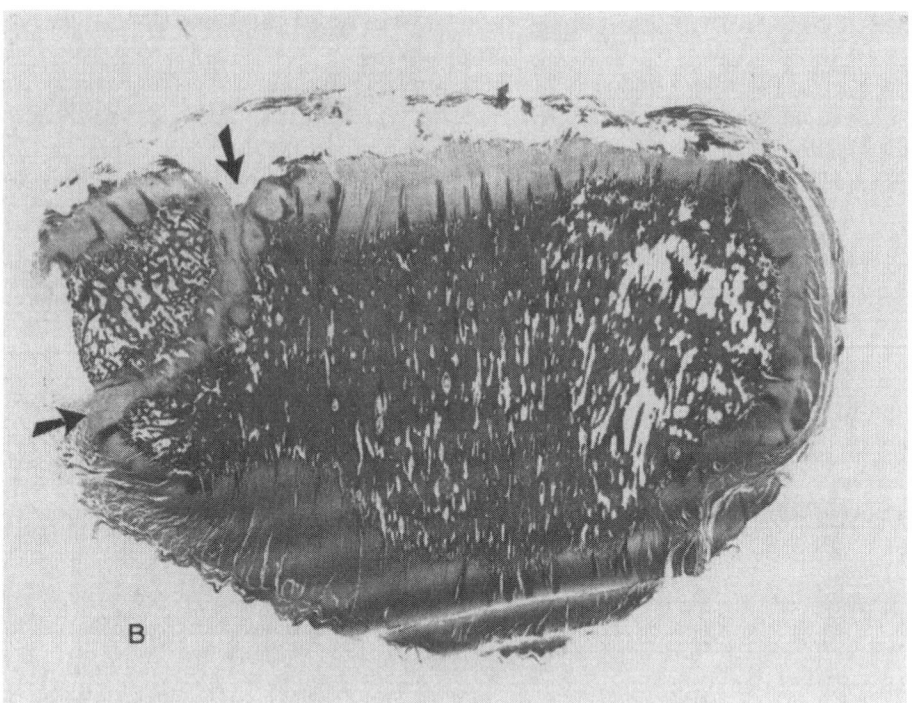

FIGURE 22-50. Lateral (A) and transverse (B) histologic sections of a bipartite patella (arrows).

Smillie thought that most bipartite patellas represented nonunion of marginal fractures due to poor blood supply.[277] However, histologic changes do not support vascular ischemia as an etiologic factor.[273]

Few patients have undergone roentgenographic studies of the patella prior to showing the bipartite patella. One patient had a normal patella 10 weeks before injury and eventual evidence of a bipartite patella.[264] In another case a roentgenogram obtained 5 years earlier did not show a bipartite patella.[260] Bourne and Bianco cited cases in which knees that appeared normal on radiograph later developed bipartite patella.[261]

Most patients with a bipartite patella are asymptomatic, despite the obvious radiographic entity (Figs. 22-51, 22-52). It is comparable to patients with Sinding-Larsen-Johansson or Osgood-Schlatter lesions in whom the radiographic changes often are fortuitous findings during evaluation of the knee. However, it is becoming increasingly evident that many patients with a bipartite patella *are* symptomatic (Figs. 22-53, 22-54). The pain associated with symptomatic bipartite patella presents in one of two characteristic ways: (1) gradual onset during activity (usually repetitive athletic activity); and (2) sudden onset after an acute injury. When onset of pain is related to direct trauma, the activity tolerance is less, and the need for treatment becomes more intense. The cause of pain is assumed to be micromotion in the abnormal synchondrosis. In one study the articular surface was intact in all but two of the operated patients, and only one patient had chondromalacia.[281]

Figure 22-54 shows a bipartite patella that was asymptomatic until the patient fell acutely, striking the knee on the ground. He developed lateral knee pain. The bipartite lesion appeared displaced, and MRI showed focal edema/hemorrhage in the lateral condyle due to chronic impingement by the fragment.

Direct or indirect trauma (e.g., "traction epiphysitis") to the interface between the main and accessory ossification centers has been a frequent hypothesis.[278,279] The cartilage interface may weaken the patella, making a stress fracture more likely at this site. Because cartilage has limited repair capacity, painful nonunion develops. When extrapolating from various studies, it appears that fewer than 2% of patients with bipartite patellas ever have sufficient symptoms to seek orthopaedic care.

Scapinelli analyzed the blood supply of the patella and showed it was compromised in the upper and outer lateral quadrants. This may account for the poor healing and tendency to form a superolateral bipartite defect or even not healing after acute or repetitive trauma.[13]

Weaver studied 21 cases of bipartite patalla. The most common physical finding was localized tenderness over the superolateral pole.[281] All the patients were athletes and experienced a gradual onset of pain while training or an onset of symptoms after a defined injury. Those patients with a traumatic onset had a much lower activity tolerance and were less likely to be managed nonoperatively.

Todd and McCally suggested that direct or indirect trauma to the interface between the main and accessory ossifications could render the area symptomatic.[278] Benedetti and Canapa thought that repetitive microtrauma to the zone of interposed cartilage was responsible for the changes of fragmented fibrocartilage calcification and necrosis.[260]

A technetium bone scan may be helpful in rendering a diagnosis of a chronic stress fracture (Fig. 22-55). When using a bone scan, the lateral view is important. Normally there is increased activity at the physeal–metaphyseal junc-

Bipartite Patella

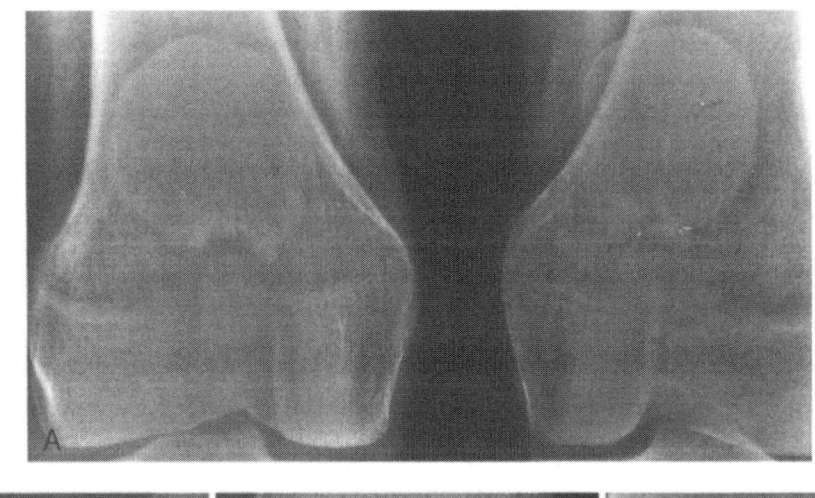

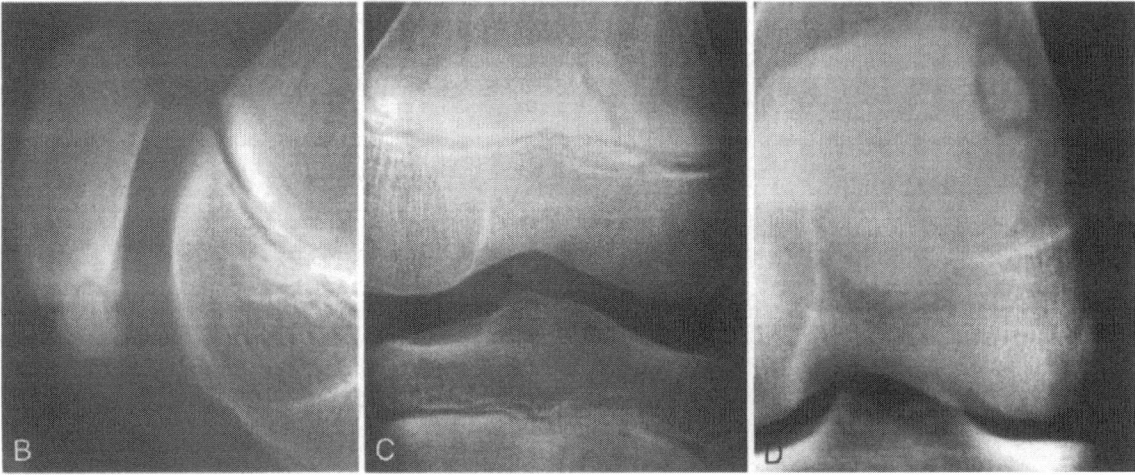

FIGURE 22-51. (A) Patient with bilateral inferior bipartite patellas. (B) Patient was treated for 4 weeks with cylinder cast immobilization. The "bipartite" patella was healing. (C, D) Anteroposterior views of superolateral bipartite patellas.

tion of the distal femur. The superolateral pole may overlie this region, such that normal uptake of the femur would obscure abnormal uptake of the patellar pole. The lateral view removes such overlap.

Initial treatment consists of immobilization for 3–4 weeks in a knee brace, knee immobilizer, or a cylinder cast. The next step is progressive muscle rehabilitation and strengthening.

Echeverria and Bersani showed that acute fracture of the superolateral patella clinically and radiographically simulated a symptomatic bipartite patella.[264] The ability to differentiate between symptomatic bipartite patella and an acute fracture has therapeutic implications. A minimally displaced acute fracture would be expected to heal uneventfully if immobilized in a cylinder cast. However, if the fracture was mistaken for a bipartite patella and isometric or isotonic

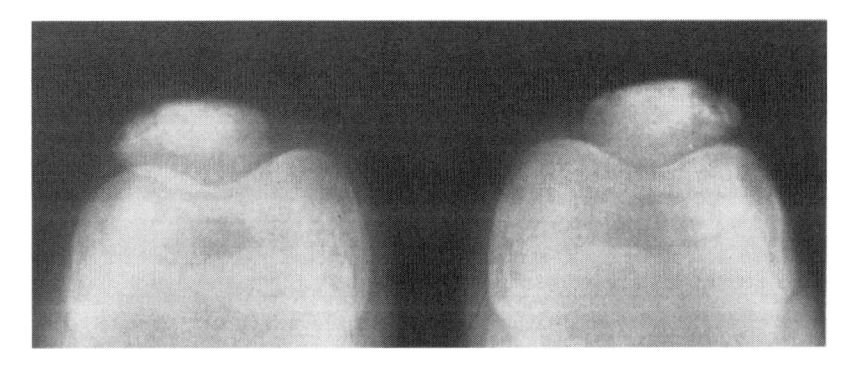

FIGURE 22-52. Bilateral bipartite patellas in an asymptomatic patient.

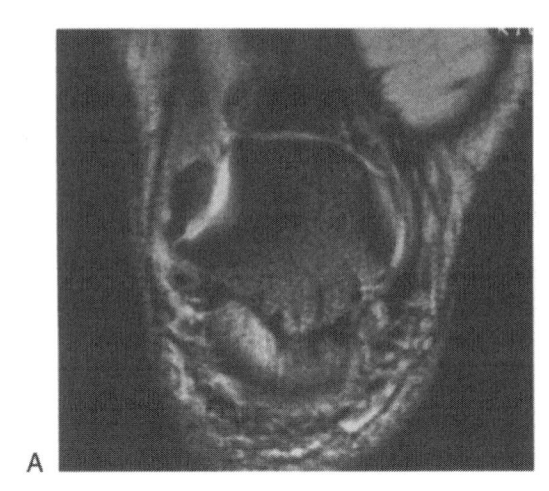

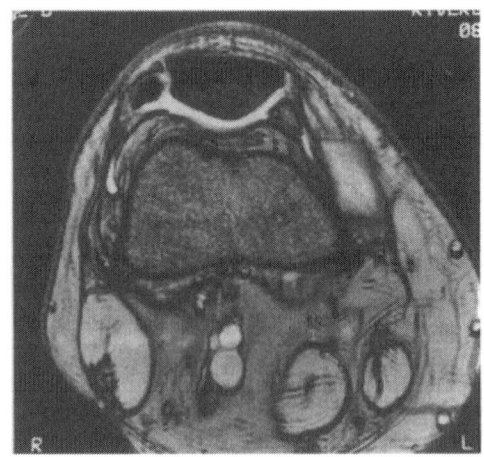

FIGURE 22-53. (A, B) MRI views of a bipartite patella.

exercises are initiated, it is theoretically possible that a fibrous nonunion could result.

Excision of the *painful*, tender accessory ossification center that fails to respond to initial nonsurgical treatment is recommended. The accessory region is often relatively small, and its removal interferes minimally with normal function of the patellofemoral joint and quadriceps mechanism. Larger fragments may involve significant portions of the articular surface. Screw or pin fixation and curettage of the cartilage between the main bulk of the patella and the accessory ossification center, rather than resection, should be considered. Such treatment, however, has not been reported in a significant number of patients. Angulation of the fragment is another reason for excision.

Weaver described painful bipartite patella in 21 patients. Sixteen were treated by fragment excision, three of whom had minor residual symptoms. The three youngest patients (10, 11, and 14 years) were treated nonsurgically.[281] Halpern and Hewitt reported improvement in a patient after excision of the accessory ossification center.[267] Similarly, Green reported three patients, one 13 years old and two each 15 years, all of whom, because of incapacitating pain, were treated with excision of the accessory ossification region. Their symptoms were relieved.[266]

Bourne and Bianco examined 16 patients with symptomatic bipartite patella.[261] In nine patients the pain began following specific trauma, and in seven the onset was insidious. All patients had pain related to activity. The average age at surgery was 14 years 6 months, with an average postoperative follow-up of 7 years. Fifteen of the patients were markedly improved; one was not. Bourne and Bianco did not note any changes of the patellofemoral articular surfaces after fragment excision. Of the 16 patients, 12 had nonoperative treatment for more than 6 months prior to surgical excision.

Dorsal Defects

Dorsal defects of the patella probably have an origin similar to that of the bipartite and multipartite patella.[263,268,269,280] Van Holsbeeck et al. thought that all of these defects represented a stress-induced disruption of normal ossi-fication patterns, rather than a posttraumatic subarticular cyst, and that the initial lesion was probably a traction lesion at the insertion of the vastus lateralis (Figs. 22-56 to 22-58).[280]

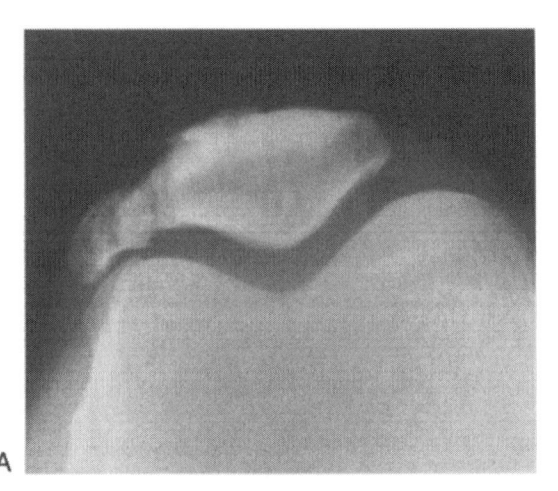

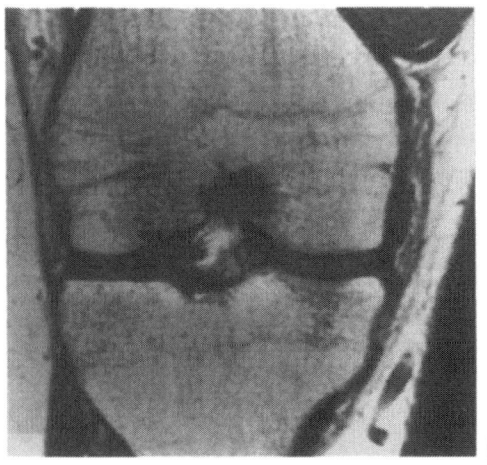

FIGURE 22-54. (A) Bipartite patella present for 6 years in a highly competitive athlete. (B) MRI shows bone bruising from chronic impingement of a fragment.

Bipartite Patella 965

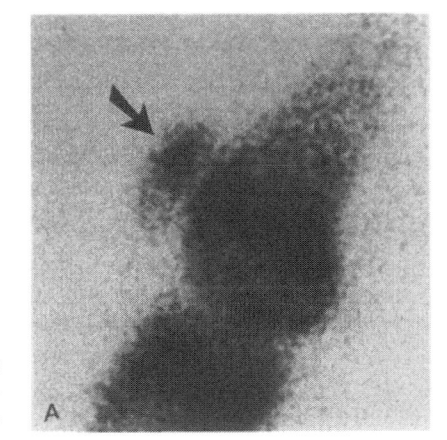

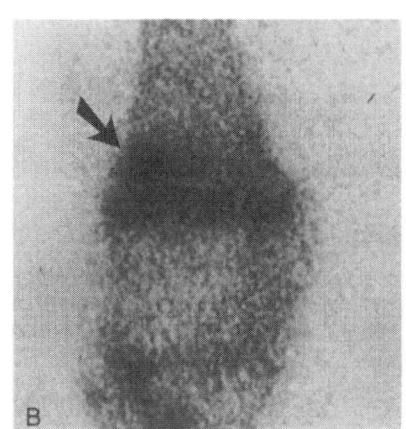

FIGURE 22-55. (A, B) "Hot" scan (arrows) of a patient with bilateral bipartite patella radiographically, Only one side was symptomatic, as corroborated by the bone scan.

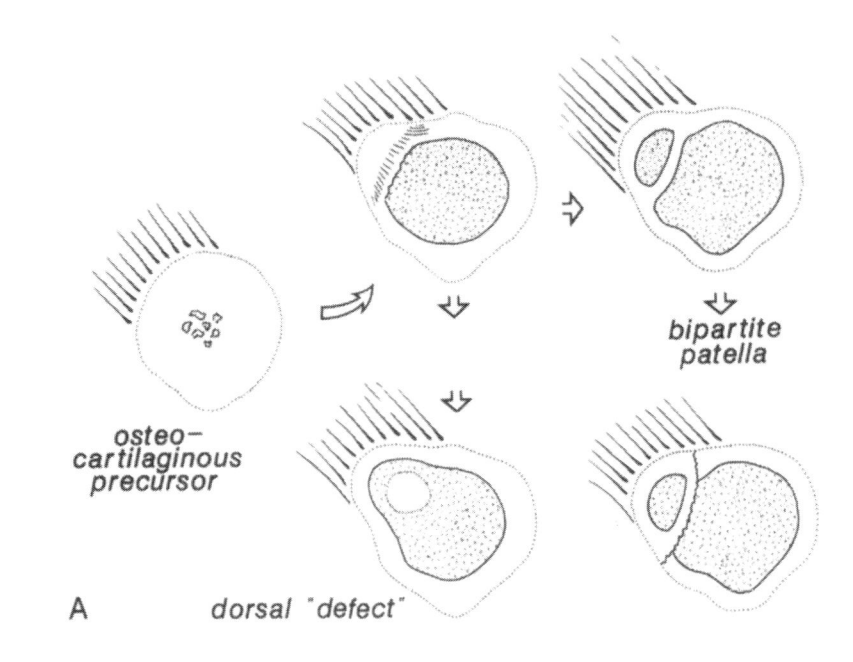

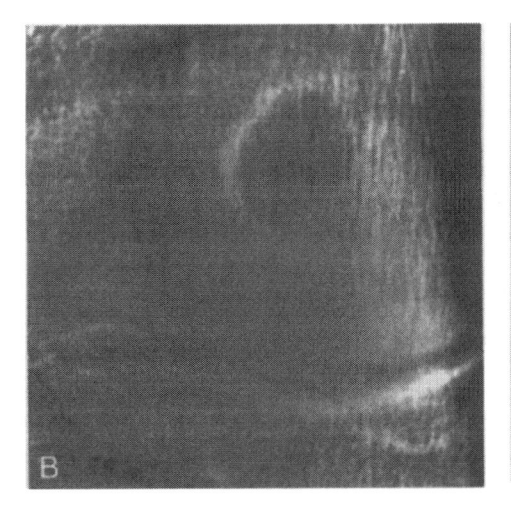

FIGURE 22-56. (A) Development of bipartite patella or dorsal defect. (B) Dorsal defect of patella. (C) Combination of dorsal defect and bipartite patella.

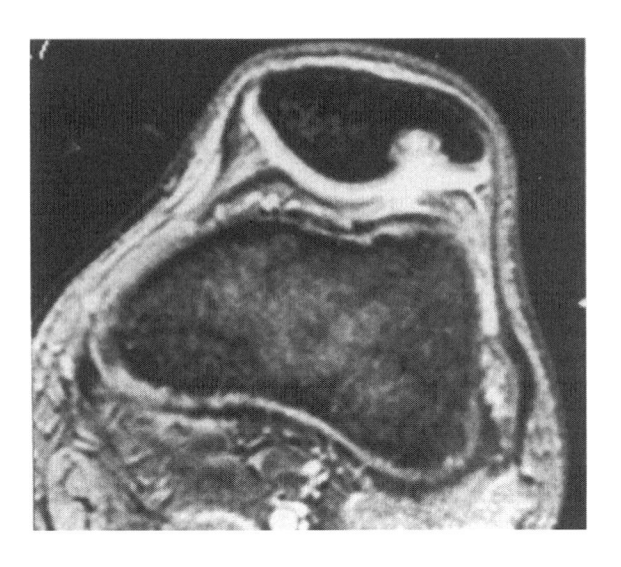

FIGURE 22-57. Dorsal defect of the patella. It was associated with maltracking.

Angiography of the patella showed a lack of arterial penetration from within the bone toward the cartilaginous superolateral margin.[279] Poor vascular supply combined with stress phenomena at the insertion of a strong vastus lateralis muscle are probably the causative mechanisms leading to irregular ossification in this region.

The concept of plastic deformity of the cartilaginous precursor of the patella allows two possibilities: (1) a deformity at the stage of the cartilaginous precursor, with subsequent formation of a multipartite patella; and (2) a deformity occurring at the stage of partial ossification of the patella, in which a displaced fragment of cartilage is partially devascularized, causing a delay in the ossification of this segment of the patella. This delay in ossification could be identified radiographically as a dorsal defect of the patella.

Fabellar Fracture

Dashefsky reported a 13-year-old boy who sustained a fracture through the sesamoid bone behind the knee.[282] This is an unusual cause for pain but certainly one that should be considered in a knee that proves difficult to diagnose and is associated with considerable posterior pain beyond obvious physical signs.

Popliteus Injury

The popliteus muscle is tendinous at the origin from the lateral side of the proximal distal femoral epiphysis. It runs intracapsularly deep to the fibular collateral ligament but external to the lateral meniscus. It has additional insertions into the periphery of the lateral meniscus and the proximal fibular epiphysis through the cruciate ligament complex.

McConkey and others[283–286] have described avulsion of the popliteus tendon. It usually follows a twisting injury of the knee, with the development of effusion and the presence of an osteochondral (epiphyseal sleeve) fracture in the lateral gutter. Open reduction and internal fixation are usually required.

Osteochondral Fractures

Osteochondral fractures of the medial or lateral femoral condylar articular surfaces may be caused by a direct blow or rapid lateral subluxation or dislocation of the patella, often accompanied by spontaneous reduction.[288,290,394,399,408] These injuries may also involve the medial surface of the intercondylar notch, although this is commonly the site of a more chronic lesion, osteochondritis dissecans. The fracture fragment may be visualized as a loose body, although it is not always easy to visualize it in young children. The separation through the subchondral bone may leave a thin layer that is difficult to visualize.

Kennedy divided these fractures into two types: (1) exogenous, in which the condyle strikes an external, direct shearing force; and (2) endogenous, in which there is a twisting injury with contact between the tibia and the condyle that causes the lesion.[10] Kennedy included an additional mechanism in which, because of patellar dislocation or subluxation, there is a fracture of the lateral femoral condyle. The

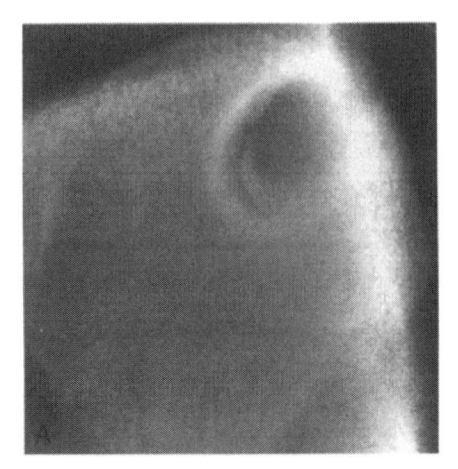

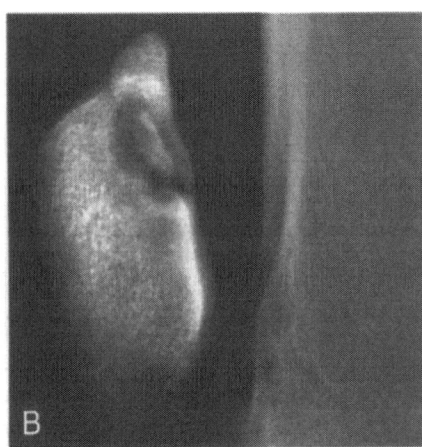

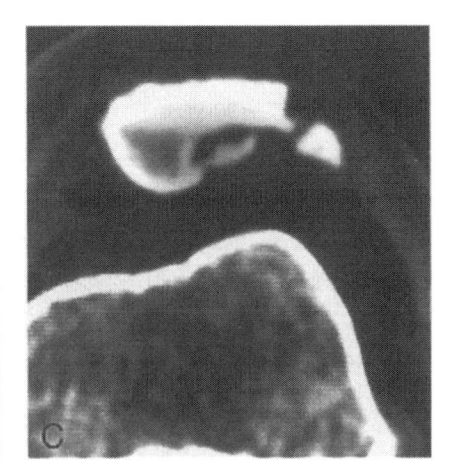

FIGURE 22-58. (A) Tomograph of a dorsal defect with enclosed ossification. (B) Lateral view. (C) CT scan.

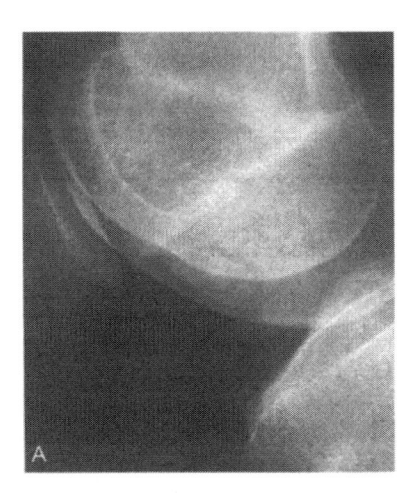

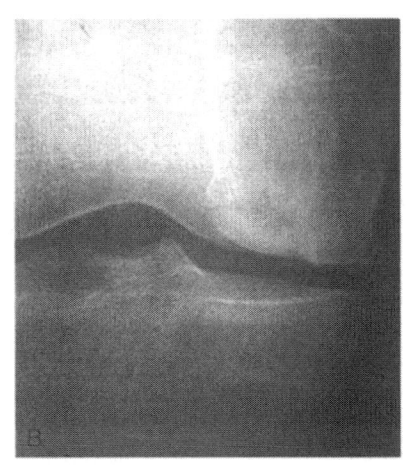

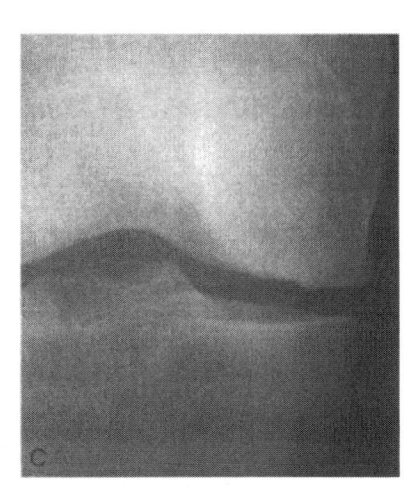

FIGURE 22-59. (A, B) Lateral and anteroposterior views of a large osteochondritis fragment in a 13-year-old girl. (C) Appearance 4 years later following operative treatment.

exogenous lesion tends to result from direct shearing trauma, whereas the endogenous lesion tends to result from a combination of rotatory and compression forces. In adults a compressive or rotatory force appears to be dissipated through the tide mark between calcified and uncalcified cartilage where the subchondral bone is not involved. In contrast, in adolescents the subchondral bone is penetrated, and an osteochondral fracture results.

Diagnosis of these injuries is sometimes difficult. Nonstandard projections may be misleading and suggest the diagnosis of a loose body, when in reality the tibial tuberosity is visualized. Because the epiphyseal regions of the young child contain more radiolucent cartilage than is seen during adolescence, the evaluation of suspected internal derangement of the knee is even more difficult. Chronic osteochondral fragmentation (osteochondritis dissecans) is more common than a meniscal tear in these age groups.

The knee should be aspirated. The presence of fat globules suggests intraarticular fracture through the subchondral plate. Treatment consists of arthroscopy or arthrotomy, evaluation of the loose fragment, and shaving of the sites of origin or reinsertion and fixation (by small metallic or polyglycolic acid-biodegradable pins) if a large fragment is found, particularly one that involves a joint surface (Fig. 22-59). A small fragment may be fixed or removed, especially if it involves a nonarticular surface. The inability to determine, with certainty, the size of the dislodged fragment preoperatively, the large weight-bearing area often discovered at operation, and the subsequent internal derangements of the knee resulting from ignored fragments warrant this approach. Replacement is indicated if the fragment or fragments are "fresh," if the osseous components are viable, and if the host area is weight-bearing and surgically accessible. A period of delay as limited as 10 days between the accident and surgery may compromise the result because the area begins to fill in with fibrous and fibrocartilaginous tissue, requiring trimming of the fragments or curetting to achieve a reasonable fit. Fixation pins should not be left protruding into the joint, as they may provoke a synovitis, pannus formation, and joint stiffness.

Osteochondritis Dissecans

Kennedy preferred to differentiate osteochondral fractures from osteochondritis dissecans.[10] The exact cause of the latter lesion is not known,[294,297] but it may represent a combination of microtrauma and ischemic disease, as proposed by Olsson's studies of similar lesions in animals (see Chapter 7). Osteochondritis dissecans is seen frequently in children during the growth spurt, particularly in children who are taller than average.[295,309]

The most frequent example of this injury pattern outside the knee is the subchondral fracture of Legg-Calvé-Perthes disease (see Chapter 11). There may be similarities: trauma leading to ischemia, attempted healing, and then subchondral fracture in the biomechanically susceptible bone.

Large, rapidly growing animals such as the giraffe, zebra, horse, elephant and cape buffalo may develop these lesions, usually during the equivalent of the adolescent growth spurt (Fig. 22-60). This is not unexpected in view of the size of the bone and articular surface and the repetitive cutting, twisting, and leaping that the knee joint is subject to during normal activity. We have found similar osteochondritic lesions in various other joints, including the large facet joints of the giraffe's cervical spine.

Green and Banks suggested that the disease starts when both subchondral bone and contiguous trabecular bone become ischemic.[297] The cartilage remains healthy because of synovial nutrition and continues to grow (thicken). The necrotic bone is gradually replaced and resorbed (Fig. 22-61). Until this occurs, osseous replacement of the thickening cartilage does not. This situation may cause loss of mechanical subchondral support of the cartilage, with subsequent softening and degeneration. Trauma, a relatively common occurrence during adolescence, may then disrupt the region and subsequently transform the lesion into a displaced fragment (Fig. 22-62).

Injured human articular cartilage tends to disrupt along the junction of calcified and uncalcified cartilage, leaving the osteochondral junction undisturbed. The child and ado-

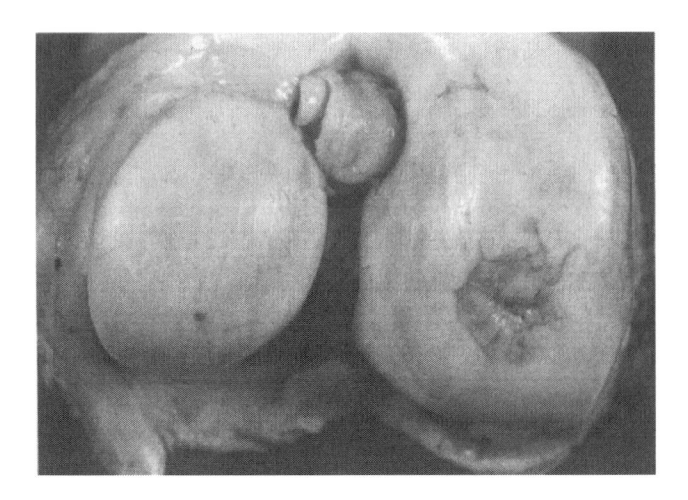

FIGURE 22-60. Osteochondritis in a juvenile (14-year-old) Indian elephant. This lesion is probably present in many animal species. The elephant is relatively unique among quadrupeds in that it walks with an upright pelvis and extended knee.

lescent have less calcified cartilage, so tangential forces, whether normal repetition or acute trauma, are directed to the subchondral region.[293] As in other areas of epiphyseal-physeal cartilage, the normal failure mode is through bone or the bone–cartilage interface, not the more resilient cartilage.

Theories invoking trauma have suggested that there was an impingement between the tibial spine on the lateral (intercondylar) aspect of the medial condyle,[296] which was further supported clinically and experimentally by Smillie.[277] The initial fracture the authors proposed was a subchondral fracture with intact articular cartilage overlying the infarcted bone, with subsequent normal use leading to eventual motion of the fragment in its bed and final propagation of the fracture through the articular surface. The fact that investigators were not able to accomplish this fracture experimentally in human cadavers does not necessarily rule out the proposed mechanism as a cause, particularly as these studies were carried out in adult cadavers, and the relation of articular cartilage, hyaline cartilage, and epiphyseal ossification in the developing knee may allow different anatomic and biomechanic mechanisms.[276] Forces transmitted through the patella also have been postulated to cause subchondral fractures eventuating in the dissecans lesion of the medial femoral condyle. Support for this theory has come from the experimental work of Aicroth.[289]

In contrast, others have strongly suggested ischemia to that area of the developing ossification center, with isolation of a necrotic fragment of bone unable to bear weight in a proper fashion. Several authors have suggested that a separate ossification center may exist for that position of the medial femoral condyle typically involved with the dissecans lesion, and that roentgenographic visualization is no more than a representation of this normal variation in epiphyseal growth and development.[10,277] Irregularity of ossification in this region may make certain children more susceptible. Olsson was able to show that irregularities in the development of the cartilage with thickening of the cartilage in the area eventually formed a dissecans lesion.[304]

Henderson and Houghton thought that osteochondral fractures are an important cause of knee morbidity in children and contribute to delayed or failed diagnosis.[299] Routine plane radiographs are often unreliable as the bony fragment may be sufficiently small to be barely visible, even to the most suspicious observer. If not diagnosed properly, osteochondral fracture may give rise to pain, instability, and locking of the knee over the short term, with subsequent irreparable damage and premature degeneration. Arthroscopy and MRI can delineate these lesions, particularly ones that are a chondral (minimally osseous) separation with little epiphyseal bone attached to the cartilage fragment.[303]

The increased use of MRI scans that demonstrate intraosseous bone bruising (accumulation of edema and hemorrhage) suggest that a focal injury may be more common than we realize (Fig. 22-61). This edema may cause localized trabecular bone cell death as a causal mechanism. The lack of vascularity means that normal chondro-osseous transfor-

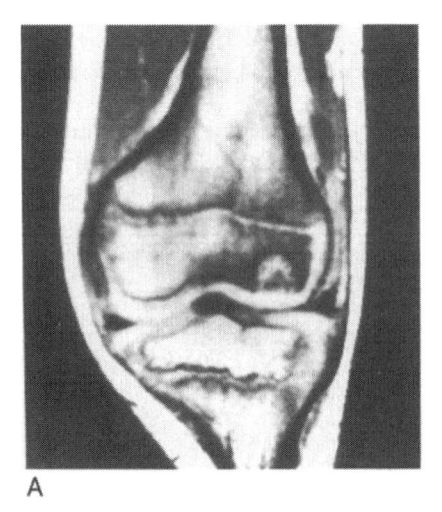

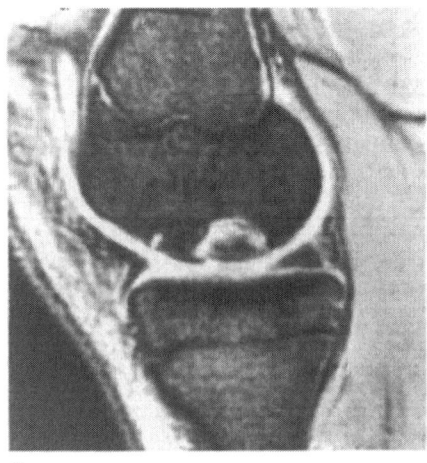

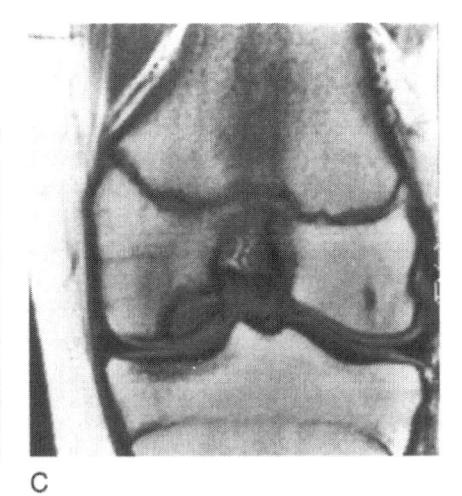

FIGURE 22-61. MRI view of early (A, B) and chronic (C) osteochondritis dissecans.

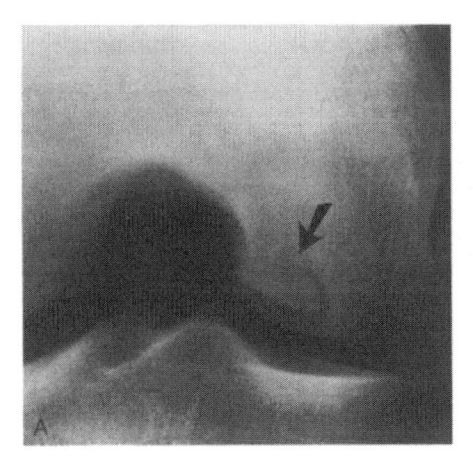

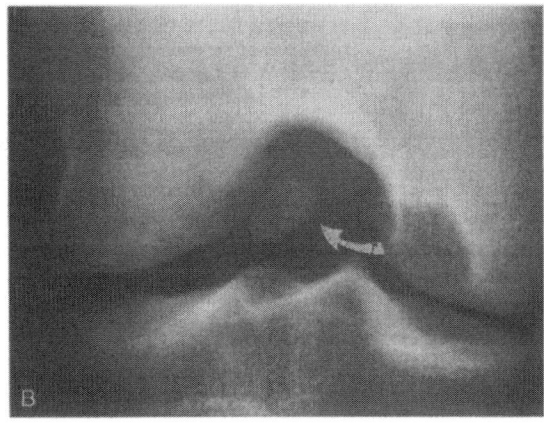

FIGURE 22-62. (A) Anteroposterior view showing undisplaced osteochondritis (arrow). (B) One week later during a basketball game the fragment displaced (arrow). It was subsequently removed.

mation cannot occur, so the cartilage focally thickens. Eventually the combination of changes is mechanically weak and nonsupportive of activity. A subchondral crack begins (as in Legge-Calvé-Perthes disease) and causes pain. If the child continues activity the fracture may propagate, loosening the fragment further and causing reactive changes such as synovitis. Healy reported a patient with a 3-year history of knee pain but no evidence of disease by routine radiography. Significant osteonecrotic lesions were evident on MRI.[298]

Adam et al. thought that MRI is the diagnostic method of choice for the determination of fragment stability and is probably the diagnostic method of choice for the early lesion that may show up on MRI but is not evident with standard radiography.[287] Their experiments suggested that MRI may reveal the various stages of the healing process of osteochondral fragments. Furthermore, MRI gives more information about the healing process and the viability of the interface than does histology. They believed that clinical studies using contrast-enhanced (e.g., gadolinium) MRI sequences were necessary to confirm these findings. The gadolinium should be injected into the joint, rather than intravenously, to give the best results.

Treatment for the young patient with a nondetatched fragment should be conservative, often with no more than restriction of symptom-producing activities. The older patient with a detached fragment (Fig. 22-63) is treated best by arthroscopy or arthrotomy with excision of the fragment and removal of joint debris.[291,302,306] Fragments that involve weight-bearing areas should be replaced and fixed.[310] In either case, the subchondral bone at the base of the defect should be drilled to stimulate a fibroblastic-fibrocartilaginous response.

Arthroscopy may be used to fix these lesions, running the pin into the condyle to a subcutaneous position so that they may be removed, if necessary, when the lesion heals. Wombwell and Nunley showed the use of Herbert screws to provide fixation of osteochondritis dissecans fragments under compression and allow early motion.[312] However, the use of these screws is not without risk. Further collapse of the lesion, especially if it is large, may cause loosening of the fixation (Fig. 22-64). Biodegradeable pins may also be used.

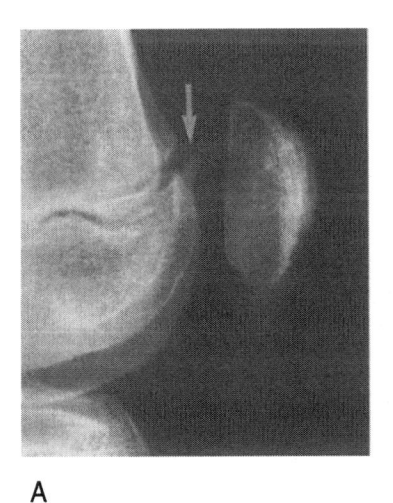

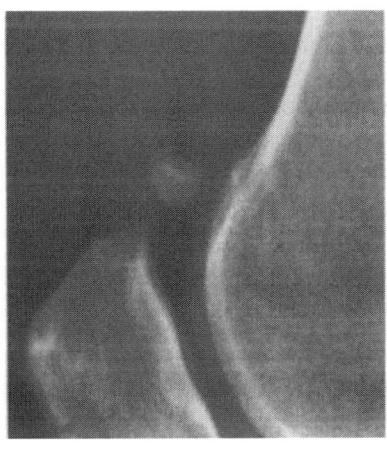

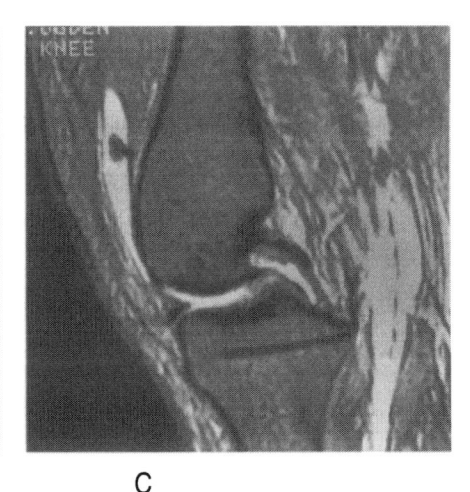

FIGURE 22-63. (A) Loose body (arrow) behind the patella. It was probably a small osteochondritis dissecans fragment. The parents refused arthroscopic removal. Eleven years later the patient presented with chronic knee pain and effusion. (B) Radiograph. (C) MRI. The fragment was finally removed arthroscopically.

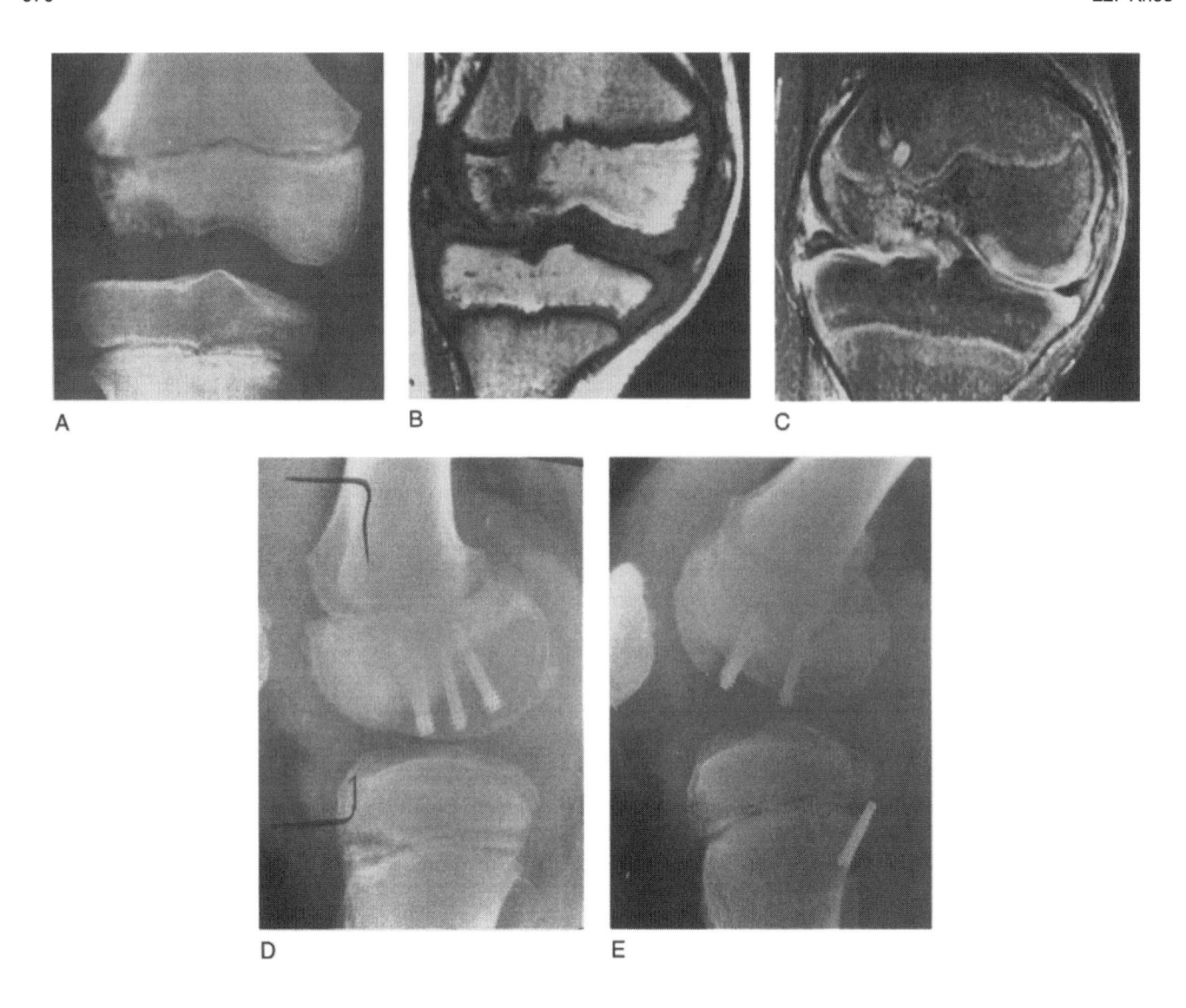

FIGURE 22-64. This 9-year-old boy presented for an evaluation of chronic knee pain and effusion. He was otherwise normal. Subsequent MRI failed to reveal any spinal or spinal cord pathology. (A) Initial presentation. There is relative radiolucency in the medial condyle. (B) MRI, however, showed extensive medial edema and changes with an unexpected area of penetration of the physis. (C) Four months later the involvement is more extensive. He was treated by arthrotomy. The joint surface was relatively intact but indented. A bone graft was inserted through a separate transepiphyseal (medial) approach. (D) The large fragment was fixed with Hebert screws. (E) Ten weeks after surgery there is collapse and penetration of the screws. While awaiting admission for removal of the screws, one completely dislodged and migrated. All screws were removed. He currently has a painful knee.

When the lesion is diagnosed before or after epiphyseal closure and there is objective evidence of looseness of the fragment and functional disability, the defect is best treated by open or arthroscopic reduction and fixation of the fragment until healing occurs. In knees with a long-standing lesion in which the loose fragment has become smaller than the crater and in which fixation and healing of the fragment would not restore a congruous joint surface, the lesion is best treated by excision of the fragment. Mosaic cartilage grafting awaits adequate outcome studies to see if it is effective and whether it should be applied to the young patient. Similarly, culture and replacement of cartilage cells is an intriguing but unproved treatment for skeletally immature patients.

Plaga et al. studied the fixation of osteochondral fractures in rabbit knees with a fibrin sealant, polydioxanone (PDS), pins, and Kirschner wires.[305] They found that all of the animals treated with Kirschner wire fixation healed versus 86% of the PDS group and only 50% of the fibrin sealant group.

Adam et al. assessed the stability of surgically induced osteochondral fragments of the femoral condyle by MRI experimentally in dogs.[287] Their MR images were compared with the histopathologic findings. They created loose and stable fragments. With the loose fragments, a well-defined line of high signal intensity was evident between the fragment and the epiphysis. Histologic examination revealed vascularized granulation tissue at the interface. Stable fragments showed a similar but irregularly defined line on MR sequences and no enhancement after injection of contrast medium. Histologic examination in these specimens showed no granulation tissue at the interface but intact bone trabeculae within the completely repaired fracture. They thought that contrast-enhanced MRI (T1-weighted sequence) allowed exact delineation of the line of separation of unstable versus stable fragments. They noted that the difference, which could not be well defined histologically, probably reflected differences of binding or distribution of protons in the healing osteochondral fragments.

Brown et al. studied the effects of osteochondral defect size on cartilage contact stress.[292] They were full-thickness osteochondral defects in the weight-bearing area of both femoral condyles. The defects were progressively enlarged from 1 mm to 7 mm. All specimens showed a tendency for contact stress concentration at the rim of the defect, and the contact stress distribution became progressively more nonuniform around the defect rim as the diameter was enlarged. They noted that these contact stress elevations at the rim were probably insufficient to inhibit defect repair or to cause degeneration of surrounding cartilage.

Twyman et al. studied 22 knees of patients who had osteochondritis dissecans diagnosed before skeletal maturity.[311] The patients were followed prospectively into middle age. One-third of them had radiographic evidence of moderate to severe osteoarthritis at an average follow-up of 33 years, with only half having either a good or excellent functional result. Osteoarthritis was more likely to occur if the defect was large or affected the lateral femoral condyle. This finding was in contrast to that of Linden's retrospective study of 23 immature knees followed for an average of 33 years in which he believed osteochondritis dissecans in children was rarely complicated by osteochondritis.[301]

A review of 83 patients with 95 involved knees followed for 2–31 years identified factors that may influence treatment and long-term prognosis.[300] Altogether 16 underwent nonsurgical treatment; 65 had surgical treatment; and 2 had nonsurgical treatment of one knee and surgical treatment of the other. Of the 22 knees that were treated nonsurgically, 15 were treated before and 7 after distal femoral epiphyseal closure. Of the 73 knees that were treated surgically, 23 were treated before epiphyseal closure and 50 after closure. A total of 77% of the knees in the surgical group and 82% of those in the conservatively treated group were rated excellent or good at long-term follow-up. The average scores in both groups were higher for knees in which the osteochondritic defect was small and in which treatment was undertaken before epiphyseal closure. In the surgical cases the results were better when the fragment healed in place, compared to the ones in which the fragment was removed. Hughston and coworkers concluded that when osteochondritis dissecans is diagnosed before epiphyseal closure the physical findings are often negative, and there is no functional disability.[300] The lesion is best treated conservatively by continuing normal activity supplemented by quadriceps-strengthening exercises, rather than by immobilization and rest.

Patella

Osteochondritis of the patella has also been described.[294] This lesion may involve varying areas of the medial and lateral articular facets, with the medial articular facet being involved more often (Figs. 22-65 to 22-67). The lesion also tends to involve the inferior, rather than the superior, half of the patella. Ischemic necrosis may be a major causal factor.[277] The patellar blood supply primarily enters the lower pole and proceeds proximally.[13] Thus if this lesion were related to defects of blood supply, one would expect more lesions in the upper pole than in the lower pole.

As discussed earlier for the femoral condyles, MRI studies show areas of focal edema following direct blow injuries. It is feasible that similar changes of focal ischemia ensue, eventually leading to microcompromise of tissue interfaces.

The indication for surgery is a loose osteochondral fragment that is either partially or completely detached from the articular surface. Excision of the affected area with drilling of the subchondral bone usually gives good results. Loose bodies should be removed.

Renu et al. followed 12 patients with osteochondritis dissecans of the patella.[307] The lesion was bilateral in three patients. All patients were initially treated conservatively,

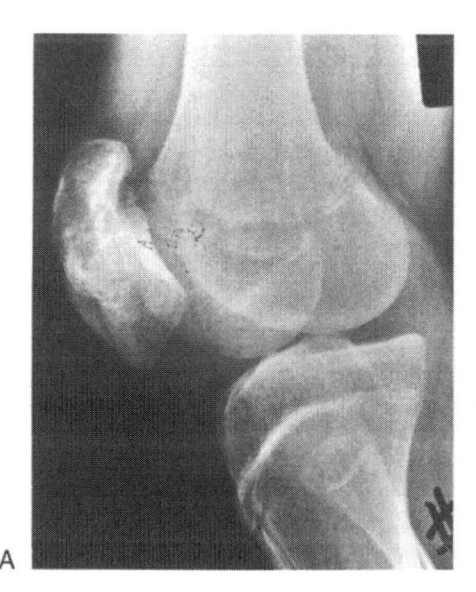

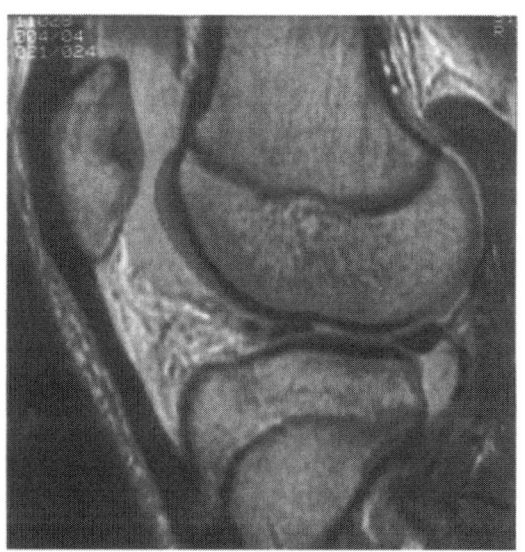

FIGURE 22-65. (A) Patellar osteochondritis dissecans. (B) MRI.

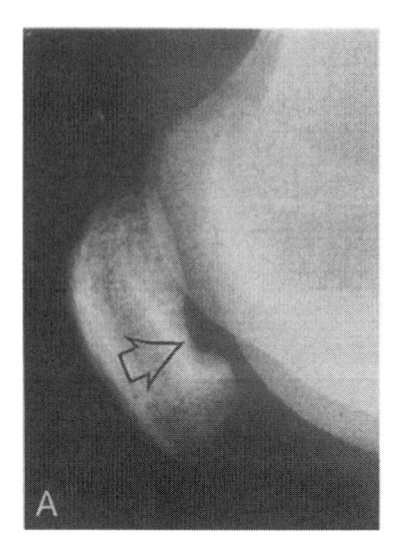

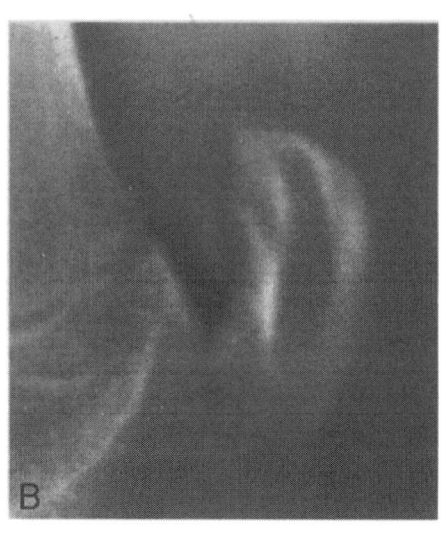

FIGURE 22-66. (A) Osteochondritis of the patella (arrow) in a 13-year-old girl with bilateral involvement. (B) Semiloose fragment.

with complete relief of symptoms in five. In the other seven patients the fragments were excised and the defect was curetted and drilled. At follow-up after 2–8 years, these patients had no restriction of activities and no pain.

Open Knee Injuries

Lacerations around the knee joint should be treated with a high degree of suspicion for penetration of an object into the knee joint.[316,317] Lacerations around the patellar tendon may not necessarily enter the joint. Instead, they may be totally within the fat pad around and behind the patellar tendon and therefore extrasynovial. For any case that is suspicious of penetration into the knee joint, a diagnosis should be made as accurately as possible because the joint should be débrided and irrigated adequately to prevent infection and serious secondary changes. If the joint has been entered by the laceration, there frequently is air within the joint (Fig. 22-68). However, there may be the appearance of an "air" arthrogram due to an associated osteochondral fracture with bleeding and fat from the underlying epiphyseal ossification center. A dye (e.g., methylene blue) may be injected into the knee joint; it usually leaks out of the laceration tract if there is a communication into the joint.

The correct diagnosis of retained foreign bodies accompanying small wounds about the knee demands a high index of suspicion. Because falls and wounds around the knee are a common occurrence in children, especially in the 4- to 8-year range, parents often defer medical advice, thinking that the pain and swelling will subside and that nothing could have entered the deep tissues or joint (see Chapter 9). Biologic structures (e.g., thorns, wood) may penetrate the skin and even the joint but may come out as the child gets up from the ground.[313–315] If the patient or parent attempts to remove them, small pieces may break off and remain within the joint or extracapsular tissues. Unfortunately, most of these objects are radiolucent. If they remain in the joint they

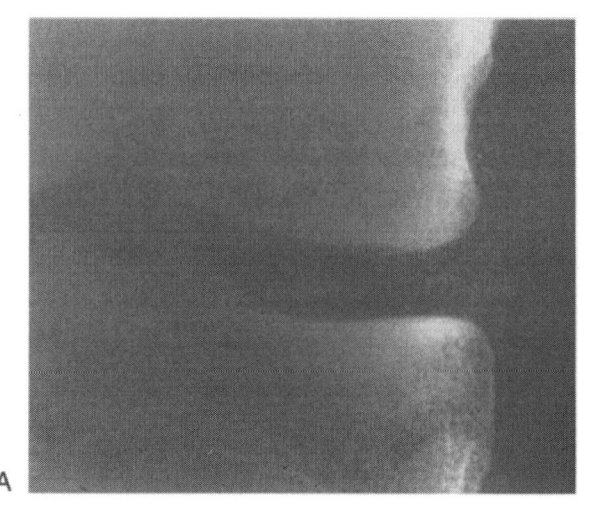

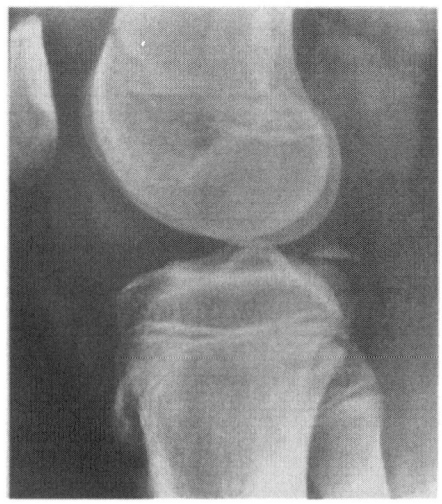

FIGURE 22-67. (A, B) Apparent loose body in the knee. It was a displaced patellar osteochondral fracture fragment.

FIGURE 22-68. (A) Example of intracapsular gas (intrasynovial). (B) Gas is confined to the fat pad (extrasynovial).

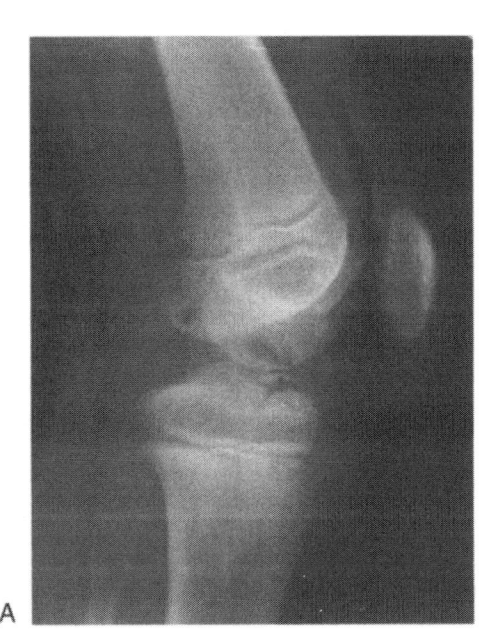

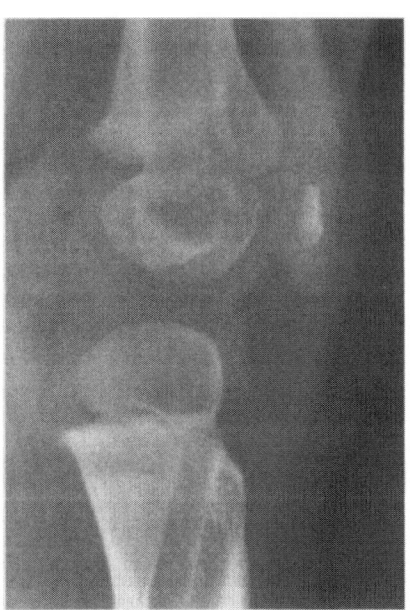

may serve as a mechanical or chemical irritant, creating a foreign body reaction or even pyarthrosis (see also organic foreign bodies in the foot, Chapter 24).

Any child presenting with a history suggestive of penetration of a foreign object into the knee may exhibit only painful range of motion and joint swelling. Elevation of temperature, white blood cell counts, or the erythrocyte sedimentation rate may be absent. If routine roentgenograms are negative, xerography is helpful. MRI is also helpful for delineating soft tissue or intraarticular foreign bodies and the surrounding areas of reactive inflammation and edema.

History and clinical examination may be entirely negative. Following local wound care, tetanus therapy, and antibiotics (if indicated), roentgenograms are mandatory. A knowledge of synovial recesses and suprapatellar pouch anatomy of the knee enables one to determine if a foreign body is lying in or communicating with the intracapsular space. Once recognized, the intracapsular foreign body *must* be removed. The desire to avoid a general anesthetic, to avoid a scar on the knee, or fear of not being able to locate a foreign body should not be contraindications, especially if one considers the potential damage to articular surfaces that may occur if the foreign body is left within the joint. Small retained fragments (e.g., glass) may become "stuck" in certain regions, such as a posterior recess, and create low grade, chronic pain and even a localized lesion with bursal fluid.

Potential problems with intracapsular foreign bodies include septic arthritis and osteomyelitis, mechanical trauma to the articular cartilage, physeal trauma, and growth disturbance as a result of the effects of any of the preceding on the physis. Articular cartilage lacerations heal poorly (often not at all) and may initiate early secondary arthritic changes.

Synovial Plications

The knee of the developing fetus is divided by thin synovial membranes into medial and lateral compartments and a suprapatellar pouch. The medial and lateral compartments of the knee joint are separated by a membranous partition that involutes so the knee joint becomes a single cavity. Failure of involution may result in a plica. The incidence of these plicae, within the general population is estimated to be 20%.[318-328]

Plicae are classified as suprapatellar, mediopatellar, or infrapatellar, according to the corresponding anatomic regions of the knee (Fig. 22-69). Any one or combination of these plicae may exist within a given knee. The most common plica of clinical significance is the suprapatellar plica, which may be subclassified into transverse, transverse with porta, medial, and lateral. Infrequently, the entire septum dividing the inferiorly placed medial and lateral compartments from the suprapatellar pouch persists into adult life as a transverse suprapatellar plica. This septum exists with an irregularly shaped opening called the porta (Fig. 22-70). A small remnant of this transverse septum may persist as a medial or lateral suprapatellar plica.

The "porta" plica may create the most problems in a growing child. The porta may effectively block fluid freely communicating between the (lower) knee joint and the suprapatellar pouch. The porta may also affect patellofemoral tracking. Such a lesion may be diagnosed with arthrography (Fig. 22-70) or MRI (Fig. 22-71). Perhaps the worst result I have seen from this type of plica was in an 11-year-old girl who underwent complete medial meniscectomy for persistent joint effusion (alleged diagnosis was hypermobile meniscus). The effusion recurred, and the same surgeon removed the lateral meniscus completely. She was referred with continuing chronic effusion. Arthrography and arthrotomy revealed a thick porta with a 4- to 5-mm opening, effectively dividing the knee into two compartments. This undoubtedly was the cause of the effusions, and it was resected with disappearance of effusion. Unfortunately, the prospects for this girl's knee was bleak, as she has no menisci. At 27 years of age she has severe degenerative osteoarthritis.

Persistence of the infrapatellar plica represents the most common plica of the knee joint.[328] It usually has a narrow

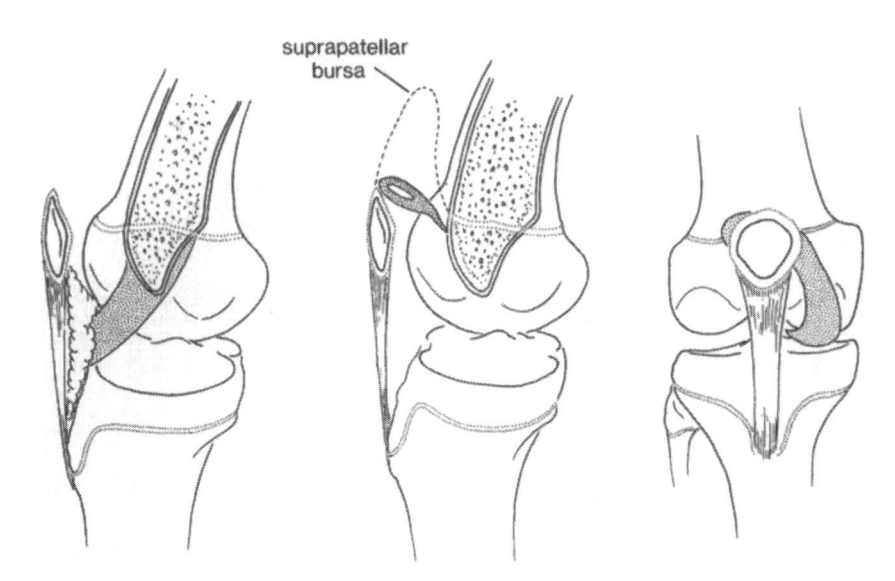

FIGURE 22-69. Synovial plica. These thickened bands of tissue remain after incomplete embryologic formation of the knee joint.

femoral origin in the intercondylar notch and widens as it sweeps through the inferior joint space to attach distally to the infrapatellar fat pad. Posteriorly, it borders but does not necessarily attach to the anterior cruciate ligament. Although the infrapatellar plica may be found in its entirety, frequently only a fenestrated septum or series of fibrous bands is all that remains.

Variable folds of the synovial membrane occasionally extend from the upper tibial fringe at the infrapatellar fat pad to the undersurface of the suprapatellar synovial plica-

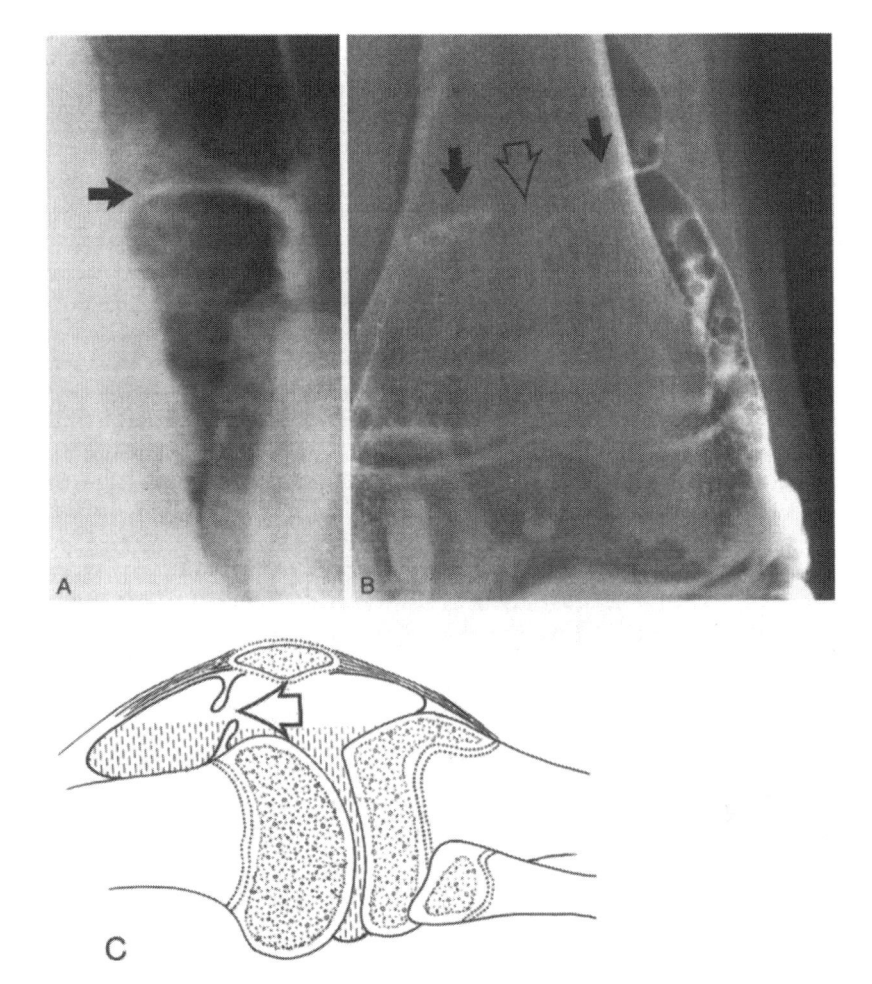

FIGURE 22-70. (A, B) Plica (solid arrows) extending across the suprapatellar pouch. It caused chronic synovitis and knee effusions for 2 years. (C) The open arrows in (B) and (C) indicate the communication.

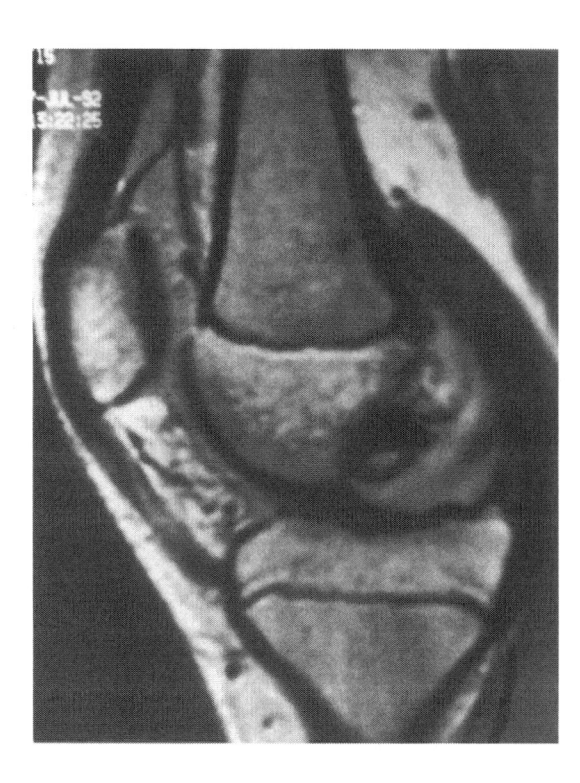

FIGURE 22-71. MRI of a symptomatic suprapatellar synovial plica.

tions.[320,323] Such a plica sometimes snaps back and forth over the condyle as the knee goes from full extension to full flexion, symptomatically duplicating the problems of a torn anterior horn of the meniscus. Most synovial folds are constantly being tensed and relaxed during joint movement. They contain a large portion of elastic fibers to facilitate the changing shape and length and may be detached easily consequent to trauma.

Most synovial plicae are asymptomatic and are likely to be incidental findings during arthroscopy, arthrotomy, arthrography, and MRI. They contain elastic tissue that allows them to slide over the femoral condyles during flexion and extension. However, inflammation with associated edema and thickening may cause symptoms when the plica becomes relatively inelastic as it snaps over the femoral condyle. Trauma usually is the precipitating cause of these inflammatory changes. The trauma may be direct or indirect. Indirect trauma may be secondary to other derangements within the knee. Alternatively, a symptomatic plica may be associated with increased demands made on the knee from excessive exercise or competitive or recreational athletics. The initial inflammatory change in a synovial plica, if not corrected, may progress to an intense synovitis with replacement of elastic tissue by fibrous elements. Erosive changes of the articular cartilage of the knee may ensue.

The size and the extent of the plicae depend on the degree of reabsorption of the various communicating bands separating the cavities.[329] Part of Johnson et al.'s study was to evaluate why plicae that had been present since birth usually were associated with the onset of symptoms that were delayed until adolescence.[324] A discrete injury preceding the pain was found in only 13% of the knees, which contrasted with the report of Hansen and Boe[322] in which there was a 50% prevalence of previous trauma. Many patients in the Johnson et al.[324] study had symptoms that were incurred during sports and appeared to have been precipitated in the structured sports activity undertaken during early adolescence. It is possible that the elasticity of the plicae diminishes with age or that the adolescent growth spurt in some way changes a mechanical relation between the synovial tissue and the movement of the femoral condyle during flexion of the knee. It is equally conceivable that the plicae do not grow and change as readily as the rest of the knee during the adolescent growth spurt.

Characteristically, the patient gives a history of trauma to the knee by a twisting injury, followed by joint effusion and pain. Symptoms are comparable to those of internal derangement of the knee: snapping, instability, pain, and swelling.

Physical examination may confirm the presence of joint effusion. Tenderness may be elicited over the femoral condyle or about the patella. Flexion and extension movements of the knee may cause crepitation of the patella; and at times an audible snap is heard as the plica courses over the femoral condyle. A symptomatic plica is often palpated as a tender band-like structure paralleling the medial border of the patella in the suprapatellar region.

The plicae syndrome has been associated with anterior pain as well as clicking, catching, locking, or pseudolocking of the knee. It may mimic acute internal derangement of the knee. Symptoms are due to the plicae bow stringing across the femoral condyle during flexion.

Single- or double-contrast arthrography is an imaging method for evaluating a possibile plica (Fig. 22-70). MRI also offers a way of assessing soft tissues such as plica (Fig. 22-71). Thickening extending from the patella, in the presence of physical findings, should indicate a plica.

Patients presenting with symptomatic plicae are initially treated with rest, antiinflammatory agents, and local heat followed by muscle strengthening/stretching exercises. Young children, whose symptoms are of short duration and most commonly associated with repetitive trauma, generally respond to conservative therapy. Patients whose symptoms are of long duration may not respond to conservative therapy and may require operative intervention. Pathologic plica may be excised by operative arthroscopy.

Johnson et al. described 30 patients with 45 involved knees who had a specific diagnosis of synovial plicae syndrome.[324] Patients were selected for arthroscopy only if the symptoms had continued unabated after a course of physical therapy. Patients were randomly selected for diagnostic arthroscopy alone or arthroscopy with division of all plicae. At the time of follow-up, the authors noted that improvement had occurred in only 29% of the knees in which the plicae had not been divided, in contrast to improvement in 83% of the patients in which the plicae had been divided. Altogether 48% of the knees that had not undergone arthroscopic division initially were treated with a subsequent arthroscopic operation to evaluate the plicae; 70% of these knees improved after subsequent division of the plicae. They concluded that synovial plicae of the knee are a definite cause of anterior pain in children and adolescents and that they respond well to division.

Meniscal Injuries

Meniscal injuries are uncommon in young children but become increasingly prevalent during adolescence. Traumatic injury of a previously intact normal medial meniscus in a child below the age of 10 is infrequent.[330-378] Smillie stated that his youngest patient was a 3-year-old girl.[277] Volk and Smith described a tear of the medial meniscus in a 5-year-old boy.[376] Schlonsky and Eyring reported lateral meniscus tears in three patients aged 4, 6, and 7 years.[369] Only one was a tear in a discoid lateral meniscus. Fairbank thought that internal derangements of the menisci in adolescents and children usually occurred only in congenitally abnormal menisci.[348]

The average annual incidence of symptomatic meniscal lesions in children increased from 0.7 to 2.5 per 10,000 during 1960–1965 to 2.5 per 10,000 during 1980–1985 in Malmö, Sweden.[330] Soccer was the predominant cause of the lesions, and the increased incidence of the diagnosis was associated with the introduction of arthroscopy rather than any change in the extent of sports exposure.

The orthopaedist must render an accurate diagnosis by ruling out lesions that mimic meniscal tear; confirm the tear with arthrography, MRI, or arthroscopy; and then, if possible, define the type and extent of the tear along with other predisposing causal factors.[341,346] Only when all information is available should any consideration of surgical removal (partial meniscectomy) be undertaken in a skeletally immature patient.

Zaman and Leonard reported the results of meniscectomy in 59 knees of 49 children.[378] In 10 children menisci had been removed from both knees, and in two knees both medial and lateral menisci had been removed. The average age at surgery was 13 years. The average length of follow-up was 7.5 years. They found three definable groups at follow-up. In group 1 the children were symptom-free as young adults; this included 25 knees, 21 of which had a definite abnormality of the meniscus. Group 2 included those with symptoms present only during sporting activity; there were 11 knees in this group, and there was no clear relation between the symptoms and an abnormality of the meniscus. In group 3 there were symptoms during normal activity; 23 patients comprised this group, and 16 had *no* abnormality of the meniscus when it was removed. The authors stressed that in one-third of all cases the meniscus was *normal* at the time of operative assessment. Despite such a finding, the normal meniscus was removed in each case. They stressed that meniscectomy in children was *not* a benign procedure, particularly in view of the fact that long-term radiologic changes were present in 43 of the knees, and only 42 were symptom-free at follow-up. Only 27% had normal radiographs at follow-up. The results in girls were worse than in boys. A definite relation existed between poor results and complete removal of normal menisci. Zaman and Leonard recommended that if a normal meniscus is found it must *not* be removed. Other sources of joint derangement such as chondromalacia, patellar subluxation, or plica syndrome should be sought as the cause of the patient's complaints.

Manzione followed 20 children and adolescence with isolated meniscal tears for an average of 5.5 years after surgery.[360] All other ligamentous injury patients were excluded. Sixty percent of the patients had unsatisfactory results.

It has been suggested that meniscectomy in pediatric patients may be followed by regeneration of a fibrocartilaginous meniscus.[347] Clinical studies, however, have yielded conflicting results. I did not find any evidence of regeneration of meniscal tissue in 11 patients who underwent MRI studies 5–9 years after *total* medial or lateral meniscectomy.

The relatively high proportion of poor results, the persistence of symptoms in many of the children, and the fact that many children with a provisional diagnosis of a meniscal lesion improve *without* operation underlines the need for careful selection before advising meniscectomy in young children. The diagnosis must be made only after careful consideration, including arthroscopy. A child presenting with symptoms of a damaged meniscus must be given a fair trial of conservative treatment before any surgery is contemplated. Indications for surgery are recurrent locking of the knee with a definite history of injury that is well documented by arthrography, MRI, or arthroscopy.

In children complete excision is certainly not the treatment of choice for torn menisci.[356,362] Every effort should be made to repair the previously normal meniscus. Patients with small tears and with tears not causing any block to movement appear to do better with nonoperative treatment. The important contributions made by the meniscus to knee stability and load transmission must not be forgotten.[352] When the meniscal tear causes abnormal knee mechanics, operative treatment is warranted. Increasing evidence demonstrates that partial meniscectomy, when possible, is the procedure of choice. In adults the concepts of meniscal preservation by partial meniscectomy are gaining acceptance owing to the decreased incidence of subsequent degenerative joint disease and the maintenance of joint stability.[343,351,355,358,359,361,365]

Surgical repair of peripheral tears is a viable alternative to meniscectomy in selected cases. The studies concerning changing vascularity in the meniscal periphery suggest that repair is a feasible procedure in the young child.[5] Only in those cases in which damage to the meniscus is extensive or totally within the body should total meniscectomy be considered in the pediatric patient.

Wroble et al. studied the long-term effects of meniscectomy in children and adolescents.[377] Thirty-nine patients younger than 16 years who had been treated with a total meniscectomy had an average follow-up of 21 years; 71% of the patients reported pain, 68% stiffness, 54% intermittent swelling, and 41% "giving way." Approximately half the patients described progression of symptoms. Only 27% were asymptomatic, and only 10% noted significant limitations; 62% had limitations in sporting activities. Altogether 12% underwent further knee surgery, and 90% of the patients had abnormal roentgenograms. Wroble et al. concluded that treatment of a torn meniscus in the child should be conservative and nonoperative whenever possible. With peripheral meniscal lesions, repair appears to provide good results and is the treatment of choice. If a lesion is not repairable, partial excision is preferable to total meniscectomy. *It is axiomatic that normal menisci not be removed*, particularly the alleged hypermobile meniscus.

Busch reviewed meniscal injuries in children.[340] The most common lesions are longitudinal (vertical) tears and peripheral detachments, with a posterior horn of the meniscus being most commonly involved. Bucket handle tears typically occur in the older teenage patients. The involvement is fairly evenly divided between the lateral and medial side, although series with a large number of lateral tears typically contain greater numbers of torn lateral discoid menisci. Spontaneous healing of meniscal tears may occur, especially in younger patients. King described four cases with demonstrable scarring of the periphery as a result of a healed meniscus tear.[357] This is in part due to the vascularity of the peripheral margin of the meniscus, particularly in the adolescent. He noted that despite the common conception that ligament injuries do not occur adolescents with open growth plates sustain anterior cruciate ligament tears that are difficult to recognize and that probably account for some of the poor results after meniscal injuries. He also pointed out that the fat pad can become abnormally fibrotic and may contain distinct fibrous bands that may mimic a torn meniscus.

Abdon et al. described a long-term follow-up study of total meniscectomy in children.[331] They studied 89 children at an average of 16.8 years after surgery. Although 74% were pleased with the outcome, only 58% had objectively satisfactory results according to two scoring systems. Significantly poor results followed lateral meniscectomy. Minor instabilities were recorded in 45% of the patients and major instability in 15%.

Vangsness et al. studied 47 patients with diaphyseal fractures of the femur.[375] Following femoral nailing, all patients had an examination under anesthesia followed by arthroscopy. There were 12 medial meniscal injuries and 13 lateral meniscal injuries. Ligamentous laxity was found in 50% of the patients. It should be recognized that the considerable energy required to cause femoral diaphyseal fractures probably damages other adjacent structures as well. Classically, it is emphasized that one must include the hip in any patient with a fractured femur to rule out and not miss a dislocated hip, but equally the knee should be adequately examined. This may be difficult in the presence of an unstable shaft but should be emphasized to the family and to the patient to allow further evaluation during the posttraumatic period. The studies have shown ipsilateral injury to knee ligaments ranging from 17% to 48% of femoral fractures in adults, with many authors emphasizing reported delays of weeks to months in the diagnosis of these lesions. No such studies have addressed the possibility of meniscal injuries in children, despite the large number of femoral fractures that occur. The seeming absence of meniscal problems or posttraumatic knee internal derangement undoubtedly relates to the differences in the degree (severity) of trauma and the mechanisms of injury that often are associated with children's femoral fractures versus those in adults.

The efficacy of meniscus transplantation in the skeletally immature knee is unproved and is not an acceptable treatment option.

Meniscal Cyst

Following a conservatively treated meniscal tear, a skeletally immature patient may develop a meniscal cyst (Fig. 22-72).[384] Kinura et al. described a 14-year-old boy with a cyst associated with a bucket handle tear of the medial meniscus.[381]

These injuries should be treated arthroscopically to decompress the cyst and repair the capsular-meniscal defect. Flynn and Kelly recommended excision of the cyst and the meniscus.[379] However, this was during prearthroscopic days, and today it is more feasible to try to resect the cyst and repair any tear. The cyst may be decompressed through the substance of the meniscus or through a separate incision over the cyst.

Glasgow et al. treated 69 patients with 72 cystic lateral menisci through arthroscopic surgery.[380] Meniscal tears were observed in all patients. Their results were good to excellent in 89% of the patients.

Mills and Henderson described 20 patients with medical meniscal cyst in a series of almost 7500 knee arthroscopies.[382] Eighty-five percent had a coexistent meniscal injury. Treatment of the cyst was by direct open resection in 12 and arthroscopic evaluation during meniscectomy in 7. They thought that medial meniscal cysts were an important but underdiagnosed cause of knee pain. Treatment should be directed toward both the meniscal lesion and the cyst, which may require direct open surgery.

Parisien reported 24 patients with meniscal cysts associated with tears of the meniscal cartilage.[383] All were treated arthroscopically with partial meniscectomy and cyst decompression.

VanderWilde and Peterson described 11 patients ranging in age from 4 to 18 years with meniscal cysts.[385] They thought that MRI was a useful tool for diagnosing the cyst (Fig.

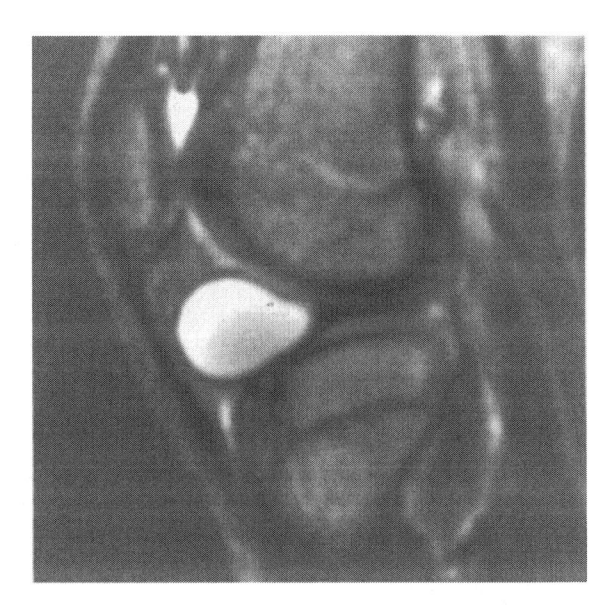

FIGURE 22-72. Meniscal cyst following a semipenetrating blow to the knee. A gear shift lever was driven against the lateral side of the patellar tendon. The skin, however, was intact.

22-72) and aiding in surgical planning. They found that there were only 17 reported cases where the patient was 20 years of age or less.

Meniscal Ossicles

Discrete ossicles, in contrast to more diffuse calcification, are rare within the human meniscus and have usually been described in case reports.[386,388–392] They most often appear in young athletes following well-documented specific injury. Often the initial radiographs appear normal, with the eventual appearance of an ossicle on subsequent radiographs. Two theories of origin of these meniscal ossicles in the human have been postulated: developmental and posttraumatic.

Lonon and Crawford were the first to report an ossicle within the medial meniscus in a person under age 19. The patient, 14 years of age,[389] had a history of antecedent trauma. The initial assumption was that the ossific finding was a loose body, but it was found to be within the substance of the posterior medial meniscus.

My group reported the development of meniscal ossicles (Fig. 22-73) in a 12-year-old boy after trauma and a 10-year-old boy who probably developed it as part of thrombocytopenia anemlia radial aplasia (TAR) syndrome (although a role for chronic trauma could not be ruled out).[391] In neither case was the ossicle present in radiographs obtained 8–10 months previously. We also assessed a definite developmental etiology for some of these lesions using a large animal model.[387]

Patients with meniscal ossification showed an age range at diagnosis of 14–76 years, with most patients in the second to third decades of life. All had some complaints of antecedent injury, recent onset of pain, or both in the involved knee. Swelling, locking, pain, and recurrent effusion were the most common complaints at the time of presentation, which was usually at least 6 months after any documented injury to the knee.

Ossicles have varied in location from the posterior periphery of the medial meniscus to a position near the tibial spines. Most reported cases described the ossicle as being in the posterior horn, even when more than one ossicle was present. Most patients had involvement of the medial meniscus.

The presence of ossicles in adolescent and young adult humans is often related to antecedent trauma, suggesting that the usually unilateral ossicle is an acquired lesion of the meniscus. Marianni and Puddu reported the same sequence of normal to a abnormal radiographs.[390] Lonon and Crawford reported a 14-year-old boy who had a "normal" roentgenogram 3 months prior to hospitalization for a "loose body" in the knee.[389] Because 17 of 23 previously reported cases reviewed by Lonon and Crawford had antecedent trauma, they concluded that most of the cases were acquired secondary to trauma and were not vestigial structures.[389]

A large animal, the tiger, with a knee approximately the same size as the human, did not have meniscal ossification at birth, but rather had a progressive chondro-osseous transformation and osseous enlargement postnatally.[387] Such a pattern certainly is consistent with the postnatal appearance of sesamoid bones within a histologically similar structure, the tendon. Progressive appearance also appears to characterize the developmental and posttraumatic ossicle in the human adolescent. It would be expected that the ossicle would not be present radiographically for several years but would eventually ossify like other sesamoid bones around the knees.

The meniscal ossicle must be differentiated from a loose body to avoid the possibility of nonessential arthrotomy or arthroscopy when a "joint mouse" is diagnosed (based on routine radiography), searched for, and not found. Operating orthopaedic surgeons may also be deceived on surgical exploration, as they search for nonexistent "loose bodies." Under fluoroscopy the ossicle moves with the tibia throughout the normal range of motion.[388]

Magnetic resonance imaging was used to analyze the meniscal ossicle in a patient with TAR syndrome.[391] This methodology, which has not been reported previously for evaluating this lesion, showed that the bone was completely within the medial meniscus. VanderWilde and Peterson have

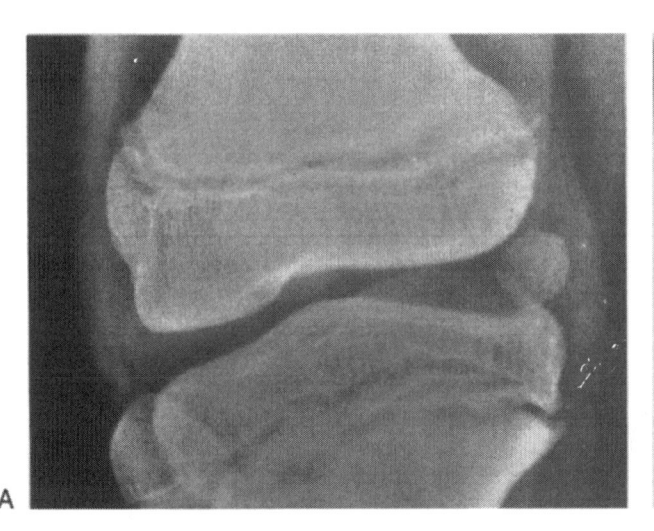

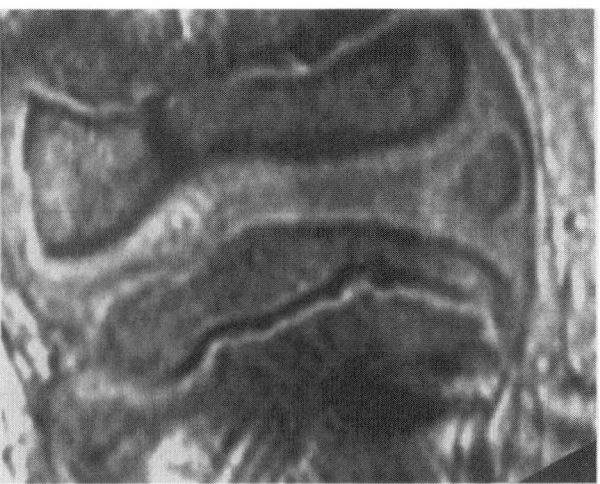

FIGURE 22-73. Patient with medial meniscal ossification. (A) Anteroposterior view. (B) MRI.

used MRI to evaluate a similar intrameniscal lesion (cyst) in children.[385] Such MRI evaluation might preclude the need for surgery.

Yao and Yao described the use of MRI to evaluate a symptomatic meniscal ossicle.[392] Interestingly, the MRI scan did not show the associated meniscal tear, which was evident only on detailed arthroscopic examination. They thought that the meniscal ossicle probably created a stress riser in the meniscus, thereby causing the tear.

Four of seven of Glass and coworkers' patients underwent surgery, and three were treated nonoperatively with complete resolution of symptoms.[388] They stated that "their" presence alone does not require their removal; only the symptomatic patient who does not respond to conservative treatment requires surgical attention. Ossicles may be present without a history of trauma and perhaps occur as a vestigial sesamoid-type phenomenon. Accordingly, their removal should be based on sufficient knee dysfunction. I advocate arthroscopic examination to assess the need for partial removal of the ossicle-containing meniscus while leaving the rest of the meniscus intact. Arthroscopy is not recommended *unless* symptoms warrant consideration of excision.

Discoid Meniscus

Smillie reported 29 cases of congenital discoid menisci in a series of 1300 meniscectomies.[414] The true incidence of this anomaly is difficult to determine, as many of these patients progress into adult life without symptoms. Discoid menisci are likely to become injured (torn) more frequently than a normal lateral meniscus.[400,403]

Some authors believe that the discoid meniscus is caused by arrested development of the meniscus in utero. Smillie thought that it was simply a reflection of persistence of the normal fetal state of development from a cartilaginous disc.[414] He noted three types: primitive, intermediate, and infantile.

Kaplan, in an extensive embryologic study, concluded that at no time in the development of the human fetus do either the lateral or the medial menisci assume a discoid form.[404,405] He performed a comparative study that included various primates and did not find any structural variation that could be termed a congenital discoid meniscus, although in several animals the lateral meniscus was almost circular. At operation on individuals with discoid menisci, he found that there was no attachment of the posterior horn to the tibial plateau. Instead of this attachment there was a continuous Wrisberg's ligament or meniscofemoral ligament that formed a link between the posterior horn in the meniscus and the medial condyle of the femur, a situation that was a normal arrangement observed in all animals except humans. He further thought that the discoid form developed gradually after birth as a result of abnormal motion of the lateral meniscus. The hypertrophied meniscus varied in shape but has been termed discoid. Discoid, or more properly circular, menisci do exist in several primates, but these circular menisci do not have the thickened, irregular central segment seen with most human discoid lateral menisci.

Nathan and Cole emphasized the importance of mechanical factors in association with failure of the posterior horn

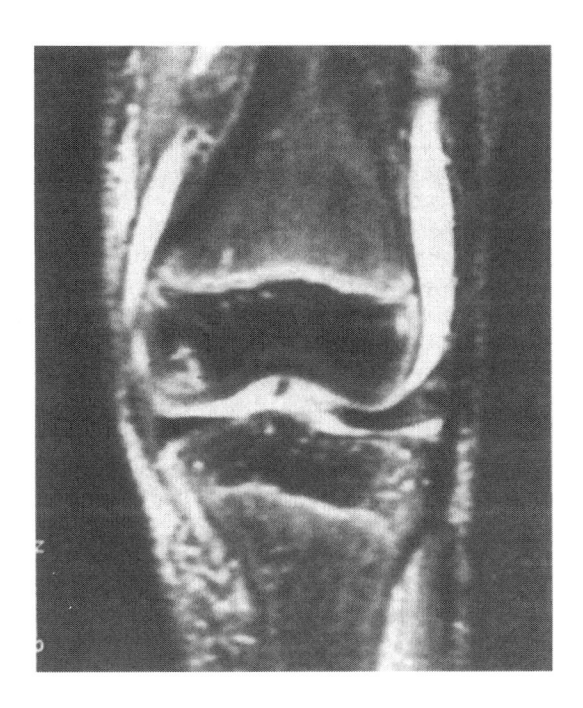

FIGURE 22-74. Focal changes in patient with discoid meniscus. Surprisingly, the epiphyseal changes were in the medial condyle.

of the discoid meniscus to attach to the lateral intercondylar tubercle of the tibia, resulting in abnormal motility, compression, and deformation into the discoid shape.[408] With continued stress, the meniscus may interfere with normal knee mechanics.

One of the most persistent symptoms of a discoid meniscus is a clicking or popping sound produced by flexion and extension of the knee joint.[406] The mechanism of the sound that is produced has not been adequately explained. Pain is the most common preoperative symptom, rather than the conventionally described "click." Radiographic findings suggestive of a discoid lateral meniscus include a squared-off lateral femoral condyle, a widened lateral joint space, and cupping of the lateral aspect of the tibial plateau.[398,411]

Stark et al. reviewed the MRI appearance (Fig. 22-74) of 27 discoid lateral menisci.[415] They were classified as the slab type ($M = 20$) or the wedge type ($M = 7$). The characteristic appearance is the slab configuration with a diffusely increased intrameniscal signal.[413]

The mere presence of such an anomaly is *not* a sufficient indication for excision, nor are symptoms such as a clicking knee.[396] In fact, some children readily "pop" the knee to gain attention. As with traumatized menisci, there should be a significant reason for removing a discoid meniscus. Chronic locking of the knee, chronic joint effusion, and chronic pain are indications.

The primary reason for partial meniscectomy of discoid meniscus is continuing pain and locking of the knee.[401,402,409,410] Washington et al. found a tear in 12 of 18 meniscectomies.[417] All but one were removed by arthrotomy and the other by meniscectomy. The knees had an excellent result at an average follow-up of 28 years.

Saucerization of the discoid meniscus has been reported by Fujikawa et al.[399] Dickhaut and DeLee, in contrast, believed that total meniscectomy is more appropriate with the Wrisberg ligament-type of discoid lateral meniscus, which lacks an adequate posterior tibial attachment, as partial meniscectomy may leave an unstable rim of meniscus.[397] Furthermore, these menisci are chronically traumatized. I believe that attempted partial resection is the most appropriate procedure initially.

Dickhaut and DeLee reported that the discoid lateral meniscus was a morphologically variable anomaly.[397] They saw 12 patients with the complete type of meniscus with intact ligament attachments as an incidental finding at arthroscopy. Ten of the twelve patients were asymptomatic without tears or laxity. They also saw six patients with the Wrisberg-ligament type of discoid lateral meniscus in which there was abnormal meniscal mobility. All patients were symptomatic and had the snapping knee syndrome; they underwent arthroscopic lateral meniscectomy. Dickhaut and DeLee thought it important to distinguish these two types, as the former should not be removed.[397] The abnormal discoid menisci have only one attachment posteriorly, the lateral meniscal femoral ligament of Wrisberg. This ligament is too short to accommodate the normal flexion and extension of the knee so there is hypermobility of the posterior portion of the lateral meniscus with secondary hypertrophic thickening of the meniscus as a result. This leads to the snapping knee.

Aichroth et al. studied 52 children with 62 discoid lateral menisci for an average follow-up of 5.5 years.[393] The average age at surgery was 10.5 years, and the mean delay in diagnosis was 24 months. Most of the children had vague and intermittent symptoms; the classic "click" was demonstrable in only 39% of the knees. Seven knees had an associated osteochondritis dissecans of the lateral femoral condyle. Forty-eight knees were treated with open total lateral meniscectomy; six underwent arthroscopic partial meniscectomy; and eight with an intact discoid meniscus found during arthroscopic examination were left alone. The authors believed that arthroscopic partial meniscectomy was recommended only when the posterior attachment of the discoid meniscus was stable and a total meniscectomy was indicated with the Wrisberg ligament-type of discoid meniscus with posterior instability.

Medial Discoid Menisci

Blacksin et al. described discoid medial menisci diagnosed by MRI.[395] Johnson and Simmons described a discoid medial meniscus with cyst formation in a 9-year-old girl.[403] The cyst mechanically blocked knee extension. Medial discoid menisci are rare.[407,410,412,414,416,418]

Popliteal Cysts

Popliteal cysts are often found in children, though infrequently during evaluation of trauma.[419,420,422] They usually represent nonarticular lesions stemming from bursal enlargement in the popliteal fossa. Figure 22-75 shows a recurrent cyst in an 8-year-old girl with joint laxity. Surgical excision was followed by recurrence. Following arthrography, the posterior capsular communication was exposed and

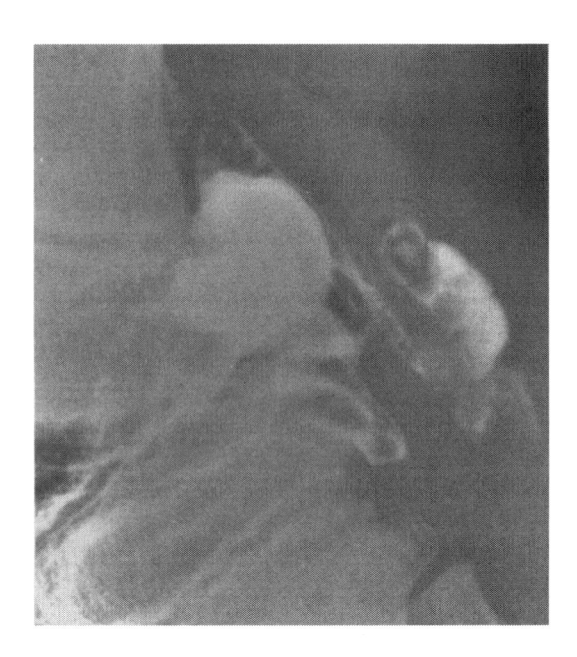

FIGURE 22-75. Popliteal cyst in an 8-year-old girl who had undergone three previous cyst excisions. Although unusual in children, the arthrogram demonstrated continuity between the cyst and the joint, but no meniscal damage was evident.

repaired. She has not had any subsequent recurrence. Most popliteal cysts, however, should be simply observed, not surgically excised.

The semimembranosus bursa may enlarge spontaneously in the child. It may also communicate with the knee joint when there is a meniscal tear (medial) or anterior cruciate ligament injury, as in adults.

Charcot Knee

In children with a sensory neuropathy, no matter what the underlying neurologic deficiency, chronic changes may result from seemingly normal use because of the inability to perceive pain in the knee region. These lesions are discussed in Chapter 11.

Hoffa Disease

Methany and Mayor[421] described chronic knee pain due to chronic impingement of the infrapatellar fat pad. This has been referred to as Hoffa disease. Treatment involves arthroscopic reduction of impinging tissues.

References

Anatomy

1. Arnoczky SP, Warren RF. Microvasculature of the human meniscus. Am J Sports Med 1982;10:90–95.
2. Bullough PG, Muneura L, Murphy J, Weinstein AM. The

strength of the menisci of the knee as it relates to their fine structure. J Bone Joint Surg Br 1970;52:564–570.
3. Cameron HU, MacNab I. The structure of the meniscus of the human knee joint. Clin Orthop 1972;89:215–219.
4. Clark CR, Ogden JA. Prenatal and postnatal development of human knee joint menisci. Iowa Orthop 1981;1:20–27.
5. Clark CR, Ogden JA, Development of the menisci of the human knee joint. J Bone Joint Surg Am 1983;65:538–539.
6. Cross MJ, Waldrop J. The patellar index as a guide to the understanding and diagnosis of patellofemoral instability. Clin Orthop 1975;110:174–176.
7. Danzig L, Resnick D, Gonsalves M, Akeson WH. Blood supply to the normal and abnormal menisci of the human knee. Clin Orthop 1983;172:271–276.
8. Grey DJ, Gardner E. Prenatal development of the human knee and superior tibial fibular joints. J Anat 1950;86:235–287.
9. Inove H, Isomaki AM, Oka M. Scanning electron microscopic studies. Acta Rheumatol Scand 1971;17:187–194.
10. Kennedy JC (ed) The Injured Adolescent Knee. Baltimore: Williams & Wilkins, 1979.
11. Lanscourt JE, Cristini JA. Patella alta and patella infera. J Bone Joint Surg Am 1975;57:1112–1115.
12. Ogden JA. Radiology of postnatal skeletal development. X. Patella and tibial tuberosity. Skeletal Radiol 1984;11:246–257.
13. Scapinelli R. Blood supply of the human patella. J Bone Joint Surg Br 1967;48:563–570.
14. Walmsley R. The development of the patella. J Anat 1939;24:360–369.

General

15. Cole PA, Ehrlich MG. Management of the completely stiff pediatric knee. J Pediatr Orthop 1997;17:67–73.
16. Eilert RE. Adolescent anterior knee pain. AAOS Instr Course Lect 1993;42:497–516.
17. Fairbank JC, Pynsent PB. Van Poortvliet JA, Phillips H. Mechanical factors in the incidence of knee pain in adolescents and young adults. J Bone Joint Surg Br 1984;66:685–693.
18. Flanagan JP, Holmes CF, Schenck RC. Part I: Use of ice, NSAID's, exercise, and braces: primary care of the acutely injured knee. J Musculoskel Med 1992;9:55–64.
19. Klimkiewicz JJ, Dormans JP. The pediatric knee. Curr Opin Orthop 1996;7:53–58.
20. Matelic TM, Aronsson DD, Boyd DW Jr, LaMont RL. Acute hemarthrosis of the knee in children. Am J Sports Med 1995;23:668–671.
21. Micheli LJ, Foster TE. Acute knee injuries in the immature athlete. AAOS Instr Course Lect 1993;42:473–481.
22. Stanitski CL. Anterior knee pain syndromes in the adolescent. J Bone Joint Surg Am 1993;75:1407–1416.
23. Stanitski CL, Harvell JC, Fu F. Observations on acute knee hemarthrosis in children and adolescents. J Pediatr Orthop 1993;13:506–510.

Diagnostic Imaging

24. Bassett LW, Grover JS, Seeger LL. Magnetic resonance imaging of knee trauma. Skeletal Radiol 1990;19:401–405.
25. Haramati N, Staron RB, Rubin S, Shreck EH, Feldman F, Kiernan H. The flipped meniscus sign. Skeletal Radiol 1993;22:273–277.
26. Koskinen SK, Taimela S, Nelimarkka O, Komu M, Kujala UM. Magnetic resonance imaging of patellofemoral relationships. Skeletal Radiol 1993;22:403–410.
27. Moes CAF, Munn JD. The value of knee arthrography in children. J Can Assoc Radiol 1965;16:226–233.
28. Ogden JA, Albright JA, Ettelson DM. An apparent loose body in the knee. Clin Orthop 1974;103:33–35.
29. Schweitzer ME, Mitchell DG, Ehrlich SM. The patellar tendon: thickening, internal signal buckling, and other MR variants. Skeletal Radiol 1993;22:411–416.
30. Speer KP, Spritzer CE, Goldner JL, Garrett WE Jr. Magnetic resonance imaging of traumatic knee articular cartilage injuries. Am J Sports Med 1991;19:396–402.
31. Stenstrom R. Diagnostic arthrography of traumatic lesions of the knee joint in children. Ann Radiol (Paris) 1975;18:391–394.
32. Yates CK, Grana WA. Patellofemoral pain in children. Clin Orthop 1990;255:36–43.
33. Zobel MS, Borrello JA, Siegel MJ, Stewart NR. Pediatric knee MR imaging: pattern of injuries in the immature skeleton. Radiology 1994;190:397–401.

Arthroscopy

34. Benfar AS, Refior AJ. Arthroscopy of the pediatric knee joint. Z Orthop 1986;124:751–754.
35. Bergstrom R, Gillquist J, Lysholm J, Hamberg P. Arthroscopy of the knee in children. J Pediatr Orthop 1984;4:542–545.
36. Casseneuve JF, Collet LM, Renand C, Flamesnil C. Posttraumatic haemarthrosis of the knee in childhood: the place of arthroscopy. Fr J Orthop Surg 1991;5:204–206.
37. Dandy DJ. Arthroscopy in the treatment of young patients with anterior knee pain. Orthop Clin North Am 1986;17:221–229.
38. Eilert RE. Arthroscopy of the knee joint in children. Orthop Rev 1976;15:61–65.
39. Eiskjaer S, Larsen ST. Arthroscopy of the knee in children. Acta Orthop Scand 1987;58:273–276.
40. Eiskjaer S, Larsen ST, Schmidt MB. The significance of hemarthrosis of the knee in children. Arch Orthop Trauma Surg 1988;107:96–98.
41. Harvell JC, Fu FH, Stanitski CL. Diagnostic arthroscopy of the knee in children and adolescents. Orthopedics 1989;12:1555–1560.
42. Hayes AG, Nageswar M. The adolescent painful knee: the value of arthroscopy in diagnosis. J Bone Joint Surg Br 1977;59:499–507.
43. Hope PG. Arthroscopy in children. J Roy Soc Med 1991;84:29–31.
44. Juhl M, Boe S. Arthroscopy in children, with special emphasis on meniscal lesions. Injury 1986;17:171–173.
45. Kloeppel-Wirth S, Koltai JL, Dittmer H. Significance of arthroscopy in children with knee joint injuries. Eur J Pediatr Surg 1992;2:169–172.
46. McCarroll JR, Rettig AC, Shelbourne KD. Anterior cruciate ligament injuries in the young athlete with open physes. Am J Sports Med 1988;16:44–49.
47. Morrissy RT, Eubanks RG, Park JP, Thompson SB. Arthroscopy of the knee in children. Clin Orthop 1982;162:103–107.
48. Niederdockl U, Hollwarth M. Hemarthrosis of the knee joint in children. Unfallchirurg 1982;8:155–158.
49. Nisonson B. Acute hemarthrosis of the adolescent knee. Physician Sportsmed 1989;17:75–87.
50. Potts H, Noble J. Arthroscopic surgery in the very young. J Bone Joint Surg Br 1989;71:541.
51. Robert H, Gouault E, Moulies D, Alian JL. L'arthroscopie du genou chez l'enfant. Rev Pediatr 1985;21:445–447.
52. Romdane HB, Neuenschwander S, Hautefort P, Gautier C, Montague JP. Pseudo-aneurysm of the popliteal artery following an arthroscopic meniscectomy: report of a pediatric case. Pediatr Radiol 1991;21:228.
53. Spiers ASD, Meacher T, Ostlere SJ, Wilson DJ, Dodd CAF. Can MRI of the knee affect arthroscopic practice? A prospec-

tive study of 58 patients. J Bone Joint Surg Br 1993;75: 49–52.
54. Suman RK, Stother IG, Illingworth G. Diagnostic arthroscopy of the knee in children. J Bone Joint Surg Br 1984;66:535–537.
55. Ure BM, Tiling T, Roddeker K, et al. Arthroscopy of the knee in children and adolescents. Eur J Pediatr Surg 1992;2:102–105.
56. Vahasarja V, Kinnuen P, Serlo W. Arthroscopy of the acute traumatic knee in children: prospective study of 138 cases. Acta Orthop Scand 1993;64:580–582.
57. Ziv I, Carroll NC. The role of arthroscopy in children. J Pediatr Orthop 1982;2:243–247.

Knee Dislocation

58. Cooper DE, Speer KP, Wickiewicz TL, Warren RE. Complete dislocation without posterior cruciate ligament disruption. Clin Orthop 1992;284:228–233.
59. Cummings RJ, Webb HW, Lovell WW, Kay G. The popliteal artery entrapment syndrome in children. J Pediar Orthop 1992;12:539–541.
60. Dart CH, J, Braitman HE. Popliteal injury following fracture or dislocation at the knee: diagnosis and management. Arch Surg 1977;112:969–973.
61. DeLee JC. Complete dislocation of the knee in a nine-year-old. Contemp Orthop 1979;1:29–30.
62. Ferris BD. Congenital snapping knee: habitual anterior subluxation of the tibia in extension. J Bone Joint Surg Br 1990;72:453–456.
63. Gartland JJ, Brenner JH. Traumatic dislocations in the lower extremity in children. Orthop Clin North Am 1976;7:687–700.
64. Green NE, Allen BL. Vascular injuries associated with dislocation of the knee. J Bone Joint Surg Am 1977;59:236–239.
65. Kendall RW, Taylor DC, Salvian AJ, O'Brien PJ. The role of arteriography in assessing vascular injuries associated with dislocations of the knee. J Trauma 1993;35:875–878.
66. Twaddle BC, Hunter JC, Chapman JR, Simonian PT, Escobedo EM. MRI in acute knee dislocation. J Bone Joint Surg Br 1996;78:573–579.
67. Walker DN, Rogers W, Schenk RC Jr. Immediate vascular and ligamentous repair in a closed knee dislocation: case report. J Trauma 1994;36:898–900.

Patellar Dislocation

68. Alioto RJ, Kates S. Intra-articular vertical dislocation of the patella: a case report of an irreducible patellar dislocation and unique surgical technique. J Trauma 1994;36:282–284.
69. Allen FJ. Intercondylar dislocation of the patella. S Afr Med J 1944;18:66.
70. Baum C, Bensahel H. Luxation recidivante de la rotule chez l'enfant. Rev Chir Orthop 1973;59:583–589.
71. Brady TA, Russell D. Inter-articular horizontal dislocation of the patella. J Bone Joint Surg Am 1965;47:1393–1396.
72. Cheesman WS. Dislocations of the patella, with rotation on its horizontal axis. Ann Surg 1905;41:107–114.
73. Colville J. An unusual case of intra-articular dislocation of the patella. Injury 1978;9:321–322.
74. Donelson RG, Tomaiuoli M. Intra-articular dislocation of the patella. J Bone Joint Surg Am 1979;61:615–616.
75. Feneley RCL. Intra-articular dislocation of the patella: report of a case. J Bone Joint Surg Br 1968;50:653–655.
76. Frangakis EK. Intra-articular dislocation of the patella: a case report. J Bone Joint Surg Am 1974;56:423–424.
77. Gilbert TJ, Johnson E, Detlie T, Griffiths HJ. Patellar dislocation, medial retinacular tears, avulsion fractures and osteochondral fragments. Orthopaedics 1993;16:732–736.
78. Goletz TH, Brodhead WT. Intra-articular dislocation of the patella: a case report. Orthopedics 1981;4:1022–1024.
79. Gore D. Horizontal dislocation of the patella. JAMA 1970;214:1119.
80. Guidera KJ, Kortright L, Barber V, Ogden JA. Radiographic changes in arthrogrypotic knees. Skeletal Radiol 1991;20: 193–195.
81. Levin GD. Vertical axis rotational dislocation of the patella. Orthop Rev 1978;7:83.
82. McManus F, Rang M, Heslin DJ. Acute dislocation of the patella in children: a natural history. Clin Orthop 1979;139: 88–91.
83. Miller PR, Klein RM, Teitge RA. Medial dislocation of the patella. Skeletal Radiol 1991;20:429–431.
84. Murakami Y. Intra-articular dislocation of the patella. Clin Orthop 1982;171:137–139.
85. Nayak RK, Bickerstaff DR. Acute traumatic patellar dislocation: the importance of skyline views. Injury 1995;26:347–348.
86. Nietsovaara Y, Aalto K. The cartilaginous femoral sulcus in children with patellar dislocation: an ultrasonographic study. J Pediatr Surg 1997;17:50–53.
87. Roger DJ, Williamson SC, Uhl RL. Difficult reductions in traumatic patellar dislocation. Orthop Rev 1992;21: 1333–1341.
88. Shaw DL, Giannoudis PV, Archer IA. Intra-articular dislocation of patella. Injury 1995;26:273–274.
89. Singleton SB, Sillman JF. Acute chondral injuries of the patellofemoral joint. Operative Tech Sports Med 1995;3:96–103.
90. Stanitski CL. Articular hypermobility and chondral injury in patients with acute patellar dislocation. Am J Sports Med 1995;23:146–150.

Patellar Subluxation

91. Ando T, Hirose H, Inoue M, Shino K, Doi T. A new method using computed tomographic scan to measure the rectus femoris: patellar tendon Q-angle comparison with conventional method. Clin Orthop 1993;289:213–219.
92. Baum C, Bensahel H. Luxation recidivante de la rotule chez l'enfant. Rev Chir Orthop 1973;59:583–592.
93. Bentley G. Articular cartilage changes in chondromalacia patellae. J Bone Joint Surg Br 1985;67:769–774.
94. Bonnard C, Nocquet P, Sollogoub I, Glorion B. Instabilite rotulienne chez l'enfant: resultat de la transposition du tiers interne du tendon rotulien. Rev Chir Orthop 1990;76:473–479.
95. Brattstrom H. Shape of the intercondylar groove normally and in recurrent dislocation of the patella. Acta Orthop Scand 1964;35(suppl 68):1–148.
96. Dabezies EJ, Schutte J. Orthopedic grand rounds: habitual patellar dislocation. Orthopedics 1981;4:224–229.
97. Fairbank JCT, Pynsent PB, van Poortvliet JA, Phillips H. Mechanical factors in the incidence of knee pain in adolescents and young adults. J Bone Joint Surg Br 1984;66:685–693.
98. Guzzanti V, Gigante A, Lazzaro A, Fabbricani C. Patellofemoral malalignment in adolescents. Am J Sports Med 1994;22: 55–60.
99. Higgenbothen CL. Children's knee problems. Orthop Rev 1981;10:37–48.
100. Insall J, Salvati E. Patella position in the normal knee joint. Radiology 1971;101:101–104.
101. Jeffreys TE. Recurrent dislocation of the patella due to abnormal attachment of the iliotibial tract. J Bone Joint Surg Br 1963;45:740–743.
102. Larson RL. The unstable patella in the adolescent and preadolescent. Orthop Rev 1985;14:156–162.

103. Lefort G, Cottalorda J, Lefebvre F, Bouche-Pillon MA, Daoud S. Les instabiltes femoro-patellaires chez l'enfant et l'adolescent. Rev Chir Orthop 1991;77:491–495.
104. Merchant AC. Classification of patellofemoral disorders. Arthroscopy 1988;4:235–241.
105. Micheli LJ, Stanitski CL. Lateral patellar retinacular release. Am J Sports Med 1981;9:330–336.
106. Moller BN, Moller-Larsen F, Frich LH. Chondromalacia induced by patellar subluxation in the rabbit. Acta Orthop Scand 1989;60:188–191.
107. Nietosvaara AY, Aalto KA. Ultrasonographic evaluation of patellar tracking in children. Clin Orthop 1993;297:62–64.
108. O'Neill DB, Micheli LJ, Warner JP. Patellofemoral stress: a prospective analysis of exercise treatment in adolescents and adults. Am J Sports Med 1992;20:151–156.
109. Reikeras O, Hoiseth A. Patellofemoral relationships in normal subjects determined by computed tomography. Skeletal Radiol 1990;19:591–592.
110. Rengeval JP. Les luxations recidivantes de la rotule chez l'enfant. Rev Chir Orthop 1980;66:216–222.
111. Stanciu C, Labelle HB, Morin B, Fassier F, Marton D. The value of computed tomography for the diagnosis of recurrent patellar subluxation in adolescents. Can J Surg 1994;37:319–323.
112. Thompson RC, Vener MJ, Griffiths HJ, Lesis JL, Oegema TR, Wallace L. Scanning electron-microscopic and magnetic resonance imaging studies of injuries to the patellofemoral joint after acute transarticular loading. J Bone Joint Surg Am 1993;75:704–713.
113. Vähäsarja V, Kinnunen P, Lanning P, Serlo W. Operative realignment of patellar malalignment in children. J Pediatr Orthop 1995;15:281–285.
114. Wiberg S, Baumgartl F. Patellar instability. In: Kennedy JC (ed) The Injured Adolescent Knee. Baltimore: Williams & Wilkins, 1979.

Ligaments

115. Abbott LC, Saunders JB, Bost FC, Anderson CE. Injuries to ligaments of the knee joint. J Bone Joint Surg 1944;26:503–521.
116. Andrews M, Noyes FR, Barber-Westin SD. Anterior cruciate ligament allograft reconstruction in the skeletally immature athlete. Am J Sports Med 1994;22:48–54.
117. Angel KR, Hall DJ. Anterior cruciate ligament injury in children and adolescents. Arthroscopy 1989;5:197–200.
118. Baxter MP. Assessment of normal pediatric knee ligament laxity using the Genucom. J Pediatr Orthop 1988;8:543–545.
119. Bertin KC, Goble EM. Ligament injuries associated with physeal fractures about the knee. Clin Orthop 1983;177:188–195.
120. Bock GW, Bosch E, Mishra DK, Daniel DM, Resnick D. The healed Segond fracture: a characteristic residual bone excrescence. Skeletal Radiol 1994;23:555–556.
121. Boynton MD, Fadale PD. The basic science of anterior cruciate ligament surgery. Orthop Rev 1993;22:673–379.
122. Bradley GW, Shives TC, Samuelson KM. Ligament injuries in the knees of children. J Bone Joint Surg Am 1979;61:588–591.
123. Brief LP. Anterior cruciate ligament reconstruction without drill holes. J Arthroscop Surg 1991;7:350–357.
124. Buckley SL, Sturm PF, Tosi LL, Thomas MD, Robertson WW Jr. Ligamentous instability of the knee in children sustaining fractures of the femur: a prospective study with knee examination under anesthesia. J Pediatr Orthop 1996;16:206–209.
125. Chick RR, Jackson DW. Tears of the anterior cruciate ligament in young athletes. J Bone Joint Surg Am 1978;60:970–973.
126. Clanton TO, DeLee JC, Sanders B, Neidre A. Knee ligament injuries in children. J Bone Joint Surg Am 1979;61:1195–1201.
127. Crawford AH. Fractures about the knee in children. Orthop Clin North Am 1976;7:639–656.
128. Crowninshield RD, Pope MH. The strength and failure characteristics of rat medial collateral ligaments. J Trauma 1976;16:99–105.
129. DeLee JC, Curtis R. Anterior cruciate ligament insufficiency in children. Clin Orthop 1983;172:112–118.
130. Dietz GW, Wilcox DM, Montgomery JB. Segond tibial condyle fracture: lateral capsular ligament avulsion. Radiology 1986;159:467–469.
131. Eady JL, Cardenas CD, Sopa D. Avulsion of the femoral attachment of the anterior cruciate ligament in a seven-year-old child. J Bone Joint Surg Am 1982;64:1376–1378.
132. Engebretsen L, Arendt E, Fritts HM. Osteochondral lesions and cruciate ligament injuries: MRI in 18 knees. Acta Orthop Scand 1994;64:434–436.
133. Engebretsen L, Svenningsen S, Benum P. Poor results of anterior cruciate ligament repair in adolescence. Acta Orthop Scand 1988;59:684–686.
134. Felenda M, Dittel KK. Bedeutung der Segond-abrissfraktur als Zeichen einer komplexen ligamentaren Kniegelenksverletzung. Akt Traumatol 1992;22:120–122.
135. Fetto JF, Marshall JL. Medial collateral ligament injuries of the knee: a rationale for treatment. Clin Orthop 1978;132:206–218.
136. Garcia A, Neer CS. Isolated fractures of the intercondylar eminence of the tibia. Am J Surg 1958;95:593–598.
137. Giorgi B. Morphologic variations of the intercondylar eminence of the knee. Clin Orthop 1956;8:209–217.
138. Goldman AB, Pavlov H, Rubinstein D. The Segond fracture of the proximal tibia. AJR 1988;15:1163–1167.
139. Goodrich A, Ballard AM. Posterior cruciate ligament avulsion associated with ipsilateral femur fracture in a ten-year-old child. J Trauma 1988;28:1393–1396.
140. Goodshall RW. The predictability of athletic injuries: an eight year study. J Sports Med 1975;3:50–54.
141. Graf BK, Lange RH, Fujisaki K, Landry GL, Sabuja RK. Anterior cruciate ligament tears in skeletally immature patients: meniscal pathology at presentation and after attempted conservative treatment. J Arthroscop Surg 1992;8:229–233.
142. Grana WA, Moritz JA. Ligamentous laxity in secondary school athletes. JAMA 1978;240:1975–1976.
143. Hall DJ, Angel KR. Anterior cruciate ligament injury in childhood and adolescence. J Bone Joint Surg Am 1990;72:1091–1092.
144. Hyndman JC, Brown DCS. Major ligamentous injuries of the knee in children. J Bone Joint Surg Br 1979;61:245.
145. Irvine GB, Dias JJ, Finlay DBL. Segond fracture of the lateral tibial condyle. J Bone Joint Surg Br 1987;69:613–614.
146. Janarv P-M, Nyström A, Werner S, Hirsch G. Anterior cruciate ligament injuries in skeletally immature patients. J Pediatr Orthop 1996;16:673–677.
147. Johansson E, Aparisi T. Congenital absence of the cruciate ligaments. Clin Orthop 1982;162:108–111.
148. Jones R, Smith SA. On rupture of the cruciate ligaments of the knee, and on fractures of the spine of the tibia. Br J Surg 1913;1:70–73.
149. Jones RE, Henley MB, Francis P. Non-operative management of isolated grade III collateral ligament injury in high school football players. Clin Orthop 1986;213:137–140.
150. Joseph KN, Pogrund H. Traumatic rupture of the medial ligament of the knee in a four-year-old boy. J Bone Joint Surg Am 1978;60:402–403.
151. Kallenberger R, von Laer L. Nonosseous lesions of the anterior cruciate ligaments in childhood and adolescence. Prog Pediatr Surg 1990;25:123–131.
152. Kannus P, Jarvinen M. Knee ligament injuries in adolescents: eight year follow-up of conservative management. J Bone Joint Surg Br 1988;70:772–776.

153. Kennedy JC, Grainger RW. The posterior cruciate ligament. J Trauma 1976;7:367–377.
154. Kennedy JC, Hawkins RJ, Willis RB, Danylchuk KD. Tension studies of human knee ligaments: yield point, ultimate failure, and disruption of the cruciate and tibial collateral ligaments. J Bone Joint Surg Am 1976;58:350–355.
155. Kerr HD. Segond fracture, hemarthrosis, anterior cruciate ligament disruption. J Emerg Med 1990;8:29–33.
156. Lee HG. Avulsion fracture of the tibial attachments of the cruciate ligaments: treatment by operative reduction. J Bone Joint Surg 1937;19:460–468.
157. Lichtor J. The loose jointed young athlete: recognition and treatment. J Sports Med 1972;1:22–23.
158. Lipscomb AB, Anderson AF. Tears of the anterior cruciate ligament in adolescents. J Bone Joint Surg Am 1986;68:19–28.
159. Matz SO, Jackson DW. Anterior cruciate ligament injury in children. Am J Knee Surg 1988;1:59–65.
160. Mayer PJ, Micheli LJ. Avulsion of the femoral attachment of the posterior cruciate ligament in an eleven-year-old boy. J Bone Joint Surg Am 1979;61:431–432.
161. McCarroll JR, Rettig AC, Shelbourne DR. Anterior cruciate ligament injuries in the young athlete with open physes. Am J Sports Med 1988;16:44–47.
162. Meyers MH, McKeever FM. Fracture of the intercondylar eminence of the tibia. J Bone Joint Surg Am 1959;41:209–222.
163. Meyers MH, McKeever FM. Fracture of the intercondylar eminence of the tibia. J Bone Joint Surg Am 1970;52:1677–1684.
164. Miller MD, Eilert RE. Management of anterior cruciate ligament deficiency in the skeletally immature individual. Operat Techn Orthop 1995;5:254–260.
165. Mylle J, Reynders P, Broos P. Transepiphyseal fixation of anterior cruciate avulsion in a child. Arch Orthop Trauma Surg 1993;112:101–103.
166. Nakhostine M, Bollen SR, Cross MJ. Reconstruction of midsubstance anterior cruciate rupture in adolescents with open physes. J Pediatr Orthop 1995;15:286–287.
167. Noyes FR, DeLucas JL, Torrik PJ. Biomechanics of anterior cruciate ligament failure: an analysis of strain-rate sensitivity and mechanisms of failure in primates. J Bone Joint Surg Am 1974;56:236–253.
168. Noyes FR, Grood ES. The strength of the anterior cruciate ligament in humans and rhesus monkeys: age-related and species-related changes. J Bone Joint Surg Am 1976;58: 1074–1082.
169. O'Donoghue DH. An analysis of end results of surgical treatment of major injuries to the ligaments of the knee. J Bone Joint Surg Am 1955;37:1–13.
170. Palmar I. On the injuries to the ligaments of the knee joint: a clinical study. Acta Chir Scand 1938;9(suppl 53):1–137.
171. Panjabi MM, Yoldas E, Oxland TR, Crisco JJ III. Subfailure injury of the rabbit anterior cruciate ligament. J Orthop Res 1996;14:216–222.
172. Parker AW, Drez D Jr, Cooper JL. Anterior cruciate ligament injuries in patients with open physes. Am J Sports Med 1994;22:44–47.
173. Pellegrini A. Traumatic calcification of the collateral tibial ligament of the left knee joint. Clin Med 1905;11:433–439.
174. Pellegrini-Stieda's disease [editorial]. AJR 1932;28:97.
175. Rinaldi E, Mazzarella F. Isolated fracture-avulsions of the tibial insertions of the cruciate ligaments of the knee. Ital J Orthop Traumatol 1980;6:77–83.
176. Robinson SC, Driscoll SE. Simultaneous osteochondral avulsion of the femoral and tibial insertions of the anterior cruciate ligament: report of a case in a 13-year-old boy. J Bone Joint Surg Am 1981;63:1342–1343.
177. Rosen MA, Jackson DW, Berger PE. Occult osseous lesions documented by magnetic resonance imaging associated with anterior cruciate ligament ruptures. Arthroscopy 1991;7: 45–51.
178. Sanders WE, Wilkins KE, Neidre A. Acute insufficiency of the posterior cruciate ligament in children. J Bone Joint Surg Am 1980;62:129–130.
179. Saperstein AL, Fetto JF. The anterior cruciate ligament-deficient knee: a diagnostic and therapeutic algorithm. Orthop Rev 1992;21:1297–1305.
180. Schaefer RA, Eilert RE, Gillogly SD. Disruption of the anterior cruciate ligament in a 4-year-old child. Orthop Rev 1993;22:725–727.
181. Segond P. Recherches cliniques et experimentales sur les épanchements sanguins du genou par entors. Prog Med 1879;7:297,319,340,379,400,419.
182. Shelton ML, Neer CS II, Grantham SA. Occult knee ligament ruptures associated with fractures. J Trauma 1971;11:853–856.
183. Skok SV, Jensen TT, Poulsen TD, Sturup J. Epidemiology of knee injuries in children. Acta Orthop Scand 1987;58:78–81.
184. Speer KP, Spritzer CE, Bassett FH III, Feagin JA Jr, Garrett WE Jr. Osseous injury associated with acute tears of the anterior cruciate ligament. Am J Sports Med 1992;20:382–389.
185. Stanitski CL. Anterior cruciate ligament injury in the skeletally immature patient: diagnosis and treatment. J Am Acad Orthop Surg 1995;3:146–158.
186. Stieda A. Über eine typische Verletzung am unteren Femurende. Arch Klin Chir 1908;85:815–818.
187. Sullivan JA. Ligamentous injuries of the knee in children. Clin Orthop 1990;255:44–50.
188. Suprock MD, Rogers VP. Posterior cruciate avulsion. Orthopaedics 1990;13:659–661.
189. Svendsen RN. High substantial rupture of the anterior cruciate ligament in a 6-year-old boy. Injury 1995;26:70–71.
190. Tipton CM, Matthes RD, Martin RK. Influence of age and sex on the strength of bone-ligament junctions in knee joints of rats. J Bone Joint Surg Am 1978;60:230–234.
191. Uhorchak JM, White PM, Scully TJ. Type III—a tibial fracture associated with simultaneous anterior cruciate ligament avulsion from the femoral origin. Am J Sports Med 1993;21:758–761.
192. Waldrop JI, Broussard TS. Disruption of the anterior cruciate ligament in a three-year-old child. J Bone Joint Surg Am 1984;66:1113–1114.
193. Wang JC, Shapiro MS. Pellegrini-Stieda syndrome. Am J Orthop 1995;21:493–497.
194. Wasilewski SA, Frankl U. Osteochondral avulsion fracture of femoral insertion of anterior cruciate ligament. Am J Sports Med 1992;20:224–226.
195. Wester W, Canale ST, Dutkowsky JP, Warner WC, Beaty JH. Prediction of angular deformity and leg-length discrepancy after anterior cruciate ligament reconstruction in skeletally immature patients. J Pediatr Orthop 1994;14:516–521.
196. Yao L, Dungan D, Sieger LL. MR imaging of tibial collateral ligament injury: comparison with clinical examination. Skeletal Radiol 1994;23:521–524.
197. Zaricznyj B. Avulsion fracture of the tibial eminence: treatment by open reduction and pinning. J Bone Joint Surg Am 1977;59:1111–1114.

Patellar Fracture

198. Bates DG, Hresko MT, Jaramillo D. Patellar sleeve fracture: demonstration with MR imaging. Radiology 1994;193; 825–827.
199. Beddow FH, Corkery PH, Slestwell GL. Avulsion of the ligamentum patellae from the lower pole of the patella. J R Coll Surg Edinb 1963;4:66–67.

200. Belman DAJ, Nevaiser RJ. Transverse fracture of the patella in a child. J Trauma 1973;13:917–918.
201. Bensahel H, Spring R. Les fractures de la rotule de l'enfant. J Chir 1970;99:45–51.
202. Berg EE. Bipolar infrapatellar tendon rupture. J Pediatr Orthop 1995;15:302–303.
203. Bishay M. Sleeve fractures of upper pole of patella. J Bone Joint Surg Br 1991;73:339.
204. Blazina ME, Korlan RK, Jobe FW, Carter VS, Carlson GN. Jumper's knee. Orthop Clin North Am 1973;4:665–673.
205. Braum W, Wiedemann M, Ruter A, Kundel K, Kolbringer S. Indications and results of nonoperative treatment of patellar fractures. Clin Orthop 1993;289:197–201.
206. Bruijn JD, Sanders RJ, Jansen BRH. Ossification in the patellar tendon and patella alta following sports injuries in children: complications of sleeve fractures after conservative treatment. Arch Orthop Traum Surg 1993;112:157–158.
207. Cahuzac JP, Lebarbier P, Picard P, Pasquie M. Les fractures parcellaires de la rotule. Chir Pediatr 1979;20:403–409.
208. Carpenter JE, Kasman R, Matthews LS. Fractures of the patella. J Bone Joint Surg Am 1993;75:1550–1561.
209. Carro LP. Avulsion of the patellar ligament with combined fracture luxation of the proximal tibial epiphysis: case report and review of the literature. J Orthop Trauma 1996;10:355–358.
210. Cipolla M, Cerullo G, Franco V, Gianni E, Puddu G. The double patella syndrome. Knee Surg Sports Traumatol Arthrosc 1995;3:21–25.
211. Crawford AH. Fractures about the knee in children. Orthop Clin North Am 1976;7:639–651.
212. Devas MB. Stress fractures of the patella. J Bone Joint Surg Br 1960;42:71–74.
213. Dickason JM, Fox JM. Fracture of the patella due to overuse syndrome in a child: a case report. Am J Sports Med 1982;10:248–250.
214. Diebold O. Über Kniescheibenbruche im Kindesalter. Arch Klin Chir 1927;14:664–673.
215. Essau P. Der inderikte Kniescheibenbruch beim Kinde. Zentralbl Chir 1932;30:2229–2231.
216. Gardiner JS, McInerney VK, Arella DG, Valdez NA. Injuries to the inferior pole of the patella in children. Orthop Rev 1990;19:643–649.
217. Grogan DP, Carey TP, Leffers DL, Ogden JA. Avulsion fractures of the patella. J Pediatr Orthop 1990;10:721–730.
218. Hallopeau P. Des certaines fractures de la rotule chez l'enfant. J Med Paris 1923;42:927–932.
219. Hanel DP, Burdge RE. Consecutive indirect patella fractures in an adolescent basketball player: a case report. Am J Sports Med 1981;9:327–328.
220. Holstein A, Lewis GB, Schultz R. Heterotopic ossification of patellar tendon. Bull Hosp Joint Dis 1964;25:191–194.
221. Houghton GR, Ackroyd CE. Sleeve fractures of the patella in children. J Bone Joint Surg Br 1979;61:165–168.
222. Iwaya T, Takatori Y. Lateral longitudinal stress fracture of the patella: report of three cases. J Pediatr Orthop 1985;5:73–75.
223. Jacquemier M, Chrestian P, Guys JM, Mailaender C, Billet P, Bouyala JM. Les fractures avulsions de la rotule de l'enfant: a propos de 3 cas. Chir Pediatr 1983;24:201–204.
224. Kaar TK, Murray P, Cashman WF. Transosseous suturing for sleeve fracture of the patella: case report. Ir J Med Sci 1993;162:148–149.
225. Kameyama O, Mori Y, Ogawa R. Sleeve fracture of the patella. Seikeigeka 1988;39:1049–1055.
226. Lenoir CAH. Contribution a l'etude de la fracture de la rotule chez l'enfant. Bordeaux, 1891.
227. Maguire JK, Canale ST. Fractures of the patella in children and adolescents. J Pediatr Orthop 1993;13:567–571.
228. Makhdoomi KR, Doyle J, Moloney M. Transverse fracture of the patella in children. Arch Orthop Trauma Surg 1993;112:302–303.
229. Khan KM, Bonar F, Desmond PM, et al. Patellar tendinosis (jumper's knee): findings at histopathologic examination, US, and MR imaging. Radiology 1996;200:821–827.
230. McLoughlin RF, Raber EL, Vellet AD, Wiley JP, Bray RC. Patellar tendinitis: MR imaging features, with suggested pathogenesis and proposed classification. Radiology 1995;197:843–848.
231. Nummi J. Fractures of the patella: a clinical study of 707 patellar fractures. Ann Chir Gynaecol 1971;63(suppl 179):1–80.
232. Peterson L, Stener B. Distal disinsertion of the patellar ligament combined with avulsion fractures at the medial and lateral margins of the patella. Acta Orthop Scand 1976;47:680–683.
233. Ray JM, Hendrix J. Incidence, mechanism of injury, and treatment of fractures of the patella in children. J Trauma 1992;32:464–467.
234. Rigault P, Mouterde P, Beneux J, Padovani JP, Raux P. Fractures osteocartilagineuses du genou chez l'enfant (a propos de 19 cas). Ann Chir Inf 1975;16:313–319.
235. Ronget D. Deux cas de fractures de la rotule meconnues chez l'enfant. Rev Orthop 1929;16:248–252.
236. Schuepp PA. Considerations sur les fracture de la rotule chez l'enfant. Thesis, Nancy, 1912.
237. Shands P, McQueen DA. Demonstration of avulsion fracture of the inferior pole of the patella by magnetic resonance imaging. J Bone Joint Surg Am 1995;77:1721–1723.
238. Spalding CB. Patellar fracture in a child two years old. Int Clin 1918;4:245–246.
239. Sugiura Y, Kaneko F. Rupture of the patella ligament with avulsion fracture of the lower pole of the patella: a case report. Orthop Surg (Tokyo) 1972;23:384–386.
240. Teitz CC, Harrington RM. Patellar stress fracture. Am J Sports Med 1992;20:761–765.
241. Torchis ME, Lewallen DG. Open fractures of the patella. J Orthop Trauma 1996;10:403–409.
242. Trillat A, Desour H. Les fractures chondro-osseuses du versant articulaire interne de la rotule. Rev Chir Orthop 1967;53:331–337.
243. Weigert M. Spontanruptur des Kniescheibenbandes bei Hochspringen. Z Orthop 1968;104:429–430.
244. Wu CD, Huang SC, Liu TK. Sleeve fractures of the patella in children: a report of 5 cases. Am J Sports Med 1991;19:525–528.

Sinding-Larsen-Johansson Lesion

245. Batten J, Menelaus MB. Fragmentation of the proximal pole of the patella. J Bone Joint Surg Br 1985;67:249–251.
246. Johansson S. En förut icke beskriven sjukdom i patella. Hygie 1922;84:161–166.
247. Kalebo P, Sward L, Karlsson J, Peterson L. Ultrasonography in the detection of partial patellar ligament ruptures (jumper's knee). Skeletal Radiol 1991;20:285–289.
248. Larsen SF. En littel ukjendt sygdom i patella. Nord Mag Laegevid 1921;19:856–858.
249. Lopez R, Lewis H. Larsen-Johansson disease; osteochondritis of the accessory ossification center of the patella: report of two cases. Clin Pediatr 1968;7:697–700.
250. Medlar RC, Lyne ED. Sinding-Larsen-Johansson disease. J Bone Joint Surg Am 1978;60A:1113–1116.
251. Sinding-Larsen MF. A hitherto unknown affection of the patella. Acta Radiol 1921;1:171–173.
252. Wolf J. Larsen-Johansson disease of the patella: seven new case reports; its relationship to other forms of osteochondritis: use

of male sex hormones as a new form of treatment. Br J Surg 1950;23:335–338.

Cerebral Palsy

253. Kaye JJ, Freiberger RH. Fragmentation of the lower pole of the patella in spastic lower extremities. Radiology 1971;101:97–100.
254. Lloyd-Roberts GC, Jackson AM, Albert JS. Avulsion of the distal pole of the patella in cerebral palsy. J Bone Joint Surg Br 1985;67:252–254.
255. Mann M. Fatigue fracture of the lower patellar pole in adolescents with cerebral movement disorders. Z Orthop 1984;122:167–172.
256. Perry J, Antonelli D, Ford W. Analysis of knee joint forces during flexed knee stance. J Bone Joint Surg Am 1975;57:961–967.
257. Roberts WM, Adams JP. The patellar-advancement operation in cerebral palsy. J Bone Joint Surg Am 1953;35:958–966.
258. Rosenthal RK, Levine DB. Fragmentation of the distal pole of the patella in spastic cerebral palsy. J Bone Joint Surg Am 1978;60:1113–1116.

Bipartite Patella

259. Adams JD, Leonard RD. A developmental anomaly of the patella frequently diagnosed as a fracture. Surg Gynecol Obstet 1925;41:601–606.
260. Benedetti GB, Canapa G. Il quadro anotomo-isologico della rotula partita. Arch Ortop 1959;72:1409–1413.
261. Bourne MH, Bianco AJ Jr. Bipartite patella in the adolescent: results of surgical excision. J Pediatr Orthop 1990;10:69–73.
262. Coonce DF, Pinstein M, Scott R. Radiology case of the month: bipartite patella. J Tenn Med Assoc 1980;73:655–657.
263. Denham RH. Dorsal defect of the patella. J Bone Joint Surg Am 1984;66:116.
264. Echeverria TS, Bersani FA. Acute fracture simulating a symptomatic bipartite patella. Am J Sports Med 1980;8:48–51.
265. George GR. Bilateral bipartite patella. Br J Surg 1935;22:555–560.
266. Green WT Jr. Painful bipartite patellae: a report of three cases. Clin Orthop 1975;110:197–200.
267. Halpern AA, Hewitt O. Painful medial bipartite patellae. Clin Orthop 1978;134:180–183.
268. Haswell DM, Berne AS, Graham CB. The dorsal defect of the patella. Pediatr Radiol 1976;4:238–242.
269. Hunter LII, Hensinger RN. Dorsal defect of the patella with cartilaginous involvement (case report). Clin Orthop 1975;110:131–132.
270. Ishikawa H, Sakurai A, Hirata S, et al. Painful bipartite patella in young athletes. Clin Orthop 1994;305:223–228.
271. Lawson JP. Symptomatic radiographic variants in extremities. Radiology 1985;157:625–631.
272. Oetteking B. Anomalous patellae. Anat Rec 1922;23:269–275.
273. Ogden JA, McCarthy SM, Jokl P. The painful bipartite patella. J Pediatr Orthop 1982;2:263–269.
274. Puddu G, Mariani P, Alzani R. Detachment of the accessory fragment in "patella partite." Ital J Orthop Traumatol 1978;42:197–203.
275. Ruggles G. Bilateral bipartite patellae. Br J Surg 1935;22:555–557.
276. Saupe H. Primare knochenmark seierung der kniescheibe. Dtsch Z Chir 1943;258:386–388.
277. Smillie IS. Injuries of the Knee Joint, 4th ed. New York: Churchill Livingstone, 1970.
278. Todd TW, McCally WC. Defects of the patellar border. Ann Surg 1921;14:775–780.
279. Tos L, Salvi V. La patologia non traumatico della rotula. Edizioni Minerva Med 1968;60:79–83.
280. Van Holsbeeck M, Vandamme B, Marchal G, Martens M, Victor J, Baert AL. Dorsal defect of the patella: concept of its origin and relationship with bipartite and multipartite patella. Skeletal Radiol 1987;16:304–311.
281. Weaver JK. Bipartite patellae as a cause of disability in the athlete. Am J Sports Med 1977;5:137–143.

Fabella

282. Dashefsky JH. Fracture of the fabella. J Bone Joint Surg Am 1977;59:698.

Popliteus Avulsion

283. McConkey JP. Avulsion of the popliteus tendon: case report. J Pediatr Orthop 1991;11:230–233.
284. Mircpulos SN, Myer TJ. Isolated avulsion of the popliteus tendon: a case report. Am J Sports Med 1991;19:417–419.
285. Naver L, Aalberg JR. Avulsion of the popliteus tendon: a rare cause of chondral fracture and hemarthrosis. Am J Sports Med 1985;13:423–424.
286. Yao L, Lee J. Avulsion of the posteromedial tibial plateau by the semimembranous tendon: diagnosis with MR imaging. Radiology 1989;172:513–514.

Osteochondral Fractures/Osteochondritis Dissecans

287. Adam G, Buhne M, Prescher A, Nolte-Ernsting C, Bohndorf K, Gunther RW. Stability of osteochondral fragments of the femoral condyle: magnetic resonance imaging with histopathologic correlation in an animal model. Skeletal Radiol 1991;20:601–606.
288. Ahstrom JP. Osteochondral fracture in the knee joint associated with hypermobility and dislocation of the patella. J Bone Joint Surg Am 1965;47:1491–1502.
289. Aicroth P. Osteochondritis dissecans of the knee: a clinical survey. J Bone Joint Surg Br 1971;53:448–454.
290. Bailey WH, Blundell GE. An unusual abnormality affecting both knee joints in a child. J Bone Joint Surg Am 1974;56:814–816.
291. Bartlett EC, Supik LF. Intraarticular arthroscopic wire fixation of bony fragments. Contemp Orthop 1989;18:369–372.
292. Brown TD, Pope DF, Hale JE, Buckwalter JA, Brand RA. Effects of osteochondral defect size on cartilage contact stress. J Orthop Res 1991;9:559–567.
293. Coleman HM. Recurrent osteochondral fractures of the patella. J Bone Joint Surg Br 1948;30:153–157.
294. Conway FM. Osteochondritis dissecans: description of the stages of the condition and its probable traumatic etiology. Am J Surg 1937;38:691–699.
295. Edwards DH, Bentle G. Osteochondritis dissecans patellae. J Bone Joint Surg Br 1977;59:58–63.
296. Fairbank HAT. Internal derangement of the knee in children and adolescents. Proc R Soc Med 1936;30:427–432.
297. Green WT, Banks HH. Osteochondritis dissecans in children. J Bone Joint Surg Am 1953;35:26–47.
298. Healy WL. Osteonecrosis of the knee detected only by magnetic resonance imaging. Orthopaedics 1991;14:703–704.
299. Henderson NJ, Houghton GR. Osteochondral fractures of the knee in children. In: Houghton GR, Thompson GH (eds)

Problematic Musculoskeletal Injuries in Children. London: Butterworths, 1983.
300. Hughston JC, Hergenroeder PT, Courtenay BG. Osteochondritis dissecans of the femoral condyles. J Bone Joint Surg Am 1984;66:1340–1348.
301. Linden B. Osteochondritis dissecans of the femoral condyles: a long-term follow-up study. J Bone Joint Surg Am 1977;59:769–776.
302. Maletuis W, Lunderg M. Refixation of large chondral fragments on the weight-bearing area of the knee joint: a report of two cases. Arthroscopy 1994;10:630–633.
303. Mezgarzadeh M, Sapega AA, Bonakdarpour A, et al. Osteochondritis dissecans: analysis of mechanical stability with radiography, scintigraphy, and MR imaging. Radiology 1987;165:775–780.
304. Olsson SE. Osteochondros hos Hund: patologi rontgendiagnostik och klinik. Sv Vet 1977;29:577–586.
305. Plaga BR, Royster RM, Donigian AM, Wright GB, Caskey PM. Fixation of osteochondral fractures in rabbit knees. J Bone Joint Surg Br 1992;74:292–296.
306. Pritsch M, Velkes S, Levy D, Greental A. Suture fixation of osteochondral fractures of the patella. J Bone Joint Surg Br 1995;77:154–155.
307. Renu JMA, Bou CV, Portet RV, Diaz JAM, Gonzalez FXA, Soler RR. Osteochondritis dissecans of the patella: 12 cases followed for 4 years. Acta Orthop Scand 1994;65:77–79.
308. Rosenberg NJ. Osteochondral fractures of the lateral femoral condyle. J Bone Joint Surg Am 1964;46:1013–1026.
309. Schenck RC, Goodnight JM. Osteochondritis dissecans. J Bone Joint Surg Am 1996;78:439–456.
310. Seitz WH Jr, Bibliani LU, Andrews DL, Levine RK. Osteochondritis dissecans of the knee, a surgical approach. Orthop Rev 1985;14:56–59.
311. Twyman RS, Desai K, Aicroth PM. Osteochondritis dissecans of the knee: a long-term study. J Bone Joint Surg Br 1991;73:461–464.
312. Wombwell JH, Nunley JA. Compressive fixation of osteochondritis dissecans fragments with Herbert screws. J Orthop Trauma 1987;1:74–77.

Open Injury

313. Kahn B. Foreign body (palm thorn) in knee joint. Clin Orthop 1978;135:104–105.
314. Karshner RG, Hanafee W. Palm thorns as a cause of joint effusion in children. Radiology 1953;60:592–594.
315. Sugarman M, Stobie DG, Quismorio FP, Terry R, Hanson V. Plant thorn synovitis. Arthritis Rheum 1977;20:1125–1128.
316. Theodorou SD, Vlachos P, Vamvasakis E. Knee joint injury by mercury from a broken thermometer. Clin Orthop 1981;160:159–161.
317. Wolfgang GL. Intraarticular foreign body of the knee: problems of recognition and treatment. Orthop Rev 1977;6:79–82.

Plica Syndrome

318. Apple JS, Martinez S, Hardaker WT, Daffner RH, Gehweiler JA. Synovial plicae of the knee. Skeletal Radiol 1982;7:251–254.
319. Blatz DJ, Fleming R, McCarroll J. Suprapatellar plica: a study of their occurrence and role in internal derangement of the knee in active duty personnel. Orthopedics 1981;4:181–186.
320. Deutsch AL, Resnick D, Dalink MK, et al. Synovial plicae of the knee. Radiology 1981;141:627–634.
321. Dupont J-Y. Synovial plicae of the knee: controversies and review. Clin Sports Med 1997;16:87–122.
322. Hansen H, Boe S. The pathological plica in the knee: results after arthroscopic resection. Arch Orthop Trauma Surg 1989;108:282–284.
323. Harty M, Joyce JJ III. Synovial folds in the knee joint. Orthop Rev 1977;6:91–92.
324. Johnson DP, Eastwood DM, Witherow PJ. Symptomatic synovial plicae of the knee. J Bone Joint Surg Am 1993;75:1485–1496.
325. Kinnard P, Levesque RY. The plica syndrome: a syndrome of controversy. Clin Orthop 1984;183:141–143.
326. Lupi L, Bighi S, Cervi PM, Limone GL, Massari L. Arthrography of the plica syndrome and its significance. Eur J Radiol 1990;11:15–18.
327. Mital MA, Hayden J. Pain in the knee in children: the medial plica shelf syndrome. Orthop Clin North Am 1979;10:713–722.
328. Muntzinger U, Ruckstuhl J, Scherrer H, Gschwend N. Internal derangement of the knee joint due to pathologic synovial folds: the mediopatellar plica syndrome. Clin Orthop 1981;155:59–64.
329. Ogata S, Uhthoff HK. The development of synovial plica in human knee joints: an embryologic study. Arthroscopy 1990;6:315–321.

Meniscus

330. Abdon CP, Swanson AG, Turner MS. Meniscectomy in children. J Bone Joint Surg Br 1985;67B:847.
331. Abdon P, Turner MS, Pettersson H, Lindstrand A, Stenstrom A, Swanson AJG. A long-term follow-up study of total meniscectomy in children. Clin Orthop 1990;257:166–170.
332. Abrams RC. Meniscus lesions of the knee in young children. J Bone Joint Surg Am 1957;35:194–197.
333. Andrish JT. Meniscal injuries in children and adolescents: diagnosis and management. J Am Acad Orthop Surg 1996;4:231–237.
334. Appel H. Late results after meniscectomy in the knee joint: a clinical and roentgenologic follow-up investigation. Acta Orthop Scand 1970;41(suppl 133):1–184.
335. Arnoczky SP, Warren RF. The microvasculature of the meniscus and its response to injury: an experimental study in the dog. Am J Sports Med 1983;11:131–141.
336. Baker BE, Peckham AC, Pupparo F, Sanborn JC. Review of meniscal injury and associated sports. Am J Sports Med 1985;13:1–4.
337. Barucha E. Meniskurisse bei Kinder. Z Orthop 1967;102:430–435.
338. Baryluk K, Oblonczek G, Zolmowski J. Kriegelenk meniskusverletzungen im Kindesalter mit Berucksiontigung der Nachuntersuchungen. Arch Orthop Unfallchir 1977;87:65–72.
339. Bhaduri T, Glass A. Menisectomy in children. Injury 1972;3:176–180.
340. Busch MT. Meniscal injuries in children and adolescents. Clin Sports Med 1990;9:661–680.
341. Butt WP, McIntyre JL. Double-contrast arthrography of the knee. Radiology 1969;92:487–493.
342. Cannon WD, Morgan CD. Meniscal repair. II. Arthroscopic repair techniques. J Bone Joint Surg Am 1994;76:294–311.
343. Cargill AO, Jackson JP. Bucket handle tear of the medial meniscus: a case for conservative surgery. J Bone Joint Surg Am 1976;58:248–251.
344. Cotta H. Kindlicher Meniscusschaden. Hefte Unfallheilkd 1976;128:59–64.

345. Cruess JV III, Ryu R, Morgan FW. Meniscal pathology: the expanding role of magnetic resonance imaging. Clin Orthop 1990;252:80–87.
346. Dalinka MK, Brennan RE, Canino C. Double contrast knee arthrography in children. Clin Orthop 1977;125:88–93.
347. Doyle JR, Eisenberg JH, Orth MW. Regeneration of knee menisci: a preliminary report. J Trauma 1966;6:50–52.
348. Fairbank HA. Internal derangements of the knee in children and adolescents. Proc R Soc Med 1937;30:427–432.
349. Fairbank TJ. Knee joint changes after meniscectomy. J Bone Joint Surg Br 1948;30:664–670.
350. Gross RH, Grana WA. Meniscus injuries in children. Adv Orthop Surg 1984;8:95–101.
351. Hamberg P, Gillquist J, Lysholm J. Suture of new and old peripheral meniscus tears. J Bone Joint Surg Am 1983;65:193–197.
352. Harway RA, Handle S. Internal derangement of the knee in an infant. Contemp Orthop 1988;17:49–50.
353. Heisel J, Schwarz B. Meniskusschaden im Kindes- und Jugendalter, Ursachen-Behandlung-Ergebnisse. Akt Traumatol 1984;14:108–114.
354. Henry JH, Craven FR. Traumatic meniscal lesions in children. South Med J 1981;74:1336–1341.
355. Hsieh HH, Walker PS. Stabilizing mechanisms of the loaded and unloaded knee joint. J Bone Joint Surg Am 1976;58:87–93.
356. Huckell JR. Is meniscectomy a benign procedure? A long-term follow-up study. Can J Surg 1965;8:254–260.
357. King AG. Meniscal lesions in children and adolescents: a review of the pathology and clinical presentation. Injury 1985;15:105–108.
358. Krause WR, Pope MH, Johnson RJ. Wilder DG. Mechanical changes in the knee after meniscectomy. J Bone Joint Surg Am 1976;58:599–604.
359. Mandiberg JJ, Lyne ED. Meniscectomies in children. Am J Sports Med 1980;8:87–93.
360. Manzione M, Pizzutillo PD, Peoples AB, Schweizer PA. Meniscectomy in children: a long-term follow-up study. Am J Sports Med 1983;11:111–117.
361. McLain LG. Sports injuries in a high school. Pediatrics 1989;84:446–450.
362. Medlar RC, Mandiberg JJ, Lyne ED. Meniscectomies in children. Am J Sports Med 1980;8:87–92.
363. O'Meara PM. Surgical techniques for arthroscopic meniscal repair. Orthop Rev 1993;22:781–790.
364. Oretrop N, Alm A, Ekstrom H, Gillquist J. Immediate effects of meniscectomy on the knee joint: the effects of tensile load on knee joint ligaments in dogs. Acta Orthop Scand 1978;49:407–415.
365. Price CT, Allen WC. Ligament repair in the knee with preservation of the meniscus. J Bone Joint Surg Am 1978;60:61–65.
366. Ritchie DM. Meniscectomy in children. Aust NZ J Surg 1965;35:239–244.
367. Saddawi ND, Hoffman BK. Tear of the attachment of a normal medial meniscus of the knee in a four-year-old child. J Bone Joint Surg Am 1970;52:809–811.
368. Schettler G. Beitrag zum Meniskusschaden im Kindesalter. Z Orthop 1972;110:443–449.
369. Schlonsky J, Eyring EJ. Lateral meniscus tears in young children. Clin Orthop 1973;97:117–122.
370. Schultiz KP. Meniscusverletzungen im Kindes- und Jugendalter. Arch Orthop Unfallchir 1973;76:195–199.
371. Smith L. A concealed injury to the knee. J Bone Joint Surg Am 1962;44:1659–1660.
372. Springorum PW. Meniskuslasionen bei Jugendlichen. Zentralbl Chir 1979;39:1581–1586.
373. Tapper EM, Hoover NS. Late results after meniscectomy. J Bone Joint Surg Am 1969;51:517–526.
374. Vahvanen V, Aalto K. Meniscectomy in children. Acta Orthop Scand 1979;50:791–798.
375. Vangsness CT Jr, DeCampos J, Merritt PO, Wiss DA. Meniscal injury associated with femoral shaft fractures. J Bone Joint Surg Br 1993;75:207–209.
376. Volk H, Smith FM. "Bucket-handle" tear of the medial meniscus in a five-year-old boy. J Bone Joint Surg Am 1953;35:234–236.
377. Wroble RR, Henderson RC, Camption ER, El-Khoury GY, Albright JP. Meniscectomy in children and adolescents: a long-term follow-up study. Clin Orthop 1992;279:188–189.
378. Zaman M, Leonard MA. Meniscectomy in children: a study of fifty-nine cases. J Bone Joint Surg Br 1978;60:436.

Meniscal Cyst

379. Flynn M, Kelly JP. Local excision of cyst of the lateral meniscus of knee with outcome recurrence. J Bone Joint Surg Br 1976;58:88–89.
380. Glasgow MMS, Allen PW, Blakeway C. Arthroscopic treatment of cysts of the lateral meniscus. J Bone Joint Surg Br 1993;75:299–302.
381. Kinura M, Hagiwara A, Hasegawa A. Cyst of the medial meniscus after arthroscopic meniscal repair. Am J Sports Med 1993;21:755–757.
382. Mills CA, Henderson IJP. Cysts of the medial meniscus. J Bone Joint Surg Br 1993;75:293–298.
383. Parisien JS Arthroscopic treatment of cysts of the menisci: a preliminary report. Clin Orthop 1990;257:154–158.
384. Passler J, Hofer HP, Fellinger M, Peicha G. Intraarticular meniscal cysts of the knee: report of two cases. Int Orthop 1991;15:357–358.
385. VanderWilde RS, Peterson HA. Meniscal cyst and magnetic resonance imaging in childhood and adolescence. J Pediatr Orthop 1992;12:761–765.

Meniscal Ossification

386. Berg EE. The meniscal ossicle: the consequence of a meniscal injury. J Arthrosc 1991;7:241–244.
387. Ganey TM, Ogden JA, Abou-Made N, Coville B, Zdyziarski JM, Olsen JH. Meniscal ossification. II. The normal pattern in the tiger knee. Skeletal Radiol 1994;23:173–179.
388. Glass RS, Barnes WM, Kells DV, Thomas S, Campbell C. Ossicles of knee menisci: report of seven cases. Clin Orthop 1975;111:163–171.
389. Lonon WD, Crawford AH. Ossicle of the medial meniscus in a child. Orthop Rev 1981;10:129–131.
390. Mariani PD, Puddu G. Meniscal ossicle: a case report. Am J Sports Med 1981;6:392–393.
391. Ogden JA, Ganey TM, Arrington JA, Leffers D. Meniscal ossification. I. Human. Skeletal Radiol 1994;23:167–172.
392. Yao J, Yao L. Magnetic resonance imaging of a symptomatic meniscal ossicle. Clin Orthop 1993;293;225–228.

Discoid Meniscus

393. Aicroth PM, Patel DV, Marx CL. Congenital discoid lateral meniscus in children: a follow-up study and evolution of management. J Bone Joint Surg Br 1991;73:932–936.
394. Bellier G, DuPont JY, Larrain M, Caudron C, Carlioz H. Lateral discoid menisci in children. Arthroscopy 1989;5:52–56.
395. Blacksin MF, Greene B, Botelho G. Bilateral diskoid medial menisci diagnosed by magnetic resonance imaging: a case report. Clin Orthop 1992;285:214–216.

396. Dickason JM, Del Pizzo W, Blazina ME, Fox JM, Friedman MJ, Snyder SJ. A series of ten discoid medial menisci. Clin Orthop 1982;168:75–79.
397. Dickhaut SC, DeLee JC. The discoid lateral meniscus syndrome. J Bone Joint Surg Am 1982;64:1068–1073.
398. Engber WD, Mickelson MR. Cupping of the lateral tibial plateau associated with a discoid meniscus. Orthopedics 1981;4:904–905.
399. Fujikawa K, Iseki F, Micura Y. Partial resection of the discoid meniscus in the child's knee. J Bone Joint Surg Br 1981;63:391–395.
400. Haveson SB, Rein BI. Lateral discoid meniscus of the knee: arthrographic diagnosis. AJR 1970;109:581–585.
401. Hayashi LK, Yamaga H, Ida K, Miura T. Arthroscopic meniscectomy for discoid lateral meniscus in children. J Bone Joint Surg Am 1988;70:1495–1500.
402. Hayashi LK, Yamaga H, Mori R, et al. Clinical and arthroscopic study of discoid lateral meniscus in infants. Central Jpn J Orthop Traumatol Surg 1987;30:639–645.
403. Johnson RG, Simmons EH. Discoid medial meniscus. Clin Orthop 1982;167:176–179.
404. Kaplan EB. The embryology of the menisci of the knee joint. Bull Hosp Joint Dis 1955;16:111–124.
405. Kaplan EB. Discoid lateral meniscus of the knee joint. J Bone Joint Surg Am 1957;39:77–87.
406. Maknoon AS. Congenital discoid meniscus (snapping knee). W Va Med J 1972;68:123.
407. Murdoch G. Congenital discoid medial meniscal cartilage. J Bone Joint Surg Br 1956;38:564–566.
408. Nathan PA, Cole SC. Discoid meniscus. Clin Orthop 1969;64:107–113.
409. Neuschwander DC. Discoid meniscus. Operat Techn Orthop 1995;5:78–87.
410. Patel D, Dinakopoulos P, Denoncourt P. Bucket handle tear of a medial discoid meniscus: arthroscopic diagnosis; partial excision. Orthopedics 1986;9:607–610.
411. Picard JJ. Aspects radiologiques des menisques discoides. J Radiol Electr 1964;45:839–841.
412. Ross JK, Tough ICK, English TA. Congenital discoid cartilage: report of a case of discoid medial cartilage, with an embryological note. J Bone Joint Surg Br 1958;40:262–267.
413. Silverman J, Mink J, Deutsch A. Discoid menisci of the knee: MR imaging appearance. Radiology 1989;173:351–354.
414. Smillie IUS. The congenital discoid meniscus. J Bone Joint Surg Br 1948;30:671–682.
415. Stark JE, Siegel MJ, Weinberger E, Shaw DWW. Discoid menisci in children: MR features. J Comp Assist Tomogr 1995;19:608–611.
416. Stern A, Hallel T. Medial discoid meniscus with cyst formation in a child. J Pediatr Orthop 1988;8:471–473.
417. Washington ER, Root L, Liner UC. Discoid lateral meniscus in children. J Bone Joint Surg Am 1995;77:1359–1361.
418. Weiner B, Rosenberg N. Discoid medial meniscus: association with bone changes in the tibia. J Bone Joint Surg Am 1974;56:171–173.

Miscellaneous

419. Gristina AG, Wilson PD, Kustan J. Popliteal cysts in adults and children: review of 90 cases. Arch Surg 1964;88:357–363.
420. Lindgren PG. Gastrocnemius-semimembranosus bursa and its relation to the knee joint. Acta Radiol Diagn 1978;19:609–622.
421. Methany JA, Mayor MB. Hoffa disease: chronic impingement of the infrapatellar fat pad. Am J Knee Surg 1988;1:134–139.
422. Sansone V, DePonti A, Pabuello GM, Del Maschio A. Popliteal cysts and associated disorders of the knee. Int Orthop 1995;19:279–284.

23
Tibia and Fibula

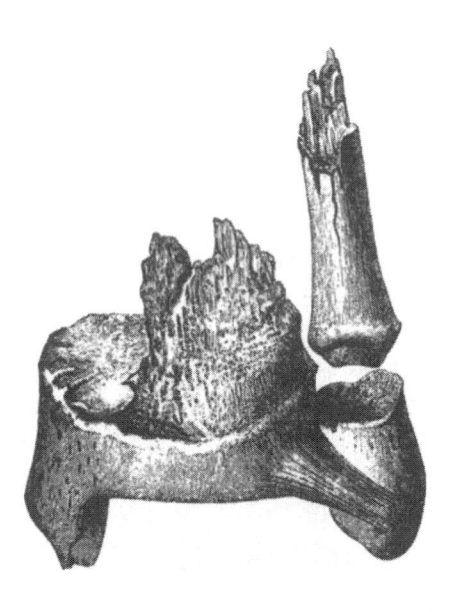

Engraving of physeal fractures of the distal tibia and fibula. (From Poland J. Traumatic separation of the Epiphyses. *London: Smith, Elder, 1898)*

Tibial trauma involving the growing child or adolescent shows considerable variation in both age-related injury and healing patterns, perhaps more so than other parts of the developing chondro-osseous skeleton. Toddler's fracture of the immature tibial and fibular diaphyses reflects the need for osteonic remodeling to accommodate the increasing demands of weight-bearing as the infant shifts from crawling to a bipedal gait. Closure patterns of both the proximal and distal tibial physes are eccentric, with certain regions undergoing the process of progressive epiphysiodesis prior to other regions. This renders selected areas susceptible to characteristic injury patterns as long as such disparity is present.

The malleoli have an array of fracture patterns that are the immature skeletal equivalent of ligamentous injury after skeletal maturation. Many of these injury patterns are undisplaced (occult) injuries that are difficult to corroborate with routine imaging procedures. The frequent emphasis or interpretation of a radiological "variant" may create a false sense of security that a true injury is absent. As will be shown, "variants" that hurt after injury may be fractured. In fact, many such variants (e.g., accessory malleoli) probably reflect antecedent avulsion similar to the appearance of an ulnar styloid "nonunion" following a distal radial fracture without obvious ulnar fracture acutely.

Anatomy

Proximal Tibia

The proximal tibial epiphysis usually forms a secondary ossification center during the first to third postnatal months. It may be present in the neonate. This centrally located ossification process progressively expands in response to both biologic growth and knee biomechanics (Fig. 23-1). If significant genu varum, a relatively normal state for the neonate, persists beyond the development of active ambulation, the secondary center may exhibit irregular marginal ossification, particularly at the medial side.[7,14] Although this area may appear involved in the child presenting with knee trauma, such ossification patterns usually represent biologic variation, not a specific injury (Fig. 23-2). In the anteroposterior view, the ossification center is slightly conical centrally as it progressively extends into the cartilaginous tibial spines. This chondro-osseous extension becomes more defined during late childhood and adolescence (Fig. 23-2), commensurate with an increasing susceptibility to avulsion fractures of the anterior tibial spine.

Throughout development the plane of the articular surface (plateau) normally tilts backward 15°–20°. Accordingly, angled anteroposterior views may be necessary to rule out the intraarticular extension of certain fractures. These views may be more helpful during adolescence when the ossification center is sufficiently developed to have the extensive subchondral bone associated with each plateau. During the reduction of proximal tibial epiphyseal and metaphyseal fractures, consideration must be given to this normal retrograde tilt. Failure to restore this angle leaves the tibia in a relative recurvatum and may have an adverse effect on subsequent development and knee mechanics, especially when the injury occurs in a young child. However, such angular

Anatomy

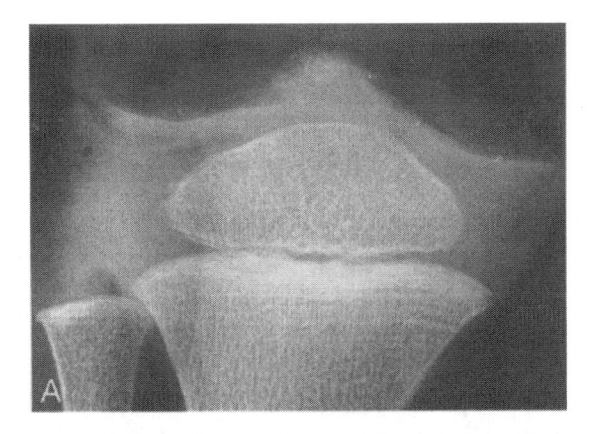

only a small area of attachment directly into the tibial physis, with the major portion of the ligament attaching directly into the metaphysis under the pes anserinus, and that such an anatomic configuration protects the proximal tibia from major epiphyseal injuries. This suggestion, however, is not anatomically true. As discussed in Chapter 22 and shown in Figure 23-3, there are dense attachments of the ligaments and capsule into the physeal perichondrium medially and laterally. During the last stages of postnatal development, the ligaments attach directly into the periosteum and the expanding epiphyseal ossification center. It is more likely that the overall anatomic configurations of the proximal

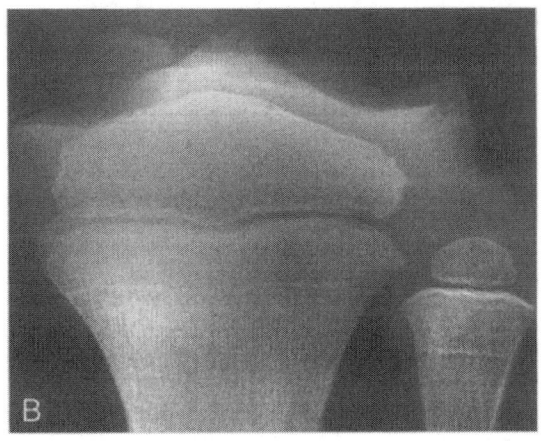

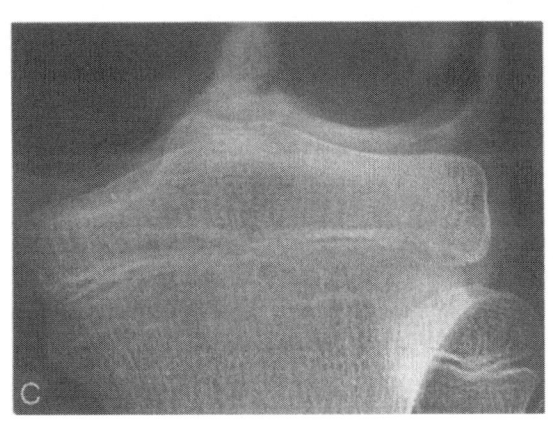

FIGURE 23-1. Radiographic development of the proximal tibia. (A) At 2 years. (B) At 5 years. (C) At 11 years.

deformities are in the plane of motion of the knee joint and thus have a propensity to improve compared to varus or valgus angulation.

Both lateral and medial collateral ligaments are firmly attached to portions of the distal femoral epiphysis, so various stresses applied to the knee are primarily dissipated through the distal femoral epiphysis and physis. The fibular collateral ligament, which has some additional attachment directly into the tibial epiphysis, primarily attaches onto the proximal fibular epiphysis, with some fibers reaching out over the lateral side of the tibial epiphysis and metaphysis.[6] It has been suggested that the medial collateral ligament has

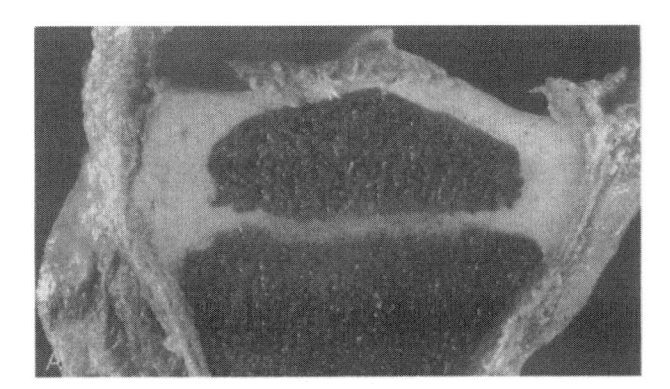

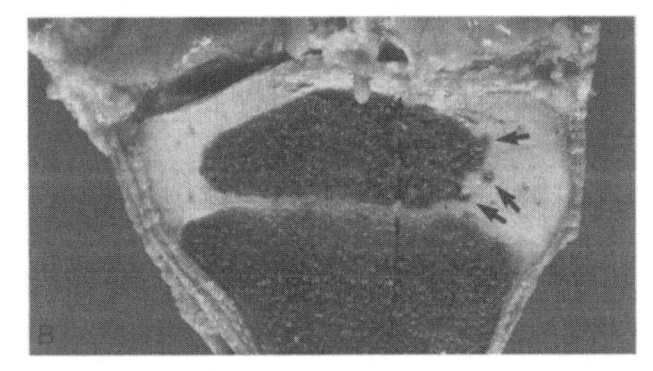

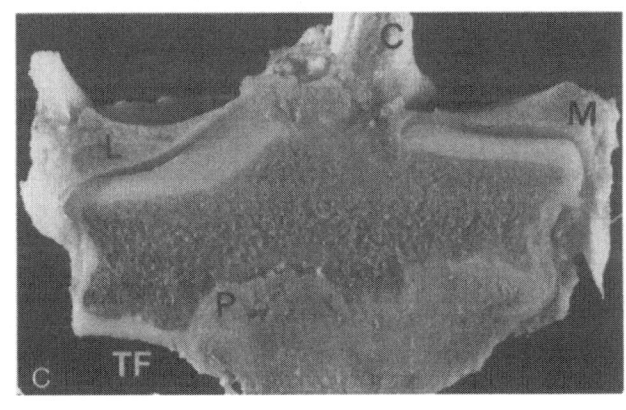

FIGURE 23-2. Chondro-osseous development of the proximal tibia. (A) Smooth contours in a 6-year-old child. (B) Irregular medial ossification (arrows) in another 6-year-old child. (C) Posterior slab from a 12-year-old child showing how tibial spine bone may extend to or beyond the articular limits and predispose the tibial spine to avulsion. Note the cruciate ligament (C), lateral meniscus (L), medial meniscus (M), physis (P), and proximal tibiofibular joint (TF).

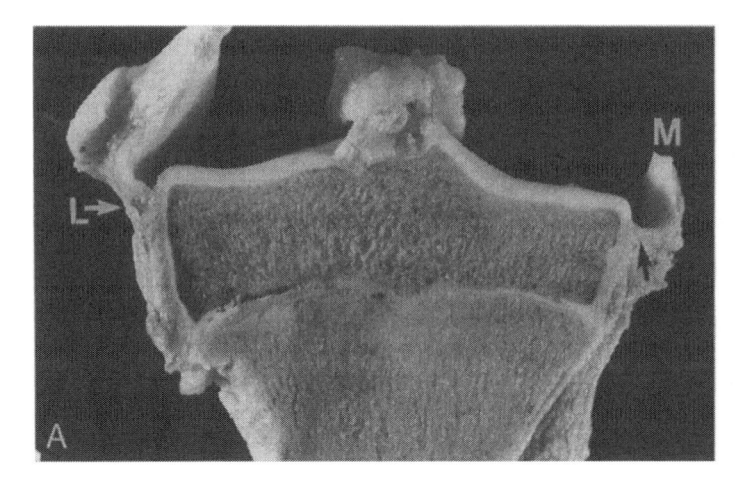

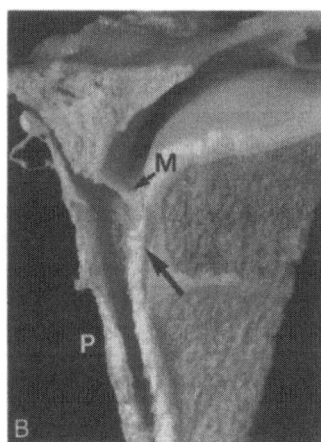

FIGURE 23-3. Attachments of capsule and ligaments directly into the proximal tibial epiphysis. (A) Section from a 14-year-old showing deep medial (M) and lateral (L) collateral ligament attachments into the cartilaginous portion of the epiphysis (specifically, the perichondrium), *not* into the metaphysis. (B) Section from a 6-year-old child showing attachments of the medial collateral ligament (M) into the epiphyseal perichondrium. In contrast, the pes anserinus (P) attaches to the metaphyseal-diaphyseal region.

tibial physis, muscular attachments (e.g., gastrocnemius, biceps, medial hamstrings), and abnormally applied biomechanical angular moment arms are, individually and collectively, the important factors in the relative failure rates of the distal femoral and proximal tibial physes.

The combination of epiphyses and external (collateral) and internal (cruciate) ligaments creates a moment arm such that when angular or rotatory stress is applied to the lower leg maximal strains occur at the end of this composite unit—the distal femoral physis. Thus the more important factor is strain dissipation throughout the entire chondro-osseous and ligamentous complex, rather than any discrete anatomic attachments of the ligaments connecting the tibia, fibula, and femur.

The tibial eminence consists of two osseous spines (tuberosities). The medial anterior spine has the attachment of the anterior cruciate ligament (ACL). No ligamentous (cruciate) tissue attaches to the apex of the lateral, posterior spine. Between and adjacent to these two elevations are the osseous attachments of the anterior and posterior horns of the medial and lateral menisci. The fibers of the fan-shaped anterior portion of the ACL coalesce with the dense anchoring fibers of the anterior horns of both the medial and lateral menisci of the tibia. The ACL does not have a singular anatomic attachment to either meniscus in this region. The posterior cruciate ligament (PCL) attaches to a shallow depression immediately behind the region of the intercondylar eminence and extends for a short distance down the posterior surface of the upper tibia. A small, stout band of this ligament (Humphrey's ligament), attaches to the posterior horn of the lateral meniscus. The PCL attachment is separate from the intercondylar eminence in the tibial spines.

Tibial Tuberosity

The tibial tuberosity (tubercle) initially develops as a morphologically discrete anterior cartilaginous extension of the proximal tibial epiphysis at about 12–15 fetal weeks (Fig. 23-4). At the end of fetal development a well-defined tuberos-

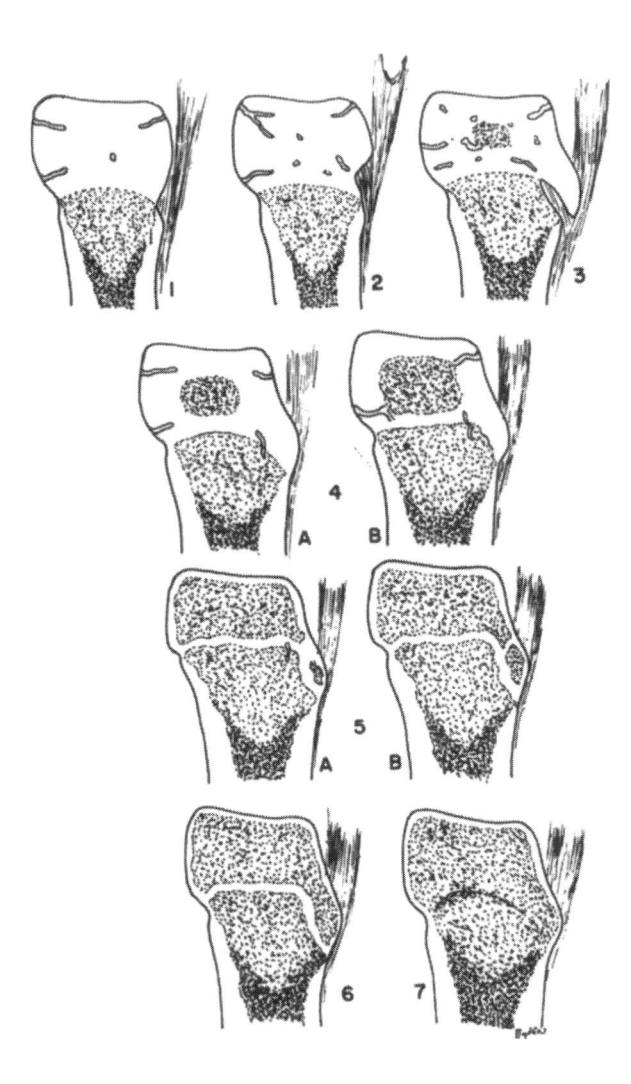

FIGURE 23-4. Development of the tibial tuberosity. 1–3 = Prenatal development. 4–7 = Postnatal development.

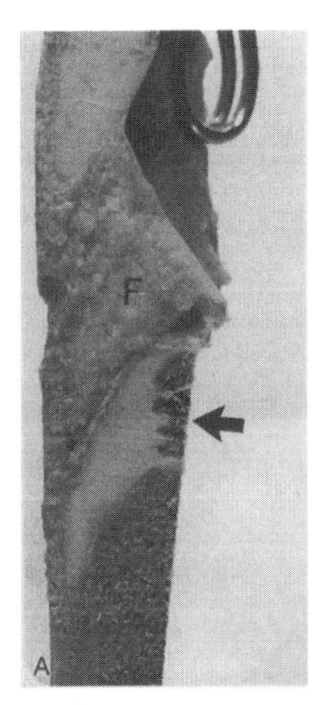

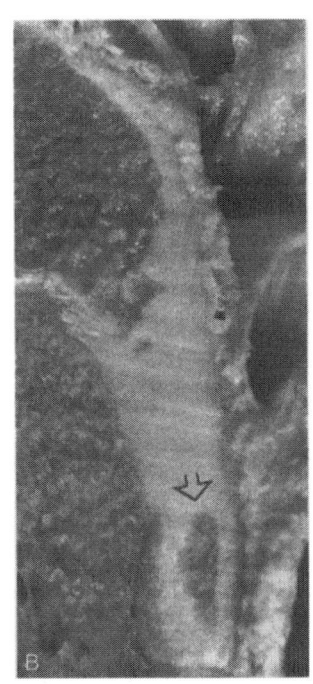

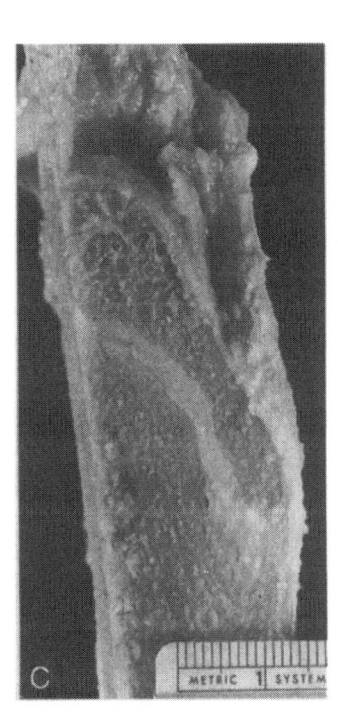

FIGURE 23-5. (A) Typical appearance of the tibial tuberosity during childhood (6 years) *prior* to the development of the tuberosity ossification center. The proximal tibial epiphyseal ossification center is present (arrow). Also note the large fat pad (F) behind the patellar tendon. (B) The ossification center initially appears in the distal portion (arrow) of the tibial tuberosity. (C) Appearance of the fused proximal tibial and tuberosity centers in a 12-year-old.

ity is present, although it is still approximately level with the main tibial physis and epiphysis. Distal "migration" is primarily a postnatal phenomenon.[8,10]

The physis underlying this tuberosity is initially composed almost completely of fibrocartilage, rather than the columnar, hypertrophic cellular structure that usually characterizes a physeal growth zone.[10,12] This cellular arrangement represents a cytoarchitectural modification to resist the normal tensile stresses imparted by the quadriceps muscles through the patellar tendon. Near the junction with the proximal tibial physis the cells begin to exhibit columnar formation (see Chapter 1). There are distinct differences in bone formation, with the tuberosity creating underlying cortical bone by membranous ossification. In essence, this is a natural model of bone elongation.

By the time a child is 7–9 years old, the tuberosity begins to develop a secondary center of ossification, which usually commences in the distal portion (Figs. 23-5, 23-6). This accessory center of ossification gradually enlarges and extends proximally toward the main secondary ossification center of the proximal tibial epiphysis. During early adolescence these two centers may be separated by a small cartilaginous bridge, but they coalesce prior to physeal closure. Concomitant with the osseous maturation that occurs within the cartilage of the tuberosity, the growth plate exhibits a progressive change from fibrocartilage to columnar physeal cartilage and gradual extension of the cell columns from the proximal tibial physis toward the tip of the tuberosity, which retains a fibrocartilaginous tissue mode until closure.

The fibrocartilaginous nature of the tuberosity physis, especially distally, is a biologic response to the imparted tensile stresses (Fig. 23-7). As the tuberosity undergoes progressive secondary ossification, normal tensile stresses more often are dissipated through the composite proximal tibial tuberosity ossification center, rather than just the tuberosity. Accordingly, the histologic structure changes to one that is more characteristic of a physis, making it more resistant to tensile (shear) failure, comparable to compression physes.

Coincident with the age range of susceptibility to the Osgood-Schlatter lesion, there are significant modifications in the histologic structure of the distal portion of the epiphysis. The cells in the region of the eventual secondary ossification center commence hypertrophy. Subsequently, ossification begins within this hypertrophic cellular mass. At this point in development, these cellular changes, anticipatory to and including actual secondary ossification, introduce biomechanically responsive tissue changes that may predispose the anterior portion of the tuberosity ossification to failure if excessive, especially repetitive, tensile stresses are applied. Bone is more likely than cartilage, to fail in tension, which is more resistant to comparable tensile forces. Major or repetitive stress increases may cause failure of small chondro-osseous interfaces that are normally subjected to constant tension. These small regions of the preossification center may be avulsed to create, with subsequent maturation of the tissue modes, a roentgenographically evident Osgood-Schlatter lesion (see later in the chapter). However, while this anterior failure pattern is occurring, the

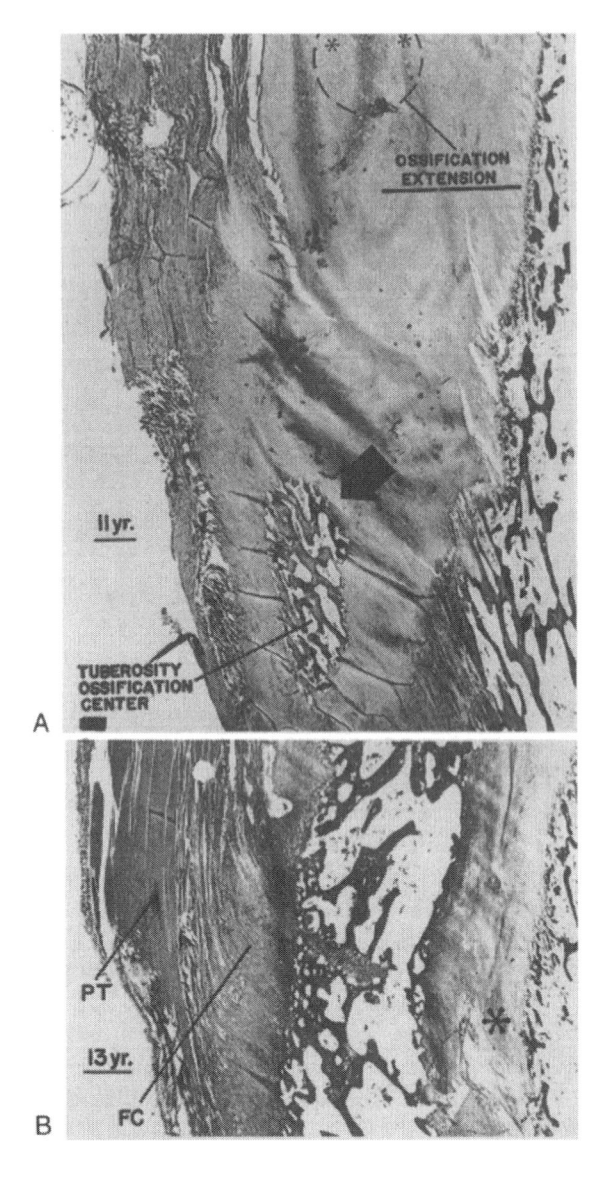

FIGURE 23-6. (A) Histologic appearance of early tuberosity ossification center (arrow) at 11 years. Extension of ossification (*) from the main tibial ossification center is evident. (B) Subsequent development, at 13 years, shows how the patellar tendon (PT) grades into the ossification center. Fibrocartilage (FC) blends from the tendon into the tuberosity ossification center. The histologic appearance here is similar to the appearance of the fibrocartilage between the tuberosity and the metaphysis.

tuberosity occur. Such failure in a tuberosity fracture commences distally and propagates proximally.

During much of development the patellar tendon has its primary attachment into the distal regions of the tuberosity and the adjoining metaphysis. However, with relative distal displacement of the tuberosity during skeletal growth and underlying portions of the distal tuberosity epiphyseal and physeal cartilage remain intact and in close apposition to the metaphysis.

The final step is physiologic epiphysiodesis. The tuberosity physis closes at 13–15 years of age in girls and at 15–18 years in boys. The physis of the proximal tibial physis closes first, starting centrally and proceeding centrifugally. The region under the tuberosity is the last to close, proceeding in a proximal to distal direction along the tuberosity. Therefore a situation similar to that of physeal closure of the distal tibia exists. Just as the fracture of Tillaux may occur because the rates of physiologic epiphysiodesis within the overall physeal area differ distally, so too may a similar limited failure of the

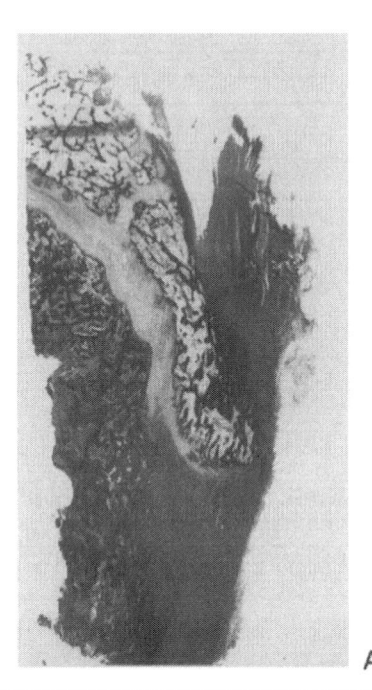

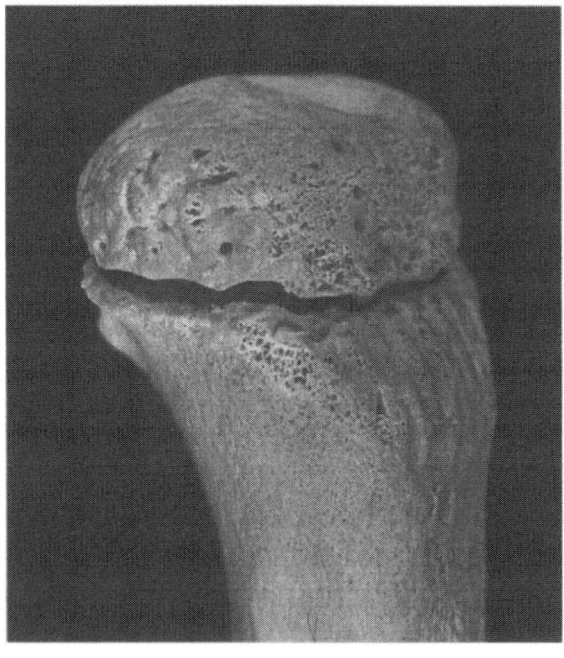

FIGURE 23-7. (A) Histologic section of the tuberosity from a 14-year-old boy showing the extent of attachment of the patellar tendon and the reactive thickening of the anterior trabecular bone of the ossification center. Note that the posterior surface of the tuberosity is relatively smooth, whereas the juxtaposed metaphyseal contour is undulated. (B) Osseous preparation (age 9 years) demonstrates the anterior metaphyseal undulation, which is a biomechanical adaptation to resist rotational shearing.

maturation, the patellar tendon develops a more extensive and proximal insertion on the anterior surface of the tuberosity.

Proximal Fibula

The proximal fibula articulates with the proximal tibial epiphysis (Fig. 23-8). The primary functions of the proximal tibiofibular joint appear to be (1) dissipation of torsional stresses applied at the ankle; (2) dissipation of lateral tibial bending moments; and (3) tensile rather than compressive weight-bearing.[6]

Some of the collateral ligaments of the proximal tibiofibular joint insert into the epiphysis (specifically, into the perichondrium) throughout most of development. This particular ligamentous insertion stabilizes the anatomy of the region and decreases the probability of fracture or displacement. A major factor in the stability of the proximal tibiofibular joint is the fibular collateral ligament. With the knee in extension, this ligament holds the fibula tautly in its normal position. With increasing flexion, the ligament relaxes and permits increasing anteroposterior subluxation. In many young children, normal joint laxity permits significant subluxation, even in tension.

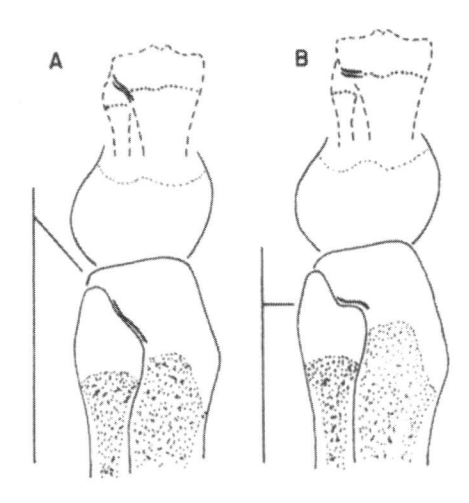

FIGURE 23-9. Two basic types of the proximal tibiofibular joint. (A) Oblique. (B) Horizontal.

There are two basic anatomic types of proximal tibiofibular joints.[6] The first is a horizontal surface (usually circular and planar) that articulates with a similar planar surface on the tibial epiphysis (Fig. 23-9). These articular surfaces are under and behind a projection of the lateral edge of the tibial epiphysis that provides some anterior stability and prevents significant forward displacement of the fibula. The second type is oblique. These articular surfaces are more variable in area, configuration, and inclination. The latter joint configurations appear to be more often associated with disruption of this joint (subluxation or dislocation).

The biomechanics of fibular rotation necessary to accommodate ankle motion are such that the more horizontal joint allows a greater degree of rotation before disruption. The horizontal type is associated with increased rotatory mobility and increased joint surface area. The oblique type is associated with less rotatory ability and less joint surface area, and it therefore appears to be more susceptible to displacement.

The proximal fibular epiphysis begins secondary ossification when the child is 2–4 years old. There are no significant variations that mimic fracture patterns, and the relatively protected location makes injury to this epiphysis among the rarest of all epiphyseal injuries. The lateral collateral ligament and biceps tendon attachments may lead to avulsion of a portion of the proximal fibula (type 3 or 4 injury) or styloid process. Proximal fibular physeal closure occurs at 15–16 years in boys and 13–14 years in girls.

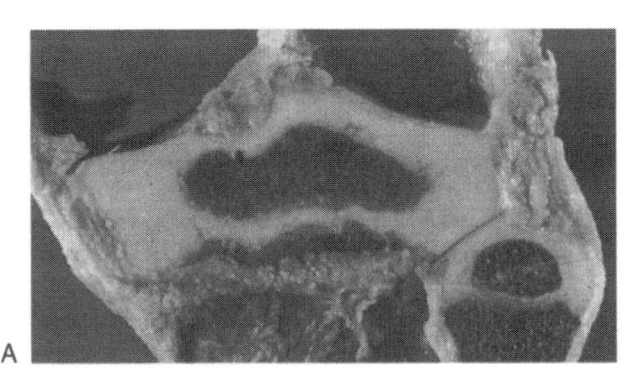

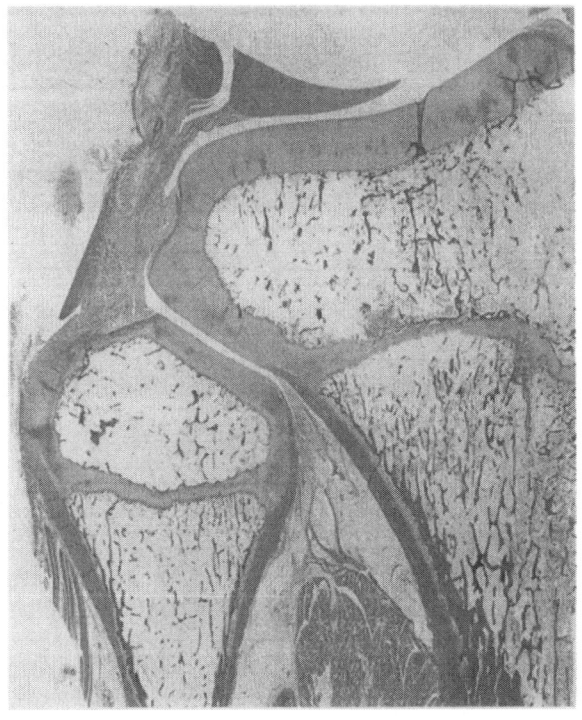

FIGURE 23-8. (A) Proximal tibiofibular relations in a 6-year-old child. (B) Histology of the the proximal tibiofibular joint in a 10-year-old.

Tibiofibular Diaphyses

The metaphyseal regions undergo typical changes, comparable to those of other long bones. However, the tibial diaphysis must undergo major changes that lead to the thickened cortex characteristic of this bone. This process requires extensive remodeling to create biomechanically responsive haversian systems. The various fracture patterns relate to the degree of development and maturation of this cortical remodeling system. The toddler's fracture of the proximal tibial metaphysis or the diaphysis, after the inception of weight-bearing, is a good example of this necessary progressive biomechanical strengthening and how it may not keep pace with the active toddler.

The extensive remodeling and bone thickening that occurs within the tibial diaphysis requires an adequate blood supply, but this vascularity probably decreases with age. We found this phenomenon in dogs of various ages, ranging from neonate to adolescence (see Chapter 1).[5,15] Such change in vascularization would explain the increasing incidence of delayed healing and even nonunion in teenagers.

Distal Tibia

The secondary ossification center of the distal tibial epiphysis usually appears during the second year. The medial malleolus ossifies as a downward prolongation from this main center but not until about 7 years in girls and 8 years in boys (Figs. 23-10 to 23-12). The medial margin, prior to and during the downward extension into the medial malleous, is often irregular. The entire distal epiphysis, including the malleolus, is ossified by 14–15 years in boys, and by 16–18 years it unites with the metaphysis. The processes occur in girls 2–3 years earlier. This physis is usually the first of the leg physes to undergo physiologic epiphysiodesis.

The initial physeal contour is transverse, although an anteromedial undulation develops within the first 18–24 months. This structural change, sometimes referred to as "Poland's hump," effectively divides the distal tibial epiphysis into lateral and medial (malleolar) areas and may have a significant effect on fracture propagation patterns.[4,11]

Accessory malleolar ossification centers (Fig. 23-13), which are often bilateral, are found in the distal region of the malleoli in some children.[2,9,13] Histologically, there is a bipolar physis between the secondary and accessory centers. Most appear to fuse to the main distal ossification center during adolescence, although they infrequently remain as a radiologically, but not necessarily anatomically, separate entity into adult life. Because these accessory centers are often found during the evaluation of acute trauma, they may be mistaken for fractures. The smooth appearance should rule out this diagnosis. Fractures may occur through this region (a type 7 growth mechanism injury), however, so an acutely symptomatic individual with an irregularity in this region, rather than a smooth-bordered ossification, should be considered and treated as a patient with a fracture (see later in the chapter).

Closure of the distal tibial physis shows a fairly characteristic pattern. Epiphysiodesis initially involves the medial portion, including the aforementioned undulation. The lateral portion begins fusion later (Fig. 23-12). The distal tibial growth plate progressively closes in a medial to lateral direction, especially posteriorly, over a 1.5-year period between 13 and 18 years. This leaves the anterolateral physis as the last region to close. If the ligaments remain intact during a severe external rotation stress to the adolescent ankle, failure may occur through the unfused lateral portion of the distal physis to cause a fracture of Tillaux or a triplane fracture.

The first region to close is the central area behind Poland's hump. Closure then radiates toward the anterior and medial portions (including much of the medial malleolus) and occurs along the posterior half, proceeding in a medial to lateral direction. The last region to close is the anterolateral segment. These closure patterns affect not only the appearance of the fracture of Tillaux but also those of the various triplane fractures.

The distal fibular physis does not close until *after* the distal tibial closure process is completed. Hence this physeal region may incur a fracture when the distal tibia appears to be skeletally mature.

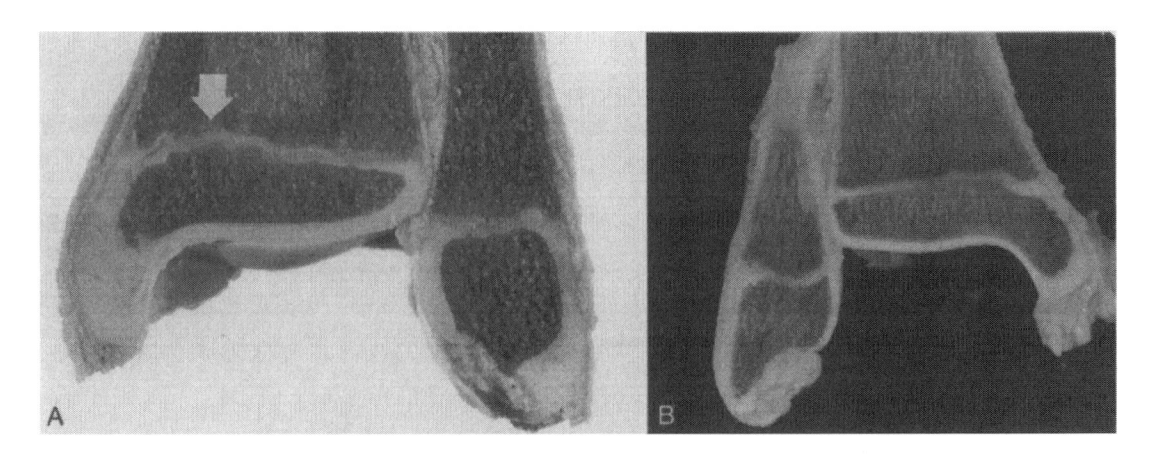

FIGURE 23-10. Appearance of the distal tibia and fibula at 6 years (A) and 11 years (B). Note how the fibular physis is level with the tibial articular surface. Also note the medial undulation in (A) (arrow). It is referred to as "Poland's hump."

Anatomy

FIGURE 23-11. Roentgenographic appearance of the distal tibia and fibula at 3 years (A), 4 years (B), 7 years (C), and 15 years (D). Note the development of the medial undulation. (D) Note that the physeal remnant is less evident medially. This medial to lateral closure pattern is undoubtedly a factor in distal tibial fracture patterns. (E) Lateral view of (B) showing how the fibular physis aligns with the tibial plafond.

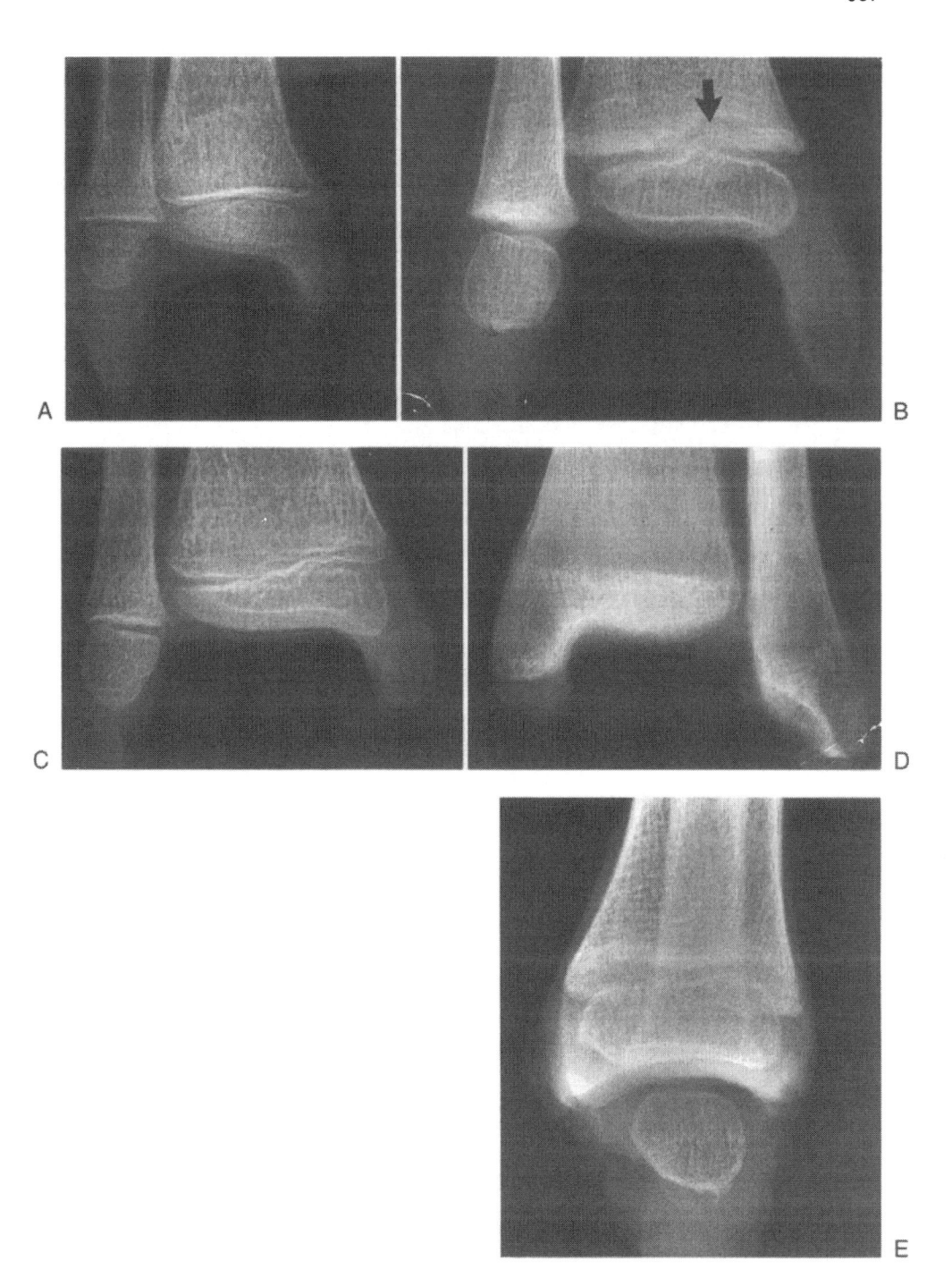

Distal Fibula

An ossification center appears in the distal fibula during the second to third years. The distal fibular epiphysis may also exhibit irregular (accessory) ossification at the tip and may show significant undulation of the physis (Fig. 23-14). Both anatomic factors may lead to a mistaken diagnosis of fracture. These accessory ossicles are more likely to be due to avulsion injuries, with the patient developing more chronic complaints, than to similar accessory ossifications of the medial malleolus.

The distal tibiofibular relations are such that the distal fibular physis is usually level with the tibial articular surface or the lower limits of the tibial ossification center (Fig. 23-10). Obviously, there are anatomic variations, just as with the ulnar plus/ulnar minor variations at the wrist.

Syndesmosis

The ankle is stabilized by the anterior and posterior tibiofibular ligaments and by the distal continuation of the

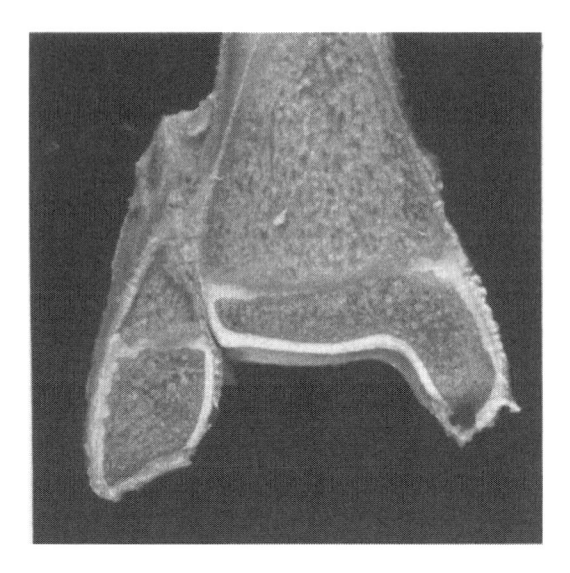

FIGURE 23-12. Slab specimen showing the closing medial and central regions and the still open lateral region.

interosseous membrane.[3] The distal tibia and fibula have an articulation that allows fibular rotation during ankle dorsiflexion-plantar flexion (Fig. 23-15). There is a variable concavity in the distal tibial metaphysis and epiphysis that serves as the distal tibiofibular joint, allowing rotation of the fibula with ankle motion. The synovium extends into this joint to the level of the tibial physis, above which the ligamentous (fibrous) syndesmosis is present.

Ahl and colleagues analyzed tibiofibular relations during the change from ankle plantar flexion to dorsiflexion.[1] They found an average widening of the ankle mortise of 1.0 mm and an average dorsal translation of the fibula of 0.9 mm. Relaxation in the syndesmosis is probably necessary to allow such change. They did not, however, discern any significant rotation of the fibula. These findings were in contradistinction to the concept that the fibula rotates around its longitudinal axis during active moments of the ankle. Ahl and colleagues[1] did not look at the anatomy of the proximal tibiofibular joint, which has significant anatomic variation that may affect the ability (or inability) of the distal fibula to rotate.[6] Stiffening or contracture of the syndesmosis after ankle injury may create chronic pain.

Tibial Spine Injuries

Avulsion of the anterior tibial spine in children is most often caused by bicycle and athletic injuries.[16-31,33-44,46-57,59-65,67-76,78-84] The incidence is 3 per 100,000. Roberts and Lovell stated that the first descriptions of intercondylar eminence fracture were in autopsy reports in 1875 and 1876.[64] In 1907 Pringle found an avulsion fracture at the end of the anterior cruciate ligament at the time of arthrotomy.[61] The injury may be encountered as an accompaniment to more serious injury to the leg. Accordingly, knee films to evaluate its presence are essential when a major fracture (e.g., femoral diaphysis) is present.

Kendall et al. reviewed fractures of the tibial spine in both children and adults and found that there was a higher incidence of associated injuries in adults compared to children, suggesting that the injury resulted from greater force and perhaps a different mechanism.[44] The difference in outcome, with it being worse in adults, was due to other associated intraarticular fractures and tears of the medial collateral ligament.

The mechanism of injury probably is tibial rotation relative to the femur coupled with hyperextension of the knee. The anterior cruciate ligament attaches to the base of the anterior spine and to a slip of the anterior horn of the medial meniscus. The ligament does not attach completely onto the tibial spine; it also attaches anterior and lateral to it.[32,38] This attachment may be stressed by a force that would probably lead to an isolated tear of the anterior cruciate ligament in a skeletally mature individual.[32,38,45,58] However, in most children, the incompletely ossified tibial spine, compared with the ligament and its dense chondral (perichondrial) attachments, is the weakest point to excessive tensile or rotational stress, so failure usually occurs through the cancellous bone underneath the subchondral plate.[32] This failure may lead to hemorrhage and edema within the trabecular bone (i.e., bone bruising).

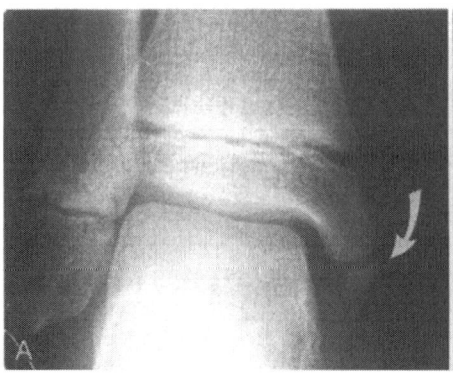

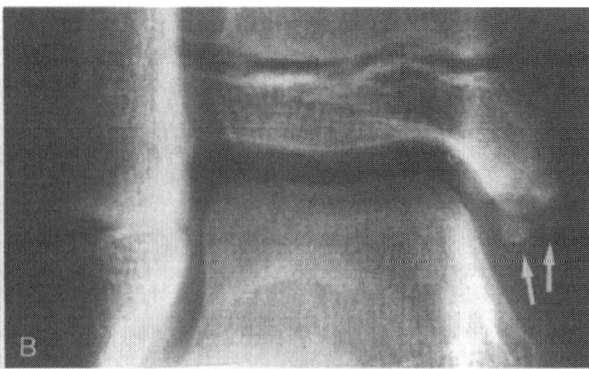

FIGURE 23-13. (A) Accessory ossification (arrow) at the medial malleolar tip. (B) Variation showing multifocal ossification (arrows).

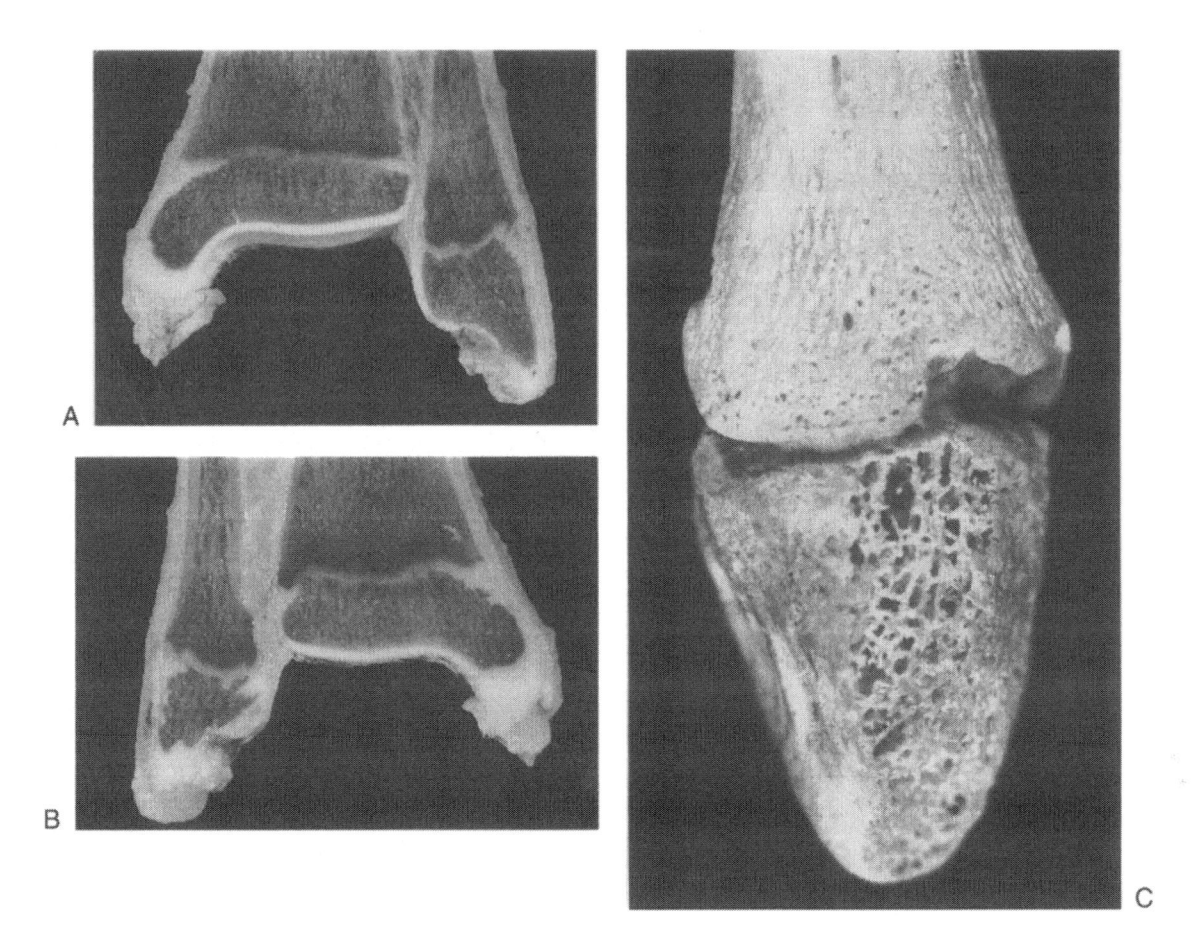

FIGURE 23-14. (A) Undulated contour of the distal fibular physis contrasted with the transverse contour of the distal tibia. (B) Irregular contour of the distal fibula. The distal tibia is also undulated and shows the characteristic medial "rise." (C) Macerated specimen showing typical "notch" of the distal fibular metaphysis. It should not be diagnosed as an injury.

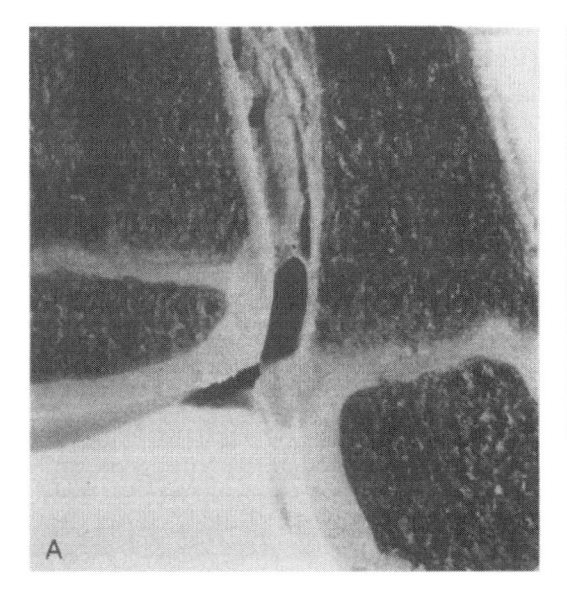

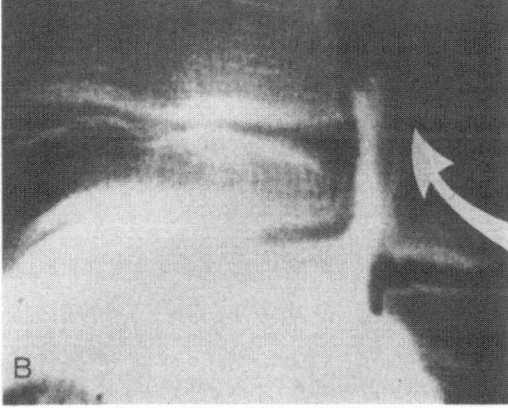

FIGURE 23-15. (A) Extension of the synovial recess between the tibia and fibula. The syndesmosis stops approximately at the level of the tibial physis. The lateral side of the tibia forms an articular surface juxtaposed to the fibula. (B) Arthrogram showing this extension toward the proximal tibiofibular joint (arrow).

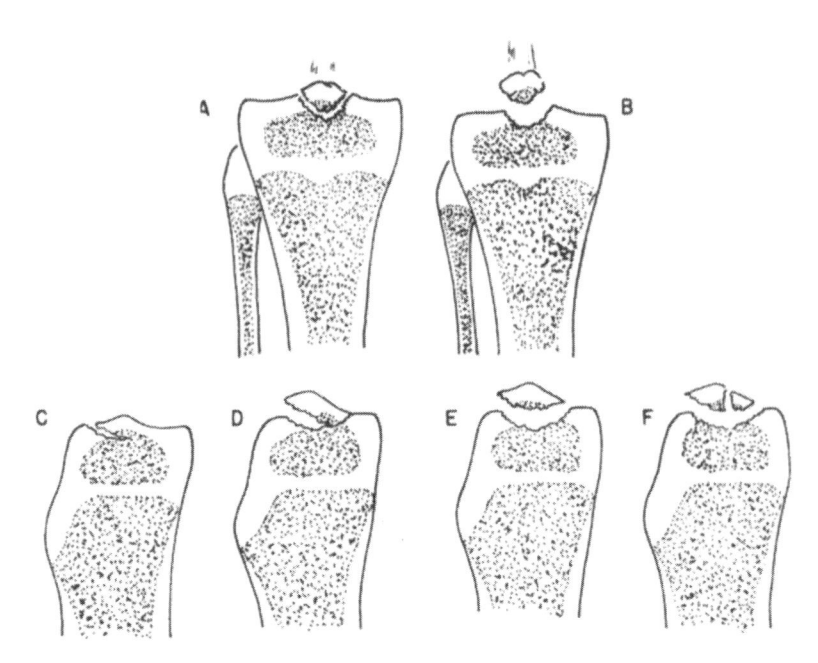

FIGURE 23-16. Classification of the types of injury to the tibial spines. These are type 7 growth mechanism injuries (see Chapter 6). (A, B) Anterior views showing undisplaced and displaced patterns. (C) Incomplete injury that is still intact posteriorly. (D) Complete fracture, hinged posteriorly but still undisplaced. (E) Displaced fragment. (F) Comminuted fragment.

Classification

Meyers and McKeever presented a classification scheme that related to the recommended treatment modalities (Fig. 23-16).[54] Type 1 is minimal displacement of the fragment from the remainder of the proximal tibial ossification center. Type 2 is a displacement (angular elevation) of the anterior one-third to one-half of the avulsed fragment to produce a beak-like appearance on the lateral roentgenogram. Type 3 is a complete separation of the avulsed segment from the remainder of the ossification center without bone-to-bone apposition. Zaricznyj further classified type 3 into A and B categories, with 3A having the fragment aligned relatively normally, albeit displaced, and 3B having the fragment angulated.[83] An additional pattern of the type lesion was a comminuted fracture. All of these types represent variations of a type 7 growth mechanism injury (see Chapter 6).

The anterior portion of the avulsed segment may angulate upward to the intercondylar notch. Displacement may be sufficient to cause the fragments to be above, rather than below, the anterior horn of either meniscus (Fig. 23-17). Such displacement is not readily evident on routine roentgengrams. Magnetic resonance imaging (MRI) may further delineate the altered anatomy.

Anatomic Variation

Robinson and Driscoll reported a case of simultaneous osteochondral avulsions of *both* femoral and tibial insertions of the anterior cruciate ligament.[65] This injury was accompanied by a tear in the medial collateral ligament. Both of the osteochondral fractures and the medial collateral ligament were repaired. Ross and Chesterman reported isolated avulsion of the posterior cruciate portion of the tibial spine; open reduction was necessary.[67]

Jones and Smith pointed out that not all fractures of the tibial spine are the result of cruciate ligament avulsion, as initially proposed by Pringle.[43,61] Kennedy and coworkers found only two cases of bone avulsion in 50 patients with specific anterior cruciate ligament injury.[45] Tears within the substance of the cruciate ligament may occur without tibial spine chondro-osseous injury (see Chapter 22).

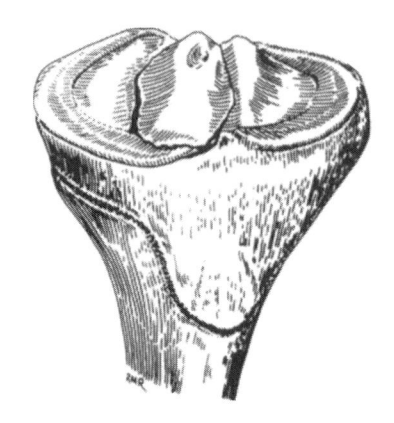

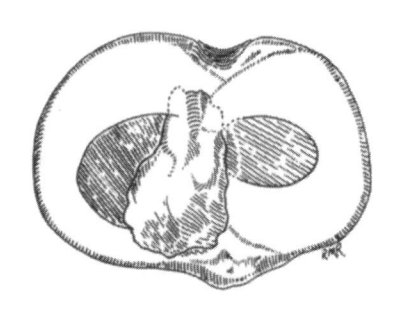

FIGURE 23-17. Mechanism by which the fragment may be displaced into the joint and above the anterior horn of the medial meniscus.

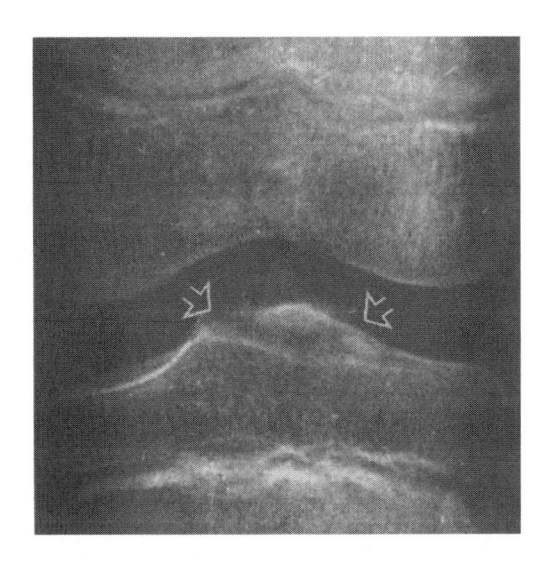

FIGURE 23-18. Undisplaced tibial spine fracture (arrows) in a 12-year-old child.

Diagnosis

Garcia and Neer reported a series of 42 tibial spine fractures in patients ranging in age from 7 to 60 years.[30] Only six patients had a positive drawer sign, and *all* had concomitant collateral ligament tears. A positive anterior drawer sign in the presence of avulsion of the tibial spine indicates the possibility of an associated tear of the collateral ligament. Varus-valgus stress films should be obtained to rule out concomitant collateral ligament injury (see Chapter 22).

It is essential to obtain anteroposterior and lateral roentgenograms to visualize the degree of displacement of the fragment adequately (Figs. 23-18, 23-19). A displaced osteochondral fragment may simulate spine avulsion (Fig. 23-20). Similarly, tuberosity ossification may mimic spine avulsion. Posterior cruciate ligament avulsion may also mimic anterior tibial spine injury in the anteroposterior view (Fig. 23-21).

Furthermore, an anteroposterior view paralleling the normal posterior tilt of the proximal tibial articular surface may help visualize minimally displaced fractures. Because these injuries are intraarticular, there may be a significant hemarthrosis.

Computed tomographic (CT) scanning may allow better appreciation of the displacement of the fragments into the intercondylar notch. MRI (Fig. 23-22) may show the extent of hemorrhage in the ossification center (i.e., more extensive damage or bone bruising), any associated ligamentous damage, any proximal damage at the femur, and the position of the fragment relative to the menisci (i.e., has it been displaced above the meniscus, is the meniscus also damaged).

Treatment

Bakalim and Wilppula used closed reduction by hyperextension in 10 cases, reporting fair to good results in seven of eight patients with adequate follow-up.[17] None of their children had any evidence of functional shortening of the anterior cruciate ligament, although some complained of anteroposterior stability. Smillie believed that closed reduction with hyperextension could be accomplished only if the fragment was large enough in width to be compressed by the condyles and fat pad.[73]

Because the intercondylar space is wide, there may be little direct opposition of the surfaces of the femoral condyles against the tibial fragment to provide sufficient compression. However, the large infrapatellar fat pad (Fig. 23-5) may act as a space-occupying, elastic cushion pushing against the fragment in hyperextension. Meyers and McKeever recommended cast immobilization with the knee in 20° of flexion, without manipulation, for all type 1 and type 2 fractures.[55] They thought that hyperextension did not improve the roentgenographic appearance in any of their patients, and that it worsened the situation in some (e.g., by converting a type 2 fracture to a type 3 fracture).

Most type 1 and type 2 fractures of the intercondylar region of the proximal tibia in children or adolescents do not require arthrotomy and open reduction. Excellent results, with no residual stability, may be anticipated from protective immobilization in extension or mild flexion (no more than 20°). Follow-up roentgenograms are obtained within 7–10

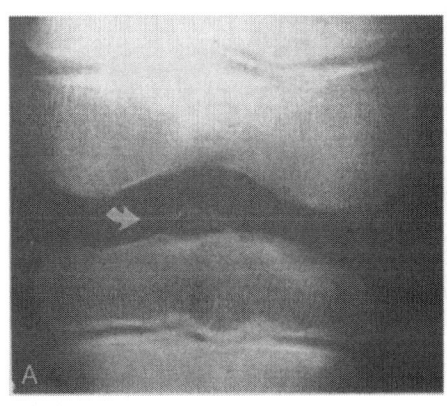

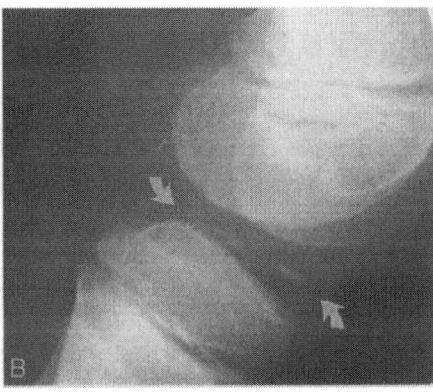

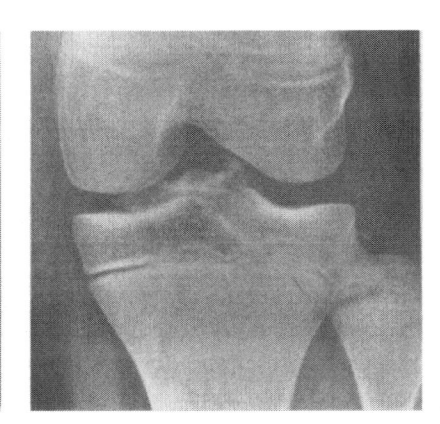

FIGURE 23-19. (A, B) Avulsion of a large fragment (arrows), best evident in the lateral view (B). (C) Large fragment extending to the medial plateau.

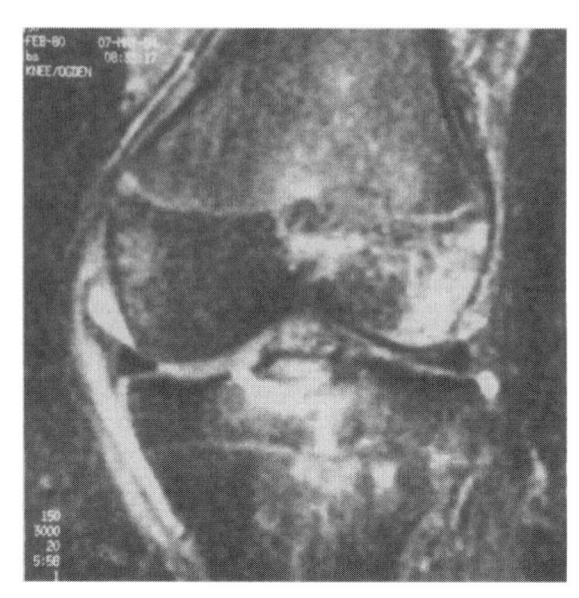

FIGURE 23-20. Apparent tibial spine fracture (top arrow) was a displaced osteochondral fragment from the patella (bottom arrow).

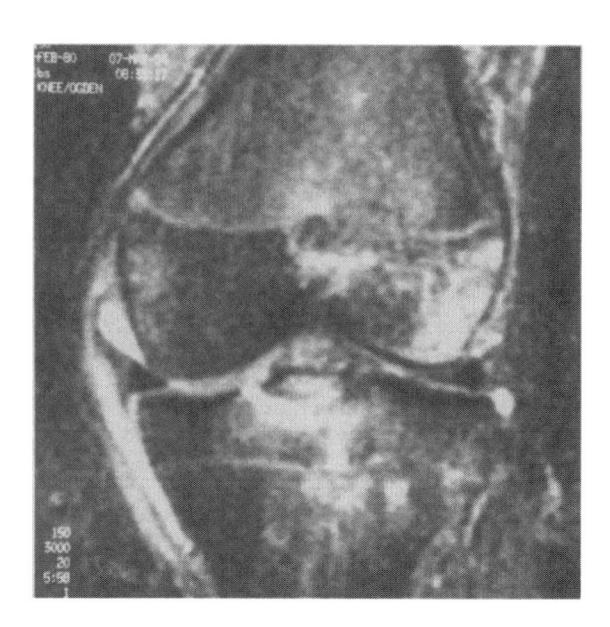

FIGURE 23-22. MRI scan of a patient with a tibial spine fracture. Note the edema in a much larger area below the tibial spine. There is also bone bruising in the medial femoral condyle and around the femoral attachment of the anterior cruciate ligament.

days to be certain the fragment is not still displaced, and the cast is maintained for 6–8 weeks. The foot is included in the cast to discourage walking and rotatory stresses that might displace the fragment.

Type 3 injuries treated by closed reduction have a high incidence of poor results, characterized by locking, chronic effusion, loss of normal range of motion, moderate pain, and complaints of intermittent collapse with strenuous activity (Fig. 23-23). Delayed union and radiographic nonunion may occur. When the fragment is completely separated from the underlying epiphyseal ossification center, arthrotomy or arthroscopy, reduction, and internal fixation are recom-

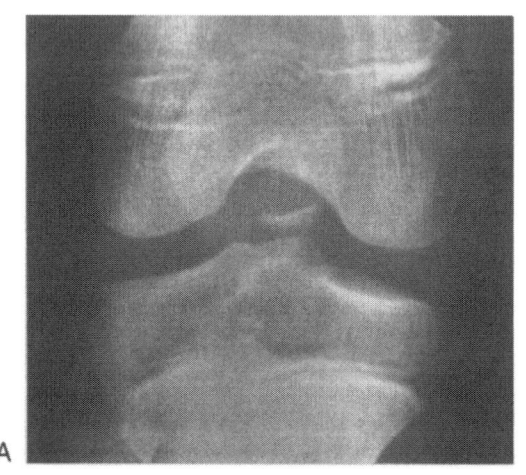

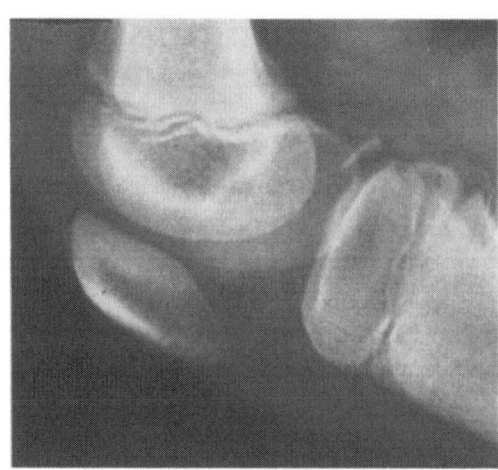

FIGURE 23-21. (A) Apparent tibial spine fracture in the anteroposterior view. (B) In the lateral view, however, it is evident that it was an avulsion of the posterior, not the anterior, cruciate ligament.

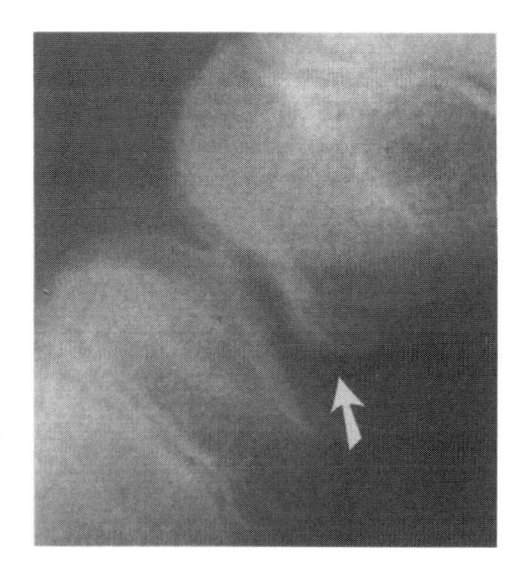

FIGURE 23-23. Overgrowth of fragment (arrow) in a patient treated initially by closed reduction. The patient was asymptomatic but had moderate anterior drawer instability.

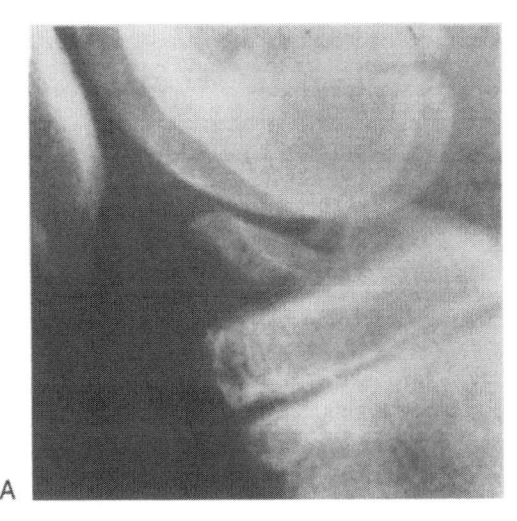

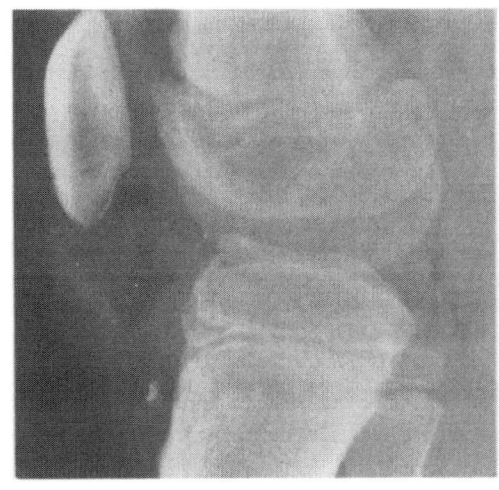

FIGURE 23-24. (A) Displaced, angulated tibial spine fracture. (B) Postoperative radiograph following arthroscopic assisted reduction under the meniscus and suture fixation.

mended (Fig. 23-24, 23-25). The best reduction, even with the knee open, was evident at 20° of flexion. The fragment is put back in anatomic position and retained by sutures that may be placed within the anterior cruciate ligament, the edges of the fragment, and the edge of the anterior horn of the medial meniscus. Metallic internal fixation may not be necessary. Removing the fragment or the anterior cruciate ligament is not indicated. Portions of the anterior horn of the medial or lateral meniscus may block reduction, but they may be retracted sufficiently to accomplish reduction of the spine to its normal anatomic position. Pin fixation may be introduced retrogradely through the anterior epiphysis, thereby avoiding the patellar tendon.

Arthroscopic surgery is playing a more important role in the treatment of fractures of the intracondylar eminence. A group of 35 patients was treated and followed for 2–7 years. There were 20 type 3A fractures and 15 type 3B fractures.[50,51] The avulsed fragment was reduced by operative arthroscopy and maintained by extension and immobilization in a cast or by percutaneous pin fixation. Involvement of the median cruciate ligament or lateral meniscus was confirmed by valgus stress radiography or arthroscopy. At follow-up, few patients suffered ligamentous laxity, lack of extension, or atrophy of the quadriceps. Pain or effusion and symptoms were minimal. Patients requiring surgical repairs of collateral ligaments for peripheral detachments of the meniscus generally required a longer period of rehabilitation. Altogether 14 patients required repair of the lateral meniscus, and 10 patients required repair of medial collateral ligaments. Seven of these patients required repair of both ligaments and meniscus. The fixation pins were directed in an inferior to superior direction from the tibial medial and lateral metaphysis. Alternatively, a cannulated screw (e.g., Herbert screw) may be used.

Chandler and Miller emphasized the importance of arthroscopy for evaluating meniscal entrapment.[24] They

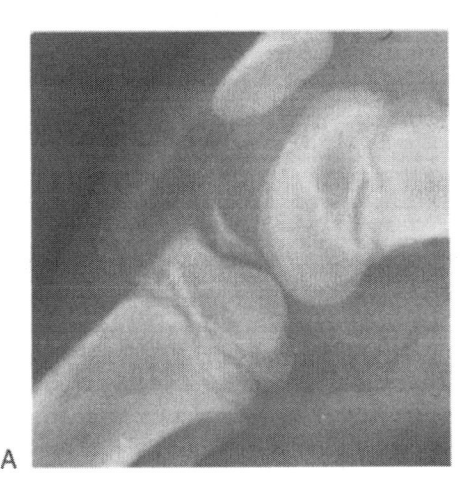

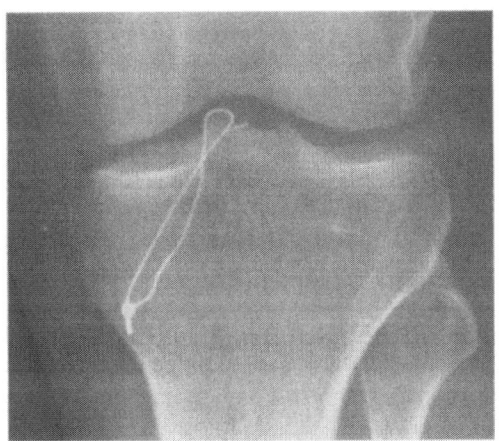

FIGURE 23-25. (A) Displaced tibial spine fracture. It was treated with arthrotomy and wiring of the fragment. (B) Appearance 9 years later. The patient participates actively and asymptomatically in intercollegiate tennis.

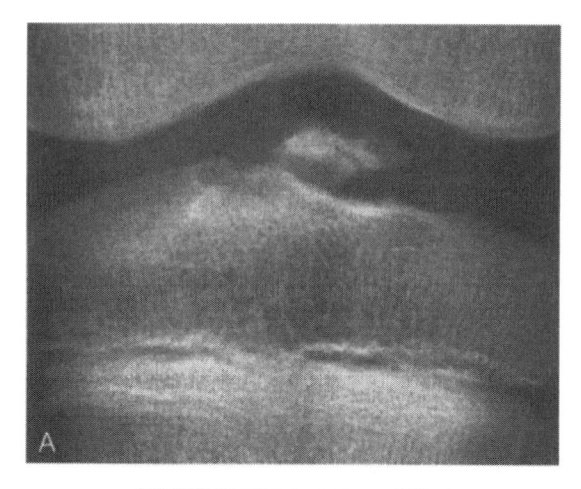

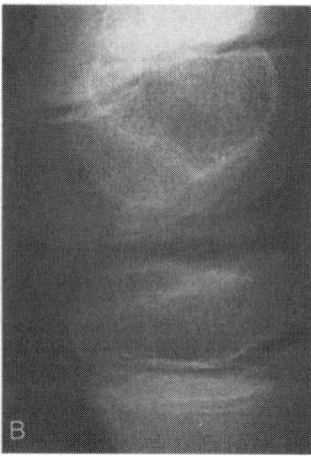

FIGURE 23-26. Overgrowth of a tibial spine fragment 7 months after the initial injury. Exploration of the knee revealed that the fragment had healed solidly through fibrous interposition, even though the roentgenogram suggested nonunion. (A) Anteroposterior view. (B) Lateral view.

noted that apparent "closed reduction" of the fragment could still be associated with incomplete reduction due to meniscal interposition.

Late Presentation

Some patients present for treatment weeks to months after the original injury (Fig. 23-26). These patients have a high likelihood of developing chronic knee instability if left untreated. Evaluation of the extent of morphologic deformity by MRI is appropriate. Arthroscopy is then undertaken. Screw fixation to stabilize the fragment, without "taking down" the fracture line, may be sufficient. Such a technique is also used for nonunion or late presentation of lateral condyle fractures (see Chapter 14). Meniscal injury or displacement should be corrected.

Results

If the type 3 fragment is not reduced and stabilized, chronic complaints may be expected owing to the presence of the intracapsular fragment with, at most, a fibrous nonunion, accompanied by knee instability. However, the physician must be wary of the radiographic appearance (Fig. 23-26). Apparent nonunion may not be true nonunion; in fact, there may be a relatively stable fibrous union. Arthrography or arthroscopy should help delineate any need for more operative procedures. Furthermore, because the anterior cruciate ligament contains blood vessels, the avulsed fragment may receive sufficient nourishment to "enlarge" considerably. Such an enlarged fragment may impair normal joint mechanics.

Lombardo described a patient who had a type II tibial spine injury treated with an extension cast.[49] Lateral radiographs 16 and 36 months after injury showed persistent radiolucency. The patient, however, was asymptomatic and athletically active. Shortly thereafter he was surfing (body board) when he felt a "pop." Radiology revealed a displaced tibial spine fracture that was reduced and attached by sutures through an arthrotomy.

Wiley and Baxter, using computed instrumental testing, found measurable degrees of residual cruciate laxity despite the absence of symptoms.[81] They were able to document, in this pediatric age group, a permanent disturbance in cruciate ligament stability, albeit functionally minor. They also found that open reduction did not always eliminate this persistent extension lag. Baxter and Wiley studied 45 patients 3–10 years after injury.[18] They gave further evidence of residual instability. Willis et al. found that most children who have sustained a tibial eminence fracture have objective evidence of anterior cruciate ligament laxity, but relatively few have subjective complaints.[82] They found that 64% of their patients examined at an average follow-up of 4 years had clinical signs of anterior cruciate ligament instability and that objective evaluation showed as much as 74% instability. Their assessment of long-term stability showed that the method of management (open versus closed methods) had no effect on eventual outcome, similar to findings in adults with anterior cruciate ligament repairs.[66,77]

McLennan reviewed 10 patients with a minimum of 6 years of follow-up who underwent "second-look" arthroscopy following the onset of new injuries or complaints.[51] Loss of reduction led to laxity, prolonged morbidity, and incongruence with the femoral condyle in both extension and flexion. There were mean peak torque deficits in the quadriceps mechanisms as measured isokinetically. Long-term morbidity was characterized by extension loss, chondromalacia, quadriceps weakness, and ligamentous instability. There was loss of reduction after closed reduction, and tibial spine fractures often were *not* adequately reduced by extension and compression from the femoral condyles because of lack of sufficient impingement on the fragment. Displaced fractures of the tibial spines required delayed surgery, appropriate tensioning, internal fixation, and aggressive rehabilitation.

Seriat-Gautier et al. reviewed 31 patients with fractures of the tibial spine with a follow-up ranging from 6 months to 7 years[70]: 10 were treated conservatively and 21 operatively. Sixteen patients had an anterior drawer sign at follow-up. Altogether 23 of these patients had clinically excellent results, 3 good, and 1 poor. Janarv et al. studied 61 children in long-term follow-up (mean 16 years).[41] Subjective knee function (Lysholm score) was excellent or good in 87% and

FIGURE 23-27. (A) Anterior displacement of the proximal tibial epiphysis, with corresponding posterior displacement (arrow) of the metaphysis. (B) Arteriogram showed complete disruption of the popliteal artery (arrow).

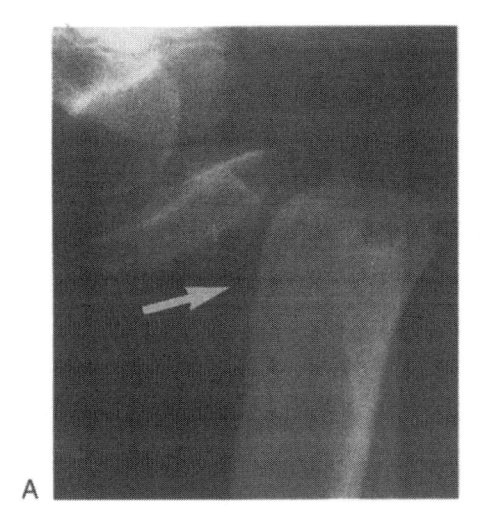

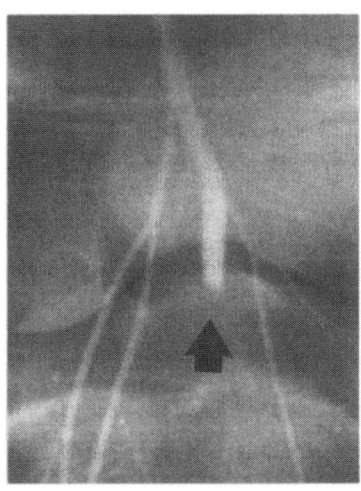

fair in 13%; 11% of the patients had a lower activity level than desired; 38% had pathologic knee laxity, but it was not reflected in subjective knee function.

Proximal Tibial Epiphyseal Injuries

Although other epiphyseal injuries are reasonably common during childhood, injury of the proximal tibial epiphysis is infrequent and probably constitutes less than 1% of all epiphyseal injuries.[85-126] In one series the average age was 14.2 years, with only one patient being younger than 10 years at the time of injury.[120]

One of the major factors controlling susceptibility to injury is the anatomic structure of the proximal tibia and the anterior downward extension of the tibial tuberosity. This arrangement appears reasonably capable of preventing posterior displacement of the epiphysis relative to the metaphysis and diaphysis. A proximal tibial growth mechanism injury usually manifests as varus or valgus displacement of the metaphyseal unit. Pure anterior or posterior displacement are much less frequent.

It is imperative to evaluate adequately the circulatory status in the region of the knee and distal to the knee, as there is a *significant incidence* of injury to the popliteal artery with this particular fracture (Fig. 23-27). The problems of ischemic complications and basic approaches to concomitant vascular injuries are discussed in Chapters 10 and 22.

Classification

All growth mechanism injury patterns may involve the proximal tibia. Type 7 injuries are essentially confined to the tibial spines, but types 1–6 may affect the proximal tibial and tibial tuberosity epiphyses and physes (Figs. 23-28 to 23-32).

Most injuries to this region are type 2 growth mechanism injuries with posterolateral or posteromedial displacement of the metaphyseal portion (Figs. 23-31, 23-32). Most type 2 injuries also exhibit a posterior displacement of the metaphysis, with the proximal-distal fracture relations essentially being in a relative recurvatum. The proximal tibial epiphysis retains its normal relation to the distal femoral physis, and the tibial shaft is displaced posteriorly with concomitant medial or lateral displacement. Because of the anatomy of the tibial tuberosity, it is unusual for a fracture to be associated with anterior displacement of the epiphyseal fragment (Fig. 23-29). The periosteum may herniate into the tension side of the injury when the fracture is reduced, whether spontaneously or by the treating physician. An infrequent type 2 injury may involve the posterior tibia in a hyperflexion injury.[114] Blanks et al.[89] showed that the pattern of closure of the proximal tibial physis was from posterior to anterior. As with other epiphyses the closure pattern affects fracture patterns. Piétu et al. reported two cases of triplane fractures of the upper end of the tibia.[114]

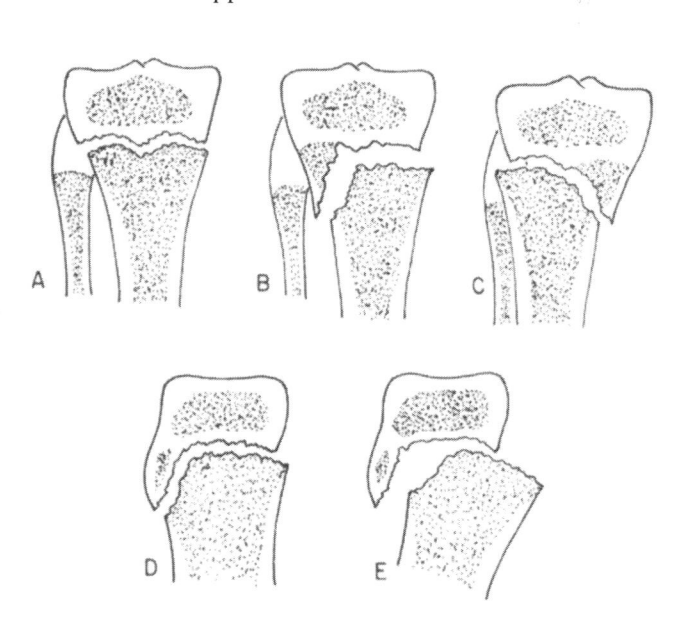

FIGURE 23-28. Type 1 (A) and type 2 (B, C) injuries. (D,E) Anteriorly undisplaced and displaced fractures. The metaphysis is usually displaced posteriorly, with additional varus or valgus angulation.

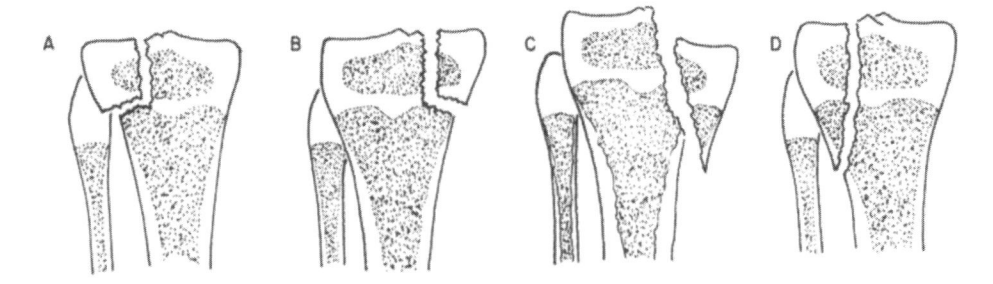

FIGURE 23-29. Type 3 (A, B) and 4 (C, D) proximal tibial injuries.

Type 1 injuries are the next most common (Fig. 23-33) and often difficult to diagnose because of their minimal displacement. Takai et al. described a 14-year-old boy who presented with knee pain, an increasing limp, and a recurvatum deformity.[122] One year earlier he had sustained what he considered to be a minor fall on the knee. Radiology showed anterior growth arrest. Most likely he had sustained an occult type 1 injury.

Because of stresses imparted by flexion contractures, the proximal tibia is consequently involved in type 1 fractures in children with neuromuscular disorders such as myelomeningocele and cerebral palsy, especially when vigorous physical therapy is undertaken to overcome joint contractures (see Chapter 11).

Type 3 injuries are less common (Fig. 23-34). The detached epiphyseal fragment is usually unstable and may be significantly displaced. Type 4 injuries also are uncommon (Fig. 23-35). It is sometimes difficult to diagnose type 4 fractures in young children when they propagate through the unossified portion of the epiphysis (Fig. 23-36). Type 5 injuries may be seen in association with proximal tibial and tibial tuberosity fractures and may be the result of crushing or microvascular disruption in that region.[105,110]

Poulsen et al. described 15 patients with proximal tibial epiphyseal fractures.[115] Five had concomitant avulsion frac-

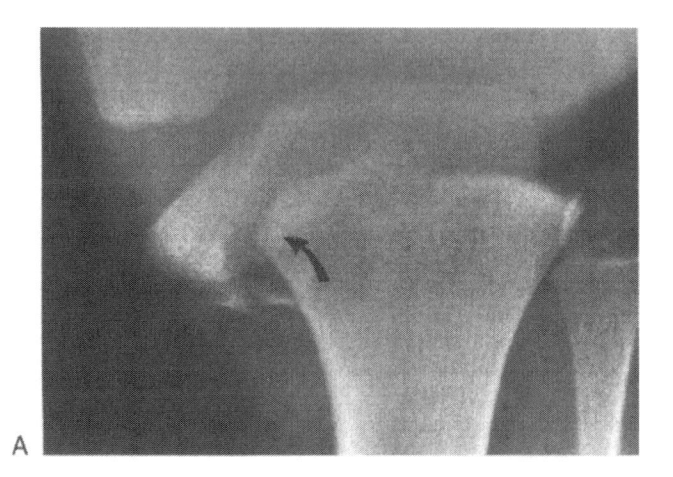

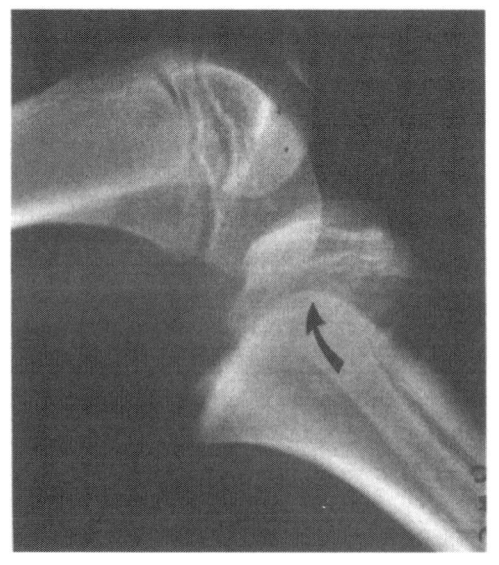

FIGURE 23-30. (A) Medially displaced type 1 injury. (B) Lateral view showing anterior displacement. The arrow indicates the site of increased pressure likely to lead to focal growth arrest.

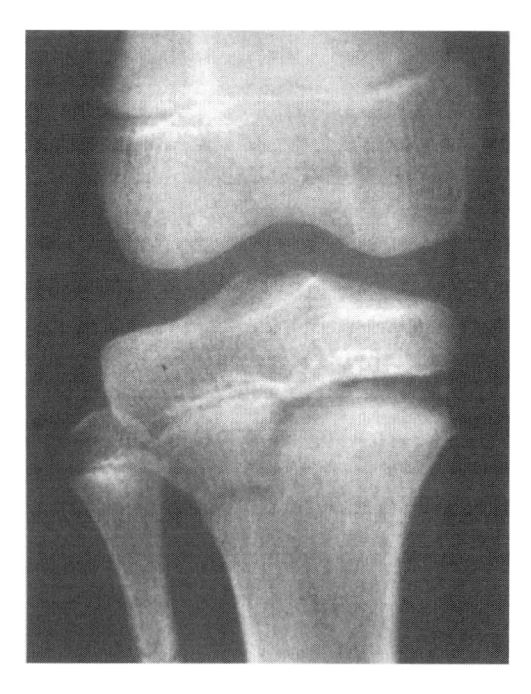

FIGURE 23-31. Lateral type 2 injury.

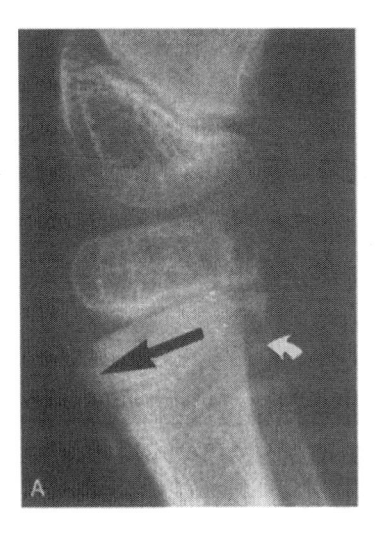

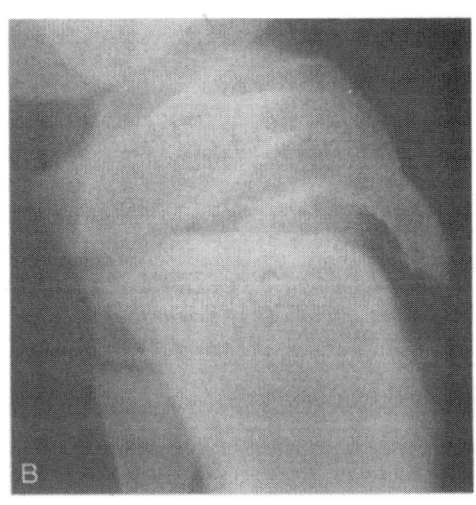

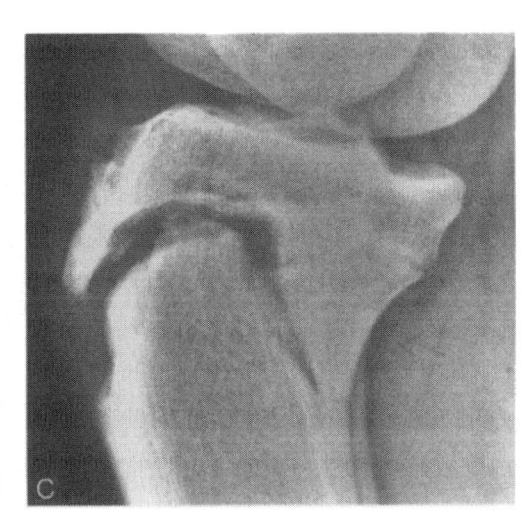

FIGURE 23-32. Unusual patterns of posterior displacement of the entire epiphysis (white arrow), along with anterior displacement of the metaphysis (black arrow). (A) Mild displacement. (B) Hyperflexion displacement with small metaphyseal fragments. (C) Hyperflexion displacement with a large posterior metaphyseal fragment.

tures of the tibial insertion of the anterior cruciate ligament, and eight patients had concomitant collateral ligamentous injuries.

Propagation of the fracture force often leads to a concomitant fracture of the fibular metaphysis or diaphysis. The entire fibula must be radiographed to rule out concomitant injury, even as far as the distal fibula. Physeal injury of the proximal fibula concomitant with tibial physeal injury is rare.

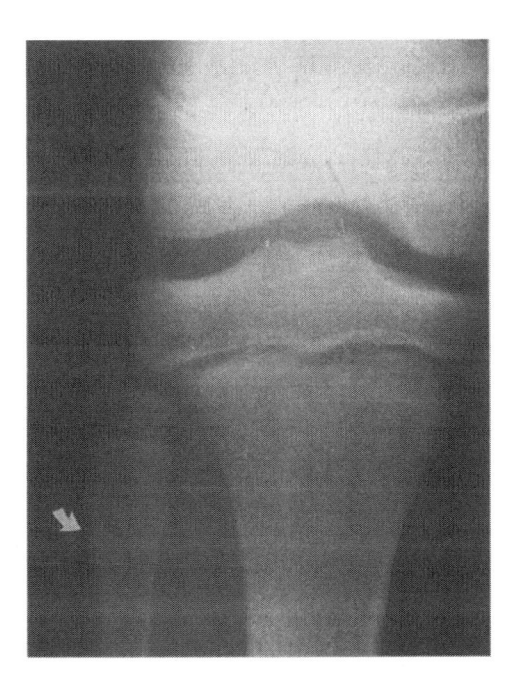

FIGURE 23-33. Type 1 growth mechanism injury of the proximal tibia. Note the fibular metaphyseal fracture (arrow).

Diagnosis

Clinical evaluation is important when diagnosing injuries to the proximal tibial epiphysis. Neurovascular status must be evaluated initially and at appropriate intervals. There is a significant incidence of damage to the popliteal artery. It is imperative that this complication be recognized as early as possible. The presence of major distal pulses should be assessed. Use of Doppler ultrasonography may be beneficial. Because of collateral circulation through the geniculate vessels, capillary filling may seem statically adequate. Such flow, however, may be insufficient for the active, growing child, leading to muscle ischemia (claudication) with normal muscular activity. Damage to the major nerves in the popliteal region is not as frequent as vascular injury. When the proximal fibula is also fractured, the peroneal nerve or one of its branches may be injured.

It is essential that careful clinical observation be used to assess the possibility of compartment syndrome after partial or temporary vascular occlusion. Reperfusion, especially if not accompanied by normal venous outflow, may lead to tissue pressure increases that may affect muscle viability.

With some of these injuries, especially when they occur during adolescence, it may be necessary to perform a roentgenographic stress test to determine if there is a type 1 or type 2 lesion, particularly if there is minimal displacement. In a series of 39 fractures of the proximal tibial epiphyseal cartilage, stress roentgenograms were essential to make the diagnosis in 3 patients.[120] On direct clinical examination, there may be marked instability of the medial side of the knee in an adolescent (particularly in a football player with a history of being tackled or clipped). Roentgenograms should be obtained with the patient in both a relaxed position and under stress to distinguish between opening of the joint (ligament injury or laxity) and opening of a physeal fracture. Alternatively, MRI may delineate "invisible" or obscure fracture propagation.

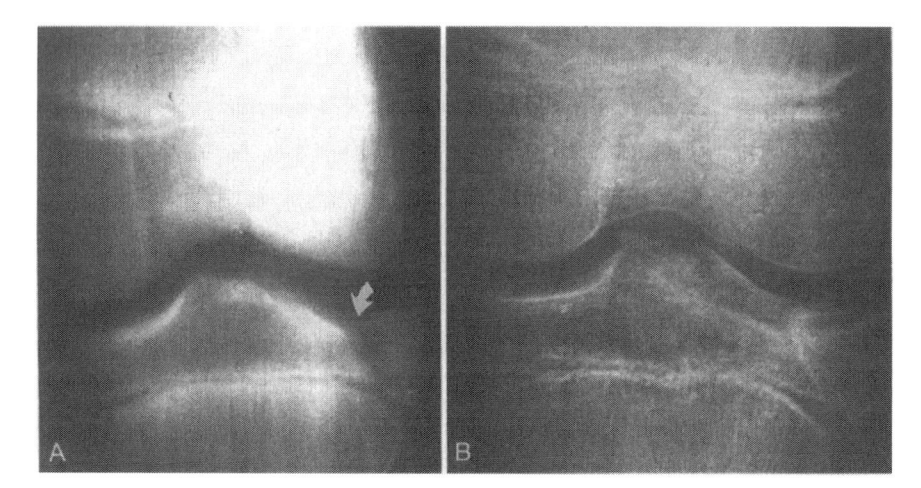

FIGURE 23-34. (A) Type 3 injury (arrow) of the lateral epiphysis. (B) Appearance 6 months after open reduction and transepiphyseal pin fixation.

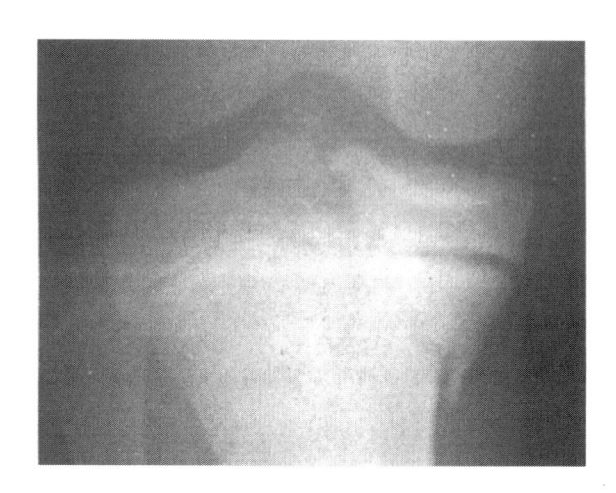

FIGURE 23-35. Type 4 injury extending into the tibial spine in a 14-year-old boy.

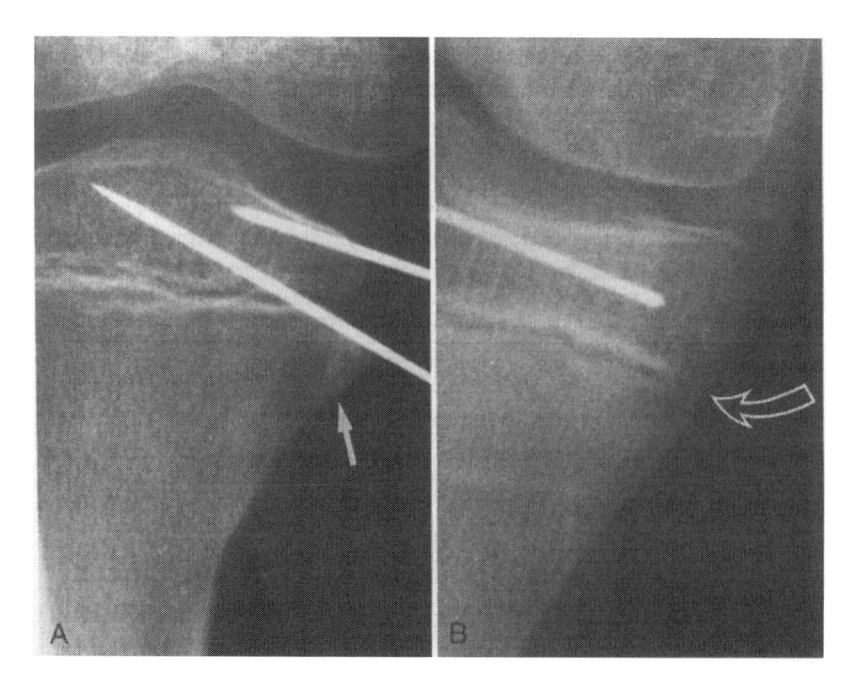

FIGURE 23-36. (A) Fixation of type 4 injury. This growth mechanism pattern was barely evident on the basis of the small metaphyseal fragment (arrow). The epiphyseal extension into the cartilage was not evident roentgenographically. (B) Upper pin migrated into the epiphysis. Pin ends should be bent 90° to prevent such a complication. Unfortunately, a peripheral bone bridge formed (arrow).

Treatment

Closed reduction should be performed initially for all type 1 and type 2 growth mechanism fractures, and the lower limb should be immobilized for a period of 4–6 weeks. It is important to obtain as accurate an anatomic reduction as possible, remembering that the direction of the proximal tibial articular surface is angled slightly downward (posteriorly) relative to the longitudinal axis of the shaft. Trying to align the joint surface epiphysis perpendicular to the shaft may result in a functional recurvatum that may not correct spontaneously with growth, especially if there is a type 5 component. A mild degree of posterior displacement of the metaphysis may be acceptable. An alternative is placing the patient in skeletal traction, with gradual correction of the displacement. Despite reduction, there is a continuing problem of instability of these fractures, even the type 2 injuries, and the difficulty experienced maintaining the initial reduction. If it is not possible to maintain adequate reduction, some type of skeletal fixation performed surgically or percutaneously under fluoroscopy (image intensification) should be attempted (Fig. 23-37). If there is a large metaphyseal fragment, it may be possible to transfix the two portions of the metaphysis to stabilize the fracture, thereby avoiding crossing the physis or epiphysis with pins. The pins are removed as soon as possible after fracture stabilization (not necessarily complete healing). Ciszewski et al. described the inability to accomplish a closed reduction of a proximal tibial physeal fracture due to the interposition of periosteum.[95]

Type 3 growth mechanism injuries require open reduction, precise anatomic placement, and internal fixation with either a compression screw or a transepiphyseal device (Fig. 23-38). Similar operative procedures are indicated for type 4 growth mechanism fractures, even when the fragments are minimally displaced, to minimize risks of premature epiphysiodesis. For a type 4 injury, fixation of both the metaphyseal and epiphyseal fragments may be necessary.

Because of the violent mechanism often causing these fractures, growth impairment may occur. Thus the parents must be warned and advised about physeal damage and the need for long-term follow-up.

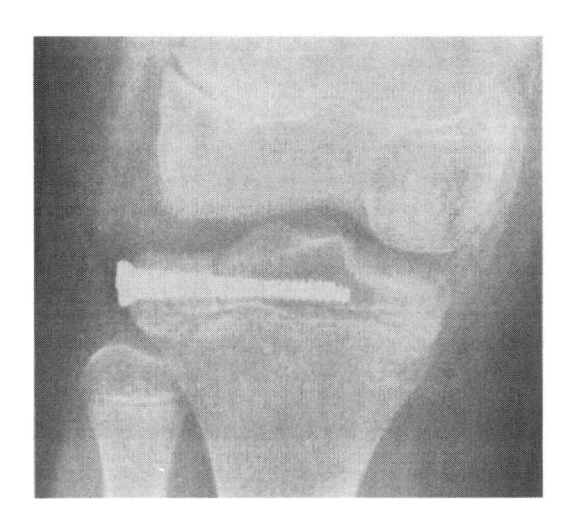

FIGURE 23-38. Transepiphyseal screw fixation of a type 3 injury.

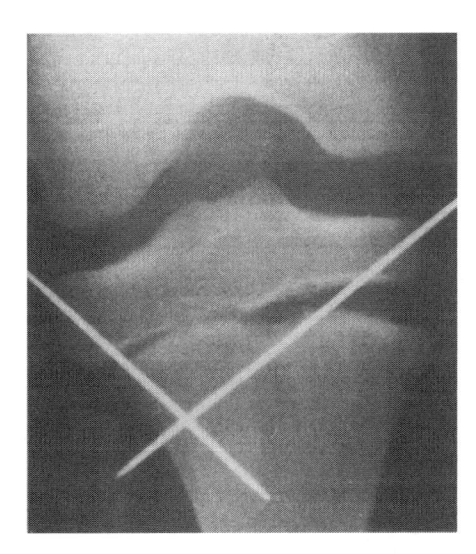

FIGURE 23-37. Fixation of a type 1 injury. The fracture has been incompletely reduced. This should *not* have been accepted, as it left the leg in mild valgus, and spontaneous correction may not occur. Accurate anatomic reduction should be the endpoint of any open procedure.

Results

In general, the results of adequately treating proximal tibial physeal fracture are generally good. Most of these injuries do not involve the joint, so postinjury knee joint mechanics are usually good. However, an increase in varus, valgus, or recurvatum position may alter mechanics and eventually predispose to joint degeneration. Of 28 fractures in 27 patients, with an average follow-up of 7.1 years, results were satisfactory in 23.[120] Unsatisfactory results in the other four patients were due to neurovascular insufficiency, growth disturbance, or traumatic arthritis.

Complications

A significant complication is a localized or complete injury to the proximal physis, which may lead to leg length equality or angular deformity (Fig. 23-39). Because many of these injuries occur during adolescence, at a time when the patient is going through the final phases of growth, major growth deformities are relatively uncommon. However, young children have sufficient growth capacity to manifest significant deformities, especially during their adolescent growth spurt. These children must be followed closely for any evidence of premature growth arrest; the physician (and parents) may be aware of the potential or actual deformity, deficiency of length, and the best methods of correction. These children may eventually require osteotomy, resection of an osseous bridge (Fig. 23-40), or leg length equalization for improvement.

Premature growth arrest with resultant varus, valgus, or curvatum deformity frequently accompanies type 3 and 4

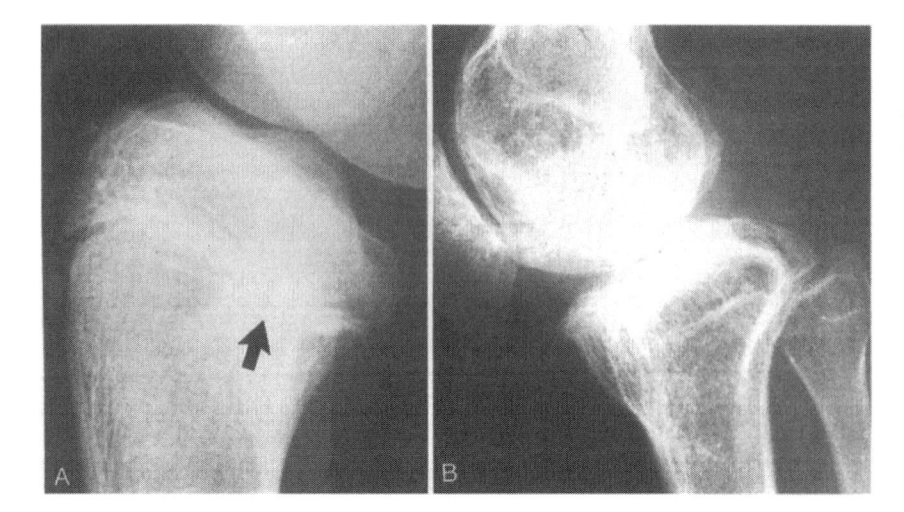

FIGURE 23-39. Growth arrest. (A) Increased posterior angulation due to a posterior osseous bridge (arrow). (B) Genu recurvatum deformity due to anterior displacement and subsequent closure.

growth mechanism injuries (Fig. 23-41) and some type 2 injuries. The parents must be warned about this possibility.

Although Shelton and Canale mentioned only four patients with unsatisfactory results, it is noteworthy that 7 of the 28 patients with these proximal tibial physeal fractures had a longitudinal growth disturbance of 1 cm or more at skeletal maturity, representing a 25% incidence of some degree of growth retardation.[120] Significantly, patients with a growth disturbance had fractures that would be classified as type 1 or type 2 patterns that supposedly, according to the Salter-Harris classification, have the least risk for this complication. It is interesting that no significant longitudinal growth disturbances were associated with type 3 or type 4 fractures. Only one patient had an unsatisfactory angular deformity of more than 7° compared to the uninjured extremity. Although eight patients had angular discrepancies of 5°–7°, angular discrepancies of less than 5° were apparently disregarded. Therefore longitudinal and angular changes consequent to this injury pattern are probably common; but because the injury occurs close to the end of skeletal growth for this physis, major morphologic changes are rare.

Olerud et al. reported genu recurvatum caused by partial growth arrest of the proximal tibial physis following treatment with a cast for correction of an angular deformity in a tibial fracture.[112] The authors resected the bony bridge and did a progressive correction with a lengthening device. They thought that growth arrest of the tibial tuberosity occurred because of excessive pressure over this area when the original cast was wedged.

Other complications are anterior compartment syndrome, peroneal nerve palsy, and associated ligamentous, meniscal, patellar tendon, and joint capsule injuries. All contribute to the biomechanics of fracture of this particular epiphysis, and all must be treated as indicated, as any of them can significantly affect the long-term result.

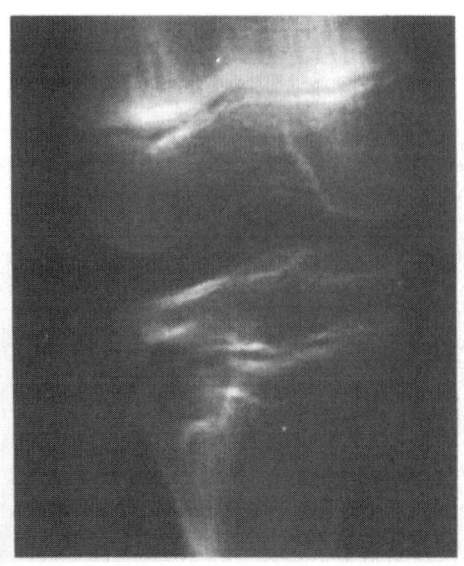

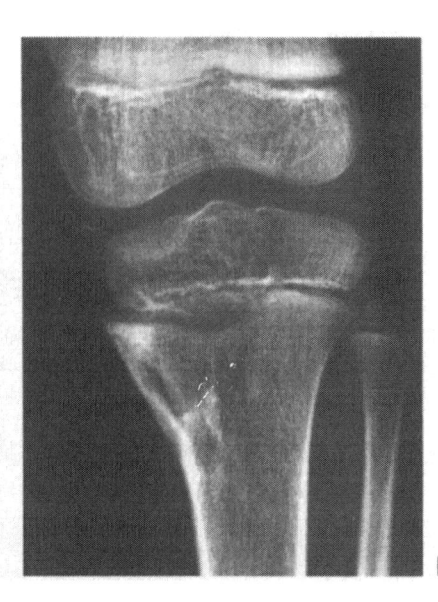

FIGURE 23-40. (A) Growth arrest of the medial physis treated by resection of the bridge and fat interposition. (B) Appearance 1 year later.

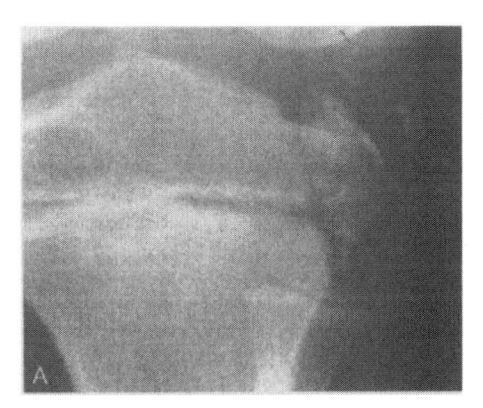

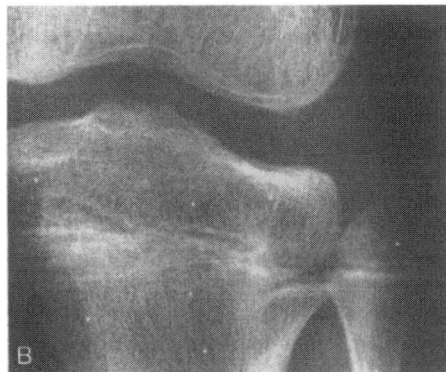

FIGURE 23-41. (A) Type 4 injury treated by closed reduction. (B) Growth arrest several months later.

Vascular Complications

The most important complication to recognize during the initial or subsequent evaluations is vascular injury.[120] Curry and Bishop reported a case in which the proximal tibial epiphysis was anteriorly displaced, the vascular injury was not recognized, and gangrene subsequently developed.[96]

Because of the posterior displacement of the distal fragment, there may be impingement, occlusion, intraluminal damage or transection of the popliteal artery. The distal fragment is closely attached to the posterior distal femur and proximal tibia, which renders limited, flexibility during displacement. Furthermore, the distal fragment may directly impinge on the vessel, leading to any of the various types of vascular injury discussed in Chapter 10. Most reported cases of proximal tibial injuries associated with vascular damage have been hyperextension injuries. Careful evaluation must be undertaken at frequent intervals to assess the possibility of vascular damage evolving as an acute or a more insidious chronic problem.

Wozasek et al. described 30 patients with proximal tibial epiphyseal fractures.[126] Three patients had peripheral ischemia and another developed delayed thrombosis of the popliteal artery. One of the patients had to undergo above-knee amputation because of the delayed diagnosis of the vascular lesion. The authors pointed out the problems of ligaments that essentially tether the popliteal artery to the back of the knee, distal femoral epiphysis, and proximal tibial epiphysis.

Arteriography is an excellent means for evaluating these injuries (Fig. 23-27B). If damage is found, appropriate repair must be undertaken reasonably rapidly. At the same time, the fracture should be stabilized by some type of skeletal fixation so the vascular repair is minimally jeopardized. Bovill reported the use of arteriography to evaluate damage to the popliteal vessels with this injury.[91] The initial films showed complete lack of filling of the normal vascular beds of the metaphyseal part of the fracture fragment and the epiphyseal plate. This vascular field defect was *still present* in an arteriogram obtained 3 months after the injury that demonstrated an increased blood supply to the vascular beds about the knee in both the distal femur and the proximal tibia but *not* in the metaphyseal fragment. The normal vascular bed was not altered in the small portion of the physis to which a triangular fragment of the metaphysis had remained attached. A subsequent arteriogram obtained *3 years after injury* showed persistent complete occlusion of the popliteal artery, with filling by collateralization. An end-to-end anastomosis of both the artery and the vein had been done at the time of injury. The pulse had decreased during the postoperative course over several weeks and became nonpalpable by 6 weeks. No attempt was made to reexplore because of the perceived amount of collateral circulation. In view of the current state of microvascular repair, reexploration probably should be undertaken to create a functioning artery, particularly in a young child. Although Bovill did not describe any vascular insufficiency 3 years after injury, the child was only 10 years old and had not gone through her growth spurt.[91] With the anticipated increased functional demands of adolescence, there might be a problem (such as ischemia associated with activity but not with rest), as in people with progressive adult-onset vascular occlusion and claudication. Claudication per se is not usually a phenomenon seen in children.

Tibial Tuberosity Injuries

Avulsion fractures of the tibial tuberosity commonly occur in boys between the ages of 14 and 16 years.* The injury has been infrequently described in girls but should be expected in the 13- to 15-year range of girls engaged in competitive sports. The distal ligamentous expansion (insertion of the quadriceps mechanism) spreads out as it approximates the anterior tibial surface. The apophysis of the tuberosity is located underneath this tendinous expansion. Because of the diffuse insertion of the quadriceps mechanism and its confluence with the more distal soft tissues (periosteum and pes anserinus), the tibial tuberosity is avulsed. Partial avulsion (chondro-osseous separation) is more common and represents the underlying failure mechanism in most cases of the Osgood-Schlatter lesion, particularly when it is of a more chronic nature (see later in the chapter).

Tibial tuberosity avulsions are also common in domestic animals.[129,138,140,144,146,155,156,169,171,179] Accordingly, they represent an unusual opportunity to study the natural history of this unique skeletal region. Such comparable, naturally

---

*Refs. 127,128,130–137,139,141–143,145,147–154,157–168,170,172–178.

occurring fractures of the immature skeleton are not frequent.

Wiss et al. described 15 patients, all with type 3 injuries.[178] Six patients had antecedent Osgood-Schlatter lesions. Two patients had type 1 osteogenesis imperfecta with this fracture pattern. Associated injuries to the meniscus were found and repaired in three patients. Two patients also had avulsion of the origin of the tibialis anterior muscle, leading to compartment syndrome in one. One patient had a nonunion, one patient had a refracture, and five patients developed bursitis over prominent screwheads, which were removed. All but two patients were eventually asymptomatic and participated in sports. There were no angular or recurvatum deformities. Four patients had a leg length discrepancy ranging from 1.0 to 1.8 cm, with two patients showing overgrowth and two showing undergrowth.

Nimityongskul et al. reviewed eight patients.[165] Six had an Osgood-Schlatter lesion. Seven underwent open reduction with internal fixation, one had closed reduction. The one patient who required a lateral meniscectomy was the only one who did not have a good recovery. One patient developed an anterior compartment syndrome, and immediate fasciotomy relieved the problem. One patient who developed a painful nonunion at the distal fracture site was relieved by excision of the distal fragment.

Classification

Tuberosity injuries were classified by Watson-Jones into three types.[172] This classification scheme did not describe propagation into the knee joint, failed to discuss the problems of such intraarticular extension, made no mention of the possibility of fragmentation (comminution) of the avulsed regions, and did not emphasize the separation of any of the avulsed portions. Accordingly, the following types and subtypes of injury have been proposed (Fig. 23-42).[166] Avulsion of the entire tuberosity-proximal tibia epiphysis may occur in the adolescent and could be considered a type 4 injury (Fig. 23-32).

In type 1 only the distal portion of the tuberosity is injured (Fig. 23-43). The simplest injury pattern (1A) is a fracture

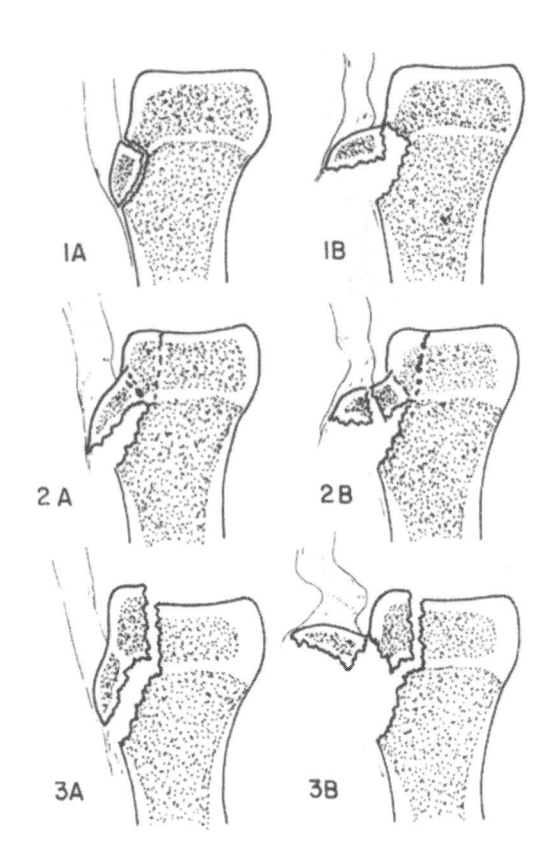

FIGURE 23-42. Patterns of tibial tuberosity fracture. See text for details.

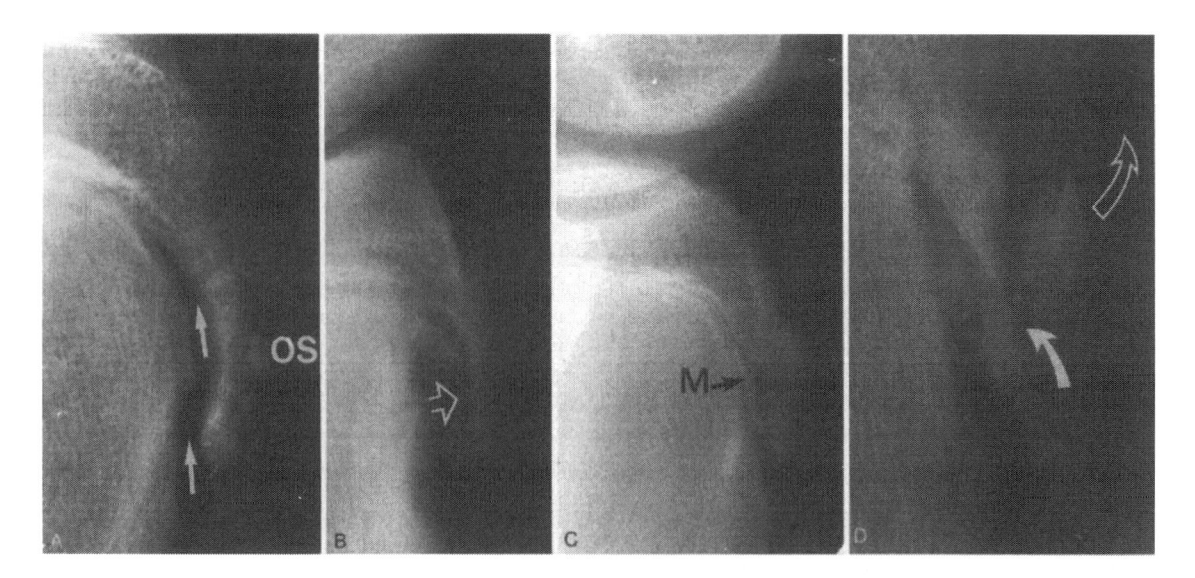

FIGURE 23-43. Type 1 injury pattern. (A) Avulsion of the entire tuberosity up to part of the proximal tibial physis (arrows). Small Osgood-Schlatter ossicle (OS) is present. (B) Displaced fracture of the entire tuberosity, with separation from the proximal tibia (arrow). (C) Variation of pattern, with fracture through the metaphysis, leaving the metaphyseal subchondral plate (M) attached. (D) Tibial tuberosity fracture of anterior portions of the ossification center (open arrow), an acute analogue of Osgood-Schlatter disease. The fracture may extend posteriorly through the ossification center (solid arrow).

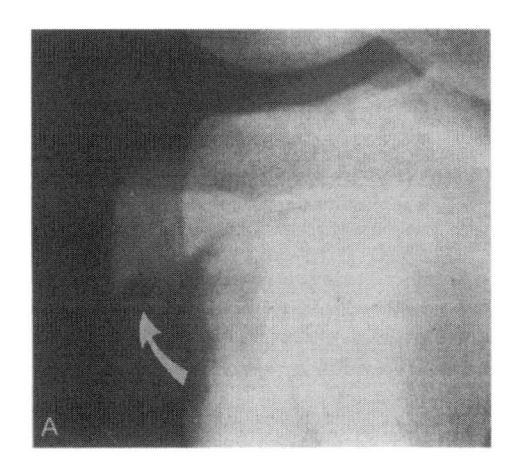

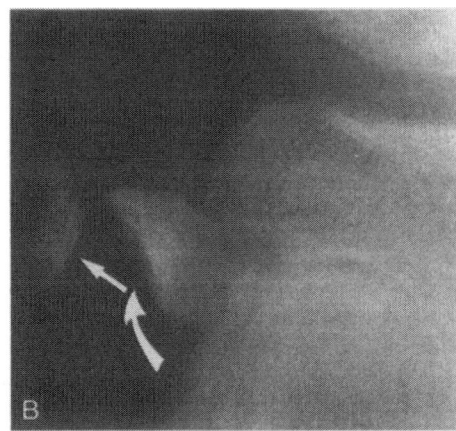

FIGURE 23-44. Type 2 injury pattern. (A) Avulsion and displacement (arrow) of the tuberosity. (B) Fragmentation (arrows).

through the tuberosity ossification center with mild anterior displacement of the fragment. On the basis of operative observations, it is likely that the soft tissue components are incompletely separated, so this injury, anatomically, is relatively stable. In the other subtype (lB) the fragment is separated from the metaphysis and may or may not also be separated from the rest of the secondary ossification center. Concomitant soft tissue injury and disruption of continuity are more likely. This type of injury occasionally requires open reduction.

A type 2 injury involves the cartilaginous junction between two secondary ossification centers and usually leads to avulsion of the distal (tuberosity) center (Fig. 23-44). This injury is probably the failure mode of adolescence that is analogous to Osgood-Schlatter lesion in the younger age group. The only difference is the extent of chondro-osseous involvement. Type 2 injuries have separation of the *entire* tuberosity ossification center, with variable propagation into the main proximal tibial ossification center. The tuberosity segment may fracture (usually a compression-impaction type of injury) at the juncture of the main tibial and tuberosity ossification centers, or it may propagate through a variably sized anterior portion of the proximal tibial ossification center; there is minimal separation of the two portions of the proximal tibia. Soft tissue disruption is contingent on the maximal degree of separation, which may not always be evident on the roentgenogram obtained in the emergency room when the knee is extended. Type 2 injuries usually require anatomic reduction by open methods.

With type 3 injuries there may be significant separation of the fragments and propagation into the knee joint, which leads to disruption of the articular surface under the anterior attachments of the medial or lateral menisci or the tibial spines (Fig. 23-45). However, the fracture may propagate into the anterior fat pad instead, so there is minimal involvement of the actual articular surface. The displaced fragment may be unitary (3A) or comminuted (3B). Open reduction is usually necessary to restore joint surface contiguity. With type 3A, some of the soft tissue extensions onto the metaphysis may be intact, especially in the region of the pes anserinus.

Fragmentation and angulation in types 2 and 3 occur in or near the region of cartilage that intervenes between the two ossification centers. The comminution evident in types 2B and 3B is significant in that the anatomically more distal fragment often becomes more proximally displaced and leads to proximal (upward) displacement of the patella (i.e., traumatic patella alta). Such proximal patellar displacement may also occur, albeit to a lesser degree, with types lB, 2A, and 3A. Because idiopathic patella alta may be associated with subluxation and chondromalacia, restoration of the preinjury anatomy is indicated to avoid these potential complications.

Concomitant Disorders

Osgood-Schlatter lesions have been described in the contralateral knee[130] and the ipsilateral knee.[147,157,165,166,178] The author's series reported ipsilateral involvement in two patients (asymptomatic prior to injury) and contralateral involvement in six patients (Fig. 23-46), all of whom had experienced symptoms 2–26 months prior to injury but had never had similar symptoms in the knee with the acute tuberosity fracture.[166]

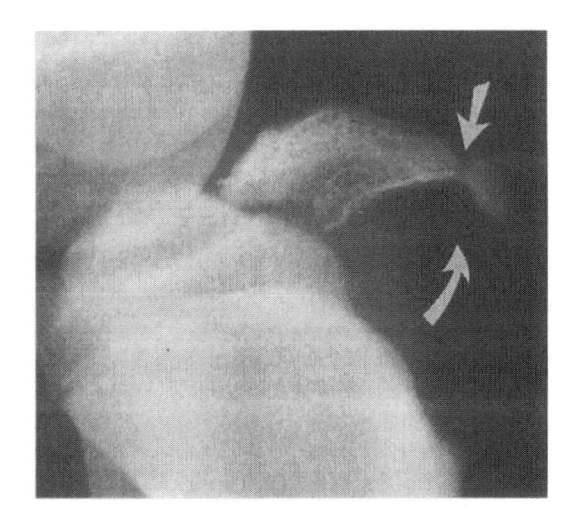

FIGURE 23-45. Type 3 injury. Upward displacement (curved arrow), with fragmentation of the distal end (straight arrow).

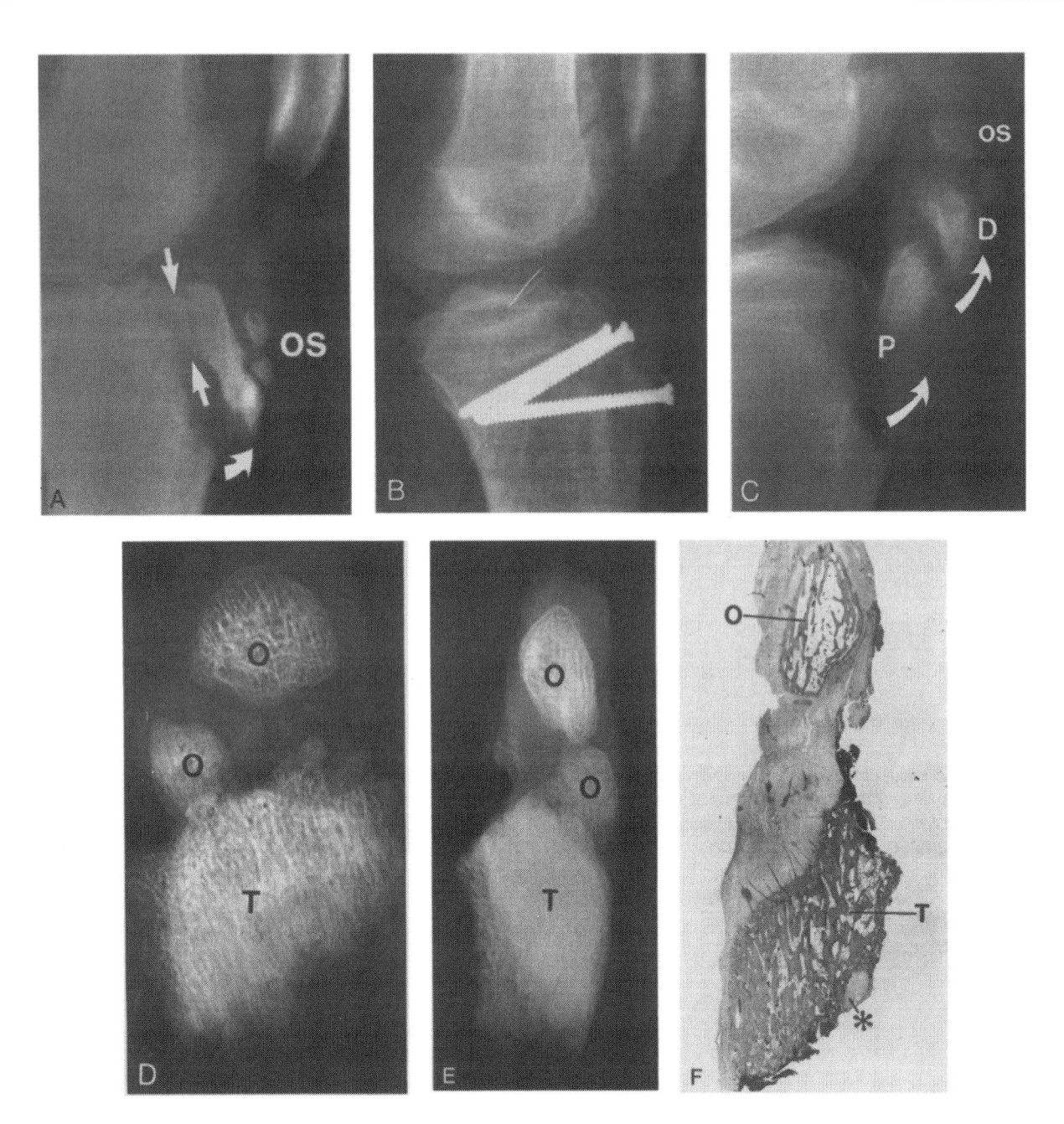

FIGURE 23-46. (A) Type 3 injury (arrows) to the left knee in a boy with a preexistent (but asymptomatic) Osgood-Schlatter lesion (OS). (B) Operative reduction. (C) Type 3 injury in the right knee in the same patient. Note the Osgood-Schlatter ossicles (OS). Also note how the distal fragment (D) has been pulled more proximally than the proximal fragment (P) (arrows). (D, E) Anteroposterior and lateral roentgenograms of the fragment removed from the (right) knee. T = tuberosity; O = Osgood-Schlatter ossicles. (F) Histologic section showing Osgood-Schlatter ossicle (O) and distal tibial tuberosity (T), with fragments of a closing tuberosity physis (*).

Pathomechanics

Tibial tuberosity ossification develops as a tongue-shaped downward protrusion of the proximal tibial epiphysis onto the anterior proximal tibial surface and a separate center of ossification that fuses with the main body of the epiphysis at the age of 16 and eventually fuses to the tibial metaphysis around the age of 18 years. Complete or partial avulsions, acute or chronic, may occur during osseous maturation. Studies have implicated the anatomic arrangement with cartilage between the tuberosity and the main proximal tibial center as the usual one susceptible to avulsion.[8,158] As shown in Figures 23-5 and 23-6, a bipolar growth plate may exist between the two centers (i.e., those of the proximal tibia and the tuberosity).

The tuberosity fracture, like the Tillaux fracture of the distal tibia, is most often seen in adolescents who are going through physiologic epiphysiodesis. This factor lessens the risk of growth abnormality, particularly genu recurvatum, consequent to premature growth arrest of the tuberosity. In any case, the prognosis must be guarded because of the potential for premature closure of the anterior portion the tuberosity or proximal tibial physis and subsequent recurvatum. The proximal tibial physis may be subjected to compression (type 5 injury), particularly if the mechanism is one of hyperextension and violent contracture of the quadriceps. However, the main proximal tibial epiphysis is usually well into physiologic epiphysiodesis when tuberosity avulsion commonly occurs. Thus significant growth damage is unlikely.

The mechanism of injury appears to be a violent active extension or passive flexion of the knee with the quadriceps muscle rigidly contracted. Preexistence of an Osgood-Schlatter lesion may increase susceptibility to injury, as the area has already shown mild tensile failure. The acutely increased tensile force is too much for the tuberosity to resist, and complete failure occurs.[158]

Balmat et al. showed that the movement that results in this injury is generally one of four: (1) springing off for a jump; (2) landing on one foot after a jump; (3) impeded extension; or (4) forced flexion.[128] When springing off for a jump, the final impulse leads to hyperextension of the knee just prior to leaving the ground. Tensile forces are thus exerted proximally and anteriorly, with the avulsion involving only the anteriotibial tuberosity. During the landing phase, avulsion fractures involve both the anterior tibial tuberosity and the proximal tibial epiphysis. The knee is normally flexed, and the latent energy stored in the quadriceps by the elasticity of the extensor complex acting as a shock absorber is transmitted by the patellar tendon to the anterior tibial tuberosity. Forces are exerted upward across the proximal epiphysis, which is thus involved in the fracture. The avulsion is often fragmented. With impeded extension, the contraction of the quadriceps encounters apposing forces that block extension of the knee. This mechanism is probable in basketball players who were blocked in their attempt to shoot. The quadriceps contractions is apposed by a strong downward force due to the opponent's countering maneuver, which causes avulsion of the anterior tibial tuberosity. With forced flexion, contraction of the quadriceps counters the force generated by flexion of the knee, which tends to produce avulsion of the anterior tibial tuberosity.

Lepse et al. reported a bilateral avulsion in a gymnast who was attempting a foward flip from a running start.[157] At takeoff from the ground with both feet firmly placed and while extending the knees for the jump, he felt the onset of acute bilateral knee pain and was unable to propel himself forward.

Diagnosis

Pain and swelling about the anterior part of the proximal end of the tibia, with an inability to extend the knee against force or gravity, are common findings. With fractures that extend into the proximal epiphysis, there is usually an associated hemarthrosis in the knee.

Roentgenography is essential for definitive diagnosis. Oblique views that adequately visualize the tuberosity ossification center may be required. Tomography may also be necessary to evaluate any extension of the fracture into the joint. However, the avulsion fracture may occur before sec-

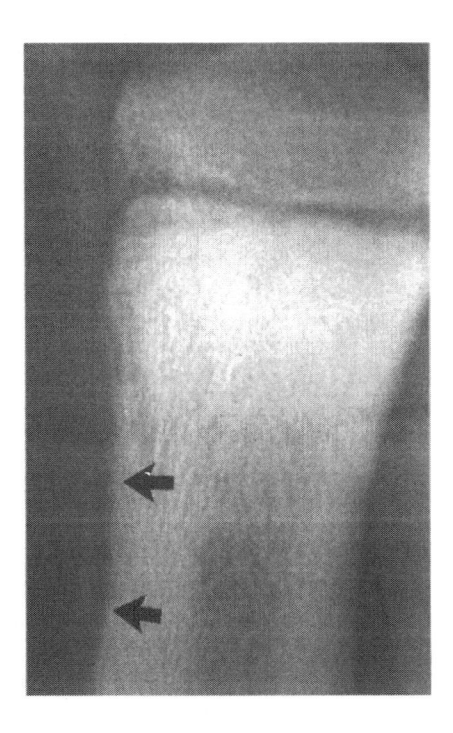

FIGURE 23-47. Reactive bone (arrows) from chronic type 1 injury in a 10-year-old jogger. It healed with discontinuation of the distance running for 8 weeks followed by directed quadriceps strengthening.

ondary ossification is present in the tuberosity. If you suspect the injury in a young patient, MRI may allow the specific diagnosis. Levi and Colemena studied 15 tuberosity fractures; included in their cases was one patient in whom the tibial tuberosity was completely cartilaginous.[158] Driessnack and Marcus reported a case of tuberosity fracture through an unossified region.[139] Treatment was no different. Diagnosis proved to be a problem because of the obvious lack of an ossification center within the tuberosity. The patella was higher than that of the opposite side.

Occasionally, these avulsions are chronic, rather than acute, and difficult to diagnose. Figure 23-47 shows the knee of a 10-year-old jogger who had complained of knee pain for several weeks and whose condition had been diagnosed as an Osgood-Schlatter lesion. The lesion was actually a type 1 chronic avulsion of the tuberosity and more distal extension of the patellar ligament.

Mayba reported a patient in whom the tibial tuberosity was avulsed, but in addition the patellar ligament was avulsed away from the fragment.[162] Frankle et al. also reported a combined situation of avulsion of the tibial tuberosity along with avulsion of the patellar ligament from the tuberosity.[142] Falster and Hasselbalch reported a combination of a tibial tuberosity avulsion combined with a ligament and meniscal tear.[141] Lipscomb et al. had reported a similar pattern of injury.[159]

Treatment

Treatment depends on the extent of displacement and must be directed at anatomic correction. In cases in which the

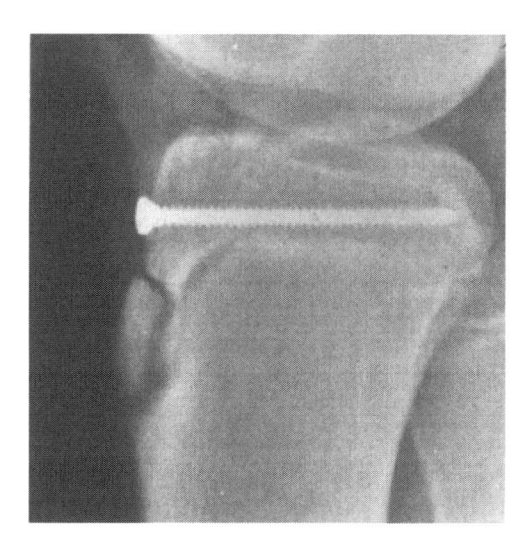

FIGURE 23-48. Transverse screw fixation of a type 3A injury.

tuberosity is still partially attached and minimally displaced, manipulative reduction is essential to restore anatomic integrity and detect the presence of herniated tissue. Watson-Jones emphasized closed reduction for these fractures whenever possible and minimized the consequences of proximal extension into the joint.[166] If closed methods are used initially, the patient must undergo roentgenography at appropriate intervals to be certain the distal fragment is not subsequently displaced significantly as swelling dissipates.

With rare exception, type 1B and all types 2 and 3 injuries should be subjected to open reduction (including evaluation of the knee), with accurate anatomic restoration of tibial surface congruity, repair of any peripheral meniscal tears, and appropriate fixation of the fragments (Fig. 23-46). Although screws are the most common method used (Figs. 23-48, 22-49), fragmentation may limit their applicability or effectiveness. Tension band wiring (Fig. 23-50) is an effective alternative method of fixation for these injuries.[162] Extensive comminution sometimes requires separate reduction of the multiple articular and tuberosity fragments. The use of the tension band wire facilitates fixation of small fragments that are too small or thin for standard screw fixation. Furthermore, early knee motion may be commenced with less fear of fragment displacement. The tension band wire supplements the screw fixation in a manner similar to tension bands applied to olecranon and patellar fractures. Tension band wiring has been advocated for tibial tuberosity avulsions in large and small animals.[129]

A large periosteal flap may be reflected along with the tuberosity at the time of injury. This concomitant injury facilitates surgical repair in that it may be easily resutured to its original position.[130] In fact, it can be attached to the pes anserinus to make a strong fixation, a factor to be taken advantage of to minimize the adjuvant use of internal metallic fixation. In two cases the periosteum was also herniated behind the tibial tuberosity, which prevented adequate closed reduction.[138] In case of displacement, it is essential to perform an open reduction to explore the area and remove any herniated tissue.

The knee joint should be explored for appropriate type 2 and all type 3 injuries. Any intraarticular damage, especially to the menisci, should be repaired. Small, comminuted fragments must be removed.

Results

The results of treating this injury are generally good to excellent. Because the growth plate is in the final stages of closure, premature growth arrest rarely occurs. Adequate quadriceps rehabilitation is essential for a good result.

Complications

Genu recurvatum is a potential problem. In our study premature epiphysiodesis was found in only one patient, and in this case the entire physis, both proximal tibia and tuberos-

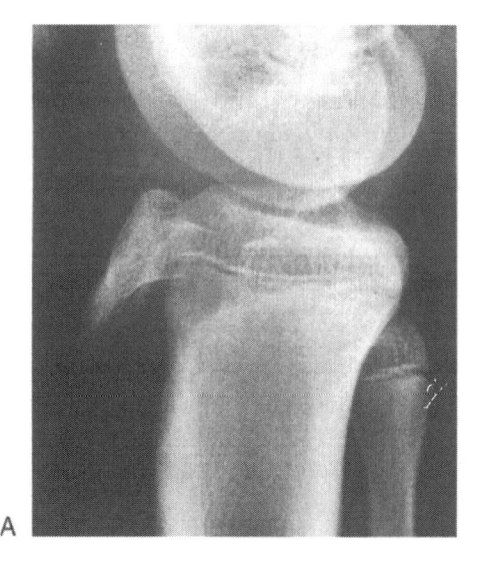

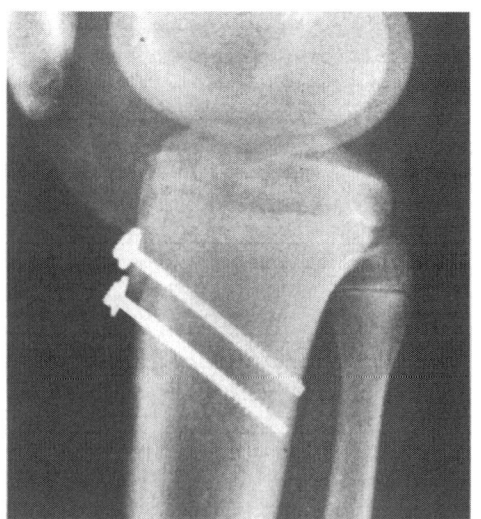

FIGURE 23-49. (A) Type 2A injury. (B) Oblique screw fixation.

Tibial Tuberosity Injuries

FIGURE 23-50. Tension band wire fixation technique. The screws compress the proximal tibial epiphyseal fragments together.

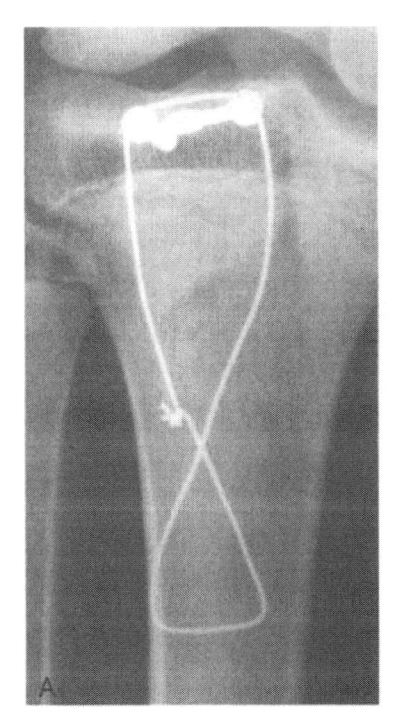

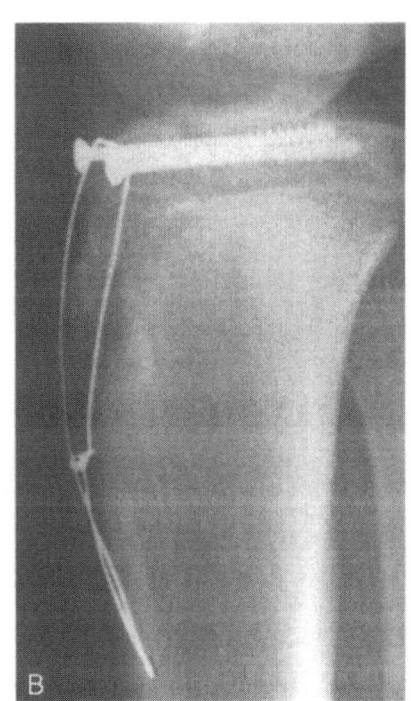

ity, was involved, probably due to a neuropathic joint (myelomeningocele) rather than to specific tuberosity physeal damage.[166] Since that study, I have seen one other case following an open injury.

Another complication is failure of the fixation. By isometric contracture, the quadriceps may pull the tuberosity off again and cause extensive ectopic bone formation (Fig. 23-51). This ectopic bone may be resected and the tendon reattached. In this case an external fixator was applied to transverse pins in the patella and metaphysis to hold the patella in an anatomic position while the tendon healed to bone. A fracture may occur through the level of screw fixation.

A rare complication is the development of avascular necrosis in the tuberosity (Fig. 23-52). Compartment syndrome has also been reported.[166,168,170,178] The lateral aspect of the tibial tubercle has a fan-shaped group of vessels originating from the anterior tibial recurrent artery. If transected, these vessels may retract laterally and distally under the fascia and into the muscle of the anterior compartment. This tissue region is significantly disrupted during the fracture mechanism. Bolesta and Fitch performed prophylactic anterior compartment fasciotomies without overt signs of compartment syndrome.[130]

Maar et al. reported a patient with bilateral tibial avulsions. He had tenderness of the tibial tubercles and point tenderness of the screw heads.[160] On one side he had developed an ossicle of bone over one of the screws. The screws were removed from both knees, along with the ossicle of bone. Six months after the surgery he was symptom-free.

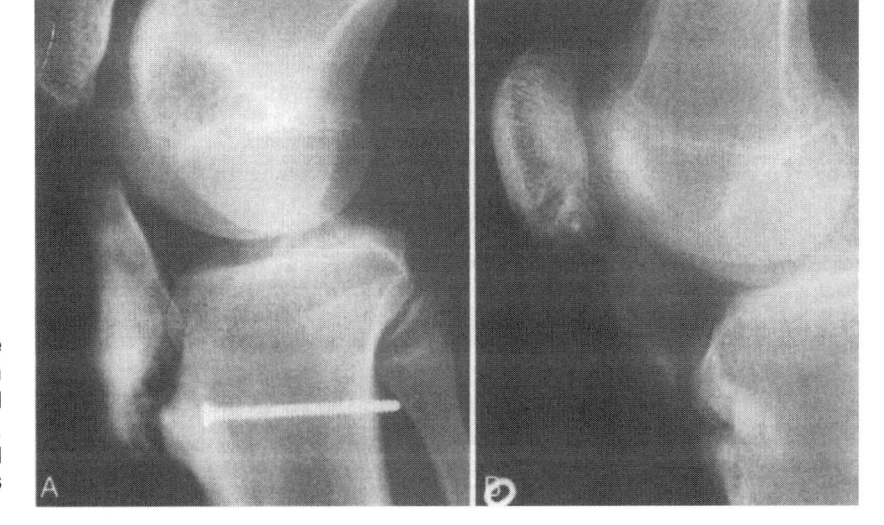

FIGURE 23-51. (A) Despite initial operative reduction, the tuberosity avulsed again when the patient removed the cast and resumed activity. The fragment displaced proximally, causing reactive bone formation, nonunion, and limited knee function. (B) The bone was resected and the patellar tendon reattached.

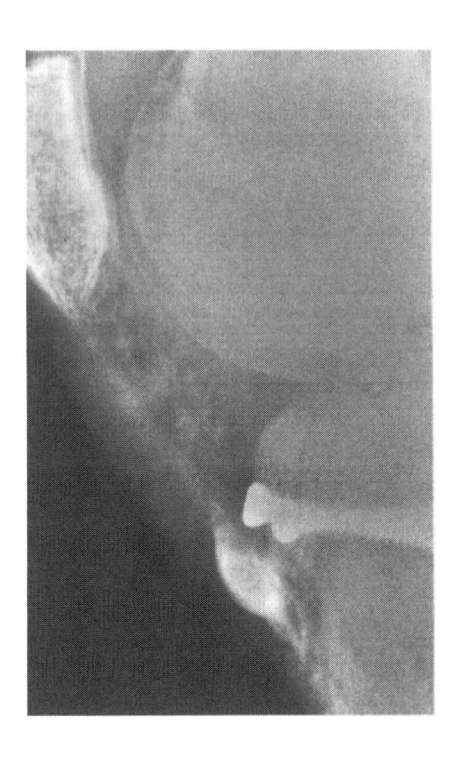

FIGURE 23-52. Sclerotic bone in the tuberosity probably indicates avascular (ischemic) necrosis of the distal secondary ossification center.

from a segment of the tibial tuberosity.[203] Increased obliquity of the angle of the patellar tendon from the patella to the insertion may also be a causative (predisposing) factor.[228] This situation is similar to the anatomy in children who tend to subluxate the patella laterally.

Cole[194] and Uhry[273] described histologic studies of sections removed from the tibial tuberosity during surgical procedures. These sections showed hemorrhage, clotting, invasion of fibroblasts and connective tissue, and other features of nonunion and increased vascularity. Figure 23-54 (see below) shows one of the most complete specimens available. The posterior portion of the patellar tendon between the ossicle and the tuberosity was frayed and in varying stages of repair. The ossicles contained viable bone with fibrocartilage at the periphery.

Anatomically, the Osgood-Schlatter lesion results from the pulling away of an anterior portion of the ossification center of the tuberosity from the remaining tuberosity (Figs. 23-53, 23-54). This traction (avulsion) may also occur when the cartilage cells are hypertrophic (i.e., preossification phase), a time when they are not roentgenographically evident. Once pulled away, the cartilage or bone may continue to grow, ossify, and enlarge, becoming radiologically evident (Figs. 23-55 to 23-57). However, because of chronic motion the intervening area may become fibrous, creating localized nonunion and a characteristic concave defect.

Osgood-Schlatter Lesion

The Osgood-Schlatter lesion may be defined as partial separation of the *anterior* portions of the chondral or chondroosseous tibial tuberosity, along with variable (partial) patellar tendon disruption.[180–206,207–232,234–240,242,244–273,275–280] Chronic, repetitive trauma is the most likely cause, although other suggested causes have included vascular damage, systemic disease, and endocrinopathy. Intense acute trauma may also cause the injury. A comparable lesion has been reported in quadrupedal mammals.[207,233,241,274]

Interestingly, when Osgood described the lesion he described avulsion of the entire tibial tuberosity, rather than the typical focal lesion associated with his name.[253] He thought that the true Osgood-Schlatter lesion was an avulsion of a small portion of the tuberosity, which was much more common than complete fracture through the tuberosity. He considered that these lesions did not cause complete loss of function, but without treatment they created a "long continued serious annoyance."

Gosselin, in 1843, may have been the first to describe osteochondritis of the tibial tubercle, describing it as "periarthritis of adolescents."[278]

Pathomechanics

Ehrenborg and Engfeldt purported that the cause of the Osgood-Schlatter lesion was traumatic and the causal mechanism was avulsion of a portion of the patellar ligament, with consequent detachment of fragments of cartilage or bone

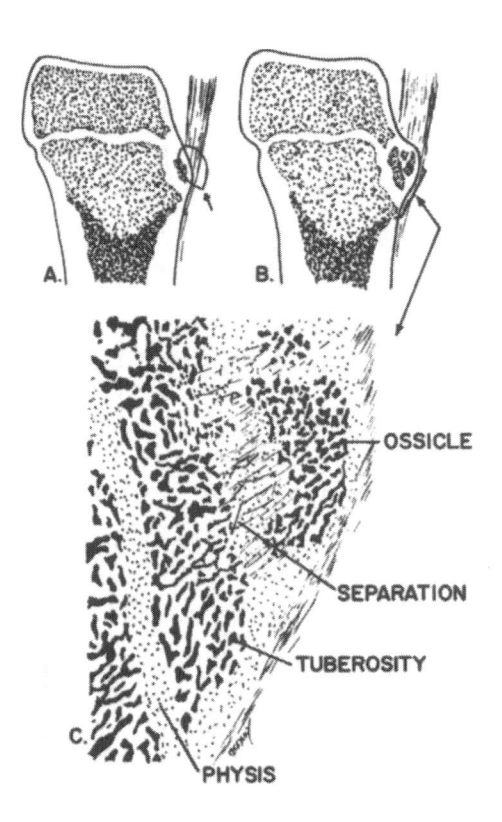

FIGURE 23-53. Development of the Osgood-Schlatter lesion. (A) Normal. (B) Involved, with fragmentation of the ossification center. (C) Enlargement shows how the ossicle pulls away from the anterior portion of the main tuberosity ossification center. The region of separation then fills in with fibrous and fibrocartilaginous tissue, which usually ossifies *only* if the tension stress is relieved.

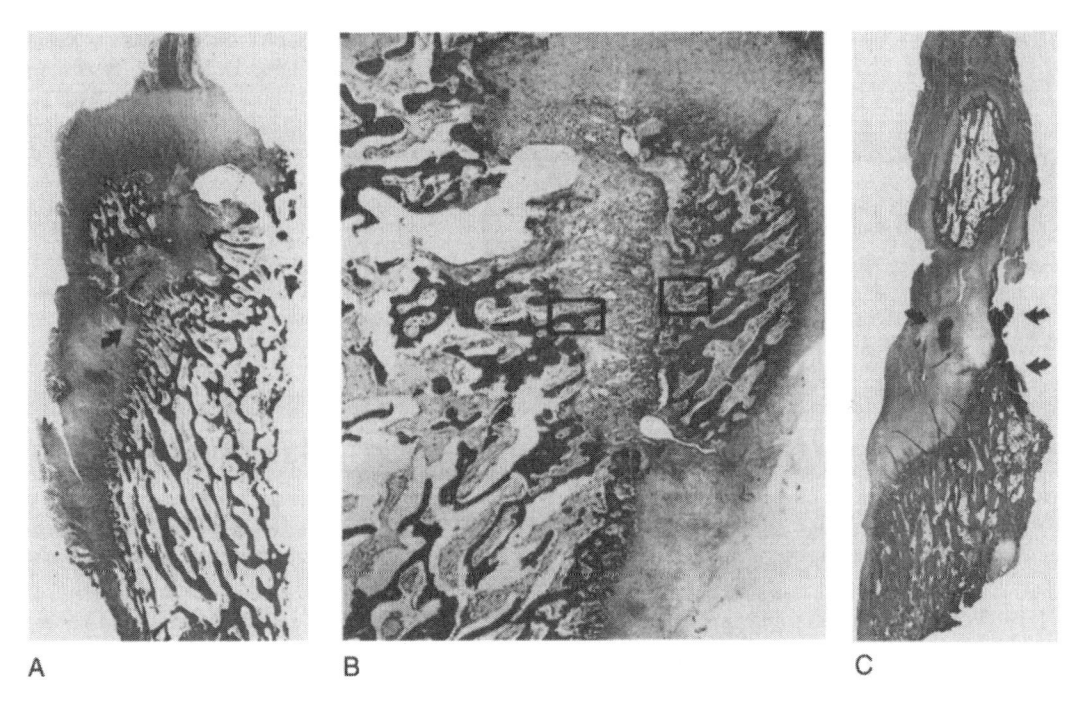

FIGURE 23-54. (A) Osgood-Schlatter (OS) ossicle separated from the rest of the ossification center of the tuberosity. There is an attempt to bridge the gap with trabecular bone (arrow). (B) Specimen of an OS lesion. The vascular spaces suggest repetitive avulsion associated with fibrocartilaginous "healing." (C) Mature OS lesion. Note the hemorrhagic areas (arrows), suggesting repetitive tensile damage.

Katoh studied quadriceps muscle force in nomal boys as well as those with Osgood-Schlatter (OS) lesions.[228] He found that an eccentric force was especially strong; and that the group of OS patients had the highest amount of lateralizing force among all groups. His finding suggested that the increased eccentric or lateralizing force in the extensor mechanism of the knee was an etiologic factor contributing to the development of the lesion.

Diagnosis

A lateral radiograph is the best method for assessing the tuberosity, but it must be a true lateral view of the tuberosity, not the tibia. The slight difference may affect the ability to see the small ossicles. The characteristic patient has an anterior concavity in the tuberosity ossification center. Most often an ossicle or ossicles of varying size are evident within

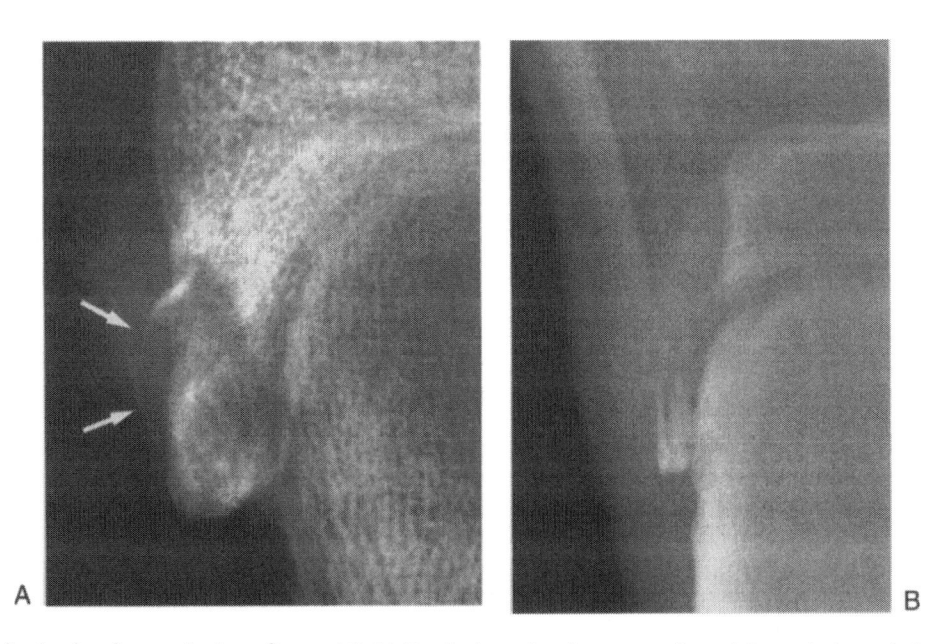

FIGURE 23-55. (A) Acute development of an Osgood-Schlatter lesion, showing separation of the anterior subchondral bone (arrows) from the tuberosity ossification center. (B) Similar fracture (acute) within the ossification center.

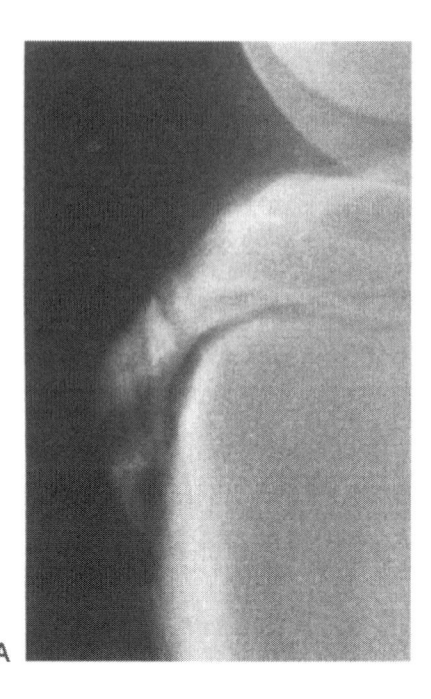

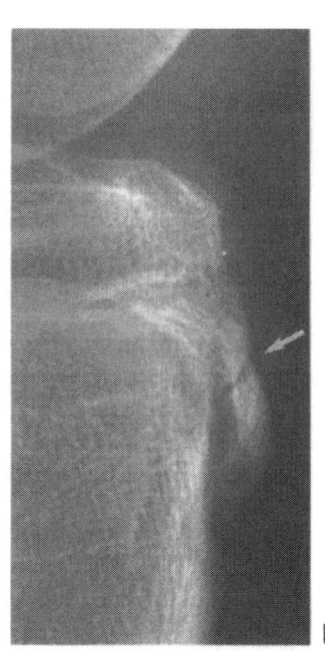

FIGURE 23-56. (A) Acute onset of tuberosity pain and swelling associated with avulsion of a large fragment of the ossification center. (B) Intraapophyseal fracture (arrow) after acute onset of pain during a baseball game (sliding into a base).

or just anterior to this concavity. If the avulsed segment is all unossified cartilage, there is a delay in the appearance of ossification. The concavity is usually present, however, and is virtually pathognomonic of the repetitive stress injury.

Computed tomography probably is unnecessary in these patients unless some other lesion (e.g., osteomyelitis, tumor) is suspected. MRI may also be used but only in selective cases. MRI can demonstrate the extensive edema in avulsed areas but can also show contiguous metaphyseal edema (Figs. 23-58, 23-59).

DeFlaviis et al. used ultrasonography (Fig. 23-60) in 82 patients with clinically suspected Osgood-Schlatter lesions and 30 normal subjects.[196] In 45 cases, comparative radiographs were obtained. Ultrasonography was equally or more effective than radiography for accurate diagnosis and was of particular value for soft tissue evaluation. The typical sonographic changes of the ossification center of the cartilage and the surrounding soft tissues were described for Osgood-Schlatter lesions and Sinding-Larsen-Johansson lesions. These signs were based mainly on cartilage swelling and edema, fragmentation of the ossification center, thickening of the patellar tendon, and bursitis (inflammation) of the infrapatellar bursa. The authors proposed that ultrasonography was a simple and reliable method for the diagnosis of osteochondrosis at either end of the patellar tendon and a suitable methodology for periodic follow-up of the course of these lesions.

They divided their cases into four types. In type 1, the ossification center was normal on sonography. The overlying cartilage, however, appeared swollen, and the subcutaneous

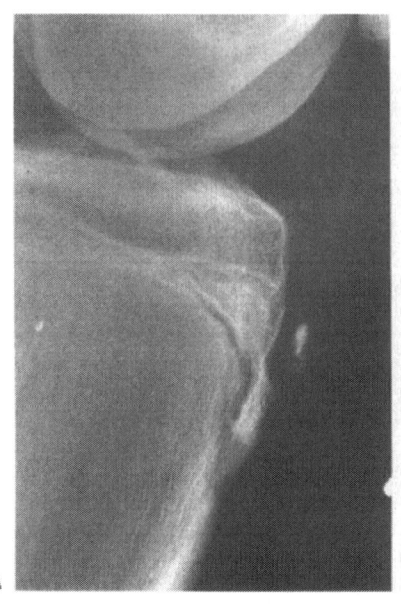

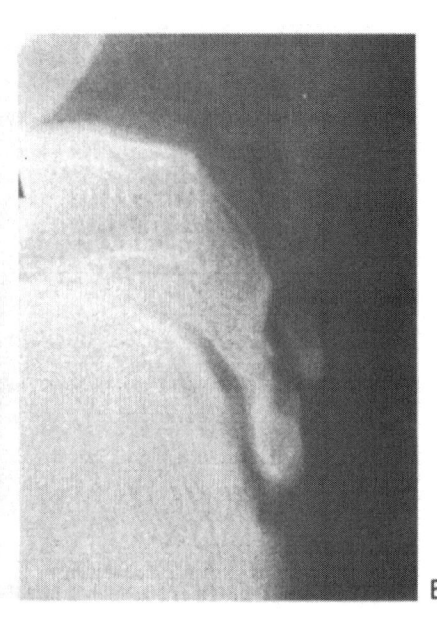

FIGURE 23-57. (A) Symptomatic patient with an early Osgood-Schlatter lesion. (B) Progressive enlargement of ossification within the avulsed cartilaginous fragment. Note the characteristic concavity left by the avulsion of the anterior portion of the chondroepiphysis.

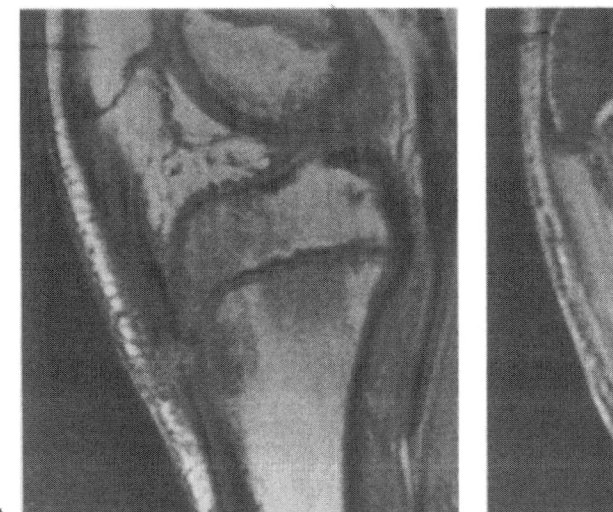

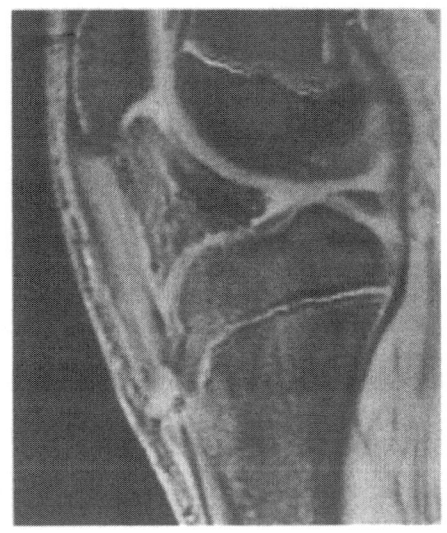

FIGURE 23-58. (A, B) T1 and T2 images showing acute edema at the insertion of the patellar tendon into the tuberosity. Also note the extensive bone bruising posterior to the tuberosity.

tissues were anteriorly displaced. These patients usually had a seemingly normal radiograph. In type 2, in addition to the aforementioned soft tissue changes, the ossification center of the tibial tuberosity becomes involved. The nucleus appeared fragmented and hypoechoic with a markedly irregular outline. In type 3, insertional tendonitis of the patellar tendon becomes evident as a diffuse thickening of the tendon that appears nonhomogeneous and vacuolated. These findings may be associated with a normal osseous aspect or in combination with fragmentation of the center (respectively, types 3A and 3B). In type 4, a fluid collection could be detected within the retrotendinous soft tissues. It was due to bursitis of the infrapatellar bursa and was clearly demonstrated by the presence of a small transonic cavity. This group also could be divided into type 4A or type 4B, depending on the absence or presence, respectively, of involvement of the ossification center.

Various methods to measure patellar position have been described. Unfortunately, many of the methods are difficult because they were designed to be done in adults (mature bone), and the incomplete ossification of the patella and tuberosity in the pediatric age group make these measurements difficult and imprecise.

Sen et al. noted that the patella has often been blamed for the Osgood-Schlatter lession because it is situated higher or lower than normal.[263] They described a new patellar angle in lateral radiographs of the knee joint. One line was drawn along the articular surface of the patella and the other from the end of the inferior articular cartilage at the patellar apex. The angle formed by these two lines averaged 33° in

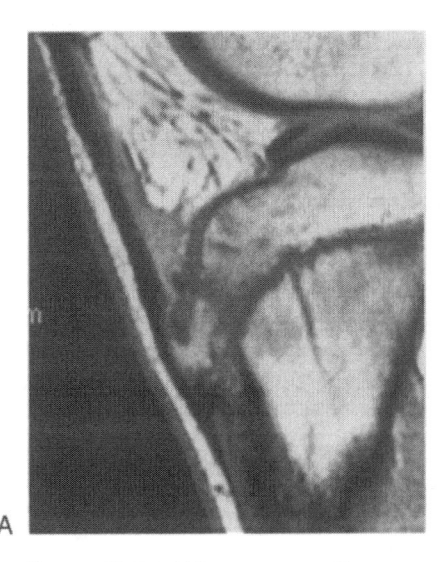

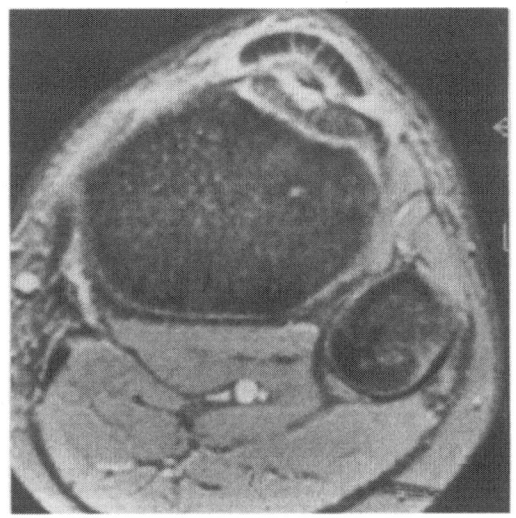

FIGURE 23-59. Edema surrounding an avulsed fragment. (A) Lateral view. (B) Transverse view.

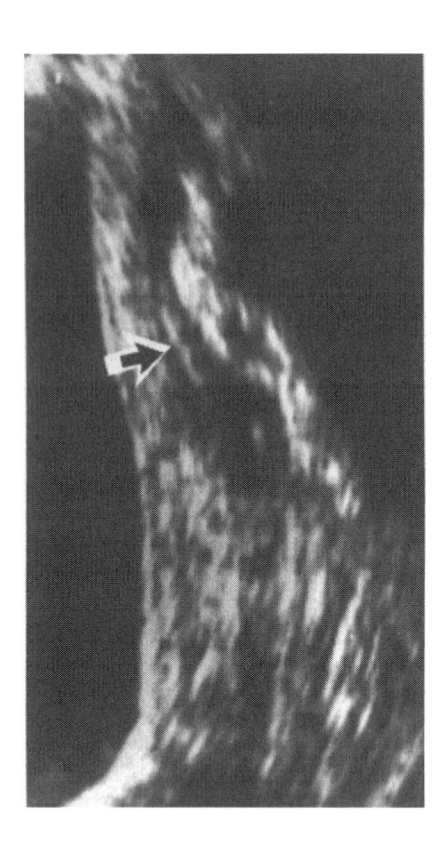

FIGURE 23-60. Ultrasonography of an acute Osgood-Schlatter lesion. The arrow indicates the avulsed anterior segment.

68 knees affected by Osgood-Schlatter lesions and 47° in 71 age-matched and 198 adult controls. The small angle in the Osgood-Schlatter lesion was proposed to be a factor in the pathogenesis of the traction apophysitis.

Gumppenberg et al. used the Blackburn and Peel method to assess the position of the patella.[215] Normal knees had an index of 0.80, whereas the Osgood-Schlatter patients measured 1.01 in boys and 0.91 in girls, increasing to 1.06 in boys with radiologic evidence of loose ossicles. These authors thought that the findings were compatible with strong pull of the quadriceps muscle, the most important etiologic factor in the patella alta associated with Osgood-Schlatter disease.

Aparicia et al. used the Caton-Deschamps index in a study of 17 patients with Osgood-Schlatter lesions.[182] They found a significant incidence of patella alta.

Yashar et al. found that skeletal age in children with Osgood-Schlatter lesions was normal.[279] They agreed that mechanical forces, not maturational delay, was the most likely etiology.

Treatment

Because chronic stress, with the formation of localized delayed union or nonunion, is a significant factor, treatment should first include discontinuation of the evocative programmed sports activities. If the lesion continues to be painful, immobilization in a cylinder cast or knee immobilizer is considered (Fig. 23-61). Patients and their parents must made aware of the probable chronic traumatic etiology and the possibility of recurrence following muscle rehabilitation. Graduated quadriceps strengthening is important to prevent recurrence.

Ignoring the symptoms of discomfort and pain, along with the oft-quoted concept of "no pain–no gain" that has now permeated the childhood level competitive and noncompetitive sports and activities, continues to subject the injury to nonhealing (tensile) forces. It may lead to severe disruption (Fig. 23-62).

This disorder represents a chronic stress fracture that is attempting to heal; therefore it is a process that requires inflammation as part of the normal biologic response. *Steroids should not be used.* Nonunions are generally painful; therefore the fracture should be treated with a method that promotes healing rather than with steroids, which discourage a crucial fracture healing stage. Several patients have had adverse reactions to steroids injected in the region of the tuberosity.[243,258,259]

Children rarely complain because of prominence of the tuberosity. They *do* complain about the restriction of activities forced on them because of pain and discomfort. It is well recognized that Osgood-Schlatter lesion is a reasonably self-limited condition and, as a rule, amenable to conservative management. Only rarely is tendon enlargement about the epiphysis continuously troublesome and persistent enough to require operative treatment. The author's experience is that patients with a distinct prominence but osseous continuity rarely have problems. In contrast, adults with a radiographic nonunion (ossicle) are much more likely to have pain with activity and are probably best treated by resection of the symptomatic ossicle (Figs. 23-63, 23-64) through a medial or lateral approach rather than splitting the patellar tendon.

Operative intervention should be used in patients rarely and only after the following conditions are met: (1) The

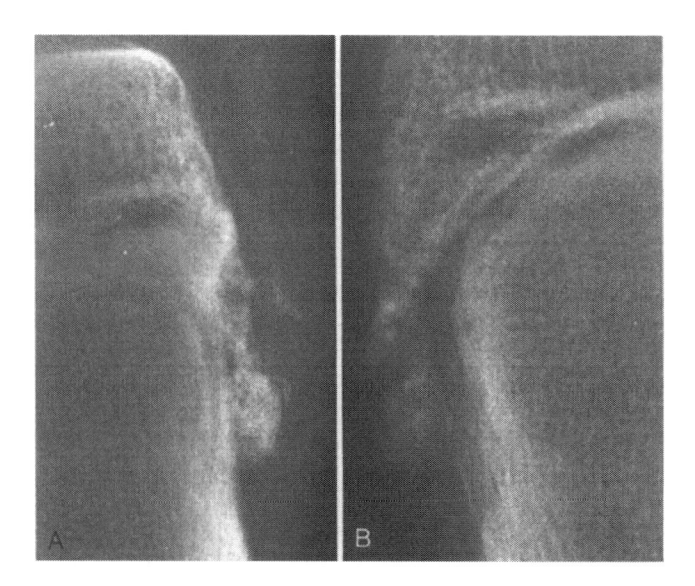

FIGURE 23-61. (A) This boy with an Osgood-Schlatter lesion had been symptomatic for several months. (B) Treatment for 5 weeks in a cylinder cast relieved the pain and resulted in roentgenologically evident healing.

Osgood-Schlatter Lesion

FIGURE 23-62. (A) Multiple ossicles from a severe case of combined Sinding-Larsen-Johansson and Osgood-Schlatter lesions. This boy, a highly competitive athlete, refused to comply with restrictions. (B) MRI. The patellar tendon is elongated and attenuated.

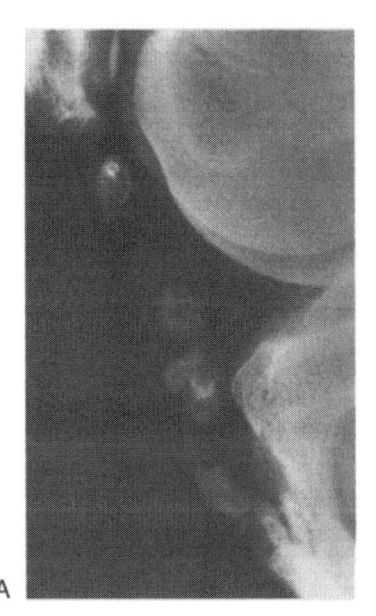

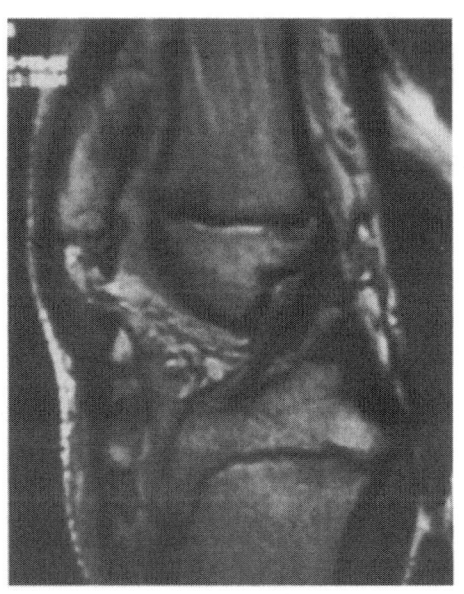

patient has had repeated episodes of severe pain with tenderness, functional disability, and deformity. (2) Even after conservative treatment with immobilization by cast or splint, the symptoms have returned. (3) The child has reached sufficient development during adolescence to justify a surgical procedure with minimal risk. These children should not be operated on until there is an established fragment (or fragments) and evident nonunion. If a localized procedure (resection of the fragment) is used, it is possible to operate on children who have not yet attained skeletal maturity. The ossicle is shelled away from the tendon.

Ferciot recommended surgical treatment of anterior tibial apophysitis and described a surgical exposure of splitting the patellar tendon.[208] I do not recommend this procedure. Instead, I prefer a lateral approach, with release of the lateral retinaculum along the patellar tendon and patella, followed

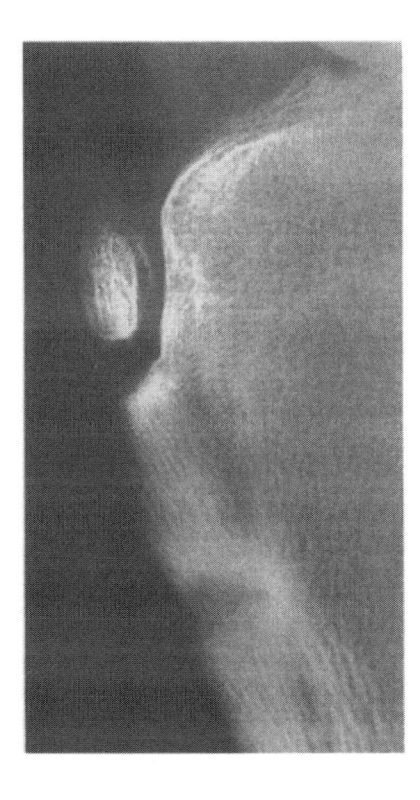

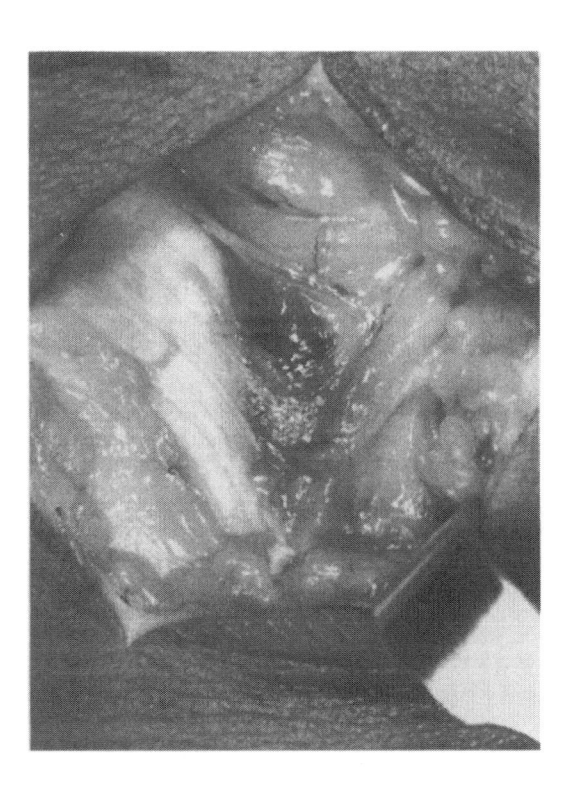

FIGURE 23-63. Chronic Osgood-Schlatter ossicle in a 16-year-old volleyball player. Because of persistent pain this fragment was selectively excised, leading to complete relief of symptoms.

FIGURE 23-64. Hemorrhagic synovial inflammation and hemorrhagic bursa in a patient with chronic pain and mature ossicles. Excision led to complete relief of pain.

by elevation of the patellar tendon from the tuberosity to expose the area of nonunion (i.e., the ossicles, which should be excised) (Fig. 23-63).

The primary operative approach is removal of the nonunion fragment (or fragments), decreasing lateralizing tensile stress, and explaining to the patient and the parents preoperatively that the prominence of the tuberosity may remain postoperatively. Attempts to remove large portions of the tuberosity are contraindicated and may lead to complications of healing and problematic knee joint mechanics.

Wray and Muddu studied 16 patients with long-standing Osgood-Schlatter lesions who underwent surgery to relieve symptoms.[278] Nine had a loose fragment under the patellar ligament when they first presented, and five developed loose fragments during the course of conservative treatment. Two patients had a prominent, irregular tuberosity that failed to unite, but neither had loose fragments. The patients with loose fragments had them removed; and the patients with irregular and prominent tubercles without fragmentation underwent multiple drilling and smoothing of the tibial tuberosity. Fourteen patients were completely free of their preoperative symptoms; two patients were improved but still had occasional pain. The authors noted that failure of a loose fragment to unite with the rest of the tibial tuberosity produced symptoms and that passive movement of a fragment and direct pressure over the fragment was painful. Removal of the fragment was indicated, which is a simple surgical procedure.

Binazzi and Lorenzi described 20 patients who underwent resection of ossicles after all types of conservative treatment had failed to alleviate the clinical symptoms.[186] None of their patients had surgery for cosmetic reasons. The average age at the time of surgery was 18 years (range 12–31 years), with an average follow-up of 12 years. Excision of the ossicle with or without excision of the tibial tuberosity produced 93% good and excellent results and no poor results.

Flowers and Bhadreshewar used a modified Ferciot procedure to excise the enlarged tuberosity (and ossicle) in 35 patients (42 knees).[210] The results showed pain relief (95%) and reduction of the osseous prominence (85%). The authors did not discuss whether patients were still skeletally immature when surgery was undertaken.

Results

The natural history of the Osgood-Schlatter lesion was studied retrospectively (69 knees in 50 patients).[234] Altogether 76% of the patients believed they had no limitation of activity, but 60% still could not kneel without discomfort. The authors found that the patients who did not have bony change, particularly ossicle formation, were far less likely to have chronic symptoms. A small number of their patients were treated in plaster, and the authors believed that this treatment did not particularly affect either the final deformity or the natural history. However, they admitted that the number of patients was too small to make any worthwhile comparison.

Lynch and Walsh reported two patients with premature fusion of the anterior part of the upper tibial epiphyseal plate.[245] These boys presented at 12 and 14 years; it is not certain when their Osgood-Schlatter lesions had started. Historically, there was no evidence that either boy had any recurvatum or hyperextension of the knee when first seen. Whether the fusion occurred as a consequence of the Osgood-Schlatter lesion or was a consequence of repetitive trauma from the aggressive pursuit of soccer (predominantly the kicking leg) is unclear.

Proximal Tibiofibular Subluxation and Dislocation

Injuries to the proximal tibiofibular joint, whether acutely symptomatic subluxations or obvious dislocations, have been considered infrequent if not rare injuries.[281–303] They are probably much more common than appreciated. In one large series and review of the literature, a major finding was that these injuries often escape initial recognition because of the lack of familiarity with them.[294] Because of generalized laxity these displacements may be more likely in children than adults.

Classification

Several types of instability or disruption of the proximal tibiofibular joint are possible. They can be classified as: (1) subluxation; (2) anterolateral dislocation; (3) posteromedial dislocation, and (4) superior dislocation (Fig. 23-65).

Idiopathic subluxation of the proximal end of the fibula, which is best defined as excessive symptomatic anteroposterior motion without complete displacement, appears to be a self-limited condition of youth, producing decreasing symptoms as the patient approaches skeletal maturity.[295] Anterolateral dislocation is the most common injury[280]; posterior dislocation is infrequent; and superior dislocation is usually an accompaniment of tibial fracture and may be considered analogous to the forearm Monteggia injury (a variant of the Maisonneuve fracture).

Diagnosis

Patients with subluxation usually complain of pain along the lateral side of the knee and lower limb. It is a chronic complaint, although it may acutely follow certain athletic events or twisting injuries. Transient paresthesia of the peroneal nerve may also occur during periods of hyperactivity. The injury may be elicited by direct pressure over the fibular head, which pushes it farther forward or medially (Fig. 23-66). It is frequently a concomitant finding in children with multiple joint hypermobility, muscular dystrophy, or Ehlers-Danlos syndrome.

The isolated anterolateral proximal fibular dislocation may be discerned by clinical examination, which reveals a mass lateral to the tibia (Fig. 23-67). The dislocation is usually evident roentgenographically, although direct pressure to accentuate the deformity, as described for subluxation, is sometimes necessary. Unfortunately, the diagnosis is initially missed in about one-third of the reported cases.

Proximal Tibiofibular Subluxation and Dislocation

FIGURE 23-65. Four patterns of proximal tibiofibular displacement. See text for details.

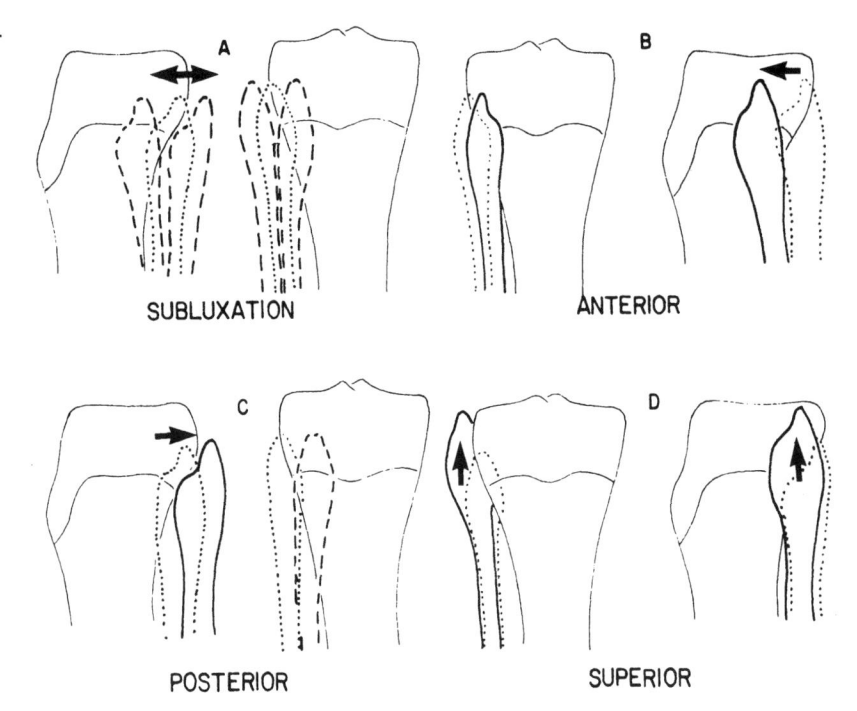

Pathomechanics

Most of these dislocations occur during athletic activity, especially with violent twisting. Some are associated with other skeletal injury, particularly fractures of the proximal tibial region (e.g., a Monteggia injury).

Treatment

In subluxation, the symptoms generally subside after rest. If not, the pain usually responds well to immobilization with a cylinder cast. Sometimes the foot must be included to prevent ankle motion, as such motion can cause mild rotation at the proximal fibula and may accentuate any synovitis.

Most patients with dislocation may be treated with closed reduction, particularly when the diagnosis is made in the acute situation. The knee should be flexed 90°–110°, the foot externally rotated, and direct pressure applied to the fibular head. Once reduction has been obtained, which is usually evident by a snapping sensation, the patient is immobilized for approximately 3 weeks. The joint is quite stable in extension, a factor that is evident in anatomic dissections in which it was impossible to displace the fibula anteriorly unless the knee was flexed 70°–80°. The foot is included to limit fibular rotation secondary to ankle motion.

Surgical approaches have been used to correct these complications, including resection of the proximal end of the fibula and arthrodesis of the joint. Arthrodesis of the proximal tibiofibular joint is complicated by a prolonged period of fusion and by eventual development of pain and instability in the ankle. The results in patients treated with arthrodesis are uniformly poor. In contrast, patients treated by resection of the fibular head usually have uneventful recoveries, and none has ever experienced the ankle pain

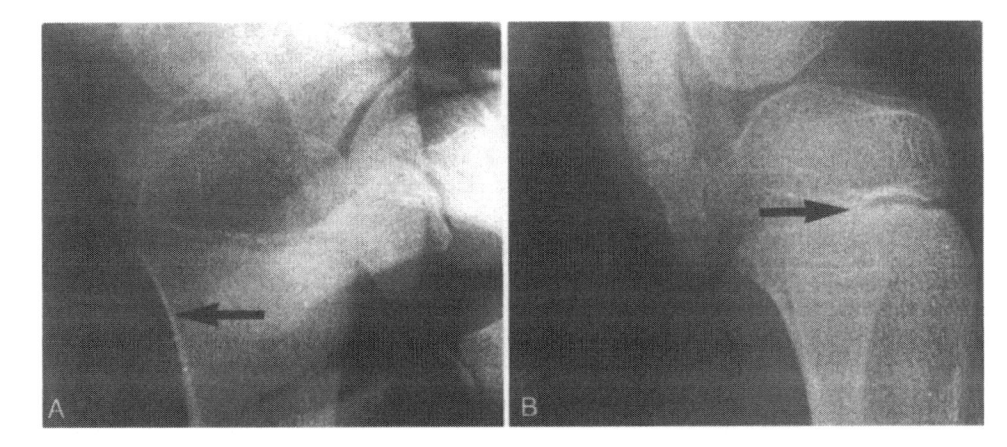

FIGURE 23-66. Anterior subluxation of the proximal fibula in a 7-year-old child with chronic pain over the lateral region of the knee. (A) Anterior stress (arrow) pushed the fibula backward. (B) Posterior stress (arrow) duplicated the pain by displacing the fibula anteriorly.

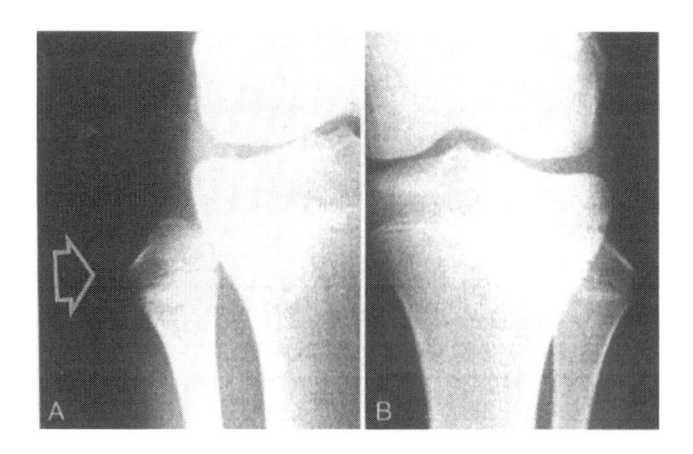

FIGURE 23-67. (A) Anterolateral dislocation (arrow). (B) Uninvolved knee.

and stability that occurred in the patients with arthrodesis. Resection of the proximal end of the fibula is not an operation to be undertaken lightly in a child still in an active growth phase, although it is possible to use it in children approaching skeletal maturity. Resection of the proximal end of the fibula might lead to cephalad migration of the fibula, as has been described by Hsu and colleagues when removing complete portions of the distal fibula for subtalar arthrodesis.[293]

Weinert and Raczka thought that stabilization might be attained using a variation of Bunnell's technique for stabilizing the distal radioulnar joint.[302] A portion of the biceps tendon may be used to construct and stabilize the superior tibiofibular joint. Shapiro et al. described a technique for reconstructing the ligamentous stability of the proximal tibiofibular joint using an iliotibial band fascial graft.[299] The technique involves isolating a strip of the iliotibial band approximately 20 cm in length and 2 cm in width, transecting it proximally and retaining its insertion to Gerdy's tubercle. The tract is tubularized and then placed through a tunnel in the proximal tibia going anteriorly to posteriorly followed by wrapping it medially around the fibula onto the lateral side, sliding up and under the lateral collateral ligament.

Results

Most patients respond satisfactorily to closed reduction but only if it is carried out within the first 1–2 weeks after the injury. Several of the dislocations developed into a chronic subluxation or arthritis of the proximal tibiofibular joint, although the latter was not a frequent complication in children. Unfortunately, many of these patients develop symptoms of "insecurity" after the injury, although this finding is much more common in adults than in children.

Wong and Weiner reported an unusual case of proximal, rather than distal, tibiofibular synostosis after trauma.[303] Other than the acute injury, however, neither patient seemed to be having chronic problems.

Posterior Dislocation

Posteromedial dislocations are more unstable after initial reduction and frequently require surgical repair. This injury is usually the result of a severe blow directly to the knee, such as that inflicted by a car bumper; the proximal part of the fibula is pushed posteriorly and medially. Severe disruption of the anterior and posterior capsular ligaments of the tibiofibular joint, along with a significant tear of part of the fibular collateral ligament, allows the biceps to draw the unsupported proximal part of the fibula posteriorly. In view

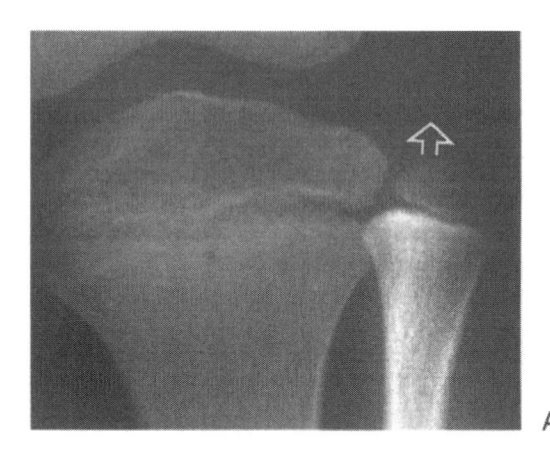

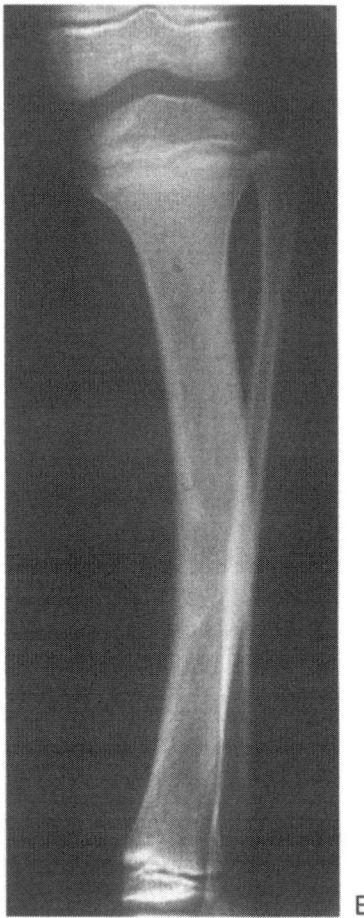

FIGURE 23-68. (A) A 12-year-old boy with multiple injuries. The proximal fibula was displaced superiorly (arrow) concomitant with a tibial diaphyseal fracture. At the time of plating of the unstable tibial fracture, the proximal fibula was reduced (closed reduction). (B) Similar proximal tibiofibular disruption that was not recognized acutely. These are Maisonneuve-equivalent injuries.

Proximal Tibial Metaphyseal Injuries

of the poor results in the few reported cases treated conservatively, a posterior dislocation should probably be treated by open reduction, capsulorrhaphy, and fibular collateral ligament repair.

Superior Dislocation

Superior dislocations are rare and are usually associated with fractures of the tibia.[282,289] Figure 23-68 shows a 12-year-old boy who sustained multiple trauma (including a severe fracture of the pelvis). He had an unstable tibial fracture with no evidence of a fibular fracture. It was impossible to control his fracture, which proved difficult to reduce even when, at the time of open reduction, compression fixation was used. It was necessary to reduce superior displacement of the proximal fibula, which was the cause of the failure to attain complete tibial reduction. This reduction was difficult, as it was attempted 2 weeks after injury. This type of injury is similar to a Monteggia injury in the forearm (also equivalent to a Maisonneuve injury variant).

Proximal Fibular Injuries

Injuries specifically involving the proximal fibular physis and epiphysis are rare (Fig. 23-69) and may be associated with significant soft tissue injury to the knee. The peroneal (fibular) nerve may be injured and must be carefully assessed clinically. If the nerve is injured, decompression may be necessary.

Because the biceps is a strong muscle, these fractures may be displaced, even if treated in a cast. Displacement of a type 1 or type 2 injury should be treated by open reduction (Fig. 23-70), as should any type 3 or type 4 injury. If the fracture involves the articular surface of the proximal tibiofibular joint, long-term degenerative changes may occur. Such joint pain should be treated by resection of the proximal fibula, not by arthrodesis.

Havránek described six patients with these injuries, three being type 2, one type 3, and two type 4 injuries.[304] Five of the six were treated with closed reduction; one patient with a type 4 injury was treated with open reduction and cerclage fixation. Havránek found that the growth plate in some of the patients fused earlier than that on the opposite side, but in none was there any adverse influence on fibular length or proximal tibiofibular congruence.

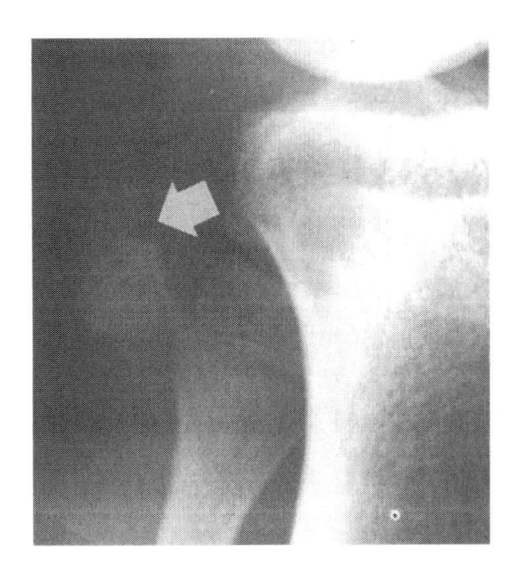

FIGURE 23-69. Type 3 fracture of the proximal fibula (arrow). This fracture complicated an acute knee dislocation and was treated by open reduction.

Proximal Tibial Metaphyseal Injuries

Fractures of the proximal tibial (Figs. 23-71, 23-72) metaphysis are relatively common in children and generally occur when children are between 3 and 8 years age.[305,308] Toddler's fractures may also involve this area (Fig. 23-73). Direct impact violence is a less common cause of fracture in this region than in the diaphysis. More commonly a twisting force, as with a fall, is likely to cause the injury.

The distal fragment may be angulated laterally, but there does not seem to be any significant loss of cortical apposition. Fragments do not usually override. The fibula may appear to escape injury, although it may sustain a green-

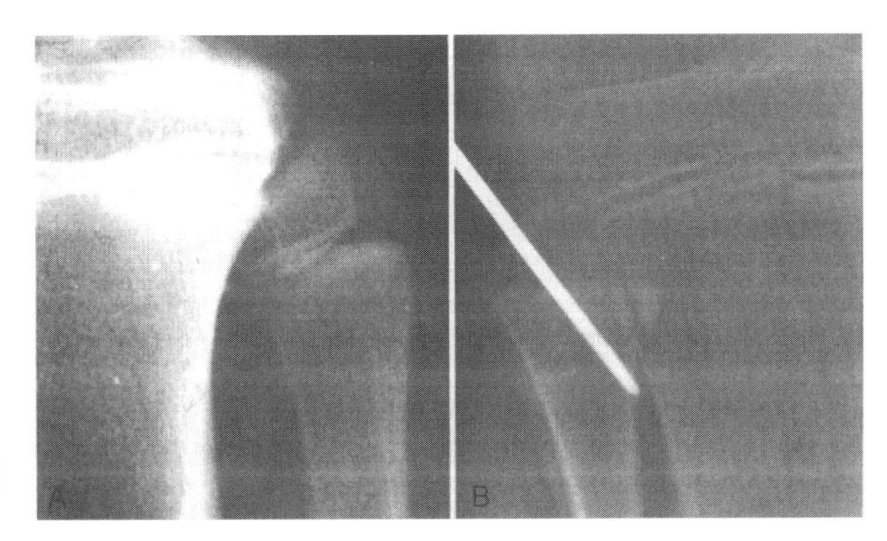

FIGURE 23-70. (A) Type 1 fibular epiphyseal fracture. (B) Pin fixation following peroneal neurolysis and open reduction.

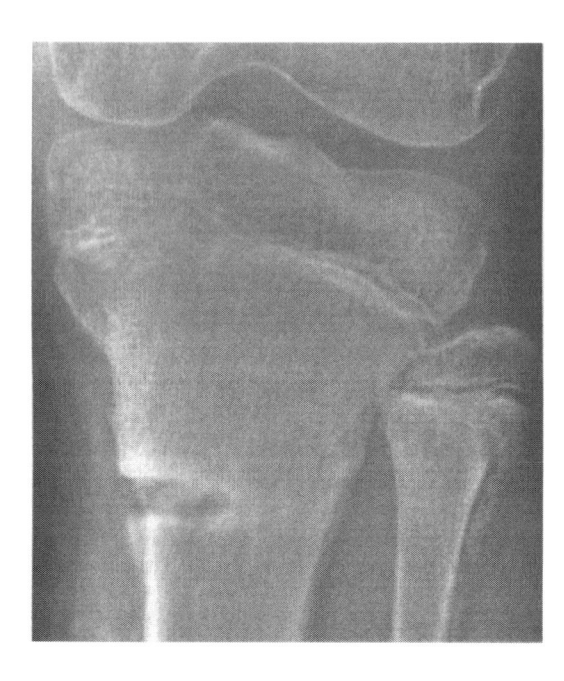

FIGURE 23-71. Type 2 proximal fibular fracture accompanying a tibial metaphyseal fracture.

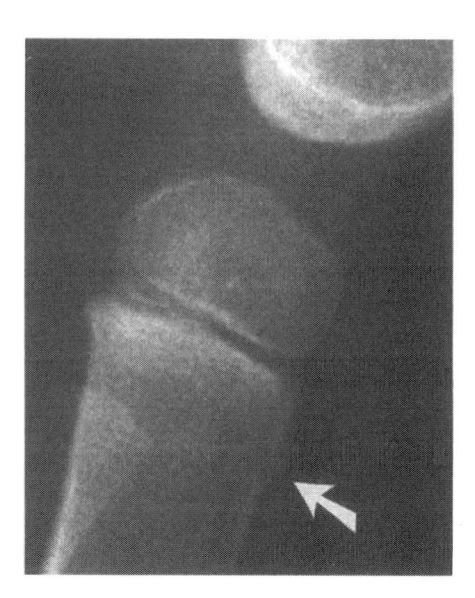

FIGURE 23-73. Toddler's fracture of the proximal metaphysis. The child had been limping for several days. Minimal buckling was evident (arrow).

stick fracture or bowing that may not be appreciated at the time of the original injury. Proximal metaphyseal fibular fractures are more likely to occur than are physeal/epiphyseal fractures.

Classification

The primary injury patterns are torus (compression) fractures and incomplete tension failure fractures (Figs. 23-74 to 23-76). Displaced, complete fractures are more common in the older child or adolescent.

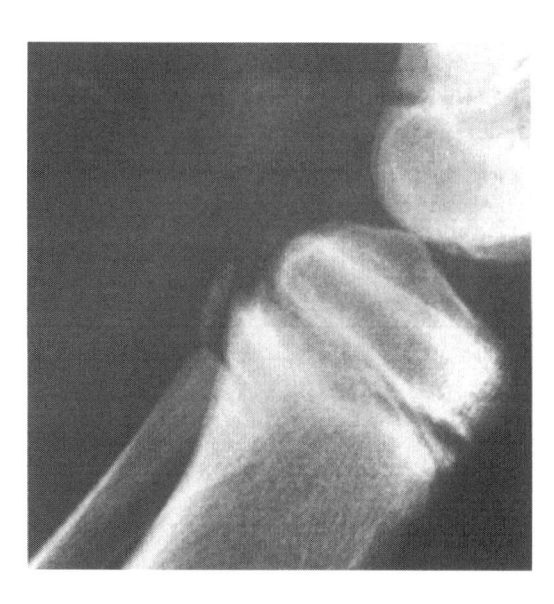

FIGURE 23-72. Appearance of a proximal tibial metaphyseal fracture 7 months after the injury.

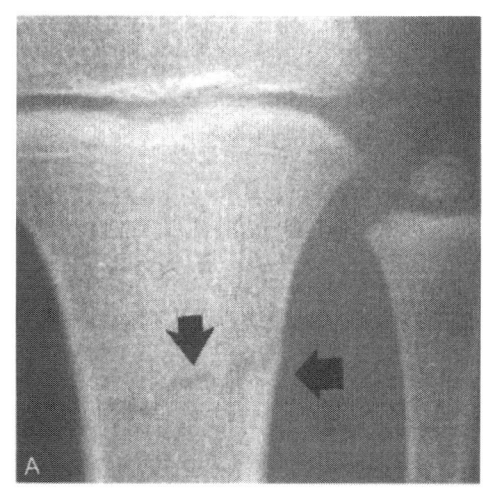

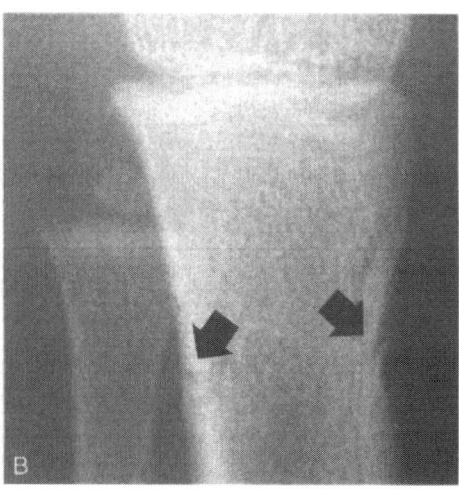

FIGURE 23-74. (A) Undisplaced proximal tibial fracture (arrow). (B) Lateral view, in which mild recurvatum (arrows) is evident.

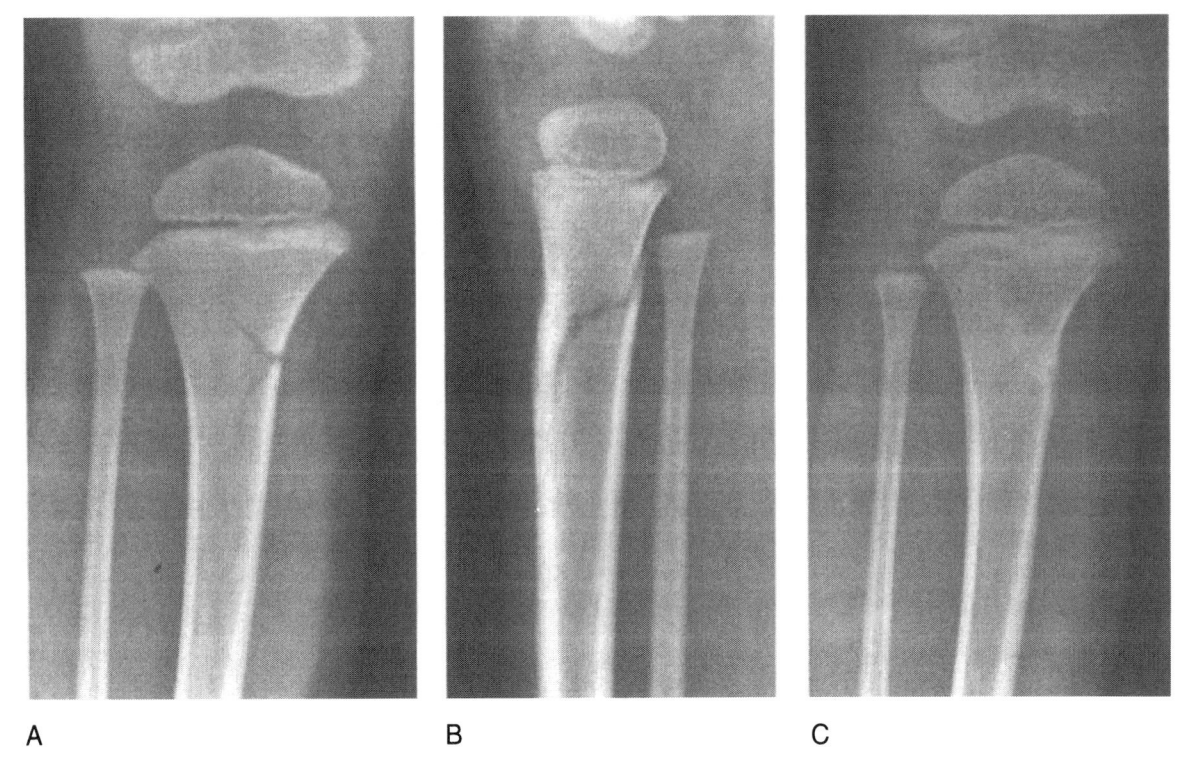

FIGURE 23-75. (A, B) Anteroposterior and lateral views of incomplete (greenstick) fracture. (C) Seven weeks later the fracture is minimally evident. *The tibia is already in valgus.*

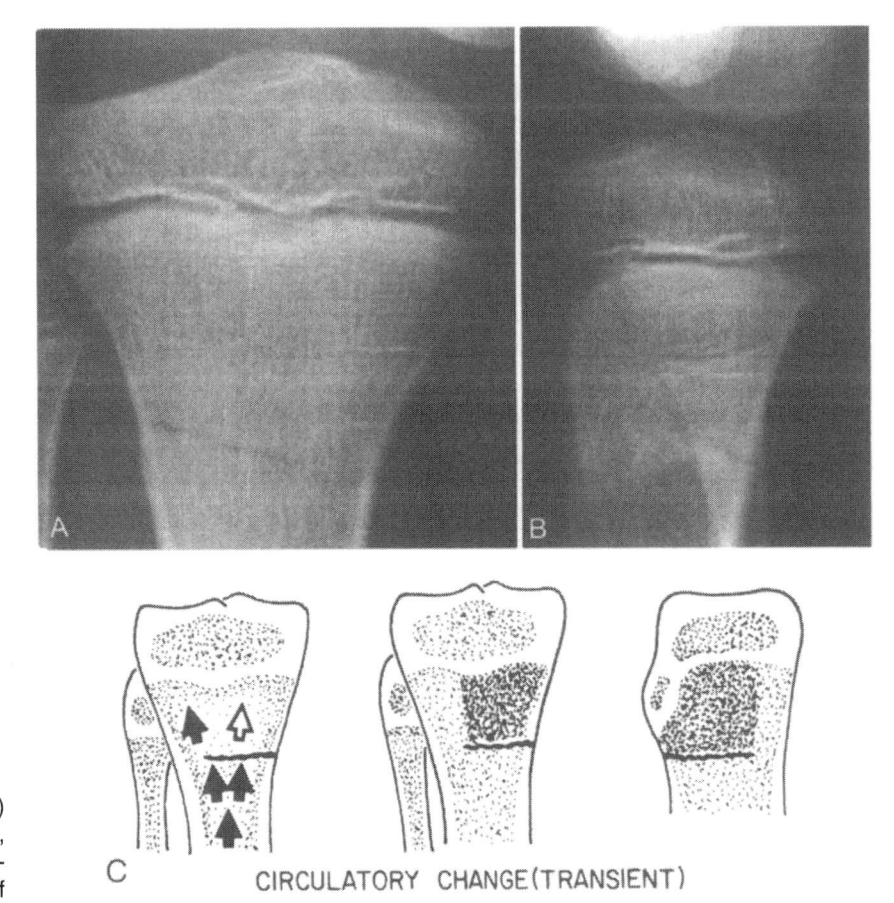

FIGURE 23-76. (A) Undisplaced fracture. (B) Two weeks later extensive sclerosis is present, suggesting temporary impairment of the metaphyseal vascular supply. (C) Schematic of the injury.

CIRCULATORY CHANGE (TRANSIENT)

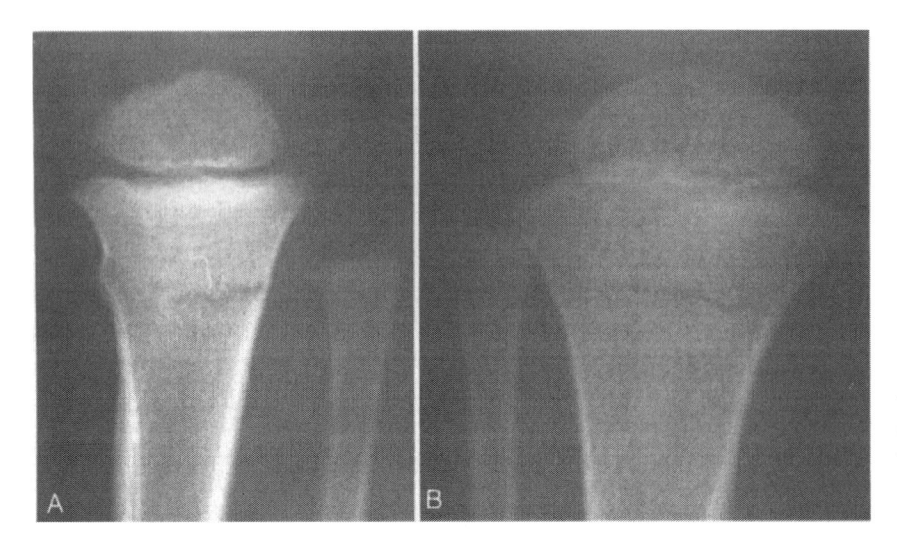

FIGURE 23-77. (A) Torus medial cortex fracture with lateral tensile failure. There is mild varus deformity. (B) Undisplaced medial tensile failure. This injury is deceptive in that it has a high risk of developing medial overgrowth and progressive valgus deformity.

The typical injury pattern associated with progressive angulation is a greenstick, transversely oriented fracture extending one-half to two-thirds of the way across the proximal tibial metaphysis. The lateral medial tibial metaphyseal cortex, when intact, may exhibit some plastic deformation. An underemphasized aspect of the injury is that the diaphyseal or metaphyseal fibula may also sustain plastic deformation or bowing. The tibial fracture may be separated 1–2 mm at the medial cortex, or it may be undisplaced. The fracture line may propagate completely across the proximal metaphysis. There may or may not be an accompanying metaphyseal fracture of the fibula. Robert et al. found that approximately 50% of their patients had concomitant fractures of the fibula; and in many cases they were greenstick fractures.[348] No matter what the fracture pattern, even if it is complete or displaced, there is a tendency for these fractures to progress to increased valgus during the weeks to months following the original injury.

Diagnosis

Roentgenographic diagnosis should include oblique views or even fluoroscopy, which may allow a better appreciation of any acute valgus deformity because of a greenstick component of the medial side (Fig. 23-77). The valgus may not be evident on the routine anteroposterior view. Magnification views may better reveal minimal cortical buckling.

The diagnosis is not always easy. Small children may limp or even refuse to bear weight on the involved extremity. Examination may reveal a tender area over the proximal tibial metaphysis.

Treatment

Treatment may include correction of any lateral (valgus) angulation by manipulative reduction and immobilization in a long leg cast for 4–6 weeks. It may be possible to reduce the greenstick component by bending the leg toward the angulation and slightly overcorrecting the deformity, as with a fracture of the radius and ulna. However, complete correction may *not* be possible because of the plastic cortical deformation. *Such retained change should not be considered the cause of any progressive medial overgrowth leading to increased valgus deformity.*

Displaced fractures in older children and adolescents should be reduced. So long as the normal longitudinal axial relations of proximal and distal fragments are maintained, mild displacement may be accepted. The reduction is checked at weekly intervals for the first 3 weeks to be certain that reduction is not lost.

Results

Fractures of the proximal tibial metaphysis in children are not generally associated with major complications such as nonunion or compartment syndrome. This observation has led to the concept of a relatively innocuous fracture pattern. However, these injuries *frequently* lead to significant valgus angulation (Fig. 23-78) through subsequent skeletal growth.[305,308–314,316–320,322–324,326–330,332,334,335,337–341,343–356,358,360–362,364,368,369] The causal mechanisms are not completely understood, particularly when associated with minimal displacement of the fracture.[325] Cozen reported four patients with relatively minor fractures of the proximal tibial metaphysis in whom valgus deformities subsequently developed.[318,319] In two patients there was no initial displacement. None of the patients was allowed out of a cast early, nor was there any radiographic evidence of malfunction in the physis.

As with overgrowth of the femur following a mid-diaphyseal injury in a skeletally immature patient, increased valgus angulation of the tibia is most likely to occur following injury in the 3- to 10-year-old age group. Although frequent, it does not occur in every case. The extent of angulation and the time of progression vary in each case. An angulation increase may begin several weeks after injury but appears to be time-limited, usually not increasing after 18–24 months following the original injury (12 months or less in most reported cases).

Valgus deformity is a time-limited phenomenon that leads to an initial angulation that is later stabilized. The deformity usually develops within 6–18 months, depending on skeletal age, implying that the deformity may occur rapidly (Fig. 23-79). Subsequently, further angular deformity (progression) is slow or is less likely to occur at all. Jackson and Cozen described 10 patients with valgus deformity.[334] The earliest deformity was observed at 10–11 weeks, but more commonly it was not seen for 20–40 weeks after the injury. All the tibial

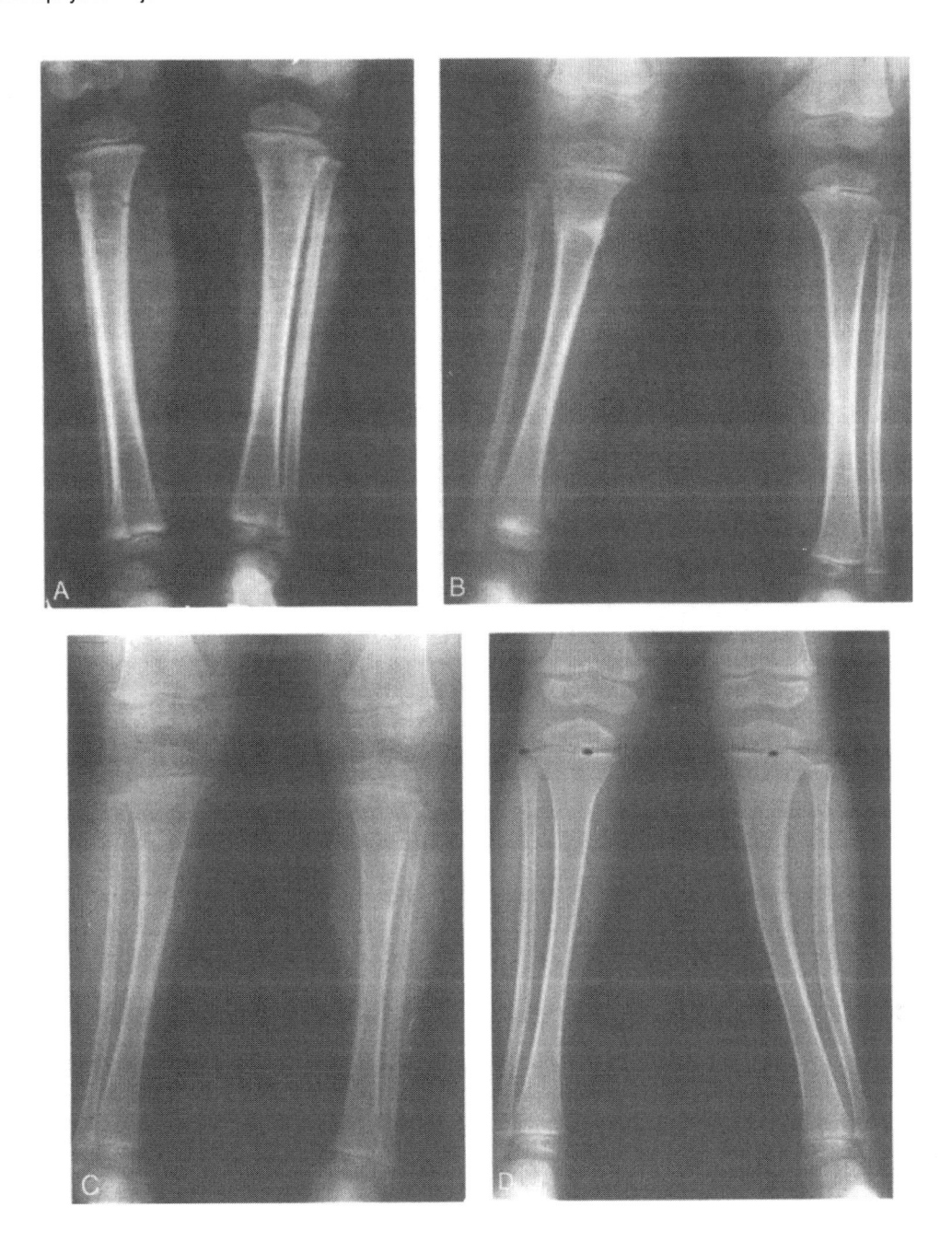

FIGURE 23-78. (A) Undisplaced fracture. (B) Healing with slight valgus deformity at 5 weeks. (C) Valgus at 15 weeks. (D) Progression of valgus at 6 months.

fractures were undisplaced. Of the 10 fractures, 8 were greenstick; the fibula was fractured in three and intact in seven. In no instance was there any evidence of injury to the proximal tibial physis, either initially or during subsequent evaluation. Of the 10 children, 8 had overgrowth of the involved tibia of 1.3 cm or more, and in each of these children there was more than 15° of genu valgum. The amount of valgus deformity ranged from 5° to 25° more than the opposite side. The two patients with the mildest deformities had less than 1.3 cm of overgrowth in the fractured tibia.

The etiology has been discussed extensively, with several theories being proposed. Taylor suggested overgrowth as the cause of valgus, but it was minimally documented.[358] Green reported a case with a proximal Harris growth slowdown line and stated that because it was not parallel to the physis there was more growth medially than laterally.[326] Ogden has suggested that the normal pattern of a more extensive medial geniculate blood supply, compared to the lateral geniculate supply, was a significant factor in such eccentric growth, a concept supported by quantitative scintigraphic studies.[343] This has been substantiated by others.[315]

Cozen thought that there was asymmetric simulation of the physis, with the tibia growing faster than the fibula, provided the fibula had not been fractured.[318–320] Ogden et al. did not find a significant difference in length measurements of the fibula versus the lateral tibia in the injured limb.[343] In most patients the fibula on the injured side grew more than the contralateral fibula.

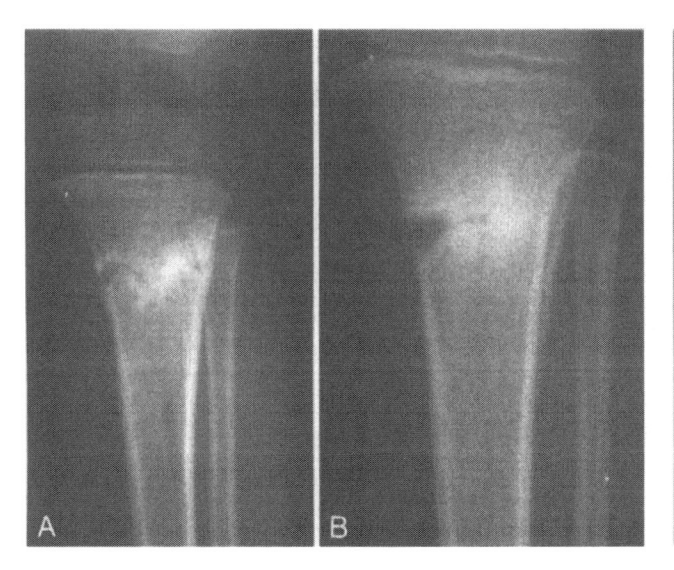

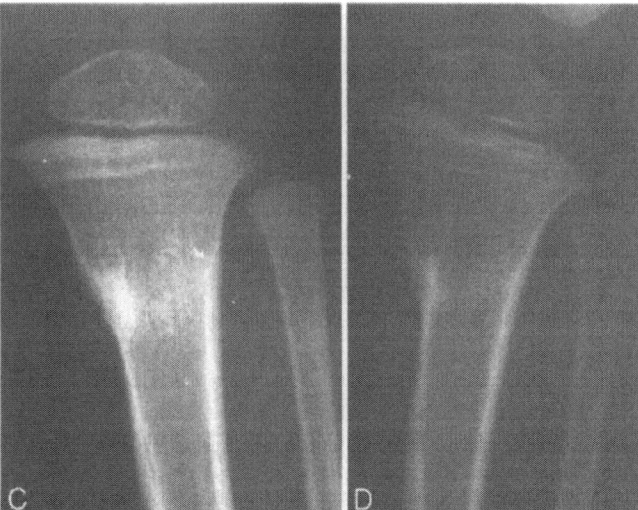

FIGURE 23-79. (A) Metaphyseal fracture in a 3-year-old child that involved medial *and* lateral cortices. No valgus deformity was evident. (B) Appearance 8 weeks after injury. Valgus deformity is already present, and the medial physis-to-physis distance is 2 mm more on the right than on the left. (C) Eight months later the medial side of the tibial shaft is 5 mm longer than the contralateral medial side, whereas the lateral measurements are equal, suggesting selective medial longitudinal overgrowth. (D) Appearance 2 years later. The parents chose not to have it treated until the child is older. (C, D) Note the eccentric growth indicated by the Harris line.

Blount suggested that there might be partial stimulation of the upper tibial metaphysis and that the iliotibial band acted as a bowstring following incomplete fracture.[313] Lehner and Dubas thought that the callus formation in the fracture site forced the fragments apart.[339] Salter and Best believed that the valgus was "preexistent"; that is, there was incomplete reduction or residual plastic deformation in the greenstick portion.[352,353] However, it certainly is recognized that nondisplaced fractures may have the same complication.

The most likely explanation is selective overgrowth of the medial portion of the proximal tibial physis. This region is normally more active in the young child as a mechanism of spontaneously changing the genu varum of infancy to the genu valgum of adolescence. Arteriography in skeletally immature cadavers (Fig. 23-80) showed increased primary and collateral (geniculate) vascularity to the medial proximal tibia compared to the vascularity of the lateral proximal tibia. This finding implies that any increased, fracture-induced arterial inflow probably brings a greater inflow medially, thus stimulating endochondral ossification on a temporary basis. This increased vascularity seems the most likely explanation for the medial overgrowth, especially as it appears to be time-limited. With the use of quantitative scintigraphy, selective increased medial activity has been demonstrated concisely.

Measurements of physis-to-physis distance along the medial and lateral sides of injured and uninjured tibias corroborate medial overgrowth, as observed by the growth slowdown lines (Fig. 23-81). Fifteen children with unilateral proximal tibial metaphyseal fractures, one child with bilateral proximal tibial metaphyseal fractures, and one bilaterally injured child with a tibial proximal metaphyseal fracture and a contralateral mid-diaphyseal tibial fracture were followed 2–7 years after injury to document increased valgus angulation of the tibia and the probable causal mechanism.[343]

Detailed measurements of the metaphyseal/diaphyseal/metaphyseal distances medially and laterally on the injured and noninjured sides were documented. In four patients there was comparable growth on the medial and lateral sides of the uninjured tibia that was equal to that of the lateral side of the injured tibia, whereas the medial distance of the injured tibia was longer than the lateral distance. In 11 patients there was overgrowth of both the medial and lateral sides of the injured tibia that was always longer on the medial than the lateral side. In the patient with bilateral metaphyseal

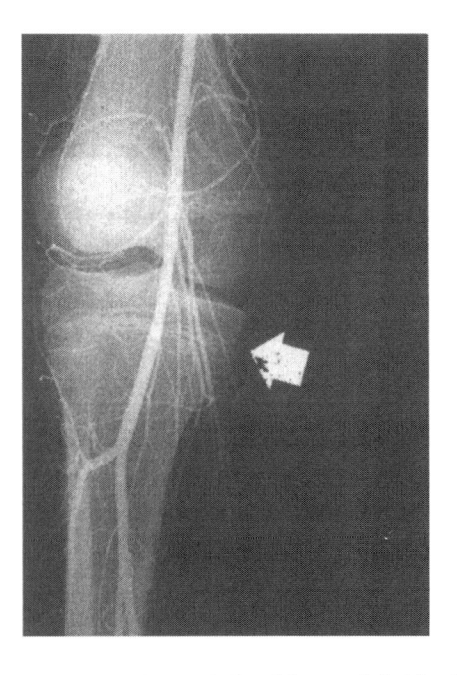

FIGURE 23-80. Increased vascularity of the medial side of the proximal tibial metaphysis.

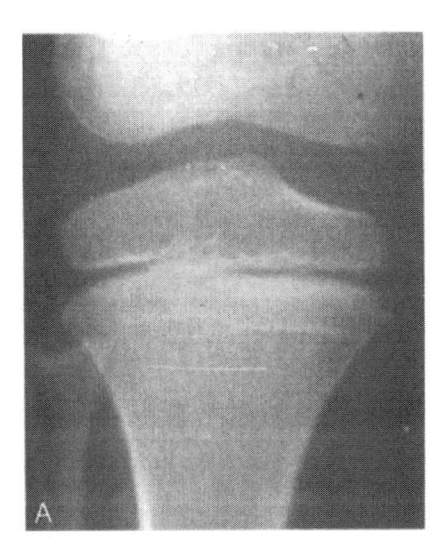

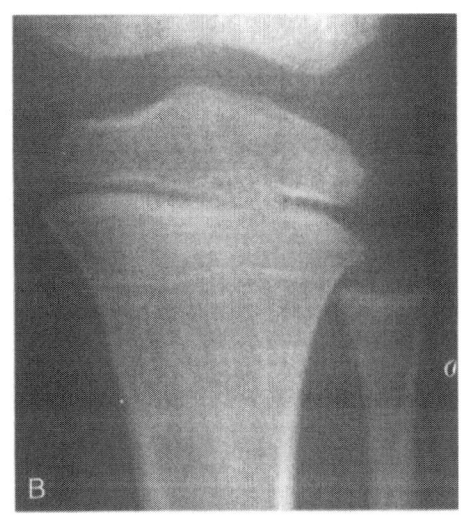

FIGURE 23-81. Growth slowdown lines show differential growth as the most likely cause of valgus. (A) Uninjured side. (B) Injured side.

fractures the medial length exceeded the lateral length in both tibias, but was asymmetric in terms of angulation and difference. In the child with metaphyseal and diaphyseal fractures, the medial side of the tibia with the metaphyseal fracture was the longest of the four measurements. In five of six patients with Harris lines, there was demonstrable distal and proximal tibial metaphyseal overgrowth, but it was always parallel to the physis and did not contribute to the valgus angulation. Thus there was not only generalized increased growth proximally and distally, there also was an eccentric proximal medial overgrowth in every patient.

Part of the fracture healing response is a temporary reactive hyperemia.[342,365,366] When hyperemia is directed at the generalized region of the metaphysis to heal the fracture, the increased vascularity of the geniculate vessels on the medial versus the lateral side undoubtedly results in a relative increase in the circulation to the medial growth plate, especially compared to the lateral side. It could stimulate temporary overgrowth, much like arteriovenous malformations and monoarticular (e.g., knee) juvenile-onset rheumatoid arthritis have been noted to stimulate overgrowth. Certainly studies corroborate an overgrowth phenomenon that, in some cases, involved even the distal tibial growth plate. They showed that there was increased growth at the lateral and the medial side of the injured proximal tibia when compared to that on the opposite side.

The data of Ogden et al. strongly suggested that the progressive valgus angulation is an *accelerated physiologic response*.[343] The age range in which children seem to be susceptible to developing the "complication" also coincides with the time period, as demonstrated by Salenius and Vankka,[14] in which they are gradually shifting from a physiologic genu varum to genu valgum. Accordingly, the physis of the proximal tibia is being normally "directed" toward the establishment of the knee valgus posture typical of most humans.

Zionts et al. used quantitative bone scintigraphy 5 months following a proximal tibial fracture that also included a complete fracture of the fibula.[368] There was demonstrable and proportionally greater uptake on the medial side than on the lateral side; and the overall uptake of the injured side was greater than that on the uninjured side. They thought that it represented a relative increase in blood flow on that side.

Experimental studies with injury to the tibial shaft have shown an active response in the physis.[365,366] This response may be partially mediated through periosteal damage.[331] The phenomenon has also been described as a complication after resection of a medial osteochondroma without an associated fracture.[360]

Aronson et al., who created metaphyseal defects and fractures in rabbits, showed that there was a phenomenon of overgrowth but could find no specific asymmetric widening of the zones of the medial versus the lateral zones of the growth plate.[307] Frey, using an experimental model in the mini-pig, thought that there was an unreduced primary valgus deformity that resulted in a secondary partial medial stimulation of the growth plate.[324] Alpar, who created diaphyseal fractures in rats,[306] noted that the growth plate cells were stimulated by a mitogenic activator (growth factor). He believed that the overgrowth of long bones in children following fracture was due to a local mitogenic stimulating factor or factors and not due to an increased blood supply. Taylor et al. showed that there was generalized cellular proliferation in the growth plates of immature rats following tibial osteotomies.[357]

The discrepancy in growth may also result from the fibula exerting a tethering effect laterally, while the medial side becomes hyperemic in response to the fracture. Taylor thought that the deformity occurred because of temporary stimulation of the tibial epiphysis and physis concomitant with a tethering effect from the fibula.[358] This deformity has been observed following fractures, but it has also occurred at the proximal tibial metaphysis consequent to surgery and osteomyelitis.

Another possible cause of the deformity might be the restraining influence of the iliotibial band, which has been described as a deforming power in poliomyelitis.[319,333] Its influence on healing fractures may be similar, although it is hypothetical.

The possibility of mild retardation of growth at the lateral side of the tibial physis must also be considered, as these frac-

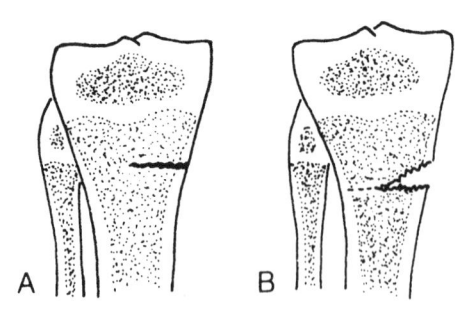

MEDIAL TENSILE / LATERAL COMPRESSIVE
FAILURE

FIGURE 23-82. (A, B) Medial failure in tension and lateral failure in compression.

tures often involve breaks in the medial cortex that may or may not extend all the way across the transverse diameter of the shaft or proximally toward the physis (Fig. 23-82). It is possible that the lateral physis absorbs more of the compression and has a temporary type 5 injury. This complication occurred in two patients in whom the anterior portion of the upper tibial epiphysis and physis closed prematurely as a complication of a tibial shaft fracture. Progressive hyperextension deformities developed in both patients.

Genu valgum might be due to the interposition of a flap of fibrous tissue consisting of the pes anserinus and the avulsed periosteum. The ensuing biomechanical disturbance would induce bowing of the shaft and asymmetric growth at both ends of the bone. Weber reported two cases of fresh fracture that were treated by surgical removal of the fibrous tissue from the gap.[364] Bassey emphasized Weber's idea of pes anserinus interposition.[310] Brougham and Nicol operated on a 2-year-old boy with a fracture of the proximal metaphysis and removed a large periosteal and soft tissue flap from the fracture site. Despite this maneuver, significant valgus deformity developed over the next 22 months.[314] They suggested that the interposed tissue was not the cause of the deformity. I agree.

The periosteum has an intrinsic tensile force within it that has an effect on physeal growth.[321,359,363,367] Damage to this structure may be a factor allowing the overgrowth. Houghton and Rooker transected the medial periosteum and created valgus deformity.[331] Kery et al. experimentally induced diaphyseal fractures in rabbits and showed that there was responsive widening of the growth plates.[336] There was more dramatic widening of the growth plate after fracture and less widening after periosteal stripping without fracture, suggesting that trauma, in and of itself, causes some type of proliferative response.

Prevention of the deformity is probably impossible. It may be plausible to immobilize these fractures in slight varus position, anticipating the propensity to valgus postion. The exact incidence of this complication is unknown, and overreduction, in anticipation, could lead to loss of the normal valgus angle.

The deformity may develop despite acceptable reduction and rapid consolidation of the fracture (Figs. 23-78, 23-79). Secondary treatment may be required to correct the valgus deformity and overgrowth.[303] Because it is progressive primarily during its initial phase, lessening of the deformity may be accomplished by means of a long leg brace. A valgus-knee orthosis may be appropriate to accelerate correction.[334] Once the deformity is well established and appears to be stable, corrective osteotomy may be considered. It should be noted that if osteotomy is undertaken, there may be a consequent recurrent deformity. Surgery that in essence duplicates the original fracture may elicit a similar physiologic response. Medial epiphysiodesis or stapling is not usually indicated unless there is an osseous bar or cartilaginous growth arrest.

Zionts and MacEwen showed that among seven patients six experienced spontaneous correction of the deformity by developing an S-shaped tibia (Fig. 23-83) to realign the growth plate.[368,369] In no patient did the deformity continue to progress for more than 17 months after injury, and in most patients the deformity was spontaneously corrected by then.[369]

In none of our patients did true tibia valgum improve spontaneously.[343] However, eccentric growth distally led to realignment of the ankle joint toward its normal parallel alignment with the floor and the knee. Furthermore, latitudinal growth (expansion) of the diaphyseal and metaphyseal cortices made the deformities less evident clinically.

Although often referred to as a deformation, this increased angulation appears to be a *natural consequence* of the injury that probably results from the mechanics of the fracture and the subsequent reparative response. To imply

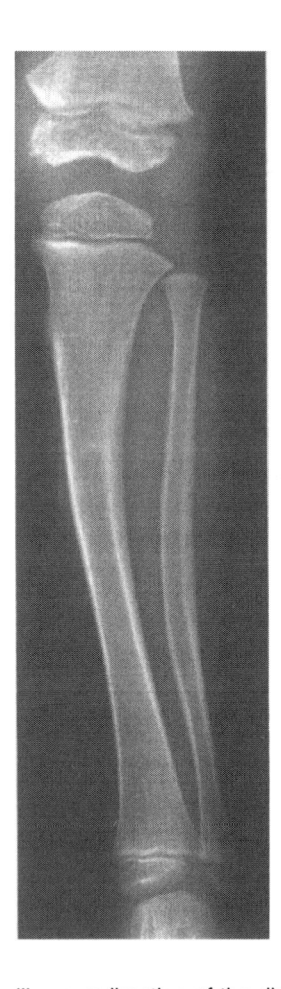

FIGURE 23-83. Curvilinear redirection of the distal tibia and fibula. This is a biologic response to realign the physes.

that the occurrence could have been unequivocally prevented or is a result of negligence on the part of the treating physician is usually inappropriate.

It is extremely important that the treating physician recognize that this problem may arise in any young patient with a proximal metaphyseal tibial fracture and, accordingly, warn the parents about the potential "problem," just as he or she would if there were specific injury to the growth plate. It should not be construed as a departure from the standard of care if this problem occurs, nor should it be construed as a deviation if the physician chooses not to complete the bowing or plastic deformation of a fracture by aggressively reversing the fracture deformity, which could create an unstable fracture. As stated previously, the angulation increase may arise even when the fracture is complete.

Proximal Fibular Metaphyseal Injuries

Proximal fibular metaphyseal injuries are usually associated with fractures of the proximal metaphysis or diaphysis of the tibia. Interventional treatment (i.e., surgery) is rarely necessary.

Diaphyseal Injuries

Injuries to the diaphyseal region vary considerably with both the age of the child and the mechanism of injury.[396] They may occur following a direct blow or a rotational, twisting force that is applied to the foot and subsequently transmitted along the tibial shaft. In the developing infant and young child, the dense cortical thickening and osteon formation have not evolved. Consequently, this region is more susceptible to injury as a child is going through the early phases of learning to walk (i.e., the toddler's fracture of the limping infant).

In infants and children, the typical injury is a spiral tibial fracture with an intact fibula. In children 3–6 years of age, a torsional stress similarly applied usually causes a spiral fracture of the tibia with or without a fracture of the fibula but more likely propagates proximally, which leads to a fracture through the proximal fibular metaphysis. It may be a greenstick fracture. As the child gets older (6–10 years), a more common injury is a simple transverse fracture, again with or without displacement and with or without injury to the fibula. This fracture usually is due to direct trauma (a tapping injury). During adolescence, athletic injuries result in more characteristic fractures in the junction of the middle and distal thirds of the tibia and fibula, frequently with the formation of a butterfly fragment. Ordinarily, the fracture fragments are held together by the thick periosteal sleeve, and displacement is minimal as most of these injuries are rotational stresses due to relatively low energy rather than direct blows with higher energy loads. There is usually intrinsic stability through the fibula with the low energy injuries.

Ahn et al. were able to produce a midshaft tibial fracture in 90% of their experimental animals.[370] This method, however, has not been used in skeletally immature animals.

Infants and Toddlers

Fracture of the tibia with an intact fibula during infancy (Fig. 23-84) and early childhood (Figs. 23-85, 23-86) is usually produced by torsional force, as when the child twists away or when the child is first learning to walk.[358] The resilience of the fibula makes it less susceptible to disruptive injury, although plastic deformation (bowing) may occur (Fig. 23-87). Because it is a torsional stress, the fibula is uniquely adapted through its joint mechanism proximally and syndesmosis distally to resist this type of stress. When deciding

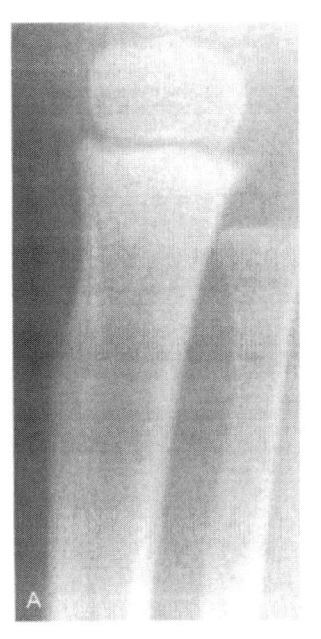

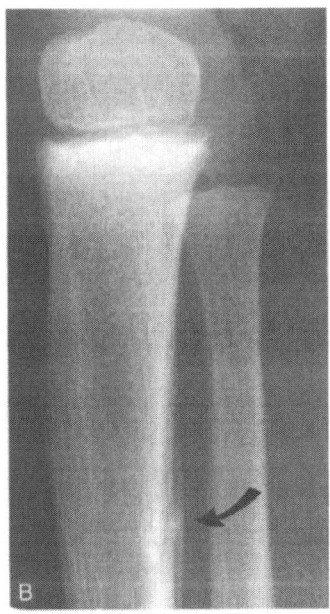

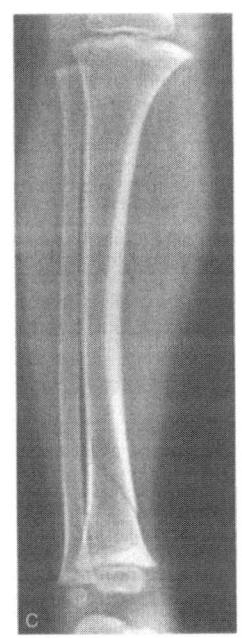

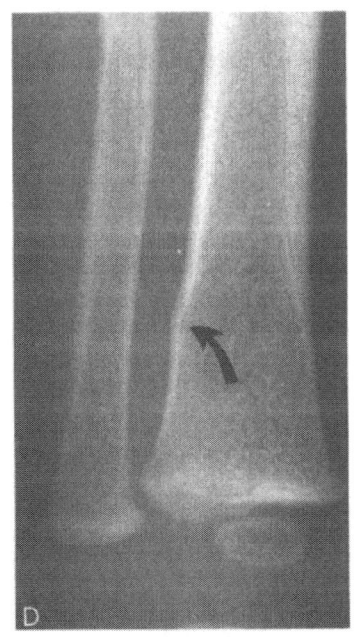

FIGURE 23-84. Toddler's fractures. (A) Normal roentgenogram 3 days after the onset of limping. No fracture is evident. (B) Two weeks later posterior callus is present (arrow). (C) Spiral fracture seen distally. (D) Minimal lateral torus injury (arrow).

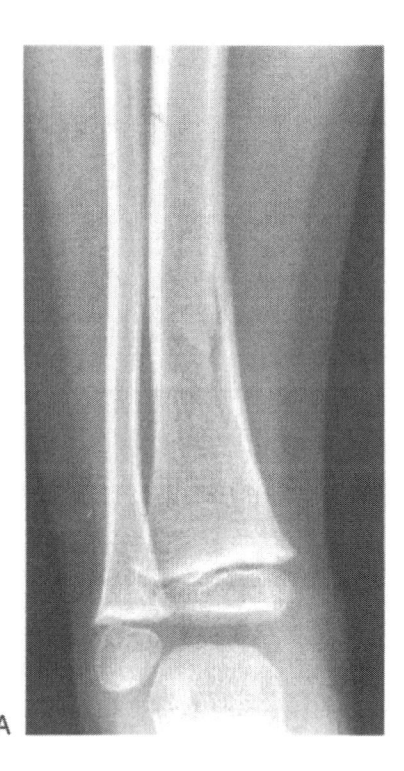

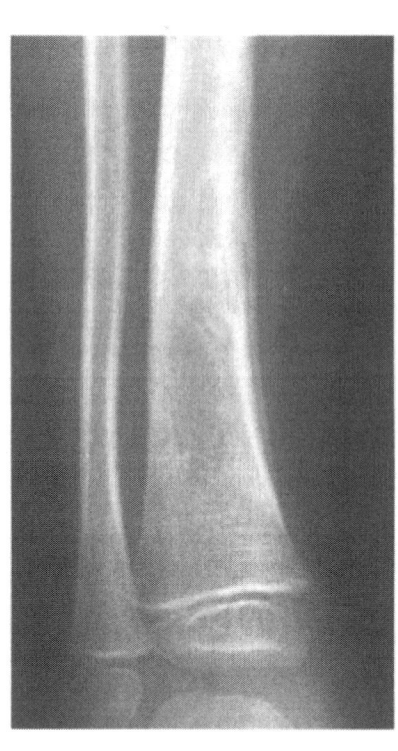

FIGURE 23-85. (A) Incomplete cortical fracture in a limping 2-year-old. (B) Appearance 7 weeks later.

on treatment, plastic deformation must be carefully assessed, as an apparently adequate reduction may be displaced by the intrinsic "spring" in the fibula.

Usually the child is irritable, cries frequently, refuses to walk or bear weight on the affected lower limb, or walks with an antalgic limp. Examination ordinarily shows no obvious

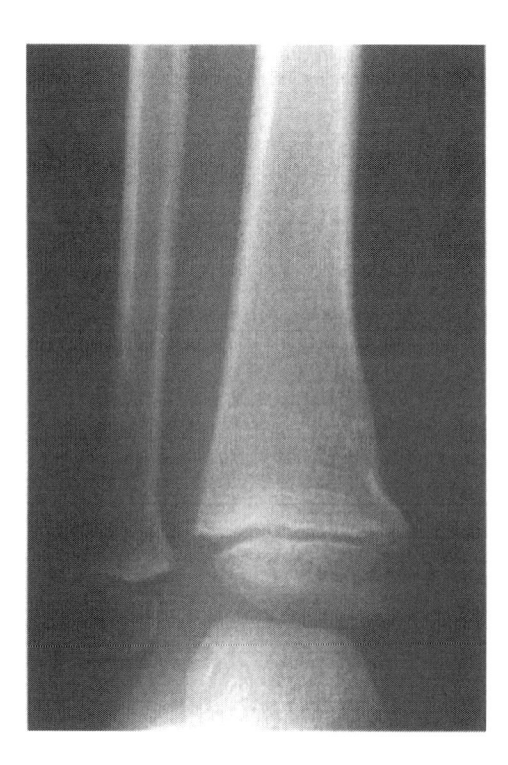

FIGURE 23-86. Buckling injury of the distal medial metaphysis. This toddler had been limping for 3 days.

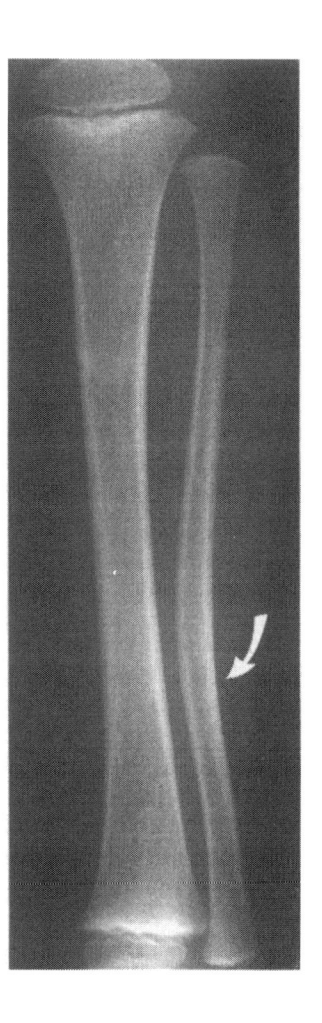

FIGURE 23-87. Another variation of toddler's fracture is greenstick bowing of the fibula (arrow), with no evidence of tibial injury.

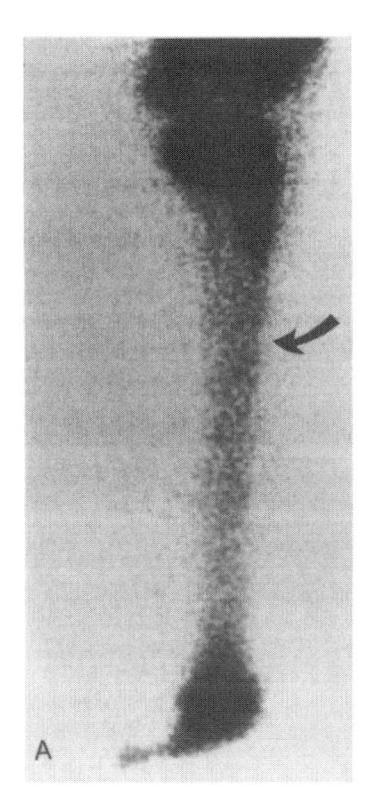

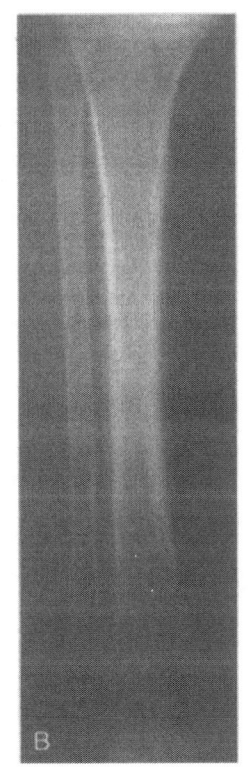

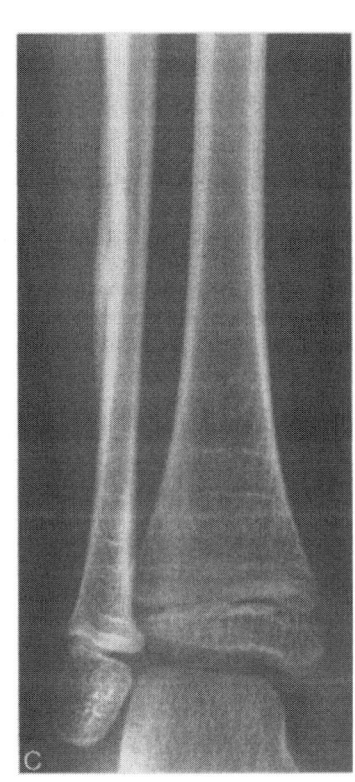

FIGURE 23-88. (A) Positive bone scan (arrow) 5 days after the onset of limping in a 15-month-old child. The routine radiographs were normal. (B) Reactive subperiosteal bone at 3 weeks. (C) Reactive bone along the fibula in an older child with limping and an initially normal film.

deformity, especially if there is minimal displacement. However, with palpation of the extremity, the area may be localized reasonably well. Although there is a tendency to evaluate the hip or foot in the limping child, the tibia should not be overlooked. The fracture may not always be evident at the time of the original injury and may not be obvious radiographically until 10–14 days later, when there is beginning callus formation or palpable thickening of the tibia (Fig. 23-88) due to the subperiosteal new bone formation. Even at this point, the hairline fracture may or may not be visualized. Care must be taken not to overinterpret the films as showing other lesions, such as osteomyelitis, eosinophilic granuloma, acute leukemia, or some other neoplastic lesion. Child abuse must be included in the differential diagnosis.

Treatment consists of immobilization in a long leg cast for 3 weeks. Treatment is often based on an empiric diagnosis. An infant suspected of having a "toddler's fracture" should be treated with effective immobilization. The child should be allowed to stand in the cast when comfortable, because it helps stimulate the bone remodeling necessary to strengthen the cortex and decrease the risk of further stress failure in the cortical bone.

Older Child

As the child grows and the midshaft tibial diaphysis progressively develops its characteristic midshaft thickening, fracture patterns change and there is a greater tendency toward fragmentation.[372,373,384,393,403,406,407] Spiral fracture patterns are relatively common (Fig. 23-89). The concomitant fibular response varies. There may be bowing, simple fracture, multiple fractures, or disruption of proximal (Fig. 23-90) or distal tibiofibular relations. Posterior displacement is also common.

Biggs et al. reviewed 65 tibial fractures in children and specifically looked at 25 that were isolated and not associated with a fracture of the fibula.[373] This one bone injury was prevalent in children under 11 years of age. They occurred after two types of force: indirect violence involving a torsional injury or an indirect twisting injury. The direct low velocity of violence tended to be a direct blow to the tibia (e.g., a football kick). In virtually all these injuries there was no change in the position of the bones over time.

Fractures of the tibia and fibula in older children and adolescents should be treated by closed reduction whenever possible, correcting both angular and rotational malalignment. The limb should be immobilized in a long leg cast, with the knee flexed to approximately 90°. Flexion is necessary to control rotation and to prevent, or at least discourage, the child from bearing weight. The child should be immobilized for a minimum of 6–8 weeks accompanied by progressive weight-bearing. Adolescents may require longer periods of casting.

During adolescence, unstable fractures may be difficult to hold and may require some sort of pins and plaster technique, closed reduction with a temporary external fixator,

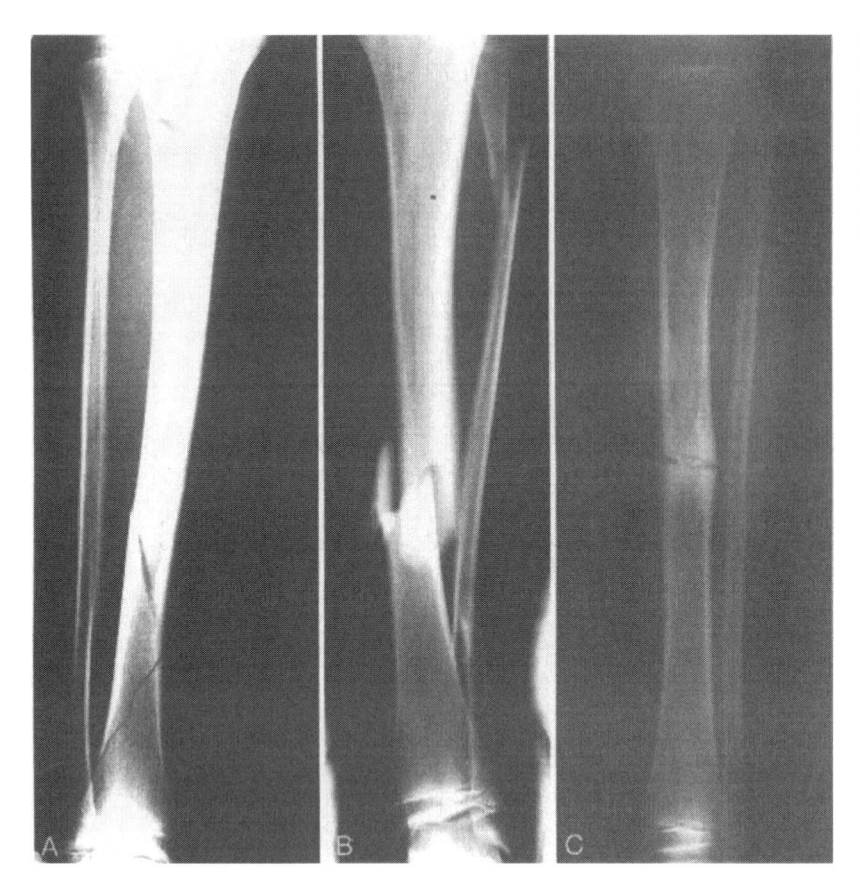

FIGURE 23-89. Typical fracture patterns of the tibial diaphysis. (A) Spiral fracture. (B) Relatively oblique injury, with concomitant double fracture of the fibula. Note that the distal tibial fragment is in valgus deformity, whereas the midfibular fragment is in varus deformity. *Both* must be corrected during treatment. (C) Transverse "tapping" fracture sustained by a direct blow to the tibia.

closed reduction with medullary pinning, or even open reduction with appropriate skeletal fixation.[381,394,405,410]

Open Injuries

Open fracture of the tibia is probably the most common open fracture in children, except for lawn mower injuries of the foot.[374,375,377,378,379,383,385,388,390,391,393,395,402,415] Management of the soft tissue trauma often takes precedence over immediate fracture treatment. Débridement must be done meticulously, with an effort to protect the periosteum, as this tissue is instrumental in fracture healing.

Various external fixators are available. Marsh et al. studied the use of unilateral external fixation until healing with a dynamic axial fixator for severe open tibial fractures.[388] Dagher and Roukoz reported on open tibial fractures with bone loss treated by the Ilizarov technique and transportation.[379] The choice of device should be at the discretion of the treating surgeon. The principles of rigid fixation applied to the adult are less necessary in the child with a more resilient skeleton.

Buckley et al. studied open fractures of the tibia in children.[374] There were 41 children with 42 open injuries of either the tibial metaphysis or diaphysis; 12 were type I, 18 type II, 6 type IIIA, 4 type IIIB, and 2 type IIIC according to the classification of Gustilo. All fractures were irrigated and débrided, and antibiotics were given for a minimum of 48 hours. Twenty fractures were initially treated with external fixation and twenty-two with immobilization in a cast. Three patients had an early wound infection, one of which was associated with osteomyelitis. All infections were treated successfully. The average time to healing of the fracture was 5 months (range 2–21 months). The time to union related to the severity of the soft tissue injury, the pattern of the fracture, the amount of segmental bone loss, the occurrence of infection, and the use of external fixation. Six patients had delayed union, and four patients had an angular malunion of more than 10°, although it spontaneously corrected in three. One patient had a progressive valgus deformity (this patient had a proximal metaphyseal fracture). Four patients treated with external fixation and end-to-end bone apposition had more than 1 cm of overgrowth. The incidences of compartment syndrome, vascular injury, infection, and delayed union were similar to those reported for open tibial fractures in adults.

Hope and Cole, describing open fractures of the tibia in children, reviewed the treatment results of 92 children; 22 with type I, 51 with type II, and 19 with type III Gustilo injuries.[385] All patients received tetanus prophylaxis, systemic antibiotics for 48 hours, and thorough débridement and irrigation of the wound. Altogether 51 wounds with minimal soft tissue injury were closed primarily; the other 41 initially were left open. In the latter group, 18 small wounds were allowed to heal secondarily, and 23 larger wounds required split-thickness skin grafts or soft tissue, local, or microvascular free-flaps. Stable fractures were reduced and immobilized in above-knee casts (71%). External fixation (28%) was used in patients with unstable fractures, extensive soft tissue injury, or multiple injuries. Short-term complications included compartment syndrome (4%), superficial infection (8%), deep infection (3%), delayed union (16%), nonunion (7.5%), and malunion (6.5%). The incidences were similar to those reported for adults. Selective primary closure of wounds did not increase the incidence of infection. External fixation was associated with a greater occurrence of delayed or nonunion than cast immobilization, but it should be remembered that this technique was used most often for the most severe injuries. Late review at 1.5–9.8 years showed a large incidence of continuing morbidity, including pain at the healed fracture site and 50% restriction of athletic activities, 23% joint stiffness, 23% cosmetic defects, and 23% minor leg length discrepancies. Hope and Cole thought that open tibial fractures in children were associated with a high incidence of early and late complications, which are much more frequent in children with Gustilo type III injuries. They found that children over the age of 8 years and particularly those closer to the end of skeletal maturation appeared to be more susceptible to delayed and nonunion than younger children. However, older children also were more likely to sustain type II and III injuries than the younger children.

Kreder and Armstrong reviewed 56 open tibial fractures in 55 children.[386] Four patients died during the treatment owing to injuries of the chest and abdomen. Four amputations were necessary. Neurovascular compromise was significant with four of eight compromised extremities in seven patients requiring amputation. Infection occurred in eight injuries. The most important variables were neurovascular injury and delay in getting the patient to surgery. A delay of more than 6 hours was correlated with a 25% infection rate compared with a 12% infection rate for those operated before 6 hours. The most significant factor affecting the union time was the age of the patient.

Cierny and Zorn described the use of the Ilizarov to transport bone for replacement in segmental defects.[375] They found that a comparison between transport versus massive cancellous grafts and tissue transfers resulted in complications in one-third of the Ilizarov patients and two-thirds of the graft patients.

Sadasivan et al. studied the anatomic variations of the blood supply to the soleus muscle and found that there were two vascular patterns.[401] Type I had a segmental posterior tibial artery. Type II had a proximally dominant posterior tibial artery. The latter pattern had fewer segmental branches into the muscle. The authors thought that a distally based flap should not be used if a type II vascular pattern was encountered and also that vascular cross-connections between the two halves of the muscle should be preserved whenever possible.

Vascularity of the Tibial Diaphysis

Oni et al. devised an experimental rabbit model, producing fractures of the tibia.[392] Soft tissue damage was assessed visually and by vascular radiography. Transverse fractures produced circumferential laceration of the periosteum and complete transection of the marrow, and spiral fractures produced longitudinal periosteal laceration and incomplete marrow damage. Oni et al. thought that the results indicated that soft tissue damage in transverse fractures may be qualitatively different from that in spiral fractures. Perfusion studies revealed that although the nutrient artery may be interrupted by fractures the main trunks on either side of and up to the fracture line may still be filled by available collateral channels.[376,408]

Wallace et al. studied quantitative early-phase scintigraphy for predicting healing of tibial fractures.[414] In previous studies, they showed a relation between fracture site activity (region A), activity in adjacent normal bone (region C), and time to union. The predicted value of the A/C ratio of the image obtained after injection of technetium was studied. They noted significant differences in absolute uptake and the A/C ratio in three different groups based on treatment but found that the differences were not related to the time to union. The prediction of fracture union with this technique was not reliable.

Triffitt et al. assessed the effects of cast immobilization on tibial diaphyseal blood flow.[411] They found that there were no significant differences in the flows to the tibial diaphysis or contiguous skeletal muscle between the immobilized and control groups after either 1 or 2 weeks. They thought that immobilization had no major effect on tibial blood flow over

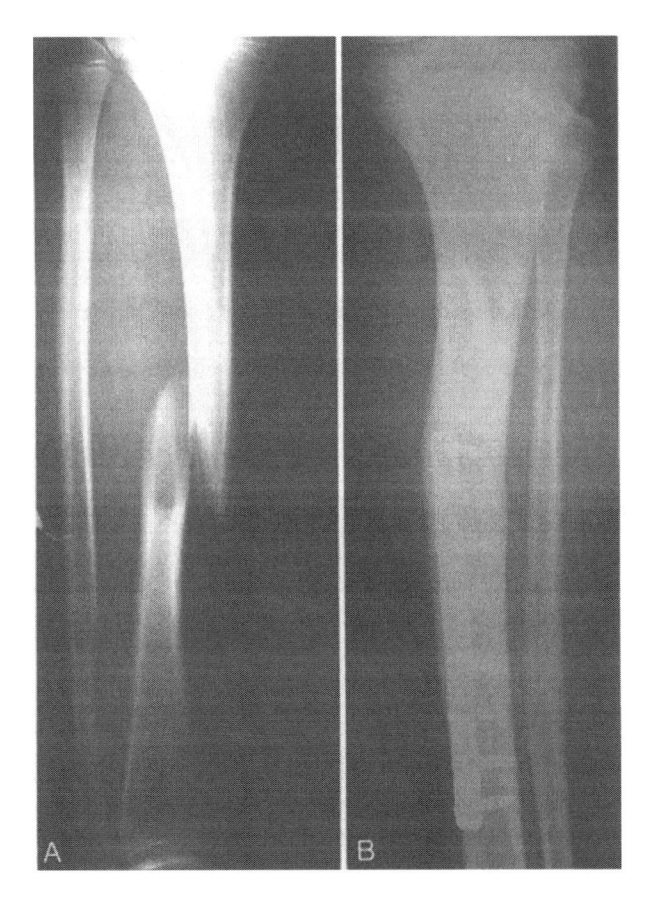

FIGURE 23-90. (A) Displaced tibial fracture. The fibula appears intact, but a proximal tibiofibular dislocation was present. (B) It was treated by open reduction of the tibia, with closed reduction of the tibiofibular dislocation. This is a pediatric version of the Maisonneuve injury.

and above the systemic effects of the fracture. In a similar study, MacDonald and Pittford studied blood flow changes in the tibia during external loading in adolescent and mature rabbits.[389] They found that when loading (weight-bearing) the tibia, the effects were an increase in blood flow on the tensile side of the injury and a decrease in flow on the compression side.

Ashcroft et al. used positron emission tomography (PET) to measure blood flow in tibial fracture patients (adults).[371] They established that there was increased tibial blood flow to the fracture site as early as 24 hours after injury, and that it reached up to 14 times that in the normal side by 2 weeks. Whether similar findings occur in children is unknown, but it is likely.

Results

In a study of 234 tibial shaft fractures that included 79 children with adequate follow-up, the average healing for 61 closed fractures was 3.26 months.[373] The average healing rate of all open fractures in children, most of whom were adolescents, was 5.47 months. The longest healing rates were in those fractures that occurred in the distal third of the tibial shaft. The next longest healing rate was in fractures located in the proximal third of the tibial shaft, and the most favorable healing rate was in midshaft fractures. Segmental fractures exhibited a slow rate of healing, even in children.

Complications

Angular union in a varus or valgus position may disrupt normal knee-ankle mechanics and should be restored to appropriate angular relations. If chronic pain occurs, corrective osteotomy may be necessary. Anteroposterior angular union may be less of a problem, although knee-ankle relations may be affected. If the fracture is in the midshaft, spontaneous correction may not occur, although new bone forms anteriorly (Fig. 23-91). It is most interesting that although the deformity of the midshaft may remain, the physes usually realign to the normal axial response patterns.[398]

Open injuries, especially with loss of some bone, may require subsequent bone grafting. However, this grafting should be done only when the soft tissue injury is healed and there is no evidence of complicating osseous or soft tissue. Quantitative bacteriology may be used to determine appropriate timing. Longer segmental loss may be treated by bone transport (either uniaxial or Ilizarov).

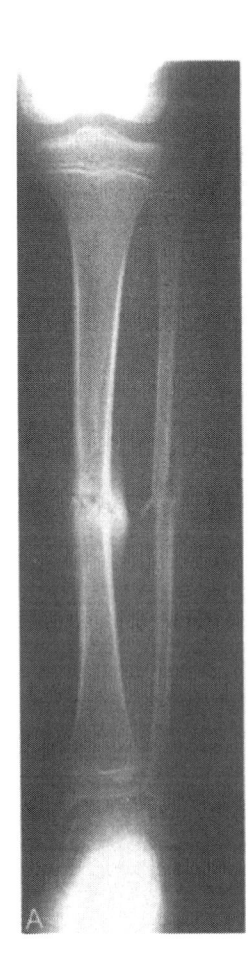

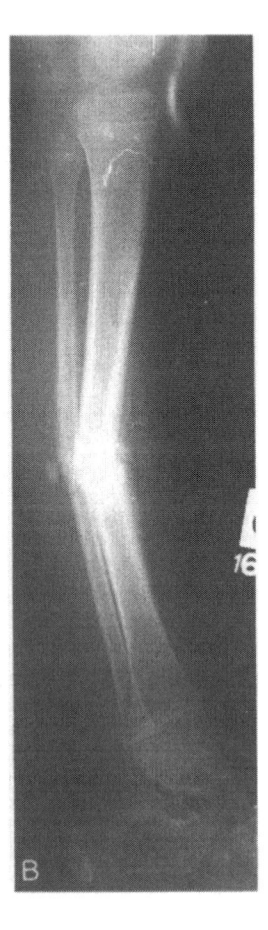

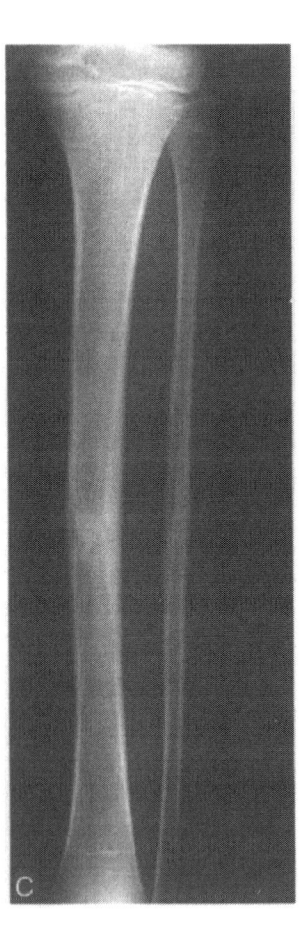

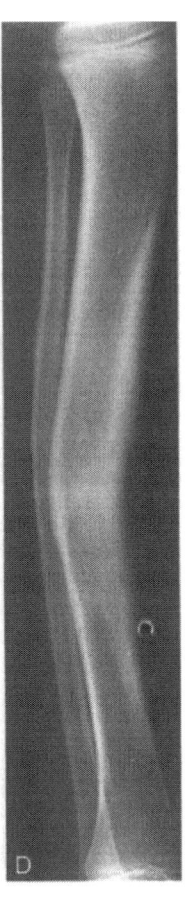

FIGURE 23-91. (A, B) Tibiofibular fractures in a child with head injury and severe spasticity. The recurvatum recurred each time closed reduction was attempted. (C, D) Thirty months later remodeling is complete in the anterior plane, and the recurvatum has improved at the fracture site. Although remodeling has produced an acceptable result, initial treatment, in view of the head injury, probably should have been an external fixator.

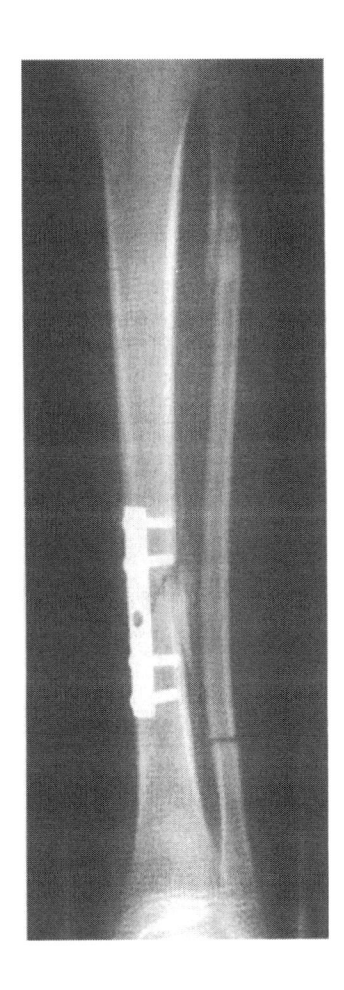

FIGURE 23-92. Early healing of the proximal fibula caused delayed healing of the tibia. It was treated by open reduction and distal fibular osteotomy.

larly indicate that healing is far from complete, despite the obvious radiographic consolidation.

Compartment Syndrome

Triffitt et al. studied compartment pressures after closed tibial fracture in adults.[412] They measured the pressures in the anterior and posterior compartments continuously for up to 72 hours in 20 patients. Pressure above 40 mmHg occurred in 7 (35%) and above 30 mmHg in 14 (70%). No patient, however, had any of the symptoms of compartment syndrome during monitoring. They found during follow-up that, *in the absence of symptoms*, the monitored pressures did *not* relate to outcome. Routine monitoring is therefore of doubtful benefit. It should be used when the complication is suspected clinically. In the future cutaneous pressure sensors may be effective for monitoring.

Ruland et al. studied the tibialis posterior muscle as a possible fifth compartment in compartment syndrome problems.[399] They found that there was no distinct fascial plane separating the tibialis posterior from the flexor digitorum longus and concluded that the tibialis posterior does not commonly rest within an isolated fascial compartment and thus does not require isolated decompression for acute compartment syndrome. The basic parameters of compartment syndrome are discussed in Chapter 10.

Delayed union is not common in children under 10 years of age. However, as the patient reaches adolescence, the tibial diaphyseal circulation and density become more like those of an adult, increasing the susceptibility to prolonged healing.[376] Early healing of the fibula may be related to delayed tibial healing (Fig. 23-92).[404,409,413] The use of electrical stimulation is still of questionable benefit in children.

Pseudarthrosis (nonunion) may occur in children, although it is rare (Fig. 23-93).[387,414] Bone grafting is the recommended method of treatment.

Rees described a complicating fracture separation of the lower femoral epiphysis in a patient who had a below-knee functional (PTB) cast for a tibial fracture.[397]

Synostosis formation is extremely rare following children's tibiofibular injuries.[367,382] The cause is unclear, especially in the type of case shown in Figure 23-94 in which a seemingly simple tibial fracture occurred. Resection may be attempted but only after the synostosis has fully matured. However, the complication may rapidly recur.

Although the fracture often appears radiographically healed, the process of microscopic remodeling in the cortex and medullary cavity may take months more to reestablish normal physiologic and biomechanical conditions. Figures 23-95 and 23-96 show the MRI appearance of fractures several months after injury. The medullary changes particu-

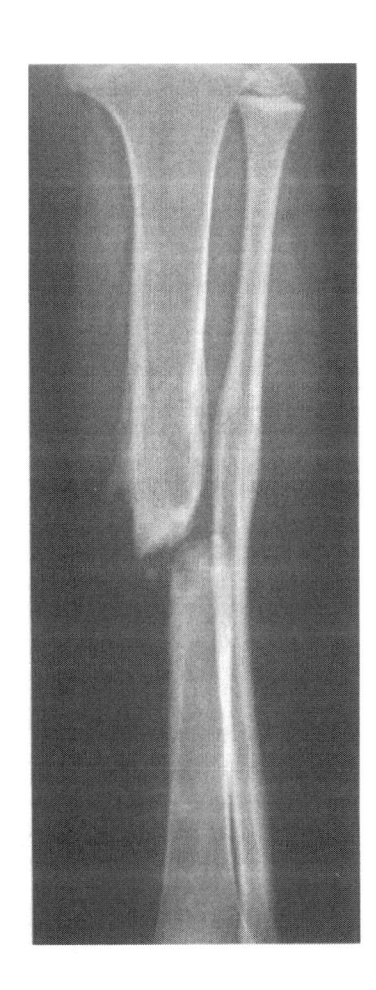

FIGURE 23-93. Pseudarthrosis of the tibia. The fibular fracture has healed.

1042 · 23. Tibia and Fibula

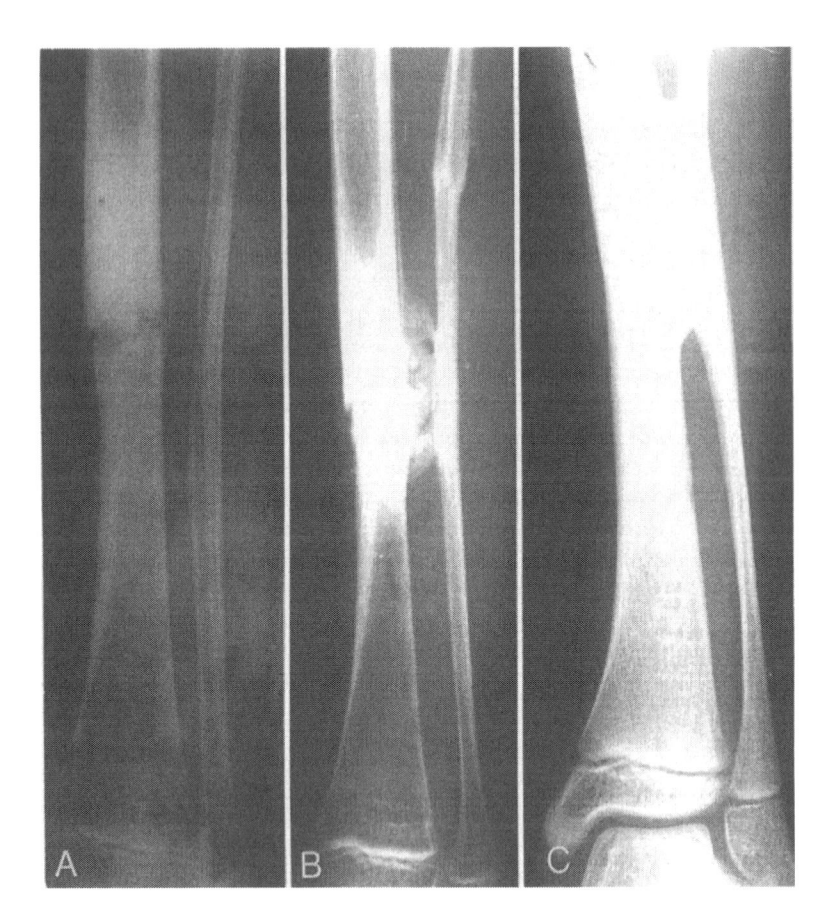

FIGURE 23-94. (A) Seemingly innocuous tibial fracture and bowed (greenstick) fibular injury. (B, C) Progressive development of a tibiofibular synostosis, a rare complication in children.

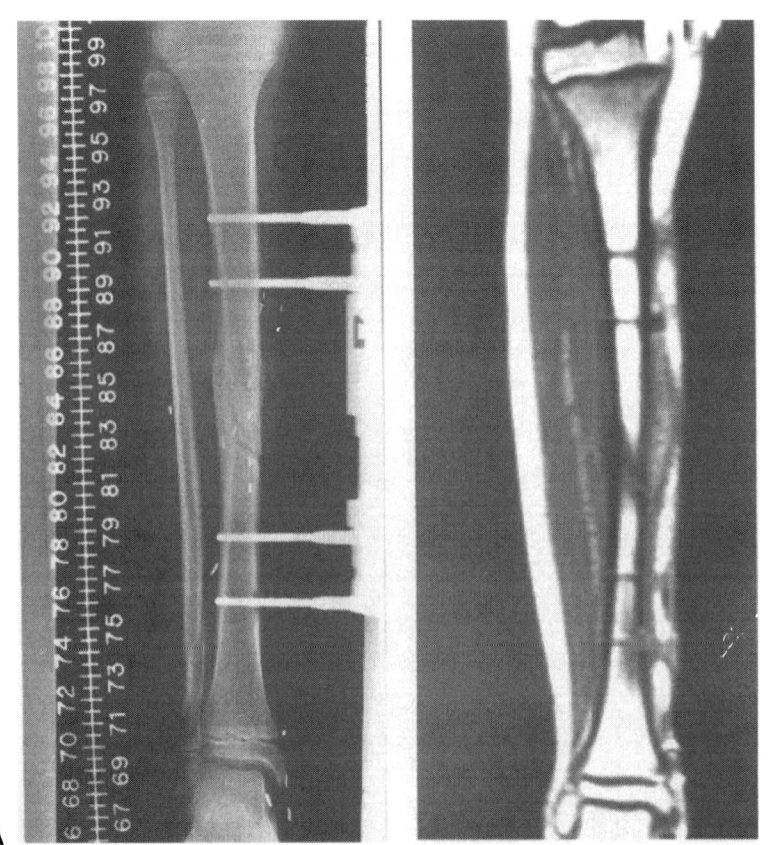

FIGURE 23-95. (A) Treatment of a tibial fracture with an external fixator. (B) MRI appearance 43 weeks after injury and 19 weeks after removal of the fixator. Note that the fracture line is still readily evident, and that altered marrow signals are still present around the fracture, despite the radiographic evidence of healing.

Distal Metaphyseal Injuries

FIGURE 23-96. (A) Healing 26 weeks after fracture. (B) Despite the radiographic appearance of healing, MRI shows limited restoration of normal physiology.

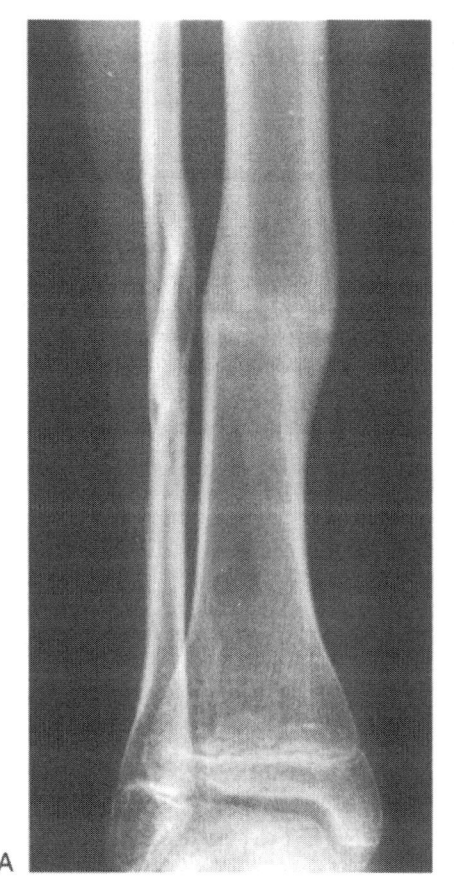

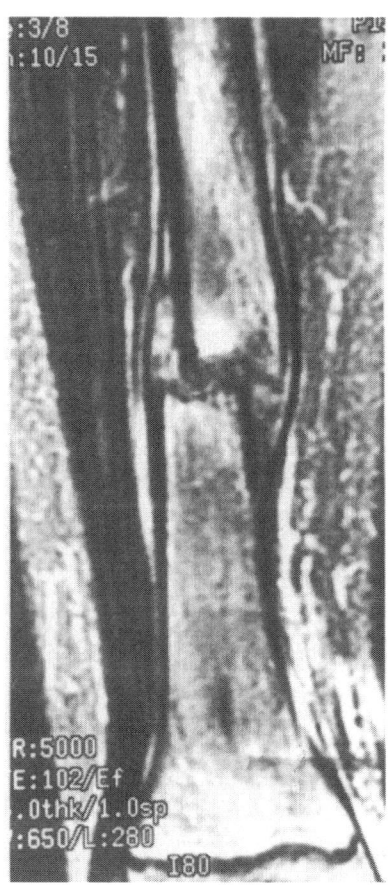

Maisonneuve Injury

The Maisonneuve injury is a combination of a distal tibial fracture (growth plate injury) and a proximal fibular fracture.[509,519,528] If an accompanying fibular fracture is not noted at the level of fracture of the distal tibia, particularly in and around the growth plate, the entire fibula must be visualized to be certain there is no disruption more proximally.

Ebraheim et al. described a Maisonneuve fracture in a pediatric patient.[380] In this case the patient had a distal physeal ankle injury (type 2) with a proximal fibular fracture. A tibial fracture with proximal tibia fibular joint disruption (Fig. 23-90) should be considered an equivalent injury.

Distal Metaphyseal Injuries

Like the proximal region, the distal metaphysis may sustain injury patterns of varying severity. Toddler's fractures may be difficult to diagnose (Fig. 23-97) and should be treated

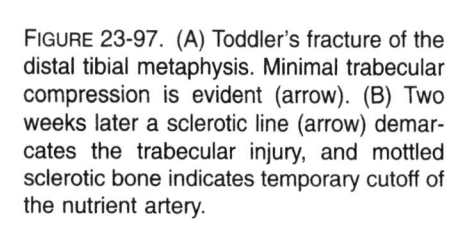

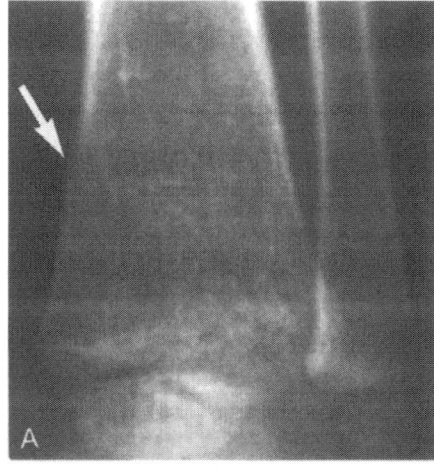

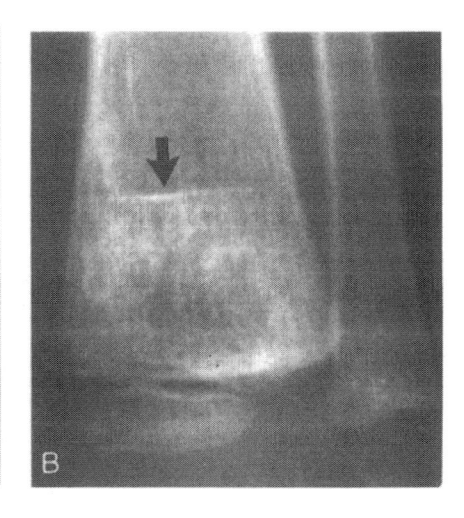

FIGURE 23-97. (A) Toddler's fracture of the distal tibial metaphysis. Minimal trabecular compression is evident (arrow). (B) Two weeks later a sclerotic line (arrow) demarcates the trabecular injury, and mottled sclerotic bone indicates temporary cutoff of the nutrient artery.

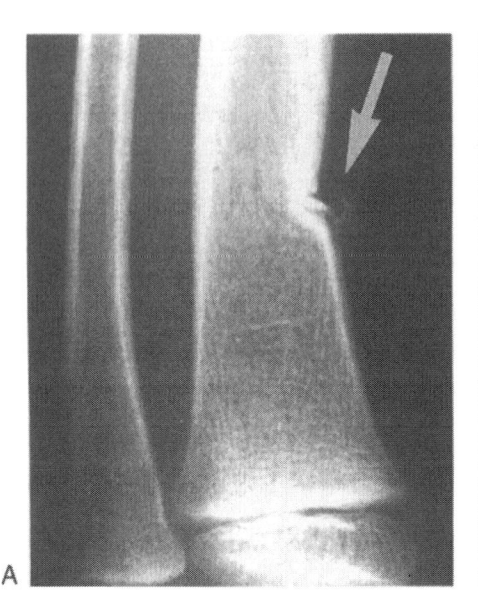

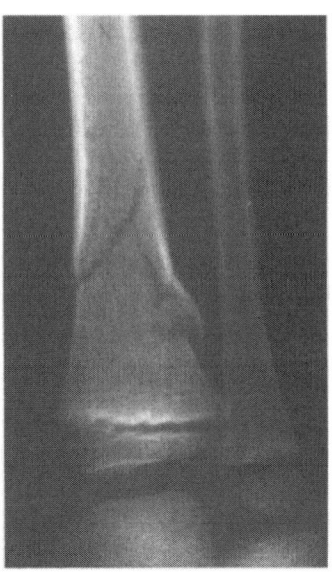

FIGURE 23-98. (A) Compression failure (arrow) of the distal metaphysis. (B) Tensile and compression failure of the distal tibia. There is minimal plastic deformation of the fibular metaphysis.

presumptively if symptoms (i.e., limping) and diagnostic findings (pain on palpation) warrant it.

Classification

Because of the differences in cortical macrostructure and microstructure grading from the thick diaphysis to the thinner metaphysis, greenstick fractures are relatively common (Fig. 23-98). More complete fractures may occur, although the thick tibial periosteum and the tendency of the fibula toward plastic deformation limit major displacement.

Treatment

With a greenstick fracture or a variably displaced, complete fracture, any angular deformity should be corrected, especially in the varus-valgus plane. Partial to complete displacement requires closed or open reduction. Some intrinsic stability remains because portions of the periosteum are intact.

Results

These injuries generally heal without significant deformity and with complete restoration of function. Synostosis, however, may occur (Fig. 23-99).

Distal Epiphyseal and Physeal Injuries

The anatomy and constricted joint motion in the ankle and foot render the distal tibial epiphysis particularly vulnerable to crushing and twisting injuries. The tibial physis is more likely to fail than are the ankle ligaments during skeletal

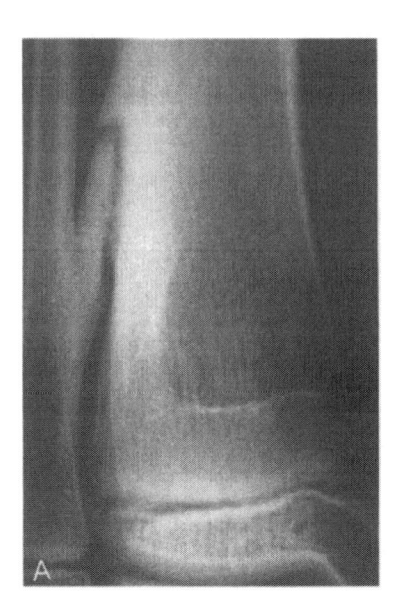

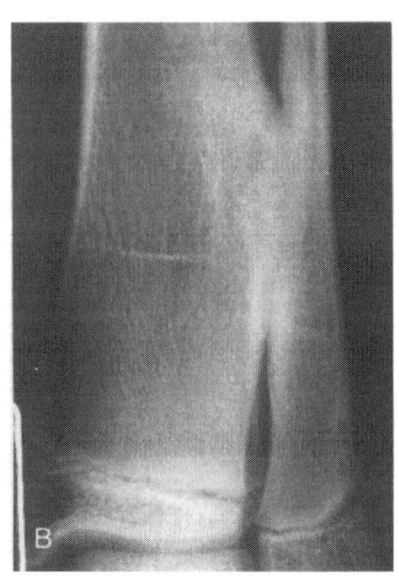

FIGURE 23-99. (A) Early synostosis formation. (B) Mature synostosis.

Distal Epiphyseal and Physeal Injuries

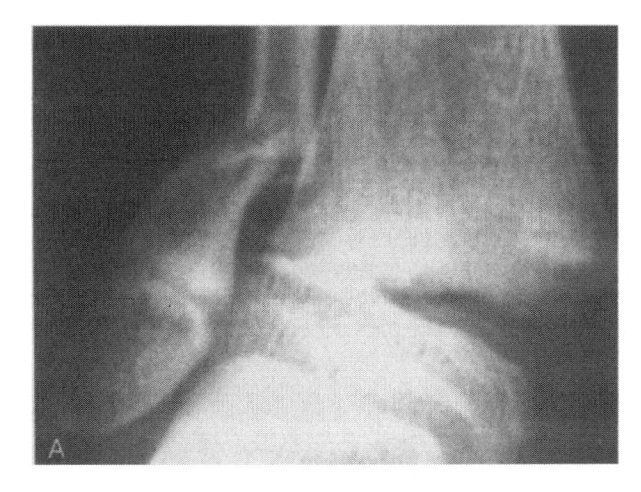

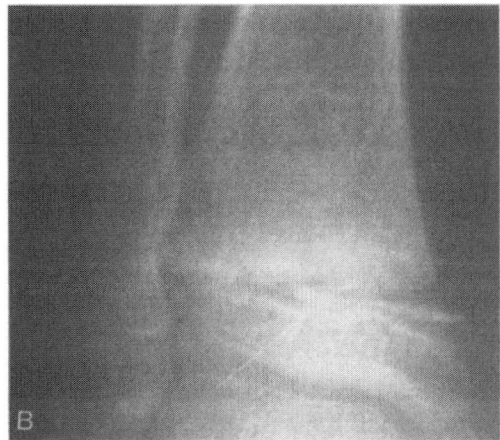

FIGURE 23-100. (A) Type 1 tibial injury associated with a fibular metaphyseal fracture. Note the thin metaphyseal bone on the tensile-failure side. (B) Appearance after closed reduction.

development. Injuries are commonly caused by indirect violence, with the fixed foot being forced into eversion, inversion, plantar flexion, internal rotation, or dorsiflexion. Fractures may also be sustained by direct violence, with the usual history being that the child was in an automobile accident, fell from a height, or was engaged in contact sports. Distal tibial injuries are more frequent in boys, with the usual age at which they occur being between 11 and 15 years, a period associated with increased emphasis on organized sports and exposure to more "fracture-prone" activities. Fractures involving the distal tibial physis are common, constituting approximately 10% of all physeal injuries.[416–612]

Classification

Fractures involving the distal tibia or fibula have been classified by many methods.[419,428,436,446,448,476,480,586] Anatomic classifications have been based, in part, on the basic growth mechanism injury schemes. However, these injuries tend to be more complicated, particularly injuries such as triplane fractures, which sometimes makes the simplistic use of such systems problematic. Mechanistic classifications, such as that of Lauge-Hansen, were devised for the analysis of adult ankle injuries and present problems in their application to children because of the alteration of fracture patterns by the biomechanical failure tendencies of various structures such as the metaphysis and physis. A modified classification based on growth mechanism injuries, rather than deforming mechanisms, is the easiest to apply to children and adolescents.

Type 1

The type 1 injury pattern is infrequent (Fig. 23-100). Diagnosis may be difficult if an obvious physeal displacement does not occur (Fig. 23-101). The pattern is infrequent in children with myelodysplasia or comparable neuropathies associated with a Charcot-like ankle joint. Unfortunately, such children tend to be pain-free (i.e., insensate). Swelling of the ankle, redness, or a fever of unknown origin should make one suspicious of this potential injury pattern. Stern and colleagues described bilateral distal tibial and fibular epiphyseal separations in patients with spina bifida.[537] These injuries must be recognized early so adequate immobilization and protection may be undertaken. Otherwise, the child

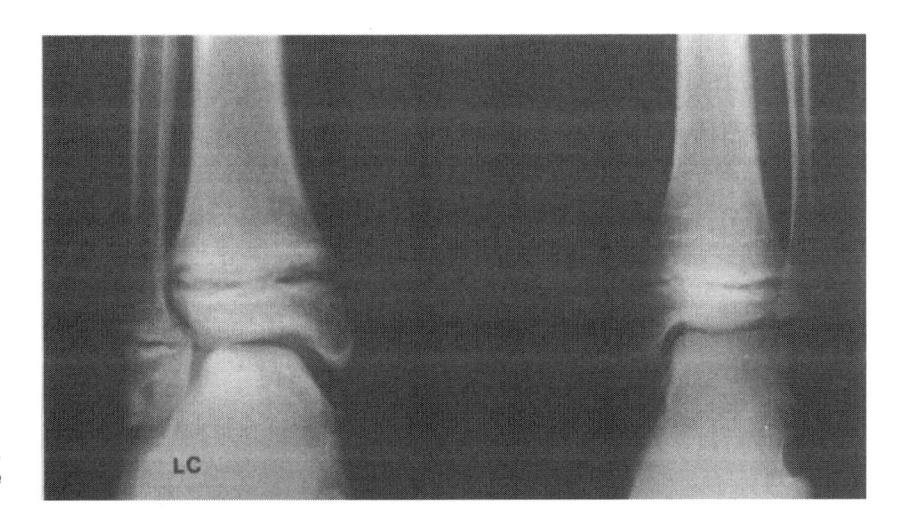

FIGURE 23-101. Widening of the right physis, compared to the left side, was the only evidence of this type 1 distal tibial fracture.

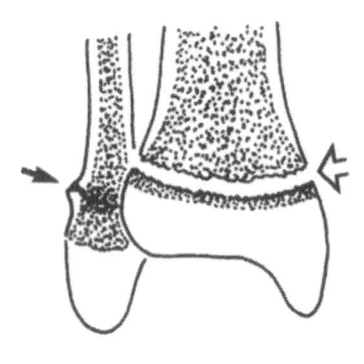

FIGURE 23-102. Type 1 tibial injury during infancy. Because of the relative failure patterns, the fracture is more likely to leave a thin transverse segment of metaphyseal bone.

bone may be included with the epiphyseal fragment (Figs. 23-102, 23-103). These fractures may be minimally displaced and difficult to diagnose roentgenographically.

Rotational displacement is an infrequent pattern of a type 1 injury.[433,471,507,524] The ankle mortise is rotated as a unit (Fig. 23-104). No ligamentous injury appears necessary for this rotation to occur, although some of the periosteal-perichondrial attachments, of necessity, must be detached. The fibula is not fractured, but, instead, is rotated along with the tibial epiphysis. The foot and ankle are externally rotated approximately 45°, even though roentgenograms seem to show 90° of rotation. The syndesmosis is minimally disrupted.

continues to walk on the fracture, frequently introducing displacement, causing excessive callus formation, and possibly impairing further growth.

The pattern is also common in young children, especially in situations such as child abuse. However, in an abuse situation, variable amounts of transversely oriented metaphyseal

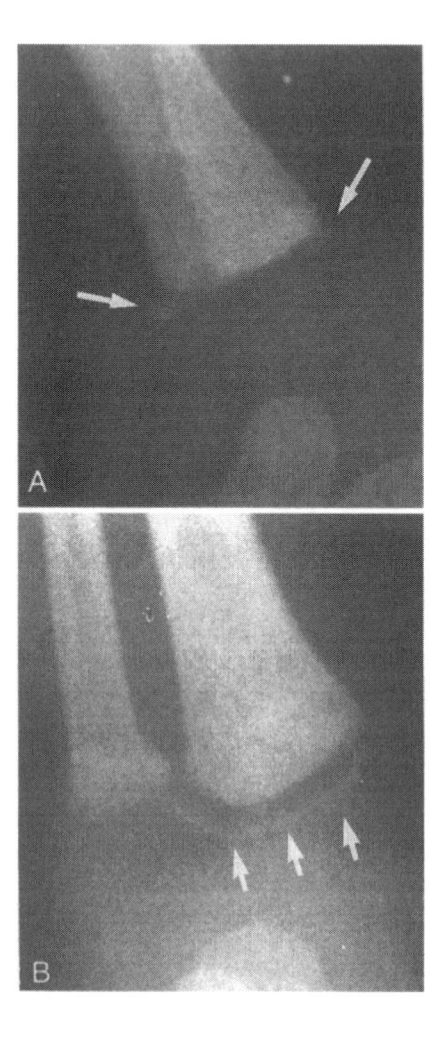

FIGURE 23-103. Injury to the distal tibia in the infant tends to be a variation of a type 1 injury, with small peripheral metaphyseal fragments (A) (arrows) or a transverse subchondral fragment (B) (arrows).

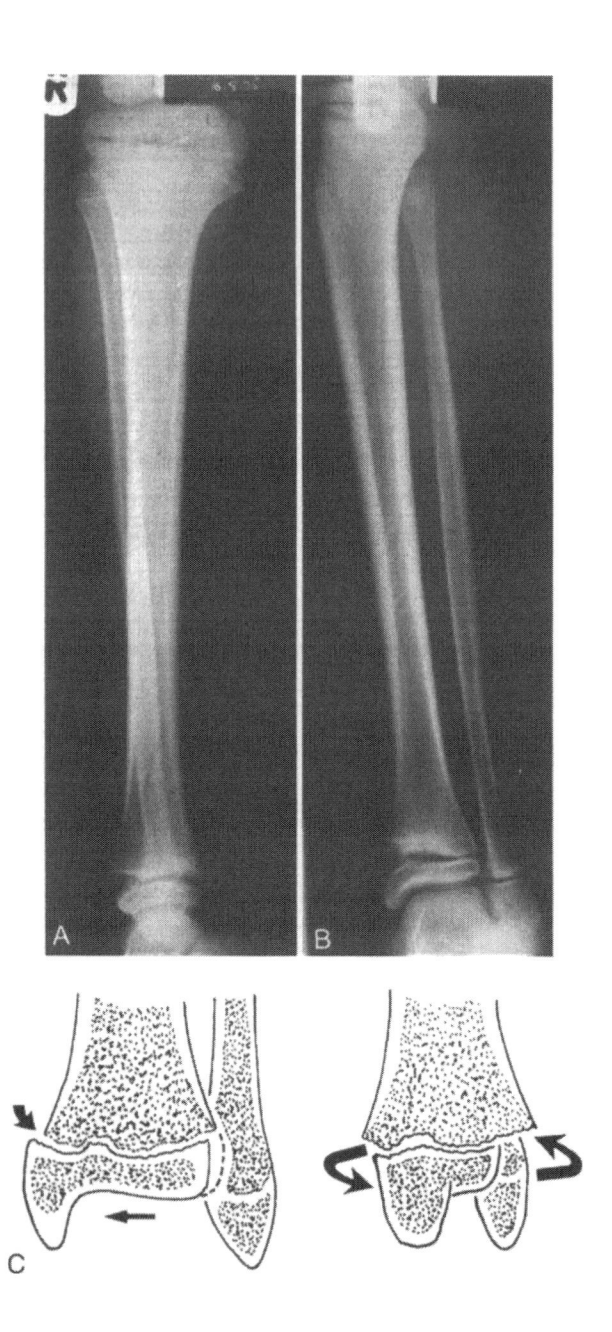

FIGURE 23-104. (A, B) Type 1 rotational injury of the distal tibia. Compare the proximal and distal ends, which show epiphyses in both lateral and anteroposterior views. (C) The injury.

Distal Epiphyseal and Physeal Injuries

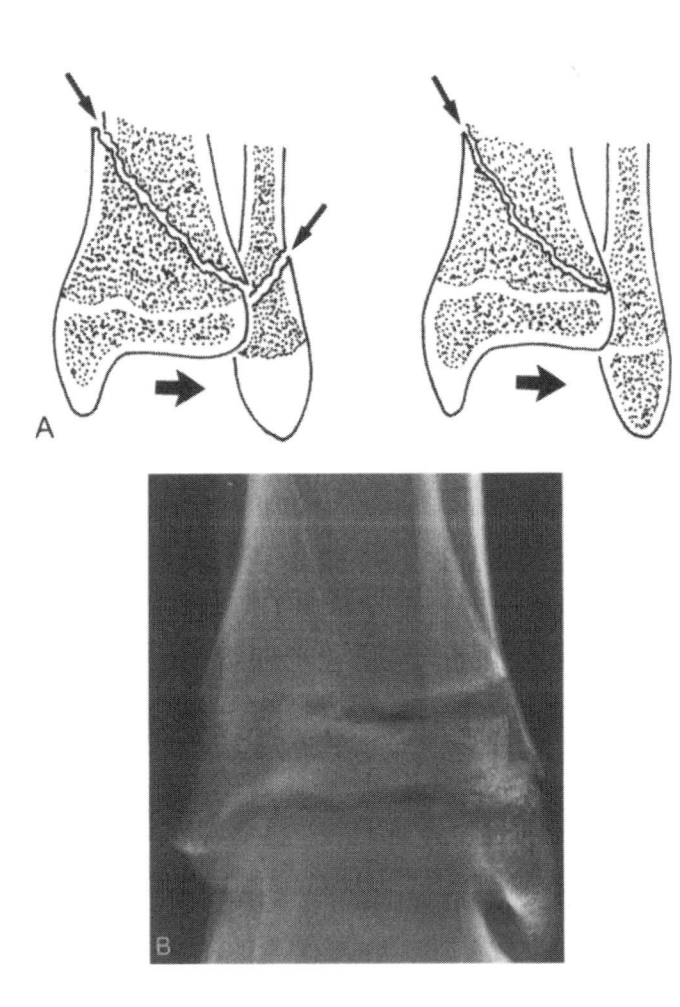

FIGURE 23-105. (A) Type 2 tibial injury with a large, medially based metaphyseal fragment. The fibula may or may not be fractured. The mechanism of injury appears to be a combination of supination and external rotation. (B) Type 2 tibial injury.

Broock and Greer duplicated the injury using amputation specimens and found that 45° of external rotation produced the same radiographic appearance.[433] The periosteum and perichondrium had to be excised, and the physis was transected transversely. However, the interosseous fragment did not have to be disrupted. The fibula was simply carried posteriorly behind the tibia by the attached ligaments of the fibula to the calcaneus. It is possible to reduce this injury by closed means.

Type 2

Type 2 injuries are the most common pattern (Figs. 23-105 to 23-108). The metaphyseal fragment may be medial, lateral, or posterior, contingent on the deforming mechanism. Accompanying fibular fractures are common and usually involve the metaphysis. Because the region of fibular metaphyseal fracture contains large amounts of thin cortical bone and is not directly weight-bearing (compression-responsive), this fracture may result in severe greenstick buckling (Fig. 23-109). Such plastic deformation may affect the reducibility of the tibial comonent of the injury. The point where the fracture changes angulation and propagates from the physis into the metaphysis is a critical area. If compression forces summate here, there may be a localized area of physeal damage, leading to premature growth arrest (Fig. 23-110). With severely displaced posterior type 2 injuries, the periosteum may be stripped from the anterior surface and pulled into the fracture gap. Reduction may only lock this tissue into the gap (Fig. 23-111).

Type 3 and Type 4

Type 3 and type 4 injuries of the medial malleolus (Figs. 23-112 to 23-115) are also relatively common and must be treated with proper respect for disruption of ankle mechanics and the articular surface, as well as for premature growth arrest and osseous bridging. Type 3 injuries may be radiologically deceiving, especially when there is incomplete ossification of the malleolar region in a young child. Sometimes oblique views of an apparent type 3 injury reveal a small metaphyseal flake, which gives the injury a type 4 pattern. Both fracture patterns usually require open reduction and accurate restoration of anatomy. The roentgenogram does not show the true extent of the cartilaginous injury, which may propagate transversely beyond the osseous limits, not unlike a sleeve fracture of the patella. Infrequently, with a type 3 injury a small piece of subchondral bone of the

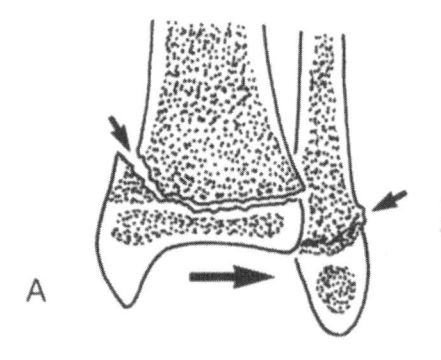

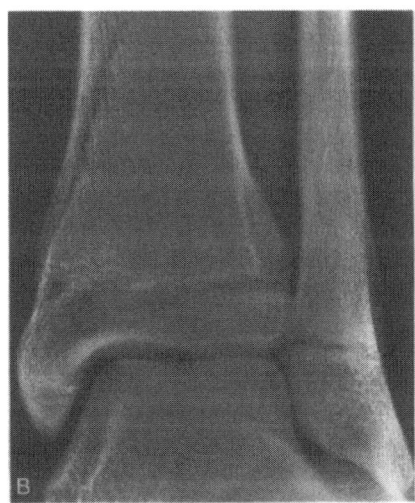

FIGURE 23-106. (A) Type 2 (supination-external rotation) tibial injury with a small medial metaphyseal fragment and compression failure of the fibular metaphysis. (B) Type 2 tibial injury with injury to the fibular physis.

FIGURE 23-107. (A) Type 2 tibial injury with a posteriorly based metaphyseal fracture. The mechanism of injury appears to be supination and plantar flexion. (B) Type 2 tibial injury. (C) Probable growth arrest 3 months later.

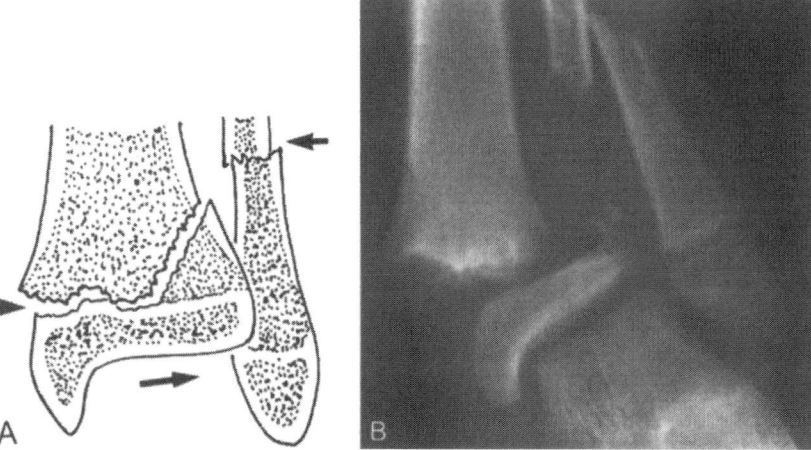

FIGURE 23-108. (A) Type 2 tibial injury with a laterally based fibular metaphyseal frature. The mechanism of the injury appears to be pronation-eversion. (B) Type 2 tibial injury.

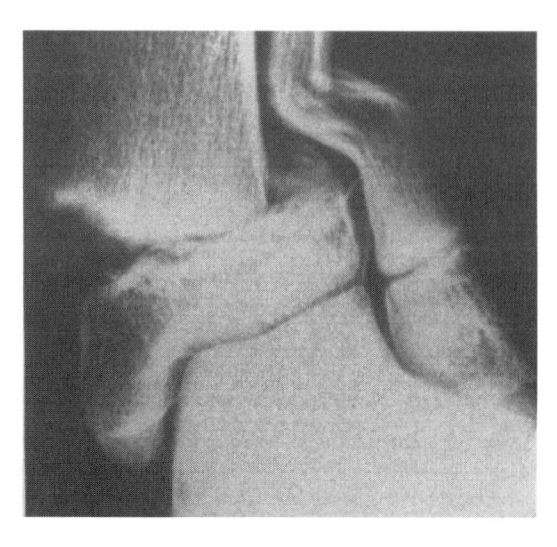

FIGURE 23-109. Pronation-eversion injury may cause severe, angular deformation of the fibula by greenstick cortical failure.

Distal Epiphyseal and Physeal Injuries

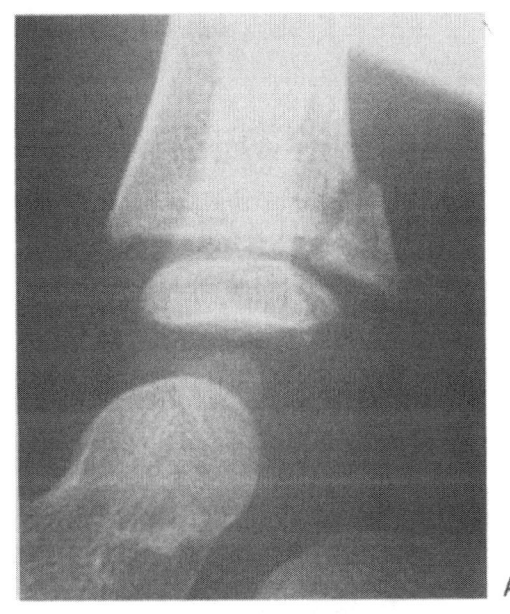

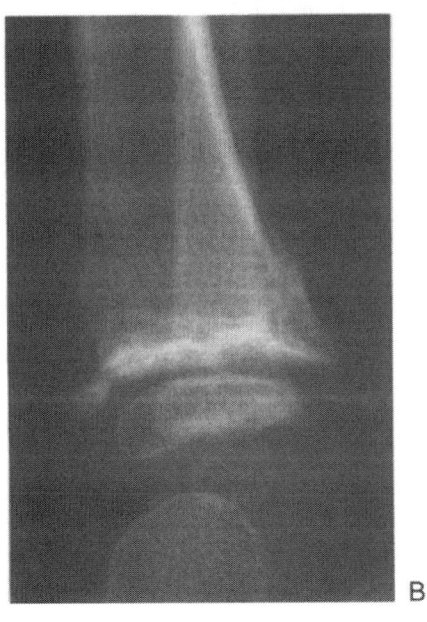

FIGURE 23-110. (A) Type 2 fracture due to child abuse. (B) Four months later the Harris line suggests growth impairment posteriorly.

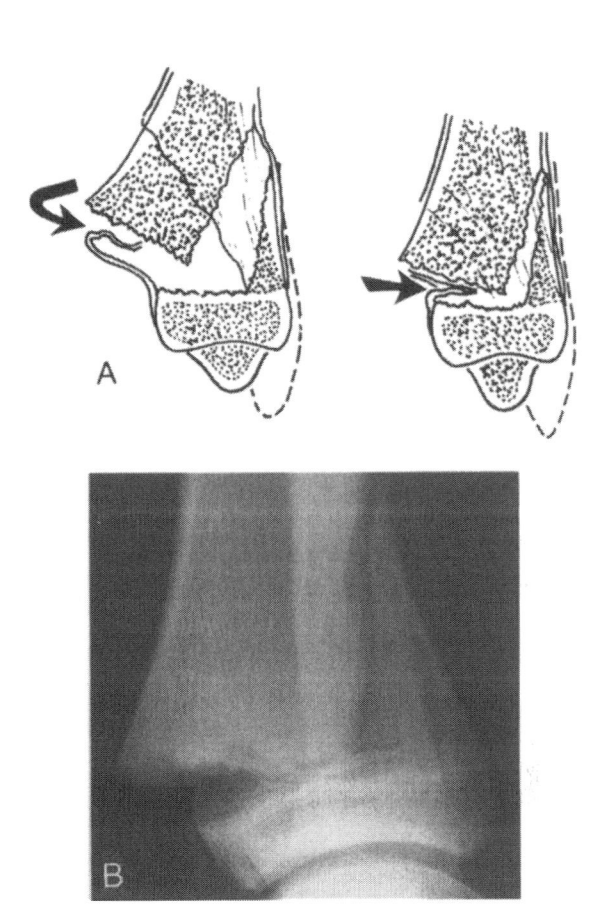

FIGURE 23-111. (A) Periosteal herniation. Anterior periosteum is being stripped from the metaphysis and pulled into the fracture gap. Reduction "locks" the periosteal flap into the fracture. (B) Roentgenogram of a posterior type 2 tibial injury.

ossification center is left, along with an intact physis. This bone devascularizes a small segment of the physis and predisposes it to premature closure, even with anatomic reduction of the fragment.

Because of the adduction-internal rotation (supination) injury mechanism that causes many of these injuries, localized growth mechanism damage may occur. This damage is difficult to ascertain at the time of the original injury but must be sought by adequate long-term follow-up until skeletal maturity. Articular damage may also occur.

Fracture of Tillaux

The Tillaux fracture, a type 3 injury (Figs. 23-116 to 23-118) involves a variably sized portion of the anterolateral tibial epiphysis.[561–580] The injury may be accompanied by a posterior metaphyseal fragment (i.e., as a variation of the triplane fracture). The segment may be extruded anteriorly and laterally. Although Paul Jules Tillaux has been given credit for describing the fracture that bears his name, Sir Astley Cooper in 1822, twelve years prior to the

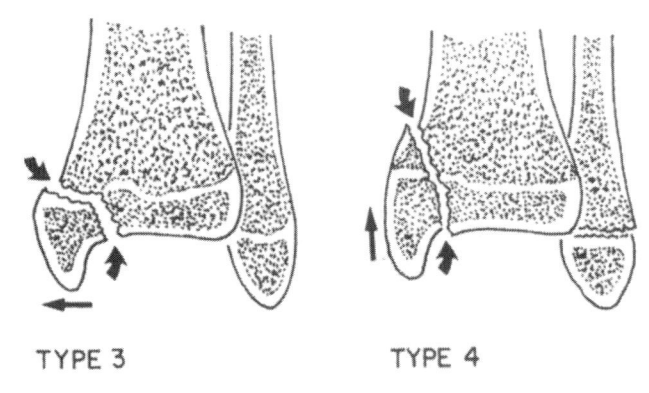

FIGURE 23-112. Failure of the medial malleolar region. The mechanism of these injuries appears to be supination and inversion. They may be type 3 or type 4 growth mechanism injuries.

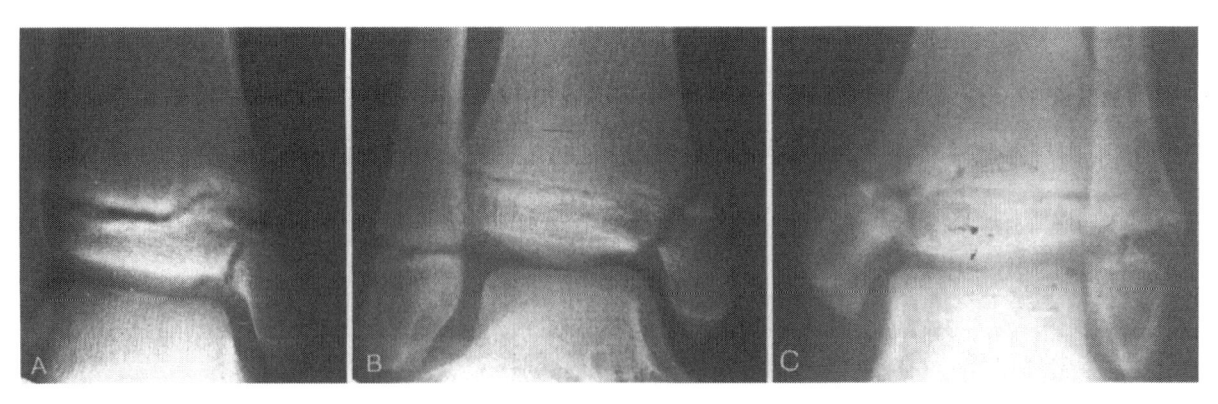

FIGURE 23-113. (A) Type 3 fracture of the medial malleolus. (B) Type 4 malleolar injury. (C) Type 4 injury of the medial malleolus with type 1 injury of the distal fibula.

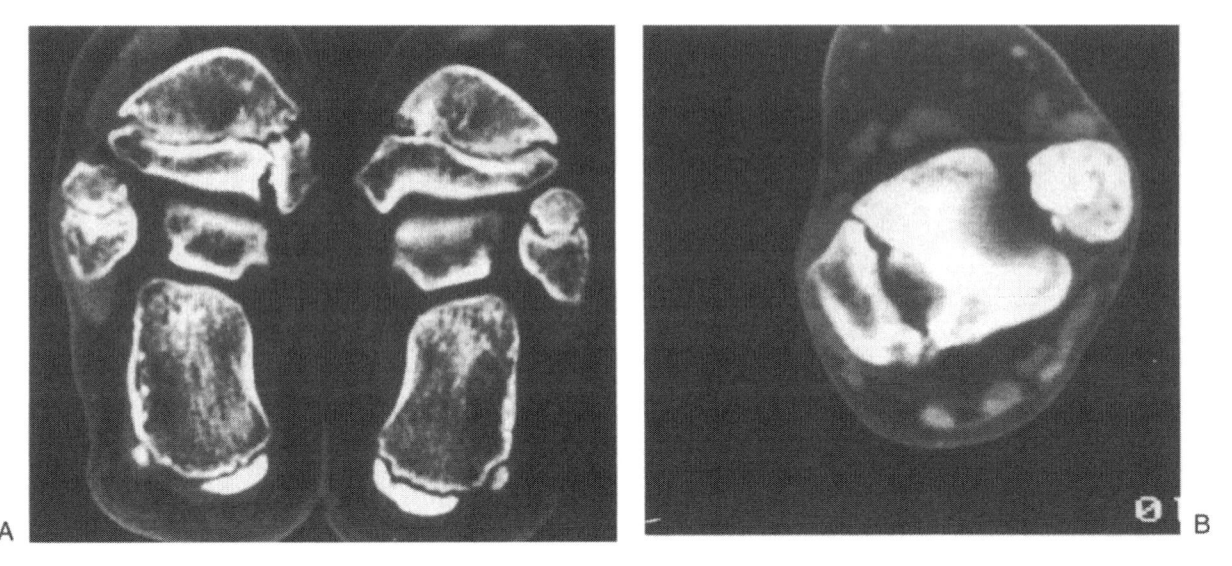

FIGURE 23-114. (A) CT scan of a type 3 fracture showing that widening may be greater at the articular surface than at the physis because of hinging. (B) Transverse cut shows the anterior to posterior extent of the injury.

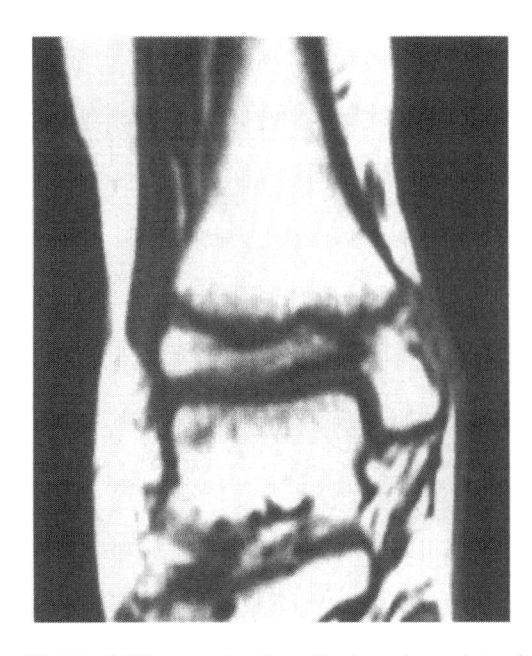

FIGURE 23-115. MRI scan of a type 3 injury shows lateral extension of the bone bruising in the plafond portion of the ossification center.

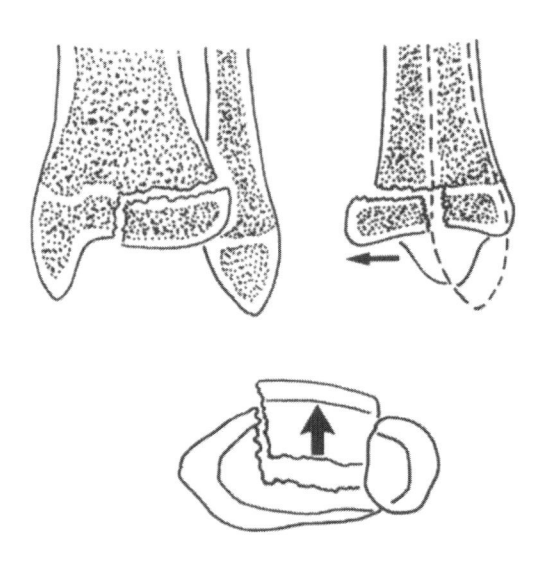

FIGURE 23-116. Fracture of Tillaux, a type 3 injury of the anterolateral distal tibial epiphysis.

Distal Epiphyseal and Physeal Injuries

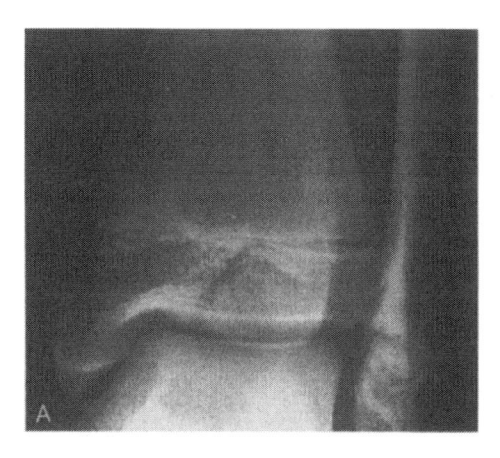

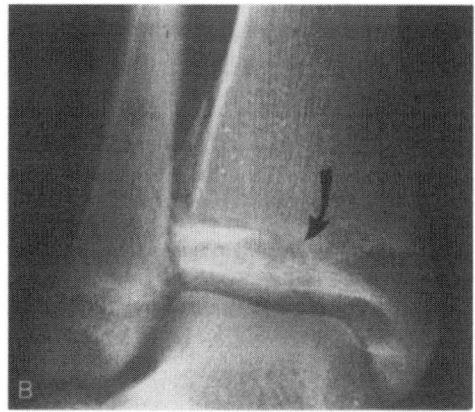

FIGURE 23-117. (A) Type 3 injury of the lateral tibia (Tillaux fracture). (B) Comparable type 4 injury (arrow).

birth of Tillaux, was the first to describe this injury pattern.[563,578,579]

Kleiger and Mankin reviewed children undergoing skeletal closure.[490] They showed that fusion occurred first in the middle portion, then on the medial side, and lastly in the lateral portion, with the entire process taking about 12–18 months (Fig. 23-119). Closure also appears to take place first posteriorly rather than anteriorly. They suggested that this anatomic closure factor was significant in the anterolateral quadrant fracture pattern.

Ankle congruity is of concern because juvenile Tillaux fractures may involve a significant portion of the weight-bearing articular surface. The extent of fracture displacement is critical when deciding whether to accept the results of closed manipulation or to proceed with open reduction and internal fixation. In general, the decision is based on the appearance of the fracture on plain radiographs. Oblique views, particularly mortise views, may be helpful. Letts pointed out the importance of taking mortise views because of the propensity of small Tillaux fractures not to be readily evident on the standard anteroposterior projection of the distal tibia and fibula.[568] However, CT has far greater accuracy than plain radiographs in delineating the degree of joint displacement, as well as fragment separation and rotation (Fig. 23-118).

Lateral rotation is usually responsible for this injury. The fracture line is vertical and extends upward from the distal articular surface. The displaced fragment may be small or large. It is believed that the injury is produced by avulsion of the lateral portion of the tibial epiphysis by the inferior tibiofibular ligaments during lateral rotation of the foot and

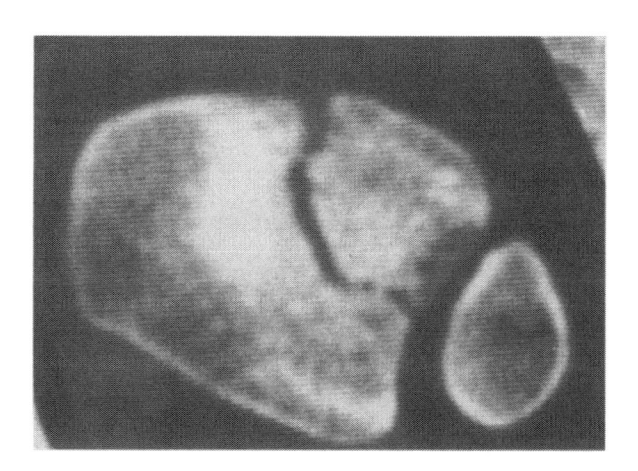

FIGURE 23-118. CT scan of a Tillaux fracture.

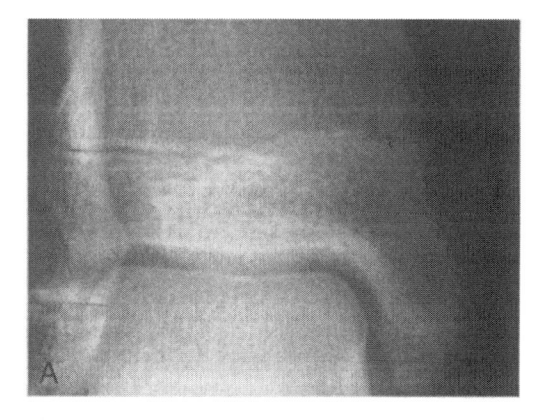

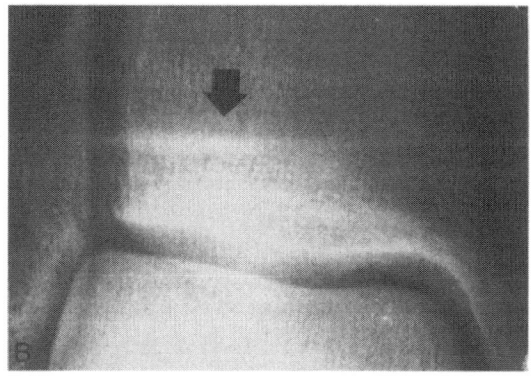

FIGURE 23-119. (A) Open lateral portion of the tibial physis. The medial portion has closed. (B) Distal tibia in an adolescent, showing complete closure and remodeling medially and residual physeal subchondral bone laterally (arrow).

ankle. However, because there are no direct ligamentous attachments to this region, it seems more likely that as the foot is externally rotated, the talus applies a compression-torque stress that propagates a crack through the articular surface up to the growth plate, which then shears. Stress roentgenograms show that displacement of the epiphyseal fragment is produced by the pull of tibiofibular ligaments. Operative observation corroborates that the lateral fragment is detached from the remainder of the epiphysis but may be partially attached to the anteroinferior tibiofibular ligament.

Vogler demonstrated a variation in which there was a Tillaux fracture with more posterior fragmentation, a medial malleolar fracture, and a greenstick fracture of the fibula.[554] He succinctly stated that "growth plate injuries" may be complex and not always classifiable.

There is general agreement that the major force of injury is external rotation, but reversing the direction by internal rotation does not always achieve satisfactory reduction. Manderson and Ollivierre recommended open reduction,[569] and the toggle maneuver may be appropriate in many of these cases. They also recommended that maximal dorsiflexion along with internal rotation may affect reduction; therefore they suggested that plantar flexion is a significant deformity force in the injury. The distal anterior tibiofibular ligament is usually intact with the Tillaux fracture.

Triplane Fracture

The triplane fracture involves transverse, sagittal, and coronal planes to create variable, comminuted type 3 and type 4 growth mechanism injuries.[581–612] Closure patterns of the distal physis affect the propagation of fracture forces. The fracture lines cross the articular surface, epiphyseal ossification center, physis, and metaphysis. The principal displaced fragment may be lateral or medial (Figs. 23-120 to 23-124). Lateral injury usually results from an external rotation mechanism, whereas medial injury is caused by adduction and direct impression. Defining the triplane nature of these fractures, which may look like a type 3 injury in the anteroposterior plane and a type 2 injury in the lateral plane, is important because of the unusual anatomy of the fragments, the large amount of disrupted articular surface, and the potential for growth deformity. The growth damage is not always a major problem, as most triplane injuries occur near skeletal maturity.

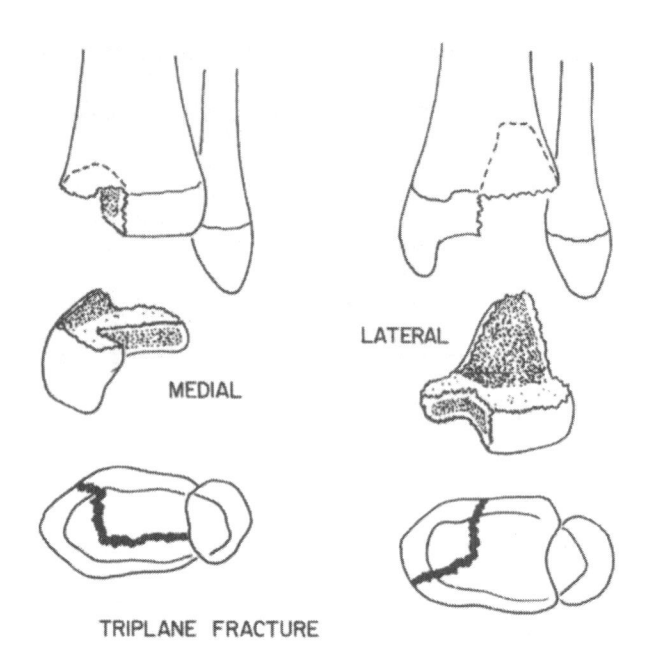

FIGURE 23-120. Medial and lateral triplane fractures.

Diagnosis of the discrete and particular anatomy of each triplane fracture must be ascertained by multiple radiographic techniques. If, on planar radiographs, a fracture line is displaced 2mm or more on any view, limited CT should be considered. Herzenberg stressed the importance of CT analysis.[473]

Cooperman and colleagues studied 5 of 15 triplane fractures on anteroposterior and lateral tomograms and found only two-fragment fractures among the five fractures.[583] One fragment consisted of the fibula, the attached posterior metaphyseal piece, and the lateral and posterior medial portion of the epiphysis. The second fragment consisted of the tibial shaft and attached medial malleolus and the remaining anteromedial portion of the epiphysis. On antero-

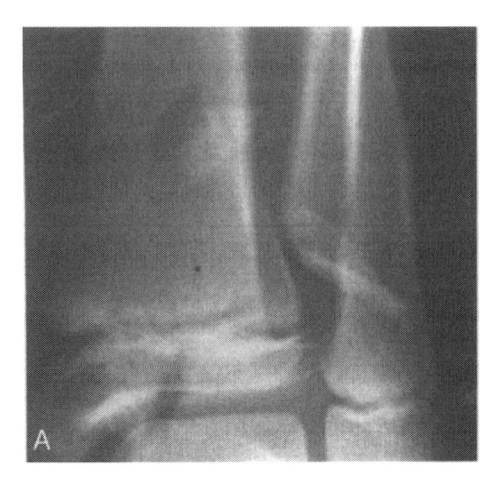

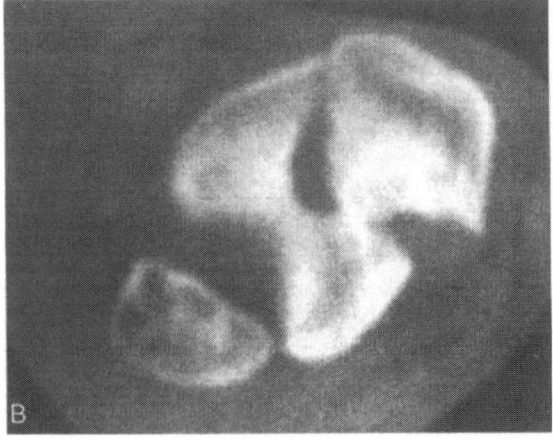

FIGURE 23-121. (A) Mortise view showing a lateral triplane fracture. This fracture is a three-part injury with a lateral type 4 fragment and a medial type 3 fragment. (B) CT scan showing rotation of the triplane component.

Distal Epiphyseal and Physeal Injuries

posterior tomograms, the sagittal type 3 fracture is seen in the anterior cuts but is lost posteriorly. This finding on the anteroposterior tomograms is consistent with either a two- or a three-fragment fracture configuration, as the posterior metaphyseal-epiphyseal part of the fracture is one piece in all triplane fractures.

If the tibial shaft and medial malleolus appear to remain in continuity anteriorly and the anterolateral epiphyseal fragment appears to be in continuity with the posterior metaphysis, a two-fragment fracture is more likely. If, however, on anteroposterior tomograms the tibial shaft does not appear to be in continuity with the medial malleolus anteriorly, and the anterolateral tibial epiphyseal piece appears to be free, a three-fragment fracture is more likely. The distinction between two- and three-fragment fractures is best

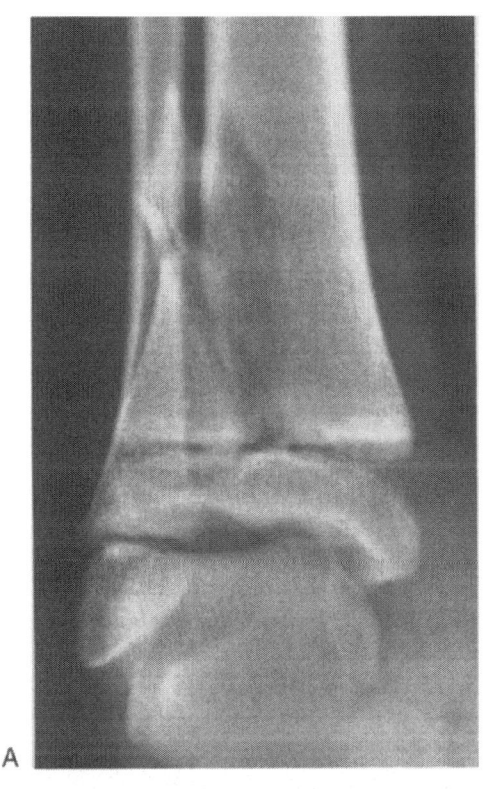

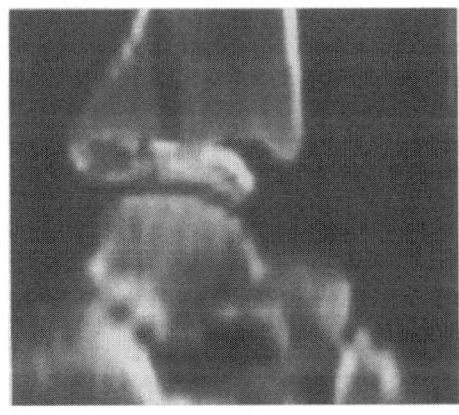

FIGURE 23-122. (A) Triplane fracture. (B) CT scan of the reconstruction.

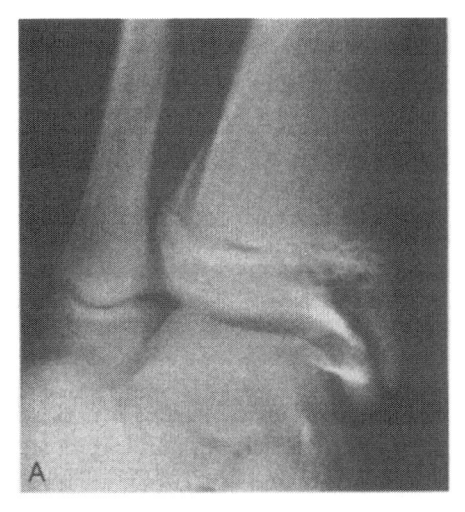

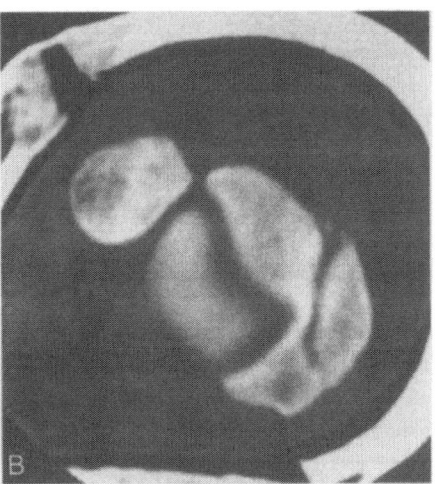

FIGURE 23-123. (A) Medial triplane fracture. (B) CT scan. This pattern may cause minimal articular disruption.

made from lateral tomographic cuts. With a two-part triplane fracture, the type 2 fracture is seen laterally and the type 4 fracture is seen medially. This finding indicates that the lateral epiphyseal and posterior metaphyseal-epiphyseal fragment piece and fibula are one unit. Medially, the fracture line extends from the metaphysis through the growth plate and epiphysis (type 4), indicating the separation of tibial shaft–medial malleolus and anteromedial portion of the epiphysis as the second fragment.

With a three-part Marmor fracture, lateral tomograms demonstrate the reverse picture. The type 4 fracture would be seen laterally through the metaphysis, growth plate, and epiphysis, as the anterolateral epiphyseal piece separates from the rest of the epiphysis. The type 2 lesion would be evident more medially; the posterior metaphyseal and medial epiphyseal piece and fibula would be the second unit, with the tibial shaft as a third unit. Additionally, the free anterolateral epiphyseal piece, if displaced, should appear anteriorly on the lateral tomograms, in contrast to a two-fragment triplane fracture. With a Marmor three-part fracture, the medial malleolus is not a part of the tibial shaft and would not be contiguous with it on lateral tomograms,

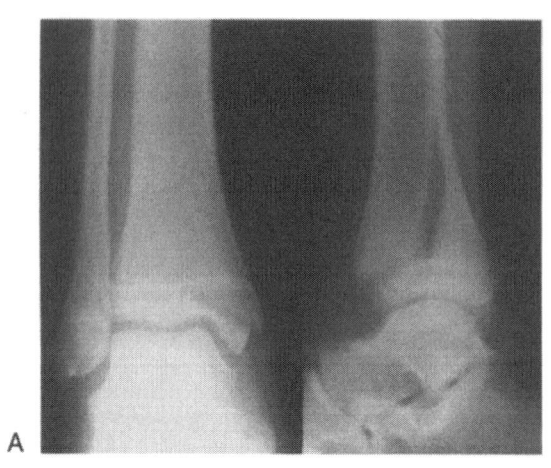

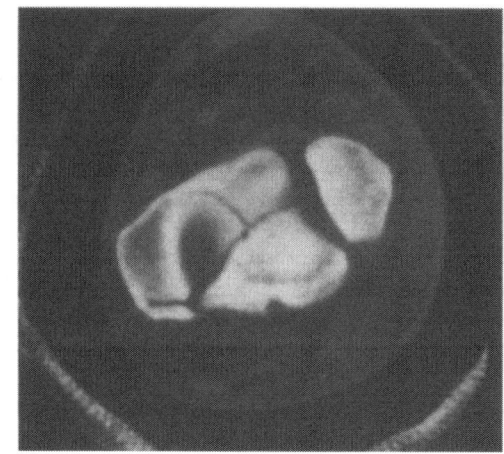

FIGURE 23-124. (A) Medial triplane injury. (B) CT scan shows that this patient, in contrast to the situation in Figure 23-123, sustained considerable intraarticular involvement.

as is the case with two-fragment fractures.[599] Such a three-fragment fracture constitutes a combined type 2, 3, and 4 growth mechanism injury. With most three-fragment fractures, the third piece (the tibial shaft) does not include any portion of the tibial epiphysis. The more comminuted fractures occur in younger patients who have unfused distal tibial epiphyses and who incur an injury involving a higher level of energy.

The most extensive work on children's triplane injuries has been done by Karrholm and associates.[478–485] Their classification is both anatomic and traumatologic and includes the use of CT to define the injury specifically. They found that triplane fractures consisted of two to four fragments in three basic fracture patterns; conventional roentgenograms did *not* differentiate between the two- and three-fragment fractures. The CT scan, however, registered the epiphyseal and metaphyseal fractures in detail, including the exact displacement of the fragments. By the use of tomography and CT scans, the epiphyseal fracture in the two-fragment triplane began more medially and had a transverse or curved shape to it, in contrast to the three-fragment type, which started more laterally and had a more perpendicular course. The metaphyseal fragment was always posterior or dorsal, with the apex located posteromedially, straight posteriorly, or sometimes posterolaterally.

Seitz et al. described a medial triplane fracture, in contrast to the usual lateral one.[604] They noted that Denton and Fischer had also reported a medial triplane fracture.[585]

Izant and Davidson reported a new pattern of triplane fracture, the four-part fracture.[593] Particularly, they reported two intraarticular metaphyseal fragments in continuity with epiphyseal fragments.

Feldman et al. described the "extraarticular" triplane fracture[590] and thought that it allowed nonoperative treatment. The classic finding is a split *within* the medial malleolus (Fig. 23-123).

Ertl et al. did a long-term follow-up of patients sustaining the triplane fracture pattern.[587] Of 23 patients, 20 were asymptomatic when they were evaluated 18–36 months after the injury; 8 of 15 were still asymptomatic when evaluated 38 months to 13 years after the fracture. Residual displacement of 2 mm or more following reduction was associated with a less than optimum result unless the epiphyseal fracture was outside the primary weight-bearing area of the ankle. Degenerative changes were evident on radiography. The patients who had epiphyseal fracture outside the weight-bearing area had intramalleolar fractures. Interestingly, Ertl et al. did some additional studies. They obtained the radiographs of 15 patients immediately after the injury and had them reviewed by three examiners who had no knowledge of the eventual anatomic diagnosis. The radiographs were interpreted as showing 11 two-fragment and 4 three-fragment fractures. In contrast, the CT scans, tomographs, and operative reports showed 11 three-fragment and 4 two-fragment fractures. Ertl et al. thought that the plain radiographs were, accordingly, unreliable for distinguishing two- from three-fragment triplane fractures.

Type 6

Type 6 injuries (Fig. 23-125) may be more common than is fully appreciated. A common mechanism of injury is catching an ankle in the spokes of a bicycle wheel. The injury may be closed or open. This injury is avulsion or compression of the periphery of the physis, specifically the zone of Ranvier, and carries a reasonably high incidence of peripheral osseous bridge formation.

Hernigou et al. described the absence of a medial malleolus.[472] Their patient initially sustained the injury at age 6 with an open fracture and loss of the medial malleolus. During a 20-year follow-up study she experienced no instability of the ankle, although she did develop degenerative arthritis. The radiograph shows significant growth arrest and ambulation. Authors have suggested that stability of the ankle is lost when the medial malleolus is fractured at the level of the joint or if there is complete disruption of the deep deltoid. Their case did not show the same degree of severe abnormality.

Distal Epiphyseal and Physeal Injuries

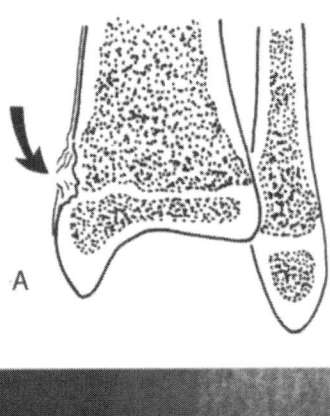

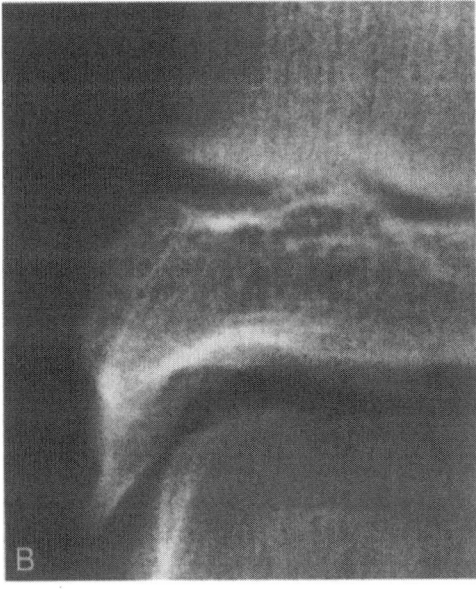

FIGURE 23-125. (A) Type 6 injury to the peripheral physis with disrupted zone of Ranvier and periosteal-perichondrial transition. This may predispose the injury to peripheral osseous bridge formation. (B) Type 6 injury of the medial malleolus.

Type 7

Type 7 injuries involve extension of the epiphyseal secondary ossification center into the malleolar region (Figs. 23-126, 23-127). Separation may occur at the junction between ossified and nonossified regions, which may be difficult to diagnose in the young child.

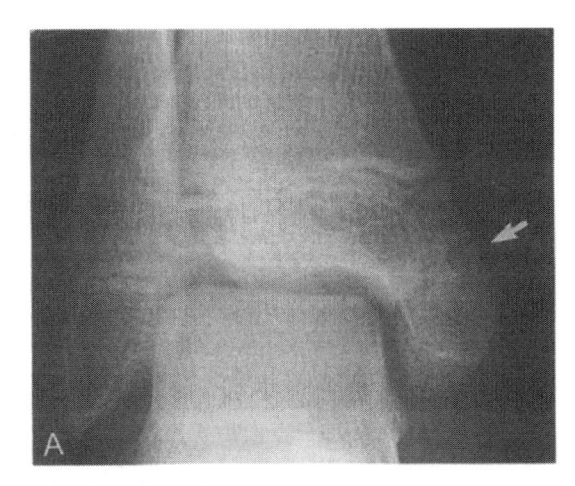

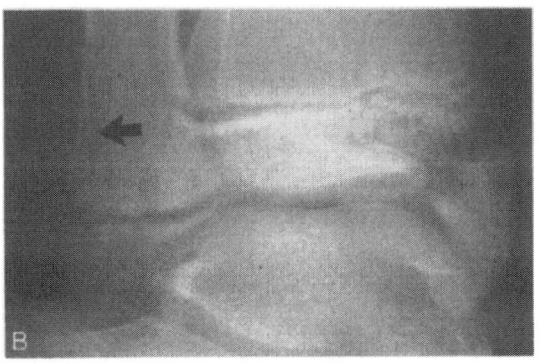

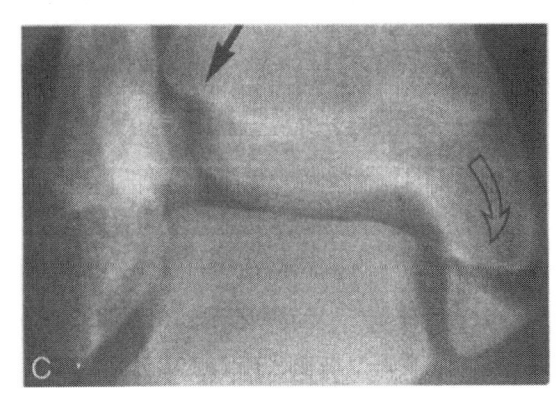

FIGURE 23-127. Type 7 injuries of the medial malleolus. (A) Undisplaced fracture (arrow). (B) Mild displacement. Note the fibular fracture. (C) Mild displacement (open arrow), with concomitant fracture of Tillaux (solid arrow).

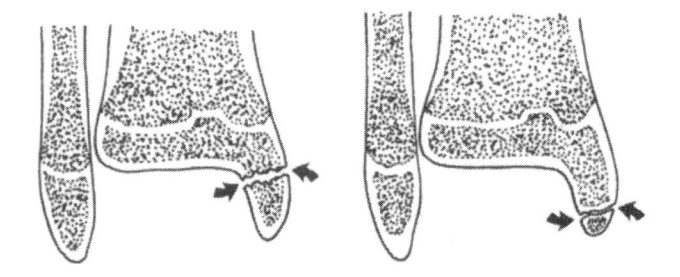

FIGURE 23-126. Type 7 injuries involving the medial malleolus. They do not usually extend to or disrupt weight-bearing areas but certainly may affect the position of the talus relative to the tibial plafond, thereby affecting talotibial contact areas.

Mechanism of Injury

Ankle fractures are usually caused by indirect violence. The fixed foot is forced into abduction, adduction, lateral or medial rotation, eversion or inversion, or plantar flexion or dorsiflexion. Pronation and supination are the positions of the foot attained by rotational movement around the axis of the talocalcaneonavicular joint. Medial and lateral rotational movements of the talus take place around the sagittal axis of the weight-bearing articular surface of the tibia. These forces are transmitted by the deltoid and lateral collateral ligaments to the epiphyses of the distal tibia and fibula, exerting tension at the physes. Ankle fractures may also be caused by direct violence, as in an automobile accident or a fall. With direct crush injuries, the fractures may be open.

Carothers and Crenshaw reviewed 54 distal tibial epiphyseal injuries.[436] These cases were derived from a series of more than 1400 ankle fractures and represented approximately 4% of all ankle fractures. These investigators classified the injuries into abduction, external rotation, plantar flexion, axial compression, and adduction injuries. Adduction injuries appeared to be more commonly associated with complications than did abduction or external rotation injuries, which were more commonly observed with fractures through the epiphysis (type 3 and type 4 growth mechanism injuries).

Carothers and Crenshaw showed experimentally that the force exerted through bone in compression is many times greater and probably more destructive than that which can be exerted through shearing.[436] There is greater tendency for compression to be applied in an adduction than an abduction injury. With external rotation or abduction injuries, a large element of shear force causes a transverse fracture through the weak point, carrying the intact epiphysis past the vertical lateral border of the tibial metaphysis and propagating toward and possibly through the fibula. With adduction injuries the medial border of the talus, after epiphyseal separation or fracture of the fibula, still exerts a compressive force through the tibial epiphysis, as its medial migration is blocked by the medial malleolus.

For the mechanism of ankle fractures in the adult, Lauge-Hansen showed that three factors should be considered: the axial load, the position of the foot at the moment of trauma, and the direction of the abnormal force. In children an additional factor determining the pattern of fracture is the state of maturity of the physes.[501,502]

Dias and Tachdjian devised a classification of physeal injuries of the ankle in children that utilizes Lauge-Hansen's categories of foot position and direction of abnormal force in correlation with a growth mechanism injury classification.[448] Four mechanisms were proposed. For each, the first term refers to the position of the foot at the time of injury, and the second refers to the direction of the injurious force on the ankle joint. The fracture patterns and the displacement of fragments are characteristic for each mechanism. When classifying an ankle fracture, one should study the roentgenograms carefully to determine the type of growth mechanism injury, the direction of the fracture line, and the direction of displacement of the epiphyseal-metaphyseal fracture fragment in relation to localized swelling and tenderness.

Supination-Inversion

With the mild injury pattern, traction by the lateral ligaments results in separation of the distal fibula (type 1 and type 2 growth mechanism injuries). Less frequently there is disruption of the lateral collateral ligaments or a type 7 growth mechanism fracture at the tip of the lateral malleolus. The distal tibia does not usually fail. However, if the inversion force persists or increases, the talus acts as a wedge to cause a type 3 or type 4 growth mechanism injury of the distal tibia.

Adduction injuries (approximately 15% of cases) are characterized by medial displacement of part or all of the distal tibial epiphysis. These injuries may include type 3 or type 4 growth mechanism fractures of the medial malleolus and may or may not be accompanied by injury to the lateral malleolus, particularly a fracture through the shaft of the fibula. Adduction injuries are associated with a much higher incidence of growth deformity. Affected children are usually young. In one series of patients, the median age was 9.5 years.[426] The talus is forcibly adducted after separation of the lower fibular epiphysis or fracture of the distal fibula. The medial border of the upper surface of the talus impinges on the medial half of the lower end of the tibia and exerts a crushing force at this point. The interarticular shearing force causes a fracture that extends from the joint surface to the zone of hypertrophic cartilage cells of the physis and then either along the physis or into the metaphysis, creating a type 3 or type 4 physeal injury. Displacement of the medial malleolus and adjacent medial epiphyseal fragment may be slight to moderate. The germinal layer of the physis may be microscopically disrupted or devascularized. Occasionally, an adduction injury displaces the entire distal tibial epiphysis medially with a medial metaphyseal fragment attached to it, as with a type 2 growth mechanism injury. The shearing force rarely splits the epiphysis completely to create a large type 4 growth mechanism injury.

Supination-Plantar Flexion

With the foot in supination, a posteriorly directed force creates a type 2 physeal fracture of the distal tibia, although a type 1 growth mechanism injury pattern may occur in the young child. Concomitant fibular injury does not usually take place. Plantar-flexion injuries occur in approximately 12% of cases. These injuries are distinguished by variable posterior displacement of the entire distal tibial epiphysis, usually without a concomitant fracture of the fibula and an associated posterior metaphyseal tibial fragment. This pattern does not appear to be associated with a significant postinjury deformity.

Supination-External Rotation

In its mild form, supination-external rotation, a type 2 jury of the distal tibia, is characterized by a long spiral fracture starting laterally at the zone of Ranvier. The metaphyseal fragment is primarily posterior, and a concomitant fibular metaphyseal fracture is typically present.

External rotation injuries are the second most common form, accounting for approximately 25% of cases. They are characterized by posterolateral displacement of the entire distal tibial epiphysis and are almost always accompanied by a posterior metaphyseal fragment from the tibia. The fracture of the fibula may be buckled (torus), but more often it is a transverse or oblique type of injury. Posterior displacement varies from 10% to 90% of the width of the metaphysis, and the epiphysis is usually accompanied in each instance by a posterior or posterolateral metaphyseal fragment. Again, this finding does not appear to be associated with major functional problems of the ankle. Posterior displacement may vary and is generally associated with an oblique fracture of the distal fibular shaft.

Pronation-Eversion and External Rotation

Pronation-eversion and external rotation, abduction injuries, are the most frequent, occurring in 40% of cases. This mechanism uses concomitant tibial and fibular fractures. A type 2 growth mechanism tibial fracture with a lateral (posterolateral) metaphyseal fragment is the most common pattern. There is lateral displacement of the entire distal tibial epiphysis. The fibular fracture is usually metaphyseal and often 4–7 cm above the physis. The fracture does not usually involve the distal fibular epiphyseal plate.

The degree of lateral displacement varies but is never extreme, as it is restrained by the fibula (unless that is also fractured). The entire distal tibial ankle mortise moves as a unit. It is frequently accompanied by a fragment of lateral metaphysis but is rarely associated with a major growth deformity. The prognosis for future growth is usually excellent, as the germinal layer is not damaged. However, there may be a disruptive (type 5) physeal injury in which the fracture propagates into the metaphysis.

Axial compression injuries and those caused by direct violence, such as a direct blow to the ankle, are associated with some posterior or posteromedial displacement. Again, these injuries do not usually produce major problems.

Treatment

Definitive treatment must usually be tailored to the specific fracture type and the reactive swelling that develops soon after injury, making closed reduction difficult. A well-padded compression dressing and posterior splint should be applied before diagnostic roentgenograms are attained. Gentle closed reduction should be carried out with the patient under a general anesthetic, as relaxation of muscles and absence of pain are essential to any minimally traumatic manipulation. The knee should be flexed to 90° with the foot in plantar flexion to relax the gastrocnemius-soleus group of muscles. Overcorrection and forcible manipulation should be avoided.

Accurate repositioning of the displaced epiphyses at the expense of forced or repeated manipulation or operative intervention is not indicated, as some realignment of the ankle may occur even late in the growing child, particularly if in the plane of motion of the ankle joint. Growth deformity at the ankle may be predicted with reasonable accuracy at the time of injury because it usually occurs in the adduction group and is accompanied by roentgenograms that demonstrate disruption of the epiphysis and physis. Many of the factors responsible for the high incidence of permanent damage probably result from the addition of a compression force through the medial side of the physis. There is evidence that massive displacement of the epiphyses results in a clinically discernible disturbance of growth or in subsequent defects in the ossification of the adjacent metaphysis.

Usually type 1 and type 2 growth mechanism injuries are treated by closed reduction and maintenance in a short leg cast. Weight-bearing is discouraged for at least 6 weeks. In some cases of instability, an open reduction and limited fixation are necessary (Fig. 23-128). Murakami et al. described a patient with a type 2 growth mechanism fracture who had an interposed periosteum and posterior tibial tendon that prevented closed reduction.[523]

With type 3 and type 4 growth mechanism fractures, accurate anatomic reduction is necessary. If it cannot be achieved by closed methods (Fig. 23-129), open surgical reduction is undertaken, and smooth Kirschner wires or a transepiphyseal fixation device is used (Figs. 23-130 to 23-132). Fixation methods should respect the degree of remaining function of the physis. With type 3 injuries, transversely oriented pins may fix the malleolus to the remainder of the tibial epiphyseal ossification center. With type 4 injuries, transversely oriented pins may be placed metaphysis to metaphysis and epiphysis to epiphysis, thereby avoiding the physis and lessening the risk of premature growth arrest.

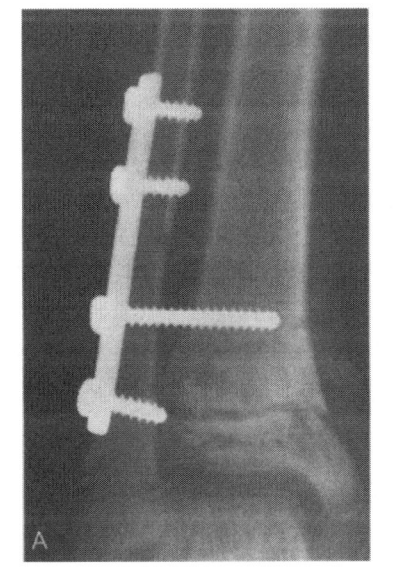

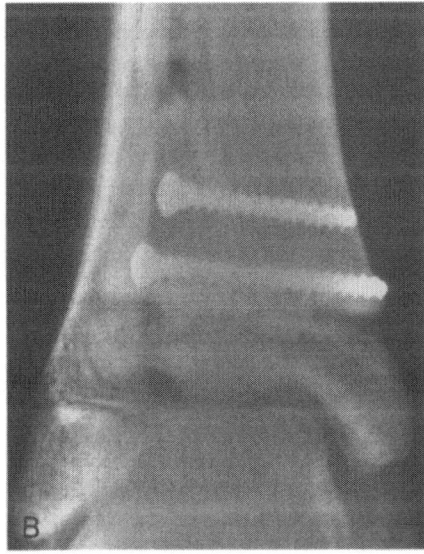

FIGURE 23-128. (A) Open reduction and internal fixation of the fibula, with a syndesmotic screw and a concomitant type 1 tibial injury. (B) Open reduction and fixation of a type 2 metaphyseal fragment.

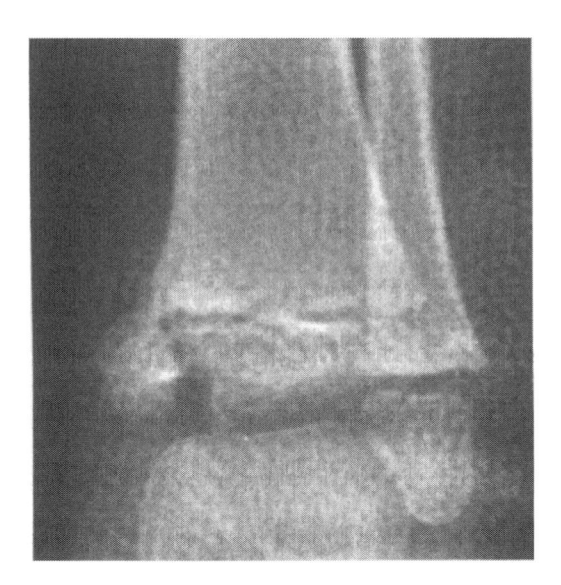

FIGURE 23-129. Unacceptable closed "reduction" of a type 3 malleolar injury.

For the displaced type 3 and type 4 injuries of the tibia, open reduction should be done to try to prevent cross-union between the metaphysis and epiphysis and to restore the congruity of the ankle mortise and articular surface. Obviously, it is not possible to improve the prognosis for growth of the damaged epiphysis by surgical treatment, and it is conceivable that the surgical approach can cause further damage to the growth center. Nevertheless, the effective restoration of congruity to the ankle joint, which may be reliably achieved by open operation, is sufficient reason for recommending open reduction in these cases. The complications of shortening and bone deformity are not nearly as important as permanent disruption of the articular surfaces of the ankle.

Georgiadas and White described modified tension band wiring of medial malleolar fractures in adults.[458] This technique may be used for certain children's fractures (e.g., type 7), as the smooth pins across the physis should not cause growth damage. However, the periosteum should not be elevated proximally toward the physis. Furthermore, subtle growth plate physeal damage may have occurred during the injury, even though the fracture appears separate from the physis. Ostrum and Litsky used tension band fixation of medial malleolar fractures.[525] In a biomechanical study they showed that tension band fixation provided the greatest resistance to pronation forces.

Toolan et al., in a study of medial malleolar fracture fixation techniques, showed that the simple use of lag screws was just as effective as more complex fixation techniques.[548] However, the lag screw is not appropriate if the physis is still open; here smooth pins are better.

The Tillaux fracture in an adolescent may be reduced by applying longitudinal axial traction and, while traction is maintained, medially rotating the hindfoot on the leg. The

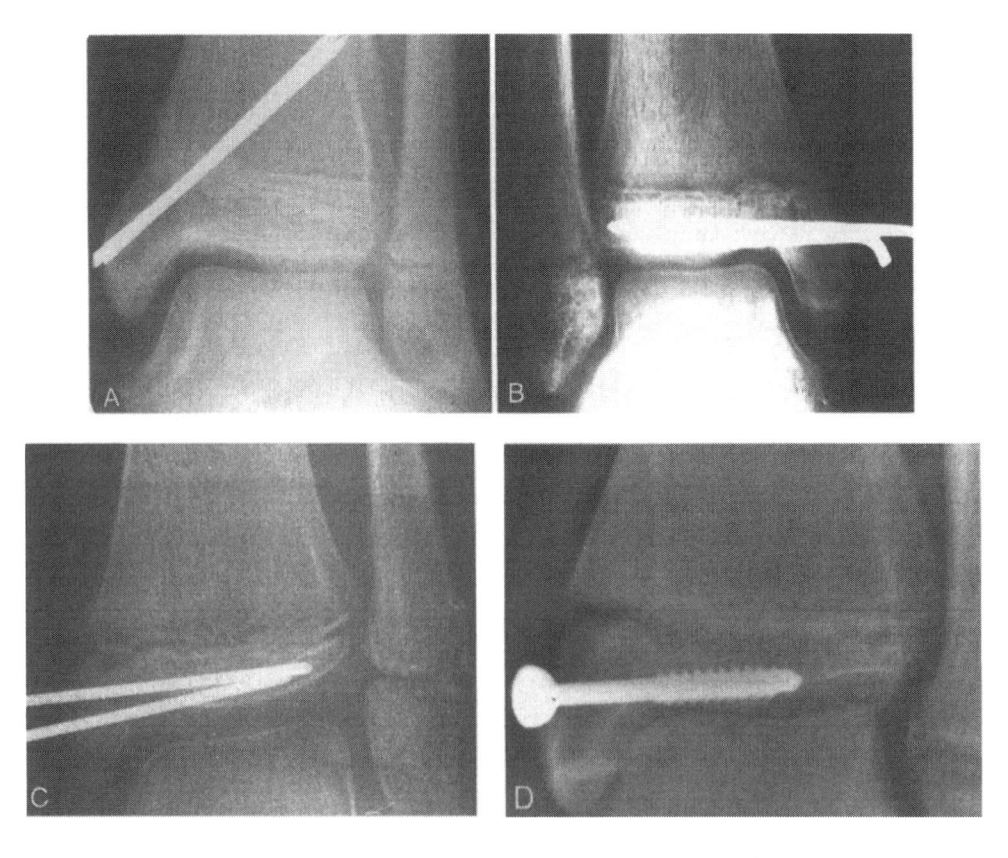

FIGURE 23-130. Methods of fixation. (A) Pins across the physis, which should be avoided whenever possible. Premature epiphysiodesis is evident. (B, C) Type 3 and type 4 injuries treated by transepiphyseal pinning. (D) Cancellous screw compressing a type 3 fragment.

Distal Epiphyseal and Physeal Injuries

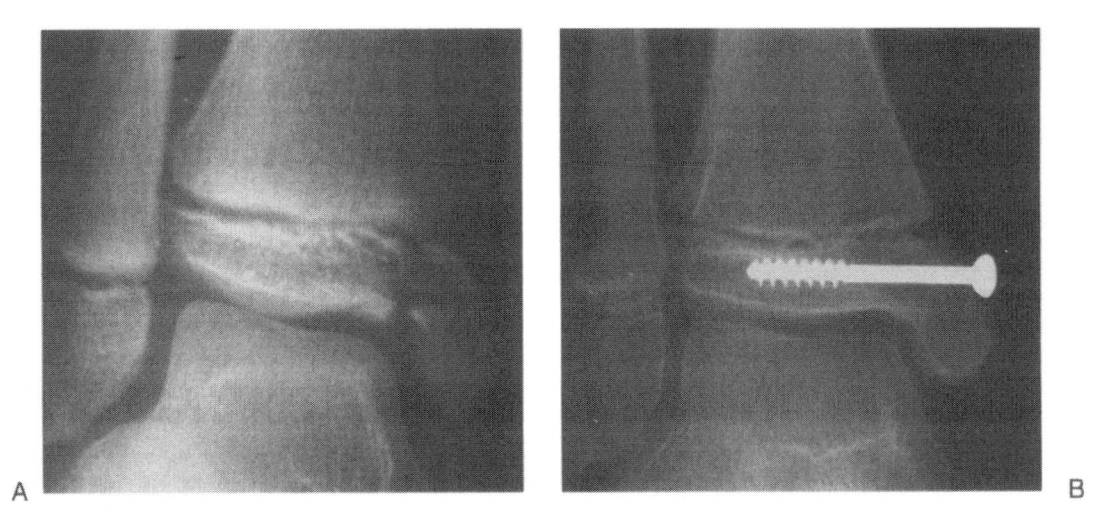

FIGURE 23-131. (A) Type 3 injury. (B) Open reduction and internal fixation. The screw is placed as centrally as possible within the ossification center.

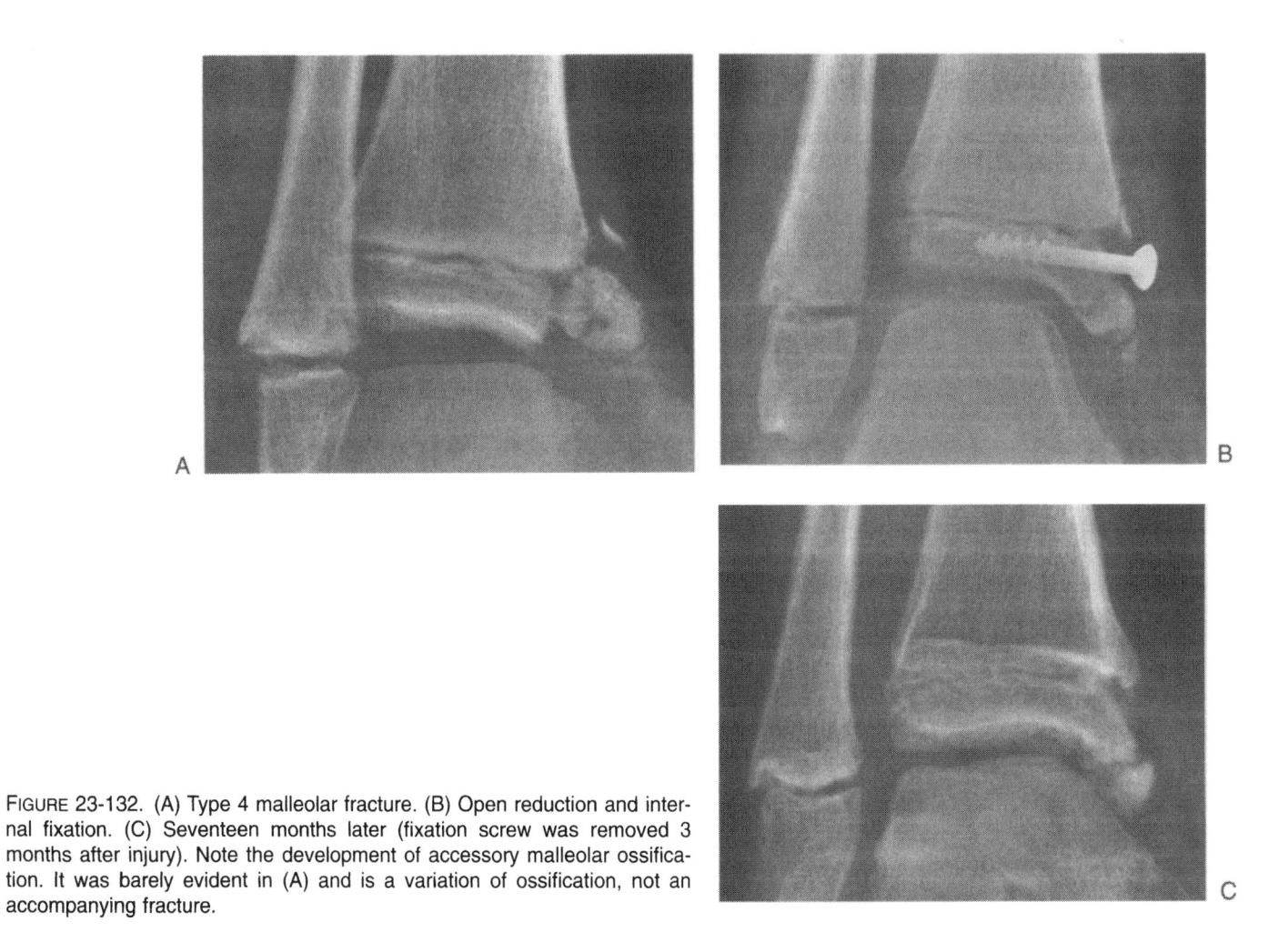

FIGURE 23-132. (A) Type 4 malleolar fracture. (B) Open reduction and internal fixation. (C) Seventeen months later (fixation screw was removed 3 months after injury). Note the development of accessory malleolar ossification. It was barely evident in (A) and is a variation of ossification, not an accompanying fracture.

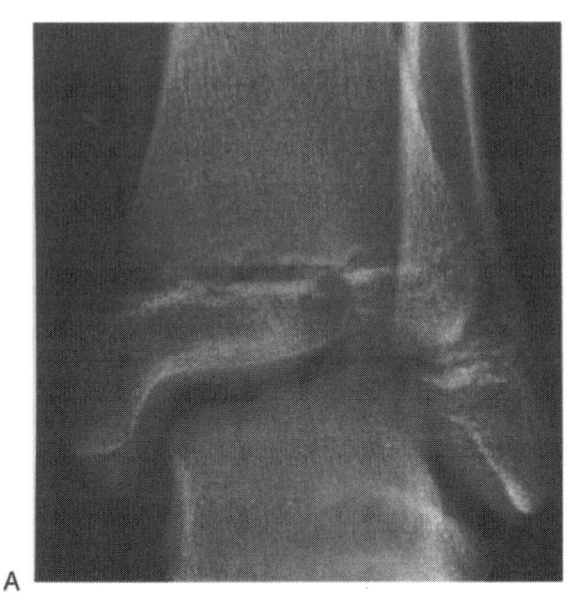

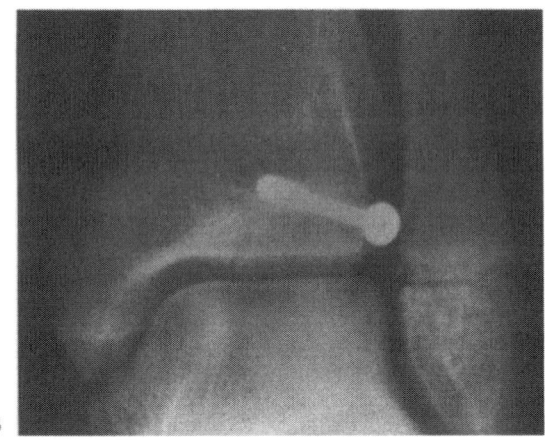

FIGURE 23-133. (A) Tillaux fracture. (B) It was reduced using a percutaneous wire followed by percutaneous screw fixation.

leg is immobilized in an above-knee cast for 6–8 weeks. The physeal injury is type 3, involving the lateral part of the distal tibial epiphysis. If the fracture fragments are displaced more than 2 mm, open reduction and internal fixation with a cancellous screw or smooth K-wires are undertaken through an anterolateral approach (Fig. 23-133). Lintecum and Blasier used a variation of open reduction to treat Tillaux fractures, performing arthrotomy reduction and then directing the screw from medial to lateral.[506] With accurate reduction, the prognosis is excellent. Deformity due to asymmetric growth from a physeal injury does not follow this fracture. Joint incongruity may be prevented by anatomic reduction.

Leitch et al. used three-dimensional reconstruction of CT scans to demonstrate the instability of the Tillaux fracture.[567] They used a single cancellous screw to accomplish reduction. It was performed by closed reduction under anesthesia with placement of the screw under fluoroscopy. The initial reduction was assessed by CT scan and three-dimensional confirmation.

Closed treatment remains the initial option for many triplane fractures, especially if significant soft tissue damage, fracture blisters, and so on are present. A cast for nondisplaced fractures or closed reduction for displaced fractures should be attempted first by internal rotation and anterior movement of the fibular metaphyseal piece. Failure to obtain or maintain an adequate closed reduction with less than 2 mm of displacement, as determined by plain radiographs, is an indication for operative treatment, which should consist of screw fixation for the metaphyseal fragment alone in two-part fractures and screw fixation for both metaphyseal and epiphyseal fragments in three-part fractures. Previously obtained tomograms (anteroposterior and lateral) and if possible a CT scan should be available prior to open reduction so proper preoperative planning may take place. Depending on the fracture configuration, two incisions may be necessary (anteromedial and anterolateral), and internal fixation both above and below the physis may be needed, particularly for the three- or four-part triplane fractures.

Interfragmentary cortical screws are preferable for fibular and epiphyseal fractures, as they may be easily removed 6–12 weeks after injury. Smooth pins are less desirable for maintenance of anatomic reduction, as they do not compress the fracture fragments adequately. Intraoperative roentgenograms are mandatory for determining the adequacy of reduction and the direction and length of the fixation devices. Regardless of postoperative immobilization, weight-bearing other than toe-touching should be delayed for 6 weeks.

Whipple et al. used arthroscopic reduction and internal fixation of triplane fractures.[612] They believed this method reduced surgical trauma, provided a method for accurate delineation of fracture fragment orientation, and ensured accurate reduction and joint continuity.

Associated fibular fractures may have to be fixed internally. Provisional fixation may be performed first. If reduction of the tibial fractures is made more difficult by the fibular fixation (e.g., periosteal interposition), the provisional fibular fixation may be released and the tibial fragments fixed internally as a first step. Fixation of the tibial components may proceed in a distal to proximal (intraarticular epiphyseal to metaphyseal) direction or vice versa, depending on the individual fracture. For some two-fragment fractures, metaphyseal fixation alone may produce an anatomic reduction.

Yablon et al. showed that incomplete reduction of the lateral malleolus was necessary to reposition the talus anatomically.[558] They thought that the lateral malleolus was the key to anatomic reduction of the biomalleolar fractures.

Type 6 injuries, which are usually acquired by catching the ankle in the spoked wheel of a bicycle, often involve an open injury. Definitive treatment must be directed at the wound to prevent osteomyelitis. The fracture itself may not require specific treatment (i.e., fixation). However, long-term observation is essential to rule out subsequent formation of an osseous bridge, which can be resected if it creates a significant deformity.

Type 7 injuries should be treated by closed reduction first, as the weight-bearing main articular surface is not usually interrupted. Transversely oriented fractures are usually

Distal Epiphyseal and Physeal Injuries

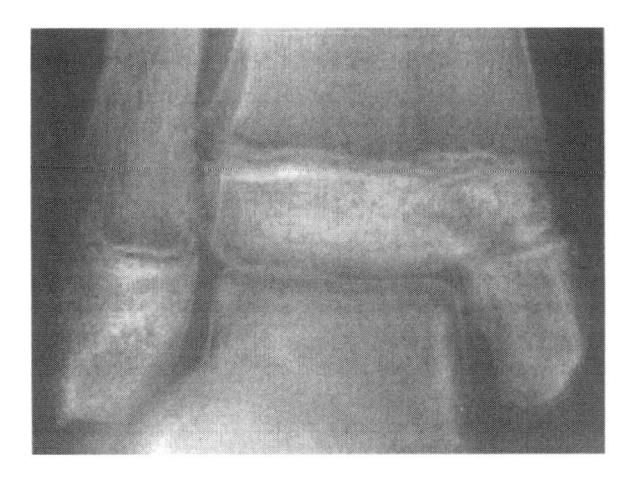

FIGURE 23-134. Transversely oriented type 7 injury treated by closed reduction.

stable (Fig. 23-134, but more obliquely oriented fractures require stabilization (Fig. 23-135).

Mechanistic Treatment

Reversal of the mechanism of injury usually reduces the fracture, even in children. Manipulation, especially in an apprehensive or uncooperative child, is best performed with the patient under adequate sedation if not general anesthesia. Relaxation of muscles and absence of pain make the manipulation less traumatic. The knee is flexed 90°, and the foot is placed in plantar flexion to relax the triceps surae muscle. An assistant applies countertraction by pulling the leg. The surgeon grasps the foot by the heel while steadying the anterior aspect of the lower tibia. Distal traction is applied in the line of the deformity and then in the direction opposite to the injurious force to reduce the fracture.

For supination-inversion injuries, longitudinal distal traction is first applied medially, and then the hindfoot is everted. The foot is immobilized in slight pronation with the ankle in neutral dorsiflexion. For type 1 or type 2 growth mechanism fractures of the distal fibular physis, immobilization is used for 3–4 weeks. The prognosis is excellent.

With supination-inversion injuries, there is a type 3 or type 4 physeal fracture of the distal tibial epiphysis. Anatomic reduction is mandatory. The separation of fracture fragments should be less than 2 mm. If the fracture cannot be reduced and anatomic reduction maintained by closed methods, open reduction is undertaken. Wires or a cancellous screw may be used for internal fixation. After closed or open reduction, an above-knee cast is applied with the knee in flexion. The cast is extended above the flexed knee to relax the pull on the Achilles tendon and to discourage weight-bearing. Immobilization is continued for 6–8 weeks, after which gradual weight-bearing is allowed. Restraint from weight-bearing for longer periods is of no value in preventing deformity once the physis has been injured. The risk of growth arrest of the medial portion of the distal tibial physis is significant. With a supination-plantar flexion fracture, longitudinal traction is first applied in plantar flexion; then, while the downward traction is maintained, the ankle is gently dorsiflexed. The limb is immobilized for 4–6 weeks in an above-knee cast, with the ankle in 5°–10° of dorsiflexion. The common type 2 physeal fracture of the distal tibial epiphysis usually has a posterior metaphyseal fragment and posterior displacement. Moderate residual deformity tends to disappear spontaneously with subsequent growth and remodeling. Posterior displacement usually corrects itself, as it is in the plane of ankle motion. The danger of managing supination-plantar flexion injury of the ankle is iatrogenic trauma caused by repeated forceful manipulation.

Supination-lateral rotation fractures of the ankle are reduced by longitudinal axial traction and medial rotation of the foot. An above-knee cast is applied with the foot and ankle in slight inversion. The period of immobilization is 8 weeks.

Pronation-eversion-lateral rotation fracture of the ankle is reduced first by longitudinal axial traction in the line of the deformity (i.e., in lateral rotation and with the hindfoot everted), and distal traction is maintained on the hindfoot,

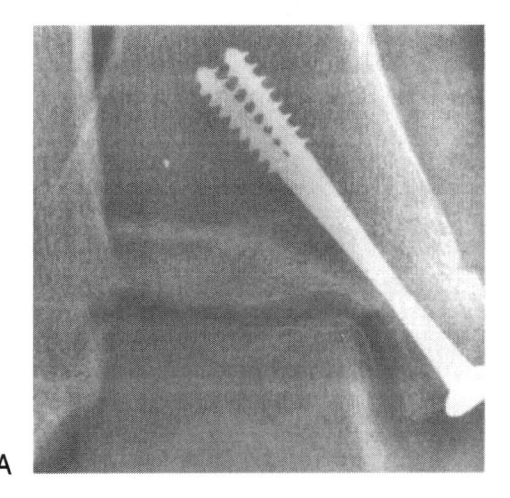

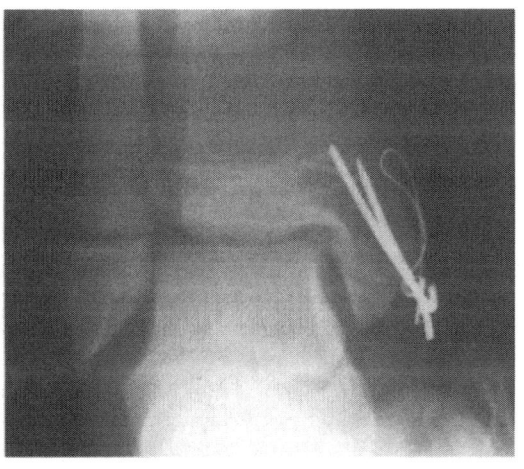

FIGURE 23-135. (A) Open reduction and fixation of oblique type 7 injury. (B) Tension band/pin fixation of type 7 injury.

which is then inverted and medially rotated. An above-knee cast is applied with the foot and ankle in inversion and medial rotation. The physeal injury is a type 2 fracture of the distal tibial epiphysis, with the metaphyseal fragment located on the lateral or posterolateral side. The displacement is lateral, producing a valgus lateral rotation deformity of the ankle. A valgus tilt of the ankle up to 15° may be accepted.

If a valgus tilt of more than 15° is present, a well-padded below-knee splint or cast may be applied. Then, after 3–4 days, gentle closed reduction is reattempted with the patient under general anesthesia. By then, the reactive swelling is usually subsiding owing to compression from the cast and elevation of the leg. If reduction fails and more than 15° of lateral angulation of the ankle persists, open reduction should be considered. Alternatively, the fracture is allowed to heal and if, after 2–3 years, the deformity persists and causes functional problems a supramalleolar osteotomy may be performed to correct the valgus deformity at the ankle.

Results

Goldberg and Aadalen stressed that injury to the distal tibial epiphysis is becoming increasingly common with the emphasis on competitive athletics and greater overall participation in athletics.[462] Of 237 fractures, 184 were followed an average of 28 months after injury. Goldberg and Aadalen identified three groups according to the risks of developing shortening of the leg, angular deformity of the bone, or incongruity of the joint. The low-risk group consisted of 89 patients, only 6.7% of whom had complications. This group included all type 1 and type 2 fibular physeal fractures, all type 1 tibial physeal fractures, type 3 and type 4 tibial physeal fractures with less than 2 mm of displacement, and epiphyseal avulsion injuries. In contrast, the high-risk group consisted of 28 patients, 32% of whom developed complications. This group included type 3 and type 4 tibial physeal fractures with 2 mm or more displacement, Tillaux fractures, triplane fractures, and comminuted tibial epiphyseal fractures. The third, unpredictable group was made up of 66 patients, 16.7% of whom had complications; it included only type 2 tibial physeal fractures. The incidence and types of the complications certainly correlated well with the type of fracture, the severity of the displacement or comminution, and the adequacy of the reduction.

Giuliani thought that each of these injuries was associated with some degree of deformity, claiming that the commonest deformity was a discrepancy in leg length, and that varus and valgus deformity appeared as late complications.[461] Hohmann concurred with this high incidence of complications, whereas other authors have stated that growth deformity usually occurs only following adduction-type fractures.[474] Johnson and Fahl believed that growth deformity could occur consequent to injuries other than adduction injuries.[476]

Type 1 and type 2 growth mechanism injuries involving the tibia or the fibula have good prognoses. However, more extensive injuries, such as type 3 and type 4 injuries with displacement, are associated with a high incidence of growth deformity with localized premature epiphysiodesis and osseous bridging. Aitken observed that many of these injuries occur in children nearing skeletal maturity, so premature ossification is not a major consequence.[416]

Complications

Fractures involving the physis should be closely followed for possible development of growth disturbance. Parents should be warned of potential complications but without causing major anxiety. As already indicated, the factors that determine the prognosis are the type of epiphyseal or physeal injury, the age of the child at the time of fracture, the integrity of the blood supply to the epiphysis, the method of reduction, and whether the fracture is open or closed.

The most significant complication is growth arrest with the formation of an osseous bridge (Figs. 23-136 to 23-140). Melchoir et al. reviewed 96 distal tibial epiphyseal fractures[518] and noted premature closure of the growth plate in 15%. Growth arrest may develop after adduction injury as a result of damage to the germinal layer of the physis,[441] but it is not always easy to predict whether this will occur. With type 3 and type 4 growth mechanism fractures the medial part of the tibial physis may fuse, whereas the lateral portion may

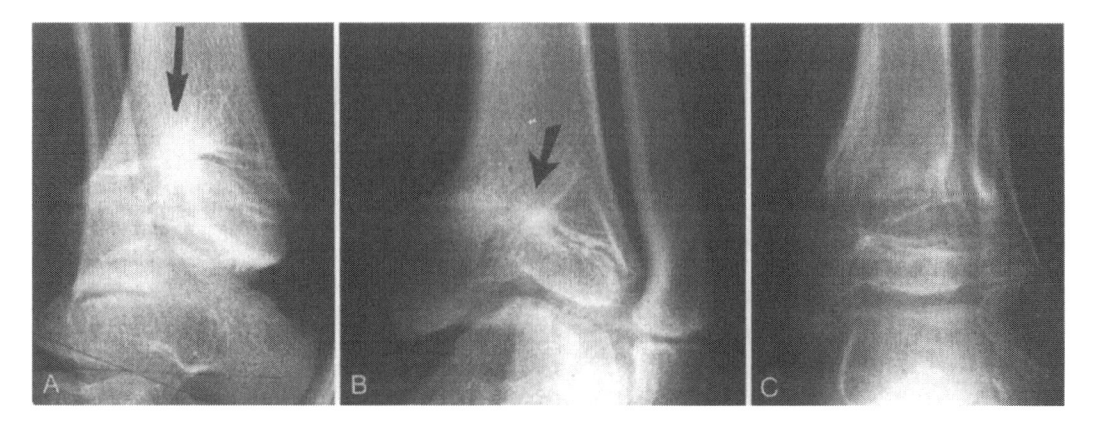

FIGURE 23-136. (A, B) Localized bridge formation (arrows). (C) After osteotomy without resection of the bridge.

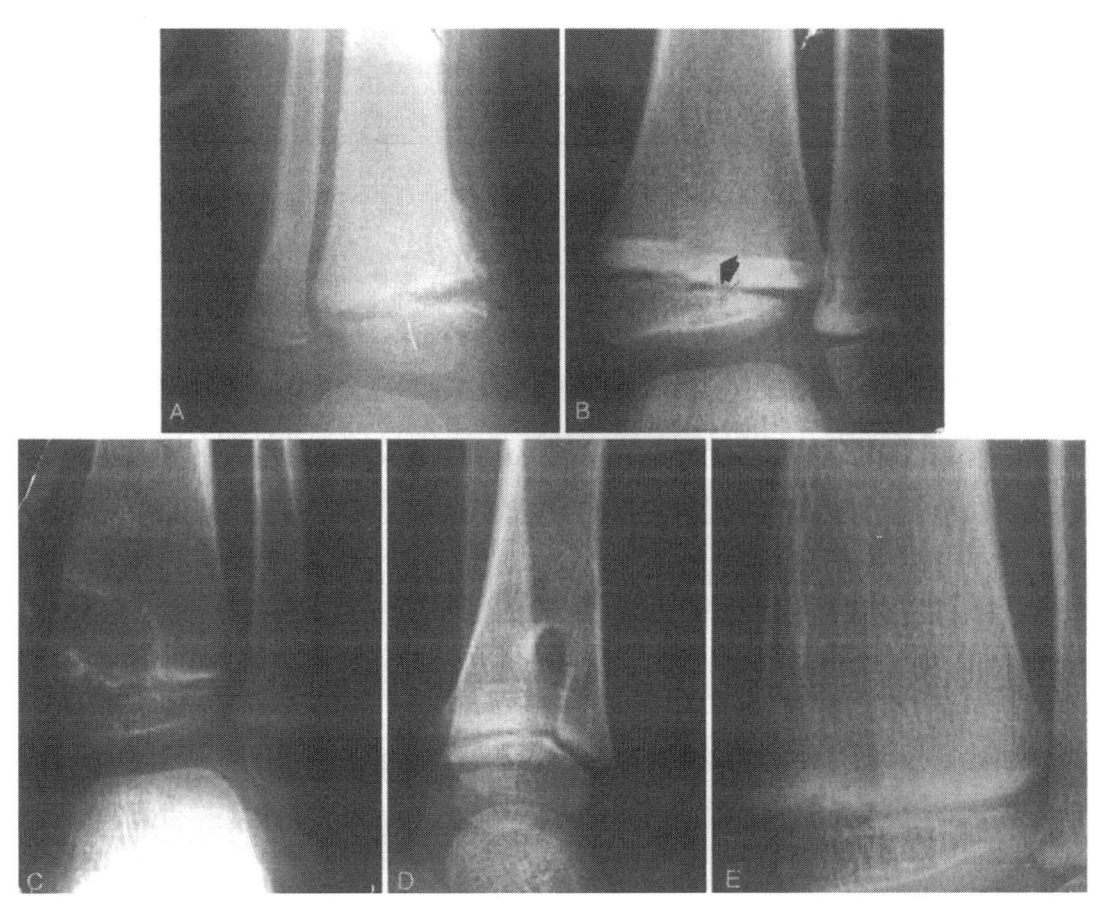

FIGURE 23-137. (A) Seemingly innocuous type 2 fracture in a 2-year-old child. (B) One year later a central bone bridge is forming. Note the "step" in the Harris line (arrow). (C, D) The bridge was resected through a metaphyseal window and filled with fat. (E) Thirty-eight months later the bridge has not reformed. Note the elongated "cavity."

continue to grow, leading to varus deformity at the ankle. The younger the patient, the worse is the subsequent deformity. Premature growth arrest of the entire distal tibial epiphysis results in shortening of the tibia.

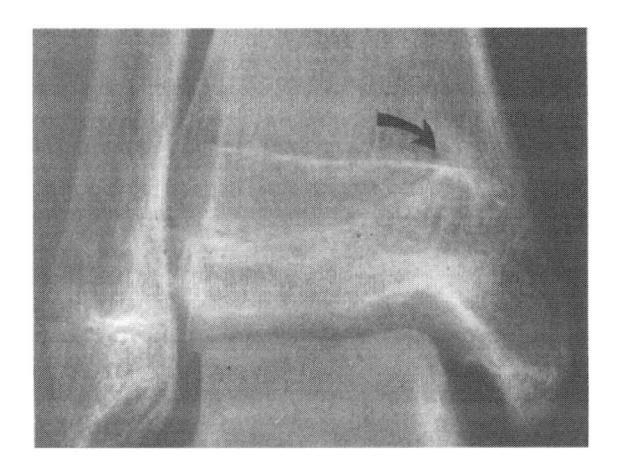

FIGURE 23-138. Growth arrest after medial malleolar fracture. Note how the growth arrest line converges with the physis at the bridge (arrow).

Bostock and Peach described a 5-year-old girl who developed a small medial bridge following closed reduction of a type 3 growth mechanism fracture. It resolved spontaneously 2.5 years later.

Langenskiöld showed that complications of traumatic premature closure are understressed, and that when they do occur, care must be taken to assess the distal fibula, as epiphysiodesis might be appropriate to prevent fibular overgrowth that can affect joint mechanics.[499] If the distal tibial physis closes prematurely, overgrowth of the distal fibula may block normal heel valgus position and cause pain. It is essential that epiphysiodesis be performed on the distal fibula to prevent such overgrowth. Shortening may also be necessary.

King and associates injected sodium diatrizoate (Hypaque) into the peroneal tendon sheath and showed that in patients with significant amounts of lateral pain there was a block in the flow of contrast medium in the sheath at the tip of the lateral malleolus because of calcaneofibular weight-bearing impingement.[705] The pain was completely relieved by excising the tip of the lateral malleolus.

Growth arrest is not usually a problem in most cases of triplane fracture, and follow-up studies for that complication are usually not necessary because of the minimal remaining growth in the tibial physis. The prognosis of triplane

1064 · 23. Tibia and Fibula

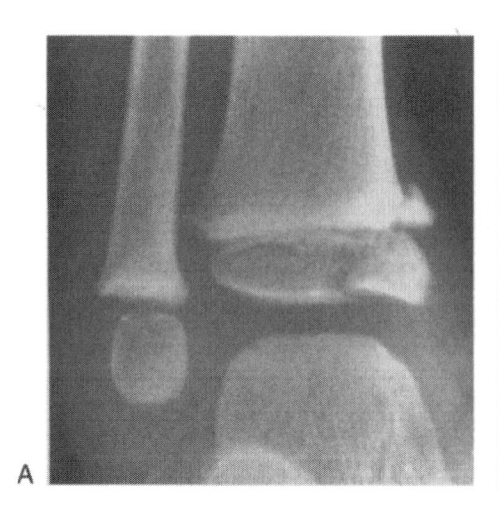

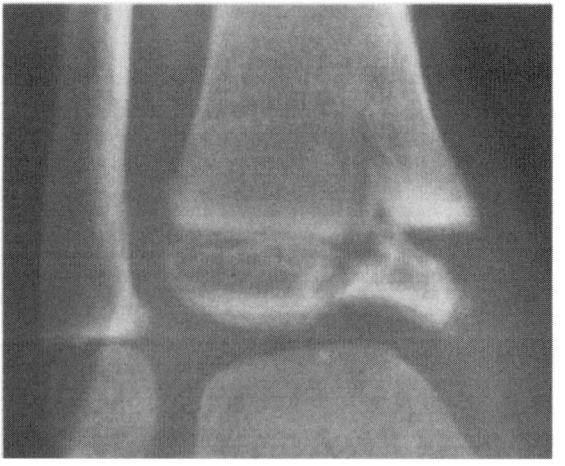

FIGURE 23-139. (A) Type 4 injury due to child abuse. (B) Early bridge formation 5 months later.

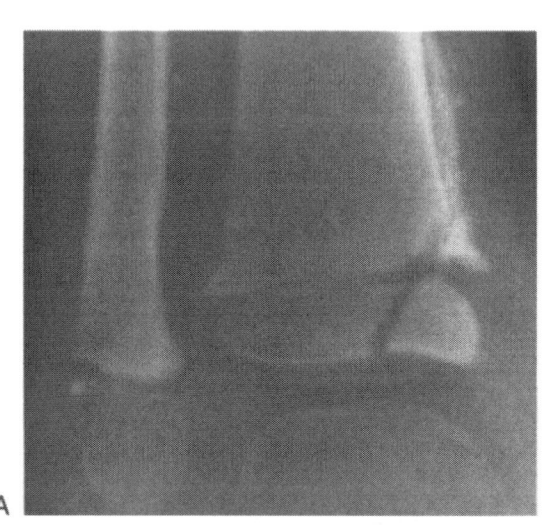

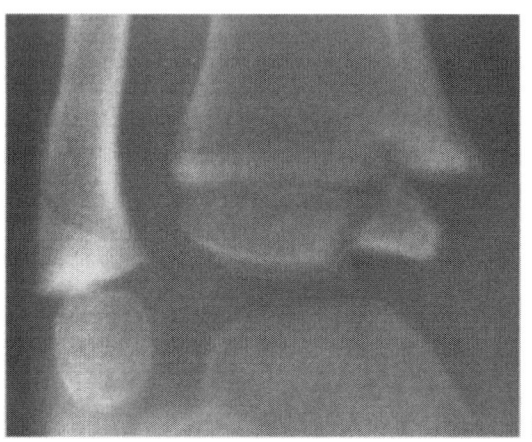

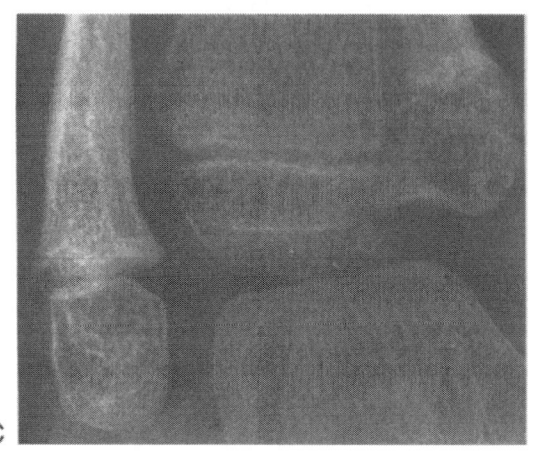

FIGURE 23-140. (A) Type 4 injury treated by closed reduction in a 23-month-old child. This was a case of child abuse, and the injury was already healing. Note the fibular physeal fracture. (B) Three months later. (C) Two years later.

fractures is thus related directly to the anatomic reduction that is attained and maintained.

The extent of fusion of the growth plate is determined by anteroposterior and lateral tomography of the ankle joint. If less than 40% of the growth plate is fused, the bone bridge may be resected and replaced with adipose tissue or cranioplast. Excision of the bone bridge should be complete (see Chapter 7).

If the extent of the bone bridge is more than 50% of the width of the physis, the varus deformity at the ankle joint may be corrected by supramalleolar osteotomy of the tibia (along with completion of the fusion). The age of the patient and the amount of shortening determine the operative procedure chosen. If surgery is postponed until ossification of the physis is complete in children and young adolescents (under 12 years for girls and under 14 years for boys), structural changes due to walking in inversion may take place in the ankle mortise. In addition, resultant shortening of the leg and overgrowth of the fibula may be of considerable magnitude. Thus it is best to perform an opening wedge osteotomy without disturbing the lateral portion of the distal tibial physis. With growth, the varus deformity recurs, and a second osteotomy may be required for correction. This possibility should be explained carefully to the parents.

In an older patient (girls over 12 years and boys over 14 years), epiphysiodesis of the distal fibular physis and of the lateral half of the distal tibial physis may be performed to prevent or lessen the development of varus deformity of the ankle. If significant ankle varus deformity has already occurred, the procedure is combined with an open-up wedge osteotomy of the medial aspect of the distal tibia.

Premature growth arrest of the entire distal tibial epiphysis usually results in shortening of the tibia. In the older patient this shortening is inconsequential clinically because of the proximity to termination of skeletal growth, whereas in the younger child leg length discrepancy may be so marked that an epiphyseal arrest of the contralateral leg is indicated. An epiphysiodesis of the distal fibula on the affected side is performed to prevent its overgrowth.

A lateral rotation deformity may result from inadequate reduction. There is a persistent posterior position of the fibula and its attached tibial fragment.

Ankle valgus deformity usually results from incomplete reduction of a pronation-eversion-lateral rotation fracture of the ankle. A valgus tilt of the ankle of more than 15°–20° does not correct itself by remodeling with skeletal growth and cannot be accepted. It should be corrected surgically. If sufficient growth potential of the distal tibial epiphysis is present, the deformity may be corrected by epiphyseal arrest of the medial side of the distal tibia. Stapling of the medial side of the physis may be performed if it is difficult to calculate the exact skeletal age of the child. Growth arrest causes further shortening of the limb.

Screw epiphysiodesis has been recommended for the management of ankle valgus in children.[444,538] It probably has limited use for posttraumatic valgus deformity but certainly may be considered as an alternative to open epiphysiodesis.

If skeletal growth is complete, osteotomy of the distal tibia and fibula is performed to correct the deformity. A wedge osteotomy of the distal tibia may cause an unsightly prominence of the medial malleolus and shortening of the limb.

Marti et al. showed various types of correction with malalignment of the distal tibia. They particularly incorporated open and closing wedge osteotomies to effect a more anatomic position.[514]

A potentially serious complication, joint incongruity, may cause early degenerative arthritis.[532] Separation of fracture fragments larger than 2 mm should not be accepted.

Lantz et al. studied the effect of concomitant chondral injuries accompanying operatively reduced malleolar fractures.[500] They believed that poor results from operative anatomic reduction were due to unrecognized injuries to the cartilaginous surfaces of the tibiotalar joint (Fig. 23-141). Patients with seemingly isolated closed malleolar fractures underwent open reduction and internal fixation using routine operative fixation techniques. In each the talar dome was inspected. Thirty-one patients, essentially 50%, had injury to the talar dome cartilage, ranging from mild "scuffing" to a free osteochondral fragment. Lantz et al. emphasized the importance of looking for these injuries at the time of malleolar fracture reduction.

Robertson[532] and Siffert and Arkin[534] described osteochondritis as a complication following a bimalleolar fracture with a crush injury of the lateral half of the epiphysis.

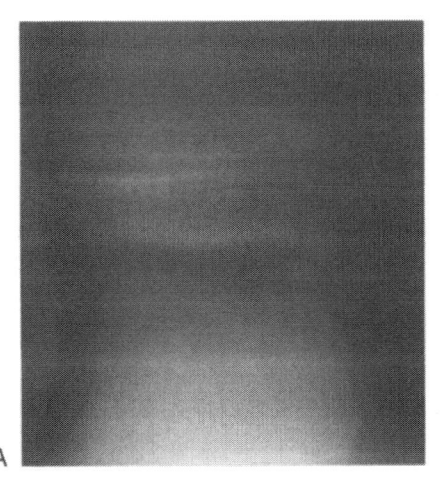

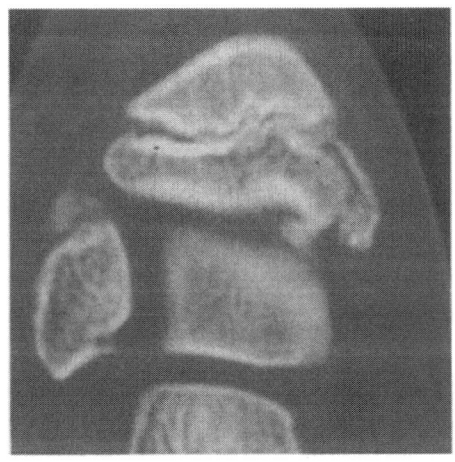

FIGURE 23-141. (A) Intraarticular fragment. (B) CT scan shows the fragment, with the probable source a medial malleolar shell fracture.

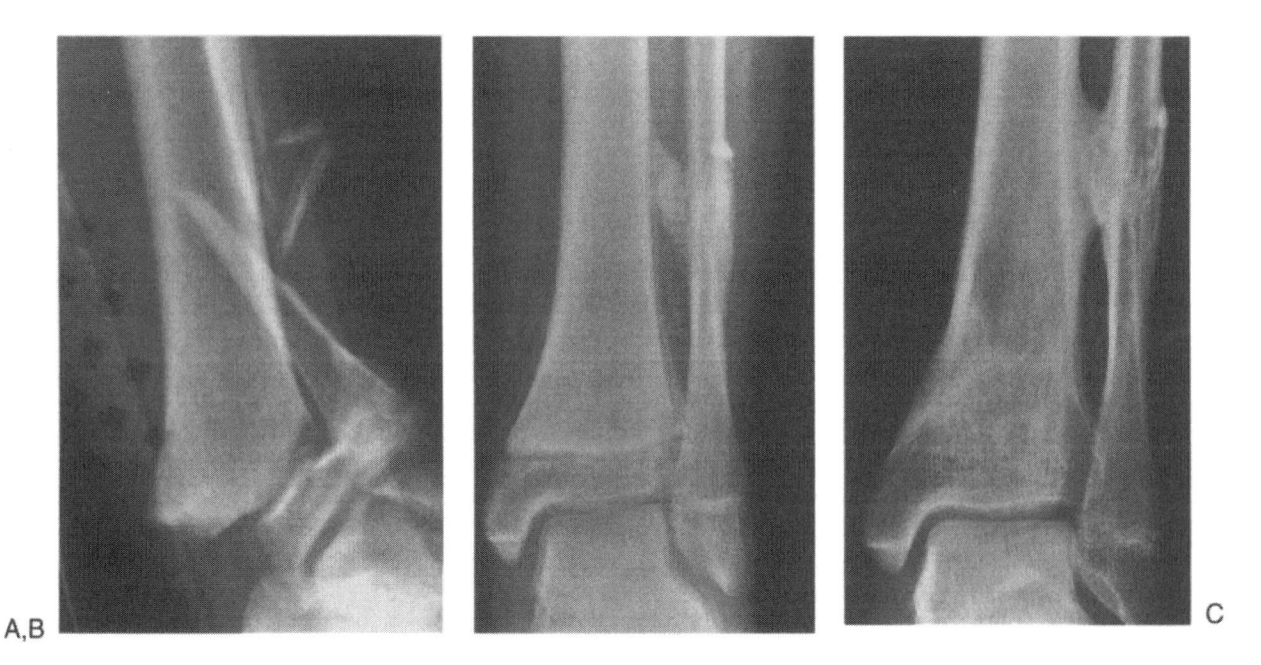

FIGURE 23-142. (A) Distal tibial physeal and fibular diaphyseal fractures. (B) Early synostosis 3 months later. (C) Mature synostosis and tibial physeal closure 15 months after injury.

Robertson's patient did not sustain a fracture but merely a "sprain." The patient was 3 years old at the time of injury, and a roentgenogram failed to reveal a type 2 fracture. The roentgenogram probably could not be used to rule it out totally if it was a pure epiphyseal displacement and reduction; however, 4 months later, when roentgenograms were obtained, there was flattening and sclerosis of the distal tibial physis, particularly laterally.

Pritsch et al., using arthroscopy of the ankle, found that adhesion of the distal tibiofibular syndesmosis was the cause of chronic ankle pain in 11 of 19 patients, and that symptoms resolved in all 11 patients after arthroscopic resection of the adhesions.[530]

Tibiofibular synostosis (Fig. 23-142) has also been reported as a rare complication of a distal tibial epiphyseal injury.[400] This condition undoubtedly results from periosteal disruptions and subsequent ectopic bone formation between the metaphyses just above the syndesmosis (see Chapter 7).

Kennedy and Weiner described a patient with distal tibial epiphyseal avascular necrosis after a severe fracture.[486] The patient subsequently had complete asymptomatic revascularization and closure of the growth plate without deformity.

Intramalleolar Injury (Accessory Ossicle)

Accessory "ossicles" of the malleoli are common in skeletally immature individuals. The lateral ossicle has been termed the "os subfibulare" and the medial ossicle the "os subtibiale."[613–660] They usually appear between 7 and 10 years of age and eventually fuse with the secondary ossification center of the malleolus at skeletal maturation. Such accessory centers of ossification rarely persist beyond skeletal maturation. In one study of normal children between 6 and 12 years of age, an accessory center of ossification was found in the medial malleolus in 20%, and in the lateral malleolus in 1%.[650] Bilaterality is common, as is involvement of both lateral and medial malleoli.

Many of these ossification variations are identified only fortuitously when radiographs are obtained to evaluate injury to the ankle or foot. Because such accessory "ossicles" are usually considered ossification variations rather than avulsion fractures, diagnostic problems may arise in the selectively symptomatic patient. There are few references to symptomatic ossicles of the malleoli.[615,621,647,651] Griffiths and Menelaus emphasized that symptomatic lateral malleolar ossicles should be evaluated with scintigraphy and treated surgically in selected cases.[632]

The medial malleolus occasionally develops a separate center or centers of ossification. The incidence and significance of accessory centers of ossification in the foot have been well investigated (see Chapter 24), but similar variations in the malleolar regions have received less attention. Most reports include a few cases and imply that such centers are infrequent. In contrast, Powell[650] and Hoed[635] described accessory ossification centers of the medial malleolus as being present in 14% of children and concluded that an accessory center of ossification of the medial malleolus and to a lesser extent the lateral malleolus is probably a relatively common developmental variation. These figures may be relatively low, as such variations are generally found only when evaluating trauma to the ankle or foot.

Hoed studied 150 healthy children; there was a separate center in the tip of the medial malleolus in 21 ankles, with the average time of appearance of this accessory ossification being 7.6 years in girls and 8.7 years in boys.[635] In another survey 20% had accessory ossification centers in one medial malleolus, and 13% had them in both medial malleoli.[619]

Selby described extra centers within the medial malleolus in 47% of girls and 17% of boys.[652] Only one study described the progressive changes within these accessory centers.[645]

Ogden and Lee reviewed 61 patients with accessory ossification involving only the medial malleolus.[647] Radiographs of both ankles were obtained in 43 of these patients, 14 of whom had involvement of both medial malleoli. In the patients with bilateral involvement, asymmetry of size and shape were common. Only 27 of the 61 patients had been specifically evaluated for acute or chronic pain of the medial malleolus. Of these, all but one were treated with cast immobilization and were subsequently relieved of their symptoms, even though the accessory center remained radiographically separate for months to years after the "injury." One patient was treated surgically with skeletal fixation.

Histologically, there is a bipolar physis between the secondary and accessory centers, not unlike the comparable region between the main tibial and tibial tuberosity ossification centers proximally or in the accessory navicular and bipartite patella. A similar accessory ossification pattern sometimes is found at the proximal end of the greater trochanter (see Chapter 21). Although there may be apparent radiographic discontinuity of bone, histologic examination shows complete continuity of surrounding cartilage. The natural history is progressive ossification and eventual fusion to the rest of the malleolar ossification center (Figs. 23-143 to 23-146).

Whether these centers represent variations of ossification or responses to repetitive occult microtrauma is conjectural. The accessory center is contained *within* the malleolar portion of the chondro-osseous epiphysis (Fig. 23-143). It is not a separate piece of ossifying cartilage. The fracture pattern, a type 7 growth mechanism injury, extends through a segment of the malleolus. An ossicle may also be avulsed as a ligament failure analogue, similar to a sleeve fracture of the patella; it is more common in the lateral malleolus than the medial malleolus. These avulsions, if not adequately diagnosed and treated, may progress to delayed union, nonunion, or a chronically painful ankle.

In a series of human embryos the os subtibiale was never found as an independent cartilaginous element.[656] O'Rahilly thought that this ossicle was a malleolar epiphysis.[648] This concept is important when assessing injury. If the accessory center is considered an apophysis, the contiguous secondary center in the malleolus becomes the physeal analogue. A fracture of the malleolar tip, whether acute or chronic, occurs on the "metaphyseal" side, comparable to the injury pattern described in the accessory navicular.[646,647]

Although most of these patients are asymptomatic, an occasional patient has localized pain, acute or chronic. Diagnostic problems particularly arise when accessory centers are found during the evaluation of acute or chronic ankle injury. As with the accessory navicular (see Chapter 24) or bipartite patella (see Chapter 22), microfracture may occur.[646] A bone scan may elucidate such an injury (Fig. 23-146) and may indicate the need for treatment.[647]

Ishii et al. used MRI to evaluate children with chronic medial malleolar injuries.[636] All had a partial avulsion fracture of the accessory ossicle and fragmentation of the ossification center. Interestingly, all three had bilateral accessory ossicle with unilateral symptomatology.

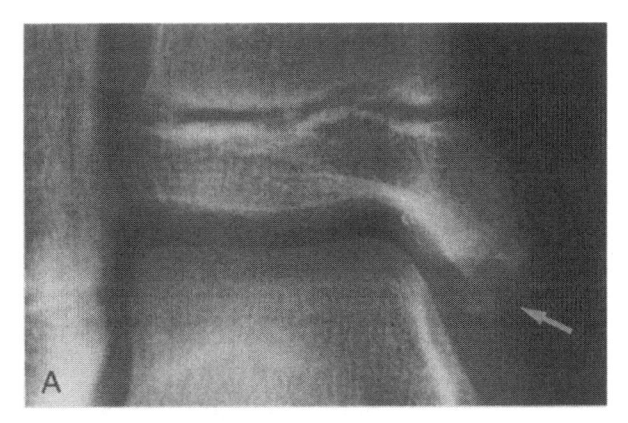

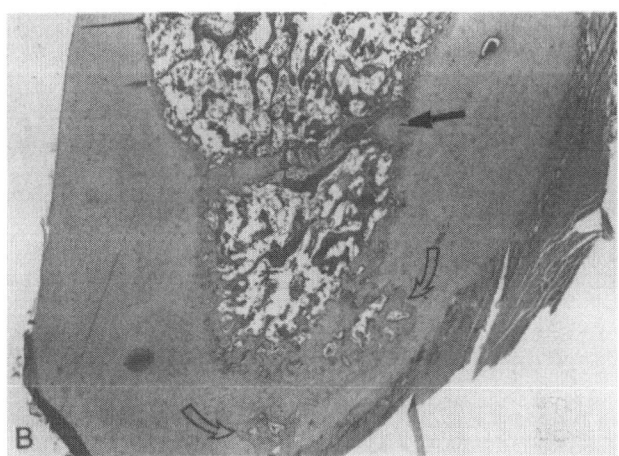

FIGURE 23-143. (A) Multifocal accessory ossification, with possible fracture (arrow). (B) Histologic section shows accessory ossification fusing with the main center (solid arrow). Two other small distal foci are present (open arrows).

The most likely explanation of symptoms is that the accessory ossification center is disrupted through the cartilaginous (chondro-osseous) continuity, resulting in a fracture, fibrous union, or a pseudarthrosis.[646] Mechanical irritation produces local pain and tenderness. A history of major trauma is infrequent. Radiographic "variants" in the patella and tarsal navicular may become acutely symptomatic through acute or chronic trauma. Furthermore, minimally painful epiphyseal injuries have been reported following repetitive stress on the physis. In these situations histologic analysis shows microfractures and chronic inflammation.

Although the accessory malleolar ossification centers are common, they rarely give rise to symptoms sufficient to warrant further radiographic examination or treatment. A center remaining unfused in adult life could cause confusion if found in an ankle that had recently been injured, and it might be regarded as evidence of antecedent, unrecognized injury at the same site. Lapidus described a 23-year-old man with a sprained ankle who gave a history of a similar injury 8 years before; radiographs showed ossicles involving both medial malleoli.[642]

If an accessory center is associated with an acute ankle injury or is found in the patient with chronic symptoms, it is

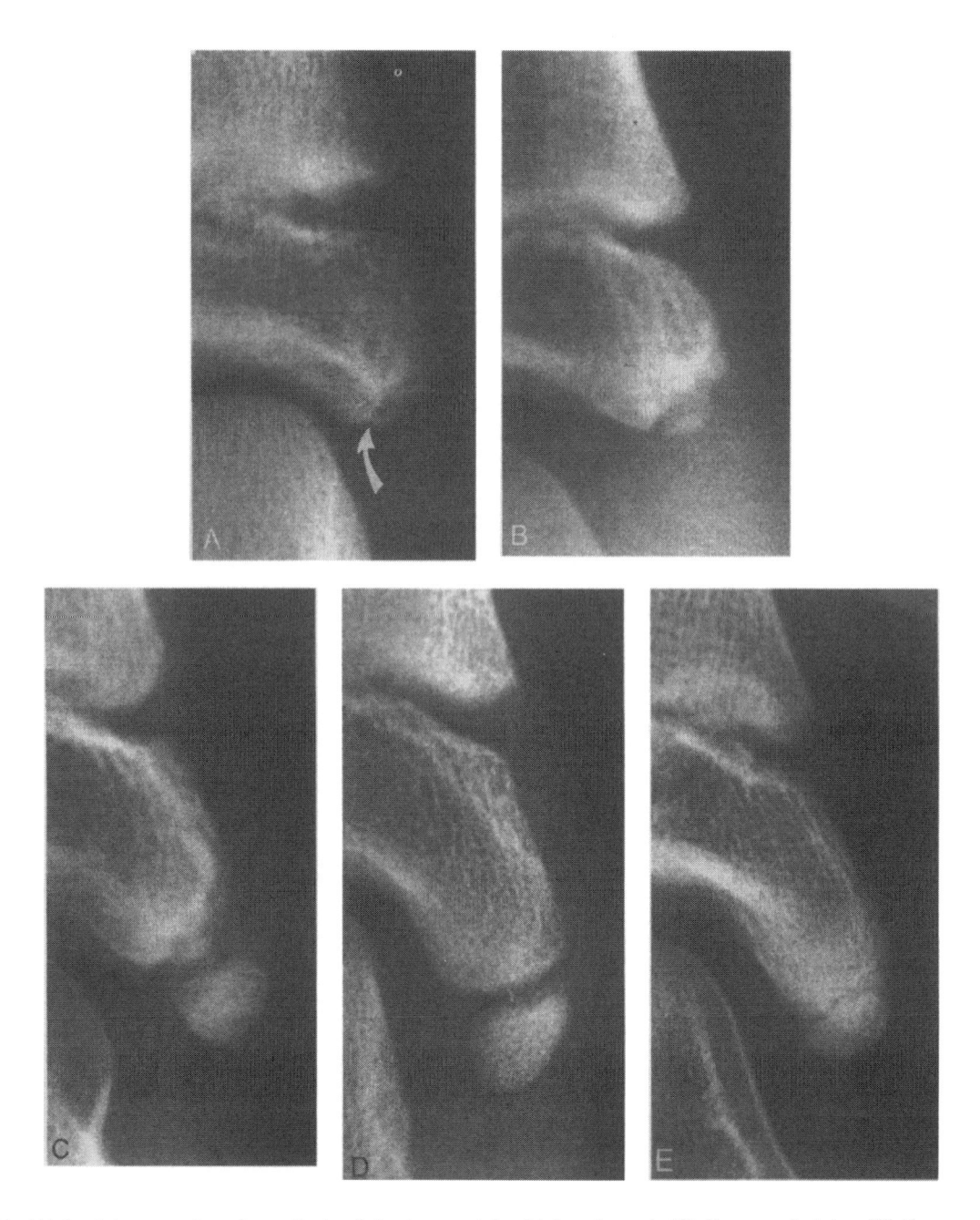

FIGURE 23-144. (A) Acutely asymptomatic malleolus following a minimal injury (arrow). (B) One month later. (C) Seven months later. (D) Two years later. (E) Three years later, with fusion to the rest of the malleolar ossification center.

appropriate to immobilize the ankle for 3–4 weeks and then to encourage mobilization and weight-bearing. Excision of the fragment should be reserved for those *few* patients with recurrent symptoms over a prolonged period and with tenderness at the site of the accessory center. In one study the rarity of the need for such surgery was indicated by the fact that only three of several thousand children with ankle injuries seen over a 26-year period required such treatment.[631] My experience is similar. Only one patient with a medial accessory ossification center required operative treatment; all the other symptomatic patients responded to temporary cast immobilization. In contrast, 5 of 11 patients with symptomatic lateral accessory ossification failed to respond to cast immobilization and subsequently had complete relief of symptoms after surgical excision.

Stanitski and Micheli showed that the enforced utilization of short leg walking casts diminished symptoms in accessory medial malleolar ossification centers.[654] They did not address the issue in lateral accessory centers. They noted that Trolle[656] thought that the os subtibiale was never an inde-

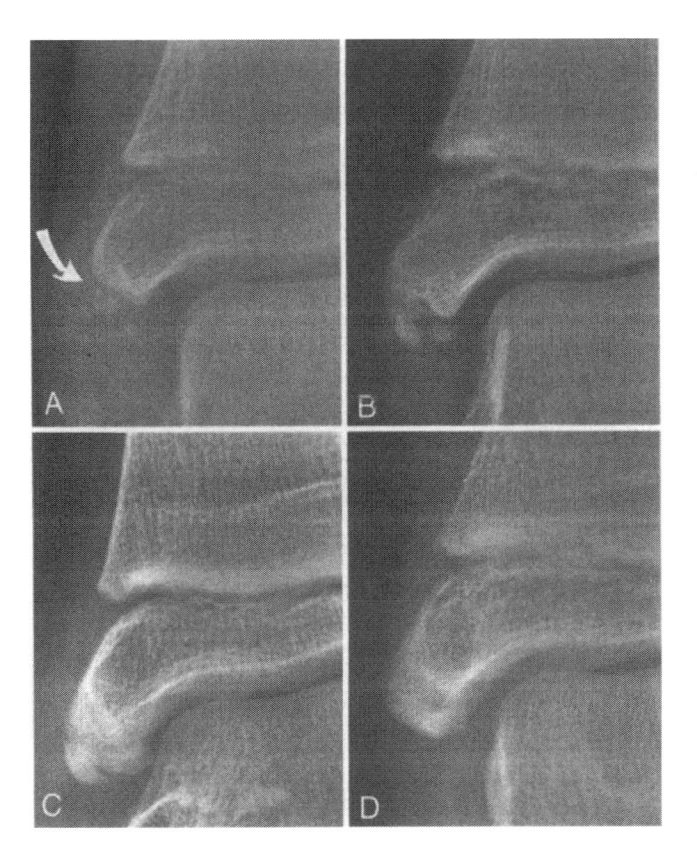

FIGURE 23-145. (A) Appearance 2 weeks after an ankle inversion injury. Is there a healing fracture (arrow)? (B) Five weeks later. (C) Three months later. (D) Six months later.

pendent element. However, in none of the patients described by Ogden and Lee [647] and Love et al.[4] was there evidence of this structure prenatally. All of the accessory centers had developed postnatally, usually after 8–10 years of age. Accordingly, one would not expect them to be present prenatally or perinatally.

Distal Fibular Injuries

Most often the distal fibular metaphysis or physis fails concomitantly with an abduction or adduction injury of the distal tibia. However, the distal fibular physis may fail, albeit infrequently, as a solitary injury.

The patterns include failure through the physis as a type 1 or type 2 growth mechanism injury (Figs. 23-147 to 23-150). This failure often occurs when the physis is undergoing normal closure, comparable to the Tillaux fracture of the distal tibia. Type 6 injuries may occur particularly when the ankle slips between the spokes of a bicycle wheel (Fig. 23-151). Type 7 injuries of the distal portion of the secondary ossification center may occur, but they should not be confused with a normal accessory ossification center at the tip (Figs. 23-152 to 23-155).

The pathomechanics usually involve an abduction-eversion injury that forces the talus and calcaneus against the fibular epiphysis. Because the physis is at the tibial articular level, transversely directed forces summate in the physis. Adduction injury mechanisms may occur but are probably much less frequent. Type 7 is from a supination-inversion mechanism.

The diagnosis may be difficult because displacement is often minimal. Comparison with the opposite side may help.

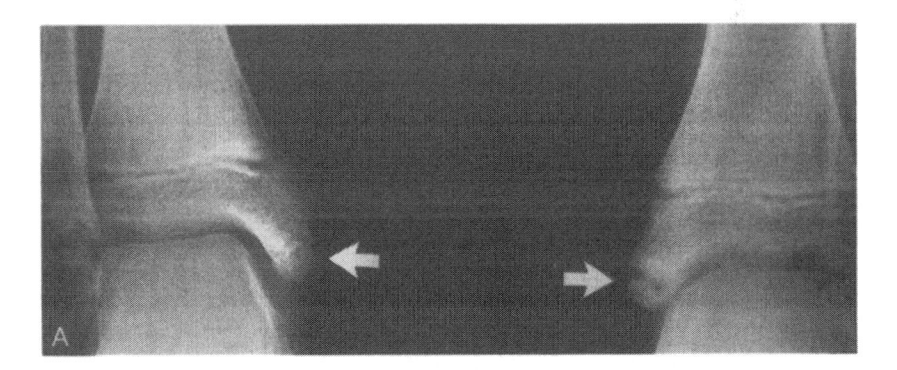

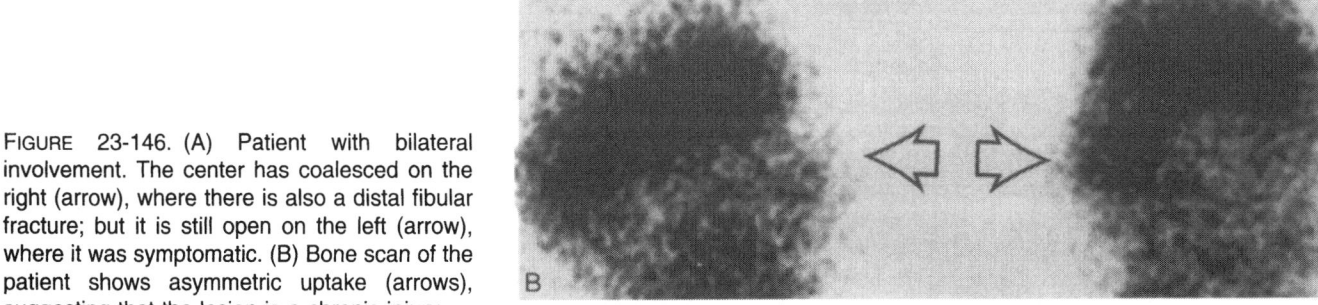

FIGURE 23-146. (A) Patient with bilateral involvement. The center has coalesced on the right (arrow), where there is also a distal fibular fracture; but it is still open on the left (arrow), where it was symptomatic. (B) Bone scan of the patient shows asymmetric uptake (arrows), suggesting that the lesion is a chronic injury.

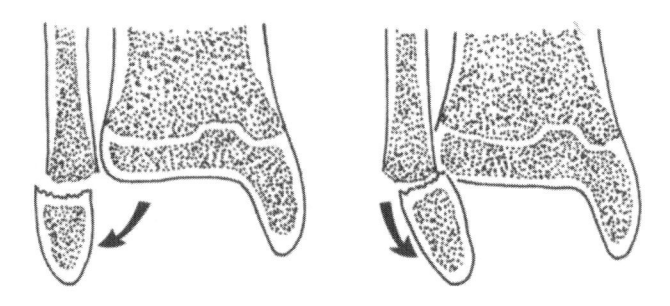

FIGURE 23-147. Type 1 fibular physeal failure patterns in abduction and adduction.

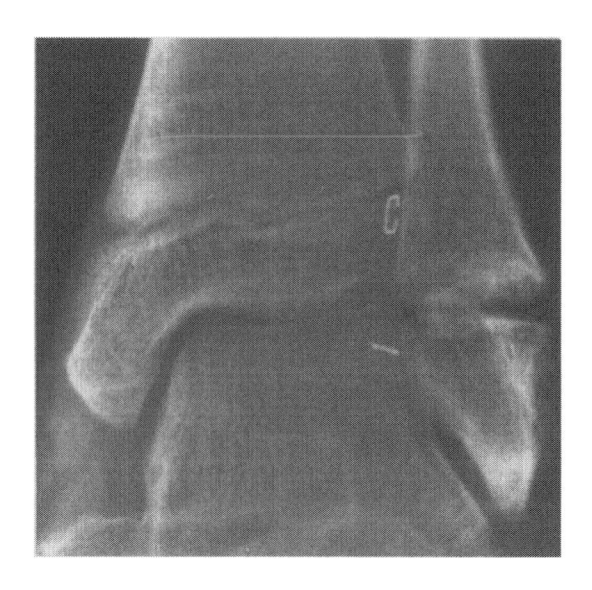

FIGURE 23-148. Type 1 injury of the fibula following an inversion injury and laceration.

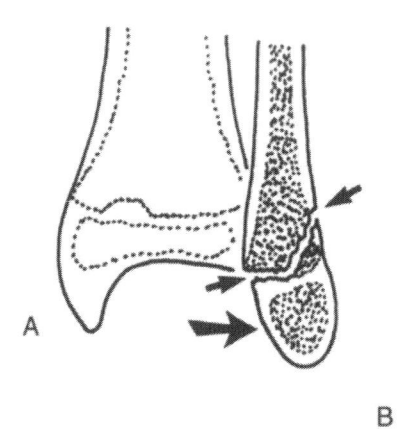

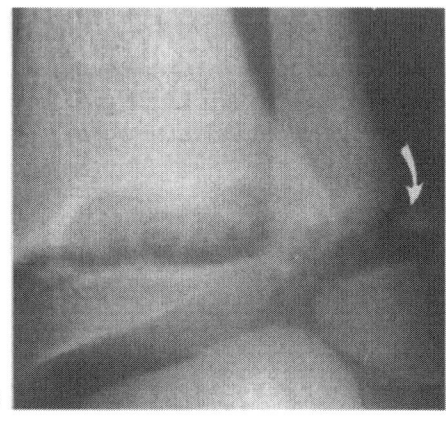

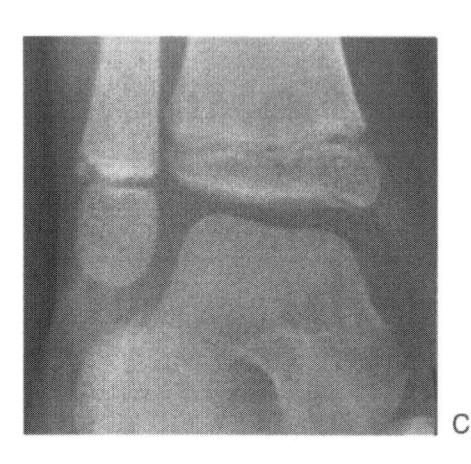

FIGURE 23-149. (A) Type 2 injury pattern of the distal fibula. (B) Roentgenogram of a patient presenting with lateral ankle pain. A type 2 fibular growth mechanism injury (arrow) is evident, but the tibial physis is widened. Subsequent evaluation showed diet-related hypocalcemic rickets. (C) Type 2 injury that spontaneously reduced, leaving a small lateral metaphyseal fragment.

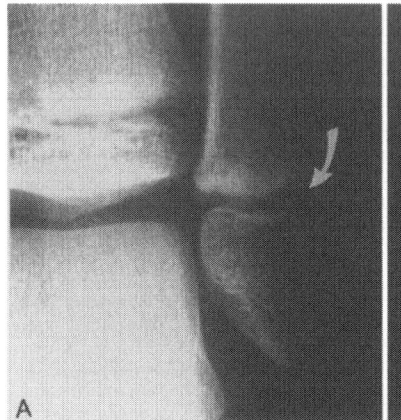

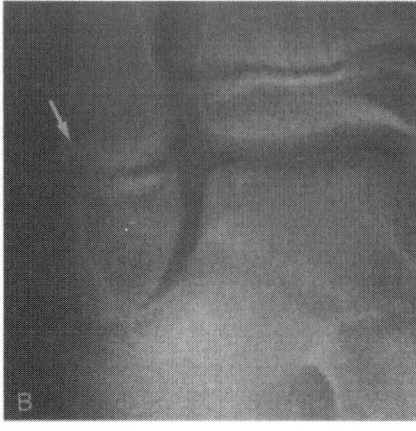

FIGURE 23-150. (A) Type 1 fracture of the distal fibula (arrow). (B) Type 2 injury (arrow) of the distal fibula. (C) Fracture through the distal fibula just after closure (comparable to a Tillaux injury). (D) Type 7 injury (arrow).

Distal Fibular Injuries

FIGURE 23-150. Continued.

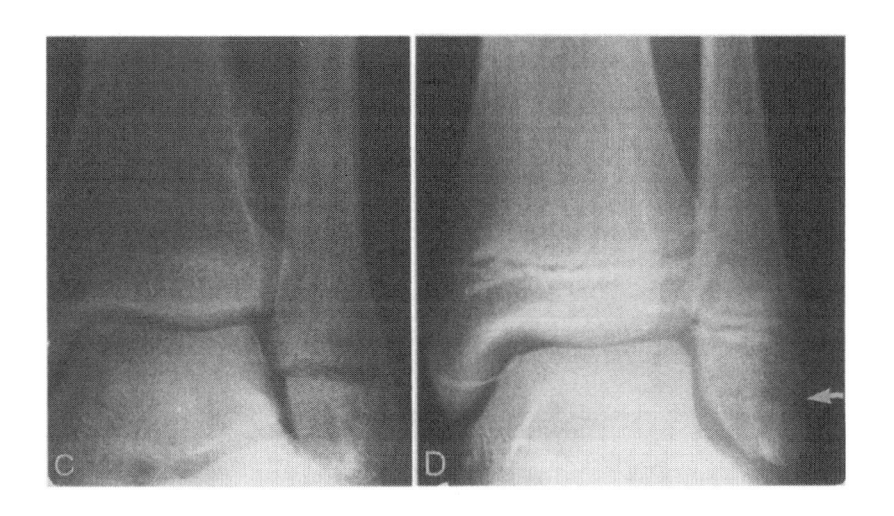

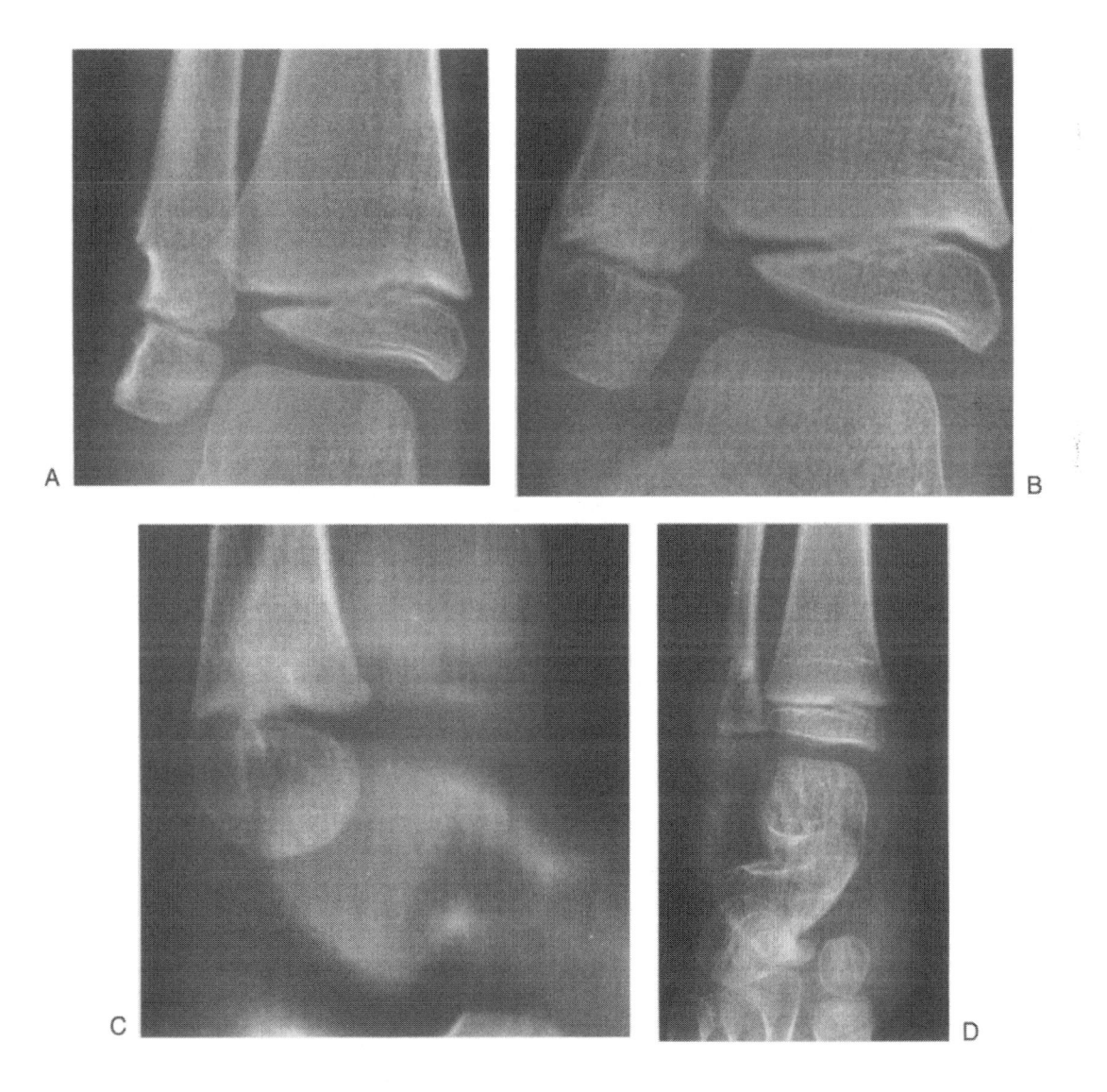

FIGURE 23-151. (A) Type 6 avulsion of the lateral side of the malleolus. This open injury was caused by a lawn mower. (B, C) Anteroposterior and lateral views of a small peripheral bridge. This child's foot was caught in the spoked wheel of a bicycle. (D) Extensive heterotopic bone along and below the lateral malleolus following an open injury.

FIGURE 23-152. Avulsion of the tip of the malleolus.

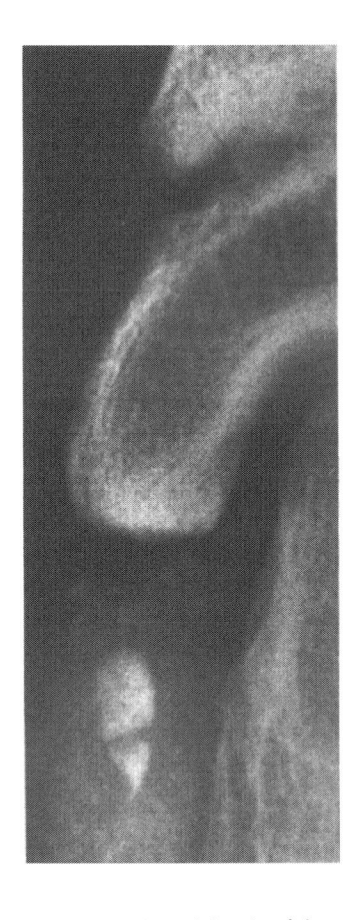

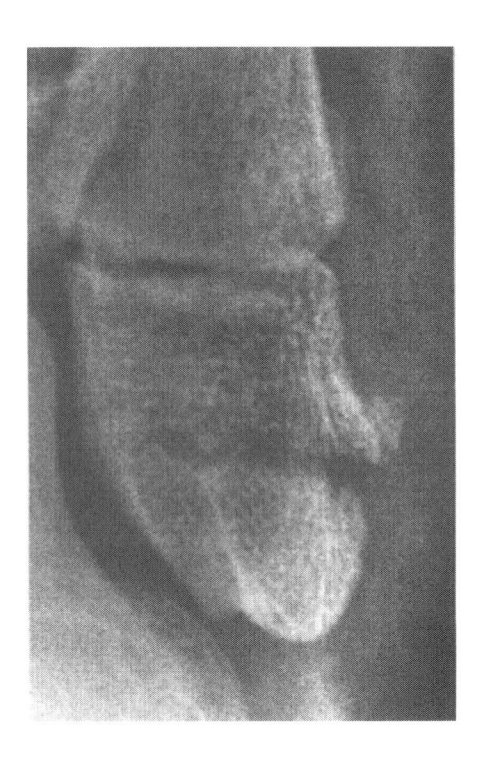

FIGURE 23-153. Type 7 fracture of the lateral malleolus.

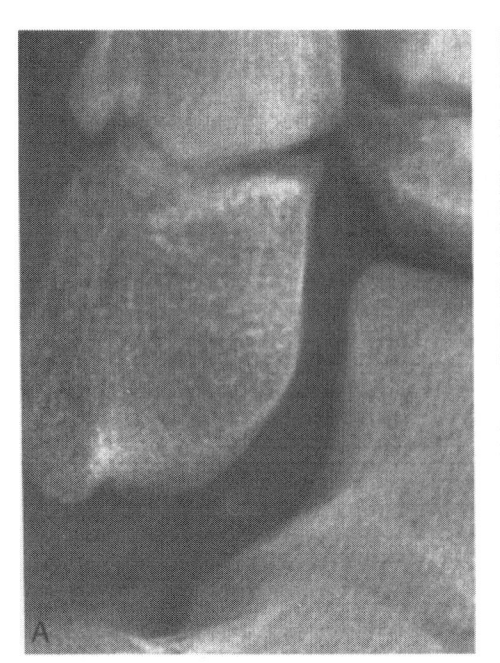

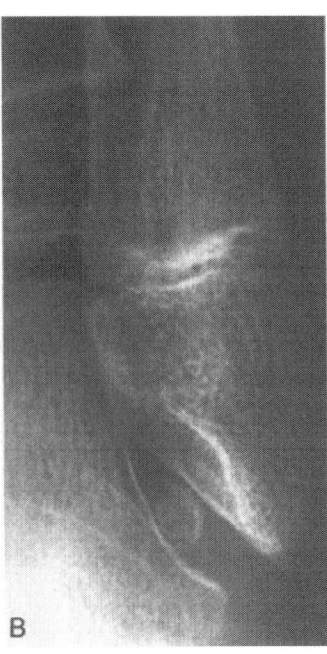

FIGURE 23-154. (A) Avulsion of the tip of the lateral malleolus. (B) Three months later. It was subsequently excised because of chronic pain.

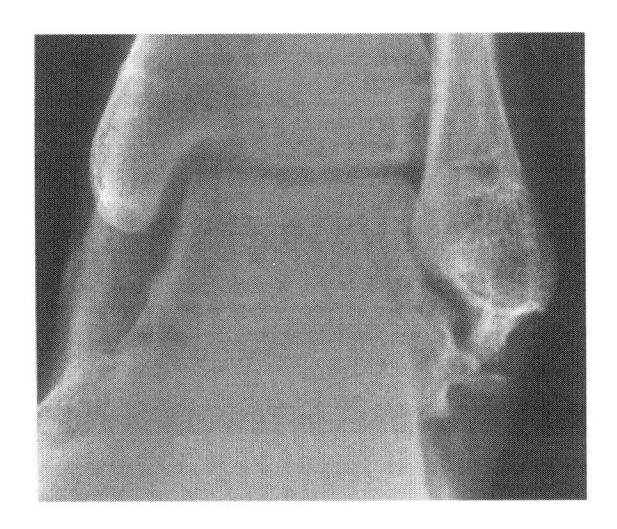

FIGURE 23-155. Chronic lateral "ligament" injuries that were more likely chondro-osseous fractures.

However, elucidation of tenderness or by direct palpation over the physis is the most accurate sign, even when a roentgenogram appears normal.

Gleeson et al. used ultrasonography to study inversional injuries. It showed subperiosteal hematoma in 23 of 40 patients,[669] which was consistent with a diagnosis of occult (type 1) physeal injury of the distal fibula.

Because these fractures are generally undisplaced, only cast immobilization, with the ankle in neutral postion, is usually necessary. The cast should be maintained for 3–4 weeks. If the region is still tender, further immobilization may be necessary. If there is any displacement, the fracture is reduced as anatomically as possible by closed manipulation. Fixation is rarely necessary.

Hamarati et al. described nonunion of pediatric fibular physeal fractures.[469] All had been treated conservatively with casting.

Villas and Schweitzer described a case of ischemic necrosis of the fibular epiphysis following an ankle sprain in a 5-year-old boy.[553]

Park et al. described a 3-year-old boy who had an open injury with loss of the lateral malleolus.[529] Seven years later he had "spontaneous regeneration" of the lateral malleolus.

Ward et al. described a lengthening osteotomy of the fibula for patients who had premature closure or a malunion that resulted in a relatively (functionally) short fibula.[555,709] They noted that fibular shortening and lateral shift of the talus often gave a poor outcome with pain, swelling, and stiffness. Lateral displacement of the talus by only 1 mm caused a 42% reduction in the tibiotalar contact area and increased stress on the articular cartilage.[654] None of the patients in this article were skeletally immature at the time the surgery was done, but the methodology may certainly be applied to children.

Berg reported four adults with symptomatic instability of the ankle and an associated os subfibulare.[613] In each instance operative exploration revealed that the ossicle had nonunion of an avulsion fracture of the anterior talofibular ligament. They believed their findings suggested that the os subfibulare represented an avulsion fracture that may or may not be associated with laxity of the anterior talofibular ligament *rather* than being a normal variant. Although each of their cases involved adults, careful review of the history showed that the injuries had probably occurred during late adolescence. They concluded that the os subfibulare, as seen on plain radiographs, should not be casually dismissed as a normal variant. In many instances it represents a chondro-osseous avulsion fracture of the anterior talofibular ligament with nonunion.

Ogden and Lee reported 19 patients with accessory ossification involving only the lateral malleolus.[647] In 15 of these patients films of both ankles were obtained, with two patients having bilateral involvement. Eleven of these patients presented with acute or chronic pain associated with tenderness at the tip of the lateral malleolus. The most characteristic injury pattern of the lateral malleolus was a sleeve fracture avulsion. Six had symptomatic relief after several weeks of cast immobilization, although the accessory ossification center remained radiographically separate for months to years. Five patients failed to obtain relief from cast immobilization and were subsequently treated with surgical exploration and excision of the fragment, which invariably was separated from the rest of the malleolus and surrounded by inflammatory tissue. All of the patients treated surgically had complete relief of symptoms.

Sometimes these injuries are not recognized as chondro-osseous fractures but are dismissed as an ankle "sprain." Continued use, despite discomfort, in an active child with a normal valgus posture to the hindfoot may create a chronic epiphysiolysis.

Schütze and Maas reviewed 130 children with ankle injury.[694] They found an osteochondral fragment avulsion from the lateral malleolus in almost 40% at surgery. In one-third of these cases the fragment was not evident on preoperative radiographs. LeFort described an isolated vertical fracture of the medial aspect of the distal fibula.[690]

Tibiofibular Ligament Injuries

Tibiofibular ligament injuries are unusual in children.[662,664,667,668,674–677,680,692,693,696–699] The injury mechanisms that would normally produce these injuries in adults often cause avulsion fractures of the tips of the tibia or fibula in children. Valgus strain applied to a child's ankle may also result in epiphyseal disruption of the distal fibula or tibia, rather than a ligament avulsion injury. There may be a fracture through the distal fibular metaphysis, which is intraarticular, because of the extent of the capsular reflection up to the region of the syndesmosis to cover the tibial lateral articular surface and the modification of the lateral malleolus in the metaphyseal region.

During late childhood and adolescence, acute inversion injuries may lead to chronic lateral ligament and capsular attenuation or disruption, adversely affecting joint mechanics.[670,688] This situation must be considered in children who participate intensely in competitive sports programs, such as gymnastics, in which acute and chronic inversion injuries are relatively common. Ankle arthrography may be helpful for

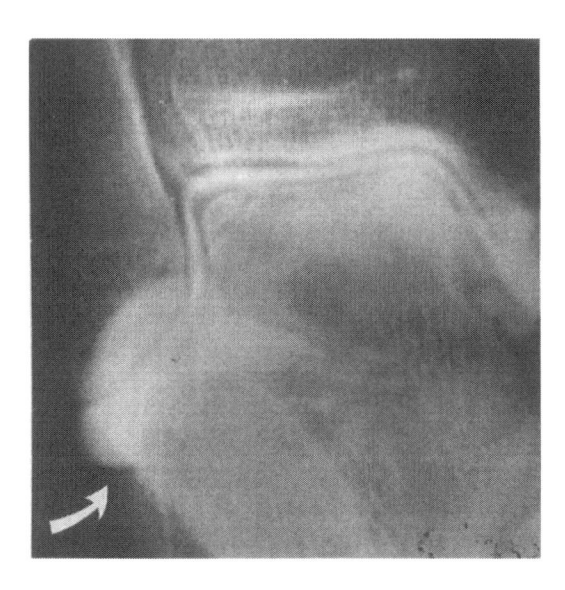

FIGURE 23-156. Ankle arthrogram showing pooling of dye laterally (arrow) at the site of chronic lateral disruption and chronic inversion in a 15-year-old female gymnast.

delineating capsular damage (Fig. 23-156). Stress views also may be helpful (Fig. 23-157). Ultrasonography also has been used to evaluate ankle soft tissue injuries in children.[669] Casting or immobilization should be used first.[687] Soft tissue repairs, especially those emphasizing peroneal tendon placement through the distal fibula,[695] should be deferred until skeletal maturity. Theoretically, if the tendon is directed through the epiphysis, tensile stress might increase in the open tibular physis during subsequent inversion and might pull off the epiphysis.

Vahvanen et al. studied lateral ligament injury of the ankle in children and presented follow-up results of primary surgical treatment.[696] They studied 40 acutely injured ankles in children. Surgery revealed a cartilaginous or osseous fragment (or both) in 19 and an isolated rupture of the anteriot talofibular ligament without any region of the bone or cartilage in another 17; There was no ligamentous lesion in 4 ankles. All lesions were surgically repaired, healed well, and were painless and functionally stable at follow-up examination. At follow-up radiographs of four ankles showed a small subfibular fragment in which bony fusion had failed; but these ankles were stable, suggesting at least soft tissue healing across what appeared to be a radiographic nonunion. Their results suggested that severe ankle sprains in children could cause isolated rupture of the anterior talofibular ligament and osteochondral lesions; they therefore advocate primary suture of ruptured lateral ligaments of the ankle in children.

Schütze and Maas investigated 130 cases of osteochondral fragments in injuries of the fibulotalar ligaments.[694] They found that 37% of the children were found intraoperatively to have an osteochondral fragment (Fig. 23-158). In one-third of them there had been no evidence on the preoperative radiograph.

Rijke et al. recommended MRI to evaluate lateral ankle ligaments following strains.[689] In cases of acute low-grade injuries, they found involvement of the interior talofibular ligaments with intact calcaneal fibular ligaments. In cases of acute high-grade sprains, the calcaneal fibular ligament

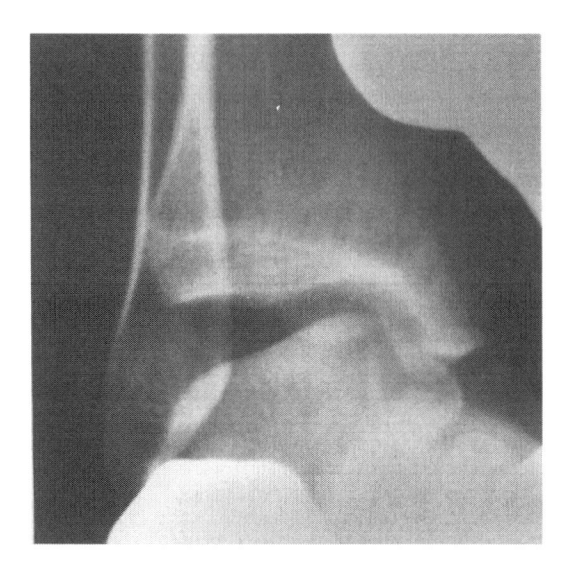

FIGURE 23-157. Stress view of a 14-year-old patient (gymnast) with chronic ankle swelling.

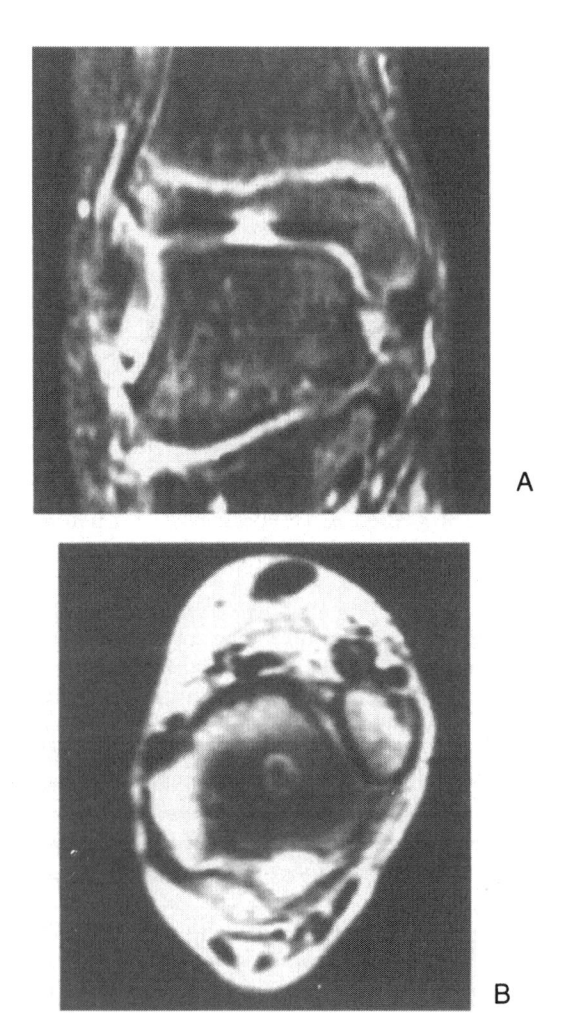

FIGURE 23-158. Osteochondritic lesion in patient with chronic ankle pain.

appeared wavy or was visualized only partially or not at all. Subacute injuries showed some ligament disruption. Chronic injuries tended not to have edema. They did emphasize that MRI findings did not directly correlate with the degree of instability and did not replace physical examination or routine radiographic studies.

Konradsen et al. studied 80 patients with grade III lateral ligament ruptures and used an air cast and immobilization.[675] All their patients were 15 years or older, so few were skeletally immature. The authors noted that rupture of lateral ligaments caused gross mechanical instability. Early immobilization resulted in a better early functional result. However, at 1 year after injury there was no statistically significant difference in outcome compared to cast-immobilized ankles. Similar results can probably be expected from skeletally immature patients.

Dittel developed a method of ligament repair for chronic fibular ligament injury of the ankle in children.[664] The procedure entails splitting the tendon of the peroneal brevis and looping it through a hole within the distal fibular epiphysis, avoiding the physis.

Scarring after ligament injuries may lead to tarsal tunnel syndrome.[661,666,678,681,682,691] Albrektsson and colleagues reported tarsal tunnel syndrome in 10 children.[661] All were girls. Only 2 of 10 had predisposing trauma. These investigators thought that these children responded best to operative treatment.

Tendon Injuries

Like ligament injuries, tendon injuries around the ankle are rare prior to skeletal maturity. In a large series, Ralston and Schmidt reported only one child with tendon jury. The patient was 14 years of age and had struck his mid-tendon; a week later, while engaged in an athletic activity, he suffered with an acute onset of pain and had a distinct and obvious rupture.[686] Treatment should initially be conservative, with the ankle immobilized in plantar flexion. The reparative capacity of the child's tendon is much greater than that of the adult.

Bellon and Horwitz used three-dimensional CT studies to evaluate tendons of the foot and ankle.[663] The technique of free rotation of density thresholds and color assignments to various structures allowed detailed evaluation of tendon anatomy. Its applicability to the clinical situation or the use of MRI with the same type of analysis may allow better elucidation of tendon anatomy and injury.

Masterson et al. presented three patients who developed unilateral pes planus after old undiagnosed lacerations of the posterior tibial tendon.[679] Transfer of the flexor hallucis longus to the distal stump of the tibialis posterior tendon produced a good result in all three patients.

Dislocation of the peroneal tendons appears to be encountered more often with the greater popularity of athletics, particularly certain athletic endeavors that tend to stress the lateral side of the ankle mechanism.[700,701] The increased impetus toward competitive gymnastics, in particular, and some of the exercise routines that increase the stress to the lateral and medial ankle ligaments are associated with a rising incidence of injuries.

Instances of recurrent dislocation of the peroneal tendon are infrequent but often disabling. However, there is no instability of the ankle or subtalar joint, and the patient often notices a "pop" in the ankle. With acute anterior dislocation of the peroneal tendons, they move from their normal posterior position and ride onto the lateral malleolus. Usually this condition occurs in patients with a predisposing anatomic normality; the groove in the fibula serving as a pulley for the tendons is absent or lax. Zoellner and Clancy reviewed the anatomy, its variations and how it affects the potential occurrence of this disorder.[701]

Physical examination reveals bow-stringing or easily dislocatable peroneal tendons and a shallow peroneal groove. I encountered an additional variation in which the muscle belly of the peroneus longus extended down through the superior peroneal retinaculum to the tip of the lateral malleolus. This muscle was obviously inflamed and created symptoms analogous to and indistinguishable from those of recurrent dislocation of the peroneal tendon.

Anomalous or accessory muscles in and around the foot and ankle are encountered frequently. There are variations in the size and origin of the muscle belly and in the length, size, course, and insertion of the tendon. Although they are usually considered curiosities, if one lies within a confined compartment or traps a vital structure, pressure on that structure may compromise function.[665,683–685,691] These anomalous accessory muscles certainly can cause pressure on the median and ulnar nerves in the carpal tunnel and in Guyon's canal.[671] Similar conditions are being increasingly recognized in the foot and ankle, even in children. Four accessory muscles have been found and described in the region of the tarsal tunnel. The peroneocalcaneus internus arises from the distal half of the fibula, and its tendon enters the compartment of the flexor hallucis longus muscle to insert into the calcaneus.[685] The tibiocalcaneus internus arises from the medial crest of the tibia, with the tendon running superficial to the neuromuscular bundle to insert into the medial surface at the calcaneus.[672] The accessory soleus muscle arises from the oblique line of the tibia. This muscle is often seen as a mass that becomes painful with exercise, suggesting a borderline blood supply.[650] The last variant, a flexor digitorum accessorius longus, was described by Sammarco and Stephans.[691] It has a variable origin including the fibula, tibia, soleus, flexor hallucis longus, flexor digitorum longus, or peroneus brevis.[649,657]

Acute dislocation manifests as a painful ankle with swelling behind the lateral malleolus. The retromalleolar region is tender, and often one or both tendons can be felt to be moving under the skin to the malleolus. Although the tendons may reduce spontaneously, dislocation can be provoked by active pronation of the foot and dorsiflexion of the ankle. Recurrent dislocation is characterized by instability at the ankle, and the peroneal tendons can be felt to be displacing over the ankle. Acute dislocation should be treated conservatively with positioning of the tendons and fixation of the ankle in slight plantar flexion by means of a below-knee cast. Treatment with an elastic bandage is inadequate. Surgical treatment is preferred for recurrent dislocation. Numerous techniques have been described for surgical treatment of the lesion. Most are directed at substitution or suturing of the superior peroneal retinaculum. The retinaculum

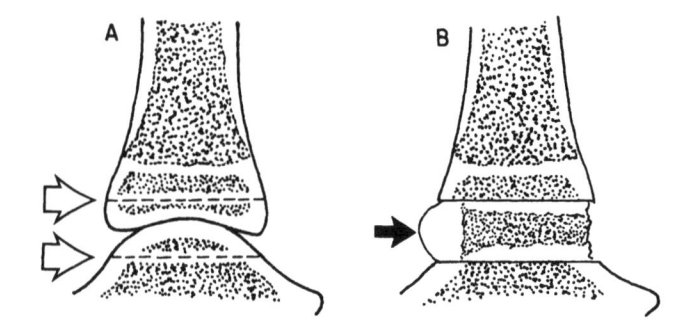

FIGURE 23-159. Arthrodesis technique for the skeletally immature patient. This method allows continued growth in the distal tibial physis. (A) Open arrows indicate levels of parallel cuts to expose subchondral trabecular bone. (B) Iliac crest graft in place (arrow) led to filling in with bone because of herniated periosteum.

may be replaced by strips in the fascia lata or skin. The tendon sheath may be sutured more tightly to the posterior edge of the lateral malleolus.

Zoellner and Clancy reported a method of fixing recurrent dislocation of the peroneal tendon by making a groove in the fibula.[701] However, operations to deepen the fossa should not be used in children until skeletal maturity, as the suggested operation may cause damage to the distal fibular physis, lead to eccentric growth arrest, or predispose to physeal disruption with subsequent inversion injury.

Arthrodesis of the Ankle

Because of significant fracture involving the articular surface (Fig. 23-159) and the major growth deformity and severe pain from osteoarthritis, arthrodesis may be necessary in some instances for a painful ankle joint, even prior to skeletal maturity. In such instances a method proposed by Chuinard and Peterson is applicable, particularly in children with functioning physes.[702] Most procedures for ankle fusion utilize bone grafts that cross the epiphyseal line and thus have limited applicability during the growth period. Several authors have employed central bone grafts and stated that growth arrest does not occur when the graft passes through the epiphyseal plate at or near the central region.[703,704,706] In contrast, Turner described gross deformities with extraarticular arthrodesis that crossed the growth plate at the ankle.[708] The graft essentially is the anterior placement of a full-thickness iliac bone graft impacted between the denuded surfaces of the tibial epiphysis and the talar ossification center.

The indications for tibiotalar fusion in children generally include pain following traumatic and septic arthritic disorders and instability from congenital anomalies or paralytic disorders.[705,707,709,710] The most appropriate procedure is Chuinard's fusion, which is aimed at obtaining fusion without damaging the growth plate. Their study showed in the long term that young patients with ankle arthrodesis function well with minimal pain or disability. The usual indication generally is disabling pain and uncontrollable instability. In children, pain is probably the most commonly reason for ankle fusion. They also noted that based on a clinical and gait analysis study the ideal position for a fused ankle is to have the foot at 90° to the tibia and the heel in neutral position. Patients with fused ankles may have relatively normal gaits because of several compensatory mechanisms that include (1) utilization of the of motion available in the unfused small joints of the foot, (2) minor alteration of the pattern of tibial foot rotation and the use of shoes with heels that allow the tibia to advance more easily in the stance stage.

References

Anatomy

1. Ahl T, Dalen N, Lundberg A, Selvik G. Mobility of the ankle mortise: a roentgen stereophotogrammetric analysis. Acta Orthop Scand 1987;58:401–402.
2. Hoed DD. A separate centre of ossification for the tip of the internal malleolus. Br J Radiol 1925;30:67–90.
3. Kaye JJ, Bohne WH. A radiographic study of the ligamentous anatomy of the ankle. Radiology 1977;125:659–667.
4. Love SM, Ganey T, Ogden JA. Postnatal skeletal development of the distal tibia and fibula. J Pediatr Orthop 1990;10: 298–305.
5. McKinistry P, Schnitzer JE, Light, TR, Ogden JA, Hoffer P. Relationship of ^{99m}Tc-MDP uptake to regional osseous circulation in skeletally immature and mature dogs. Skeletal Radiol 1982;8:115–121.
6. Ogden JA. The anatomy and function of the proximal tibiofibular joint. Clin Orthop 1974;101:186–191.
7. Ogden JA. Radiology of postnatal skeletal development. IX. Proximal tibia and fibula. Skeletal Radiol 1984;11:169–177.
8. Ogden JA. Radiology of postnatal skeletal development. X. Patella and tibial tuberosity. Skeletal Radiol 1984;11:246–257.
9. Ogden JA, Lee J. Accessory ossification patterns and injuries to the malleoli. J Pediatr Orthop 1990;10:306–316.
10. Ogden JA, Hempton RF, Southwick WO. Development of the tibial tuberosity. Anat Rec 1975;182:431–445.
11. Ogden JA, McCarthy SM. Radiology of postnatal skeletal development. VIII. Distal tibia and fibula. Skeletal Radiol 1984;10: 209–220.
12. Ogden JA, Southwick WO. Osgood-Schlatter's disease and tibial tuberosity development. Clin Orthop 1976;116:180–189.
13. Powell HDW. Extra centre of ossification for the medial malleolus in children. J Bone Joint Surg Br 1961;43:107–113.
14. Salenius P, Vankka E. The development of the tibiofemoral angle in children. J Bone Joint Surg Am 1977;57:259–261.
15. Schnitzer JE, McKinstry P, Light TR, Ogden JA. Qualification of regional chondro-osseous circulation in the maturing canine tibia and femur. Am J Physiol 1982;242:H365–H375.

Tibial Spine

16. Aimes A, Mimram R. Les fractures recentes de l'epure tibiale. Rev Chir Orthop 1959;45:895–904.
17. Bakalim G, Wilppula E. Closed treatment of fracture of the tibial spines. Injury 1974;5:210–212.
18. Baxter MP, Wiley JJ. Fractures of the tibial spine in children: an evaluation of knee instability. J Bone Joint Surg Br 1988;70:228–230.
19. Berg EE. Pediatric tibial eminence fractures: arthroscopic cannulated screw fixation. Arthroscopy 1995;11:328–331.
20. Borch-Madsen P. On symmetrical bilateral fracture of the tuberositas tibiae and eminentia intercondyloides. Acta Orthop Scand 1954;24:44–49.

21. Bradley GW, Shives TC. Ligament injuries in the knees of children. J Bone Joint Surg Am 1979;61:1195–1201.
22. Brunelli G. Fractures of the intercondylar tibial eminence. Ital J Orthop Traumatol 1978;4:5–12.
23. Burnstein DB, Viola A, Fulkerson JP. Entrapment of the medial meniscus in a fracture of the tibial eminence. Arthroscopy 1988;4:47–50.
24. Chandler JT, Miller TK. Tibial eminence with meniscal entrapment. Arthroscopy 1995;11:499–502.
25. Clanton TO, DeLee JC, Sanders B, Neidre A. Knee ligament injuries in children. J Bone Joint Surg Am 1979;61:1195–1201.
26. Falstie-Jensen S, Sondergard-Peterson PE. Incarceration of the meniscus in fractures of the intercondylar eminence of the tibia in children. Injury 1984;15:236–238.
27. Finochetto R, Azulay D. Fracture de l'epine du tibia. Semin Med 1959;76:211–213.
28. Frick M. Les fractures des epines tibiales chez l'enfant. Theses Medicine, Marseille, 1979.
29. Fyfe IS, Jackson JP. Tibial intercondylar fractures in children: a review of the classification and the treatment of malunion. Injury 1981;13:165–169.
30. Garcia A, Neer CS II. Isolated fractures of the intercondylar eminence of the tibia. Am J Surg 1958;95:593–598.
31. Germaneau J, Cahuzac JP, Lebardier P, Pasquie M, Bondonny JM. Les fractures des epines tibiales de l'enfant. Chir Pediatr 1980;21:161–166.
32. Girgis FG, Marshall JL, Al Monajem AR. The cruciate ligaments of the knee joint: anatomical, functional and experimental analysis. Clin Orthop 1975;106:216–231.
33. Goudarzi YM. Zur operativen Behandlung von Abrissfrakturen der Eminentia intercondylica in Kindersalter. Akt Traumatol 1985;15:66–70.
34. Gronkvist H, Hirsch G, Johansson L. Fractures of the anterior tibial spine in children. J Pediatr Orthop 1984;4:465–468.
35. Haring M, Schenk R. Zur transepiphysaren verschraubung des intercondylaren eminentiaausrisses am wachsenden skelett. Unfallchirurg 1981;84:204–208.
36. Hayes JM, Masear FM. Avulsion fracture of the tibial eminence associated with severe medial ligamentous injury in an adolescent: a case report and literature review. Am J Sports Med 1984;12:330–333.
37. Hertel P. Ergebnisse der operativen behandlung von Eminentiaausrissen des Kniegelenkes im Kindesalter. Unfallchirurg 1981;83:397–404.
38. Horne JG, Parsons CJ. The anterior cruciate ligament: its anatomy and a new method of reconstruction. Can J Surg 1977;20:214–220.
39. Hupfauer W. Die bruche der Eminentia intercondylica. Z Unfall 1968;71:35–42.
40. Hyndman JC, Brown DC. Major ligamentous injuries of the knee in children. J Bone Joint Surg Br 1979;61:245.
41. Janarv P-M, Westload P, Johansson C, Hirsch G. Long-term follow-up of anterior tibial spine fractures in children. J Pediatr Orthop 1995;15:63–68.
42. Janosch R. Verletzungen bei Kindern bis zurn 14 Lebensjahr. Beitr Z Monaltschr Unfallheilkd 1981;150:91–94.
43. Jones R, Smith SA. On rupture of the crucial ligaments of the knee, and on fractures of the spine of the tibia. Br J Surg 1913;1:70–79.
44. Kendall NS, Hsu SY, Chan KM. Fracture of the tibial spine in adults and children: a review of 31 cases. J Bone Joint Surg Br 1992;74:848–852.
45. Kennedy JC, Weinberg HW, Wilson AS. The anatomy and function of the anterior cruciate ligament: as determined by clinical and morphological studies. J Bone Joint Surg Am 1974;56:223–235.
46. Keys GW, Walters J. Nonunion of intercondylar eminence fracture of the tibia. J Trauma 1988;28:870–871.
47. Kühl W. Die operative Behandlung von Abriss frakturen der Eminentia intercondylica mittles furst förmig gekreuzten transepiphysären Kirschner-Drähten. Unfallchirurgie 1987;13:315–319.
48. Kuner EH, Haring M. Zur transepiphysären Verschraubung des osteochondralen Eminentiaausrisses. Unfallchirurg 1980;83:495–498.
49. Lombardo SJ. Avulsion of a fibrous union of the intercondylar eminence of the tibia. J Bone Joint Surg Am 1994;76:1565–1568.
50. McLennan J. The role of arthroscopic surgery in the treatment of fractures of the intercondylar eminence of the tibia. J Bone Joint Surg Br 1982;64:477–480.
51. McLennan JG. Lessons learned after second look arthroscopy in type III fractures of the tibial spine. J Pediatr Orthop 1995;15:59–62.
52. McNair PJ, Marshall RN, Matheson JA. Important features associated with anterior cruciate ligament injury. NZ Med J 1990;103:537–539.
53. Meyers MH. Isolated avulsion of the tibial attachment of the posterior cruciate ligament of the knee. J Bone Joint Surg Am 1975;57:669–672.
54. Meyers MH, McKeever FM. Fracture of the intercondylar eminence of the tibia. J Bone Joint Surg Am 1959;41:209–222.
55. Meyers MH, McKeever FM. Fracture of the intercondylar eminence of the tibia. J Bone Joint Surg Am 1970;52:1677–1684.
56. Molander ML, Wallin G, Wikstad I. Fracture of the intercondylar eminence of the tibia. J Bone Joint Surg Br 1981;63:89–91.
57. Nichols JN, Tehranzaden J. A review of tibial spine fractures in bicycle injury. Am J Sports Med 1987;2:172–174.
58. Noyes FR, Delucas JL, Torvik PJ. Biomechanics of anterior cruciate ligament failure: an analysis of strain-rate sensitivity and mechanisms of failure in primates. J Bone Joint Surg Am 1974;56:236–253.
59. Oostrogel HJ, Klasen HJ, Reddingius RE. Fractures of the intercondylar eminence in children and adolescents. Arch Orthop Trauma Surg 1988;107:242–247.
60. Pellaci F, Mignani G, Valdiserri L. Fractures of the intercondylar eminence of the tibia in children. Ital J Orthop Traumatol 1986;12:1441–1446.
61. Pringle JA. Avulsion of the spine of the tibia. Ann Surg 1907;46:169–173.
62. Rigault P, Moulies D, Padovani JP, Lesaux D. Les fractures des epines tibiales chez l'enfant. Ann Chir Infant 1976;17:237–144.
63. Rinaldi E, Mazzarella F. Isolated fracture: avulsions of the tibial insertions of the cruciate ligaments of the knee. Ital J Orthop Traumatol 1980;6:77–83.
64. Roberts JM, Lovell WW. Fractures of the intercondylar eminence of the tibia. J Bone Joint Surg Am 1970;52:827.
65. Robinson SC, Driscoll SE. Simultaneous osteochondral avulsion of the femoral and tibial insertions of the anterior cruciate ligament: report of a case in a thirteen-year-old boy. J Bone Joint Surg Am 1981;63:1342–1343.
66. Rosenberg TD, Franklin JL, Barlowin GN, Nelson KA. Extensor mechanism function after patellar tendon graft harvest for anterior cruciate ligament reconstruction. Am J Sports Med 1992;20:523–526.
67. Ross AC, Chesterman PJ. Isolated avulsion of the tibial attachment of the posterior cruciate ligament in childhood. J Bone Joint Surg Br 1986;68:747.
68. Roth P. Fracture of the spine of the tibia. J Bone Joint Surg 1928;10:509–513.

69. Seitz W, Hoffmann S. Die bruche der Eminentia intercondylica im Kindesalter. Z Kinderchir 1974;14:104–109.
70. Seriat-Gautier B, Frick M, Pieracci M. Fractures des épines tibiales l'enfant. Rev Chir Orthop 1983;69:221–231.
71. Sever JW. Fractures of the tibial spine combined with fractures of the tuberosities of the tibia. Surg Gynecol Obstet 1922;35:558–561.
72. Sharrard JC. The management of fractures of the tibial spine in children. Proc Soc Med 1959;52:905–910.
73. Smillie IS. Injuries of the Knee Joint, 4th ed. New York: Churchill Livingstone, 1970.
74. Smith JB. Knee instability after fractures of the intercondylar eminence of the tibia. J Pediatr Orthop 1984;4:462–464.
75. Sorrel A, Jonier L, Compagnon C. De l'arrachement du massif des épines tibiales et de la fracture isolee de leur pointe (a propos de 6 cas personnels). Mem Acad Chir 1941;67:507–519.
76. Sullivan DJ, Dines DM, Hershon SJ, Rose HA. Natural history of type III fracture of the intercondylar eminence of the tibia in an adult: a case report. Am J Sports Med 1989;17:132–133.
77. Tibone JE, Antich TJ. A biomechanical analysis of anterior cruciate ligament reconstruction with patellar tendon. Am J Sports Med 1988;16:332–335.
78. Trillat A, Maunier-Kuhn A. Les fractures des épines tibiales. Rev Chir Orthop 1966;52:261–275.
79. Von Laer L, Brunner R. Einteilung und Therapie der Ausribfrakturen der Eminentia intercondylica im Wachstumsalter. Unfallchirurg 1984;87:144–150.
80. Wagner H. Die biologishe Reaktion des knochengewebes und des Epiphysenknorpels auf die Verschranburg. Z Orthop 1972;110:914–919.
81. Wiley JJ, Baxter MP. Tibial spine fractures in children. Clin Orthop 1990;225:54–60.
82. Willis RB, Blokker C, Stoll TM, Paterson DC, Galpin RD. Long-term follow-up of anterior tibial eminence fractures. J Pediatr Orthop 1993;13:361–364.
83. Zaricznyj B. Avulsion fracture of the tibial eminence: treatment by open reduction and pinning. J Bone Joint Surg Am 1977;59:1111–1114.
84. Zifko B, Gandernak T. Zur Problematik in der Therapie "Eminentiaausrissen" bei Kindern and Jugendlichen. Unfallheilkunde 1984;87:267–272.

Proximal Tibial Epiphysis

85. Aitken AP. Fractures of the proximal tibial epiphyseal cartilage. Clin Orthop 1965;41:92–97.
86. Aitken AP, Ingersoll RE. Fractures of proximal tibial epiphyseal cartilage. J Bone Joint Surg Am 1956;38:787–796.
87. Bak K. Separation of the proximal tibial epiphysis in a gymnast. Acta Orthop Scand 1991;62:293–294.
88. Bergenfeldt E. Beitrage zur kenntnis der traumatischen epiphysenlösungen an den langen Röhrenknochen. Acta Chir Scand 1933;24(suppl 28):1–422.
89. Blanks RH, Lester DK, Shaw BA. Flexion type Salter II fracture of the proximal tibia. Clin Orthop 1994;301:256–259.
90. Bohler J. Zur Behandlung der traumatischen Epiphysenlösung am oberen Schienbeinende. Chirurg 1951;22:81–89.
91. Bovill EG. Arteriographic visualization of the juxtaepiphyseal vascular bed following epiphyseal separation. J Bone Joint Surg Am 1973;45:1260–1262.
92. Burkhart SS, Peterson HA. Fractures of the proximal tibial epiphysis. J Bone Joint Surg Am 1979;61:996–1002.
93. Bylander B, Aronson S, Egund N, Hansson LI, Selvik G. Growth disturbance after physeal injury of distal femur and proximal tibia studied by roentgen stereophotogrammetry. Arch Orthop Trauma Surg 1981;98:25–35.
94. Cahill BR. Stress fracture of the proximal tibial epiphysis. Am J Sports Med 1977;5:186–187.
95. Ciszewski WA, Buschmann WR, Rudolph CN. Irreducible fracture of the proximal tibial physis in an adolescent. Orthop Rev 1989;18:891–893.
96. Curry GJ, Bishop DL. Diastasis of the superior tibial epiphysis complicated by gangrene. J Bone Joint Surg 1937;19:1093–1098.
97. Ferrari GP, Fama G, Maran R. Un caso di "frattura triplana" dell' epifisi prossimale della tibia. Chir Organi Mov 1988;73:165–169.
98. Gall F. Nachuntersuchung con Epiphysenbrüchen. Langenbecks Arch Klin Chir 1958;289:372–378.
99. Gibson A. Separation of the upper epiphysis of the tibia. Ann Surg 1923;77:485–487.
100. Gill JG, Chakrabarti HP, Becker SJ. Fractures of the proximal tibial epiphysis. Injury 1983;14:324–331.
101. Glaser F, Newmann K, Muhr G. Verletzungen der proximalen tibiaepiphyse. Unfallchirurg 1987;90:412–420.
102. Greenfield GQ Jr. Proximal tibial epiphyseal fracture. Orthopedics 1980;3:747–750.
103. Hresko TM, Kaspar SR. Physeal arrest about the knee associated with non-epiphyseal fractures in the lower extremity. J Bone Joint Surg Am 1989;71:698–703.
104. Kaplan EB. Avulsion fracture of proximal tibial epiphysis. Bull Hosp Joint Dis 1973;24:119–122.
105. Kestler OC. Unclassified premature cessation of epiphyseal growth about the knee joint. J Bone Joint Surg 1947;29:788–797.
106. Kuner S, Siebler G, Kuner EH. Verletzungen im Bereich der proximalen tibiaepiphyse. Z Unfallchir 1988;81:181–186.
107. Mazingarbe A, Truong V. Lésions traumatiques de l'épiphyse tibiale superieure chez l'enfante ou l'adolescent. J Chir 1979;116:8–9, 497–504.
108. McGuigan JA, O'Reilly MJ, Nixon JR. Popliteal arterial thrombosis resulting from disruption of the upper tibial epiphysis. Injury 1984;16:49–50.
109. Merloz P, de Cheveigne C, Butel J, Robb JE. Bilateral Salter-Harris type II upper tibial epiphyseal fractures. J Pediatr Orthop 1987;7:466–467.
110. Morton KS, Starr DE. Closure of the anterior portion of the upper tibial epiphysis as a complication of tibial-shaft fracture. J Bone Joint Surg Am 1964;46:570–574.
111. Nolan RA. Tibial epiphyseal injuries. Contemp Orthop 1978;1:11–16.
112. Olerud C, Danckwardt-Lilliestrōm G, Olerud S. Genu recurvatum caused by partial growth arrest of the proximal tibial physis: simultaneous correction and lengthening with physeal distraction. Arch Orthop Traum Surg 1986;106:64–68.
113. Pappas AM, Anas P, Toczylowski HM. Asymmetrical arrest of the proximal tibial physis and genu recurvatum deformity. J Bone Joint Surg Am 1984;66:575–581.
114. Piétu G, Cistac F, Letenneur J. Triplane fractures of the upper end of the tibia. Fr J Orthop Surg 1991;5:104–107 [also published in Rev Chir Orthop 1991;77:121–124].
115. Poulsen TD, Skak SV, Toftgaard L, Jensen T. Epiphyseal fractures of the proximal tibia. Injury 1989;20:111–113.
116. Quell M, Vecsei V. Beitrag zur Behandlung der Epiphysenlösung am oberen Schienbeinende. Unfallchirurg 1987;90:79–85.
117. Rivero H, Bolden R, Young LW. Proximal tibial physis fracture and popliteal artery injury. Radiology 1984;150:390.
118. Rogers LF, Jones S, Davis AR, Dietz G. "Clipping injury" fracture of the epiphysis in the adolescent football player: an occult lesion of the knee. AJR 1974;121:69–78.
119. Ryu RK, Debenham JO. An unusual avulsion fracture of the proximal tibial epiphysis. Clin Orthop 1985;194:181–184.

120. Shelton WR, Canale ST. Fractures of the tibia through the proximal tibial epiphyseal cartilage. J Bone Joint Surg Am 1979;61:167–173.
121. Silberman WW, Murphy JL. Avulsion fracture of the proximal tibial epiphysis. J Trauma 1966;6:592–594.
122. Takai R, Grant AD, Atar D, Lehman WB. Minor knee trauma as a possible cause of asymmetric proximal tibial physis closure. Clin Orthop 1994;307:142–145.
123. Thompson GH, Gesler JW. Proximal tibial epiphyseal fracture in an infant. J Pediatr Orthop 1984;4:114–117.
124. Von Stubenbauch L. Über die traumatische (subcutane) Epiphysenlösung am oberen Tibiaende. Arch Klin Chir 1931;164:621–623.
125. Welch PH, Wynne GF. Proximal tibial epiphyseal fracture separation. J Bone Joint Surg Am 1963;45:782–784.
126. Wozasek GE, Moser KD, Capousek M. Trauma involving the proximal tibial epiphysis. Arch Orthop Trauma Surg 1991;110:301–306.

Tibial Tuberosity

127. Abesser EW. Zur Fraktur der Tuberositas tibiae. Zentralbl Chir 1954;79:1997–2002.
128. Balmat P, Vichard P, Pem R. The treatment of avulsion fractures of the tibial tuberosity in adolescent athletes. Sports Med 1990;9:311–316.
129. Blanks RH, Lester DK. Flexion type Salter II fracture of the tibia with growth arrest. Clin Orthop 1994;301:260–263.
130. Bolesta MJ, Fitch RD. Tibial tubercle avulsions. J Pediatr Orthop 1986;6:186–192.
131. Brandesky G, Salem G. Die Fraktur der Tuberositas tibiae. Chirurg 1961;32:517–520.
132. Brinkmann WH, Niedenzu H. Epiphysenlösungen und ausrisse der Schienbeinrautigkeit und des Tibiakopfes. Monatsschr Unfallheilkd 1966;69:116–124.
133. Buhari SA, Singh S, Wong HP, Low YP. Tibial tuberosity fractures in adolescents. Singapore Med J 1993;34:421–424.
134. Cancelmo RP. Isolated fracture of anterior tibial tubercle. AJR 1962;87:1064–1065.
135. Chow SP, Lam JJ, Leong JCY. Fracture of the tibial tubercle in the adolescent. J Bone Joint Surg Br 1990;72:231–234.
136. Christie MJ, Dvonch VM. Tibial tuberosity avulsion fracture in adolescents. J Pediatr Orthop 1981;1:391–394.
137. Deliyannis SN. Avulsion of the tibial tuberosity: report of two cases. Injury 1973;4:341–344.
138. Dingwall JS, Sumner-Smith G. A technique for repair of avulsion of the tibial tubercle in dogs. J Small Anim Pract 1971;12:665–671.
139. Driessnack RP, Marcus NW. Fracture of an unossified tibial tubercle. J Pediatr Orthop 1985;5:728–730.
140. Ehrhardt D. Ein Beitrag zur Abrissfraktur der Tuberositas tibia bein Hund. Monatsschr Vet 1966;23:938–941.
141. Falster O, Hasselbalch H. Avulsion fracture of the tibial tuberosity with combined ligament and meniscal tear. Am J Sports Med 1992;20:82–83.
142. Frankle U, Wasilewski SA, Healy WL. Avulsion fracture of the tibial tubercle with avulsion of the patellar ligament. J Bone Joint Surg Am 1990;72:1411–1413.
143. Gaudier M. De l'arrachement de la tuberosité antérieure du tibia. Rev Chir Paris 1905;3:305–309.
144. Gerring EL, Davies JV. Fracture of the tibial tuberosity in a polo pony. Equine Vet J 1982;14:158–159.
145. Gebuhr P, Lyndrup P. Avulsion fractures of the tibial tuberosity in adolescents. Acta Orthop Belg 1987;53:59–62.
146. Goverts JT. Avulsie van de tuberositas tibiae bij de hond. Tidj Dierg 1986;111:1257–1259.
147. Hand WL, Hand CR, Dunn AW. Avulsion fractures of the tibial tubercle. J Bone Joint Surg Am 1971;53:1579–1583.
148. Hartley JE, Ricketts DM. An unusual proximal tibial epiphyseal injury. Injury 1993;24:568–569.
149. Henard DC, Bobo RT. Avulsion fractures of the tibial tubercle in adolescents: a report of bilateral fractures and a review of the literature. Clin Orthop 1983;177:182–187.
150. Hulting B. Roentgenologic features of the fractures of the tibial tuberosity. Acta Radiol 1957;48:161–174.
151. Ione G, Kuboyama K, Shido T. Avulsion fractures of the proximal tibial epiphysis. Br J Sports Med 1991;25:52–56.
152. Kameyama O, Okamoto T, Kumamoto M, et al. The avulsion fracture of the tibial tuberosity as a result of violent muscle contracture. Biomechanics 1983;8:157–161.
153. Kaplan EB. Avulsion fracture of proximal tibial epiphysis: case report. Bull Hosp Joint Dis 1963;24:123–122.
154. Kruger-Franke M, Schroers U. Apophysenaussris der Tuberositas tibiae beim skifahren. Sportvertlet Sportsch 1990;4:193–195.
155. Lamothe P, Guay P, Bordeleau M. Correction chirurgicale d'un arrachement de la tubérosité tibiale chez un bovin. Can Vet J 1972;13:138–140.
156. Leighton RL. Avulsion of the tibial tubercle. Vet Med 1978;73:755–759.
157. Lepse PS, McCarthy RE, McCullough FL. Simultaneous bilateral avulsion fracture of the tibial tuberosity. Clin Orthop 1988;229:232–235.
158. Levi JH, Colemena CR. Fracture of the tibial tubercle. Am J Sports Med 1976;4:254–263.
159. Lipscomb AB, Gilbert PP, Johnston RK, et al. Fracture of the tibial tuberosity with associated ligamentous and meniscal tears: a case report. J Bone Joint Surg Am 1984;66:790–792.
160. Maar DC, Kernek CB, Pierce RO. Simultaneous bilateral tibial tubercle avulsion fracture. Orthopedics 1988;11:1599–1601.
161. Maekawa M, Kobayashi A, Tokunaga J, Fukumoto K, Ueno H, Ohno K. Symmetrical bilateral fracture of the tibial tuberosity. Rinsho Seikei Geka 1981;15:195–197.
162. Mayba II. Avulsion fracture of the tibial tubercle apophysis with avulsion of patellar ligament. J Pediatr Orthop 1982;2:303–3305.
163. Mirbey J, Besancenot J, Chambers RT, Durey A, Vichard P. Avulsion fractures of the tibial tuberosity in the adolescent athlete. Am J Sports Med 1988;16:336–340.
164. Mirly HL, Olix ML. Bilateral simultaneous avulsion fractures of the tibial tubercle. Orthopedics 1996;19:66–68.
165. Nimityongskül P, Montague WL, Anderson LD. Avulsion fracture of the tibial tuberosity in late adolescence. J Trauma 1988;28:505–509.
166. Ogden JA, Tross RB, Murphy MJ. Fractures of the tibial tuberosity in adolescents. J Bone Joint Surg Am 1980;62:205–215.
167. Osmond-Clarke H. Discussion on fracture of the tibia involving the knee-joint. Proc Soc Med 1935;28:1035–1037.
168. Pape JM, Goulet JA, Hensinger RN. Compartment syndrome complicating tibial tubercle avulsion. Clin Orthop 1993;295:201–204.
169. Pettit GD, Slatter DH. Tension band wires for fixation of an avulsed canine tibial tuberosity. JAVMA 1973;163:242–244.
170. Polakoff DR, Bucholz RW, Ogden JA. Tension band wiring of displaced tibial tuberosity fractures in adolescents. Clin Orthop 1986;209:161–165.
171. Power JW. Avulsion of the tibial tuberosity in the greyhound. Aust Vet J 1976;52:491–495.
172. Roberts JD. Avulsion fractures of the proximal tibial epiphysis. In: Kennedy JC (ed) The Injured Adolescent Knee. Baltimore: Williams & Wilkins, 1979.

173. Ryu RK, Debenham JO. An unusual avulsion fracture of the proximal tibial epiphysis. Clin Orthop 1985;194:181–184.
174. Schwarzkopf W. Ausrisse der Schienbeinrauhigkert beikindern und jugendlichen. Zentralbl Chir 1983;108:200–205.
175. Sibley SW. Fracture of the tubercle of the tibia by the musculoaction of the rectus femoris. Med Times Gaz 1853;6:268–270.
176. Silberman WW, Murphy JL. Avulsion fracture of the proximal tibial epiphysis. J Trauma 1966;6:592–594.
177. Usui M, Ando H, Tangiku T. Three cases of avulsion fracture of the proximal tibial epiphysis in sports activities. Chubuseisaishi [Cent Jpn J Orthop Traumatol] 1983;26:2167–2172.
178. Wiss DA, Schilz JL, Zionts L. Type III fractures of the tibial tubercle in adolescents. J Orthop Trauma 1991;5:475–479.
179. Withrow S, DeAngelis M, Arnoczky S, Rosen H. Treatment of fractures of the tibial tuberosity in the dog. JAVMA 1976;168:122–124.

Osgood-Schlatter Lesion

180. Altschul W. Neuer Beitrag zur Aetiologie der Schlatterschen. Beitr Klin Chir 1922;125:198–207.
181. Anders F. Zur Aetiologie der Aseptischen Knochennekrosen. Beitr Orthop Traumatol 1955;2:91–104.
182. Aparicia G, Abril JC, Calvo E, Alvarez L. Radiologic study of patellar height in Osgood-Schlatter disease. J Pediatr Orthop 1997;17:63–66.
183. Asada T, Kato A. Zur Aetiologie der sogenannten Schlatterschen Krankheit. Z Orthop 1927;48:191–199.
184. Beddow FH. Treatment of 103 patients with Osgood-Schlatter disease. J Bone Joint Surg Am 1960;48:384.
185. Benassi V, Lorenzi GL. Sulla malattia di Osgood-Schlatter. Chir Organi Mov 1960;48:202–204.
186. Binazzi R, Felli L, Vaccari V, Borrelli P. Surgical treatment of the unresolved Osgood-Schlatter lesion. Clin Orthop 1993;289:202–204.
187. Bortolotti C. Del morbo di Schlatter. Chir Organi Mov 1923;7:601–608.
188. Bosworth DM. Autogenous bone pegging for epiphysitis of the tibial tubercle. J Bone Joint Surg 1934;16:829–838.
189. Bowers KD. Patellar tendon avulsion as a complication of Osgood-Schlatter's disease. Am J Sports Med 1981;9:356–359.
190. Brandt H. Beitrag zur operativen Behandlung der Osgood-Schlatters schen Ehrkrankung. Z Orthop 1965;100:340–345.
191. Broome GHH, Houghton GR. Anatomical note: a congenital abnormality of the tibial tuberosity representing the evolution of traction epiphyses. J Anat 1989;165:275–278.
192. Carter DR, Caler WE. A cumulative damage model for bone fracture. J Orthop Res 1985;3:84–90.
193. Cohen B, Wilkinson RW. The Osgood-Schlatter lesion: a radiological and histological study. Am J Surg 1958;95:731–742.
194. Cole JP. A study of Osgood-Schlatter disease. Surg Gynecol Obstet 1937;65:55–71.
195. D'Ambrosia RD, MacDonald GL. Pitfalls in the diagnosis of Osgood-Schlatter disease. Clin Orthop 1975;110:206–209.
196. DeFlaviis L, Nessi R, Scaglione P, Balconi G, Albisetti W, Derchi LE. Ultrasonic diagnosis of Osgood-Schlatter and Sinding-Larsen-Johansson diseases of the knee. Skeletal Radiol 1989;18:193–197.
197. Dillehay GL, Deschler T, Rogers LF, Neuman HL, Hendrix KW. The ultrasonic characterizations of tendons. Invest Radiol 1984;19:338–341.
198. Douglas G, Rang M. The role of trauma in the pathogenesis of the osteochondroses. Clin Orthop 1981;158:28–32.
199. Dunlop J. The adolescent tibial tubercle. Am J Orthop Surg 1912;9:313–316.
200. Ehrenborg G. The Osgood-Schlatter lesion: a clinical and experimental study. Acta Chir Scand 1962;53(suppl 288):1–36.
201. Ehrenborg G. The Osgood-Schlatter lesion: a clinical study of 170 cases. Acta Chir Scand 1962;124:89–105.
202. Ehrenborg G, Engfeldt B. Histologic changes in the Osgood-Schlatter lesion. Acta Chir Scand 1961;121:328–337.
203. Ehrenborg G, Engfeldt B. The insertion of the ligamentum patellae on the tibial tuberosity: some views in connection with the Osgood-Schlatter lesion. Acta Chir Scand 1961;121:491–499.
204. Ehrenborg G, Engfeldt B, Olsson SE. On the aetiology of the Osgood-Schlatter lesion. Acta Chir Scand 1961;122:445–457.
205. Ehrenborg G, Lagergren C. Roentgenologic changes in the Osgood-Schlatter lesion. Acta Chir Scand 1961;121:315–327.
206. Ehrenborg G, Lagergren C. The normal arterial pattern of tuberositas tibae in adolescents and growing dogs. Acta Chir Scand 1961;121:50–60.
207. Ehrenborg G, Olsson SE. Avulsion of the tibial tuberosity in the dog. Acta Chir Scand 1962;123:28–37.
208. Ferciot CF. Surgical management of anterior tibial epiphysis. Clin Orthop 1955;5:204–206.
209. Fisher RL. Treatment of unresolved Osgood-Schlatter's disease. Orthop Rev 1980;9:93–96.
210. Flowers MJ, Bhadreshewar DR. Tibial tuberosity excision for symptomatic Osgood-Schlatter disease. J Pediatr Orthop 1995;15:292–297.
211. Fornage BD, Rifkin MD, Touche DH, Segal PM. Sonography of the patellar tendon: preliminary observations. AJR 1984;143:179–182.
212. Gillert LH, Waschulewski H. Ossifikationsstörungen und aseptische Osteonekrosen der Tibiaapophyse (Morbus Lannelogue Osgood-Schlatter) unter dem Aspekt des dualistischen Prinzips der Osteogenese. Z Orthop 1968;105:14–36.
213. Glynn MK, Regan BF. Surgical treatment of Osgood-Schlatter's disease. J Pediatr Orthop 1983;3:216–219.
214. Gösta E, Bengt E. Histologic changes in the Osgood-Schlatter lesion. Acta Orthop Scand 1961;121:328–337.
215. von Gumppenberg S, Jakob RP, Englehardt P. Beeinflusst der M. Osgood Schlatter die position der patella? Z Orthop 1984;122:798–802.
216. Haglund P. Om utvecklingen av tuberositas tibiae och en typisk kada a densamma i uppraxtaren (Schlatters sjukdom). Allm Svensk Lakartidn 1905;32:497–502.
217. Haglund P. Zur Frage der Schlatterschen Krankheit (Fraktur, wachstums Anomalie oder Apophysitis). Z Orthop 1910;27:475–479.
218. Hodgson ES, Kaplan YS, Edmonds NRV. Unusual presentation of Osgood-Schlatter's disease. Br J Ind Med 1980;37:90.
219. Holstein A, Lewis GB, Schulze R. Heterotopic ossification of the patellar tendon. J Bone Joint Surg Am 1968;45:656.
220. Horbst L. Mikroskopische Befunde bei der Sogenannten Schlatter-Osgoodschen Erkrankung (Apophysitis Tibiae) und bei Osteochondritis des Monbeines nebst vergleichenden Mitteilungen einschlagiger Befunde in Wachstumsfugen Jugendlicher. Arch Orthop Unfallchir 1933;33:229–241.
221. Hughes ESR. Osgood-Schlatter's disease. Surg Gynecol Obstet 1948;86:323–341.
222. Hughes ESR, Sunderland S. The tibial tuberosity and the insertion of the ligamentum patellae. Anat Rec 1946;96:439–447.
223. Hulting B. Roentgenologic features of fracture of the tibial tuberosity (Osgood-Schlatter's disease). Acta Radiol 1957;48:161–174.
224. Jakob RP, von Gumppenberg S, Englehardt P. Does Osgood-Schlatter disease influence the position of the patella? J Bone Joint Surg Br 1981;63:579–582.
225. Jeffreys TE. Genu recurvatum after Osgood-Schlatter disease. J Bone Joint Surg Br 1965;47:298–299.

References

226. Jentzer A, Perrott A. Remarques sur la maladie d'Osgood-Schlatter. Rev Orthop 1941;27:176–179.
227. Kannus P, Nittymake S, Jarvinen M. Athletic overuse injuries in children. Clin Pediatr 1988;7:333–337.
228. Katoh K. An analysis of quadriceps muscle force in boys with Osgood-Schlatter disease. J Jpn Orthop Assoc 1988;62:523–533.
229. Ketelbant R. Faut-il intervenir chirurgicalement dans la maladie d'Osgood-Schlatter? Scalpel 1954;107:797–802.
230. King AG, Blundell-Jones G. A surgical procedure for the Osgood-Schlatter lesion. Am J Sports Med 1981;9:250–253.
231. Kirchner A. Zur Frage der Juvenilen Frakturen der Tuberositas Tibiae, Tuberositas Navicularis und des Tuber Calcanei. Arch Klin Chir 1907;84:898–905.
232. Klopfer P. Aetiologie und operative Therapie der Osgood-Schlatter's schien Tibiaapophysenstörung. Arch Orthop Unfallchir 1952;45:39–46.
233. Kold SE. Traction apophysitis in a yearling colt resembling Osgood-Schlatter disease in man. Equine Vet J 1990;22:60–61.
234. Krause BL, Williams JPR, Catterall A. Natural history of Osgood-Schlatter disease. J Pediatr Orthop 1990;10:65–68.
235. Kridelbaugh WW, Wyman AC. Osgood-Schlatter's disease. Am J Surg 1948;75:553–561.
236. Kujala UM, Kvist M, Heinonen O. Osgood-Schlatter disease in adolescent athletes. Am J Sports Med 1985;13:236–241.
237. Laine HR, Harjula A, Peltokallio P. Ultrasound in the evaluation of the knee and patellar region. J Ultrasound Med 1987;6:33–36.
238. Lanning P, Heikkinen E. Ultrasonic features of the Osgood-Schlatter lesion. J Pediatr Orthop 1991;11:538–540.
239. LaZerte GD, Rapp IH. Pathogenesis of Osgood-Schlatter's disease. Am J Pathol 1958;34:803–815.
240. Levine J, Kashyap S. A new conservative treatment of Osgood-Schlatter disease. Clin Orthop 1981;158:126–128.
241. Lewis JCM. Osgood-Schlatter disease in an African lion in the Middle East. Br Vet J 1989;145:494–495.
242. Lightowler CH, Cambas CE. Enfermedad de Osgood-Schlatter y lesiones asociadas en la especie canina. Rev Milit Vet 1978;25:3–6, 8–13.
243. Liselotte M, Schott HJ. Local hydrocortisone therapy of Schlatter's disease and its local side effects. Med Klin 1961;56:1834–1836.
244. Lutterotti M. Beitrag zur Genese der Schlatterschen Krankheit. Z Orthop 1947;77:160–165.
245. Lynch MC, Walsh HPJ. Tibia recurvatum as a complication of Osgood-Schlatter's disease: a report of 2 cases. J Pediatr Orthop 1991;11:543–444.
246. Makins GH. Three cases of separation of the descending process of the upper tibial epiphysis in adolescents. Lancet 1905;83:213–217.
247. Mital MA, Matza RA, Cohen J. The so called unresolved Osgood-Schlatter lesion. J Bone Joint Surg Am 1980;62:732–739. [Correspondence to the editor concerning this article subsequently appeared in J Bone Joint Surg Am 1981;63:170–171.]
248. Nagura S. Die Patologie und das Wesen der Schlatterschen Krankheit. Arch Klin Chir 1940;198:650–657.
249. Namey TC, Daniel WW. Scintigraphic study of Osgood-Schlatter disease following delayed clinical presentation. Clin Nucl Med 1980;5:551–553.
250. Ogden JA. Osgood-Schlatter disease. In: Netter F, Hensinger R (eds) CIBA: The Musculo-Skeletal System, vol II, 1990.
251. Ogden JA, Southwick WO. Osgood-Schlatter's disease and tibial tuberosity development. Clin Orthop 1976;116:180–189.
252. Ollerenshaw R. Some observations on Osgood-Schlatter disease. Med J 1925;2:944–949.
253. Osgood RB. Lesions of the tibial tubercle occurring during adolescence. Boston Med Surg J 1903;148:114–118.
254. Parsons FG. Observations on traction epiphysis. J Anat 1904;38:248–253.
255. Parsons FG. Further remarks on traction epiphysis. J Anat 1908;42:388–395.
256. Rapp IH, LaZerte GD. The pathologic and clinical aspects of Osgood-Schlatter disease. J Bone Joint Surg Am 1958;40:965.
257. Reichelt A. A new concept of the aetiology and pathogenesis of juvenile osteochondrosis of the tibial apophysis (Osgood-Schlatter's disease). Egypt Orthop J 1972;7:131–140.
258. Reichmister J. Injection of the deep infrapatellar bursa for Osgood-Schlatter's disease. Clin Proc Child Hosp DC 1969;25:21–24.
259. Rostron PKM, Calver RF. Subcutaneous atrophy following methylprednisolone injection in Osgood-Schlatter epiphysitis. J Bone Joint Surg Am 1979;61:627–628.
260. Schlatter C. Verletzungen des schnabelformigen Fortsatzes der oberen Tibiaepiphyse. Beitr Klin Chir 1903;38:87–96.
261. Schlatter C. Unvollstandige Abrissfrakturen der Tuberositas Tibiae oder Wachstumsanomalien? Beitr Klin Chir 1908;59:518–526.
262. Scotti DM, Sadhu VK, Heimberg F, O'Hara AG. Osgood-Schlatter's disease, and emphasis on soft tissue changes. Skeletal Radiol 1979;4:21–25.
263. Sen RK, Sharma LR, Thakur SR, Lakhampah VP. Patellar angle in Osgood-Schlatter disease. Acta Orthop Scand 1989;60:26–27.
264. Sherry DD, Petty RE, Tredwell S, Schroeder ML. Histocompatibility antigens in Osgood-Schlatter disease. J Pediatr Orthop 1985;5:302–305.
265. Singh K, Prakash V. Osgood-Schlatter disease. Indian J Orthop 1981;15:32–37.
266. Soren A. Treatment of Osgood-Schlatter disease. Am J Orthop 1968;10:70–71.
267. Soren A, Fetto JF. Pathology, clinical presentation and treatment of Osgood-Schlatter disease. Orthopaedics 1984;7:230–234.
268. Stirling RI. Complications of Osgood-Schlatter's disease. J Bone Joint Surg Br 1952;34:149–150.
269. Sutro CJ, Pomeranz MM. Osgood-Schlatter's disease. Arch Surg 1944;48:406–411.
270. Sweetnam R. Corticosteroid arthropathy and tendon rupture. J Bone Joint Surg Br 1969;51:397–398.
271. Thomson JEM. Operative treatment of osteochondritis of the tibial tuberosity. J Bone Joint Surg Am 1956;38:142–148.
272. Trail IA. Tibial sequestrectomy in the management of Osgood-Schlatter disease. J Pediatr Orthop 1988;8:554–557.
273. Uhry E. Osgood-Schlatter disease. Arch Surg 1944;48:406–414.
274. Venturini A. Osgood-Schlatter disease in the dog. Clin Vet 1908;103:98–101.
275. Wall JJ. Compartment syndrome as a complication of the Hauser procedure. J Bone Joint Surg Am 1979;61:185–191.
276. Willner P. Osgood-Schlatter's disease: etiology and treatment. Clin Orthop 1969;62:178–179.
277. Windhager R, Engel A. Zur operativen Behandlung des Morbus Osgood-Schlatter. Z Orthop 1988;126:179–184.
278. Wray DG, Muddu BN. Operative treatment for longstanding Osgood-Schlatter's disease. J R Coll Surg Edinb 1982;27:200–203.
279. Yashar A, Loder RT, Hensinger RN. Determination of skeletal age in children with Osgood-Schlatter disease by using radiographs of the knee. J Pediatr Orthop 1995;15:298–301.
280. Zimbler Z, Merkow S. Genu recurvatum: a possible complication after Osgood-Schlatter disease. J Bone Joint Surg Am 1984;66:1129–1130.

Proximal Tibiofibular Joint

281. Agoropoulos Z, Papachristou G, Velikas E, Wretos S. Isolierte traumatische Dislokation des oberen Tibia-Fibular Gelenks. Chirurg 1976;47:149–151.
282. Burgos J, Alvarez-Montero R, Gonzalez-Herranz P, Rapariz JM. Traumatic proximal tibiofibular dislocation. J Pediatr Orthop Part B 1997;6:70–72.
283. Christensen S. Dislocation of the upper end of the fibula. Acta Orthop Scand 1966;37:107–109.
284. Clews AG. Dislocation of the upper end of the fibula. Can Med Assoc J 1968;98:169–170.
285. Cossa JF, Evrard C, Poilleux F. Un des inconvenients du judo: luxation isolee de l'articulation peroneo-tibiale superieure. Rev Clin Orthop 1968;54:211–214.
286. Crothers OD, Johnson JTH. Isolated acute dislocation of the proximal tibiofibular joint: case report. J Bone Joint Surg Am 1973;55:181–183.
287. Delaney RJ, MacDonald IB, MacNab I. Simple dislocation of the superior tibio-fibular joint: report of two cases. Can Med Assoc J 1956;74:906–908.
288. Dennis JB, Rutledge BA. Bilateral recurrent dislocations of the superior tibiofibular joint with peroneal nerve palsy. J Bone Joint Surg Am 1958;40:1146–1148.
289. Ender J. Zur Behandlung schwerer Schienbeinkopfbruche. Arch Orthop Unfallchir 1965;57:16–25.
290. Falkenberg P, Nygaard H. Isolated anterior dislocation of the proximal tibiofibular joint. J Bone Joint Surg Br 1983;65:310–311.
291. Giachino AA. Recurrent dislocations of the proximal tibiofibular joint. J Bone Joint Surg Am 1986;68:1104–1106.
292. Ginnerup P, Sorensen VK. Isolated traumatic luxation of the head of the fibula. Acta Orthop Scand 1978;49:618–620.
293. Hsu LCS, O'Brien JP, Yau ACMC, Hodgson AR. Valgus deformity of the ankle in children with fibular pseudarthrosis. J Bone Joint Surg Am 1974;56:503–510.
294. Ogden JA. Subluxation and dislocation of the proximal tibiofibular joint. J Bone Joint Surg Am 1974;56:145–154.
295. Ogden JA. Subluxation of the proximal tibiofibular joint. Clin Orthop 1974;101:192–197.
296. Owens R. Recurrent dislocation of the superior tibio-fibular joint: a diagnostic pitfall in knee joint derangement. J Bone Joint Surg Br 1968;50:342–345.
297. Parkes JC II, Zelko RR. Isolated acute dislocation of the proximal tibiofibular joint: case report. J Bone Joint Surg Am 1973;55:177–180.
298. Pellegrino J, Maupin JM, Casanova G, et al. La luxation anterieure isolee de l'extremite superieure du perone (a propos de deux cas dont un irreductible). Rev Chir Orthop 1971;57:547–554.
299. Shapiro GS, Fanton GS, Dillingham MF. Reconstruction for recurrent dislocation of the proximal tibiofibular joint. Orthop Rev 1993;22:1229–1232.
300. Shelbourne KD, Pierce RO, Ritter MA. Superior dislocation of the fibular head associated with a tibia fracture. Clin Orthop 1981;160:172–174.
301. Sujbrandij S. Instability of the proximal tibiofibular joint. Acta Orthop Scand 1978;49:621–626.
302. Weinert CR, Raczka R. Recurrent dislocation of the superior tibiofibular joint. J Bone Joint Surg Am 1986;68:126–128.
303. Wong K, Weiner DS. Proximal tibiofibular synostosis. Clin Orthop 1978;135:45–47.

Proximal Fibular Epiphysis

304. Havránek P. Proximal fibular physeal injury. J Pediatr Orthop Part B 1996;5:115–118.

Proximal Tibial Metaphysis

305. Aadalen R. Proximal tibial metaphyseal fractures in children. Minn Med 1979;62:785–788.
306. Alpar EK. Growth plate stimulation by diaphyseal fracture: autoradiography of DNA synthesis in rats. Acta Orthop Scand 1986;57:135–137.
307. Aronson DD, Stewart MC, Crissman JD. Experimental tibial fractures in rabbits stimulating proximal tibial metaphyseal fractures in children. Clin Orthop 1990;255:61–67.
308. Bahnson DH, Lovell WW. Genu valgum following fractures of the proximal tibial metaphysis in children. Orthop Trans 1980;4:306–307.
309. Balthazar DA, Pappas AM. Acquired valgus deformity of the tibia in children. J Pediatr Orthop 1984;4:538–541.
310. Bassey LO. Valgus deformity following proximal metaphyseal fractures in children: experiences in the African tropics. J Trauma 1990;30:102–107.
311. Bennek J, Steinert V. Knochenwachstum nach deform verheilten Unterschenkelschaftfrakturen bei Kindern. Zentralbl Chir 1966;91:633–639.
312. Best TN. Valgus deformity after fracture of the upper tibia in children. J Bone Joint Surg Br 1973;55:222.
313. Blount WP. Fractures in Children. Baltimore: Williams & Wilkins, 1954.
314. Brougham DI, Nicol RO. Valgus deformity after proximal tibial fractures in children. J Bone Joint Surg Br 1987;69:482.
315. Bylander B, Hansson LI, Karrholm J, Naversten Y. Scintimetric evaluation of post-traumatic and postoperative growth disturbance using ^{99m}Tc MDP. Acta Radiol Diagn 1983;24:85–96.
316. Caillon F, Rigault P, Padovani JP, Janklevicz P, Langlais J, Touzet PH. Les traumatismes de l'extremite superieure du tibia chez l'enfant. Chir Pediatr 1990;31:322–332.
317. Coates R. Knock knee deformity following upper tibial "greenstick" fractures. J Bone Joint Surg Br 1977;59:516.
318. Cozen L. Fracture of the proximal portion of the tibia in children followed by valgus deformity. Surg Gynecol Obstet 1953;97:183–188.
319. Cozen L. Knock knee deformity after fracture of the proximal tibia in children. Orthopedics 1959;1:230–234.
320. Cozen L. Valgus deformity after proximal tibial metaphysical fracture. Clin Orthop 1956;27:31–34.
321. Crilly RG. Longitudinal overgrowth of chicken radius. Anat Rec 1972;112:11–18.
322. Curarino G, Pinckney LE. Genu valgum after proximal tibial fractures in children. AJR 1981;136:915–918.
323. Dal Monte A, Manes E, Cammarota V. Post-traumatic genu valgum in children. Ital J Orthop Traumatol 1983;9:5–11.
324. Frey P. Growth disturbance following metaphyseal bending fractures of the proximal tibia: an experimental study in the mini pig. Z Kinderchir 1990;45:291–297.
325. Gentile G. Measurement of valgus deformity in the lower limb. Ital Orthop Trauma 1978;4:183–195.
326. Green NE. Tibia valga caused by asymmetrical overgrowth following a nondisplaced fracture of the proximal tibial metaphysis. J Pediatr Orthop 1983;3:235–237.
327. Hansen BA, Greiff J, Bergmann F. Fractures of the tibia in children. Acta Orthop Scand 1978;47:448–453.
328. Harcke HT, Zapf SE, Mandell GA, Sharkey CA, Cooley LA. Angular deformity of the lower extremity: evaluation with quantitative bone scintigraphy. Radiology 1987;164:437–440.
329. Herring JA, Moseley C. Posttraumatic valgus deformity of the tibia. J Pediatr Orthopp 1981;1:435–439.
330. Hertel P, Schweiberer L. Spezielle Frakturen in Kindersalter. In: Breitner U (ed) Chirurgische Operationslehre, vol 6. Berlin: Urban & Schwarzenberg, 1976:58–59.

331. Houghton GR, Rooker GD. The role of the periosteum in the growth of long bones: an experimental study in the rabbit. J Bone Joint Surg Br 1979;61:218–220.
332. Ippolito E, Pentimalli G. Post-traumatic valgus deformity of the knee in proximal tibial metaphyseal fractures in children. Ital J Orthop Traumatol 1984;10:103–108.
333. Irwin CE. The iliotibial band. J Bone Joint Surg Am 1949; 31:141–146.
334. Jackson DW, Cozen L. Genu valgum as a complication of proximal tibial metaphyseal fractures in children. J Bone Joint Surg Am 1971;53:1571–1578.
335. Jordan SE, Alonso JE, Cook FF. The etiology of valgus angulation after metaphyseal fractures of the tibia in children. J Pediatr Orthop 1987;7:450–457.
336. Kery L, Lenart G, Szasz I. Effect of diaphyseal injury on the proximal growth zone of the tibia in rabbits. Acta Orthop Scand 1980;51:743–753.
337. Klapp F, Eitel F, Dambe LT. Fehlwachstum nach metaphysären Verletzungen im Wachstumsalter. Hefte Unfallheilkd 1978; 138:282–285.
338. Koch A, Kehrer B, Tschappeler H. Fractures of the proximal tibia metaphysis. Ther Umsch 1983;40:978–980.
339. Lehner A, Dubas J. Sekundare Deformierungen nach Epiphysenlösungen und epiphysenliniennahen Frakturen. Helv Chir Acta 1954;21:388–393.
340. Mechin JF, Moulies D, Barrett JL. Les deviations en valgus apres fracture metaphysaire haute du tibia chez l'enfant, a propos de 20 cas. Ann Orthop Ouest 1986;8:41–44.
341. Michel CR, Berard J. Le genu valgum unilateral evolutif du jeune enfant: etiologie et problemes therapeutiques. Ann Alger Chir 1981;25:23–21.
342. Morgan JD. Blood supply of growing rabbit's tibia. J Bone Joint Surg Br 1959;41:185–203.
343. Ogden JA, Ogden DA, Pugh L, Raney EM, Guidera KJ. Tibia valga following proximal metaphyseal fractures in childhood: a normal biologic response. J Pediatr Orthop 1995;15:489–497.
344. Parsch K, Manner G, Dippe K. Genu valgum nach proximaler Tibiafraktur beim Kind. Arch Orthop Unfallchir 1977;90:289–297.
345. Potthoff H. Beitrag zur Behandlung der Proximalen metaphysaren: Tibia fraktur in Kindesalter. Akt Traumatol 1982;12:127–128.
346. Rettig H, Oest O. Das genu recurvatum als Folge derproximalen Tibiaapophysenverletzung und die resultierende Valgusfehlstellung nach Fraktur im proximalen Tibiabereich. Arch Orthop Unfallchir 1971;71:339–344.
347. Richard Y, Morcos R, Trias A. Genu valgum secondary to proximal metaphyseal fracture of the tibia. Rev Chir Orthop 1982;68:419–423.
348. Robert M, Khouri N, Carlioz H, Alain JL. Fractures of the proximal tibial metaphysis in children: review of a series of 25 cases. J Pediatr Orthop 1987;7:444–449.
349. Rooker GD, Coates RL. Deformity after greenstick fractures of the upper tibial metaphysis. In: Houghton GR, Thompson GH (eds.) Problematic Musculoskeletal Injuries in Children. London: Butterworths, 1983.
350. Rooker GD, Salter RB. Prevention of valgus deformity following fracture of the proximal metaphysis of the tibia in children. J Bone Joint Surg Br 1980;62:527.
351. Salenius P, Vankka E. The development of the tibiofemoral angle in children. J Bone Joint Surg Am 1977;57:259–261.
352. Salter R, Best T. Pathogenesis and prevention of valgus deformity following fractures of the proximal metaphyseal region of the tibia in children. J Bone Joint Surg Br 1972;54:767–773.
353. Salter RB, Best T. The pathogenesis and prevention of valgus deformity following fractures of the proximal metaphyseal region of the tibia in children. J Bone Joint Surg Am 1973;55:1324.
354. Schutze U, Mischkowsky T, Gotze V, Amberger H. Diagnostik und Therapie der lateralen Bandruptur am oberen Sprunggelenk. Z Kinderchir 1982;36:128–130.
355. Skak SV. Valgus deformity following proximal tibial metaphyseal fracture in children. Acta Orthop Scand 1982;53:141–147.
356. Steel H, Sandrow R, Sullivan P. Complications of tibial osteotomy in children for genu varum or valgum. J Bone Joint Surg Am 1971;53:1629–1635.
357. Taylor JF, Warrell E, Evans RA. Response of the growth plates to tibial osteotomy in rats. J Bone Joint Surg Br 1987;69:664–669.
358. Taylor SL. Tibial overgrowth: a cause of genu valgum. J Bone Joint Surg Am 1963;45:659.
359. Van de Sandt H. The influence of transverse section of the periosteum on the growth of the rabbit femur. Thesis, Catholic University, Nijmegen, The Netherlands, 1977.
360. Verhelst MP, Spaas FM, Fabry G. Progressive valgus deformity of the knee after resection of an exostosis at the proximal medial tibial metaphysis: a case report. Acta Orthop Belg 1975;41:689–694.
361. Visser JD, Veldhuizen AG. Valgus deformity after fracture of the proximal tibial metaphysis in childhood. Acta Orthop Scand 1982;53:663–667.
362. Von Laer L, Jani L, Cuny T, Jenny P. Die proximale Unterschenkelshaftfraktur im Wachstumsalter. Unfallheilkunde 1982;85:215–225.
363. Warrell E, Taylor JF. The role of periosteal tension in the growth of long bone. Anat Rec 1979;128:179–184.
364. Weber BG. Fibrous interposition causing valgus deformity after fracture of the upper tibial metaphysis in children. J Bone Joint Surg Br 1977;59:290–292.
365. Wray JB, Goodman HO. Post-fracture vascular phenomena and long-bone overgrowth in the immature skeleton of the rat. J Bone Joint Surg Am 1961;43:1047–1055.
366. Wray JB, Lynch CJ. The vascular response to fracture of the tibia in the rat. J Bone Joint Surg Am 1959;41:1143–1148.
367. Yabsley RH, Harris WR. The effect of shaft fractures and periosteal stripping on the vascular supply to epiphyseal plates. J Bone Joint Surg Am 1965;47:551–565.
368. Zionts LE, Harcke HT, Brooks KM, MacEwen GD. Posttraumatic tibia valga: a case demonstrating asymmetric activity at the proximal growth plate on technetium bone scan. J Pediatr Orthop 1987;7:458–462.
369. Zionts LE, MacEwen GD. Spontaneous improvement in posttraumatic tibia valga. J Bone Joint Surg Am 1986;68A:680–687.

Diaphysis

370. Ahn Y, Friedman RJ, Parent T, Draugh RA. Production of a standard closed fracture in the rat tibia. J Orthop Trauma 1994;8:111–115.
371. Ashcroft GP, Evans NTS, Roeda D, et al. Measurement of blood flow in tibial fracture patients using positron emission tomography. J Bone Joint Surg Br 1992;74:673–677.
372. Bennett J, Steinert V. Knochenwachstum nach deform Verheilten Unterschenkel Schaftrakturen bei Kindern. Zentralbl Chir 1966;91:633–639.
373. Briggs TWR, Orr MM, Lightowler CDR. Isolated tibial fractures in children. Injury 1992;23:308–310.
374. Buckley SL, Smith G, Sponseller PD, Thompson JD, Griffin PP. Open fractures of the tibia in children. J Bone Joint Surg Am 1990;72:1462–1469.

375. Cierney G, Zorn KE. Segmental tibial defects: comparing conventional and Ilizarov methodologies. Clin Orthop 1994;301:118–123.
376. Cole WG. Arterial injuries associated with fractures of the lower limbs in childhood. Injury 1981;12:460–463.
377. Court-Brown CM, Wheelwright EF, Christie J, McQueen MM. External fixation for type III open tibial fractures. J Bone Joint Surg Br 1990;72:801–804.
378. Cramer KE, Limbird TJ, Green NE. Open fractures of the diaphysis of the lower extremity in children. J Bone Joint Surg Am 1992;74:218–232.
379. Dagher F, Roukoz S. Compound tibial fractures with bone loss treated by the Ilizarov technique. J Bone Joint Surg Br 1991;73:316–321.
380. Ebraheim NA, Andreshak TG, Jackson WT. Epiphyseal and Maisonneuve fractures in a pediatric patient. Contemp Orthop 1996;32:175–178.
381. Feldkamp G, Mischkowski T, Daum R. Indikationen zur Osteosynthese kindlicher Unterschenkelschaftbrüche. Unfallchirurgie 1976;2:23–26.
382. Grobelski M. Congenital tibiofibular synostosis. Chir Narzadow Ruchu Ortop Pol 1965;30:79–83.
383. Gustilo RB, Anderson JT. Prevention of infection in the treatment of one thousand and twenty-five open fractures of the long bones. J Bone Joint Surg Am 1976;58:453–458.
384. Hansen BA, Greiff J, Bergmann F. Fractures of the tibia in children. Acta Orthop Scand 1976;47:448–453.
385. Hope PG, Cole WG. Open fractures of the tibia in children. J Bone Joint Surg Br 1992;74:546–553.
386. Kreder HJ, Armstrong P. A review of open tibia fractures in children. J Pediatr Orthop 1995;15:482–488.
387. Lewallen RP, Peterson HA. Nonunion of long bone fractures in children: a review of 30 cases. J Pediatr Orthop 1985;5:135–142.
388. Marsh JL, Nepola JV, Wuest TK, Osteen D, Cox K, Oppenheim W. Unilateral external fixation until healing with the dynamic axial fixator for severe open tibial fractures. J Orthop Trauma 1991;5:341–348.
389. McDonald F, Pittford TR. Blood flow changes in the tibia during external loading. J Orthop Res 1993;11:36–48.
390. Mollan RA, Bradley B. Fractures of the tibial shaft treated in a patellar-tendon-bearing cast. Injury 1978;10:124–127.
391. Odland MD, Gisbert VL, Gustilo RB, Ney AL, Blake DP, Bubrick MP. Combined orthopedic and vascular injury in the lower extremities: indications for amputation. Surgery 1990;108:660–664.
392. Oni OOA, Stafford H, Gregg PJ. An experimental study of the patterns of periosteal and endosteal damage in tibial shaft fractures using a rabbit trauma model. J Orthop Trauma 1989;3:142–147.
393. Osterwalker A, Beeler C, Huggler A, Matter P. Längenwachstum an der unteren Extremität nach jugendlichen Schaftfrakturen. Unfallheilkunde 1979;82:451–457.
394. Pearce MS. Calcaneal pin traction in the management of unstable tibial fractures. Aust NZ J Surg 1993;63:279–283.
395. Prokopova LV, Salame MM. Lechenie diafizarnykh perelomov kostei goleni u detei. Vestu Khir 1990;145:76–79.
396. Rahmanzadeh R, Hahn F. Tibial shaft fractures in children. Orthopäde 1984;13:293–297.
397. Rees D. Fracture separation of the lower femoral epiphysis as a complication of the Sarmiento below-knee functional cast: a case report. Injury 1984;16:117.
398. Reynolds DA. Growth changes in fractured long-bones: a study of 126 children. J Bone Joint Surg Br 1981;63:83–88.
399. Ruland RT, April EW, Meinhard BP. Tibialis posterior muscle: the fifth compartment? J Orthop Trauma 1992;6:347–351.
400. Rupp RE, Podeszwa D, Ebraheim NA. Danger zones associated with fibular osteotomy. J Orthop Trauma 1994;8:54–58.
401. Sadasivan KK, Ogden JT, Albright JA. Anatomic variations of the blood supply of the soleus muscle. Orthopedics 1991;14:679–683.
402. Schuppert W, Majer WA, Becker M. Besonderheiten in der Behandlung drittgradiger offener Unterschenkelfrakturen in Kindesalter. Langenbecks Arch Chir 1986;369:772–779.
403. Shannak AO. Tibial fractures in children: Follow-up study. J Pediatr Orthop 1988;8:306–310.
404. Shenolikr A, Hoddinott C. Tibiofibular impaction: obstruction to tibial fracture reduction. J Bone Joint Surg Br 1995;77:158–159.
405. Sim E. Intramedullary wiring for tibial shaft fractures in children before epiphyseal closure: indications and technique experience of 38 patients. Arch Orthop Trauma Surg 1991;110:87–92.
406. Stanford TC, Rodriguez RP Jr, Hayes JT. Tibial shaft fractures in adults and children. JAMA 1966;195:111–114.
407. Swaan JW, Oppers VM. Crural fractures in children. Arch Chir Neurol 1972;23:259–272.
408. Taylor GI, Wilson KR, Rees MD, Corlett RJ, Cole WG. The anterior tibial vessels and their role in epiphyseal and diaphyseal transfer of the fibula: experimental study and clinical applications. Br J Plast Surg 1988;41:451–469.
409. Teitz CC, Carter DR, Frankel VH. Problems associated with tibial fractures with intact fibulae. J Bone Joint Surg Am 1980;62:770–776.
410. Tolo CT. External skeletal fixation in children's fractures. J Pediatr Orthop 1983;3:435–442.
411. Triffitt PD, Cieslak CA, Gregg PJ. Cast immobilization and tibial diaphyseal blood flow: an initial study. J Orthop Res 1992;10:784–788.
412. Triffitt PD, König D, Harper WM, Barnes MR, Allen MJ, Gregg PJ. Compartment pressures after closed tibial shaft fracture: their relation to functional outcome. J Bone Joint Surg Br 1992;74:195–198.
413. Vidal J, Buscayret C, Fassio B, Connes H, Escare P, Dimeglio A. Les perone: cet oublie des fractures de jambe. Ann Chir 1976;30:769–772.
414. Wallace AL, Strachan RK, Blane A, Best JJK, Hughes SPF. Quantitative early phase scintigraphy in the prediction of healing of tibial fractures. Skeletal Radiol 1992;21:241–245.
415. Yasko AW, Wilber JA. Open tibial fractures in children. Orthop Trans 1989;13:547–548.

Distal Tibia and Fibula Epiphysis

416. Aitken AP. The end results of the fractured distal tibial epiphysis. J Bone Joint Surg 1936;18:685–691.
417. Albee WA. Compound separation of the lower epiphysis with fracture of the fibula. Trans Maine Med Assoc 1886;9:117–119.
418. Von Ansorg P, Graner G. Behandlung und Ergebnisse nach Epiphysenverletzungen am distalen Unterschenkel im Wachstumsalter. Beitr Orthop Traumatol 1980;27:95–102.
419. Ashhurst APC, Bromer RS. Classification and mechanism of fractures of the leg bones involving the ankle. Arch Surg 1922;4:51–72.
420. Baldrian V. Fehlformen nach traumatischer Epiphysenschadigung am distalen Unterschenkelende. Z Orthop Chir 1933;58:82–91.
421. Bartl R. Die traumatische Epiphysenlösung am distalen Ende des Schienbeines und des Wadenbeines. Hefte Unfallheilkd 1957;54:228–235.
422. Beck E. Die Bedeutung der Periostinterposition bei der Epiphysenlösung. Teil I. Unfallheilkunde 1982;85:226–231.

423. Beck E. Die Bedeutung der Periostinterposition bei der Epiphysenlösung. Part II. Unfallheilkunde 1982;85:232–243.
424. Beck E, Engler I. Zur Prognose der Epiphysenverletzungen am distalen Schienbeinende. Arch Orthop Unfallchir 1969;65:47–62.
425. Bensahel H, Huguenin P. Les fractures de la cheville et du pied de l'enfant. Ann Pediatr 1981;28:437–442.
426. Bensahel H, Huguenin P. Les fractures de la cheville et du pied de l'enfant. Ann Chir 1981;35:114–119.
427. Bergenfeldt E. Beitrage zur Kenntnis der traumatischen Epiphysenlösungen an den langen Röhrenknochen der Extremitäten; eine klinischröntgenologische Studie. Acta Chir Scand 1933;73:409–419.
428. Bishop PA. Fractures and epiphyseal separation fractures of the ankle: a classification of 332 cases according to the mechanism of their production. AJR 1932;28:49–62.
429. Blasier RD. Direct reduction with indirect fixation of distal tibial physeal fractures, a report of a technique. Clin Orthop 1991;267:141–142.
430. Bostock SH, Peach BGS. Spontaneous resolution of an osseous bridge affecting the distal tibial epiphysis. J Bone Joint Surg Br 1996;78:662–663.
431. Boussevain AC, Raaymakers EL. Traumatic injury of the distal tibial epiphysis: an appraisal of forty cases. Reconstr Surg Traumatol 1970;17:40–46.
432. Bowen DR. Epiphyseal separation-fracture. Interstate Med J 1915;22:607–610.
433. Broock GJ, Greer RB. Traumatic rotational displacements of the distal tibial growth plate. J Bone Joint Surg Am 1970;52:1666–1668.
434. Burrows HJ. Brockman's operation for talipes varus resulting from defective tibial growth. Proc R Soc Med 1937;30:207–212.
435. Cameron HU. A radiologic sign of lateral subluxation of the distal tibial epiphysis. J Trauma 1975;15:1030–1031.
436. Carothers CO, Crenshaw AH. Clinical significance of a classification of epiphyseal injuries at the ankle. Am J Surg 1955;89:879–885.
437. Cass JR, Peterson HA. Salter Harris type IV injuries of the distal tibial epiphyseal growth plate with emphasis on those involving the medial malleolus. J Bone Joint Surg Am 1983;65:1059–1070.
438. Chadwick CJ. Spontaneous resolution of varus deformity at the ankle following adduction injury of the distal tibial epiphysis. J Bone Joint Surg Am 1982;64:774–776.
439. Chironi P. Considerazioni sulla frattura isolata de margine esterno dell' epifisi tibiale inferiore. Minerva Ortop 1955;6:123–125.
440. Colton CL. Injuries of the epiphyses at the ankle. In: Wilson JN (ed) Watson-Jones Fractures and Joint Injuries. Edinburgh: Churchill Livingstone, 1976.
441. Conklin MJ, Kling TF. Careful management of pediatric ankle fractures. J Musculoskel Med 1992;9:43–59.
442. Cornil V, Coudray P. Fractures du cartilage de conjugaison, fractures juxta-epiphysaires et fractures des extremites osseuses. Arch Med Exp 1904;16:257–279.
443. Crenshaw AH. Injuries of the distal tibial epiphysis. Clin Orthop 1965;41:98–107.
444. Davids JR, Valadie AL, Ferguson RL, Bray EW, Allen BL Jr. Surgical management of ankle valgus in children: use of a transphyseal medial malleolar screw. J Pediatr Orthop 1997;17:3–8.
445. DeValentine SJ. Epiphyseal injuries of the foot and ankle. Clin Podiatr Med Surg 1987;4:279–310.
446. Dias LS. Fractures of the tibia and fibula. In: Rockwood CA Jr, Wilkins KE, King RE (eds) Fractures in Children, 3rd ed. Philadelphia: Lippincott, 1994.
447. Dias LS, Giegerich CR. Fractures of the distal tibial epiphysis in adolescence. J Bone Joint Surg Am 1983;65:438–444.
448. Dias LS, Tachdjian MO. Physeal injuries of the ankle in children. Clin Orthop 1978;136:230–235.
449. Dingeman RD, Shaver GB Jr. Operative treatment of displaced Salter-Harris III distal tibial fractures. Clin Orthop 1978;135:101–103.
450. Dotter WE, McHolick WJ. The results of treatment of traumatic injuries to the distal tibial epiphyseal cartilage. Guthrie Clin Bull 1953;22:165–173.
451. Dugan G, Herndon WA, McGuire R. Distal tibial physeal injuries in children: a different treatment concept. J Orthop Trauma 1987;1:63–67.
452. Duhaime M, Gauthier B, Labelle P, Simoneau R. Traumatismes epiphysaires de l'extrémité distale du tibia. Un Med Can 1972;101:1827–1831.
453. Fischer JF. Beitrag zur Stauchungsverletzung der distalen Tibia-epiphyse. Zentralbl Chir 1964;89:1372–1379.
454. Foucher JT. Recherches sur la disjonction traumatique des epiphyses. Moniteur Sci 1860;290:713–744.
455. Frain P. Les decollements epiphysaires de l'extrémité inferieure de tibia. J Chir (Paris) 1966;91:113–124.
456. Frick H, Thori H. Die radiolischen Zeichen der Sprunggelenks: verletzungen im Kindesalter. Monatsschr Kinderheilkd 1987;135:550–558.
457. Geigy CF. Beitrag zur traumatischen Epiphysenlösung distalen Unterschenkelendes. Schweiz Med Wochenschr 1937;67:626–634.
458. Georgiadis GM, White DB. Modified tension band wiring of medial malleolar ankle fractures. Foot Ankle 1995;16:64–68.
459. Gerner-Smidt M. Ankelbrud hos born. Copenhagen: Nytt Nordiskt Forlag, 1963.
460. Gill GG, Abbott LC. Varus deformity of ankle following injury to distal epiphyseal cartilage of tibia in growing children. Surg Gynecol Obstet 1941;72:659–663.
461. Giuliani K. Spätzustande nach traumatische-mechanischen Schadigungen der Epiphyse am distalen Tibiaende. Arch Orthop Unfallchir 1952;45:386–3392.
462. Goldberg VM, Aadalen R. Distal tibial epiphyseal injuries: the role of athletics in 53 cases. Am J Sports Med 1978;6:263–268.
463. Gosselin M. Recherches cliniques et experimentales sur les fractures malleolaires. Bull Acad Med (Paris) (Series 2), 1872;1:817–842.
464. Grace DL. Irreducible fracture separations of the distal tibial epiphysis. J Bone Joint Surg Br 1983;65:160–162.
465. Gregg JR, Das M. Foot and ankle problems in the preadolescent and adolescent athlete. Clin Sports Med 1982;1:131–147.
466. Greiff J, Bergmann F. Growth disturbance following fracture of the tibia in children. Acta Orthop Scand 1980;51:315–320.
467. Gueretin JJ. Recherches sur le decollement spontanee traumatique des epiphyses. Presse Med 1837;1:297–302.
468. Hamanishi C, Tanaka K, Fujio K. Correction of asymmetric physeal closure. Acta Orthop Scand 1990;61:58–61.
469. Haramati, Roye DP, Adler PA, Ruzal-Shapiro C. Non-union of pediatric fibula fractures: easy to overlook, painful to ignore. Pediatr Radiol 1994;24:248–290.
470. Harrington KD. Degenerative arthritis of the ankle secondary to long-standing lateral ligament instability. J Bone Joint Surg Am 1979;61:354–361.
471. Henke JA, Kiple DL. Rotational displacement of the distal tibial epiphysis without fibular fracture. J Trauma 1979;19:64–66.
472. Hernigou P, Goutallier D. Absence of the medial malleolus: a case report with a 20-year follow-up. Clin Orthop 1991;267:141–142.

473. Herzenberg JE. Computed tomography of pediatric distal tibial growth plate fractures: a practical guide. Techniques Orthop 1989;4:53–64.
474. Hohmann G. Zur Korrektur frischer und veratteter Fälle von Verletzung der distalen Tibiaepiphyse. Arch Orthop Unfallchir 1952;45:395–406.
475. Hynes D, O'Brien T. Growth disturbance lines after injury of the distal tibial physis. J Bone Joint Surg Br 1988;70:231–233.
476. Johnson EW, Fahl JC. Fractures involving the distal epiphysis of the tibia and fibula in children. Am J Surg 1957;93:778–781.
477. Jonsson K, Fredin HO, Cederlund CG, Bauer M. Width of the normal ankle joint. Acta Radiol Diagn (Stockh) 1984;25:147–149.
478. Karrholm J, Hansson LI, Laurin S. Computed tomography of intraarticular supination: eversion fractures of the ankle in adolescents. J Pediatr Orthop 1981;1:181–187.
479. Karrholm J, Hansson LI, Laurin S. Supination-eversion injuries of the ankle in children: a retrospective study of radiographic classification and treatment. J Pediatr Orthop 1982;2:147–159.
480. Karrholm J, Hansson LI, Laurin S. Pronation injuries of the ankle in children: retrospective study of radiographical classification and treatment. Acta Orthop Scand 1983;54:1–17.
481. Karrholm J, Hansson LI, Laurin S, Selvik G. Post-traumatic growth disturbance of the ankle treated by the Langenskiöld procedure: evaluation by radiography, roentgen stereophotogrammetry, scintimetry and histology: case report. Acta Orthop Scand 1983;54:721–729.
482. Karrholm J, Hansson LI, Selvik G. II. Roentgen stereophotogrammetric analysis of growth pattern after supination adduction ankle injuries in children. J Pediatr Orthop 1982;2:25–37.
483. Karrholm J, Hansson LI, Selvik G. I. Roentgen stereophotogrammetric analysis of growth pattern after supination eversion ankle injuries in children. J Pediatr Orthop 1982;2:271–279.
484. Karrholm J, Hansson LI, Selvik G. Changes in tibiofibular relationships due to growth disturbances after ankle fractures in children. J Bone Joint Surg Am 1984;66:1198–1210.
485. Karrholm J, Hansson LI, Selvik G. Longitudinal growth rate of the distal tibia and fibula in children. Clin Orthop 1984;191:121–128.
486. Kennedy JP, Weiner DS. Avascular necrosis complicating fracture of the distal tibial epiphysis. J Pediatr Orthop 1991;11:234–237.
487. Kimberley AB. Malunited fractures affecting the ankle joint. Surg Gynecol Obstet 1936;62:79–84.
488. Kleiger B. The mechanism of ankle injuries. J Bone Joint Surg Am 1956;38:59–70.
489. Kleiger B, Barton J. Epiphyseal ankle fractures. Bull Hosp Joint Dis 1964;25:240–245.
490. Kleiger B, Mankin HJ. Fracture of the lateral portion of the distal tibial epiphysis. J Bone Joint Surg Am 1964;46:25–32.
491. Kling T, Bright R, Hensinger R. Distal tibial physeal fractures in children that may require open reduction. J Bone Joint Surg Am 1984;66:647–657.
492. Kling TF. Operative treatment of ankle fractures in children. Orthop Clin North Am 1990;21:381–392.
493. Koval KJ, Lehman WB, Koval RP. Rotational injury of the distal tibial physis. Orthop Rev 1989;9:987–990.
494. Kump WL. Vertical fractures of the distal tibial epiphysis. AJR 1966;97:676–681.
495. Lambotte A. Fractures epiphysaires inferieures de la jambe. In: Chirurgie Operatoire des Fractures. Paris: Masson & Cie, 1913.
496. Landin LA, Danielsson LG. Children's ankle fractures: classification and epidemiology. Acta Orthop Scand 1983;54:634–640.
497. Landin LA, Danielsson LG, Jonsson K, Pettersson H. Late results in 65 physeal ankle fractures. Acta Orthop Scand 1986;57:530–534.
498. Langenskiöld A. The possibilities of eliminating premature partial closure of an epiphyseal plate caused by trauma or disease. Acta Orthop Scand 1967;38:267–279.
499. Langenskiöld A. Traumatic premature closure of the distal tibial epiphyseal plate. Acta Orthop Scand 1967;38:520–531.
500. Lantz BA, McAndrew M, Scioli M, Fitzrandolph RL. The effect of concomitant chondral injuries accompanying operatively reduced malleolar fractures. J Orthop Trauma 1991;5:125–128.
501. Lauge-Hansen N. Fractures of the ankle: analytic historic survey as basis of new experimental, roentgenologic, and clinical investigations. Arch Surg 1948;56:259–317.
502. Lauge-Hansen N. Fractures of the ankle. II. Combined experimental-surgical and experimental-roentgenologic investigations. Arch Surg 1950;60:957–985.
503. Letts RM. The hidden adolescent ankle fracture. J Pediatr Orthop 1982;2:161–164.
504. Lievre L. Du decollement epiphysaire traumatique de l'extremite inferieure du tibia. Thesis, G. Steinheil, Paris, 1903.
505. Lindsjo U. Operative treatment of ankle fractures. Acta Orthop Scand 1981;52(suppl 189):1–131.
506. Lintecum N, Blasier RD. Direct reduction with indirect fixation of distal tibial physeal fractures. J Pediatr Orthop 1996;16:107–112.
507. Lovell ES. An unusual rotatory injury of the ankle. J Bone Joint Surg Am 1968;50:163–165.
508. MacNealy GA, Rogers LF, Hernandez R, Poznanski AK. Injuries of the distal tibial epiphysis: systematic radiographic evaluation. AJR 1982;138:683–689.
509. Maisonneuve MJG. Recherches sur la fracture du perone. Arch Gen Med 1840;7:165–167.
510. Mallet J. Les epiphysiodeses partielles traumatiques de l'extremite inferieure du tibia chez l'enfant. Rev Chir Orthop 1975;61:5–16.
511. Mandell J. Isolated fractures of the posterior tibial lip at the ankle as demonstrated by an additional projection, the "poor" lateral view. Radiology 1971;101:319–322.
512. Marti R, Besselaar PP, Raaymakers E. Fehlstellungen Verletzungen der distalen tibia und Fibulaepiphysen. Orthopäde 1991;20:367–373.
513. Marti R, Raaymakers E. Sekundareingriffe bei fehlverheilten Frakturen des oberen Sprunggelenkes. Orthopäde 1990;19:400–408.
514. Marti R, Raaymakers E, Nolte P. Malunited ankle fractures, the late results of reconstruction. J Bone Joint Surg Br 1990;72:709–713.
515. Marti R, Saxer U, Sussenbach F. Prearthrotische Folgezustande nach Epiphysenfugenverletzungen am distalen Unterschenkel. Z Orthop 1974;112:653–656.
516. McFarland B. Traumatic arrest of epiphyseal growth at the lower end of the tibia. Br J Surg 1931;19:78–83.
517. Meenan NM, Lorke DE, Westerhoff M, Jungbluth KH. Die isolierte Fraktur des Voldmannschen Dreicksein eigenständiges Verletzungsbild. Unfallchirurgie 1993;19:98–107.
518. Melchoir B, Badelon O, Peraldi P, Bensahel H. Les fractures: decollements epiphysaires de l'extremite inferieure du tibia. Chir Pediatr 1990;31:113–118.
519. Merrill KD. The Maisonneuve fracture of the fibula. Clin Orthop 1993;287:218–223.
520. Michelson JD, Magid D, Ney DR, Fishman EK. Examination of the pathologic anatomy of ankle fractures. J Trauma 1992;32:65–70.
521. Mosca VS. The management of displaced distal tibial injuries involving the physis. Techniques Orthop 1989;4:65–73.

522. Mouterde P, Rigault P, Padovani JP, Finidori G. Les traumatismes de cartilage de conjugaison de l'extremite inferieure du tibia. Chir Pediatr 1979:20:115–122.
523. Murakami S, Yamamoto H, Furuya K, Tomimatsu T. Irreducible Salter-Harris type II fracture of the distal tibial epiphysis. J Orthop Trauma 1994;8:524–526.
524. Nevelos AB, Colton CL. Rotational displacement of the lower tibial epiphysis due to trauma. J Bone Joint Surg Br 1977;59:331–332.
525. Ostrum RF, Litsky AS. Tension band fixation of medial malleolus fractures. J Orthop Trauma 1992;6:464–468.
526. Owen E. Cases of injury to the epiphysis: arrested development of tibia. Lancet 1891;2:767–771.
527. Paleari GL. Sul meccanismo di produzione dei distacchi antero-esterni dell' epifisi distale della tibia. Arch Ortop 1960;73:1146–1151.
528. Pankovich AM. Maisonneuve fractures of the fibula. J Bone Joint Surg Am 1976;58:337–342.
529. Park H-W, Kim H-J, Park B-M. Spontaneous regeneration of the lateral mallelous after traumatic loss in a three-year-old boy. J Bone Joint Surg Br 1997;79:66–67.
530. Pritsch M, Lokjec F, Sali M, Valkes S. Adhesions of distal tibial syndesmosis. Clin Orthop 1993;289:220–222.
531. Reynolds DA. Growth changes in fractured long-bones: a study of 126 children. J Bone Joint Surg Br 1981;63:83–88.
532. Robertson DE. Post-traumatic osteochondritis of the lower tibial epiphysis. J Bone Joint Surg Br 1964;46:212–213.
533. Scurran BL. Fractures in children. Clin Podiatr 1985;2:365–377.
534. Siffert RS, Arkin AM. Post-traumatic aseptic necrosis of the distal tibial epiphysis. J Bone Joint Surg Am 1950;32:691–694.
535. Spiegel PG, Cooperman DR, Laros GS. Epiphyseal fractures of the distal ends of the tibia and fibula. J Bone Joint Surg Am 1978;60:1046–1050.
536. Stampfel O, Zoch G, Scholz R, Ferlic P. Ergebnisse der operativen Behandlung von Verletzungen der distalen Tibiaepiphyse. Arch Orthop Unfallchir 1976;84:211–220.
537. Stern MB, Grant SS, Isaacson AS. Bilateral distal tibial and fibular epiphyseal separation associated with spina bifida. Clin Orthop 1967;50:191–196.
538. Stevens PM, Belle RM. Screw epiphyseodesis for ankle valgus. J Pediatr Orthop 1997;17:9–12.
539. Stringa G. Osteointesi con vite sul distacco epifiserio parsiate anteroexterne inferiore tibiale. Arch Putti Chir Organi Mov 1951;1:139–147.
540. Suessenbach F, Weber BG. Epiphysenfugenverletzungen am Distalen Unterschenkel. St Gallen, Switzerland: Verlag Hans Huber Bern Satz und Druck, Zollikofer & Company AG, 1970.
541. Sullivan JA. Ankle and foot injuries in the pediatric athlete. AAOS Instr Course Lect 1993:42:545–551.
542. Sussenbach F, Marti R. Achsenabweichungen nach Epiphysenfugenverletzungen am Unterschenkel. Orthop Prax 1981;9:738–45.
543. Tessari L, Tagliabue D. I distacchi epifisori distale di tibia. Gaz Int Med Chir 1961;66:1545–1549.
544. Thomas JL. Epiphyseal plate sparing fixation for Salter Harris IV ankle fractures. J Foot Surg 1989;28:120–123.
545. Titze A. Verletzungen im Breich des Sprunggelenkes und der Fusswurzel beim Kind und Jugendlichen. Verh Dtsch Orthop Ges 1957;44:283–288.
546. Titze A. Erfahrungen bei der Korrektur jugendlicher Wachstumsstörungen. Z Orthop 1958;89:88–93.
547. Titze A. Sprunggelenkverletzungen bei Kindern. Kinderchir 1967;4:400–405.
548. Toolan BC, Koval JK, Kummer FJ, Sanders R, Zuckerman JD. Vertical shear fractures of the medial malleolus: a biomechanical study of five internal fixation techniques. Foot Ankle 1994;15:483–489.
549. Torg JS, Ruggiero RA. Comminuted epiphyseal fracture of the distal tibia. Clin Orthop 1975;110:215–217.
550. Torretta F, Brambilla S, Fava G, Lanzoni L. Frequency of painful pronation in childhood injuries. Chir Ital 1982;34:469–424.
551. Vajaradul Y, Laupattarakasem W, Surangsrirat W. Fractures around the ankle joint. J Med Assoc Thai 1981;64:555–561.
552. Van Assen J. Missbildung des distalen Unterschenkelendes nach Schadigung der Epiphysensheiben. Z Orthop Clin 1934;60:454–459.
553. Vilas C, Schweitzer D. Avascular necrosis of the distal fibular epiphysis: a new condition. J Pediatr Orthop 1996;14:497–499.
554. Vogler HW. Unusual juvenile ankle fracture: explanation and a surgical repair. Foot Surg 1990;29:516–520.
555. Ward AJ, Ackroyd CE, Baker AS. Late lengthening of the fibula for malaligned ankle fractures. J Bone Joint Surg Br 1990;72:714–717.
556. Weiner DS. Avascular necrosis complicating fracture of the distal tibial epiphysis. J Pediatr Orthop 1991;5:125–128.
557. Wiggins HH. Pronation-dorsiflexion fractures with involvement of distal tibial epiphysis. AAOS Instruct Course Lect 1975;24:309.
558. Yablon IG, Heller FG, Shouse L. The key role of the lateral malleolus in displaced fractures of the ankle. J Bone Joint Surg Am 1977;59:169–173.
559. Zderkiewicz W. Traumatic epiphysiolysis of the distal ends of the tibia and fibula and its sequelae. Narzd Ruchu 1961;25:425–431.
560. Zuppinger H. Ueber Torsionsfrakturen speziell des Unterschenkels. Beitr Klin Chir 1900;27:735–743.

Tillaux Fracture

561. Dingeman RD, Shaver G. Operative treatment of displaced Salter-Harris III distal tibial fractures. Clin Orthop 1978;135:101–103.
562. Duchesneau S, Fallat LM. The Tillaux fracture. J Foot Ankle Surg 1996;35:127–133.
563. Felman AH. Tillaux fractures of the tibia in (adolescents). Pediatr Radiol 1989;20:87–89.
564. Hasler C, Hardegger F. Fraktur des tubercule de Tillaux-Chaput—ein Fall aus der Kindertraumatologie. Z Unfallchir 1993;86:149–154.
565. Kleiger B, Mankin HJ. Fracture of the lateral portion of the distal tibial epiphysis. J Bone Joint Surg Am 1964;46:25–32.
566. Kump WL. Vertical fractures of the distal tibial epiphysis. AJR 1966;97:676–681.
567. Leitch JM, Candy PJ, Patterson DC. Three-dimensional imaging of a juvenile Tillaux fracture. J Pediatr Orthop 1989;9:602–603.
568. Letts RM. The hidden adolescent ankle fracture. J Pediatr Orthop 1982;2:161–164.
569. Manderson EL, Ollivierre CO. Closed anatomic reduction of a juvenile Tillaux fracture by dorsiflexion of the ankle. Clin Orthop 1992;276:262–266.
570. McWilliams DJ. Fracture of fibular aspect of lower tibial epiphysis. Ulster Med J 1962;31:185–187.
571. Molster A, Soreide O, Solhaug JH, Raugstad TS. Fractures of the lateral part of the distal tibial epiphysis (Tillaux or Kleiger fracture). Injury 1976;8:260–263.
572. Morris RH, Downing FH. Report of a case of vertical fracture through lower tibial epiphysis during period of bone growth and operation for correction of resultant deformity. N Engl J Med 1936;215:272–274.

573. Protas JM, Kornblatt BA. Fractures of the lateral margin of the distal tibia. Diagn Radiol 1981;138:55–58.
574. Schlesinger I, Wedge JH. Percutaneous reduction and fixation of displaced juvenile Tillaux fractures: a new surgical technique. J Pediatr Orthop 1993;13:389–391.
575. Spinella AJ, Turco VJ. Avulsion fracture of the distal tibial epiphysis in skeletally immature athletes (juvenile Tillaux fracture). Orthop Rev 1988;17:1245–1249.
576. Stefanich RJ, Lozman J. The juvenile fracture of Tillaux. Clin Orthop 1986;210:219–227.
577. Sundberg SB, Clark B, Foster BK. Three dimensional reformation of skeletal abnormalities using computed tomography. J Pediatr Orthop 1986;6:416–420.
578. Tillaux PJ. Recherches cliniques et experimentales sur les fractures malleolaires. Bull Acad Med Paris 1872:817–832.
579. Tillaux PJ. Traite d'Anatomie Topographique avec Applications a la Chirurgie. Paris: Asselin & Hozeau, 1878, 1892.
580. Yao J, Huurman WW. Tomography in a juvenile Tillaux fracture. J Pediatr Orthop 1986;6:349–351.

Triplane Fracture

581. Clement DA, Worlock PH. Triplane fracture of the distal tibia: a variant in cases with an open growth plate. J Bone Joint Surg Br 1987;69:412–415.
582. Cone RO, Nguyen V, Flournoy JG, Guerra J. Triplane fracture of the distal tibial epiphysis: radiographic and CT studies. Radiology 1984;153:763–767.
583. Cooperman DR, Spiegel PG, Laros GS. Tibial fractures involving the ankle in children: the so-called triplane epiphyseal fracture. J Bone Joint Surg Am 1978;60:1040–1046.
584. Deckard J. Fractures-décollements épiphysaires de l'extrémite du tibia chez l'enfant. These medicine, Paris, 1982.
585. Denton JR, Fischer SJ. The medial triplane fracture: report of an unusual injury. J Trauma 1981;21:991–995.
586. Dias LD, Giegerich CR. Fractures of the distal epiphysis in adolescence. J Bone Joint Surg Am 1983;65:438–444.
587. Ertl JP, Barrack RL, Alexander AH, Vanbuecken K. Triplane fracture of the distal tibial epiphysis. J Bone Joint Surg Am 1988;70:967–976.
588. Fama G, Ferrari GP. Un raro tipo di distacco epifisario misto dello epifisi distale della tibia: la frattura triplana. Atti Sertot XXIV 1982;2:299–304.
589. Feldman DS, Otsuka NY, Hedden DM. Extra-articular triplane fracture of the distal tibial epiphysis. J Pediatr Orthop 1995;15:479–481.
590. Feldman F, Singson RD, Rosenburg ZS, et al. Distal triplane fractures: diagnosis with CT. Radiology 1987;164:429–435.
591. Ferrari GP, Fama G, Maran R. Un caso di "frattura triplana" dell epifisi prossimale della tibia. Chir Organi Mov 1988;73:165–169.
592. Goodwin M, D'Ambrosia RD. Triplane fracture of the distal tibial epiphysis. Orthopedics 1981;4:85–90.
593. Izant TH, Davidson RS. The four part triplane fracture: a case report of a new pattern. Foot Ankle 1989;10:170–175.
594. Kärrholm J. The triplane fracture: four years of follow-up of 21 cases and review of the literature. J Pediatr Orthop Part B 1997;6:91–102.
595. Khouri N, Ducloyer PH, Carlioz H. Fractures triplanes de la cheville à propos de 25 cas et revue générale. Rev Chir Orthop 1989;75:394–404.
596. Kornblatt N, Neese DJ, Azzolini TJ. Triplane fracture of the distal tibia: unusual case presentation and literature review. J Foot Surg 1990;29:421–428.
597. Lynn MD. The triplane distal tibial epiphyseal fracture. Clin Orthop 1972;86:187–190.
598. MacNealy GA, Rogers LF, Hernandez R, Poznanski AK. Injuries of the distal tibial epiphysis: systemic radiographic evaluation. Ann J Radiol 1982;138:683–689.
599. Marmor L. An unusual fracture of the tibial epiphysis. Clin Orthop 1970;73:132–135.
600. Morton LD. The triplane distal tibial epiphyseal fracture. Clin Orthop 1972;86:187–190.
601. Murray K, Nixon GW. Epiphyseal growth plate: evaluation with modified coronal CT. Radiology 1988;166:263–265.
602. Peiro A, Aracil J, Martos F, Mut T. Triplane distal tibial epiphyseal fracture. Clin Orthop 1981;160:196–200.
603. Rapariz JM, Ocete G, González-Herranz P, et al. Distal tibial triplane fractures: long-term follow-up. J Pediatr Orthop 1996;16:113–118.
604. Seitz WH, Andrews DL, Shelton ML, et al. Triplane fractures of the adolescent ankle: a report of three cases. Injury 1985;16:547–553.
605. Spiegel PG, Mast JW, Cooperman DR, Laros GS. Triplane fractures of the distal tibial epiphysis. Clin Orthop 1984;188:74–89.
606. Spiegel PG, Mast JW, Cooperman DR, Laros GS. Triplane fractures of the distal tibial epiphysis. In: Techniques in Orthopaedics. Baltimore: University Park Press, 1984.
607. Tinnemans JG, Severijnen RS. The triplane fracture of the distal tibial epiphysis in children. Injury 1981;12:393–396.
608. Torg JS, Ruggiero RA. Comminuted epiphyseal fracture of the distal tibia. Clin Orthop 1975;110:215–217.
609. Turra S, Ferrari GP, Taglialavoro G. I distacchi epifisari traumatici dell'arto inferior: classificazione, controllo a distanza e prognosi. Riv Ital Ortop Traumatol Pediatr 1987;3:15–23.
610. Van Laarhoven CJ, Vander Werken C. Quadriplane fracture of the distal tibia: a triplane fracture with a double metaphyseal fragment. Br J Accid Surg 1992;23:497–499.
611. Von Laer L. Classification, diagnosis and treatment of transitional fractures of the distal part of the tibia. J Bone Joint Surg Am 1985;67:687–698.
612. Whipple TL, Martin DR, McIntyre LF, Meyers JF. Arthroscopic treatment of triplane fractures of the ankle. Arthroscopy 1993;9:456–463.

Accessory Malleolar Ossification

613. Berg EE. The symptomatic os subfibulare: avulsion fracture associated with recurrent instability of the ankle. J Bone Joint Surg Am 1991;73:1251–1254.
614. Bircher E. Neue Falle von Varietaten der Handwurzel und des Fussgelenkes. a) Os Trigonum traumaticum? b) Os subtibiale. Fortschr Roentgen 1918;26:85–93.
615. Bjornson RG. Developmental anomaly of the lateral malleolus simulating fractures. J Bone Joint Surg Am 1956;38:128–130.
616. Brostrom L. Sprained ankles. I. Anatomical lesions in recent sprains. Acta Chir Scand 1964;128:483–495.
617. Brostrom L. Sprained ankles. III. Clinical observations in recent ligament ruptures. Acta Chir Scand 1965;130:560–569.
618. Brostrom L. Sprained ankles. VI. Surgical treatment of "chronic" ligament ruptures. Acta Chir Scand 1966;132:551–565.
619. Caffey J. Pediatric X-ray Diagnosis, 5th ed. Chicago: Year Book, 1967.
620. Coral A. Os subtibiale mistaken for a recent fracture. BMJ 1986;292:1571–1572.
621. Coral A. The radiology of skeletal elements in the subtibial region: incidence and significance. Skeletal Radiol 1987;16:298–303.
622. De Cuveland, Heuck F. Osteochondropathie eines akzessorischen Knochenkernes am Malleolus tibiae (des sog. os subtibiale). Fortschr Roentgen 1953;79:728–783.

623. De Cuveland, Heuck F. Uber akzessorische Knochenkerne an der unteren Fibulaepiphyse und Os subfibulare ant und post. Z Orthop 1955;85:421–424.
624. Edwards WG, Lincoln CR, Bassett FH, Goldner JL. The tarsal tunnel syndrome. JAMA 1969;207:716–720.
625. Fairbank HAT. A separate centre of ossification for the tip of the internal malleolus. Arch Radiol 1923;27:238–240.
626. Fairbank HAT. Some affections of the epiphyses. Proc R Soc Med Sect Orthop 1926;18:1–11.
627. Ferrero DG, Basso DA. Su alcuni casi di lesioni traumatiche rare della regione tibio-astragalica. Minerva Chir 1950;5:384–387.
628. Francis CC, Werle PP. Appearance of center of ossification from birth to 5 years. Am J Phys Anthropol 1939;24:273–299.
629. Goodhard G. The apophyses of the lateral malleolus. Radiol Clin Biol 1952;39:330–338.
630. Grace DL. Lateral ankle ligament injuries, inversion and anterior stress radiography. Clin Orthop 1984;183:153–159.
631. Grasmann M. Zur Kenntinis des Os Subtibiale. Munch Med Wochenschr 1932;79:824–828.
632. Griffiths JD, Menelaus MB. Symptomatic ossicles of the lateral malleolus in children. J Bone Joint Surg Br 1987;69:317–319.
633. Gruber W. Uber einen am malleolus externus artikularender Knochen. Arch Pathol Anat Physiol J Klin Med 1863;27:205–207.
634. Gueretin J. Recherchés sur le decollement spontané traumatique de épiphyses. Presse Med 1837;1:297–302.
635. Hoed DD. A separate center of ossification for the tip of the internal malleolus. Br J Radiol 1925;30:67–69.
636. Ishii T, Miyagawa S, Hayashi K. Traction apophysitis of the medial malleolus. J Bone Joint Surg Br 1994;76:802–806.
637. Jani L, Baumgartner R. Injury to the talofibular ligament in children. In: Chapchal G (ed) Injuries of the Ligaments and Their Repair. Stuttgart: Georg Thieme, 1977.
638. Johnson RP, Collier BD, Carrera DF. The os trigonum syndrome: the use of bone scan in diagnosis. J Trauma 1984;24:761–764.
639. Keats TE. An Atlas of Normal Roentgen Variants That May Simulate Disease. Chicago: Year Book, 1979.
640. Kohler A. Borderlands of the Normal and Early Pathologic in Skeletal Roentgenology, 10th ed. New York: Grune & Stratton, 1956.
641. Kruger E. Beobachtungen an einem grossen, gelenkartig an den Innenknochel gelagarten Os subtibiale. Monatsschr Unfallheilkd 1956;59:41–45.
642. Lapidus PW. Os subtibiale: inconstant bone over the tip of the medial malleolus. J Bone Joint Surg 1933;15:766–771.
643. Leimbach G. Beitrage zur Kenntnis der inkonstanten Skeletelamente des Tarsus (Akzessorische Fusswurzelknochen): (Untersuchunger an 500 kontgenbildern der Chir. Universitatsklinik zn Jena). Arch Orthop Trauma Surg 1937;38:431–448.
644. Lindenbaum BL. Loss of the medial malleolus in a bimalleolar fracture: a case report. J Bone Joint Surg Am 1983;65:1184–1185.
645. Mouchet A. Point d'ossification du sommet de la malleole tibiale. Bull Mem Soc Chir Paris 1923;49:798–803.
646. Ogden JA, Ganey TM, Ogden DA. The histopathology of injury to the accessory malleolar ossification center. J Pediatr Orthop 1996;16:61–62.
647. Ogden JA, Lee J. Accessory ossification patterns and injuries of the malleoli. J Pediatr Orthop 1990;10:306–316.
648. O'Rahilly R. A survey of carpal and tarsal anomalies. J Bone Joint Surg Am 1953;35:626–642.
649. Ostrum RF, Litsky AS. Tension band fixation of medial malleolus fractures. J Orthop Trauma 1992;6:464–468.
650. Powell HD. Extra center of ossification of the medial malleolus in children: incidence and significance. J Bone Joint Surg Br 1961;43:107–113.
651. Sandor L. Zur traumatischen Genese des Os subtibiale. Beitr Orthop Traumatol 1977;24:558–561.
652. Selby S. Separate centers of ossification of the tip of the internal malleolus. AJR 1961;86:496–501.
653. Shands AR Jr. Accessory bones of foot: x-ray study of feet of 1,054 patients. South Med Surg 1931;93:326–334.
654. Stanitski CL, Micheli LJ. Observations on symptomatic medial malleolar ossification centers. J Pediatr Orthop 1993;13:164–168.
655. Trolle D. De to acceroriske knogler: Os subtibiale og ossubfibulare i relation til diagnosen af malleolaerfracturer. Nord Med 1945;25:247–249.
656. Trolle D. Accessory Bones of the Foot. Copenhagen: Ejner Munksgaard, 1948.
657. Tsuruta T, Shiokawa Y, Kato A, et al. Radiological study of the accessory skeletal elements in the foot and ankle. Nippon Seikeigeka Gakki Zasshi 1981;55:357–370.
658. Washulewski H. Os subtibiale I and II: os subfibulare. Rontgenpraxis 1941;13:468–473.
659. Watkins WW. Anomalous bones of the wrist and foot in relation to injury. JAMA 1937;108:270–273.
660. Zerna M. Das sogenannte os subtibiale: eine seltene anomalie. Zentralbl Chir 1970;95:1481–1485.

Ligaments and Tendons

661. Albrektsson B, Rydholm A, Rydholm U. The tarsal tunnel syndrome in children. J Bone Joint Surg Br 1982;64:215–217.
662. Baumgartner R, Jani L, Herzog B. Verletzungen des Ligamentum fibulo-talare im Kindesalter. Helv Chir Acta 1975;42:443–447.
663. Bellon RJ, Horwitz SM. Three-dimensional computed tomography studies of the tendons of the foot and ankle. J Digit Imag 1992;5:46–50.
664. Dittel KK. Chronic fibular ligament injury of the ankle in young children: a new method of ligament repair. Arch Orthop Trauma Surg 1986;105:191–192.
665. Dunn AW. Anomalous muscles simulating soft-tissue tumors in the lower extremities: report of three cases. J Bone Joint Surg Am 1965;47:1397–1400.
666. Edwards WG, Lincoln CR, Bassett FH, Goldner JL. The tarsal tunnel syndrome: diagnosis and treatment. JAMA 1969;207:716–720.
667. Ehrensperger J. Die fibularen Bandverietzungen am Sprunggelenk des Kindes und des Jugendlichen. Ther Umsch 1983;40:989–995.
668. Ehrensperger J. Das Spruggelenksarthrogramm bei Verletzungen des Bandapparates beim Kind und Jugendlichen. Z Kinderchir 1985;40:203–208.
669. Gleeson AP, Stuart MJ, Wilson B, Phillips B. Ultrasound assessment and conservative management of inversion injuries of the ankle in children. J Bone Joint Surg Br 1996;78:484–487.
670. Griffiths H, Wandtke J. Tibiotalar tilt: a new slant. Skeletal Radiol 1981;6:193–197.
671. Hayes CW Jr. Anomalous flexor sublimis muscle with incipient carpal tunnel syndrome: case report. Plast Reconstr Surg 1974;53:479–483.
672. Hecker P. Study on the peroneus of the tarsus: preliminary notes. Anat Rec 1923;26:79–82.
673. Heim M, Blankstein A, Israeli A, Horoszowski H. Which x-ray views are required in juvenile ankle trauma. Arch Orthop Trauma Surg 1990;109:175–176.

674. Klotter HJ, Muller HA, Pistor G, Schild H, Dahnert W. Zur Diagnostik und Therapie der fibularen Bandverletzung im oberen Sprunggelenk bei Kindern. Akt Traumatol 1983;13:217–221.
675. Konradsen L, Holmer P, Sondergaard L. Early mobilizing treatment for grade III ankle ligament injuries. Foot Ankle 1991;12:69–73.
676. Lies A, Scheurer I. Flake fraktures am oberen Sprunggenlenk: Kann die operative Versorgung die posttraumatische Arthrose verhindern? Hefte Unfallheilkd 1985;174:14–20.
677. Linhart WE, Wildburger R, Holarth M, Sauer H. Ergebnisse nach operativer Behandlung von Bandrupturen am Kindlichen Sprunggelenk. Z Kinderchir 1987;42:246–249.
678. Mann RA. Tarsal tunnel syndrome. Orthop Clin North Am 1974;5:109–115.
679. Masterson E, Jagannathan S, Borton D, Stephens MM. Pes planus in childhood due to tibialis posterior tendon injuries. J Bone Joint Surg Br 1994;76:444–446.
680. Monk CJE. Injuries of the tibia-fibular ligaments. J Bone Joint Surg Br 1969;51:330–337.
681. Mosimann W. Das tarsaltunnelsyndrom: Klinik und Ergebnisse der operativen Therapie anhand von 39 eigenen Beobachtungen. Schweiz Arch Neurol Neurochir Psychiatry 1969;105:19–54.
682. Mumenthaler M, Probust CH, Mumentahler A, et al. Das tarsaltunnelsyndrom. Schweiz Med Wochenschr 1964;94:373–378.
683. Nathan H, Gloobe H, Yosipovitch Z. Flexor digitorum accessorius longus. Clin Orthop 1975;113:158–161.
684. Nichols GW, Kalenak A. The accessory soleus muscle. Clin Orthop 1984;190:279–280.
685. Perkins JD Jr. An anomalous muscle of the leg: peronaeocalcaneus internus. Anat Rec 1914;8:21–25.
686. Ralston EL, Schmidt ER Jr. Repair of the ruptured Achilles tendon. J Trauma 1971;11:15–21.
687. Ramey H, Jakob RB. Die funktionelle Behandlung der frischen fibularen Bandläsion mit der Air-Cast-Schiene. Schweiz Z Sportsmed 1983;31:53–56.
688. Ramsey PL, Hamilton W. Changes in tibiotalar area of contact caused by lateral talar shift. J Bone Joint Surg Am 1976;58:356–357.
689. Rijke AM, Goitz HT, McCue FC, Dee PM. Magnetic resonance imaging of injury to the lateral ankle ligaments. Am J Sports Med 1993;21:528–534.
690. Roberts CS. Le Fort's fracture. Surg Rounds Orthop 1989;3:58–60.
691. Sammarco GJ, Stephens MM. Tarsal tunnel syndrome caused by the flexor digitorum accessorius longus. J Bone Joint Surg Am 1990;72:453–454.
692. Schlemminger R, Burchhardt H, Leppin K, Stankovic R. Zur problematik der Aubenband läsion am Sprunggelenk bei Kindern und Jugendlichen. Monatsschr Kinderheilkd 1987;135:150–154.
693. Schneider A, von Laer L. Die Diagnostik der fibularen Band läsion am oberen Sprunggelenk im Kindesalter. Unfallheilkunde 1981;84:133–138.
694. Schütze F, Maas U. Osteochondrale Mitbeteiligung bei fibulotalaren Bandrupturen. Z Kinderchir 1989;44:91–93.
695. Snook GA, Chrisman OD, Wilson TC. Long-term results of the Chrisman-Snook operation for reconstruction of the lateral ligaments of the ankle. J Bone Joint Surg Am 1985;67:1–7.
696. Vahvanen V, Westerlund M, Nikku R. Lateral ligament injury of the ankle in children. Acta Orthop Scand 1984;55:21–25.
697. Von Laer L. Distorsio pedis beim Kind. Orthopäde 1986;15:251–259.
698. Von Laer L, Jani L, Ackermann C. Die Technik und Interpretation der gehaltenen Sprunggelenksaufnahmen beim Distorsionstrauma im Kindesalter. Orthop Praxis 1980;12:1018–1023.
699. Watson AWS. Sports injuries during one academic year in 6799 Irish school children. J Sports Med Phys Fitness 1984;12:65–71.
700. Wobbes T. Dislocation of the peroneal tendons. Arch Chir Neerl 1975;27:209–215.
701. Zoellner G, Clancy W. Recurrent dislocation of the peroneal tendon. J Bone Joint Surg Am 1979;61:292–294.

Miscellaneous

702. Chuinard EG, Petersen RE. Distraction-compression bone graft arthrodesis of the ankle. J Bone Joint Surg Am 1963;45:481–490.
703. Hatt RN. The central bone graft in joint arthrodesis. J Bone Joint Surg 1940;22:393–402.
704. Hefti FL, Baumann JU, Morscher EW. Ankle joint fusion: determination of optimal position by gait analysis. Arch Orthop Trauma Surg 1980;96:187–195.
705. King J, Burke D, Freeman MAR. The incidence of pain in the rheumatoid hindfoot and the significance of calcaneofibular impingement. Int Orthop 1978;2:255–257.
706. Mazur JM, Cummings RJ, McCluskey WP, Lovell WW. Ankle arthrodesis in children. Clin Orthop 1991;268:65–69.
707. McMaster JH, Scranton PE Jr. Tibiofibular synostosis: a cause of ankle disability. Clin Orthop 1975;111:172–174.
708. Turner H. Deformities of the foot associated with arthrodesis of the ankle joint performed in early childhood. J Bone Joint Surg 1934;16:423–425.
709. Weber BG. Lengthening osteotomy of the fibula to correct a widened mortise of the ankle after fracture. Int Orthop 1981;4:289–293.
710. Wiltse LL. Valgus deformity of the ankle: a sequel of acquired or congenital abnormalities of the fibula. J Bone Joint Surg 1972;54:595–606.

24

Foot

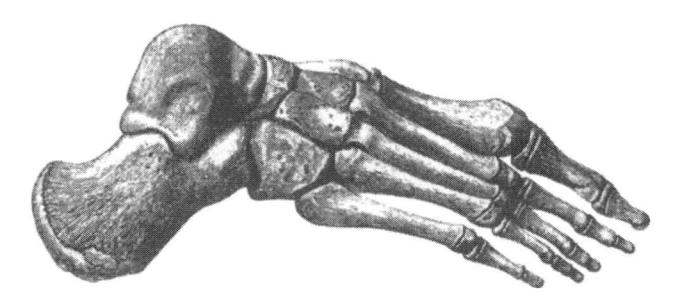

Engraving of a skeletally immature foot. (From Poland J. Separation of the Epiphyses. London: Smith, Elder, 1898)

Injury to the child's foot is probably the most underemphasized aspect of musculoskeletal trauma to the growing skeleton in the orthopaedic literature. However, similar to childhood hand injuries (see Chapter 17), detailed analyses of the most common reasons for presentation to a physician's office or urgent/emergency care setting are related to the need for analysis of trauma to the foot.

Specific chondro-osseous involvement constitutes only a small portion of the presenting problems. Children and adolescents are often barefooted. Accordingly, soft tissue injuries such as lacerations and puncture wounds are extremely common. Even in these seemingly benign injuries it is essential to adequately elucidate both the possibility and actuality of concomitant deeper fascial, muscular, tendinous, periosteal or chondroosseous damage. A laceration extending to and disrupting the periosteum or a joint capsule still constitutes an open injury, even if there is no radiographic evidence of actual fracture. The risk of deep infection or osteomyelitis is part of such injuries.

Anatomy

The calcaneus and talus are usually the only nonlongitudinal tarsal bones ossified at birth. The cuboid primary ossification center appears shortly after birth (9 months). The lateral cuneiforms appears within the first year, followed by the middle and medial cuneiforms (3–4 years). The tarsal navicular is the last to begin primary ossification, at around 3 years. Thus all the primary ossification tarsal centers are usually present by the time a child is 5 years old (Fig. 24-1).[5,7] The extent of ossification, both primary and secondary, affects the ability to diagnose skeletal injury in the limping child or a child who has had a crushing-type injury.[24] Unfortunately, fracture-separation of the nonossified epiphyseal cartilage from the contiguous expanding secondary ossification center is not usually evident when utilizing routine radiography (see Chapters 5, 7).

Primary ossification in the talus, calcaneus, and navicular chondral anlagen does not always begin in the center of the anlage. Ossification in each bone may begin and proceed eccentrically within the anlage. This eccentricity probably has little effect following trauma because of the extent of chondro-osseous transformation when most of the injuries occur.

Each of the tarsal bones progressively enlarges its primary ossification center throughout childhood and adolescence. However, typical radiographic tarsal osseous contours, especially those of the calcaneus and talus, do *not* usually resemble those of an adult until the child enters the second decade of life (Fig. 24-2). Recognition of these progressive changes becomes important when interpreting radiographs, computed tomographic (CT) scans, and magnetic resonance imaging (MRI) scans.[10–12,22] Osseous contours characteristic of the adult, on which many measurements such as Bohler's angle are based, are not always present in young children. *Accordingly, such radiographic measurements must not be relied on for diagnosis or fracture reduction in a child under 10 years of age*, although measurements based on MRI studies showing the true cartilaginous contours may be more reliable.[24]

Talus

Talar ossification occurs initially in the head and neck and subsequently extends *retrograde* into the body (Fig. 24-3). The anatomic area most indicative of ischemic necrosis following talar trauma in an adult (i.e., the subchondral zone at the ankle joint) is the last region into which primary ossification eventually extends. Reliance is placed on Hawkins sign to determine that ischemic change *cannot* occur until there is sufficient ossification expansion. As with

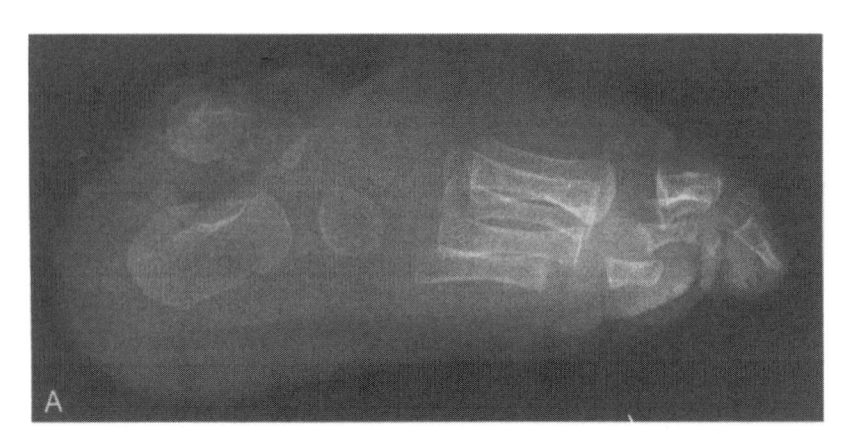

FIGURE 24-1. Lateral roentgenograms of feet from cadavers aged 7 months (A), 3 years (B), and 11 years (C). Note the variable extent of ossification in the tarsal and subtalar regions.

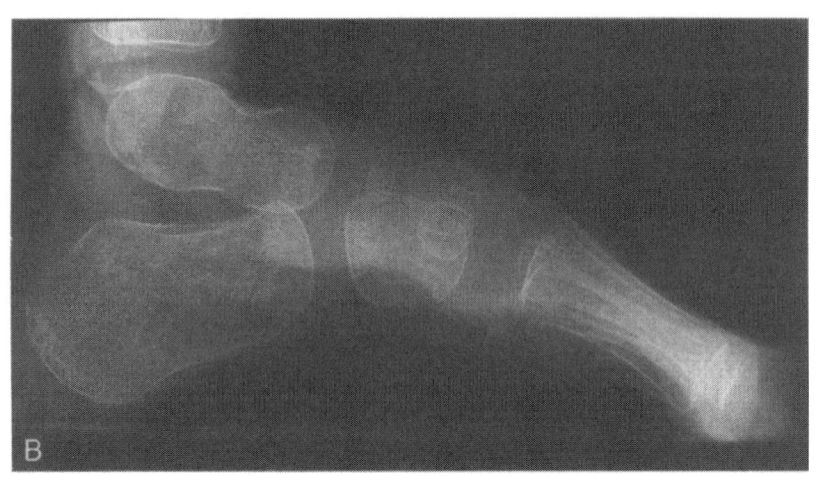

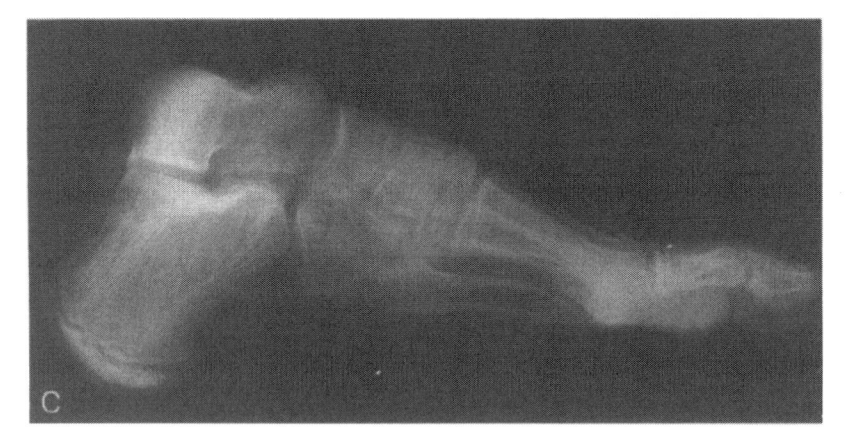

the Legg-Calvé-Perthes lesion, the younger the child and the less ossification present, the less likely there is to be significant ischemic damage of the bone, followed by deformation, if there is a talar neck fracture. Furthermore, should ischemia occur, it is less likely to cause significant subsequent osseous deformation.

The sinus tarsi is the entry for much of the blood supply of both the talus and the calcaneus. It should be minimally disturbed during any exposure for open reduction of injuries to either the talus or calcaneus, no matter what the age of the patient. The blood flow to the talus is supplied by the lateral artery of the sinus tarsi (a branch of the perforating peroneal artery) and the medial tarsal canal artery (a branch of the posterior tibial artery). These branches form an anastomotic sling in the subtalar region and supply most of the talus.[8,15] The process of formation of the talar ossification center is dependent on an adequately functioning vascular supply. As normal ossification matures (i.e., enlargement of the primary center), the patterns of circulation may be altered.

Two-thirds of the talus is usually covered with articular cartilage. There are no direct muscular attachments on the talus. Ischemic necrosis is the main reason for disability following fractures of the talus. The talar neck has a variable arterial blood supply, but it is relatively constant. There is an anastomosis between the central arteries of the talus, which is

Anatomy

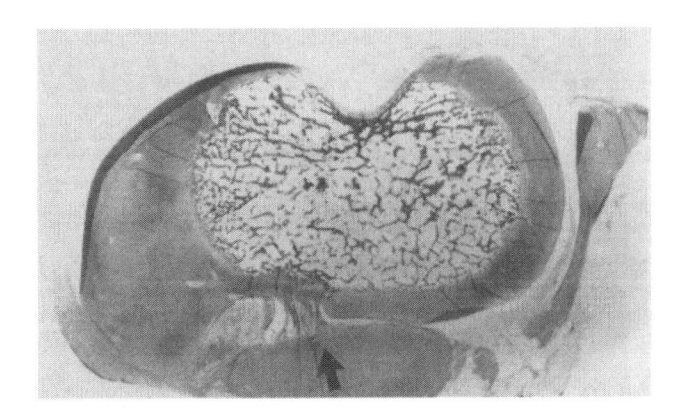

FIGURE 24-3. Development of the talus: ossification at 5 years. Note that the head and neck have ossified first and then extended to the superior surface of the neck. Talocalcaneal ligament is evident (arrow).

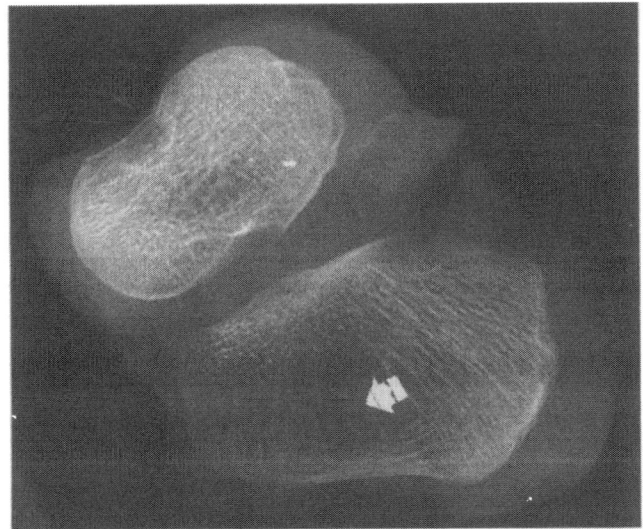

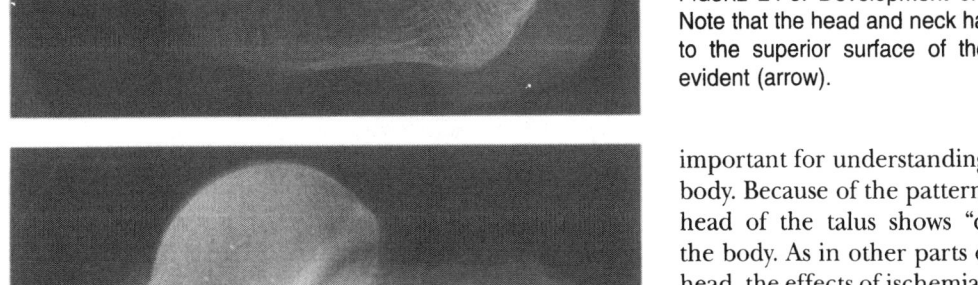

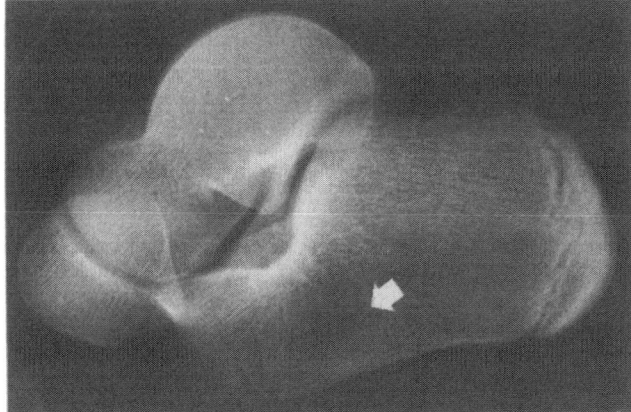

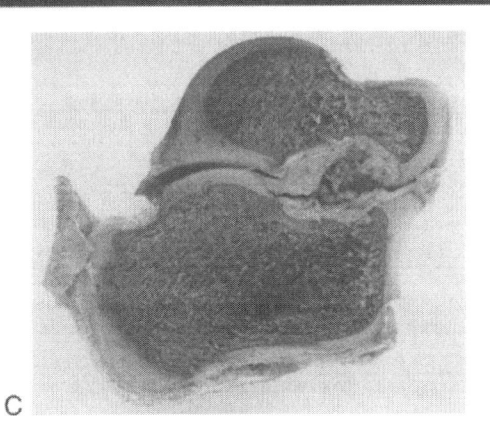

FIGURE 24-2. Talocalcaneal units at 6 years (A) and 14 years (B). The basic cartilaginous contours resemble the final, mature shape, even though the osseous contours do not. In (A) the superior osseous surface of the calcaneus has a "flat" Bohler's angle, whereas in (B) the final contour is near skeletal maturity. In both, there is a normal region of trabecular rarefaction (arrows), which is an area of extensive trabecular remodeling as the basic cancellous bone orientation shifts from oblique (A) to horizontal (B). (C) Talus and calcaneus from a 5-year-old boy injured in a motor vehicle accident. Ossification is proceeding retrograde into the talar "dome" area. The talocalcaneal contours do not resemble those of an adult pattern. Ward's triangle area is evident in the calcaneus (black area deficient in trabecular bone).

important for understanding patterns of necrosis within the body. Because of the patterns of progressive ossification, the head of the talus shows "delayed" ossification relative to the body. As in other parts of the body, such as the femoral head, the effects of ischemia are contingent on the degree of chondro-osseous transformation. Thus the more skeletally transformed talar body is more susceptible to injury than is the less ossified talar head in a young child.

Calcaneus

Calcaneal ossification normally progresses from a single primary center. This ossification center has a cortical shell inferiorly along with a periosteal sleeve, and it subsequently expands centrifugally toward all the other cartilaginous borders (Fig. 24-4). Variations of ossification may occur but may not be evident until the child presents for evaluation of trauma.[16] Initial ossification is usually directly under the talus and then expands posteriorly, superiorly, and anteriorly.

Calcaneal ossification particularly expands to develop a mechanically responsive cortical shell surrounding a trabecular network with bone that is continually remodeling during growth in response to dynamic weight-bearing stresses, especially in the posterior region. The infant and young child have a superior cartilaginous "cortex" that imparts protective resilience to the developing bone and makes certain "adult" calcaneal fracture patterns are infrequent. Stress fractures, especially in the toddler, may occur if mechanical demands exceed the rate of the normal biomechanical remodeling response.[5] During the second decade the subchondral plate extends to the contours of the surrounding cartilage, at which time radiologic landmarks such as Bohler's angle become adequately defined.

Because of the extensive remodeling in the primary ossification center, calcaneal "cysts" may occur. They are not always true cystic lesions of bone but, instead, may be biologic variances of trabecular patterning and remodeling that are reflected on a radiograph. Similar cystic lesions have been described in the talus;[17] they may pathologically fracture, bringing the child or adolescent to medical attention. Their incidental finding does *not* imply a need for surgery and bone grafting.

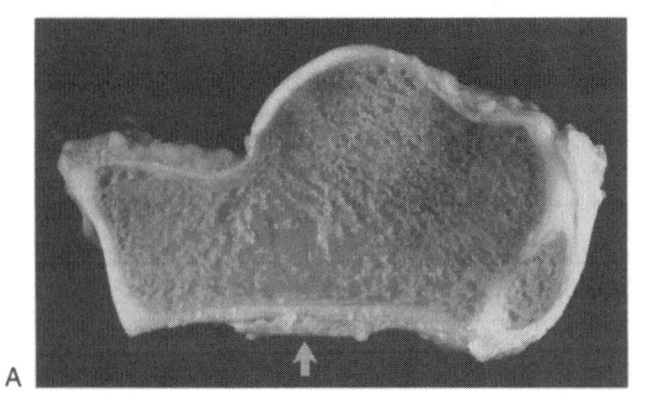

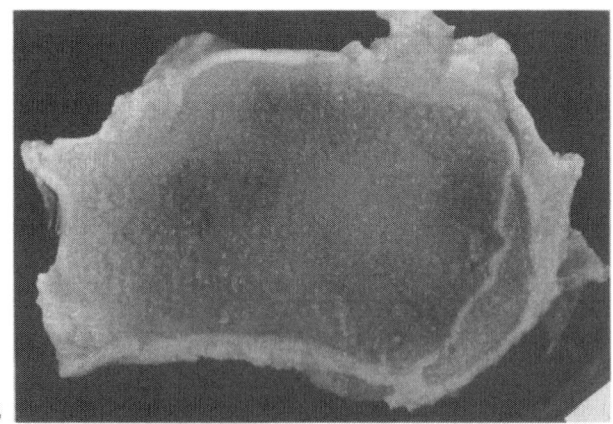

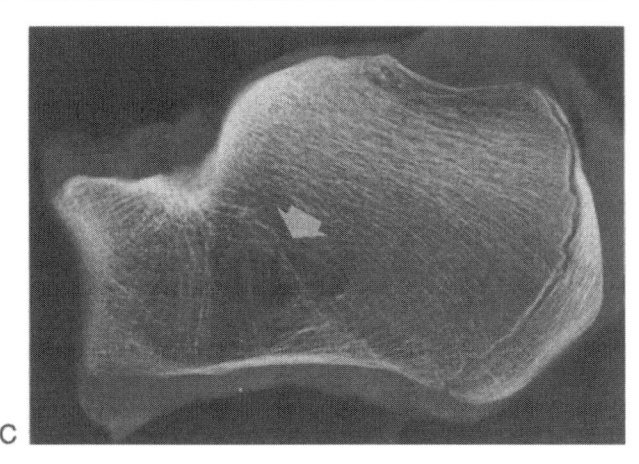

FIGURE 24-4. (A) Slab section of the calcaneus at 9 years. Secondary ossification is evident in the apophysis. Note the paucity of bone in Ward's triangle (arrow). (B) Slab section of calcaneus from a 13-year-old showing undulation of the physeal contour and configuration of the secondary ossification center. (C) Roentgenogram of the same morphologic slab. Arrow indicates normal area of trabecular thinning surrounded by tensile and compressive trabecular patterns. Note also the relatively sclerotic appearance of portions of the secondary ossification center.

The calcaneus is the only tarsal bone in which a physis and secondary center of ossification develop consistently (Fig. 24-4). It is the mechanism of posterior elongation of the calcaneus,[10,12,13] a process that is especially evident in quadrupedal mammals. Damage to the calcaneal growth potential obviously affects this elongation capacity (see Lawn Mower injuries, below; see also Chapter 9).

Secondary ossification of the calcaneal apophysis, which is variable, appears when the child is between 6 and 10 years old and may be multifocal, which must be considered when attempting to diagnose a potential fracture.[14,21] This apophyseal region may be the site of developmental problems, such as a Sever's lesion, although such osteochondroses should be considered the result of repetitive microtrauma.[5] Relative sclerosis of the secondary center is probably normal and reflects the need for increased amounts of responsive, remodeling bone to accommodate the repetitive impact of childhood and adolescent activities. The physeal–metaphyseal juncture is variably undulated in response to the tensile, compressive, and shearing forces generated in this area during normal activity. It is not appropriate to conceive of this calcaneal region as a pure traction apophysis, as is usually done, because the summated forces of the Achilles tendon and plantar fascia and musculature, plus the direct impact compression during heel strike, make the calcaneal "apophysis" primarily (functionally) a compression physis, rather than a "pure" traction physis comparable to the tibial tuberosity. Histologic analysis of this region corroborates a primary compression, rather than tension, cytoarchitecture.[9]

Closure of the calcaneal physis usually occurs between 12 and 16 years in girls and 15 and 18 years in boys. In the neonate there is a thick continuity of fibers between the Achilles tendon and the plantar fascia. As the skeleton matures there is a diminution of these fibrous connections.[23]

The Achilles tendon eventually inserts into the calcaneus. A bursa intervenes between tendon and bone. The enthesis (insertion) forms a complex insertional region protecting against repetitive use.[20] The bursal wall may develop fibrocartilage, probably as a result of micromechanical demands.

Other Tarsal Bones

Each of the midfoot tarsal bones—navicular, cuboid, cuneiforms—usually forms from a single ossification center that is relatively central within the chondral anlage. The chondro-osseous transformation is similar to the secondary ossification process in an epiphysis of a long bone (Fig. 24-5). Marginal variability should not be overinterpreted as a fracture. Preexistent vascularity within the cartilage canals is essential. Disruption of the blood supply may play a role in the development or propagation of an osteochondrosis (e.g., Kohler's lesion in the tarsal navicular).

Whereas these bones are relatively cuboidal in shape, the tarsal navicular may have a curvilinear extension medially and proximally. It is uncertain whether this pattern is congenital or biomechanically acquired. This anatomic shape is associated with pes planovalgus. A secondary ossification center may develop within this cartilaginous extension and is usually referred to as the accessory navicular. As discussed later, the tarsal navicular is a site of potential injury due to repetitive stress.

Variations of ossification are relatively common in each of these small tarsal bones. Accordingly, any attribution of morphologic change to trauma must be done carefully. Variations in ossification may occur and may be unusual or unanticipated sites of injury.

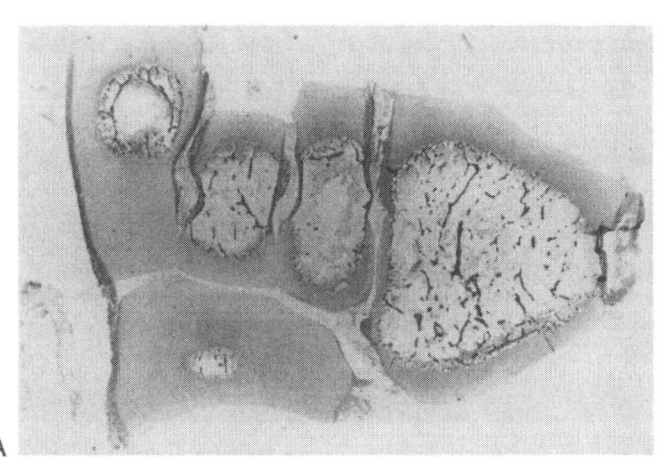

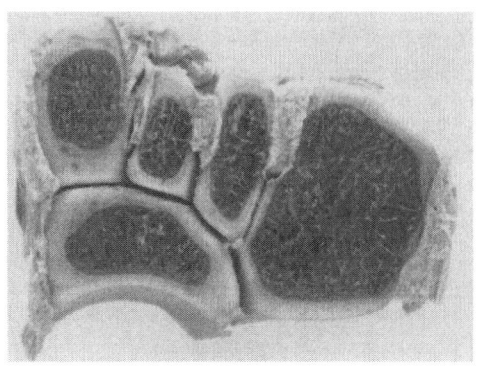

FIGURE 24-5. Early (A) and midchildhood (B) development of the midfoot.

Metatarsals

Secondary centers appear in the metatarsal epiphyses at around 5 years of age. The secondary ossification center at the proximal end of the first metatarsal may be bipartite. A pseudoepiphysis frequently forms at the distal end of the first metatarsal (Fig. 24-6). As in the hand, the four lateral metatarsals develop their secondary ossification centers distally, and pseudoepiphyses may be evident proximally. The fifth metatarsal develops an additional secondary ossification center at the proximal, lateral portion, near the peroneus brevis insertion (Fig. 24-7). This small secondary center becomes evident in children between 10 and 14 years of age and is often confused with an avulsion injury.[26]

Phalanges

The phalanges progressively form secondary ossification centers, usually by the time a child is 5 years old. There may be considerable structural variation in these centers. They may be bipartite, discoid, conical, or fissured.[5] The great toe is occasionally triphalangeal. The fifth toe may have only two phalanges, and the middle phalanx in any toe may lack epiphyseal (secondary) ossification. Sesamoid bones appear under the first metatarsal-phalangeal joint and may be bipartite or tripartite (Fig. 24-8).[25] Sometimes it is difficult to distinguish between an unusual sesamoid bone and a possible occult type 3 or 4 proximal phalangeal physeal injury.

Maturation and Variation

The rates of growth and maturation of the skeletal components of the foot not only exhibit differences between the sexes but are physiologically accelerated when compared with the corresponding rates of maturation of the longitudinal bones of the arm and leg. Factors that might disturb

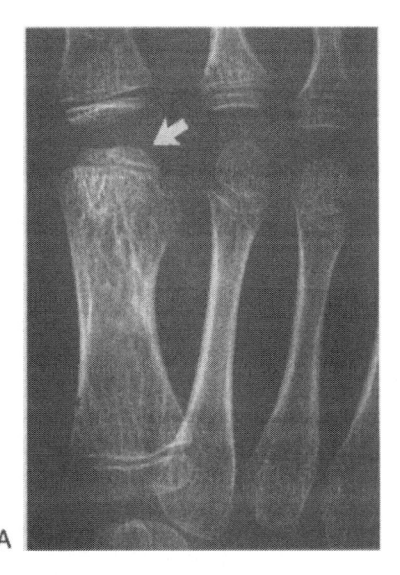

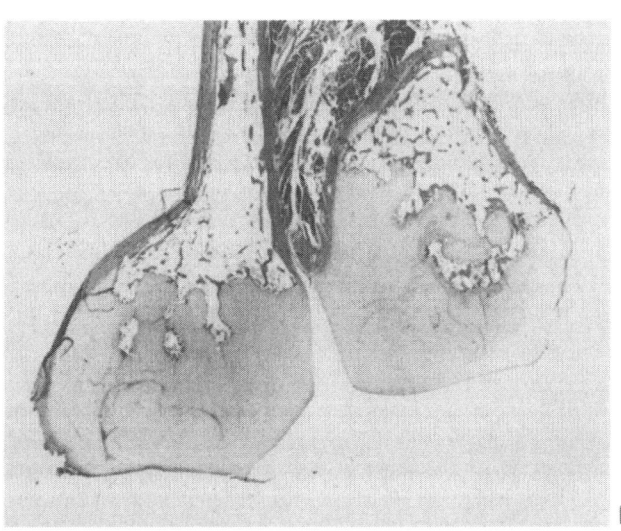

FIGURE 24-6. (A) Pseudoepiphysis (arrow) of the distal first metatarsal. (B) Histology of proximal pseudoepiphyses of the second and third metatarsals (see Chapter 1 for further discussion).

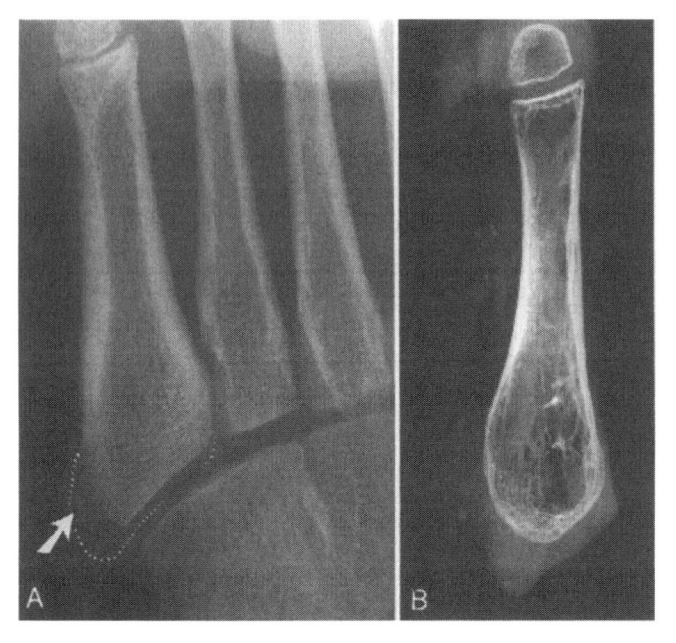

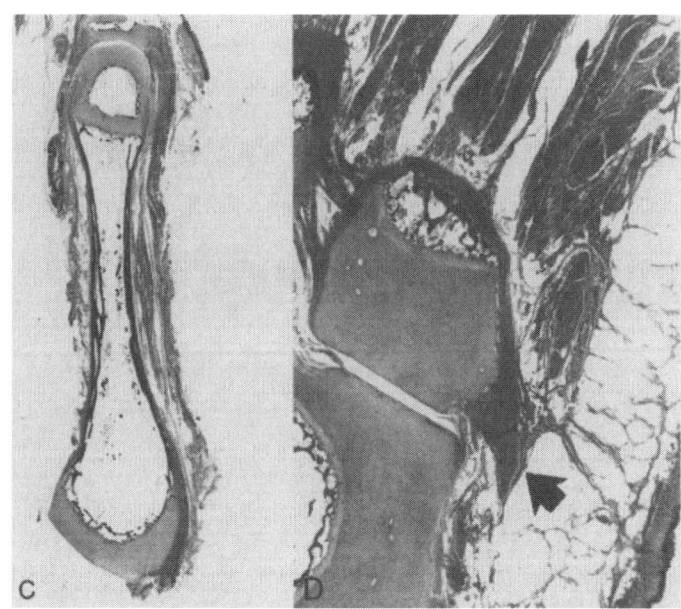

FIGURE 24-7. (A) Actual shape of the fifth metatarsal in a 9-year-old boy is indicated by the dotted line and arrow. (B) Anatomic specimen showing the proximal cartilage. (C) Histologic section of the proximal epiphysis. (D) Histologic section showing the structure of the proximal epiphysis and attached tendon (arrow).

growth, maturation, and the ultimate length of the foot are proportionally less in the older child than they might be for similar growth mechanism injuries to the long bones. The extent of longitudinal growth in the metatarsals and phalanges that might correct malalignment is not comparable to that of the major long bones. Longitudinal growth patterns are not reliable for correcting significant malalignment, particularly when the complication may have an effect on the normal weight-bearing capacity and arch patterns of the foot.

The developing foot has many anatomic variations and ossification patterns that are often difficult to distinguish from injury (i.e., radiologically obvious fractures). More than 20% of all children have at least one of the multiple structural roentgenographic variations recognized by radiologists.[6] The common accessory bones are illustrated in Figure 24-9. These accessory bones are rarely acutely injured. Infrequent case reports usually involve adults.[16] The most common accessory bones are the accessory navicular and the os trigonum, but they are really secondary ossification centers within the overall cartilaginous precursor of each particular bone. These anatomic variations are discussed in more detail because of their frequent association with skeletal trauma.

Accessory Navicular

The tarsal navicular may develop a secondary ossification center that becomes radiographically evident by the age of 10–12 years and does not always unite with the primary ossification center during adolescence. This accessory tarsal navicular, which may also be referred to as the prehallux or os tibiale externum, occurs in as many as 10% of children. The ossification is located at the medial side of the navicular and extends proximally along the medial margin of the talus (Fig. 24-10). This accessory center usually coalesces with the primary center of ossification of the navicular to form a cornuate-shaped navicular during late adolescence. Although this ossification center appears to be separate radiographically, it is important to realize that it forms completely within epiphyseal cartilage that is anatomically continuous with the rest of the tarsal navicular.

Os Trigonum

The os trigonum develops within the posterior cartilage of the talus, appearing in children 8–11 years old as a radiographically (but not anatomically) separate center of ossification (Figs. 24-11, 24-12).[9] This osseous structure usually fuses to the body of the talus during late adolescence. The connecting, radiolucent cartilage may be misinterpreted as a fracture line. The os trigonum may impinge directly on the posterior tibial epiphysis, especially when the ankle is in maximal plantar flexion, and thereby sustains an injury. This microfracture occurs most often during the period of fusion to the body of the talus. The os trigonum may persist as a radiographically separate ossicle in the adult.

Plantar Foot Padding

The bipedal gait of the child requires the foot to function as an impact shock absorber and a rigid lever for push-off during normal gait. Disruption of soft and skeletal tissues interferes with such processes and may have an adverse effect on the child's ability to walk comfortably. Accordingly, the soft tissues of the plantar surface in a child assume just as much importance in diagnosis and treatment as the specific skeletal injuries.

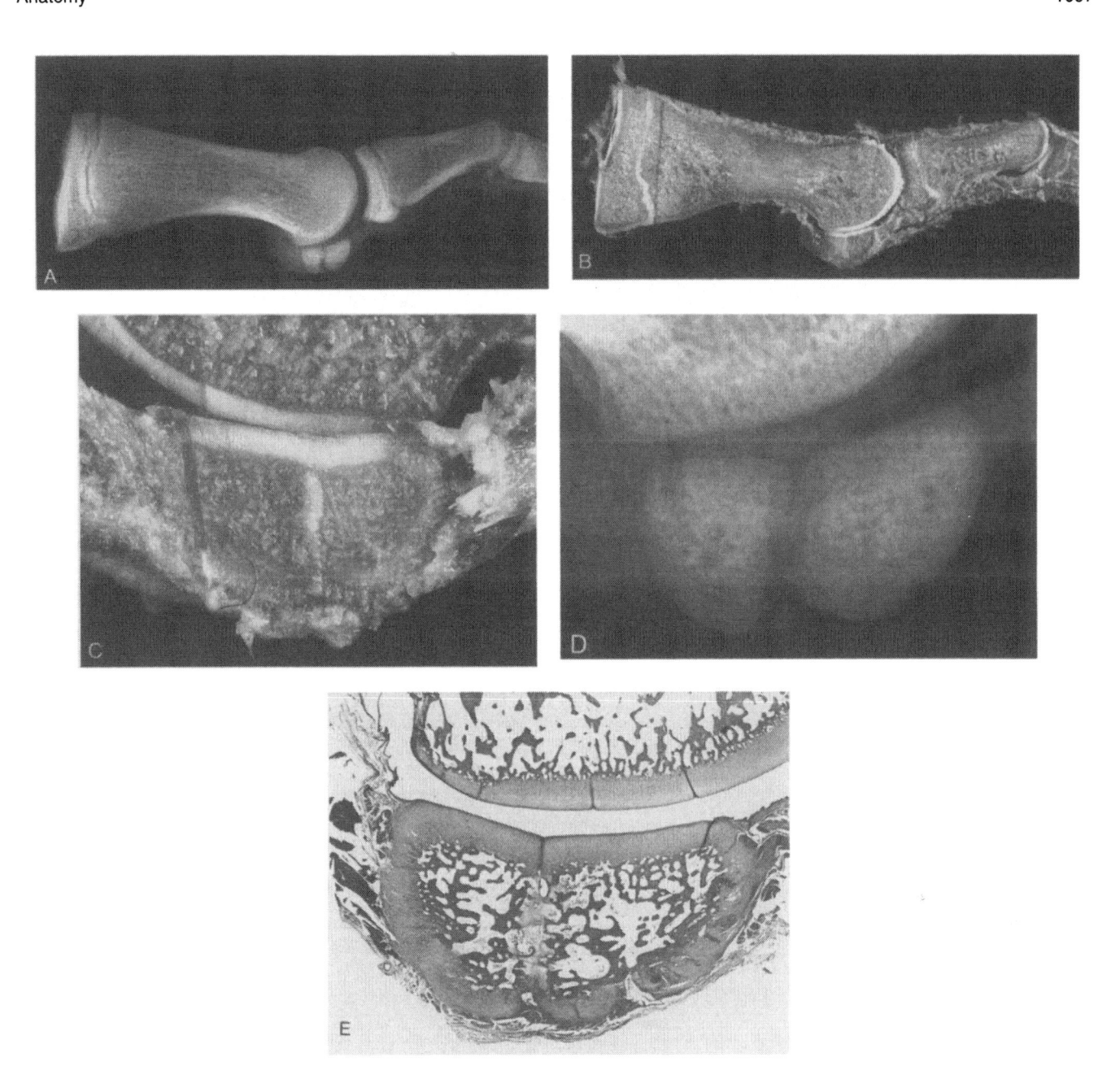

Anatomy 1097

FIGURE 24-8. Bifid sesamoid. (A) Radiography of the first toe. (B) Longitudinal section shows that the two centers are contained within *one* cartilaginous precursor. Magnification views show morphology (C), radiology (D), and histology (E).

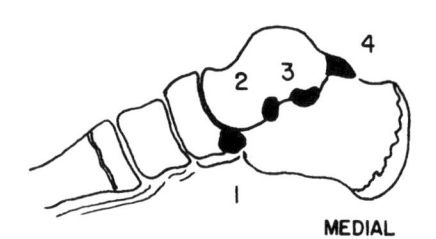

FIGURE 24-9. Common accessory tarsal ossification locations. 1 = os tibiale; 2 = os sustentaculi; 3 = talus secundarius; 4 = os trigonum; 5 = calcaneus secundarius; 6 = os intercuneiforme; 7 = os intermetatarseum; 8 = os vesalianum; 9 = os fibulare. Many of these ossifications have apparent radiologic discontinuity but anatomic (cartilaginous) continuity.

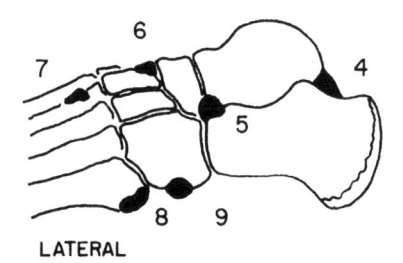

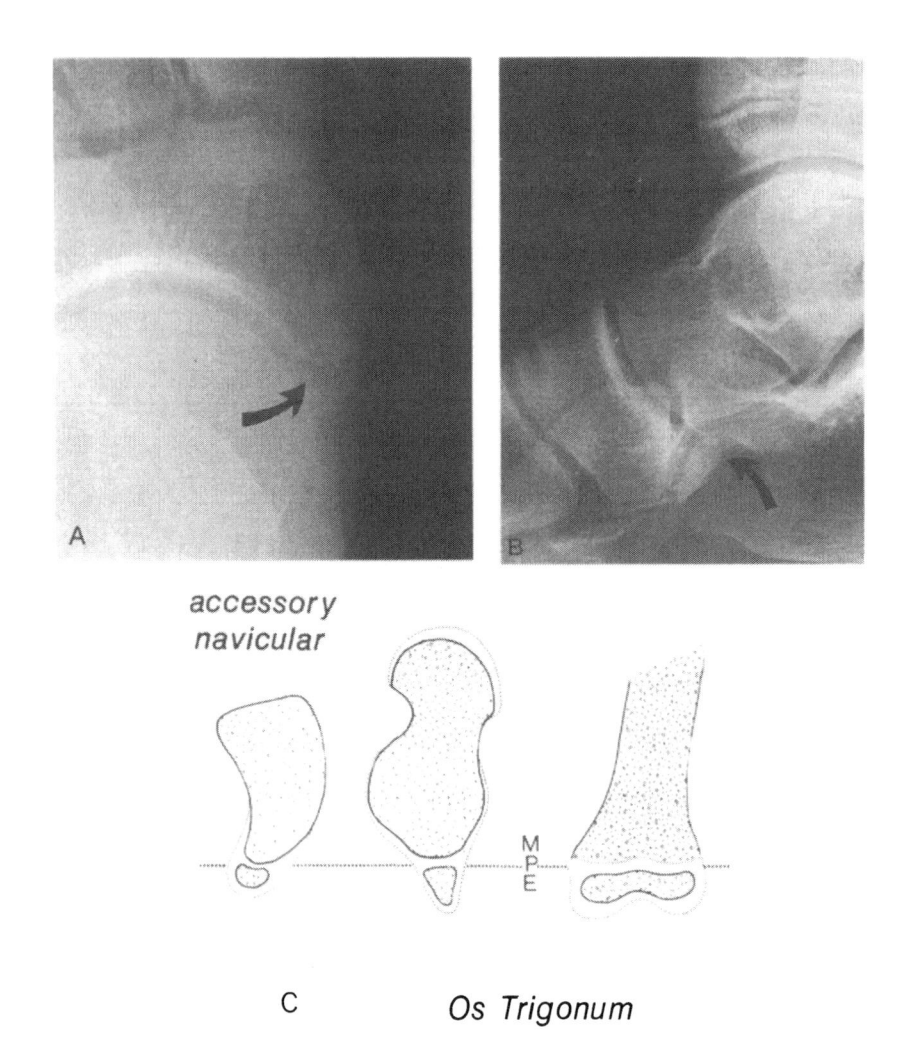

FIGURE 24-10. (A, B) Accessory navicular (arrow). (C) Cartilaginous continuity despite radiologic discontinuity of the accessory navicular and the os trigonum. Note how they correspond developmentally to the regions of a long bone. M = metaphysis; P = physis; E = epiphysis.

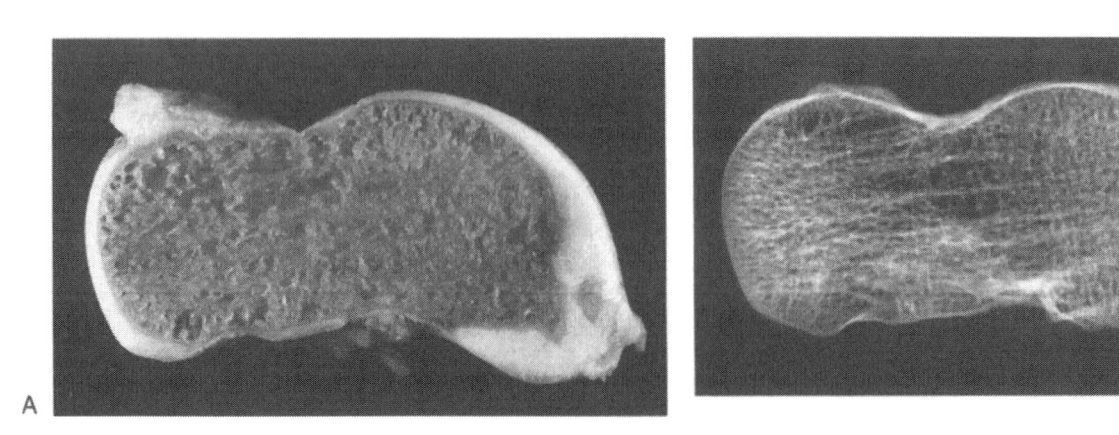

FIGURE 24-11. (A) Slab section of talus from a 9-year-old boy. Accessory ossification (os trigonum) is evident posteriorly within the remaining unossified cartilage. (B) Roentgenogram of the specimen revealed two accessory bones.

Anatomy

and hypothenar eminences, ischial tuberosity, and prepatellar region). The fibroelastic architecture in each of these regions, and especially the plantar surfaces, binds the fat cells into demarcated volumes. Atrophy may result in fragmentation of these elastic compartments. Trauma accomplishes the same, both from acute disruption and subsequent fibrosis within the septa, adversely affecting the cellular biomechanics.[6]

This elastic padding is set into oscillations that result in a temporary loss of contact with the ground at the beginning of a step (toe-off).[1] Plantar pads (and palmar pads in quadrupeds) are highly resilient, returning about 70% of the energy used to deform them in their elastic recoil; the remaining energy is presumably lost.[1,2] Collagenous elements connect the calcaneus to the skin and compartmentalize the reactive fat within the pad; accordingly directing any displacement when the pad is subjected to compressive loading and ascertaining that the subcalcaneal fat pads provide cushioning, thereby reducing the peak force at the instance of heel strike.[4]

The fibrous structure of the human calcaneal fat pad in fetuses and adults is a thick, fibrous outercoat that demarcates a "primary vesicle."[4] Major fibrous septae connect this outer coat to the periosteum or perichondrium of the calcaneus. These septae are curvilinear. The septae tend to be oblique on the plantar surface, S-shaped at the junction of side and plantar, and whorl-shaped along the sides of the calcaneus. Between birth and adulthood, undoubtedly in response to progressive weight-bearing, the relatively large, demarcated chambers are further subdivided into small reactive "cells" composed of anatomically defined vesicles that are especially rich in elastic fibers.[4]

As is discussed later under calcaneal trauma and lawn mower and propeller injuries, loss of some or all of the fat pad creates a significant problem for effective, pain-free weight-bearing. Any type of flap (e.g., rotation, free) brings in a layer of fat and dermal elements. No flap duplicates the anatomy of the intricate normal fibrous septae that cushion weight-bearing impact.

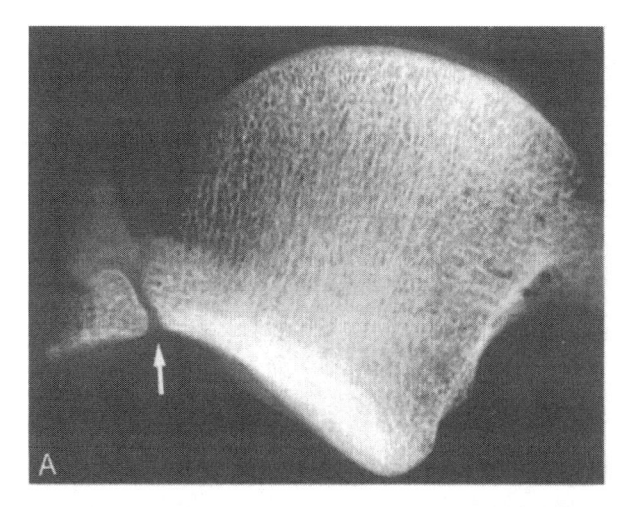

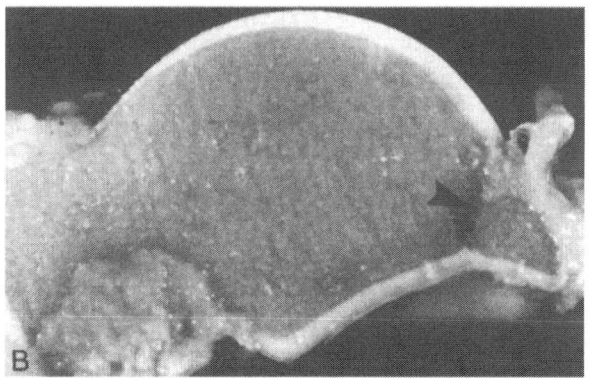

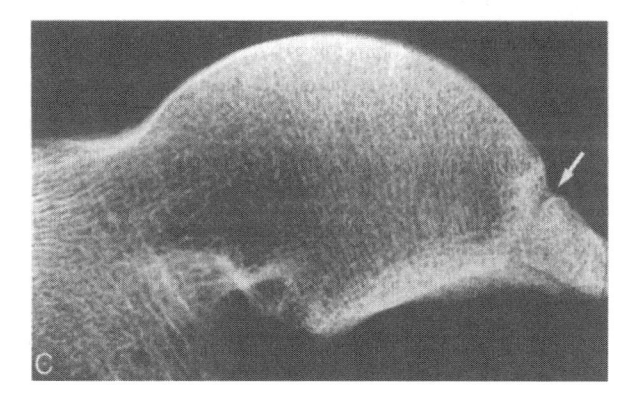

FIGURE 24-12. Os trigonum. (A) Roentgenogram of talar specimen from a 12-year-old child showing accessory ossification separated from the main talar ossification center by a cartilaginous bridge (arrow). (B) Morphologic section of a talar specimen from a 14-year-old, showing early consolidation of the accessory and main talar ossification centers. (C) Roentgenogram of specimen in (B) (arrow).

The fat pads of the sole of the foot have adapted to weight-bearing by a process of localizing small, compression-responsive compartments of fat cell groups (Fig. 24-13). These may be significantly disrupted or altered by scar formation or open injuries.

The heel fat pad thus contains elastic, encapsulated adipose tissue that is capable of physiologically resisting the compressive and shear forces of ambulation.[19] Similar tissue combinations are found in other areas (fingertips, thenar

Foot Growth

Blais et al. provided growth charts and parameters of the growing foot comparable to their studies on growth of the leg.[3] They noted that at 12 years of age the average length of the foot was about the same for girls and boys. Boys, however, continued their foot growth for another 2 years. They also noted that the feet of both boys and girls grew at a rapidly decreasing rate from infancy through 5 years: From the age of 5 years there is an annual increase in length of roughly 0.9 cm. There is also a tendency for the foot to be relatively closer to its adult dimension than in other areas of skeletal growth. Thus factors that would inhibit growth at a particular age, as trauma, would affect the ultimate length of the foot proportionately less than would similar disturbances in the long bones at the same age. Even if all centers of growth were damaged as early as a skeletal age of 10 years in girls and 12 years in boys, an average reduction of only 10% would be expected.[3] This pattern of growth should be considered carefully before undertaking epiphysiodesis to improve foot size asymmetry.

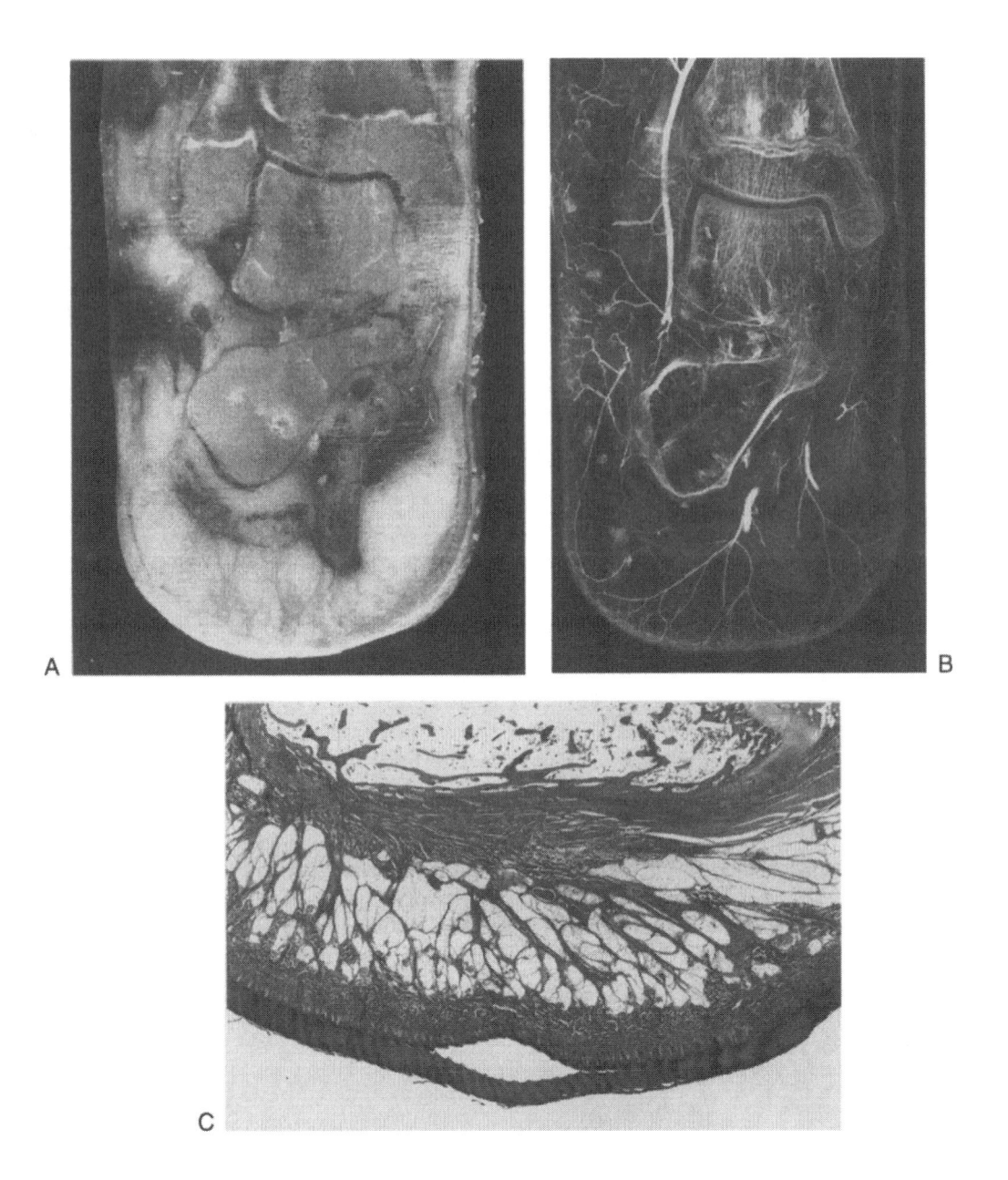

FIGURE 24-13. (A) Slab section of the hindfoot showing an extensive fat pad underneath the calcaneus. (B) Injection showing the vascularity of the fat pad. (C) Histologic section of loculations in the fat pad.

Pedal Nerves

Sensation on the dorsum of the foot is supplied by the saphenous nerve medially, the superficial peroneal nerve dorsally, and the sural nerve laterally. A small area of the dorsum and the web space between the first and second toes is supplied by the superficial branch of the deep peroneal nerve.

Traumatic injuries of the lateral foot and ankle place the sural nerve and its branches at risk. Few anatomic studies detail the course of this nerve. Lawrence and Botte found considerable variation in the nerve in its branches but were able to describe a "typical" nerve trunk that lay in close proximity to the Achilles tendon.[13] Approximately 25% of their specimens had an anastomotic branch coursing into the sinus tarsi. The importance of this nerve is that direct or indirect trauma may result in neuroma formation, entrapment syndrome, reflex sympathetic dystrophy, or causalgia.

Tendons

When assessing whether tendons are damaged, it is important to realize that there may be structural variations, such as bifurcation of the extensor digitorum longus. Such variations must be considered during any evaluation.[18]

Foot Injuries

Fractures

Phalangeal and metatarsal fractures occur frequently in children, although their real incidence is not well documented. In contrast, injuries to the other chondro-osseous components of the child's foot (i.e., the tarsal bones) seem to be less common, although they have received greater emphasis in the literature.[27,30-34,37-42,49,51,52,53,57-60,63] Flexibility and resilience appear to render the immature foot less susceptible than leg bones to major skeletal injury.[28] Forces of indirect violence are usually transmitted more proximally to the distal tibia and fibula.

Crawford reviewed 175 foot injuries in children who presented to an emergency room.[31] Ninety percent of the children had metatarsal fractures, with phalangeal fractures being the next most common injury pattern. The navicular was the most commonly fractured tarsal bone, followed by the talus, calcaneus, and cuboid. In 8% of the skeletally immature patients there were coexistent fractures, sometimes initially unrecognized, of the tibia, fibula, or both.

Children's foot injuries during sports are unusually rare. Accordingly, "protective" athletic shoes are rarely protective of repetitive injury. Similarly, orthotics tend to be an area of potential abuse.[56]

Children's foot fractures often result from direct violence, such as a crush from a heavy object that lands on the foot, being run over by vehicular wheels or a lawn mower, and falling or jumping from a height.[55] Concomitant soft tissue injury becomes a significant component of such trauma. Accordingly, initial treatment must often be directed toward the swelling and associated cutaneous, muscular, neural, and vascular problems. Potential circulatory and neurologic complications must be evaluated thoroughly during the days following trauma. The potential for compartment syndromes must be evaluated closely.

Compression dressings, elevation, and icing constitute the initial treatment for many of these injuries. Definitive fracture treatment (closed manipulation or open reduction) often should be rendered later (24–72 hours after injury), when soft tissue swelling has subsided and vascular and skin status permit it. The fracture or fractures may then be more effectively reduced and immobilized.

The management of open fractures of the foot is no different from that of any other anatomic site. In fact, because of mechanisms such as lawn mower or vehicular damage, aggressive treatment is usually mandatory. Broad-spectrum antibiotic coverage is used initially contingent on any allergies of the patient and the most likely regional bacterial flora (e.g., a farm setting versus the seacoast).

Athletic footwear suggests a need for *Pseudomonas* coverage as part of "broad-spectrum antibiotics." Tetanus booster may be appropriate, contingent on the date of the last immunization and the injury milieu.

Contaminated and traumatized tissues must be meticulously débrided. *Adequate tissue débridement is the essential initial step toward avoiding complications.* The wound is dressed open and the child brought back to the operating room for subsequent dressing changes and further débridement, depending on the overall appearance of the marginal and deeper tissues. This approach allows continued evaluation of the viability of the exposed and deep soft tissues. Appropriate anesthesia allows adequate assessment in a reactive child.

A significant area of subtle chondro-osseous trauma and soft tissue injury and avulsion occurs with spoked wheel injuries, which are principally due to bicycle injuries. The likelihood is that this injury occurs to a child riding on the back of a bicycle and has a foot caught between some of the support bars and the spoked wheel.[50] These injuries become more common as societies place greater emphasis on the use of the bicycle as a means of mobility. Subrahmanyam et al. described 12 children who had been riding on the back of a bicycle and who had a common problem of injury to the great toe.[55] The injuries included fractures and, at the worst, traumatic amputation of the great toe along with soft tissue laceration of the sole of the foot.

In a review of patients with crush injuries to the foot, only 46% had a good functional outcome, 29% had fair results, and 25% had poor results.[48] These statistics may be worse in children because of the increased incidence of mutilating injuries (e.g., lawn mower accidents) and the damage to growth regions. Poor results are more likely to occur if treatment is not initiated immediately, if soft tissue coverage is delayed, or if patients developed neuritis or reflex sympathetic dystrophy.

Osteochondroses

The osteochondroses represent a variety of bone disorders associated with a lack of continued normal chondro-osseous transformation. They are also associated with fragmentation and sclerosis of a preexisting secondary ossification center of an epiphysis or the primary ossification center of a nontubular tarsal bone.

The tarsal and metatarsal bones have several associated osteochondroses, such as Sever's (calcaneus), Kohler's (navicular) Iselin's (proximal fifth metatarsal), and Freiberg's (second metatarsal). Although they are often considered radiologic variants, their significance to any pain complaints should always be considered during both diagnosis and treatment. Each of the entities, as it affects the foot, is addressed in the specific anatomic sections of this chapter.

An acute injury to the foot may be associated with a normal radiograph of the tarsal navicular at the time of acute injury, only to have a subsequent radiograph show ischemic changes. These changes may be detected early by bone scan and MRI in patients who subsequently develop Kohler's disease. These "osteochondroses" represent *elastic* injury to the bone (see Chapters 1, 5, 7).

Foot Compartment Syndrome

Fakhouri and Manoli assessed the problem of foot compartment syndrome in patients (principally adults) with calcaneal and metatarsal fractures and Lisfranc fracture-dislocations.[35] The possibility of this complication in injured children certainly must be anticipated and assessed, as the soft tissue attachments and compartment delineations do not vary significantly throughout the period of skeletal maturation.

Compartment syndromes in the foot usually result from high-energy and crushing injuries. Many calcaneal fractures in children involve much less injury; therefore, the risk of this complication is less likely to be considered, although it should not decrease the physician's index of suspicion in the child or adolescent.[29]

The most serious and frequently neglected aspect of treatment of foot fractures is the extent of soft tissue injury. A circular cast probably should not be applied initially to children with moderate to severe swelling secondary to a crush injury. Instead, these children usually require splinting, observation, elevation, and icing, watching for the potential development of compartment syndrome.

Pain disproportionate to the injury may not be a reliable clinical finding of compartment syndrome in an apprehensive child who has sustained injuries to the foot. Many of the injuries (i.e., the fractures) that cause accompanying compartment syndrome *already* produce considerable pain. Nerve damage due to crushing may remove pain as a significant finding. In Fakhouri and Manoli's study, only half of the conscious patients had pain, which was further accentuated by passive motion of the toes.[35] Sensory deficits may be due to neural ischemia from the compartment syndrome or direct nerve damage from the initial injury. *The most consistent physical finding is tense swelling of the foot.* As with other compartment syndromes, tissue pressure measurement is still the ideal method for diagnosis, with elevation above 30 mmHg being the basic, but not unequivocal, limit.[45,54] Persistent measurements above this level should be carefully assessed by physical examination but *not* used as an arbitrary indication for decompression.

Because of the skeletal resilience of the developing foot, there may not be an obvious fracture, even though the foot is tense and swollen. I treated a 2-year-old whose foot was run over by an automobile tire. No fractures were evident, although compartment pressures in the emergency room were 90 mmHg. Immediate compartment releases were undertaken, and the child has had no residual problems. Several other children also had tense swelling of the foot, without radiologically evident fracture; they also underwent decompression.

It is important that a treating physician not assume that feet with open fractures are spontaneously decompressed and do not require fasciotomies. Compartment syndromes may also accompany open fractures.[62]

Myerson[46,47] and Manoli and Weber[44] identified nine compartments in the foot. Three of the compartments are confined to either the hindfoot (calcaneal) or the forefoot (interosseous and one adductor). This complex anatomy increases the problems of making an accurate diagnosis and undertaking specific fasciotomy. Myerson[46,47] and Manoli and Weber[44] used MRI scans to demonstrate the extension of hematoma into the calcaneal compartment. In the immature foot many of these compartments are small; and bleeding from a trabecular bone may rapidly raise the interstitial pressure to a level at which the microcirculation ceases to function effectively.

Fasciotomy in the child may be best accomplished through two dorsal incisions and an additional medial incision. The dorsal incisions are parallel to the second and fourth metatarsals.[61] The incisions should be carried down to the bones with minimal dissection. The overlying fascia may then be identified and the interosseous compartments released. The medial incision should be from the proximal end of the first metatarsal to the posterior portion of the heel. There is also significantly less need for skin grafting to attain delayed closure. Rapid dissolution of the edema brings wound edges together in the child. Delayed primary closure is usually realistic.

An anatomic communication between the compartments of the foot and the deep posterior compartment of the leg has been described.[44] This communication has important implications for treatment of leg and foot trauma, as compartment syndromes may occur in an adjacent part when only one of them has been specifically injured. Patients may develop compartment syndromes of the foot as well as the leg.[35] Patients with foot compartment syndrome may have leg fractures without a specific chondro-osseous injury to the foot.[35] The long-term sequelae of foot compartment syndrome generally include plantar contracture, cavus deformity, clawing of the toes, chronic pain, dysfunction, sensory disturbances, and stiffness.[36]

Roentgenographic evaluation should be undertaken in any child with heel or foot pain, with or without a history of trauma. Such pain may be the first symptom of a systemic disease such as leukemia or a more localized stress injury process such as a Sever's lesion or toddler's fracture (usually involving the calcaneus).

For any patient who has sustained a foot injury as a consequence of a fall from a height, it is imperative that the back be evaluated clinically and radiographically. Compression fractures of the spine, though less common in children than in adults, may occur and certainly should be recognized even if they do not affect the treatment. The most likely anatomic region of injury is the lumbar spine, although the thoracolumbar junction may also be a focal point of injury. Nearby fractures (e.g., distal tibia) may occur as well.

Radionuclide scanning may help in the diagnosis of persistent foot pain following injury and may enable the diagnosis of stress fractures and fractures of the sesamoids and subtalar arthritis to be diagnosed earlier. This test is extremely reliable for screening when radiographs are normal despite persistent symptoms in the limping child.

Talus

The talus is fractured very infrequently in the child.[72,75,88,98,100,104,108,111,115,121,126,127] The most common injury is a vertical fracture, with variable displacement, through the talar neck (Figs. 24-14, 24-15). However, unusual fracture

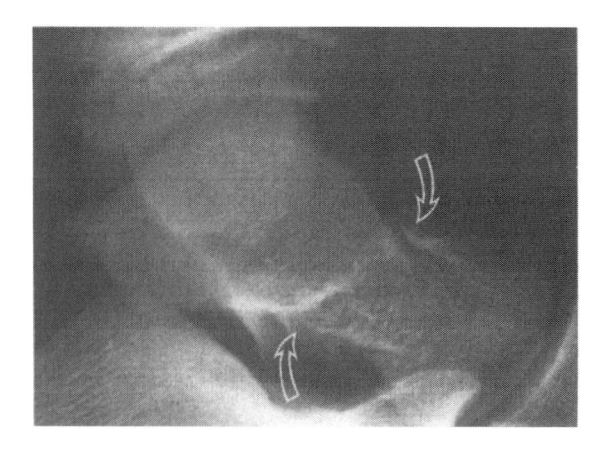

FIGURE 24-14. Displaced, oblique fracture of the talar neck (arrows) in a 10-year-old child.

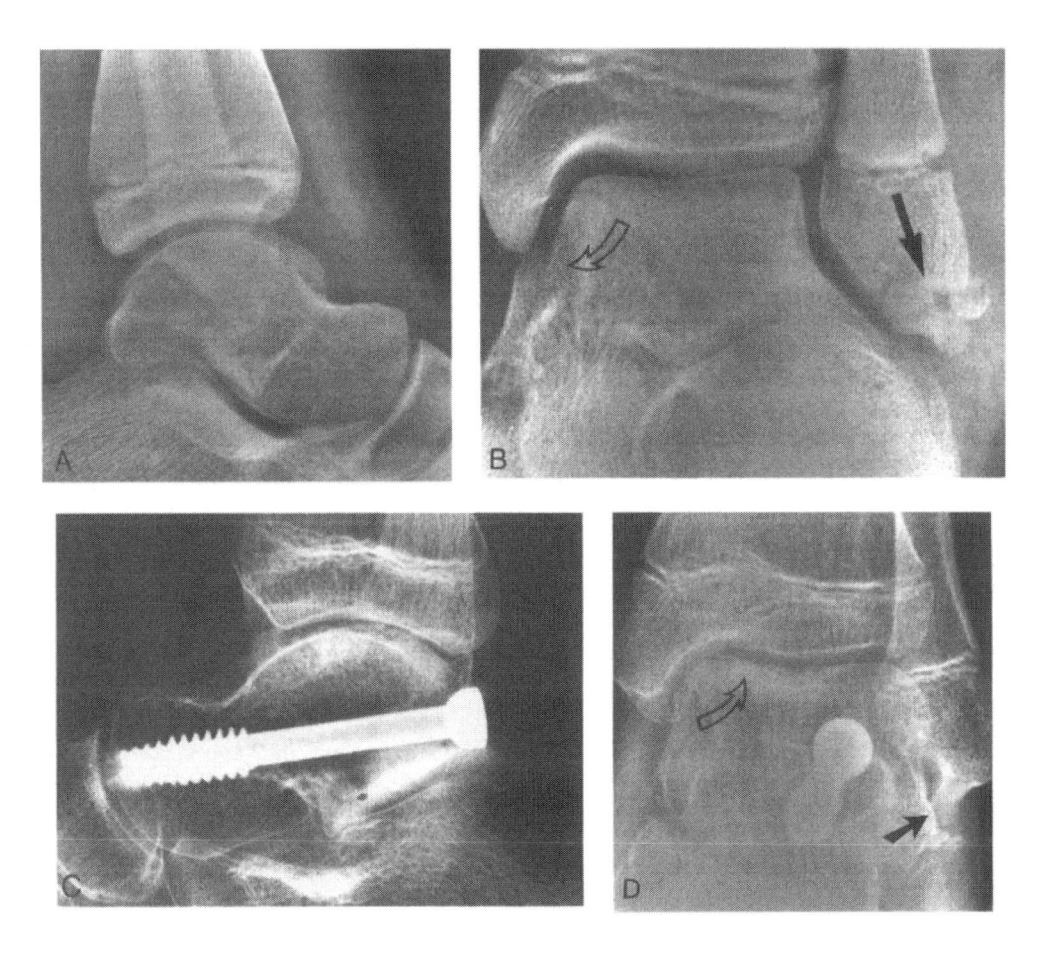

FIGURE 24-15. (A) Lateral view of a talar fracture with minimal displacement. (B) Anteroposterior view shows displacement (open arrow). Also note the fragmentation of the lateral malleolus, suggesting ligament injury analogue (solid arrow). (C) Open reduction and internal fixation. (D) Evidence of subchondral cyst formation (open arrow). There is linear ossification within the lateral collateral ligament (solid arrow).

patterns may occur because of immature ossification. In particular, sleeve ("shell") fractures may cause separation of cartilage from bone (Fig. 24-16), a pattern not always evident radiologically unless there is a thin piece of subchondral bone. The usual mechanisms of injury are twisting trauma, being crushed (as by an automobile tire), and damage from a lawn mower.

Patterns of fracture are contingent on the extent of formation of the ossification center and the skeletal maturity of the subtalar region. The most severe injuries resemble adult patterns, but they do not generally occur (or at least become readily radiologically evident) until the talus and calcaneus are relatively mature, when the treatment and risks essentially are no different from those in an adult.

Visualization of minimally displaced fractures is not always easy, especially when evaluating a chondro-osseous avulsion (Fig. 24-15). A variable-sized piece of the subchondral bone may be attached to the cartilage. The adjacent trabecular bone may sustain microfractures and focal hemorrhage that extends 1 cm or more into the ossification center. The cartilaginous fracture may also extend, at an angle, into the cartilage and may even reach the external margin. Such extension may involve the articular surfaces. I have noted these occult injuries in a significant number of feet in children who have had a traumatic amputation (Fig. 24-16).

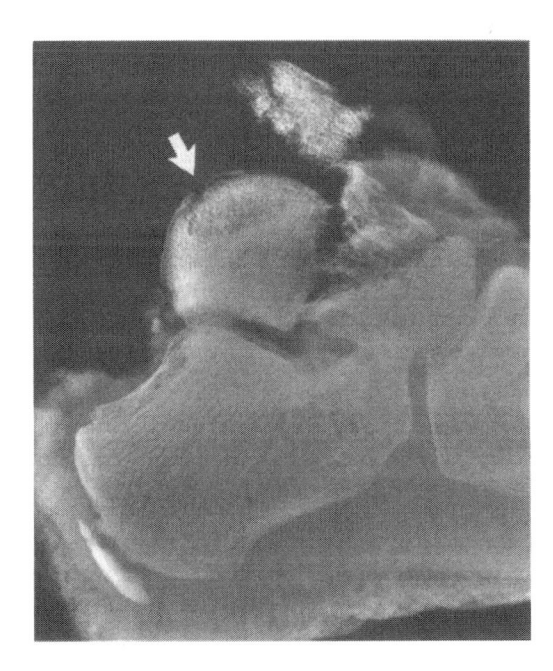

FIGURE 24-16. Traumatic amputation specimen showing a comminuted fracture of the talus. The principal injury involves the talar neck. A thin subchondral fracture is evident as well (arrow) involving the articular surface.

Even detailed specimen radiography has not always elucidated the specific pathologic anatomy, whereas anatomic and histologic studies have shown the true histopathology. Accordingly, strong consideration should be given to obtaining an MRI scan of the foot if clinical examination suggests skeletal trauma when the radiograph is "negative." Such MRI should evaluate all of the tarsal and metatarsal bones for occult injury.

Furthermore, although the osseous contours of the talus and calcaneus do not duplicate the adult patterns, fractures are more likely to occur in the bone and the cartilage. Accordingly, cartilage deformity (e.g., subtalar injury) may occur but may not be radiologically evident.

Fracture Patterns

Talar neck fractures may be divided into three patterns: (1) vertical fracture of the talar neck; (2) vertical fracture of the talar neck and dislocation or subluxation of the subtalar joint; (3) vertical fracture of the neck and dislocation of the talar body from both the ankle and the subtalar joint.

Talar body fractures may be divided into five patterns: (1) transchondral or compression fractures of the talar dome; (2) shearing fractures, which may be coronal, sagittal, or horizontal involving the entire talar body; (3) fractures of the posterior tuberosity of the talus; (4) fractures of the lateral process of the talus; (5) crush fractures of the talar body. Hawkins considered fractures of the lateral process of the talus the second most common fracture of the talar body.[89] The lateral process serves as an attachment for the lateral ligaments of the foot and ankle.

Treatment

If the talar fracture is undisplaced or minimally displaced, treatment consists of immobilization in a non-weight-bearing cast once the soft tissue swelling has subsided. A padded, splinted compression wrap may be used temporarily until a cast can be effectively applied. Continued clinical evaluation is essential to evaluate the decrease of soft tissue edema (i.e., to continue to evaluate the foot for complications such as compartment syndrome).

When the head of the fractured talus is displaced, closed reduction is undertaken initially and the foot immobilized appropriately to avoid recurrence of the deformity. Most often the foot should be casted with the forefoot in mild plantar flexion (20°–30°) in a non-weight-bearing cast for 6–8 weeks.

If the reduction is unstable, the fragments may be transfixed, either by percutaneous pinning under an image intensifier or by open reduction (Fig. 24-15).[97] Surgical exposure should be minimal to lessen the risk of potential or further vascular damage. It is best to use a lateral approach to decrease the risk of injury to the medial arterial supply. There should be minimal stripping of the peritalar and subtalar soft tissues.

Considering the remodeling potential of the child's talus, less harm may be done by accepting minor displacement with a closed reduction than by potentially attenuating the blood supply through repeated manipulation or extensive open reduction. Displacement or angulation that could lead to permanent deformity should be avoided. A CT scan or MRI may be helpful to define fully the extent of the injury, particularly to nonossified cartilage, if one is planning operative exposure and reduction. It is important to restore disrupted joint surfaces (ankle, subtalar, talonavicular) to minimize any long-term problems of joint dysfunction.

Ischemic Necrosis

Ischemic necrosis is the main cause of disability following fractures of the talus, even in children.[92,118] The sustentaculum has a limited but relatively constant arterial blood supply. There is an anastomosis between the sustentacular arteries of the talus, which is important for understanding patterns of necrosis within the body. Because of patterns of progressive ossification, the head of the talus shows delayed ossification relative to the body. As in other parts of the body such as the femoral head, the effects of ischemia are contingent on the degree of chondro-osseous transformation. Thus the more skeletally transformed talar body is more susceptible to injury than is the talar head in a young child.

Ischemic (avascular) necrosis of the talus may occur in children.[90] Development of the talar ossification center may be temporarily or permanently impaired, depending on the amount of ischemia. In the older child (over 10 years), ischemic necrosis becomes increasingly probable because of the amount of the vascular dependent bone mass. Most cases of ischemic necrosis of the talus in children become evident within 6–9 months following injury. Letts and Gibeault reviewed children with fractures of the neck of the talus.[98] Ischemic necrosis of the body developed in three (25%). In two of the three patients the antecedent talar fracture was recognized only retrospectively, after the ischemic necrosis became evident.

Hawkins sign is the usually accepted radiographic indicator of the presence or absence of ischemic necrosis in the skeletally mature patient.[90] After 6–8 weeks of immobilization, a subchondral zone of radiolucency appears in the dome of the talus and around other tarsal bones (Fig. 24-17). This radiolucency reflects osteopenia caused by disuse (i.e.,

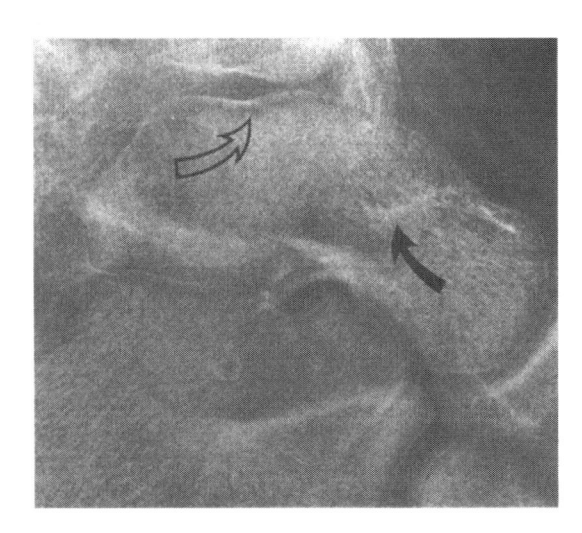

FIGURE 24-17. Hawkins sign (open arrow) in a 13-year-old with a healing talar neck fracture (*solid arrow*).

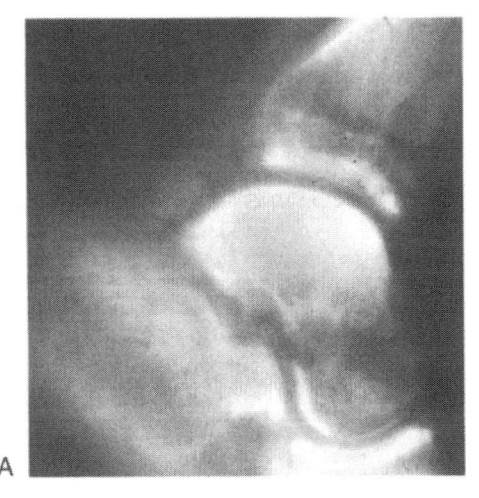

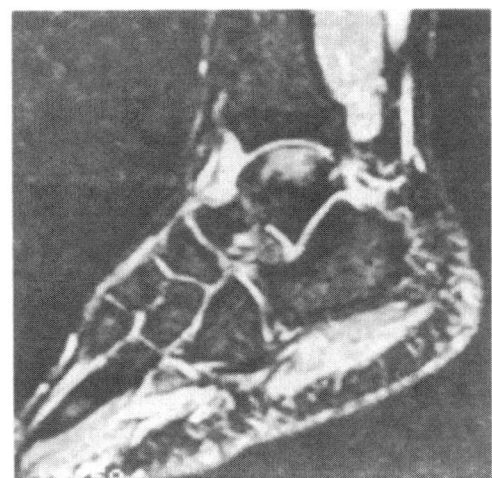

FIGURE 24-18. Ischemic necrosis after a talar neck fracture. (A) Tomographic appearance. Note the disuse osteoporosis in the distal tibial metaphysis and talar head. The avascular body cannot undergo such osseous turnover and thus becomes "sclerotic" relative to the vascularized areas. (B) MRI appearance 4 weeks after injury.

non-weight-bearing) and requires an intact blood supply. If it does not develop in the talar dome, ischemic necrosis is probable. However, this phenomenon requires sufficient expansion of the ossification center toward the articular surface to create a pattern of subchondral physiology that would be reflected by a well-defined osseous plate and a relative osteopenia below it. Accordingly, children under 10 years of age are less likely to demonstrate this finding, although they may exhibit a similar phenomenon within the enlarging ossification center. A comparison view may be helpful. A smaller talar ossification center on the injured side may reflect a lack (delay) of chondro-osseous transformation (similar to unilateral Perthes disease).

Several risk factors are associated with the subsequent development of ischemic necrosis. Displaced fractures of the neck, crush injuries, and dislocations of the talus carry the highest risk of subsequent development of ischemic necrosis. Injuries treated with open reduction and internal fixation are often complicated by ischemic necrosis, but these procedures are usually necessary after comminution and severe trauma, which has undoubtedly affected the intrinsic circulation. Neither the age of the patient nor the time from injury to the time of reduction influences the risk of developing ischemic necrosis in the child.[98] Anatomic studies suggest more severe crushing, chondro-osseous disruption, and vascular compromise than may be appreciated on a radiograph.

In young patients there is a tendency to decrease the duration of immobilization, especially in comparison to the treatment of a similar talar injury in an adult. Osteopenia resulting from disuse may not have time to develop. Absence of the Hawkins sign of subchondral lucency in the child should *not* be interpreted rigidly as indicating ischemic necrosis, although it should raise suspicion. A technetium bone scan may allow early diagnosis of this complication and should be considered for any child as part of the follow-up after allowing initial healing and remodeling (at least 2–3 months).

If bone scan, roentgenographic, or MRI changes suggest ischemic necrosis (Fig. 24-18), the child or adolescent may be protected with a weight-relieving orthosis for several months. As with Legg-Calvé-Perthes disease, the critical period is not when the vascular insult occurs but months later, when dead bone is being replaced and the initial replacement trabecular bone formation and patterns are randomly oriented, not stress-oriented, as they would be with normal, progressive trabecular maturation within the expanding talar ossification center.

Henderson compared the reliability of the Hawkins sign versus MRI.[91] He thought that MRI was more sensitive than plain radiographs, CT, or radionuclide bone scans for predicting early osteonecrosis. In one of his cases, however, a false-negative MRI scan was obtained shortly after injury, and a radiograph 8 weeks after the injury indicated the necrosis. It was thought that the nonunion of the talar neck fracture had resulted in the false-negative scan.

Whether it is necessary to prohibit weight-bearing during management of childhood talar ischemic necrosis has not been settled. However, because unsatisfactory results have followed both weight-bearing and no weight-bearing, the conservative approach is to keep the child from bearing weight until there is evidence of revascularization. This goal is usually difficult, but every effort should be made to talk to the child and the parents about the importance of this approach. Altered growth (Fig. 24-19) should be monitored until skeletal maturity.

Chronic Deformity

Talectomy has been described as a salvage procedure for older children and adults with complications of fracture or severe fracture dislocation of the talus. Gunal described a technique of removing a central portion of the distal tibia including the articular surface and shifting the medial malleolus toward the lateral malleolus to narrow the gap to accommodate the calcaneus.[84] This particular procedure should be done only after distal tibial skeletal maturity; otherwise the risk of a transphyseal osseous bridge is high. Morris et al. described a modified Blair fusion of the ankle and subtalar joints.[109]

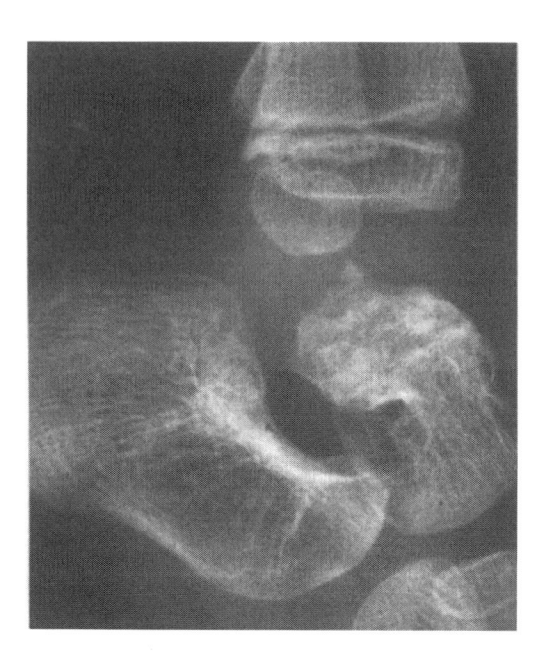

FIGURE 24-19. Appearance of the talus 18 months after this infant fell seven stories. The calcaneus also exhibits abnormality in the subtalar region.

FIGURE 24-20. Avulsion fracture (arrow) from the side of the talus. As in other areas, the trabecular bone adjacent to ligamentous attachments is much more likely to fail than the ligament itself during an acute inversion injury in a child.

Avulsion Injury

Inversion and eversion injuries may cause chondral or osteochondral fractures of the medial or lateral talus.[89] These chondro-osseous fractures are ligament avulsion analogues (Fig. 24-20). Persistent pain around a malleolus, especially the lateral malleolus, warrants close examination with oblique radiographs to adequately visualize the region between the talus and malleolus. Sometimes tomography is indicated. Because these fragments can be completely cartilaginous, they may not be visible until many months after the injury, when they may subsequently ossify (Fig. 24-15).

Even if the fracture is only suspected and not demonstrated radiologically, the child should be immobilized in a short leg cast for 3–4 weeks to enhance healing of the injury. If there is persistent pain with ankle motion following such treatment, excision of the fragment may be necessary. True ligament injury is less likely until the middle of the second decade. If a large fragment is avulsed, internal fixation may be indicated.

Stress fracture of the lateral process of the talus may occur in a young runner. This incomplete fracture of the lateral process extends into the subtalar joint and is surrounded by significant amounts of reactive sclerosis. Areas of bone formation are reactive to the repetitive stress and most likely lead to fracture through the more dense bone.

Impingement Syndrome

Chronic, excessive plantar flexion and dorsiflexion of the ankle, as occurs during highly competitive sports such as gymnastics, may cause attenuation of the anterolateral ligaments and capsule as well as reactive bone formation. It is referred to as an "impingement" syndrome (Fig. 24-21).[114] The accepted cause of this lesion is chronic, repetitive contact between the anterior tibial articular surface and the talar neck. Restriction of athletic activity is appropriate when the child has pain. Infrequently, surgical excision of the reactive bone and soft tissue repair is required to relieve the pain.

Dome Fracture (Osteochondritis Dissecans)

An osteochondral dome fragment (Fig. 24-22) may involve the medial or the lateral margin, although the lateral side is affected more frequently.[64,66,68,71,76,80,82,90,96,99,101,102,112,113,130,131,132] Because the fracture pattern requires adequate subchondral bone development in the dome, it is an unlikely injury in the child under 10 years of age. In the series reported by Berndt and Harty only 16 of 201 patients were under 16 years of age[67]; 21 of 29 patients reported by Canale and Belding were adolescents.[71]

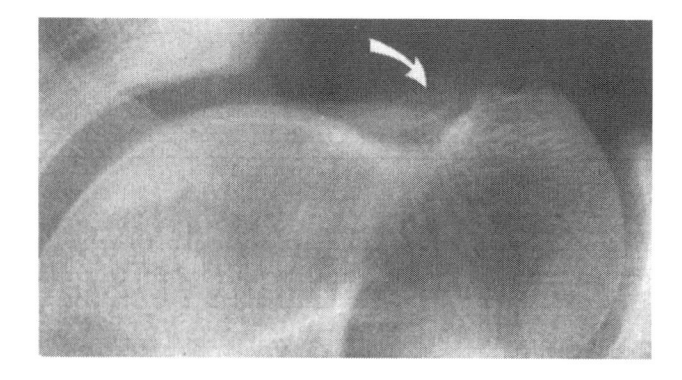

FIGURE 24-21. Reactive spur of the anterior talus (arrow) due to chronic impingement between the anterior tibia and the talar neck in a 14-year-old gymnast. This area had been intermittently painful since she was 11 years old.

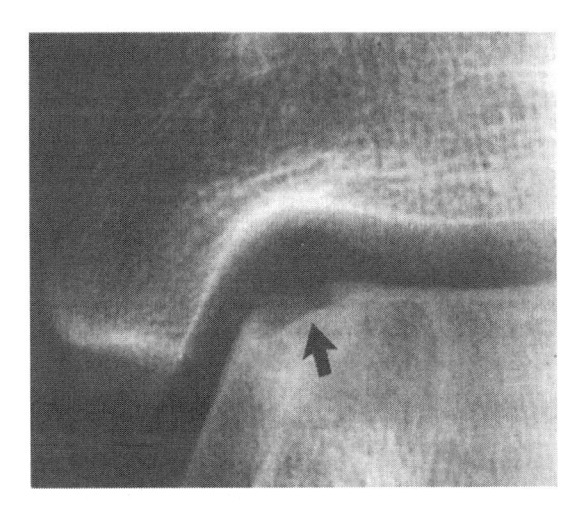

FIGURE 24-22. (A) Osteochondral fracture of the medial talar dome (arrow). The fragment is displaced, but there was no restriction of ankle motion.

Early symptoms are generally minimal and often attributed to a sprain. It is unusual for this lesion to be diagnosed at the time of injury. Lateral lesions tend to be thin and are likely to become displaced into the joint, causing chronic symptoms. Medial lesions are usually larger but tend to be less symptomatic.

Gerard et al. studied 102 cases of talar dome osteochondral lesions.[80] The lateral lesions were almost always traumatic osteochondral fractures. The medial lesions, however, could not be regularly associated with a definite traumatic origin. Repetitive low-grade trauma could produce a stress fracture, as in other areas.

The diagnosis often requires an adequate mortise view, as the injury may lie behind the lateral malleolus on a routine anteroposterior view. It is important to ascertain the extent of displacement and whether the fragment is rotated so the articular cartilage apposes bone. CT scanning may assist in the determination of lesion size (Fig. 24-23). Tomography is also helpful. MRI may better define the overall size of the lesion and demonstrate the contiguous altered hemodynamics and intraosseous edema.

Anderson and Lyne described osteochondral fractures of the dome of the talus in 24 patients who were examined by plain radiography, MRI, CT, and scintigraphy.[65] They thought that scintigraphy was important in the assessment of patients who had a clinical history compatible with osteochondral fracture but seemingly normal radiographs. They also thought that patients who have positive scintiscans should be assessed additionally by MRI. They were surprised at how commonly an osteochondral fracture of the talus was found in patients who complained of chronic disability after an ankle sprain. They particularly thought that MRI made possible an earlier and more certain diagnosis of the fracture.

An MRI scan often shows a much larger area of the talar involvment than is usually evident on the radiograph.[65] Particularly, there may be decreased signal intensity in the cancellous bone surrounding the fracture due to hemorrhagic and inflammatory reactions during the acute stage and probably due to the deposition of fibrous tissue with the more chronic injuries.

Loomer et al. reviewed 92 patients with osteochondral lesions of the talus.[101] All patients reported pain as the primary symptom. Physical examination was not helpful for the diagnosis. Using bone scans and CT, as well as an increased awareness of the potential diagnosis, these authors reported a sevenfold increase in the diagnostic frequency of talar osteochondral lesions when comparing the period 1981–1986 with 1987–1992. They noted that bone scans are an excellent screening tool and had 99% sensitivity for depicting osteochondral lesions. CT demonstrated a previously unclassified lesion, the radiolucent defect, which accounted for approximately 77% of the lesions in their series. They thought that the radiolucent defect most likely progressed from an undisplaced, often recognized osseous injury.

This fracture may be treated initially with non-weight-bearing cast immobilization followed by protected weight-bearing in a patellar tendon-bearing cast or orthosis. However, the probable need for surgical excision of the fragment, curettage of the base, or both, should be emphasized to the family. Of 15 children treated with cast immobilization, only 3 had good results; 7 subsequently underwent surgery.[58] Excision of the fragment and curettage of the underlying defect may be necessary when the symptoms persist after adequate conservative treatment.[64,75,81] Furthermore, the fragment may be rotated.[94] Should this occur, open reduction is indicated. Large fragments should be replaced and small ones removed.

The surgical approach to the lateral lesion is anterolateral arthrotomy. This procedure generally is not difficult. The posteromedial lesion, however, is less accessible and may require an osteotomy of the medial malleolus for adequate exposure.[81] The level of the osteotomy is obviously contingent on whether the tibial physis is open, as is the choice of fixation (Fig. 24-24). If the tibial growth plate is open, upward screw fixation through the medial malleolus into the

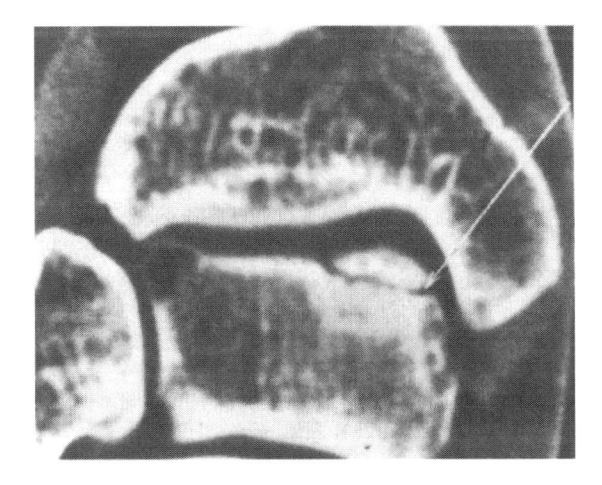

FIGURE 24-23. CT scan of a medial talar osteochondral lesion. There is considerable reactive sclerotic bone underneath the medial fragment, which can prevent revascularization and impair healing.

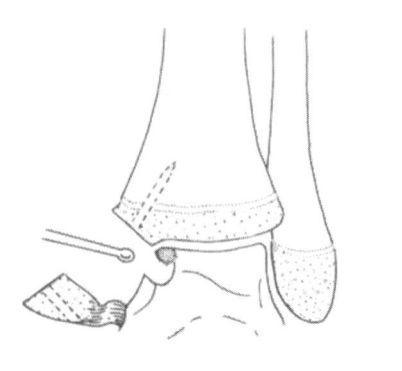

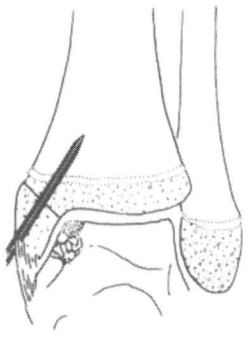

FIGURE 24-24. Method for osteotomizing the medial malleolus to expose and graft a medial talar dome lesion.

metaphysis is not the ideal fixation method, as it would be in the skeletally mature patient. Smooth Kirschner wires should be used instead. Early postoperative motion is emphasized, but weight-bearing should be restricted for 6–8 weeks. An alternative approach to the medial lesion has been proposed that does not require osteotomy of the medial malleolus.[101] The role of arthroscopy in this lesion is yet to be defined, but should be considered for a small lesion.

Os Trigonum Injury

Early studies of the os trigonum suggested that it was a distinct but infrequent ossicle, separate from the posterior border of the talus and containing a groove for the tendon of the flexor hallucis longus. This concept of separateness was not evident in an anatomic study of several cases acquired from skeletally immature individuals, in which the secondary ossification center or os trigonum was indeed present within the overall block of talar cartilage (Figs. 24-11, 24-12) and thus analgous to the apophyseal region of the calcaneus or similar to accessory malleolar ossification.[9,83] The natural history is probably one of eventual fusion with the rest of the talus, similar to the accessory navicular to form a cornuate-shaped navicular.

As the secondary ossification center enlarges, a narrowing synchondrosis develops between the two ossifying regions. This chondro-osseous junction may be injured as either a chronic stress fracture or less frequently as an acute fracture comparable to injury patterns involving the accessory navicular.

The unfused appearance, especially in patients beyond the normal age of skeletal maturity, has no correlation with symptoms. Pain often is present in professional dancers and may be due to tenderness or osseous impingement rather than micromotion within a stress fracture of the os trigonum.[87] Symptoms of os trigonum impingement include recurrent pain with stiffness, tenderness, and swelling behind the ankle and the region anterior to the Achilles tendon. They are especially noticeable during toe pointing while dancing (Fig. 24-25).[103]

The os trigonum may be confused with a fracture.[105] Careful inspection of the os trigonum usually reveals that it

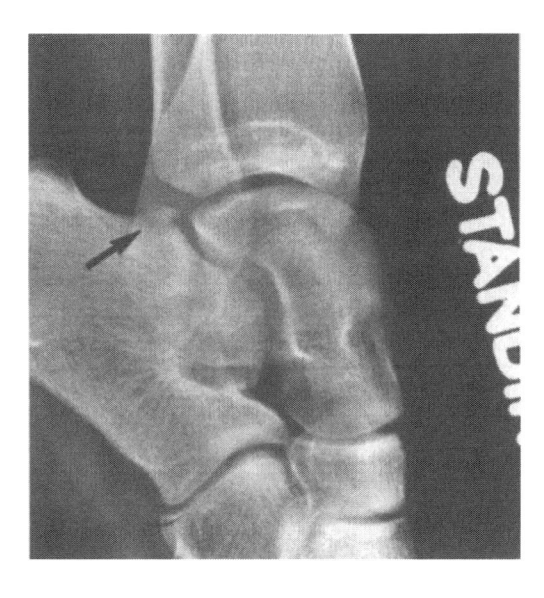

FIGURE 24-25. "En pointe" ballet position showing impaction injury mechanism of the os trigonum (arrow).

has smooth edges, instead of the irregular edges of a fracture (Fig. 24-26). In the young child initial ossification may be multifocal and irregular. However, such rigid statements may be misleading, as there may be a microfracture, particularly in young dancers, comparable to the microfracture of the accessory navicular.[65,74] Repetitive stress to this region certainly may cause chondro-osseous failure.

Whereas many patients with hindfoot pain have symptoms due to a variety of nonosseous causes, the region of the os trigonum may incur an undisplaced fracture.[79,81,95,107] Such an injury may occur acutely or more frequently chronically as a chondro-osseous microseparation similar to that described in pathologic specimens from patients with painful accessory navicular or bipartite patellas.[96,110]

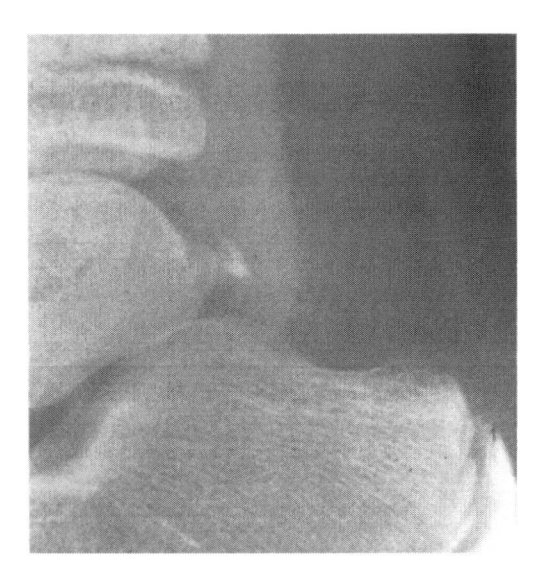

FIGURE 24-26. Acute fracture through the posterior portion of the talus, an infrequent injury that must be distinguished from the developmental os trigonum.

Radionuclide bone scanning may be valuable for assessing the significance of a symptomatic variant by providing physiologic information.[41,70,93,96] If the bone scan is positive, the specific variant should be treated as an undisplaced fracture with probable microscopic delayed union or nonunion. MRI demonstration of the lesion has been reported.[128]

Initial treatment is conservative, with cast immobilization (short leg) for 3–4 weeks. In those instances in which pain does not subside with adequate treatment, exploration and excision of the fragment may be considered. Complete relief of pain usually follows such an excision. Marotta and Micheli described 12 patients who underwent surgical incision of an impinging os trigonum.[103] Postoperatively, the pain due to impingement was alleviated in all 16, although 8 of the 12 continued to have occasional discomfort.

Congenital Deformity

Schreiber and colleagues described a 15-year-old girl with a 4-year history of pain and swelling whose radiograph showed a bipartite talus.[117] During arthrography, contrast medium flowed from the ankle joint through the cleft and into the subtalar joint. No surgery was done. Weinstein and Bonfiglio reported a similar case that required excision of the large posterior fragment.[129] It is possible that these cases were due to unrecognized injury with pseudarthrosis formation (Fig. 24-27), rather than an embryonic segmentation abnormality. If a fracture at the chondro-osseous interface was unrecognized and not treated, a fibrous union could result (i.e., similar to the development of an os odontoideum). Subsequent ossification would occur in the separated fragment similar to the phenomenon in the scaphoid.

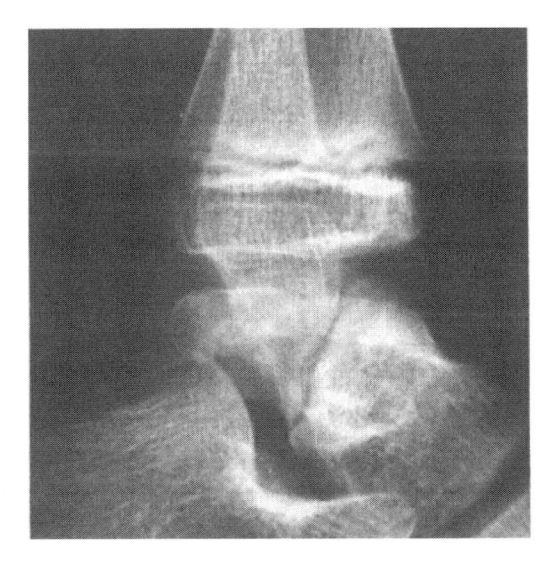

FIGURE 24-27. Lateral view of a radiographically divided talus in a 9-year-old boy. He had fallen four stories at age 19 months. At that time he had no obvious talar fracture, although the foot was swollen.

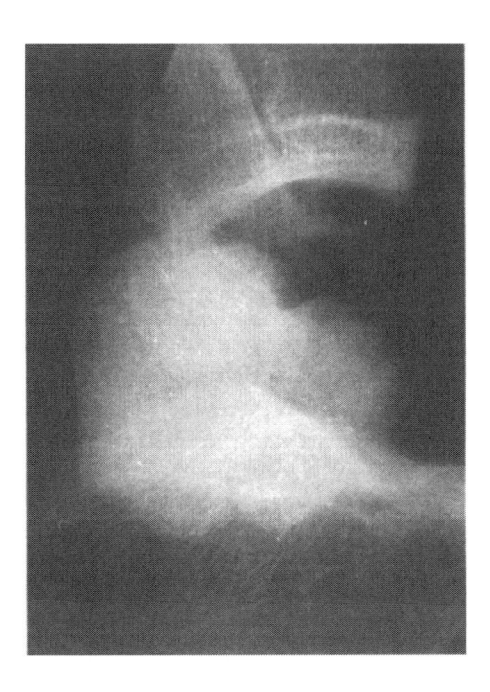

FIGURE 24-28. Acute ankle dislocation in a 14-year-old gymnast. A distal tibial fracture is also present.

Peritalar and Subtalar Dislocations

Peritalar and subtalar disruptions (subluxation or dislocation) are unusual in young children, but become more likely during adolescence (Fig. 24-28).[69,73,77,86,106,119,120,122] Initial radiographs may not show the severity of disruption, as incomplete spontaneous reduction may occur. There is a high association with talar fractures. These may not be readily evident until the dislocation is reduced.[123,124] Consider the possibility of a sleeve fracture if an osseous fracture is not readily evident on the radiograph.

Dimentberg and Rosman reported five children with peritalar dislocations.[77] In two patients the dislocation was missed, causing a delay in management because more attention was focused on concomitant obvious fractures. Smith et al. mentioned 10 isolated cases of this injury in patients less than 19 years of age,[119] and since then other case reports have been described.[69,73,85,122] All patients had at least one associated fracture in the same foot, and two patients had multiple fractures in the involved foot. None of the patients had a fracture through the talar neck. Three patients underwent closed reduction. Other patients, because of a 2- to 3-week delay in diagnosis, required open reduction. In the cases with delayed diagnosis, attention was initially focused on the more obvious fractures. Closed reduction may be successful, especially in children. Impediments to reduction are primarily the toe tendons, the peroneal or posterior tibial tendon, the tibialis anterior tendon, interposed joint capsules, or impaction fractures. Four of the five children had acceptable results with respect to pain and gait, leading Dimentburg and Rosman to suggest that, at least in children, the long-term results are favorable.[77]

The most significant concern in the acute situation is the vascular status of the foot. Careful neurologic and vascular evaluation is necessary. If the foot is pulseless, an initial attempt at reduction should be undertaken in the emergency room. Post-reduction observation should be directed at assessing not only the return of good palpable pulses but also adequate capillary filling and the possible occurrence of compartment syndrome. Doppler flow studies are important. Ischemic necrosis of the talus is likely.

The injury is often open, requiring appropriate débridement in the operating room. Fixation of any fractures must be contingent on the extent of osseous and soft tissue damage. Long-term complications may require talectomy, peritalar arthrodesis, or both.

There are variations of the configurations of the sustentacular facets.[78] Foot mobility and susceptibility to arthritis may be associated with a long, continuous facet rather than two separate "anterior" facets. Facet variations in the sustentaculum tali influence subtalar joint stability. How much such variations influence the injury in children is difficult to predict. Similar facet configurations are present in fetal calcanei and are not developmental responses to physical activities. Obviously, injury to these regions could affect further development. With the continuous facet configuration "Bohler's angle" was 127°, whereas the angle in the normal three-facet articulation was 150°.

Wester et al. followed 24 patients for up to 36 years and believed that the long-term history was not significant in regard to pain.[130] They recommended initial conservative treatment and additional imaging with CT and MRI if symptoms persisted. None of the cases they followed for an extended period developed significant osteoarthrosis. In another study of 17 patients with subtalar dislocations, 4 of whom were children, the results were good in 6, fair in 6, and poor in 5.[116] The patients under age 18 had fair or good results.

Injuries to the Calcaneus

Fractures of the calcaneus appear to be the most frequently encountered tarsal injuries in children.* Wiley and Profitt reported 34 os calcis fractures in 32 children over a 12-year period.[205] In most reports the children were older than 6 years. Schantz and Rasmussen reported 80 calcaneal fractures in 78 children, 16 of whom were 5 years old or younger.[191]

It seems to be a common belief that the cancellous bone of the child is more dense than that in adults and is thus responsible for the child's not sustaining the comminution patterns seen in adults. Thomas, however, found that comminution and depression were common in young patients.[202] It is the largely cartilaginous nature of the child's calcaneus combined with the increased elasticity of the bone that probably dissipates applied forces throughout the foot and leg without concentrating on the calcaneus.

Children less than 3 years of age may sustain calcaneal fractures following relatively minor trauma. It may be difficult to make a roentgenographic diagnosis in such young children.[149,164,170,198] Occult calcaneal fracture should be

---

* Refs. 141–144,148,149,151–153,158–160,162,167,168,176,179, 185–195,200–203,205,206.

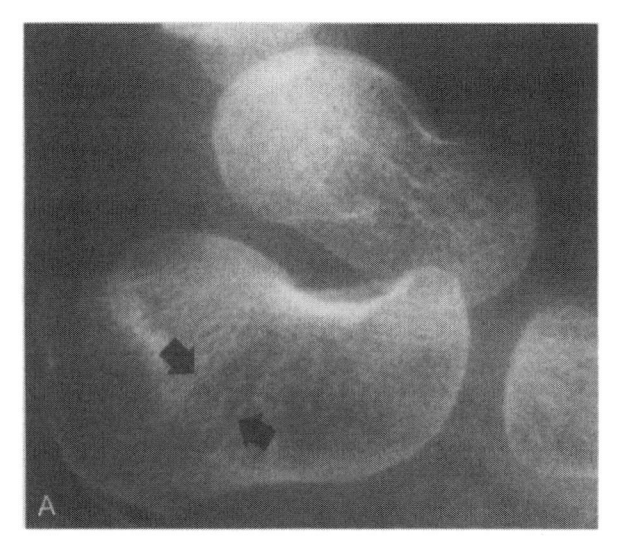

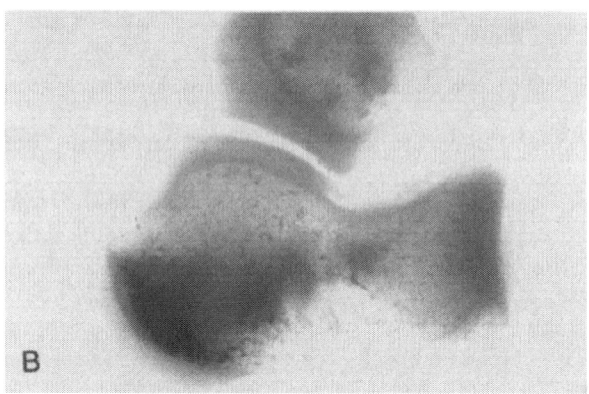

FIGURE 24-29. (A) Linear lucency (arrows) in 2-year-old boy with a limp. This fracture was not evident until the third week following symptom onset. (B) Calcaneus from a 3-year-old child killed in an automobile accident. A calcaneal fracture was not readily evident, but there was considerable hemorrhage (black area) localized adjacent to the apophysis as well as areas of microscopic calcaneal trabecular damage.

part of the differential diagnosis of a limping child and certainly must be considered as one type of "toddler's fracture" in a young child learning to walk (Fig. 24-29). Calcaneal stress fractures are less frequent in older children and are more likely in the neurologically impaired child with osteoporosis secondary to immobilization or limited weight-bearing.[139,199]

Zlatkin et al. reported stress fractures of the calcaneus that occurred distal to the site of a healing fracture of the tibia or fibula in five patients.[207] Three of the patients were under 10 years of age. Such stress fractures should be considered during any phase following the original injury and immobilization if there is new or persistent discomfort.

Calcaneal "cysts" are relatively common and usually comprise a normal area not filled with trabecular bone (Fig. 24-30). The child with a unicameral bone cyst of the os calcis may present with heel pain. The pain may be due to a fracture through the thinned cortical bone, similar to such occult fractures in cystic lesions elsewhere in the long bones.[153]

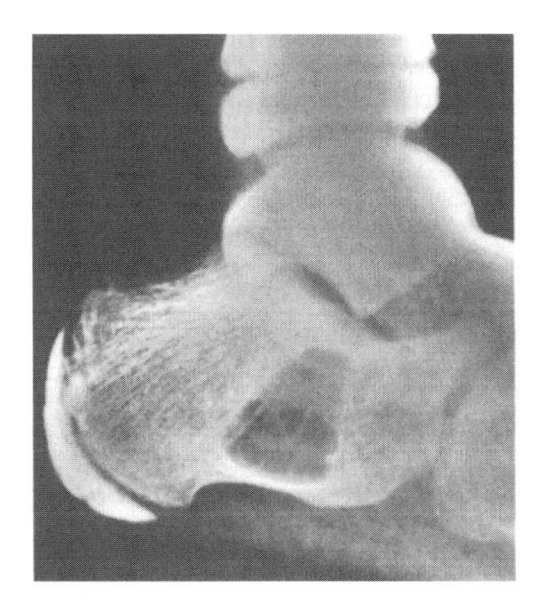

FIGURE 24-30. Calcaneal cyst found during the evaluation of chronic foot pain in an adolescent soccer player.

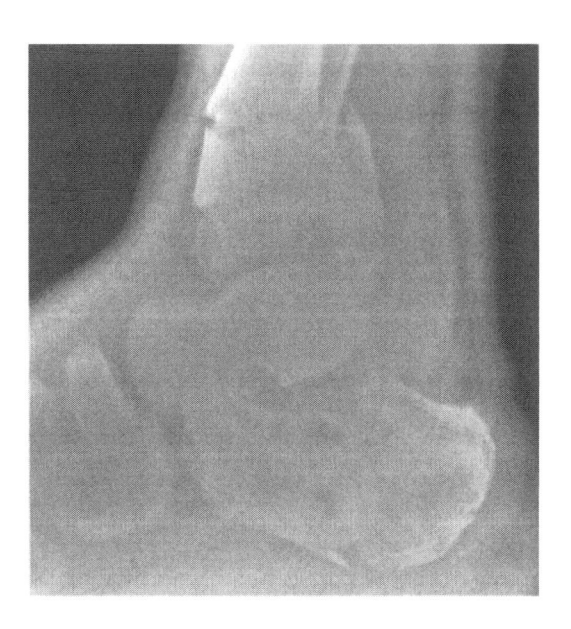

FIGURE 24-32. Concomitant fractures of the distal tibia and fibula and the calcaneus after a three-story fall.

The differential diagnosis of heel pain must include infection, developmental variations such as immature tarsal coalitions, inflammations, rheumatologic disease, malignant disease (e.g., leukemia), neurologic conditions, and tarsal tunnel syndrome. Occult soft tissue or osseous infections in children resulting from puncture or other wounds must also be considered, as they are relatively common.

Falls from a height may cause comminuted calcaneal fractures (Figs. 24-31 to 24-33). Careful evaluation is necessary to rule out other fractures in the leg or spine. However, the incidence of associated spine fractures is much less than that in adults. In the series of Wiley and Profitt only two patients sustained significant accompanying injuries, one of whom had a wedge compression fracture of L5. This was the only associated spinal injury in the entire series.[205] Wiley and Profitt noted that in the child under 10 years of age simple falls usually caused the calcaneal injury.[205] In contrast, the adolescent group simulated fracture mechanisms in adults, with a much greater incidence of falls from a height and severe twisting injuries. Open injuries to the calcaneus occur commonly in children because of lawn mower injuries.

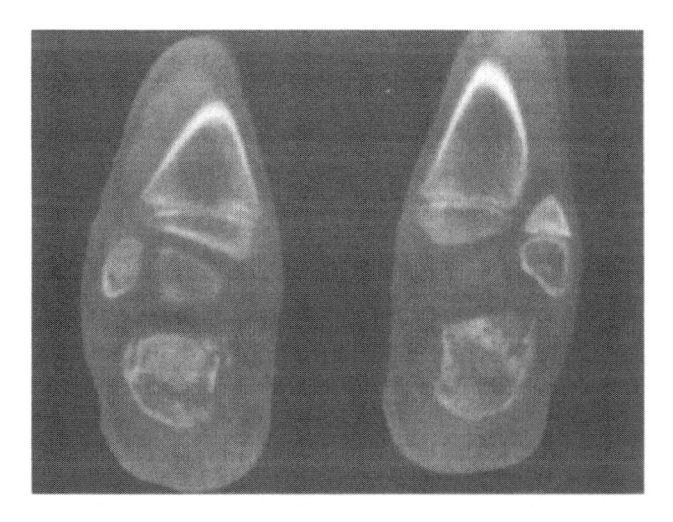

FIGURE 24-31. CT scans of bilateral calcaneal fractures in a child who fell approximately 30 feet from a ski lift.

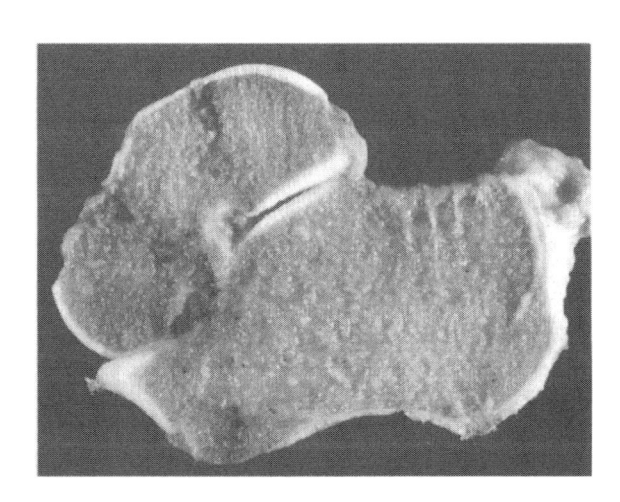

FIGURE 24-33. Talar fracture and anteroinferior calcaneal injury in a 13-year-old after a fatal fall. It shows the linear impact image pattern.

Classification

There are several classification schemes for calcaneal fractures in adults.[188] The one devised by Wiley and Profitt (Fig. 24-34) is most applicable to children.[205]

Fractures *not* involving the subtalar joint are classified as type 1. They include the (a) beak fracture, (b) vertical fracture, (c) horizontal fracture, (d) avulsion of the medial border, and (e) anterior process fracture. Representative cases are illustrated in Figures 24-35 to 24-37.

Fractures involving the subtalar joint are classified as type 2. Most have little or no displacement and are subtyped as follows: (a) undisplaced, (b) tongue fracture, (c) centrolateral fracture with displacement, (d) sustentaculum tali, and

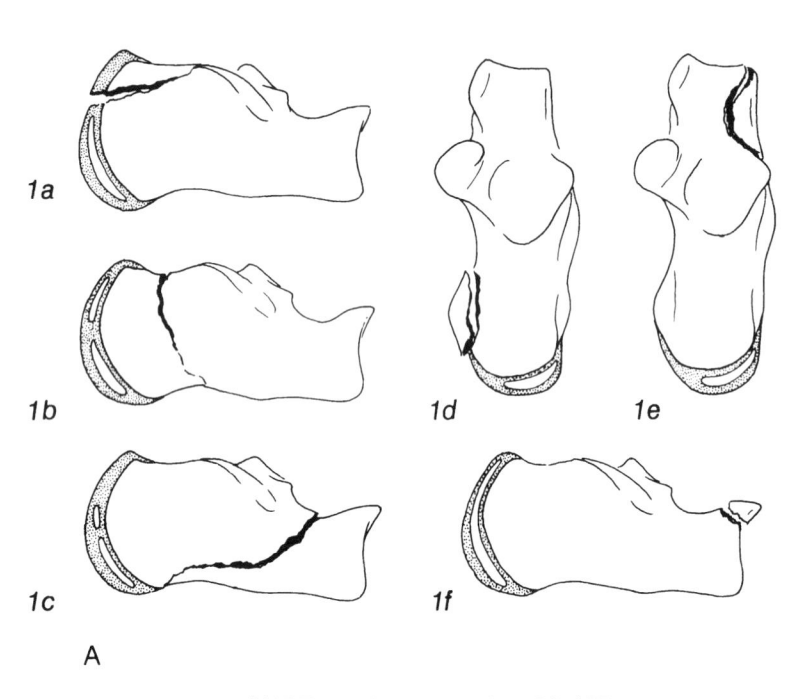

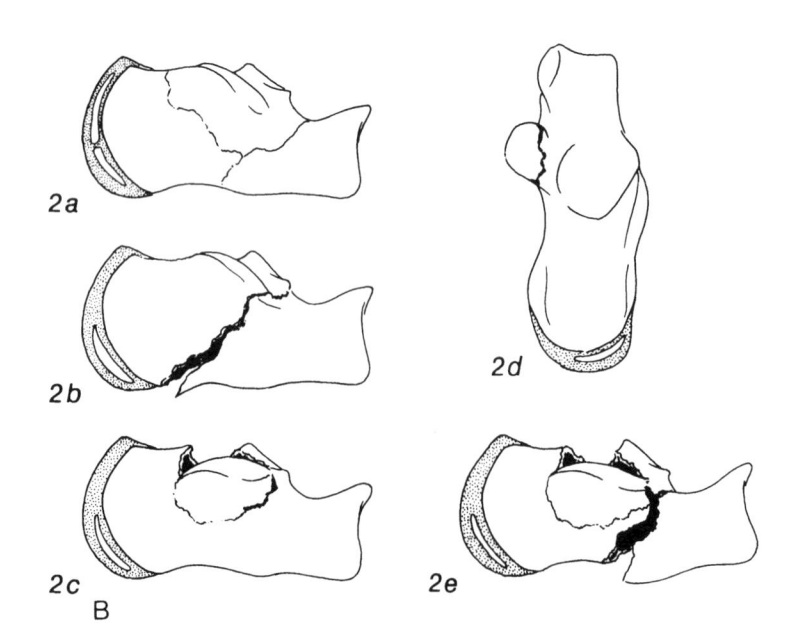

FIGURE 24-34. Modified Wiley's classification of nonarticular (A) and articular (B) calcaneal fractures in the skeletally immature patient. See text for details.

Injuries to the Calcaneus

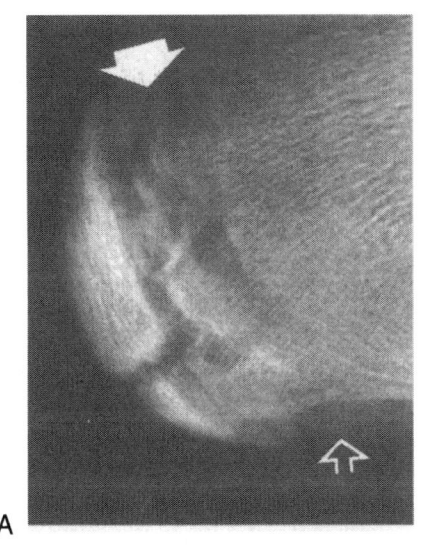

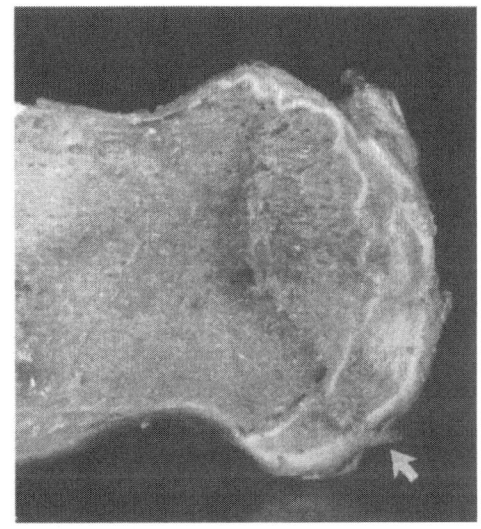

FIGURE 24-35. (A) Type 1b injury. It is analogous to a metaphyseal fracture. Crushing injury to the heel has caused fragmentation (white arrow) and new subperiosteal bone formation (open arrow). The calcaneal secondary ossification center exhibits a normal gap, not necessarily an extension of the fracture. (B) Slab section of type 1b injury (traumatic below-knee amputation). This fracture did extend across the apophyseal ossification center (arrow).

(e) grossly comminuted. Representative cases are illustrated in Figures 24-38 to 24-43.

Carr assessed the mechanism and pathoanatomy of the intraarticular calcaneal fracture.[141] This fracture is produced by axial loading. A combination of shear and compression forces produce two characteristic primary fracture lines. Shearing forces produce a fracture dividing the calcaneus into medial and lateral portions. This fracture line typically splits the posterior facet and may extend anteriorly to involve the anterior and cuboid facets. Compression forces divide the calcaneus into anterior and posterior portions. This fracture line may extend medially to involve the middle facet. Loss of calcaneal height and length are readily explained by this mechanism. This fracture pattern is more likely in the older child or adolescent.

Diagnostic Imaging

Injury to the child's calcaneus is often subtle, and the fracture may be overlooked during the initial radiographic examination (Figs. 24-34, 24-35). Furthermore, as

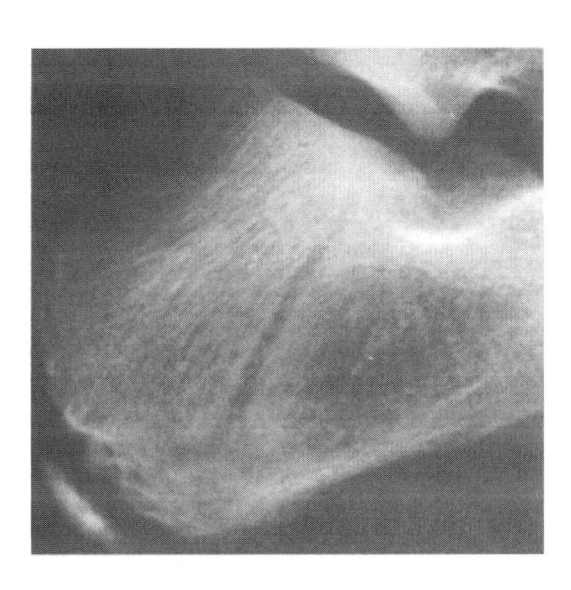

FIGURE 24-36. Type 1c fracture.

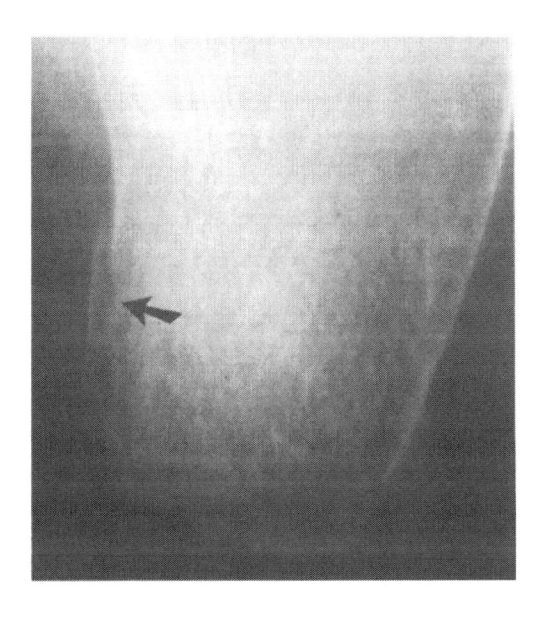

FIGURE 24-37. Type 1d fracture with avulsion of the medial cortex (arrow).

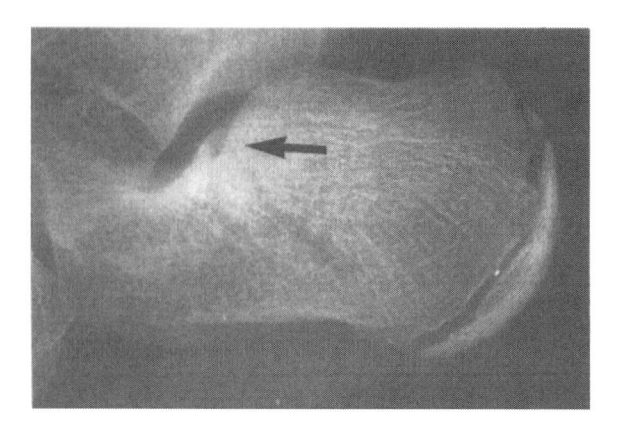

FIGURE 24-38. Type 2a injury of the subtalar joint (arrow).

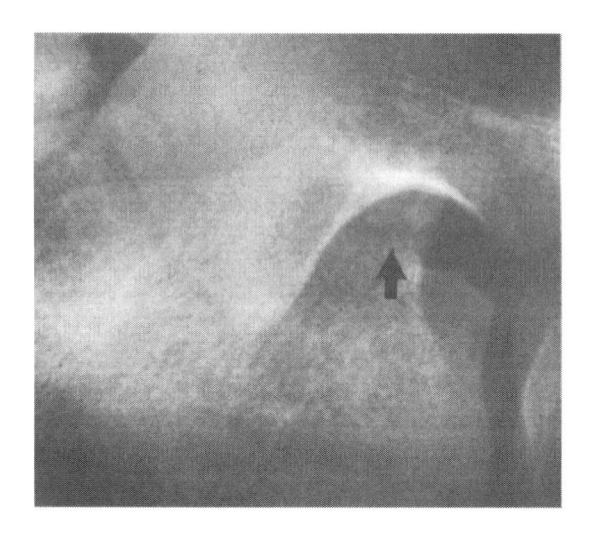

FIGURE 24-39. Type 2d injury of the sustentaculum tali (arrow).

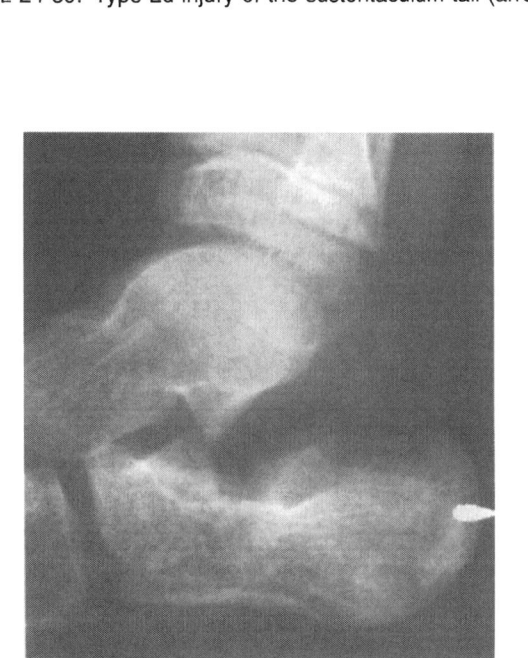

FIGURE 24-40. Type 2e fracture with significant depression in an 11-year-old child.

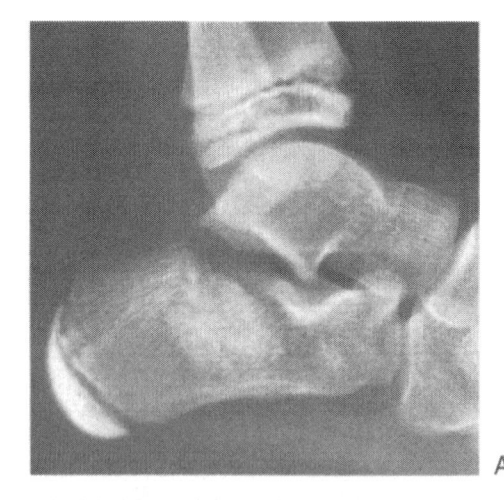

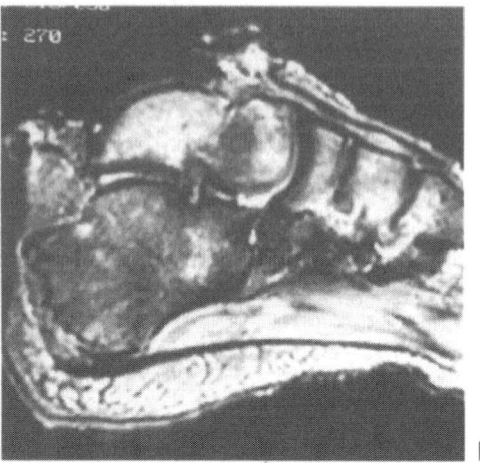

FIGURE 24-41. (A) Type 2c calcaneal fracture. (B) MRI showed talar neck bone bruising (probable occult fracture) and focal areas of hemorrhage within the calcaneus.

illustrated in certain intracartilaginous fractures, sleeve chondro-osseous disruptions may not be readily evident radiographically.

Schmidt and Weiner reported 59 fractures of the calcaneus in patients younger than 20 years of age; in 16 the calcaneal fracture was initially unrecognized.[194] There was a delay in diagnosis, particularly in the younger children, because (1) the specific injury was not suspected by the physician, (2) the child withheld admitting the injury for fear of punishment, and (3) the diagnosis was missed on the initial radiographs. In contrast, a delay in diagnosis was much less common in patients older than 10 years. Obviously, the greater the extent of bone relative to cartilage, the greater the likelihood of detecting the injury radiographically during the initial evaluation.

Injuries to the Calcaneus

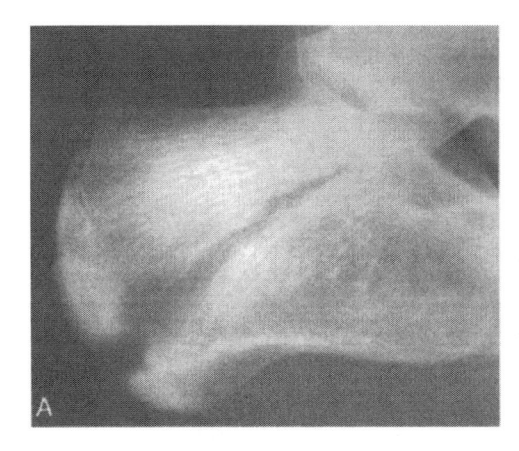

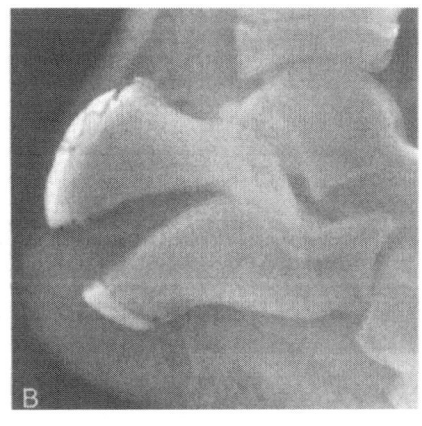

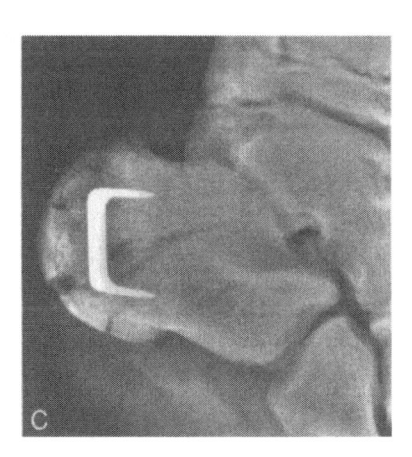

FIGURE 24-42. (A) Type 2b fracture extending from the subtalar joint to the calcaneal apophysis, which is traumatically split. (B, C) Similarly involved case treated by open reduction and internal fixation.

Involvement of the posterior subtalar joint is probably as common in children as it is in adults.[205] Minor involvement of the posterior subtalar joint is usually identified by disruption of the lateral wall of the os calcis, producing a longitudinal sliver of bone on the axial radiograph.

The optimal radiographic demonstration in a child depends on the type of calcaneal fracture. Obviously, it is clinically difficult to predict the specific pattern on the basis of the physical examination. Consequently, several views may be obtained following trauma to the calcaneal region.[185]

1. *Lateral projection:* The foot is placed with the lateral side resting directly on the cassette. The x-ray beam should be centered 1 cm below the medial malleolus.
2. *Axial projection:* The patient is placed supine with the heel on the cassette and the ankle maximally dorsiflexed. The x-ray beam should be centered on the sole of the foot at an angle 45° to the horizontal plane. The film should be slightly overexposed to obtain a good view of the subtalar joint.
3. *Straight dorsoplantar projection:* The foot is placed flat on the cassette. The x-ray beam should be centered on the calcaneocuboid joint.
4. *Oblique dorsoplantar projection:* With the patient in the semirecumbent position, the knee is flexed to allow the plantar surface to contact the film. The knee is tilted medially. The x-ray beam should be centered on the cuboid navicular region.

In the lateral view a great deal of emphasis is placed on the tuber-joint angle (Bohler's angle). This angle is formed by a line parallel to the articular surfaces of the calcaneus, with a line drawn from the posterior lip of the posterior facet to the superior margin of the tuberosity. However, these areas are among the last to ossify in the developing foot, so in young children this sign is unreliable, even if the subtalar joint is involved.[138,140] Even a child just entering the second decade normally has an angular pattern different from that of an adult. It tends to be a flat angle, duplicating the "appearance" of a depressed fracture in an adult.

Analysis by CT may be superior to planar films for demonstrating additional fracture components.[181,187] CT scanning may allow improved preoperative planning by better defining the size and location of fracture fragments to determine the site of the incision and the type of surgery required; it also provides improved postoperative follow-up. Two- and three-dimensional CT with volume (voxel) reconstruction may further elucidate fracture anatomy and may also provide a detailed analysis of causes for chronic

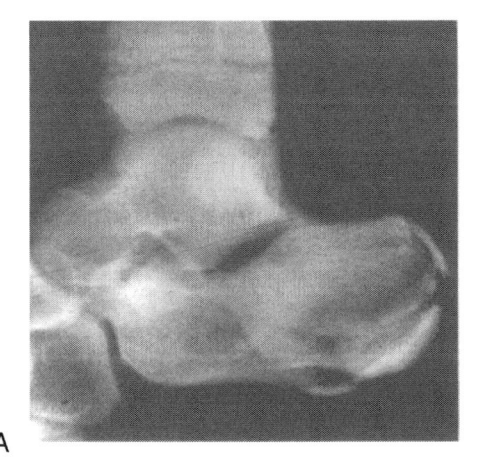

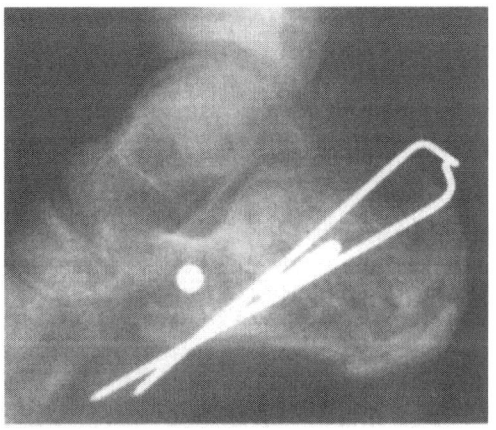

FIGURE 24-43. (A) Type 2 injury with depression. It was treated with open reduction and internal fixation, with excellent results.

pain and identification of significant soft tissue injury, such as peroneal tendon displacement.

Koval and Sanders reviewed the acceptable ways of evaluating calcaneal fractures radiologically.[161] They thought that simple studies such as Bohler's view still had a significant role in diagnosis and management. They emphasized that CT scanning has increased the understanding of these fractures and, with the addition of three-dimensional reconstruction, allowed more adequate preoperative planning. Obviously, the extent of utilization of such procedures in the child is contingent on the degree of chondro-osseous transformation. They believed that tomograms were rarely indicated because they did not provide additional information when CT scanning is readily available.

The MRI technique is also useful, especially for delineating occult injury patterns, including bone bruising (Fig. 24-41). Ebraheim et al. showed that among 21 cases of intraarticular calcaneal fracture there were 8 cases of peroneal tendon subluxation or dislocation.[150] MRI proved to be the most useful method for delineating this type of involvement. The youngest patient in their series was 23 years old. Comparable injuries have not been described in children but obviously need to be assessed as a possibility, as proper management of tendon disruption may reduce subsequent tendon dysfunction and may also alter calcaneal fracture management.

In 10 children between the ages of 19 and 41 months who were evaluated for acute onset of limping, bone scintigraphy showed abnormal uptake in the calcaneus.[198] Many fractures of the os calcis are not detected in children, particularly young children and toddlers, because scintigraphy is not routinely carried out and because of the rapid recovery of function and subsidence of pain in young children after such an injury. In toddlers and infants it may be necessary to do a bone scan to detect occult injury when they refuse to bear weight normally.

Treatment

Initial treatment is directed toward the soft tissue trauma, which may be extensive. The foot and ankle are immobilized in a well-padded compression dressing, and the leg and foot are elevated for 2–3 days. Measurement of compartment pressures should be considered (see Foot Compartment Syndrome, above).[174]

Approximately 10% of patients with calcaneal fractures develop compartment syndromes; and of these, approximately half develop clawing of the lesser toes and other foot deformities including stiffness and neurovascular dysfunction.[177] Tense swelling and severe pain are the hallmarks of an impending compartment syndrome, and the diagnosis is confirmed by a multistick invasive evaluation, particularly of the calcaneal compartment in the hindfoot. Fasciotomy is recommended to prevent the development of ischemic contracture. If necessary, open reduction and internal fixation of a calcaneal fracture should be performed on a delayed basis, after the fasciotomy wounds are closed.

A cast should not be applied until the bulk of the soft tissue swelling has subsided, at which time the intrinsic stability of the fracture can be better evaluated. A compressive dressing is often more appropriate as the initial treatment. Significant displacement is uncommon in children, as the extensive surrounding cartilage, perichondrium, and periosteum help to maintain intrinsic stability. Excessive manipulation is usually unnecessary, although manual molding of the cast may improve fragment positions.

The foot should be splinted or casted in a neutral position or mild dorsiflexion. However, if this position causes fragment distraction or a tendency for the proximal fragment to drift into an equinus position relative to the rest of the foot, it may be necessary to use plantar flexion initially. Furthermore, failure to wait for soft tissue swelling to subside may limit the ability to bring the foot out of plantar flexion to a neutral position.

These fractures should heal sufficiently within 4–6 weeks to allow cast removal and early range of motion. Weight-bearing should not be allowed for 8–12 weeks, especially if the subtalar joint or Achilles tendon insertion is involved. A protective orthosis may be appropriate to allow graded range of motion.

Most cases can be treated nonoperatively, including those with mild deformities of the subtalar joint.[201-205] Follow-up assessment revealed satisfactory results in cases with extraarticular fractures or minor posterior subtalar joint involvement. Patients with more marked joint displacement had persistent limitation of subtalar joint motion but an *absence* of discomfort or pain.

Schmidt and Weiner noted that displacement was much less common and that approximately two-thirds of all children's calcaneal fractures, with the exception of major bone loss, healed without any functional sequelae. Of their 32 patients, *none* of the closed fractures was treated by open reduction. The only surgery involved débridement of open fractures.[194] Satisfactory results probably relate to the growth potential and remodeling of the osteocartilaginous os calcis, particularly in those under 10 years of age.

Because of the remodeling potential, it may not be necessary to place as much emphasis on rigid closed reduction in children as in adults. However, this situation must be assessed on an individual basis. Patients older than 10 years must be watched closely because their anatomy is more comparable to that of an adult than to that of a young child, and their remodeling potential is decreasing. In the teenager with depression of Bohler's angle, it is appropriate to consider open reduction and surgical fixation, as one would in an adult.

Sandermann et al. described two patients with significant displaced intraarticular calcaneal fractures in children 6–10 years of age who did well with closed reduction and casting.[190] Because most injuries are due to a direct blow rather than a vertical fall, calcaneal fractures during childhood usually do not involve the joints. DeBeer et al. reported eight patients with nine calcaneal fractures. Six were intraarticular and six extraarticular.[145] They found little relevance of this differentiation to treatment or prognosis. All were treated conservatively, and all had good results.

Significant displacement that does not respond to manipulation may be treated with open reduction and appropriate internal or external fixation (Figs. 24-42, 24-43).

Levin and Nunley addressed the management of soft tissue problems associated with calcaneal fractures.[165] They divided these injuries into several types. Type 1 was a closed fracture treated by open reduction and internal fixation, with an inability to close the incision. Type 2 was a wound breakdown after open reduction. Type 3 was an open fracture with traumatic large soft tissue loss but adequate bone stock. Type 4 was traumatic loss of soft tissue and bone. Type 5 was calcaneal osteomyelitis. Type 6 was chronic, unstable soft tissue over the

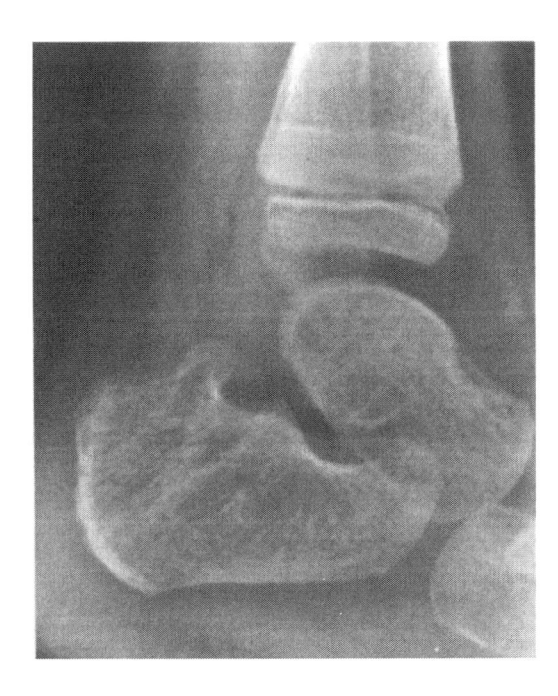

FIGURE 24-44. Posterior facet growth abnormality after fracture caused by a fall of about 20 feet.

calcaneus. They described a variety of methods for closing the areas, presenting several treatment algorithms. Because inability to close an operative incision is often due to the severe swelling that accompanies these injuries, leaving the wound open and covering it with an allograft, epigard, split-thickness skin graft, and so on and then going back for a delayed primary closure may be a realistic approach. The use of any flap must be coordinated with the concept of vascular territories (angiosomes, venosomes). Certainly flaps that may be used effectively include dorsalis pedis, abductor, and peroneal artery-based flaps. Free flaps are also feasible.

Growth Sequelae

When a segment of the calcaneus is removed traumatically, reactive bone may form similar to transdiaphyseal or transmetaphyseal fractures of long bones. Because there often is soft tissue loss with or without skin grafting, this reactive bone may become painful with weight-bearing. Pieces of calcaneal apophyseal cartilage may be separated during the trauma ("sleeve" injuries). During débridement of tissues these small fragments may be left. Direct cartilage-to-cartilage healing is unlikely. The cartilaginous fragment eventually ossifies, creating an ossicle or protuberance that may become painful.[147]

Damage to the physis of the calcaneal apophysis may disrupt the posteriorly directed growth of the bone, which may affect the heel pad and heel strike during ambulation. The overall shape of the calcaneus may be distorted due to such physeal damage. Altered facet growth may follow subtalar damage (Fig. 24-44).

Fracture of the Anterior Process

The anterior process of the calcaneus, which articulates with the cuboid, does not appear radiographically before the age of 10 years. It is a saddle-shaped promontory of varied length that articulates inferiorly with the cuboid. The bifurcate ligament originates from the anterior process and attaches to the navicular and the cuboid.

The postulated mechanisms of injury to this process are forced abduction of the forefoot, inversion, plantar flexion, and direct trauma. Because of the mechanistic similarity to an injury producing a sprain of the anterior talofibular ligament, this injury is often misdiagnosed as an ankle sprain. Careful examination should delineate point tenderness anterior and inferior to the insertion of this ligament.

Fracture of the anterior process is more common than appreciated and is often misdiagnosed as an ankle sprain, which explains the tendency of the ossicle to be present as an unrecognized finding.[135,137,146,154,157,183] There is no secondary ossification center in this region to cause confusion with a fracture (Fig. 24-45). Rarely, a small, rounded accessory ossicle, the calcaneus secondarius, occurs in this region. However, in view of the tendency of this area to be injured, it is likely that the os secondarius is really the end result of a nonunion (i.e., an acquired disorder, similar to the os trigonum or accessory navicular).

A routine anteroposterior roentgenogram of the foot may fail to show the fracture. Similarly, this area may not be seen well on a routine lateral roentgenogram. Oblique roentgenograms are helpful. The roentgenogram should be made with the x-ray beam directed 10°–15° superior and posterior to the middle of the foot. This angle projects the process over the neck of the talus, allowing the fracture to be more easily visualized.

Degan and associates reported that 18 of 25 patients with anterior process fractures on the calcaneus were treated successfully by closed reduction and cast immobilization, although symptoms persisted for variable periods after removal of the cast.[146] The other seven patients required fragment excision, with two not being relieved of their symptoms even after excision. Included in their cases requiring surgical excision was a 13-year-old boy whose fracture was not diagnosed until almost a year after the injury.[146]

In children there is an excellent chance that closed reduction can alleviate symptoms. If the fracture is relatively acute, healing usually occurs. However, in the more chronic case,

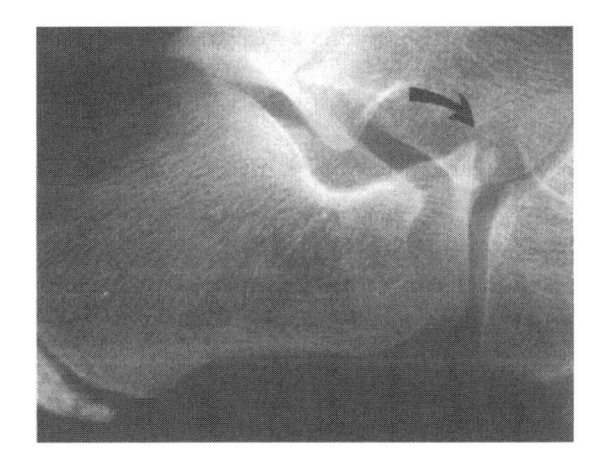

FIGURE 24-45. Anterior process fracture (arrow). It healed after 4 weeks in a cast.

an ossicle may persist, even though symptoms are relieved. If immobilization fails to alleviate pain, ossicle excision is indicated.[146] Drvaric and Schmitt reported a 5-year-old child who sustained a fracture involving the anterior process of the calcaneus that required open reduction.[148]

Norfray et al. described an avulsion fracture involving the dorsolateral aspect of the calcaneus at the origin of the extensor digitorum brevis muscle.[178] The youngest patient in their series was 17 years of age. This fracture was associated with inversion injury to the ankle. The fracture may be visualized by standard dorsoplantar foot or anteroposterior ankle views. The fracture may be confused with the os peroneum or with a fracture of the anterior process of the calcaneus. Treatment is conservative: elevation, supportive bandage, and early activity.

Stress Fractures

Calcaneal stress fractures have been described in children.[134,139,169,193,199] If a young child refuses to bear weight or limps, the calcaneus must be examined closely, as a stress fracture may have occurred (Fig. 24-29). Depending on the degree of primary ossification, it may be difficult to diagnose. Treatment is based on symptoms. Moss and Carty studied four toddlers who presented with an acute limp.[175] None had fractures present on routine radiography, but all had positive bone scans. The patients ranged in age from 15 to 30 months.

The diagnosis of calcaneal fractures in toddlers is made difficult by several factors. The cause of the injury is often trivial, with the injury sustained during normal play activity. The child may adopt a typical posture of hip and knee flexion with failure to dorsiflex the foot. Poor verbalization and localization of pain in young children may cause the clinician not to suspect calcaneal injury and therefore not to request the most appropriate radiographic examination. Finally, owing to the high percentage of cartilage and the immature trabecular pattern of the calcaneus in children, fractures often produce minimal, if any, of the bony changes detectable by roentgenography. The result is that the underlying cause for the acute limp remains undiagnosed, and the patient rapidly recovers.

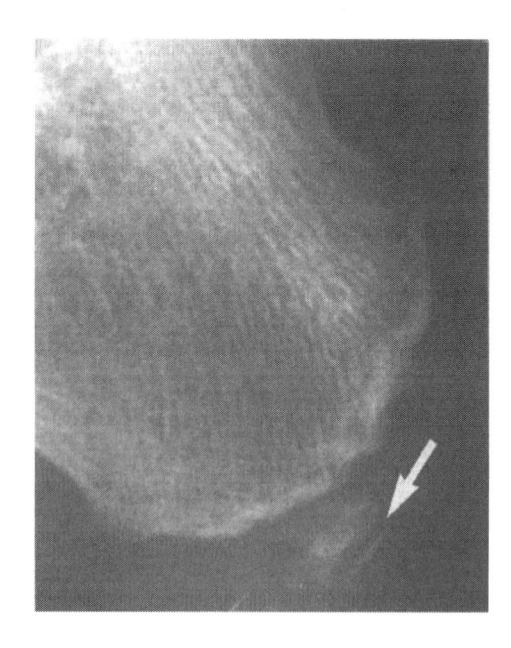

FIGURE 24-46. Fragmentation of a secondary ossification center (arrow) after direct impact on the heel following a 24-foot fall.

Apophyseal Fractures

Damage to the calcaneal apophysis in open injuries (e.g., from a lawn mower) is common and may lead to significant disruption of posterior calcaneal growth.[204] Damage may also be due to direct impact from a fall (Fig. 24-46).[182] Disruption of all or part of the apophysis of the calcaneus as a closed injury was initially described by Ehalt.[151] The physeal undulation and multiple contiguous joints undoubtedly protect the apophysis from most shearing mechanisms that cause physeal injury in other areas. Nonetheless, fracture may occur. The case illustrated in Figure 24-47 occurred in an adolescent, suggesting that this area may be susceptible

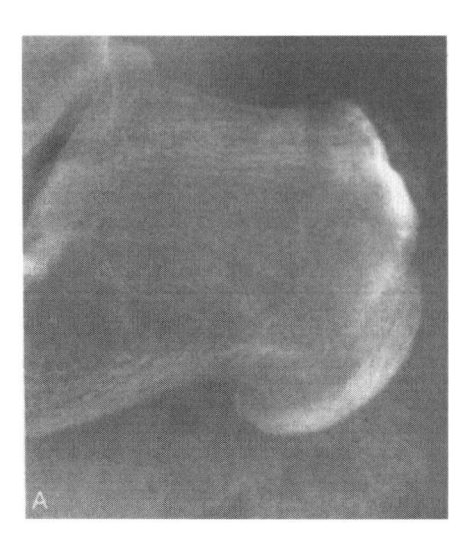

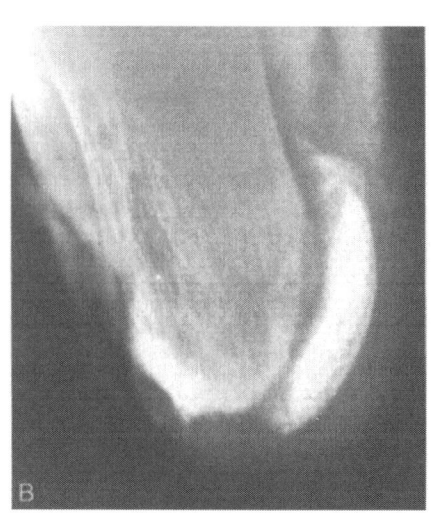

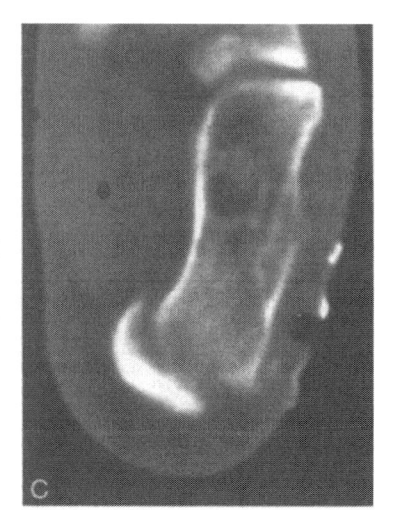

FIGURE 24-47. Fracture of the calcaneal apophysis in an adolescent. (A) Lateral view of the heel showing inferior displacement. (B) Axial view showing medial displacement. (C) CT view of the displacement.

FIGURE 24-48. Growth plate (apophysis) fractures. (1) Type 1 physeal injury. (2) Type 2 physeal injury. (3) Type 3 physeal injury. (4) Type 4 physeal injury.

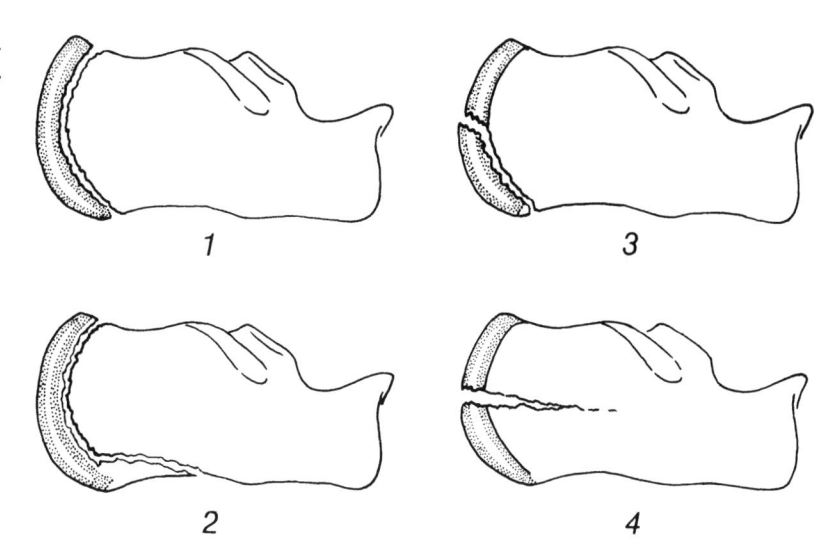

during closure, much like the capital femur or tibial tuberosity (see Chapters 21, 23).

The injury is likely to be a type 1 growth mechanism injury, similar to a slipped capital femoral epiphysis, or a type 4 growth mechanism injury (Figs. 24-47, 24-48). In one case a radiograph obtained when the patient first complained of pain showed a radiolucency adjacent to the apophysis.[136] She continued gymnastics and subsequently had acute onset of pain. The radiograph showed avulsion of the superior apophyseal fragment. It was reduced and internally fixed.

Walling et al. described 11 patients with open or closed fractures of the calcaneal apophysis.[204] The patterns of fracture varied, although all could be classified by a scheme similar to that used for physeal injuries in the long bones. Open injuries involved young children and were associated with subsequent maldevelopment of the posterior (nonarticular) portion of the calcaneus due to growth mechanism damage. The other susceptible age group, adolescents, contained two patients with slipped calcaneal apophysis as a type 1 injury similar to slipped capital femoral epiphysis and three patients with a splitting fracture through the apophysis and physis into the main part of the calcaneus (a type 4 injury). Microscopic physeal injury was also observed in the calcaneus of a fatally injured boy.

Closed reduction should be attempted. If it fails, open reduction may be indicated for the acute injury. However, manipulation of a "slipped apophysis" may not be sufficient if the injury is chronic. Long-term results are unknown.

Alvarez Fernandez et al. reported epiphysiolysis of the great tuberosity of the calcaneus.[133] The more superior portion was avulsed. It was treated closed, and the girl subsequently avulsed it a second time.

Havránek and Hájková reported a patient with bilateral fractures that principally involved the lower two-thirds of the calcaneal apophysis.[156] The fractures were reduced using a tension band wiring concept (Fig. 24-43).

Apophysitis

Heel pain is a common complaint in the child and adolescent, particularly in the athlete.[134,155,160,163,170,171,184] Sever originally described the condition as an inflammatory injury to the apophysis.[196] He did not classify it as osteochondritis, as suggested by subsequent authors. More recently, the cause has been attributed to overuse and repetitive microtrauma, especially in the young athlete.[134,163,166,171-173]

Liberson et al. reviewed 35 children with Sever's lesions and 6 calcanei from children who were accident victims.[166] These authors studied the radiolucent apophyseal regions and found evidence of ongoing reparative processes. They thought that these regions were areas of stress fractures, attempted healing, and remodeling.

There is controversy concerning the radiographic findings of calcaneal apophysitis.[197] Sever described radiologic findings that included "epiphyseal enlargement" and "cloudiness along the plate."[196] Increased sclerosis of the secondary ossification center has been described (Fig. 24-49). Micheli and Ireland agreed that the radiographic appearance is usually normal in patients with calcaneal apophysitis.[173] Sclerosis and irregular radiolucencies extending across the epiphyseal ossification center may be part of the normal multifocal ossification process. It seems much more likely that, comparable to pain in the accessory navicular, it is a compression-type microfracture within the "metaphyseal" portion of the calcaneus, *not* in the secondary ossification center. Accordingly, changes such as radiolucency in the "metaphysis" may be more significant (Figs. 24-50, 24-51).

Patients should be treated with a physical therapy program of lower extremity stretching, especially the heel cords with ankle dorsiflexion stretch. Soft orthoses (e.g., heel cups) may be helpful. Persistent pain may benefit from a brief period (2–3 weeks) of cast or brace immobilization.

Injuries to the Navicular

The tarsal navicular may be injured (Fig. 24-52) but is rarely displaced.[210,214,223,227] Crawford noted that the "dorsal chip fracture" is the most common navicular fracture in children (Fig. 24-53).[31]

Orava et al. described a stress avulsion fracture of the tarsal navicular that they thought came about through repetitive cyclic compressive loading secondary to impingement of the

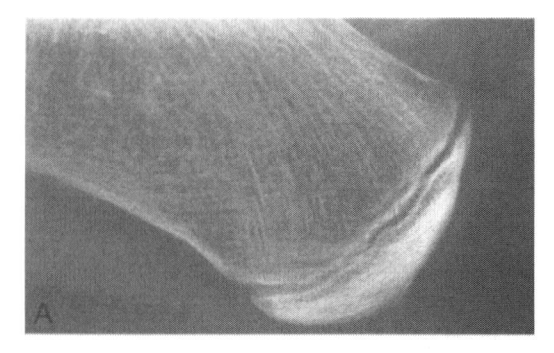

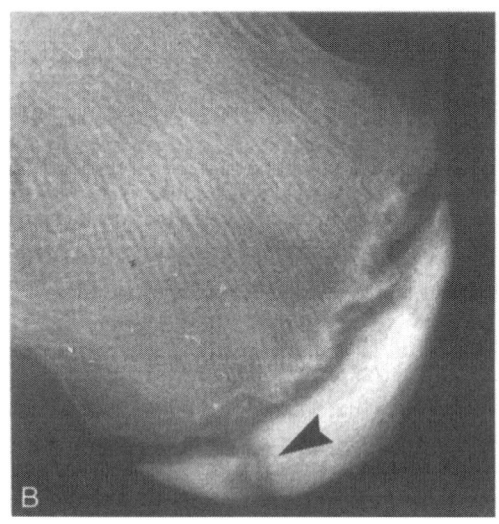

FIGURE 24-49. (A, B) Sclerotic appearance of the secondary ossification centers compared with the "metaphysis." Arrowhead in (B) points to a common area of radiolucency between sections of the often multifocal ossification center. Both findings are probably normal variations and not pathognomonic of Sever's lesion.

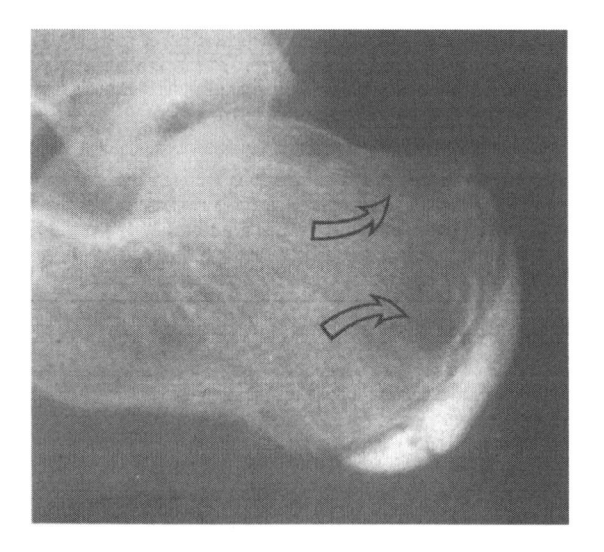

FIGURE 24-50. Radiograph of an adolescent with heel pain. Radiolucencies are apparent in the "metaphysis" (arrows) and are probably more significant than the sclerotic secondary center.

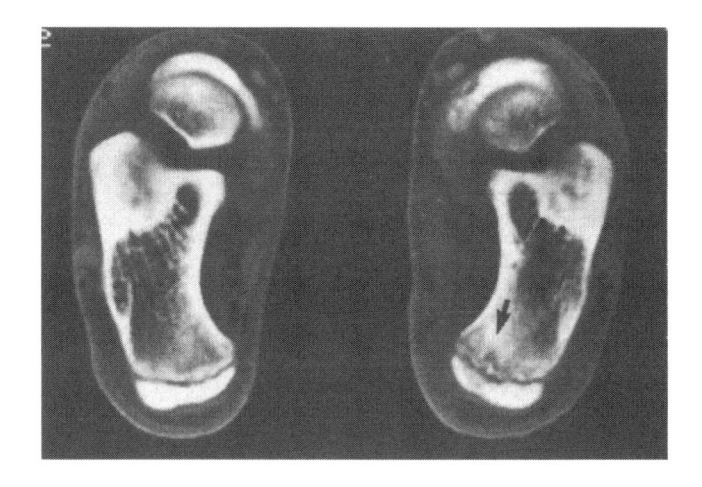

FIGURE 24-51. CT scan of a unilateral Sever's lesion. Note the metaphyseal changes (arrow). Similar radiolucent irregularity and widening may occur in a gymnast's wrist from repetitive impact and shearing.

tarsal navicular.[221] This resulted in a small dorsal triangular fragment best seen in a weight-bearing lateral view. Bone scan or tomography helped confirm the diagnosis. Operative treatment was recommended in highly symptomatic cases and among top athletes because of the short recovery time. Their patients ranged in age from 15 to 22 years, but many had been symptomatic for a considerable time prior to diagnosis. This lesion was similar to Kohler's disease in the younger child.

Alfred et al. described a 17-year-old girl who had an approximately 2-month history of intermittent pain in both feet.[208] She was participating actively in basketball and multiple conditioning exercise programs. The radiograph suggested a probable cortical crack. Bone scan was positive. These authors thought that biplane or CT scans also could pinpoint such elusive diagnoses that do not occur commonly.

Treatment consists in application of a short leg cast, with no weight-bearing permitted. Percutaneous fixation with K-wires may be necessary to keep fragments aligned, but it is an unusual circumstance.

Kohler's Injury

The tarsal navicular may be the site of a localized, chronic trauma-related process. This particular chondro-osseous stress injury has been termed Kohler's lesion (Fig. 24-54) and is often found during evaluation of a painful foot in a child.[209,216,228] It is certainly much more common than well-defined fractures, but it is a subacute injury, not a "disease."

Waugh studied the ossification of the tarsal navicular and its relation to Kohler's lesion, obtaining radiographs of the feet of boys and girls at intervals of 2–5 years.[228] About 25% displayed "abnormal ossification," but in all of them, a normal navicular eventually developed. This finding led to the concept that fragmentation of the ossification center of the navicular was a normal variant and that irregularities of ossification had no consistent relation to symptoms. However, if a child has point tenderness over the navicular associated with irregular ossification (especially if the other side exhibits

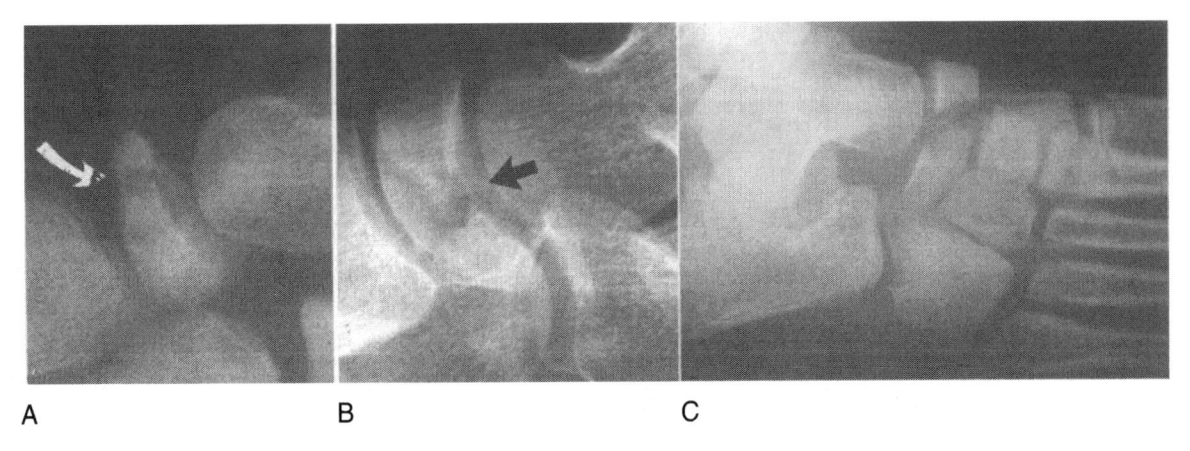

FIGURE 24-52. (A) Navicular fracture (arrow) in a 5-year-old child, sustained in a fall from a skateboard. (B) Navicular fracture (arrow) in a 12-year-old child following a crushing injury. (C) Navicular fracture in an 11-year-old boy. The medial cuneiform is also fractured.

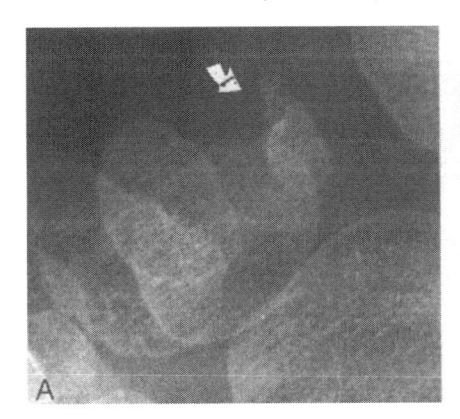

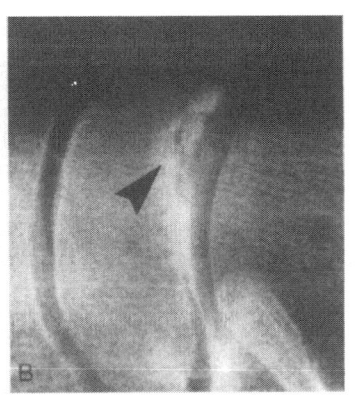

FIGURE 24-53. (A) Six-year-old child with pain over the dorsum of the foot (arrow) following a fall. (B) Eleven-year-old child with point tenderness over the navicular (arrowhead). She had activity-related discomfort, particularly with gymnastics. (C) Similar injury in an adolescent.

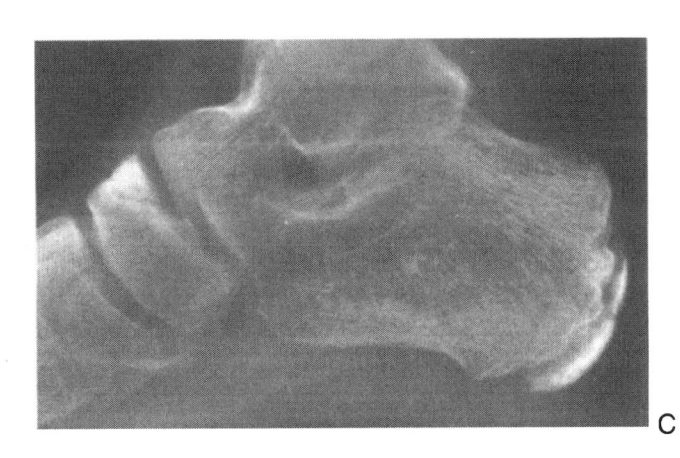

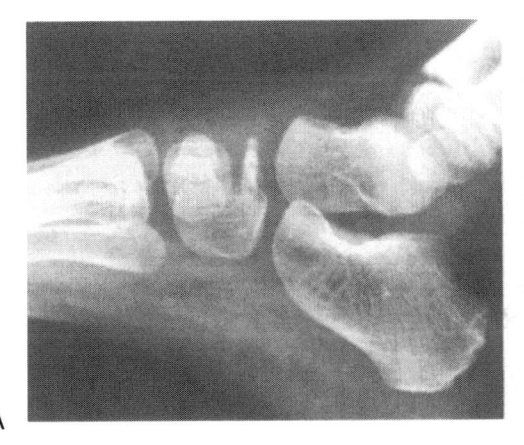

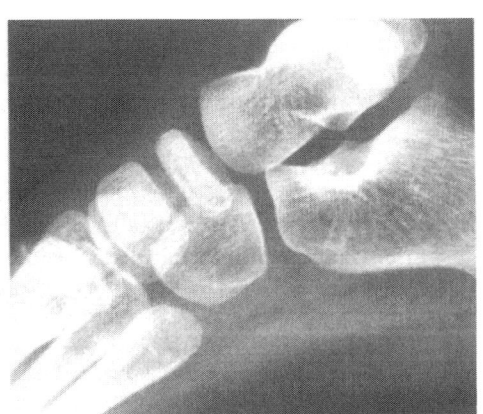

FIGURE 24-54. (A) Kohler's lesion. Collapse is evident. (B) Two years later there has been almost complete recovery.

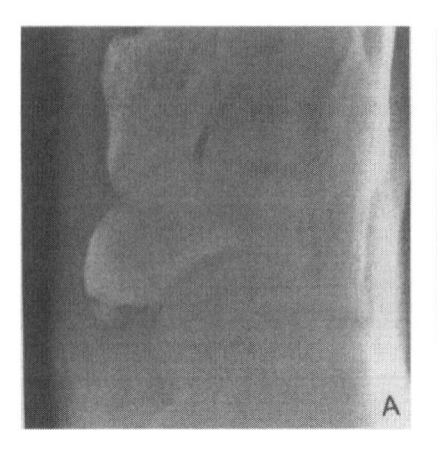

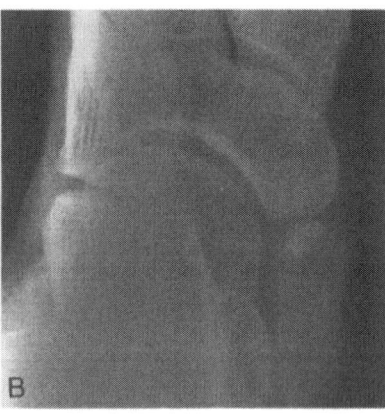

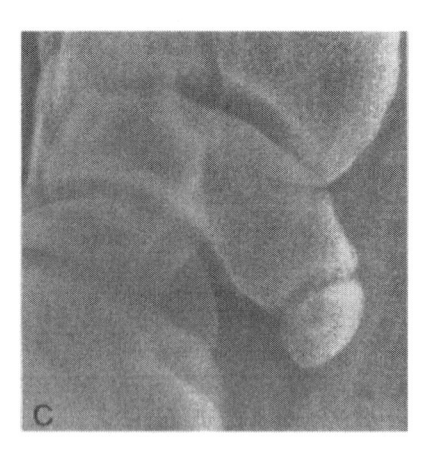

FIGURE 24-55. Progressive ossification of an intermittently symptomatic accessory navicular at 8 years (A), 10 years (B), and 12 years (C).

normal ossification), he or she should be treated with 3–4 weeks of immobilization in a cast, with no weight-bearing.

Ippolito et al. followed 12 patients with Kohler's injury for a follow-up averaging 33 years after diagnosis.[215] All patients were asymptomatic at their final evaluation. Neither alteration of the navicular shape nor osteoarthritis was observed radiographically. The treatment the patients had as children had varied, lasting an average of 8 months. Casts for a period of 3 months that permitted weight-bearing rendered patients pain-free, whereas arch supports only decreased the local pain, which lasted an average of 7 months. They showed that the amount of time required for a complete radiographic restoration ranged from 6 to 13 months (average 8 months).

Accessory Navicular

The accessory navicular may be the source of pain in older children and adolescents, particularly those participating in athletics.[211,213,217–220,222,225,226,229,230] There are three types of accessory navicular: type 1 is an ossicle in the substance of the posterior tibial tendon; type 2 has a synchondrosis within the navicular (Fig. 24-55; also see Fig. 24-10); and type 3 is the cornuate navicular, which probably represents the end-stage of chondro-osseous maturation and coalescence of type 2. The pull of the posterior tibial tendon and the degree of foot pronation are factors that produce tension, shear, or compression forces at the synchondrosis in the type 2 accessory naviculars.[224] They also cause chronic microscopic chondro-osseous failure, usually within the main portion of the navicular, creating a fracture pattern analogous to a type 1 or 2 growth mechanism injury (Fig. 24-56).

Such structural alterations are not always visible on standard roentgenograms but may be detected by a pronated oblique film, which removes the superior position of the other tarsal bones. Radionuclide bone scanning may delineate a positive scan on the symptomatic side in patients with bilateral radiographic findings. The nonsymptomatic side should be "cold" on the scan. MRI may detect the occult fracture, especially in the young child (Fig. 24-57).

The initial treatment should be conservative and directed at support underneath the longitudinal arch with a scaphoid pad, a contoured arch support (orthosis), or a molded short leg cast to lessen stress in the midfoot. If symptoms persist (which is likely) or recur, surgical treatment is recommended. It consists of excising the accessory navicular along with its synchondrosis, making the osteotomy through the main portion of the navicular just beyond (lateral to) the synchondrosis. It is not necessary to transpose the posterior tibial tendon, as originally described by Kidner. Resected specimens usually show evidence of acute or chronic injuries (or both) and reactive inflammation.

In a study of 22 skeletally immature patients with 39 accessory tarsal navicular bones seen over a 4-year period, 25

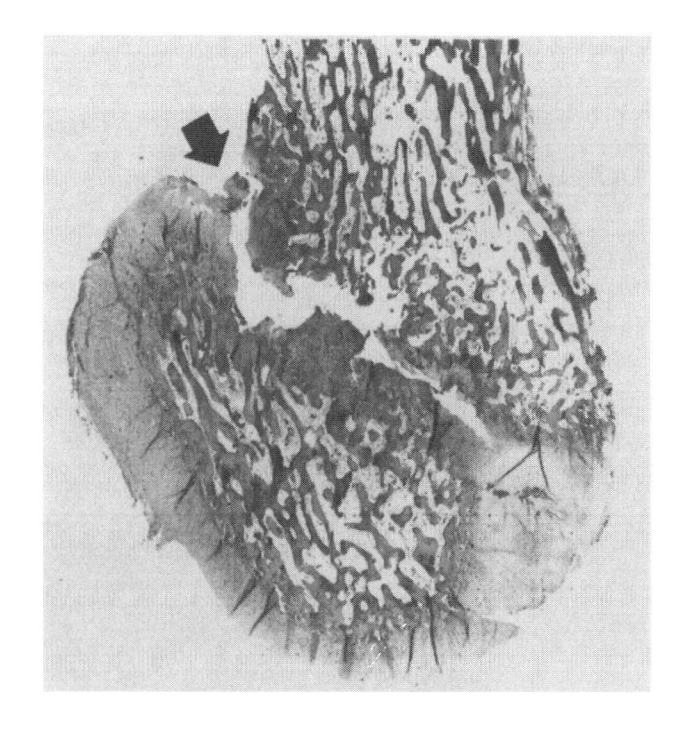

FIGURE 24-56. Symptomatic accessory navicular in an 11-year-old. Note the lucencies in the "metaphysis." Resected specimen shows an incomplete fracture (arrow) between the accessory navicular and the main portion of the navicular.

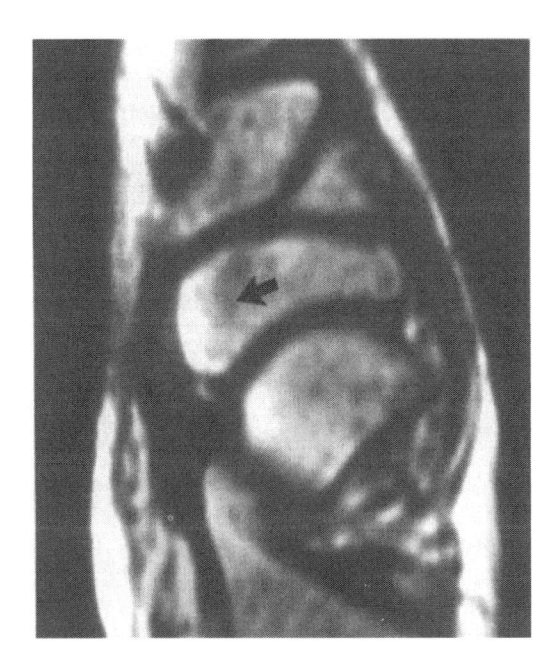

FIGURE 24-57. MRI showing intraosseous edema (arrow) and an angulated fragment with beginning secondary ossification.

of the feet had continued symptoms after failure of conservative treatment and were treated by excision of the accessory bone, the synchondrosis, and prominent portions of the main navicular ossification process.[212] There was no attempt to reroute the posterior tibial tendon. All 25 feet were completely relieved of the preoperative pain.

Injuries to the Other Tarsal Bones

The remainder of the tarsal bones appear relatively free of injury, except when accompanying extensive fracture-dislocations of the tarsometatarsal junction. These fractures are generally accompanied by extensive soft tissue swelling, especially on the dorsum of the foot. The fractures may be small and difficult to detect (Fig. 24-58).[231,239] The apparent lessened involvement of these bones may relate to our inability to diagnose injuries involving cartilage or chondro-osseous interfaces.[240]

Treatment is usually directed at closed reduction, with emphasis on the primary injury. Infrequently, open reduction, restoration of volume anatomy, and bone grafting are appropriate.

Mubarek reported osteochondrosis of the lateral cuneiform, which presented as a cause of limp in a child 2.5 years of age (at the time of initial presentation).[238] The child received no treatment, and the problem gradually resolved. Roentgenographic findings are similar to those seen when other cuneiforms or Kohler's injury of the navicular is involved: There is initially a decrease in osseous size (compared to the other side), irregularity, and increased density; and reossification eventually commences.

Several other authors have reported involvement of the other two cuneiforms.[232-237,241] Minimal treatment was given in all cases, with restitution of normal radiographic osseous anatomy over time.

Tarsometatarsal Injury

Tarsometatarsal (Lisfranc) joint injuries in the pediatric population usually occur in the older child.[241-264] Wiley described the most extensive pediatric series (18 children) and confirmed that such injuries are probably not uncommon, often misdiagnosed, and, like the adult variety, easily overlooked.[263] The "bunk bed" first metatarsal fracture (discussed in a subsequent section) is a "lesser" variation of the Lisfranc injury pattern that tends to occur in younger children.

Originally described during the Napoleonic era because a rider's feet remained in the stirrup during falls from horses, these injuries have been reported in children and young adults engaged in basketball, running, sailboarding,

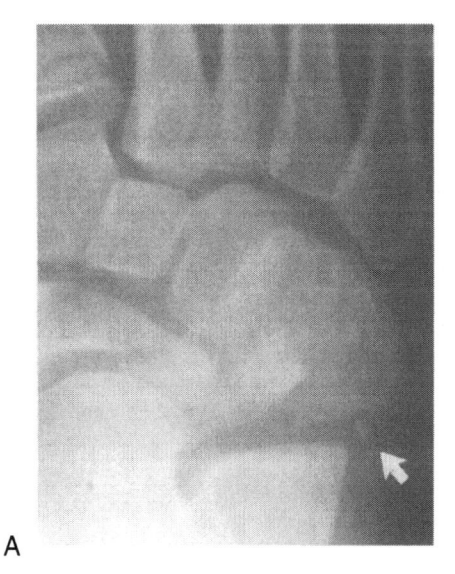

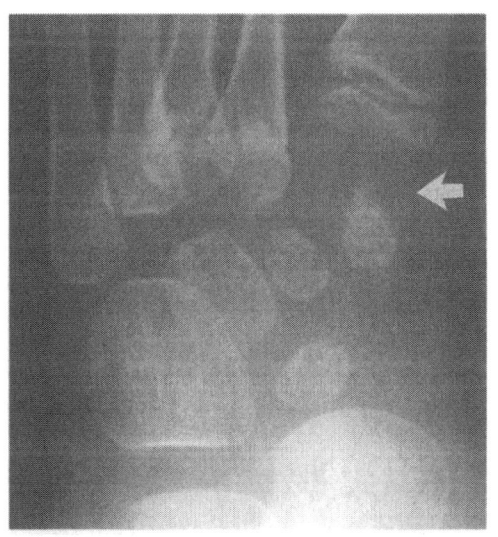

FIGURE 24-58. Fractures of cuboid (arrow) (A) and medial cuneiform (arrow) (B).

baseball, soccer, and gymnastics. Mantas and Burks describe the infrequency of the Lisfranc injury in the athlete.[252] They saw 15 patients with sports-related Lisfranc injuries, most sustained during gymnastics and football.[252] Each of the injuries was a mild subluxation of the second metatarsal base and diastasis between the first and second metatarsal bases rather than more severe injuries. They note that nearly 20% of all Lisfranc injuries escape identification on the initial radiographs.

Most patients sustain the injury with a combination of forced plantar flexion and rotation with or without abduction of the forefoot. Wiley described three basic injury mechanism patterns: (1) impact in the tiptoe position; (2) heel-to-toe compression; and (3) a backward fall with the forefoot fixed.[262,263]

The amount of force imposed on the foot to produce this injury may be considerable; accordingly, extensive soft tissue injury is usually present. Compartment syndrome must be considered and carefully evaluated. In Wiley's series only four of the injuries were the result of direct trauma. The other 14 were the result of indirect injuries, 10 of which occurred after jumping in the tiptoe position and two after tobogganing accidents in which the foot had been held out trying to brake the sled.[263]

There may not be obvious deformity because spontaneous reduction, often incomplete, usually occurs. Marked local pain and tenderness, accompanied by an inability to bear any weight, should lead to a suspicion of injury in this area. A subtle clinical sign is mid-foot ecchymosis on the plantar surface.[257] If evident, these patients should undergo further evaluation (e.g., stress radiographs or MRI) to rule out a Lisfranc injury.

With a partial dislocation usually the lateral four metatarsals are shifted laterally, whereas with a complete Lisfranc dislocation there is a diverted dislocation with the lateral four shifting laterally and the great toe shifting medially.

Vuori and Aro reviewed 66 patients with Lisfranc joint injury.[261] Among them, 12 had a total dislocation, 47 had a partial dislocation, *and 7 had a subtle injury.* They found no apparent relation between the mechanism of injury and the type of Lisfranc joint disruption. All but 3 patients had associated metatarsal fractures, most commonly involving the second metatarsal. Almost 40% of the patients also had fractures, dislocations, or fracture-dislocations of the mid-tarsal bones (cuneiforms, cuboid, navicular). Multiple metatarsal fractures and mid-tarsal bone injuries were more likely in children. In 23 patients (35%) treatment was focused on the multiple metatarsal fractures or mid-tarsal bone injuries without a full appreciation of the concomitant Lisfranc joint incongruity.

Rarely is the injury a simple dislocation of the metatarsals (Fig. 24-59). There are usually accompanying fractures, most often involving the second metatarsal (Fig. 24-60). This situation occurs because of the more proximal fixed position of the base of the second metatarsal and the ligamentous attachments of its base. The metatarsals are generally displaced in a plantar and lateral direction, rupturing the plantar ligaments. These fractures may be chondro-osseous separations, which are evident only as a small, linear piece of bone. Delineating these small pieces of bone may be difficult with routine radiographic techniques.

Anteroposterior, lateral, and oblique views of the foot are essential. A fracture of the base of the second metatarsal should alert the examiner to the possibility of a tarsometatarsal subluxation or dislocation. Similarly, fractures of the cuboid or the cuneiforms should make one suspect this injury. Spontaneous reduction, after dissipation of the deforming force, may leave an associated fracture as the only clue.

Norfray et al. pointed out that Lisfranc fracture-dislocations may be difficult to recognize radiographically, particularly in children.[254] Evaluation of the Lisfranc joint can be simplified by meticulously studying the alignment of the metatarsal bases with their corresponding tarsal bones. They noted that subtle abnormalities could be identified using such observation, including metatarsal subluxations identified only on a single projection, associated tarsal subluxations and dislocations, irreducible metatarsal subluxations after closed manipulation, and recurrent metatarsal subluxations. Other subtle signs to look for include widening between the proximal second and third metatarsals or

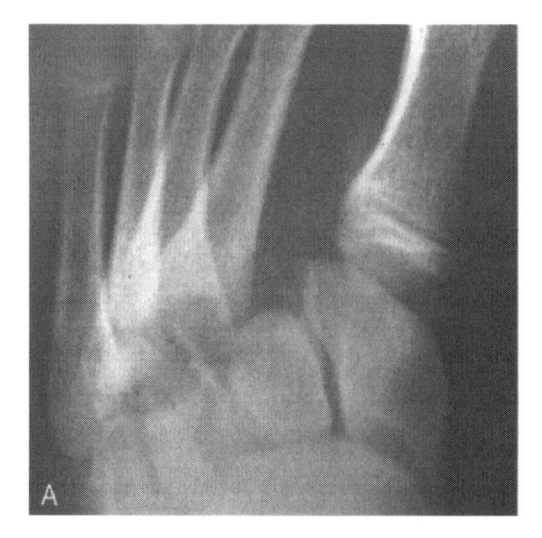

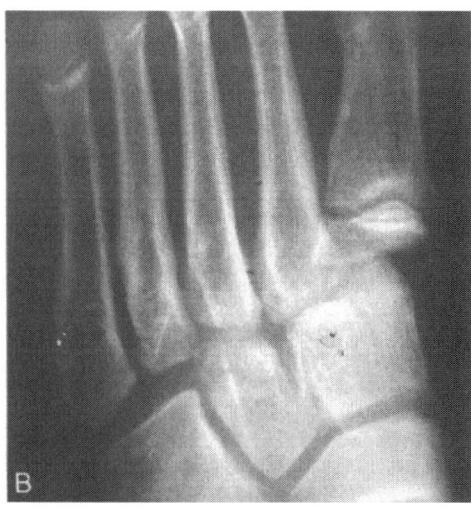

FIGURE 24-59. (A) Lisfranc's dislocation. (B) Reduction.

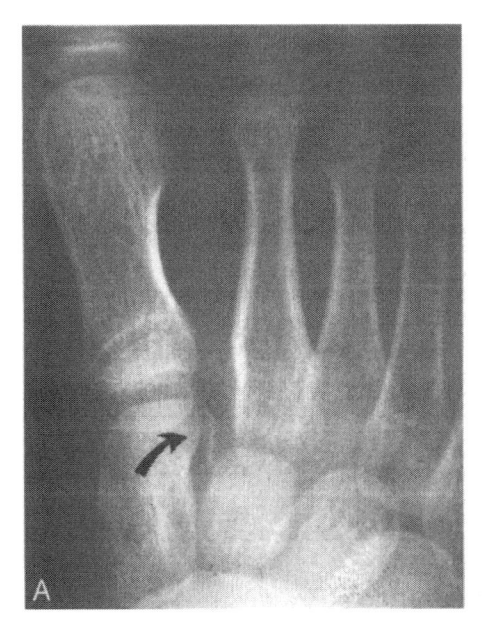

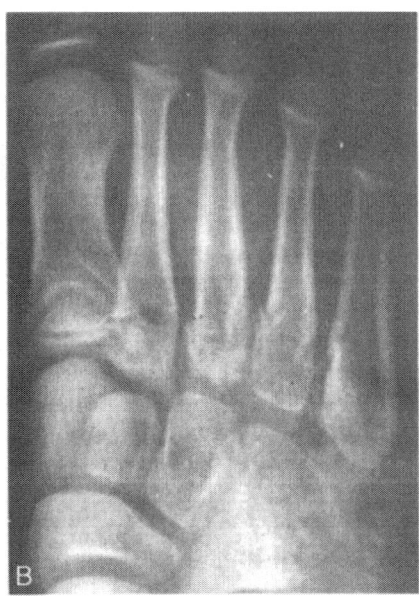

FIGURE 24-60. (A) Lisfranc's dislocation with fragment (arrow) from either the medial cuneiform or the second metatarsal. (B) Reduced Lisfranc's dislocation with fractures of the second and third metatarsals.

slight widening between the first and second metatarsals with a small avulsion fracture.

Fluoroscopy with anesthesia is necessary in some cases to determine the stability of the tarsometatarsal joint.[253] The pronation abduction test is used for such injuries; tenderness over the joint during gentle passive pronation and abduction usually indicates an injury.

The MRI technique may be useful for delineating the extent of injury. In one study this method, in contrast to routine radiology, showed joint malalignment in all 22 cases and disruption of Lisfranc's ligament in 8 of 11 patients.[255] The other 3 had an avulsion fracture of the second metatarsal or medial cuneiform bones. Subtle tarsal and metatarsal fractures were evident in 10 of the 11 patients, in contrast to the regative findings on radiographs.

The major consideration during treatment is the extensive swelling of the dorsum of the foot associated with this injury, regardless of whether gross displacement occurs. The viability of the skin and soft tissue must be observed closely. Decompression of the dorsum of the foot may be necessary. Extensive soft tissue injury, particularly involving disruption of major vessels, may require amputation. Evaluation of tissue compartment pressures is prudent.

Treatment is relatively straightforward. Undisplaced or minimally displaced tarsometatarsal dislocations may be managed with elevation and pressure dressings initially and application of a short leg cast for 3–4 weeks. For any injury with more than minimal displacement, adequate reduction is required. Closed reduction should be attempted first, as it is usually successful. Supplemental pin fixation (percutaneous) may be necessary to stabilize the reduction (Fig. 24-61). The key to reduction is stabilizing the fracture of the proximal second metatarsal.

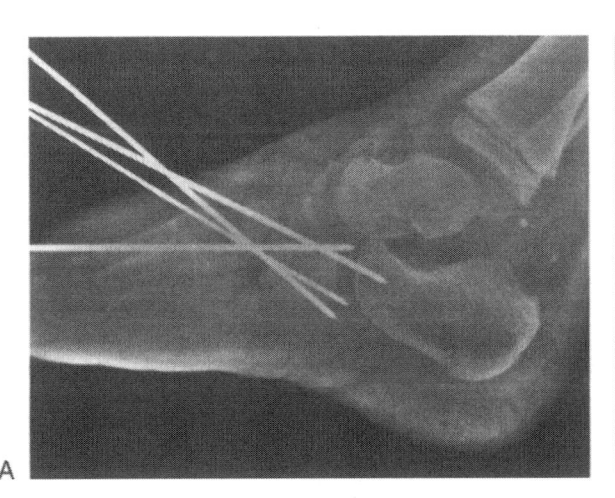

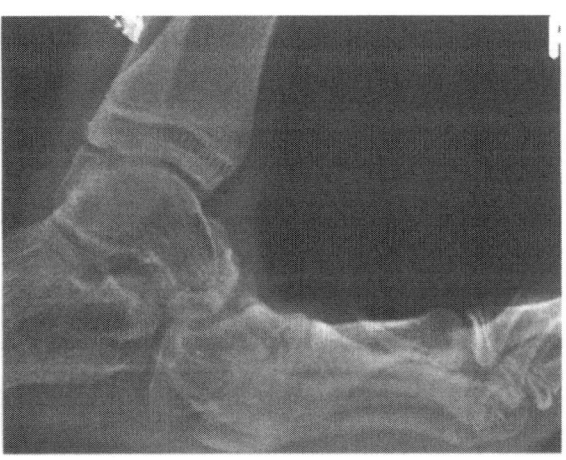

FIGURE 24-61. Open Lisfranc injury following the child's foot being run over by a school bus. It was treated by débridement, fasciotomies, and delayed fixation. (B) Poor result 5 years later.

Myerson thought that treatment with casting was appropriate only for patients who had acute, stable injuries with no radiographic diastasis.[253] If the joint is unstable, however, open reduction and internal fixation provide the best results. If the approach is surgical, exposure of the tarsometatarsal joint is usually through a longitudinal incision over the second metatarsal. This approach permits removal of the interposed soft tissue or bone fragments blocking reduction. Myerson used transarticular screw fixation to secure the reduction of the second metatarsal head, which invariably is dislocated dorsolaterally. The screw is inserted obliquely through the medial wall of the medial cuneiform into the base of the second metatarsal to reduce it into its mortise.

Sangeorzan et al. recommended rigid fusion with multiple screws for salvage of Lisfranc's tarsometatarsal joint injury in the patient with significant pain (all patients were adults).[258] This procedure has not been described for children; but obviously, with long-term follow-up of these injuries it may become indicated more often. Any fixation devices must avoid the physis of the first metatarsal.

The short-term results are usually good despite extensive disruption of the tarsometatarsal joint complex. Wiley noted that 14 of 18 patients were asymptomatic 3–8 months after injury, whereas the other 4 had persistent discomfort up to a year following injury. Wiley thought that long-range follow-up was necessary.[263]

Vascular complications have been reported in adults with this joint injury but have not been described in children, with the exception of a 16-year-old in Wiley's series.[263] This adolescent had radiologic evidence of early ischemic necrosis of the second metatarsal head 4 months after the injury.

Babst et al. reviewed 30 patients, the youngest being 6 years of age.[244] The average follow-up was 3.8 years. Bad results clearly correlated with the quality of reduction. An open procedure was usually necessary to achieve anatomic reduction, especially in the older patients. Certainly, attempts should be made to do a closed reduction *initially* in children.

Injuries to the Metatarsals

In a review of 388 children with foot injuries, 62 metatarsal fractures and 7 tarsal fractures were identified in 60 children. The most common fracture was of the fifth metatarsal (45%), with most of these patients over 10 years old. In children under 5 years of age first metatarsal fractures accounted for 73%, whereas in children older than 5 years this injury pattern constituted only 12% of all injuries.[273] Overall 6.5% of all foot fractures and 20.0% of first metatarsal fractures were *not* diagnosed during the initial evaluation.[288] Child abuse may be associated with foot fractures.[280]

Solitary fractures of the metatarsal diaphyses are usually undisplaced. Most often the first or fifth metatarsal is involved, with the displacement not significant. Less commonly, the second or third metatarsal is injured. However, when the latter is involved, the injury may be a stress fracture.[269,272,278] Such a possibility should be considered in any child who complains of persistent pain along the longitudinal arch. Because these fractures may not be visible using routine roentgenographic techniques, a bone scan should be considered. Such injuries may be associated with child abuse.

Pseudoepiphyses are relatively common in the first metatarsal (Fig. 24-62) and are present distally. Similarly, apparent accessory ossification centers have been reported in the proximal ends of the third and fourth metatarsals;

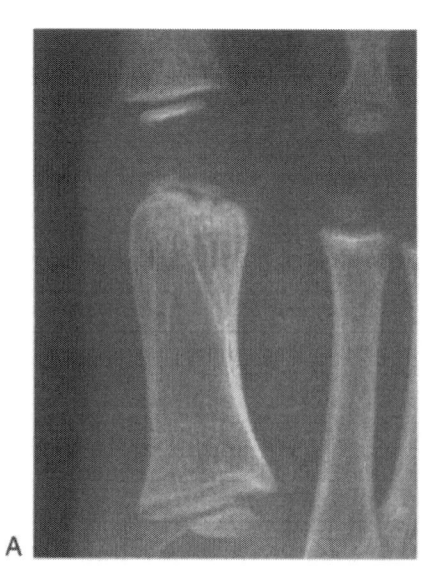

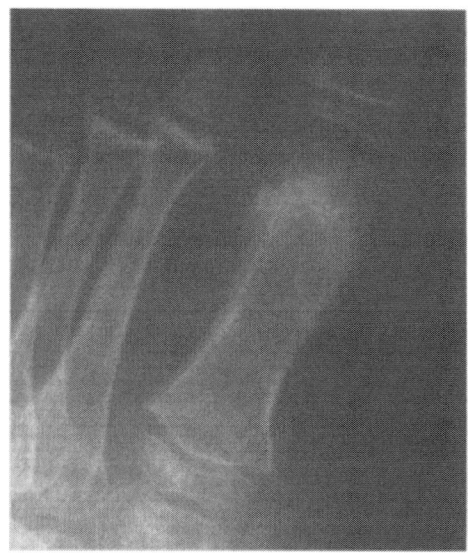

FIGURE 24-62. (A) Distal pseudoepiphyseal ossification. This process is normal and is not indicative of injury. (B) Fracture through the pseudoepiphyseal region.

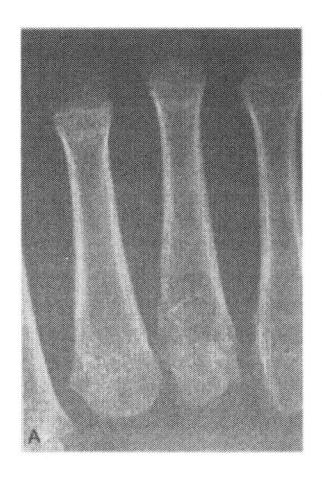

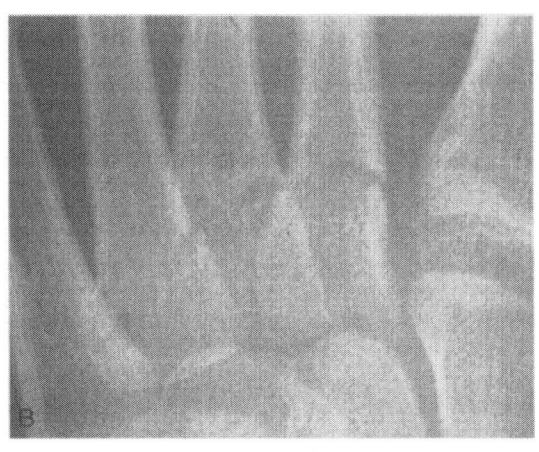

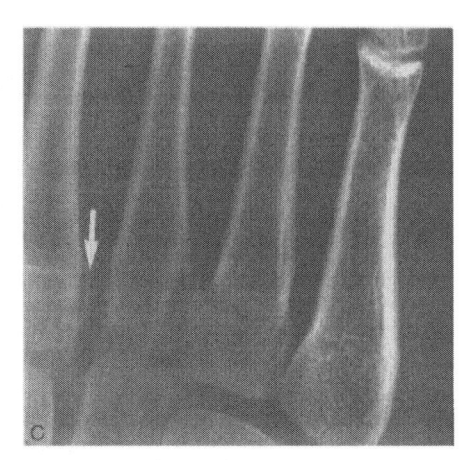

FIGURE 24-63. (A) Fracture of the proximal third metatarsal following direct impact. (B) Fractures of the proximal second, third, and fourth metatarsals after a twisting injury. (C) Multiple metaphyseal fractures (third and fourth) with avulsion from the lateral side of the second (arrow). It is a Lisfranc injury analogue.

they should not be misinterpreted as fractures, although the latter may occur (Fig. 24-62).

Proximal metatarsal fractures are usually caused by direct impact or twisting injuries (Fig. 24-63). They tend to be undisplaced and heal well after treatment directed at the accompanying soft tissue injuries. Always assess the possibility of a Lisfranc injury variant. When multiple proximal fractures are present, there may be concomitant disruption of at least one tarsometatarsal joint (Fig. 24-63C). There may also be widening of the space between the first and second proximal metatarsals. Because of the strong interosseous membranes and ligaments between the metatarsals, displacements are unusual, except between the first and second metatarsals.

With multiple metatarsal fractures, the first metatarsal often is fractured proximally, and the remaining metatarsals are fractured distally (Fig. 24-64). Mid-diaphyseal metatarsal injuries are often caused by direct impact from heavy objects (Fig. 24-65). They generally are undisplaced and heal well. The most serious and complex metatarsal injuries are caused by lawn mowers (Fig. 24-66).[290] The extent of concomitant soft tissue and osseous damage is rarely evident on the initial examination. Adequate débridement and continuing evaluation of soft tissue viability are essential.

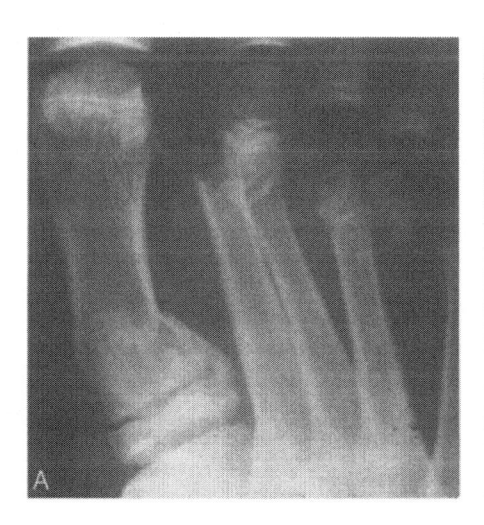

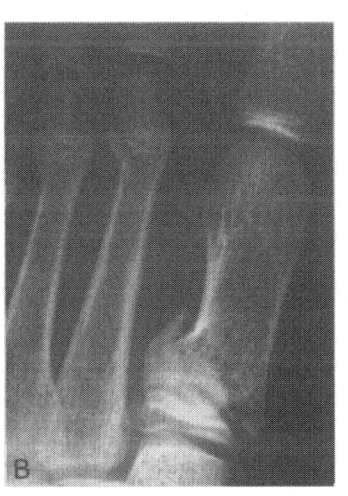

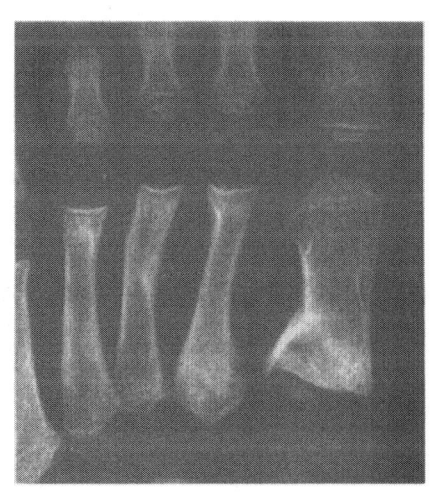

FIGURE 24-64. (A) Fractures of the proximal first metatarsal and distal second, third, and fourth metatarsals. (B) Type 2 physeal injury of the proximal first metatarsal, with concomitant fracture of the distal second and third metatarsals. This barefoot girl fell off a skateboard. (C) Healed proximal first and more distal second and third metatarsal fractures.

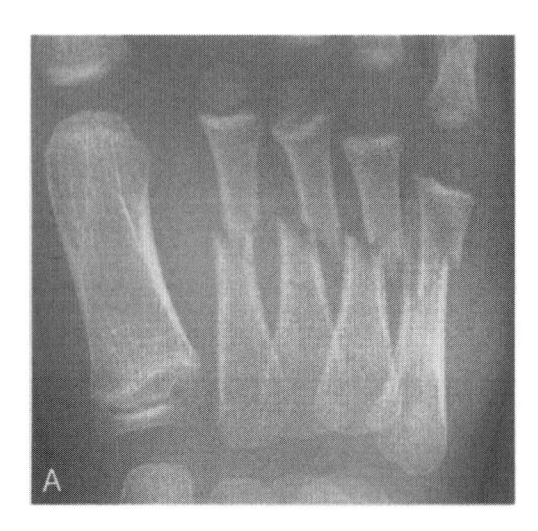

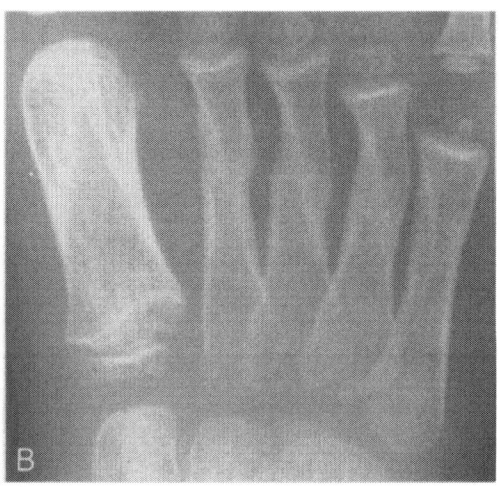

FIGURE 24-65. (A) Multiple fractures of the second to fifth diaphyses following the direct impact of a heavy object. (B) Healing and remodeling 4 months later.

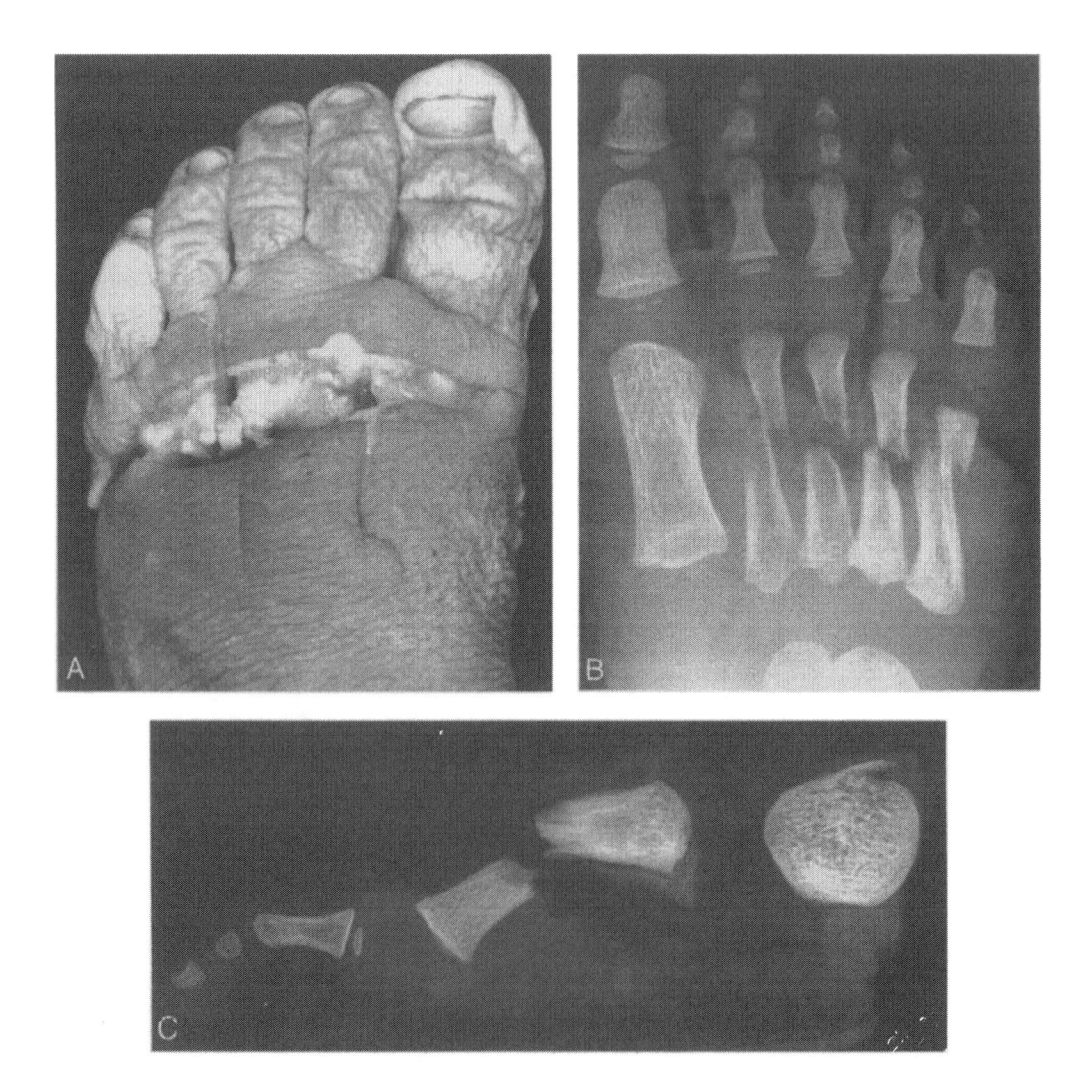

FIGURE 24-66. (A) Open diaphyseal injuries caused by a lawn mower. (B) Radiograph of the specimen. (C) Lateral radiograph of the third ray. (D) Histologic appearance of the fracture (arrow).

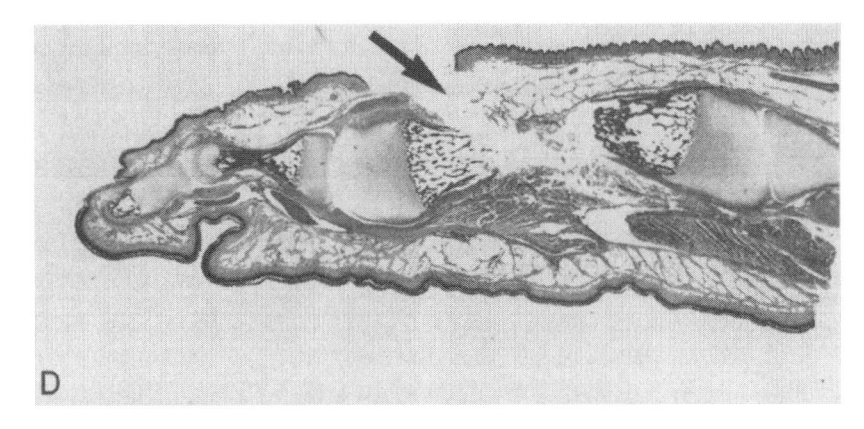

FIGURE 24-66. *Continued*

The distal metatarsal necks, with a relatively small diameter, are susceptible to injury (Figs. 24-67, 24-68).[277] These distal fractures may involve the metaphysis or the physis. The metatarsal heads may be malaligned, exhibiting increased valgus and plantarward deviation. Correction of angular displacement is important because the amount of longitudinal growth and remodeling may not be sufficient to correct the angular change (thus causing a subtle alteration of foot mechanics). The distal fifth metatarsal appears particularly susceptible to injury (Fig. 24-69). The distal epiphyses infrequently sustain fractures through the physes (Fig. 24-70).

As is true for all injuries of the child's foot, radiographic evaluation in multiple planes is essential to determine the site of fracture and the extent of anatomic displacement. The anteroposterior and oblique views generally reveal the extent of the fracture, but the lateral view is necessary to assess plantar displacement of the distal fragment (or fragments). The exposure is generally set to provide penetration of the larger tarsal bones, which results in overexposure of the smaller metatarsal bones and phalanges. Therefore when injuries of the forefoot are suspected, the radiologic technician should provide optimal exposure of this area, rather than the midfoot or hindfoot. A bone scan may reveal occult injury.[287]

Initial management is contingent on the severity of the injury. Marked swelling and soft tissue injury are often present. The interossei and short plantar muscles are contained in closed fascial compartments. Fasciotomy may be indicated if the intracompartmental swelling is severe. The long-term result of failure to perform fasciotomy of the interossei, in the presence of increased tissue pressure, is fibrosis and an intrinsic minus foot with claw toes.

Fortunately, treatment of most fractures of the metatarsals in children is generally simple and requires only immobilization in a short leg walking cast. For fractures that require reduction, Chinese finger traps may be used: The respective toes of the injured metatarsals are placed in the finger traps, followed by manipulative reduction and application of a well-molded cast. A slipper cast with free ankle motion is an

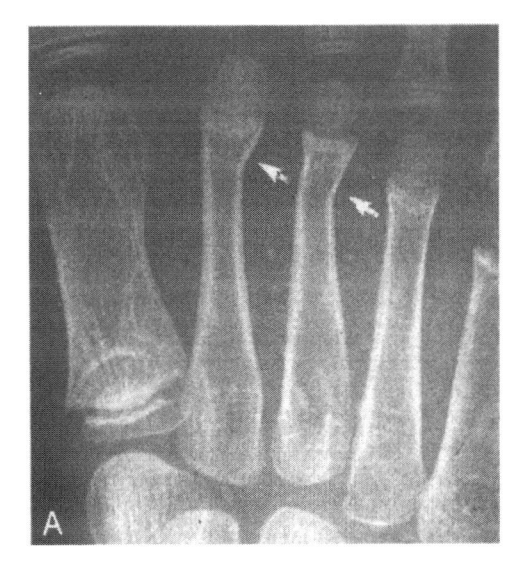

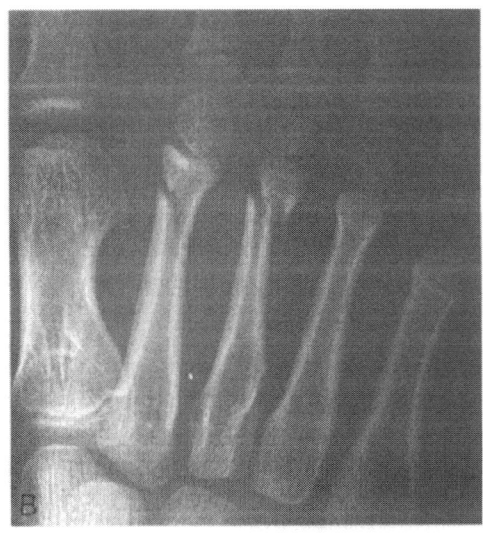

FIGURE 24-67. (A) Greenstick fractures (arrows) of the second and third metatarsal heads. (B) Distal metatarsal fractures. The second one is a greenstick, and the third is displaced.

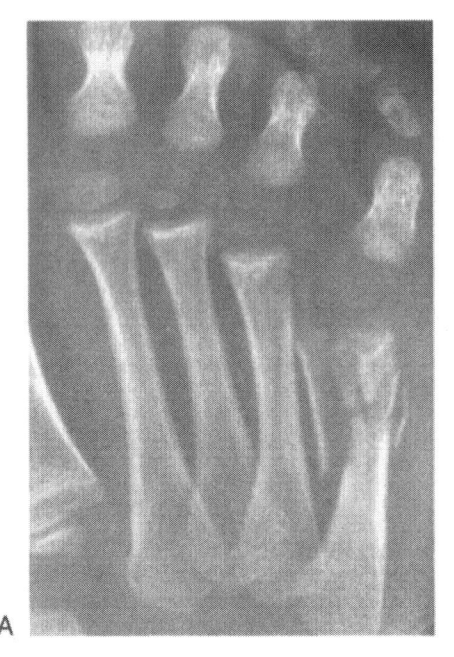

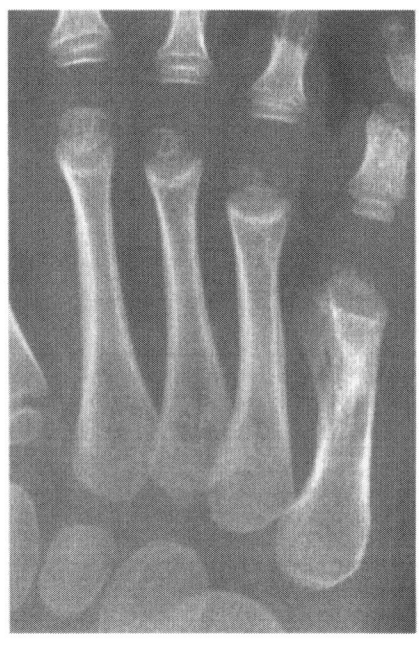

FIGURE 24-68. (A) Comminuted distal fifth metatarsal fracture. (B) Mild growth deformity 5 months later.

acceptable method of treatment, especially for the first few days, when tissue swelling may be extensive. A short leg cast may be applied later. If the reduction is unstable, percutaneous pin fixation or internal fixation may be necessary (Fig. 24-71).[274] Angulation of the distal ends may be permissible, depending on the age of the child. This is the area of most rapid growth in these bones (the second to fifth metatarsals). When open reduction is required, the standard approach is dorsal exposure.

Varus or valgus malalignments should be corrected during reduction. When the fractures involve the distal metatarsal heads, they should be reduced as accurately as possible to correct plantar displacement. The transverse ligaments between the distal first and second metatarsals may also be disrupted, and reapproximation of this region by closed reduction and a well-molded cast may prevent a splayfoot and functional loss of the transverse and longitudinal arches.

As soft tissue swelling subsides, radiography should be repeated at appropriate intervals to be certain the reduction is maintained. Proper alignment is necessary because growth and remodeling may not be sufficient to correct angular (plantar flexion) deformity and abnormal weight distribution.

Physeal involvement may lead to altered growth (Fig. 24-72).[276] Premature bridging may be eccentric. Splitting of the physis may lead to a bifid physis. Complete disruption of growth may lead to a short metatarsal. If damage to the growth plate causes premature epiphysiodesis, the length discrepancy may be treated by callotasis lengthening.[285,289]

First Metatarsal

The first metatarsal may be injured proximally, either in the metaphysis or at the proximal growth plate.[293] If there is damage to the physis, shortening of the medial side of the foot and deficiency of the longitudinal arch may occur (Fig. 24-73). Because of the locations of the physes at the proximal end of the first and distal ends of the second through fifth metatarsals, trauma may affect rates of growth differentially by direct injury or relative response to the increased blood flow caused by the injury.

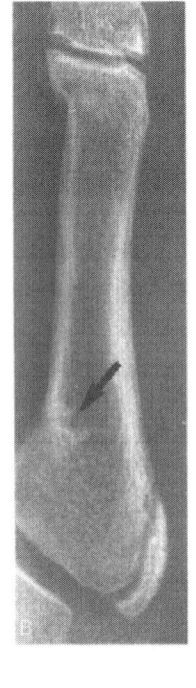

FIGURE 24-69. (A) Crush fracture of the distal fifth metatarsal. (B) One week later sclerosis is evident in an accompanying, but undiagnosed, proximal injury (arrow).

Injuries to the Metatarsals   1131

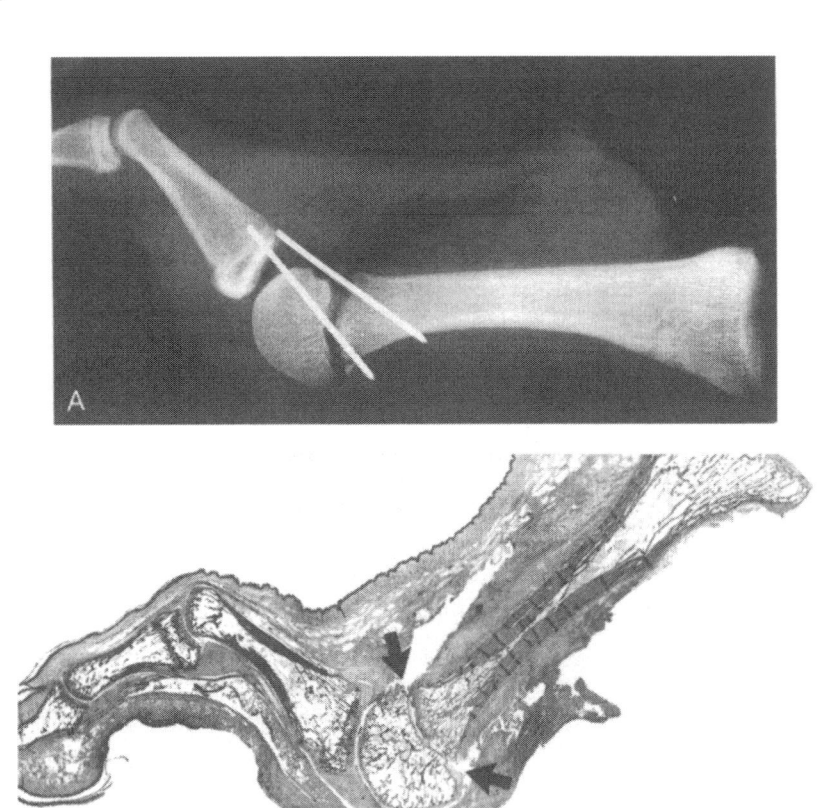

FIGURE 24-70. Distal physeal fracture. (A) Fixation done prior to amputation revision. (B) Histologic section showing the fracture (arrows).

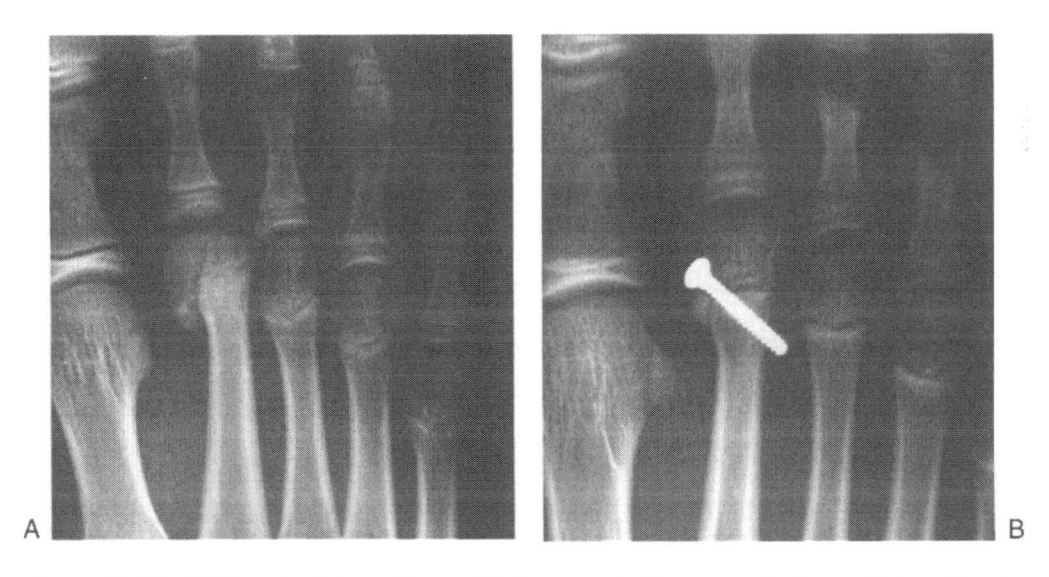

FIGURE 24-71. (A) Type 4 epiphyseal injury. (B) It was treated by open reduction and internal fixation.

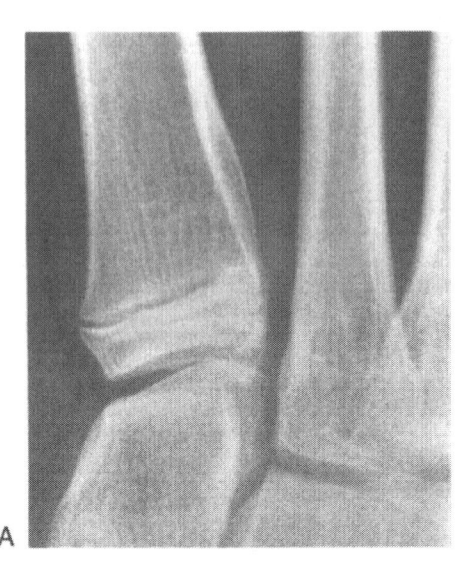

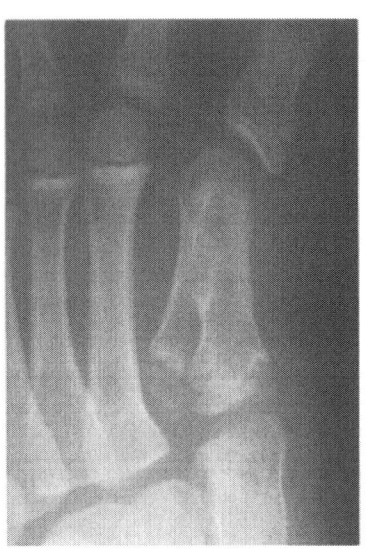

FIGURE 24-72. (A) Lateral bone bridge in the first metatarsal. (B) Previous type 4 growth mechanism injury treated closed has led to a bifid proximal first metaphysis 3 years later.

Avulsion fractures (type 7 injuries) from the first metatarsal head are analogous to ligament injuries in the adult. Such fragments may need to be stabilized (Fig. 24-74).

Bunk Bed Fracture

Young children (10 years or less) may sustain a variation of the Lisfranc injury specifically affecting the first ray.[281,293] By jumping from a height (especially a bunk bed) and landing on the first metatarsal head, these children sustain variable fractures of the lateral (or less commonly medial) side of the proximal first metatarsal and some damage to the medial (first) cuneiform (Fig. 24-75). These fractures sometimes involve the proximal physis (type 2 injury). The diagnosis may be made retrospectively after a sclerotic healing fracture becomes evident. Unfortunately, reported follow-up of only a few weeks was available.[250] There should be long-term observation for growth arrest in such injuries.

Fifth Metatarsal

Avulsion fracture of the proximal, lateral fifth metatarsal is usually caused by a strong inversion force or sudden twisting of the foot. The main problem with this fracture is often the inability to make the diagnosis. Chronic traction apophysitis is referred to as Iselin's disease.[267,279,284]

Dameron described the anatomic variations of this region. He found no radiographic evidence of a secondary ossification center prior to the age of 8 years.[270,271] This center becomes evident between 9 and 11 years in girls and 11 and 14 in boys, uniting by 12 years in girls and 15 years in boys. Other structures that may cause difficulty in the differential diagnosis include the os peroneum (located in the peroneus longus

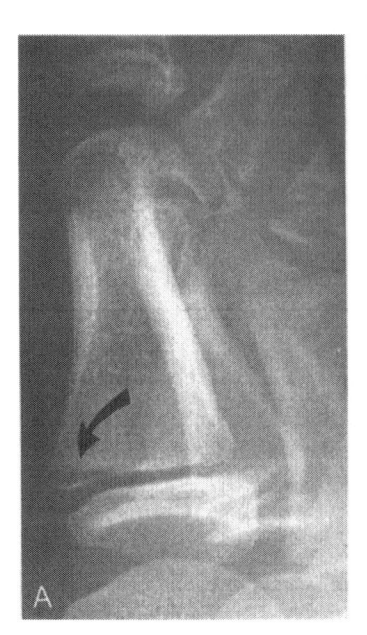

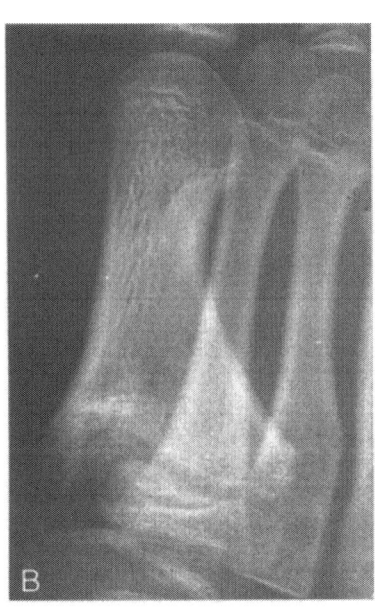

FIGURE 24-73. (A) Fracture (arrow) through the proximal physis of the first metatarsal. Extensive subperiosteal bone has formed. (B) Three years later. The fracture has not extensively remodeled, irregularity of the physis confirms growth arrest, and the metatarsal is shorter than the others.

Injuries to the Metatarsals

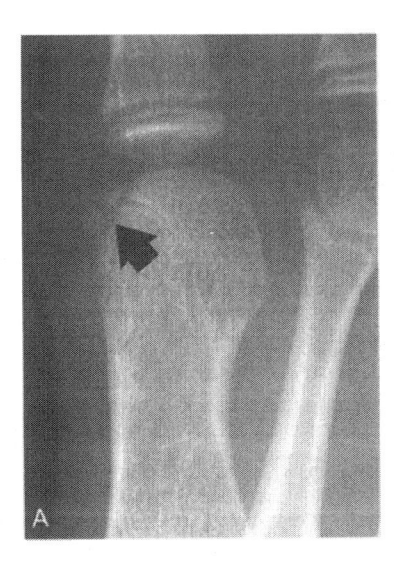

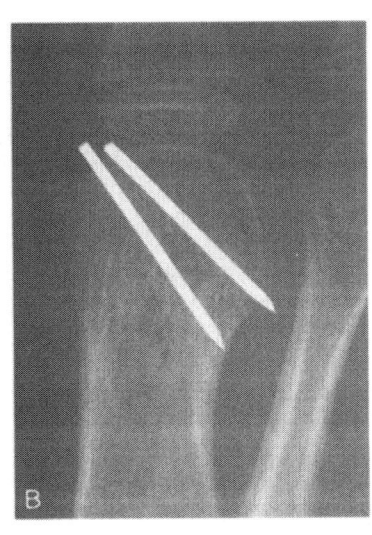

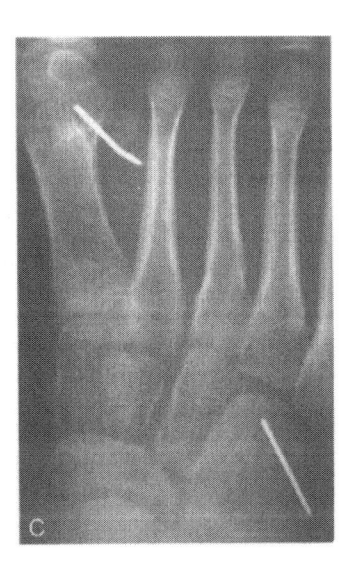

FIGURE 24-74. (A) Type 7 avulsion fracture (arrow). (B) Fixation with smooth pins. (C) Oblique view showing extent of pin migration in 7 months.

tendon and evident in 15% of roentgenograms) and the os vesalianum (Fig. 24-9), which is thought to be either an ossicle in the peroneus brevis or part of the metatarsal and present in fewer than 1% of radiographs.

Several patterns of fracture may occur (Fig. 24-76). First, the entire chondro-osseous epiphysis may be avulsed from the metaphysis, although the degree of separation is usually minimal. Second, the fracture may extend into the metaphysis with varying degrees of comminution. Third, the developing secondary ossification center or the preossification center may be split.

A fracture is usually perpendicular to the shaft. More distal fractures (i.e., the Jones fracture) are approximately 1.5 cm distal to the base.[265,282,283,292] Because the peroneus brevis attaches 0.50–0.75 cm distal to the tuberosity, it is unlikely that it produces or displaces this fracture. It is more likely that the abductor digiti minimi and the calcaneometatarsal ligament are factors.

Bone scanning may be useful for delineating a fracture from a radiologic variant (Fig. 24-77). Focal increased radionuclide uptake, especially in comparison to the opposite side, suggests a fracture.

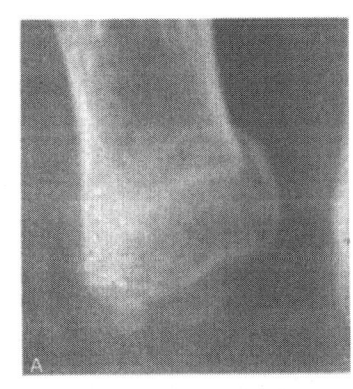

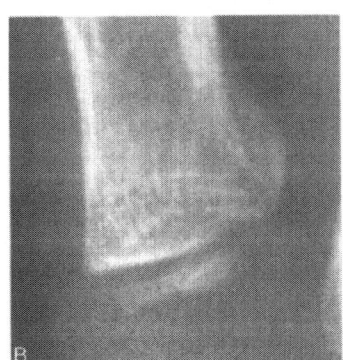

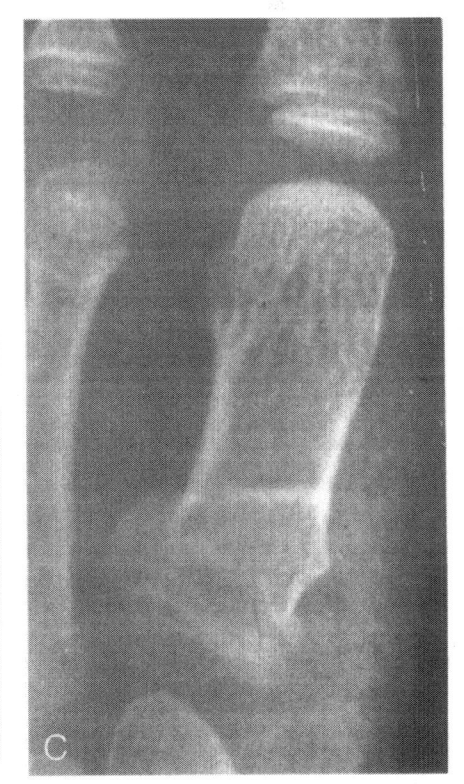

FIGURE 24-75. Bunk bed fractures. (A) Acute injury. (B) Seven months later. (C) Impacted injury.

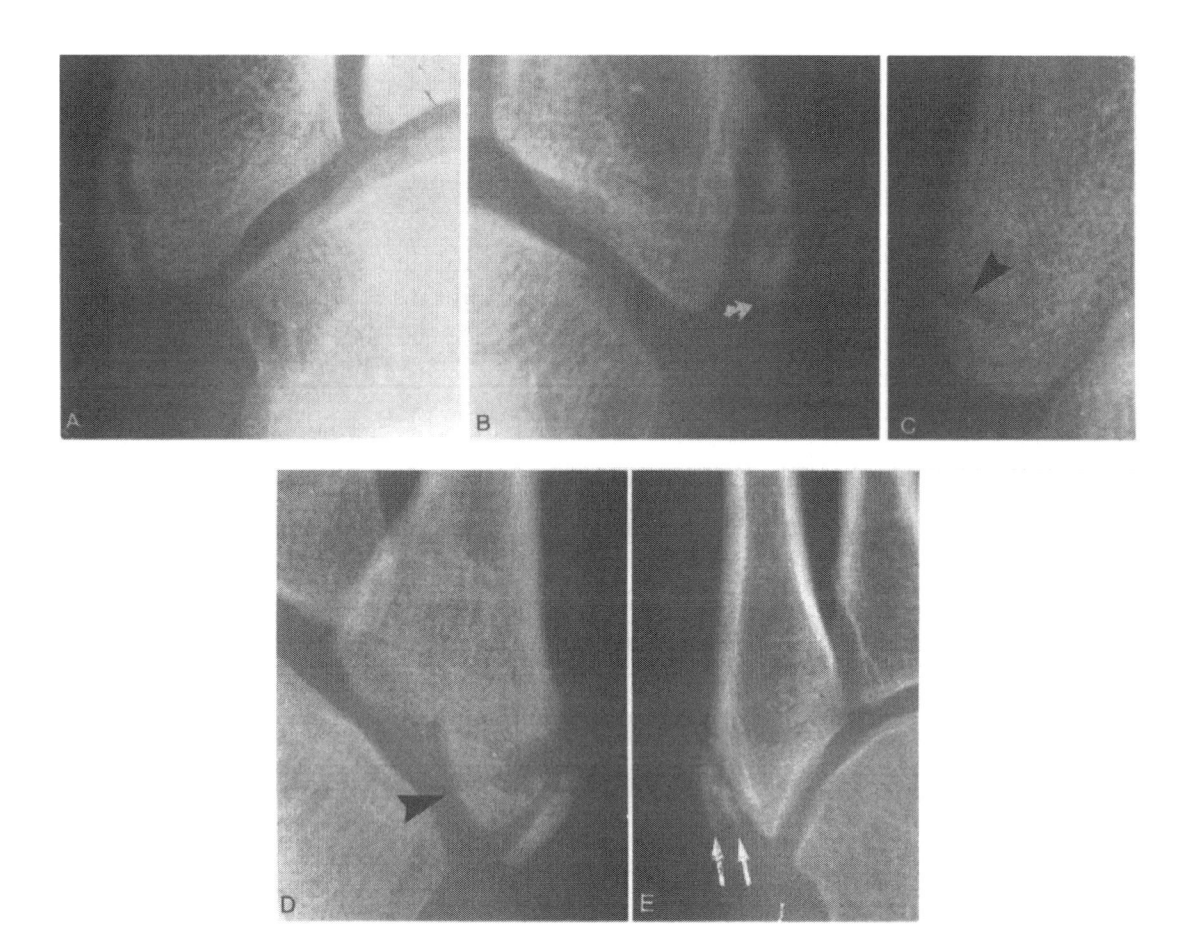

FIGURE 24-76. (A) Normal appearance of the fifth metatarsal. (B) Avulsion of the epiphysis (arrow), with some fragmentation. (C) Fracture into the metaphysis prior to secondary ossification (arrowhead). (D) Similar fracture (arrowhead) after the appearance of the secondary center. (E) "Splitting" fracture (arrows) of the secondary center.

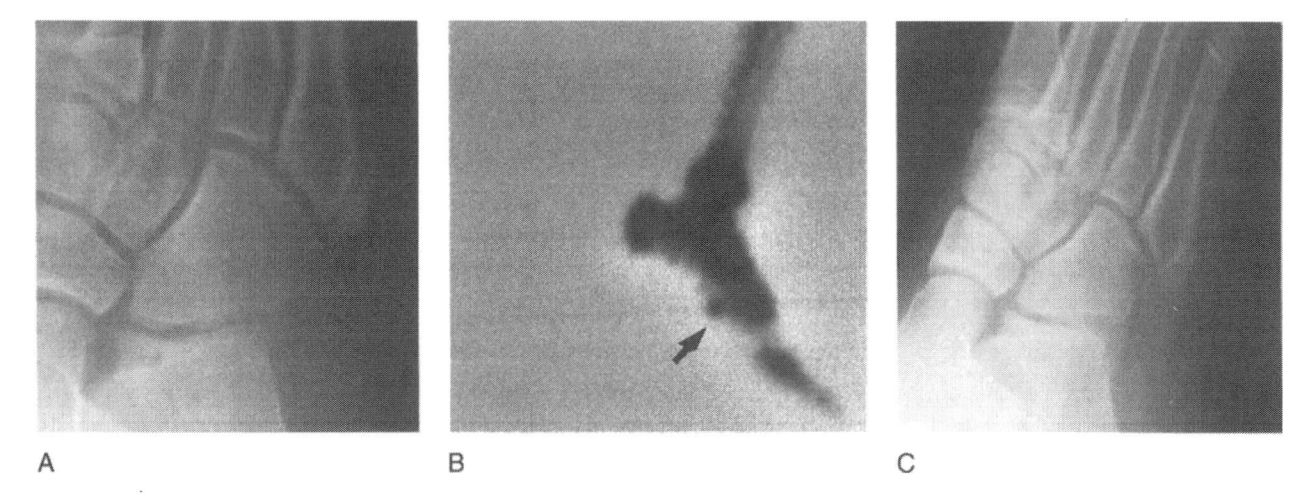

FIGURE 24-77. (A) Acute inversion injury. Is it a fracture or a normal ossification center? (B) Bone scan showed focal uptake (arrow), so it is a fracture. (C) Result after 4 weeks in a short leg cast.

Injuries to the Metatarsals

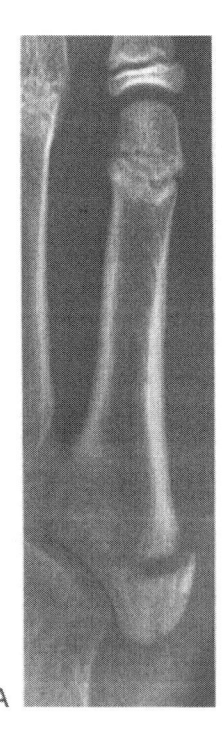

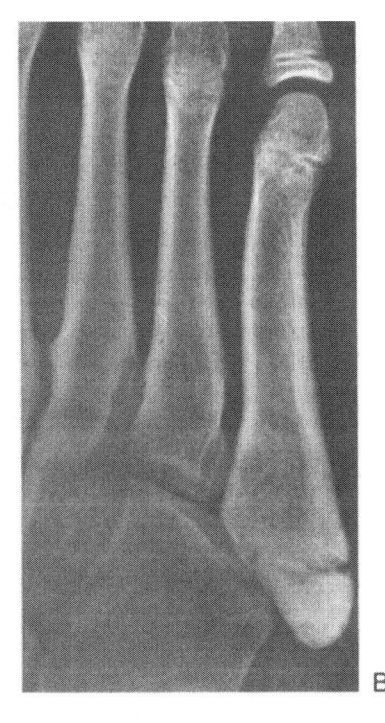

FIGURE 24-78. (A) Displaced fracture of the proximal fifth metaphysis. It was reduced by direct pressure and casted in eversion. (B) Result 9 weeks later.

Treatment of all types should consist of immobilization in a short leg walking cast for 3–4 weeks (Fig. 24-78). Open reduction is rarely indicated, as significant distraction of the avulsed portion is unusual (Fig. 24-79). Chronic pain from a nonunion may indicate a need for fragment excision.

Growth deformities are rare, although overgrowth, similar to an Osgood-Schlatter injury, may occur and cause enlargement of this region (Fig. 24-80). This is more likely in an athlete who continues to play despite pain. Such enlargement may cause discomfort in shoes, and the patient may benefit from excisional surgery. Nonunion of this fracture is rare.

Stress Fractures

Stress fractures of the metatarsals, although less common than in adults, do occur and most often involve the second or third metatarsal.[269,270] Childress reported a stress fracture of the metatarsal in a 7-year-old child.[268] These injuries are probably more common than observed because extensive workup (e.g., bone scan) is rarely done. These injuries are relatively common in children who experience a sudden increase or change in physical activity. In the pediatric population, this group is likely to include maturing adolescents as they begin to participate in intensive training for a particular sport, especially if they have been relatively inactive during the preceding months. However, the injury pattern should not be overlooked in the differential diagnosis of the limping toddler.

Initial radiographs are often normal. The development of subperiosteal callus 2–3 weeks after the onset of pain and tenderness can retroactively establish the diagnosis (Fig. 24-81). Bone scanning has been advocated if conventional radiographs do not demonstrate any abnormality. However, my preference is a 2-week trial of immobilization in a short leg walking cast if history, signs, and symptoms suggest a stress fracture. At the time of cast removal, radiographs often reveal the subperiosteal callus.

A short first metatarsal was once thought to predispose to a fracture of the second metatarsal, but Harris and Beath found no such evidence in their study.[276] Oudjhane et al. studied 500 consecutive radiographic examinations of acutely limping infants and toddlers and reported that 20% had a fracture as the underlying cause.[180] Among these patients, 11 had occult or stress fractures of the metatarsals.

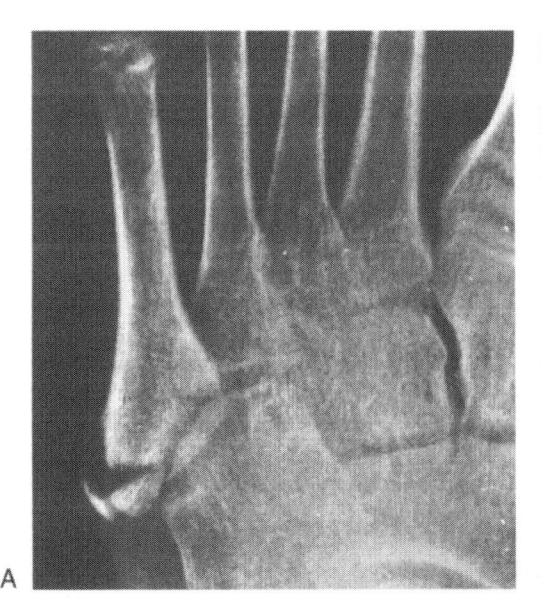

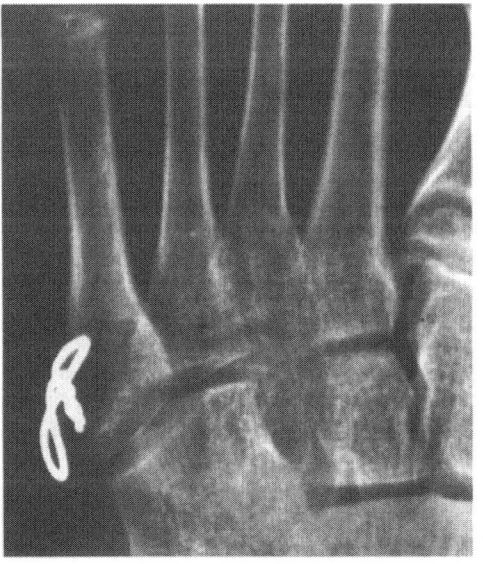

FIGURE 24-79. Tension band fixation of a fifth metatarsal apophyseal avulsion. (A) Fracture. (B) Wiring.

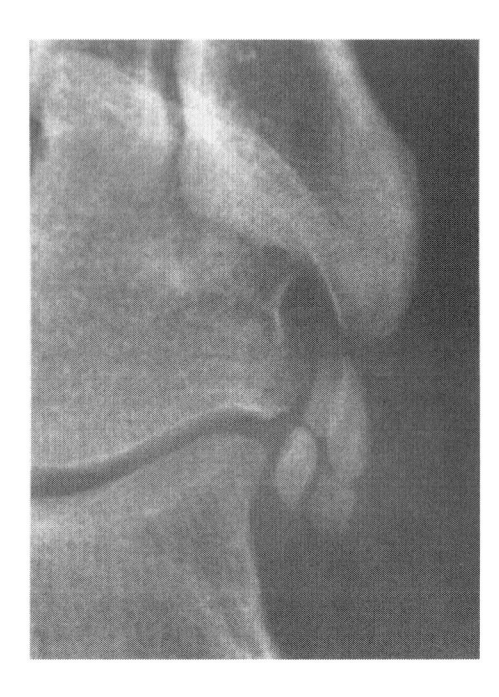

FIGURE 24-80. Multifocal os vesalianum present in a 14-year-old gymnast with repetitive ankle inversion injuries. It is equivalent to an Osgood-Schlatter lesion.

Freiberg's Lesion

The Freiberg lesion is an osteochondrosis of the second metatarsal head (Fig. 24-82). Three of the six original cases reported by Freiberg had a defined history of trauma, and subsequent reports by Smillie and Braddock supported a traumatic etiology.[275] However, there is no accepted correlation between injury to the metatarsal heads and the subsequent appearance of Freiberg's lesion.[266,291] It is probable that the more proximal, rigid fixation of the second metatarsal alters its mechanics relative to the other metatarsals and predisposes it to injury through repetitive impact.

Using detailed scintigraphic collimation, Mandell and Harcke demonstrated a pattern of a photopenic defect with a hyperactive collar and thought that this finding supported the existence of avascular necrosis during infarction.[286] The photopenia was appreciated only on pinhole collimation images. The subsequent revascularization phase with diffuse increase in uptake was also demonstrated.

Braddock experimentally produced a comminuted fracture of the second metatarsal epiphysis in anatomic (autopsy) specimens (age range 4–12 years and young adults) by loading the skeletally immature foot while held in plantar flexion.[266] In contrast, the method produced fractures of the phalanges in younger children or adults. He postulated that the epiphysis was especially vulnerable at an age that correlated with the age at which Freiberg's infraction commonly occurs.

Immobilization is the initial treatment. Occasionally, small osteochondral fragments are fractured from the rest of the distal metatarsal and may call for open reduction if there is significant joint involvement. Elevation of the depressed metatarsal head with bone grafting may be done in severe cases.

Dislocations

Dislocations of the metatarsophalangeal or interphalangeal joints are unusual in children and are ordinarily easily reduced.[294–297,307] The dislocation may be overlooked.

Sesamoids

Leventen discussed sesamoid disorders and treatment, but principally in adults.[316] The maturing of sesamoids of the great toe is rather constant, ossifying during the eighth year in girls and the twelfth year in boys. Usually both sesamoids are present, although congenital absence may involve the medial sesamoid. One or both sesamoids may be multipartite. Partition of the medial sesamoid occurs about 10 times more often than partition of the lateral sesamoid. The partite sesamoid usually shows a smooth outline, which helps differentiate the more irregular outline characteristic of a sesamoid fracture.

The metatarsal sesamoids of the great toe are significantly vulnerable to injury from acute impact trauma and repetitive weight-bearing stresses.[308,311,318,320,321] Injuries to the sesamoids may result in plantar forefoot pain, which can cause severe disability in both the athlete and the nonathlete. Unfortunately, owing to the small size and limited visualization on routine foot radiographs, both clinician and radiologist may ignore the sesamoids and thus overlook them as a significant cause of disabling foot pain. Variable patterns of ossification are common. Partite sesamoids range in incidence from 10% to 33%.[313]

Walling and Ogden described a specimen of a bipartite sesamoid that revealed anatomic cartilaginous continuity in the presence of radiographic osseous discontinuity.[323] Epiphyseal cartilage was present between the two ossific foci, strongly supporting the bipartite ossification process as a developmental variation rather than a posttraumatic phenomenon or fracture. The gaps in the histologic section suggest that a mild separation may have occurred under tensile stress during the development of chondro-osseous transformation.

Burton and Amaker reported a stress fracture of the medial sesamoid in a 7-year-old who participated in ballet.[309] Despite discontinuation of ballet and conservative treatment with orthotics, the child remained symptomatic. MRI showed loss of normal signal intensity in both the T1- and T2-weighted images when compared to that of the lateral sesamoid. Because of continued symptomatology even when walking, the patient underwent resection of the sesamoid, which histologically showed a fibrous nonunion through a fracture. Her symptoms were completely relieved following the resection. These authors noted that young dancers are particularly susceptible to acute, transverse, and stress fractures of the sesamoids; and that typically the symptoms began insidiously and then became progressively intolerable. Van Hal et al. were the first to report stress fractures of the sesamoid bones of the toe; they described four patients, all of whom eventually required surgical resection.[322] Others have also reported stress fractures or osteochondritis in active adolescents.[310,314,315,317,319]

Because radiographs do not distinguish a fractured sesamoid from a bipartite or multipartite sesamoid, addi-

FIGURE 24-81. Stress fractures. (A) Evident fracture in the third metatarsal. (B) Two weeks later fractures of the fourth and fifth metatarsals are also evident. (C) Stress fractures of the fourth metatarsal. (D) Healed stress fractures of the fourth and fifth metatarsals.

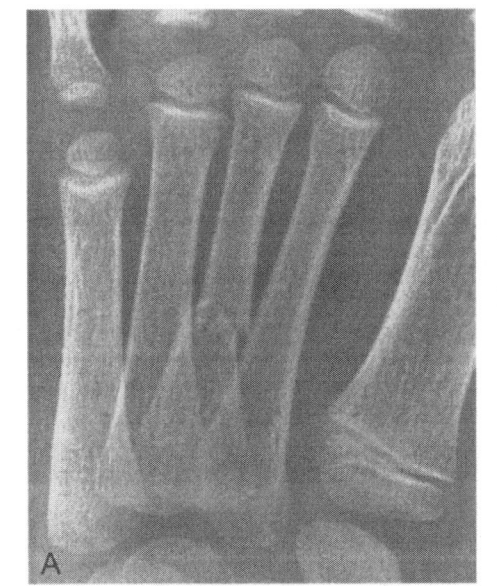

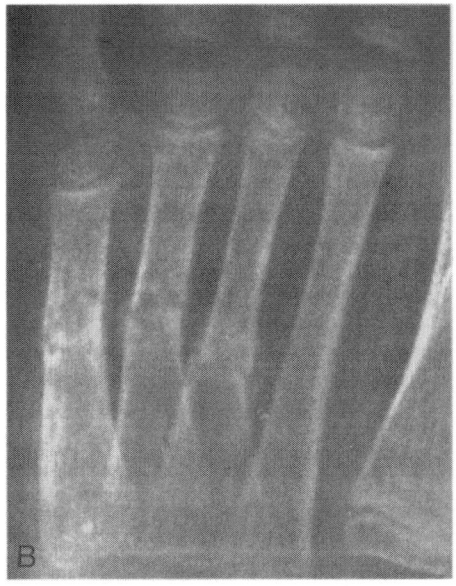

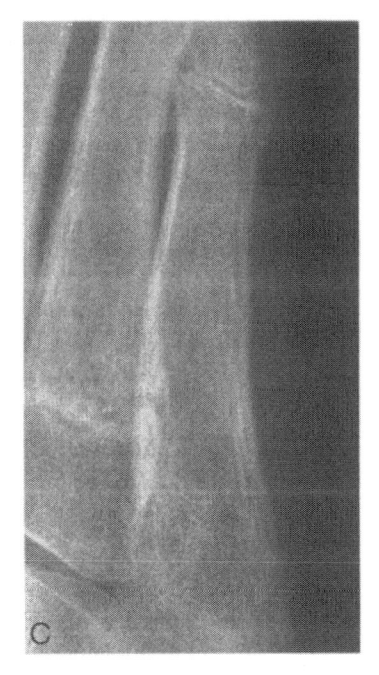

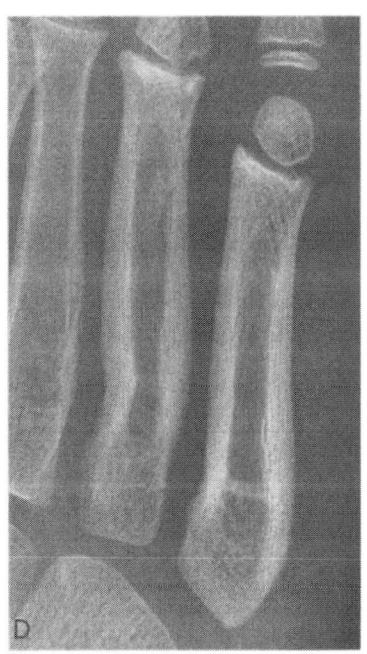

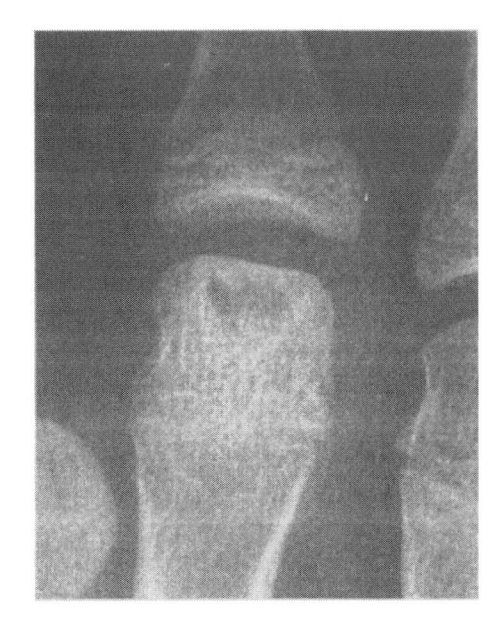

FIGURE 24-82. Freiberg's injury of the distal end of the second metatarsal epiphyseal ossification center. This injury is stress-related.

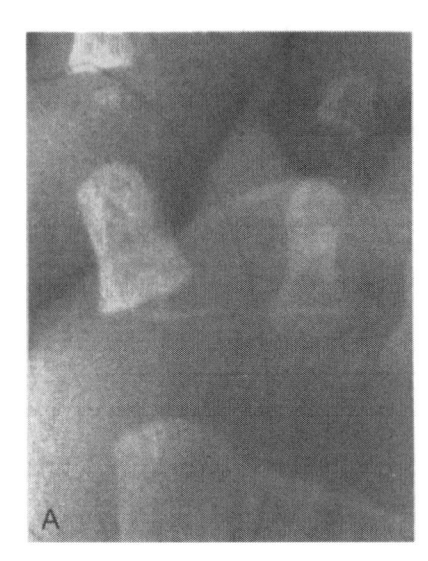

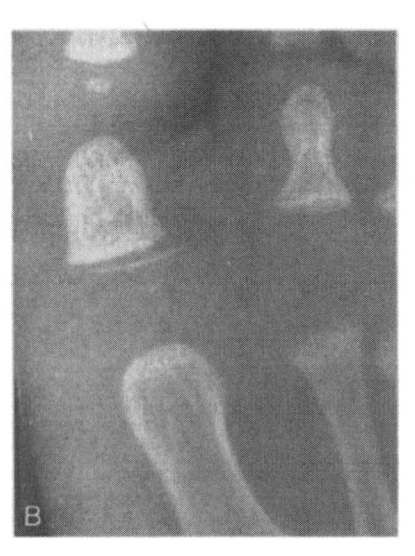

FIGURE 24-83. (A) Medially displaced physeal fracture of the first proximal phalanx. (B) Reduction.

tional imaging may be necessary. A hot bone scan is suggestive of bone turnover and injury, as with injuries to the accessory navicular or the accessory ossicles of the medial and lateral malleoli. MRI also may be influential in making the diagnosis by looking for changes in signal intensity that may be due to ichemia or to edema and hemorrhage. These authors believed that MRI could not distinguish between a stress fracture and ischemic necrosis of the sesamoid. However, they thought that this distinction was moot because both were usually treated by excision if symptoms persisted.

Infrequently, a sesamoid develops osteomyelitis.[312] It is usually due to a puncture wound.

Injuries to the Phalanges

Fractures

Fractures of the phalanges are relatively common, especially to the first toe (Figs. 24-83 to 24-85).[298,299] Type 3 epiphyseal injuries are common and require open reduction if they are significantly displaced. Sometimes only a small portion of the epiphyseal ossification center is involved as a type 7 injury (Fig. 24-86). Damage may seem innocuous but may involve regions of the physis and thus cause subsequent growth deformity. Physeal injuries may also involve the more distal phalangeal epiphyses (see Stubbed Toe, below).

The phalangeal shaft may be affected by angular deformation (Fig. 24-87). More distally, an unstable condylar fracture (Figs. 24-88 to 24-90) may be as problematic as one in the hand.

Fractures of the first toe require close observation and relatively accurate reduction. Malalignment may affect the normal weight-bearing axes of the foot. The deformity should be reduced anatomically, especially if the joint is involved, and may require percutaneous K-wire fixation or open reduction. As in the fingers, care should be taken to prevent rotational malunion.

Open reduction should be considered if an unstable type 3 fragment is present. Skeletal traction may be necessary to maintain reduction. Varus or valgus malalignment should be avoided.

Although most toe physeal fractures involve the great toe, the other toes may be affected.[307] Mozena and Kroepel reported a fracture involving the proximal phalanx of the fourth toe in a 15-year-old boy.[302] The separation was similar to the ulnar deviation seen in the proximal phalanx of the fifth digit in the hand. The method of placing a pencil in the interspace may be used to reduce it.

A common mechanism of injury to any of the lateral four toes is crushing. When the first toe is injured, a crushing force may also be implicated. It is also common for the first toe to be

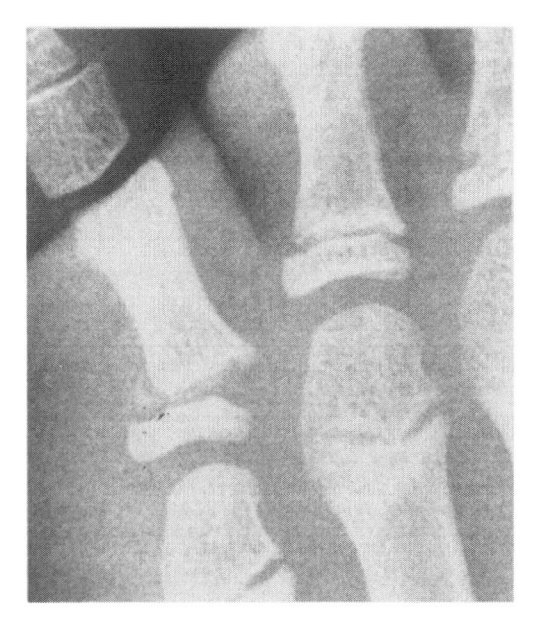

FIGURE 24-84. Displaced type 2 physeal injury.

Injuries to the Phalanges 1139

FIGURE 24-85. (A) Angulated type 2 physeal injury. (B) Complete growth arrest occurred.

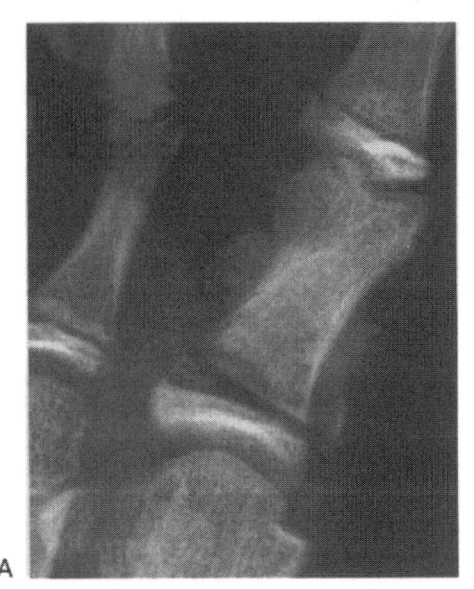

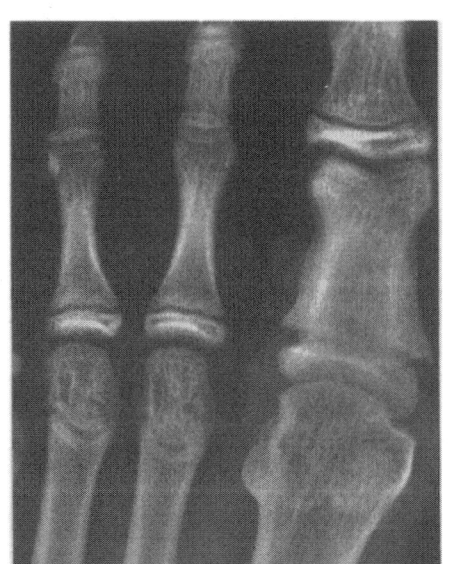

FIGURE 24-86. Type 7 avulsion injuries of the secondary ossification center of the first toe. (A) Proximal phalanx. (B) Distal phalanx. As the toe was forced into a varus position (open arrow), the fracture "propagated" obliquely across the joint to involve the medial proximal phalanx (solid arrows).

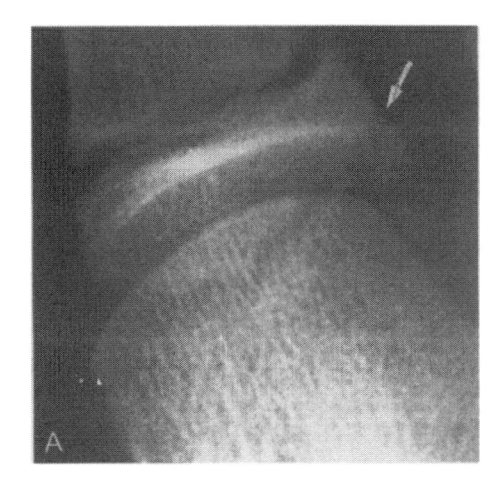

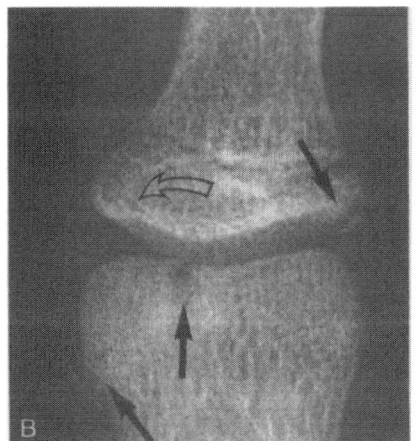

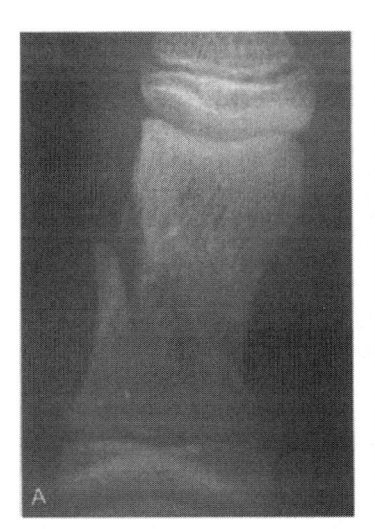

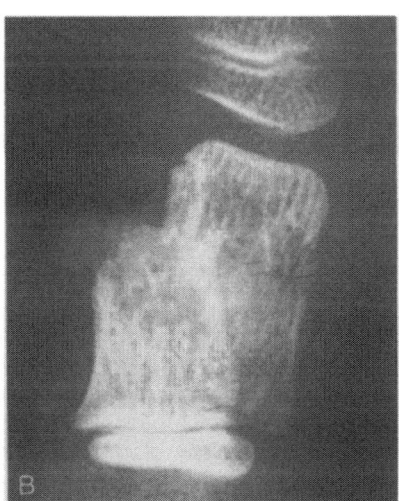

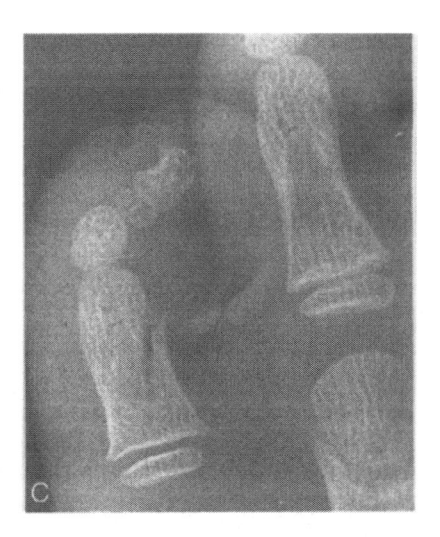

FIGURE 24-87. (A) Shaft fracture with mild angulation. (B) Moderate angular deformity accompanying a shaft fracture. (C) Undisplaced fracture of the phalanx of the fifth toe.

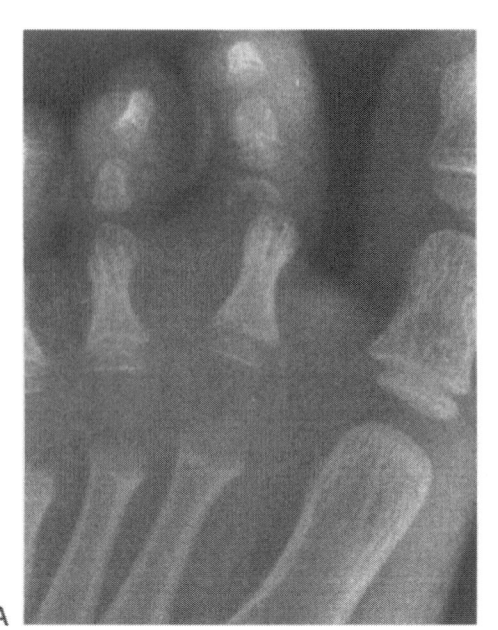

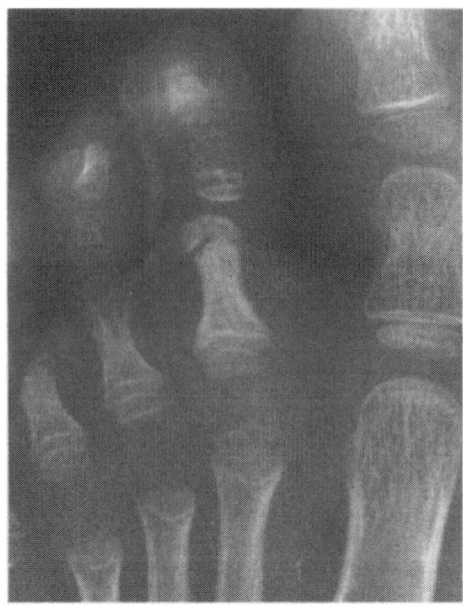

FIGURE 24-88. (A) Displaced condylar fracture. (B) Result 3 weeks after closed reduction.

angulated relative to the rest of the foot, an accident pattern that often occurs when a table leg or similar object is jammed against the first toe or between the toes, or when the child is walking barefooted and hyperflexes the toe.

Fractures involving the lateral four toes seldom require more than symptomatic treatment. Reduction is usually not necessary; most can be adequately treated by taping the injured toe to adjacent, uninjured toes. Cotton, lamb's wool, or some other suitable soft material should be placed between the toes to prevent maceration.

Shiraishi et al. reported three patients with stress fractures of the proximal phalanx of the great toe and thought that the condition resulted after repeated forced dorsiflexion of the first metatarsal phalangeal joint with changing steps in athletes who repeatedly run and jump.[306] It should be suspected in any young athlete who complains of pain in the first metatarsal phalangeal joint in whom there is no history of specific trauma. Shiraishi et al. thought that a fissure was diagnostic of the injury. However, they also noted that this fissure was present in approximately 6% of Japanese children, who are usually symptom-free. Accordingly, the injury may be categorized as radiologic variants that may be present with or without pain.

Stubbed Toe

Children may strike the tip of the toe, sustaining a fracture from a forceful hyperflexion that subsequently reduces spontaneously, a factor that may make diagnosis difficult.[301] The mechanism is similar to a mallet finger.

Fractures of the distal phalanx of the great toe, which usually involve the physis, may be associated with osteomyelitis.[305] The injury mechanism causes small breaks in the dorsal skin that allow bacterial penetration (Fig. 24-91). Pinckney and colleagues described the stubbed great toe as a cause of occult open fracture and infection in six children who sustained type 1 growth mechanism fractures of the distal phalanx.[304] Engber and Clancy have seen a similar phenomenon in the phalanges of the fingers.[300] Noonan et al. reported three cases of stubbed toe. All had lacerated skin

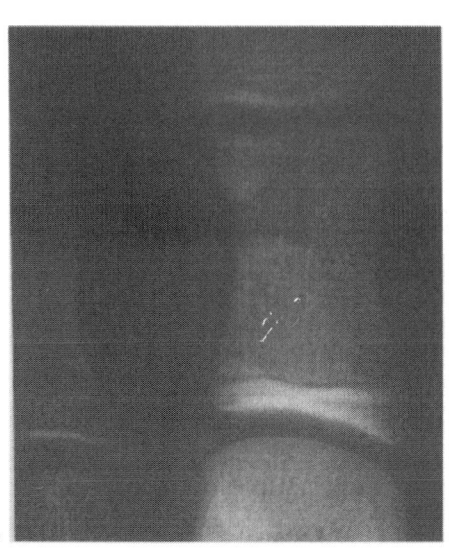

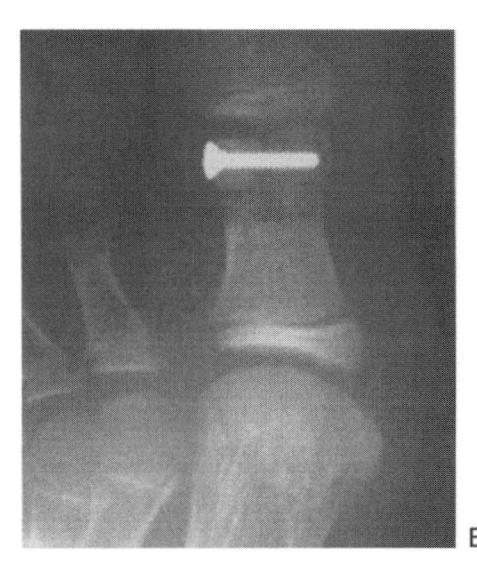

FIGURE 24-89. (A) Unicondylar distal fracture. (B) Result of reduction and fixation.

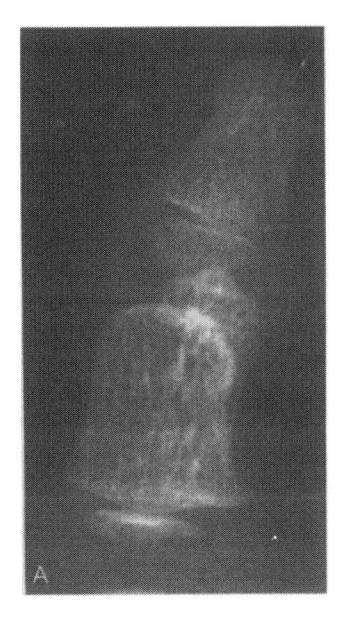

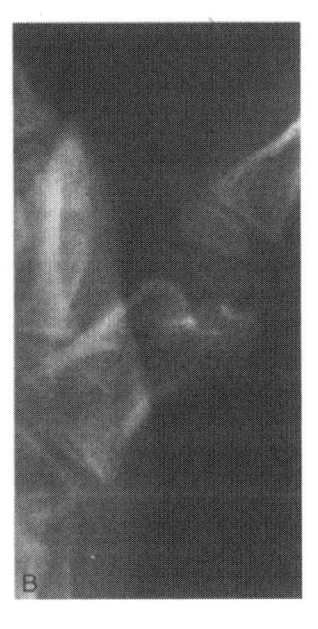

FIGURE 24-90. Unstable, displaced condylar fracture. (A) Anteroposterior view. (B) Lateral view. It had healed in an unreduced position. The patient presented for evaluation of a dorsal mass.

around the bed of the nail and a physeal fracture of the distal phalanx.[303] All became infected, and all three developed partial closure of the physis.

The relation of the bone, physis, and nail in the distal segment of the toe explains the risk of infection. The skin is attached directly to the periosteum, with no intervening layer of subcutaneous tissue (Fig. 24-92). The skin between nail and bone is thinnest directly above the physis, where only the germinal matrix of the nail and the specialized inner layers of the epidermis and a shallow layer of dermis are present. Because of this close apposition of skin and bone, any fracture through the physis, especially with displacement, is likely to extend through the adjacent skin and thereby establish an open fracture. Such a break in the skin or in the depth of the germinal zone of the nail bed may be hidden from view if it reaches the surface through the nail fold, or it may be visible just proximal to the nail fold on the dorsal surface of the toe.

Clinical signs such as bleeding from the nail fold or a laceration proximal to the nail or bleeding underneath the nail, are significant, corroborating the open nature of the injury. Any fracture of the distal physis, whether involving the stubbed great toe or any other of the four toes, should be considered an open injury, even in the absence of absolute clinical or historical evidence. The child should be treated with prophylactic antibiotics to cover the most likely skin microorganisms and common gram-negative bacteria (e.g., *Pseudomonas*). Initial antibiotics are given orally. Parenteral antibiotics are reserved for children who do not respond well and subsequently develop a distinct infection, at which point it is necessary to determine the organism causing the infection and its appropriate antibiotic susceptibilities. Adequate drainage and débridement are essential to prevent chronic osteomyelitis.

Plantar Wounds

Puncture wounds to the foot are common presenting problems in pediatric emergency departments.[379] Although seemingly benign, the consequences of puncture wounds to the foot may include cellulitis, retained foreign bodies, or even osteomyelitis. Despite an apparently benign initial presentation, puncture wounds to the foot in a child may result in

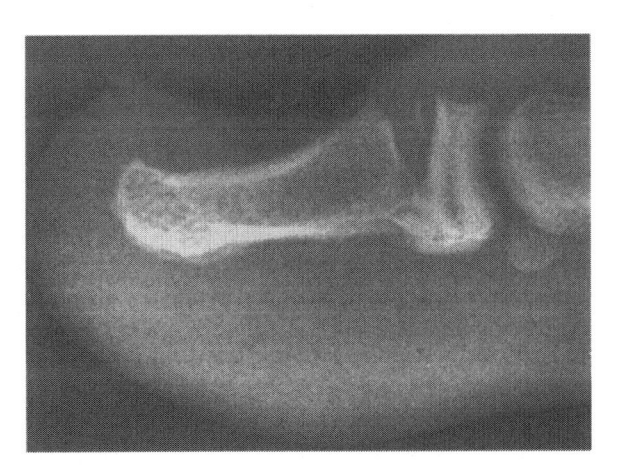

FIGURE 24-91. "Stub" toe fracture of distal phalangeal physis. Note the thin line of metaphyseal bone indicating a type 2 growth mechanism fracture.

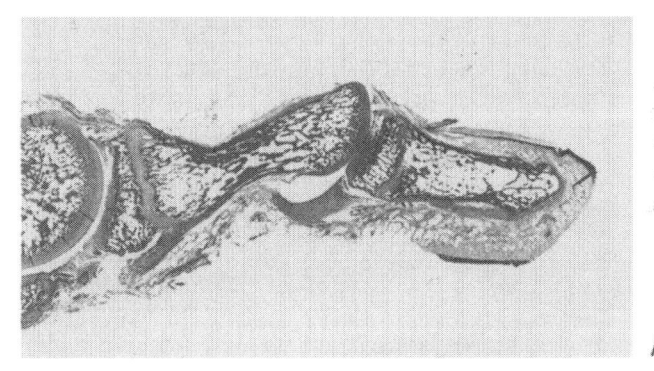

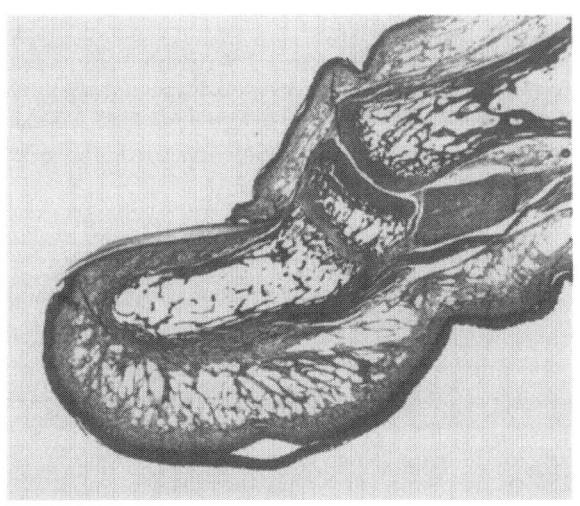

FIGURE 24-92. (A) Interrelation of the physis and the nail bed (arrow). (B) Simulated hyperextension injury shows the nail bed being driven toward the physis.

significant, sometimes severe morbidity. In most climates the highest incidence of injury occurs from May through October, although a greater seasonal incidence may occur in more temperate climates. The patient is most often under 10 years of age; and in most cases a nail is responsible for the injury. Tree branches, thorns, glass, wood splinters, metal objects, plastics, gravel, dirt, straw, or wire comprise the remaining objects reported to cause puncture wounds of the foot.

The barefoot child or adolescent frequently sustains a penetrating wound (puncture, laceration) to the foot or toes.[324–385] Although skin penetration may appear insignificant (especially with a sharp puncture), these wounds often require adequate débridement, tetanus toxoid (when indicated), a broad-spectrum antibiotic, and frequent reexamination during the first week after injury. Many children initially present several days after the injury and may not even recall a specific injury. Penetration may extend to the periosteum or the cortical bone and may eventually lead to osteomyelitis, rather than soft tissue infection (cellulitis). The calcaneus and metatarsal heads are particularly susceptible because of the normal mechanics of walking and running. Sharp objects may migrate if not removed.

The pathophysiology and management of any puncture wound are dependent on the probable material that punctured the foot (if identification is possible), location of the wound, depth of penetration, time from puncture to presentation for care, and overall health status of the patient. The geography is also important. Wounds in soil increase the risk of *Clostridium* infection. Wounds incurred in water carry an increased risk of *Aeromonas* or *Vibrio* species. Several authors have reviewed localized and systemic infection due to a variety of *Vibrio* species present in warm freshwater and saltwater.[354,383] Wallace showed that many species of nontuberculous mycobacteria are prevalent within the aquatic environment and may be readily recovered from both freshwater and saltwater.[380]

Many foot infections are caused by gram-negative, rather than gram-positive, microorganisms. Although *Pseudomonas aeruginosa* is an unusual causative agent of hematogenous osteomyelitis in children, it is a relatively common cause of foot infections following open wounds.[329] These microorganisms are found in soil and may be normal inhabitants of the skin. Therefore they may be reasonably expected to cause infection if the skin barrier is broached. Specific bacteriologic diagnosis by culturing the fluid from spontaneous drainage, aspirations, surgical incisions, and adequate débridement is essential.

Managing the Puncture Wound

In general, the appearance of the wound and the mechanism of injury dictate the most appropriate treatment. Because proper initial treatment is critical for preventing subsequent complications, wound cleansing, probing and débridement, radiographs, prophylactic antibiotics, updated tetanus immunization, and arrangement for follow-up care are essential. Any traumatic puncture wound must be considered dirty and contaminated to some degree by soil, debris, clothing, or bacteria. All puncture wounds therefore should undergo mechanical cleansing or irrigation with copious amounts of sterile saline. Irrigation by syringe with fluid forced in under pressure has been shown to be effective for decreasing the potential contamination within a wound. Iodophor solutions, tincture of green soap, and surfactants have been used for mechanically cleansing and soaking puncture wounds. In contrast, the use of hexachlorophene should be avoided, as it may harbor *Pseudomonas* when stored in open containers. In addition, although this chemical may impair the growth of gram-positive organisms, it may facilitate the growth of gram-negative organisms. Débridement of a wound is dictated by the mechanism of injury and the appearance of the wound site. The edges surrounding the wound are débrided as necessary. A wound is cleansed, probed, and any foreign body or devitalized tissue removed. Radiographic studies are left to the discretion of the treating physician. Many materials are radiolucent and therefore difficult to detect on standard radiography.

The problem of managing deep lacerations of the plantar surface of the foot in children has received little attention. There is no unanimity of opinion about management.[385] Chisholm and Schlesser divided management approaches into two basic categories: within 24 hours and after 24 hours.[333]

Patients presenting less than 24 hours after injury constitute a relatively low risk group for complications. Any wounds should be inspected, and if the plantar surface of the foot is grossly soiled, a detergent wash may be done, followed by appropriate débridement.

Deep wounds should be carefully cleaned and explored. Profuse irrigation and débridement are necessary. Intraoperative radiography with probes may better demonstrate the true depth of the wound and whether skeletal or tendon injury may have occurred.

Puncture wounds should not be closed, particularly if the wound is contaminated or if the puncture, by probing, penetrates to the deep fascia.

Interestingly, the time to presentation, which is also prognostic of the potential for poor outcome, is not a major factor in children, who tend to be brought to the emergency department by a concerned parent or guardian relatively soon after the injury. Late presenters tend to have ignored the original wound and generally present because of subclinical infections, increasing pain, swelling, drainage, or a combination.

Because superficial puncture wounds usually heal well, the depth of penetration becomes the most critical factor. Punctures of the metatarsal phalangeal joint area may also be at higher risk for serious wound complications because of the greater likelihood of such injuries on the weight-bearing portion of the foot penetrating deeper, possibly entering bone, cartilage, or joint.

Superficial irrigation of the puncture site of the dermis that is exposed is acceptable. The injection of fluid under pressure into a closed wound tract may be contraindicated because of foreign bodies, bacteria, or both. The concept of coring does not seem to be associated with any reduction of complications.

There are no good studies showing that the use of prophylactic antibiotics prevents wound complications. Until benefit is demonstrated in a well-detailed prospective study, antibiotics are probably best reserved for treating established wound infections. Adequate mechanical cleansing or débridement are much more important to the prognosis.

Tetanus immunization must be updated as indicated by the patient's history. A leading cause of tetanus infection is the minor wound. Approximately 95% of patients reported with tetanus during 1982 to 1984 had *not* received a primary series of tetanus immunizations. The use of tetanus anatoxin is controversial. The administration of 500 units of tetanus immune globulin should be considered if the patient has never been immunized, is incompletely immunized, or the immunization status is uncertain.

Chondro-osseous Infection

The early diagnosis of osteomyelitis prior to roentgenographic changes (which may take 7–10 days to appear) can often be made with bone scans (e.g., technetium, gallium, or labeled leukocytes). Johanson reported an average delay before diagnosis of 3 weeks from the time of onset of symptoms.[360] In the series of Brand and Black the average delay from injury to diagnosis was 23 days.[329] Atypical osteomyelitis of the foot in children, particularly that caused by *Pseudomonas aeruginosa*, should be suspected when any puncture wound has occurred and the symptoms and signs of infection do not abate within 2–4 days after beginning therapy.

The typical history is that of a patient with an onset of local pain and swelling 2–5 days after a puncture wound. Roentgenograms initially show no osseous reaction. There usually is partial resolution of the inflammation with the initial therapeutic regimen, but symptoms and signs of infection either return or do not fully subside. If cultures from spontaneous drainage or from the surgical drainage incision reveal *Pseudomonas*, the organisms should not be considered a contaminant, particularly if the culture shows a mixture of organisms. If treatment with oral antibiotics is unsuccessful, symptoms probably persist, and subsequent roentgenograms demonstrate osseous changes 8–21 days after injury. A more aggressive therapeutic course, including surgery, is then instituted, although the infection is relatively advanced by this stage.

Jacobs and coworkers found that the initial administration of parenteral antibiotics alone (especially those effective against *Pseudomonas*) for 1–14 days did *not* result in clinical improvement.[356,357] Eradication of *Pseudomonas* osteomyelitis occurred *only after thorough surgical débridement and curettage of tissue*. Following such débridement, antibiotic therapy effective against *Pseudomonas* was continued for an average of 10 days. These investigators thought that only 1–2 weeks of this antibiotic therapy was necessary after thorough surgical débridement, rather than the "arbitrary 6 weeks."

The appropriate antibiotic, especially for *Pseudomonas* osteomyelitis, depends on sensitivity studies. Many new antibiotics have been and are being introduced. Approval for use in children should be verified. Consultation with an infectious disease specialist may be obtained. The length of antibiotic therapy varies from case to case, but significant bone involvement is generally an indication for parenteral therapy combined with surgical drainage.

Baltimore and Jensen described puncture wound osteochondritis of the foot caused by *Pseudomonas maltophilia* and stressed the importance of establishing the specific etiology with this organism, as it affects treatment considerations (i.e., antibiotic choices).[326] In most cases the source of *Pseudomonas* appears to be the layer of foam rubber cushion found in sneakers, but it has not been reliably found on the surfaces of such shoes[345,349] *P. maltophilia* tends to be found in warm, moist environments. This particular organism typically displays an unusually broad pattern of resistance to antimicrobial agents. Combined surgical débridement and antimicrobial therapy are recommended. In particular, it is resistant to aminoglycosides, penicillins (first and second generation), imipenem, and aztreonam.

Doberstein et al. reported group B β-hemolytic streptococcus as a cause of osteomyelitis of the calcaneus, in contrast to the more common staphylococcal causation.[340]

Midani and Rathmore described a 10-year-old who stepped on a catfish spine and developed a *Vibrio* osteomyelitis. *Vibrio* is the more common saltwater catfish spine organism, not *Aeromonas hydrophilia*, which is the common infectious organism with freshwater catfish spine injury.[365]

Murray et al. reported two children who developed osteochondritis caused by *Serratia* after foot puncture wounds.[369] They noted that *Serratia* species are unique among the Enterobacteriaceae, but similar to *Pseudomonas*, in their production of three extracellular hydrolytic enzymes: deoxyribonuclease, gelatinase, and lipase. These enzymes are probably important in the pathogenesis of infection after foot puncture wounds and probably contribute to the predominance of *Pseudomonas* and the recurrence of *Serratia*.

Despite treatment, permanent skeletal changes, such as premature epiphysiodesis of the proximal phalanx of the first toe, may occur (Fig. 24-93). The infection involves the peripheral growth regions (zone of Ranvier), which are intracapsular in this epiphyseal-physeal unit (Fig. 24-94). This involvement leads to progressive epiphysiodesis as extensive peripheral osseous bridges form.

Barton et al. looked at the long-term radiologic outcome of *Pseudomonas* osteomyelitis of the feet of 27 patients.[327] Fifteen patients returned for follow-up 1–8 years after

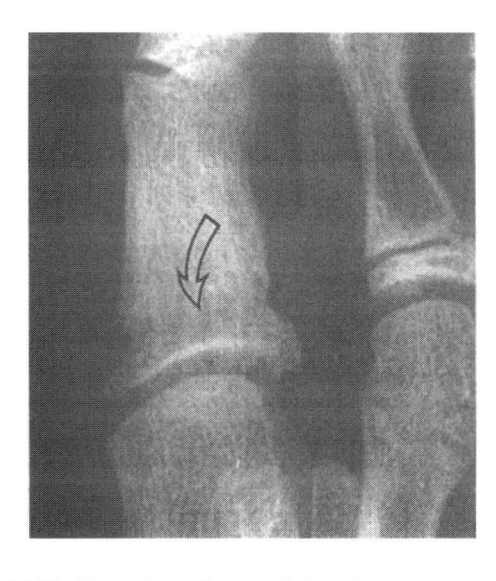

FIGURE 24-93. Premature closure of the physis of the proximal phalanx following puncture wound infection.

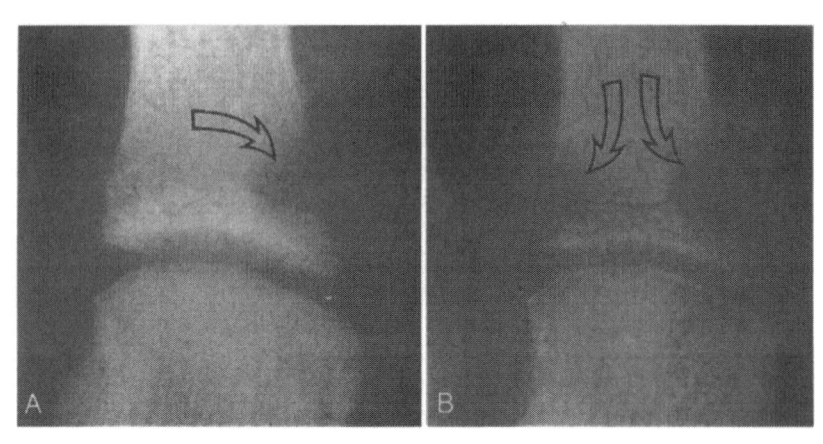

FIGURE 24-94. Osteomyelitis secondary to a small puncture wound. (A) Appearance 3 weeks after the original injury (arrow). (B) Despite débridement, further destruction continued (arrows). (C) Surgical specimen showing peripheral destruction of the physis (arrow). AC = articular cartilage; P = physis.

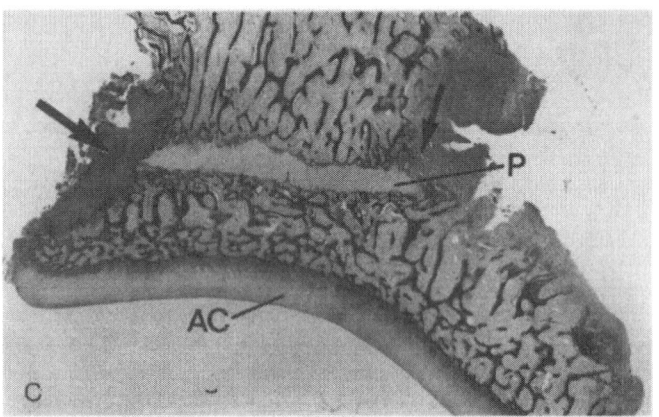

hospitalization. Poor radiologic outcome, ranging from bony deformity to joint space abnormality, was noted in four patients. Clinical abnormality was noted in only one adolescent boy, and he had the most severe radiologic sequelae. The long-term functional significance of these radiologic anomalies awaits further delineation and detailed outcome studies.

Foreign Bodies

Foreign bodies are common causes of injury in children. There may be no clear history of penetrating injury, and radiographs may be negative, which challenges the physician to formulate an effective treatment plan. Localized inflammation, edema, and tenderness should raise a degree of suspicion that a retained foreign body is the source, particularly if there is an extended period from a defined injury.

The presence of a foreign body in a puncture wound tract is one of the most difficult diagnostic and management dilemmas. Fitzgerald and Cowan found foreign bodies complicating puncture wounds in 26 of 887 patients, with 50% being pieces of a tennis shoe or sock introduced into the wound tract.[346] They also found that five of nine patients with an unresolved culture-positive cellulitis, who were treated with the appropriate antibiotic, had an unrecognized foreign body.[338] These authors reviewed some of the theories of the source of *Pseudomonas*. They noted that cultured inner, middle, and outer layers of sneaker soles from patients with puncture wound osteomyelitis revealed *Pseudomonas* in seven of eight cases.[345] In contrast, *Pseudomonas* was recovered only 9% of the time when they cultured nonpunctured, donated gym shoes; and the organism was absent in new controls. They postulated that *Pseudomonas* colonized in the warm, damp environment of the sneaker sole and was inoculated by small pieces of foam when the child stepped on the puncturing nail or other sharp object.

Porat et al. reported a patient who, 6 months before presentation, had stepped on a palm thorn that penetrated the plantar aspect of his heel.[370] Medical treatment with repetitive antibiotics and antiinflammatory drugs was unsuccessful. Surgical treatment included removal of the thorn, tenosynovectomy around tendons, excision of a granuloma, and curettage of an osteomyelitic lesion of the calcaneus. Surgical excision of these foreign bodies is strongly recommended (Fig. 24-95).

Localization of small foreign bodies for removal is not always easy. If the foreign body is radiopaque, a simple technique may be used. A marker is placed over an entry wound. Three or four needles of differing gauges are then placed in the probable vicinity of the lesion, and another radiograph is obtained. The needle closest to the foreign body is then identified.

According to Cracchiolo, wooden foreign bodies are difficult to detect radiographically or with xerography.[337] However, wood may produce a variety of reactions depending on the tissue within which the foreign body comes into contact. Chronic tendonitis may occur if the material is lodged in or near a tendon sheath. Periosteal reactions may also occur along metatarsal shafts or the tarsal bones.

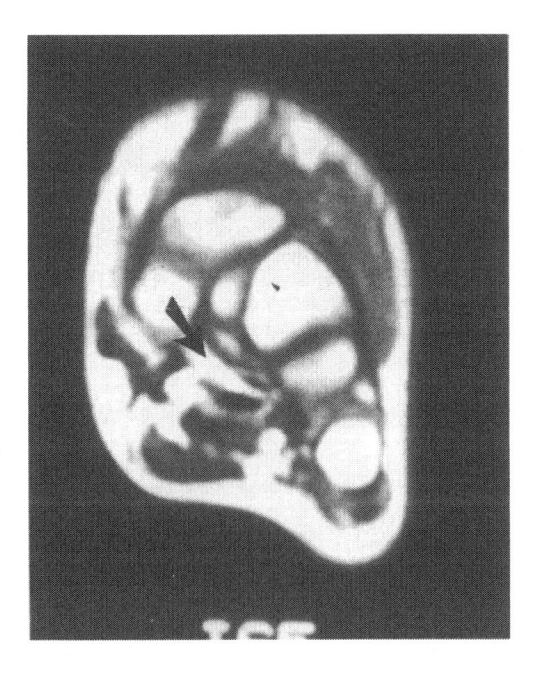

FIGURE 24-95. This 11-year-old stepped on a palm thorn, which was "pulled out" in the emergency room. She presented with a swollen, erythematous foot 3 weeks later. MRI revealed the end of the thorn (arrow) surrounded by an abscess, along with the penetration tract. It was removed.

Simmons et al.[375] and Swishuk et al.[377] reported cases of young boys who had MRI-identified lesions that were initially interpreted as tumors and were found to have wood lodged in a cavity caused by an abscess.

Kobs et al. were able to delineate a retained piece of wood fragment through ultrasonographic localization on the plantar aspect of the foot.[362] This allowed localization and subsequent removal. Crawford also recommended the use of ultrasonography for radiolucent and radiodense objects.[31]

Charney et al. showed that xerography was superior to radiography for detecting nonmetallic foreign bodies,[332] particularly material such as glass. They studied 66 kinds of glass fragment and showed that fragments as small as 0.5 mm when unobscured by bone and as small as 2.0 mm when superimposed on bone could be detected by xerography and often by radiography. They further found that the literature regarding wooden foreign bodies was conflicting and often inconclusive. Woesner and Sanders were able to detect a wooden fragment placed in a water phantom but were unable to detect the same fragment when it was implanted in an experimental animal.[384] In contrast, these same examiners were able to show that xerography visualized the wood in the animal tissue. After being embedded in soft tissue for more than 48 hours wood splinters and wooden toothpicks become waterlogged and are much more difficult to detect by xerography. Woesner and Sanders implanted a number of different materials and showed a varying degree of visibility.[384] These authors also showed that gravel, tile, and clay were highly visible, along with glass, on regular radiography. In contrast, wooden and plastic foreign bodies may or may not be seen on standard radiographs, which relates to the configuration of the implanted material, orientation relative to bone, and the direction of the x-ray beam. Standard projections remain the most clinically practical means of screening for foreign bodies. If none is found and there is still a high index of suspicion, xerography should be implemented next.

Pins and needles are the most commonly encountered foreign bodies. The object is usually superficial, but it may migrate into deeper tissues with weight-bearing. Although it is stated that removal is often not necessary unless there is bone, joint, or neurovascular involvement, if a sharp object continues to migrate it may eventually cause problems. I believe that these objects should be removed if detected using limited surgical exposure and triangulation to determine the site of the object. The indications for removal include persistent discomfort with or without weight-bearing and chronically draining or infected wounds. Electromagnetic metal detectors are also sometimes used. My preference is again to use radiography, CT scanning, or MRI to try to visualize the most likely location of an object three-dimensionally and to have C-arm equipment available in the operating room. Deep wooden foreign bodies may be asymptomatic for some time, but they eventually become symptomatic as an inflammatory reaction develops. The reaction is different depending on the tissue involved and the material involved. Glass-induced wounds frequently cause more extensive lacerations than the superficial location might suggest. Tendon and neurovascular function must be carefully evaluated for all glass-induced lacerations. A fragment of glass within a joint may cause damage to the articular surface.

Lawn Mower Injuries

The most destructive injuries to the child's foot result from crushing by an automobile tire or laceration by a power lawn mower.[386,389,392,395,397,398,400,423,426] These injuries require considerable judgment regarding the extent of tissue damage, especially at the time of initial evaluation in the acute setting. Of the 18 children reported by Ross and associates, 11 children were riding on the mower with their parent at the time of injury.[413] The spinning blades carry tremendous destructive forces, cutting through soft tissue and bone alike.[409] Furthermore, fragments of dirt, grass, and debris enter the wound under pressure.

When the physes are involved, conservative initial débridement is recommended. However, there should be no reservation about removing areas that become infected or that appear nonviable (Figs. 24-96 to 24-98). If an epiphysis and its attached physis are stripped of virtually all soft tissue connections, the fragment is only going to serve as a sequestrum, and the potential for growth is extremely limited.

The surgeon often must use ingenuity and knowledge of anatomy and biomechanics to reconstruct the most functional foot possible with the remaining viable structures. Extensive trauma to the heel with loss of weight-bearing sensate skin after lawnmower injuries, especially when coupled with loss of some of the posterior portion of the calcaneus or its apophysis (or both), presents a major reconstructive challenge. The loss of bone limits the capacity of the calcaneus to bear weight in a normal fashion. In the

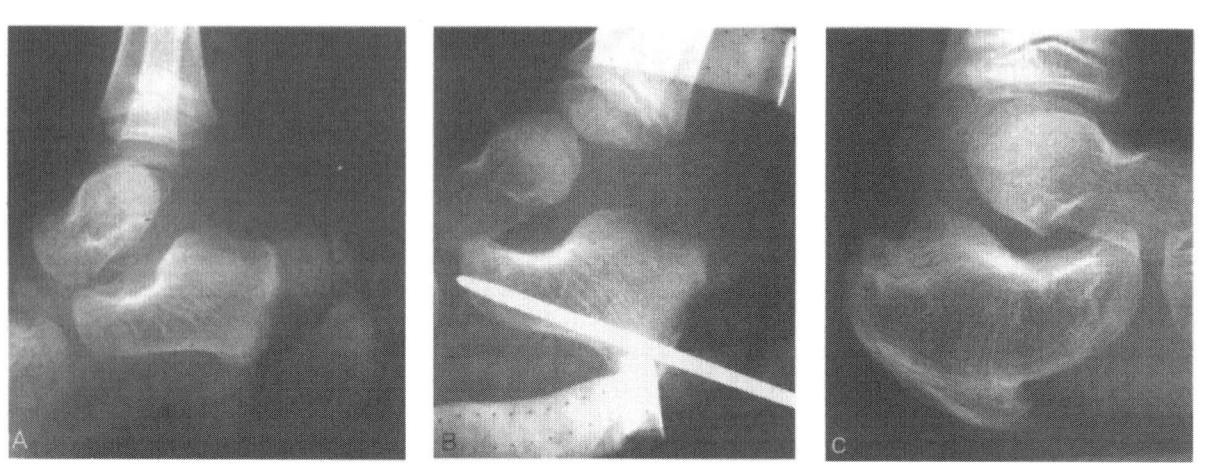

FIGURE 24-96. Heel damage after lawn mower injury. (A) Open injury. (B) Fixation of damaged apophysis and remaining heel pad. (C) Deformity of the calcaneus consequent to growth impairment.

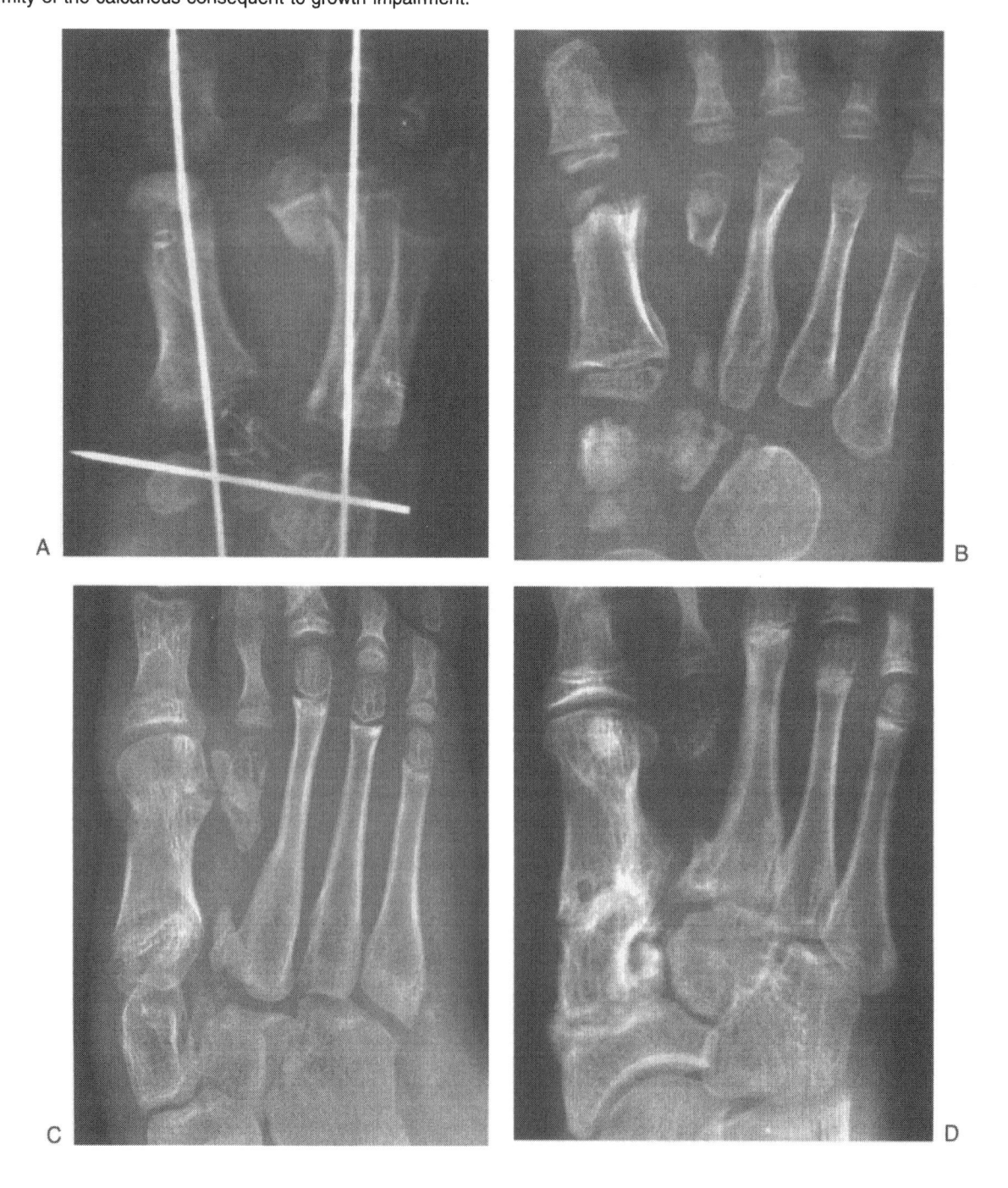

FIGURE 24-97. Lawn mower injury. (A) Stabilization of fractures during the period of repeated débridement. The remainder of the second metatarsal was at the accident scene. Soft tissue and osseous healing occurred without infection. (B) Ten days later. (C) Five years later. (D) Seven years later. Note the progressive changes in the midfoot with spontaneous fusion.

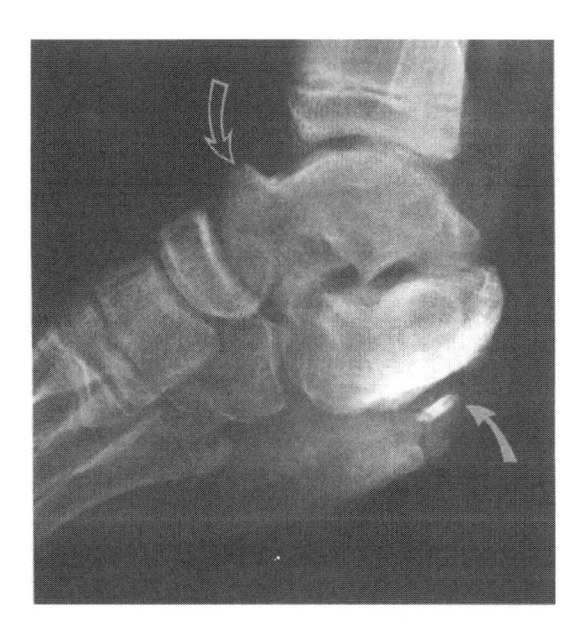

FIGURE 24-98. Lawnmower injury to the heel. The talar exostosis (open arrow) was probably related to altered foot mechanics (loss of distal Achilles tendon). A painful ossicle formed (solid arrow), probably from an avulsed piece of calcaneal apophysis that subsequently ossified.

young child any type of damage to the apophysis that results in the underdevelopment of this area may create a similar effect. The ideal heel reconstruction to lessen the soft tissue problems associated with this type of injury should have several characteristics, the most important of which is durability.[399,405] Local sensation in the reconstructed heel provides protection against repetitive traumatic breakdown. Other factors include a satisfactory cosmetic appearance and an ability to fit into a regular shoe.

For foot injuries with gross tissue loss, split skin grafts do not usually provide adequate coverage for weight-bearing or tendon gliding; and they cannot be used where joint or bone are exposed. There are limitations to the use of local flaps, particularly relative to size and mobility. Furthermore, raising a flap inflicts an additional injury to the already severely traumatized foot. The advantage of microvascular flaps over distant pedicle flaps, such as the cross leg flap, is that the former may solve the problem of coverage in a single stage more conveniently with fewer donor site problems.[387,388,394,412,414,415,424] For providing coverage with any flap, it is essential that the complex wound of the foot be converted to a surgically clean, excised area with stable skeletal structures. There is little to justify the use of emergency free flaps. Adequate débridement and delayed reconstruction is much more appropriate, particularly in the obviously contaminated wound of a lawn mower injury.

The ideal flap for reconstruction of a foot wound should include thin, durable, hairless skin with potential for reinnervation. The lateral arm flap may meet these demands. The thicker the flap, the more likely it is that there will be fissuring at the edges due to shear forces in the bulky flap. This may be solved by flap thinning and tightening in combination with scar excision and Z-plasties.

Several techniques are available for heel reconstruction. Skin grafts, local flaps, and flaps transferred from a distant site have been used.[391,392,396,401-404,417] In the presence of an exposed calcaneus stripped of periosteum, split-thickness skin grafting would probably be unsuccessful. Furthermore, a split-thickness skin graft is generally not sufficiently durable to provide lasting heel coverage, especially in an active child or adolescent.

The plantar surface of the foot may provide donor sites useful for heel reconstruction. Local random skin flaps have been transferred to the heel[391]; they are often sensate or rapidly become so through the ingrowth of adjacent cutaneous sensory nerves.[408] However, the use of a random skin flap may be precluded by the extent of heel injury. The dorsalis pedis flap reaches the medial or lateral side of the heel but does not easily reach the plantar surface.[406,407]

Neurovascular island flaps from the foot allow heel reconstruction with immediate sensation. These flaps include the transposition of innervated skin from the toe,[419] dorsum,[401] or plantar surface[411] of the foot. The sensate flexor digitorum brevis musculocutaneous flap has proved useful for treating adults with heel injuries.[396,418,420] The flap is stable when subjected to the stress of weight-bearing, is not bulky, and has a satisfactory appearance. Moreover, donor site morbidity is minimal.

If local tissue is unavailable, heel reconstruction may be accomplished by cross-foot or cross-leg flaps.[408,422] Immobilization is then prolonged. Complications of cross-extremity procedures, including flap necrosis, infection, pressure ulceration, and neuropathy, have been described.[372] Children tolerate the immobilization and rehabilitation periods better than adults.

Free tissue transfers for heel reconstruction have also been described. The latissimus dorsi musculocutaneous flap and scapular flap both provide satisfactory reconstruction.[416,421,425]

Serafin and associates listed the indications for lower extremity reconstruction with vascularized tissue transferred from a distant site as: (1) large avulsion injuries; (2) failure of conventional reconstructive techniques; (3) treatment of extensive chronic osteomyelitis; (4) deficiency of soft tissue cover and skeletal support; (5) restoration of form and contour with minimal secondary deformity at the donor site; and (6) extensive isolated soft tissue loss.[416]

Rajacic et al., assessing a number of flaps for use in children with avulsions of the dorsum of the foot, found that the relatively high failure rate (approximating 15%) was caused mainly by postoperative arterial occlusion.[410] They suggested that an anastomosis be placed as far proximal to the injury as possible, preferably with suturing to an uninjured artery. Proper assessment of blood flow from the proximal arterial stump after transection and education of nursing staff and monitoring of blood circulation in free flaps lessens the risk of failure. They also found that the most common reasons for subsequent procedures included excessive bulk of the flaps, contractures and overriding of the toes, instability of the ankle joint, and adhesion of tendons to the flap. Bulkiness may be avoided by careful selection of the flap, proper tailoring of the flap to the contours of the area, and suturing under slight transverse tension. They found that in patients in whom the skin defect included the dorsal aspect of the toes a wavy or undulating design of the distal edge of the flap could prevent overriding of the toes.

Stevenson and colleagues described a flap utilizing the flexor digitorum brevis and its overlying muscle, fat, and skin with local transposition to the heel.[420] This muscle is nourished by calcaneal branches from the lateral plantar vessels, and the skin is innervated by a branch of the lateral plantar nerve. The ability to use this flap is contingent on the extent of injury, as many of the posterior injuries damage the blood and nerve supplies to the sole of the foot. A meticulous examination of the sensory capacity of the area *prior to* any consideration of the flap is necessary.

Because of the nature of the injury and the high risk of deep tissue contamination, replantation is usually not a feasible procedure. However, if a reasonably clean, sharp amputation has occurred, such a procedure may be considered.[390,392]

Tarsal Tunnel

Albrektsson et al. evaluated 10 children with tarsal tunnel syndrome.[427] Six of the children walked with the affected foot in supination. The pain was usually described as a burning sensation in the sole and more pronounced in the medial part. Some patients also reported a feeling of numbness in the foot. All patients reported paresthesias in the sole, often radiating to the toes on percussion over the tibial nerve behind the medial malleolus. This sign was a prerequisite for the diagnosis. Nine patients had tenderness over the tarsal tunnel. All underwent surgery. At follow-up nine patients were symptom-free, and the tenth had improved. The operative technique involved division of the lanciate ligament and exposure of the tibial nerve and the medial and lateral plantar nerves, freeing them from any adhesions or constricting bands. Interestingly, all the patients reported in this series were girls. Three patients reported recurrent episodes of sharp pain in the foot. Similarly, pain by day leading to total inability to put weight on the foot has not been reported in adults but has occurred in four children. It is easy to confuse this syndrome with reflex sympathetic dystrophy (RSD). Because of the presence of hyperesthesia and the relief obtained temporarily after a sympathetic block, RSD is usually preceded by an injury but can occur without one.

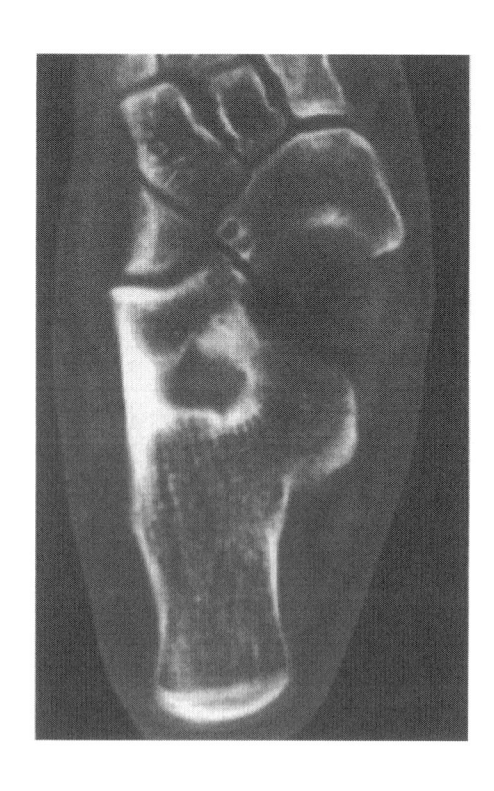

FIGURE 24-100. This patient had foot pain. Even though a coalition is not evident, the apposed bone and cysts suggest at least a fibrocartilaginous coalition.

Plantar Tendons

Tendon injuries are relatively uncommon in children,[432] but a high index of suspicion must be maintained in both the child with chronic pain in the foot or ankle and the child with a sharp laceration in these regions. Repetitive injury in sports such as gymnastics may stretch retinacular tissues, allowing subluxation or dislocation of tendons.[428,429,431,435,436]

Wicks and associates[437] discussed tendon injuries caused by laceration about the foot and ankle in children. They found that injuries to the Achilles, anterior tibial, and posterior tibial tendons resulted in significant deformity when not promptly recognized and repaired.

Masterson et al. described pes planus due to tibialis posterior tendon injuries and recommended treatment by a flexor hallucis longus tendon transfer.[434] Others have found similar biomechanical disruption.[430,432,433] The possibility of tibialis posterior tendon injury and lacerations around the medial malleolus should always be kept in mind. Damage to tendon sheaths or contiguous bursal tissue may lead to post-traumatic calcification.[442]

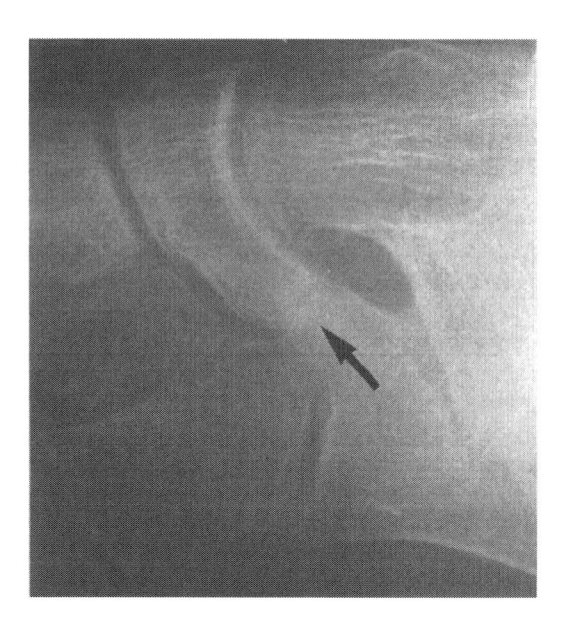

FIGURE 24-99. Calcaneonavicular bar with painful pseudarthrosis (arrow).

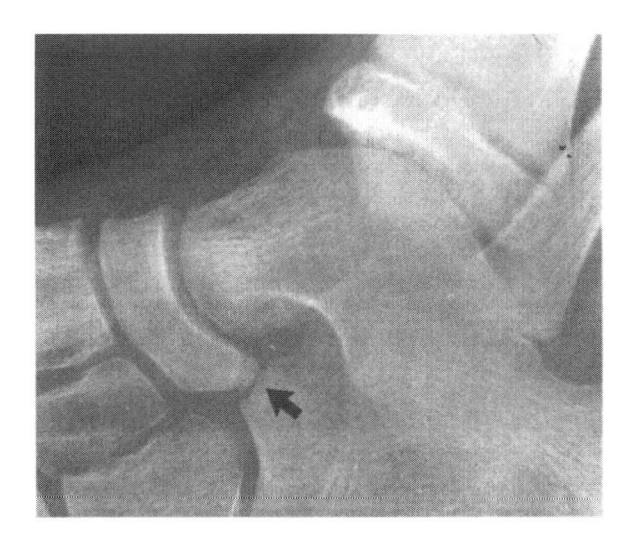

FIGURE 24-101. During evaluation for peroneal spasm a calcaneus secandarius (arrow) was found, rather than a coalition. It was eventually treated by resection and soft tissue interposition when conservative treatment failed.

Ligaments

Chronic ankle ligament injury in children is underemphasized, probably due to the concept that physeal or epiphyseal failure of the malleoli is the more likely injury. Avulsion of the talus or malleolus may be the only evidence of such ligament failure. However, mid-substance failure of ankle ligaments may occur and require repair methods that do not interfere with physeal growth.[438] See Chapter 23 for a further discussion of ankle ligament injuries.

Congenital Deformity

Foot pain following childhood injury may be the result of rendering a congenital defect symptomatic (Figs. 24-99 to 24-101). Tarsal coalitions particularly must be ruled out in children with painful flat feet.[439-441,443-446,448-451] They most commonly are calcaneonavicular and talocalcaneal bars (Fig. 24-99). As these coalitions mature (i.e., progressively calcify and ossify), resilience lessens. Cartilaginous or fibrocartilaginous bars are reasonably flexible, whereas osseous maturation decreasingly removes motion and increases the likelihood of trauma-induced pain or even fracture. Onset of symptoms is more likely during the second decade, when chondro-osseous maturation "stiffens" the previously resilient deformity (Fig. 24-100). Richards et al. reported a fracture through a calcaneonavicular bar in a patient with bilateral tarsal coalition.[448] The fracture healed, but the symptoms persisted.

Children with sensory neuropathic conditions such as myelomeningocele, Lesch-Nyhan syndrome, congenital insensitivity to pain, and syringomyelia may have nonpainful, chronic damage to the ossifying portions of the foot bones. Over time, these insidious disruptions of the normal chondro-osseous transformation processes may lead to significant deformity due to crushing or premature growth arrest.

Children with sensory neuropathies are particularly prone to occult puncture wounds with deep abscess formation or osteomyelitis. Parents and patients must be educated frequently on the importance of proper shoe fit and daily observation of the feet for areas of redness or swelling.

Children may develop subungual exostoses, especially of the great toe.[447] They often become symptomatic following an athletic injury. They are isolated lesions. Removal is necessary because of pain.

References

Anatomy

1. Alexander RM, Bennett MB, Ker RF. Mechanical properties and function of the paw pads of some mammals. J Zool (Lond) 1986;209:405–419.
2. Bennett MB, Ker RF. The mechanical properties of the human subcalcaneal fat pad in compression. J Anat 1990;171:131–138.
3. Blais MM, Green WT, Anderson M. Lengths of the growing foot. J Bone Joint Surg Am 1956;38:998–1000.
4. Blechschmidt E. The structure of the calcaneal padding. Foot Ankle 1983;2:260–283.
5. Brower AC. The osteochondroses. Orthop Clin North Am 1983;14:99–117.
6. Buschmann WR, Jahss MH, Kummer F, et al. Histology and histomorphometric analysis of the normal and atrophic heel fat pad. Foot Ankle 1995;16:254–258.
7. Caffey J. Pediatric X-ray Diagnosis, 6th ed. Chicago: Year Book, 1972.
8. Gelberman RH, Mortensen WW. The arterial anatomy of the talus. Foot Ankle 1983;4:64–72.
9. Grogan DP, Walling AK, Ogden JA. Anatomy of the os trigonum. J Pediatr Orthop 1990;10:618–622.
10. Harris EJ. The relationship of the ossification centers of the talus and calcaneus of the developing bone. J Am Podiatr Assoc 1976;66:76–81.
11. Howard CB, Benson MK. The ossific nuclei and the cartilage anlage of the talus and calcaneum. J Bone Joint Surg Br 1992;74:620–623.
12. Hubbard AM, Meyer JS, Davidson RS, Mahboubi S, Harty MP. Relationship between the ossification center and cartilaginous anlage in the normal hind foot in children: study with MR imaging. AJR 1993;161:849–853.
13. Lawrence SJ, Botte MJ. The sural nerve in the foot and ankle: an anatomic study with clinical and surgical implications. Foot Ankle 1994;15:490–494.
14. Kurz AD. Apophysis of the os calcis. Am J Orthop Surg 1917;15:659–661.
15. Mulfinger GL, Trueta J. The blood supply of the talus. J Bone Joint Surg Br 1970;52:160–167.
16. Ogden JA. Anomalous multifocal ossification of the os calcis. Clin Orthop 1982;162:112–118.
17. Ogden JA, Griswold DM. Solitary cyst of the talus. J Bone Joint Surg Am 1972;54:1309–1311.
18. O'Neal ML, Ganey TM, Ogden JA. Asymmetric bifurcation of the extensor digitorum longus tendon in a case of congenital digitus minimus varus. Foot Ankle 1994;15:505–507.
19. Prichasuk S, Mulpruek P, Siriwongpairat P. The heel-pad compressibility. Clin Orthop 1994;300:197–200.
20. Rufai A, Ralphs JR, Benjamin M. Structure and histopathology of the insertional region of the human Achilles tendon. J Orthop Res 1995;13:585–593.

21. Schopfner CE, Coin CG. Effect of weight-bearing on the appearance and development of the secondary calcaneal epiphysis. Radiology 1968;86:201–206.
22. Smith RW, Staple TW. Cat-scan evaluation of the hindfoot—anatomical and clinical study. Clin Orthop 1983;177:34–38.
23. Snow SW, Bohne WHO, DiCarlo E, Chang VK. Anatomy of the Achilles tendon and plantar fascia in relation to the calcaneus in various age groups. Foot Ankle 1995;16:418–421.
24. Vanderwilde R, Staheli LT, Chew DE, Melagon V. Measurement on radiographs of the foot in normal infants and children. J Bone Surg Am 1988;70:407–414.
25. Walling AK, Ogden JA. Case Report 666: Bipartite medial sesamoid. Skeletal Radiol 1991;20:233–235.
26. Wilson RC, Moyles BG. Surgical treatment of the symptomatic os peroneum. J Foot Surg 1987;26:156–158.

General Considerations

27. Bensahel H, Huguerin P. Les fractures de la cheville et du pied de l'enfant. Ann Pediatr 1981;28:437–442.
28. Bordelon RL. Hypermobile flatfoot in children: comprehension, evaluation and treatment. Clin Orthop 1983;181:7–14.
29. Bonutti PM, Bell GR. Compartment syndrome of the foot. J Bone Joint Surg Am 1986;68:1449–1451.
30. Cehner J. Fractures of the tarsal bones, metatarsals, and toes. In: Weber BG, Brunner C, Freuler F (eds) Treatment of Fractures in Children and Adolescents. New York: Springer, 1980.
31. Crawford AH. Fractures and dislocations of the foot and ankle. In: Green NE, Swiontkowski MF (eds) Skeletal Trauma in Children. Saunders: Philadelphia, 1993.
32. DeValentine SJ. Epiphyseal injuries of the foot and ankle. Clin Podiatr Med Surg 1987;4:279–310.
33. DeValentine SJ. Foot and Ankle Disorders in Children. New York: Churchill Livingstone, 1992.
34. Ehrensperger J. Frakturen des kindlichen und jugendlichen Fusses. Ther Umsch 1983;40:996–1000.
35. Fakhouri AJ, Mandi A II. Acute foot compartment syndromes. J Orthop Trauma 1992;6:223–228.
36. Heim M, Martinowitz U, Horoszowski H. The short foot syndrome: an unfortunate consequence of neglected raised intra-compartment pressure in a severe hemophilic child: a case report. Angiology 1986;37:128–131.
37. Huguenin BH. Les fractures de la cheville et du pied de l'enfant. Ann Chir 1981;35:114–119.
38. Huguenin BH. Les fractures de la cheville et du pied de l'enfant. Ann Pediatr 1981;28:437–442.
39. Izant RJ, Rohmann BF, Frankel VH. Bicycle spoke injuries of the foot and ankle in children: an underestimated "minor" injury. J Pediatr Surg 1969;4:654–656.
40. Jonasch E. Fussenbeinbruche bei Kindern. Hefte Unfallheilkd 1979;134:170–175.
41. Kurz W, Gundel T, Hartmann H. Fusswurzelfrakturen im Kindesalter. Zentalbl Chir 1984;109:984–990.
42. Linhart WE, Hollwarth ME. Frakturen des kindlichen Fusses. Orthopäde 1985;15:242–250.
43. Loeffler RD, Ballard A. Plantar fascial spaces of the foot and a proposed surgical approach. Foot Ankle 1980;1:11–14.
44. Manoli A, Weber TG. Fasciotomy of the foot: An anatomical study with special reference to release of the calcaneal compartment. Foot Ankle 1990;10:267–275.
45. Matsen FA. Compartmental syndrome: a unified concept. Clin Orthop 1975;113:8–14.
46. Myerson MS. Acute compartment syndromes of the foot. Bull Hosp Joint Dis Orthop Inst 1987;47:251–256.
47. Myerson MS. Diagnosis and treatment of compartment syndrome of the foot. Orthopaedics 1990;13:711–717.
48. Myerson MS, McGarvey WC, Henderson MR, Hakim J. Morbidity after crush injuries to the foot. J Orthop Trauma 1994;8:343–349.
49. Oudjhane K, Newman B, Oh KS, Young LW, Girdany BR. Occult fractures in preschool children. J Trauma 1988;28:858–860.
50. Sankhala SS, Gupta SP. Spoke wheel injuries. Indian J Pediatr 1987;54:251–256.
51. Schuberth JM. Principles of fracture management in children. Clin Podiatr Med Surg 1987;4:267–277.
52. Schuberth JM. Fractures of the foot. In: DeValentine SJ (ed) Foot and Ankle Disorders in Children. New York: Churchhill Livingstone, 1992.
53. Schwarz N, Gabauer M. Die Fraktur des Springbeines beim Kind. Unfallheilkunde 1983;86:212–221.
54. Silas SI, Herzenberg JE, Myerson MS, Sponseller PD. Compartment syndrome of the foot in children. J Bone Joint Surg Am 1995;77:356–360.
55. Subrahmanyam M, Date VN, Samant NA, Patil AJ, Arwade DJ. Bicycle injuries in children. J Indian Med Assoc 1980;75:224–221.
56. Sullivan JA. Ankle and foot injuries in the pediatric athlete. AAOS Instr Course Lect 1993;42:545–551.
57. Tachdjian MO. Pediatric Orthopaedics. Philadelphia: Saunders, 1972.
58. Tachdjian MO. The Child's Foot. Philadelphia: Saunders, 1985.
59. Tomaschewski HK. Ergebnisse der Behandlung des posttraumatischen Fehlwuchses des Fusses bei Kindern und Jugendlichen. Beitr Orthop Traumatol 1975;22:90–96.
60. Trott AW. Fractures of the foot in children. Orthop Clin North Am 1976;7:677–686.
61. Willis RB, Rorabeck CH. Treatment of compartment syndromes in children. Orthop Clin North Am 1990;21:401–412.
62. Ziv I, Mosheiff R, Zelgowski A, Liebergal M, Lowe J, Segal D. Crush injuries of the foot with compartment syndrome: immediate one-stage management. Foot Ankle 1989;9:285–289.
63. Zwipp H, Renft TH. Fehlverheilte Kindliche Frakturen im Fuss bereich. Orthopäde 1991;20:374–380.

Talus

64. Alexander AH, Lichtman DM. Surgical treatment of transchondral talar dome fractures (osteochondritis dissecans): long-term follow-up. J Bone Joint Surg Am 1980;62:646–652.
65. Anderson DV, Lyne ED. Osteochondritis dissecans of the talus: case report on two family members. J Pediatr Orthop 1984;4:356–357.
66. Anderson IF, Crichton KJ, Grattan-Smith T, et al. Osteochondral fractures of the dome of the talus. J Bone Joint Surg Am 1989;71:1143–1152.
67. Berndt AL, Harty M. Transchondral fractures (osteochondritis dissecans) of the talus. J Bone Joint Surg Am 1959;41:988–1020.
68. Bourrel P, Maitre B, Palinacci JC, Gouri JL, Jardin M. Osteochondrite de l'astragale: a propos de 9 observations. Rev Chir Orthop 1972;58:609–622.
69. Buckingham WW Jr. Subtalar dislocation of the foot. J Trauma 1973;13:753–756.
70. Burkus JK, Sella EJ, Southwick WO. Occult injuries of the talus diagnosed by bone scan and tomography. Foot Ankle 1984;4:316–324.
71. Canale ST, Belding RH. Osteochondral lesions of the talus. J Bone Joint Surg Am 1980;62:97–102.
72. Canale ST, Kelly FB. Fractures of the neck of the talus: long-term evaluation of 71 cases. J Bone Joint Surg Am 1978;60:143–156.

References

73. Christensen SB, Lorentzen JE, Krogose O, Sneppen O. Subtalar dislocation. Acta Orthop Scand 1977;48:707–711.
74. Contompasis J. Common adolescent dance injuries. Clin Podiatr Med Surg 1984;1:631–644.
75. Davidson AM, Steele HD, MacKenzie DA, Penny JA. A review of cases of transchondral fracture of the talus. J Trauma 1967;7:378–415.
76. Davy A. A propos de 3 cas d'osteochondrite dissequante de l'enfant. Ann Chir 1961;15:311–316.
77. Dimentburg R, Rosman M. Peritalar dislocations in children. J Pediatr Orthop 1993;13:89–93.
78. Draijer F, Havemann D, Bielstein M. Verletzungs analyse Kindlicher Talus Frakturen. Unfallchirurgie 1995;98:130–132.
79. Ecker L, Ritter MA, Jacobs BS. The symptomatic os trigonum. JAMA 1967;201:882–884.
80. Gerard Y, Bernier JM, Ameil M. Lesions osteochondrales de la poulie astragalienne. Rev Chir Orthop 1989;75:466–478.
81. Gottlieb A. Posttraumatic os trigonum. J Int Coll Surg 1956;26:80–82.
82. Greenspoon J, Rosman M. Medial osteochondritis of the talus in children: review and surgical management. J Pediatr Orthop 1987;7:705–708.
83. Grogan DP, Walling AK, Ogden JA. Anatomy of the os trigonum. J Pediatr Orthop 1990;10:618–622.
84. Gunal I. Talectomy for osteoporotic and neuropathic feet: 7 cases followed for 20 years. Acta Orthop Scand 1994;65:349–350.
85. Gunal I, Atilla S, Arac S, Gürsoy Y, Karagözlü H. A new technique of talectomy for severe fracture-dislocation of the talus. J Bone Joint Surg Br 1993;75:69–71.
86. Haliburton RA, Barber JR, Fraser RL. Further experience with peritalar dislocation. Can J Surg 1967;10:322–324.
87. Hamilton WG. Stenosing tenosynovitis of the flexor hallucis longus tendon and posterior impingement upon the os trigonum in ballet dancers. Foot Ankle 1982;3:74–80.
88. Havermann D, Schroder L, Egbers H-J. Talus Frakturen beim Kind. Hefte Unfallheilkd 1984;164:702–705.
89. Hawkins LG. Fractures of the lateral process of the talus. J Bone Joint Surg Am 1965;47:1170–1175.
90. Hawkins LG. Fractures of the neck of the talus. J Bone Joint Surg Am 1970;52:991–995.
91. Henderson RC. Post-traumatic necrosis of the talus: the Hawkins sign versus magnetic resonance imaging. J Orthop Trauma 1991;5:96–99.
92. Jensen I, Wester JU, Rasmussen F, Lindequist S, Schantz K. Prognosis of fracture of the talus in children: 21 (7–34) year follow-up of 14 cases. Acta Orthop Scand 1994;65:398–400.
93. Johnson RP, Collier BD, Carrera GF. The os trigonum syndrome: use of bone scan in the diagnosis. J Trauma 1984;24:761–764.
94. Kenny CH. Inverted osteochondral fracture of the talus diagnosed by tomography. J Bone Joint Surg Am 1981;63:1024–1025.
95. von Laer L. Distorsio pedis beim Kind. Orthopade 1986;15:251–259.
96. Lawson JP. Symptomatic radiographic variants in the extremities. Radiology 1985;157:625–631.
97. Lemaire RG, Bustin W. Screw fixaton of fractures of the neck of the talus using a posterior approach. J Trauma 1980;20:669–673.
98. Letts RM, Gibeault D. Fractures of the neck of the talus in children. Foot Ankle 1980;1:74–77.
99. Letts RM, Greenspoon J, Rosman M. Medial osteochondritis of the talus in children: review and new surgical management. J Pediatr Orthop 1987;7:705–708.
100. Linhart WE, Höllwarth M. Talus Frakturen bei Kindern. Unfallchirurg 1985;88:168–175.
101. Loomer R, Fischer C, Lloyd-Smith R, Sisler J, Cooney T. Osteochondral lesions of the talus. Am J Sports Med 1993;21:13–19.
102. Ly PN, Fallat LM. Transchondral fractures of the talus: a review of 64 surgical cases. J Foot Ankle Surg 1993;32:352–374.
103. Marrotta JJ, Micheli LJ. Os trigonum impingement in dancers. Am J Sports Med 1992;20:533–538.
104. Mazel C, Rigault P, Padovani JP, et al. Les fractures de l'astragale de l'enfant: a propos de 23 cas. Rev Chir Orthop 1986;72:183–195.
105. McDougall A. The os trigonum. J Bone Joint Surg Br 1955;37:257–265.
106. Meinhard BP, Girgis I, Moriarty RV. Irreducible talar dislocation with entrapment by the tibialis posterior and the flexor digitorum longus tendons. Clin Orthop 1993;286:222–224.
107. Meisenbach R. Fracture of the os trigonum: report of two cases. JAMA 1927;89:199–200.
108. Mindell ER, Cisek EE, Kartalian G, Dziob JA. Late results of injuries to the talus. J Bone Joint Surg Am 1963;45:221–245.
109. Morris HD, Hand WL, Dunn AW. The modified Blair fusion for fractures of the talus. J Bone Joint Surg Am 1971;53:1289–1297.
110. Ogden JA, Lee J. Accessory ossification patterns and injuries of the malleoli. J Pediatr Orthop 1990;10:306–316.
111. Pathi K. Fracture of the neck of the talus in children. J Indian Med Assoc 1974;63:157–158.
112. Pereles TR, Koval KJ, Feldman DS. Fracture dislocation of the neck of the talus in a ten-year-old child: a case report and review of the literature. Bull Hosp Joint Dis 1996;55:88–91.
113. Pick MP. Familial osteochondritis dissecans. J Bone Joint Surg Br 1955;37:142–145.
114. Quirk R. Talar compression syndrome in dancers. Foot Ankle 1982;3:65–68.
115. Rendu A. Fracture intra-articulaire parcellaire de la poulie astragalienne. Lyon Med 1932;150:220–221.
116. Ruiz Valdivieso T, Miguel Vielba JA, Hernandez Garcia C, et al. Subtalar dislocation. Int Orthop 1996;20:83–86.
117. Schreiber A, Differding P, Zollinger H. Talus partitus: a case report. J Bone Joint Surg Br 1985;67:430–431.
118. Schuind F, Andrianne Y, Burny M, Donkerwolcke M, Saric O. Avascular necrosis after fracture or dislocation of the talus: risk factors, prevention. In: Arlet J, Ficat RP (eds) Bone Circulation. Baltimore: Williams & Wilkins, 1984.
119. Smith GR, Winquist RA, Allan TNK, Northrop CH. Subtle transchondral fractures of the talar dome: radiological perspective. Radiology 1977;124:667–673.
120. Smith H. Subastragalar dislocation. J Bone Joint Surg 1937;19:373–380.
121. Sneppen O, Christensen SB, Krogsoe O, et al. Fracture of the talus. Acta Orthop Scand 1977;48:317–327.
122. Spak I. Fractures of the talus in children. Acta Chir Scand 1954;107:553–566.
123. St. Pierre RK, Velazco A, Fleming LL, Whitesides T. Medial subtalar dislocation in an athlete: a case report. Am J Sports Med 1982;10:240–244.
124. Stephens NA. Fracture-dislocation of the talus in childhood. Br J Surg 1956;43:600–604.
125. Sullivan CR, Jackson SC. Fracture dislocation of the talus in children. Acta Orthop Scand 1958;90:302–309.
126. Szyszkowitz R, Reschauer R, Seggl W. Eighty-five talus fractures treated by ORIF with five to eight years of follow-up study of 69 patients. Clin Orthop 1985;199:97–107.
127. Valentine BC, Buoye SF, Naples JJ. Talar fracture/dislocation in the adolescent patient. J Foot Ankle Surg 1995;34:379–383.
128. Wakeley CJ, Johnson DP, Watt I. The value of MR imaging in the diagnosis of the os trigonum syndrome. Skeletal Radiol 1996;29:133–136.

129. Weinstein SL, Bonfiglio M. Unusual accessory (bipartite) talus simulating fracture. J Bone Joint Surg Am 1975;57:1161–1163.
130. Wester JU, Jensen IE, Tasmussen F, Lindequist S, Schantz K. Osteochondral lesions of the talar dome in children: a 24 (7–36) year follow-up of 13 cases. Acta Orthop Scand 1994;65:110–112.
131. Yuan HA, Cady RB, DeRosa C. Osteochondritis dissecans of the talus associated with subchondral cysts. J Bone Joint Surg Am 1979;61:1249–1251.
132. Zinman C, Wolfson N, Reis ND. Osteochondritis dissecans of the dome of the talus. J Bone Joint Surg Am 1988;70:1017.

Calcaneus

133. Alvarez Fernandez JL, Vaquero MV, Cimiano JG. Epiphyseolysis of the great tuberosity of the calcaneum: brief report. J Bone Joint Surg Br 1989;71:321.
134. Andrish JT. Overuse syndrome of the lower extremity in youth sports. In: Boileau RA (ed) Advances in Pediatric Sports Sciences. Champaign, IL: Human Kinetics Publishers, 1984.
135. Bachman S, Johnson RR. Torsion of the foot causing fracture of the anterior calcaneal process. Acta Chir Scand 1953;105:460–462.
136. Birtwistle SJ, Jacobs L. An avulsion fracture of the calcaneal apophysis in a young gymnast. Injury 1995;26:409–410.
137. Bradford CH, Larsen I. Sprain-fractures of the anterior lip of the os calcis. N Engl J Med 1951;244:970–972.
138. Bruckner J. Variations in the human subtalar joint. J Orthop Sports Phys Ther 1987;8:489–494.
139. Buchanan J, Greer RB III. Stress fractures in the calcaneus of a child: a case report. Clin Orthop 1978;135:119–120.
140. Bunning PSC, Barnett CH. A comparison of adult and foetal talocalcaneal articulations. J Anat 1965;99:71–76.
141. Carr JB. Mechanism and pathoanatomy of the intraarticular calcaneal fracture. Clin Orthop 1993;290:36–40.
142. Chapman HG, Galway HR. Os calcis fractures in childhood. J Bone Joint Surg Br 1977;59:510–513.
143. Cole RJ, Brown HP, Stein RE, Pearce RG. Avulsion fracture of the tuberosity of the calcaneus in children. J Bone Joint Surg Am 1995;77:1568–1571.
144. Crosby LA, Fitzgibbons T. Computerized tomography scanning of acute intra-articular fractures of the calcaneus. J Bone Joint Surg Am 1990;72:852–859.
145. DeBeer JD, Maloon S, Hudson DA. Calcaneal fractures in children. S Afr Med J 1989;76:53–54.
146. Degan TJ, Morrey BF, Braun DP. Surgical excision for anterior-process fractures of the calcaneus. J Bone Joint Surg Am 1982;64:519–524.
147. Drayer-Verhagen F. Arthritis of the subtalar joint associated with sustentaculum tali facet configuration. J Anat 1993;183:631–634.
148. Drvaric DM, Schmitt EW. Irreducible fracture of the calcaneus in a child. J Orthop Trauma 1988;2:154–157.
149. Dworczynski W, Pomierna I. Zlamanie kosci pietowej u 32-miesiecznego dziecka. Chir Narzadow Ruchu Ortop Pol 1981;46:107–109.
150. Ebraheim NA, Zeiss J, Skie MC, Jackson WT. Radiologic evaluation of peroneal tendon pathology associated with calcaneal fractures. J Orthop Trauma 1991;5:365–369.
151. Ehalt W. Verletzungen bei Kindern und Jugendlichen. Stuttgart: Enke, 1961.
152. Essex-Lopresti P. The mechanism, reduction, technique and results in fractures of the os calcis. Br J Surg 1952;39:395–419.
153. Garceau GJ, Gregory CF. Solitary unicameral bone cysts. J Bone Joint Surg Am 1954;36:267–280.
154. Gellman M. Fracture of the anterior process of the calcaneus. J Bone Joint Surg Am 1951;33:382–386.
155. Glancy J. Orthotic control of ground reaction forces during running (a preliminary report). J Orthop Prosthet 1984;38:12–40.
156. Havránek P, Hájková H. Beiderseitige dislozierte intraartikulare Kalkaneus Fraktur beim Kind. Zentralbl Chir 1990;115:625–629.
157. Hunt DD. Compression fracture of the anterior articular surface of the calcaneus. J Bone Joint Surg Am 1970;52:1637–1642.
158. Jaschke W, Hiemer W. Funktionelle Behandlung von Fussenbeinfrakturen ohne Gelenkbeteiligung im Kindesalter. Akt Traumatol 1983;13:235–238.
159. Jonasch E. Fussenbeinbruche bei kindern. Hefte Unfallheilkd 1979;134:170–177.
160. Katoh Y, Chao EYS, Murray BF, Laughman RK. Objective technique for evaluating painful heel syndrome and its treatment. Foot Ankle 1983;3:227–237.
161. Koval KJ, Sanders R. The radiologic evaluation of calcaneal fractures. Clin Orthop 1993;290:41–46.
162. Kurz W, Gundel T, Hardtmann H. Fusswurzelfrakturen im Kindesalter. Zentralbl Chir 1984;109:984–990.
163. Kvist M, Kujälä U, Heinönen O, Kölu T. Osgood-Schlatter and Sever's disease in young athletes. Duodecim 1984;100:142–150.
164. Laliotis N, Pennie BH, Carty H, Klenerman L. Toddler's fracture of the calcaneum. Injury 1993;24:169–170.
165. Levin LS, Nunley JA. The management of soft tissue problems associated with calcaneal fractures. Clin Orthop 1993;290:151–156.
166. Liberson A, Lieberson S, Mendes DG, et al. Remodeling of the calcaneal apophysis in the growing child. J Pediatr Orthop 1995;4:74–79.
167. Linhart WE, Höllworth ME. Frakturen des Kindlichen Fusses. Orthopäde 1985;15:242–250.
168. Marti R. Fractures of the calcaneus. In: Weber BG, Brunner C, Freuler R (eds) Treatment of Fractures in Children and Adolescents. New York: Springer, 1980.
169. Massada JL. Ankle overuse injuries in soccer players. J Sports Med Phys Fitness 1991;31:447–451.
170. Matteri RE, Frymoyer JW. Fracture of the calcaneus in young children: report of three cases. J Bone Joint Surg Am 1973;55:1091–1094.
171. McKenzie DC, Taunton JE, Clement DB, et al. Calcaneal epiphysitis in adolescent athletes. Can J Appl Sport Sci 1981;6:123–125.
172. Micheli LJ. Pediatric and Adolescent Sports Medicine. Boston: Little, Brown, 1984.
173. Micheli LJ, Ireland ML. Prevention and management of calcaneal apophysitis in children: an overuse syndrome. J Pediatr Orthop 1987;7:34–38.
174. Mittlmeier TM, Mächler G, Lob G, Mutschler W, Bauer G, Vogl T. Compartment syndrome of the foot after intraarticular calcaneal fracture. Clin Orthop 1991;269:241–248.
175. Moss EH, Carty H. Scintigraphy in the diagnosis of occult fractures of the calcaneus. Skeletal Radiol 1990;19:575–577.
176. Mrzena V, Popelka S. Kalkaneusfrakturen bei Kindern. Acta Chir Orthop Traumatol Cech 1984;51:530–535.
177. Myerson M, Manoli A. Compartment syndromes of the foot after calcaneal fractures. Clin Orthop 1993;290:142–150.
178. Norfray JF, Rogers LF, Adamo GP, Groves HC, Heiser WJ. Common calcaneal avulsion fracture. AJR 1980;134:119–123.
179. Olson TR, Seidel MR. The evolutionary basis of some clinical disorders of the human foot: a comparative survey of the living primates. Foot Ankle 1983;3:322–341.
180. Oudjhane K, Newman B, Oh KS, Young LW, Girdauy BR. Occult fractures in preschool children. J Trauma 1988;28:858–860.

References

181. Pablot SM, Daneman A, Stringer DA, Carroll N. The value of computed tomography in the early assessment of comminuted fractures of the calcaneus: a review of three patients. J Pediatr Orthop 1985;5:435–438.
182. Paley KJ, Milem CA, Ebraheim NA, Merritt TR. Severe displacement of a calcaneal apophyseal fracture. J Foot Ankle Surg 1994;33:180–183.
183. Patt AD. Fracture of the promontory of the calcaneus. Radiology 1956;67:386–387.
184. Puddu G, Ippolito E, Postacchini F. A classification of Achilles tendon disease. Am J Sports Med 1976;4:145–150.
185. Rasmussen R, Schantz K. Radiologic aspects of calcaneal fractures in childhood and adolescence. Acta Radiol Diagn 1986;27:575–580.
186. Rigault P, Padovani JP, Kliszowski H. Les fractures du calcaneum chez l'enfant (a propos de 26 cas). Ann Chir Infant 1973;14:115–119.
187. Rosenberg ZS, Feldman F, Singson RD. Intra-articular calcaneal fractures: computed tomographic analysis. Skeletal Radiol 1987;16:105–113.
188. Ross SD. The operative treatment of complex os calcis fractures. Techn Orthop 1987;2:55–61.
189. Rowe CR, Sakellarides HT, Freeman PA, Sorbie C. Fractures of the os calcis. JAMA 1963;184:920–923.
190. Sandermann J, Torp FT, Thomsen PB. Intraarticular calcaneal fractures in children: report of two cases and a survey of the literature. Arch Orthop Trauma Surg 1987;106:129–131.
191. Schantz K, Rasmussen F. Calcaneus fracture in the child. Acta Orthop Scand 1987;58:507–509.
192. Schellenberg P, Mebold A. Die juvenile calcaneus Fraktur. Akt Traumatol 1980;10:251–254.
193. Schindler A, Mason DE, Allington NJ. Occult fracture of the calcaneus in toddlers. J Pediatr Orthop 1996;16:201–205.
194. Schmidt TL, Weiner DS. Calcaneal fractures in children: an evaluation of the nature of the injury in 56 children. Clin Orthop 1982;171:150–155.
195. Schofield RO. Fractures of the os calcis. J Bone Joint Surg 1936;18:566–580.
196. Sever JW. Apophysis of the os calcis. NY State J Med 1912;95:1025–1028.
197. Shopfner CE, Coin CG. Effect of weightbearing on appearance and development of secondary calcaneal epiphysis. Radiology 1966;86:201–206.
198. Starshak RJ, Simons GW, Sty JR. Occult fracture of the calcaneus: another toddler's fracture. Pediatr Radiol 1984;14:37–40.
199. Stein RE, Stelling FH. Stress fracture of the calcaneus in a child with cerebral palsy. J Bone Joint Surg Am 1977;59:131.
200. Stephenson JR. Displaced fractures of the os calcis involving the subtalar joint: the key role of the superomedial fragment. Foot Ankle 1983;4:91–101.
201. Stuflesser H, Kundert HP, Dexel M. Fersenbein Frakturen: Langzeitergebnisse nach operativen und nach konservativer Erstbehandlung und orthopädietechnische Versorgung. Akt Traumatol 1979;9:277–282.
202. Thomas HM. Calcaneal fracture in childhood. Br J Surg 1969;56:664–666.
203. Trott AW. Fractures of the foot in children. Orthop Clin North Am 1976;7:677–686.
204. Walling AK, Grogan DP, Carty CT, Ogden JA. Fracture of the calcaneal apophysis. J Orthop Trauma 1990;4:349–355.
205. Wiley JJ, Profitt A. Fractures of the os calcis in children. Clin Orthop 1984;188:131–138.
206. Zayre M. Fracture of the calcaneus: a review of 110 fractures. Acta Orthop Scand 1969;40:530–542.
207. Zlatkin MB, Bjorkengren A, Sartoris DJ, Resnick D. Stress fractures of the distal tibia and calcaneus subsequent to acute fractures of the tibia and fibula. AJR 1987;149:329–320

Navicular

208. Alfred RH, Belhobeck G, Bergfeld JA. Stress fractures of the tarsal navicular: a case report. Am J Sports Med 1992;20:766–768.
209. Borges JLP, Guille JT, Bowen JR. Köhler's bone disease of the tarsal navicular. J Pediatr Orthop 1995;15:596–598.
210. Eichenholtz SN, Levine DB. Fractures of the tarsal navicular bone. Clin Orthop 1964;34:142–157.
211. Francillon MR. Untersuchungen zur anatomischen und klinischen Bedeutung des os Tibiale externum. Z Orthop Chir 1932;56:61–72.
212. Grogan DP, Gasser SI, Ogden JA. The painful accessory navicular: a clinical and histopathologic study. Foot Ankle 1989;10:164–169.
213. Haglund P. Über Fraktur des Tuberculum ossis navicularis in den Jugendjahren und ihre Bedeutung als Ursache einer typische Form von Pes valgus. Z Orthop Chir 1906;26:347–353.
214. Hunter LY. Stress fractures of the tarsal navicular bone. Am J Sports Med 1981;9:217–219.
215. Ippolito E, Ricciardi PT, Falez F. Köhler's disease of the tarsal navicular: long-term follow-up of 12 cases. J Pediatr Orthop 1984;4:416–417.
216. Karp MG. Kohler's disease of the tarsal scaphoid. J Bone Joint Surg 1937;19:84–96.
217. Kidner FC. The prehallux (accessory scaphoid) in its relation to flat-foot. J Bone Joint Surg 1929;11:831–837.
218. Latten W. Histologische Beziehungen zwischen Os tibiale und Kahnbein nach Untersuchungen an einem operierten Falle. Dtsch Chir 1927;205:320–325.
219. Lawson JP, Ogden JA, Sella EJ, Barwick KW. The painful accessory navicular. Skeletal Radiol 1984;12:250–262.
220. MacNicol MF, Voutsinas S. Surgical treatment of the symptomatic accessory navicular. J Bone Joint Surg Br 1984;66:218–226.
221. Orava S, Karpakka J, Hulkko A, Takala T. Stress avulsion fracture of the tarsal navicular: an uncommon sports related overuse. Am J Sports Med 1991;19:392–395.
222. Ray S, Goldberg VM. Surgical treatment of the accessory navicular. Clin Orthop 1983;177:61–66.
223. Sangeorzan BJ, Benirschke SK, Mosca V, Mayo KA, Hansen ST Jr. Displaced intra-articular fractures of the tarsal navicular. J Bone Joint Surg Am 1989;71:1504–1510.
224. Sella EJ, Lawson JP. Biomechanics of the accessory navicular synchondrosis. Foot Ankle 1987;8:156–163.
225. Sella EJ, Lawson JP, Ogden JA. The accessory navicular synchondrosis. Clin Orthop 1986;209:280–285.
226. Sullivan JA, Miller WA. The relationship of the accessory navicular to the development of the flat foot. Clin Orthop 1979;144:233–237.
227. Torg JS, Pavlou H, Cooley LH, et al. Stress fractures of the tarsal navicular. J Bone Joint Surg Am 1982;61:700–712.
228. Waugh W. The ossification and vascularization of the tarsal navicular and their relation to Kohler's disease. J Bone Joint Surg Br 1959;40:765–777.
229. Zadek I. The significance of the accessory tarsal scaphoid. J Bone Joint Surg 1926;8:618–626.
230. Zadek I, Gold AM. The accessory tarsal scaphoid. J Bone Joint Surg Am 1948;30:957–968.

Other Tarsals

231. Blumberg K, Patterson RJ. The toddler's cuboid fracture. Radiology 1991;179:93–94.
232. Buchman J. Osteochondritis of the internal cuneiform. J Bone Joint Surg 1933;15:225–232.

233. Elghawabi MH. Fractures of the cuneiform bones: classification and treatment. Egypt Orthop J 1972;7:206–211.
234. Haboush EJ. Bilateral disease of the internal cuneiform bone with an associated disease of the right scaphoid bone (Köhler's). JAMA 1933;100:41–42.
235. Hicks BTG. Case report: osteochondritis of the tarsal second cuneiform bone. Br J Radiol 1953;26:214–215.
236. Leeson MC, Weiner DS. Osteochondrosis of the tarsal cuneiforms. Clin Orthop 1985;196:260–264.
237. Meilstrup DB. Osteochondritis of the internal cuneiform, bilateral: case report. AJR 1947;58:329–330.
238. Mubarek SJ. Osteochondrosis of the lateral cuneiform: another cause of limp in a child. J Bone Joint Surg Am 1992; 74:285–289.
239. Nicastro JF, Haupt HA. Probable stress fracture of the cuboid in an infant: a case report. J Bone Joint Surg Am 1984;66: 1106–1108.
240. O'Neal, Ganey TM, Ogden JA. A fracture of the bipartite medial cuneiform synchondrosis. Foot Ankle 1995;16:37–40.
241. Siffert RS. Classification of the osteochondroses. Clin Orthop 1981;158:10–18.
242. Simonian PT, Vahey JW, Rosenbaum DM, Mosca VS, Staheli LT. Fracture of the cuboid in children: a source of leg symptoms. J Bone Joint Surg Br 1995;77:104–106.

Tarsometatarsal

243. Aitken AP, Poulson D. Dislocations of the tarsometatarsal joint. J Bone Joint Surg Am 1963;45:246–260.
244. Babst R, Simmen BR, Regazzoni P. Klinische Bedeutung und ein Behandlungskonzept der Lisfrancluxation und luxationsfraktur. Helv Chir Acta 1989;56:603–607.
245. Bonnel F, Barthelemy M. Traumatismes de l'articulation de Lisfranc: entores graves, luxations, fractures. J Chir (Paris) 1976;3:573–592.
246. Cassebaum WH. Lisfranc fracture dislocations. Clin Orthop 1963;30:116–129.
247. Collett HS, Hood TK, Andrews RE. Tarsometatarsal fracture dislocations. Surg Gynecol Obstet 1958;106:623–626.
248. Easton ER. Two rare dislocations of the metatarsals at Lisfranc's joint. J Bone Joint Surg 1938;20:1053–1056.
249. Foster SC, Foster RR. Lisfranc's tarsometatarsal fracture-dislocation. Radiology 1976;120:79–83.
250. Hardcastle PH, Reschauer R, Kitsha-Lissberg E, Schoffman W. Injuries to the tarsometatarsal joint, incidence, classification and treatment. J Bone Joint Surg Br 1982;64:349–356.
251. Main BJ, Jowett RL. Injuries of the mid-tarsal joint. J Bone Joint Surg Br 1975;57:89–97.
252. Mantas JP, Burks RT. Lisfranc injuries in the athlete. Clin Sports Med 1994;13:719–730.
253. Myerson M. Tarsometatarsal joint injury: subtle signs hold the key. Physician Sports Med 1993;21:97–107.
254. Norfray JF, Geline RA, Steinberg RI, Galinski AW, Gilula A. Subtleties of Lisfranc fracture—dislocations. AJR 1981;137: 1151–1156.
255. Priedler KW, Brossman J, Daenen B, et al. MR imaging of the tarsometatarsal joint: analysis of injuries in 11 patients. AJR 1996;167:1217–1222.
256. Rainaut JJ, Cedard C, D'Hour JP. Les luxations tarsometatarsiennes. Rev Chir Orthop 1966;52:449–462.
257. Ross G, Cronin R, Hanzenblas J, Juliano P. Plantar ecchymosis sign: a clinical aid to diagnosis of occult Lisfranc tarsometatarsal injuries. J Orthop Trauma 1996;10:119–122.
258. Sangeorzan BJ, Veith RG, Hansen ST. Salvage of Lisfranc's tarsometatarsal joint by arthrodesis. Foot Ankle 1990;10:193–200.
259. Stein RE. Radiological aspects of the tarsometatarsal joints. Foot Ankle 1983;3:286–289.
260. Trillat A, Lerat JL, LeClerc P, Schuster P. Tarsometatarsal fracture dislocation. Rev Chir Orthop 1976;62:685–702.
261. Vuori JP, Aro HT. Lisfranc joint injuries: trauma mechanisms and associated injuries. J Trauma 1993;35:40–45.
262. Wiley JJ. The mechanism of tarso-metatarsal joint injuries. J Bone Joint Surg Br 1971;53:474–482.
263. Wiley JJ. Tarso-metatarsal joint injuries in children. J Pediatr Orthop 1981;1:255–260.
264. Wynne AT, Southgate GW. Delayed tarsometatarsal joint dislocation following forefoot injury. Orthopedics 1986;9:52–54.

Metatarsals

265. Acker JH, Drez D Jr. Non-operative treatment of stress fractures of the proximal shaft of the fifth metatarsal (Jones' fracture). Foot Ankle 1986;7:152–155.
266. Braddock GT. Experimental epiphysial injury and Freiberg's disease. J Bone Joint Surg Br 1959;41:154–159.
267. Canale ST, Williams KD. Iselin's disease. J Pediatr Orthop 1992;12:90.
268. Childress HM. March foot in a seven-year-old child. J Bone Joint Surg 1946;28:877–878.
269. Cwiklicki Z. [Stress fractures of the third metatarsal bone in a child.] Chir Narzadow Ruchu Ortop Pol 1965;30:333–334.
270. Dameron TB. Fractures and anatomical variations of the proximal portion of the fifth metatarsal. J Bone Joint Surg Am 1975;57:788–792.
271. Dameron TB. Fractures of the proximal fifth metatarsal: selecting the best treatment option. J Am Acad Orthop Surg 1995;3:110–114.
272. Drez D Jr, Young JC, Johnston RD, Parker WD. Metatarsal stress fractures. Am J Sports Med 1980;8:123–125.
273. Falkenberg MP, Dickens DR, Menelaus MB. Osteochondritis of the first metatarsal epiphysis. J Pediatr Orthop 1990;10: 797–799.
274. Franke K, Paul B. Indications for osteosynthesis of metatarsal fractures. Zentralbl Chir 1984;109:20–22.
275. Freiberg A. Infraction of the second metatarsal bone. Surg Gynecol Obstet 1914;19:191–193.
276. Harris RI, Beath T. The short first metatarsal. J Bone Joint Surg Am 1949;31:553–565.
277. Harrison M. Fractures of the metatarsal head. Can J Surg 1968;11:511–514.
278. Hulkko A, Orava S. Stress fractures in athletes. Int J Sport Med 1987;8:221–226.
279. Iselin H. Wachstums beschewerden zur Zeit der Knochernen Entwicklung der Tuberositas metatarsi quint. Dtsch Z Chir 1912;117:529–535.
280. Jaffee AC, Lasser DH. Multiple metatarsal fractures in child abuse. Pediatrics 1977;60:642–643.
281. Johnson GF. Pediatric Lisfranc injury: "bunk bed" fracture. AJR 1981;137:1041–1044.
282. Jones R. Fracture of the base of the fifth metatarsal bone by indirect violence. Ann Surg 1902;35:697–701.
283. Kavanaugh JH, Brower TD, Mann RV. The Jones fracture revisited. J Bone Joint Surg Am 1978;60:776–782.
284. Lehman RC, Gregg JR, Torg E. Iselin's disease. Am J Sports Med 1986;14:494–496.
285. Magnan B, Bragantini A, Regis D, Bartolozzi P. Metatarsal lengthening by callotasis during the growth phase. J Bone Joint Surg Br 1995;77:602–607.
286. Mandell GA, Harcke HT. Scintigraphic manifestations of infarction of the second metatarsal (Freiberg's disease). J Nucl Med 1987;28:249–251.
287. Maurice HD, Newman JH, Watt I. Bone scanning of the foot for unexplained pain. J Bone Joint Surg Br 1987;69: 448–452.

288. Owen RJT, Hickey FG, Finlay DB. A study of metatarsal fractures in children. Injury 1995;8:537–538.
289. Saxby T, Nunley JA. Metatarsal lengthening by distraction osteogenesis: a report of two cases. Foot Ankle 1992;13:536–539.
290. Shereff MJ. Complex fractures of the metatarsals. Orthopedics 1990;13:875–882.
291. Smillie IS. Freiberg's infraction (Kohler's second disease). J Bone Joint Surg Br 1957;39:580–582.
292. Stewart IM. Jones fracture of the base of the fifth metatarsal. Clin Orthop 1960;16:190–198.
293. Trafton PG. Epiphyseal fracture of the base of the first metatarsal: a case report. Orthopedics 1979;2:256–257.

Metatarsal-Phalangeal Dislocation

294. Giannikas AC, Papachristou G, Nikforidis P, Garofalidis G. Dorsal dislocation of the first metatarsophalangeaal joint: report of four cases. J Bone Joint Surg Br 1966;57:384–386.
295. Henderson CE, Denno GJ Maj LN. Simultaneous open dislocation of the metatarsophalangeal and interphalangeal joints of the hallux: a case report. Foot Ankle 1986;6:305–308.
296. Jahss MH. Traumatic dislocations of the first metatarsophalangeal joint. Foot Ankle 1980;1:15–21.
297. Jahss MH. Chronic and recurrent dislocations of the fifth toe. Foot Ankle 1980;1:275–278.

Phalanges

298. Banks AS, Cain TD, Ruch JA. Physeal fractures of the distal phalanx of the hallux. J Am Podiatr Med Assoc 1988;78:310–313.
299. Buch BD, Myerson MS. Salter-Harris type IV epiphyseal fracture of the proximal phalanx of the great toe: a case report. Foot Ankle 1995;16:216–219.
300. Engber WD, Clancy WG. Traumatic avulsion of the fingernail associated with injury to the phalangeal epiphyseal plate. J Bone Joint Surg Am 1978;60:713–715.
301. Jahss MH. Stubbing injuries to the hallux. Foot Ankle 1981;1:327–332.
302. Mozena JD, Kroepel LR. Digital fractures in children. J Am Podiatr Assoc 1985;75:288–292.
303. Noonan KJ, Saltzman CL, Dietz FR. Open physeal fractures of the distal phalanx of the great toe. J Bone Joint Surg Am 1994;76:122–125.
304. Pinckney LE, Currarino G, Kennedy LA. The stubbed great toe: a cause of occult compound fracture and infection. Pediatr Radiol 1981;138:375–377.
305. Rathmore MH, Tolymat A, Paryani SG. Stubbed great toe injury: a unique clinical entity. Pediatr Infect Dis J 1993;12:1034–1035.
306. Shiraishi M, Mizuta H, Kubota K, Sakuma K, Takagi K. Stress fracture of the proximal phalanx of the great toe. Foot Ankle 1993;14:28–34.
307. Weinstein RN, Insier HP. Irreducible proximal interphalangeal dislocation of the fourth toe: a case report. Foot Ankle 1994;15:627–629.

Sesamoids

308. Bizarro AH. On the traumatology of the sesamoid structures. Ann Surg 1921;74:783–787.
309. Burton EM, Amaker BH. Stress fracture of the great toe sesamoid in a ballerina: MRI appearance. Pediatr Radiol 1994;24:37–38.
310. Chillag K, Grana WA. Medial sesamoid stress fracture. Orthopaedics 1985;8:819–821.
311. Feldman F, Pochaczevsky R, Hecht H. The case of the wandering sesamoids and other sesamoid afflictions. Radiology 1970;96:275–283.
312. Freund KG. Haematogenous osteomyelitis of the first metatarsal sesamoid. Arch Orthop Trauma Surg 1989;108:53–54.
313. Helal B. The great toe sesamoid bones: the lus or lost souls of Ushaia. Clin Orthop 1981;157:82–87.
314. Ilfeld FW, Rosen V. Osteochondritis of the first metatarsal sesamoid. Clin Orthop 1972;85:38–41.
315. Irvin CM, Witt CS, Zielsdorf LM. Traumatic osteochondritis of lateral sesamoid in active adolescents. J Foot Surg 1985;24:219–221.
316. Leventen EO. Sesamoid disorders and treatment. Clin Orthop 1991;269:236–240.
317. Ogata K, Sugioka Y, Urano Y, Chikama H. Idiopathic osteonecrosis of the first metatarsal sesamoid. Skeletal Radiol 1986;15:141–145.
318. Potter HG, Pavlov H, Abrahams TG. The hallux sesamoids revisited. Skeletal Radiol 1992;21:437–444.
319. Pretterkleiber ML, Wanivenhaus A. The arterial supply of the sesamoid bones of the hallux: the course and source of the nutrient arteries as an anatomical basis for surgical approaches to the great toe. Foot Ankle 1992;13:27–31.
320. Richardson EG. Injuries to the hallucal sesamoids in the athlete. Foot Ankle 1987;7:229–244.
321. Taylor JAM, Sartoris DJ, Huang G-S, Resnick DL. Painful conditions affecting the first metatarsal sesamoid bones. Radiographics 1993;13:817–830.
322. Van Hal ME, Kene JS, Lange TA, Clancy WG. Stress fractures of great toe sesamoids. Am J Sports Med 1982;10:122–128.
323. Walling AK, Ogden JA. Case report 666: bipartite medial sesamoid. Skeletal Radiol 1991;20:233–235.

Plantar Wounds

324. Alfred RH, Jacobs R. Occult foreign bodies of the foot. Foot Ankle 1984;4:209–211.
325. Baack BR, Kucan JO, Zook EG, Russell RC. Hand infections secondary to catfish spines; case reports and literature review. J Trauma 1991;31:1432–1436.
326. Baltimore RS, Jenson HB. Puncture wound osteochondritis of the foot caused by *Pseudomonas maltophilia*. Pediatr Infect Dis J 1990;9:143–144.
327. Barton LL, Hoddy DM, Rathore MH, Friedman AD, Graviss ER. Long term radiologic outcome of *Pseudomonas* osteomyelitis of the foot. Pediatr Infect Dis J 1990;9:476–478.
328. Bowers DG Jr, Lunch JB. Xeroradiography for non-metallic foreign bodies. Plast Reconstr Surg 1977;60:470–471.
329. Brand RA, Black H. *Pseudomonas* osteomyelitis following puncture wounds in children. J Bone Joint Surg Am 1974;56:1637–1642.
330. Burton DS, Nagel DA. *Serratia marcescens* infections in orthopaedic surgery: a review of the literature and a report of two cases. Clin Orthop 1972;89:145–149.
331. Cahill N, King JD. Palm thorn synovitis. J Pediatr Orthop 1984;4:175–179.
332. Charney DB, Manzi JA, Turlik M, Young M. Non-metallic foreign bodies in the foot: radiography versus xeroradiography. J Foot Surg 1986;25:44–49.
333. Chisholm CD, Schlesser JF. Plantar puncture wounds: controversies and treatment recommendations. Ann Emerg Med 1989;18:1352–1357.

334. Chusid MG, Jacobs WM, Sty JR. *Pseudomonas* arthritis following puncture wounds of the foot. J Pediatr 1979;94:429–431.
335. Congeni BL, Weiner DS, Izsak E. Expanded spectrum of organisms causing osteomyelitis after puncture wounds of the foot. Orthopedics 1981;4:531–533.
336. Conway WF, Hayes CW, Murphy WA. Case report 568: total resorption of the lateral sesamoid secondary to *Pseudomonas aeruginosa* osteomyelitis. Skeletal Radiol 1989;18:483–484.
337. Cracchiolo A III. Wooden foreign bodies in the foot. Am J Surg 1980;140:585–587.
338. Das De S, McAllister TA. *Pseudomonas* osteomyelitis following puncture wounds of the foot in children. Injury 1981;12:334–339.
339. Denton JR. *Pseudomonas aeruginosa* foot infections from puncture wounds. Orthop Rev 1985;14:102–106.
340. Doberstein C, MacEwen GD, Lee MS. Group B β-hemolytic *streptococcal* osteomyelitis of the heel. Clin Orthop 1988;231:225–228.
341. Edlich RF, Rodeheaver GT, Horowitz JH, Morgan RF. Emergency department management of puncture wounds and needlestick exposure. Emerg Clin North Am 1986;4:581–593.
342. Feigin RD, McAlister WH, San Joaquin VH, Middelkamp JN. Osteomyelitis of the calcaneus. Am J Dis Child 1970;119:61–65.
343. Felman AH, Fisher MS. The radiographic detection of glass in soft tissue. Radiology 1969;92:1529–1531.
344. Felman AH, Fisher MS. Detection of glass in soft tissue by x-ray. Pediatrics 1970;45:478–486.
345. Fisher MC, Goldsmith JF, Gilligan PH. Sneakers as a source of *Pseudomonas aeruginosa* in children with osteomyelitis following puncture wounds. J Pediatr 1985;106:607–609.
346. Fitzgerald RH, Cowan JD. Puncture wounds of the foot. Orthop Clin North Am 1975;6:965–972.
347. Floman Y, Katz S. Osseous lesions simulating a bone tumor due to an unsuspected fragment of wood in the foot. Injury 1975;6:344–345.
348. Frey C. Marine injuries: prevention and treatment. Orthop Rev 1994;17:645–649.
349. Fritz RH, Crosson FJ Jr. Concerning the source of *Pseudomonas* osteomyelitis of the foot. J Pediatr 1977;91:161–162.
350. Ginsburg MJ, Ellis GL, Flom LL. Detection of soft-tissue foreign bodies by plain radiography, xerography, computed tomography and ultrasonography. Ann Emerg Med 1990;19:701–703.
351. Goldstein EJ, Ahonkai VI, Cristofaro RL, et al. Source of *Pseudomonas* in osteomyelitis of heels. J Clin Microbiol 1980;12:711–713.
352. Gordon SL, Evans C, Greer RB. *Pseudomonas* osteomyelitis of the first metatarsal sesamoid of the great toe. Clin Orthop 1974;99:188–189.
353. Hagler DJ. *Pseudomonas* osteomyelitis: puncture wounds of the feet. Pediatrics 1971;48:672–673.
354. Hill MK, Sanders CV. Localized and systematic infection due to *Vibrio* species. Infect Dis Clin North Am 1987;1:687–705.
355. Howard RJ, Lieb S. Soft tissue infections caused by halophilic marine *Vibrios*. Arch Surg 1988;123:245–249.
356. Jacobs RF, Adelman L, Sack CM, Wilson CB. Management of *Pseudomonas* osteochondritis complicating puncture wounds of the foot. Pediatrics 1982;69:432–435.
357. Jacobs RF, McCarthy RE, Elser JM. *Pseudomonas* osteochondritis complicating puncture wounds of the foot in children: a 10-year evaluation. J Infect Dis 1989;160:657–661.
358. Janda JM, Bottone EJ. *Pseudomonas aeruginosa* enzyme profiling: predictor of potential invasiveness and use as an epidemiological tool. J Clin Microbiol 1981;14:55–60.
359. Jennett WB, Watson JA. The radio-opacity of glass foreign bodies. Br J Surg 1958;46:244–246.
360. Johanson PH. Pseudomonas infections of the foot following puncture wounds. JAMA 1968;204:262–264.
361. Klein B, McGahan JP. Thorn synovitis: CT diagnosis. J Comput Assist Tomogr 1985;9:1135–1136.
362. Kobs JK, Hansen AR, Keefe B. A retained wooden foreign body in the foot detected by ultrasonography. J Bone Joint Surg Am 1992;74:296–298.
363. Lang AG, Peterson HA. Osteomyelitis following puncture wounds of the foot in children. J Trauma 1976;16:993–999.
364. MacKinnon AE. *Pseudomonas* osteomyelitis following puncture wounds. Postgrad Med J 1975;51:33–34.
365. Midani S, Rathmore M. *Vibrio* species infection of a catfish spine puncture wound. Pediatr Infect Dis J 1994;13:333–334.
366. Miller EH, Semian DW. Gram-negative osteomyelitis following puncture wounds of the foot. J Bone Joint Surg Am 1975;57:535–537.
367. Minnefor AB, Olson MI, Carver DH. *Pseudomonas* osteomyelitis following puncture wounds of the foot. Pediatrics 1971;47:598–601.
368. Molla A, Mastumuru Y, Yamamuto T, Okamura R, Maeda H. Pathogenic capacity of proteases from *Serratia marcescens* and *Pseudomonas aeruginosa* and their suppression by chicken egg white ovomacroglobulin. Infect Immun 1987;55:2509–2525.
369. Murray MM, Welch DF, Kuhls TL. *Serratia* osteochondritis after puncture wounds of the foot. Pediatr Infect Dis J 1990;9:523–525.
370. Porat S, Mosheiff R, Okun J. Palm thorn osteomyelitis of the calcaneus: a case report of triple pathology. J Pediatr Orthop Part B 1992;1:85–87.
371. Puhl RW, Altman MI, Seto JE, Nelson GA. The use of fluoroscopy in the detection and excision of foreign bodies in the foot. J Am Podiar Assoc 1983;73:514–517.
372. Reigler HF, Routson FW. Complications of deep puncture wounds of the foot. J Trauma 1979;19:18–22.
373. Rickoff SE, Bauder T, Kerman BL. Foreign body localization and retrieval in the foot. J Foot Surg 1981;20:33–34.
374. Rockett MS, Gentile SC, Gudas CJ, Brage ME, Zygmunt KN. The use of ultrasonography for the detection of retained wooden foreign bodies in the foot. J Foot Ankle Surg 1995;34:478–484.
375. Simmons BP, Southmayd WU, Schwartz HS, Hall JE. Wood, an organic foreign body of bone: a case report. Clin Orthop 1975;106:276–278.
376. Stucky W, Loder RT. Extremity gunshot wounds in children. J Pediatr Orthop 1991;11:67–71.
377. Swischuk LE, Jorgenson F, Jorgenson A, Capen D. Wooden splinter induced "pseudotumors" and "osteomyelitis-like lesions" of bone and soft tissue. AJR 1974;122:176–179.
378. Tandberg D. Glass in the hand and foot. JAMA 1982;248:1872–1874.
379. Verdile VP, Freed HA, Gerard J. Puncture wounds of the foot. J Emerg Med 1989;7:193–199.
380. Wallace RJ Jr. Nontuberculous mycobacteria and water: a love affair with increasing clinical importance. Infect Dis Clin North Am 1987;1:677–685.
381. Weber CA, Wetheimer SJ, Ognijan A. *Aeromonas hydrophilia*: its implications in freshwater injuries. J Foot Ankle Surg 1995;34:442–446.
382. Weston WJ. Thorn and twig induced pseudotumours of bone and soft tissues. Br J Radiol 1963;36:323–326.
383. Wickbolt LG, Sanders CV. *Vibrio vulnificus* infection. J Am Acad Dermatol 1983;9:243–251.
384. Woesner ME, Sanders I. Xeroradiography; a significant modality in the detection of non-metallic foreign bodies in soft tissues. AJR 1972;115:636–640.

385. Yancey HA Jr. Lacerations of the plantar aspect of the foot. Clin Orthop 1977;122:46–52.

Lawn Mower Injuries

386. Anger DM, Ledbetter BR, Stagikelis PJ, Calhoun JH. Injuries of the foot related to the use of lawn mowers. J Bone Joint Surg Am 1995;77:719–725.
387. Banic A, Wulff K. Latissimus dorsi free flaps for vital repair of extensive lower leg injuries in children. Plast Reconstr Surg 1987;79:769–775.
388. Barclay TL, Sharp DT, Chisholm EM. Cross-leg fasciocutaneous flaps. Plast Reconstr Surg 1983;72:843–850.
389. Bergman AB. Power lawn mowers are dangerous weapons. Northwest Med 1965;64:261–263.
390. Chavoin JP, Dupin B, Gourdou JF, Lagarrigue J, Gayrard M. Microchirurgie. II. Reimplantation d'un pied apres amputation traumatique total. Rev Med Toulouse 1978;14:31–35.
391. Curtin JW. Functional surgery for the intractable conditions of the sole of the foot. Plast Reconstr Surg 1977;59:806–811.
392. Dawson RL. Complications of the cross-leg flap operation. Proc R Soc Med 1972;65:626–629.
393. DeMuth WE. A summer warning: lawn mowers can maim. JAMA 1973;225:355–365.
394. Furnas DW. The cross-grain flap for coverage of foot and ankle defects in children. Plast Reconstr Surg 1976;57:246–247.
395. Grosfeld JL, Morse TS, Eyring EJ. Lawn mower injuries in children. Arch Surg 1970;100:582–583.
396. Hartrampf CR, Scheflan M, Bostwick J. The flexor digitorum brevis muscle island pedicle flap: a new dimension in heel reconstruction. Plast Reconstr Surg 1980;66:264–270.
397. Herowitz JH, Nichter LS, Kenney JG, Morgan RF. Lawnmower injuries in children: lower extremity reconstruction. J Trauma 1985;25:1138–1146.
398. Johnstone BR, Bennet CS. Lawnmower injuries in children. Austral NZ J Surg 1989;59:713–718.
399. Kerr PS, Silver DA, Telford K, Andrews HS, Atkins RM. Heel-pad compressibility after calcaneal fractures; ultrasound assessment. J Bone Joint Surg Br 1995;77:504–505.
400. Letts RM, Mandirosian A. Lawn mower injuries in children. J Can Med Assoc 1977;116:1151–1153.
401. Lister G. Use of an innervated skin graft to provide sensation to the reconstructed heel. Plast Reconstr Surg 1978;62:157–161.
402. Love S, Ogden JA. Corrective procedures for soft tissue and osseous post-traumatic deformities of the child's foot and ankle. Tech Orthop 1987;2:80–87.
403. Love SM, Grogan DP, Ogden JA. Lawn mower injuries in children. J Orthop Trauma 1988;2:94–101.
404. Maisels DO. Repairs of the heel. Br J Plast Surg 1961;14:117–125.
405. Matsumura H, Malrino K, Watanabe K. Reconstruction of the sole and heel in infancy and childhood followed up for more than 10 years. Ann Plast Surg 1995;34:488–492.
406. McGraw JB. Selection of alternative local flaps in the leg and foot. Clin Plast Surg 1979;6:227–246.
407. McGraw JB, Furlow LT. The dorsalis pedis arterialized flap. Plast Reconstr Surg 1975;55:177–185.
408. Mir Y, Mir L. Functional graft of the heel. Plast Reconstr Surg 1954;14:444–450.
409. Park WH, DeMuth WE, Wounding capacity of rotary lawn mowers. J Trauma 1975;15:36–38.
410. Rajacic N, Lari AR, Khalaf ME, Kersnic M. Free flaps for the treatment of avulsion injuries in the feet. J Pediatr Orthop 1994;14:522–525.
411. Reiffel RS, McCarthy JG. Coverage of heel and sole defects: a new subfascial arterialized flap. Plast Reconstr Surg 1980;66:250–260.
412. Reigstad A, Hetland KR, Bye K, Waage S, Rokkum M, Husby T. Free flaps in the reconstruction of foot injury. 4 (1–7) year follow-up of 24 cases. Acta Orthop Scand 1994;65:103–106.
413. Ross PM, Schwentker EP, Bryan H. Mutilating lawn mower injuries in children. JAMA 1963;236:480–481.
414. Saltz R, Hochberg J, Given K. Muscle and musculocutaneous flaps of the foot. Clin Plast Surg 1991;18:627–638.
415. Serafin D, Georgiade NG, Smith DH. Comparison of free flaps with pedicled flaps for coverage of defects of the leg or foot. Plast Reconstr Surg 1977;59:492–499.
416. Serafin D, Sabatier RE, Morris RL, Georgiade NG. Reconstruction of the lower extremity with vascularized composite tissue: improved tissue survival and specific indications. Plast Reconstr Surg 1980;66:230–241.
417. Shanahan RE, Gingrass RP. Medial plantar sensory flap coverage of heel defects. Plast Reconstr Surg 1979;64:295–298.
418. Skef Z, Ecker HA Jr, Graham WP. Heel coverage by a plantar myocutaneous island pedicle flap. J Trauma 1983;23:466–472.
419. Snyder GB, Edgerton JT. The principle of the island neurovascular flap in the management of ulcerated anesthesic weightbearing areas of the lower extremity. Plast Reconstr Surg 1965;36:518–528.
420. Stevenson TR, Kling TF, Friedman RJ. Heel reconstruction with flexor digitorum brevis musculocutaneous flap. J Pediatr Orthop 1985;5:713–716.
421. Takami H, Takahashi S, Ando M. Microvascular free musculocutaneous flaps for the treatment of avulsion injuries of the lower leg. J Trauma 1983;23:473–477.
422. Taylor GA, Hopson WL. The cross-foot flap. Plast Reconstr Surg 1975;55:677–681.
423. Thurston AJ. Foot injuries caused by power lawnmowers. NZ Med J 1980;B1:131–133.
424. Tsutomu I, Harü H, Yamada A. Microvascular free flaps for the treatment of avulsion injuries in the feet of children. J Trauma 1982;22:15–19.
425. Urbaniak JR, Koman LA, Goldner RD, Armstrong NB, Nunlet JA. The vascularized cutaneous scapular flap. Plast Reconstr Surg 1982;69:772–778.
426. White WL. The menace of the rotary lawn mower. Am J Surg 1957;93:674–675.

Tarsal Tunnel

427. Albrektsson B, Rydholm A, Rydholm U. The tarsal tunnel syndrome in children. J Bone Joint Surg Br 1982;64:215–217.

Tendon Injuries

428. Brage ME, Hansen ST. Dramatic subluxation/dislocation of the peroneal tendons. Foot Ankle 1992;13:423–431.
429. Butler BW, Lanthier J, Wertheimer SJ. Subluxing peroneals: a review of the literature and case report. J Foot Ankle Surg 1992;32:134–139.
430. Citron N. Injury of the tibialis posterior tendon: the cause of acquired valgus foot in childhood. Injury 1985;16:610–612.
431. Eckert WR, Davis EA. Acute rupture of the peroneal retinaculum. J Bone Joint Surg Am 1976;57:670–673.
432. Griffiths JC. Tendon injuries about the ankle. J Bone Joint Surg Br 1965;47:686–689.
433. Johnson KA. Tibialis posterior tendon rupture. Clin Orthop 1983;177:140–147.
434. Masterson E, Jagannathan S, Borton D, Stephens MM. Pes planus in childhood due to tibialis posterior tendon injuries. J Bone Joint Surg Br 1994;76:444–446.

435. Ouzounian TJ, Myerson MS. Dislocation of the posterior tibial tendon. Foot Ankle 1992;13:215–219.
436. VanWellen PAJ, Boeck HE, Opdecam P. Non-traumatic dislocation of the tibialis posterior tendon in a child: a case report. Arch Orthop Trauma Surg 1993;112:243–244.
437. Wicks MH, Harbison JS, Paterson DC. Tendon injuries about the foot and ankle in children. Aust NZ J Surg 1980;50:158–161.

Ankle

438. Dittel KK. Chronic fibular ligament injury of the ankle in young children: a new method of ligament repair. Arch Orthop Trauma Surg 1986;105:191–192.

Congenital Injuries

439. Beckly DE, Anderson PW, Pedegana LR. The radiology of the subtalar joint with special reference to talo-calcaneal coalition. Clin Radiol 1975;26:333–341.
440. Grogan DP, Holt GR, Ogden JA. Talocalcaneal coalition in patients who have fibular hemimelia or proximal femoral focal deficiency. J Bone Joint Surg Am 1994;65:1363–1370.
441. Harris RI, Beath T. Etiology of peroneal spastic flat foot. J Bone Joint Surg Br 1948;30:624–634.
442. Hatori M, Sakurai M, Watanabe N, Oomamiuda K. Calcific bursitis in a three-year-old boy: a case report. Foot Ankle 1995;16:295–298.
443. Jack EA. Bone anomalies of the tarsus in relation to "peroneal spastic flat foot." J Bone Joint Surg Br 1954;36:530–542.
444. Klein DM, Merola AA, Spero CR. Congenital vertical talus with a talocalcaneal coalition. J Bone Joint Surg Br 1996;78:326–327.
445. Leonard MA. The inheritance of tarsal coalition and its relationship to spastic flat foot. J Bone Joint Surg Br 1974;56:520–526.
446. Morgan RC Jr, Crawford AH. Surgical management of tarsal coalition in adolescent athletes. Foot Ankle 1986;7:183–193.
447. Multhopp-Stevens H, Walling AK. Subungual (Dupuytren's) exostosis. J Pediatr Orthop 1995;15:582–584.
448. Richards RR, Evans JG, McGoey PF. Fracture of a calcaneonavicular bar: a complication of tarsal coalition; a case report. Clin Orthop 1984;185:220–221.
449. Snyder RB, Lipscomb AB, Johnston RK. The relationship of tarsal coalitions to ankle sprains in athletes. Am J Sports Med 1981;9:313–317.
450. Takakura Y, Sugimoto K, Tanaka Y, Tamai S. Symptomatic talocalcaneal coalition: its clinical significance and treatment. Clin Orthop 1991;269:249–256.
451. Tanaka Y, Takakura Y, Akiyams K, et al. Fracture of the tarsal navicular associated with calcaneonavicular coalition: a case report. Foot Ankle 1995;12:800–802.

Index

A

Abdominal trauma
   multiple injury protocol, 73
   paralytic ileus with, 311–312
   pelvic fractures and, 807–808
   thoracic spinal injuries and, 748
   thorax and rib trauma and, 427–428
Abduction injuries, distal femoral epiphyseal injuries as, 906
Abrasions, fractures associated, with, closed reduction cast application, 90–91
Accessory tarsal navicular
   anatomical development, 1096, 1098
   injury to, 1122–1123
Accidents
   hyperactivity and, immature skeletal injury incidence and, 42
   immature skeletal injuries, statistics on, 38–40
Acetabular fractures, 810–816
   central injuries, 811
   hip injury, fragments with, 845–846
   peripheral fractures, 810–811
   triradiate injuries, 811–816
Acetabular protrusion, membranous bone formation and, 2
Achilles tendon
   calcaneus, 1094
   pedal nerves, 1100
Acidosis, tourniquet use and, 273
Acquired coagulopathies, bone injury and, 321
Acquired immunodeficiency syndrome (AIDS), hemophiliac diseases, fracture injuries and risk of, 377
Acquired limb deficiencies, sports-related injuries and, 405
Acromial clavicle. *See* Distal (acromial) clavicle
Acromion
   distal (acromial) clavicle fracture and, 438, 440
   scapular fractures and, 443–445
Activity levels, immature skeletal injuries, 44
Acute skeletal trauma, magnetic resonance imaging (MRI), 136–139
Adduction injury, distal femoral epiphyseal injuries as, 906
Aerophagia, chest trauma and, 425
Age factors
   bridge development, diagnostic imaging and, 223–224
   foot growth, 1099
   fracture treatments
      closed reduction techniques, 89
      sedation and anesthesia procedures, 105
   growth mechanism injury, 147–148
   hip injuries, ischemic necrosis incidence and, 847–848
   immature skeletal injury and, 42–43
   skeletal growth, diagnostic imaging for age evaluation, 129–130
   sports-related injuries, stress fracture risk, 408
Airway, breathing, circulation (ABC) approach, multiple injury protocol, 72–73
Airway status, multiple injury protocol
   assessment and stabilization, 71
   Pediatric Trauma Score (PTS), 76
Allis reduction technique, posterior hip dislocation, 838–839
Allografting, bridge resectioning, 234
All-terrain vehicles, immature skeletal injuries, 46
ε-Aminocaproic acid (EACA), hemophiliac diseases, fracture injuries, treatment of, 375–377
Amputation
   characteristics of, 293–295
   complications, 299–301
   débridement prior to, 271–272
   epiphyseal grafting, 299–300
   finger tip injuries, 690–691
   foot injuries, talus, 1103
   hand injuries, 693–696
      autoamputation, 695
      phalangeal lengthening, 695
      replantations and transplantation, 693–695
      thermal injuries, 695
   overgrowth, 295–299
   prostheses, 300
   reflex sympathetic dystrophy (RSD) therapy, 328
Anaerobic infection, gas gangrene, 286–287
Anatomic development
   anatomy at birth, 456–462
   clavicle, 420–422
   femur, 857–861
      diaphysis, 860
      distal femur, 860–863
      femoral neck, 857–859
      greater trochanter, 858–860
      lesser trochanter, 859–860
      proximal femur, 857–858
      proximal vascularity, 860
   fibula
      distal fibula, 996–997, 999
      proximal fibula, 995
      syndesmosis, 997–999
      tibiofibular diaphyses, 995–996
   foot, 1091–1100
      accessory navicular development, 1096, 1098
      calcaneus, 1093–1094
      growth patterns, 1099–1100
      maturation and variation, 1095–1096
      metatarsals, 1095–1096
      os trigonum, 1096, 1098–1099
      pedal nerves, 1100
      phalanges, 1095, 1097
      plantar foot padding, 1096–1097

Anatomic development (*cont.*)
    talus, 1091–1093, 1098
    tarsal bones, 1094–1095, 1097
    tendons, 1100
  hip, 831–832
  immature skeletal injuries
    articular injuries, 49–50
    cervical injuries, 50
    childhood *vs.* adult trauma, 47–48
    diaphyseal injuries, 48–49
    epicondylar injuries, 49–50
    epiphyseal region, 49
    intercondylar (intraepiphyseal) injuries, 50
    malleolar, 51
    metaphyseal injuries, 48–50
    physeal region, 49
    subcapital injuries, 50
    supracondylar injuries, 50
    transcondylar injuries, 50
  knee joint, 929–932
    ligaments and capsule, 932–933
    meniscus, 932
    patella, 929–932
  pelvis, 790–794
  ribs, 419
  scapula, 422
  skeletal development, 3–13
  spine, 708–717
  sternum, 419–420
  tibia
    distal tibia, 996–998
    proximal tibia, 990–992
    syndesmosis, 997–999
    tibial tuberosity, 992–995
    tibiofibular diaphyses, 995–996
  wrist and hand, 650–653
    functional anatomy, 653–654
    injury incidence, 654–655
Androgens, growth mechanism injury, physeal biomechanics and, 196
Anesthesia, fracture treatment and, 105–108
Angiography
  arterial injury diagnosis, 315
  magnetic resonance imaging (MRI) with, vascular injury, 140
  scintigraphy (radionuclide imaging) and, 139–140
Angulation
  as bone injury complication, 334–335
  bridge resectioning and, 232
  diagnostic imaging, postreduction evaluation, 122
  diaphyseal humeral fractures, 478–479
  distal radioulnar injuries, 622–623
  extra-octave fracture, 680–682
  femoral shaft fractures, 883–884
    complications from, 893–894
  of fracture fragments
    closed reduction techniques, 89
    correction of, 87
  growth mechanism injury
    management of deformation, 219, 226
    type 8 fracture pattern, 188
  immature skeletal injury, residual angulation remodeling, 259
  limb length equalization, 235
  proximal humeral physeal fracture, 473
  proximal radial fractures, 586–588
  proximal tibial metaphyseal injuries, 1030–1031
  radioulnar fracture as, 606
  radius and ulna, 571
  tibiofibular diaphyseal injuries, 1040–1041
Animal studies, spinal injury pathology, 722–724
Anisomelia, limb length evaluation, diagnostic imaging, 130
Ankle injury
  arthrodesis, 1076
  computed tomography (CT) imaging, 135
  distal fibular injuries, 1069–1073
  intramalleolar injury (accessory ossicle), 1067–1069
  syndesmosis development, 997–999
  tendon injuries, 1075–1076
  tibiofibular ligament injuries, 1073–1075
  Tillaux fracture, congruity issues, 1051–1052
  See also Distal tibial fractures
Anorexia nervosa, sports-related injuries and, 403
Antecedent injury, role of, in sports-related injuries, 403
Anterior cruciate ligament (ACL) injuries to, 946, 948–950
  tibia
    anatomic development, 992
    tibial spine injuries, 1000
Anterior spinal artery syndrome, diagnosis, 726
Anteroinferior iliac spine (AIIS), pelvic avulsion fractures, 818–822
Anterosuperior iliac spine (ASIS), pelvic avulsion fractures, 818–822
Antibiotics
  bites and sting wounds, 279
  débridement, with open injury and, 272
  examination prior to using, 271
  open injury infection and, 281–282
  gas gangrene, 287
Antiseizure medications, sedation and anesthesia procedures in presence of, 105
Apophyseal injury
  calcaneus, 1094
    treatment and repair, 1117–1118
  ischial tuberosity avulsion, 822–824
  spinal injuries, lumbar injury, 760–765
  sports-related injuries, 407
Apophysitis
  in calcaneus, 1119
  metatarsal injury, 1132–1133
Arbeitsgemeinschaft für Osteosynthesefragen (AO) technique
  complications, management of, 102
  fracture treatment using, 99
Arm growth, diagnostic imaging
  limb length evaluation, 130–134
  postnatal growth evaluation, 128–129
Arterial injury
  complications from, 313–320
    compartment syndrome, 316–318
    vasospasm, 315–316
    Volkmann's contracture, 318–320
  diagnosis of, 314
  transection, 313
  trauma involving, 313–320
    compartment syndrome, 316–318
    vasospasm, 315–316
    Volkmann's contracture, 318–320
Arterial oxygen tension, fat embolism and, 322
Arteriography
  arterial injury diagnosis, 314–315
  proximal tibial epiphyseal injuries, vascular injury assessment, 1011
Arthritis, distal tibial fracture complications, 1065
Arthrodesis, ankle, 1076
Arthrography
  child abuse and fracture injuries, 383–384
  elbow injuries, capitellum, 561
  lateral condyle injuries, 515–516
  magnetic resonance imaging (MRI) in, 137
  Monteggia lesions, 601–602
  proximal femoral fractures, 868
  techniques for, 135
Arthrogryposis, joint stiffness, 360–362
Arthroscopy
  distal tibial injuries, 1060–1061
  knee injuries, 935–936
    osteochondritis dissecans, 968–971
  tibial spine injuries, 1002–1005
Articular cartilage, intraarticular fractures, cartilage repair, 260–261
Articular joints
  growth mechanism injury, type 5 fracture patterns, 172–180
  immature skeletal injury and, characteristics of, 49–50

Index

Assessment rating system, multiple injuries, 76
Asthma, fracture treatment, sedation and anesthesia procedures, 105
Ataxia, head trauma complications, 324
Athletics
  bone injuries and
    apophyseal injury, 407
    causation, 403
    epiphyseal injury, 406–407
    exercise routines, 403–404
    fitness and, 404
    incidence and epidemiology, 399–402
    osteochondroses, 407
    physeal injury, 405–407
    physiologic alteration, 403
    preparticipation screening, 402–403
    repetitive injuries, 406–407
    stress fractures, 407–414
    team physicians' role concerning, 402
  congenital/acquired limb deficiencies, 405
  exertional compartment syndrome, 405
  growth mechanism injury and, 149–150
    type 1B injury, repetitive use and, 157–158
    type 3 fracture pattern, 176
  head injury, 404
  muscle injury, 405
  spinal injury, 404–405
Atlantoaxial joint
  anatomy of, 708
  rotatory subluxation, 734–736
Atlantooccipital dislocation, characteristics of, 732
Atlas
  fractures of, 731–733
  rotatory subluxation, atlantoaxial joint, 734
Atlas-dens interval (ADI), Down syndrome and compression risk, 721
Atraumatic osteolysis of the distal clavicle (AODC), sports-related injuries, 407
Autoamputation, sensory neuropathy and, 695
Automatic garage door opening/closing devices, immature skeletal injuries, statistics on, 39
Automobile accidents. See Motor vehicle accidents
Autonomic dysreflexis, spinal cord injury, 767–768
Avulsion injuries
  collateral knee ligaments, 946–947
  distal (acromial) clavicle fracture and, 441
  distal fibular injuries, 1069–1073
  elbow dislocation, 548
  growth mechanism injuries, type 9 fracture patterns, 192–194
  lesser tuberosity avulsion, 474
  Osgood-Schlatter lesions, 1018–1020
  patellar fractures, sleeve fractures, 953–957
  pelvic fractures, 816–824
    iliac crest, 817–818
    iliac spines, 818–822
    ischial tuberosity, 822–824
  scaphoid fractures, 659–660
  talus, 1103, 1106
  tibial spine injuries, 998, 1000–1011
  tibial tuberosity injuries, 1011–1013
  wringer injuries, 292
Axial compression, biomechanics of bone and, 28–30
Axis
  body and neural arch fractures, 740–741
  dens injuries, 736–738
  rotatory subluxation, atlantoaxial joint, 734–735

B

Bacterial growth patterns
  open injury infection, 280
  plantar foot padding wounds, 1141–1145
Baker's cyst, pseudothrombophlebitis with, 321
Bankart lesion, glenohumeral joint dislocation, 464
Barton's fracture, distal radial injury, 625
Baseball, sports-related injuries with, 401
Battered child syndrome
  fracture injury with, 380–381
  pathology, 384–385
  proximal humeral physeal fracture, 466
  radiology and, 383–384
  See also Child abuse
Beds
  bunk bed fracture, 1132–1133
  falls from, immature skeletal injuries, 47
Bennett's fracture
  thumb involvement, 667
  wringer injuries and, 292
Bicycles
  crush-burn injuries, 290
  foot injuries, 1101
  immature skeletal injuries, 46
Bier block procedure, fracture treatment using, 106–107
Bigelow reduction technique, posterior hip dislocation, 838–840
Bimetallic corrosion, internal fixation devices, 103
Biodegradable materials
  growth mechanism injury, physeal injuries, management of, 212
  internal fixation of fractures using, 100
Bioelectric phenomena, fracture repair patterns, remodeling, analysis of, 256–257
Biomechanics
  immature skeletal injury
    childhood vs. adult trauma, 48
    healing and repair patterns, 243–264
  physis, growth mechanism injury and, 193, 195–196
  proximal tibial epiphyseal injuries, 1010–1011
  of skeletal development, 24–30
Bioresorbable implants, internal fixation fracture treatment using, 100
Bipartite patella, mechanisms of, 960–964
Birth trauma
  brachial plexus injuries, 446
  clavicle injury
    diagnosis, 432
    incidence, 430–431
    injury mechanism, 431–432
    treatment, 433–434
  distal femoral epiphyseal injury, 896–898
  fracture patterns
    type 1C fracture injury, 159–161
    type 1 fracture injury, 157
  glenohumeral joint dislocation, 466–468
  hip dislocation, 850–851
  pelvic fractures and, 810
  proximal femoral fractures, 866–868
  pulled elbow, 556
  spinal cord injury, 731
  spinal injury from, 731
Bites
  hand injuries, 691–692
  open injury from, 279–280
Blackburn and Peel technique, Osgood-Schlatter lesion diagnosis, 1022
Bladder injury, pelvic fractures and, 808–810
Blair fusion, chronic talar deformity, 1105
Blastema. See Reparative tissue
Blood loss
  fracture injuries, associated vascular injury, 88
  shock as complication of, 312–313
    multiple injury protocol, 72

Blood loss (cont.)
  significance in children, 311–312
Blood pressure
  initial response protocols and maintenance of, 71
    shock, treatment of, 72
  Pediatric Trauma Score (PTS), multiple injury protocol, 76
Blount's disease
  intraepiphyseal osteotomy, 198
  osteochondroses, fracture injuries, 365
  type 5 fracture patterns, 173
  See also Varus deformities
Body type, sports injury incidence and, 399–400
Bohler's angle
  calcaneus injuries, radiographic imaging, 1115–1116
  peritalar and subtalar dislocations, 1110
Bone bruising
  distal femoral epiphyseal injuries and, 905–906
  growth mechanism injury, type 7 fracture pattern, 187–189
  immature skeletal injury as, 54, 56
  knee injuries, diagnosis, 934–935
  magnetic resonance imaging (MRI), 136–138
  type 8 injury pattern, 189, 197
  sports-related injuries, stress injuries and, 409
Bone density, mineralization and, 23–24
Bone fatigue, biomechanics of, 29–30
Bone grafting
  lateral condyle injuries, complications, 520–521
  pseudarthrosis, 331–332
Bone growth and development
  control of, 16
  endochondral ossification, 2–3
  estimation, limb length equalization, 234–235
  femoral shaft fractures, complications from, 892–893
  growth mechanism injury, incidence and epidemiology, 209–210
  limb length equalization, 235–236
  membranous bone formation, 1–2
  metaphyseal changes, 16–17
  physeal growth patterns, 16
  physiologic epiphysiodesis, 17–18
  saltation concept, 16
  See also Longitudinal growth; Overgrowth
Bone loss, in open fractures, 276–277
Bone marrow
  fat embolism incidence and, 322
  magnetic resonance imaging (MRI) of, 136

  in thalassemia patients, 377–378
Bone mineral density (BMD)
  cerebral palsy and fractures with, 371
  immature skeletal injury, fracture healing and repair, 259
Bone scans
  bipartite patella, 962–964
  metatarsal injury, 1133–1134
  os trigonum injuries, 1108–1109
  talus injury, ischemic necrosis, 1105
Bone shortening, limb length equalization, 235
"Booby-trap" fracture, phalangeal neck fractures as, 681–684
Botulism, open injury infection, 288
Bowel injury, pelvic fractures, 807–808
  avulsion fractures, 818
Bowing injuries
  diagnostic imaging, 124–125
  femoral shaft fractures, complications from, 893–894
  immature skeletal injury as, 51, 53
  metacarpal fractures, 669–670
  Monteggia lesions, 598
  osteogenesis imperfecta and, 357–358
Boxer's fracture, characteristics, 672, 674–675
Brachial plexus, trauma to, 445–448
  glenohumeral joint dislocation, 465
Brain stem auditory evoked potentials (BAEPs), head trauma, multiple injury protocol, 79
Break-dancing, immature skeletal injuries from, 45
Bridge development
  diagnostic imaging, 220–221, 223–224
  distal femoral epiphyseal injuries and, 902–904
  distal tibial injuries, 1062–1066
  growth mechanism injury
    diagnostic imaging, 221
    physeal injuries, management of, 211
  immature skeletal injury, fracture healing and repair patterns, 258
  physeal growth alteration, 212–219
    central (type 3) bridge formation, 218–219, 225–226
    experimental bridging, 216–217
    formation mechanisms, 214–216
    histopathology, 217–223
    linear (type 2) bridge formation, 218, 224–225
    mapping of, 224, 226
    natural bridge formation, 212
    nondisruptive bridging, 213–214
    peripheral (type 1) bridge formation, 217–218, 223
  resectioning of, 228–234
    acute fat replacement, 234
    allografting, 234

    central (type 3) bridge, 230–232
    distraction epiphysiolysis, 233–234
    epiphyseal transplantation, 2334
    general principles, 230–233
    linear (type 2) bridge, 229–230
    peripheral (type 1) bridge, 228–229
    postoperative care, 234
  surgical treatment, 226–228
    indomethacin, 227–228
    interposition materials, 226–227
  type 4 fracture injury, 169–170
  type 5 fracture injury, 173–180
Brown-Sequard lesions, spinal cord injury, 768
Bryant's traction
  femoral shaft fractures, 882–883
  proximal femoral fractures, birth trauma, 868
Bucket handle injury, pelvis, characteristics of, 805
Buckle fracture, diagnostic imaging, 125
Bunk bed fracture, metatarsal injury, 1132–1133
Burns
  fracture treatment with complications involving, 87
    external fixators, indications for, 94–96
  growth mechanism injury, 182, 184
    type 6 fracture patterns, 181
  hand injuries, 695–696
  joint stiffness and, 361
Burst fractures, lumbar spine injuries, 756–758

C

Caffey's disease, membranous bone formation and, 2
Calcaneus
  anatomic development, 1093–1094
  apophysitis, 1119–1120
  fractures
    anterior process fracture, 1117–1118
    apophyseal fractures, 1118–1119
    classification, 1112–1115
    compartment syndrome, 1101–1102
    diagnosis, 1112–1116
    growth sequelae, 1117
    patterns of, 1110–1112
    stress fracture, 1118, 1120
    treatment, 1116–1117
Calcaneus secundarius, calcaneus fractures and, 1117
Calcific deposition
  hand injuries and, 656
  tendon injuries, 699
Calcitonin therapy, hypercalcemia, 329
Callus formation
  immature skeletal injury, fracture repair, 244–246

myelodysplasia and fracture injury and, 368–369
osteogenesis imperfecta and, 357–358
Cancellous bone
  immature skeletal injuries, fracture repair, 249
  immature skeletal injury, reparative phase, 254–255
Capillary refill, arterial injury and, 314
Capital femur injury
  complications, 875–876
  slipped capital femoral epiphysis (SCFE), 843–845
Capitellar deformities
  elbow injuries, 560–562
  lateral condyle injuries, 521–523
  radial head dislocations, 591, 594
  sports-related injuries, 406–407
Capsule. *See* Joint capsule
Carbonated beverages, rickets and, 351–352
Cardiac tamponade
  multiple injury protocol, chest trauma and, 73
  thorax and rib trauma, 427
Cardiogenic shock, as trauma complication, 311
Carpal fractures
  diagnosis, 661–663
  incidence, 657
Carpal primary ossification, anatomical development, 650–651
Carpal subluxation and dislocation, wrist injuries, 657
Carpometacarpal (CMC) joint dislocation, characteristics of, 664–665
Cartilage
  biomechanics of, 26–28
  bridge resection using, 227
  complications involving, 338
  distal femoral epiphyseal injuries, complications involving, 908–910
  endochondral ossification, bone replacement, 3–4
  epiphyseal cartilage, 9–10
    diagnostic imaging, 123
  growth mechanism injury
    physeal biomechanics and, 195–196
    type 6 fracture patterns, 181
    type 7 injury patterns, 186–187
  immature skeletal injury
    continuous passive motion (CPM), 262
    fracture repair, inflammatory phase, development of, 248–249
    hematoma formation, 251
    repair patterns, 259–262
    reparative phase in, 254
  knee injuries, osteochondritis dissecans, 967–971

metaphyseal circulation and maturation of, 20, 22
skeletal vasculature and, 19–20
spinal, 710–711
talus bone, 1092–1093
  injuries, 1103–1104
triradiate cartilage
  acetabular fractures and, 811–816
  pelvic development, 790–792
zones of, in physis, 13
Casts and casting
  arterial injury with, 313
  bipartite patella, 963–964
  closed reductions with
    application, 90–91
    complications, 91
    removal of, 91
    See also Pins and cast insertions
  diaphyseal humeral fractures, 478–479
  distal femoral metaphyseal injuries, 896
  distal metaphysis (supracondylar) injuries, 486–488
  distal radioulnar injuries, 620–621
  femoral shaft fractures, 886–888
  fixation treatments, supplementation of, 93
  foot injuries
    calcaneus injuries, 1116
    tarsometatarsal injuries, 1125–1126
  head injury, fracture treatment using, 88–89
  metatarsal injury, 1135
  Osgood-Schlatter lesions, 1022–1024
  padding for, 91
  Sinding-Larsen-Johansson (SLJ) lesions, 958–960
  spinal injury, atlas fractures, 733–734
  tibial spine injuries, 1003–1005
  tibiofibular diaphyseal injuries, vascular complications with, 1039–1040
Cast syndrome, as bone injury compilation, 337–338
Causation, role of, in sports-related injuries, 403
Cellular proliferative disorders, physeal fracture patterns, type 1B injuries, 157
Cellular reactivity, immature skeletal injury
  fracture repair, inflammatory phase, 248
  physiologic response assessment, 251–253
Cellulitis, open injury infection, clostridial cellulitis, 287–288
Central nervous system (CNS)
  rehabilitation treatment, 104–105
  tourniquet use, effects on, 273
Central (type 3) bridge formation

physeal growth alteration, 218–219, 225–226
resectioning techniques, 230–232
Cephalosporin, open wound infection treatment using, 282
Cerebral palsy
  fractures with, 370–372
  proximal tibial epiphyseal injuries, 1006–1007
  Sinding-Larsen-Johansson (SLJ) lesions, 959–960
Cerebral swelling, multiple injury protocol, diagnostic imaging of head trauma and, 78–79
Cervical region
  atlas fractures and, 733
  birth injury, 731
  diagnostic imaging of, 727
  end-plate injury, 744–748, 762
  immature skeletal injury to, 50
  lower cervical fracture-dislocation, 741–743
  multiple injury protocol, diagnostic imaging of head trauma and, 78–79
  spinal cord injury, 767–768
  subluxation, 729
  upper cervical fracture-dislocation, 740–741
  vasculature in, 711–713
Chance fracture, characteristics of, 751–754
Charcot arthropathy, growth mechanism injury, type 5 fracture pattern, 173, 177
Charcot joint
  ankle injuries, 1045–1047
  knee injuries, characteristics of, 980
Chemonucleolysis, disk herniation, 763
Chemotherapy, growth mechanism injury from, 179–180, 182
CHEOPS scale, fracture treatment
  nitrous oxide administration and, 108
  sedation and anesthesia procedures, 105–108
Chest and shoulder girdle. *See* Sternum; Thorax; specific areas, e.g. Ribs
Chest trauma
  multiple injury protocol, 73
  thorax and ribs, 422–429
    cardiac tamponade, 427
    diaphragm and abdominal injury, 427–428
    first rib fracture, 425–426
    hemothorax, 427
    pancreas, 428
    pneumothorax, 427
    pulmonary contusion, 426–427
    slipping rib syndrome, 428–429
    splenic injury, 428
    subcutaneous emphysema, 427

Chest trauma (*cont.*)
   thoracic outlet syndrome, 426
   tracheobronchial tree injury, 427
Child abuse
  chest and rib trauma and, 422–425
  fracture injuries, 379–386
    incidence of, 379–380
    pathology, 384–385
    radiology, 383–384
    soft tissue injury, 385–386
  fracture patterns
    type 1C fracture injury, 159–161
    type 1 fracture injury, 157
  growth mechanism injury
    classification, 149
    diagnostic imaging, 152
    incidence and epidemiology, 209
  hand injuries, 656
  osteogenesis imperfecta and, 356–358
  proximal humeral physeal fracture, 466
  scapular fractures and, 443–445
  spinal injury and, 731
  transcondylar injuries, 497, 499–500
  See also Battered child syndrome
Chinese finger traps, metatarsal injuries, 1129–1130
Chloral hydrate, fracture treatment using, 107
Chondral divot fracture, open injury as, 279
Chondroepiphyses
  endochondral ossification, vascularization of, 3
  physis characteristics and, 11–13
  wrist and hand anatomy, 651
  See also Epiphyses
Chondro-osseous fractures
  bone injury complications, 328–336
    angulation, 334–335
    epiphysiolysis, 332
    exostosis and osteochondroma, 334
    fracture recurrence, 332
    hypercalcemia, 328–329
    hypertension, 336
    myositis ossificans (heterotopic ossification), 329–330
    pin migration, 336–337
    postfracture cyst, 332–334
    pseudarthrosis, 331–332, 336
    synostosis, 330–331
    traction complications, 336
  compartment syndrome, 317
  dysplasias and, 354–355
  foot injuries, 1101
  growth mechanism injury
    healing patterns, 198–200
    type 7 fracture pattern, 185–187
  intramalleolar injury (accessory ossicle), 1067–1069
Chopart level, amputation, 295

Chronic arterial insufficiency, arterial injury and, 315
Circulation, assessment of
  immature skeletal injury, fracture repair, inflammatory phase, 246–249
  multiple injury protocol, 71–72
    shock, treatment of, 72
  See also Vascular injury
Circumferential lamellar bone, remodeling characteristics of, 21, 23
Clavicle
  anatomical characteristics of, 420–422
  growth patterns in, 421–422
  membranous ossification in, 2
  trauma to, 430–442
    complex injury, 435
    complications, 434–435
    congenital pseudarthrosis, 435–436
    diagnosis, 431
    diagnostic imaging, 432–433
    distal (acromial) clavicle, 438–442
    injury mechanism, 431–432
    pathologic anatomy, 431
    proximal (sternal) clavicle, 436–438
    remodeling, 434
    treatment, 433–434
Clavicular "duplication," distal (acromial) clavicle fracture, 441–442
Clinical findings
  predictive value of, *vs.* radiographic findings, 116–117
  sports-related injuries, stress injuries and, 410
Closed reduction
  advantages of, 89–90
  basic principles, 87
  cast application techniques, 90–91
  cast complications, 91
  cast removal, 91
  distal (acromial) clavicle fracture, 441
  distal metaphysis (supracondylar) injuries, 490
  distal radial injury, 628–629
  distal radioulnar injuries, 618–619
  distal tibial injuries, 1060–1061
  distal ulnar injuries, 634–635
  divergent elbow dislocation, 549–550
  femoral shaft fractures, 886–888
  fixation treatments combined with, 93
  growth mechanism injury, physeal injuries, management of, 211–212
  head injury fracture treatment, 88–89
  intercarpal disruptions, 664
  interphalangeal dislocation, 678
  patellar sleeve fractures, 957
  pelvic fractures, 805
  phalangeal neck fractures, 682–684

  proximal humeral physeal fracture, 472
  proximal phalangeal fracture, 680
  proximal radial fractures, 586–588
  proximal (sternal) clavicle injury, 437–438
  proximal tibial epiphyseal injuries, 1007–1009
  proximal tibiofibular joint dislocation, 1025–1026
  radioulnar fractures, 611–612
  slipped capital femoral epiphysis (SCFE), 869–870
  thumb dislocation, 665–666
  tibial spine fractures, 1001–1005
  tibial tuberosity injuries, 1015–1017
  type 2 fracture patterns, 163–166
Clostridial infection, open injury and, 284–288
  atypical infection, 287–289
  botulism, 288
  clostridial cellulitis, 287
  gas gangrene, 285–287
  tetanus, 287
Clot formation, immature skeletal injury, fracture repair, inflammatory phase, 246–249
Clotting factor deficiencies, bone injury complications from, 321
Clubfoot, fracture injury with, 361
Coagulation disorders, fracture injuries with, 374–377
Coagulation phase, wound healing, immature skeletal injury, 244
Coccyx, injuries to, 763, 766–767
Collagen
  amputation involving, overgrowth, 296
  biomechanics of, 28–30
  hip injuries, voluntary habitual dislocation with collagen disorders, 851
  immature skeletal injury, fracture repair, inflammatory phase, development of, 248–249
  osteogenesis imperfecta and involvement of, 356–358
  skeletal development and, 15–16
Collateral ligaments
  injuries to, 945–947
  knee dislocations and reconstruction of, 937–938
  proximal fibula, anatomic development, 995
Colorization
  Doppler sonography, 140
  magnetic resonance imaging (MRI), 136
Comatose children, fracture treatment in, external fixators, indications for, 94–96
Comminuted fracture

Index

acute fat replacement, 234
calcaneus, 1110–1112
growth mechanism injuries, physeal injuries, management of, 211–212
immature skeletal injury as, 51, 53
type 3 fracture injury, 167, 170
type 4 fracture injury, 172–175
Comparison views, diagnostic imaging, importance of, 118
Compartment syndrome
  arterial injury and, 314–318
  diagnosis of, 316–317
  distal metaphysis (supracondylar) injuries and, 494–495
  foot injuries, 1101–1102
    calcaneus injuries, 1116
    tarsometatarsal injury, 1123–1124
  fracture treatment and, 88
  initial response protocol and, 71
  multiple injury protocol, 74
  open injury, muscle involvement, 273
  proximal tibial epiphyseal injuries
    complications, 1010–1011
    diagnosis of, 1007
  radioulnar fractures, 608
  sports-related injuries and exertional compartment syndrome, 405
  tibial tuberosity injuries, 1017–1018
  tibiofibular diaphyseal injuries, 1041–1042
  venomous snake bites, 279
Complex clavicular injury, characteristics of, 435
Complex metacarpophalangeal (MCP) joint dislocation, diagnosis of, 675–676
Complications
  amputation, 299–300
  arterial injury, 313–320
    compartment syndrome, 316–318
    vasospasm, 315–316
    Volkmann's contracture, 318–320
  cartilage, 338
  cast complications, 338
  cast syndrome, 337–338
  characteristics of, in children, 311–312
  chondro-osseous complications, 328–336
    angulation, 334–335
    epiphysiolysis, 332
    exostosis and osteochondroma, 334
    fracture recurrence, 332
    hypercalcemia, 328–329
    hypertension, 336
    myositis ossificans (heterotopic ossification), 329–330
    pin migration, 336–337
    postfracture cyst, 332–334
    pseudarthrosis, 331–332, 336
    synostosis, 330–331
    traction complications, 336

clavical injury, 434
  proximal (sternal) clavicle injury, 438
diaphyseal humeral fractures, 479
distal femoral epiphyseal injuries, 908–910
distal metaphysis (supracondylar) injuries, 491–494
distal radial injury, 629–632
  exostosis, 631–632
  growth disturbance, 629–631
  neurologic problems, 629
  synostosis, 631
  ulnar styloid complications, 631–632
distal radioulnar injuries, 621–624
distal tibial injuries, 1062–1066
distal ulnar injuries, 635
elbow dislocation, 550–551
fat fractures, 337
fat necrosis, 337
femoral shaft fractures, 892–895
  angulation/bowing, 893–894
  bone length/overgrowth, 892–893
  growth arrest, 895
  muscle function, 895
  myositis, 895
  nerve injury, 895
  refracture, 895
  rotation, 894–895
  vascular injury, 892
foreign bodies, 336
fracture blisters, 338
fracture treatments, 100–104
  closed reductions, 91
  hardware removal, 101–103
  summary of, 87–88
hemorrhagic complications, 321–323
  acquired coagulopathies, 321
  disseminated intravacsular coagulation (DIC), 321–322
  fat embolism, 322–323
  hereditary coagulopathies, 321
hip injuries, 846–850
  ischemic necrosis (osteonecrosis), 846–849
  myositis ossificans, 850
  neurologic deficits, 850
  osteoarthritis, 850
  osteochondrosis, 850
  recurrent dislocation, 849–850
immature skeletal injury and, 58, 60
infection, 338
lateral condyle injuries, 520–523
Monteggia lesions, 602
myelodysplasia and fracture injury and, 369–370
neurologic complications, 323–328
  head injury, 323–324
  muscle immobilization, 328
  peripheral nerve injuries, 324–326

reflex sympathetic dystrophy (RSD), 326–328
olecranon fractures, 578, 580
pelvic fractures, 805–810
proximal femoral fractures, 873–876
proximal humeral physeal fracture, 473
proximal radial fractures, 588–590
proximal tibial epiphyseal injuries, 1009–1011
proximal tibial metaphyseal injuries, 1030–1035
radioulnar fractures, 614–615
shock, 312–313
tibial spine injuries, 1004–1005
tibial tuberosity injuries, 1016–1018
tibiofibular diaphyseal injuries, 1040–1042
  open injuries, 1038–1039
venous disorders, 320–321
Composite wiring, hand injuries and, 656
Compression
  arterial injury, 313
  clavicle injury and, 434
  distal metaphysis (supracondylar) injuries, 485–486
  distal radial fractures, neurologic complications, 629
  fracture treatment with, external fixators using, 96
  growth mechanism injuries
    type 5 fracture patterns, 172–180
    type 9 fracture patterns, 192–194
    type 2 injury patterns, 162–166
  immature skeletal injury, reparative phase in, 254
  multiple injury protocol, abdominal trauma and, 73
  pelvic fractures, 805
  skeletal biomechanics and, 26–30
  spinal injury, lower cervical fracture-dislocation, 742–744
Computed tomography (CT)
  ankle tendon injuries, 1075–1076
  brachial plexus injuries, 447
  calcaneus injuries, 1115–1116
  glenohumeral joint dislocation, 464–465
  growth mechanism injury
    diagnosis, 152
    diagnostic imaging, 221
    physeal injuries, management of, 211
  hip injuries, posterior dislocation, 837
  knee injuries, 933–935
  Monteggia lesions, 601–602
  multiple injury protocol, 75
    head trauma assessment, 78–79
  Osgood-Schlatter lesions, 1020–1022
  pelvic fractures, diagnosis, 796–798

Computed tomography (*cont.*)
  proximal (sternal) clavicle injury, 436–437
  pulmonary contusion assessment, 426
  spinal injury, 727–728
  talus fractures, 1104
    dome fracture, 1107–1108
    ischemic necrosis, 1105
  techniques for, 135–136
  triplane distal tibial fracture, 1052–1054
  Volkmann's contracture diagnosis, 319
Conditioning, role of, in sports-related injuries, 403
Congenital abnormalities
  bipartite scaphoid, 661
  as complication, 311–312
  foot injuries and, 1149
  medial condyle injuries and, 502
  pseudoarthrosis, clavicle injury and, 435–436
  radial head dislocations, 591–594
  spinal injuries, 719–720
  sports-related injuries and, limb deficiencies, 405
  talus bone, 1109
Congenital sensory neuropathy
  foot injuries and, 1149
  fractures with, 373–376
  growth mechanism injury, type 5 fracture pattern, 173, 177
Consciousness, assessment of, Pediatric Trauma Score (PTS), 76
Conservatism, in children's fracture treatment, limits of, 86
Continuity lesions, arterial injury, 313
Continuous passive motion (CPM), immature cartilage injury, repair and healing of, 262
Contouring processes, characteristics of, 10
Contractures
  burn injuries, hand injuries, 696
  elbow dislocations, 551
  tendon injury, 697
Contusions
  arterial injury, 313
  See also Lacerations
Convergent dislocation. *See* Translocation
Cooley's anemia, fracture injuries with, 378
Copper deficiency, fracture injury and, 354
Coracoid process
  glenohumeral joint dislocation, transfer procedure, 464
  scapular fractures and, 443–444
  separation, distal (acromial) clavicle fracture and, 441

"Corner fractures," type 1B injury as, 157
Corner signs, diagnostic imaging of, 123
Coronoid process
  fractures of, 580–582
  growth and development, 567–568
Cortical bone
  biomechanics of, 28
  diagnostic imaging, irregularities in, 124
  immature skeletal injuries, fracture repair, 249
  sports-related injuries, stress injuries and, 410
Coxa plana, osteochondroses, fracture injuries, 365
Coxa valga, slipped capital femoral epiphysis (SCFE), 869–870
Coxa vara, proximal femoral fractures
  birth trauma, 868
  complications, 873–876
  treatment and repair, 872
Crack propagation, sports-related stress injuries, 410
Cranial bone, membranous bone formation, 1–2
Craniopharyngioma, fracture injuries and, 353–354
Crouched-knee gait, Sinding-Larsen-Johansson (SLJ) lesions, 960
Cruciate insufficiency syndrome, anterior cruciate ligament (ACL) injury, 949
Cruciate ligaments
  injuries to, 946–950
    anterior cruciate ligament (ACL), 946, 948–950
    posterior cruciate ligament (PCL), 950
  knee dislocations, reconstruction with, 937–941
  tibial spine injuries involving, 1000
    complications, 1004–1005
Crush-burn injuries
  characteristics of, 290
  foot injuries, 1101
Crushing injuries
  characteristics of, 290–292
  compartment syndrome and, 318
  scapular fractures, 443
Cubitus varus, distal metaphysis (supracondylar) injuries, 495
Cuboid bones, anatomical development, 1094–1095
Cuneiform bones
  anatomical development, 1094–1095
  injuries to, 1123
Curretage, physeal growth alteration
  experimental bridging, 216–217
  limb length equalization, 235
Cystic fractures

hip injuries, acetabular fragments, 846
  pathology of, 362–364
Cystography, pelvic fractures and urologic injury diagnosis, 809–810
Cysts
  Baker's cyst, 321
  calcaneus, 1093–1094
    incidence of, 1110–1111
  meniscal cysts, 977–978
  pathologic fractures and, 362–364
  popliteal cysts, 980

D
Débridement
  crushing injuries, 290
  foot injuries, 1101
    peritalar and subtalar dislocations, 1110
  wound care, open fractures, 271–272, 274
    bone loss, 276–277
    botulism infection, 288
    gas gangrene, 287
    infection, 280–282
Decubiti development, spinal cord injury, 770
Degloving injuries, characteristics of, 290–291
Delayed union
  distal radioulnar injuries, 621–622
  as fracture treatment complication, 101
  incidence of, with open fracture débridement, 272
  lateral condyle injuries, 518–522
  proximal femoral fractures, 873–876
  radioulnar fractures, 614–615
  tibial spine fractures, 1002–1005
  tibiofibular diaphyseal injuries, 1041
Demand ischemia. *See* Chronic arterial insufficiency
Dens
  anatomy of, 708–712
  animal studies of, 723–724
  fracture injuries, 736–738
  os odontoideum and, 738–740
  preexisting disease/deformities in, 719
  rotatory subluxation, atlantoaxial joint, 735
Dentocentral cartilage, anatomy of, 710–711
Dentocentral synchondrosis chondrosis, anatomic features, 711
Diabetes, fracture injuries and, 353–354
Diagnostic imaging. *See* Radiographic imaging
Diaphragm, thorax and rib trauma and, 427–428

Diaphysis
- amputation involving, 298–299
- as anatomic region, 3–5
- biomechanics of, 26–28
- birth fractures in, 348
- composition of, 5, 7
- diagnostic imaging, 125
- endochondral ossification, bone replacement of cartilage, 3–4
- femoral anatomy, 860
- fractures involving
  - comminution of, 87
  - gunshot injury, 289
- growth mechanism injuries, type 9 injury pattern, 191–194
- humeral fractures, 475–480
  - complications, 479
  - diagnosis, 477
  - injury mechanism, 475, 477
  - pathologic anatomy, 476–477
  - supracondylar process, 479–480
  - treatment, 477–479
- humerus and, 459
- immature skeletal injury, 42
  - characteristics of, 48–49
  - fractures in infancy, 349–350
  - remodeling following, 58
  - reparative phase, 255
- membranous bone formation and regeneration of, 2
- metacarpal fractures, 669–673
- myelodysplasia and fracture injury in, 368–369
- open fractures and, 270
- radioulnar fractures
  - classification, 605–607
  - compartment syndrome, 608
  - complications, 614–615
  - diagnosis, 606–607
  - neurovascular injury, 608
  - rotation, 608–610
  - treatment, 610–613
- tibiofibular injuries, 1035–1043
  - anatomic development, 995–996
  - compartment syndrome, 1041–1043
  - complications, 1040–1041
  - infants and toddlers' injuries, 1035–1037
  - Maisonneuve injury, 1043
  - older children's injuries, 1037–1038
  - open injuries, 1038–1039
  - treatment, 1040
  - vascular injury, 1039–1040
- ulnar development, 570–571
- vasculature of, 21

Diastatic fractures, multiple injury protocol, diagnostic imaging of head trauma, 78

Diastolic pressure, compartment syndrome diagnosis, 318

Diazepam, fracture treatment using, 107

Digital cuff impedance plethysmography, arterial injury diagnosis, 315

Digital subtraction angiography, arterial injury diagnosis, 315

Disability evaluation, immature skeletal injury and, 60

Discoid meniscus, characteristics of, 979–980

Discoid physis, characteristics of, 10–11

Discontinuity lesions, arterial injury, 313

Disk herniation, in children, 761, 768

Dislocation
- ankle tendon injuries, 1075–1076
- atlantooccipital dislocation, 732
- carpal subluxation and dislocation, 657
- cartilage injury, repair mechanisms, 262
- cerebral palsy and fractures with, 371–372
- elbow injuries, 543–556
  - classification, 544–545
  - complications, 550–552
  - diagnosis, 548
  - divergent dislocation, 549–550
  - pathomechanics, 545–548
  - recurrent dislocation, 553
  - translocation (convergent dislocation), 550
  - treatment, 548–549
  - unreduced dislocations, 554
- foot injuries
  - metatarsal injury, 1136
  - peritalar and subtalar dislocations, 1109–1110
- hip injuries, 831–833
  - anterior dislocation, 840–842
  - bilateral traumatic dislocation, 835–836
  - central dislocation, 833, 842
  - classification of, 833–836
  - inferior dislocation, 833, 836, 842
  - obstetric dislocation, 850–851
  - posterior dislocation, 833, 836–840
  - recurrent dislocation, 849–850
  - voluntary habitual dislocation, 851
- immature skeletal injury, 55, 57
- interphalangeal dislocation, 677–678
- knee joint, 936–941
  - habitual dislocation, 941
  - intraarticular dislocation, 940–941
  - patellar dislocation, 938–940
  - subluxation, 938
- Lisfranc's dislocation, 1124–1126
- metacarpophalangeal (MCP) joint, 672, 675–677
- misdiagnosis of fracture, type 1 fracture injury, 157
- open injuries and, 284
- proximal tibiofibular joint
  - classification, 1024
  - diagnosis, 1024–1026
  - injury mechanisms, 1025
  - posterior dislocation, 1026–1027
  - superior dislocation, 1027
  - treatment, 1025–1026
- thumb injury, 665–666

Displacement
- calcaneus injuries, 1116
- distal metaphysis (supracondylar) injuries, 482–484
  - treatment, 486–487
- in distal ulnar injuries, 634
- fracture patterns, type 1 fracture injury, 157
- growth mechanism injury, physeal injuries, management of, 211
- hip anatomy and, 831–832
- lateral condyle injuries, 515–520
- patellar sleeve fractures, 954–957
- proximal fibular injuries, 1027
- proximal humeral physeal fracture, 470–471, 472–473

Disseminated intravascular coagulation (DIC), bone injury and, 321–322

Distal (acromial) clavicle
- dislocation, 442
- injury to, 438–442
  - acromioclavicular dislocation, 442
  - associated fractures, 441
  - clavicular "duplication," 441–442
  - diagnosis, 439
  - pathology, 438–440
  - radiology, 439, 441
  - subcoracoid displacement, 441–442
  - treatment, 441

Distal femoral epiphyseal injuries
- complications, 908–910
- diagnosis, 906–907
- growth mechanism injuries as, 898–905
- incidence, 896
- injury mechanisms of, 905–906
- obstetric injury, 896–897
- treatment, 907–908

Distal femoral metaphyseal injuries
- anterior cruciate ligament (ACL) injury and, 950
- characteristics of, 895–896

Distal femur
- anatomy, 860–863
- physeal growth alteration, bridge formation, 215

Distal fibula
- anatomic development, 996–997, 999
- injuries, characteristics of, 1069–1073

Distal fifth fractures (Boxer's fracture), characteristics, 672, 674–675

Distal humerus
- anatomy of, 459–462

Distal humerus (cont.)
  epiphyses in, 8–10
  injury to, 459–462
  unreduced elbow dislocations, 554
Distal interphalangeal (DIP) joint, interphalangeal dislocation, 677–678
Distal metacarpal fractures, epiphyseal region, 670–674
Distal metaphyseal injuries, classification and treatment, 1043–1044
Distal metaphysis, supracondylar injuries, 480–495
  classification, 480
  complications, 491–494
  diagnosis, 483–485
  displacement, 483–484
  elbow dislocation, 495
  extension type injury, 480–482
  flexion type injury, 481, 483, 487
  myositis, 495
  pathologic anatomy, 480–483
  radiologic examination, 483
  surgical release, 494–495
  treatment, 485–491
  unstable fractures, 487–490
  varus-valgus deformities, 491–494
  Volkmann's ischemia, 493–494
Distal phalangeal injury
  fractures, 689
  thumb injuries and, 668–669
Distal radial fractures, 624–632
  classification, 624–627
  complications, 629–632
    exostosis, 631–632
    growth disturbance, 629–631
    neurologic problems, 629
    synostosis, 631
    ulnar styloid complications, 631–632
  diagnosis, 626–627
  lunate subluxation with, 663
  pathomechanics, 626–627
  scaphoid fractures and, 657–658
  transcarpal injuries, 662
  treatment, 627–629
Distal radioulnar joint
  anatomical development, 571–572
  fractures, 615–624
    complications, 621–624
    diagnosis, 618
    Galeazzi fracture-dislocation and, 635–638
    pathomechanics, 617–618
    treatment, 618–621
Distal tibia, anatomic development, 996–998
Distal tibial fracture
  epiphyseal and physeal injury
    classification, 1045–1055
    complications, 1062–1066
    injury mechanisms, 1055–1057
    treatment, 1057–1062
  Tillaux fracture, 1048, 1050–1052
  triplane fracture, 1052–1054
  See also Maisonneuve injury
Distal ulnar injuries, incidence and classification, 632–635
Distraction epiphysiolysis
  bridge resectioning, 233–234
  limb length equalization, 236–237
Divergent dislocation, elbow dislocations, 549–550
Dog bites, open injury from, 279
Dome fracture, talar injuries, 1106–1108
Doppler sonography
  foot injuries, peritalar and subtalar dislocations, 1110
  proximal tibial epiphyseal injuries, 1007
  techniques, 140
  venous disorder diagnosis, 321
Dorsal defects, patella injuries, 964, 966
Down syndrome, spinal injury and, 720–721
DPT sedation compound, fracture treatment using, 107
Dual energy x-ray absorptiometry (DEXA), bone density analysis, 23–24
Ductility, skeletal biomechanics and, 28
Dysplasias, fracture injury and, 354–355

E
Eccentric injury, diagnostic imaging, 127–128
Ecchymosis, predictive value of vs. radiographic findings in children, 117
Economic factors, fracture treatment, 87–88
Ectopic bone formation
  head trauma complications, 323–324
  tibial tuberosity injuries, 1017
Edema, in compartment syndrome, 316
Ehler-Danlos syndrome
  carpal subluxation and dislocation, 657
  proximal tibiofibular joint dislocation, 1024
Elbow injuries
  arterial injury with, 313
  chondro-osseous anatomy, 542–543
  compartment syndrome, fracture treatment and, 88
  computed tomography (CT) imaging, 135
  dislocation, 543–556
    classification, 544–545
    complications, 550–552
    diagnosis, 548
    divergent dislocation, 549–550
    pathomechanics, 545–548
    recurrent dislocation, 553
    translocation (convergent dislocation), 550
    treatment, 548–549
    unreduced dislocations, 554
  distal metaphysis (supracondylar) injuries and dislocation of, 495
  epicondyle, 561
  fixation of, biodegradable materials for, 100
  floating elbow, 523–525
  heterotopic ossification, 330
  lateral condyle injuries, 510, 514
  little league elbow, 559–561
  "little league elbow," 400, 406–407
  medial epicondyle injuries, 503, 505–508
  pulled elbow, 555–559
    diagnosis, 556–557
    treatment, 558–559
  ultrasonography (US), 140
Electrical injuries, growth mechanism injury and, 176–178, 181
Electronegativity, fracture repair patterns, remodeling, analysis of, 257
Elongation mechanics
  altered physeal growth, growth acceleration, 212–213
  in bone tissue, 28
EMLA cream, fracture treatment using, 106–107
Enders nails/rods
  femoral shaft fractures, 890–891
  fracture treatment using, 99–100
Endochondral ossification
  bone development, 2–4
  immature skeletal injury
    hematoma formation, 250–251
    reparative phase, 254–255
  in physis, 8–10
Endochondral tissue formation, bone development, 1
Endocrinopathy, fracture injury and, 353–354
Endosteal callus, in overriding fractures, 86
Endosteum
  immature skeletal injury, childhood vs. adult trauma, 47–48
  metaphyseal vasculature and, 21
End-plate development, endochondral ossification, 3
End-plate injury. See Cervical region, end-plate injury
Endurance, role of, in sports-related injuries, 403
Engelmann's disease, dysplasias and, 354
Epicondylar region
  elbow dislocations, 548–549, 561–562

immature skeletal injury to, characteristics of, 49
injury to, 461–462
lateral epicondyle injuries, 523–524
medial epicondyle injuries, 503, 505–508
Epilepsy, fractures with, 373
Epiphyseal cartilage
diagnostic imaging, 123
intraarticular fractures, cartilage repair, 260–261
Epiphyseal grafting, amputation, 299–300
Epiphyseal ossification center
biomechanics in, 24–30
cartilage canals and vasculature of, 19–23
distal femur, 860–863
growth mechanism injury in
electrical injuries, 178
frostbite, 179
type 4A injury pattern, 169–171
type 7 fracture pattern, 187–190
immature skeletal injury
childhood vs. adult trauma, 47–48
diagnostic issues in, 42
joint disruption, 57
physeal growth alteration, bridge formation, 215–216
physis development and, 11–13
Epiphyseal slip, proximal femoral fractures, complications, 873–876
Epiphyseal transplantation, bridge resectioning, 234
Epiphysiodesis
amputation and, overgrowth, 297–298
bone growth and, 17–18
bridge resectioning, 233–234
diagnostic imaging of, longitudinal inequality assessment, 133–134
distal femoral epiphyseal injuries, complications involving, 910
distal tibia development, 996–998
distal tibial fractures, 1065
irradiation and, 180
limb length equalization, 235
physeal growth alteration, bridge formation, 215
tibial tuberosity
anatomic development, 994–995
injuries, 1016–1017
type 4 fracture injury, 170–172, 175
type 3 fracture patterns, 166–170
type 5 fracture patterns, 173
Epiphysiolysis
as bone injury complication, 332
bridge resectioning, 233–234
endocrinopathy and, 353–354
growth mechanism injury
type 5 fracture pattern, 173
type 8 fracture pattern, 188, 190

physeal growth alteration, experimental bridging, 216–217
proximal femoral fractures, birth trauma and, 866–868
rachitic fractures, 350–351
scurvy and, 352
See also Distraction epiphysiolysis
Epiphysis
amputation involving, 295
overgrowth, 296
as anatomic region, 3–5
biomechanics in, 25–26
birth fractures in, 348
characteristics of, 8–10
child abuse and fracture pathology, 385
distal radial fractures, 624–632
classification, 624–627
complications, 629–632
diagnosis, 626–627
pathomechanics, 626–627
treatment, 627–629
distal tibial injury
classification, 1045–1055
complications, 1062–1066
injury mechanisms, 1055–1057
treatment, 1057–1062
fractures involving, fixation treatments, 93
growth mechanism injury, 149–150
circulation and ischemia, 198
experimental trauma studies, 196–197
frostbite, 178–179
physeal biomechanics and, 193, 195–196
type 1 fracture injury, 153–161
type 2 fracture injury, 163–166
type 3 fracture injury, 166–170
type 4 fracture injury, 167, 169–175
type 5 fracture injury, 173–180
type 7 fracture injury, 183, 185–190
immature skeletal injury and characteristics of, 49
fractures in infancy, 349–350
remodeling following, 58
magnetic resonance imaging (MRI) of, 136
metacarpal fractures, 670–674
olecranon fractures, 577–578
regeneration, 219–220
sports-related injuries to, 406–407
tibia, anatomic development, 991–992
tibial tuberosity, anatomic development, 993–995
vasculature, development of, 18–20
wrist and hand anatomy, 651
Equestrian sports, immature skeletal injuries, 44–45
Erb's palsy
brachial plexus injuries, 447

clavicle injury and, 432
Monteggia lesions, 605
Esmarch bandages, fracture treatments using, 106
Essex-Lopresti injuries, Galeazzi fracture-dislocation and, 635
Ewing's sarcoma, membranous bone formation and, 2–3
Exercise, sports-related injuries and, 403–404
Exertional compartment syndrome, sports-related injuries and, 405
Exostosis
as bone injury complication, 334
distal radial fractures, 631–632
foot, congenital deformities, 1149
pelvic avulsion fractures, 820–822
Explosions, hand injuries, 693
Extension fractures
distal metaphysis (supracondylar) injuries, 480–482
lumbar spine injuries, 756–758
Extensor tendons
chronic patellar subluxation and abnormalities of, 941–944
injury to, 698–699
External fixation (external fixators)
femoral shaft fractures, 892
fracture treatment
associated soft tissue/vascular injury, 88
biologic factors, 87
complications, 102–103
indications for, 93
multiple injuries, use with, 91–92
techniques for, 94–96
head trauma
basic principles of, 89
multiple injury protocol, 79–80
tibiofibular diaphyseal injuries, 1038–1039
Extracellular matrices, immature skeletal injury, fracture repair, inflammatory phase, 248–249
Extradural hematomas, head trauma, multiple injury protocol, 79
Extra-octave fracture, characteristics of, 680–682
Extremity films, predictive value of, *vs.* clinical findings, 116–117

F
Fabellar fracture, characteristics of, 966
Facet joints
anatomic development, 713
fractures of, 750
peritalar and subtalar dislocations, 1110
Falls, immature skeletal injuries from, statistics on, 46–47

Fasciotomy, compartment syndrome, 318
  foot injuries, 1102
Fast imaging steady-state precession (FISP)
  magnetic resonance imaging (MRI), 136
  sports-related injuries, stress injury diagnosis, 412
Fast low-angle shot (FLASH)
  magnetic resonance imaging (MRI), 136
  sports-related injuries, stress injury diagnosis, 412
Fast spin echo (FSE), magnetic resonance imaging (MRI), 136
Fat embolism
  bone injury and, 322–323
  disseminated intravascular coagulation (DIC) with, 321–322
Fat-fluid level, diagnostic imaging, 119
Fat fractures, as bone injury complication, 337
Fat necrosis, as bone injury complication, 337
Fat pads
  bridge resection using, 226–227, 231–232
    acute fat replacement, 234
  diagnostic imaging, 119–120
  foot anatomy, 1096, 1099–1100
  patellar anatomy, 929–932
Femoral condyles, distal femoral epiphyseal injuries and, 905
Femoral fractures
  central acetabular fractures and, 811
  child abuse and, 380–382
  distal femoral epiphyseal injuries, 896–910
    classification, 898–905
    complications, 908–910
    concomitant ligament injury, 910
    diagnosis, 906–907
    injury mechanisms, 905–906
    obstetric injury, 896–898
    treatment, 907–908
  distal femoral metaphyseal injuries, 895–896
  femoral neck fractures
    complications, 875–876
    treatment, 870–872
  floating knee, 910–912
  hip injuries and, 843
  proximal femoral fracture
    acute slipped capital femoral epiphyseal (SCFE) injury, 868–870
    classification, 863–864
    complications, 873–876
    diagnosis, 872
    femoral neck fractures, 870–872

  incidence and epidemiology, 861, 863
  injury mechanisms, 870–871
  ipsilateral proximal/diaphyseal fracture, 876
  neonates, 866–868
  stress fractures, 876
  transphyseal injury, 864–866
  treatment, 872–873
shaft fractures, 880–895
  angulation/bowing, 893–894
  bone length/overgrowth, 892–893
  complications, 892–895
  diagnosis, 881
  external fixation, 892
  growth arrest, 895
  immediate casting, 886
  injury mechanisms, 881
  intramedullary rodding, 889–890
  muscle function, 895
  myositis, 895
  nerve injury, 895
  nontrochanteric rodding, 890–891
  Pavlik harness, 887
  plate fixation, 891–892
  refracture, 895
  rotational deformity, 894–895
  surgical procedures, 887–892
  traction, 882–886
  treatment, 881–892
  vascular injury, 892
subtrochanteric fractures, 878–880
triradiate cartilage fracture, 813–816
trochanteric injuries
  greater trochanter, 876–877
  lesser trochanter, 877–878
Femoral head fractures
  birth trauma and, 867–868
  hip injuries and, 843
Femur, anatomy of, 857–861
  diaphysis, 860
  distal femur, 860–863
  femoral neck, 857–859
  greater trochanter, 858–860
  lesser trochanter, 859–860
  proximal femur, 857–858
  proximal vascularity, 860
Fenestrations, in metaphyses, 6–9
Fetal injury
  discoid meniscus, 979–980
  immature skeletal injury, fracture repair, inflammatory phase, 248
  intrauterine fractures, 346–348
  See also Birth trauma
Fibrinolysins, intraarticular fractures, cartilage repair, 260
Fibroblast growth factor (FGF), immature skeletal injury, fracture repair, inflammatory phase, 249
Fibrocellular tissue, bone development, 1

Fibrous tissue, skeletal development and, 30–32
Fibula
  anatomy of
    distal fibula, 996–997, 999
    proximal fibula, 995
    syndesmosis, 997–999
    tibiofibular diaphyses, 995–996
  See also Tibiofibular diaphyses
Fibular fractures
  distal fibular injuries, 1069–1073
  epiphyseal fracture, knee dislocations and, 936–938
  proximal fibular injuries, 1027
  metaphyseal injury, 1035
"Fight bite," hand injuries, 691
Fingers
  finger tip injuries, 690–691
  fracture treatment, 655–656
  rotational deformities, 656
  See also Phalanges
First rib fracture, characteristics of, 425–426
"Fishtail" deformity, lateral condyle injuries, 522
Fitness, sports-related injuries and, 404
Fixation techniques
  cast complications, 338
  diaphyseal humeral fractures, 477–479
  distal femoral epiphyseal injuries, 907–908
  distal tibial fractures, 1057–1061
  femoral shaft fractures, 884–888
    external fixation, 892
    intramedullary nailing and rodding, 889–890
    nontrochanteric rodding, 890–891
    plate fixation, 891–892
  fracture treatment
    basic concepts, 91–93
    complications, 101–104
    economic factors in, 87–88
    external fixators, 94–97
    hardware removal, complications with, 101–103
    indications for, 92
    internal fixation devices, 97–100
    percutaneous fixation, 93–94
    pin and cast insertions, 93
  fracture treatments, closed reduction techniques, 89–91
  growth mechanism injury
    physeal injuries, management of, 211–212
    type 4A fracture, 169–170
  halo fixation, spinal injury, 730–731
  hemophiliac diseases, fracture injuries, treatment of, 377
  hip injuries, posterior hip dislocation, 840
  hypercalcemia and, 328–329

immature skeletal injury
  fracture motion, 257–258
  physiologic response, 253
initial response protocols using, 71
knee injuries, osteochondritis dissecans, 969–971
lateral condyle injuries, 516–520
lawn mower injury, 293
Monteggia lesions, 600
muscle atrophy with, 328
olecranon fractures, 578–580
open injury care, 275–276
  antibiotics for infection, 282
patellar dislocation, chronic patellar subluxation and, 943–944
pelvic fractures, 805–806
proximal radial fractures, 585–588
proximal (sternal) clavicle injury, 437–438
proximal tibial epiphyseal injuries, 1009
pseudarthrosis, 331–332
scaphoid fractures, 660–661
spinal injury, 730–731
tibial spine injuries, 1002–1005
tibial tuberosity injuries, 1016–1017
vasospasm and, 316
See also Casts; External fixation; Internal Fixation; Pins and screws, and so on
Flail chest, multiple injury protocol, 73
Flexion
  distal metaphysis (supracondylar) injuries, 481, 483, 485–487
  distal radial injury, 627–629
  lumbar spine injuries, 756–758
  pulled elbow treatment, 558
  spinal injuries, 718–719
  thoracic spine injury, 750, 752
Flexor tendons, injury to, 697–698
Floating elbow, characteristics of, 523–525
Floating knee, incidence and epidemiology, 910–912
Fluid restriction, head injury and, 71
Fluoroscopic imaging
  fracture treatment
    basic principles, 87
    screw fixation techniques, 97–98
  techniques for, 134–135
Foot, anatomic development, 1091–1100
  accessory navicular development, 1096, 1098
  calcaneus, 1093–1094
  growth patterns, 1099–1100
  maturation and variation, 1095–1096
  metatarsals, 1095–1096
  os trigonum, 1096, 1098–1099
  pedal nerves, 1100
  phalanges, 1095, 1097
  plantar foot padding, 1096–1097

talus, 1091–1093, 1098
tarsal bones, 1094–1095, 1097
tendons, 1100
Football, sports-related injuries with, 401
Foot injuries
  apophysitis, 1119
  calcaneus, 1110–1119
  compartment syndrome, 1101–1102
  congenital deformity, 1149
  fractures, 1100–1101
    bunk bed fracture, 1132–1133
    calcaneus, 1110–1119
    navicular injuries, 1119–1120
    phalanges, 1138–1141
    stress fractures, 1135–1137
    talus, 1102–1108
  Kohler's injury, 1120–1122
  lawn mower injuries, 1145–1148
  ligaments, 1149
  metatarsals, 1126–1138
    bunk bed fracture, 1132–1133
    dislocations, 1136
    fifth metatarsal, 1133–1135
    first metatarsal, 1130, 1131
    Freiberg's lesion, 1136–1137
    sesmoids, 1136–1138
    stress fractures, 1135–1137
  navicular injuries, 1119–1123
    accessory navicular, 1122–1123
  osteochondroses, 1101
  os trigonum injury, 1108–1109
  phalanges, 1138–1141
    fractures, 1138–1141
    stubbed toe, 1140–1141
  plantar tendons, 1148
  plantar wounds, 1141–1145
    chondro-osseous infection, 1143–1144
    foreign bodies, 1144–1145
    puncture wounds, 1141–1143
  talus, 1102–1110
    congenital deformity, 1109
    fractures, 1102–1108
    os trigonum injury, 1108–1109
    peritalar and subtalar dislocations, 1109–1110
  tarsal bones, 1123
  tarsal tunnel, 1148
  tarsometatarsal injury, 1123–1126
Foreign objects
  as bone injury complication, 336
  crush-burn injuries, 290
  diagnostic imaging, 121
  hand injuries, 692–693
  insertion in casts, complications from, 91
  knee injuries, 972–973
  open injury and, 279–280
  plantar foot padding wounds, 1144–1145

Four-part fracture, triplane distal tibial fracture, 1054
Fracture blisters, as bone injury complication, 338
Fracture bracing, fracture treatment using, 91
Fracture classification, immature skeletal injury, 51–54
  physical changes and, 54
Fracture fragments
  angular deformity, 219
  arterial injury from, 313
  closed reduction techniques, cast application, 90–91
  fracture reductions, basic principles regarding, 87–88
  growth mechanism injury
    physeal injuries, management of, 211–212
    type 4 fracture patterns, 173–175
    type 9 fracture patterns, 191–194
    type 2 injury patterns, 161–166
    type 3 injury patterns, 166–170
    type 7 injury patterns, 186–187
  hip injuries, acetabular fragments, 845–846
  immature skeletal injury
    relationship of, 54, 57
    reparative phase, 255
  lateral condyle injuries, 510–514
  open injury, gas gangrene, 286–287
  patellar fractures, sleeve fractures, 954–957
  pelvic fractures and, bowel injury, 807–808
  proximal humeral physeal fracture, 466, 468–471
  proximal radial fractures, treatment and repair, 588
  Thurston-Holland fragments, screw fixation techniques for, 97–98
"Fracture illness," fixation treatment of fractures and, 91
Fracture injuries
  brachial plexus injuries and incidence of, 448
  carpal fractures, 657
  compartment syndrome and, 316
  complications. *See* Complications
  computed tomography (CT) imaging, 135–136
  in deformed limbs, 311–312
  diaphysis composition and, 5
  elbow injury, dislocation associated with, 543–544
  in epiphyses, 9–10
  foot injuries, 1100–1101
    bunk bed fracture, 1132–1133
    calcaneus, 1110–1119
    navicular injuries, 1119–1120
    phalanges, 1138–1141

Fracture injuries (*cont.*)
    stress fractures, 1135–1137
    talus, 1102–1108
  growth mechanism injury
    burn injury, 182, 184
    diagnostic imaging, 152–153
    electrical injury, 176–178, 181
    frostbite, 178–179, 182
    histology, 151–152
    irradiation, 180–182
    management principles, 210–211
    osteochondroma formation, 183–184
    physeal injuries, management of, 211–212
    type 1 injury, 153–161
    type 2 injury, 161–166
    type 3 injury, 166–170, 176
    type 4 injury, 167, 169–175
    type 5 injury, 172–180
    type 6 injury, 181–183
    type 7 injury, 183, 185–190
    type 8 injury, 188–192
    type 9 injury, 191–194
  hand injuries, incidence of, 654–655
  head trauma as complication, 323–324
  hip injuries, associated injuries, 843–846
    actebular fragments, 845–846
    capital femoral epiphysis separation, 843–845
    femoral fracture, 843
    femoral head fracture, 843
  immature skeletal injuries
    age as factor in, 42–43
    childhood *vs.* adult trauma, 48
    closed *vs.* open fractures, 54, 57
    fracture fragments, relationship of, 54, 57
    longitudinal growth and, 42
    remodeling after, 57–60
    statistics and, 40
  knee injuries
    fabellar fracture, 966
    osteochondral fracture, 966–967
    patellar fractures, 951–957
  olecranon fractures, 575–582
    classification, 575–576
    complications, 578, 580–581
    diagnosis, 576–578
    gymnastic injury, 580
    pathomechanics, 576
    treatment, 578–579
  pediatric growth disorders
    birth fractures, 348–349
    child abuse, 379–386
    congenital pseudarthroses, 364
    dysplasias, 354–355
    endocrinopathy, 353–354
    Gaucher's disease, 352–353
    hematologic disorders, 374–379
    infants, fracture injury in, 349–350
    intrauterine fractures, 346–348
    joint laxity/dislocation, 359
    joint stiffness, 359–361
    lead exposure, 352
    metabolic disorders, 354
    multiple fractures of unknown etiology, 358–359
    neurologic disorders, 365, 367–374
    osteochondroses, 364–366
    osteogenesis imperfecta, 355–358
    osteosclerotic disorders, 359
    pathologic fractures, 361–364
    prematurity, 349
    rickets, 350–352
    scurvy, 352
    vitamin A deficiency, 352
  pelvic fractures, classification of, 798–805
  phalanges, 678–679
  postfracture cysts and, 332–334
  proximal femoral fracture
    acute slipped capital femoral epiphyseal (SCFE) injury, 868–870
    classification, 863–864
    complications, 873–876
    diagnosis, 872
    femoral neck fractures, 870–872
    incidence and epidemiology, 861, 863
    injury mechanisms, 870–871
    ipsilateral proximal/diaphyseal fracture, 876
    neonates, 866–868
    stress fractures, 876
    transphyseal injury, 864–866
    treatment, 872–873
  radius and ulna, incidence, 574–575
  recurrence as complication of, 332
  scaphoid fractures, 657–661
  scintigraphy (radionuclide imaging) of, 139
  spinal cord injuries and incidence of, 770
  spinal injuries
    atlas fractures, 731–733
    cervical fracture-dislocation, 740–744
    dens injuries, 736–738
    developmental spine's response to, 717–719
    occipital fracture, 732
  tibial spine injuries, 998, 1000–1005
    anatomic variation, 1000
    classification, 1000
    diagnosis, 1001–1002
    treatment, 1001–1005
  ulna, incidence of, 574–575
Fracture repair and treatment
  anesthesia, 105–108
    Bier block, 106–107
    hematoma block, 106
    regional block anesthesia, 107
    skin anesthesia, 107
    spinal/epidural anesthesia, 107
  associated soft tissue and vascular injuries, 88
  basic principles of, 86–88
  calcaneus injuries, 1116–1117
  clavicle fractures, 433–434
  closed reduction, 89–91
    cast application, 90–91
    cast complications, 91
    cast removal, 91
  compartment syndrome, 88
  complications of fixation, 100–104
    hardware removal, 101–103
    tourniquet use, 103–104
  diagnostic imaging, postreduction evaluation, 122
  diaphyseal humeral fractures, 477–479
  distal (acromial) clavicle, 441
  distal femoral epiphyseal injuries, 907–908
  distal metaphysis (supracondylar) injuries, 485–491
  distal radial injury, 627–629
  distal radioulnar injuries, 618–621
  distal tibial fractures, 1057–1062
  distal tibial injuries, 1044
  distal ulnar injuries, 634–635
  extra-octave fracture, 680–682
  femoral shaft fractures, 881–892
  hand injury, 655–656
  head injury, 88–89
  hip injuries
    Allis reduction, 838–839
    Bigelow reduction, 838–840
    posterior dislocation, 837–840
    postreduction care, 840
    Stimson reduction, 838
  immature skeletal injury, 244–259
    bridge development, 258
    fracture motion, 257–258
    hematoma, 250–251
    inflammatory phase, 245–249
    long-term changes, 259
    mechanical healing properties, 258–259
    periosteum, 249–250
    physeal healing, 256
    physiologic response, 251–253
    remodeling phase, 256–257
    reparative phase, 253–255
    residual angulation remodeling, 259
  lateral condyle injuries, 515–520
  lawn mower injuries, 1145–1148
  mallet finger deformities, 687–689
  medial epicondyle injuries, 507–508
  middle phalangeal fractures, 685–687
  Monteggia lesions, 599–602

olecranon fractures, 578
patellar fractures, 951–957
pelvic fractures, 805–810
   vascular injury, 806–807
proximal femoral fractures, 872–873
proximal humeral physeal fracture, 472–473
proximal radial fractures, 585–588
proximal (sternal clavicle), 437–438
proximal tibial epiphyseal injuries, 1007–1009
proximal tibial metaphyseal injuries, 1030–1035
radioulnar fractures, 610–613
rehabilitation, 104–105
   multiple injuries, 104
   psychological rehabilitation, 104–105
   single fractures, 104
sedation, 107–108
   nitrous oxide, 108
skeletal fixation
   basic concepts, 91–93
   external fixators, 94–97
   internal fixation devices, 97–100
   percutaneous fixation, 93–94
   pin and cast insertions, 93
slipped capital femoral epiphysis (SCFE), 869–870
spinal injury, 730–731
   atlas fractures, 733–734
   halo fixation, 730–731
   rotatory subluxation, atlantoaxial joint, 735–736
subtrochanteric fractures, 879–880
talus fractures, 1104
tarsometatarsal injuries, 1125–1126
tibial spine fractures, 1001–1005
tibial tuberosity injuries, 1015–1017
tibiofibular diaphyseal injuries, 1038–1040
transcondylar injuries, 500–502
See also Closed reduction; Fixation techniques; Open reduction; specific techniques, e.g. Casts and casting
Freiberg's lesion, metatarsal injury, 1136–1137
Fretting corrosion, internal fixation devices, 103
Frostbite
   growth mechanism injury from, 178–179, 182
   hand injuries, 696

G
Gadolinium, magnetic resonance imaging (MRI) using, 137
Galeazzi fracture-dislocation
   characteristics of, 635–638
   radioulnar fractures, 606

Galvanic corrosion, internal fixation devices, 103
Gamekeeper's thumb, characteristics of, 666–667
Gas gangrene, open injury and, 285–287
Gate control pain theory, reflex sympathetic dystrophy (RSD), 327–328
Gaucher's disease, fracture injuries and, 352–353
Gene expression, immature skeletal injury, fracture repair, inflammatory phase, 249
Genitourinary injury, pelvic fractures and, 808
Genu recurvatum
   femoral shaft fractures, 883–884
   proximal tibial epiphyseal injuries, 1009–1011
   tibial tuberosity injuries, 1016–1018
Genu valgum, proximal tibial metaphyseal injury, 1034
Germinal zone
   type 3 fracture injury in, 167, 170
   type 4 fracture injury in, 167, 169–175
   type 5 fracture injury in, 173–180
Glasgow Coma Score
   multiple injury protocol and, head trauma and, 77–78
   multiple injury protocol using
     airway assessment and stabilization, 71
     Pediatric Trauma Score (PTS), 76–77
Glenohumeral joint dislocation
   humeral fractures and, 462–466
     brachial plexus injury, 465
     luxatio erecta, 465–466
     proximal humeral physeal fracture and, 471
Glenoid region
   hypoplasia, scapular fractures and, 444
   scapular fractures and, 443–445
Gradient Recalled Acquisition in the Steady State (GRASS), 136
   bridge development, diagnostic imaging, 223
Gradient recalled echo (GRE), magnetic resonance imaging (MRI), 136
Gram-negative bacteria, open injury infection, 282
Gram-positive bacteria, open injury infection, gas gangrene, 286–287
Granulation phase, wound healing, immature skeletal injury, 244
Greater trochanter, injuries, 876–877
Greenstick fracture
   biomechanics of bone and, 28–30
   clavicle injury as, 434
   diagnostic imaging, 125

distal radial injury, ulnar involvement, 625–626
distal radioulnar injuries, 615–617
   complications, 622
   treatment, 618–621
distal tibial injuries, 1044
immature skeletal injury, 51, 54–55
   statistics on, 40
metatarsal injuries, 1129
Monteggia lesions, 598
postfracture cysts and, 333
proximal metaphysis, 475–476
proximal radial fractures, 582–584
proximal tibial metaphyseal injuries as, 1028–1030
radioulnar fractures, 606–608
   treatment, 612–613
reduction of, sedation and anesthesia for, 106–107
rib fractures as, 422–423
type 2 injury patterns, 162–166
Greulich method
   longitudinal inequality assessment, 130–131
   skeletal age estimation, 130
Grisel syndrome, subluxation, 729
Growth factors
   fracture treatments, closed reduction techniques, 89
   immature skeletal injury, fracture repair, inflammatory phase, 248–249
Growth hormones, immature skeletal injury, fracture repair, inflammatory phase, 249
Growth mechanism injury
   anterior cruciate ligament (ACL) injury and, 950
   classification, 150–151
   distal femoral epiphyseal injury as, 898–905
   distal metacarpal fractures, 670–674
   distal radial fractures, complications, 629–631
   distal radioulnar injuries, 624
   distal tibial fractures as, 1062
     complications, 1062–1066
   distal ulnar injuries, 632–635
   epiphyseal-physeal injury
     circulation and ischemia, 198
     distal radial injuries, 624–632
     experimental physis trauma, 196–197
     healing patterns, 198–200
     hemiepiphyses, 197–198
     intraepiphyseal ostotomy, 198
     physis biomechanics, 193, 195–196
     transphyseal pins, 197
   femoral shaft fractures
     complications, 895
     post-surgical growth problems, 890

Growth mechanism injury (cont.)
  foot injuries
    apophyseal calcaneus injury, 1117–1118
    calcaneus injuries, 1117
    metatarsal injury, 1130–1131
  fracture/failure patterns
    burn injury, 182, 184
    diagnostic imaging, 152–153
    electrical injury, 176–178, 181
    frostbite, 178–179, 182
    histology, 151–152
    irradiation, 180–182
    osteochondroma formation, 182–184
    synostosis with type 9 injuries, 330–331
    type 1 injury, 153–161
    type 2 injury, 161–166
    type 3 injury, 166–170, 176
    type 4 injury, 167, 169–175
    type 5 injury, 172–180
    type 6 injury, 181–183
    type 7 injury, 183, 185–190
    type 8 injury, 188–192
    type 9 injury, 191–194
  as fracture treatment complication, 101
  incidence of, 147
  lateral condyle injuries, 521–522
  management and arrest
    angular deformity, 219
    diagnostic imaging, 220–224
    epiphyseal regeneration, 219–220
    fracture management, 210–212
    incidence and epidemiology, 209–210
    limb length equalization, 234–237
    physeal growth alteration, 212–219
    physeal mapping, 224–226
    resection technique, 228–234
    surgery, 226–228
  middle phalangeal fractures, 686–687
  pelvic avulsion fractures, 818
  pelvic region, triradiate cartilage fracture, 812–816
  proximal femoral fractures, complications, 873–876
  proximal humeral physeal fracture, 466, 468–471
  proximal radial fractures, 582–584
  proximal tibial epiphyseal injuries, 1005–1011
  proximal tibial metaphyseal injury, 1031–1035
  sex-related patterns of, 147
  spinal injury, 721–723
    cervical end-plate injury, 745–748
    thoracic spinal injuries, 749–750
  See also Injury mechanisms
Growth plate. See Physis

"Guillotine injuries," replantation techniques, 300–303
Gunshot injury
  hand injuries, 693
  open fractures, 288–289
  spinal injuries, 719

H
Habitual dislocations. See Recurrent dislocations
Hair strangulation, hand and finger injuries, 700
Halo fixation
  atlantooccipital dislocation, 732
  spinal injury, 730–731
    lower cervical fracture-dislocation, 742–744
Hamate fracture, characteristics of, 662–663
Hand injuries
  amputations, 693–696
    autoamputation, 695
    phalangeal lengthening, 695
    replantations and transplantation, 693–695
    thermal injuries, 695
  anatomic development and, 650–653
  bite injuries, 279, 691–692
  burns, 695–696
  diagnostic imaging, 655
  fracture repair, positioning guidelines, 653–654
  frostbite, 696
  functional anatomy, 653–654
    injury incidence, 654–655
  hair strangulation, 700
  nerve injuries, 699–700
  open injuries, 692–693
  sting wounds, 279
  tendons, 696–699
    calcification, 699
    extensor tendons, 698–699
    flexor tendons, 697–698
  treatment and repair, 655–656
  See also Metacarpals; Phalanges; Thumb; Thumb injury; Wrist injury
Harris "growth slowdown/arrest" lines
  diagnostic imaging, 125–128
  growth mechanism injury, 221
  metaphyseal growth and, 17
Haversian systems
  biomechanics in, 26–28
  in diaphysis, 5
  immature skeletal injury, fracture repair, inflammatory phase, 246–249
Hawkin's sign, talus fractures, ischemic necrosis, 1104–1105
Head trauma
  complications, 323–324

  epidemiology of, 323
  fracture treatment, 88–89
    external fixators, indications for, 94–96
    neurologic complications, 373
    immature skeletal injury statistics including, 39–40
    multiple injuries involving, 77–80
      diagnostic imaging, 78–79
      fracture care, 79–80
      Glasgow coma scale, 77–78
      posttrauma care, 80
      treatment protocols, 79
  neurologic consequences, 323
    fractures and, 373
  sports-related injuries and, 404
  statistics on, 77
  See also Skull fractures
Heat loss, from trauma, 311
Heel trauma, lawn mower injuries, 1147–1148
Heinig view (radiography), clavicle injury, proximal (sternal) clavicle injury, 436
Hematogenous osteomyelitis
  open wound infection, 283
  Volkmann's contracture and, 320
Hematologic disorders, fracture injuries with
  coagulation disorders, 374–377
  leukemia, 378–379
  sickle cell anemia, 378
  thalassemia, 377–378
Hematoma block procedure, fracture treatment, sedation using, 106
Hematomas
  child abuse and fracture injury with, 380
  pathology, 384–385
  as complication, 311–312
  immature skeletal injury
    fracture repair, 245–246, 250–251
    physiologic response assessment, 252–253
    reparative phase, 253–255
  medial epicondyle injuries, 507–508
  nail bed injuries, 690
Hemiepiphyses, growth mechanism injury, 197–198
Hemoglobinopathies, fracture treatment in presence of, 105–106
Hemophiliac diseases
  bone injury complications from, 321
  fracture injuries with, 374–377
Hemorrhagic complications
  bone injury, 321–323
    acquired coagulopathies, 321
    disseminated intravascular coagulation (DIC), 321–322
    fat embolism, 322–323
    hereditary coagulopathies, 321

Index

in compartment syndrome, 316
pelvic fractures, vascular injury and, 807
Hemothorax
  multiple injury protocol, chest trauma and, 73
  thorax and rib trauma, 427
Heparin, disseminated intravascular coagulation (DIC) therapy, 322
Herbert screws, knee injuries, osteochondritis dissecans, 969–970
Hereditary coagulopathies, bone injury and, 321
Hernia, pelvic fractures and, 808
Herpes B virus, bites and sting wounds, 279
Heterotopic ossification
  amputation and, overgrowth, 296–298
  distal metaphysis (supracondylar) injuries, 495
  elbow dislocations, 551–552
  femoral shaft fractures, 895
  head trauma complications, 323–324
  hip injuries, 850
  Monteggia lesions, 602
  proximal radial fractures, 589
Heuter-Volkmann's law, angular deformity, 219
Hill-Sachs lesion, glenohumeral joint dislocation, 464–465
Hip injuries
  anatomical development, 831–832
  anterior dislocation, 840–842
    anterior obturator, 833
    anterior pubic, 833
  associated injuries, 843–846
    acetabular fragments, 845–846
    capital femoral epiphysis separation, 843–845
    femoral fracture, 843
    femoral head fracture, 843
  central dislocation, 833, 842
  chronic hip pain, 850
  complications
    ischemic necrosis (osteonecrosis), 846–849
    myositis ossificans, 850
    neurologic deficits, 850
    osteoarthritis, 850
    osteochondrosis, 850
    recurrent dislocation, 849–850
  dislocation
    anterior dislocation, 840–842
    bilateral traumatic dislocation, 835–836
    central dislocation, 833, 842
    classification of, 833–836
    inferior dislocation, 833, 836, 842
    obstetric dislocation, 850–851
    posterior dislocation, 833, 836–840
    recurrent dislocation, 849–850
  incidence, 832–833
  inferior dislocation, 833, 836, 842
  medial dislocation, 833
  peripheral acetabular fractures, 810–811
  posterior dislocation
    Allis reduction, 838–839
    Bigelow reduction, 838–840
    diagnosis, 834, 836–837
    injury mechanism, 833, 836
    posterior iliac dislocation, 833–835
    posterior ischial dislocation, 833, 835–836
    postreduction care, 840
    Stimson reduction, 838
    treatment, 837–840
    vascular injury with, 848
  slipped capital femoral epiphysis (SCFE), 833, 843–845
    treatment, 838–840
  snapping hip syndrome, 850–851
Histologic analysis, growth plate failures, 151–153
Hobbs view (radiography), clavicle injury, proximal (sternal) clavicle injury, 436
Hockey, immature skeletal injuries, 44
Hoffa disease, characteristics of, 980
Hormones, growth mechanism injury, physeal biomechanics and, 196
Hospital admission statistics, immature skeletal injuries, 39–40
Human immunodeficiency virus (HIV), hemophiliac diseases, fracture injuries and risk of, 377
Humeral fractures
  birth injury, 466–468
  child abuse and, 382
  diaphyseal fractures, 475–480
    complications, 479
    diagnosis, 477
    injury mechanism, 475, 477
    pathologic anatomy, 476–477
    supracondylar process, 479–480
    treatment, 477–479
  distal metaphysis (supracondylar) injuries, 480–495
    classification, 480
    complications, 491–494
    diagnosis, 483–485
    displacement, 483–484
    elbow dislocation, 495
    extension type injury, 480–482
    flexion type injury, 481, 483, 487
    myositis, 495
    pathologic anatomy, 480–483
    radiologic examination, 483
    surgical release, 494–495
    treatment, 485–491
    unstable fractures, 487–490
  floating elbow, 523–525
  glenohumeral joint dislocation, 462–466
    brachial plexus injury, 465
    luxatio erecta, 465–466
  intercondylar injuries, 495–497
  lateral condyle injuries, 509–523
    complications, 520–523
    diagnosis, 515–516
    late case, 518–519
    pathomechanics, 510, 514
    treatment, 515–520
  lateral epicondyle injuries, 523–524
  medial condyle injuries, 502–505
  medial epicondyle injuries, 503, 505–508
  proximal humeral physeal fracture, 466, 468–474
    complications, 473
    diagnosis, 471
    diagnostic imaging, 471–472
    lesser tuberosity avulsion, 474
    shoulder fusion, 474
    stress injury, 473–474
    treatment, 472–473
  proximal metaphysis, 474–476
  transcondylar injuries, 497–502
Humerus, anatomical characteristics, 456–462
Hyaline cartilage, bridge resection using, 227
Hyperactivity, immature skeletal injury incidence and, 42
Hyperbaric oxygen therapy, open injury infection, gas gangrene, 287
Hypercalcemia
  as bone injury complication, 328–329
  dysplasias and, 354
Hyperemia, proximal tibial metaphyseal injuries, 1033–1035
Hyperextension injuries
  distal femoral epiphyseal injuries, 898–899, 906, 908
  distal femoral epiphyseal injuries and, 902, 905–907
  spinal injury, diagnostic imaging, 727
Hyperflexion injury
  diagnosis, 726
  preexisting disease/deformities with, 719–720
  spinous processes, 744
  thoracolumbar junction, 751–752
Hypertension, as bone injury complication, 336
Hypertrophic cartilage zone, in physis, 13–14
Hypervitaminosis A, fracture injuries and, 352
Hypoestrogenism, role of, in sports-related injuries, 403
Hypophosphatemia, rickets and, 351

Hypotension, femoral shaft fractures, traction for, 881–882
Hypothyroidism, fracture injuries and, 353–354

I

Ibuprofen, immature skeletal injury, fracture repair, inflammatory phase, 249
Iliac crest and spine
   anatomical development of, 793–794
   iliac wing fractures, 799
   pelvic avulsion fractures, 817–822
Iliofemoral ligament
   anterior hip dislocation, 841–842
   hip injuries and, 831–832
Iliopsoas tendon, hip injuries and, 832
Ilizarov devices
   tibiofibular diaphyseal injuries, open injuries, 1039
   unreduced elbow dislocations, 554
Immature skeleton
   failure of, diagnostic imaging, 124–125
   healing and repair patterns
      cartilage repair, 259–263
         nerve regeneration and repair, 263–264
         osseous fracture repair, 244–259
         skeletal muscle repair, 264
         wound healing, 243–244
   injury to
      activity levels and, 44
      adult skeletal trauma compared with, 47–48
      age effects on, 42–43
      anatomic locations, 48–51
      automobile injuries, 45–46
      bicycle injuries, 46
      common mechanisms of, 45–47
      complications, 58–60
      disability evaluation, 60
      falls, 46–47
      infant walkers, 46
      joint disruption, 55–58
      off-road vehicle injuries, 46
      parental involvement, 41
      patient history, 41
      patterns and statistics on, 38–40
      periosteum, 54–56
      physical change, 54
      prevention of, 40–41
      remodeling, 57–59
      seasonal factors in, 43–44
      special features of, 42
      sports and recreational injuries, 44–45
      susceptibility in children, 41–42
      type of fracture, 51–54
      vending machines, 47

Immobilization. *See* Fixation techniques; Traction
Immunoprophylaxis, open injury infection
   gas gangrene immunization, 287
   tetanus immunization, 287
Impacted fracture, immature skeletal injury as, 51–52
Impingement syndrome
   distal ulnar injuries, 634–635
   talus fractures, 1106
Impotence, pelvic fractures and urethral injury, 810
Incision techniques, débridement, with open injury, 272
Indomethacin, bridge resection using, 227–228
Infants and neonates
   birth fractures, 348–349
      premature infants, 349
   brachial plexus injuries, 446–447
   clavicle injury
      diagnosis, 432
      incidence, 430–431
      injury mechanism, 431–432
      treatment, 433–434
   compartment syndrome in, 316
   distal femoral epiphyseal injury, 896–898
   fracture patterns
      in infancy, 349–350
      type 1C fracture injury, 159–161
      type 1 fracture injury, 157
   glenohumeral joint dislocation, 466–468
   myelodysplasia and fracture injury in, 368
   osteogenesis imperfecta in, 356–358
   premature infants, birth fractures in, 349
   proximal femoral fractures in, 863–864, 866–868
   radial head dislocations, 591–594
   spinal cord injury, 370
   tibiofibular diaphyseal injuries, 1035–1037
   See also Birth trauma; Fetal injury
Infant walkers, immature skeletal injuries with, 46
Infection
   amputation in children, 295
   bites and sting wounds, 279
      hand injuries, 691–692
   as bone injury complication, 338
   distal radioulnar injuries, 622–624
   as fracture treatment complication, 101
   nail bed injuries, 690
   open injuries, 280–288
      antibiotics for, 281–282

      botulinism, 288
      clostridial cellulitis, 287–288
      clostridial infections, 284–285, 287–289
      gas gangrene, 285–287
      hematogenous osteomyelitis, 283
      joint involvement, 284
      late infection, 283–284, 288
      osteomyelitis, 282–285
      tetanus, 287
      toxic shock syndrome, 282
   plantar foot padding wounds, 1141–1145
Infectious disease, casts, complications from, 91
Inflammatory phase, immature skeletal injury
   fracture repair patterns, 245–249
   wound healing, 244
Initial response protocol, for multiple injury, 71–73
   airway assessment and stabilization, 71
   circulation assessment and stabilization, 71–72
   orthopaedic injury, 75–76
   pain management, 72
   physical evaluation, 72–73
   shock, treatment of, 72
Injury mechanisms
   clavicle injury and, 431–432
   diaphyseal humeral fractures, 475, 477
   distal femoral epiphyseal injuries and, 905–906
   distal fibular injuries, 1069–1073
   distal radial injury, 626–627
   distal radioulnar fractures, 617–618
   distal tibial fractures, 1055–1057
      pronation-eversion and external rotation, 1057
      supination-external rotation, 1056–1057
      supination-inversion, 1056
      supination-plantar flexion, 1056
   femoral shaft fractures, 881
   fracture reductions, 87
   gunshot injury, 289
   hip injuries, posterior dislocation, 833, 836
   immature skeletal injuries, 45–46
   lateral condyle injuries, 510, 514
   Monteggia lesions, 596–598
   Osgood-Schlatter lesions, 1018–1020
   proximal femoral fractures, 870–872
   proximal humeral physeal fracture, 466
   proximal radial fractures, 584–585
   proximal tibiofibular joint dislocation, 1025
   pulled elbow, 555–556
   spinal cord injury, 763–765, 767–768

spinal injury, 721–723
tibial spine injuries, 998, 1000–1005
tibial tuberosity injuries, 1014–1015
transcondylar injuries, 497–502
See also Growth mechanism injury
Insulin-like growth factor-I (IGF-I), immature skeletal injury, fracture repair, inflammatory phase, 249
Insulin-like growth factor-II (IGF-II), immature skeletal injury, fracture repair, inflammatory phase, 249
Intercarpal disruptions, diagnosis of, 663–664
Intercellular cartilaginous matrix, growth mechanism injury, physeal biomechanics and, 195
Intercondylar region
  fractures in, 683–684
  humeral fractures and, 495–498
  immature skeletal injury to, 50
Intermedullary nailing technique
  fracture treatment using, 99–100
  head trauma, 89
  proximal radial fractures, 587–588
Internal bleeding, multiple injuries and, 71
Internal fixation
  children's fractures, biologic factors, 87
  distal tibial injuries, 1060–1061
  fracture treatment
    alignment using, 97
    biodegradable materials, 100
    complications, 101–104
    indications for, 91, 93
    intermedullary techniques, 99–100
    plate fixation, 98–99
    screw fixation, 97–98
    techniques, 97–100
  growth mechanism injury, physeal injuries, management of, 211
  head trauma, 89
Interphalangeal injuries
  dislocation, characteristics of, 677–678
  incidence of, 654–655
  thumb dislocation, 666
Interposition materials, bridge resection using, 226–227
Interstitial gas shadows, diagnostic imaging, 119
Intertrochanteric fractures, proximal femoral fractures and, 873
Intervertebral disc
  anatomic development, 717
  calcification, subluxation and, 729
Intraarticular dislocation
  calcaneus injuries, 1116
  patella, 940–941
Intraarticular fractures
  cartilage repair, 260

coronoid process, 581–582
hip injuries, acetabular fragments, 846
lateral condyle injuries, 510–514
medial epicondyle injuries, 506–508
osteochondral knee fractures, 966–967
Intraarticular gas shadows, diagnostic imaging, 119
Intracapsular fat-fluid levels, diagnostic imaging, 119
Intracompartmental pressure monitoring, compartment syndrome, 317
Intracranial pressure (ICP)
  fracture treatment with, external fixators, indications for, 94–96
  head trauma, multiple injury protocol, 80
Intraepiphyseal osteotomy, growth mechanism injury, 198
Intramalleolar injury (accessory ossicle), characteristics of, 1066–1069
Intramedullary nailing and rodding
  femoral shaft fractures, 888–890
  head trauma, multiple injury protocol, 80
  osteogenesis imperfecta and, 357–358
Intraoperative imaging, fracture treatment, basic principles, 87
Intraosseous effusions, growth mechanism injuries, type 5 fracture pattern, 176
Intraosseous infusion
  compartment syndrome, 316
  initial response protocols using, 71
  circulation, assessment of, 71–72
Intrauterine fractures, epidemiology, 346–348
Intrinsic-plus position, wrist and hand injury repair, 653, 655–656
Ipsilateral proximal/diaphyseal femoral fractures, characteristics of, 876
Irradiation, growth mechanism injury from, 179–180, 182
Ischial tuberosity
  anatomical development of, 793
  avulsion fractures, 817, 822–824
  type 3 fracture injury in, 167, 169
Ischemic necrosis
  arterial injury and, 314
    compartment syndrome, 318–319
    Volkmann's contracture, 318–320
  capital femur injury, slipped capital femoral epiphysis (SCFE), 844–845
  dens fractures, 738
  distal metaphysis (supracondylar) injuries and, 494–495

femoral shaft fractures, surgical treatment, complications with, 888–892
foot injuries, talus fractures, 1104–1105
growth mechanism injuries
  physeal damage, 198
  type 5 fracture pattern, 176
  type 7 fracture pattern, 187
  type 8 injury pattern, 189, 197
hip injuries, 846–849
  posterior hip dislocation, 840
immature skeletal injury, fracture repair, inflammatory phase, 246–249
knee injuries, osteochondritis dissecans, 968–971
necrosis with
  burn injury, 182
  scintigraphy (radionuclide imaging) of, 139
osteochondroses, fracture injuries, 364–365
physeal growth arrest, experimental bridging and, 217
proximal femoral fractures, 868
  complications, 873–876
  treatment methods, 872–873
proximal radial fractures, 589
replantation techniques, 300–303
scaphoid fractures, 659
talus region, 1091–1093
tibial tuberosity injuries, 1017–1018
Ischiopubic osteochondrosis, pelvic fractures, 824
Ischiopubic rami
  fracture of, 799–802
  triradiate cartilage fracture and, 811–816
Ischium, anatomical development of, 792–793
Iselin's disease, metatarsal injury, 1132–1133

J

Jaw thrust maneuver, multiple injury protocol, airway assessment and stabilization, 71
"Jefferson fracture," spinal injury pathology, 723
Joint capsule
  fibrous tissue in, 30–31
  hip anatomy and, 831–832
  knee anatomy and, 932
Joint disruption. *See* Dislocations
Joint evaluation, magnetic resonance imaging (MRI) using, 137
Joint incongruity, distal tibial fracture complications, 1065
Joint injuries

Joint injuries (cont.)
  glenohumeral joint dislocation, 462–466
    brachial plexus injury, 465
    luxatio erecta, 465–466
  growth mechanism injury, burns, 182
  hip anatomy and, 831–832
  joint laxity/dislocation
    epidemiology, 359, 362
    knee ligament injuries and, 944–946
    posterior hip dislocation, 836
  tarsometatarsal injury, 1123–1126
  See also Hip injury; Knee injury; specific joints, e.g. Elbow injury
Joint stiffness
  burn injuries, hand injuries, 696
  elbow dislocations, 551
  epidemiology in children, 359–362
  poliomyelitis and fractures witih, 370
Juvenile rheumatoid arthritis
  joint stiffness, osteoporosis and fracture with, 361
  membranous bone formation and, 2
  spinal injury and, 721

K
Kienbock's disease, carpal fractures, 662
Kingella kingae, as musculoskeletal pathogen, 280
Kirner's deformity, phalangeal fractures, 679
Kirschner pins, growth mechanism injury, type 4A fracture, 169–170
Klippel-Feil syndrome
  rotatory subluxation, atlantoaxial joint, 735
  spinal injuries, 719–720
  sports-related injuries and, 400
  spinal injury, 405
Klumpke's palsy, brachial plexus injuries, 446–447
Knee injuries
  arterial injury with, 313
  arthroscopy, 935–936
  bipartite patella, 960–964
  Charcot knee, 980
  chronic subluxation, 941–944
  compartment syndrome, fracture treatment and, 88
  computed tomography (CT) imaging, 135
  diagnostic imaging, 933–935
  dislocations, 936–941
    habitual dislocation, 941
    intraarticular dislocation, 940–941
    patellar dislocation, 938–940
    subluxation, 938
  dorsal defects, 964, 966
  examination guidelines, 932–933
  floating knee, 910–912
  fractures
    fabellar fracture, 966
    osteochondral fracture, 966–967
    patellar fractures, 951–957
  Hoffa disease, 980
  ligament injury, 944–950
    collateral ligaments, 945–946
    cruciate ligaments, 946–950
    Pellegrini-Stieda lesion, 946
    Segond lesion, 946
  meniscal cyst, 977–978
  meniscal injuries, 976–977
  meniscal ossicles, 978–980
    discoid meniscus, 979–980
    medial discoid menisci, 980
  open injuries, 972–973
  osteochondritis dissecans, 967–972
  popliteal cysts, 980
  popliteus injury, 966
  Sinding-Larsen-Johansson (SLJ) lesion, 957–960
    neuromuscular disorders, association with, 959–960
    proximal pole lesion, 959
  synovial plications, 973–975
Knee joint, anatomy of, 929–932
  ligaments and capsule, 932–933
  meniscus, 932
  patella, 929–932
Kohler's lesion, navicular trauma, 1120–1122
Kozlowski's spondylometaphyseal dysplasia, fracture injuries with, 354
Kremser's disease, ischial tuberosity avulsion and, 822–824
K-wire (Kirschener wire) fixation
  distal femoral epiphyseal injuries, 908
  distal metaphysis (supracondylar) injuries, 487–491
  femoral shaft fractures, 883–884, 886–888
  fracture treatment using, 94
    vs. biodegradable materials, 100
  growth mechanism injury, physeal injuries, management of, 212
  proximal radial fractures, 587–588
  proximal (sternal) clavicle injury, 437–438
  talus dome fracture, 1108
  unreduced elbow dislocations, 554
Kyphosis
  spinal cord injury, 767–768
    late sequelae, 768–770
  thoracic spinal injuries, 749

L
Labral injury, hip injuries, acetabular fragments, 846
Lacerations
  fracture treatment with associated, closed reduction cast application, 90–91
  knee injuries, 972–973
  pelvic fractures, vascular injury and, 807
  plantar foot padding wounds, 1142–1143
  tendon injury, 696–697
    flexor tendons, 697–698
Lamellar signs, diagnostic imaging of, 123–124
Lappet formation
  growth mechanism injury and, physeal biomechanics, 193, 195–196
  type 1B injury as, 157
Larson syndrome
  carpal subluxation and dislocation, 657
  joint laxity/dislocation, 359
Lateral condyle injuries
  classification, 509–514
  complications, 520–523
    growth damage, 521–522
    nonunion, 520–521
    split capitellar fracture, 522–523
  diagnosis, 515–516
  distal femoral epiphyseal injuries and, 900–904
  distal metaphysis (supracondylar) injuries, 493–494
  late case, 518–519
  pathomechanics, 510, 514
  treatment, 515–520
Lateral epicondyle injuries, humeral fractures, 523–524
Lateral femoral condyle, patellar dislocation and involvement of, 940
Latitudinal growth, physis characteristics and, 11–14
Lauge-Hansen's categories, distal tibial fractures, 1056
Lawn mower injury
  foot injuries, 1145–1148
    calcaneus injuries, 1112
    metatarsal injuries, 1127–1128
  incidence of, 292
  joint involvement, 284
  open injuries, débridement, 271–272
  soft tissue coverage techniques for, 275
  treatment of, 293
Lead exposure
  fracture injuries and, 352
  gunshot injury, open fractures and, 289
"Left behind" cartilage, physeal growth alteration, histopathology, 217, 219

Index

Legal issues, diagnostic imaging, predictive value of, *vs.* clinical findings, 117
Legg-Calvé-Perthes disease
  distal metacarpal fractures, 672
  hip injury necrosis compared with, 846–847
  knee injuries, osteochondritis dissecans, 967–971
  osteochondroses, fracture injuries, 365
  talus fractures, ischemic necrosis, 1105
  talus region ossification, 1092–1093
  type 5 fracture pattern, 175
Leg growth
  diagnostic imaging
    limb length evaluation, 130–134
    postnatal growth evaluation, 128–129
  femoral shaft fractures, complications from, 892–893
  proximal femoral fractures, complications, 873–876
  proximal tibial epiphyseal injuries, 1009–1011
Leptomeningeal cyst, multiple injury protocol, diagnostic imaging of, 78
Lesh-Nyhan syndrome, congenital foot deformity, 1149
Lesser trochanter, injuries, 877–878
Lesser tuberosity avulsion, proximal humeral physeal stress fracture, 474
Leukemia
  fracture injuries with, 378–379
  spinal injury and, 721
Lhermitte's sign, spinal cord injury, 765
Ligaments
  cruciate ligaments, injury to, 946–950
  distal femoral epiphyseal injuries, complications involving, 910
  elbow dislocation, 544, 546
  fibrous tissue in, 30–31
  foot ligaments, injury to, 1149
  hip anatomy and, 831–832
  interphalangeal dislocation, 677–678
  knee capsule anatomy and, 932–933
  knee injuries, 944–950
    collateral ligaments, 945–946
    cruciate ligaments, 946–950
    dislocations, 937–941
    Pellegrini-Stieda lesion, 946
    Segond lesion, 946
  meniscal, 932
  pelvic fractures and injury to, 807–808
  repair and healing of, 262–263
  spinal injuries, 718–719
    diagnostic imaging of, 727

lower cervical fracture-dislocation, 741–744
thumb injury, collateral ligament involvement, 666–667
tibia, anatomic development, 991–992
tibiofibular ligament injuries, 1073–1075
wrist and hand anatomy, 652–653
See also Ligamentum teres; Y ligament; specific ligaments, e.g. Cruciate ligaments
Ligamentum capitum femoris, hip injuries and, 832
  femoral head fractures, 843
Ligamentum teres, femoral head fracture, hip injury and, 843
Limb length evaluation. *See* Longitudinal growth
Linear (type 2) bridge formation
  physeal growth alteration, 218, 224–225
  resectioning techniques, 229–230
Lipohemarthrosis. *See* Fat-fluid level
Lisfranc injuries
  characteristics of, 1123–1126
  metatarsal injury and, 1127
Lisfranc level, amputation, 295
"Little league elbow"
  epiphyseal injury with, 406–407
  incidence of, 400, 559
"Little league shoulder syndrome," proximal humeral physeal stress fracture, 473–474
Liver disease, fracture injury and, 354
Liver injury
  multiple injury protocol, abdominal trauma and, 73
  pelvic fractures and, 808
Localization problems, diagnostic imaging, 121
Longitudinal fracture, immature skeletal injury as, 51–52
Longitudinal growth, inequality assessment
  altered physeal growth
    acceleration of, 212–213
    slowdown in, 212–213
  control of, 16
  diagnostic imaging, 130–134
  equalization procedures
    bone lengthening, 235–236
    bone shortening, 235
    distraction epiphysiolysis, 236–237
    epiphysiodesis, 235
    growth estimation, 234–235
    physeal stimulation, 236
    stapling, 235
  femoral shaft fractures, complications from, 892–893
  immature skeletal injury and, 42
  pelvic fractures, 805–806

physeal growth, 16
physis and, 10–14
proximal tibial epiphyseal injuries, 1009–1011, 1010–1011
treatment of, 134
Longitudinal ossific striations, physeal growth alteration, nondisruptive bridging, 213–214
Long-term fracture changes, immature skeletal injury, fracture healing and repair, 259
Loose casts, distal radioulnar injuries, 621
Lordosis, spinal cord injury, 767–770
Lumbar spine
  anatomic development, 714
  apophyseal injury, 760–765
  injuries to, 752–758
  spondylolysis, 759
Lumbosacral region, injury to, 763, 765–766
Lunate
  anatomical development, 651
  subluxation, diagnosis of, 663–664
Luxatio erecta
  glenohumeral joint dislocation, 465–466
  See also Hip injuries, inferior dislocation
Lysinuric protein intolerance, osteoporosis and, 354

M

Machinery injuries, hand injuries, 693
Madelung-type deformity
  distal radial fractures, 629, 631
  distal radioulnar injuries, 624
  proximal radial fractures, 588
Magnetic resonance imaging (MRI)
  ankle tendon injuries, 1075–1076
  anterior cruciate ligament (ACL) injury, 949
  brachial plexus injuries, 447
  calcaneus injuries, 1116
  colorization of, 136
  elbow injuries, capitellum, 561
  epiphyseal cartilage, 123
  first rib fracture, 426
  fracture repair patterns, remodeling, analysis of, 256–257
  fracture treatment, basic principles, 87
  glenohumeral joint dislocation, 464–465
  growth mechanism injury
    bridge development, 223
    growth plate fracture/failure analysis, 153
    physeal injuries, management of, 212
    type 2 fracture pattern, 161–162

Magnetic resonance imaging (cont.)
    type 7 fracture pattern, 188
    type 8 fracture pattern, 189, 197
  hip injuries
    ischemic necrosis evaluation, 849
    posterior dislocation, 837
  Keinbock's disease, 662
  knee injuries
    examination and diagnosis, 932–935
    knee dislocations, 936–941
    osteochondritis dissecans, 968–971
  lateral condyle injuries, 515–516
  meniscal cysts, 977–978
  meniscal ossicles, 978–980
  Monteggia lesions, 601–602
  multiple injury protocol
    airway assessment and stabilization, 71
    imaging protocols, 75
  patellar injury
    dislocation, 938–941
    osteochondritis dissecans, 971–972
  pelvic fractures, diagnosis, 797–798
  peripheral nerve injury diagnosis, 326
  physeal growth arrest, histopathologic analysis, 217
  scaphoid fractures, 658–659
  soft tissue injury concomitant with fracture, effectiveness of, 119
  spinal cord injury, 763–765, 767–768
  spinal injury, 727–728
    disk herniation, 763
  sports-related injuries and muscle injury, 405
    stress injury diagnosis, 412
  talus fractures, 1104
    dome fracture, 1107–1108
    ischemic necrosis, 1105
  tarsometatarsal injuries, 1125–1126
  techniques for, 136–139
  tibial spine injuries, 1004
  tibial tuberosity injuries, 1015
  tibiofibular ligament injuries, 1074–1075
  transverse lines of Park (Harris lines), 126–128
  Volkmann's contracture diagnosis, 319–320
  wrist and hand injury, 655
  See also SCIWORA (spinal cord injury without obvious radiologic abnormality)
Maisonneuve fracture
  proximal tibiofibular joint, 1024, 1026
  tibiofibular diaphyseal injuries, 1043
Malleolar region
  distal tibia
    development, 996, 998
    fractures, fixation techniques, 1057–1061
  growth mechanism injury
    acute fat replacement, 234
    physeal injuries, management of, 211
    type 5 fracture pattern, 173, 179
    type 7 fracture pattern, 185
  immature skeletal injury to, 51
  intramalleolar injury (accessory ossicle), 1066–1069
Mallet finger deformities, 686–689
Malrotation, phalangeal fractures, 679
Malunion
  cerebral palsy and fractures with, 371
  diaphyseal humeral fractures, 479
  incidence of, with open fracture débridement, 272
  lateral condyle injuries, 521–522
  middle phalangeal fractures, 685–687
  phalangeal neck fractures, 682–684
  proximal phalangeal fracture, 680
Mammllary processes, characteristics of, 10
Mandible, membranous ossification in, 2
Manipulation techniques
  closed reduction of fractures, cast application and, 90–91
  distal tibial injuries, 1061–1062
Marmor fractures, triplane distal tibial fracture, 1053–1054
Matev's sign, elbow dislocations, complications involving, 551
Matrix flow phenomenon, cartilage injury, repair mechanisms, 262
Measles, casts, complications from, 91
Mechanical hindrance, immature skeletal injury and, 60
Mechanical injury, cartilage, repair mechanisms, 261
Mechanical properties, immature skeletal injury, fracture healing and repair patterns, 258–259
Medial collateral ligament (MCL)
  injuries to, 948
  tibial spine injuries involving, 1000
Medial condyle injuries
  distal femoral epiphyseal injuries and, 900–904
  humeral fractures, 502–505
Medial discoid menisci, characteristics of, 980
Medial epicondyle injuries
  elbow dislocations, 548–549
  humeral fractures, 503, 505–508
Median nerve, elbow dislocations, complications involving, 551
Mediastinum, rib fractures and, 423
Medullary callus, immature skeletal injury, reparative phase, 255
Membranous bone formation
  anatomical regions, 1–2
  immature skeletal injury, reparative phase, 254–255
  tumor formation and, 2–3
Membranous osseous tissue formation, bone development, 1–2
Menarche, delay in, role of, in sports-related injuries, 403
  stress fracture incidence and, 409
Meniscus (menisci)
  anatomy of, 932
  meniscal cyst, 977–978
  meniscal injuries, 976–977
  meniscal ossicles, 978–980
    discoid meniscus, 979–980
    medial discoid menisci, 980
  tibial spine injuries, meniscal entrapment and, 1003–1004
Meralgia paresthetica, characteristics of, 825
Mesenchymal cellular condensations
  bone development, 1
  endochondral ossification, 2–4
  membranous bone formation, 2
Metabolic disorders, fracture injury and, 354
Metabolism
  compartment syndrome and muscle energy, 318
  multiple injury protocol, 73–74
  trauma's impact on, 311
Metacarpals
  diaphyseal fracture, 669–670
  distal (epiphyseal) fracture, 670–674
  distal fifth fractures (Boxer's fracture), 672
  fracture treatment, 655–656
  growth mechanism injury, natural bridging, 212
  metacarpophalangeal dislocation, 672–677
  proximal injury, 669
Metacarpophalangeal (MCP) joint
  bite injuries, 691–692
  burn injuries, 696
  carpometacarpal (CMC) dislocation and, 664–665
  dislocation, 672, 675–677
  thumb dislocation, 665–666
Metaphyses
  amputation involving, overgrowth, 298–299
  as anatomic regions, 3–5
  biomechanics in, 25–26
  bone growth and, 16–17
  calcaneus, 1094
  child abuse and pathology in, 384–385
  diagnostic imaging, cortical irregularities, 124
  distal radial region, 574
    radioulnar injury, 615–624
  distal tibial injuries, 1043–1044
  endochondral ossification, bone replacement of cartilage, 3–4

fractures involving
  closed reduction of, 89–90
  comminution of, 87
  external fixation, pin and cast insertions, 96
  gunshot injury, 289
  growth mechanism injuries
    healing patterns, 198–199
    overgrowth in, 213
    physeal injuries, management of, 211–212
    type 2 fracture pattern, 161–163
    type 5 fracture pattern, 173, 178
    type 8 fracture pattern, 188–192
  histology of, 5–8
  in humerus, 458–459
  immature skeletal injury
    characteristics of, 48–50
    fractures in infancy, 349–350
    reparative phase, 255
  magnetic resonance imaging (MRI) of, 136
  myelodysplasia and fracture injury in, 368–369
  physeal growth arrest and
    experimental bridging (resection), 216–217
    tenting, 215
  proximal radial fractures, 582
  rachitic changes, 350
  sclerosis of, due to fracture, 20, 22
  ulnar fractures, 576
  vasculature development in, 18, 20–23
Metatarsals
  anatomical development, 1095–1096
  growth mechanism injury, natural bridging, 212
  injuries to, 1126–1138
    bunk bed fracture, 1132–1133
    dislocations, 1136
    distal injuries, 1129–1130
    fifth metatarsal, 1129–1130, 1133–1135
    first metatarsal, 1127, 1130, 1131
    Freiberg's lesion, 1136–1137
    sesmoids, 1136–1138
    stress fractures, 1135–1137
    tarsometatarsal injuries and, 1124–1126
Methylmethacrylate (cranioplast), bridge resection using, 226–227, 232
Microbridging, physeal growth alterations, 213–215
Microdeformations, during skeletal development, 24
Microfracture mechanism, biomechanics of bone and, 29–30
Microvascular anastomosis
  arterial injury repair, 315
  open injury care using, 275

Midazolam, fracture treatment using, 107
Middle phalanx, fractures of, diagnosis and treatment, 684–687
Missed fractures, multiple injury and, 75–76
Mithramycin, hypercalcemia therapy, 329
Modified Injury Severity Score (MISS), pelvic injury, 795
Modulus of elasticity, skeletal biomechanics, 26–28
Monteggia lesions
  characteristics of, 594–595
  classification, 594–596
  complications, 602–605
  diagnosis, 598
  pathomechancs, 596–599
  radioulnar fractures, 606
  treatment, 599–602
Morbidity statistics, immature skeletal injuries, 38–40
Moseley graphic analysis, longitudinal inequality assessment, 131–134
Motor function, spinal injury diagnosis, 725–726
Motor vehicle accidents
  immature skeletal injuries
    injury mechanisms in, 45–46
    statistics on, 39–40
  multiple injury protocol in, shock treatment and, 72
Multiple injuries
  disseminated intravacsular coagulation (DIC) with, 321–322
  fracture treatment
    complicating factors in, 87
    conservatism, limits of, 86
    external fixators, indications for, 94–96
    plate fixation techniques, 98–99
    rehabilitation treatment, 104–105
    sedation and anesthesia procedures, 105, 107–108
    survival rates, 91–92
  growth mechanisms, type 4 fracture patterns, 172, 175
  head trauma complications, 323–324
  pediatric growth disorders, fractures of unknown etiology, 358–359
  protocol for
    abdominal trauma, 73
    assessment rating, 76
    associated soft tissue/vascular injury, 74
    chest trauma, 73
    compartment syndrome, 74
    head injury, 77–80
    imaging studies, 74–75
    initial response protocol, 71–73
    metabolic considerations, 73–74

    orthopaedic injury, 75–76
    overview, 69–71
    pediatric intensive care, 77
    pediatric trauma score, 76–77
    respiratory distress syndrome, 74
    proximal radial fractures, 582
Multiple joint hypermobility, proximal tibiofibular joint dislocation, 1024
Muscle injury
  arterial injury and
    compartment syndrome, 317–318
    Volkmann's contracture, 318–320
  as bone injury complication, 328
  diaphyseal humeral fractures, 476–477
  distal femoral metaphyseal injuries, 895–896
  femoral shaft fractures, complications from, 895
  immature skeletal injury, 264
  magnetic resonance imaging (MRI) in, 137, 139
  open wound care and, 273
  proximal humeral physeal fracture, 470–471
  sports-related injuries and, 405
  tendon and ligament repair and healing, 262–263
  tibiofibular diaphyseal injuries, compartment syndrome, 1041
Muscle relaxants, growth mechanism injury, physeal injuries, management of, 211
Muscle strength, sports-related injuries and, 404
Muscle transplantation, for Volkmann's contracture, 320
Muscular dystrophy
  fractures with, 372–373
  proximal tibiofibular joint dislocation, 1024
Myelodysplasia
  fat embolism as complication, 322
  fracture injury with, 367–370
  physeal fracture patterns, type 1B injuries, 157
Myelomeningocele
  congenital foot deformity, 1149
  distal femoral epiphyseal injuries and, 902
  growth mechanism injury, type 5 fracture pattern, 173
  proximal tibial epiphyseal injuries, 1006–1007
  tibial tuberosity injuries, 1017
Myositis ossificans. *See* Heterotopic ossification

N
Nail bed injuries
  diagnosis and treatment, 689–691
  subungual hematoma, 690

Nail patella syndrome, fractures and, 354
Nancy nails/rods, fracture treatment using, 99–100
Navicular bones
  anatomical development, 1094–1096
  injuries
    accessory navicular, 1122–1123
    characteristics of, 1119–1123
    Kohler's injury, 1120–1122
Necrosis. *See* Ischemia
Neonates. *See* Infants and neonates
Nerve injury
  autoamputation and, 695
  bone injury, 323–328
    head injury, 323–324
    muscle immobilization, 328
    peripheral nerve injuries, 324–326
    reflex sympathetic dystrophy (RSD), 326–328
  dens fractures, 737–738
  diaphyseal humeral fractures, 479
  distal metaphysis (supracondylar) injuries, 495
  distal radial fractures, 629
  elbow dislocations, complications, 550–551
  femoral fractures, distal femoral metaphyseal injuries, 895–896
  femoral shaft fractures
    complications, 895
    Russell's skin traction and, 885
  foot, 1100
    compartment syndrome, 1102
    congenital deformities, 1149
  fracture injury complications
    peripheral nerve injuries, 324–326
    Volkmann's contracture and assessment of, 320
  hand injuries including, 699–700
  hip injuries
    acetabular fragments, 846
    anterior dislocation, 841–842
    complications involving, 850
    posterior dislocation, 836
  lateral condyle injuries, complications, 522–523
  medial epicondyle injuries, 509
  Monteggia lesions, 602, 605
  pelvic fractures, 808
    diagnosis, 796–798
  proximal humeral physeal fracture, 470–471
  proximal tibial epiphyseal injuries, 1010
  radioulnar fractures, 608
  spinal cord injury, 769–770
  spinal injury
    diagnosis, 724–725
    lower cervical fracture-dislocation, 743–744

See also specific nerves
Nerve regeneration and repair
  immature skeletal injury, 263–264
  peripheral nerve injury and, 325
Nerve root injury, fractures and, 373–374
Nerve transfer therapy, brachial plexus injuries, 447
Neuritis, as bone injury complication, 324
Neurocentral chondroses
  anatomic development, 713
  atlas fractures and, 733
Neurologic disease
  fracture injury with, 365, 367–374
    cerebral palsy, 370–372
    congenital sensory neuropathy, 373–376
    epilepsy, 373
    head injury, 373
    muscular dystrophy, 372–373
    myelodysplasia, 367–370
    nerve root injury, 373–374
    poliomyelitis, 370
    prevention, 365
    spinal cord injury, 370
  fracture treatment, sedation and anesthesia procedures in presence of, 105
Neurometric degeneration, as bone injury complication, 324
Neuromuscular disorders
  proximal tibial epiphyseal injuries, 1006–1007
  Sinding-Larsen-Johansson (SLJ) lesions, 959–960
NEX number, magnetic resonance imaging (MRI), 136
Nitrous oxide, fracture treatment using, 108
Nonbridging, physeal growth alteration, 213
Nondisruptive bridging, physeal growth alterations, 213–215
Nonossifying fibromas, pathologic fractures, 363–364
Nontrochanteric rodding, femoral shaft fractures, 890–891
Nontubular bones, endochondral ossification, 3, 5
Nonunion (pseudarthrosis)
  as bone injury complication, 331–332
  cerebral palsy and fractures with, 371
  clavical fractures, 434
  clavicle injury and congenital pseudoarthrosis, 435–436
  congenital pseudarthroses, 364, 366
    clavicle injury and, 435–436
  dens fractures, 738
  distal radioulnar injuries, 621–622
  elbow dislocations, 551–553

  as fracture treatment complication, 101
  incidence of, with open fracture débridement, 272
  intrauterine fractures, 347–348
  lateral condyle injuries, 518–521
  metacarpal fractures, 670, 672–673
  myelodysplasia and fracture injury and, 368–369
  osteogenesis imperfecta and, 357–358
  proximal femoral fractures, 873–876
  radioulnar fractures, 614–615
  scaphoid fractures, 659–661
  talus bone, 1109
  tibial spine fractures, 1002–1005
  tibiofibular diaphyseal injuries, 1041
Nuclear magnetic resonance (NMR) spectroscopy, immature skeletal injury, physiologic response assessment, 251–253
Nutrient canals, diagnostic imaging, 123–124
Nutritional fitness, sports-related injuries and, 404

O

Obesity, venous disorder in children and, 319–321
Oblique fracture, immature skeletal injury as, 51–52
Obstetric/gynecologic injury. *See* Birth trauma
Occipital fracture, characteristics of, 732
Occlusion
  arterial injury and, 313–314
  compartment syndrome and, 316
Occult injury
  diagnostic imaging, growth mechanism failure, 152
  diagnostic imaging and, 115
  fracture patterns, type 1 fracture injury, 155–161
  magnetic resonance imaging (MRI), 136–137
  missed fracture, multiple injury and, 75–76
Odontoid, anatomy of, 712
Off-road vehicles. *See* All-terrain vehicles
Olecranon fractures
  elbow dislocations, 553
  epidemiology, 575–582
    classification, 575–576
    complications, 578, 580–581
    diagnosis, 576–578
    gymnastic injury, 580
    pathomechanics, 576
    treatment, 578–579
  lateral condyle injuries, 510, 514
  transcondylar injuries and, 500
Olecranon osteotomies, fixation of, biodegradable materials for, 100

Olecranon process, growth and development, 567–569
Open injuries
  basic wound care, 270–279
    bone loss, 276–277
    débridement, 271–272
    muscle injury, 273
    periosteum care, 273–274
    puncture wounds, 273
    skeletal stabilization, 275–276
    soft tissue coverage, 274–275
    tourniquet use, 273
    vascular bone transplant, 277–279
    wound examination, 270–271
  bite and sting wounds, 279–280
  calcaneus fractures, 1112
  characteristics of, 269–270
  crushing and avulsion injuries, 290–292
    degloving, 290–291
    wringer injuries, 292
  foot injuries as, 1101
  foreign bodies, 279–280
  gunshot injury, 288–289
  hand injuries, 692–693
  incidence of, 269
  infection, 280–288
    antibiotics for, 281–282
    botulism, 288
    clostridial cellulitis, 287–288
    clostridial infections, 284–285, 287–289
    gas gangrene, 285–287
    hematogenous osteomyelitis, 283
    joint involvement, 284
    late infection, 283–284, 288
    osteomyelitis, 282–285
    tetanus, 287
    toxic shock syndrome, 282
  knee injuries, 972–973
  lawn mower injury, 292–293
  tibiofibular diaphyses, 1038–1039
Open reduction
  capital femur injury, slipped capital femoral epiphysis (SCFE), 844–845
  distal (acromial) clavicle fracture, 441
  distal femoral epiphyseal injuries, 907–908
  distal metaphysis (supracondylar) injuries, 490–491
  distal radial injury, 629
  distal radioulnar injuries, 619–621
  distal tibial fractures, 1057–1061
  femoral head fracture, hip injury and, 843
  fixation treatments combined with, 93
  fracture treatment
    indications for, 92
    internal fixation, 97
    tourniquet use, 103–104
  growth mechanism injuries, physeal injuries, management of, 211–212
  lateral condyle injuries, 516–520
  Monteggia lesions, 600–601
  patellar sleeve fractures, 957
  proximal humeral physeal fracture, 472
  proximal phalangeal fracture, 680
  proximal radial fractures, 586–588
  proximal (sternal) clavicle injury, 437–438
  proximal tibial epiphyseal injuries, 1009
  radioulnar fractures, 612
  scaphoid fractures, 660–661
  tibial tuberosity injuries, 1016–1017
  transcondylar injuries, 500–502
  type 3 fracture injury, 167
  type 4 fracture injury, 170–172
Open reduction and internal fixation (ORIF), fracture treatment using, indications for, 91
Organized sports, sports-related injuries with, 401–402
Oropharynx, assessment of, multiple injury protocol, airway assessment and stabilization, 71
Orthopaedic injury, multiple injury protocol, 75–76
  initial treatment, 75
  missed fractures, 75–76
Orthotics, foot injury incidence and, 1101
Os acetabuli, pelvic development, 791–792
Osgood-Schlatter lesions
  diagnosis, 1019–1022
  epidemiology, 1018
  fibrous tissue development and, 32
  growth mechanism injury, 149–150
    type 7 fracture pattern, 185–186
  injury mechanisms, 1018–1020
  Sinding-Larsen-Johansson (SLJ) lesions, 959–960
  sports-related injuries, 406–407
  tibial tuberosity anatomic development, 993–995
  tibial tuberosity injuries
    incidence, 1011–1014
    injury mechanisms, 1015
    treatment, 1022–1024
Osmotic pressure, compartment syndrome and, 316
Os odontoideum, spinal injury and, 738–740
Osseous ring of Lacroix
  metaphyses and, 7–9
  physis development and, 10–12
Osseous tissue formation, bone development, 1
Ossicle formation
  intramalleolar injury (accessory ossicle), 1066–1069
  meniscal ossicles, 978–980
  Osgood-Schlatter lesions, 1022–1024
Ossification centers
  bipartite patella, 960–964
  calcaneus, 1093–1094
  carpal regions, 650–651
  in chondroepiphyses, 8–10
  in clavicle, 420–422
  diagnostic imaging, growth and development evaluation, 128, 130
  foot bones, anatomic development, 1091–1093
  humerus, 456, 458
  lateral condyle injuries, 510, 513
  medial epicondyle, 461–462
  Osgood-Schlatter lesions, 1020–1022
  pelvis, 790–791
  radius and ulna, 572–574
  in scapula, 421–423
  spine, 708–709
Ossification ring of Lacroix, growth mechanism injury, experimental trauma studies, 196–197
Osteoarthritis, hip injuries, 850
Osteoblasts, immature skeletal injury, fracture repair, inflammatory phase, 248–249
Osteocartilaginous exostosis, osteochondroma formation and, 183–184
Osteochondral fractures
  cartilage, repair mechanisms, 262
  growth mechanism injury, type 7 fracture pattern, 185–187
  immature skeletal injury, cartilage repair, 260
  knee injuries as, 966–967
  metacarpophalangeal (MCP) joint dislocation, 676–677
Osteochondritis dissecans
  distal tibial fracture complications, 1065–1066
  growth mechanism injury, type 7 fracture pattern, 186–187
  knee injuries, 967–971
  patella, 971–972
  plantar foot padding wounds, 1143–1145
Osteochondroma
  as bone injury complication, 334
  growth mechanism injury and, 182–184
  pathologic fractures, 364–365
Osteochondroses
  epiphyses, 8–10
  foot injuries, 1101
    Freiberg's lesion, 1136–1137
  fractures and, 364–365
  hip injuries, 850

Osteochondroses (*cont.*)
  ischiopubic osteochondroses, 824
  "Little league elbow," 560
  scintigraphy (radionuclide imaging) of, 139–140
  sports-related injuries, 407
  tarsal bones, 1094–1095
Osteoclastic resorption, remodeling process and, 23
Osteogenesis imperfecta
  child abuse and, 379–380
  fracture injury, 355–358
Osteogenic sarcoma, pathologic fractures with, 361, 364
Osteogenic tissue, immature skeletal injury, physiologic response, 253
Osteolytic reactions, biodegradble materials, internal fixation of fractures using, 100
Osteomyelitis
  lawn mower injury, 293
  longitudinal inequality related to, diagnostic imaging for assessment of, 130–134
  membranous bone formation and, 2
  open wound infection, 282–285
    hematogenous osteomyelitis, 283
    late infection, 283–284, 289
    plantar foot padding wounds, 1143–1144
  posttraumatic, external skeletal fixation and, 96–97
  scintigraphy (radionuclide imaging) of, 139
Osteonecrosis. *See* Ischemic necrosis
Osteopenia, spinal injury and, 721
Osteopetrosis, epidemiology of, 359–361
Osteoporosis
  burn injuries and, 361
  growth mechanism injury, burns, 182
  metaphyseal vasculature and, 20, 22
  muscular dystrophy and fractures due to, 372–373
  spinal cord injury, late fractures, 770
  spinal injury and, 721
  in thalassemia patients, 378
Osteosclerotic disorders, fracture injuries, 359–361
Osteosynthesis, femoral shaft fractures, 888–892
Osteotomy
  distal metaphysis (supracondylar) injuries, 491, 493
  osteogenesis imperfecta and, 357–358
  talus dome fracture, 1107–1108
Ostochondritis dissecans, joint disruption, 57
Os trigonum
  anatomical development, 1096, 1098–1099
  injury to, 1108–1109

Overgrowth
  amputation and, 296–297
  amputation in children and, 295–299
  distal radioulnar injuries, 621–622
  femoral shaft fractures, complications from, 892–893
  fracture treatment and, 87
    plate fixation techniques, 98
  growth mechanism injury, altered physeal growth, 212–213
  limb length equalization, physeal stimulation, 236
  metatarsal injury, 1135–1136
  proximal tibial metaphyseal injuries, 1031–1035
  tibial spine injuries, 1004
Overriding fractures
  diaphyseal humeral fractures, 477–478
  treatment of, in children, 86
Overuse syndromes, pediatric athletes, incidence of, 400
"Oxford Method," skeletal age estimation, 129–130
Oxygen free radicals, immature skeletal injury, fracture repair, inflammatory phase, release during, 247–249
Oxygen tension variations, immature skeletal injury, reparative phase, 254

P
Paget-Schroetter syndrome, incidence in children, 320
Pain
  compartment syndrome diagnosis, 317
  hip injuries, chronic hip pain, 850
  knee pain, with hip injuries, 836
  management
    fracture treatment, sedation and anesthesia for, 105–108
    growth mechanism injury, 211–212
    multiple injury protocol, 72
Pancreatic injury
  multiple injury protocol, abdominal trauma and, 73
  thorax and rib trauma and, 428
Panner's lesion, sports-related injuries, epiphyseal injury, 406–407
Parental involvement, immature skeletal injury, 41
Pars interarticularis, spondylolysis, 758–759
Partial-thickness injury, immature skeletal injury, cartilage repair, 260
Pasteurella multocida, bites and sting wounds, 279
Patella
  anatomy of, 929–932
  bipartite patella, 960–964

  deformity, cerebral palsy and, fractures with deformity, 371–372
  dislocation of, 938–941
  dorsal defects, 964, 966
  fracture injuries, 951–957
    sleeve fracture, 953–957
    stress fracture, 953
  habitual dislocation, 941
  intraarticular dislocation, 940–941
  Osgood-Schlatter lesions and position of, 1021–1022
  osteochondritis dissecans, 971–972
  Sinding-Larsen-Johansson (SLJ) lesions, 957–960
Patellofemoral pain syndrome, chronic patellar subluxation and, 942–944
Pathologic fractures
  clavicle injury and, 432
  epidemiology of, 361–364
  in thalassemia patients, 378
  type 1 fracture injury, 157–158
Patient history
  immature skeletal injury, 41
  role of, in sports-related injuries, 402–403
Pauwel's angle, proximal femoral fractures, 872, 875–876
Pavlik's harness
  femoral shaft fractures, 887
  proximal femoral fractures, birth trauma, 868
Pearson attachment, femoral shaft fractures, 884
Pedal nerves, development and injury to, 1100
Pedestrian accidents, immature skeletal injuries
  injury mechanisms, 46
  statistics on, 39–40
Pediatric growth disorders
  fracture injury
    birth fractures, 348–349
    child abuse, 379–386
    congenital pseudarthroses, 364
    dysplasias, 354–355
    endocrinopathy, 353–354
    Gaucher's disease, 352–353
    hematologic disorders, 374–379
    infants, fracture injury in, 349–350
    intrauterine fractures, 346–348
    lead exposure, 352
    metabolic disorders, 354
    multiple fractures of unknown etiology, 358–359
    neurologic disorders, 365, 367–374
    osteochondroses, 364–366
    osteogenesis imperfecta, 355–358
    osteosclerotic disorders, 359
    pathologic fractures, 361–364
    prematurity, 349
    rickets, 350–352

scurvy, 352
vitamin A deficiency, 352
joint laxity/dislocation, 359, 362
joint stiffness, 359–361
Pediatric intensive care, multiple injury protocol and, 77
Pediatric Trauma Score (PTS), multiple injuries, 76–77
Pedicle flaps, open injury care using, 274–275
Pedicle fractures, lumbar spine injuries, 756–758
Pellegrini-Stieda lesion, ligament injury, 946–947
Pelvic fractures
  acetabular fractures, 810–816
    central injuries, 811
    peripheral fractures, 810–811
    triradiate injuries, 811–816
  anterior arch fractures, 802–804
  avulsion fractures, 816–824
    iliac crest, 817–818
    iliac spines, 818–822
    ischial tuberosity, 822–824
  bucket handle injury, 805
  classification of, 798–805
  complications, 805–810
  diagnosis, 796–798
  iliac wing fracture, 799
  ischiopubic osteochondrosis, 824
  ischiopubic rami, 799–802
  lateral compression injuries, 805
  management guidelines, 805–810
    external fixators, indications for, 95
    vascular injury, 806–807
  meralgia paresthetica, 825
  pubic symphysis, 824
  ring fractures
    diagnosis, 795–796
    stable fractures, 798–804
  stress fracture, 824
  symphysis separation, 800, 802–803
    sacroiliac joint separation, 802–804
  vertical shear fractures, 803, 805
Pelvis, anatomic development, 790–794
Pentobarbital, fracture treatment using, 107
Percutaneous fixation
  distal metaphysis (supracondylar) injuries, 490
  fracture treatment with
    complications, 102–103
    indications for, 93
    techniques for, 93–94
  growth mechanism injury, physeal injuries, management of, 211–212
  metatarsal injuries, 1130–1131
  phalangeal fractures, 679
  proximal humeral physeal fracture, 472–473
  proximal radial fractures, 588

radioulnar fractures, 612–613
talus fractures, 1103–1104
Periarticular structures, growth mechanism injury, burns, 182
Perilunate instability, intercarpal disruptions, 663
Periodic acid-Schiff (PAS) reaction, intraarticular fractures, cartilage repair, 260–261
Periosteal callus
  immature skeletal injury, formation of, 250
  in overriding fractures, 86
Periosteal stripping
  distal (acromial) clavicle fracture and, 439–440
  fracture patterns
    type 1 fracture injury, 155–156
    type 2 injury patterns, 162–166
  immature skeletal injury, fracture repair, 249–250
  open fractures, 270
  open injury care, débriding and, 273–274
  scurvy and, 352
  synostosis and, 331
Periosteum
  as anatomic region, 5, 7
  biomechanics in, 26–28
  bone loss and salvaging of, 276–277
  diaphyseal vasculature in, 21
  fibrous tissue in, 30–32
  growth mechanism injury
    burns, 182
    physis biomechanics and, 195–196
    type 9 fracture patterns, 191–194
  humeral growth and, 456, 468
  immature skeletal injury
    characteristics of, 54–57
    childhood vs. adult trauma, 47–48
    fracture repair, 245, 249–250
    remodeling following, 58
    reparative phase in, 253–255
  limb length equalization, physeal stimulation, 236
  in metaphyses, 6–9
  physeal growth alteration, experimental bridging, excision and, 216–217
  proximal tibial metaphyseal injury and, 1034–1035
  roentgenographic response to, 122
Peripheral nerve injuries
  as fracture injury complication, 324–326
  hand injuries including, 699–700
Peripheral (type 1) bridge formation
  physeal growth alteration, 217–218, 223–224
  resectioning techniques, 228–229
Periphysis, components of, 13

Peterson injury patterns
  classification, 150–151
  metaphyseal fracture pattern, 189–190
  vascular etiology in, 175, 180
Phalangeal lengthening, hand amputations, 695
Phalangeal neck fractures, characteristics of, 681–684
Phalanges
  foot
    anatomical development, 1095, 1097
    fractures, 1138–1141
    injuries, 1138–1141
    stubbed toe, 1140–1141
  hand
    distal phalanx injury, 689
    extra-octave fracture, 680–682
    finger tip injuries, 690–691
    fractures, 678–679
    fracture treatment, 655–656
    intercondylar fractures, 683–684
    interphalangeal dislocation, 677–678
    mallet finger injury, 686–689
    middle phalanx injuries, 684–687
    nail bed injuries, 689–690
    phalangeal neck fracture, 681–683
    proximal phalanx fractures, 679–680
    thumb injuries and, 668–669
Phosphaturia, rickets and, 351
Physeal ghost, skeletal vasculature and, 18–19
Physical changes, immature skeletal injury and, 54
Physical evaluation
  multiple injury protocol, 72–73
  predictive value of vs. radiographic findings in children, 116–117
Physical fitness, sports-related injuries and, 404
Physical maturity, sports injury incidence and, 399–400
Physical rehabilitation, fracture treatment, 104–105
  fixation and, 88
  multiple injury, 104
  psychological factors, 104–105
  single fractures, 104
Physiology
  immature skeletal injury, childhood vs. adult trauma, 48
  role of, in sports-related injuries, 403
Physis
  amputations involving, replantation techniques, 303
  as anatomic region, 3–5
  biomechanics in, 24–28
    growth mechanism injury and, 193, 195–196

Physis (cont.)
  birth fractures in, 348
  bone development, 3–4
  bone growth and, 15–16
  bridge resectioning technique, 228–234
    acute fat replacement, 234
    allografting, 234
    central (type 3) bridge, 230–232
    distraction epiphysiolysis, 233–234
    epiphyseal transplantation, 234, 2334
    general principles, 230–233
    linear (type 2) bridge, 229–230
    peripheral (type 1) bridge, 228–229
    postoperative care, 234
  calcaneus, 1094
  characteristics of, 10–13
  child abuse and pathology in, 384–385
  diagnostic imaging of, 123–124
    longitudinal inequality assessment, 132–134
  distal fibula development, 997, 999
  distal radial fractures, 624–632
    classification, 624–627
    complications, 629–632
    diagnosis, 626–627
    pathomechanics, 626–627
    treatment, 627–629
  distal tibial injury
    classification, 1045–1055
    complications, 1062–1066
    injury mechanisms, 1055–1057
    treatment, 1057–1062
  endochondral ossification in, 5–6
  epiphysiodesis and, 17–18
  fractures involving, 87
    fixation treatments, 93
    gunshot injury, 289
    lawn mower injury, 293
    percutaneous fixation treatment of, 94
    pin and cast insertions, 96
  growth alterations, 212–219
    acceleration, growth mechanism injury and, 212–213
    arrest/slowdown, growth mechanism injury and, 212–214
    arterial injury and, 315
    bridge formation, 214–216
    central bridging (type 3), 218–219, 225–226
    experimental bridging, 216–217
    histopathology, 217–223
    linear bridging (type 2), 218, 224–225
    natural bridging, 212
    nonbridging, growth arrest and, 213
    nondisruptive bridging, 213–214
    peripheral (type 1) bridge

formation, 217–218, 223–224
  growth mechanism injury
    experimental trauma studies, 196–197
    frostbite, 178–179
    healing patterns, 198–199, 200
    incidence of, 147–150
    irradiation, 180, 182
    lower extremity, incidence in, 209
    magnetic resonance imaging (MRI) of, 136–137
    management of, 211–212
    type 1 fracture pattern, 153–161
    type 2 fracture pattern, 162–166
    type 3 fracture pattern, 162–170
    type 5 fracture pattern, 173–180
    type 6 fracture pattern, 181, 183
    type 8 fracture pattern, 189–192
  hormonal response of, 16
  hypertrophic zones of, 12, 14
  immature skeletal injury
    characteristics of, 49
    initial healing in, 256
    remodeling following, 58
  limb length equalization, stimulation of, 236
  mapping of, 224, 226
  myelodysplasia and fracture injury in, 368–369
  rachitic changes, 350
  sports-related injuries, 406–407
  sports-related injuries to, 405–407
    repetitive injuries, 406
  tibial tuberosity, anatomic development, 993–995
  ulnar development in, 567–570
  vasculature of, 18–23
  wrist and hand anatomy, 651
Pin and cast insertions
  biodegradable materials in, 100
  bipartite patella, 964
  complications following, 336–337
  distal (acromial) clavicle fracture, 441
  femoral shaft fractures
    intramedullary nailing and rodding, 889–890
    nontrochanteric rodding, 890–891
    traction with, 882–884
  fracture fixation using, 93
    complications, 101
    external fixators, use of, 95–97
  growth mechanism injury
    physeal injuries, management of, 211–212
    transphyseal pins, 197
    type 4A fracture, 169–170
  halo fixation, spinal injury, 730–731
  intercondylar fractures, 683–684
  proximal radial fractures, 587–588
  slipped capital femoral epiphysis (SCFE), 869–870

tibial spine injuries, 1003–1005
"Ping-pong ball" fracture, multiple injury protocol, diagnostic imaging of, 78
Plantar foot padding
  anatomical development, 1096, 1099–1100
  injuries, 1141–1145
    chondro-osseous infection, 1143–1144
    foreign bodies, 1144–1145
    puncture wounds, 1141–1143
Plantar tendons, injury to, 1148–1149
Plasminogen administration, venous disorder therapy, 321
Plaster of Paris (POP) beads, débridement, with open injury and, 272
Plastic deformation
  bone biomechanics and, 28–30
  diagnostic imaging, 124–125
  patellar dorsal defects, 966
  pelvic development and, 794–795
  radioulnar fracture as, 606–607
Plate fixation
  femoral shaft fractures, 891–892
  fracture treatment using, 98–99
    complications, 101–103
Platelet-derived growth factor (PDGF), immature skeletal injury, fracture repair, inflammatory phase, 249
Platelet formation, immature skeletal injury, fracture repair, inflammatory phase, 248–249
Playground, immature skeletal injuries on, 45
Plica syndrome, synovial plications, 973–975
Pluripotential cells, immature skeletal injury
  physiologic response, 253
  reparative phase, 253–255
Pneumothorax
  multiple injury protocol, chest trauma and, 73
  thorax and rib trauma, 427
"Poland's hump," distal tibia development, 996
Poliomyelitis, fractures with, 370
Polymethylmethacrylate (PMMA) antibiotic beads, débridement, with open injury and, 272
Polymorphonuclear neutrophils (PMNs)
  elastase, osteomyelitis, 283
  immature skeletal injury, wound healing, 244
  multiple injury protocol, 74
Polyvalent gas gangrene serum, open injury infection, immunization with, 287

Index

Popliteal artery entrapment syndrome, knee dislocations, 937
Popliteal cysts, characteristics of, 980
Popliteus injury, knee injuries and involvement, 966
"Porta" plica, synovial plications, 973–975
Positive anterior drawer sign, anterior cruciate ligament (ACL) injury, 948–949
Positive end-expiratory pressure (PEEP), pulmonary contusion assessment, 426–427
Positron emission tomography, tibiofibular diaphyseal injuries, vascular complications with, 1040
Posterior chondroses, anatomic development, 713
Posterior cruciate ligament (PCL)
 injuries to, 950
 tibia, anatomic development, 992
Postfracture cysts, as bone injury complication, 332–334
Postoperative care, bridge resectioning, 234
Postreduction evaluation, diagnostic imaging, 122
Posttrauma care
 fracture treatments, external fixators, posttraumatic osteomyelitis, 96–97
 head trauma, multiple injury protocol, 80
Posttraumatic joint stiffness, immature skeletal injury and, 58
Posttraumatic pulmonary insufficiency, multiple injury protocol, 74
Prevention procedures, immature skeletal injury, 40–41
Primary bone
 immature skeletal injury
  childhood vs. adult trauma, 47–48
  union of, 258
  remodeling characteristics of, 21, 23
Primary osteons
 biomechanics of, 27–28
 remodeling characteristics of, 21, 23
Pritchett tables, longitudinal inequality assessment, 130–131
Progeria, dysplasias with, 355
Pronation-eversion and external rotation, distal tibial fractures, 1057, 1061–1062
Prostheses
 amputation in children and, 295, 300
 sports-related injuries and limb deficiencies, 405
Proteoglycan matrix, immature skeletal injury, cartilage repair, 259–260
Proximal femoral fracture
 acute slipped capital femoral epiphyseal (SCFE) injury, 868–870
 classification, 863–864
 complications, 873–876
 diagnosis, 872
 femoral neck fractures, 870–872
 incidence and epidemiology, 861, 863
 injury mechanisms, 870–871
 ipsilateral proximal/diaphyseal fracture, 876
 neonates, 866–868
 stress fractures, 876
 transphyseal injury, 864–866
 treatment, 872–873
Proximal fibula
 anatomic development, 995
 injuries, 1027
 metaphyseal injury, 1035
 See also Maisonneuve injury
Proximal focal femoral deficiency (PFFD)
 dysplasias with, 355
 intrauterine fractures, 347–348
Proximal humeral physis
 anatomy of, 456–462
 fracture
  characteristics of, 466, 468–474
  complications, 473
  diagnosis, 471
  diagnostic imaging, 471–472
  injury mechanisms, 466
  lesser tuberosity avulsion, 474
  pathologic anatomy, 466, 468–471
  shoulder fusion, 474
  stress injury, 473–474
  treatment, 472–473
Proximal interphalangeal (PIP) joint
 bite injuries, 691–692
 interphalangeal dislocation, 677–678
Proximal metacarpals, injury to, 669–671
Proximal metaphysis, fractures of, 474–476
Proximal phalangeal physeal injury
 fracture, proximal portion, 679–680
 metacarpophalangeal (MCP) joint dislocation, 676–677
Proximal phalanx, thumb injuries and, 668–669
Proximal pole lesions, Sinding-Larsen-Johansson (SLJ) lesions, 959
Proximal radius
 anatomy and development of, 568–570
 fractures, 582–589
  classification, 582–585
  complications, 588–589
  diagnosis, 584–585
  pathomechanics, 584–585
  treatment, 585–588
 physeal growth alteration, bridge formation, 215
Proximal (sternal) clavicle, injury to, 436–438
Proximal tibia
 anatomic development, 990–992
 epiphyseal injuries, 1005–1011
  classification, 1005–1007
  complications, 1009–1011
  diagnosis, 1007
  treatment, 1007–1009
 metaphyseal injuries, 1027–1035
  classification, 1028–1030
  diagnosis, 1030
  treatment, 1030–1035
 physeal growth alteration, bridge formation, 215
 physeal injury, anterior cruciate ligament (ACL) injury and, 950
Proximal tibiofibular joint, dislocation and subluxation
 classification, 1024
 diagnosis, 1024–1026
 injury mechanisms, 1025
 posterior dislocation, 1026–1027
 superior dislocation, 1027
 treatment, 1025–1026
Proximal ulna
 development of, 567
 fracture patterns, 575–577
Pseudarthrosis. See Nonunion
"Pseudodislocation," distal (acromial) clavicle, 438
Pseudoepiphysis
 metatarsals, 1095
  injuries and incidence of, 1126–1127
 spherical growth plate and, 11
 wrist and hand anatomy, 652–653
Pseudomeningocele, thoracic spinal injuries, 749
"Pseudo-Monteggia" legion, radial head dislocations, 592
Pseudoparalysis, clavicle injury and, 432
Pseudosubluxation, characteristics of, 728–729
Pseudothrombophlebitis, compression and, 321
Psychological fitness, sports-related injuries and, 404
Psychological rehabilitation, fracture treatment and, 104–105
Pubis, anatomical development of, 792–793
Pulled elbow, 555–559
 diagnosis, 556–557
 immature skeletal injury, 57
 injury mechanisms, 555–556
 treatment, 558–559
Pulmonary contusion, rib fractures and, 426–427

Pulmonary damage, femoral shaft fractures, post-surgical complications, 890
Pulselessness, compartment syndrome diagnosis, 317
Puncture wounds
  bites and sting wounds as, 279
  examination of, 271
  with open injury, 273
  plantar wounds, 1141–1143
Push-pull evaluation, femoral shaft fractures, casting methods and, 886
Pyknodysostosis, epidemiology of, 359–361
Pyle method
  longitudinal inequality assessment, 130–131
  skeletal age estimation, 130

Q

Quadriceps tendon
  intraarticular patellar dislocation, 941
  patellar fractures and, 951–957
Quantitative bacterial counts
  bone loss monitoring, 276–277
  soft tissue coverage techniques, 275

R

Radial head dislocations
  fractures and, 354–355
  incidence and epidemiology, 589, 591–594
  Monteggia lesions, 600, 602
  proximal radial fractures, 589
Radial nerve injury, Monteggia lesions, involvement of, 596
Radial styloid, ossification of, 573–574
Radiographic imaging
  bipartite patella, 962–964
  bridge resectioning, 228
  calcaneus injuries, 1112–1116
  child abuse and fractures injuries, 382–383
  clavicle injury, 432–433
    proximal (sternal) clavicle injury, 436–437
  developing skeleton, radiology of, 122–128
    cortical irregularities, 124
    epiphyseal cartilage, 123
    growth plate (physis), 123
    immature bone failure, 124–125
    nutrient canals, 123–124
    transverse line of Park (Harris lines), 125–128
  distal (acromial) clavicle fracture and, 439, 441
  distal metaphysis (supracondylar) injuries, 483–484
  distal radial fractures, 626–627, 627
  distal radioulnar injuries, 618
  distal ulnar injuries, 632–635
  elbow dislocation, 548
  femoral shaft fractures, 881–882
    therapeutic assessment, 887–888
  foot injuries
    compartment syndrome, 1102
    metatarsal injuries, 1135–1136
  fracture treatment, basic principles, 87
  general guidelines, 115–122
    adequate films, 117–118
    comparison views, 118
    fat pads, 120–121
    foreign bodies, 121
    interstitial and intraarticular gas shadows, 119
    intracapsular fat-fluid level, 119
    localization problems, 121
    postreduction evaluation, 122
    predictive value of, vs. clinical findings, 116–117
    roentgenographic response to trauma, 121–122
    skull films, 118
    soft tissue injury, 118–119
  glenohumeral joint dislocation, 462–466
  growth and development evaluation, 128–134
    limb length evaluation, 130–134
    ossification center development, 128
    postnatal arm and leg growth, 128–129
    skeletal age estimation, 129–130
  growth mechanism injury
    frostbite, 178–179, 182
    management and arrest, 220–221, 223–224
    physis, failure in, 152–153
  hand injuries, 655
  hip injuries, posterior dislocation, 837
  immature skeletal injury, physiologic response assessment, 251–253
  knee injuries, 933–935
  lateral condyle injuries, 515–516
  limb length evaluation, measurement techniques, 130
  medial epicondyle injuries, 507–508
  metacarpophalangeal (MCP) joint dislocation, 675–676
  Monteggia lesions, 598
  multiple injury protocol, 74–75
    head trauma and, 78–79
  Osgood-Schlatter lesions, 1019–1022
  patellar dislocation, 938–941
    chronic patellar subluxation and, 942–944
  patellar fractures and, 951–952
  pelvic fractures, 796–798
  physeal growth alteration, bridge formation, detection with, 213, 215
  proximal femoral fractures, 867–868
    ischemic necrosis, 873–876
  proximal humeral physeal fracture and, 471–472
  proximal radial fractures, 584–585
  proximal tibial epiphyseal injuries, diagnosis of, 1007
  proximal tibial metaphyseal injuries, 1030
  pulled elbow, 556–558
  radial head dislocations, 593–594
  radioulnar fractures, 607
  reflex sympathetic dystrophy (RSD), 327
  scaphoid fractures, 658
  Sinding-Larsen-Johansson (SLJ) lesions, 957–960
  special techniques, 134–140
    arthrography, 135
    computed tomography (CT), 135–136
    fluoroscopy, 134–135
    magnetic resonance imaging, 136–139
    scintigraphy (radionuclide imaging), 139–140
    sonography, 140
    SPECT (single positron emission computed tomography) scanning, 140
    stress films, 135
    vascular radiology, 140
  spinal injury, 726–728
  sports-related injuries, stress injuries and, 410–412
  talus fracture
    dome fracture, 1107–1108
    ischemic necrosis, 1105
  tibial spine injuries
    diagnosis, 1001–1002
    treatment, 1002–1005
  tibial tuberosity injuries, 1015
  transcondylar injuries, 500–502
  wrist and hand, 655
  See also Computed tomography (CT); Magnetic resonance imaging (MRI)
Radioisotope-labeled fibrinogen, venous disorder diagnosis, 321
Radionuclide imaging. See Scintigraphy
Radiopaque markers, diagnostic imaging of physis, 123
Radioulnar fractures
  classification, 605–607
  compartment syndrome, 608
  complications, 614–615
  diagnosis, 606–607
  distal injuries, 615–624

Index

complications, 621–624
diagnosis, 618
pathomechanics, 617–618
treatment, 618–621
neurovascular injury, 608
rotation, 608–610
treatment, 610–613
Radius
Bennett's fracture analogue, 667
Galeazzi fracture-dislocation and, 635–638
growth and development, 567–571
Monteggia lesions, involvement of, 594–598
See also Distal radial injury; Proximal radius; Radial head dislocations; Radioulnar fractures
Rami. *See* Ischiopubic rami
Recombinant human bone morphogenetic protein (rhBMP-2), immature skeletal injury, fracture repair, inflammatory phase, 249
Rectal injury, pelvic fractures and, 808
Recurrent dislocations
elbow dislocations, 551–553
hip injuries, 849–850
voluntary habitual dislocation, 851
patellar dislocation, 941–944
pulled elbow, 559–560
Recurrent fractures
cerebral palsy and fractures with, 371
epidemiology, 332
femoral shaft fractures, 895
in thalassemia patients, 378
Reflex function, spinal injury diagnosis, 725–726
Reflex sympathetic dystrophy (RSD)
as bone injury complication, 326–328
tarsal tunnel syndrome and, 1148
Regional block anesthesia, fracture treatment using, 107
Remodeling
calcaneus injuries, 1116
clavicle injury, 434
distal metaphysis (supracondylar) injuries, 486–487
distal radial injury, 628–629
distal radioulnar injuries, 619–621
fracture treatment, closed reduction techniques, 89–90
immature skeletal injury, 57–60
fracture healing and repair patterns, 256–257
periosteum, 250
residual angulation remodeling, 259
phalangeal neck fractures, 682–684
proximal humeral physeal fracture, 472–473
radioulnar fractures, 610
skeletal development and, 21, 23

talus fractures, 1104
tibiofibular diaphyseal injuries, 1041
Renal osteodystrophy, rickets and, 351
Reparative tissue, immature skeletal injury
fracture healing, reparative phase, 253–255
physiologic response assessment, 252–253
Repetitive injuries
autoamputation and, 695
first rib fracture and, 426
foot injury incidence and, 1101
medial condyle injuries as, 503–505
pelvic avulsion fractures, 816–817
plantar tendons, 1148–1149
spondylolysis, 759
sports-related injuries as, physeal injuries, 406–407
Replantation
amputation and, 294
characteristics of, 300–303
hand injuries, 693–695
techniques for, 300–303
Resectioning technique, bridge resectioning, 228–234
acute fat replacement, 234
allografting, 234
central (type 3) bridge, 230–232
distraction epiphysiolysis, 233–234
epiphyseal transplantation, 2334
general principles, 230–233
linear (type 2) bridge, 229–230
peripheral (type 1) bridge, 228–229
postoperative care, 234
Respiratory distress syndrome, multiple injury protocol, 74
Respiratory infection, fracture treatment, sedation and anesthesia procedures, 105
Rett syndrome, fractures with, 372
Rhabdomyolysis, multiple injury protocol, soft tissue and vascular injury, 74
Rib injuries
anatomical characteristics and, 419
cardiac tamponade, 427
child abuse and fractures of, 382
diaphragm and abdominal injury, 427–428
first rib fracture, 425–426
hemothorax, 427
multiple injury protocol, chest trauma and, 73
pancreas, 428
pneumothorax, 427
pulmonary contusion, 426–427
slipping rib syndrome, 428–429
splenic injury, 428
subcutaneous emphysema, 427
thoracic outlet syndrome, 426

tracheobronchial tree injury, 427
Rickets
fracture patterns with, 350–352
type 1 injuries, 157–158
hypertrophic zone of physis and, 13
"Ring" apophysis
cervical end-plate injury, 745–748
spinal development, 714, 716
Ring (polyaxial) fixators, fracture treatment using, 94–96
Ring sequestrum, external fixators, risk of, 94–95
Roland-Galeazzi fracture-dislocation, characteristics of, 635
Rollerblading, immature skeletal injuries, 44
Rotational deformity
distal tibial fractures
complications, 1065
pronation-eversion and external rotation, 1056–1057
supination-external rotation, 1056–1057
distal tibial injuries, 1046–1047
femoral shaft fractures, complications from, 894–895
metacarpal fractures, 669
Rotational techniques
basic principles, 87
distal metaphysis (supracondylar) injuries, 489
radioulnar fractures, 608–610
Rotatory subluxation, atlantoaxial joint, 734–736
Rule infractions, role of, in sports-related injuries, 403
"Rule of thirds," rotational techniques, radioulnar fractures, 609
Russell's skin traction, femoral shaft fractures, 885

S

Sacroiliac joint, pelvic fractures, vascular injury and, 807
Sacrum, injuries to, 763, 766–767
Salicylates, head trauma complications, management with, 324
Saltation concept, of bone growth, 16
physeal growth alteration, nondisruptive bridging, 213–214
Salter-Harris injury patterns
growth mechanism injury classification, 149–150
incidence and epidemiology, 209–210
tibial tuberosity injuries, 1012–1013
type 1 injury
bridge formation, 215
classification, 8–10, 149–150
distal radial injuries as, 625–626
distal tibial injuries, 1045–1047

Salter-Harris injury patterns (*cont.*)
   distal ulnar injuries as, 632–635
   failure patterns, 153–161
   management of, 211
   type 1A patterns, 153–157
   type 1B patterns, 157–159
   type 1C patterns, 159–161
  type 2 injury
   bridge formation, 215
   classification, 8–10, 149–151
   distal radial injuries as, 625
   distal tibial injuries, 1047–1049
   distal ulnar injuries as, 632–635
   failure patterns, 161–166
   management of, 211
   physeal healing, immature skeletal injury, 256
   type 2A injury, 161–163
   type 2B injury, 163–166
   type 2C injury, 164–166
   type 2D injury, 165–166
  type 3 injury
   bridge formation, 214
   classification, 150–151
   distal radial injuries as, 625, 627
   distal tibial injuries, 1047–1050
   distal ulnar injuries as, 632–635
   failure patterns, 166–170, 176
   management of, 211
   physeal healing, immature skeletal injury, 256
  type 4 injury
   bridge formation, 214
   classification, 150–151
   distal radial injuries as, 625, 627
   distal tibial injuries, 1047–1050
   distal ulnar injuries as, 632–635
   failure patterns, 167, 169–175
   management of, 211
   physeal healing, immature skeletal injury, 256
   type 4A patterns, 167, 169–171
   type 4B patterns, 170, 172–174
   type 4C patterns, 172, 174
   type 4D patterns, 172, 175
  type 5 injury
   classification, 150–151
   fracture/failure patterns, 165, 172–180
   management of, 211–212
  type 6 injury
   bridge formation, 214
   classification, 150–151
   distal tibial fractures, 1054–1055
   failure patterns, 181–183
   management of, 212
  type 7 injury
   classification, 150–151
   distal radial injuries as, 625, 627
   distal tibial fractures, 1055
   distal ulnar injuries as, 632–635
   fracture/failure patterns, 183, 185–190
   management of, 212
  type 8 injury
   classification, 150–151
   failure patterns, 188–192
  type 9 injury
   classification, 150–151
   failure patterns, 191–194
Scaphoid bone
  anatomical development, 650–651
  fractures of, 657–661
Scapula
  anatomical characteristics of, 422–423
  endochondral ossificaton in, 3
  trauma to, 442–445
   glenoid hypoplasia, 444
   scapular winging, 445
   scapulothoracic dissociation, 444–445
Scapulothoracic dissociation, scapular fractures and, 444–445
Scar formation, wound healing, immature skeletal injury, 244
Scheuerman's disease
  endochondral ossification and, 3
  thoracic spinal injuries, 750, 762
Schmidt syndrome, fracture injuries and, 353–354
Schwann cells, nerve regeneration and repair, 263–264
Sciatic nerve injury, bone injury and, 325–326
Scintigraphy (radionuclide imaging)
  calcaneus injuries, 1116
  child abuse and fracture injuries, 383–384
  foot injuries, compartment syndrome, 1102
  growth mechanism injury, bridge formation, diagnosis, 221
  growth plate failure analysis, 152
  multiple injury protocol, 75
  proximal tibial metaphyseal injury, 1033–1035
  reflex sympathetic dystrophy (RSD), 327
  scaphoid fractures, 658
  sports-related injuries, stress injuries and, 412
  talus dome fracture, 1107–1108
  techniques, 139–140
  tibiofibular diaphyseal injuries, 1039–1040
SCIWORA, (spinal cord injury without obvious radiologic abnormality)
  child abuse and fracture injury with, 380–382
  diagnostic imaging, 729
  fracture patterns, type 1 fracture injury, 156–157
  immature skeletal injury statistics and, 40
  magnetic resonance imaging (MRI), 136
  spinal cord injury, 763–765, 767–768
  spinal injury, pathology, 722, 724
Sclerotic bone
  immature skeletal injury, fracture repair, inflammatory phase, 247–249
  physeal growth alteration
   bridging histopathology, 217–219, 221–226
   nondisruptive bridging, 213–214
  spondylolysis, 758–759
Scoliosis
  spinal cord injury, 767–770
  spinal injury and, 720
  thoracic spinal injuries, 749–750
Screening procedures, role of, in sports-related injuries, 402–403
Screw fixation
  anterior cruciate ligament (ACL) injury, 950
  biodegradable materials in, 100
  bipartite patella, 964
  distal tibial injuries, 1060–1061
  fracture treatment using, 97–98
   complications, 102–103
  growth mechanism injury, physeal injuries, cancellous screws for, 211
  knee injuries, osteochondritis dissecans, 969–970
  tarsometatarsal injuries, 1126
Scurvy, fracture injuries and, 352
Seasonal patterns, immature skeletal injuries, 43–44
Seat-belt restraints
  immature skeletal injuries
   injury mechanisms, 45–46
   statistics on, 39–40
  lumbar spine injuries, 752–758
  multiple injury protocol, abdominal trauma and, 73
Secondary bone, characteristics of, 21
Secondary cartilage, membranous bone formation, 2
Secondary ossification center
  calcaneus, 1094
  fracture patterns
   type 1C fracture injury, 159–161
   type 1 fracture injury, 157
   type 7 fracture pattern, 185
  hip injuries and, 831–833
  metatarsals, 1095–1096
  pelvis, 790–792
  phalanges, 1095, 1097
  proximal fibula, anatomic development, 995
  spinal development, 714–716

cervical end-plate injury, 746–748
tibial tuberosity, anatomic development, 993–995
wrist and hand anatomy, 651–652
Secondary osteons, remodeling process and, 23
Sedation
　diagnostic imaging, evaluating need for, 116
　fracture treatment and, 105–108
Segond lesion, ligament injury, 946, 948
Septic arthritis, open injury infection, 284
Serratia marcescens
　late infection osteomyelitis, 283–284, 289
　muscle involvement, with open injury, 273
Sesamoid bones
　injury to, 1136, 1138
　phalanges, 1095, 1097
Sever's legion
　calcaneus, 1094
　　apophysitis, 1119
　sports-related injuries, 406–407
Shapiro injury patterns, classification, 150
Shark bites, open injury from, 279–280
Sharpey's fibers
　development of, 31–32
　patellar anatomy, 929–932
Shock
　complications from, 312–313
　multiple injury protocol and, 72
　　head trauma and, 77
　pelvic fractures, vascular injury and, 806–807
Shopping carts, immature skeletal injuries on, 45
Short term inversion recovery (STIR) sequence
　bridge development, diagnostic imaging, 223
　magnetic resonance imaging (MRI), 136
　peripheral nerve injury therapy, 326
　sports-related injuries, stress injury diagnosis, 412
Shoulder dystocia, clavicle injury and, 430–431
Shoulder fusion, proximal humeral physeal fracture, 474
Sickle cell anemia, fracture injuries with, 378
Silicone rubber, bridge resection using, 227
"Silver fork" deformity, distal radioulnar injuries, 618
Simple radiologic sign, defined, 118
Sinding-Larsen-Johansson (SLJ) lesion
　patellar anatomy, 931

patellar injuries, 957–960
　neuromuscular disorders, association with, 959–960
　proximal pole lesion, 959
Single fractures, rehabilitation following, 104
Size categorization, multiple injury protocol, Pediatric Trauma Score (PTS), 76
Skateboarding, immature skeletal injuries, 44
Skeletal development
　anatomy and physiology
　　anatomic regions, 3–13
　　biomechanics, 24–30
　　bone density, 23–24
　　bone development, 1–3
　　bone growth, 16–18
　　collagen, 15–16
　　fibrous tissue, 30–32
　　remodeling, 21, 23
　　tensegrity, 13–15
　　vasculature, 18–21
　burn injury and, 182
　diagnostic imaging, 122–128
　　age evaluation, 129–130
　　cortical irregularities, 124
　　end of growth evaluation, 134
　　epiphyseal cartilage, 123
　　evaluation of growth and development, 128–134
　　growth plate (physis), 123
　　immature bone failure, 124–125
　　limb length evaluation, 130–134
　　multiple views, necessity of, 116
　　nutrient canals, 123–124
　　postnatal arms and legs, growth evaluation, 128–129
　　transverse line of Park (Harris lines), 125–128
　end of, diagnostic imaging of, 134
　foot bones, 1095–1096, 1098–1099
　spinal cord injury, 768–770
　spinal injury, diagnostic imaging of skeletal growth centers, 727
　sports-related injuries and, 400
　See also Immature skeleton
Skeletal fixation. *See* Fixation techniques
Skeletal injuries
　articular injuries, 49–50
　cervical injuries, 50
　childhood *vs.* adult trauma, 47–48
　diaphyseal injuries, 48–49
　epicondylar injuries, 49–50
　epiphyseal region, 49
　intercondylar (intraepiphyseal) injuries, 50
　magnetic resonance imaging (MRI), 137, 139
　malleolar, 51
　metaphyseal injuries, 48–50

physeal region, 49
　subcapital injuries, 50
　supracondylar injuries, 50
　transcondylar injuries, 50
Skiing, immature skeletal injuries, 45
Skin anesthesia, fracture treatment, 107
Skin fibroblast cultures, child abuse and fracture analysis, 380
Skin grafting
　crushing injuries, 290
　lawn mower injuries, 1143–1148
Skin injury or loss, fracture treatment with, external fixators, indications for, 94–96
Skin surface pressures, closed reduction of fractures
　cast application and, 90–91
　casts, complications from, 91
SKIWORA (skeletal injury without obvious radiologic abnormality)
　fracture patterns, type 1 fracture injury, 156–161
　immature skeletal injury statistics and, 40
Skull fractures
　child abuse and fracture injury with, 381
　diagnostic imaging
　　effectiveness of, 118
　　predictive value of clinical findings *vs.* radiographic findings, 116–117
　multiple injury protocol, diagnostic imaging, 78–79
　treatment of, 79–80
　　basic principles, 88–89
Sleeve (shell) fracture
　coronoid process, 581–582
　distal femoral epiphyseal injuries and, 905
　foot injuries, calcaneus injuries, 1117
　growth mechanism injury
　　type 7 fracture pattern, 185–186
　　type 9 fracture patterns, 192–194
　immature skeletal injury as, 54–56
　magnetic resonance imaging (MRI), 137
　olecranon process, 580
　patellar fractures as, 953–957
　ulnar region, 576
Slipped capital femoral epiphysis (SCFE)
　proximal femoral fractures, acute condition, 868–870
　titanium pins for treatment of, advantages and disadvantages, 91
Slipping rib syndrome, characteristics of, 428–429
Snapping hip syndrome, characteristics of, 850–851
Soccer, immature skeletal injuries, 44

Soft tissue injury
  amputation and, 294
  arterial injury with, 313
  avulsion injury, 290–291
  child abuse and fracture injury with, 385–386
  diagnostic imaging, shadowing and, 118–119
  foot injuries
    calcaneus injuries, 1116–1117
    compartment syndrome, 1101–1102
    metatarsals, 1129–1130
    tarsal bones, 1123
  fracture treatment in presence of, 88
    external fixators, 95–97
    fixation techniques and, 91
    sedation and anesthesia procedures, 106
  growth mechanism injury, physeal injuries, management of, 212
  hemophiliac diseases, fracture injuries, treatment of, 377
  lawn mower injuries, 1147–1148
  multiple injury protocol, 74
  open fractures, 270
  open injury care, 274–275
  Osgood-Schlatter lesions, 1020–1022
  patellar dislocation, 938–941
  spinal injury, diagnosis, 725
  tibiofibular diaphyseal injuries, 1039–1040
  tibiofibular ligament injuries, 1073–1075
  wringer injuries and, 292
  See also Cartilage; Ligaments; Tendons
Somatotrophic hormone (STH), growth mechanism injury, physeal biomechanics and, 196
Sonography
  growth mechanism failure diagnosis, 152
  techniques, 140
Spare-part surgery, epiphyseal grafting, amputation, 299–300
Spasticity
  cerebral palsy and fractures due to, 370–372
  fracture treatment, complications involving, 87
  head injury
    complications, 324
    fracture treatment, 88–89
SPECT (single positron emission computed tomography) scanning
  physeal growth alteration, 221
  spondylolysis diagnosis, 759
  sports-related injuries, stress injuries and, 412
  techniques, 140
Spherical physis
  characteristics of, 10–13
  growth mechanism injury, type 7 fracture pattern, 185
Spica immobilization, femoral shaft fractures, 886–888
Spina bifida, myelodysplasia and fracture injury with, 367–368
Spinal canal, anatomic development, 714
Spinal cord injury
  birth injury, 731
  dens fractures, 737–738
  diagnosis, 763–764, 767
  Down syndrome and compression risk, 721
  fractures with, 370–371
  injury mechanisms, 763
  late sequelae, 768–770
  spinal shock, 764–765
  treatment, 767–768
Spinal/epidural anesthia, fracture treatment using, 107
Spinal injury
  abuse injuries, 731
  atlas fractures, 732–734
  axis, body and neural arch fractures, 740
  birth injury, 731
  calcaneus fractures and, 1112
  cervical fracture-dislocation
    lower region, 741–744
    upper region, 740–741
  Chance fracture, 751–754
  child abuse and fracture injury with, 380–381
  computed tomography (CT) imaging, 135
  dens fracture, 736–738
  developing spine's response to, 717–721
    Down syndrome, 720–721
    gunshot injury, 719
    pathologic fractures, 721
    preexisting disease/deformity, 719–720
    scoliosis, 720
  diagnosis of, 724–728
    radiographic imaging, 726–728
  disk herniation, 761, 763, 765
  facet fractures, 750
  foot injuries with, 1102
  fractures with, 370–371
  Grisel syndrome, 729
  halo fixation technique, 731
  lumbar apophyseal injury, 760–763
  lumbar region, 754–758
  lumbosacral region, 763, 765–766
  magnetic resonance imaging (MRI), 136
  occipital fracture, 732
  occipitoatlantal dislocation, 732
  os odontoideum, 738–740
  pathobiology of, 721–724
    animal fractures, 722–724
  Scheuermann's disease, 750
  SCIWORA studies, 729–730
  spinous processes, 744–748
  spondylolisthesis, 759–760
  spondylosis, 758–759
  sports-related injuries and, 404–405
  stress fractures, 760
  subluxation, 728–729
    rotatory subluxation of the atlantoaxial joint, 734–736
  thoracic spine, 748–750
  thoracolumbar junction, 750–752
  transverse and spinous process, 758
  treatment guidelines, 730–731
Spinal muscular atrophy. *See* Werdnig-Hoffman disease
Spinal shock
  diagnosis, 726
  spinal cord injury, 764–765
Spine, anatomical development, 708–717
Spinous process, injury to, 758
Spiral fracture
  immature skeletal injury as, 51–52
  tibiofibular diaphyseal injuries, 1037–1038
Spleen injury
  multiple injury protocol, abdominal trauma and, 73
  thorax and rib trauma and, 428
Splenectomy, Gaucher's disease, fracture injuries and, 353
Splint applications, closed reduction techniques, 90
Split capitellar fracture, lateral condyle injuries, 522–523
Split-thickness skin grafts
  crush-burn injuries, 290
  lawn mower injury, 293
  open injury care using, 275
Spoiled gradient-echo (SPGR) imaging
  physeal trauma, 137
  vs. magnetic resonance imaging (MRI), 136
Spondolytic spondylolisthesis, sports-related injuries, 405
Spondylolisthesis
  characteristics of, 759–760
  Scheuerman's disease, 750–751
Spondylolysis, spinal injuries, 758–759
  Scheuerman's disease, 750
Spongiosa formation, metaphyseal cortex, 5–8
Sports injuries
  apophyseal injury, 407
    lumbar apophyseal injury, 761
  causation, 403
  congenital/acquired limb deficiencies, 405

epiphyseal injury, 406–407
exercise routines, 403–404
exertional compartment syndrome, 405
fitness and, 404
immature skeletal injuries, 44–45
incidence and epidemiology, 399–402
Lisfranc injuries in, 1123–1124
olecranon process
  gymnastic injury, 580
  gymnastics, 580
Osgood-Schlatter lesions, 406–407, 1018–1024
osteochondroses, 407
pelvic fractures
  avulsion fractures, 816–817
  ischiopubic osteochondrosis, 824
  meralgia paresthetica, 825
physeal injury, 405–407
physiologic alteration, 403
preparticipation screening, 402–403
proximal humeral physeal stress fracture, 473–474
repetitive injuries, 406–407
snapping hip syndrome, 850–851
spinal injuries
  lumbar apophyseal injury, 760–765
  preexisting disease/deformities and, 719–720
spondylolysis, 758–759
stress fractures, 407–414
  diagnosis, 410
  pathomechanics, 410
  radiologic imaging, 410–412
  toddler's fracture, 412–414
  treatment, 412
team physicians' role concerning, 402
S-shaped tibia, proximal tibial metaphyseal injury, 1033–1035
Stair-climbing, immature skeletal injuries from, 47
Staphylococcal infection, open injury infection, 281–282
  bites and sting wounds, 279
  joint involvement, 284
  late infection osteomyelitis, 284
Stapling, limb length equalization, 235
Sternum
  anatomical characteristics of, 419–420
  trauma to, 429–430
Steroid therapy
  multiple injury protocol, pneumonia risk and, 74
  pathologic fractures, 363–364
  reflex sympathetic dystrophy (RSD), 328
Stimson reduction technique, posterior hip dislocation, 838
"Stinger" injury, sports-related injuries, 405

Sting wounds, open injury from, 279–280
Straight-leg traction, femoral shaft fractures, 885–886
Strain
  biomechanics of, in bone, 28–30
  during skeletal development, 24
Stress films, techniques for, 135
Stress fractures
  foot injuries
    calcaneus, 1117
    metatarsal injury, 1135–1137
    talus, 1106
  growth mechanism injury, type 7 fracture pattern, 185–186
  ischiopubic junction, 792–793
  medial condyle injuries as, 503–505
  osteogenesis imperfecta and, 357–358
  patellar fractures as, 953
  pelvic fractures, 824
  proximal femoral fractures, 876
  proximal humeral physeal fracture, 473–474
  roentgenographic response to, 121–122
  scapular fractures as, 443
  scintigraphy (radionuclide imaging) of, 139
  spinal injury, 760
    sacral injuries, 763, 767
  sports-related injuries, 407–414
    diagnosis, 410
    epiphyseal injuries, 406–407
    grading of, 412
    pathomechanics, 410
    physiology and, 403
    radiologic imaging, 410–412
    skeletal abnormalities and, 400
    treatment, 412
  toddler's fracture as, 412–414
Stress mechanisms
  biomechanics of bone and, 28–30
  immature skeletal injury, mechanical fracture healing and repair properties, 258–259
  reflex sympathetic dystrophy (RSD), 326
  during skeletal development, 24–25
Stress test, proximal tibial epiphyseal injuries, diagnosis of, 1007
Stubbed toe, characteristics and treatment, 1140–1141
Subcapital region, immature skeletal injury to, 50
Subchondral bone, in epiphyses, 8–10
Subcoracoid displacement, distal (acromial) clavicle fracture, 441–442
Subcutaneous emphysema, thorax and rib trauma, 427
Subluxation

atlantoaxial joint, rotatory subluxation, 734–736
diagnostic imaging of, 727
knee subluxation, 938
Monteggia lesions, 601
patella, chronic subluxation, 941–944
proximal tibiofibular joint
  classification, 1024
  diagnosis, 1024–1026
  injury mechanisms, 1025
  posterior dislocation, 1026–1027
  superior dislocation, 1027
  treatment, 1025–1026
spinal injury, 728–729
rotatory subluxation of the atlantoaxial joint, 734–736
Subtrochanteric fractures, characteristics and management of, 878–880
Sucking, rotational finger deformities and, 656
Superior mesenteric artery (SMA) syndrome, as bone injury complication, 338
Supination-external rotation, distal tibial fractures, 1056–1057, 1061
Supination-inversion injury pattern, distal tibial fractures, 1056, 1061
Supination-plantar flexion injury pattern, distal tibial fractures, 1056
Supracondylar process, diaphyseal humeral fractures, 479–480
Supracondylar region
  distal metaphysis (supracondylar) injuries, 480–495
    classification, 480
    complications, 491–494
    diagnosis, 483–485
    displacement, 483–484
    elbow dislocation, 495
    extension type injury, 480–482
    flexion type injury, 481, 483, 487
    myositis, 495
    pathologic anatomy, 480–483
    radiologic examination, 483
    surgical release, 494–495
    treatment, 485–491
    unstable fractures, 487–490
  humerus and, 459
  immature skeletal injury to, 50
Surface renderings, fracture imaging, 136
Surgery
  femoral shaft fractures, 888–892
    external fixator, 892
    intramedullary rodding, 889–890
    nontrochanteric rodding, 890–891
    plate fixation, 891–892
  fracture treatment using, fixation techniques and, 91
  lateral condyle injuries, 515–520

Surgery (*cont.*)
  lawn mower injuries, 1145–1148
  meniscal injuries, 976–977
  Osgood-Schlatter lesions, 1022–1024
  patellar dislocation, chronic patellar subluxation and, 943–944
  talus dome fracture, 1107–1108
  tendon injury, flexor tendons, 697–698
Surgical release, distal metaphysis (supracondylar) injuries and, 494–495
Surgical techniques, physeal bridging
  indomethacin, 227–228
  interposition materials, 226–227
Susceptibility, for immature skeletal injury, 41–42
Suspension traction, femoral shaft fractures, 884
Swan-Ganz catheter, pulmonary contusion assessment, 426
Swan-neck deformity, spinal injury, lower cervical fracture-dislocation, 743–744
Syme level ankle disarticulation, amputation, 295
  complications, 299–300
Symphysis pubis
  anatomical development of, 794
  separation of, 800, 802–803
    sacroiliac joint separation, 802–804
  stress fractures, 824
Syndesmosis
  anatomic development, 997–999
  distal tibial fracture complications, 1066
Synostosis
  as bone injury complication, 330–331
  distal radial fractures, 631
  distal tibial injuries, 1044
  proximal radial fractures, 588–589
  radioulnar fractures, 614
  tibiofibular diaphyseal injuries, 1041–1042
Synovial plications, knee injuries and, 973–975
Syringomyelia, spinal cord injury, 769–770

T
Talectomy procedure, talus deformity, 1105
Talus
  anatomic development, 1091–1093
  injuries to, 1102–1110
    avulsion injury, 1106
    chronic deformity, 1105
    congenital deformity, 1109
    dome fracture, 1106–1108
    fractures, 1102–1108

    impingement syndrome, 1106
    os trigonum injury, 1108–1109
    peritalar and subtalar dislocations, 1109–1110
Tanner-Whitehouse technique, skeletal age estimation, 130
Tarsal bones
  anatomical development, 1094–1095, 1097
  congenital coalitions, 1149
  injury to, 1123
Tarsal tunnel syndrome, incidence and epidemiology, 1148
Tarsometatarsal injury, characteristics of, 1123–1126
Team physician, role of, in sports-related injuries, 402
Technetium bone scanning, bipartite patella, 962–964
Tendons
  ankle injuries and involvement of, 1075–1076
  calcification, 699
  development and injury to, 1100
  fibrous tissue in, 30–31
  hip injuries and, 832
  injuries to, 696–699
    extensor tendons, 698–699
    flexor tendons, 697–698
  patellar tendons, 929–932
  plantar tendons, 1148–1149
  repair and healing of, 262–263
  tibial tuberosity development, patellar tendon, 994–995
  See also specific tendons
Tensegrity structures, skeletal development and, 13–15
Tensile-induced fibrous hyperplasia, type 1B fracture, repetitive use injuries, 158
Tensile strength, skeletal biomechanics, 26–28
Tension pneumothorax, thorax and rib trauma, 427
Tetanus, open injury infection, 287
Tethering effect, distal ulnar injuries, 635
Thalassemia, fracture injuries and, 377–378
Thenar flaps, finger tip injuries, 691
Thermal injury, hands, 695
Thermoregulation, sports-related injuries and, 404
Thomas splint, femoral shaft fractures, 885
Thoracic outlet syndrome, characteristics of, 426
Thoracic spinal injuries
  characteristics of, 748–750
  spinal cord injury, 767–768

Thoracic vertebra, anatomic development, 713–714
Thoracolumbar junction
  anatomic development, 714
  fractures of, 718–719
  injury to, 750–752
Thorax, trauma to, 422–429
  cardiac tamponade, 427
  diaphragm and abdominal injury, 427–428
  first rib fracture, 425–426
  hemothorax, 427
  pancreas, 428
  pneumothorax, 427
  pulmonary contusion, 426–427
  slipping rib syndrome, 428–429
  splenic injury, 428
  subcutaneous emphysema, 427
  thoracic outlet syndrome, 426
  tracheobronchial tree injury, 427
Three-point fixation
  mallet finger deformities, 687–689
  radioulnar fractures, 612
Thrombocytopenia anemia radial aplasia (TAR) syndrome, meniscal ossicles, 978
Thumb injury
  Bennett's fracture analogue, 667
  collateral ligament injury, 666–667
  dislocation, 665–666
  interphalangeal dislocation, 666
  phalangeal fracture, 668–669
  See also Hand injuries
Thurstan-Holland fragments
  diagnostic imaging of, 123
  growth mechanism injuries
    healing patterns, 199
    type 2 injury pattern, 162–166
  immature skeletal injury, physeal healing, 256
  proximal phalangeal fracture, 680
  screw fixation techniques for, 97–98
  thumb injuries, 668–669
  triradiate cartilage fracture, 814–816
Tibia
  anatomy of
    distal tibia, 996–998
    proximal tibia, 990–992
    syndesmosis, 997–999
    tibial tuberosity, 992–995
    tibiofibular diaphyses, 995–996
  See also Tibiofibular diaphyses
Tibial fractures
  casting of, compartment syndrome monitoring, 88–89
  proximal tibial epiphyseal injuries, 1005–1011
    classification, 1005–1007
    complications, 1009–1011
    diagnosis, 1007

Index

treatment, 1007–1009
proximal tibial metaphyseal injuries, 1027–1035
  classification, 1028–1030
  diagnosis, 1030
  treatment, 1030–1035
tibial spine injuries, 998, 1000–1005
  anatomic variation, 1000
  classification, 1000
  diagnosis, 1001–1002
  treatment, 1001–1005
tibial tuberosity injuries, 1011–1018
  classification, 1012–1013
  complications, 1016–1018
  concomitant disorders, 1013–1014
  diagnosis, 1015
  injury mechanisms, 1014–1015
  treatment, 1015–1016
Tibial tuberosity
  anatomic development, 992–995
  injuries, 1011–1018
    classification, 1012–1013
    complications, 1016–1018
    concomitant disorders, 1013–1014
    diagnosis, 1015
    injury mechanisms, 1014–1015
    treatment, 1015–1016
Tibiofibular diaphyses
  anatomic development, 995–996
  injury of, 1035–1043
    anatomic development, 995–996
    compartment syndrome, 1041–1043
    complications, 1040–1041
    infants and toddlers' injuries, 1035–1037
    Maisonneuve injury, 1043
    older children's injuries, 1037–1038
    open injuries, 1038–1039
    treatment, 1040
    vascular injury, 1039–1040
  ligament injuries, 1073–1075
  See also Proximal tibiofibular joint
Tibiotalar fusion, ankle arthrodesis, 1076
Tillaux fracture
  distal tibial injuries, 1048, 1050–1052
    repair and treatment, 1058–1060
  tibial tuberosity development, 994
  type 3 injury, 167
Tissue glue, fixation treatments using, 100
Tissue injury, physeal growth arrest and, 217
Titanium pins, fracture treatment using, slipped capital femoral epiphysis (SCFE), 91
Toddler's fracture
  characteristics of, 412–414
  foot injuries, calcaneus, 1117

proximal tibial metaphyseal injuries as, 1027–1028
tibiofibular diaphyseal injuries, 1035–1037
Toes
  anatomical development, 1095, 1097
  injuries, 1138–1141
    fractures, 1138–1141
    stubbed toe, 1140–1141
  See also Phalanges
Torticollis, rotatory subluxation, atlantoaxial joint, 734–735
Torus fracture
  biomechanics of bone and, 28–31
  diagnostic imaging, 125
  distal femoral metaphyseal injuries, 895–896
  distal radioulnar injuries, 615–618
    treatment, 618–621
  immature skeletal injury, statistics on, 40
  immature skeletal injury as, 54–55
  proximal tibial metaphyseal injuries as, 1028–1030
Total bone mineral (TBM), immature skeletal injury, fracture healing and repair, 259
Tourniquet use
  bridge resectioning, 228
  open fracture reduction, complications, 103–104
  puncture wounds, 273
Toxic shock syndrome
  cast complications, 338
  open wound infection, 282
Trabeculae
  bone density analysis, 23–24
  fractures, magnetic resonance imaging (MRI), 136–137
  growth mechanism injury
    physeal biomechanics and, 195
    type 8 fracture pattern, 189
  growth of, 17
  immature skeletal injury, reparative phase, 254–255
  metaphyses, 6–9
  remodeling process and, 23
Trachea, assessment of, multiple injury protocol, airway assessment and stabilization, 71
Tracheobronchial tree, thorax and rib trauma and injury to, 427
Traction
  arterial injury with, 313
  complications following, 336
  distal femoral epiphyseal injuries, 907–908
  distal metaphysis (supracondylar) injuries, 486–491
  femoral shaft fractures, 882–886

fracture treatment using, economic factors in, 87–88
head injury, treatment using, 88–89
posterior hip dislocation, 840
proximal femoral fractures, birth trauma, 868
subtrochanteric fractures, 879–880
vasospasm and, 316
Trampolines, immature skeletal injuries on, 45
Transcervical fractures, proximal femoral fractures as, 864
Transcondylar region
  distal metaphysis (supracondylar) injuries and, 493–494
  humeral fractures, 497–502
  immature skeletal injury to, 50
Transcutaneous electric nerve stimulation (TENS), reflex sympathetic dystrophy (RSD), 327–328
Transforming growth factor-β (TGF-β), immature skeletal injury, fracture repair, inflammatory phase, 249
Translocation, elbow dislocation, 550
Transphyseal collagen, characteristics of, 16
Transphyseal injury, proximal femoral fractures as, 864–866
Transphyseal pins, growth mechanism injury, 197
Transplantation, hand injuries, 693–695
Transverse fracture
  immature skeletal injury as, 51–52
  type 3 fracture injury, 166–170
Transverse ligament, rotatory subluxation, atlantoaxial joint, 734
Transverse lines of Park, diagnostic imaging, 125–128
Transverse process
  anatomic development, 713
  injury to, 758
Trauma
  amputation stump, overgrowth from, 299
  brachial plexus, 445–448
  child abuse and fracture injury with, 380–386
  clavicle, 430–442
    complex injury, 435
    complications, 434–435
    congenital pseudarthrosis, 435–436
    diagnosis, 431
    diagnostic imaging, 432–433
    distal (acromial) clavicle, 438–442
    injury mechanism, 431–432
    pathologic anatomy, 431
    proximal (sternal) clavicle, 436–438
    remodeling, 434

Trauma (cont.)
- treatment, 433–434
- developing spine's response to, 717–721
  - Down syndrome, 720–721
  - gunshot injury, 719
  - pathologic fractures, 721
  - preexisting disease/deformity, 719–720
  - scoliosis, 720
- growth mechanism injury and osteochondroma formation, 182–184
  - type 7 fracture pattern, 187–190
- hand injuries, incidence of, 654–655
- immature skeletal injuries
  - age as factor in, 42–43
  - fracture repair, effects of, 249
  - statistics on, 38–40
- longitudinal inequality, diagnostic imaging for assessment of, 130–134
- multiple injury and
  - orthopaedic injuries and, 75–76
  - Pediatric Trauma Score (PTS), 76–77
- pelvic injury, incidence of, 795–796
- postfracture cysts and, 332–334
- roentgenographic response to, 121–122
- scapula, 442–445
  - glenoid hypoplasia, 444
  - scapular wringing, 445
  - scapulothoracic dissociation, 444–445
- shock from, 312–313
- soft tissue injury, fracture treatment with associated injury, 88
- spinal injury, os odontoideum, 738–740
- sternum, 429–430
- thorax and ribs, 422–429
  - cardiac tamponade, 427
  - diaphragm and abdominal injury, 427–428
  - first rib fracture, 425–426
  - hemothorax, 427
  - pancreas, 428
  - pneumothorax, 427
  - pulmonary contusion, 426–427
  - slipping rib syndrome, 428–429
  - splenic injury, 428
  - subcutaneous emphysema, 427
  - thoracic outlet syndrome, 426
  - tracheobronchial tree injury, 427

Treatment algorithm, amputation in children, 294–295

Triangular fibrocartilaginous complex (TFCC)
- carpal subluxation and dislocation, 657
- distal radial fractures, 626, 631–632
- Galeazzi fracture-dislocation and, 635, 637–638
- wrist and hand injury, 655

Triceps fascia, Monteggia lesions, 601

Triplane fracture
- distal tibial injuries, 1052–1054
  - complications, 1063–1065
- growth mechanism injury, physeal injuries, management of, 211

Triquetrum fractures
- carpal bones, 661–663
- scaphoid bone, 660–661

Triradiate cartilage
- acetabular fractures and, 811–816
- pelvic development, 790–792

Trochanter
- anterior hip dislocation, 841–842
- femoral anatomy
  - greater trochanter, 858–860
  - lesser trochanter, 859–860
- injuries to, 876–878
- surgical treatment, 890

Tubular bones, endochondral ossification, 3

Tubular insertions, fracture treatment with, external fixators using, 96

Tumors
- diagnostic imaging, acute injury evaluation, discovery during, 116
- irradiation, growth mechanism injury, 179–180, 182
- scintigraphy (radionuclide imaging) of, 139

U

Ulna
- anatomy and development of, 567–569
- Bennett's fracture analogue, 667
- Monteggia lesions, involvement of, 594–598
- *See also* Distal ulnar injuries; Proximal ulna; Radioulnar fractures

Ulnar impingement syndrome, distal ulnar injuries, 634–635

Ulnar nerve
- elbow dislocations, complications involving, 550–551
- lateral condyle injuries, 522–523

Ulnar styloid process, distal radial fractures, 625–627
- complications, 631–632

Ultrasonography
- multiple injury protocol, 75
- Osgood-Schlatter lesions, 1020–1022
- proximal tibial epiphyseal injuries, 1007
- scaphoid fractures, 658
- Sinding-Larsen-Johansson (SLJ) lesions, 957–960
- techniques, 140
- tendon injury, 696–697

Undiagnosed fractures, scintigraphy (radionuclide imaging) of, 139

Undulations, distal femoral epiphyseal injuries
- classification, 898–905
- complications, 908–910

Uniaxial fixators, fracture treatment using, 94–96

Unilateral frames, external fixators, fracture treatment using, 95

Unreduced dislocations, characteristics of, 554

Unstable fractures, distal metaphysis (supracondylar) injuries, 487–488

Upper respiratory infection, rotatory subluxation, atlantoaxial joint, 735

Urethral injury, pelvic fractures and, 808–810

Urologic injury, pelvic fractures and, 808–810

V

"Vacuum" phenomenon
- epiphyseal cartilage, diagnostic imaging, 123
- hip injuries, voluntary habitual dislocation with collagen disorders, 851

Valgus deformity
- distal femoral epiphyseal injuries, 899–900
- distal metaphysis (supracondylar) injuries, 489, 491–494
- distal tibial fractures, complications, 1065
- femoral shaft fractures, intramedullary nailing and rodding, 889–890
- growth mechanism injuries, overgrowth in, 213
- growth mechanism injury, type 8 fracture pattern, 188
- immature skeletal injury, residual angulation remodeling, 259
- lateral condyle injuries, 522
- metatarsal injuries, 1130
- proximal femoral fractures, 870–872
- proximal tibial epiphyseal injuries, 1009–1011
- proximal tibial metaphyseal injuries, 1030–1035

Varus deformity
- distal femoral epiphyseal injuries, 899–900
- distal metaphysis (supracondylar) injuries, 489, 491–494
- distal tibial fractures, 1063–1065
- irradiation, 180

metatarsal injuries, 1130
proximal femoral fractures, 870–872
proximal humeral physeal fracture, 473
proximal tibial epiphyseal injuries, 1009–1011
type 5 fracture patterns, 173
Vascular bone transplant, open fracture and, 277–279
Vascular foramina, spinal anatomic development, 714
Vascular injury
 clavicle injury and, 434
  proximal (sternal) clavicle injury, 438
 diagnostic imaging of, 140
 distal metacarpal fractures, 671–672
 distal metaphysis (supracondylar) injuries, 486–487, 495
 distal radioulnar injuries, 621
 elbow dislocations, 550–551
 femoral shaft fractures
  complications from, 892
  post-surgical complications, 890
 first rib fracture and, 425–426
 foot injuries, peritalar and subtalar dislocations, 1109–1110
 fracture treatment with associated injury, 88
  fixation techniques and, 91
  tourniquet use, 103–104
 growth mechanism injuries
  frostbite, 179
  physeal damage, 198
  physeal injuries, management of, 212
  type 5 fracture pattern, 175–176, 180
  type 8 pattern, 188–192
 gunshot injury, open fractures and, 289
 hip injuries
  anterior hip dislocation, 842
  ischemic necrosis (osteonecrosis), 846–849
 knee dislocations, 936–941
 lateral condyle injuries, 514
 metacarpophalangeal (MCP) joint dislocation, 676–677
 multiple injury protocol, 74
 Osgood-Schlatter lesions, 1018–1020
 pelvic fractures, 806–807
 proximal femoral fractures, complications, 873–876
 proximal tibial epiphyseal injuries complications, 1011
  diagnosis of, 1007
 proximal tibial metaphyseal injuries, 1033–1035
 radioulnar fractures, 608
 scapular injury and, 445

spinal cord injury, 767–768
 thoracic spinal injuries and, 748–750
 wringer injuries and, 292
 See also Arterial injury; Blood loss; Venous disorders
Vascular radiology, techniques, 140
Vasculature
 biomechanics of, in bone, 27–28
 carpal scaphoid, 650–651
 distal femur, anatomy of, 861–863
 femoral anatomy, 860
 in fibrous tissue, 30–31
 hand injuries, 654
 immature skeletal injury, wound healing patterns, 243–244
 meniscal, 932
 physeal growth alteration, histopathology, 217, 220–221
 physeal growth arrest, experimental bridging and, 217
 skeletal development and, 18–21
 spinal cord, 717
 spinal region, 711–713
 talus bone, 1092–1093
 tarsal bones, 1094–1095
 tibiofibular diaphyseal injuries, 1039–1040
 Volkmann's contracture and vascular supply, 320
Vasodilators, vasospasm treatment using, 316
Vasospasm, arterial injury, 315–316
 continuity lesions, 313
Vending machines, immature skeletal injuries from, 47
Venography, venous disorder diagnosis, 321
Venous disorders
 as bone injury complication, 319–321
 incidence in children, 320–321
Ventricular septic defect, as trauma complication, 311
Vertebrae
 anatomic development, 713–715
 birth injury, 731
 diagnostic imaging of, 727
 spinal cord injury and development of, 768–770
 subluxation, 729
Vertebral body height/sagittal diameter ratio, values for, 716
Vertebral height/disk space height ratio, values for, 716
Vitamin C deficiency, scurvy and, 352
Vitamin D deficiency
 rickets, fractures with, 350–352
 sports-related injuries and, 403
Vitamin K deficiency, bone injury complications from, 321
Volkmann's contracture

arterial injury and, 318–320
 compartment syndrome and, 316–317
 diagnostic imaging and, 140
 distal metaphysis (supracondylar) injuries and, 494–495
 distal radioulnar injuries, 621
 incidence of, 318
Volkmann systems, immature skeletal injury, fracture repair, inflammatory phase, 246–249
Volume rendering, fracture imaging, 136
von Willebrand's disease, bone injury complications from, 321

W

Waist fractures, scaphoid bone, 657–658
Water immersion, of casts, complications from, 91
Wedge fractures
 lumbar spine, 752–758
 thoracic spinal injuries, 748
Werdnig-Hoffman disease, fractures due to, 373
Winging, scapular injury, 445
Wolff's law, angular deformity, 219
Wound care
 immature skeleton repair, 243–244
 open fractures
  bone loss, 276–277
  débridement, 271–272, 274
  examination, 270–271
  periosteal stripping, 273–274
  puncture wounds, 273
  skeletal stabilization, 275–276
  soft tissue coverage, 274–275
  tourniquet use, 273
  vascular bone transplant, 277–279
Woven-fibered bone, remodeling characteristics of, 21, 23
Wringer injuries, growth mechanism injury, type 9 fracture patterns, 191–194
Wrist injury
 anatomic development and, 650–653
 carpal fractures, 657, 661–663
 carpal subluxation and dislocation, 657
 carpometacarpal joint dislocation, 664–665
 diagnostic imaging, 655
 functional anatomy, 653–654
 injury incidence, 654–655
 intercarpal disruptions, 663–664
 scaphoid fractures, 657–658
 treatment and repair, 655–656
 type 1B fracture injury, repetitive use and, 157–158
 See also Hand injury; Scaphoid bone
"Wrong-side" fractures

"Wrong-side" fractures (*cont.*)
  growth plate failures, 152
  physeal growth arrest, histopathologic analysis, 217
  type 1C patterns, 160–161
  type 3 injury, 167, 170
  type 4 injury, 170, 174

X

Xerographic imaging, plantar foot padding wounds, 1145

X-ray studies, closed reduction of fractures, post-reduction films, importance of, 90–91

Y

Y ligament, hip injuries and, 831–832

Z

Zone of Ranvier
  distal metacarpal fractures, 672
  fibrous tissue in, 31–32
  growth mechanism injury
    burn injury, 182, 184
    circulation and ischemia, 198
    experimental trauma studies, 196–197
    healing patterns, 198–199
    osteochondroma formation, 183
    physeal injuries, management of, 211–212
    type 1 fracture patterns, 154–155, 159
    type 2 fracture patterns, 162–166
    type 6 fracture patterns, 181, 183
  physeal bone growth and, 16
    bridging and growth arrest, 214–215
  physis characteristics and, 10–13
  vasculature of, 20–23

Zuker transplantation procedure, for Volkmann's contracture, 320